St. Louis Regional Poison Center, Cardinal Glennon Memorial Hospital for Children, 1465 S. Grand Ave., St. Louis, MO 63104, 314 772-5200.

MONTANA

Montana Poison Control System, Cogswell Building, Helena, MT 59620, 406 442-2480, 800 525-5042.

NEBRASKA

Mid-Plains Regional Poison Center, Children's Memorial Hospital, 8301 Dodge, Omaha, NE 68114, 402 390-5400, 800 642-9999 (Statewide), 800 228-9515 (Surrounding states).

NEVADA

Southern Nevada Memorial Hospital, 1800 W. Charleston Blvd., Las Vegas, NV 89102, 702 385-1277.

Washoe Medical Center, 77 Pringle Way, Reno, NV 89520, 702 785-4129.

NEW HAMPSHIRE

New Hampshire Poison Center, Mary Hitchcock Hospital, 2 Maynard St., Hanover, NH 03756, 603 646-5000, 800 562-8236 (Statewide).

NEW JERSEY

Jersey Shore Medical Center, Fitkin Hospital, 1945 Corlies Ave., Neptune, NJ 07753, 201 775-5500, 800 822-9761 (Statewide).

NEW MEXICO

New Mexico Poison Drug Information & Medical Center, University of New Mexico, Albuquerque, NM 87131, 505 843-2551, 800 432-6866 (Statewide).

NEW YORK

Long Island Regional Poison Control Center, Nassau County Medical Center, 2201 Hempstead Turnpike, E. Meadow, NY 11554, 516 542-2324, 516 542-2323.

New York City Poison Center, Department of Health, Bureau of Laboratories, 455 First Ave., New York City, NY 10016, 212 340-4494, 212 764-7667.

Finger Lakes Poison Center, LIFELINE, University of Rochester Medical Center, Rochester, NY 14642, 716 275-5151, 716 275-2700.

NORTH CAROLINA

Duke University Medical Center Poison Control Center, P.O. Box 3007, Durham, NC 27710, 919 684-8111.

NORTH DAKOTA

Bismarck Hospital Emergency Department, 300 N. 7th St., Bismarck, ND 58501, 701 223-4357.

St. Luke's Poison Center, St. Luke's Hospitals, Fifth St. at Mills Ave., Fargo, ND 58122, 701 280-5575.

OHIO

Central Ohio Poison Center, Children's Hospital of Ohio, 700 Children's Dr., Columbus, OH 43205, 614 228-1323.

Children's Medical Center, One Children's Plaza, Dayton, OH 45404, 513 222-2227, 800 762-0727 (Statewide).

OKLAHOMA

Oklahoma Poison Control Center, Oklahoma Children's Memorial Center, P.O. Box 26307, Oklahoma City, OK 73126, 405 271-5454, 800 522-4611 (Statewide).

OREGON

Oregon Poison Control and Drug Information Center, University of Oregon Health Sciences Center, Portland, OR 97201, 503 225-8968, 800 452-7165 (Statewide).

PENNSYLVANIA

Philadelphia Poison Information, 321 University Ave., Philadelphia, PA 19104, 215 922-5523, 215 922-5524.

Pittsburgh Poison Center, Children's Hospital, 125 DeSoto St., Pittsburgh, PA 15214, 412 681-6669, 412 647-5600.

PUERTO RICO

Pharmacy School, Medical Sciences Campus, San Juan, PR 00936, 809 753-4849.

RHODE ISLAND

Rhode Island Poison Center, Rhode Island Hospital, Annex Bldg. 422, 593 Eddy St., Providence, RI 02902, 401 277-5727.

SOUTH CAROLINA

National Pesticide Telecommunications Network, Medical University of South Carolina, 171 Ashley Ave., Charleston, SC 29403, 803 792-4201, 800 845-7633 (Outside SC).

SOUTH DAKOTA

McKennan Poison Center, McKennan Hospital, 800 E. 21st St., Sioux Falls, SD 57101, 605 336-3894, 800 952-0123 (Statewide), 800 843-0505 (NE, MN, IA).

Rapid City Regional Poison Control Center, 353 Fairmont Blvd., P.O. Box 6000, Rapid City, SD 57709, 605 341-3333, 800 742-8925.

TENNESSEE

Vanderbilt University Hospital, 21st and Garland, Nashville, TN 37232, 615 322-6435.

TEXAS

Southeast Texas Poison Center, The University of Texas Medical Branch, Eighth & Mechanic Sts., Galveston, TX 77550, 713 765-1420.

UTAH

Intermountain Regional Poison Control Center, 50 N. Medical Dr., Salt Lake City, UT 84132, 801 581-2151.

VERMONT

Vermont Poison Center, Medical Center Hospital of Vermont, Burlington, VT 05401, 802 658-3456.

VIRGINIA

Blue Ridge Poison Center, University of Virginia Hospital, Charlottesville, VA 22903, 804 924-5543, 800 446-9876 (Out-of-state), 800 552-3723 (Statewide).

WASHINGTON

Seattle Poison Center, Children's Orthopedic Hospital and Medical Center, 4800 Sand Point Way, NE, Seattle, WA 98105, 206 634-5252, 800 732-6985.

Spokane Poison Center, Deaconess Hospital, W. 800 5th Ave., Spokane, WA 99210, 509 747-1077, 800 572-5842 (Statewide).

WEST VIRGINIA

The West Virginia Poison System, West Virginia University School of Pharmacy, 3110 Mac Corkle Ave., S.E., Charleston, WV 25304, 304 348-4211, 800 642-3625 (Statewide).

WISCONSIN

Madison Area Poison Center, University Hospital & Clinic, 600 Highland Ave., Madison, WI 53792, 608 262-3702.

WYOMING

Wyoming Poison Center, DePaul Hospital, 2600 E. 18th St., Cheyenne, WY 82001, 307 635-9256, 800 442-2704.

CLINICAL PHARMACOLOGY AND THERAPEUTICS IN NURSING

CLINICAL PHARMACOLOGY AND THERAPEUTICS IN NURSING

SECOND EDITION

MATTHEW B. WIENER, B.S., Pharm.D.
Clinical Research Pharmacist
National Jewish Hospital and Research Center/
National Asthma Center
Adjunct Associate Professor of Clinical Pharmacy
School of Pharmacy
University of Colorado

GINETTE A. PEPPER, R.N., M.S., G.N.P.
Doctoral Candidate in Nursing and Pharmacology
University of Colorado Health Sciences Center
Teaching Associate
Gerontological Nurse Practitioner Program
School of Nursing
University of Colorado

McGRAW-HILL BOOK COMPANY
New York St. Louis San Francisco Auckland Bogotá Hamburg
Johannesburg London Madrid Mexico Montreal New Delhi
Panama Paris São Paulo Singapore Sydney Tokyo Toronto

NOTICE

As new medical and nursing research and clinical experience broaden our knowledge, changes in treatment and drug therapy are required. The editors and the publisher of this work have made every effort to ensure that the drug dosage schedules herein are accurate and in accord with the standards accepted at the time of publication. Readers are advised, however, to check the product information sheet included in the package of each drug they plan to administer to be certain that changes have not been made in the recommended dose or in the contraindications for administration. This recommendation is of particular importance in regard to new or infrequently used drugs.

CLINICAL PHARMACOLOGY AND THERAPEUTICS IN NURSING

Copyright © 1985, 1979 by McGraw-Hill, Inc. All rights reserved. Printed in the United States of America. Except as permitted under the United States Copyright Act of 1976, no part of this publication may be reproduced or distributed in any form or by any means, or stored in a data base or retrieval system, without the prior written permission of the publisher.

1 2 3 4 5 6 7 8 9 0   RMTRMT   8 9 8 7 6 5

ISBN 0-07-070163-6

This book was set in Sabon by University Graphics, Inc.
The editors were Karol M. Carstensen and Jo Satloff;
the designer was Scott Chelius;
the production supervisor was Phil Galea.
New drawings were done by J & R Services, Inc.
Rand McNally & Company was printer and binder.

Library of Congress Cataloging in Publication Data
Main entry under title:

Clinical pharmacology and therapeutics in nursing.

Includes bibliographies and index.
1. Pharmacology. 2. Therapeutics. 3. Nursing.
4. Pharmacy—Information services—United States—
Directories. I. Wiener, Matthew B. II. Pepper,
Ginette A. [DNLM: 1. Drug Therapy—nurses' instruction.
2. Pharmacology, Clinical—nurses' instruction.   QV 38
C6417]
RM300.C53   1985   615′.024613   84-26188
ISBN 0-07-070163-6

TO OUR FAMILY AND FRIENDS
WHO ARE, AFTER ALL,
OUR BEST MEDICINE.

CONTENTS IN BRIEF

CONTENTS

UNIT III
NEUROTRANSMISSION & THE
AUTONOMIC NERVOUS SYSTEM

UNIT V
CLINICAL PHARMACOLOGY & THERAPEUTICS OF COMMON DISORDERS

LIST OF CONTRIBUTORS

Margaret Ball, B.S., M.S., R.D.
Assistant Professor
School of Nursing
University of Colorado Health Sciences Center
Denver, Colorado
Chapter 25

Rosemary R. Berardi, Pharm.D.
Clinical Pharmacist, Gastroenterology
Veterans Administration Medical Center, and
    Associate Professor of Pharmacy
College of Pharmacy
University of Michigan
Ann Arbor, Michigan
Chapter 32

James R. Bonk, Ph.D., R.N., C.S., C.A.C.
Research Assistant II
Department of Family and Community Medicine
College of Medicine
University of Arizona
Tucson, Arizona
Chapter 49

Eleanor H. Boyd, Ph.D.
Formerly, Assistant Professor of Pharmacology and
    Toxicology, and of Nursing
University of Rochester
Schools of Medicine and Dentistry, and of Nursing
Rochester, New York
Unit III

Patricia K. Brannin, R.N., M.S.N., R.T., A.N.P.
Formerly, Director of Education, Quality Assurance, and
    Research
National Jewish Hospital/National Asthma Center
Denver, Colorado
Chapter 22

Beverly A. Burton, R.N., A.N.P.
Independent Author and Consultant
Formerly, Nurse Manager
Internal Medicine Clinic
University of Colorado
School of Medicine
Denver, Colorado
Chapter 21

Michael A. Carter, R.N., D.N.Sc., F.A.A.N.
Dean and Professor
College of Nursing
University of Tennessee
Center for Health Sciences
Memphis, Tennessee
Chapter 26

Moses Chow, Pharm.D.
Director, Drug Information
Hartford Hospital
Hartford, Connecticut, and
    Associate Professor of Clinical Pharmacy
University of Connecticut
Storrs, Connecticut
Chapter 43

Richard A. F. Clark, M.D.
National Jewish Hospital and Research Center
Denver, Colorado
Chapter 38

Brenda Font Clarke, R.N., M.S.
Staff Development Coordinator
Medical-Psychiatric Nursing
The Methodist Hospital
Houston, Texas
Chapter 19

Ira A. Cohen, Pharm.D.
Assistant Professor of Pharmacy
College of Pharmacy
The University of Michigan, and
    Clinical Pharmacist, Adult Internal Medicine
Veterans Administration Medical Center
Ann Arbor, Michigan
Chapter 32

JoAnn Ganje Congdon, R.N., M.S.
Lecturer, Adult-Gerontology Division
University of Colorado
School of Nursing
Denver, Colorado
Chapter 35

John B. Constantine, M.D.
Leahey Eye Clinic
Lowell, Massachusetts
Chapter 39

Joel Covinsky, Pharm.D.
Professor and Director
Clinical Pharmacology and Metabolic Support Service
School of Medicine
University of Missouri-Kansas City
Kansas City, Missouri
Chapter 44

Vaughn C. Culbertson, Pharm.D.
Assistant Professor of Pharmacy
School of Pharmacy
University of Colorado
Health Sciences Center
Denver, Colorado
Chapter 21

Anne G. Davis, Pharm.D.
Assistant Professor of Pediatrics
University of Colorado
Department of Pediatrics
Denver, Colorado
Chapter 18

Janet K. Dickerson, R.N.
Research Assistant
Department of Internal Medicine
University of Arizona
Tucson, Arizona
Chapter 6

Dorothy L. Diehl, R.N., B.S.N., C.C.R.N.
Clinical Nurse—Critical Care
Memorial Hospital Medical Center of Long Beach
Long Beach, California
Chapter 41

Roswell Lee Evans, Pharm.D.
Associate Professor of Clinical Pharmacy
University of Missouri, and
    Clinical Pharmacist
Western Missouri Mental Health Center
Kansas City, Missouri
Chapter 34

Ronald P. Evens, Pharm.D.
Assistant Director of Clinical Research
Medical Department
Bristol Laboratories
A Division of Bristol-Myers Co.
Syracuse, New York
Chapter 26

Judith Underwood Grothe, R.N., B.S.N.
Proprietor, Avalon Health Care Consultants
Lakewood, Colorado
Formerly, Director of Pharmacological Research
Medical Care and Research Foundation
Denver, Colorado
Chapter 9

Ann E. Gunnett, R.N., M.S.N., N.P.
Assistant Professor of Nursing
School of Nursing
University of Maryland
Baltimore, Maryland
Chapter 20

Arthur F. Harralson, Pharm.D.
Director, Pharmacokinetics Service
Memorial Hospital Medical Center
Assistant Clinical Professor
University of California and University of
    Southern California
Long Beach, California
Chapter 41

John M. Hoopes, Pharm.D.
Associate Professor
Departments of Clinical Pharmacy and Family Medicine
University of Maryland
Baltimore, Maryland
Chapter 20

Suzanne L. Howell, R.N., M.N.
Assistant Professor in Nursing
Loretto Heights College
Denver, Colorado
Chapter 48

Robert J. Ignoffo, Pharm.D.
Associate Clinical Professor
Division of Clinical Pharmacy
University of California at San Francisco
San Francisco, California
Chapter 37

Betty Jennings, C.N.M., M.S.N., R.N.
Assistant Professor
University of Colorado
School of Nursing
Denver, Colorado
Chapter 7

Cary E. Johnson, Pharm.D.
Associate Professor of Pharmacy
University of Michigan
College of Pharmacy
Clinical Pharmacist, Pediatrics
University of Michigan Hospitals
Ann Arbor, Michigan
Chapter 36

Catherine Johnson, R.N., B.S.N.
Head Nurse, Surgical Intensive Care Unit and Cardiac
    Surgical Unit
Mount Sinai Medical Center
Miami, Florida
Chapters 28 and 29

Sande Jones, R.N., M.S.
Education Coordinator
Department of Nursing Education
Mount Sinai Medical Center
Miami Beach, Florida
Chapters 28 and 29

Amy M. Karch, R.N., M.S.
Assistant Professor of Cardiovascular Nursing
University of Rochester School of Nursing
Rochester, New York
Unit III

Leigh K. Kaszyk, R.N., M.S.
Clinical Specialist
Penrose Cancer Hospital
Colorado Springs, Colorado
Formerly, Senior Instructor
University of Colorado
School of Nursing
Denver, Colorado
Chapter 24

Roger Lander, Pharm.D.
Assistant Professor of Clinical Pharmacy
University of Missouri-Kansas City
Kansas City, Missouri
Chapter 44

Sheldon Lefkowitz, M.S., R.Ph.
Assistant Director for Clinical Pharmacy Services
Mount Sinai Medical Center
Miami, Florida
Chapters 28 and 29

Arthur G. Lipman, Pharm.D.
Professor for Clinical Pharmacy and Chairman,
    Department of Pharmacy Practice
University of Utah
Salt Lake City, Utah
Chapter 17

Anita G. Lorenzo, Pharm.D.
Assistant Professor
Department of Pharmacy Practice
College of Pharmacy
University of Illinois at Chicago
Chicago, Illinois
Chapters 24 and 30

Beth Lyman, R.N., M.S.N.
Nurse Clinician
Metabolic Support Service
Truman Medical Center West
Kansas City, Missouri
Chapter 44

Joan K. Magilvy, Ph.D., R.N.
Assistant Professor
University of Colorado Health Sciences Center
School of Nursing
Denver, Colorado
Chapter 49

Richard J. Martin, M.D.
Assistant Professor of Medicine
University of Colorado Health Sciences Center
Director, Sleep Disorders Center
Director, Adult Special Care Unit
National Jewish Hospital and Research Center
Denver, Colorado
Chapter 22

Celeste Martin Marx, Pharm.D.
Associate Professor
Massachusetts College of Pharmacy and Allied Health
    Sciences
Clinical Pharmacist,
Brigham and Woman's Hospital
Boston, Massachusetts
Chapter 35

Mary Harkness Mayers, R.N., M.S.N., J.D.
House Counsel
Greater Southeast Community Hospital
Washington, D.C.
Chapter 8

Ruth Merryman, Pharm.D.
University of Texas M.D. Anderson
Hospital and Tumor Institute at Houston
Department of Pharmacy
Houston, Texas
Chapter 19

Kathleen Mooney, Ph.D., R.N.
Associate Professor
University of Utah College of Nursing
Salt Lake City, Utah
Chapter 17

Mary A. Murphy, C.P.N.P., Ph.D.
Pediatric Nurse Practitioner
Child Development Unit
Children's Hospital
Denver, Colorado
Chapter 18

Thomas J. Nester, Pharm.D.
Assistant Professor
Ohio State University
College of Pharmacy
Columbus, Ohio
Chapter 43

Laura K. Neilley, R.N., M.S., C-A.N.P.
Associate Director of Nursing
National Jewish Hospital/National Asthma Center
Denver, Colorado
Chapter 33

Virginia E. Parker, F.N.P., M.S.
Medical College of Virginia
Virginia Commonwealth University
Richmond, Virginia
Chapter 42

Rita J. Payton, R.N., M.S., D.A.
Associate Dean and Professor of Nursing
University of Tulsa College of Nursing
Tulsa, Oklahoma
Chapter 8

Ginette A. Pepper, R.N., M.S., G.N.P.
Doctoral Candidate in Nursing and Pharmacology
University of Colorado Health Sciences Center
Teaching Associate, Gerontological Nurse Practitioner
  Program
University of Colorado School of Nursing
Denver, Colorado
Chapters 1, 2, 3, 4, 5, and 7

Lynne Johnson Phillips, R.N., M.S.N.
Administrator
Home Health Care of America
Englewood, Colorado
Chapter 25

Robert W. Piepho, Ph.D., F.C.P.
Associate Dean and Professor
University of Colorado
School of Pharmacy
Denver, Colorado
Chapter 33

Kathleen Simons Piggott, R.N.-C., M.S.
Assistant Professor
Seattle University
School of Nursing
Seattle, Washington
Chapter 20

Agatha A. Quinn, R.N., M.A.
Assistant Professor in Nursing
Loretto Heights College
Denver, Colorado
Chapter 31

Jane C. Regnier, R.N.
Cardiology Research Nurse
Division of Cardiology
Hartford Hospital
Hartford, Connecticut
Chapter 43

Thomas P. Reinders, Pharm.D.
Associate Professor of Pharmacy
Medical College of Virginia
Virginia Commonwealth University
Richmond, Virginia
Chapter 42

Nancy A. Richart, B.A., R.N.-C.
Director of Nursing Education
Western Missouri Mental Health Center
Kansas City, Missouri
Chapter 34

David S. Roffman, Pharm.D.
Associate Professor
Clinical Pharmacy Department
School of Pharmacy
Baltimore, Maryland
Chapter 40

Grace Carboni Ruggiero, R.N., B.S., B.A.
Peninsula Hospital Medical Center
Burlingame, California
Chapter 48

Mary Jo Sagaties, R.N., M.S.N., F.N.P.-C.
Nurse Practitioner/Ophthalmic Photographer
Leahey Eye Clinic
Lowell, Massachusetts
Chapter 39

Rosalie Sagraves, Pharm.D.
Associate Professor
Clinical Pharmacy Division
College of Pharmacy
The University of Texas at Austin
Austin, Texas
Chapter 46

Patricia A. Saran, R.N., B.S.N.
Nurse Clinician, General Surgery
The University of Michigan
Ann Arbor, Michigan
Chapter 32

Gilda Saul, R.N., C.C.R.N.
Head Nurse
Blum Intensive Care Center
Mount Sinai Medical Center
Miami Beach, Florida
Chapter 45

Rosemary A. Simkins, R.N., M.N.
Associate Director of Nursing, Pediatrics
National Jewish Hospital/National Asthma Center
Denver, Colorado
Chapter 27

Ross A. Simkover, Pharm.D.
Assistant Director, Drug Information
The University of Illinois College of Pharmacy
Chicago, Illinois
Chapters 6, 48, and 49

Ralph E. Small, Pharm.D.
Associate Professor of Pharmacy and Pharmaceutics
Assistant Professor of Medicine
Medical College of Virginia
Virginia Commonwealth University
Richmond, Virginia
Chapter 26

Barbara Gould Smith, C.R.N.A.
Nurse Anesthetist
South Denver Anesthesiology
Denver, Colorado
Chapter 47

Vincent C. Speranza, B.S., Pharm.D.
Director of Pharmacy Services
North West Regional Hospital
Margate, Florida
Chapter 45

Robert J. Stagg, Pharm.D.
Assistant Clinical Professor
Division of Clinical Pharmacy
University of California
San Francisco, California
Chapter 37

Martha H. Stoner, Ph.D., R.N.-C., A.N.P.
Assistant Professor
School of Nursing
University of Colorado Health Sciences Center
Denver, Colorado
Chapter 23

Elvira Szigeti, R.N., M.N.
Associate Professor in Nursing
Loretto Heights College
Denver, Colorado
Doctoral Candidate in Nursing
University of Texas at Austin
Austin, Texas
Chapter 46

H. Katheryn Tatum, R.N., M.S.
Head Nurse, Dialysis Unit
University Hospital
University of Colorado Health Sciences Center
Denver, Colorado
Chapter 31

Sue Ann Thomas, R.N., Ph.D.
Associate Professor
School of Nursing, and
    Clinical Director
Psychophysiological Clinic
School of Medicine
University of Maryland
Baltimore, Maryland
Chapter 40

Anna M. Tichy, R.N., Ph.D.
Professor and Head of the Department of Maternal-Child
    Nursing
College of Nursing
University of Illinois at Chicago
Chicago, Illinois
Chapter 30

Theodore G. Tong, Pharm.D.
Director, Arizona Poison Information Center
Professor of Pharmacy Practice
University of Arizona
Tucson, Arizona
Chapters 48 and 49

Marcia G. Tonnesen, M.D.
Assistant Professor
Department of Dermatology
University of Colorado School of Medicine, and
    Chief of Dermatology Service
Veterans Administration Medical Center
Denver, Colorado
Chapter 38

John F. Tourville, Pharm.D.
LT, MSC, USN
Clinical Pharmacist
Naval Hospital Bethesda
Bethesda, Maryland
Chapter 7

Carol S. Viele, R.N., M.S.
Assistant Clinical Professor of Nursing
Clinical Nurse Specialist in Hematology/Oncology
University of California at San Francisco
San Francisco, California
Chapter 37

Mary J. Waskerwitz, B.S.N., C.P.N.P.
Pediatric Nurse Practitioner
University of Michigan
Department of Pediatrics
Section of Hematology-Oncology
Ann Arbor, Michigan
Chapter 36

Matthew B. Wiener, B.S., Pharm.D.
Clinical Research Pharmacist
National Jewish Hospital and Research Center/
National Asthma Center
Adjunct Associate Professor of Clinical Pharmacy
School of Pharmacy
University of Colorado
Denver, Colorado
Chapters 1, 5, and 27

PREFACE

The purpose of this book is to advance the role of the nurse in promoting rational drug therapy. This requires an understanding of the various clinical disorders and how drugs are most effectively and safely used to treat them. Also important are the application of pharmacokinetic principles in clinical decision making, recognition of the significance of drug-induced diseases, and appreciation of how psychosocial factors affect drug outcome.

The overall philosophy and organization of this edition are unchanged from the first edition. The editors and authors maintain that pharmacology is learned best and most efficiently in the context in which it is to be used, so the book is organized by clinical entity (diseases and symptoms) rather than by drug group. However, the presentations of the clinical entities have been abridged in the second edition to focus on those aspects directly relevant to rational drug therapy. Nursing process is again the organizing framework for the nursing implications of drug therapy. The explanations of pharmacokinetics and psychosocial factors have been expanded in this edition, and a chapter has been added to centralize the presentation of developmental considerations in pharmacology. Other new chapters include those on ethical and legal aspects, edema, and community health care. The chapters in the first edition on drug abuse, stress, myocardial infarction, and sources of drug information have been deleted and this content has been included in other chapters. Many chapters have been entirely rewritten, both to incorporate advances in pharmacology and nursing care and to improve clarity and consistency in style and organization.

Authorship of the chapters is again interdisciplinary, with clinically experienced nurses teamed with clinical pharmacists, physicians, pharmacologists, or other specialists. A few chapters were authored solely by nurses with unique education and experience, such as a nurse anesthetist, a nurse lawyer, a nurse ethicist, and so forth. Each chapter in the text features learning objectives, a case study, discussions of nursing process, and consideration of associated drug-induced diseases. Learning exercises keyed to the objectives and case studies are located in the Instructor's Manual. To facilitate use of the textbook as a reference, generic drug names are indicated in boldface print and the index has been expanded and revised to be more congruent with the needs of the intended audience. Information on investigational drugs has been included if it is anticipated

that these agents will significantly impact on future therapy of a disorder.

Unit I introduces an updated discussion of nursing process as applied to drug therapy. This unit is designed to orient beginning students to this important aspect of nursing practice. However, several tables have been added that students may consult throughout their education and even as graduate nurses for quick reference regarding abbreviations, dosage calculation, and basic drug administration techniques. Other new features in this unit are expanded discussions of nursing diagnosis, proper recording and documentation, what to do when medication errors occur, how to handle a medication order which the nurse judges to be erroneous or unsafe, and a self-assessment of dosage calculation skills.

While the content in Unit II on the general principles of pharmacology is also basic information, much of this knowledge has been developed in the past few years and is of interest to learners at many levels. Chapter 5 lays the groundwork for a holistic approach to pharmacotherapy, including the basics of pharmacokinetics, pharmacodynamics (drug-receptor interactions), genetics, biorhythms, placebo effect, compliance, and other physical, psychologic, and sociologic considerations. The presentation of adverse effects of drugs in Chapter 6 focuses on principles and appropriate nursing actions, with an expanded discussion of the mechanisms of drug interactions. Chapter 7 presents a life-span developmental approach to pharmacokinetics, adverse drug reactions, and relevant nursing care. Nursing perspectives on law, ethics, drug development, and drug research complete the content of this unit.

Unit III introduces fundamental information about the physiology and pharmacology of neurotransmission and the autonomic nervous system. This knowledge is essential for a complete understanding of the clinical uses and adverse effects of numerous drugs, including many of the newer agents used to treat cardiovascular and respiratory disorders.

Unit IV describes the nursing process related to common signs and symptoms of diseases. Many of these conditions are commonly managed by nurses or self-managed by patients using nonpharmacologic approaches, drugs prescribed for PRN use, and/or nonprescription drugs. Knowledge necessary for the nursing judgments required in these conditions and for patient education in self-care is the emphasis of this unit.

The largest unit in the book is Unit V, which includes the pharmacotherapy of medical and psychiatric diseases. The chapters on cardiovascular disorders, which comprised a separate unit in the first edition, have been incorporated into this unit. The discussion of infectious diseases is expanded and divided into two chapters to cover this rapidly developing area of drug therapy.

The drug therapy relevant to four clinical nursing specialties is included in Unit VI, rather than with previous discussions of diseases and symptoms, because the specialties are wellness or prevention oriented, involve specialized technical skills, or require a unique approach to the client. Chapter 46 addresses the special needs of women associated with drug therapy in the areas of fertility, pregnancy, and menopause. Nursing process related to the drugs administered to patients as they progress through the operative experience is the focus of Chapter 47. Chapter 48 is introduced with a discussion of medication administration skills required in emergency and intensive care settings, followed by a presentation of drug therapy in several acute, life-threatening conditions: cardiopulmonary arrest, shock, burns, poisoning, and overdose. The final chapter addresses aspects of drug and chemical exposure of particular concern to nurses with a community focus: immunization, environmental and occupational health, and drug abuse.

While the text is designed to fulfill the learning needs of the basic nursing student, the explosion of basic and clinical pharmacologic knowledge and changes in the nursing role make the text useful to any nurse who last studied pharmacology more than five years ago. It has been well received by faculty and learners employing the text in undergraduate and graduate programs, in formal continuing education programs, and in self-directed independent study. The organization by clinical entity makes the text particularly useful to nurse practitioners in their education and practice.

ACKNOWLEDGMENTS

The preparation of a contributed text involves the efforts of a large number of individuals. The editors are deeply grateful to the contributors to the first edition who were able and eager to revise chapters or to write new chapters for the second edition in the areas of their current practice and teaching. While recognizing our indebtedness to all of the contributors to the first edition who laid the foundation for this volume, we sincerely welcome the numerous contributors who joined the text in the second edition. In addition, acknowledgment is due Suzanne Kaemper, R.N., M.N., and Ruth Harboe, R.N., M.S., for reviewing the neoplastic disorders chapter and to Omeera Anne Harrison, R.N., Ed.D., for her helpful suggestions on the respiratory chapter. We would like to thank Chip Mason, M.D., for reviewing the immune and inflammatory disorder chapter and Jim Cook, M.D., for his comments on the infectious disease chapters. The editors also thank the American Society of Hospital Pharmacists, Inc., for permission to use the compilation of Drug Information Centers which appears inside the front cover.

Special thanks are also due to Judy Franconi and Ellen Teter for secretarial support and to Karen Culvey whose unsurpassed skills and good humor were a major factor in the completion of this undertaking. The editors and contributors also owe a great debt to Karol Carstensen and Jo Satloff for their guidance, support, and commitment to the project. Our sentiments toward family and friends are expressed in the dedication, but particularly worthy of mention are our spouses, Terry Pepper and Madeline Wiener, and our children, Adam and Joshua Wiener and Julie, Teddy, Willy, and Vickie Pepper.

Ginette A. Pepper
Matthew B. Wiener

UNIT I

THE NURSING PROCESS IN CLINICAL PHARMACOLOGY & THERAPEUTICS

1

INTRODUCTION

GINETTE A. PEPPER
MATTHEW B. WIENER

LEARNING OBJECTIVES

Upon mastery of the contents of this chapter, the reader will be able to:

1. Define the terms *drug, pharmacology, clinical pharmacology,* and *therapeutics.*
2. Differentiate over-the-counter drugs and prescription drugs; chemical name, generic name, and trade name; illicit drugs, social drugs, and controlled substances; drug group and prototype drug; therapeutic effect and adverse effect.
3. Identify the generic and trade name of a drug from the common form of notation.
4. List forces and events which have influenced the development of the nursing role in drug therapy.
5. Outline a decision-making process appropriate to the nursing role in drug therapy.

Nurses practice in a variety of settings that require the application of pharmacology, but the specific nursing activities related to medications vary from setting to setting. In the hospital a significant proportion of the staff nurses' time may be spent administering medications and observing their effects. The intensive care nurse makes continuous evaluations of patients' responses to drugs in life-threatening circumstances. Nurses in research may study the effects of drugs in animals, tissues, cells, or human subjects. During surgical procedures and childbirth the nurse anesthetist administers the anesthetic, intravenous fluids, and other medications and monitors the patient's response. When a child with epilepsy or another disease must take medications chronically, the school nurse helps teachers, parents, and the student to identify approaches that are least disruptive to the learning process. In some states nurse practitioners prescribe medications under the supervision of a physician. Assisting people to overcome the physical and psychosocial concomitants of drug abuse is the goal of nurses in drug and alcohol treatment programs. The occupational health nurse assesses the possible deleterious effects of gases and other chemicals to which workers are exposed. Community health nurses organize immunization clinics, advise clients about the rational use of nonprescription drugs, and teach them about their diseases and the medications prescribed by their physicians. Nurses also use pharmacology in their practice in poison control centers, outpatient clinics, hospices, psychiatric hospitals and clinics, emergency rooms, and many other settings.

THE NURSE'S ROLE

Nurses require an understanding of the principles of pharmacology not only to administer medications, but also for numerous other functions. They observe for desired and unwanted drug effects, collaborate with physicians and other health professionals, educate patients and other consumers, and intervene to promote the drug's beneficial effects and minimize adverse drug reactions. In spite of the diversity of these activities, it is common to refer to a single *role of the nurse* in drug therapy. This is because the same method of logical decision making should be the basis for nursing actions in drug therapy regardless of the setting or nursing specialty. This decision-making method is the *nursing process* which underlies all rational nursing practice. The nursing process is the application of *scientific method* to nursing care, and it guides the nurse or student through established problem-solving steps (see Table 1-1). The nursing process parallels the scientific method, although it embodies a system of humanistic values and ethical principles while the scientific method is reputed to be value-free.

Collaboration

All patient care requires the input of a variety of health care professionals. As in other therapeutic modalities, adequate, safe drug therapy requires the interaction of groups of health professionals, most notably nurses, pharmacists, physicians, and pharmacologists, if therapy is to achieve its intended effect: enabling the patient to reach a maximal health potential with minimal adverse effects.

As a partner in the delivery of health care, the nurse *shares* roles and functions but never relinquishes responsibility for the outcome of therapeutic intervention. Thus, the

3

nurse operates with other professionals in a system of checks and balances to ensure patient safety. The nurse must be prepared to intervene and discuss rational therapeutics with other health care providers in order to execute this aspect of health care delivery.

The nurse has the most constant and consistent access to the patient, particularly the inpatient, and serves as the "last line of defense" in protecting the patient from adverse effects of drug therapy. Consequently, the nurse can never assume that all is well but must verify that *all* aspects of drug therapy, from the initial order, through administration, to final evaluation of drug effect, have been correctly and completely executed. Patient safety and well-being demand that the nurse view drugs and drug therapy with the questioning attitude that characterizes scientific method.

Requisite Knowledge Base

The nursing process in drug therapy requires a correspondence of pathophysiology and pharmacology knowledge. This involves an understanding of normal anatomy and physiology, the structural and functional derangements that occur in various diseases, and the mechanisms responsible for the clinical manifestations of diseases. The nurse must fully recognize the principles governing how drugs are absorbed, distributed, metabolized, and excreted; the various factors which alter these processes; and the consequences of any alteration. Professional responsibility dictates comprehension of the many ways in which drugs produce their therapeutic and adverse effects, the nature of these drug effects, how biophysical and psychosocial factors affect drug response, and the means by which drug effects can be evaluated. Further, the nurse must understand the ethical and legal principles that impact on drug therapy.

Although literally thousands of drugs are currently marketed, there are about 50 or 60 major drug groups that encompass most of the therapeutically useful drugs. Although the nurse or student cannot know all of the individual drugs, it is feasible to learn about these major groups.

With this knowledge base, nurses can acquire a more extensive understanding of the individual drugs commonly employed in their practice setting or clinical specialty.

The nurse's grasp of the principles underlying drug therapy is far more useful than a rote memorization of facts about particular drugs—principles may easily be converted to clinical application as long as the nurse practices. Pharmacology will become more complex as new drugs are introduced each year, and the nurse's role in providing meaningful health care will continue to expand, requiring the depth of the nurse's knowledge of pharmacology to be comparable with that of the physician and pharmacist, although the scope and focus will differ. Rather than struggle to know *all* about drugs, nurses need a knowledge of the general mechanisms of drug therapy to be able to ask intelligent questions about drugs, interpret the answers, and thus convert their knowledge into patient care. Nurses should also cultivate a commitment to continuing, lifelong education in pharmacology. It is never safe to assume one knows all that is necessary about any drug; even the most fundamental scientific principles can evolve as science advances!

The purpose of Unit I of this text is to introduce the nursing process as it is unique to drug therapy. The fundamental principles of clinical pharmacology can be found in Unit II. Subsequent chapters relate specific drugs to the diseases and symptoms which they are used to treat.

WHAT IS PHARMACOLOGY?

From the preceding discussion it may be apparent that terms such as *pharmacology* and *drug* are used differently by scientists and health care professionals than by the layperson. *Pharmacology* is the study of the properties of chemicals and all aspects of their interactions with living organisms. Pharmacologists may study, for example, how acetylcholine (a chemical normally found in nerves) exerts its physiologic effects in a certain tissue derived from healthy rats. While this study may eventually lead to a development that affects

TABLE 1-1 Relation of the Nursing Process to Scientific Method of Problem Solving and the Problem-Oriented Record (POR)

SCIENTIFIC METHOD	NURSING PROCESS	PROBLEM-ORIENTED RECORD (POR)

1. Defining the problem
  a. Recognizing the general problem area
  b. Surveying the literature
  c. Defining the specific problem
	1. Assessment
	  a. Data collection
	  b. Data analysis
	  c. Nursing diagnosis (judgment)
		1. Data base
		2. Problem list

2. Proposing hypotheses
3. Testing hypotheses
	2. Management
	  a. Planning
	    (1) Goals
	    (2) Priorities
	    (3) Specific approaches
	  b. Implementation
		3. Initial assessment and plan

4. Analyzing data	3. Evaluation	4. Progress notes

treatment of a disease in humans, much pharmacologic research is basic research that has no direct therapeutic application. *Clinical pharmacology is the study of drug effects in humans,* while *therapeutics* concerns agents and procedures used in the prevention, diagnosis, and treatment of diseases. *Pharmacotherapeutics* specifically addresses the use of drugs as therapeutic agents. On the other hand, *pharmacy* is a profession and an academic discipline concerned with the preparing and dispensing of agents for therapeutic use and the dissemination of drug information.

A *drug* can be broadly defined as any chemical other than food that affects living processes. This would include not only chemicals used to prevent, diagnose, or treat disease, but also substances (such as birth control pills) employed purposely to alter normal function. Also considered drugs are pollutants, food additives, nicotine, caffeine, ethanol, and analogous chemicals. Natural sources of drugs are plants, animals (including microorganisms), and minerals, while a large number of drugs are chemically synthesized. The terms *medication* and *pharmacologic agent* are generally used interchangeably with the term *drug.*

DRUG NOMENCLATURE

Drugs are often classified according to their legal status. Drugs which are not considered safe for unsupervised use are called *prescription* drugs, since they are dispensed only by the order of practitioners licensed by law to prescribe (i.e., physicians, dentists, veterinarians, and, in a few states, podiatrists, nurse practitioners, and physician's assistants). *Nonprescription,* or *over-the-counter,* drugs are purchased and used at the discretion of the consumer. In a special class of prescription drugs are the *controlled substances,* which are agents with the potential for abuse or development of drug dependence. Special prescription procedures apply to controlled substances, and a few are legally available only for research. *Social drugs* are those used for their subjectively pleasant psychologic or physical effects. Caffeine, ethanol, and tobacco are legal social drugs, while prescription drugs employed for nontherapeutic purposes and illegally obtained controlled substances are considered *illicit* social drugs, or *street drugs.*

Drugs may also be classified to designate the chemical or pharmacologic relationship of a group of drugs, such as the penicillins, phenothiazines, general anesthetics, antiarrhythmics, etc. One drug, usually the first or most useful agent, may become the representative, or *prototype,* of the drug group, which permits recognition and comparison of the characteristics of the entire class. For example, chlorpromazine (Thorazine) is the prototype of the phenothiazine antipsychotic drugs.

Individual drugs each have at least three names. One is the *chemical name,* which is a precise description of the arrangement of atomic groups in the drug's chemical structure. These names are generally too complex for common use. The nonproprietary name, or *generic name,* of a drug

is assigned when a chemical agent demonstrates potential therapeutic usefulness. If the drug may be marketed, a United States Adopted Name (USAN) is then selected by the USAN Council. If the drug is entered in the *United States Pharmacopeia,* the official compendium, the generic name may become the *official name.* The manufacturer will also assign a *trade name,* or *proprietary name,* to the drug. If more than one manufacturer makes the drug, each will give the drug its own trade name. The use of the generic name is encouraged by most institutions, since this avoids the problem of the same generic drug being available under numerous trade names. Unfortunately, generic names are often long, difficult to spell, and hard to pronounce, so the drug is often referred to by the trade name. By convention the generic name is written with the first letter in the lowercase, often followed in parentheses by the trade name (also called *brand name*), which has the first letter capitalized. This notation form is used throughout this textbook.

For example, a widely recognized drug is commonly known as Valium, which is its trade name. Pharmacologically it is a member of the antianxiety drug group, although the older name *sedatives* is also used. Chemically it belongs to a group of drugs called the benzodiazepines. The chemical name of this specific drug is 7-chloro-1,3-dihydro-1-methyl-5-phenyl-2H-1,4 benzodiazepin-2-one. The generic name is diazepam, and in this text this drug will be cited as *diazepam* or *diazepam (Valium).* There are some 27 trade names for this drug internationally, but in the United States only Valium and Valreleace are used, due to the period of patent protection afforded the drug developer. A drug with numerous proprietary names is hydrochlorothiazide, a diuretic available under the trade names HydroDIURIL, Oretic, Esidrix, and others. Most institutional pharmacies will purchase only one brand of hydrochlorothiazide (usually the least expensive), so to avoid confusion, the nurse should use the generic name, since the trade name could change numerous times during the year.

COST VERSUS BENEFIT

Drug effects are categorized as therapeutic effects and adverse effects. The *therapeutic effect* is the desired, beneficial action for which the drug is administered. *Adverse effects* are the undesired and sometimes dangerous effects of a drug. The terms *toxic effect* and *side effect* are sometimes used as though they were synonymous with adverse effect, but toxicity and side effects are two distinct subtypes of adverse drug reactions (see Chap. 6). If a drug exerts the desired effect, it is called *efficacious* or is said to possess *efficacy.* Drugs which produce relatively insignificant adverse effects are said to be *safe.*

Every drug available for use has a potential for adverse effects; every situation in which drugs are used requires a balancing of the anticipated beneficial effects of the therapeutic measure and the potential adverse effects of that form of therapy. Each time a drug is taken, the cost-to-benefit ratio, in terms of patient well-being and in terms of dollars, must be analyzed carefully. Cost-to-benefit analysis is an important component of nursing process in drug therapy.

Drug utilization can be studied by looking at the sales of prescription and nonprescription drugs. For example, the top-selling prescription drugs in 1982 included an antianxiety agent, an antibiotic, and an antiulcer drug. These products are safe and effective when used properly, but in many cases they are used incorrectly; for example, the antibiotic ampicilin may be used for treatment of the common cold. Benzodiazepines (e.g., Valium, Librium) are antianxiety agents indicated for the relief of anxiety and tension. Use of such drugs requires the clinician to consider several questions about the rationale of therapy: Is anxiety a normal physiologic mechanism or an abnormal state? Should anxiety always be suppressed, or do mild anxiety states enable us to function more effectively? Is a drug the answer, or would nondrug intervention in the form of an effective nurse-patient relationship be more appropriate? Such questions are difficult to answer. What is required is a complete knowledge of the individual patient being treated, a willingness on the part of health care practitioners to initially test nondrug forms of therapy, and a healthy skepticism, or therapeutic nihilism, which encourages the practitioner to weigh the costs and the benefits of drug therapy for each patient and for each drug. Drugs are vital and necessary tools in the treatment of health disorders. They must be used appropriately and sensibly, not as panaceas for human ills, but as adjuncts to other types of therapeutic intervention.

The dynamic science of medicine is dealing with many unanswered questions. Ideally, underlying disease states rather than symptoms should be treated. But for many disease entities, pathophysiologic mechanisms are unknown and treatment is empiric or based on a symptom. Truly rational drug therapy cannot occur until the pathologic processes associated with a disease, the physiologic mechanisms by which drugs exert their effects, and the potential for adverse effects are fully known. Until then, caution must be the rule in all drug therapy.

HISTORICAL PERSPECTIVE

The history of the nursing role in drug therapy has been one of contrasts and controversy. Doubtless this pattern will continue in the future, as the profession articulates its unique contribution within an evolving health care system. The general history of pharmacology, which is chronicled in many medical pharmacology texts, corresponds to the history of science and the development of the profession of medicine. Similarly, the role of the nurse in drug therapy is an accurate reflection of the development of the nursing profession.

Records of ancient times from China, India, Sumer, and Greece, some of which date as far back as 4000 B.C., record the accumulation of local drug lore. Healers who performed

the care and comfort functions of nursing are known to have used herbs in illness treatment and health maintenance. This practice continued among lay nurses at least up to the development of modern nursing. However, because of the silence of the records, it is thought that organized nursing by trained practitioners was virtually unknown prior to the Christian era.

The history of nursing first became continuous with the advent of Christianity and its emphasis on care of the poor and sick. The accumulated knowledge from the Greeks was taught to nuns and monks who performed medicine and nursing of the ill in hospitals throughout western Europe. Little scientific development took place during this time. By the twelfth century three distinctive Christian orders for the care of the sick had evolved: the military nursing orders originating in the Crusades, secular orders, and regular orders such as the Augustinian Sisters of the Hôtel-Dieu de Paris. Herein lie the military and religious roots that have had a great impact on the nursing role in drug therapy.

The same events that broke the dominance of religion in the world and brought the Renaissance in science and art dealt a setback to the development of nursing as a respected, educated, and autonomous profession. Copernicus (1473–1543) and Vesalius (1514–1564) typified the revolution in science with the conviction that natural, and not divine, forces dominated the universe and that these forces could be understood by direct observation. A young physician named Philippus Aureolus Theophrastus Bombastus von Hohenheim (1493–1541), who later called himself Paracelsus, founded modern pharmacology by insisting that drugs should be subjected to critical investigation. The Reformation caused the closing of many hospitals, the education of women virtually ceased, and there was a significant decline in humane and charitable work. Nursing tasks fell to women from the lowest classes, to perform along with household cleaning and laundry.

Florence Nightingale (1820–1910), recognized as the founder of modern nursing, also defined the role of the nurse in drug therapy. Because of her training with nuns and deaconesses and her experience in the Crimean War, religious and military influences are evident in her adoption of such terms as *physician's orders* and *obedience*. Nightingale devoted little attention to pharmacology, since most drugs of the time were ineffective, but among her voluminous writings are directions that (1) nurses should have nothing to do with the prescribing of medications or stimulants; (2) the administration of medicines as ordered, including enemas, injections, leeches, and suppositories, is a legitimate nursing function; (3) medicines and treatments must be given at fixed times each day; (4) nurses should understand the origin of symptoms and why a particular therapy has been prescribed; (5) nurses must observe the effects of medicines; and (6) as science and medicine develop, nurses should take on more tasks, do research, and learn new and improved methods.

While Nightingale did encourage obedience to the physician's orders, she stressed that it must be *educated obedience* based upon an understanding of the anticipated course of the disease. The nurse was expected to recognize that physicians' orders were "conditional" and that if any of the required conditions (of the patient or the environment) were altered, the nurse should not execute the order. However, for about 100 years nursing practice emphasized some of Nightingale's specifications more than others, perhaps because *Notes on Nursing,* the classic work on nursing care which she wrote for the layperson, was commonly used as a nursing text (Nightingale, 1859). Many of the less familiar exhortations are found in her other works, which were addressed to policymakers and educators of nurses. Thus, almost ritualistic obedience to the physician's order, adherence to a fixed dosage schedule, and observation primarily for adverse effects were characteristic of the nursing role in drug therapy for the first half of the twentieth century. Expansion of the nursing role to include evaluation for therapeutic as well as adverse effects, assessment of the appropriateness of a drug order in a specific situation, consumer education, and research were in response more to social and political forces following World War II than to Nightingale's influence or the phenomenal growth of pharmacologic knowledge.

In the 1950s nurses began to critically evaluate the role of the profession in health care and to differentiate *dependent* nursing functions, which required the direction of the physician, from *independent* functions, which were entirely under the direction of the nurse. The need for research to develop a scientific basis for nursing care was recognized. Audits of the quality of nursing care were initiated, starting a trend which continued over the next two decades as private insurance companies and governmental agencies assumed financial responsibility for growing health care costs. Regulations and standards of care were developed as a basis for these quality assurance programs. The elderly population increased, establishing a demand for standards applicable to nursing homes as well. Documentation of accurate and effective drug therapy was common to such standards.

Civil suits against nurses increased in numbers in the postwar era, and no longer was the physician held responsible for the errors of the nurse. Nurses were even held liable for harm suffered by patients when the nurses followed orders that were contraindicated; thus nurses became legally responsible for their own actions.

In response to a shortage of physicians and the perception of the value of traditional nursing functions in health maintenance, nurse practitioners were trained to assume primary care responsibilities. By 1984 nurse practitioners had prescriptive authority in at least eleven states if they practice under the supervision of a physician or use approved protocols. Other forces which have shaped the development of the nursing role in drug therapy over the last three decades are the increasing effectiveness and specificity of drugs, the epidemic of drug abuse and misuse, the development of critical care units, the consumer movement, the women's movement, and the holistic health movement.

NURSING PROCESS IN DRUG THERAPY

Most discussions of the nursing process address its use in the so-called independent functions of nursing. This should not imply that the implementation of a physician's direction (i.e., "following the doctor's order") does not involve problem solving. Merely because it is a collaborative function which is initiated by the physician, and is under the control of the physician, does not mean a task is nonnursing or relieves the nurse of the responsibility for scientific judgment. If nursing is "the diagnosis and treatment of human responses to actual or potential health problems" (American Nurses Association, 1980), then assisting a person to follow the advice of the physician is a part of nursing and requires the nursing process. This is true whether the nurse educates the person on how to take a drug, actually administers the drug, or only observes the response to the drug.

Therapeutic interventions are initiated as a result of the identification of a health problem, which is called a *diagnosis.* Because the problems addressed by the health professions differ, an adjective may be placed before the term, as in *nursing diagnosis, medical diagnosis,* and *casework diagnosis* (by social workers). The advice or prescription of the health care professional to a patient or client may be called the *orders,* or prescription, and can also be designated by the area of origin, as in *medical orders* and *nursing orders.* Because a recognized function of nursing is assisting persons with self-care deficits in activities of daily living, nurses often help people implement the orders of another professional when these people lack the necessary knowledge or skill to do so for themselves.

This view of medical prescriptions and orders as advice to the patient, which the nurse assists the patient to implement, is at variance with the traditional and militaristic view of orders as commands of physicians which nurses must obey. However, it reflects certain modern values that are denied by the traditional view. These include:

1. Patients have the legal and moral right to give informed consent for any therapeutic intervention.

2. Medicine and nursing are autonomous professions which collaborate toward the optimal well-being of the client.

3. Nurses have sole legal and ethical responsibility for all their decisions and actions.

The implications of this discussion should not be misunderstood. *Nurses may not omit any medical order unless it is clearly contraindicated.* This principle is inherent in the legal and social contract between the professions. Further, students and nurses must recognize that this conceptual view is not universally accepted. Other opinions fall on a continuum between two extremes. There are those that still subscribe to the traditional view of medical orders as commands from a superior officer to be obeyed without question, including all its hierarchical, coercive, and militaristic overtones. At the other extreme, there are those who would banish the term *order* from the health care vocabulary and with it all practices and terms that imply hierarchy, coercion, or dependency on the part of the consumer.

Elements of the Nursing Process

While there are a variety of definitions of the elements of the nursing process, the specific breakdown of the steps is not as important as the systematic progression through certain phases to the objective. The most common division of the nursing process into four steps—assessment, planning, implementation, and evaluation—emphasizes the most important aspects of problem solving in nursing. In application to drug therapy, the planning and implementation steps are so closely related that these can be combined into a step called *management*. Thus, this textbook will discuss the nursing process in these three steps: assessment, management, and evaluation.

Assessment is the systematic collection and interpretation of data. The nurse gathers accurate data about the *patient,* the *drug,* and the *influencing environmental factors.* This information is used to identify patient problems or patient states that relate to nursing care, i.e., the nursing diagnosis. On the basis of these data the nurse determines before administration whether a drug order is safe and effective for a particular patient.

The planning component of *management* includes defining objectives, establishing priorities, and selecting the best approach. Implementation is the action phase of the nursing process, in which the plan is carried out by the nurse or someone designated by the nurse. In drug therapy, management involves deciding whether and how best to administer the drug, what measures will complement the desired drug action, and which will control undesirable actions, followed by the actual performance of these measures.

In *evaluation* the nurse determines if the plan was effective or why it was not, according to the goals established during the formation of the plan, and makes appropriate modifications in the plan.

Chapters 2 to 4 will consider each step of the nursing process in relation to pharmacotherapeutics.

REFERENCES

Abu-Saad, H.: *Nursing: A World View,* St. Louis: Mosby, 1979.

Ackerknecht, E. H.: *Therapeutics from the Primitives to the 20th Century,* New York: Hafner, 1973.

American Nurses Association: *Nursing: A Social Policy Statement,* Kansas City: ANA, 1980.

Gordon, M.: *Nursing Diagnosis: Process and Application,* New York: McGraw-Hill, 1982.

LaMonica, E. L.: *The Nursing Process: A Humanistic Approach,* Reading, Mass.: Addison-Wesley, 1979.

Langeman, E. C. (ed.): *Nursing History: New Perspectives, New Possibilities,* New York: Teachers College, 1983.

Levine, R. R.: *Pharmacology: Drug Actions and Reactions,* 2d ed., Boston: Little, Brown, 1978.

Marriner, A.: *The Nursing Process: A Scientific Approach to Nursing Care,* St. Louis, Mosby, 1979.

Mayer, S. E., K. L. Melmon, and A. G. Gilman: "Introduction; the Dynamics of Drug Absorption, Distribution, and Elimination," in A. G. Gilman, L. S. Goodman, and A. Gilman (eds.), *Goodman and Gilman's The Pharmacological Basis of Therapeutics,* 6th ed., New York: Macmillan, 1980.

Mitchell, P. H.: "Science, Research, and the Helping Process in Nursing: An Overview," in P. H. Mitchell and A. Loustau (eds.), *Concepts Basic to Nursing,* 3d ed., New York: McGraw-Hill, 1981.

Nightingale, F.: *Notes on Nursing: What It Is, and What It Is Not,* London: Harrison, 1859.

Seymer, L. R.: *Selected Writings of Florence Nightingale,* New York: Macmillan, 1954.

Stitzel, R. E.: "Development of Pharmacological Thought," in C. R. Craig and R. E. Stitzel (eds.), *Modern Pharmacology,* Boston: Little, Brown, 1982.

Yura, H., and M. B. Walsh: *The Nursing Process,* 3d ed., New York: Appleton-Century-Crofts, 1978.

2

NURSING ASSESSMENT AND PHARMACOTHERAPEUTICS

GINETTE A. PEPPER

LEARNING OBJECTIVES

Upon mastery of the contents of this chapter, the reader will be able to:

1. List at least six patient variables which may alter the effect of drug therapy.
2. Describe the content of and approach to obtaining a medication history.
3. Explain what a nurse needs to know about a specific drug in order to carry out the nursing process.
4. List the major parts of a medication order.
5. Recognize the meanings of abbreviations commonly used in medication orders.
6. Describe the common dosage routes and dosage forms.
7. Differentiate between a routine order, PRN order, single order, stat order, verbal order, and protocol.
8. Explain five systems of measurement used in drug orders.
9. List three important factors in assessing the environment in relation to drug therapy.
10. Explain how data analysis and nursing diagnosis vary depending upon the type of drug order.
11. Describe five sources of drug information.
12. Give examples of nursing diagnoses related to drug therapy.
13. Formulate clinical drug questions appropriately.

The effectiveness of nursing care is directly dependent upon the quality of the data collection and accuracy of the conclusions drawn from the data. Within nursing process, *assessment* has three important components: *data collection, analysis of the data,* and *nursing diagnosis.* Table 1-1 shows how these steps fit into the total nursing process. In this chapter each step will be considered in relation to drug therapy.

DATA COLLECTION

Nurses gather data relative to drug therapy from the same sources used for all nursing assessments: interview and observation of the patient; interview of relatives and friends; physical examination; measurement of physical variables (height, weight, vital signs, fluid intake and output, etc.); evaluation of laboratory, x-ray, and other diagnostic test results; consultation with other health care professionals; and use of textbooks, journal articles, and references. The medication history is an important part of the data base. The basic areas of assessment important to drug therapy are data about the *patient,* data about the *drug,* and data about the *environment.*

Assessing the Patient

The effect of a medication does not depend solely upon the drug and dosage but also upon individual patient variables. In fact, it is because of the variability in patient response that the nursing process is so important in drug therapy. If every patient given the same dose of the same drug had exactly the same response, there would be no need for problem solving. Although the majority of patients will respond in the "normal" or "average" way to a drug, some portion of patients exhibit unusual responses. Research helps the clinician to identify the characteristics of patients that are associated with abnormal responses. Based on this knowledge, the assessment phase of the nursing process is aimed at detecting or predicting those with atypical responses so that plans can be made to prevent or limit deleterious effects and to tailor drug therapy to individual patients.

The individual patient variables which have been found through research and clinical experience to be associated with atypical drug response are summarized in Table 2-1. These variables are further discussed in general in Unit II and as they specifically relate to individual drugs in Units III to VI.

9

TABLE 2-1 Patient Variables That May Affect Drug Response

VARIABLE TO ASSESS	REASON
Age	Very young and very old people have altered drug disposition* and sensitivity.†
Gender	Drug disposition* and sensitivity differ.†
Body build (weight, height, lean body mass, obesity)	Smaller people need smaller doses. Body composition affects drug disposition.*
Disease states	Diseases—especially renal, hepatic, gastrointestinal, and cardiac—can alter drug disposition.* Diseases can increase susceptibility to adverse effects of some drugs or impair action of the drugs. Stage of the disease is also important, since drug response may vary at different stages.
Concurrent drug use	Drug interactions can alter drug disposition* and sensitivity.†
Allergies (drugs, food, animals, clothing, pollen, etc.)	Cross allergies can occur between drugs and between drug and nondrug allergens.
Pregnancy	Drug disposition is altered.* Fetal effects must be considered.
Lactation	Content in milk and effects on infants must be considered.
Race, family history of drug reactions	Some variations in drug disposition* are inherited and may be more prevalent in certain races.
Diet and fluids	Oral absorption and other drug disposition* and sensitivity may be increased or decreased.†
Environmental pollutants	Drug disposition* and sensitivity are altered.†
Psychosocial factors (health-illness beliefs, attitudes, prior experiences with medicines, social support, culture, economic status, etc.)	These factors affect whether the patient takes the drug and drug sensitivity.†
Psychomotor and cognitive functioning	Ability to self-administer drugs is affected.

*Drug disposition may be altered in absorption, distribution, metabolism, and/or excretion. See Pharmacokinetic Phase in Chap. 5.

†Sensitivity relates to alteration at the site of action. See Pharmacodynamic Phase in Chap. 5.

The Medication History

While it has been shown that prior and current drug use will have an effect on a patient's present condition, a complete drug history is too often unavailable. Due to the volume of data needed in assessment for drug therapy, it is important that the information be collected in a systematic way, but often nursing histories provide meager information about the patient's medication history. In some institutions the clinical pharmacist uses an assessment tool, known as the *medication history*, that can serve as a valuable source of information about a specific patient's prior drug use (see Fig. 2-1). Where clinical pharmacists are not available, nurses should include a thorough medication history in the initial patient assessment.

The medication history should compile all relevant data relating to the patient's drug use, including all prescription drugs, nonprescription drugs (analgesics, antacids, laxatives, vitamins, cough and cold preparations, etc.), caffeine-con-taining products (cola drinks, coffee, tea), alcohol, tobacco, and illicit drugs (marijuana, opiates, barbiturates, etc.). "Back-fence medications," or those drugs which the patient has obtained from relatives or friends, should also be considered. Since the area of drug therapy and drug use may be an emotion-charged one for the patient, it is necessary to develop a good nurse-patient rapport for this interview, to appropriately combine nondirective and directive techniques, and to avoid letting personal bias about drug use influence data collection. The vocabulary will need to be appropriate to the patient, and the use of specific brand names and simple terms such as "sleeping pills" for hypnotics and "pain pills" for analgesics may facilitate communication.

It is best to begin with open-ended questions like "Are you taking any medication?" As the interview progresses, the questions should be more specific; the basic objective should be to obtain a complete medication history including

PATIENT MEDICATION HISTORY

Name_____

Phone_____Address_____

Age_____Sex_____Race_____Height_____Weight_____

BP_____Pulse_____Temperature_____Occupation_____

PROBLEM(S)	ACUTE	CHRONIC
Head		
Eyes/ears/nose/throat		
Respiratory		
Cardiovascular		
Gastrointestinal		
Genitourinary		
Endocrine		
CNS, neurological		
psychological		
Bones/joints/muscles		
Blood/lymph		
Dermatology		
General		

ALLERGIES	TYPE OF UNDESIRABLE EFFECT	DATE OF OCCURRENCE
Penicillin		
Sulfa		
Aspirin		
Narcotics		
Other		

MEDICATION HISTORY

Prescription medications	DOSAGE	DURATION

Nonprescription medication	DOSAGE	FREQUENCY	DURATION
Alcohol			
Tobacco			
Caffeine			
Street drugs			
OTC medications			

DRUG-RELATED PROBLEMS

_____
_____
_____

PHARMACIST'S CONSULTATION

_____
_____
_____

Date _____

Time of interview _____ Interviewer _____

FIGURE 2-1

A Format for Recording the Patient Medication History. Note that it includes prescription, nonprescription, and social drugs.

the drugs, frequency (how often the drugs were taken *and* how often the prescriber recommended use), dosage, duration of use, what the drugs were used for, expected and actual outcomes, and any problems associated with the drugs' use. In many cases the patient will not remember the drug name or may never have known what the name was. Therefore, the nurse may need to ask the patient or a family member to bring in all the medications that the patient is currently taking, for purposes of identification.

Persons who use illicit drugs are afraid of legal implications and only a good nurse-patient relation will encourage the patient to give a complete history. Further information related to allergies or reactions to food, clothing, chemicals, and drugs is important, including when the reaction occurred and the nature of the reaction. Often patients will have experienced a reaction that was not allergic in nature but assumed that any adverse reaction is caused by allergy (see Chap. 6). In obtaining the medication history, the nurse collects valuable information about the teaching needs of the patient, such as information about patient drug compliance, understanding of the therapeutic regimen, and understanding of the need for continuing prescribed medications and medical follow-up.

Many patients see more than one prescriber simultaneously. This may include physician, podiatrist, nurse practitioner, dentist, or medical subspecialist, such as a dermatologist. This may lead to *polydrug therapy*, the utilization of more than one medication at one time. While polydrug therapy is not always avoidable, early identification of potentially dangerous situations through utilization of the medication history can spare the patient much discomfort and expense.

Assessing the Drug

Nursing assessment in pharmacotherapeutics requires knowledge of the pharmacology of the drug and accurate interpretation of the medical order.

Pharmacology of the Drug

Knowledge of the drug's mechanism of action, pharmacokinetics, clinical effects and uses, adverse effects, dosage, routes of administration, and indications for patient education are needed to execute the nursing process in drug therapy. Since there are so many drugs available and it is impossible to know all this information about every drug, it is often necessary to consult a reference about unfamiliar drugs. Sources of drug information are discussed later in this chapter.

Students and some nurses find that outlining the pharmacology of a drug or drug group on a file card affords a portable and accessible reference for unfamiliar or seldom-used drugs until their characteristics can be committed to memory. An example of the organization of a drug reference card is shown in Fig. 2-2. However, nursing process requires

Generic name: indomethacin Drug category: NSAID

Trade names(s): Indocin, Indocin SR

Clinical action and uses: Anti-inflammatory, analgesic, antipyretic. Used in moderate to severe RA (incl. acute), OA, ankylosing spondilitis, acute painful shoulder, acute gouty arthritis. Investigational for closure of patent ductus in neonate and to prevent premature labor.

Mechanism of action: Inhibits prostaglandin formation.

Pharmacokinetics: Food decreases rate but not extent of absorption. Peak level = 2 h. $t_{1/2}$ = 4.5 h. Metabolized by liver to inactive metabolites. Albumin bound = 90%. Excreted 10–20% unchanged in urine.

Adverse Drug Reactions: GI = anorexia, N&V, abdominal pain, ulcer formation. CNS = headache (25–50%), dizziness, confusion. Blood dyscrasias. Edema. Cross-allergy to aspirin possible. Contraindicated in pregnancy, psychiatric disorders, epilepsy, parkinsonism, GI ulcers, renal disease. Drug interactions: probenecid, furosemide. May mask infection.

Usual dose: 50–200 mg/day in 2–3 doses. Maximum dose 400 mg/day. Not recommended for children under 4.

Patient education: 1. Take with meals, milk, or antacid ($AlOH_3$, $MgOH_2$). 2. Use caution in driving or operating machinery. 3. Notify physician if rash, persistent headache, black stools, swelling, or weight gain occur.

FIGURE 2-2

An Example of a Medication Card for Quick, Portable Reference. (Abbreviations: NSAID = nonsteroidal anti-inflammatory drug, SR = sustained-release, RA = rheumatoid arthritis, incl. = including, OA = osteoarthritis, $t_{1/2}$ = half-life, GI = gastrointestinal, N&V = nausea and vomiting, CNS = central nervous system, $AlOH_3$ = aluminum hydroxide, $MgOH_2$ = magnesium hydroxide) that the drug information on the card be analyzed in light of specific patient characteristics and an individualized plan for care be developed. Otherwise, nursing is practiced by recipe or rule of thumb rather than rational problem solving.

The Medication Order

Medication ordered for patients by a licensed prescriber is recorded on a prescription form or a physician's order form in the medical record. Generally, the term *prescription* is associated with ambulatory health care facilities (clinics and physicians' offices); *physicians' orders*, or *chart orders*, or *medication orders*, relate to the inpatient situation (see Fig. 2-3). Prescriptions are presented directly to a pharmacist, who dispenses the drug to the patient. On the other hand, medication orders are usually controlled by the nursing staff, who are required to ensure that ordered medications are obtained and administered.

The physician's order should be carefully screened for accuracy and legibility. If there is any ambiguity about the intent of the order, it should be clarified with the prescriber.

When medication orders are transmitted orally by the prescriber, they should be reduced to writing immediately and read back to the prescriber in order to double-check the requisition. Oral transmission should be discouraged in all but emergency situations because of the increased possibility of medication error. For this reason most students are prohibited from accepting verbal and phone orders.

Components of the Medication Order

The medical order has seven important components:

1. Name of the patient for identification—The full name is best, to avoid confusing patients with others who have similar names. A name stamp is often used. (Other forms of identification on the order sheet are hospital number, age, sex, date of birth, and date of admission.)
2. Date and time of the order—These are important in establishing the discontinuation date and for a more accurate transcription.
3. Name of the drug—The name may be brand or generic, unless hospital policy dictates generic. Dosage form is also indicated if more than one form is available.
4. Dosage—The amount of the drug to be given at each dose is given in metric units at most institutions.
5. Route—If not specified, the route is assumed to be oral.
6. Time and frequency—The exact times or the number of times per day may be stipulated. (In the second case, hospital policy and/or specific qualities of the drug will determine specific times.) Rather than stipulate a time, the order may describe the conditions under which the drug may be given and the maximum frequency of use.
7. Signature of the prescriber—The signature should be legible so that nurses know whom to contact if further information is needed.

In order to interpret the medication order, the nurse must understand the types of medication orders, common routes of administration, and available dosage forms. Further, the nurse should be aware of the abbreviations which are officially approved within the institution and request validation with the prescriber of any others, since the usage of abbreviations may vary widely. Common medical abbreviations used in drug orders are shown in Table 2-2.

Types of Medication Orders

Standard Order The standard order, or *routine order,* is of two types: that with a termination date and that without a termination date. If no specified termination date is given, the drug orders are written with the intention that the drug be given until discontinued by the prescriber. Some institutions have policies that dictate that all drug orders or those in certain categories are automatically discontinued after a stated period of time and that they must be rewritten by the prescriber for the drug to be continued (e.g., narcotics, antibiotics).

Single and Stat Orders The *single order* is written to be given only once, at some specific time or at the earliest convenient time. An example is the preoperative medication order. The *stat order* is written to be given only once and immediately. *Stat* comes from the Latin *statim,* meaning "immediately." Since these orders must be handled differently, requiring immediate action by nursing and pharmacy personnel, they are meant to be reserved for emergency situations.

PRN Order The PRN order is given according to the nurse's judgment regarding the patient's needs for the drug. The term comes from the Latin *pro re nata,* meaning "as occasion arises" or "as needed." These medications are given on a "when necessary" basis, and the order may stipulate the appropriate circumstances, such as "for mild pain," or may leave the circumstances to the judgment of the nurse or the outpatient. Common examples are PRN pain medication and PRN antiemetics. PRN orders usually stipulate the maximum frequency with which the drug can be administered. In critical care units, PRN orders may be written in which dosages are dependent upon sophisticated measurements, such as the number of premature ventricular contractions or the direct arterial blood pressure.

Protocol Protocols are guides for analyzing and treating a disease process or symptom complex. For example, the pediatric nurse practitioner might have a protocol applicable when clinical and laboratory findings are indicative of tonsillitis caused by group A, β-hemolytic streptococcus. In coronary care units, certain drug treatments for life-threatening arrhythmias are often established. These may sometimes be referred to as *standing orders.* Protocols can be highly specific and directive or more general and flexible, depending

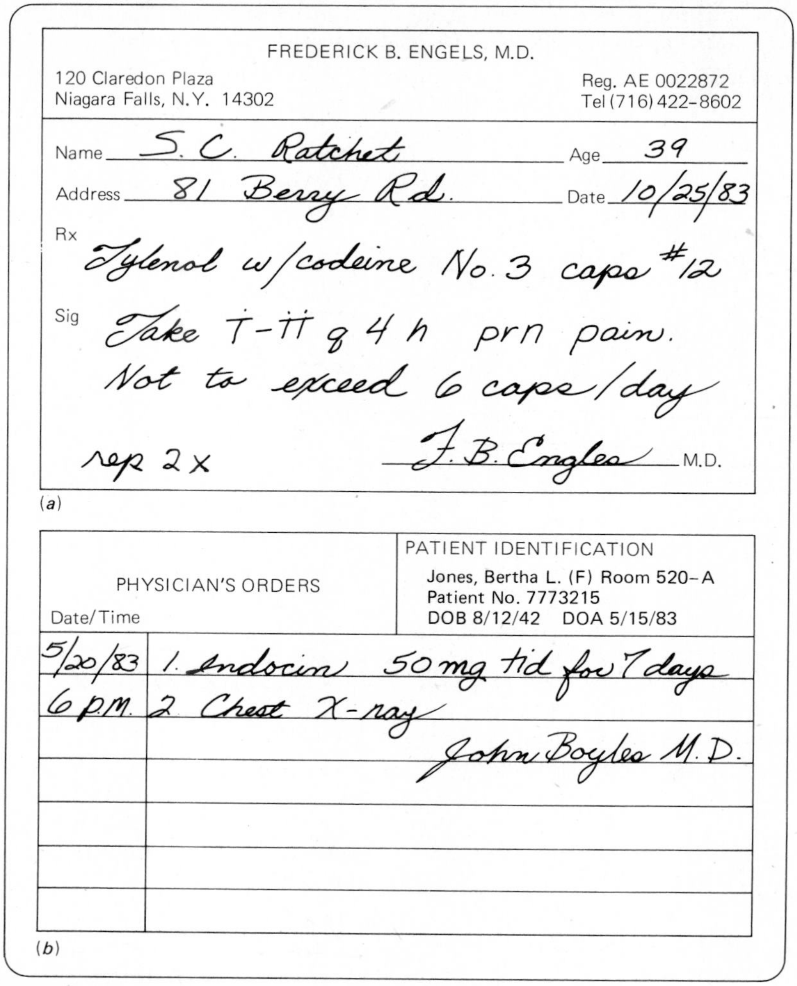

FREDERICK B. ENGELS, M.D.

120 Claredon Plaza   Reg. AE 0022872
Niagara Falls, N.Y. 14302   Tel (716) 422–8602

Name   *S. C. Ratchet*   Age   *39*

Address   *81 Berry Rd.*   Date *10/25/83*

Rx

Tylenol w/codeine No. 3 caps #12

Sig

Take I–II q 4 h prn pain.
Not to exceed 6 caps/day

rep 2 x   *F. B. Engles* ___ M.D.

(a)

PHYSICIAN'S ORDERS	PATIENT IDENTIFICATION
Date/Time	Jones, Bertha L. (F) Room 520–A Patient No. 7773215 DOB 8/12/42 DOA 5/15/83

5/20/83	*1. Indocin 50 mg tid for 7 days*
6 PM	*2 Chest X-ray*
	John Boyles M.D.

(b)

FIGURE 2-3

The method of communicating the physician's order depends upon the setting: (a)
In the outpatient setting the prescription form is used, and (b) in the inpatient setting the order is written on an order form in the chart.

on the situation, the skill and training of the nurses, and the availability of physician supervision.

With a protocol it is important for the nurse to critically assess the patient for factors that might contraindicate application of the protocol (e.g., allergies, impaired drug elimination, and diseases). When a protocol has been established to allow rapid response to emergency situations, this analysis must be anticipatory, that is, done before the emergency arises, since there may not be time for consideration when the situation does occur.

Clearly, PRN orders and protocols require *more discretion* on the part of the nurse than do regular, single, and stat orders. The mechanics of the use of the nursing process will be different for orders that require more independent judg-

ment than for those that require less. This difference is discussed in the Analysis of Data and Nursing Diagnosis sections of this chapter.

Dosage Measurement Units

Five types of measurements are used in medication orders. *Metric units* are preferred for most drugs (see Table 2-3). Some older drugs (e.g., nitroglycerin, morphine, atropine, and codeine) are still ordered in the *apothecary system* (see Table 2-4), although prescribers can use metric units to order these drugs. *Household measures* (see Table 2-5) are common for outpatient prescriptions and over-the-counter drugs, as patients are more likely to have devices to measure

TABLE 2-2 Abbreviations Commonly Used in Drug Orders

aa	of each	L or l	liter	q2h, q3h, etc.	every 2 h, every 3 h, etc.
ac	before meals	Ⓛ	left	qn or qnoc	every night
ad	right ear	LA	long-acting	qod	every other day
ad lib.	freely, at pleasure	lb or #	pound(s)	qs	as much as needed
A.M. or a.m.	morning	♍	minim(s)	qs ad	add a sufficient amount to make
APAP	acetaminophen	m²	square meter(s)	Ⓡ	right
aq	water	mcg or μg	microgram(s)	rep	repeat, refill
as	left ear	meq or mEq	milliequivalent(s)	Rx	treatment, prescription
ASA	aspirin	mg	milligram(s)	s̄	without
au	both ears	Mg	magnesium	s̈s or ss	one-half
bid	twice per day	min	minute(s)	sat	saturate
c̄	with	mL or ml	milliliter(s)	SC, SQ, or subq	subcutaneous
Ca	calcium	mm	millimeter(s)	s or sec	second(s)
cap	capsule(s)	MOM	milk of magnesia	sig	write on label
cc or cm³	cubic centimeter(s)	MR×1	may repeat once	SL or sl	sublingually
Cl⁻	chloride	Na	sodium	SOS	if necessary
cm	centimeter(s)	ng	nanogram(s)	Sp	spirits
comp	compound	NOC or noc	at night	span	spansule(s)
d	day	NPO or npo	nothing by mouth	SR	sustained-release
/d	per day	NR or nr	no refill, do not repeat	stat	immediately
dc or D/C	discontinue	NS or N/S	normal saline (0.9%)	Supp	suppository
DS	double strength	¼ NS	¼ normal saline (0.2%)	Syr	syrup
D₅W	5% dextrose in water	½ NS	½ normal saline (0.4%)	T, Tbl, or tbsp	tablespoon(s)
EC	enteric coated	OD	right eye	tsp or t	teaspoon(s)
elix	elixir	OS	left eye	tab	tablet(s)
et	and	os	mouth	TCN	tetracycline
ext	extract	OTC or otc	over-the-counter	tid	three times daily
fl	fluid	OU or ou	both eyes	tinct or tr	tincture
g, gm, or Gm	gram(s)	oz or ℥	ounce(s)	TO	telephone order
gr	grain(s)	p̄	after	U	unit(s)
gtt	drop(s)	pc	after meals	ung	ointment
h or hr	hour(s)	PCN	penicillin	ut dict.	as directed
H₂O₂	hydrogen peroxide	per	by, through	vag	vaginal
HCTZ	hydrochlorothiazide	φbarb	phenobarbital	VO	verbal order
HCO₃⁻	bicarbonate	PO or po	by mouth	w/	with
hs	at bedtime	PR or R	by rectum	×	times, multiply
IM	intramuscular	PRN or prn	as needed	%	percent
in. or ″	inch(es)	pt	pint(s)	i, ii, iii, iv, v	Roman numerals 1, 2, 3, 4, 5
IV	intravenous	pulv	powder	With analgesics:	
IVPB	intravenous "piggyback"	q	every	No. 1 or #1	with 8 mg codeine
K	potassium	qam or qAM	every morning	No. 2 or #2	with 15 mg codeine
KCl	potassium chloride	qd	every day	No. 3 or #3	with 30 mg codeine
kg	kilogram	qh	every hour	No. 4 or #4	with 60 mg codeine
		qid	four times daily		

TABLE 2-3   Metric System of Measurement*

MASS (WEIGHT)		VOLUME
1000 ng (nanograms) = 1 μg (microgram)		1000 mL (milliliters)† = 1 L (liter)
1000 μg	= 1 mg (milligram)	
1000 mg	= 1 g (gram)	
1000 g	= 1 kg (kilogram)	

*See Table 3-2 for interconversion with other systems of measurement.
†1 cubic centimeter (cc or cm³) = 1 mL.

these units in their homes. (However, error is common with household measurement, since teaspoons and tablespoons vary in size and a cup can be either a teacup, which is 6 oz, or a measuring cup, which is 8 oz. Many clinicians prefer to supply measuring devices to minimize this source of error. See Chap. 7 for pediatric drug administration.) The units of measurement for some drugs are based on their physiologic activity, rather than on mass or weight. Some drugs with biologic sources (e.g., insulin, heparin, penicillin G, hormones) are supplied in *units* which are determined by bioassay for pharmacologic activity. Electrolytes are usually supplied in *milliequivalents*.

Dosage Routes

The *dosage route* is the means of access to the site of action or systemic circulation. In other words, it defines where or how the drug is administered. The preferred route of administration will depend upon the disease being treated, the chemical and pharmacologic properties of the drug, and patient acceptance. Drugs are given to achieve systemic or local effects. Access to the general circulation is required for *systemic effects*. Topical application to skin or mucous membranes is the major way to achieve *local effects*, although inhalation and injection into a specific site can also be used. Table 2-6 defines common dosage routes.

Drug routes are also classified as enteral and parenteral. *Enteral routes* are those that involve administration through the gastrointestinal tract (oral, sublingual, buccal, and rectal). *Parenteral routes* include all other routes, but in common usage the term designated injected routes (intravenous,

intraarterial, intramuscular, subcutaneous, intradermal, etc.).

Dosage Forms

The dosage form is defined as the configuration and composition of the preparation which is administered to the patient. In addition to the active drug, a dosage form will contain substances that alter palatability, solubility in body fluids, shape or size, and rate and extent of absorption. Selection of dosage form will depend upon the chemical and pharmacologic characteristics of the drug, the desired drug action, and patient acceptance. Table 2-7 defines some common dosage forms for administration by various routes.

Assessing the Environment

Because too many people consider drug action to be exclusively a biologic phenomenon, environment is an important determinant of drug response that is often disregarded. Many components of the institutional environment are under the control of nursing, and community-based nurses can supply valuable data about the home environment.

Equipment and Materials

The nurse assesses the equipment available for drug administration, patient education, and other activities related to drug therapy so that resources are used to best advantage. Even in large hospitals the pharmacy and central supply service cannot stock all the drugs and equipment on the market. In the hospital it is the responsibility of the pharmacy

TABLE 2-4   Apothecary System of Measurement*

MASS (WEIGHT)		VOLUME	
60 gr (grains) = 1 ʒ (dram)		60 ℳ (minims) = 1 fʒ (fluid dram)	
8 ʒ	= 1 ℥ (ounce)	8 fʒ	= 1 f℥ (fluid ounce)
12 ℥	= 1 lb (pound)	16 f℥	= 1 pt (pint)

*In this system the symbol or abbreviation usually precedes the Roman numeral or fraction, as in gr¼, ʒiii. See Table 3-2 for interconversion with other systems of measurement.

TABLE 2-5   Household System of Measurement*

MASS (WEIGHT)	VOLUME	
16 oz (ounces) = 1 lb (pound)	20 gtt (drops)	= 1 mL (milliliter)
	3 tsp (teaspoons)	= 1 tbsp (tablespoon)
	2 tbsp	= 1 oz (fluid ounce)
	6 oz	= 1 teacup
	8 oz	= 1 glassful
	16 oz	= 1 pt (pint)

*See Table 3-2 for interconversion with other systems of measurement.

TABLE 2-6   Common Dosage Routes

ROUTE	DEFINITION	ROUTE	DEFINITION
Systemic Routes			
Oral*	Taken by mouth and swallowed. Some drugs are chewed or dissolved in the mouth prior to being swallowed.	Intravenous	Injected or infused into a vein.
		Intramuscular	Injected into a muscle.
Sublingual	Held under the tongue until absorbed into blood supply of mouth.	Subcutaneous	Injected into fat layer that lies below the dermal layers.
Buccal	Held in pocket of the cheek until absorbed into blood supply of mouth.	Hypodermoclysis	Infused into fat layer that lies below the dermal layers with an enzyme that breaks down connective tissue so large volumes can be infused.
Rectal*	Inserted or instilled into rectum.		
Inhaled†	Taken in with inspired air as gas or small droplets.	Percutaneous	Applied to skin for systemic absorption.
Local Effects (Topical)			
Dental, throat	Applied to mucous membranes or mouth structures directly or as dosage form dissolves in mouth.	Otic	Instilled into ear.
		Nasal	Sprayed or dropped into nose.
Dermatologic	Applied to skin (or mucous membrane) for local effects.	Vaginal‡	Applied, inserted, or instilled into vagina.
		Urethral	Inserted or instilled into urethra.
Ophthalmic	Applied to eye structure(s).		
Local Effects (Not Topical)			
Intraarterial	Injected or infused into an artery to attain high concentration in end organ.	Intraocular	Injected into globe of eye.
		Intraspinal	Injected into spinal canal.
Intradermal	Injected into skin layers, usually for diagnosis.	Intrathecal	Injected or instilled into cerebrospinal fluid of subarachnoid space.
Intraperitoneal‡	Instilled or injected into peritoneal cavity.	Intrapleural	Injected into pleural space of lungs.
Intracardiac	Injected into heart to attain high levels of emergency drugs.	Intralesional	Injected into a wound or incision.
		Sublesional	Injected beneath a wound or incision.
Intraarticular	Injected into a joint.		

*Drugs may be given by this route for their local effects on the intestinal mucosa or their chemical, anti-infective, or mechanical effects in the intestinal lumen.
†Drugs may be given by this route for their local effects.
‡Drugs may be given by this route for systemic effects.

TABLE 2-7   Major Dosage Forms

ROUTE	FORM	DESCRIPTION/TYPE
Oral (solid)	Capsule	Powder or liquid drug encased in a hard or soft gelatin. *Sustained-release* forms (capsules or tablets) have small beads of drug, which are coated so that they dissolve at various times.
	Tablet	Compressed or molded drug. May be coated and colored. *Enteric coated tablets* have a covering to keep them from dissolving until reaching the small intestine. *Chewable tablets* contain flavorings. *Effervescent tablets* have chemicals which release gas when in water so they produce a foam.
	Powder	Fine solid particles prepared as single-dose packets or in bulk, to be mixed with liquid or food before administration.
Oral (liquid)	Solution[c]	Drug dissolved in water or another solvent.
	Elixir or tincture	Solution containing alcohol.
	Suspension	Dispersion of insoluble particles of drug in liquid.
	Emulsion	Combination with liquid in oil.
	Syrup	Drug in aqueous sucrose.
Dermatologic	Ointment[a]	Semisolid preparation of drug in a water-resistant base such as petroleum jelly.
	Cream	Semisolid preparation of drug in a water-removable base.
	Paste	Semisolid preparation containing a large proportion of powder.
	Lotion	Insoluble powder dispersed in water or alcohol.
	Plaster	Solid or semisolid adhesive mass on a suitable backing.
	Liniment	Insoluble powder in an oil or alcohol base.
	Aerosol[b]	Suspension of fine solid or liquid particles in gas.
	Powder	Fine solid particles.
Parenteral (intravenous, intramuscular, subcutaneous, intraspinal, etc.)	Solution[c] for injection	Same as an oral solution except sterile, buffered, etc.
Intramuscular	Repository	Drug in oil or another solvent or with an additive that makes it absorb slowly.
Dental and throat	Lozenge	Solid sucrose which releases drug as it is dissolved in mouth.
Vaginal, rectal, or urethral	Suppository	Drug in a solid oil or gelatin base that melts at body temperature. Shaped for insertion into appropriate body cavity.
Vaginal[d]	Solution for irrigation[e]	Solution for surface rinsing.
Ophthalmic	Ocusert[f]	Silicone rubber disk impregnated with a drug.

[a]Ophthalmic ointments are available which are sterile and specially prepared for the eye.

[b]Aerosols for inhalation are also available.

[c]Ophthalmic solutions, otic solutions, nose drop solutions, etc., are available. Each is specially formulated for the appropriate route of administration.

[d]Other vaginal dosage forms also available include compressed tablets, foams, effervescent tablets, and gels.

[e]Solutions for bladder irrigation, wound irrigation, gastric irrigation, etc., are also available.

[f]Other new dosage forms include transdermal forms, oral solids with drugs encased in semipermeable membranes, and wax with a drug matrix.

and therapeutics (P & T) committee to develop policies for use of the medication in the institution. This committee is a subcommittee of the medical board and is composed of at least a physician, a nurse, a pharmacist, and an administrator. This committee develops a formulary system of which drugs will be stocked in the pharmacy, to avoid duplication and to save money. Expensive equipment for drug administration (such as infusion pumps) and for monitoring of drug effects may need to be allocated to cases where the drug therapy clearly requires this level of technology. Cost to the patient should not be ignored in choosing equipment and procedures. In the outpatient environment and at discharge from the hospital, the nurse must assess if the patient has the required financial resources, transportation, and knowledge to obtain the drugs and equipment for measuring dosages, administering the drug, and monitoring drug effects.

Drug Distribution Systems

The procedure by which a drug is obtained for administration to patients in institutional settings, or the *drug distribution system,* is another important environmental variable which the nurse should assess. There are three major types of drug distribution systems, which vary according to utilization of nursing time, types of checks and counterchecks of the drug order provided, speed with which a drug order can be implemented, and incidence of error.

Floor Stock   With the floor stock drug delivery system, the order on the chart is interpreted by the nursing personnel. Then the nurse selects the appropriate medication from a supply of drugs kept on the nursing unit and administers it to the patient. While this system permits rapid implementation of orders, it requires nurses to evaluate orders and select drugs without any routine input by pharmacists. This system is associated with a high incidence of error.

Individual Patient Prescriptions   The second type of drug delivery system is analogous to that in outpatient settings, since the physician's order is sent to the pharmacy, where a supply of the medication sufficient for several days is dispensed and labeled for the individual patient. This individual patient prescription system permits review of the order by the pharmacist. The label on the drug container affords the nurse a second check on drug choice prior to administration. Errors are less numerous than with floor stock systems, although implementation of the order may be delayed by the need to transmit it to the pharmacy.

Unit Dose System   The most accurate and controlled system of drug delivery is the unit dose system. This method requires that a copy of the physician's order be sent to the pharmacy, which dispenses *individual doses* (generally a 6- to 24-h supply) of each medication ordered. These medications are usually stored in a medication cart which has a separate drawer for each patient and can be rolled to the patient's room when drugs are administered. This system also permits the preparation of parenterals in the pharmacy under laminar air flow, which decreases risk of contamination by microorganisms.

Some institutions use combinations of the three systems. Other variations include a system in which a pharmacy technician administers all routine medications and one in which selected patients are instructed in self-administration and administer their own medications.

Physical and Psychosocial Environment

In the hospital the nurse must assess factors that influence drug outcome: the strange environment; unfamiliar people, noises, and procedures; and lack of physical activity. These can increase patient anxiety and the requirement for some types of medications, such as analgesics, laxatives, and hypnotics.

The interpersonal relations between the patient and significant others in the environment may influence the effectiveness of some drugs. For example, the patient on an antipsychotic drug may cope well for a period of time, but if there are severe family stresses, the drug may become inadequate.

Knowledge of the family or friends available for assistance and emotional support will be needed for discharge planning. This data should be gathered early, since discharge planning begins long before the discharge order is written. The attitudes, values, and abilities of these significant others will influence the patient's willingness to follow the prescriptions of health professionals.

Legal and Ethical Considerations

Nursing is practiced within a legal and ethical environment (see Chap. 8). These environmental factors dictate the standards and limits of practice. Nurses must be apprised of the laws, institutional policies, and ethical code in their own areas of practice and of how these relate to the nurses' role in drug therapy.

ANALYSIS OF DATA

After data about the patient, the drug, and the environment are collected, these must be collated and analyzed for actual and potential problems. For most drug therapy the nurse considers the following questions:

1. What is the medical diagnosis for which the drug is prescribed and the goals of therapy?

2. Are there any patient or environmental factors which contraindicate the drug, the dosage, the route, or the dosage form?

3. If the patient has received the drug previously, what is the evidence that the expected therapeutic effect is being achieved? Is there evidence of adverse effects from previous doses?

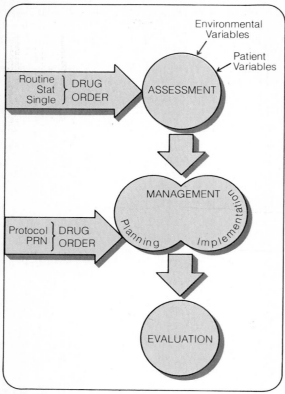

FIGURE 2-4

The entry point of a medication order into the nursing process depends upon the type of order. With routine orders, stat orders, and single orders, the drug order enters the nursing process at the outset of assessment, when the nurse assesses the drug ordered, the patient, and the environment. Data analysis results in a judgment on the safety and efficacy of the drug order in the patient situation. However, with protocol and PRN orders, the purpose of assessment is to diagnose the patient problem and its causes. The order is only one of several alternative approaches to the problem and therefore enters the nursing process during the planning step of management.

4. What are the potential adverse effects in this patient which have implications for nursing care?

5. Are there factors which will influence administration of the drug and the patient's ability and willingness to take the drug?

The beginning nurse needs to consciously and systematically consider each of these questions; with experience this analysis process becomes more automatic.

These five questions are sufficient for the data analysis with standard, single, and stat orders but not for PRN orders and protocol. *A diagnosis must be made by the nurse prior to the administration of a drug based on a PRN order or*

protocol. Further, the PRN or protocol drug will be administered only if it is the best available method to treat the diagnosed problem. Figure 2-4 illustrates the nursing process with different types of orders.

NURSING DIAGNOSIS

A nursing diagnosis is a specification of the patient's problem with reference to nursing care. A complete nursing diagnosis contains the etiology of the problem and the defining signs and symptoms, as well as a statement of the problem (Gordon, 1982). Nurses diagnose actual or potential problems in health maintenance and in human responses to disease.

Physicians diagnose disease processes and write prescriptions and medical orders for drugs to treat or prevent diseases. Nurses assist patients who lack the necessary skill or knowledge to follow the prescription or medical order. This assistance can take many forms, such as administering the drug, implementing measures to promote therapeutic drug effects, and evaluating drug effects, which will be discussed in Chaps. 3 and 4. There are two forms of assistance relevant to the assessment phase of nursing process. First, because most patients lack the knowledge necessary, the nurse must *judge* if the drug is appropriate to the medical diagnosis and therapeutic goals and is not otherwise contraindicated. The first three questions listed above under Analysis of Data are pertinent to this judgment. Second, the nurse will make nursing diagnoses regarding (1) potential health problems resulting from adverse drug effects and (2) patient education or counseling needs related to the order. The last two questions under Analysis of Data are pertinent to making these nursing diagnoses.

As indicated previously, PRN orders and protocols require that the nurse make a diagnosis, and the order is usually only one of the methods to be considered for treating the diagnosed problem. The diagnosis for which a PRN drug is administered is often a nursing diagnosis, such as "sleep pattern disturbance due to unfamiliar environment, manifested by difficulty falling asleep." However, execution of PRN orders or protocols can also be based on a medical diagnosis made by a nurse, such as the emergency administration of lidocaine for a life-threatening ventricular arrhythmia. Nurse practitioners also make medical diagnoses in the execution of protocols.

In summary, for *all* types of orders, the nurse makes a *judgment* on whether the order is safe and effective in the specific patient situation. In addition, for all orders nurses make *nursing diagnoses* regarding potential adverse effects and teaching requirements. Carrying out the PRN or protocol requires that an appropriate diagnosis (medical or nursing) be made. The distinction is important, since students, nurses, patients, and other health care providers must recognize the complexity of the decision-making process with PRN orders and protocol.

For example, Bertha Jones, aged 49, reports to the emergency room with an acutely tender and swollen right ankle, claiming that she must have injured it at a recent family reunion picnic. Following a history, physical examination, and laboratory testing, Dr. Boyles diagnoses acute gouty arthritis and prescribes indomethacin (Indocin) 50 mg tid for 7 days to decrease the inflammation and 300 mg acetaminophen with 30 mg codeine (Tylenol with codeine) q4h PRN for pain. Ms. Jones is incredulous that her problem could be "only arthritis." The nurse assesses the prescription and judges that the order is not contraindicated but diagnoses (1) deficit in knowledge about the disease and drugs, (2) potential stomach irritation and headache (common adverse effects of indomethacin), and (3) altered comfort from pain, manifested by a subjective statement, protection of the ankle, and fearfulness. For the third diagnosis the nurse has the option of one or more of the following interventions: application of ice, application of heat, elevation of the ankle, administration of the PRN pain medication, teaching the patient to use crutches, distraction, etc.

A final step in nursing assessment is validation of the nursing diagnosis with the patient. Failure to do this results in nursing care done *to patients* rather than *with patients*. In the example above, the nurse could validate the nursing diagnoses by saying to Ms. Jones, "I have identified three things I can assist you with: understanding gout and the drugs Dr. Boyles ordered, how to prevent adverse effects from the drugs, and how to control your pain until the medication improves your condition. Do you agree? Is there anything else I can help you with?" If Ms. Jones were to respond, "That doctor is crazy! I don't have gout. I'm going to see my orthopedist tomorrow!" the nurse would know that reformulation of the nursing diagnosis was required.

SOURCES OF DRUG INFORMATION

Nurses frequently consult references to analyze data or to augment data collection in drug therapy. Numerous resources are available. The nursing process is most efficient once the nurse or student knows what reference to consult for a specific question.

Compendiums

Compendiums include encyclopedic information about drugs or some aspect of drugs, such as side effects or drug interactions. *The United States Pharmacopeia and The National Formulary* are recognized as the official compendiums in the United States. Some of the compendiums are handbooks specifically designed for nurses and emphasize administration, observation, and patient education but may be weak in pharmacokinetics and pharmacodynamics.

Factors to consider when choosing a compendium are frequency of revision, organization, scope of information, and the viewpoint of the authors. If revised less than annually, the reference could be significantly outdated prior to purchase. Alphabetic organization allows for rapid reference, while organization by drug group promotes understanding of an entire class of drugs. Resources prepared by manufacturers are less likely to contain critical or comparative information. Some sources include both prescription and nonprescription drugs, and others focus only on one or the other.

Listed below are a selection of compendiums that may be useful to nurses and students.

Dukes, M. N. G.: *Meylers' Side Effects of Drugs,* Vols. 1–8, Excerpta Medica. [Annual supplements.]

Hospital Formulary, Bethesda, MD: American Society of Hospital Pharmacists. [Loose-leaf. Continually updated.]

Kastrup, E. K. (ed.): *Facts and Comparisons,* Philadelphia: Lippincott. [Monthly update available. Comprehensive. Prescription and nonprescription agents included. Monographs on drug groups as well as individual agents. Loose-leaf and microfilm.]

Loebl, S., G. Spratto, and E. Heckheimer: *The Nurse's Drug Handbook,* 3d ed., New York: Wiley, 1983. [Updated about every third year. Alphabetic listing.]

Mangini, R. J. (ed.): *Drug Interaction Facts,* Philadelphia: Lippincott, 1983. [Loose-leaf. Describes significance, effects, mechanism, and management of drug interactions.]

Nursing 85 Nurses' Drug Handbook, 5th ed., Springhouse, PA: Intermed Communications, 1984, [Listed by drug group. Annual revision. Interdisciplinary authorship.]

Penna, R. P. (ed.): *Handbook of Nonprescription Drugs,* 7th ed., Washington, DC: American Pharmaceutical Association, 1981.

Physician's Desk Reference, Oradell, NJ: Medical Economics. [Annual revision. Compiled by drug manufacturers. Not a critical guide.]

Skidmore, L. C.: *Medication Cards for Clincal Use.* Bowie, MD: Brady, 1982. [Individual reference cards for about 150 common drugs.]

Textbooks

Textbooks are most helpful in gaining an understanding of broad pharmacologic principles and drug groups, although they can be used as references about specific drugs. Considerations in selecting a textbook are focus (basic pharmacology or therapeutics), level of presentation, and copyright date.

Avery, G. S. (ed.): *Drug Treatment: Principles and Practices of Clinical Pharmacology and Therapeutics,* Sydney, Australia: ADIS, 1980. [Large. Therapeutics-oriented.]

Falconer, M. W., et al.: *The Drug, the Nurse, the Patient,* 7th ed., Philadelphia: Saunders, 1982. [Appendix reference of individual drugs.]

Gilman, A. G., L. S. Goodman, and A. Gilman: *Goodman and Gilman's The Pharmacological Basis of Therapeutics*, 6th ed., New York: Macmillan, 1980. [Large, medically oriented. A classic basic pharmacology text.]

Katzung, B. C.: *Basic and Clinical Pharmacology*, Los Altos, CA: Lange Medical Publications, 1984. [Updated every 2 years. Good correlation of pathophysiology and pharmacology.]

Journals

Drug information will be found in pharmacology journals, pharmacy journals, medical journals, and nursing journals. Nurses will probably find articles in the journals listed below to be most applicable to clinical practice. These journals include regular features on drug administration, updates on new drugs, and feature articles about drug groups and drug administration. Journals of clinical specialty areas are also useful.

American Journal of Nursing

Canadian Nurse

Drugs

New England Journal of Medicine

Nursing '84

Nurse Practitioner

RN

In addition, the following publish critical reviews and research summaries:

Clin-Alert

Facts and Comparisons Newsletter

Medical Letter on Drugs and Therapeutics

Nurses' Drug Alert (now included as a supplement to *American Journal of Nursing*)

Rational Drug Therapy

Resource Consultants

Pharmacists in hospitals, clinics, and retail pharmacies; poison control centers; and drug information centers are important consultants for nurses' drug therapy questions. *Drug information centers* are resources for information on all aspects of drugs for health professionals. They provide clinically relevant drug information in response to patient-specific and general requests from health practitioners in hospitals, in skilled care facilities, and from the community at large. The overall goal of drug information centers is to promote the effective and safe use of drugs in the diagnosis and treatment of disease through selection, evaluation, and dissemination of drug literature. Existing drug information

centers and details of some of the services they provide are given on the inside front cover of this book.

Poison control centers provide information about poisons, particularly regarding poisonous substances in products that might be accidentally ingested, and the treatment for such poisonings. The availability of such vital information is of great help in the emergency treatment of poisoning victims. A list of poison control centers is given on the inside back cover of this book.

Formulating a Drug Question   In order to get maximal benefit from consultation with pharmacists and other drug specialists, the nurse must recognize that the form and content of the question determines the clinical relevance of the response. For example, if the question is whether a total daily dose of 4 g of methyldopa (Aldomet) is excessive, the nurse should supply information about the specific patient situation, such as age of the patient, weight of the patient, patient's renal and hepatic function, disease(s) being treated, other medications being taken, past responses to the drug, route of administration, and dosage interval schedule. Similarly, a question about the compatibility of two drugs in an intravenous (IV) medication should be accompanied by information about the amounts of each drug to be mixed, the type of solution in which the drugs will be mixed, the container to be used (glass bottle, plastic IV bag, plastic syringe), the route of administration (IV infusion, IV push, "piggyback" infusion), and the duration and frequency of administration. The key to formulating good drug information questions is supplying all relevant information about the patient, the drug order, and the drug administration situation.

Package Inserts

The package insert, the printed material that is enclosed in a drug package, is the Food and Drug Administration (FDA)–approved official label for drug products in the United States. The recommended dosage ranges given in the insert have been judged safe and effective by the FDA, but they may be exceeded if this is deemed necessary by the prescriber. Still, the official label does carry legal weight, and a prescriber should be able to justify a decision to exceed the recommended dosage. Unfortunately, the package insert does not provide information regarding implications for nursing practice or patient teaching. It does give good information about proper reconstitution of medications (addition of a fluid to a powder to make a liquid dosage form) when this is required.

The pharmaceutical manufacturer of the product about which there is a question is often a valuable resource. Many manufacturers maintain toll-free telephone numbers or will accept collect calls on questions concerning their products. In most pharmaceutical companies a health professional is usually in charge of a product, and inquiries should be directed to the "physician in charge" of the specific product.

REFERENCES

Bell, S. K.: "Guidelines for Taking a Complete Drug History," *Nursing 80,* **10**:10–11, 1980.

Gordon, M.: *Nursing Diagnosis: Process and Application,* New York: McGraw-Hill, 1982.

Hudak, C. M.: *Clinical Protocols: A Guide for Nurses and Physicians,* Philadelphia: Lippincott, 1976.

Levine, R. R.: *Pharmacology: Drug Actions and Reactions,* 2d ed., Boston: Little, Brown, 1978.

Mitchell, P. H, and A. Loustau (eds.), *Concepts Basic to Nursing,* 3d ed., New York: McGraw-Hill, 1981.

Parker, W.: "Medication Histories," *Am J Nurs,* 76:1769–1772, 1976.

NURSING MANAGEMENT IN PHARMACOTHERAPEUTICS: PLANNING AND IMPLEMENTATION

GINETTE A. PEPPER

LEARNING OBJECTIVES

Upon mastery of the contents of this chapter, the reader will be able to:

1. List the components of planning and implementation in pharmacotherapeutics.

2. State the general goals of management in pharmacotherapeutics.

3. Write a nursing care plan related to a patient's drug therapy, including goals and approaches.

4. List the "five rights" of giving a medication.

5. Describe practices that promote accurate drug administration.

6. Explain how the nurse assures that the drug is being administered to the right patient.

7. State from memory the approximate equivalents in the metric, household, and apothecary systems.

8. Accurately calculate conversions between measurement systems, common dosages, and intravenous (IV) rates (or, if unable to calculate accurately, formulate a plan of self-study to acquire this skill).

9. State the factors which should be considered in establishing a rational dosage schedule for a drug.

10. Explain the principles of drug administration technique and safety for the following routes: oral (for liquids and solids), sublingual and buccal, topical, otic, intradermal, subcutaneous, intramuscular, and intravenous.

11. Give an example and effective approaches for each type of teaching goal.

12. Describe behavioral approaches to patient education.

13. Explain how the nursing care plan should reflect measures for support of the therapeutic effect, prevention or minimization of adverse effects, and patient observation.

14. List five guidelines for recording of drug therapy.

15. Explain nursing responsibilities related to medication errors.

16. Describe the nursing management of the contraindicated medical order.

Management involves action. It is the most visible step in the nursing process, and the public tends to identify nurses as the "ones who give the pills and shots." However, nursing care is not merely the observable act but is also the data collection, analysis, diagnosis, and planning on which the act is based. Data collected must be used to individualize care or it is merely a useless exercise, as was chauvinistically noted in 1859 in a humorous statement by Florence Nightingale:

> In dwelling on the vital importance of *sound* observation, it must never be lost sight of what observation is for. It is not for the sake of piling up a lot of miscellaneous information or curious facts, but for the sake of saving life and increasing health and comfort. The caution may seem useless, but it is surprising how many men (and some women do it too) practically behave as if the scientific end were the only one in view, or as if the sick body were but a reservoir for stowing medicines into, and the surgical disease only a curious case the sufferer has made for the attendant's special information. This is really no exaggeration. [*Notes on Nursing*, p. 70]

Management is composed of two closely related parts; *planning* and *implementation*. Planning has three steps:

goal setting, establishing priorities, and selecting the best approach. Implementation involves drug administration, patient teaching, patient observation, measures to support the drug effect and to limit adverse effects, recording and documentation, and proper response to medication errors and contraindicated orders.

PLANNING

Planning must be a conscious and purposeful activity. It is not intuitive or automatic. Sometimes the nurse make make the effort to sit down and concentrate on a patient problem in order to competently plan. While this may seem to expend time better spent with patients, it avoids time wasted in giving unplanned care that may turn out to be inappropriate, ineffective, or even harmful.

An example is the problem of the patient who refuses medication. Without adequate assessment and planning, the usual approaches are to cajole, coerce, or bribe the patient into taking the drug, which are time-consuming and often ineffective. Analyzing the reason why the patient refused medication may reveal that the patient feels powerless in the hospital environment and is attempting to exert control by this act. The goal of management for the diagnosis of powerlessness is to increase the patient's sense of competence and control. One method to accomplish this is to give the patient control in decisions affecting his or her care. This might include making the patient aware of the right and responsibility to give *informed consent* for therapy and of the reciprocal responsibility of the nurse to provide adequate information and to abide by the decision of the patient. (If the patient refuses any medical therapy, it is a nursing responsibility to inform the physician. This responsibility is explained to the patient, but never in a punitive or coercive way, such as "If you don't take this drug, I will call your doctor.") When the nurse focuses on the problem (feeling of powerlessness) rather than the symptom (refusal to take the medication), the probability of success is increased.

Goal Setting

A goal is a statement of the desired or expected outcome of management. Goals are crucial to evaluation; in order to judge the success of nursing management, it is necessary to know what outcome was anticipated.

There are both medical and nursing goals related to drug therapy. *Medical goals* are established by the physician in collaboration with the health care team. Part of the nursing role in drug therapy is to ascertain what these medical goals are and to assess, plan, implement, and evaluate drug therapy in light of these goals. Nurses should independently initiate measures to promote the medical goal, *or therapeutic end point,* and to observe for drug effects. *Nursing goals* are related to nursing diagnoses but are also established in collaboration with the health care team. Medical goals and nursing goals should be compatible; some may be identical.

Types of Goals

The three types of medical and nursing goals are diagnostic, therapeutic, and teaching. *Diagnostic goals* are those related to collecting additional information to ascertain patient status or to identify adverse effects of therapy. *Therapeutic goals* are directed at correcting, preventing, or alleviating a problem. *Teaching goals* aim at increasing the patient's understanding of a problem and ability to give truly informed consent and follow the therapy. Examples of medical and nursing goals of each type are shown in Table 3-1. Note that a goal is stated in measurable terms and contains a deadline, which is a projection of when the goal should be accomplished or evaluated. However, it is not always possible to state a specific deadline for diagnostic and preventative goals.

General Nursing Goals

Nursing care is deficient if the only component of the written nursing care plan that reflects pharmacotherapeutics is a statement such as "Give antibiotic as ordered." Care plans by nurses and students should reflect consideration of the following general nursing goals in pharmacotherapeutics:

1. Accurate and appropriate administration
2. Support of the desired therapeutic response
3. Prevention of adverse effects
4. Observation for the desired therapeutic response
5. Early detection of nonpreventable adverse effects
6. Education of patients for participation in the management of their own drug therapy
7. Accurate recording of drug administration and patient response
8. Appropriate management of medication errors and contraindicated orders

These general goals are translated into patient-specific nursing goals, based upon the data collection and nursing diagnosis. Figure 3-1 is a portion of the care plan for a patient with a urinary tract infection taking the drug methenamine mandelate (Mandelamine). The care plan demonstrates several specific goals which correlate with the general goals above.

Establishing Priorities

Establishing priorities is one of the more difficult types of decisions made in health care delivery. When there is a severe threat to life or future functioning, prioritizing is relatively simple. However, a patient's physical or psychologic problems may require some action or medication that is contraindicated by another of the patient's problems. Further, it is not possible to manage all patient problems simultaneously; some must wait until both the patient and the care provider have the resources to deal with them. The health care team must weigh the importance of one problem

TABLE 3-1   Examples of Goals for Pharmacotherapeutics

MEDICAL GOALS	NURSING GOALS
Diagnostic	
Rule out secondary hypertension.	Identify sources of anxiety.
Diagnose etiology of melena.	Detect anticholinergic adverse drug reactions.
Therapeutic	
Return hematocrit to normal range in 6 months.	Maintain daily urine pH reading at 5 or less.
Maintain weekly prothrombin clotting test results at 2–2½ times control level.	Have patient abstain from alcohol for next 3 weeks.
Reduce diastolic blood pressure below 95 mmHg without adverse drug reactions by next appointment.	Establish a regular pattern of soft-formed stools by January 15.
Teaching	
Take prescription as ordered until next appointment.	Be able to prepare and self-administer insulin injections by April 1.
Give informed consent for use of investigational drug by tomorrow.	Prior to discharge, list signs of digitalis toxicity and appropriate action if these occur.

against the other(s) and select the one with the highest priority.

Selecting the Best Approach

Identification of all feasible approaches is necessary for effective planning. This often requires consultation with other health care providers and use of written references. In selecting the best approach for a given patient situation, the nurse must consider four criteria: (1) probability of success in fulfilling the goal, (2) feasibility, (3) risk to the patient, and (4) acceptability to the patient. After comparing the possible approaches on the basis of these criteria, a specific specific plan is devised. This is communicated to the nursing staff via a written nursing care plan (see Fig. 3-1).

IMPLEMENTATION

Nurses may personally implement the care plan or designate someone else to do so. Implementing a nursing care plan relevant to drug therapy involves the entire scope of nursing functions: teaching, drug administration, communication, collaboration, observation, supervision, and examination. Further, nurses involved in administrative positions (directors of nursing, supervisors, head nurses, etc.) participate in administrative decisions in the selection of overall procedures and equipment to get the medication safely and efficiently to the patient. Although this facet of management is beyond the scope of this text, it is well for the student or nurse to be aware of this process, as patient well-being may require a change in institutional policy, procedures, equipment acquisition, or supply purchases. However, this chapter will focus on nursing functions involved in the implementation of drug therapy for the *individual patient*.

Drug Administration

The "Five Rights"

In some settings as much as half of nursing time is spent in drug administration. The fundamental responsibilities of the nurse in drug administration are subsumed in the *five rights* of giving medications:

Right drug
Right patient
Right dose
Right time
Right route

In spite of the recent rapid expansion of the nursing role in drug therapy, the five rights remain the *absolute minimum requirements* in nursing pharmacotherapeutics. The nurse must assure that each right is given consideration before medication administration or assure that the patient or other person who will administer the drug can do this.

Certain general practices are conducive to accomplishing the five rights. Each time an order is recopied, the risk of error in transcription is increased, so institutions establish procedures to minimize this risk. However, rarely is the original order used as the nurses' reference in administering a drug. Usually drug orders are transcribed onto an official working document, such as a medication Kardex, medica-

NURSING CARE PLAN

Name _J. Mann_ Age _63_ Medical Diagnosis _Osteoarthritis; angina; UTI_
Hypertension

Date	Nursing Diagnosis	Goals	Approaches
8/29/83	Ineffective coping with restrictions imposed by diseases indicated by denial, depressed mood.	Identify coping mechanisms effective in past life	Primary nurse will meet with pt's wife on 8/30 to discuss this. Complete nursing history with pt, esp. section on coping.
	Altered pattern of urinary elimination due to E. Coli infection manifested by dysuria, frequency, laboratory reports.	Promote effectiveness of Mandelamine (most active at urine pH < 5.0).	Give Mandelamine (ordered 1 g qid) around the clock (see below). Test urine pH bid (9A-9P). Ask nutritionist to provide urine-acidifying diet: Cranberry juice or prune juice vs citrus juice; limit milk and milk products; as much meat as low sodium diet allows. Minimum of 8 glasses juice or water qd. Measure I & O. If urine pH not consistently < 5.0 by 9/1/83, ask Dr. for order for ascorbic acid.
		Evaluate effectiveness of Mandelamine.	Check for dysuria and frequency daily. Urine culture in 1 week.
		Prevent gastric irritation from Mandelamine.	Give Mandelamine pc or with snack (8A-1P-6³⁰P-1A with crackers). Follow with full glass H₂O.
		Observe for complications of UTI (severe pyelonephritis, sepsis, renal impairment) and Mandelamine (GI distress, skin rash, bladder irritation).	Contact Dr if ① still febrile by 9/2 ② poor urine output, ③ increased serum creatinine. Question pt. daily about stomach pain, nausea, pruritis, increased dysuria. Tell pt. to report these symptoms. Record results on flow sheet in chart.

FIGURE 3-1

Portion of a Nursing Care Plan for a Patient Receiving Methenamine Mandelate (Mandelamine) for a Urinary Tract Infection.

tion tickets, medication sheets in a loose-leaf notebook, or a computer printout. Special precautions are taken to assure accuracy of this document, and it is used as the nurses' official work sheet for drug administration. In this discussion the term *drug administration record* will be used generally to refer to this official working document. Where medication tickets (also called med cards) are the working document, a procedure must be established to check the tickets against a master list each shift, to assure none have been misplaced.

Drugs are always prepared and administered directly from the drug administration record, and not from memory or from the nurse's or student's personal work sheet. It is wise to compare the drug administration record to the original order in the chart each shift for the first 24 hours after an order is written. Orders on the drug administration record should be printed (rather than written in longhand) and are recopied whenever they become soiled or illegible. A second person should check the new copy to assure that it was transcribed properly. The drug administration record should not be left on the medication cart in the hall while the nurse takes the drug(s) into the patient's room; the cart should be rolled into the room or the drug administration record must be carried into the room. Unless it is a drug dose in the unit dose system and is labeled by a pharmacist, *nurses should never give a medication poured or drawn up by someone else.*

A quiet area free from distractions is crucial to accurate preparation of drugs. *Whenever there is doubt about any aspect of a medication order, the nurse should question the prescriber and/or the pharmacist.* In addition to these general precautions, certain practices are also specific to accomplishing each of the individual five rights.

Right Drug   Frequent checks of drug selection promote administration of the right drug. The traditional "three check method" is used with floor stock and individual patient prescription distribution systems. This involves checking the bottle label against the drug administration record (1) when the drug is removed from storage, (2) when it is poured into the medication cup or drawn into the syringe, and (3) when it is returned to the storage place. In unit dose systems the label remains on the individual dose until the moment of administration and is checked against the drug administration record (1) when the drug is removed from storage and (2) in the patient's room just prior to administration.

Knowing the patient's diagnoses, the medical objectives for that patient, and the pharmacology of the drugs also reduces errors in drug selection. *No drug should be given to a patient until the nurse understands why it has been prescribed for that patient.*

Awareness that many drugs have similar names will increase the nurse's vigilance in interpreting orders and in comparing the drug administration record to the drug label. Consider the following three groups that contain drug names that look and sound similar:

Digoxin, Digitoxin, Desoxyn

Keflin, Keflex, Kantrex, Kelex

Esimil, Estinyl, Ismelin

Some of these are generic names and others are trade names, but if they were hastily written (especially in longhand) or not interpreted carefully, the patient could end up getting dangerously high doses of a drug or a very different drug than was ordered. *Illegible handwriting is a major cause of drug errors.*

Whenever a patient expresses surprise or questions a medication, the nurse should recheck the order and drug selection. Sometimes patients' cues that they suspect the drug is wrong are as subtle as the statement, "The doctor must think I'm a lot sicker today."

Right Patient   In order to assure that the right patient gets a medication, *the nurse should always compare the patient's armband with the drug administration record.* Further, whenever the patient's abilities permit, *the nurse should ask the patient to state his full name as a second check.* If there are two patients on the unit with similar names, the drug administration record should be flagged with a warning. *Never identify a patient by asking, "Are you so-and-so?"* An astounding number of patients have received someone else's medication when they responded to another's name because they misheard the question or were dozing or confused or even because they hoped to get an extra dose of narcotics.

Right Dose   Most medications are currently labeled in the metric system, but doses are sometimes ordered in household or apothecary units. The nurse should, therefore, memorize the accepted *approximate equivalents* shown in Table 3-2, as well as the equivalents within each system (see Tables 2-3, 2-4, and 2-5).

The most common dosage calculations done by nurses for adult patients are (1) conversions within and between the measurement systems, (2) identifying the amount of a solution or number of tablets or capsules to administer, and (3) figuring the rate of an IV (in terms of drops per minute). Far less common are calculations to prepare or dilute a solution (because the pharmacist usually does this), but nurses may require this knowledge in smaller or rural settings, in home health care, and for patient teaching. Table 3-3 is a quick reference to the formulas often used for these five common calculations. Pediatric dosage calculation is discussed in Chap. 7.

A major goal in drug administration is *consistently accurate dosage calculation.* Students vary tremendously in the amount of study required to accomplish this. The first step is assessment of one's own ability to calculate dosages; this is followed by a plan to correct any deficits identified. Table 3-4 is a self-assessment of common types of dosage calculation problems, designed as a pretest or for use after studying Table 3-3. (Answers are included and the Appendix to this chapter shows the calculations.) In "real life" dosage calculations, *patient safety requires that every calculation be correct.* Therefore, the reader who does not answer *all* the questions on the self-assessment correctly should seek a formal course or study one of the available publications on dosage calculations (see References).

Use of formulas does not guarantee the right dose, however. The nurse should compare the dose ordered to the

TABLE 3-2   Approximate Metric Conversions*

APOTHECARY TO METRIC	
Mass (Weight)	
1 gr (grain)	= 60 mg (milligrams)†
$\frac{1}{100}$ gr	= 0.6 mg
$\frac{1}{150}$ gr	= 0.4 mg
15 (or 16) gr	= 1 g (gram)
2.2 lb (pounds)‡	= 1 kg (kilogram)

HOUSEHOLD TO METRIC			APOTHECARY TO METRIC		
		Volume			
1 tsp (teaspoon)	=	5 mL (milliliters)	1 ♏ (minim)	=	0.6 mL
1 tbsp (tablespoon)	=	15 mL	15 (or 16) ♏	=	1 mL
1 oz (ounce)	=	30 mL	1 ʒ (dram)	=	4 mL
1 pint	=	500 mL (0.5 L)	8 ʒ	=	30 mL
1 qt (quart)	=	1000 mL (1 L)			

*Relationships between the units in the metric, apothecary, and household systems are shown in Tables 2-3, 2-4, and 2-5, respectively. The above conversions are commonly accepted equivalents, although they are only approximate.

†Or 64 or 65 mg.

‡Avoirdupois pounds.

usual dosage listed in published references. If more than one or two capsules, tablets, or vials are required for a single dose, it is wise to recheck the order and the calculations. This is also true if a small fraction of the dosage form is required. Particularly troublesome are decimals, which, if misplaced, can result in dosages that are 10, 100, or even 1000 times too large or only a fraction of the effective dose. Misplaced decimals occur as a result of miswritten, misread, or incorrectly transcribed orders, as well as from calculation errors.

Prior to dosage calculation, it is a good practice to estimate the dosage so the estimate can be compared to the calculated dosage. As a simple example, consider the order for 80 mg of a drug which comes in 100 mg per 2 mL. The nurse can estimate that the dosage should be between 1 and 2 mL by reasoning that, since 2 mL contains 100 mg, 1 mL will contain half that amount, or 50 mg, so 80 mg (which is between 50 and 200 mg) will require more than 1 mL but less than 2 mL. Whenever possible, all calculations should be checked by another nurse or pharmacist. For small children and also with insulin, heparin, and other drugs with narrow margins of safety, this double check of the calculation and the prepared dose should be routine.

Right Time   The total daily dosage of a drug is often given in several divided doses through the day, to achieve more consistent blood levels for maintenance of therapeutic effects and/or to prevent adverse effects that occur with high blood levels. For some drugs this consistency in blood levels is more important than for others. For example, some antibiotic and antiarrhythmic drugs require a consistent blood level and the patient must awaken during the night to take them. Relatively even spacing of doses throughout the waking hours is adequate for most drugs. Although time of administration is comparatively unimportant for drugs taken once per day, these drugs should be taken at approximately the same time each day, since therapeutic failure or toxic effects can occur when there are wide deviations in the time of daily administration. Drugs which must be taken on an empty stomach, those that must be taken with food, and ulcer drugs whose peak effects are desirable when stomach acid secretion is highest must be timed with respect to usual meal times. Hence, *both the pharmacology of the drug and the patient's daily routine must be considered in establishing a dosing schedule.*

Since Florence Nightingale mandated that dosage times be fixed, inpatient settings have designated routine times for drug doses, and in many places it is even considered a medication error if the drug is not given within 30 min of the routine time. Since little was known until recently about blood level patterns, schedules were arbitrarily established for institutional convenience (to avoid shift changes and other busy times). Drugs were routinely given at 9 A.M., 1 P.M., 5 P.M., and 9 P.M. (or 8 A.M., 12 noon, 4 P.M., and 8 P.M.,

TABLE 3-3 Quick Reference for Drug Calculation

Formula 1 Conversion to Metric System*

General Formula:

$$\frac{\text{Nonmetric value no. 1}}{\text{Unknown metric equivalent of no. 1}} :: \frac{\text{Nonmetric value no. 2}}{\text{Known metric equivalent of no. 2}}$$

Formula Statement: The ratio of a nonmetric value to its unknown metric equivalent is proportional to the ratio, *stated in the same units,* of a nonmetric value to its known metric equivalent.

Example: Convert 10 gr to milligrams.

   Step 1: Identify the ratio between a value in grains and its known metric equivalent. (In this case 1 gr = 60 mg.)
   Step 2: Substitute into the formula and solve. (Ratio-proportion problems are solved by setting the product of the means equal to that of the extremes and solving for the unknown.)

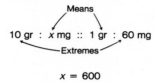

10 gr : x mg :: 1 gr : 60 mg

$$x = 600$$

Formula 2 Drug Dosage Calculation†

General Formula:‡

$$\frac{\text{Dose ordered}}{\text{Drug strength available}} \times \frac{\text{Dosage form (capsule, tablet, liquid) containing strength available}}{} = \frac{\text{Amount to administer}}{}$$

Formula Statement: The prescribed drug dose (*D*) divided by the available drug strength (*S*) times the quantity of the dosage form containing the available drug strength (*F*) equals the amount of the drug to administer.

Abbreviated Formula:

$$\frac{D}{S} \times F = \text{Amount to administer}$$

Example (Solid Dosage Form): The physician orders 600 mg of ibuprofen (Motrin). Available tablets contain 300 mg.

   Step 1: Make sure all values are in the same system of measurement (preferably metric).
   Step 2: Substitute into the formula and solve.

$$\frac{600\ \text{mg}}{300\ \text{mg}} \times 1\ \text{tablet} = \text{Amount to administer}$$

$$2\ \text{tablets} = \text{Amount to administer}$$

Example (Liquid Dosage Form): The drug ordered is morphine sulfate 10 mg IM. The available 2-mL vial contains 15 mg.

$$\frac{10\ \text{mg}}{15\ \text{mg}} \times 2\ \text{mL} = \text{Amount to administer}$$

$$\frac{20\ \text{mg} \cdot \text{mL}}{15\ \text{mg}} = 1.33\ \text{mL} = \text{Amount to administer}$$

Example (Percent Solutions): The nurse is to give 5 g of magnesium sulfate. It is available as a 25% solution. (Note: A 25% solution contains 25 g per 100 mL.)

$$\frac{5\ \text{g}}{25\ \text{g}} \times 100\ \text{mL} = \text{Amount to administer}$$

$$\frac{500\ \text{g} \cdot \text{mL}}{25\ \text{g}} = 20\ \text{mL} = \text{Amount to administer}$$

TABLE 3-3 Quick Reference for Drug Calculation (*Cont.*)

Formula 3 Intravenous Fluid Rate Calculation

General Formula:

$$\frac{\text{Drop factor}}{60 \text{ min/h}} \times \text{Ordered volume per hour} = \text{Drops per minute}$$

Formula Statement: The drops per minute to be administered intravenously equals the drop factor (drops per milliliter delivered by the administration set) divided by 60 min/h times the ordered hourly volume.§

Example: The physician orders 3000 mL of fluid to be infused in 24 h. The drop factor is 20 gtt/mL.

Step 1: Compute the milliliters infused per hour.

$$\frac{300 \text{ mL}}{24 \text{ h}} = 125 \text{ mL/h}$$

Step 2: Substitute into the formula and solve.

$$\frac{20 \text{ gtt/mL}}{60 \text{ min/h}} \times 125 \text{ mL/h} = \text{about } 42 \text{ gtt/min}$$

Using a Constant: For any type of administration set, the term $\dfrac{\text{drop factor}}{60 \text{ min/h}}$ is a constant and need not be computed each time. In the example above, the constant is ⅓. Dividing the ordered hourly volume by 3 (which is the same as multiplying by ⅓) is a calculation shortcut if the denominator of the constant is a whole number.

Constants for Common Administration Sets

MANUFACTURER	DROP FACTOR, gtt/mL	CONSTANT	DIVIDE HOURLY VOLUME BY†
Abbott	15	¼	4
Baxter	10	⅙	6
Cutter	20	⅓	3
McGaw	13	—*	—*
Travenol	10	⅙	6
All pediatric (microdrip)	60	1	1
All blood (macrodrip)	10	⅙	6

*Not applicable; denominator of constant is not a whole number.
†To get drops per minute.

Formula 4 Preparation of Solutions from Solids

General Formula:

$$\frac{\text{Concentration of}}{\text{drug desired}} \times \frac{\text{Volume of}}{\text{solution desired}} = \frac{\text{Mass of}}{\text{drug required}}$$

Formula Statement: The mass of drug required to make a solution equals the desired concentration times the desired volume.

Example: Prepare 500 mL of 0.9% saline solution from salt tablets weighing 0.5 g each.

Step 1: Substitute into the formula and solve. Remember 0.9% = 0.9 g per 100 mL.)

$$\frac{0.9 \text{ g}}{100 \text{ mL}} \times 500 \text{ mL} = 4.5 \text{ g}$$

Step 2: Use formula 2 above to identify the amount of drug required.

$$\frac{4.5 \text{ g}}{0.5 \text{ g}} \times 1 \text{ tablet} = 9 \text{ tablets}$$

Step 3: Put the tablets in a container, and add enough water to make 500 mL.

31

TABLE 3-3 Quick Reference for Drug Calculation (*Cont.*)

Formula 5 Dilution of Solutions

General Formula:

$$\frac{\text{Strength}}{\text{desired}} : \frac{\text{Strength}}{\text{available}} :: \frac{\text{Amount of}}{\text{solute to use}} : \frac{\text{Amount of}}{\text{solution desired}}$$

Formula Statement: The ratio of the strength of solution desired to the strength of the solution from which it is to be diluted is proportional to the ratio of the amount of solute (stronger solution) to use to the amount of solution desired.

Example: Prepare a 4% Burow's solution from a 1:15 solution.

Step 1: If no desired amount of solution is specified, select a reasonable amount based on need. (In this case 500 mL was to be made.)

Step 2: Substitute into the formula and solve as a ratio-proportion (see formula 2 above).

$$\frac{4 \text{ g}}{100 \text{ mL}} : \frac{1 \text{ g}}{15 \text{ mL}} :: x \text{ mL} : 500 \text{ mL}$$

$$\frac{x \text{ g} \cdot \text{mL}}{15 \text{ mL}} = \frac{2000 \text{ g/mL}}{100 \text{ mL}}$$

$$x = 300$$

Step 3: Pour 300 mL of the 1:15 Burow's solution into a container. Add 200 mL of water to make 500 mL of a 4% solution.

---

*This ratio-proportion formula can be adapted to the calculation of conversions between any two measurement systems or even within one system.

†Pediatric dosage calculation is considered in Chap. 7.

‡The alternate formula, which can be solved as a ratio-proportion, is

$$\frac{\text{Drug strength}}{\text{available}} : \frac{\text{Dosage form containing}}{\text{strength available}} :: \frac{\text{Dosage}}{\text{ordered}} : \frac{\text{Amount to}}{\text{administer}}$$

§For IVs running less than 1 h, the following formula may be more convenient:

$$\frac{\text{Drop factor}}{\text{Time span of infusion}} \times \frac{\text{Volume to}}{\text{be infused}} = \text{Drops per minute}$$

or at other times) if ordered qid, and at one, two, or three of those times if ordered qd, bid, or tid, respectively. Historically then, the frequency of dosing was the sole determinant of the dosing schedule. This routine was followed so fervently that some nurses taught patients to use the 9-1-5-9 schedule at home, as though there were some scientific rationale for selecting these times!

Advances in pharmacologic knowledge have caused the reappraisal of these rigid routines. Institutions still have routine dosage schedules, but these are increasingly being implemented in a rational way. For example, although drugs ordered bid are routinely given in many institutions at 9 A.M. and 9 P.M., both doses of a twice-daily diuretic (a drug that increases urine output) should be given early in the day (e.g., 9 A.M. and 1 P.M.) so the need to urinate will not interfere with the patient's sleep. Rational use of routine dosing schedules is still a major way to prevent omissions and other drug errors. Once the optimal dosing schedule for a given drug and patient is established, every reasonable effort should be made to meet the schedule.

Right Route Some routes of administration require specially manufactured dosage forms. For example, regular topical ointments or solutions are not safe for ophthalmic or otic administration. Benzathine penicillin G or procaine penicillin G should not be given intravenously, and no solution should be injected unless it is specifically marked *for injection.*

Improper administration technique or poor choice of equipment can result in a drug intended for one route being given by another. Too short needles turn an intramuscular injection into a subcutaneous injection; improper injection angle may cause deposit into the muscle of a drug meant to be absorbed subcutaneously; placing a dressing over a topi-

TABLE 3-4   Dosage Calculation Self-Assessment*

1. The order reads, "Amoxicillin suspension 250 mg tid." The label on the drug states that the concentration of the liquid is 125 mg per 5 mL. The only available measuring device is a pediatric dosing spoon calibrated in household units. (*a*) How much should be given in each dose? (*b*) If the recommended child dosage is 40 mg/kg/day and this order was written for a 33-lb child, does the dosage exceed the recommended level? ...
2. The nurse must give phenobarbital gr iss stat. On hand are tablets containing 65 mg and 100 mg. How many of which tablets should be given? (Choose the easiest and safest approach.)
3. The order reads, "Give 500 mcg dexamethasone q6h × 48 h." On hand are 0.25-mg tablets. How many tablets should be given per dose?
4. The physician orders 30 meq of potassium chloride to be added to an intravenous (IV) solution. Available is a vial containing 40 meq in 20 mL. How much of the potassium chloride solution should be added to the IV?
5. From a vial labeled tobramycin 80 mg per 2 mL, what volume should the nurse administer per dose if the order reads, "Tobramycin 70 mg IM tid"?
6. The physician orders nitroglycerin SL gr 1/200, to be kept at the patient's bedside. Available dosage strengths include 0.15-mg, 0.3-mg, 0.4-mg, and 0.6-mg tablets. Which strength should be used?
7. From a vial labeled heparin 40,000 U/mL, the nurse must give 15,000 U. What volume should be administered?
8. The nurse must inject 4 g of magnesium sulfate IM stat. On hand are 10-mL vials of 50% solution. What volume should the nurse administer?
9. The IV order reads, "1000 mL D₅W to run for 8 h." The administration set delivers 20 gtt/mL (drop factor). (*a*) How many drops per minute should this IV infuse? (*b*) How many drops per minute should this IV infuse if a microdrip set (60 gtt/mL) is used?
10. The doctor orders mezlocillin 4 g by intermittent IV "piggyback" q6h. The dose is diluted in 100 mL. (*a*) If the drop factor is 20 gtt/mL and the IV is infused over 45 min, how many drops per minute should the IV infuse? (*b*) If the drop factor is 10 gtt/mL and the IV is infused over 30 min, how many drops per minute should the IV infuse?

Answers: 1.(*a*) 2 tsp (*b*) Yes   2. one 100-mg tablet (giving 1½ of the 65-mg tablets would involve splitting a tablet, a practice which should be avoided) 3. 2 tablets 4. 15 mL 5. 1.75 mL 6. 0.3 mg 7. 0.38 mL (actually 0.375 mL, but 0.005 mL is too small to measure in usual syringes) 8. 8 mL (should be divided into two IM injections 9. (*a*) 42 (*b*) 125 10. (*a*) 44 (*b*) 33.

*The Appendix to this chapter shows the calculations of these dosage problems.

cal drug can promote its absorption; and inadequate fluid with an oral medication can permit it to lodge in the esophagus. Table 3-5 is a quick reference for important principles of drug administration. It is *not* meant as an initial source for learning medication technique; nursing fundamentals texts (see References), audiovisual presentations, and hands-on experience in learning laboratories are recommended. This table summarizes major principles and serves as a reference.

Some Other "Rights"

Suggestions have been made for adding a sixth, or even seventh, responsibility to the five rights. Right administration technique, right approach to the patient (developmental and psychosocial), right patient assessment, and right patient teaching have been recommended. These considerations are covered elsewhere in this chapter. The right drug storage and proper drug reconstitution are also nursing responsibilities.

Drug Storage   Drugs stored too long or under improper conditions can lose potency and even be harmful. Temperature, air, light, moisture, and even the containers in which drugs are stored can affect stability. Therefore, medications should not be transferred from the containers in which they are dispensed. They should not be stored in the sunlight or near a source of heat (stove, window, heat outlet, lights). Only those medications that specifically require a cool or cold storage place should be refrigerated, since moisture condensation resulting when the drug is removed from the refrigerator for administration could impair its stability. Most published drug references include drug storage requirements, and this information should be part of patient education.

The *expiration date* is a conservative indication of the date beyond which a drug may not have the specified potency. Antibiotics and biologicals (drugs from animal sources) always receive an expiration date, although manufacturers now put expiration dates on most drugs. Nurses should check the expiration dates of floor stock drugs, including those on the emergency carts, and rotate new quantities of drugs so that the drugs with the earliest expiration dates are used first. Regardless of the expiration date, nurses should not give any drug that looks discolored, has an unusual precipitate, or smells abnormal.

Reconstituted Drugs   Many drugs are supplied as powders to preserve stability and must be reconstituted into a liquid form by addition of a diluent (solvent). *It is imperative to use the diluent recommended by the manufacturer and to use appropriate aseptic techniques when reconstituting drugs.* After reconstitution many drugs are stable for as long as 1

TABLE 3-5 Quick Reference for Medication Administration Principles*

ROUTE	INDICATIONS/USES	ADMINISTRATION	PRECAUTIONS
Oral (*a*) Solid	Preferred route for convenience, safety, and cost.	1. A full glass of water taken with oral solid drugs will reduce stomach irritation and speed absorption. 2. If possible, patient should sit to take solid dosage forms, since they can lodge in esophagus if patient is recumbent. 3. Check with pharmacist or published reference to ascertain if food affects drug absorption. If it impairs absorption, administer drug 1 h before or 2 h after meals. Some drugs' absorption is enhanced by food. Drugs which irritate stomach are usually administered with meals. 4. Lying on right side promotes stomach emptying and speeds drug absorption. 5. Chewable tablets must be masticated thoroughly and followed with water. 6. Lozenges should be allowed to dissolve and should not be chewed.	1. Solid oral drugs should not be given to those who are unconscious, have impaired swallowing ability, or are at risk of vomiting. 2. *Do not crush* tablets or capsules of enteric coated, long-acting, or sustained-release dosage forms.
(*b*) Liquid	1. For children, elderly, and others unable to swallow solid forms. 2. For drugs for which small particle size is desirable (antacids, absorbent antidiarrheals, etc.). 3. When drug must be given by nasogastric or gastrostomy tube. 4. When unusual dosages or small dosage increments are needed.	1. See above regarding effects of food and positioning. 2. Shake all liquid forms thoroughly. 3. Follow dose with a drink of fluid. (For antacids this should be only 30–90 mL, to retard stomach emptying. Lying on left side also promotes gastric retention of antacids.) 4. Read volume level at bottom of meniscus. 30 — 20 — 15 — 10 — Read volume here at eyelevel 5 —	1. Since most liquid dosage forms do not need to dissolve, they may absorb faster and more completely than solids. Watch for change in effect if dosage form is switched. 2. Do not use kitchen spoons to measure, as these may vary in volume. 3. Pour liquids toward side of bottle opposite label.
(*c*) Powder	1. For unusual dosage levels, tube feedings, children, and others who have difficulty swallowing. 2. For bulk laxatives, potassium.	1. Mix with a small portion of food or juice. (Check compatibility.) Powder may adhere to container; redissolve if necessary. Bulk laxatives (e.g., Metamucil) may need to be mixed with 120–240 mL of fluid. 2. Follow with a full glass of fluid.	Powders are rarely used, except for laxatives and potassium, since pharmacist must measure and package most other drugs.
Sublingual/buccal	For rapid onset of a drug which is not active if swallowed (e.g., nitroglycerin, glucagon).	Instruct patient to hold drug under tongue (sublingual) or between cheek and upper gum (buccal). Patient should not drink or swallow saliva for 3 min, or until burning sensation is gone.	Make sure patient is able to understand directions for use.

34

ROUTE	INDICATIONS/USES	ADMINISTRATION	PRECAUTIONS
Topical	1. For local effects to skin or mucous membranes. 2. For systemic absorption of some drugs (nitroglycerin ointment, scopolomine patch, etc.).	1. Apply in a thin layer with clean fingertips, a glove, gauze squares, a tongue blade, or an applicator swab. Use a *sterile* glove or finger cot if skin is broken. Avoid cotton balls, which get trapped in medication. 2. Use a patting rather than rubbing application motion, as it is less traumatic to tissue. With pruritis avoid being too gentle, as this exacerbates itching. 3. Shake lotions and emulsions. Lotions may be warmed in a pan of warm water. 4. Do not use fingers to remove medication from jar, as this will contaminate entire container.	1. Drug may stain clothing. 2. Occlusive dressings (e.g., plastic wrap) will increase absorption of drug. 3. Use gloves if there is danger of drug absorption by nurse. 4. Some agents cannot be applied to injured skin. 5. Drug may cause irritation or rash. Rotate sites of application of drugs given for percutaneous absorption. 6. Ointment or patches may need replacement after a shower.
Rectal	1. For local conditions such as hemorrhoids and constipation. 2. For systemic absorption in infants and with seizures, coma and nausea and vomiting, and gastrointestinal disease. 3. Rectal solutions give more consistent absorption than other dosage forms.	1. *Suppository insertion*—Have patient lie in left lateral Sims position. Lubricate tip of suppository and gloved finger. Touching rectum may cause reflex contraction of sphincter, so do not insert suppository until sphincter relaxes again. Placement of drug depends on its purpose. Suppositories and enemas for evacuation should be placed well into rectum. Rectal drugs for systemic absorption are generally placed just beyond anorectal ridge inside internal sphincter, since drugs absorbed from this site are less subject to metabolism prior to entering systemic circulation than those absorbed higher in rectum. Regardless of purpose, rectal drugs should be placed *in contact with mucosa.* 2. Patient should retain rectal drug for 20–30 min if given to promote defecation and for at least 60 min if given for systemic absorption. Lying down promotes retention.	1. Assure that patient understands purpose of medication, since many people believe all rectal drugs are to promote evacuation. 2. Observe for perirectal irritation. 3. Solid oral dosage forms (e.g., capsules and tablets) can be given rectally, but they are often erratically absorbed, as are most suppositories. Pierce capsules with a needle prior to rectal insertion. 4. Make sure patients know to remove wrappers from suppositories prior to insertion. 5. Some suppositories need to be refrigerated, or they will be too soft to insert. 6. Feces in rectum will impede drug absorption. A cleansing enema may be indicated prior to a retention enema or a suppository given for systemic effect.

ROUTE	INDICATIONS/USES	ADMINISTRATION	PRECAUTIONS
Otic	For local anesthetics for earache. Also for anti-inflammatory and antibacterial drugs for local effect.	1. Warm medicine to body temperature by placing bottle (in a plastic bag to protect label) in a cup of warm water. 2. Patient should lie on side or tilt head so affected ear is up. Due to anatomic differences, procedure is varied for adults and infants. For adults, auricle is lifted *up* (cephalically) and *back* (posteriorly). For infants (shown below), auricle is pulled *down* and *back*. Drops are instilled toward wall of canal, rather than toward sensitive eardrum. 3. Patient should remain on side for 15 min following instillation.	1. Assure that medication is not too hot or too cold. 2. Hand holding dropper should be *braced on patient's head* to avoid injury if patient moves suddenly. 3. Manipulation of auricle may be painful in otitis.
Intradermal	For local skin anesthesia or diagnostic testing of immune response.	1. Numerous sites on forearm, back, and upper posterior arm can be used for intradermal skin testing. Forearm is usually preferred, unless extensive testing is done. 2. Use short-bevel, 26-gauge × ⅜-in. needle.	1. Avoid sites where clothing might affect local tissue reaction. 2. Volume is limited to 0.1–1.0 mL. 3. Some drugs can precipitate anaphylaxis, so have emergency drugs (epinephrine) available. Notify physician if respirations or heart rate increase after injection. 4. Chart exact position and time of injection of any diagnostic skin tests. 5. *Alcohol sponges should not be used to wipe site of any injection after needle is withdrawn.* Not only does this cause pain, but it also interferes with clot formation.

TABLE 3-5   Quick Reference for Medication Administration Principles* (*Cont.*)

ROUTE	INDICATIONS/USES	ADMINISTRATION	PRECAUTIONS
Intradermal (continued)		3. *Intradermal procedure*—After the site cleansed with alcohol or iodine dries, pull skin taut and insert needle at a 10–15° angle with bevel up. Insertion will be so shallow that needle outline will be visible. Inject drug slowly and note blanching and wheal formation. Withdraw needle rapidly and wipe site with dry gauze. Circle injection site with a pen.	

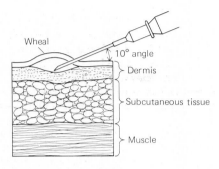

Subcutaneous (SC)	For slower systemic absorption than IM. Used for insulin, vaccines, heparin, and narcotic analgesics.	1. While any site with adequate subcutaneous tissue and free of bony prominences, major blood vessels, and large nerves is acceptable, usual sites are abdomen, flank, outer aspects of upper arm, and anterior thigh.	1. Sites should be rotated to limit tissue damage. Keep a chart of site rotation. 2. Rarely are volumes in excess of 1.5 mL given SC. 3. When insulin-dependent persons are hospitalized, nurses should use sites not accessible to self-administration. 4. Concentrated solutions can cause sterile abscesses. 5. Needle length and insertion angle will depend on amount of subcutaneous tissue patient has. Thin people will require "pinching up" of subcutaneous tissue. Needle may be inserted at 90° angle in obese people. 6. A sudden increase in activity can increase subcutaneous absorption. 7. Do not use alcohol wipes to swab site after injection.

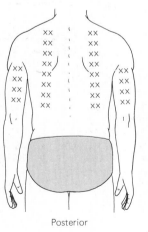

Anterior   Posterior

2. Typical needles are 25–27 gauge × ½–⅝ in.

TABLE 3-5 Quick Reference for Medication Administration Principles* (*Cont.*)

ROUTE	INDICATIONS/USES	ADMINISTRATION	PRECAUTIONS
Subcutaneous (continued)		3. *Subcutaneous procedure*—After site cleaned with alcohol or iodine dries, (*a*) insert needle at a 45° angle to skin surface or (*b*) pinch up tissue and insert needle at 90° angle to pocket formed. Aspirate, and (if no blood returns) inject solution slowly. Remove needle rapidly, maintaining angle of insertion. Wipe area with dry gauze.	

45° angle — Dermis — Subcutaneous tissue — Muscle
(a)

Angle of the pocket — 20 to 45° angle — Dermis — Subcutaneous tissue — 90° angle — Muscle
(b)

ROUTE	INDICATIONS/USES	ADMINISTRATION	PRECAUTIONS
Intramuscular (IM)	1. For more rapid onset than SC. Accepts larger volumes and is more tolerant to irritating drugs than SC route. 2. Repository forms available for some drugs (last weeks to months).	1. *Intramuscular procedure*—After site is cleaned and dry, stabilize muscle and insert needle rapidly at a 90° angle to belly of muscle. Aspirate, and (if no blood appears in syringe) slowly inject drug. Remove needle rapidly and wipe area with dry gauze. If not contraindicated, massage or exercise muscle for 2 min.	1. A few drugs [e.g., diazepam (Valium), digoxin, chlordiazepoxide (Librium), haloperidol (Haldol), phenytoin (Dilantin), and other drugs with propylene glycol as solvent] do not absorb well by IM route. 2. Generally IM route is limited to 5 mL per injection, although in deltoid muscle and in infants the limit is 2 mL. Volumes are usually limited to 3 mL in the anteriolateral thigh. 3. Inadequate needle length often results in inadvertent SC injection, causing slowed absorption and tissue damage. Proper selection of needle length depends on available muscle mass and amount of subcutaneous fat to be penetrated. Needles should be long enough to leave ¼–½ in. of the needle shaft exposed, in case it breaks from hub. Amount of subcutaneous fat can be estimated by "pinch test" of tissue overlying muscle; needle length must be half the amount pinched to penetrate to muscle. Weight and body build can also be used:

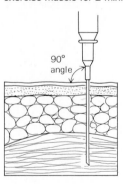

90° angle

BUILD	WEIGHT, lb	NEEDLE LENGTH, in.
Frail	70–90	1–1½
Average	90–170	1½–2
Muscular	170–200	2–3
Obese	> 200	3–5

TABLE 3-5   Quick Reference for Medication Administration Principles* (*Cont.*)

ROUTE	INDICATIONS/USES	ADMINISTRATION	PRECAUTIONS
Intramuscular (continued)	3. *Indications for various IM sites: Deltoid*—for greater blood supply and faster absorption; for small-volume drugs. Accessible and preserves modesty. Brachial and axillary nerves and blood vessels are superficial near lower deltoid.	2. *Deltoid site*—Typical needle is 23–25 gauge × ⅝–1 in. Site is located in middle third of width of arm, bordered above by a line two finger breadths below acromion process and below by a line two fingers above insertion of deltoid.	Finally, site also affects required needle length (see Administration column). 4. Selection of needle gauge depends on viscosity. Needle of 20 or 22 gauge may be needed for viscous drugs like penicillin G benzathine, but 23–25 gauge may work for most drugs. 5. Decrease pain and/or subcutaneous tissue damage by (*a*) numbing site with ice, (*b*) tapping site sharply just prior to needle insertion, (*c*) changing needle after solution is drawn up from vial or ampule, (*d*) using "air lock technique," in which 0.2 mL of air is drawn into syringe to prevent leakage into subcutaneous tissue, or (*e*) using Z-track technique. 6. For dorsogluteal site (*a*) *quadrant method* of finding site can result in dangerous misplacement of needle and (*b*) pain can be limited by having patient lie prone with toes turned inward or lie in lateral Sims position (these positions relax muscle). 7. In infants and emaciated adults, grasp muscle and elevate it from bone, major nerves, and blood vessels. 8. Do not mix drugs in a syringe unless verified compatible by a pharmacist or published reference.
	Dorsogluteal—for larger volumes (up to 5 mL). Not for children less than 2 years old. Avoid in children 2–5 years old and emaciated. Close to sciatic nerve and gluteal artery.	3. *Dorsogluteal site*—Typical needle is 20–23 gauge × 1½–3 in. Site is located above a diagonal line drawn between superior iliac spine and greater trochanter of femur.	

Acromion process

Insertion of the deltoid

Approximate location of radial nerve and brachial artery

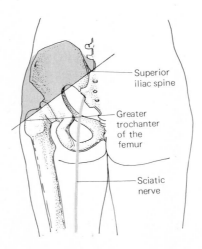

Superior iliac spine

Greater trochanter of the femur

Sciatic nerve

TABLE 3-5 Quick Reference for Medication Administration Principles* (*Cont.*)

ROUTE	INDICATIONS/USES	ADMINISTRATION	PRECAUTIONS
Intramuscular (continued)	*Ventrogluteal*—for larger volumes (up to 5 mL). Most removed from major nerves and blood vessels. Accessible when patient is in a variety of positions. Can be used for children or adults.	4. *Ventrogluteal site*—Typical needle is 20–23 gauge × 1½–3 in. Locate site by placing palm of hand over greater trochanter of femur with thumb pointing toward patient's abdomen. When index finger is placed over anterior iliac spine and middle finger is spread back as far as possible along iliac crest, ventrogluteal site is in V-shaped space between fingers. Needle should be directed slightly cephalically into greatest mass of muscle.	

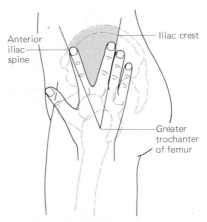

	Anteriolateral thigh—for infants, in whom vastus lateralis and rectus femoris muscles are well-developed. Accessible for self-administration. Sciatic nerve runs along posterior thigh.	5. *Anteriolateral thigh site*—Typical needle is 20–23 gauge × 1½ in. for adults and 22–25 gauge × ⅝–1 in. for infants and children. Site is mid-third of distance from greater trochanter to knee and in area between midline of anterior thigh and midline of lateral thigh.	

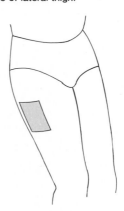

ROUTE	INDICATIONS/USES	ADMINISTRATION	PRECAUTIONS
Intravenous (IV)	For rapid onset and constant blood levels with continuous infusion. Useful for large volumes and drugs too irritating for IM or SC injection.	1. Venipuncture for IVs should be done only by trained personnel, preferably a designated IV team on each shift. 2. Bottles or bags for continuous IVs should be labeled with contents and a "time tape" that indicates amount of fluid which should remain at various times. IVs are checked at least hourly (every 30 min if they contain drugs and every 15 min for blood products). Checking an IV involves checking IV order, container contents, container fluid level, flow rate, location of needle's bevel in vein, effects of drugs, and presence of phlebitis or infiltration. 3. Do not mix drugs in an IV solution unless they are verified as compatible by a pharmacist or published reference. If incompatible drugs are given via intermittent infusions through same IV site, flush tubing thoroughly with saline before and after each drug and use different infusion sets ("piggybacks") for each drug. Stop main IV when piggyback runs. 4. Take drop factor into consideration when setting rate on an infusion controller or pump if standard tubing is used. 5. Make sure needle and tubing are stabilized with tape. Chevron method of taping produces a good anchor for butterfly needles and angiocaths.	1. Risks include phlebitis, infiltration, fluid overload, and drug overdosage. Infusion pumps or controllers are recommended for drugs with narrow margins of safety. 2. To assess for phlebitis, pinch IV line just above venipuncture and then compress flash chamber. This will dilate vein and cause pain if vein is inflamed. 3. To assess for infiltration, use a small penlight against skin over insertion site. Infiltration will appear as a diffuse glow under skin while normal will be only a small halo of light. 4. Do not give IV fluids that are discolored or contain precipitates or particles. 5. Arm boards should be well padded and secured with a minimal amount of tape. Apply tape with tape-to-tape method or over gauze. 6. Administer IV medications diluted unless manufacturer specifies that an undiluted bolus may be given.

Tape wrapped chevron style

Butterfly needle wings

---

*The following medication administration techniques are discussed in other chapters: nasal sprays and drops (Chap. 21), intravenous bolus (Chap. 48), Z-track (Chap. 36), inhalants (Chaps. 27 and 47), rectal creams and ointments (Chap. 30), ophthalmic ointments and drops (Chap. 37), vaginal (Chap. 46), dermatologic (Chap. 38), intraspinal (Chap. 47), and insulin administration (Chap. 35).

month, while some are stable for only a few hours. It is important that the dose be completely administered within the required time. Any remaining drug should be thrown out, unless another dose is due before the suggested time limit expires. In this case the container should be labeled with the date and time reconstituted, the potency (e.g., 5000 U/mL), and the initials of the nurse. Some drugs are so unstable that the container must be protected from light (wrapped in tinfoil) during IV infusion and a new infusion must be prepared every few hours. When outpatients receive reconstituted drugs (e.g., many antibiotic suspensions), the time limit for use should be emphasized as part of patient education.

Patient Teaching

Teaching is possibly the most important part of the nursing role in drug therapy, since a major portion of prescription and nonprescription drugs are self-administered by patients in their own homes. The teaching-learning process runs parallel to the nursing process and consists of the following steps:

1. Identify the need for teaching.
2. Establish realistic learning goals.
3. Select teaching methods.
4. Implement teaching.
5. Evaluate effect of teaching.

Identification of the need for teaching may occur when the patient asks a question, such as "What are those little yellow pills supposed to do?" or "Why does my blood-thinner pill look different each day?" or "Will I continue to be so drowsy on these pills that I can't go to work?" The need for teaching may also be independently identified by the professional, recognizing that all patients in some categories (e.g., newly diagnosed diabetics) require education or that a patient has individual learning needs (e.g., the patient has misconceptions about his or her drug therapy). The consumer rights and responsibilities (Table 3-6) established by the Food and Drug Administration and the National Council on Patient Information and Education identity the minimal content of patient education.

Realistic learning goals must take into consideration the patient's recognition of a need for education, readiness to learn, health-illness values, and general cognitive function and education. Learning goals should be stated concisely and clearly in behavioral terms, such as "State drug schedule verbally" and "Demonstrate correct subcutaneous heparin injection technique." The goals must be stated precisely enough that all the members of the nursing team who may be involved with teaching will understand the exact objectives of the teaching.

Patient teaching can then proceed either on a formal or incidental basis. Incidental teaching occurs as the need arises, such as when the patient asks a question, while for-

TABLE 3-6   Consumer Rights and Responsibilities Regarding Prescription Drugs*

Rights	Responsibilities
1. To be informed of:	1. To inform the care provider regarding:
The name of the drug prescribed	Allergic reactions or adverse effects of drugs taken in the past
What the drug is supposed to do	What drugs, including nonprescription drugs, are taken on a regular basis
Specifically when and how to take the drug	
How long to continue to take the drug	Pregnancy, heavy smoking, heavy drinking, or use of recreational drugs
Any foods, beverages, or medicines which should be avoided when taking the drug	Treatment for another condition by another health care provider
The possible adverse effects and how to recognize them	2. To consult the care provider before stopping the drug, changing the dosage, or deviating from the recommendations of the prescriber
What to do if adverse effects occur	
Any approved generic version of the drug	3. To refrain from taking any medications while hospitalized, unless specifically authorized by the attending physician
How to store the drug	
2. To receive available written information about the drug	4. To store medications properly and out of the reach of children
	5. To refrain from taking medications prescribed for someone else or letting another person use his or her medicine
	6. To report any unexpected symptoms to the care provider
	7. To read and follow the label directions and never take a drug at night without turning on the light to read the label

*Free consumer brochures are available by writing to RX Drugs, Department 69, Pueblo, CO 81009.

mal teaching involves setting aside a time strictly for teaching. This may be in groups or with individuals and their families.

Teaching Goals

Learning objectives have been classified into three domains: *cognitive* (understanding and knowledge), *affective* (feelings and attitudes), and *psychomotor* (physical skills). Teaching related to drug therapy involves all three. The patient with severe diabetes must know about the effects of the disease process, the necessity for lifelong therapy, and how diet and exercise affect insulin need (cognitive). This patient must also make a major psychosocial adjustment and come to accept the disease and the restrictions it imposes (affective). Finally, the patient must learn to inject insulin and to check urine and blood for sugar levels (psychomotor).

The nurse needs to adjust the approaches to the needs of the patient and the type of objective (see Table 3-7). Most patients will need the instructions in writing for reinforcement. Some may be able to learn by reading a pamphlet, while others may need very concrete learning experiences, such as the opportunity to actually self-administer the drug in the hospital. Nurses should collect a library of teaching supplies such as drug-company models and publications, pamphlets from organizations like the American Heart Association and the American Diabetic Association, and information sheets such as those in *Drug Information for Patients* (Griffith, 1978), which can be photocopied and handed to patients. Nurses should also be familiar with books about drugs written for the lay person (see References), since some patients will have sophisticated questions based on use of this information.

Behavioral Approaches

Some educational approaches focus on patient behavior, rather than on patient knowledge. Assertiveness programs have been initiated for adults and children and teach the person to be an active rather than passive health care consumer.

Patient contracts are also effective in altering patient behavior. While the contract may be written or verbal, it is necessary that both the nurse and the patient participate in its formulation and understand the mutuality of obligations. Steps in patient contracting include:

1. Identify the problem
2. Set goals
3. Explore resources and develop a plan
4. Divide the responsibility and set a time limit
5. Evaluate the contract and modify it as needed

For example, the problem might be identified as high blood pressure readings related to the patient's failure to take his or her antihypertensive drugs and follow a low-sodium reducing diet. Jointly the patient and the nurse agree that their goals are that the patient will lose 5 lb and take both doses of medication daily and that he or she should not have to lose any work time due to clinic appointments. The patient agrees to keep a daily record of food intake and drug administration, and the nurse schedules appointments in the laboratory and clinic around the patient's work schedule and agrees to facilitate the appointments so that the patient leaves the clinic in time to drive across town to work by the beginning of the afternoon shift. They agree to review their progress in 1 month and that the contract will be in force for 3 months.

Patient Observation

Part of nursing planning is establishing observational parameters to evaluate for the therapeutic and adverse effects of medications. Taking the apical pulse prior to every dose of digoxin (or related drug) and prior to β blockers (e.g., propranolol, metoprolol, pindolol) is an example of patient observation for *potential adverse effects* of these drugs, which include bradycardia and arrhythmias. Weighing the patient daily, measuring urine output each shift, and auscultating lung sounds every 4 h are examples of actions for

TABLE 3-7 Effective Teaching Methods for Cognitive, Affective, and Psychomotor Goals

COGNITIVE	AFFECTIVE*	PSYCHOMOTOR
Explanation (lecture)	Discussion (nurse-patient-family)	Demonstration by teacher (nurse)
Discussion	Group session	Practice (with appropriate equipment in real or simulated situation)
Programmed instruction	Visits by former patients or representatives from support groups (such as ostomy club)	Return demonstration by learner
Audiovisual aids (as a supplementary or primary source)		Written directions with pictures
Written instructions		Films, slides, tapes
Pretest/posttest		

*When attitudes are not strongly formed, methods used in the other two domains may be effective.

which nursing orders might be written on a care plan to evaluate for the *therapeutic effects* of digoxin, which improves the strengh of cardiac pumping. Figure 3-1 gives other examples of planned observation for drug effects.

Support and Prevention

Actions taken by the nurse may support the drug therapy by maximizing the beneficial effects and preventing or minimizing the side effects so that the therapy is tolerated better. For example, elderly men on drugs with atropine-like side effects often experience difficulty voiding, may be dizzy, may be constipated, and may have a dry mouth. The nursing actions that might minimize these effects include encouraging the patient to stand to void (for better drainage of the bladder), assisting when the patient gets out of bed (to avoid falls), encouraging high fluid intake and physical activity (to prevent constipation), and suggesting that the patient take frequent sips of water or frequently perform oral hygiene routines (to combat the dryness of mouth). An example of nursing action that may potentiate the therapeutic drug effect is staying with the patient to talk and give emotional support for a few minutes after administering an analgesic. Another example of nursing intervention to support the desired therapeutic effect is teaching the patient on diuretics for high blood pressure how to decrease salt intake. These activities must be a *planned* part of the nursing care related to drug therapy.

Recording and Documentation

Most institutions have an established medication record, which the nurse initials when a dose is administered or on which the nurse writes the time that the dose is given. This gives a rapid reference for assessing the drug history of the patient, as well as documenting the drug therapy for legal reasons. *It is imperative that the drug record be complete and accurate.* Some assessment and evaluation data, such as apical pulse taken prior to digoxin and β blockers, are usually recorded directly on the medication record.

Medication given on a PRN basis should be entered into the narrative notes with an indication of the reason the drug was given and the effect of the drug, as well as the dose and route of the drug. If the drug is injected, the site of administration is recorded to facilitate rotation of the injection site.

Data documenting the desired therapeutic effect or the development of adverse reactions should be specifically described in the nurses' progress notes. Action taken related to observation, prevention, or treatment of adverse reactions should also be reported to document that these measures are being done and to give baseline data. Flow sheets also can be a useful format for recording this information. When a drug is discontinued, it is important to note the reason for this, such as allergy or other adverse effect or failure to achieve the desired therapeutic effect.

Response to Medication Errors

Even the most conscientious nurse makes an occasional medication error. Some nurses claim that they have never made a drug error, but there is research evidence that a large proportion of the errors go unnoticed by the erring nurse or anyone else (Barker and McConnel, 1962). *Most medication errors are preventable by making habitual those practices discussed for the five rights.* There are five nursing responsibilities related to medication errors: (1) to prevent and detect errors in drug therapy, (2) to report any errors made or detected to the physician and appropriate nursing supervisors, (3) to monitor for adverse effects resulting from the error and to institute medical care as ordered, (4) to accurately and thoughtfully complete the incident report, and (5) to seek to eliminate the cause(s) of the error.

Incident Reports Incident reports are legal records of any error or accident that is potentially harmful to a patient. Usually one copy is placed in the patient record and one is analyzed by an administrative committee concerned with safety. Information about the event may also be entered onto the record of the student or nurse and is sometimes used punitively (such as for dismissal if "too many" errors occur). Incident reports can also help identify administrative policies and procedures that need to be changed to avoid errors.

Incident reports usually require a reconstruction of the event, include a summary of the physician's examination of the patient, and ask for suggestions on prevention of similar events. Most errors are multicausal and could have been prevented at several points in their history; incident reports are most helpful for future prevention if they reflect this attitude.

The Need for Continuing Education Pharmacologic knowledge quickly becomes outdated. Available evidence indicates that as the time since graduation from nursing school increases, the knowledge deficit about drug hazards increases and that continuing education can improve the quality of nursing care related to drug therapy (Markowitz et al., 1981; Westfall and Speedie, 1981). Since many drug errors are attributable to lack of current and comprehensive drug information, continuing updates of pharmacologic knowledge are a professional responsibility.

MANAGING THE CONTRAINDICATED ORDER

As described in Chap. 2, the result of nursing assessment in drug therapy is either a nursing diagnosis or a judgment about the safety and effectiveness of the drug order in the given patient situation. All previous discussion in this chapter relates to orders which are judged safe and effective to implement. However, a few orders are not safe to implement and pose a danger to the patient. *A nurse must defer implementation of a contraindicated medical order until it is replaced, modified, or justified.*

What is the proper course of action when the nurse judges an order to be unsafe or not effective? First, it must be stated that there is no clear line of distinction between a contraindicated drug and a safe and effective drug. For example, some drugs are absolutely contraindicated in pregnancy but still will be ordered if the potential benefits outweigh the risks. Dosages and drug uses are sometimes accepted medical therapy long before they are approved by the Food and Drug Administration for inclusion as part of the official drug labeling. However, the nurse is correct in requesting an explanation by the prescriber when a drug is ordered for an unlabeled use, in doses in excess of approved levels, or in the presence of a contraindication. The nurse should make this request for information privately (public confrontations are threatening and often result in defensiveness), courteously, and in the spirit of scientific inquiry and shared responsibility, keeping in mind that the best interests of the patient are the ultimate goal of both medicine and nursing. If the physician cannot offer a sound medical reason for the order but will not change it, the nurse should refuse to implement it and suggest the physician administer the drug. The reasons for refusal to carry out the order must be stated clearly and confidently. It is important to document in writing the actions taken by the nurse prior to the refusal and the rationale for the actions. The nursing supervisor should be notified of the situation.

Many nurses are reticent to question a doctor because of fear of being in error or being rebuffed. Most nurses find it helpful to seek validation of their concerns from a pharmacist and to discuss the problem with other nurses prior to addressing the physician.

When an order is not unsafe but is of no apparent therapeutic value, the nurse should call this to the attention of the physician, documenting the basis for this conclusion. While the drug may be doing no immediate harm, it does increase the risk of adverse effects and drug interactions, not to mention health care costs. When the nurse asks confident and knowledgeable questions about drug therapy, the patient is the ultimate benefactor.

APPENDIX: EXPLANATION OF SOLUTIONS TO DOSAGE CALCULATION SELF-ASSESSMENT* (Table 3-4)

1. **a.** First compute the dosage required (formula 2):

$$\frac{250 \text{ mg}}{125 \text{ mg}} \times 5 \text{ mL} = 10 \text{ mL}$$

*Formula numbers relate to formulas in Table 3-3.

Then convert to household units (modified formula 1):

| Unknown nonmetric value | : | Metric value no. 1 | :: | Known nonmetric value | : | Metric value no. 2 |

$$x : 10 \text{ mL} :: 1 \text{ tsp} : 5 \text{ mL}$$

$$10 \text{ mL} \cdot \text{tsp} = 5x \text{ mL}$$

$$2 \text{ tsp} = x$$

b. Compute total daily dosage administered:

$$3 \times 250 \text{ mg} = 750 \text{ mg}$$

Convert weight to kilograms (modified formula 1):

| Nonmetric value no. 1 | : | Unknown metric value | :: | Nonmetric value no. 2 | : | Known metric value |

$$33 \text{ lb} : x \text{ kg} :: 2.2 \text{ lb} : 1 \text{ kg}$$

$$2.2x = 33 \text{ kg}$$

$$x = 15 \text{ kg}$$

Compute recommended dosage:

$$15 \text{ kg} \times 40 \text{ mg/kg/day} = 600 \text{ mg/day}$$

Compare 750 mg to 600 mg.

2. Convert grains to milligrams (formula 1):

| Nonmetric value no. 1 | : | Unknown metric value no. 1 | :: | Nonmetric value no. 2 | : | Known metric value no. 2 |

$$1\frac{1}{2} \text{ gr} : x :: 1 \text{ gr} : 64 \text{ mg}$$

$$x = 64 \times 1\frac{1}{2} \text{ mg}$$

$$x = 96 \text{ mg}$$

Since apothecary-to-metric conversions are approximate, the 100-mg tablet would be indicated.

3. Convert micrograms to milligrams (modified formula 1).

| μg value no. 1 | : | Unknown mg equivalent of no. 1 | :: | μg value no. 2 | : | Known mg equivalent of no. 2 |

$$500 \ \mu\text{g} : x :: 1000 \ \mu\text{g} : 1 \text{ mg}$$

$$1000x = 500 \text{ mg}$$

$$x = 0.5 \text{ mg}$$

Compute dosage (formula 2):

$$\frac{D}{S} \times F = \text{Amount to administer}$$

$$\frac{0.5 \text{ mg}}{0.25 \text{ mg}} \times 1 \text{ tablet} = \text{Amount to administer}$$

$$2 \text{ tablets} = \text{Amount to administer}$$

4. Calculate dosage (formula 2):

$$\frac{D}{S} \times F = \text{Amount to administer}$$

$$\frac{30 \text{ meq}}{40 \text{ meq}} \times 20 \text{ mL} = \text{Amount to administer}$$

$$15 \text{ mL} = \text{Amount to administer}$$

5. Calculate dosage (formula 2):

$$\frac{D}{S} \times F = \text{Amount to administer}$$

$$\frac{70 \text{ mg}}{80 \text{ mg}} \times 2 \text{ mL} = \text{Amount to administer}$$

$$1.75 \text{ mL} = \text{Amount to administer}$$

6. Convert grains to milligrams (formula 1):

$$\begin{matrix} \text{Nonmetric} \\ \text{value no. 1} \end{matrix} : \begin{matrix} \text{Unknown} \\ \text{metric} \\ \text{equivalent} \\ \text{of no. 1} \end{matrix} :: \begin{matrix} \text{Nonmetric} \\ \text{value no. 2} \end{matrix} : \begin{matrix} \text{Known metric} \\ \text{equivalent} \\ \text{of no. 2} \end{matrix}$$

$$\frac{1}{200} \text{ gr} : x :: 1 \text{ gr} : 60 \text{ mg}$$

$$x = \frac{60}{200} \text{ mg}$$

$$x = 0.3 \text{ mg}$$

7. Compute dosage (formula 2):

$$\frac{D}{S} \times F = \text{Amount to administer}$$

$$\frac{15,000 \text{ U}}{40,000 \text{ U}} \times 1 \text{ mL} = \text{Amount to administer}$$

$$0.375 \text{ mL} = \text{Amount to administer}$$

$$\text{(round to 0.38 mL)}$$

8. Compute dosage (formula 2):

$$\frac{D}{S} \times F = \text{Amount to administer}$$

$$\frac{4 \text{ g}}{50 \text{ g}} \times 100 \text{ mL} = \text{Amount to administer}$$

$$8 \text{ mL} = \text{Amount to administer}$$

9. **a.** Compute flow rate in mL/h.

$$\frac{1000 \text{ mL}}{8 \text{ h}} = 125 \text{ mL/h}$$

Calculate flow rate in gtt/min. (formula 3):

$$\text{Flow rate} = \frac{\text{Drop factor}}{60 \text{ min/h}} \times \text{ordered hourly volume}$$

$$= \frac{20 \text{ gtt/mL}}{60 \text{ min/h}} \times 125 \text{ mL/h}$$

$$= \frac{2500 \text{ gtt}}{60 \text{ min}} = 41.7 \text{ gtt/min}$$

$$\text{(round to 42 gtt/min)}$$

b. Calculate flow rate in gtt/min (formula 3):

$$\frac{60 \text{ gtt/mL}}{60 \text{ min/h}} \times 125 \text{ mL/h} = \text{Drops per minute}$$

$$125 \text{ gtt/min} = \text{Drops per minute}$$

10. **a.** Compute flow rate in mL/h (modified formula 1):

$$100 \text{ mL} : 45 \text{ min} :: x \text{ mL} : 60 \text{ min}$$

$$45x = 6000 \text{ mL/h}$$

$$x = 133$$

Compute flow rate in gtt/min (formula 3):

$$\frac{\text{Drop factor}}{60 \text{ min/h}} \times \text{hourly volume} = \text{Drops per minute}$$

$$\frac{20 \text{ gtt/mL}}{60 \text{ min/h}} \times 133 \text{ mL/h} = \text{Drops per minute}$$

$$\frac{2660 \text{ gtt}}{60 \text{ min}} = \text{Drops per minute}$$

$$44 = \text{Drops per minute}$$

b. Compute using alternate to formula 3:

$$\frac{\text{Drop factor}}{\text{Time span}} \times \text{volume to be infused} = \text{Drops per minute}$$

$$\frac{10 \text{ gtt/mL}}{30 \text{ min}} \times 100 \text{ mL} = \text{Drops per minute}$$

$$\frac{1000 \text{ gtt}}{30 \text{ min}} = \text{Drops per minute}$$

$$33 = \text{Drops per minute}$$

REFERENCES

General

Barker, K. N., and W. E. McConnel: "How to Detect Medication Errors," *Mod Hosp,* **99**:95, 1962.

Cohen, M. R.: "Medication Errors," *Nursing 81,* **11**:105, 1981.

Davis, N. M., and M. R. Cohen: "20 Tips for Avoiding Medication Errors," *Nursing 82,* **12**:65–72, 1982.

George, G.: "If Patient Teaching Tries Your Patience, Try This Plan," *Nursing 82,* **12**:50–56, 1982.

Long, G.: "The Effect of Medication Distribution Systems on Medication Errors," *Nurs Res,* **31**:182–184, 1982.

Loustau, A.: "The Management Process: Planning, Intervention, Evaluation," in P. H. Mitchell and A. Loustau (eds.), *Concepts Basic to Nursing,* 3d ed., New York: McGraw-Hill, 1981.

———— "Patient-Clinic Teaching: An Application of the Nursing Process," in P. H. Mitchell and A. Loustau (eds.), *Concepts Basic to Nursing,* New York: McGraw-Hill, 1981.

Markowitz, J. S., G. Pearson, B. G. Kay, and R. Loewenstein: "Nurses, Physicians, Pharmacists: Their Knowledge of Hazards of Medications," *Nurs Res,* **30**:366–370, 1981.

"Motivating Children to Become Assertive Health-Care Consumers," *Nursing 82,* **12**:941, 1982.

Newton, M.: "Guidelines for Handling Drug Errors," *Nursing 77,* **7**:62–65, 1977.

Nightingale, F.: *Notes on Nursing, What It Is and What It Is Not,* London: Harrison, 1859.

Redman, B.: *The Process of Patient Teaching in Nursing,* 4th ed., St. Louis: Mosby, 1980.

Rich, P. L.: "Making the Most of Your Charting Time," *Nursing 83,* **13**:34–39, 1983.

Safren, M. A., and A. Chappnis: "A Critical Incident Study of Hospital Medication Errors," *Hospitals,* **34**:32, 1980.

Sandroff, R.: "Booby-Trapped Orders," *RN,* **44**:24–31, 1981.

Sloan, M. R., and B. T. Schommer: "Want to Get Your Patient Involved in His Care? Use a Contract," *Nursing 82,* **12**:48–49, 1982.

Westfall, L. K., and S. M. Speedie: "The Effect of Inservice Education Provided by Consultant Pharmacist on the Behavior of Nurses in Long-Term Care Facilities," *Drug Intell Clin Pharm,* **15**:777–781, 1981.

Youngren, D.: "Improving Patient Compliance with a Self-Medication Teaching Program," *Nursing 81,* **11**:60–61, 1981.

Drug Administration Techniques

Brill, E. L., and D. F. Kilts: *Foundations for Nursing,* New York: Appleton-Century-Crofts, 1980.

Bruya, M. A.: "Administering Injectable Medications," in K. C. Sorenson and J. Luckmann (eds.), *Basic Nursing: A Psychophysiologic Approach,* Philadelphia, Saunders, 1979.

————: "Administering Topical Medications," in K. C. Sorenson and J. Luckmann (eds.), *Basic Nursing: A Psychophysiologic Approach,* Philadelphia: Saunders, 1979.

————: "Medication Principles and Oral Administration," in K. C. Sorenson and J. Luckmann (eds.), *Basic Nursing: A Psychophysiologic Approach,* Philadelphia: Saunders, 1979.

Burke, E. L.: "Insulin Injection: Site and Technique," *Am J Nurs,* **72**:2194–2196, 1972.

Coblio, N. A.: "Don't Combine Those Drugs (Until You Check This Table!)," *Nursing 81,* **11**:48–49, 1981.

Cockshott, W.: "Intramuscular or Intralipomatous Injections?" *N Engl J Med,* **307**:356–357, 1982.

Giovannitti, C., and T. Schwinghammer: "Food and Drink: Managing the Right Mix for Your Patient," *Nursing 81,* **11**:26–31, 1981.

Giving Medications, Springhouse, PA: Springhouse Intermed, 1982.

Greenblatt, D., and J. Kock-Weser: "Intramuscular Injections of Drugs," *N Engl J Med,* **295**:542–546, 1976.

Hickman, R. A.: "When You Have to Reconstitute Meds," *RN,* **44**:40–43, 1981.

How to Give an Intramuscular Injection, New York: Pfizer Laboratories, 1982.

Lenz, C. L.: "Make Your Needle Selection Right to the Point," *Nursing 83,* **13**:48–50, 1983.

Lenz, S., A. Zawacki, and J. Johnson: "Reducing Discomfort from IM Injections," *Am J Nurs,* **76**:800–803, 1976.

Managing IV Therapy, Springhouse, PA: Springhouse Intermed, 1983.

Narrow, B. W., and K. B. Buschle: *Fundamentals of Nursing Practice,* New York: Wiley, 1982.

Newton, D. W., and M. Newton: "Needles, Syringes, and Sites for Injectable Medications," *Am Pharm Assoc J,* NS **17**:685–687, 1977.

Newton, D. W., and M. Newton: "Route, Site, and Technique: Three Key Decisions in Giving Parenteral Medication," *Nursing 79,* 9:18–25, 1979.

Pitel, M.: "The Subcutaneous Injection," *Am J Nurs,* **71**:76–79, 1971.

Plein, J., and E. Plein: *Fundamentals of Medications,* 2d ed., Hamilton, IL: Drug Intelligence Publication, 1974.

"Quick and Easy: 50 Tips for Improving Care," *Nursing 81,* **11**:51–64, 1981.

"Report on Intravenous Therapy National Survey," *Nursing 81,* **11**:80–82, 1981.

Rosenberg, J. M., and P. Sangkachad: "Take with Meals . . . Or Not?" *RN,* pt I, **44**:46–52, 1981; pt. II, **44**:60–65, 1981.

Saperstein, A. B., and M. A. Frazier: "Administration of Medications," in A. B. Saperstein and M. A. Frazier (eds.), *Introduction to Nursing Practice,* Philadelphia: Davis, 1980.

Slawson, M., and S. Slawson: "To Crush or Not to Crush, That Is the Question," *J Nurs Care,* **14**:22–24, 1981.

Smith, S. F., and D. Duell: *Nursing Skills and Evaluation: A Nursing Process Approach,* Los Altos, CA: National Nursing Review, 1982.

Wordell, D. C.: "Should You Crush That Tablet," *Nursing 82,* **12**:78, 1982.

Dosage Calculation

Blume, D. M.: *Drugs and Solutions,* 3d ed., Philadelphia: Davis, 1980.

Carr, J. J ., N. L. McElroy, and B. L. Carr, "How to Solve Dosage Problems in One Easy Lesson," *Am J Nurs,* **76**:1934–1936, 1976.

Eisenbach, R.: *Calculating and Administering Medications,* Philadelphia: Davis, 1977.

Engram, B.: "Computing IV Flow Rates," *Nursing 81,* **11**:89–92, 1981.

Hart, K. L.: *The Arithmetic of Dosages and Solutions: A Programmed Presentation,* 5th ed., St. Louis, Mosby, 1981.

Jessee, R. W., and R. W. McHenry: *Self-Teaching Tests in Arithmetic for Nurses,* 9th ed., St. Louis: Mosby, 1975.

Medici, G. A.: *Dosage Calculations: A Guide for Current Clinical Practice,* Englewood Cliffs, N.J.: Prentice-Hall, 1980.

Norville, M. A. F.: *Drug Dosages and Solutions,* Bowie, MD: Brady, 1982.

Radcliff, R. K., and S. J. Ogden: *Calculation of Drug Dosages: A Workbook,* 2d ed., St. Louis, Mosby, 1980.

Readey, H., and M. Teague, et al.: *Introduction to Nursing Essentials: A Handbook,* St. Louis, Mosby, 1977.

Richardson, L. I., and J. K. Richardson: *The Mathematics of Drugs and Solutions with Clinical Applications,* 2d ed., New York: McGraw-Hill, 1980.

Sackheim, G. I., and L. Robins: *Programmed Mathematics for Nurses,* 4th ed., New York: Macmillan, 1979.

Scott, M. A.: *Calculations of Medications: Using the Proportion,* New York: Appleton-Century-Crofts, 1982.

Worley, E.: *Pharmacology and Medications,* 4th ed., Philadelphia: Davis, 1982.

Consumer Drug Information

American Society of Hospital Pharmacists: *Medical Teaching Guide—A Guide for Patient Education,* American Hospital Formulary Service, 1983.

Benowicz, R. J.: *Nonprescription Drugs and Their Side Effects,* New York: Berkely, 1982.

Graedon, J.: *The People's Pharmacy,* New York: Avon, 1976.

Griffith, H. W.: *Drug Information for Patients,* Philadelphia: Saunders, 1978.

Long, J. W.: *The Essential Guide to Prescription Drugs,* 3d ed., New York: Harper & Row, 1982.

Pantell, R. H., and D. A. Bergman: *The Parent's Pharmacy,* Reading, MA: Addison-Wesley, 1982.

Public Citizen Health Research Group: *Over the Counter Pills That Don't Work,* Washington: Public Citizens Health Research Group (Dept 27, 2000 P Street, 20036), 1983.

Wolfe, S. M.: *Pills That Don't Work,* New York: Warner, 1981.

Zimmerman, D. R.: *The Essential Guide to Nonprescription Drugs,* New York: Harper & Row, 1983.

4

NURSING EVALUATION AND PHARMACOTHERAPEUTICS

GINETTE A. PEPPER

LEARNING OBJECTIVES

Upon mastery of the contents of this chapter, the reader will be able to:

1. List five kinds of evaluation in which nurses participate that might concern pharmacotherapeutics.
2. Explain evaluation as a component of nursing process with individual patients.
3. State the three types of criteria on which evaluation of care is based.
4. Describe the evaluation of diagnostic, therapeutic, and teaching goals in nursing pharmacotherapeutics.
5. List several quality assurance issues and problems relevant to the nursing role in drug therapy.
6. Assess the impact of current research on the nursing role in drug therapy.

Evaluation is extremely important in nursing. Nurses evaluate (1) the effectiveness of the health care of individual patients, (2) the overall quality of care in hospitals, clinics, nursing homes, and wards, (3) the quality of care given by other nurses and health care providers (e.g., personnel evaluation by supervisors and peer audits), and (4) personal knowledge, skill, and professional development needs. In addition, evaluation research determines the effectiveness of nursing care delivery systems and educational programs, as well as the usefulness of nursing care approaches for populations of patients. Pharmacotherapeutics is frequently considered in all of these kinds of evaluation.

EVALUATION IN NURSING PROCESS

Within the nursing process, evaluation is the analysis of the progress of a patient toward predetermined health goals. *The purpose of evaluation is modification of the nursing care if the patient is not progressing as expected.* The reason a nursing intervention was ineffective is not always because the wrong approach was selected; therapeutic failure is just as likely to result if some important data are not detected during assessment, if the diagnosis is in error, if the goal is set too high or too low, or if the intervention is improperly implemented. A frequently overlooked reason for therapeutic failure is that the patient did not understand or did not concur with the goals and methods imposed by the health professionals. Hence, evaluation involves analyzing *whether a plan succeeded* and, if necessary, *why it failed.*

Evaluation is an ongoing process. The nurse does not wait until the full course of therapy is complete and then decide whether it has been helpful or harmful. Rather, the nurse constantly compares the patient's status to an anticipated course of progress. In the event there is deviation from the expected course which threatens patient well-being, the intervention is immediately modified or discontinued. Thus, if a nurse is administering an intravenous medication and the patient becomes apprehensive, diaphoretic, and has a rapid pulse and labored respirations, the infusion is stopped immediately. Similarly, if verbal attempts to soothe and distract a patient in pain have no effect within a reasonable amount of time, another approach is sought.

Evaluation is not separate and distinct from the other phases of the nursing process but interacts with them, as represented in Fig. 4-1. Assessment furnishes baselines against which progress can be evaluated. The goals established during planning are the guidelines for evaluation and the determinants of whether the intervention is considered a success. If goals are clearly stated in measurable terms (with deadlines) during the initial step of management, and approaches are selected to monitor therapeutic and adverse effects of drugs as part of nursing care, evaluation is readily accomplished.

49

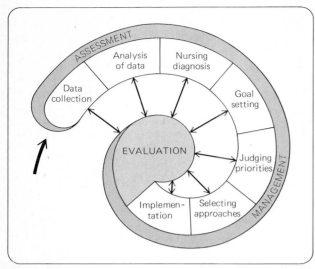

FIGURE 4-1

Conceptualization of the nursing process as a spiral promotes representation of the interaction of evaluation with every step of the nursing process.

Evaluating Goal Attainment

The three types of goals discussed in Chap. 3, diagnostic, therapeutic, and teaching, vary in management and evaluation. One difference in evaluation relates to the types of criteria most commonly used to judge whether or not the goal was attained.

Criteria for Evaluation

There are three types of criteria for evaluating effectiveness and quality of care: structure, process, and outcome. These criteria are relevant to evaluating individual patient care and to quality assurance programs.

Structural criteria refer to the qualities or qualifications of the health care providers, the equipment and supplies, and the characteristics of the health care facility. Some examples of structural criteria are that there is a trained intravenous therapy team available on all shifts to do venipunctures and that needles for intramuscular injection are stocked on each ward in the following inch lengths: 1, 1½, 2, 2½, 3, and 4. Structural criteria are more common in quality assurance programs than in individual patient care evaluation.

Process criteria relate to what is done for the patient and how it is done. Some examples of process criteria are that a medication history is performed and recorded, that the proper needle length is used for an intramuscular injection, and that the proper drug and dosage for a given disease are prescribed and administered.

Outcome criteria address the status of the patient after the intervention, such as that the patient will state he or she is comfortable, that the diastolic blood pressure is main-

tained below 90 mmHg, or that the prothrombin time is 2 to 2½ times the control level. There is no requirement that outcome criteria be based on objective data; in many cases the patient's subjective appraisal is an important and valid criterion.

Outcome goals are obviously the most direct means of evaluating care, but some outcomes are difficult to measure. It is presumed that proper structure and process correlate with the desired outcome.

Therapeutic Goal Evaluation

Outcome criteria are appropriate for the evaluation of therapeutic goals which anticipate improvement in the patient's condition. The *expected therapeutic time course* is crucial to evaluating drug effects, since some drugs achieve full therapeutic benefit in minutes while others require weeks. Therefore, the nurse evaluates the therapeutic effect of drugs according to whether the anticipated effects occur in the expected amount of time. If not, the nurse contacts the prescriber, who must discontinue the drug, adjust the dosage, add another drug, or revise the goal and reevaluate at a later time.

With some drugs the goal is prevention of a potential problem or maintenance of the current patient status, rather than a change in the patient's condition. Outcome criteria are difficult to measure for problems which are potential rather than actual. Therefore, preventative therapeutic goals are generally evaluated by process criteria such as whether a child receives all recommended immunizations prior to starting school. Generally, maintenance goals cannot be considered with respect to a typical time course, so goals like "This diabetic patient's daily fasting blood sugar should not exceed 150 mg/dL" are evaluated by a combination of outcome and process criteria. Outcome criteria are used to judge maintenance of the therapeutic goal (blood sugar level), and process criteria evaluate the way in which the effect is monitored (daily fasting blood sugar).

Patient Teaching Goal Evaluation

Except for goals in the affective domain, learner goals for patient education are readily stated in terms of measurable behaviors (passing a written test, verbally stating some information, demonstrating a psychomotor skill) and can be evaluated by outcome criteria. It should be noted, however, that these behaviors are often surrogates for the behaviors actually desired, because the desired behaviors may be difficult to measure. For example, it is important that the patient on digoxin recognize the symptoms of digitalis toxicity and call the prescriber if these occur, but the ability to pass a written test is no guarantee the patient will actually do the right thing if the symptoms arise.

Measurement of Compliance   The term *compliance* is used in the literature of the health fields to denote adherence by the patient to the prescribed medication routine. A significant proportion of patients who receive a prescription do not take it properly, and lack of patient education is thought to be one cause of this *noncompliance*. Since it is impossible to evaluate whether a drug is effective unless it is known whether the patient took the drug as the prescriber intended, attempts have been made to develop valid and reliable ways to evaluate drug compliance.

Patient reports of how a drug was taken are sometimes unreliable, so pill counts (the patient brings the medication bottles to the clinic or office, and the number of pills used is counted) and pharmacy refill records may be used. More direct measurements include testing the amount of the drug or its breakdown products in the blood or urine and adding a tracer substance to the medication that causes the urine to fluoresce under certain lighting or that can be detected in the blood. The theoretical and ethical concerns about the concept of patient compliance are discussed in Chaps. 5 and 8.

Diagnostic Goal Evaluation

Diagnostic goals in pharmacotherapeutics are typically potential problems and often involve the recognition of adverse drug effects. Outcome criteria for a goal such as "Detect any dizziness, drowsiness, or confusion from diazepam" would be virtually unmeasurable, since if none of these potential problems were detected, it could be because they actually did not occur or because they were overlooked. Therefore, process criteria are used to evaluate diagnostic goals. Process criteria for most diagnostic goals in nursing pharmacotherapeutics can be evaluated by the following questions: Were the adverse effects *for which this patient is at greatest risk* identified? Were plans made to monitor laboratory tests and/or the patient's clinical condition for evidence of these adverse effects? Were these observational plans executed properly and the data obtained analyzed?

Sometimes the diagnostic goal involves establishing or refining a nursing diagnosis, such as "Identify sources of stress." Process criteria in evaluating these goals will emerge as a result of the testing and standardization of nursing diagnoses (Gordon, 1982). Until this is accomplished, nursing texts and journals are the best sources of process criteria for establishing a certain diagnosis.

QUALITY ASSURANCE

The rise of consumerism and increased accountability of the various professionals for their own practice, as well as government involvement as a financial supporter of health care, have given impetus to the concept of quality assurance programs in the health professions and in health care institutions. Just as individual patient care evaluation identifies whether the therapeutic plan is working so it can be modified as needed, quality assurance programs evaluate the care provided by a professional or an institution, so methods to improve the care of whole groups of patients can be identified.

Measurement Issues and Problems

A number of questions have arisen about the way in which quality of care should be measured in these programs. Experts disagree on whether the evaluation criteria should address only outcome variables or if structure and process variables are also valid indicators. The best source of the data for evaluation is also disputed; some feel that the medical record is a comprehensive and inexpensive source of data, and others contend that the actual care should be observed. Whether the criteria of evaluation should represent minimal, average, or ideal standards and whether the assessment of quality of care should focus on the average practitioner or those who render substandard or unorthodox care are other issues.

A fundamental question in quality assurance programs concerns the components of quality care. Recently, Lohr and Brook (1981) have defined quality of care as consisting of both "technical care" and "art of care" components. Technical care refers to the actual services rendered in curing an illness, and art of care to humanistic behaviors in delivering the care. These authors postulate that the two factors interact so that high levels of both greatly augment quality of care. The role of the nurse in drug therapy is highly compatible with this conceptualization, and there is evidence that psychosocial factors, particularly a warm and caring approach to the patient, contribute to positive drug outcomes (see Chap. 5).

Drug Utilization Review

The *drug utilization review* (DUR) program is a form of quality assurance specific to drug use in health care settings. DUR is aimed at combating overuse of medications, promoting rational drug therapy, reducing cost, and preventing adverse reactions. After the DUR committee studies the existing patterns of drug use in the setting, the DUR program may involve nurses along with other health professionals in the development of standards of appropriate drug use.

RESEARCH AND EVALUATION

Research and evaluation in nursing process are closely allied activities. The nurse who analyzes the effects of a nursing intervention on a single patient's response to a medication is doing evaluation, while the nurse who analyzes the effect of the same intervention on the response to the same drug by a group of similar patients is doing research. Further, the nurse who meticulously documents nursing activities and drug outcomes in the medical record not only improves individual patient care, but also furnishes a rich source of information to future research.

There are two significant problems associated with research that impact the nursing process in pharmacotherapeutics. First, there is a dismaying lack of research on topics relevant to the nursing role in drug therapy. Studies of measures to support the therapeutic drug effect, of approaches to preventing or minimizing adverse drug effects, of effective medication administration, of techniques to detect adverse effects, of patient education, and of the psychosocial aspects of drug therapy are few. Second, the dissemination to nurses of technologic and research information in pharmacology is slow. Continuing education programs on advances in the field are lacking. Until recently a new drug or new indication for an old drug literally went unreported for years in the nursing journals, and many were never reported. The expanding role of nursing in drug therapy will require greater emphasis on this topic in nursing research and the nursing literature.

REFERENCES

Corn, F., and K. Magill: "The Nursing Care Audit: A Tool for Peer Review," *Superv Nurse,* 5:20–28, 1974.

Gordon, M.: *Nursing Diagnosis: Process and Application,* New York: McGraw-Hill, 1982.

Lohr, K. N., and R. H. Brook: "Quality Assurance and Clinical Pharmacy: Lessons from Medicine," *Drug Intell Clin Pharm,* 15:757–765, 1981.

Marriner, A.: *The Nursing Process: A Scientific Approach to Nursing Care,* St. Louis, Mosby, 1979.

Mitchell, P. H., and A. Loustau (eds.), *Concepts Basic to Nursing,* 3d ed., New York: McGraw-Hill, 1981.

Nehring, V., and B. Geach: "Patient's Evaluation of Their Care: Why They Don't Complain," *Nurs Outlook,* 21:317–321, 1973.

Pardee, G., D. O. Hoshaw, C. S. Huber, et al., "Patient Care Evaluation Is Every Nurse's Job," *Am J Nurs,* 71:1958–1960, 1971.

Ramey, I. G.: "Setting Nursing Standards and Evaluating Care," *J Nurs Adm,* 3:27–35, May–June, 1973.

GENERAL PRINCIPLES OF CLINICAL PHARMACOLOGY & THERAPEUTICS

5

BIOPHYSICAL AND PSYCHOSOCIAL PRINCIPLES OF DRUG ACTION

GINETTE A. PEPPER
MATTHEW B. WIENER

The observed clinical effects of a drug are dependent not only on its unique mechanism of action, but also on a number of factors affecting all drugs. These genetic, physiologic, pathologic, biorhythmic, social, and psychologic variables influence dosage requirements and whether the desired beneficial effect or unwanted adverse effects occur. Proper nursing assessment, management, and evaluation build on these biophysical and psychosocial principles.

BIOPHYSICAL FACTORS

LEARNING OBJECTIVES

Upon mastery of the contents of this section, the reader will be able to:

1. Differentiate three phases of drug action.
2. List four pharmacokinetic processes.
3. Explain how alterations in dosage formulation affect disintegration and dissolution.
4. Define bioequivalence and its implications for drug therapy.
5. Define bioavailability, volume of distribution, clearance, and half-life in terms of the relevant pharmacokinetic processes.
6. Explain the clinical significance of the difference between first-order kinetics and zero-order kinetics of drugs.
7. Describe the membrane characteristics and physiochemical drug characteristics which govern the transport of drugs across biologic membranes.
8. Define the four mechanisms by which drugs cross biologic membranes.
9. Describe the variables that may alter drug absorption and the principles that determine these alterations.
10. Explain the clinical significance of first-pass metabolism.
11. Describe the variables that may alter drug distribution and the principles that determine these alterations.
12. Define metabolism and name the most important site of metabolism.
13. Differentiate phase I nonsynthetic and phase II conjugation reactions.
14. Explain the characteristics of the microsomal enzyme system.
15. Describe the variables that may alter drug metabolism and the principles that determine these alterations.
16. Explain the implications for clinical practice of pharmacogenetics and chronopharmacology.
17. Describe the variables that may alter renal excretion and the principles that determine these alterations.
18. Describe enterohepatic recirculation.
19. Characterize receptors and drug-receptor interactions.
20. Define agonist, competitive antagonist, noncompetitive antagonist, physiologic antagonist, chemical antagonist, and partial agonist.
21. Differentiate potency, efficacy, and selectivity.
22. Explain what a dose-response curve is.
23. Define steady state, maintenance dose, and loading dose.
24. Explain the use of plasma drug concentrations in evaluating drug therapy.
25. State the implications of pharmacokinetics for nursing assessment and evaluation of drug therapy.

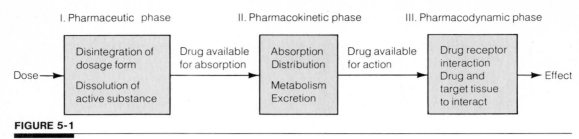

FIGURE 5-1

Pharmacologic Model of Drug Action.

The fate of a drug can be conceptualized as a sequence of three phases—pharmaceutics, pharmacokinetics, and pharmacodynamics—although in reality the phases are interrelated and proceed concurrently (see Fig. 5-1). Because therapeutic interactions between the drug and the biologic system require the drug to be in solution, the *pharmaceutic* phase involves the disintegration and dissolution of solid dosage forms. The *pharmacokinetic* phase includes the processes which result in the delivery of a drug to its site of action (absorption and distribution) and those which terminate drug effect (metabolism and excretion). The sites and mechanisms by which drugs produce their biologic effects compose the *pharmacodynamic* phase.

PHARMACEUTIC PHASE

The first step which determines onset of the action of the drug is its release from the dosage form, which is referred to as *liberation, or disintegration*. All drugs must be in solution to cross biologic membranes, so dissolution often becomes the rate-limiting step for drug action (see Fig. 5-2). Drugs already in solution (injectable and oral solutions) do not require dissolution, but drug particles liberated into body fluids in the gastrointestinal tract, body cavities, or tissues from oral suspensions, capsules, tablets, suppositories, implants, and intramuscular suspensions must go into solution before absorption.

In addition to the active drug, most dosage forms contain pharmaceutic additives included to improve formulation (stability, size, shape, ease of manufacture, patient acceptance, absorbability, etc.). These additives can alter the disintegration and dissolution, especially with solid oral dosage forms. Manufacturers also modify drugs to improve solubility. Acids and bases are often formulated as salts (e.g., **warfarin sodium**, **sodium penicillin**, **quinidine sulfate**, **propoxyphene hydrochloride**), which are usually more soluble than the parent compounds. Because the exposed surface area of the drug is greater with smaller particles, some drugs with poor solubility (e.g., **sulfadiazine**) are manufactured as microcrystalline particles.

On the other hand, solubility characteristics can be manipulated to delay disintegration and dissolution and thereby prolong duration of action or alter the location of disintegration. Large crystals (macrocrystals) delay dissolution and prolong the absorption of drugs like **nitrofurantoin** (Macrodantin). *Enteric coated tablets* have a special covering to prevent their disintegration in the stomach, usually to decrease gastric irritation from the drug. *Sustained-release* drugs are in dosage forms modified to liberate the drugs over an extended period of time. With *depot preparations* (also called repository preparations), the physical state of the drug is altered so that it goes into solution slowly when injected intramuscularly, and the drug is effective for several weeks. Examples of drugs given as depot preparations include **benzathine penicillin G** (Bicillin), the antipsychotic **fluphenazine decanoate** (Prolixin Decanoate), and the female hormone **medroxyprogesterone acetate** (Depo-Provera).

A recent trend in the pharmaceutical industry is the development of new dosage delivery systems for old drugs, such as **pilocarpine**, **progesterone**, **nitroglycerin**, **scopolamine**, **aspirin**, and **theophylline**. Many of these recently

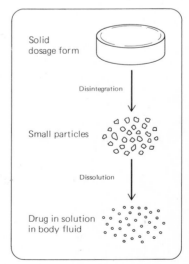

FIGURE 5-2

The pharmaceutic phase involves drug disintegration and dissolution of solid dosage forms. Once a drug is in solution in the gastrointestinal tract or other body fluid, it is available for absorption and distribution.

marketed systems involve the manipulation of drug liberation and dissolution to attain prolonged or localized effects. **Pilocarpine**, a drug used to treat glaucoma, has been incorporated into a silicone rubber insert (Ocusert Pilo-20 and Pilo-40), which is placed behind the eyelid and provides a consistent rate of drug release for a week. A similar device, the Progestasert, is placed in the uterus and delivers doses of hormone adequate to achieve contraception for up to a year. Another new system uses what look like regular tablets, but they consist of solid cores of drug surrounded by a semipermeable membrane, which delivers a drug at a predetermined rate, based on the principle of osmosis. Such long-acting systems are available for **theophylline** (Theo-24) and **aspirin** (Zorprin). One new slow-release transdermal system liberates **scopolamine** for 72 h to control motion sickness (Transderm-Scop), and another, which releases **nitroglycerin** for 24 h (Transderm-Nitro), is used to treat angina.

Factors which affect drug dissolution rates include pH and agitation, so disease states, drugs, and conditions which affect gastric acidity and intestinal motility (e.g., old age, pregnancy, antacids) may affect solubility of oral drugs. The amount of fluid ingested with an oral medication will also affect drug dissolution.

Bioequivalence The methods and materials used in the manufacture of a drug can markedly affect absorption and therapeutic effect. Identical amounts of the same active drug in different preparations may not yield equal therapeutic response (i.e., are not *bioequivalent*). In 1977 the Food and Drug Administration began to require data on bioequivalence. Manufacturers of solid oral dosage forms of a new drug product must demonstrate its rate and extent of absorption compared with a standard preparation, usually an oral solution or an intravenous dosage form. Once a product is marketed, it becomes the standard. If additional manufacturers want to market the same product, they must demonstrate bioequivalence to the standard.

PHARMACOKINETIC PHASE

Pharmacokinetics is defined as the time course over which a drug is absorbed, distributed, metabolized, and excreted. Clinical pharmacokinetics is the application of pharmacokinetics to the safe and effective management of individual patients. Pharmacokinetic principles are an important tool in guiding prescribers in rational drug selection, dosage selection, and dosage adjustment. These principles can also direct prescribers, nurses, and other clinicians in monitoring patient response for adverse and therapeutic effects.

Pharmacokinetic Models
Pharmacokinetics involves the *quantification* of the processes of drug disposition in the body. When scientists attempt to quantify processes in complex systems such as the human body, it is necessary to make assumptions that simplify the real system, or else it would be impossible to obtain rigorous measurement. Based on these assumptions, a *model* is constructed that is a simplified representation of the complex real system. To the extent that the model reflects the behavior of the real system, it facilitates understanding and quantitative representation.

In pharmacokinetics it has been useful to represent the body as a series of connected compartments. These compartments do not refer to any anatomic reality but represent regions of the body which behave similarly with respect to drug disposition. There are currently two models commonly used in pharmacokinetics (see Fig. 5-3). The *one-compartment model* depicts the body as a single, homogenous unit and assumes that drugs distribute rapidly and uniformly throughout the body. The pharmacokinetic behavior of many drugs will more closely approximate a *two-compartment model* that consists of a central compartment (which includes plasma) and the peripheral tissue area. As technology advances and with the aid of computers, perhaps the body can be represented by a multiple-compartment model, which may generate pharmacokinetic information that better explains disposition of various drugs and the effects of disease states and other patient factors.

Basic Pharmacokinetic Parameters
Pharmacokinetics involves the evaluation of factors which influence the magnitude of drug effects as a function of time. These factors consist of the input of the drug into the biologic system, the drug's distribution characteristics within the system, and output from the system through drug elimination (see Fig. 5-4). The *quantification* of these factors employs the basic parameters of pharmacokinetics.

Bioavailability
Bioavailability is rate and extent of absorption, which determine the fraction of unchanged drug that reaches the systemic circulation following administration by any route. Drugs given intravenously have 100 percent bioavailability. The reasons bioavailability may be less by other routes include insolubility of the dosage formulation; presystemic metabolism in the gut, gut wall, or portal circulation through the liver; and incomplete absorption. Bioavailability affects the time of onset of drug effect, the time and magnitude of peak effect, and the duration of effect (see Fig. 5-5).

Volume of Distribution
The portion of a drug dose that enters the systemic circulation is distributed to various body compartments, depending upon the characteristics of the drug. Some drugs remain in the blood, bound to plasma constituents, and some distribute to total body water, while lipid-soluble drugs accumulate in body fat. Plasma, total body water, and body fat are real physiologic volumes to which drugs can distribute, but some

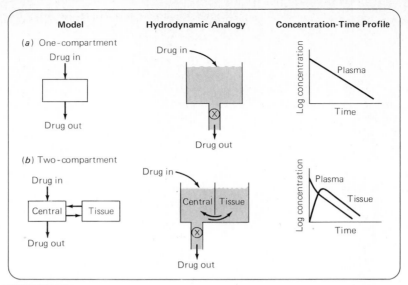

FIGURE 5-3

The one-compartment and two-compartment pharmacokinetic models of drug disposition following intravenous administration of a drug. Also illustrated are the hydrodynamic analogies and concentration-time drug profiles. If the model is appropriate for a given drug and patient, the patient's plasma levels after an intravenous dose will follow a pattern similar to the one shown. (*Source:* From M. Mayersohn: ''Fundamental Principles of Pharmacokinetics,'' in K. A. Conrad and R. Bressler (eds.), *Drug Therapy for the Elderly,* St. Louis, Mosby, 1982. Used by permission.)

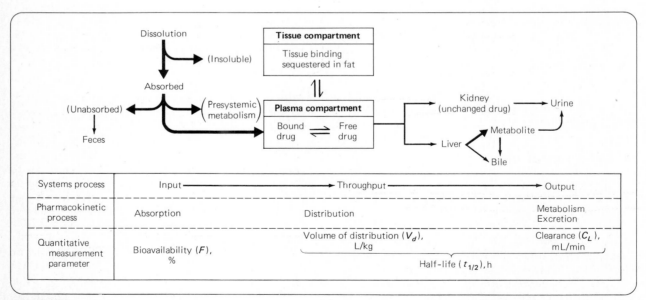

FIGURE 5-4

Summary of the fate of a drug in the biologic system, showing the parameters used to quantify each of the pharmacokinetic processes. Input of the drug into the system through absorption must be preceded by dissolution. Bioavailability is the measure of net input (dose minus amount of drug that is unsolubilized, unabsorbed, or metabolized prior to entering the systemic circulation). Throughput is quantified by volume of distribution, which represents the relative concentration of drug in various body compartments. The two modes of drug output, metabolism and excretion, are measured as clearance. Volume of distribution and clearance together determine how long a drug remains within the body system, expressed as *(elimination) half life.*

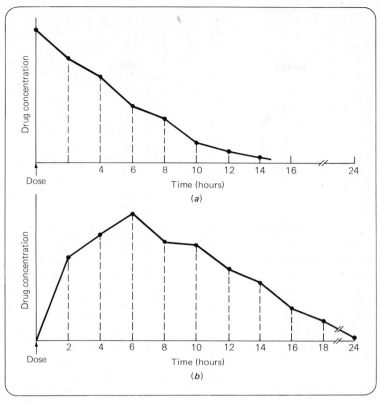

FIGURE 5-5

Bioavailability (F), or fraction of the drug absorbed, is calculated by measuring the plasma levels following (a) an intravenous (IV) dose and (b) an oral dose. These are plotted on graphs, and the areas under the curves (AUCs) are calculated and then compared. The calculation can be done by cutting the AUCs from the graph paper and then weighing the paper on an analytical balance, by counting the squares on the graph paper, or by using an appropriate computer program. Bioavailability is computed by the formula:

$$F = \frac{\text{AUC for oral dose}}{\text{AUC for IV dose}}$$

drugs also bind extensively to cell surfaces and intracellular macromolecules. The volume to which a drug seems to distribute is called the *apparent volume of distribution* (V_d).[1]

For a drug which distributes only to plasma water, the V_d for a 70-kg man is 3 L (the volume of plasma), or about 0.04 L/kg, and in the same individual a drug distributed to total body water would have a V_d of 40 L, or approximately 0.6 L/kg. For drugs distributed to fat, the apparent volume of distribution is greater than the entire fluid volume of the body (> 0.6 L/kg); drugs with extensive binding to tissue structures can have apparent volumes of distribution greater than total body volume (> 1.0 L/kg). Thus, apparent volume of distribution is an *abstraction* useful in quantifying the distribution characteristics of a drug. Volume of distribution affects duration of drug action, since drugs with large V_d are less frequently exposed to sites of elimination and require less-frequent dosing.

Clearance

The rate of elimination of a drug, by all routes, relative to the concentration in the plasma is called the clearance (C_L). Clearance is expressed in terms of milliliters of blood from which the drug is completely removed per minute. The liver

---

[1]One method of calculating V_d is by dividing the amount of drug administered intravenously by the drug concentration in the plasma 1 h after the drug is given:

$$V_d = \frac{\text{total amount of drug administered}}{\text{concentration of drug in plasma}}$$

TABLE 5-1   Major Route of Elimination for Selected Drugs

Renal Clearance		Hepatic Clearance		
		LOW (<100 mL/min/70 kg)	MEDIUM (100–500 mL/min/70 kg)	HIGH (>500 mL/min/70 kg)
Amikacin	Furosemide	Amobarbital	Acetaminophen	Amitriptyline
Amoxicillin	Gentamicin	Chlordiazepoxide	Aspirin	Chlorpromazine
Ampicillin	Hydrochlorothiazide	Diazepam	Erythromycin	Imipramine
Bumetanide	Lithium	Digitoxin	Prazosin	Lidocaine
Carbenicillin	Methotrexate	Indomethacin	Quinidine	Meperidine
Cefoperazone	Nadolol	Phenobarbital		Metaproterenol
Cephalexin	Netromycin	Phenytoin		Morphine
Cephalothin	Penicillin	Theophylline		Propoxyphene
Chlorothiazide	Procainamide	Tolbutamide		Propranolol
Cimetidine	Tetracycline	Warfarin		
Clonidine	Tobramycin			
Disopyramide	Vancomycin			

and the kidneys are the major sites of drug elimination. *Renal clearance* is clearance of the active drug (or metabolites) by the kidney. *Hepatic clearance* occurs by biotransformation of the drug to one or more metabolites and/or by excretion into the bile. The upper limit of hepatic clearance is determined by liver blood flow (1.5 L/min), and drugs can be divided into low-, medium-, and high-hepatic-clearance drugs (see Table 5-1). Clearance affects the time the drug remains in the body and, hence, the dosage required.

Elimination Half-Life

The elimination half-life, or plasma half-life, ($t_{1/2}$) is the time required for the concentration of drug in the blood to decrease by 50 percent (see Fig. 5-6). The time course of a drug in the body is directly proportional to its volume of distribution and indirectly proportional to its clearance.[2] Thus, half-life increases when the volume of distribution increases or the clearance decreases and vice versa.

Although it is the concentration of drug at the target organ that determines a drug's effect, plasma concentrations are used to compute half-life and other pharmacokinetic measurements, since samples of plasma are readily obtained. Once distribution is complete, plasma concentration is in

equilibrium with drug concentrations in tissue compartments and, thus, generally reflects the relative concentration at the target organ. However, plasma drug sampling is an invasive procedure and is not without risk to the patient. Other body fluids that have been sampled are saliva and urine, although the results have not always been satisfactory.

Most drugs are eliminated at a *constant proportion* per unit of time and demonstrate decline in plasma levels after an intravenous dose, as illustrated in Fig. 5-6. These drugs are said to have nonsaturable kinetics or *first-order kinetics*.

---

[2]Half-life is computed by the formula:

$$t_{1/2} = \frac{0.693 V_d}{C_L}$$

where V_d is the volume of distribution and C_L is the total clearance. A related parameter, the elimination rate constant K_{el}, a major determinant of dosage interval or time to reach steady state, is computed by the formula:

$$K_{el} = \frac{C_L}{V_d} \quad \text{or} \quad K_{el} = \frac{0.693}{t_{1/2}}$$

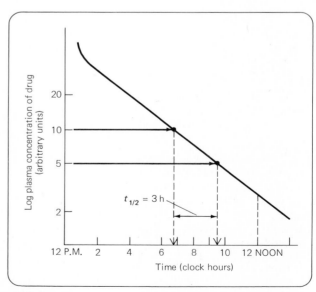

FIGURE 5-6

The disappearance curve for drugs with first-order kinetics is linear if plasma concentration is plotted on a logarithmic scale. In this case, the plasma concentration drops by 50 percent (10 units to 5 units) between about 6:45 P.M. and 9:45 P.M. Thus, the half-life ($t_{1/2}$) of the drug is about 3 h.

However, a few drugs (**phenytoin, ethanol, dicumarol, aspirin**) demonstrate dose-dependent kinetics, or *zero-order kinetics,* in which the plasma levels following large doses decline at a *constant amount* per unit of time. This is because there is a limited amount of the enzymes necessary to metabolize the drug and these become saturated at higher dosages. A small increase in dosage of these drugs can cause large increases in plasma levels and result in toxicity.

Table 5-2 reflects the pharmacokinetic parameters of some commonly prescribed medications.

Biotransport of Drugs

Common to all pharmacokinetic processes is the movement of drugs across biologic membranes. Drugs must cross membranes to be absorbed into the circulation, to gain access to receptor sites, and to reach the sites of metabolism and excretion. Several qualities of membranes and the physiochemical characteristics of drugs influence whether and how they will cross biologic membranes.

Membrane Properties

Cell membranes are thought to have a mosaic structure composed of lipids and proteins. The lipid bilayer has fluidlike properties and is the major constituent. Globular proteins are embedded in the lipid matrix and have ionic and polar groups protruding from one or both sides of the membrane. These proteins may be capable of shifting rapidly to form openings or pores. Lipid-soluble "carrier" proteins have also

TABLE 5-2 Pharmacokinetic Parameters for Some Common Drugs[a]

DRUG	TRADE NAME	HALF-LIFE, h	BIOAVAIL-ABILITY, %	C_L, mL/min/kg	V_d, L/kg	BOUND IN PLASMA, %	EFFECTIVE CONC	TOXIC CONC
Acetaminophen	Tylenol	2.0	65	5.0	0.95	0	10–20 μg/mL	>300 μg/mL
Amikacin	Amikin	2.0	[b]	1.1	0.21	4		
Ampicillin	(Many)	1.2	25–70[c]	3.9	0.28	18		
Amitriptyline	Elavil	15–24	[d]	6.1	8.3	96	160–240 ng/mL	>1 ng/mL
Aspirin	(Many)	0.25	68	9.3	0.15	49	0–100 μg/mL[e] 150–300 μg/mL[f]	
Carbamazepine	Tegretol	15–27	>70	0.58	1.4	82	5–10 μg/mL	>9 μg/mL
Cephalothin	Keflin	0.57	[b]	6.7	0.26	71		
Cimetidine	Tagamet	2.0	70	12.0	2.1	19		
Diazepam	Valium	20–90[g]	100	0.38	1.1	98	>600 ng/mL[h]	
Digoxin	Lanoxin	42	75	1.8	6.5	25	>0.8 ng/mL	>1.8 ng/mL
Doxepin	Adapin, Sinequan	17	27	14	20		30–150 ng/mL	
Ethosuximide	Zarontin	33		0.26	0.72	0	40–100 μg/mL	
Furosemide	Lasix	0.85	63	2.2	0.11	96		
Gentamicin	Garamycin	2–3	[b]	0.73	0.25	<10		
Imipramine	Tofranil	13	47	20	15.0	89–94	>225 ng/mL	>1 μg/mL
Lidocaine	Xylocaine	1.8	[b]	9.2	1.1	51	2–5 μg/mL	6–10 μg/mL
Lithium	Eskalith (others)	22	100	0.35	0.79	0	0.7 meq/L	2.0 meq/L
Meperidine	Demerol	3.7	52	17.0	4.2	58		
Nadolol	Corgard	16.0	34	2.9	2.1	20		
Nortriptyline	Aventyl, Pamelor	31	51	7.2	18	95	50–139 ng/mL	
Phenobarbital	Numerous	86		0.093	0.88	51	10–25 μg/mL	>30 μg/mL
Phenytoin	Dilantin	[i]	98		64	89	>10 μg/mL	>20 μg/mL
Primidone	Mysoline	8	92	0.78	0.59	0.9	5–10 μg/mL	>10 μg/mL
Procainamide	Pronestyl	2.9	75–95	8.6–9.8	1.9	16	3.5 μg/mL	9–14 μg/mL
Propranolol	Inderal	3.9	36	12.0	3.9	93.3	20 ng/mL	
Protriptyline	Vivactil	78	77–93	3.6	22	92	70–250 ng/mL	
Quindine sulfate	(Many)	6.0	80	4.7	2.7	71	2–5 μg/mL	>14 μg/mL
Tolbutamide	Orinase	5.9	93	0.30	0.15	93	80–240 μg/mL	
Theophylline	(Many)	2–10[g]	97	0.69	0.5	56	>10 μg/mL	>20 μg/mL
Warfarin	Coumadin	37	100	0.045	0.11	99	2.2 μg/mL	

[a]See pertinent chapters for more information. [b]Not given orally. [c]Varies widely among studies. [d]Varies widely due to first-pass metabolism. [e]Analgesic-antipyretic effect. [f]Anti-inflammatory effect. [g]Age-dependent. [h]Seizure control. [i]Zero-order kinetics; $t_{1/2}$ depends on dose.

been proposed as components of membranes. The majority of substances crossing membranes must diffuse through the lipid layer, although a few may traverse through pores or be transported by carrier systems.

Physiochemical Properties of Drugs

The molecular size, lipid solubility, and ionization of a drug affect its ability to cross biologic membranes.

Solubility   The more *lipid-soluble* a drug is, the faster it will cross biologic membranes. The tendency of a drug to distribute itself between water and lipid when both phases are present can be expressed as a ratio between the concentration in the lipid phase and the concentration in the water phase once equilibrium is attained. This ratio is known as the *oil/water partition coefficient*. Drugs with high oil/water partition coefficients are considered lipid-soluble, fat-soluble, or *lipophilic* (Greek for "lipid-loving"). Those with low oil/water partition coefficients often contain polar groups in their chemical structures, and are considered water-soluble, or hydrophilic ("water-loving"). Water-soluble drugs generally cross biologic membranes slowly or not at all.

Size   Large molecules cross biologic membranes poorly, even if they are lipid-soluble. Therefore, most drugs used clinically are in the molecular weight range of 100 to 1000.

Ionization   Most drugs are weak acids or weak bases and can exist in either the ionized or the nonionized form. *Nonionized drugs are more lipid-soluble and readily cross biologic membranes*, so the rate of drug transport across a membrane will be dependent on the proportion of the drug in its nonionized state. (See Fig. 5-7.)

The proportion of a drug in the nonionized state is, in turn, related to two factors: its ionization constant and the pH of the aqueous medium in which it is dissolved. The *ionization constant* (pK_a), or dissociation constant, is defined as the pH at which a chemical is 50 percent ionized and 50 percent nonionized. Each acid and base has a characteristic ionization constant. For example, **aspirin**, an acid, has a pK_a of 3.5. This means that if the pH of the aqueous medium in which aspirin is dissolved is more than 3.5, the drug will be *primarily* ionized and relatively lipid-insoluble. At pH levels less than 3.5, aspirin will be predominantly nonionized and lipid-soluble and will cross membranes readily. As a basic drug with a pK_a of 7.9, **morphine** is *predominantly* ionized at pH levels below 7.9 but nonionized at levels above 7.9. *In general, it can be said that weak acids tend to be nonionized and to cross biologic membranes readily at lower pH. Weak bases tend to be nonionized and to cross biologic membranes at higher pH.*

This characteristic causes the phenomenon of *ion trapping*, which results when the pH is different on the two sides of the membrane. For example, the pH of the stomach is around 2, while plasma pH is 7.4. **Aspirin** is nonionized in the stomach and crosses the membrane into the plasma, where it becomes ionized and lipid-insoluble. Thus, it is "trapped" in the plasma. This phenomenon is used therapeutically in the treatment of drug overdose and poisoning. Alkalization of the urine promotes ionization of the acid **phenobarbital** ($pK_a = 7.4$) and facilitates its excretion by trapping it in the urine.

It is important to remember that the ionized and nonion-

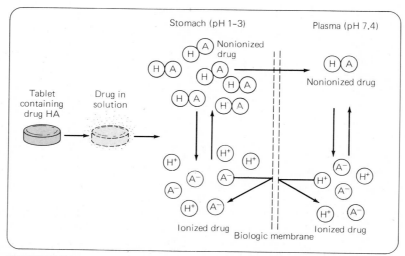

FIGURE 5-7

Weak acids tend to remain nonionized in the stomach and are able to permeate biologic membranes to enter the bloodstream. Weak bases tend to ionize in the stomach and are unable to permeate the membranes in this form.

ized forms of a drug are in equilibrium. Thus, if a drug is 98 percent ionized at a given pH, the 2 percent nonionized drug can still be absorbed, permitting another 2 percent of the remaining drug to become nonionized. Eventually, most of the drug can be absorbed.

Transport Mechanisms

Pharmacologic agents cross membranes by one of four mechanisms (see Fig. 5-8): passive diffusion, filtration, pinocytosis, and carrier-mediated transport.

Passive Diffusion   By far the most important mechanism of drug transport across membranes is passive diffusion, which proceeds with the concentration gradient and is moderated by physiochemical characteristics of the drug. Thus, smaller, lipid-soluble, nonionized drugs diffuse readily; larger, water-soluble, or ionized drugs do not.

Filtration   Filtration through pores of cell membranes occurs only with small molecules and electrolytes with molecular weights less than 100. This mechanism may be important in the passage of the cationic form of **lithium** (Li$^+$) when it is administered therapeutically for manic

depression, but is an uncommon transport mechanism for drugs into cells. On the other hand, the large pores in capillary membranes pose a barrier only to very large molecules.

Pinocytosis   Pinocytosis involves the engulfment of a large molecule and its transport across the membrane in a vesicle. Although it is of little importance for current therapeutic agents, it is projected that stimulation of this mechanism will be useful in the future treatment of inborn errors of metabolism. The deficient enzymes, which are large protein molecules, could be administered and gain access to the cell interior by pinocytosis.

Carrier-Mediated Transport   For some physiologic substances, such as glucose, organic acids, amino acids, and certain vitamins, there are carriers within cell walls which facilitate membrane transport. Drugs which chemically resemble these physiologic substances can be transported by the carriers. When the transport is against the concentration gradient and requires energy expenditure, the mechanism is called *active transport.* Carrier-mediated transport with the concentration gradient and not requiring energy is called *facilitated diffusion.* Examples of drugs which undergo carrier-mediated transport into the urine in the kidney tubule are the diuretic **furosemide** (Lasix) and the **penicillin** and **cephalosporin** antibiotics.

Absorption

In order to cause a pharmacologic effect, a drug must generally be absorbed, that is, transferred from the site of administration into the bloodstream. Exceptions are those drugs injected intravascularly, those injected into a body space for local effect, drugs applied topically for effect on skin and mucous membrane, and agents administered for their actions within the intestinal lumen. Route of administration, age, pregnancy, and disease affect the rate and extent of drug absorption because of physiologic variation in principles that affect membrane transport in general (solubility and ionization) and because of differences in the following specific principles:

1. Amount of absorptive surface area
2. Concentration gradient
3. Contact time with the absorptive surface
4. Extent of presystemic metabolism

The greater the surface area available for absorption, the more rapidly absorption occurs. The concentration gradient is the driving force of passive diffusion, so the larger the difference in concentration of drug on the two sides of the membrane, the faster the drug will move from the area of high concentration to that of low concentration. Extent of blood flow to the absorptive site is important in maintaining the concentration gradient, since the blood flow will carry

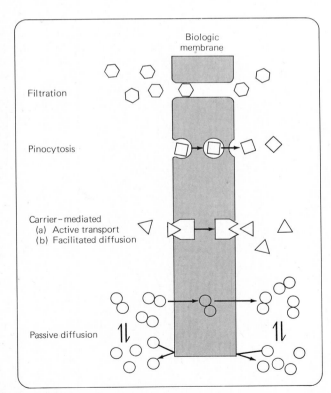

FIGURE 5-8

Drugs cross biologic membranes primarily by passive diffusion but may also cross by filtration, pinocytosis, and carrier-mediated mechanisms.

the newly absorbed drug away and sustain a gradient across the membrane until absorption is complete. With drugs injected into tissue, the amount of circulation also contributes to absorptive surface area; drugs are more rapidly absorbed from highly vascular muscle tissue than from less-vascular subcutaneous fat. Extended contact of a drug with the absorptive surface increases bioavailability.

Presystemic Metabolism Drugs can be metabolized before reaching the systemic circulation. This is particularly prominent when drugs are administered orally. Figure 5-9 summarizes the potential sites of presystemic metabolism of an orally administered drug. These include gastrointestinal acid and enzymes, bacterial action, and enzymes in the cells of the walls of the intestine. All of the venous blood from the areas of the gastrointestinal tract where drug absorption takes place, except the mouth and lower rectum, passes through the liver via the portal system prior to entering the systemic circulation. Drugs which are highly cleared by the liver (see Table 5-1) will undergo considerable metabolism before entering the general circulatory pool, a phenomenon

known as *first-pass metabolism.* In general, drugs that undergo first-pass metabolism will (1) require much larger oral doses than parenteral doses to achieve the same effect and (2) show considerable variation in the blood levels attained from a specified dosage, since there is large variation between individuals in liver metabolic capacity and even variation in the same individual at different times. Thus, dosage requirements for drugs which undergo first-pass metabolism will vary widely between individuals.

Effect of Route Administration

Absorption from the Gastrointestinal Tract Drugs absorbed through the mucous membranes of the mouth bypass first-pass metabolism. The *buccal* and *sublingual* routes are useful for drugs, such as **nitroglycerin** and **isoproterenol**, which are highly metabolized by the liver. Tablets must be formulated to dissolve quickly, and only drugs which are effective in very small amounts can be administered by these routes because, although circulation to the mouth

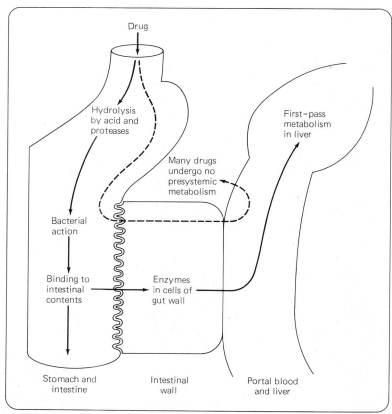

FIGURE 5-9

Sites of presystemic metabolism of an orally administered drug, including the first-pass phenomenon.

is good, the absorption surface is small and contact time is limited.

Lipid-soluble substances such as ethanol and acid drugs, which are relatively nonionized at the low gastric pH, are absorbed in the stomach due to its rich blood supply. However, the absorptive surface is small in comparison with the intestine, so even acid drugs are predominantly absorbed in the intestine. Slowed *gastric emptying time*—which is caused by hot meals, vigorous exercise, pain, emotion, high gastric acidity, and drugs such as **morphine, amphetamines,** and **anticholinergics** (see Table 12-5)—will slow the absorption of most drugs, because transit to the intestine is delayed. Gastric emptying time is speeded by lying on the right side, ingestion of dilute solutions, mild exercise, and hunger. Some drugs (e.g., **propranolol, metoprolol, trazodone, keto-conazole**) are better absorbed when taken with food, but most are best absorbed taken on an empty stomach with a full glass of water.

Because of its many villi and microvilli, which yield an extensive surface area, the small intestine is the most important absorptive site for orally administered drugs, even though presystemic metabolism limits the bioavailability of some drugs. Peristalsis in the stomach and intestine is important to the mixing of intestinal contents to encourage disintegration and dissolution of solid dosage forms and to increase contact of the soluble fraction of a drug with the absorptive surface.

Drugs given by the *rectal route* avoid first-pass metabolism if they are administered in the lower rectum. Although it has good blood supply, the rectum has limited surface area, and dissolution of drugs also occurs slowly. Unless drugs are administered in solution, rectal absorption is often erratic and unpredictable.

Absorption from the Lungs Drugs delivered as gases or aerosols to the lungs by the inhalational route are rapidly absorbed because of the large surface area, rich blood supply, and high permeability of the alveolar epithelium. Anesthetics, bronchodilators, and nicotine in tobacco smoke are examples of drugs administered by this route.

Absorption from the Skin The outer horny layer of the skin forms an effective barrier to most drug absorption because it is low in lipid and water content, resulting in a close-packed structure. Dermatologic preparations are generally administered for their local effects, and little absorption takes place. Placing an occlusive dressing over the site of drug application, as is done with nitroglycerin paste, improves absorption. The more lipid-soluble the drug is and the larger the surface area to which the drug is applied, the more rapidly it will be absorbed by the *topical route*.

Absorption of Injectables Drugs given by intravascular routes (*intravenous* and *intraarterial*) do not require absorption. Neither do drugs injected directly at the desired site of activity (e.g., *intraspinal, intradermal, intraarticular, intra-cardiac*), although unwanted effects can result if the drug is absorbed into the circulation from the local injection site. However, *intramuscular* and *subcutaneous* injections are given for their systemic effects and must be absorbed. The rate of absorption will be influenced by the pH and composition of the solution, quality of the connective tissue, and circulation to the area. Because of high perfusion and the ability to diffuse laterally in the tissues, intramuscular injections absorb more rapidly and can consist of larger volumes than subcutaneous injections. Addition of the enzyme hyaluronidase, which breaks down connective tissue, allows large volumes to be given subcutaneously, a procedure called *hypodermoclysis*.

Effect of Age and Pregnancy

Drug absorption in infants, children, elderly adults, and pregnant women is discussed in Chap. 7.

Effect of Disease

Disease states such as congestive heart failure and shock decrease blood perfusion to all absorptive sites and slow drug absorption. Gastric emptying rates are slower in patients with gastric ulcers, although some surgical procedures for this disease (e.g., partial gastrectomy) will significantly speed gastric emptying. Decreased first-pass metabolism occurs with some liver diseases and surgical procedures (e.g., portal shunts), resulting in increased bioavailability of certain drugs. Diarrhea decreases intestinal transit time and may retard drug absorption.

Distribution

Following absorption, drugs are distributed via the blood to inert plasma and tissue binding sites, to the site of action, and to the organs of elimination. Gender, age, body build, and diseases alter drug distribution, based on the general principles of membrane transport and the specific principles of drug distribution summarized as follows:

1. Volume of blood flow to organs
2. Plasma and tissue protein binding
3. Tissue solubility and mass
4. Special membrane barriers

The apparent volume of distribution is a reflection of protein binding, tissue solubility, and tissue mass.

Blood Flow Uptake of drug is faster in well-perfused tissues such as kidney, liver, heart, and brain than it is in poorly perfused tissues such as adipose and muscle. Therefore, drug concentrations equilibrate rapidly between the blood and the organs with high blood flow and then equilibrate more slowly with other tissues. Redistribution is responsible for the termination of the observed clinical effect of some drugs given by intravenous bolus. For example, when intravenous barbiturates are given alone for anesthesia, the patient awakens within a few minutes, even though the half-life of these drugs is many hours. It is the decay of the initially high brain levels as the drug is redistributed to adipose tissue, rather than drug elimination, that terminates the anesthetic effect. A similar phenomenon is seen with the intravenous antiarrhythmic **lidocaine**.

Protein Binding   Drugs bind to proteins throughout the body. The importance of this binding is that it ties up the drug and decreases the concentration of free (i.e., unbound) drug in the plasma. Since only free drug is available to cross membranes to sites of drug action, the bound drug is lost to pharmacologic action. The loss is only temporary, however, since the binding is reversible and bound drug is in equilibrium with the free fraction. When free drug is eliminated, some of the bound drug is released from the protein binding, which thus functions like a storage, or biologic "sustained-release," mechanism.

Drug binding to the plasma proteins *albumin* and α_1-*acid glycoprotein* is a very important aspect of drug distribution. Albumin tends to bind acidic drugs, such as **warfarin, penicillins, phenylbutazone, sulfonamides,** and **tolbutamide.** Two independent sites have been identified on human albumin, and different drugs tend to bind at each site. Basic drugs bind mainly to α_1-acid glycoprotein; these include **meperidine, chlorpromazine, dipyridamole, imipramine,** and **quinidine.** A few drugs, like **propranolol**, bind to both proteins.

Drugs bound to plasma proteins are not pharmacodynamically active but are resistant to elimination (except high-hepatic-clearance drugs and those eliminated by renal tubular secretion). One type of drug interaction occurs when two drugs given concurrently have small volumes of distribution and are highly bound to the *same* site on a plasma protein; these drugs will compete for the binding site, resulting in a greater proportion of free drug (see Chap. 6).

Tissue Solubility and Mass   In addition to tissue protein binding, the solubility of the drug in the tissue and how much tissue mass there is will determine the amount of drug which accumulates outside the vascular space. **Diazepam,** a fat-soluble drug, accumulates in adipose tissue and has a very large V_d. In an obese person the V_d of fat-soluble drugs is even larger, because of the greater potential reservoir for drug deposition.

Special Membrane Barriers   Certain organs have unique membrane structures that potentially alter drug distribution. The *placental barrier* and *blood-milk barrier* are discussed in Chap. 7. Recently, the existence of a *blood-testicular barrier* has been recognized. The unique morphology of the tunica propria greatly limits the passage of water-soluble drugs into the seminiferous tubules, where spermatogenesis takes place, although there is little barrier to the passage of lipid-soluble drugs.

Many of the drugs in current use could not be employed therapeutically if some barrier to the passage of chemicals into the central nervous system did not exist, since they would cause unacceptable adverse effects. The capillary boundary between the plasma and brain cells is less permeable to water-soluble drugs than is the case in other tissues. This has been termed the *blood-brain barrier*. The blood-brain barrier consists of firmly joined capillary endothelial cells and a glial sheath closely adherent to the capillary wall. Glia are the connective tissue of the brain, and the sheath effectively interposes a second membrane between the plasma and the brain interstitium. Drugs can enter the brain through the cerebrospinal fluids, and it is sometimes necessary to administer water-soluble drugs, such as the **penicillin** antibiotics, by the *intrathecal route* to treat central nervous system infections (see Chap. 33, "Neurologic Disorders").

Effect of Gender, Age, Pregnancy, and Body Build

Age and pregnancy alter drug distribution by changing body composition, blood flow, and levels of plasma proteins, as discussed in Chap. 7. Gender and body build also affect body composition. Women and obese people have a larger proportion of their body weight as fat than do men and lean people, resulting in increased volume of distribution and prolonged half-life for lipid-soluble drugs. Similarly, with water-soluble drugs women and obese people will demonstrate smaller volumes of distribution, shorter half-lives, and higher blood levels for weight-adjusted doses.

Effect of Disease

Diseases which decrease perfusion, such as congestive heart failure and hypovolemic shock, alter drug distribution. Starvation, hepatic disease, and renal disease alter the amount or binding characteristics of plasma albumin, resulting in increased free drug. On the other hand, the levels and drug binding of α_1-acid glycoproteins increase in an infection or inflammatory process. Starvation decreases fatty tissue and may release the accumulated drug into the blood, resulting in toxicity. Edematous conditions also alter the fat/water ratio of the body and affect the volumes of distribution of drugs. In meningitis and encephalitis the blood-brain barrier is less competent; this may be exploited therapeutically with the systemic administration of water-soluble antibiotics to treat the infection.

Metabolism

Metabolism, or *biotransformation*, is the process whereby the body converts a drug by chemical reaction into a compound different from that originally administered. While some water-soluble drugs can be excreted by the kidneys in an unchanged form, many fat-soluble drugs could stay in the body for years if they were not metabolized to more easily excreted forms. Metabolism does not necessarily yield a compound without pharmacologic activity, but generally results in one that is less fat-soluble and, as a result, more readily excreted.

Metabolic processes are often complex and can yield several different *metabolites* (the products of metabolic reactions). These metabolites may differ quantitatively or qualitatively in pharmacologic activity, compared with the administered drug. Some metabolites are inactive, but others are more active, equally active, or less active than the parent drug. In fact, *prodrugs* are inactive as administered and must be metabolized before they have any therapeutic effect.

Most drug metabolism occurs in the liver, although the lungs, kidneys, skin, intestine, and plasma, as well as other tissues, also demonstrate metabolic activity. Metabolic reactions are catalyzed by enzyme systems, which include protein enzymes and various cofactors such as vitamin coenzymes (pyridoxine, niacin derivatives, etc.) and ions such as Ca^{2+} and Mg^{2+}.

Types of Metabolic Reactions

Although there are many specific reactions by which drugs are chemically altered, it is possible to identify two main types: *phase I, or nonsynthetic, reactions* and *phase II, or conjugation, reactions* (see Fig. 5-10).

Phase I Nonsynthetic Reactions Phase I reactions convert the drug to a more polar metabolite by introducing or unmasking polar (charged) functional groups through oxidation, reduction, or hydrolysis. If the phase I metabolite is sufficiently polar, it can be excreted, but many phase I products are not eliminated before undergoing a subsequent phase II reaction. Phase I metabolites may be active or inactive but are usually more water-soluble than the parent drug.

Phase II Conjugation Reaction Parent drugs or phase I metabolites can be coupled with endogenous derivatives of carbohydrates and amino acids (e.g., glucuronic acid, sulfate, glycine, acetate) to yield polar molecules, which are usually inactive and readily excreted in the bile or urine. Some of these reactions are glucuronidation, sulfation, glycine conjugation, and acetylation. Some drug conjugates are thought to contribute to hepatotoxic reactions.

Microsomal Enzymes

Many drug-metabolizing enzymes are located in the membranes of the smooth endoplasmic reticulum in the cells of the liver and other tissues. When these membranes are extracted for research by certain laboratory procedures, they form vesicles called *microsomes*. An important class of enzymes located in these membranes is responsible for the metabolism of many exogenous chemicals, including drugs, insecticides, food additives, and environmental pollutants. Because these *microsomal enzymes* insert a single oxygen atom into the structure of the metabolite, they are called the *mixed-function oxidases (MFOs)*, or the *monooxygenases*. This class of enzymes is responsible for many phase I nonsynthetic reactions and one phase II conjugation reaction (glucuronidation).

The necessary constituents of the system include two enzymes, a flavoprotein called NADPH cytochrome *c* reductase, and a hemoprotein called cytochrome P450. Also required are a lipid, molecular oxygen, and reduced nicotinamide adenine dinucleotide phosphate (NADPH) as a source of electrons.

Characteristic of this enzyme class is its nonspecificity, since it metabolizes many different exogenous substances, but only fat-soluble drugs can be metabolized by this system. Certain drugs and chemicals can stimulate or inhibit the production and activity of cytochrome P450–dependent enzymes. There are several types of cytochrome P450, and different drugs and chemicals affect different types.

Principles of Drug Metabolism

Many variables are associated with altered drug metabolism, including age, pregnancy, diet and nutrition, genetic inheritance, biologic rhythms, chronicity of drug use, and diseases. Such alterations are determined by changes in either of two principles:

1. Intrinsic metabolizing capacity of liver enzymes
2. Magnitude of liver blood flow

For drugs which are not avidly metabolized by the liver (i.e., low-clearance drugs; see Table 5-1), the hepatic clear-

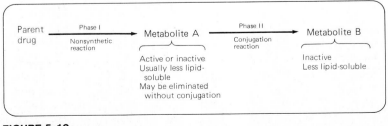

FIGURE 5-10

Types of Metabolic Reactions.

ance is determined by the *intrinsic activity of the liver enzymes* and the extent of plasma protein binding, since only free drug can be metabolized. Factors which alter enzyme activity will result in changes in the clearance of low-hepatic-clearance drug. On the other hand, only the extent of *liver blood flow* limits the clearance of high-hepatic-clearance drugs. So avidly do the hepatic enzymes clear these drugs that even the fraction bound to plasma proteins is released and metabolized. Only factors which alter liver blood flow will affect the clearance of high-hepatic-clearance drugs.

Pharmacogenetic Effects

The investigation of hereditary influences on drug response is called *pharmacogenetics*. Studies of identical and frateral twins have shown definite genetic influence on drug response. Some of these differences are due to altered activity of drug-metabolizing enzymes, and others are related to other pharmacokinetic and pharmacodynamic processes (see Table 5-3).

One of the most prevalent genetically determined alterations involves the phase II conjugation reaction *acetylation*. Based on an autosomal recessive inheritance, about half the United States population are slow acetylators, which

means that in this group of people drugs metabolized by this mechanism are slowly eliminated from the body. As a result, slow acetylators are more likely to develop toxicity from drugs like **isoniazid** (INH), **hydralazine** (Apresoline), and **procainamide** (Pronestyl) and often require lower doses. A syndrome resembling lupus erythematosus (joint pain, arthritis, pleuritic pain), which is a side effect of hydralazine and procainamide, is also more likely to develop in slow acetylators on these drugs. On the other hand, fast acetylators may not respond to lower dosages and with isoniazid can develop hepatotoxicity, probably caused by the conjugated metabolites.

Glucose-6-phosphate dehydrogenase (G6PD) is an enzyme which helps to protect red blood cells from hemolysis when exposed to oxidizing drugs, such as **aspirin, primaquine**, and **nitrofurantoin**. G6PD deficiency is more common in blacks and in certain Mediterranean and Asian groups (Sardinians, Sephardic Jews, Greeks, and Iranians), who often have more severe drug reactions. This deficiency and the sickle trait in general follow the same pattern of geographic distribution as falciparum malaria; erythrocytes with these genetic changes are less susceptible to infection by malaria. Because the pattern of inheritance is a sex-linked incomplete codominant, males are more frequently and severely affected, although heterozygous females can exhibit

TABLE 5-3 Some Genetically Determined Alterations in Drug Response

ABNORMALITY	INHERITANCE	PREVALENCE	DRUGS INVOLVED	RESPONSE
Abnormal pseudocholinesterase	Codominant	1 in 2820	Succinylcholine	Prolonged paralysis following surgery
Fast and slow acetylators	Autosomal recessive	50% slow acetylators; 50% fast acetylators	Isoniazid (INH) Hydralazine Procainamide Sulfamethazine (and some other sulfonamides) Dapsone (DDS)	Slow acetylators may show toxic adverse effects; fast acetylators may not get therapeutic effects or may get hepatic toxicity from metabolites
Glucose-6-phosphate dehydrogenase (G6PD) deficiency	Sex-linked incomplete codominant	10–15% in U.S. male blacks; also higher incidence in those of Mediterranean descent	Nitrofurantoin Aspirin Probenecid Primaquine Quinidine Sulfonamides Many other drugs (Also vitamin K, fava beans, infection, ketoacidosis, etc.)	Hemolytic anemia, which is self-limited
Malignant hyperthermia (altered calcium in cell membrane)	Autosomal dominant	1 in 20,000	Drugs used in anesthesia (halothane, succinylcholine)	Extreme muscle rigidity and hyperthermia during surgery

a milder form of the disease. After the initial hemolytic episode the disease is usually self-limiting, since young erythrocytes are less susceptible to hemolysis and the hemolysis will result in a higher proportion of young cells in the circulation.

Chronopharmacologic Effects

Many biologic processes, including response to drugs, exhibit a time structure or rhythmicity. The rate of drug absorption, hepatic clearance, half-life, duration of action, and magnitude of drug effect have all been shown to differ depending upon the time of day a drug is administered. Drugs which have demonstrated circadian variation in magnitude of therapeutic effects and toxicity include **halothane, barbiturates, lidocaine, histamine, antihistamines, corticosteroids, amphetamines, apomorphine, morphine, salicylates,** and **penicillin.** Additionally, drugs can alter normal biologic rhythms such as sleep patterns and cortisol secretion. *Chronopharmacology* is the study of the relationship of drug effects and biologic rhythm characteristics.

Much of the rhythmicity in drug response is probably related to hormone cycles, particularly of the adrenal hormones. In animals there is diurnal variation in hepatic drug metabolism, but this circadian rhythm is abolished by adrenalectomy. Hepatic drug-metabolizing enzyme activity seems highest when plasma cortisol levels are lowest (6 P.M. to 6 A.M.) and vice versa, but more research in humans is needed. There is also evidence to suggest that levels of estrogens and progestogens, which are hormones exhibiting rhythmicity, affect drug metabolism.

Once there is a sufficient research base, the clinical value of chronopharmacology will lie in the design of optimal dosage schedules. Attempts have been made to plan cancer chemotherapy so that dosages are given at the conjunction of the time of peak susceptibility of the tumor cells with the time the patient is most resistant to toxicity. Corticosteroids are given in the morning, to simulate normal circadian cycles and to minimize adrenal suppression. Travelers who want to avoid "jet lag" are advised to avoid caffeine and alcohol. Another example is **amitriptyline** (Elavil), an antidepressant with a very long half-life that can be administered as a single bedtime dose. One rationale for bedtime administration is that **amitriptyline** is more slowly absorbed at night than it is after a morning dose. While the average blood level (which is what determines the effectiveness of **amitriptyline**) is the same with either dosage schedule, the peak blood level (which determines its adverse effects) is much higher with a morning dose (Nakano and Hollister, 1983).

Effect of Age and Pregnancy

As discussed in detail in Chap. 7, age and pregnancy affect liver blood flow and the intrinsic activity of the hepatic drug-metabolizing enzymes.

Effect of Nutrition and Diet

Both lipid and protein, as well as vitamin cofactors and iron, are required for the production and function of microsomal enzymes, so malnutrition impairs enzyme activity. For example, prolonged protein malnutrition extends the effects of barbiturates. A balanced diet promotes drug metabolism.

Dietary constituents can also cause induction (increased activity) of hepatic microsomal enzymes. Known inducers include charcoal-broiled meat, ethanol, caffeine, and cruciferous vegetables (cabbage, broccoli, brussels sprouts).

Effect of Drugs and Pollutants

Drugs and pollutants, such as cigarette smoke, insecticides, and food additives, can increase or decrease the activity of the microsomal enzymes for metabolizing drugs administered concomitantly. These drug interactions of enzyme induction and enzyme inhibition are discussed in detail in Chap. 6, "Adverse Drug Reactions."

On chronic administration some drugs induce their own metabolism (see Table 5-4). This autoinduction is one cause of the *tolerance* (increasing dosage requirement to get the same pharmacologic effect) that occurs with sedative-hypnotic drugs.

Effect of Disease

Obviously, hepatic disease can alter both blood flow and intrinsic metabolizing activity, resulting in altered drug metabolism (see Chap. 32, "Hepatobiliary Disorders"). Thyroid disease, pulmonary disease, and surgery also affect drug metabolism. Hypothyroid states and acute hypoxemia are associated with decreased hepatic enzyme activity, and chronic hypoxemia and operative procedures appear to increase liver blood flow and the activity of hepatic microsomal drug-metabolizing enzymes.

Excretion

Excretion is the process whereby drugs and their metabolites are transferred from the interior to the exterior of the body.

TABLE 5-4   Drugs That Induce Their Own Metabolism

Carbamazepine (Tegretol)
Chlordiazepoxide (Librium)
Chlorpromazine (Thorazine)
DDT (insecticide)
Glutethimide (Doriden)
Meprobamate (Equanil)
Pentobarbital (Nembutal)
Phenobarbital (Luminal)
Phenylbutazone (Butazolidin)
Phenytoin (Dilantin)
Probenecid (Benemid)
Tolbutamide (Orinase)

The major organ of excretion is the kidney, although biliary excretion is important for a few drugs. The lungs are the primary excretion route for gaseous anesthetics, and the intestines, sweat, saliva, and milk constitute minor routes of drug excretion.

Renal Excretion

Renal clearance of drugs is determined by the general principles of transfer of drugs across membranes and the following principles:

1. Extent of glomerular filtration
2. Susceptibility to tubular secretion
3. Extent of reabsorption by passive diffusion
4. Extent of active tubular reabsorption

Age, pregnancy, and disease are variables which alter excretion.

The two processes involved in excretion by the kidneys are glomerular filtration and tubular secretion; reabsorption generally occurs by passive diffusion (see Fig. 5-11). *Glomer-ular filtration* is the major process by which drugs exit the plasma and enter the tubular urine. Most drugs are passively filtered into the tubules, but those bound to plasma proteins, are poorly filtered and remain in the plasma. Therefore, extent of plasma protein binding and renal blood flow determine glomerular filtration.

Some drugs are removed by active transport from the plasma and introduced into the tubular lumen by a process called *tubular secretion*. Strong organic acids (**penicillins, diuretics,** and **salicylates**) are strong organic bases (**mecamylamine, tolazoline, histamine,** and **morphine**) are removed from the plasma by special carriers located in the proximal convoluted tubule of the nephron. Even plasma protein–bound drugs can be eliminated by tubular secretion. Drugs and endogenous chemicals compete for the limited number of tubular secretion sites, resulting in reduced clearances of one or both substances. The competition between endogenous uric acid and **thiazide diuretics** can precipitate gouty arthritis. On the other hand, this competition for the carrier is used therapeutically to prolong the half-life of certain antibiotics when **probenecid** is given with the **penicillins** or **cephalosporins**.

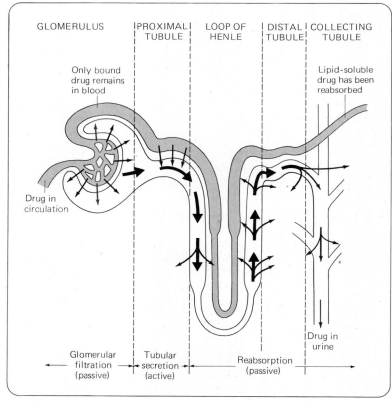

FIGURE 5-11

Schematic representation of renal excretion of drugs, including sites of glomerular filtration, tubular secretion, and passive reabsorption.

As the filtrate passes into the loop of Henle, distal tubule, and collecting duct, large amounts of water are reabsorbed, establishing a concentration gradient, which drives the *passive reabsorption* of fat-soluble, nonionized drugs and metabolites across the lipoprotein tubular membrane and back into the blood. Ionized or water-soluble drugs and metabolites remain in the tubule and are excreted in the urine. Urine pH usually varies from 4.5 to 8.0 in the maintenance of physiologic blood pH, and drugs such as **antacids** in high doses, **sodium bicarbonate, ascorbic acid, acetazolamide** (Diamox), **ammonium chloride,** and **tromethamine** (Tham) alter urine pH. Therefore, drugs and metabolites which are weak acids (pK_a of 3.0 to 7.5) or weak bases (pK_a of 7.5 to 10) can be ionized or nonionized in the tubule, depending on urinary pH. Alternating urinary pH by giving an acidifying or alkalizing drug is done therapeutically to promote the excretion of some cancer chemotherapeutic agents and in cases of poisoning or overdose. For example, **amphetamine,** a base with a pK_a of 9.8, is nonionized and largely reabsorbed when the tubular urine is alkaline, but is ionized and excreted rapidly in acid urine.

Active tubular reabsorption of some ions, glucose, organic acids, and other endogenous substances does occur, but this mechanism is of minor significance for drug elimination. However, some drugs used for gout cause their therapeutic effects by blocking active tubular reabsorption of urates [e.g., **sulfinpyrazone** (Anturane), **probenecid,** high-dose **aspirin** ($>$ 5 g/day)].

Biliary Excretion

Most drugs which are excreted in the bile are secreted by an active carrier-mediated process. **Probenecid, digoxin, glutethimide** (Doriden), **diethylstilbestrol,** and some other conjugated metabolites are eliminated in part by biliary excretion. A few drug conjugates undergo *enterohepatic recirculation* when the conjugate is hydrolyzed by intestinal bacteria, allowing much of the drug to be reabsorbed. Such drugs usually have prolonged effects, since the cycle (secretion into bile → hydrolysis by intestinal bacteria → reabsorption → secretion into bile, etc.) continues until the drug is eliminated in the urine (as a metabolite or in unchanged form) or is gradually eliminated in the feces.

Effect of Age and Pregnancy

Renal excretion of drugs in infants and elderly adults is less efficient than that in young adults, and in pregnancy renal excretion is accelerated due to increased renal blood flow (see Chap. 7). Neonates and pregnant women may have impaired biliary excretion.

Effect of Disease

Relatively few unchanged drugs and active metabolites depend on renal clearance for elimination, but a few of these (**digoxin,** aminoglycoside antibiotics, some antihypertensive drugs, **cimetidine**) will produce serious toxic symptoms if the dosage is not adjusted in the presence of renal impairment. The *creatinine clearance test* is a good indicator of renal function and is often used as the basis for dosage adjustment. Hepatic or biliary disease can impair biliary excretion (see Chaps. 31 and 32).

PHARMACODYNAMIC PHASE

Pharmacodynamics includes the biochemical and physiologic effects of drugs and their mechanisms of action. The fundamental pharmacologic principle underlying pharmacodynamics is that *drugs cannot impart any new function to a cell.* Drugs act by modulating existing capacities or by affecting disease-induced alterations in function. The majority of drugs exert their effects by combining with cellular macromolecules called *receptors.* Drugs whose mechanism of action does not involve combining with a receptor have either a chemical effect (e.g., the neutralization of stomach acid by antacids and the neutralization of **heparin** by **protamine**), a mechanical effect (e.g., with bulk forming **laxatives**), or a generalized membrane effect (e.g., gaseous with **anesthetics**).

Drug-Receptor Concept

Receptors

Even though the analogy of a lock and key has been used to represent the relationship of receptors and drugs, receptors are not identifiable organelles, but are thought to be specific chemical configurations. Most receptors are portions of proteins; they may be an area of a cell membrane, a transport protein, a structural protein, an enzyme which is inhibited by drugs, or the nucleic acid of a cell.

An important group of receptors are those cellular proteins which function physiologically as receptors for endogenous regulatory substances such as the hormones, neurotransmitters, and autacoids (e.g., histamine, kinins, angiotensin, prostaglandins). Many of these have been classified on the basis of the responses elicited by various drugs. Hence, there are cholinergic receptors (with muscarinic and nicotinic subtypes), adrenergic receptors (with α_1, α_2, β_1, and β_2 subtypes),[3] histamine receptors (with H_1 and H_2 subtypes), and many others. The receptors for endogenous regulators are themselves subject to homeostatic control. Changes in drug response during chronic drug therapy may be due to changes in the numbers or characteristics of the receptors. For example, tardive dyskinesia (abnormal movements of the facial area) with long-term antipsychotic drug therapy is attributed to increased numbers of dopamine receptors in certain basal ganglia.

---

[3] α and β are the Greek letters alpha and beta, respectively.

Drug-Receptor Interaction

The reversible binding of a drug to a receptor is thought to initiate a change in the configuration of the receptor, which triggers a chain of events resulting in the pharmacologic effect. This interaction can be represented:

$$\text{Drug} + \text{receptor} \rightleftharpoons \frac{\text{Drug-receptor}}{\text{complex}} \rightarrow \rightarrow \rightarrow \text{Effect}$$

The intermediary steps between the formation of the drug-receptor complex and the effect, which may be simple or complicated, are called *receptor-effector coupling*. These intervening steps are not well understood, but they can involve "secondary messengers" [e.g., cyclic adenosine 3′,5′-monophosphate (cyclic 3′,5′-AMP) or guanosine triphosphate (GTP)]. This topic is currently the subject of intensive research by pharmacologists.

Structure-Activity Relationship

The ability of the drug to combine with the receptor, or its afinity for the receptor, is related to its chemical structure, often referred to as its *structure-activity relationship* (SAR). The chemical structure of the drug (the "key") must fit into the receptor (the "lock"). In some cases small alterations in the structure of the drug can alter its affinity for the receptor and thus the action or toxicity of the drug. It is the responsibility of the medicinal chemist (researcher) to create compounds or modify existing compounds that will have improved therapeutic indices.

Selectivity

It is therapeutically advantageous to administer drugs which work selectively at one receptor. The **phenothiazines**, which block dopamine receptors, cholinergic receptors, α-adrenergic receptors, and histamine receptors, have numerous adverse effects because of this nonselectivity. An important goal in current drug development is to identify drugs which demonstrate greater selectivity for a receptor. For example, **atenolol** (Tenormin) and **metoprolol** (Lopressor) are relatively more selective for β_1 receptors than the older drug **propranolol** (Inderal), which blocks β_1 and β_2 receptors and often causes bronchoconstriction as a result of the β_2 blockade of receptors on the bronchi.

Relation between Dose and Response

One theory suggests that drug response is proportional to the number of receptors occupied. Thus, response to a drug in the lower dosage ranges increases in direct relation to dose. As the dose further increases, the incremental response declines (the curve flattens), since there are relatively fewer available receptor sites. The typical dose-response curve is shown in Fig. 5-12*a*. To make mathematical manipulation easier and to better depict relationships, dose-response curves are usually plotted with dosage on a logarithmic scale, which results in an S-shaped curve with a linear segment, as shown in Fig. 5-12*b*.

Agonists

Drugs which elicit the physiologic response when bound to the receptor are called *agonists*. The degree of "fit" between the chemical structure of the drug and that of the receptor is called *affinity* and determines how strongly a drug will bind to the receptor. Drugs which bind to the same receptor produce varying degrees of effect, that is, have different *intrinsic activity*. Agonists bind well to their receptors and

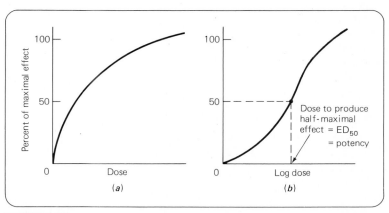

FIGURE 5-12

(*a*) A dose-response curve. (*b*) A sigmoidal dose-response curve results when dosage in *a* is plotted on a logarithmic scale. ED$_{50}$ is the dose which achieves 50 percent of the maximal response and is the indicator of drug potency.

produce significant response (i.e., have high affinity and high intrinsic activity). *Partial agonists* have less intrinsic activity than do full agonists.

Antagonists

Agents which bind well to the receptor and produce no receptor response (i.e., have high affinity and no intrinsic activity) are called *antagonists*. Since antagonists prevent any drugs that do have intrinsic activity from reaching the receptor sites, they are sometimes called *blockers*. There are two main types of pharmacologic antagonists: the competitive and the noncompetitive.

Competitive Antagonists *Competitive antagonists,* or *surmountable antagonists,* bind reversibly with the same receptors as the agonists. Increasing the concentration of agonists overcomes competitive antagonism. As shown in Fig. 5-13*a*, the dose-response curve for the agonist is shifted to the right (toward higher dosage requirement) in the presence of the competitive antagonist, since more agonist is required to achieve the same effect.

Noncompetitive Antagonists *Noncompetitive antagonists* or *insurmountable antagonists,* inactivate the receptor by binding irreversibly with it or by altering its conformation to make it unavailable to the agonist. The efficacy of the agonist is decreased, and addition of agonist has no effect (see Fig. 5-13*b*).

Other Types of Antagonism In addition to pharmacologic (competitive and noncompetitive) antagonism mediated at the same receptor site as the agonist, there are physiologic antagonism, chemical antagonism, and biochemical antagonism. *Physiologic antagonism,* or *functional antagonism,* occurs when two drugs counterbalance each other, working at different receptors. *Chemical antagonism* is the chemical reaction of two drugs to form an inactive product. *Biochemical antagonism* is pharmacokinetic in nature; the antagonist decreases the concentration of the agonist drug at the receptor by altering its absorption, distribution, metabolism, or excretion.

Potency, Efficacy, Slope

The dose-response curve elucidates several characteristics of drugs (see Fig. 5-14). *Potency* relates to the amount of the drug required to achieve the desired effect. It is determined by the affinity of the drug for the receptor and its pharmacokinetic parameters. From a clinical viewpoint potency has little significance, since it doesn't really matter whether it takes 2 mg or 400 mg of a drug to achieve an effect, as long as the effective dose is not so large that it is awkward to administer. Potency should *not* be confused with safety, value, or effectiveness.

Efficacy, effectiveness, or *maximal efficacy* relates to the

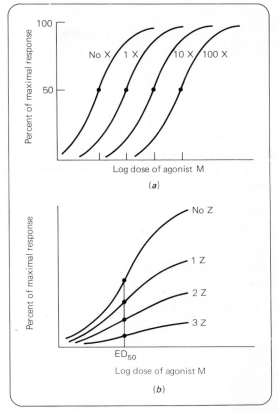

FIGURE 5-13

(*a*) Competitive antagonism. Dose-response curves for drug M, which is an agonist, with increasing doses of competitive antagonist, drug X. Dosage of drug M must be increased to maintain maximal effect.

(*b*) Noncompetitive antagonism. Dose-response curves for drug M with increasing doses of noncompetitive antagonist, drug Z. As dose of drug Z increases, maximal response of drug M declines. Increasing concentration of drug M cannot overcome the antagonism.

greatest response a drug can elicit. Maximal efficacy, also called *powerfulness,* is a clinically important drug characteristic in the selection of a drug for a specific purpose. **Morphine** would be selected over **aspirin** for the treatment of severe pain, since the maximal efficacy of aspirin does not include the higher ranges of pain. Thus, it can be said that with respect to severe pain, aspirin is less powerful (i.e., less efficacious) than morphine.

A steep *slope* of the dose-response curve implies that toxicity may result from relatively small increments in dosage above the effective dosage. The **benzodiazepine sedative-hypnotics** have a flat dose-response curve and are rarely associated as the single agent in death from overdosage. However, the **barbiturates** have a steeper curve and have often

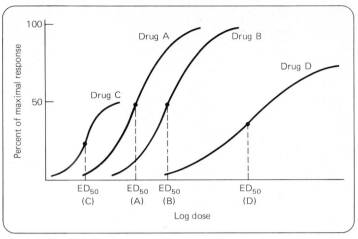

FIGURE 5-14

Comparison of Potency, Efficacy, and Slope of Dose-Response Curves of Four Drugs. Drugs A and B are equally efficacious (give same level of response), but drug B is less potent than drug A (i.e., has a lower ED_{50}). Drug C is more potent than drug A but less powerful (drug C and drug D are partial agonists due to low level of response achieved). Drug D is less potent and less effective than drug A. The gradual slope of the dose-response curve for drug D implies, but does not prove, a wide margin of safety between therapeutic and toxic dosage levels.

been implicated in overdosage deaths. The slope gives a limited indication of the margin of safety of a drug; the *therapeutic index*[4] (see Chap. 6) more directly reflects drug safety.

DOSAGE REGIMEN AND DRUG EVALUATION

Pharmacodynamics guides the rational selection of the drug to be used to achieve a defined therapeutic goal. Pharmacokinetics is important in establishing a dosage regimen (selecting dosage level and dosage interval) and guides the interpretation of blood concentrations of drugs.

Dosage Level and Interval

Single Dose

Several important concepts can be visualized by examining the drug concentration curve (called the *plasma level profile*) after a single oral dose, as shown in Fig. 5-15. After the dose

is administered, there is a *latency* period prior to the onset of action, which occurs when sufficient drug has been absorbed to reach the *minimum effective concentration* (MEC) in the plasma. With antibiotics the term *minimum inhibitory concentration* (MIC) is used instead. The plasma level gradually rises until the *peak plasma level* is reached and plasma levels begin to decline.

Because pharmacokinetic processes are continuous, as soon as a portion of the drug is absorbed and distributed, metabolism and excretion begin. Therefore, some drug elimination occurs even before the peak level is reached, and some drug may be absorbed even after the peak has been passed. After the peak level is reached, elimination occurs more rapidly than absorption. If too large a dose is given, the *toxic level* may be reached. This is the plasma concentration at which toxic effects generally first occur, although there is wide interindividual variation of the level at which people manifest toxicity. The range of drug concentration between the minimum effective concentration and the toxic level is the *therapeutic range* of a drug. The *duration of action* is the time interval during which the plasma level exceeds the minimum effective concentration and during which the clinical effect may be observed.

The plasma level profile of an intravenous bolus is shown in Fig. 5-6 (although the decline would be slightly curved if the plasma level were on an arithmetic rather than logarithmic scale). The rapid initial decline reflects distribution,

---

[4]The median effective dose (ED_{50}) is the dose of a drug that will produce a specific beneficial effect in 50 percent of the population, and the median lethal dose (LD_{50}) is the dose that will produce death in 50 percent of the population (usually laboratory animals). The therapeutic index (TI) is the ratio of toxic effects to beneficial effects:

$$TI = \frac{LD_{50}}{ED_{50}}$$

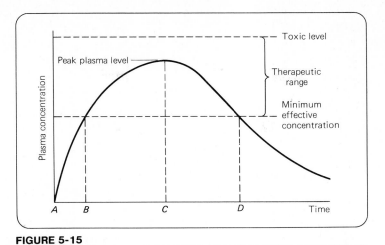

FIGURE 5-15

A Typical Plasma Level Profile for an Orally Administered Drug. (*A*) The dose is administered. (*B*) Onset of action is delayed until the drug is absorbed and the minimum effective concentration is reached. (*A–B* interval) Latency. (*C*) Peak plasma level ($C_{P_{max}}$) corresponds to maximal drug effect. (*D*) Drug effect is terminated when the plasma concentration falls below the minimum effective level. (*B–D* interval) Duration of action.

but the plasma level profile otherwise reflects drug elimination.

Multiple Doses

Few drugs, except analgesics, sedative-hypnotics, and other treatments for episodic symptoms, are administered as single doses. Most drugs are given one or more times per day for several days or longer. About four half-lives are required for complete elimination of a drug, so any drug given more often than this will *accumulate* in the plasma. Most drugs will continue to accumulate until a blood level is reached where elimination equals the dosage. (Recall that drugs subject to first-order kinetics are eliminated at a constant fraction per unit time. Hence, as the plasma level increases, the amount of drug eliminated per unit time also increases.) When drug elimination is equal to drug absorption and the average plasma concentration is stable, it is said that a *steady state* has been reached. (see Fig. 5-16.)

The steady state is more closely approximated as each half-life passes. (In two half-lives the plasma concentration is 75 percent of the steady state plasma concentration; in three half-lives, 87.5 percent; in four half-lives, 93.5 percent.) Thus it requires four to five half-lives to approximate steady state.

It also requires four to five half-lives for a drug to reach a new steady state plasma level whenever the dose is increased or decreased. For drugs such as the heart drug **dig-itoxin**, the sedative **phenobarbital**, and the antihypertensive **guanethidine**, the half-life may be several days to a week or more. Thus, almost a month may pass before steady state is attained after a dosage change or before the drug has been eliminated from the body sufficiently to prevent pharmacologic effects after it is discontinued.

It is sometimes necessary to make decisions concerning drug dosage after only one or two half-lives; in these cases blood levels can be determined and allowances can be made for the increases that would have occurred if there had been time to approximate steady state.

Unless the drug is administered by constant intravenous infusion, there will be fluctuations in plasma level during the intervals between doses. Immediately before a dose the *trough level* will occur, and after a dose the plasma concentration will reach its highest or *peak level*.

Maintenance Dose

The goal in designing a dosage regimen is to select the dosage level that will achieve and maintain the desired plasma level and the dosage interval that will prevent toxic concentrations during the peak levels and loss of effect during the trough levels. *To minimize fluctuations in blood levels, drugs are usually given at intervals of once per half-life*, except when this would result in more than four doses per day. Drugs with narrow therapeutic ranges may be given more frequently than once per half-life. When the half-life is longer than 24 h, the drug is usually given daily. There are several methods of estimating or computing maintenance dose. One precise method is based on a knowledge of the drug's clearance, since steady state plasma levels will be maintained if the dose replaces the amount of drug cleared during the dosage interval.

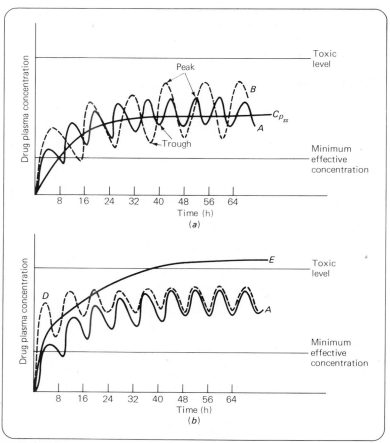

FIGURE 5-16

Effects of Dose, Dosage Interval, and Loading Dose on Plasma Level Profile. Line A in both graphs (a and b) represents a drug with a $t_{1/2}$ of 9 h, which is administered every 8 h at a dosage of 10 mg. Steady state is approximated in 4 to 5 half-lives. Line B represents the same drug administered every 12 h at a dosage of 15 mg. Steady state is achieved at the same time regardless of dosing interval. The mean steady state plasma concentration (C_{pss}) is the same for both dosage regimens, but the peaks and troughs are greater for line B. If the drug were administered by continuous intravenous infusion, the plasma level profile would be the same as the line labeled C_{pss}. Line D represents the same medication with the use of a loading dose (two 20-mg oral doses) prior to the maintenance dose of 10 mg every 8 h. Steady state is approximated more rapidly than with dosing regimen A. Line E represents the mean steady state concentration (C_{pss}) that would have been attained had the dosage remained 20 mg every 8 h.

Loading Dose

A large *loading dose*[5] (or several large initial priming doses) is sometimes given to quickly achieve a therapeutic blood level, which is then maintained by a constant infusion or intermittent oral dosage schedule.[6] This may be desirable when drugs have long half-lives and reach steady state slowly or when rapid response is needed. The loading dose is calculated on the basis of body size, volume of distribution of the drug, and desired steady state plasma concentration. However, use of loading doses is not without hazards, especially if there is impaired drug clearance, and is recommended only in serious conditions.

Evaluation of Plasma Drug Levels

Pharmacokinetic principles and techniques can contribute significantly to improving drug efficacy and preventing adverse reactions in the individual patient. For certain drugs the measurement of drug levels in the blood, urine, or saliva is a valuable addition to traditional methods used to predict the optimum dosage of a drug and to evaluate drug effects. (See Table 5-2 for listings of therapeutic levels of some drugs.) However, at no time should clinical observations be neglected because measurements of blood levels are available. Neither should clinical observations be discounted because they are not congruent with blood levels. Indications for measuring the levels of a drug in a body fluid (usually plasma) are the use of those drugs with narrow therapeutic ranges, zero-order kinetics, or wide interindividual differences in pharmacokinetics; the ascertainment of drug compliance; the observation of the patient who is at risk due to poor organ function; and the management of poisoning and overdose.

In order for the monitoring of plasma concentrations of a drug to be feasible and useful, several criteria must be met. The therapeutic effect must be related to the concentration of the drug in the plasma, and the therapeutic range must be known. For some drugs like **diazepam** (Valium), the plasma level does not correlate adequately with its (antianxiety) effects. Many drugs have not been sufficiently studied, so their effective plasma levels and the factors which affect those levels are not known. Further, it is necessary to have available a laboratory assay procedure for the drug in the plasma that is sensitive and specific and that can be performed in a reasonable amount of time and at reasonable expense. If some other parameter is more easily measured or is a more direct reflection of drug activity, it is preferable to measurement of plasma levels. For example, the prothrombin time test of clotting function is a direct and accurate measurement of **warfarin** activity; plasma levels of **warfarin** would not contribute further to evaluation of its effect.

Interpretation of Plasma Levels

Established therapeutic plasma concentration ranges for drugs are not absolute, since a few patients exhibit toxicity with plasma levels in the typical therapeutic range. Occasionally the laboratory assay procedures are in error and the laboratory report is an inaccurate reflection of patient status. Interpretation of the laboratory report requires a clear understanding of what the test purports to measure: If there are active metabolites, are these measured? Does the assay detect only free drug or total drug? The nurse must be aware of both the value and the limitations of plasma drug levels and use them as an additional parameter in evaluation of drug effects, rather than as the sole standard.

It is important that the nurse minimize sources of error in the determination of a plasma level. Obtaining the blood sample at the wrong time can invalidate the results, so the nurse must be aware of the correct time for sampling of the specific drug, which is based on its pharmacokinetic characteristics. For example, for **phenytoin**, **procainamide**, **quinidine**, and the **salicylates**, the blood should be drawn just prior to the next dose to be administered, but for **digoxin**, sampling should be done at least 8 h after the last dose; and for **lithium**, 12 h after the last dose.

NURSING PROCESS IMPLICATIONS

A number of physiologic and pathologic variables discussed in this chapter can alter the pharmaceutics, pharmacokinetics, and pharmacodynamics of drugs. The nurse must *assess* the patient for these biophysiologic factors.

The usual dosage level cited in reference books may be inappropriate for some patients. In assessing the appropriateness of a drug dose for a patient, the nurse should consider the factors in Table 5-5.

Proper drug administration will promote drug dissolution and drug absorption and will help preserve the anticipated pharmacokinetic profile. Oral drugs should be administered with an 8-oz glass of water, unless contraindicated. Tablets for sustained release or those which are enteric coated should not be crushed, as this could result in rapid

---

[5]Loading dose is computed by the formula:

$$\text{Loading dose} = \frac{V_d \times C_p}{F}$$

where V_d is the volume of distribution, C_p is the desired plasma concentration, and F is the bioavailability of the preparation.

[6]Maintenance dose is computed by the formula:

$$\text{Maintenance dose} = \frac{C_L \times C_{pss}}{F} \times \tau$$

where C_L is the total clearance, C_{pss} is the plasma concentration at steady state, F is the bioavailability of the preparation, and τ (tau) is the dosing interval.

TABLE 5-5 Use of Pharmacokinetic Parameters and Patient Factors to Assess Dosage Regimen

DRUG PHARMACOKINETICS	PATIENT FACTOR(S)	CONSIDERATIONS
Drug is variably absorbed after oral administration.	Gastrointestinal disease Concomitant drug therapy with antacids or other drugs which alter absorption	Consider liquid dosage forms, which may be more completely absorbed. Time drug administration 1 h prior to or 2 h after other drugs or meals (unless there is evidence that absorption is improved by food). Consider pharmacokinetic studies to document bioavailability. Increased dosage may be required. Duration of action is prolonged by slow absorption.
Drug is highly (>90%) bound to plasma albumin.	Renal or hepatic disease. Advanced age Infancy Pregnancy Malnutrition Concomitant drug therapy with another highly albumin-bound drug	High-hepatic-clearance drugs require lower dosages when binding is decreased. Other drugs will have the same steady state levels as the free drug unless clearance is impaired. Interpretation of blood levels of the drug must consider altered binding. Observe for excess effect of the primary or interacting drug, especially when there is a change in therapy.
Drug is lipid-soluble and distributed to body fat.	Obesity Being female Pregnancy Advanced age	Volume of distribution and half-life are increased. Less-frequent dosage is possible.
	Infancy, youth Starvation, malnutrition	Converse of above.
Drug is water-soluble and distributed to body water.	Infancy, youth Pregnancy Edematous conditions	Increased volume of distribution and half-life decrease blood concentrations.
	Obesity Advanced age Being female Dehydration	Converse of above.
Drug is primarily eliminated unchanged by renal mechanisms.	Renal disease or disorders of fluid balance. Advanced age Infancy	Decreased dosage may be required; adjust according to creatinine clearance, especially if drug has a narrow therapeutic range. Half-life and plasma concentrations are increased. Follow blood levels if available.
Drug is primarily eliminated by liver metabolism.	Hepatic disease Advanced age Pregnancy Infancy Drug or environmental enzyme inhibitors Slow acetylation	Consider type of metabolic reaction; phase I nonsynthetic is often more impaired. Half-life and plasma concentration may be increased. Toxicity may result. Decreased dosage may be indicated. Follow blood levels (if available) or clinical effect. If there are active metabolites, these may be more slowly formed, resulting in decreased effect.
	Drug or environmental enzyme inducers Rapid acetylation	Half-life and plasma concentration may be decreased. If there are active metabolites, these may be formed more rapidly, increasing effect. Increased dosage may be required. Follow blood levels if drug has a narrow therapeutic range.

absorption of drug meant to be slowly released over several hours.

The patient will need to be educated about the expected time course of drug effect. Many drugs require several days or even longer to reach maximum effect, and the person who is not aware of this may prematurely discontinue the drug, believing it is ineffective. For single-dose administration it is sometimes helpful for the patient to know the usual latency and peak times and the duration of action. Many patients expect the onset of action of drugs like oral analgesics to occur much more rapidly than it does. The nurse can take this latency into account and try to administer the drug as soon as possible after there is indication that the drug will be required.

Establishing the dosage schedule, selecting the dose to be administered within a prescribed range, and choosing the form or route of administration are decisions often made by nurses. The rationale for the nurse's decision in these situations may be found in the pharmacokinetics of the drug, as well as in individual patient variables. Knowledge of the half-life of the agent should help to determine the dosage schedule. If the drug is ordered qid and hospital policy generally indicates this should be 9 A.M., 1 P.M., 5 P.M., and 9 P.M., the nurse should consider the therapeutic range of the drug and the possible consequences of fluctuation in drug level. For example, the blood level of **theophylline** and some antiarrhythmics will drop below the minimum effective concentration during the 12-h night period if no drug is administered, causing therapeutic failure. Such drugs should be placed on an every-6-hour schedule.

Observation for *evaluation* of drug effect should be planned according to the half-life of the drug. Dosage increments should not be made until the steady state level has been approximated. The full effect of a drug is not appreciated until after 4 to 5 half-lives, so patient observation for therapeutic or adverse effects needs to be vigilant during this period.

Changes in dosage form or even manufacturer may affect drug response by alteration of bioequivalence or bioavailability, so the nurse should inquire about these changes when there is a sudden difference in drug response. Many consumers are aware of the cost savings afforded by use of generic drugs rather than brand name products and request that all their prescriptions be written by generic name. Health care providers need to explain that occasionally drugs are not bioequivalent and, therefore, the prescriber may prefer a specific brand, but nurses should assist the patient in obtaining a satisfactory explanation if a more expensive brand name is prescribed when a less costly generic equivalent is available.

It is important to remember that laboratory blood levels of drugs are almost always reported in levels of total drug. Alteration of plasma protein binding, changes in the partitioning of the drug in various physiologic compartments, and changes in receptor responsiveness all may affect the validity of the usual therapeutic blood level for an individual

patient. If the reported laboratory results are unusual or incongruent with the patient's clinical condition, it is good practice to have the laboratory repeat the measurements on the sample. If the results are still difficult to interpret, it may be necessary to take another sample and repeat the measurement.

PSYCHOSOCIAL FACTORS

LEARNING OBJECTIVES

Upon mastery of the contents of this section, the reader will be able to:

1. Describe the relevance of health values, social support, social roles, and clinician-patient interaction to a holistic approach to drug therapy.

2. Explain what a positive placebo response does indicate and what it does not indicate.

3. Describe nursing measures to promote compliance and the placebo response.

Psychosocial factors play a major role in drug response. However, current knowledge about the psychosocial basis of drug therapy is primarily intuitive and theoretical; clinical studies are relatively few and often inconclusive. The information is diffusely spread among the literature on a variety of concepts, models, and theories. This discussion will summarize the major psychosocial concepts relevant to drug therapy, placing them within a holistic framework.

A Holistic Model of Drug Action

The model in Fig. 5-17 represents a holistic view of drug action. While pharmacologic factors (pharmaceutics, pharmacokinetics, and pharmacodynamics; see Fig. 5-1) generally establish the range of potential responses to a drug, biophysical, psychologic, and social factors modulate drug effect and are responsible for tremendous variability in drug response. Some of the variables which have been found to influence drug effect are listed on the model, although their assignment to a domain is somewhat arbitrary. For example, genetic inheritance influences psychologic and physical processes; perceptions are as much physical and social as psychologic; etc. The purpose of a holistic model of drug action is to illustrate that drug response is a manifestation of the *total being*, rather than merely a biologic response to a pharmacologic stimulus.

The psychosocial variables which have been studied fall into two main categories: those that influence if or how the drug is actually taken and those that have a qualitative or quantitative influence on drug effect, exclusive of any inherent pharmacologic characteristics of the drug. The former make up what has been labeled *patient compliance*, the lat-

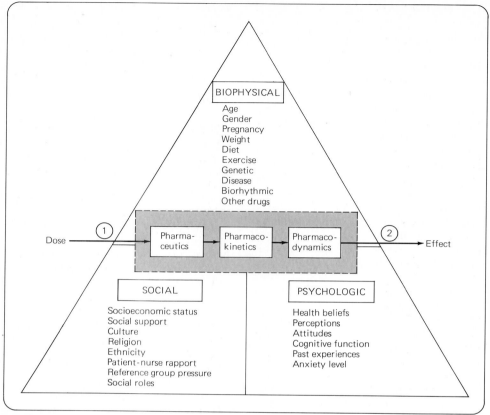

FIGURE 5-17

A holistic model of drug action, which incorporates biophysical and psychosocial aspects. The numerals represent the points at which (1) patient compliance and (2) placebo effect intervene. (Modified from G. A. Pepper: ''A Holistic Model of Drug Action in the Elderly,'' unpublished paper, 1980. Used by permission.)

ter what is called the *placebo effect*. Both terms carry negative or value-laden connotations (often subconscious) for nurses and physicians, but represent two crucial phenomena in clinical pharmacology and therapeutics. As described below, research studies have indicated that many psychosocial variables (e.g., social support, patient-clinician interaction, and perceptions of the value of the drug) influence both social support and placebo effect, while some psychosocial variables are related to only one of the phenomena.

PATIENT COMPLIANCE

Compliance is defined as the extent to which the patient's behavior (in terms of taking medications, following diets, or executing other lifestyle changes) coincide with the clinical prescription (Sackett and Haynes, 1976). It is estimated that noncompliance occurs in 15 to 93 percent of medical pre-

scriptions. Noncompliance is like any symptom in that it can be caused by a wide variety of problems. Intervention may be ineffective until the cause of the noncompliance is diagnosed.

Opposition to Terminology Many people object to the term *compliance* because it connotes a hierarchical relationship between the health care professional and the patient, with the professional establishing the goals and "sending down" the prescription to a patient, who is expected to "follow the orders." This authoritarian relationship is in direct contrast to ideals for the nurse-patient relationship that stress egalitarianism and collaborative exchange (Stanitis and Ryan, 1982). Use of the alternative terms *therapeutic alliance* or *adherence* has been suggested in response to this disparity. Whatever the terminology, the nurse must make a conscious effort to respond to the individual and not to the label "noncompliant." Legal and ethical principles (see

Chap. 8) also guide the nurse to avoid coercion and to seek truly informed consent.

Health Belief Model

While the "health belief model" was originally developed to account for preventive health behaviors, it is commonly employed to explain patient compliance with the prescribed drug regimen (Becker et al., 1977). Components of the model are the individual's perceptions about the threat posed by the disease, the individual's perceptions about the benefits and risks of the prescribed therapy, and factors that can modify these perceptions. The model predicts that a person will comply with a prescribed therapy if she or he perceives the disease as a personal threat and thinks that the problems posed by the therapy are outweighed by the probable effectiveness of the therapy. Factors such as age, race, peer pressure, past experiences, and mass media reports can alter the perceptions of the threat and of the potential benefits of the therapy.

The treatment of high blood pressure affords a good example of how this model describes the determinants of compliance. Hypertension is a disease with few symptoms, although a significant percentage of those with high blood pressure go on to develop strokes, heart attacks, and heart failure. Because patients may perceive the likelihood of these complications as remote or may not consider high blood pressure to be serious, they may judge it to be of little threat. In addition, the therapy for high blood pressure causes a number of discomforting adverse effects, such as frequent urination, drowsiness, stuffy nose, lethargy, and sexual dysfunction, which can be more troublesome than the disease. Therefore, it is no surprise that noncompliance is common among hypertensive patients. This trend may be compounded by modifying factors. Therapy is lifelong and may be expensive, so socioeconomic status is potentially important. The patient may have had a bad experience with the medication previously or know someone else who has. Older people with impaired memories have trouble remembering to take medications. On the other hand, modifying factors can alter the perceptions of the patient and promote compliance. Experience with a parent who died from a stroke might convince a patient that he or she is vulnerable and the disease is serious. Public service announcements on television or the opinion of coworkers can also encourage the patient to take the drug.

Research studies have generally supported the health belief model. Perception of the seriousness of the disease, personal susceptibility to the disease, and the potential value of the therapy, as well as past experiences, all affect compliance. The amount of knowledge a person has about the disease and drug can affect initial compliance, but the perceived benefits of therapy are more important in chronic therapy. Knowledge alone will not ensure compliance. Demographic factors (age, gender, socioeconomic status, intelligence, and education) and diagnosis are not systematically related to compliance, so there is no easy way to identify the person likely to be noncompliant, although a psychiatric diagnosis, health beliefs inconsistent with the dominant medical model, and a prior problem of noncompliance are risk factors.

Social Roles

The behavior that is expected of an individual by others, as defined by social status and culture, is called the person's social role. One of many roles we engage in is the sick role, which includes a set of exemptions and obligations expected of an ill person. One of the obligations is to follow the health care providers' directions to get well. Noncompliance may result from unwillingness to adopt the sick role or from conflict between the sick role and other social roles. For example, working parents may be unable to divest themselves of the roles of employee, parent, and homemaker, so they may continue to work and care for the family rather than go to bed and take the prescribed medicine.

Social Support

Social support is defined as information leading the individual to believe he or she is cared for, esteemed, and a member of a network of mutual obligations (Cobb, 1976). Social support is associated with compliance. While the instrumental aspects of social support promote compliance (reminding the patient to take a drug, actually administering the drug, or expressing belief in the value of the medication), the most important part of social support seems to be exclusive of any direct assistance with the medication.

Patient-Clinician Interaction The relationship between the patient and clinician (nurse, physician, or pharmacist) potentially affords a unique social support system. If the patient perceives the interaction as warm, stable, and mutual, compliance is improved. Better supervision of drug therapy and asking the patient for feedback on drug effects also promote compliance. Nonverbal cures are important in the interaction; long waits to see the clinician, crowded waiting rooms, inconvenient clinic hours, and a rushed demeanor do not give patients a message that they are esteemed, and these cues are associated with noncompliance.

Extent of Behavior Change Required

The greater the change in lifestyle required by the therapeutic prescription, the more common is noncompliance. Complex drug regimens, with numerous drugs taken at different times, and chronic medication therapy require a considerable change in behavior. Because a group of new habits must be developed, compliance is easily compromised. Even more problematic are those prescriptions that involve changing established habits, such as diet changes and giving up smoking or other social drug use.

PLACEBO EFFECT

Historically, only a few of the drugs in general use had specific pharmacologic effects, but the recent availability of drugs with proven therapeutic efficacy has stimulated interest in the placebo effect as a psychobiologic phenomenon. Wold (1959) defined the *placebo effect* as "any effect attributable to a pill, potion, or procedure, but not to its pharmacodynamics or specific effects." Therefore, *even drugs with proven specific pharmacologic effects have associated placebo effects.* Surgery and other procedures have a placebo component as well.

The placebo effect pervades therapeutics. It is a part of every drug's effect. Diseases and symptoms improved by *placebos* (pharmacologically inert "dummy" medications such as saline injections or lactose pills) include peptic ulcers, essential hypertension, pain, depression, anxiety, cough, headache, angina, rheumatoid arthritis, intermittent claudication, asthma, and warts. While an average of 30 to 40 percent of patients with these and other conditions will respond to a placebo, the response rate is sometimes as high as 80 percent. Effects of placebo treatment are not limited to subjective improvement, but are also reflected in objective physiologic and psychologic measurements such as blood pressure, blood count, spirometric measurements of lung function, extent of gastric acid secretion, amount of rapid eye movement (REM) sleep, accuracy of time estimation, etc. Even adverse effects are caused by placebos (called *nocebo* or *negative placebo response*); gastrointestinal distress, dizziness, drowsiness, parasthesias, addiction and withdrawal, mental confusion, elevated eosinophil and leukocyte counts, and even anaphylaxis and death have been reported. Investigational drugs are compared against a placebo to see if their specific pharmacologic effects or adverse effects exceed those of the placebo (see Chap. 9). *The placebo effect can promote, antagonize, or even reverse the effects of an active drug.*

Recent research suggests that one mechanism of placebo analgesia is release of endogenous pain-relieving hormones, the endorphins (Levine et al., 1978). However, still unexplained is the placebo effect in non-pain conditions and how the administration of a placebo initiates endorphin release. The potency of placebo analgesia appears to be equivalent to 4 to 6 mg of **morphine** intravenously (Levine et al., 1981).

Misconceptions and Attitudes about Placebos
Many health care providers misunderstand the placebo effect and often react negatively to any patient who responds to a placebo. In a study of the knowledge and use of placebos by physicians and nurses in a university teaching hospital (Goodwin et al., 1979), the value of placebos in the relief of

postoperative pain was significantly underestimated. Although research studies show that an average of 36 percent of patients do receive adequate pain relief from a placebo on the day after abdominal surgery, one-fifth of the physicians and nearly two-thirds of the nurses expected 5 percent or less would get adequate relief. Other common misconceptions are that "real" or "organic" pain does not respond to a placebo and that placebo response can be used to diagnose psychogenic problems. Many physicians and nurses reported use of placebos to diagnose "psychologic problems" or to judge "if the pain was real." In reality, *placebo response indicates nothing about the origin of a symptom.* Placebos tend to be administered to patients who are disliked or considered undeserving of active medication.

Extensive research to identify a placebo-reactive personality type has resulted in no consistent pattern, but many nurses and physicians persist in the erroneous belief that only those who are neurotic, suggestible, psychologically defective, or weak-willed will respond to placebos. In fact, situational factors are far more important than personality traits in the determination of placebo effect, and *under the right circumstances anyone could experience a placebo response.*

Situational Factors Associated with Placebo Effect
When the prescriber is warm and enthusiastic, likes the patient, and is confident of the effectiveness of the prescribed therapy, the placebo response is promoted. Expressions of confidence in the therapy by other health care providers, in addition to the prescriber, are also beneficial. The drug recipient's heightened level of anxiety is probably important in motivating the expectations of therapeutic success and hope of getting well. Faith of the patient in medical technology in general, and in the specific therapy, is extremely important. A strong social support network, including a favorable perception of the patient-clinician interaction, also contributes to the placebo effect. The size, color, form, and route of a medication influence the placebo response.

The placebo effect is a part of all drug therapy. It constitutes a clear and prevalent manifestations of holism in drug action and is worthy of the understanding and respect of clinical nurses and nurse researchers. *It should be purposely promoted for the patients' benefit.*

NURSING PROCESS IMPLICATIONS

Appropriate intervention to improve compliance and to promote the placebo effect requires a complete assessment of psychosocial factors. Past experience plays an important role in determining behavior. What diseases has the individual experienced either personally or in a close family member? Does the person have biases about medications that are helpful and those that are dangerous? If the patient has previously taken the drug or knows someone else on the medication, how well did it work? Were there unpleasant effects?

Patients should be encouraged to express their fears of addiction, carcinogenesis, and impaired functioning. Medications can have special meaning to a patient based on personal experience. For example, if a patient's parent died shortly after being placed on **digoxin**, the patient may feel the prescription for this heart drug means that his or her condition is terminal.

Current life events can also impact drug therapy. The anxious patient is unlikely to remember instructions, and extreme anxiety may require an adjustment in drug choice. Cognitive, psychomotor, and memory function should be tested, especially in the elderly. The patient enters the health care system with particular presenting symptoms and expectations for their resolution; these must be identified and addressed, since the goals of the health care system may be incongruent with these expectations.

Culture and Ethnicity

In our heterogenous society, nurses should not overlook the impact of culturally determined values and expectations on compliance and drug response. These beliefs affect decisions about what symptoms constitute illness, how illnesses are caused, and how they should be treated. A person's health belief system may be a curious mixture of modern bioscience, folk medicine beliefs, and assumptions from the popular health culture. For example, one mother used her skills with an otoscope, acquired in a course given by a pediatric nurse practitioner, to diagnose her daughter's ear infection, which she then reported to a *curandera* for treatment advice. (The *curandera* is a woman healer in the Mexican folk culture who uses both spiritual and herbal treatments.)

Religious beliefs may play a role similar to that of culture in compliance and drug response. Under no circumstances, however, should the nurse assume that membership in an ethnic, religious, or cultural group means that an individual accepts the beliefs and values ascribed to the group; each patient should be assessed as an individual.

Recent research indicates that ethnicity is also a factor in drug response, especially to psychoactive drugs. Preliminary evidence suggests that this may be due to both psychosocial and biophysical differences in ethnic groups (Levine et al., 1980; Yamamoto et al., 1979).

Promoting Compliance and the Placebo Effect

Once the cause of noncompliance is identified, the patient and clinician can jointly consider several ways to ameliorate the problem. First, the dosage regimen itself should be assessed by the health care team. Decreased complexity of dosage regimen is desirable, and drug cost should be weighed. Use of drugs with long half-lives permits dosing once or twice a day and optimizes compliance. Many adults prefer capsule dosage forms, and others object to childproof packaging. Labels should have the drug name, strength, purpose, and detailed dosing information.

Patient education must be integrated into the care of the patient. Most patients express a desire to know more about their disease and drugs. Although education may only marginally improve compliance, it should also improve safety and efficacy. The informed patient is capable of "rational noncompliance" (as when toxicity develops), and the enthusiastic description of drug mechanism promotes the placebo effect.

A variety of behavior modification techniques have been used to improve compliance. These seem most effective when the patient is taught to systematically observe the antecedents and consequences of taking medication. The written contract between the patient and the clinician is a useful technique (see Steckel, 1982; Barofsky, 1977; and Chap. 3).

Communication and a supportive nurse-patient relationship are the keys to consciously promoting the placebo component of all medication's efficacy through verbal and nonverbal means. Drug action can be explained briefly, and minor side effects can be cited in a positive light as evidence the drug is working. Talking with the patient as drugs are administered and seeking patient appraisal of the effects of prior doses are also beneficial.

If a pure placebo ("dummy medication") is ordered (and an order is required as for any medication), the nurse should chart the placebo and observe for the desired therapeutic effect and any adverse effects. Attempts by health care providers to use a placebo to diagnose the psychogenic origin of symptoms or to retaliate for undesirable behavior should be challenged. The ethical dilemma posed by the order for a pure placebo is considered in Chap. 8.

APPENDIX: USING PHARMACOKINETIC PRINCIPLES

The three examples that follow show the clinical application of pharmacokinetic principles.

Example 1—Developing a Pharmacokinetic Profile

R. V. P., a 35-year-old asthmatic patient, was given an intravenous (IV) bolus of 250 mg of **aminophylline** for severe respiratory difficulties. The medical staff ordered a **theophylline** pharmacokinetic study because of an increase in clinical symptoms and erratic theophylline levels.

The pharmacokinetic study generated information on how the patient metabolized theophylline (clearance, half-life, and volume of distribution). With this information it was possible to make predictions concerning maintenance dosages. The pharmacokinetic information was generated after a dose of a short-acting theophylline preparation; this could have been a solution, tablet, IV bolus, or IV infusion (which would have to have been discontinued while the study was conducted). A long-acting (sustained-release) or continuous IV infusion could not be used to generate pharmacokinetic information, since the elimination of the theophylline would be masked by the continuous absorption of more theophylline. To develop a pharmacokinetic profile for an individual patient, two types of information are required: the serum theophylline levels and the times the samples for levels are taken.

Before the IV bolus was given, a sample was taken; this was considered time 0. Multiple samples (usually 4 or 5) were obtained (usually over the next 3 to 5 h). The samples were taken every hour, but they could have been taken at any time as long as the exact times were recorded. If a study follows dosage with a short-acting oral theophylline preparation, at least 7 samples are taken, usually at approximately time 0, 0.5, 1, 2, 3, 4, and 5 h. The more samples that are obtained, the better the probability that the conclusions generated will be correct. With theophylline a one-compartment model of the body and elimination by first-order pharmacokinetics are assumed.

When the logarithm values of serum theophylline concentrations are plo-ted against time, a straight line can be generated (see figure). The straight line can be drawn by looking at the data points and then drawing the line, but the most accurate method is to use a hand-held calculator or a computer program that will fit the data points to the best possible straight line, using the method of least squares. Such programs generate the slope of the line, which is equal to the elimination rate constant (K_{el}). From this the half-life can be calculated.

The levels drawn from this study of R. V. P. were:

TIME, h	LEVEL, μg/mL
0	5.6
0.5	16.1
1.0	13.6
2.0	10.4
4.0	5.8

The study gave the following pharmacokinetic information:

Elimination rate constant (K_{el}) = 0.317 h^{-1}
Half-life = 2.18 h
Clearance = 175.1 mL/kg/h

The patient is a rapid metabolizer of theophylline and would benefit from a sustained-release preparation, since this would minimize serum theophylline fluctuations and allow for less-frequent dosing.

Example 2—Computing the Loading Dose

M. B. W. was admitted to the hospital with the first attack of asthma. The emergency room physician wanted to give a loading dose of theophylline. M. B. W. was not yet on any theophylline preparation. What loading dose for this 10-kg child would have resulted in a serum theophylline concentration of 10 μg/mL, assuming a volume of distribution of 0.45 L/kg? Aminophylline is theophylline ethylenediamine and it is 80 percent theophylline. (See footnote 5.)

$$\text{Loading dose} = \frac{V_d \times C_p}{F}$$

$$= \frac{4.5 \text{ L} \times 10 \text{ mg/L}}{0.8}$$

$$= 56.25 \text{ mg}$$

The loading dose should have been approximately 56 mg of aminophylline by IV bolus over 20 min. A theophylline level then should have been taken 2 h after the dose.

Example 3—Adjusting the Maintenance Dose

M. B. W. was placed on sustained-release theophylline (Slo-Phylline Gyrocaps) 60 mg sprinkled over applesauce every 8 h. His peak level after 1 week of therapy was 6 μg/mL, and his mother still complained of hearing him cough and wheeze. It was decided to increase his theophylline level to 12 μg/mL. What should the new dose of theophylline have been?

A simple method for adjusting the dose of drugs that fit the one-compartment and first-order pharmacokinetics

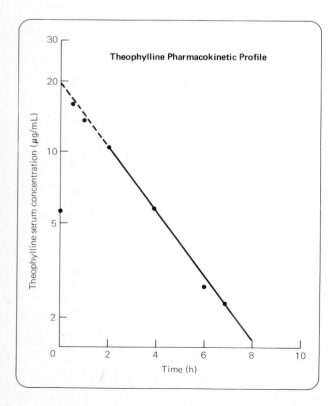

Theophylline Pharmacokinetic Profile

model is using the formula:

$$\frac{L_1}{L_2} = \frac{D_1}{D_2}$$

where L_1 is the first level obtained at the first dose, D_1; L_2 is the new level desired; and D_2 is the new dosage. In our example the patient was on 180 mg of theophylline a day and had a level of 6 μg/mL.

$$\frac{6\ \mu g/mL}{12\ \mu g/mL} = \frac{180\ mg}{X}$$

$$X = 360\ mg$$

Since Slo-Phylline Gyrocaps are available as 125-mg capsules, the new dose should be 125 mg sprinkled over food every 8 h.

REFERENCES

Barofsky, I. (ed.): *Medication Compliance: A Behavioral Management Approach,* Thorofare, N.J.: Slack, 1977.

Bauer, L. A.: "Clinical Pharmacokinetics," *Nurse Prac,* 7:42–48, 1982.

Becker, M. H., D. P. Haefner, S. V. Kasl, J. P. Kirscht, L. A. Maiman, and I. M. Rosenstock: "Selected Psychosocial Models and Correlates of Individual Health-Related Behaviors," *Med Care,* **15** (Suppl. 5):27–43, 1977.

Benet, L. Z.: "Pharmacokinetics 1. Absorption, Distribution and Excretion," in B. G. Katzung (ed.), *Basic and Clinical Pharmacology,* Los Altos, Calif.: Lange, 1982.

———, and L. B. Sheiner: "Appendix 2: Design and Optimization of Dosage Regimens: Pharmacokinetic Data," in A. G. Gilman, L. S. Goodman and A. Gilman (eds.), *Goodman and Gilman's The Pharmacological Basis of Therapeutics,* 6th ed., New York: Macmillan, 1980.

Benson, H., and M. Epstein: "The Placebo Effect: A Neglected Asset in the Care of Patients," *JAMA,* **232**:1225–1227, 1975.

Billars, K. S.: "You Have Pain? I Think This Will Help," *Am J Nurs.* **70**:2143–2145, 1970.

Borgman, R. J.: "Bioavailability, Dosage Regimens and New Delivery Systems," in C. R. Craig and R. E. Stitzel (eds.), *Modern Pharmacology,* Boston: Little, Brown, 1982.

Bourne, H. R.: "Rational Use of Placebo," in K. L. Melmon and H. F. Morrelli (eds.), *Clinical Pharmacology: Basic Principles in Therapeutics,* 2d ed., New York: Macmillan, 1978.

Byck, R.: "Psychologic Factors in Drug Administration," in K. L. Melmon and H. F. Morrelli (eds.), *Clinical Pharmacology: Basic Principles in Therpauetics,* 2d ed., New York: Macmillan, 1978.

Chrisman, N. J.: "Nursing in the Context of Social and Cultural Systems," in P. H. Mitchell and A. Loustau (eds.), *Concepts Basic to Nursing,* 3d ed., New York: McGraw-Hill, 1981.

Cobb, S.: "Social Support as a Moderator of Life Stress," *Psychoso Med,* **38**:300–314, 1976.

Correia, M. A., and N. Castognoli: "Pharmacokinetics. 2. Drug Biotransformation," in B. G. Katzung (ed.), *Basic and Clinical Pharmacology,* Los Altos, Calif.: Lange, 1982.

Fleming, W. W.: "Mechanisms of Drug Action," in C. R. Craig and R. E. Stitzel (eds.), *Modern Pharmacology,* Boston, Little, Brown, 1982.

Gilman, A. G., S. E. Mayer, and K. L. Melmon: "Pharmacodynamics: Mechanisms of Drug Action and the Relationship between Drug Concentration and Effect," in A. G. Gilman, L. S. Goodman, and A. Gilman (eds.), *Goodman and Gilman's The Pharmacological Basis of Therapeutics,* 6th ed., New York: Macmillan, 1980.

Given, C. W., B. A. Given, and L. E. Sismondi: "The Association of Knowledge and Perception of Medicine with Compliance and Health Status among Hypertension Patients: A Prospective Study," *Res Nurs Health,* **1**:76–84, 1978.

Goodwin, J. S., J. M. Goodwin, and A. V. Vogel: "Knowledge and Use of Placebos by House Officials and Nurses," *Ann Intern Med,* **91**:106–110, 1979.

Gram, T. E.: "Metabolism of Drugs," in C. R. Craig and R. E. Stitzel (eds.), *Modern Pharmacology,* Boston: Little, Brown, 1982.

Gryll, S. L., and M. Katahn: "Situational Factors Contributing to the Placebo Effect," *Psychopharmacology,* 57:253–61, 1978.

Jacobs, K. W. "Classification of Placebo Drugs: Effect of Color," *Percept Mot Skills,* 19:367–372, 1979.

Jospe, R. A.: *The Placebo Effect in Healing,* Lexington, Mass.: Lexington, 1978.

Kaplan, B. H., J. C. Cassel, and S. Gore: "Social Support and Health," *Med Care,* 15:47–58, 1977.

Kasl, S. V., and S. Cobb, "Health Behavior, Illness Behavior and Sick Role Behavior," *Arch Environ Health,* 12:531–541, 1966.

Levine, J. D., N. C. Gordon, and H. L. Felds: "The Mechanism of Placebo Analgesia," *Lancet,* 2:654–657, 1978.

———, C. G. Newlon, R. Smith, and H. L. Fields: "Analgesic Response to Morphine and Placebo in Individuals with Post Operative Pain," *Pain,* 10:379–389, 1981.

Levine, P., P. H. Rack, K. S. Vaddati, and J. J. Allen: "Ethnic

Differences in Drug Response," *Postgrad Med J,* **56** (Suppl. 1):46–49, 1980.

Levine, R. R.: *Pharmacology: Drug Actions and Reactions,* 2d ed., Boston: Little, Brown, 1978.

Mayer, S. E., K. L. Melmon, and A. G. Gilman: "Introduction: The Dynamics of Drug Absorption, Distribution and Elimination," in A. G. Gilman, L. S. Goodman, and A. Gilman (eds.), *Goodman and Gilman's The Pharmacological Basis of Therapeutics,* 6th ed., New York: Macmillan, 1980.

Mayersohn, M.: "Fundamental Principles of Pharmacokinetics," in K. A. Conrad and R. Bressler, *Drug Therapy for the Elderly,* St. Louis: Mosby, 1982.

McCaffery, M.: "Would You Administer a Placebo for Pain?" *Nursing 82,* **12**:80–85, 1982.

Nakano, S., and L. E. Hollister: "Chronopharmacology of Amitriptiline," *Clin Pharmacol Ther* 33:453–459, 1983.

Pender, N. J.: *Health Promotion in Nursing Practice,* New York: Appleton-Century-Crofts, 1982.

Pepper, G. A.: "A Holistic Model of Drug Action in the Elderly," unpublished paper, University of Colorado, 1980.

Perry, S. W., and G. Heidrich: "Placebo Response: Myth and Matter," *Am J Nurs* 81720–725, 1981.

Reinberg, A.: "Advances in Human Chronopharmacology," *Chronobiologia,* 3:151–166, 1976.

——, and F. Halberg: "Circadian Chronopharmacology," *Ann Rev Pharmacol,* **11**:455–487, 1971.

Rickels, K. (ed.): *Non-Specific Factors in Drug Therapy,* Springfield, Ill.: Thomas, 1968.

Roberts, H. M., and H. P. Bourne: "Drug Receptors and Pharmacodynamics," in B. G. Katzung (ed.), *Basic and Clinical Pharmacology,* Los Altos, Calif.: Lange, 1982.

Rosenberg, J. M., H. L. Kirschbaum, and R. S. Levinson: "Finding the Therapeutic Window," *RN,* **43**:42–51, 1980.

——, and P. Sangkachad: "Take With Meals . . . Or Not?" *RN,* pt. I, **44**(5):46–52; pt. 2, **44**(6):60–65, 1981.

Rowland, M.: "Drug Administration and Regimens," in K. L. Melmon and H. F. Morrelli (eds.), *Clinical Pharmacology: Basic Principles in Therapeutics,* 2d ed., New York: Macmillan, 1978.

Sackett, D. L., and R. B. Haynes (eds.): *Compliance With Therapeutic Regimens,* Baltimore: Johns Hopkins University Press, 1976.

Shapiro, A. K.: "Placebo Effects in Medicine, Psychotherapy, and Psychoanalysis," in A. E. Bergin and S. L. Garfield (eds.), *Handbook of Psychotherapy and Behavior Change: An Empirical Analysis,* New York: Wiley, 1971.

Sheiner, L. B., and T. N. Tozer: "Clinical Pharmacokinetics: The Use of Plasma Concentrations of Drugs," in K. L. Melmon and H. F. Morrelli (eds.), *Clinical Pharmacology: Basic Principles in Therapeutics,* 2d ed., New York: Macmillan, 1978.

Siddik, A. H., M. A. Trush, and T. E. Gram: "Drug Absorption and Distribution," in C. R. Craig and R. E. Stitzel (eds.), *Modern Pharmacology,* Boston: Little, Brown, 1982.

Sjoqvist, F., O. Borga, and M. L. E. Orme: "Fundamentals of Clinical Pharmacology," in G. S. Avery (ed.), *Drug Treatment: Principles and Practice of Clinical Pharmacology and Therapeutics,* 2d ed., Sydney: ADIS, 1980.

Smolensky, M. H., and A. Reinberg: "The Chrono-Therapy of Corticosteroids: Practical Application of Chronobiologic Findings to Nursing," *Nurs Clin North Amer,* **11**:569–638, December 1976.

Stanitis, M. A., and J. Ryan: "Non-compliance: An Acceptable Diagnosis?" *Am J Nurs,* 82:941–942, 1982.

Steckel, S. G.: "Predicting, Measuring, Implementing, and Following up on Patient Compliance," *Nurs Clin North Am,* 17:491–497, September 1982.

Stitzel, R. F.: "Excretion of Drugs," in C. R. Craig and R. E. Stitzel (eds.), *Modern Pharmacology,* Boston: Little, Brown, 1982.

Thomson, P. S., and J. C. Willis: "Compliance Changes in a Black Lung Clinic," *Nurs Clin North Am,* 17:513–521, September 1982.

Vessell, E. S.: "Genetic and Environmental Factors Affecting Drug Disposition in Man," *Clin Pharmacol Ther,* 22:659–667, 1977.

Vogel, A. V., J. S. Goodman, and J. M. Goodwin: "The Therapeutics of Placebo," *American Family Practitioner,* 22:105–109, 1980.

Vrhovac, B.: "Placebo and Its Importance in Medicine," *J Clin Pharmacol,* 15:161–165, 1977.

Wold, S.: "The Pharmacology of Placebos," *Pharmacology Rev,* **11**:689–704, 1959.

Yamamoto, J., D. Fung, S. Lo, and S. Reece: "Psychopharmacology for Asian Americans and Pacific Islanders," *Psychopharmacol Bull,* **15**:29–31, 1979.

6

ADVERSE DRUG REACTIONS

JANET K. DICKERSON
ROSS A. SIMKOVER

LEARNING OBJECTIVES

Upon mastery of the contents of this chapter, the reader will be able to:

1. Define the term *adverse drug reaction.*
2. Explain the significance of drug-induced disease.
3. Describe how the risk-to-benefit ratio is determined.
4. List nine types of adverse drug reactions and give an example of each.
5. Describe the nursing care in four types of drug allergy reactions.
6. Identify patients who are at high risk for adverse drug reactions on the basis of 10 predisposing factors.
7. Describe measures which can be taken to decrease the probability of adverse drug reactions in high-risk patients.
8. State the pharmacologic mechanism and appropriate nursing assessment and management of drug interactions which affect each of the following: absorption, metabolism, distribution, excretion, and pharmacodynamics of drugs.
9. Describe two types of drug incompatibilities.
10. Identify data pertinent to adverse drug reactions to be included in the patient medication history.
11. List four mechanisms of drug-food interactions.
12. State two types of drug-laboratory interactions.
13. Define *additive, synergistic,* and *antagonistic* in the context of drug interactions.

An adverse drug reaction is any unintended or undesired consequence of drug therapy. The term *adverse drug reaction* (ADR) is used to describe a broad range of untoward drug effects, from mild *side effects* to severe and potentially lethal *toxic effects* and *hypersensitivity* reactions (see Table 6-1). ADR also applies to instances of *drug interaction* and *errors in the administration* of drugs.

Even if a drug has been tested favorably in large groups

of patients, the small possibility of unwanted complications cannot be excluded in individuals or in atypical patient groups such as the elderly or those with certain diseases. This is particularly true of *new* drugs, as evidenced by the withdrawal from the market in recent years of several newly released agents as a result of ADRs undetected during the investigational phase. (See Chap. 9 for discussion of drug development and testing.)

SIGNIFICANCE OF ADRs

Studies have shown that the incidence of ADRs is quite high. Of the total number of patients admitted to the hospital, some 3 to 5 percent are admitted for adverse drug reactions. Among hospitalized patients, 10 to 20 percent acquire ADRs during their hospitalization. Deaths secondary to ADRs are estimated to occur in 0.4 to 12.9 percent of total fatalities. When this information is extrapolated to all hospital admissions yearly, one-seventh of all hospital days are devoted to the care of drug toxicity at an approximate cost of $3 billion annually.

In addition to these direct costs of treating the patient who has a drug reaction, the economic consequences of ADRs include the indirect expense involved in efforts to detect and prevent such reactions. *Detection costs* are those involved in finding early evidence of a drug-induced problem, as in the monitoring of the blood cell counts of patients who are receiving cytotoxic drugs for the treatment of cancer. *Prevention costs* are expenses incurred in reducing the possible occurrence of an ADR, as by the administration of potassium supplements to patients receiving thiazide diuretics or the administration of **pyridoxine** (vitamin B_6) to patients receiving **isoniazid** (INH) therapy for tuberculosis.

Drug-Induced Diseases (Iatrogenic Effects)

Iatrogenic effects are literally problems that are caused by the physician, but most often the term connotes *drug-induced diseases.* Many drugs, either as an extension of

87

TABLE 6-1 Classification of Adverse Drug Reactions

Drug allergy (hypersensitivity)
Unwanted, inseparable secondary effects (side effects)
Extension of pharmacologic effect
Toxic effects
Idiosyncratic reactions
Teratogenic effects
Carcinogenic effects
Drug dependence
Drug interactions
Administration errors

their pharmacologic properties or as a result of an allergic reaction, have the potential to produce disease states independent of the condition for which the patient is being treated. For example, deafness or partial hearing loss can occur from the use of **aminoglycoside antibiotics**, especially if serum levels exceed the therapeutic concentrations. The antihypertensive medications **reserpine**, **methyldopa**, and **clonidine** can cause depression. Elevated blood pressure can be induced or aggravated by **oral contraceptives** or **corticosteroids**. It is not uncommon for a drug-induced disease to be more serious than the patient's original illness, requiring a decision about whether or not to continue therapy. Because the nurse must consider drugs as causes of disease, as well as treatments of disease, each chapter of this text contains a discussion of drug-induced diseases pertinent to the topic of the chapter.

Risk-to-Benefit Ratio

The risk of ADRs is a concomitant of modern drug therapy. Few reactions are life-threatening, but almost all drugs, no matter how efficacious, can cause a serious ADR in some patients. For this reason, an evaluation of the risk-to-benefit ratio must be made for *individual* patients. The beneficial, intended effects of the drugs administered are weighed against the potential undesirable ADRs which may occur in the individual.

Assessing Risk

To evaluate a drug risk for a specific patient, the potential for an adverse effect or medical problem without drug therapy must be compared with the potential for the same problem with drug therapy. For example, the mortality rate from pregnancy in young American women is 20 per 100,000 women. In contrast, young women on birth control pills have a lower mortality rate (12 per 100,000 women), mainly due to fewer pregnancies. Women smokers over 35 years of age on oral contraceptives suffer a fourfold increased risk of cardiovascular disease. Thus, risk of a given drug may vary for different persons, based upon a variety of patient, environmental, and drug factors.

Assessing Potential Benefit

To evaluate drug benefit for specific individuals, the goals of therapy along with many social, psychologic, and economic factors must be assessed. The *goal of drug therapy* is the outcome that can reasonably be expected, based upon evidence derived from studies of patients with similar disease states. Goals are further modified by patient and situational characteristics. For example, a young woman might consider using a diaphragm for contraceptive purposes, but effectiveness of a diaphragm is dependent upon user motivation and carefulness of use. For the unmotivated person, an oral contraceptive might be more beneficial. Similarly, an expensive drug is of no benefit to a patient who cannot afford to buy it.

Not only must the health care providers assess the advantages and disadvantages of a specific therapy for the patient, but alternate therapy should be examined for its inherent risks and benefits. *Ultimately, the therapy with the greatest benefits and the least number of risks should be chosen.* The use of a potentially toxic drug for a minor illness is unacceptable. As an example, when **chloramphenicol** was first available, it was indiscriminately used in the treatment of minor infections, resulting in many serious cases of agranulocytosis (absence of certain white blood cells). This drug is now reserved for the treatment of infections caused by organisms not susceptible to less-toxic drugs. In life-threatening illness, a severe ADR may be acceptable, such as those ADRS which accompany antineoplastic drugs used to treat cancer. Likewise, drug dependence on narcotic analgesics is not a limitation in a patient with a painful terminal disease.

Therapeutic Index

One way to quantify the risk-to-benefit ratio is called the *therapeutic index*. The therapeutic index (TI) is a ratio of the dosage which is lethal in 50 percent of the animals tested to the dosage required to produce the specified therapeutic effect in 50 percent of the humans tested. The lower the TI, the more toxic the drug. However, the TI does not take into account that serious adverse effects can occur at doses significantly less than those lethal to animals and that some ADRs are not dose-dependent (such as drug allergy).

Basic to an understanding of the significance of ADRs is the concept of risk versus benefit. All drugs have adverse effects, and there is no completely safe drug; yet, there are very few drugs whose benefits do not outweigh their risks when properly prescribed and monitored. Most ADRs can be predicted, based on the pharmacology of the drug, and prevented by establishing a therapeutic end point for drug effect and observing the patient for this effect. The nurse who consistently evaluates drug effects in patients contributes a great deal to the prevention of adverse drug reactions.

FACTORS AFFECTING ADRs

Many patient factors contribute to the ability of an individual to tolerate drugs. Among such factors are genetic makeup, weight, age, and sex. Epidemiologic studies have suggested a higher occurrence of ADRs in females and the elderly, with white women having a higher incidence of ADRs than black women.

Patient characteristics, environment, disease, and drug administration factors all affect the occurrence, magnitude, and clinical significance of ADRs (see Table 6-2).

CLASSIFICATION OF ADRs

Drug Allergy (Hypersensitivity)

Allergic reactions to drugs are the result of the body's *immune response* to a drug following prior exposure to the same drug or an antigenically similar drug. A hypersensitivity reaction requires that the drug serve as a stimulus to the body's production of antibodies. Subsequent to the initial exposure, or *sensitization,* to such a drug, the body's immune system recognizes the drug as foreign (antigenic) and produces antibodies in response to its presence, thereby initiating the allergic reaction.

Drug allergies pose a major therapeutic problem, as it is difficult to predict such reactions, even after a good medical history has been taken. The antigenic property may be in the drug itself or may be in its metabolites or in the so-called inert ingredients used in drug manufacture.

The exact reasons why a given patient develops an immunologic reaction to a drug often remain unknown, although

TABLE 6-2   Factors That Predispose to ADRs

FACTOR*	PHYSIOLOGIC / PHARMACOLOGIC ALTERATION	RESULT	NURSING ASSESSMENT AND INTERVENTION
Age Neonate	Deficient drug-metabolizing enzymes Decreased renal plasma flow	Accumulation of drug Decreased elimination of drug and toxic metabolites	Assess renal function by laboratory parameters, urine output. Give pediatric drug doses based upon age, weight, surface area. Observe for drug toxicity.
Geriatric	Decreased blood flow to kidney, liver Increased blood flow to brain and heart (relative to kidney, liver)	Decreased elimination, metabolism of drugs Increased central nervous system and cardiac drug toxicity Altered distribution and tissue levels of drugs	Assess cardiac, kidney status. Give drugs that cross blood-brain barrier with care, or use alternative drugs. Monitor blood levels of cardiac drugs. Decrease drug dose for elderly; use less-toxic drugs.
Gender	Different fat-to-lean ratios, size, metabolic and hormonal functions	Altered distribution of drugs Unknown effect on drug metabolism and receptor function	Assess weight, body composition. Be aware of potential differences.
Weight	Abnormal thinness or obesity	Altered distribution and tissue levels of drugs	Assess nutritional status. Obtain dietary consultation. Avoid IM or SC administration of drugs in the thin. Increase drug dosage as appropriate for obese patients.
Pregnancy	Altered stomach-emptying time, protein binding, elimination Drug penetration of placenta	Altered pharmacokinetics Potential birth defects	Evaluate drug response. Avoid drugs in pregnancy when possible.
Breast-feeding	Drug secretion in breast milk	Potential adverse reaction in child	Avoid drug use when child's risk is greater than mother's benefits. Observe child for symptoms of drug effect.
Genetics	Altered enzyme activity or deficiency	Increased drug- or toxic metabolite–induced disease	Obtain adequate health and medication history. Observe for unusual, delayed, or rapid drug response.
Renal disease	Decreased renal filtration, secretion	Accumulation of drugs and metabolites	Monitor kidney function by urine output, serum urea nitrogen, and creatinine. Avoid drugs excreted unchanged by kidneys, or decrease dose. Assess for drug toxicity.

TABLE 6-2 Factors That Predispose to ADRs (*Cont.*)

FACTOR*	PHYSIOLOGIC/PHARMACOLOGIC ALTERATION	RESULT	NURSING ASSESSMENT AND INTERVENTION
Liver disease	Decreased liver enzyme production	Accumulation of drug	Assess liver function status by clinical lab (transaminases, alkaline phosphatase, LDH). Observe for increased or decreased drug effect. Give lower doses of drugs if ADR develops, or discontinue medicine.
Environment Caffeine, smoking, insecticides	Induction of liver enzymes	Increased drug metabolism	Obtain good social, occupational history. Observe for decreased drug effect.
Adjuvants used in food and drug manufacture	Allergy to or irritation from adjuvant	Dermatologic, respiratory, or immune reaction	Consider "inert" ingredients used in drug and food processing when assessing any atypical reaction.
Drug administration Dosage level	Variable concentration at site of action	Possible ADR in one person with a dose that is effective in another	Assess appropriateness of dose to weight, age, underlying disease, and degree of debilitation.
Storage	Inactivation or degradation of a drug into a less-active or toxic substance because of improper storage	Decreased therapeutic response or ADR	Check with pharmacist or package insert about proper storage. Do not give any drug which looks or smells abnormal or is past expiration date.
Route	Increased immune response associated with topical and injected routes. Possible high blood levels from injected drugs	Allergic ADR, most common with topical route. Severe ADR, more common with injected routes	Use enteral routes if possible. Give IV drugs diluted and slowly. Observe for redness and rash with topical therapy.
Multiple therapy	Concomitant presence of several drugs in GI tract, blood, receptor sites	Increased number of drug interactions	Avoid unnecessary drugs. Observe carefully when multiple drugs are required.
Drug errors	Wrong drug, dose, route, or time	Therapeutic failure, toxicity, or other ADR	Administer medication properly. Educate patient thoroughly. Know drugs, diseases, usual indications, and doses. Consult published references, another nurse, a pharmacist, or a physician if order seems inappropriate.

*More comprehensive discussions of these topics are found in the following chapters: age (Chap. 7), pregnancy and breast-feeding (Chap. 7), genetics (Chap. 5), renal disease (Chap. 31), liver disease (Chap. 32), and environment (Chap. 49).

certain factors do seem to influence the probability of sensitization. In general, the likelihood that an allergic ADR will occur increases with the number of courses of treatment. For drugs given in single courses over a long period of time, allergic ADRs are more likely to occur in the first 2 to 3 weeks of treatment, although ADRs may occur up to several years after treatment. Numerous drugs have been implicated as causative agents—**aspirin**, the **penicillins**, and the **sulfonamides** (including sulfonamide antibiotics, sulfonylurea hypoglycemics, thiazide diuretics, and carbonic anhy-drase inhibitors) account for 80 to 90 percent of all allergic ADRs.

Types of Drug Allergies
Drug allergies can be classified into four types (see Fig. 6-1), based upon the immunologic mechanism.

Type I Reactions (Immediate, or Anaphylactic) These are due to IgE, or reaginic, antibodies, which are bound to the cell membrane of mast cells or circulating basophils. Com-

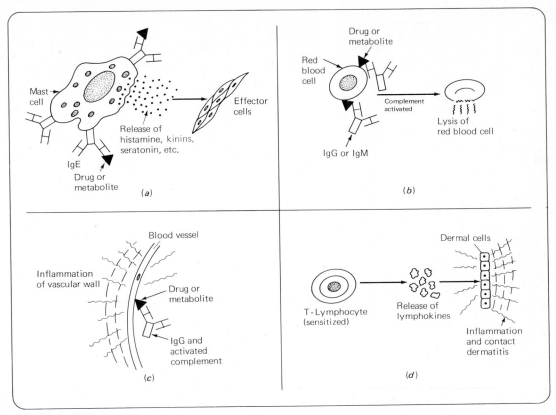

FIGURE 6-1

Schematic Representation of the Types of Drug Allergy Reactions. (*a*) Type I (immediate, or anaphylactic) reaction: acts on effector cells in vessels and smooth muscle, resulting in anaphylaxis, urticaria, angioneurotic edema. (*b*) Type II (cytotoxic, or autoimmune) reaction: causes lysis of red blood cells, resulting in hemolytic anemia. (*c*) Type III (complex-mediated, or vasculitic) reaction: acts on the vascular wall. (*d*) Type IV (delayed hypersensitivity, or fixed-drug) reaction: causes contact dermatitis.

bination of the antigen with the antibody releases histamine and other vasoactive amines. Anaphylactic shock, urticaria (hives), and angiodema (a localized swelling) are the clinical manifestations of this type of reaction.

Anaphylactic reactions may be generalized, acute, life-threatening allergic reactions characterized by hypotension, bronchospasm, laryngeal edema, and severe itching, either in combination or as isolated features, or they may be localized reactions characterized by rash or itching, bronchial asthma, vomiting, abdominal pain, or diarrhea.

Anaphylaxis is most common with drugs given intramuscularly or intravenously, although oral, percutaneous, or even respiratory exposure may produce the response. Allergic symptoms need not necessarily have occurred during previous courses of treatment. Indeed, anaphylactic shock reaction to **penicillin** has been known to occur with the seventeenth course of treatment, the previous 16 courses having been given without incident. On the other hand, there may be no history of prior exposure to the drug.

The typical type I, or immediate, reaction develops rap-idly (reaching a maximum within 5 to 30 min). Anaphylactic reactions are life-threatening situations requiring immediate intervention to relieve symptoms rather than attempts to determine the cause of the reaction. Laryngeal edema and bronchospasm can cause severe respiratory difficulty. **Epinephrine**, 0.3 to 1.0 mg, administered subcutaneously may be helpful in alleviating the reaction. Antihistamines (e.g., **diphenhydramine** (50 mg orally or parenterally) may also be used alone or as an adjuvant to epinephrine.

Type II Reactions (Cytotoxic, or Autoimmune)   In Type II reactions, the antigen is present on the surface of cells, and combination with IgG or IgM antibodies activates the complement system, causing cell destruction. Type II reactions are responsible for many allergic blood dyscrasias. Examples are hemolytic anemia induced by **quinidine** and **rifampin**, thrombocytopenia due to the **thiazide diuretics** and other drugs, and agranulocytosis due to **aminopyrine** and **phenylbutazone**. In these situations the drug forms an antigenic complex on the surface of the cell, which is destroyed by the antibody. The body tissue is damaged or destroyed, although an innocent bystander to an immunologic response to a drug. These reactions usually subside within several months after the drug is discontinued, although supportive therapy and immunosuppression with corticosteroids or other drugs is sometimes required in severe acute autoimmune responses.

Type III Reactions (Complex-Mediated, or Vasculitic)

The serum sickness syndrome, mediated by complement-fixing IgG or IgM, is the most common example of a type III reaction. Circulating antigen-antibody complexes are deposited on the walls of small blood vessels, producing an inflammatory response. Serum sickness is a less-acute allergic reaction than anaphylaxis and has been associated with various drugs, including the antibiotics **penicillin** (especially the long-acting **procaine penicillin**), **streptomycin**, and the **sulfonamides**. Other vasculitic reactions include erythema multiforme, a relatively mild skin disorder, and the more severe Stevens-Johnson syndrome, which frequently has been associated with **sulfonamides** and manifests as erythema multiforme, arthritis, nephritis, myocarditis, and central nervous system abnormalities. Severe vasculitic reactions may require corticosteroids during the acute phase.

Type IV Reactions (Delayed Hypersensitivity, or Fixed-Drug)

These are cell-mediated reactions due to T lymphocytes. Contact dermatitis is the typical example and is due to external sensitization to drugs like **penicillin, sulfonamides, phenothiazines** (antipsychotic medications), and **local anesthetics**. Treatment is usually local application of calamine lotion or a similar soothing topical medication.

Management of Drug Allergies

It is important to recognize that more than one type of hypersensitivity reaction may produce a particular clinical manifestation. Thus urticaria (erythematous, well-circumscribed wheals) may be a type I reaction or may occur as part of the serum sickness syndrome. Also, although an allergic reaction probably underlies many drug reactions, the precise mechanisms for many are unknown. This is true of many drug rashes, fever due to drugs, several types of drug-induced jaundice, systemic lupus erythematosus, and kidney disease.

Hypersensitivity reactions can often be avoided by comprehensive drug and food allergy history taking. Due to continuous patient contact and communication, the nurse may be in the best position for allergic reaction monitoring. Many hypersensitivity reactions can be diagnosed early, before they can cause serious illness, by monitoring the white blood count for eosinophilia and checking the patient's skin for rashes.

Hypersensitivity reactions almost always require that the drug be discontinued immediately, and treatment of the symptoms of the reaction may be needed. With some mild drug allergy reactions, the physician may choose to continue the offending drug while simultaneously treating the allergic symptoms. In this instance, the nurse must carefully monitor and document the progress of the patient and watch for worsening symptoms of allergy.

Unwanted, Inseparable Secondary Effects (Side Effects)

A side effect is best described as an undesirable, but often unavoidable, extension of the pharmacologic effects of the drug. Side effects are the most frequently encountered ADRs and can occur with the administration of normal therapeutic doses of drugs. Most drugs have several actions, generally only one of which is the desired action; the other actions are considered side effects. For example, a diuretic may promote the urinary excretion of sodium and water (desired effect), but it also may cause the excretion of potassium, increase the blood level of uric acid, and raise the blood level of glucose (undesired or side effects).

A knowledge of the pharmacologic actions of drugs permits the nurse to predict these side effects and to intervene to prevent or reverse these reactions. For example, **codeine** and other narcotics have both analgesic and constipating effects. If a patient is receiving codeine for pain, the nurse should check that the patient has regular bowel movements and, if not, suggest that the diet be modified or a laxative be ordered. However, some narcotics are used to treat diarrhea and, in this case, the constipating effect is the desired action, rather than a side effect.

Probably the most challenging type of ADR from the point of view of the nurse is these unwanted, inseparable secondary effects. Sometimes the drug dose can be decreased to avoid side effects, but at other times these reactions may accompany the administration of the drug as long as the drug dosage is adequate to achieve the therapeutic effect. The ingenuity of the nurse may be greatly challenged in assisting the patient to have the highest degree of comfort possible in spite of side effects. At times the patient may be so uncomfortable the drug must be discontinued.

Extension of Pharmacologic Effect

Extension of the primary, expected action of the drug can produce an undesirable effect, as in diarrhea caused by the overuse of laxatives, or hypoglycemia (low blood sugar) following the administration of **insulin**. The cytotoxic agents used in cancer chemotherapy cause a variety of serious ADRs because they lack the specificity to affect only tumor cells.

Nursing management of this type of ADR requires withholding the drug and notifying the physician of the undesirable symptom. An extension of pharmacologic effect could become an emergency, requiring immediate treatment (e.g., intravenous administration of 50% dextrose solution for hypoglycemia secondary to an insulin reaction). At times, only minor adjustments in therapy (decreasing the dose, for example) are necessary. Therapy must be stopped if the ADR becomes life-threatening. Nursing interventions may be directed at decreasing the impact of these ADRs. For example, decreased platelet and white blood cell counts from cancer chemotherapy require extensive nursing intervention to decrease the patient's risk of bleeding and susceptibility to infections.

Toxic Effects

The toxic effects of a drug are directly related to the systemic or local concentration of the drug in the body. Such effects are usually predictable and may be expected in any patient whenever a threshold level of the drug has been exceeded. Each drug has characteristic toxic effects. Overdosage may result from an excess dose taken accidentally or deliberately, or it may be due to accumulation of the drug as a result of some abnormality which interferes with normal metabolism or excretion of the drug. For example, the toxicity of **morphine**, a narcotic used for pain relief, is enhanced in the presence of liver disease (because of inability to detoxify the drug) or myxedema (severe hypothyroidism). In the presence of renal failure, such drugs as the antibiotics **gentamicin** (Garamycin) and **kanamycin** (Kantrex), the heart drug **digoxin**, and **potassium**, which are normally excreted by the renal route, may accumulate and produce toxic effects. Occasional instances of toxicity have resulted from accidental introduction of toxic substances via an inappropriate route of administration, such as thromboembolic phenomena resulting from the intraveous administration of **procaine penicillin G.**

Toxic manifestations are often of a life-threatening nature, and the drug should not be given once a toxic reaction is observed. After a thorough assessment of the patient, the nurse should contact the physician, who may decrease the dose or discontinue the drug entirely. At times it is necessary to continue to treat the toxic symptoms until the drug is metabolized or eliminated.

Idiosyncratic Reactions

An idiosyncratic reaction is an unusual response to a drug by a patient. Idiosyncratic reactions are involved in fewer than 5 percent of all drug reactions. However, reactions currently labeled "idiosyncratic" may actually be reactions of another classification. As more patients are studied, such reactions may be reclassified.

A typical idiosyncratic reaction is the stimulation which occurs following the administration of **phenobarbital**. The usual response to phenobarbital is sedation; persons exhibiting an idiosyncratic reaction to this drug often are jittery, nervous, and excitable—quite the opposite of the expected effect of the drug.

The nurse cannot be overly suspicious in the evaluation of this type of drug response. Too often a patient's complaint is labeled "neurotic" because the complaint does not fit the expected consequence of disease or therapy. Today, even with drug testing and clinical trials prior to release of drugs for widespread use, the potential for unusual, as-yet-unrecognized drug effects is very great. Management of the idiosyncratic reaction will depend upon the character of the reaction, but often the drug must be withheld until the physician is notified.

Teratogenic Effects

Teratogenic effects are drug-induced birth defects which follow drug therapy in pregnant females. To avoid these possible effects, most pregnant women are advised not to take any medications without checking with their obstetricians. (See Chap. 7.)

Drug Dependence

Drug dependence is the use of drugs causing behavior that reinforces the need for the drug. Heroin addiction is an obvious example of such an ADR, but drug dependence also can involve the habitual use of such over-the-counter drugs as nasal decongestants or laxatives. (See Chap. 49.)

Drug-Induced Cancer (Carcinogenesis)

Acute side effects of drugs are usually well documented through toxicity studies and clinical trials. Long-term side effects, including cancer, are much more difficult to evaluate and still remain largely unknown (see Chap. 37). One of the most widely publicized incidences of drug-induced cancer involved the agent **diethylstilbesterol** (DES). In 1971 an unusual form of vaginal cancer detected in females aged 14 to 22 years was linked to intrauterine exposure to DES.

Drug Interactions

Drug interactions account for more than 50 percent of reported adverse drug reactions. Drugs interact not only with other drugs but also with laboratory tests and foods. Drug interactions can be beneficial, as with the concurrent use of **probenecid** (Benemid) and **penicillin** in the treatment of venereal disease because probenecid retards the excretion of penicillin, or they can be harmful, as when a hypertensive crisis occurs in a person who takes a **monoamine oxidase** (**MAO**) **inhibitor** and then drinks Chianti wine. Drugs also have pharmacokinetic and pharmacodynamic interactions with disease states, as discussed in Chap. 5. These interactions may contraindicate a drug in a particular patient.

Since it is impossible to memorize each interaction, health professionals must be aware of the mechanisms of drug interaction. Numerous patient and drug factors may affect whether a potential interaction occurs and whether it is *clinically significant*. Clinically significant drug interactions are defined as those which cause either a decrease of therapeutic response to a drug or undesirable effects such as toxicity or extension of the pharmacologic effect of a drug.

In reviewing the clinical data on drug interactions, the nurse should be concerned with these considerations:

Is the reported drug interaction fact or theory? Many reactions theoretically can occur but sometimes only under very special circumstances; health professionals are most concerned with whether or not a drug interaction truly occurs and whether it is clinically significant.

Was the original report based on animal studies or human studies? Animal studies are of limited predictive value in human beings because of species differences; it can never be assumed that drug interactions observed in animals will necessarily occur in human beings.

What was the source of the data? Many reports of drug interactions are based on anecdotal or single, isolated case reports without sufficient follow-up. Some early reports of drug interaction with implied far-reaching consequences have not been confirmed in subsequent studies.

What were the conditions of drug administration? The specific circumstances under which the drugs are given are frequently more important than the theoretical existence of the interaction. Important conditions might include liver and kidney function of the patient, other drug therapy, doses, route, diet, disease states, etc.

Table 6-3 describes a model based on the nursing process to identify and manage potentially significant drug interactions. It consists of five steps to determine how and why an interaction can occur. With this knowledge, based on sound scientific principles, the nurse can devise appropriate patient care plans to decrease the risk for interactions and enhance the benefits to the patient of potent drug therapy.

Drug-Drug Interactions

Drug-drug interactions occur when the effects of one drug are altered by the prior or concurrent administration of another or the same drug. Drug-drug interactions may arise at any point in the process of drug action where a mechanism of drug disposition can be acted upon by other drugs, thus increasing or decreasing the active serum drug level in a clinically significant manner. These significant points include:

1. The pharmaceutic phase: A drug may become inactivated by incompatibilities with other compounds prior to administration.
2. The pharmacokinetic phase:

   Absorption—Other drugs may block, slow, or hasten the process.

TABLE 6-3 A Nursing Process Model for Assessment and Intervention in Clinically Significant Drug Interactions

STEPS IN PREVENTING POTENTIAL DRUG INTERACTIONS	NURSING INTERVENTIONS AND SKILLS
1. Identify mechanisms of drug action and drug disposition.	Base interventions upon sound knowledge of drug pharmacokinetics and pharmacodynamics.
2. Assess factors that could alter drug action.	Assess coexisting therapy to identify where drugs might compete for or antagonize action and thus interact. Assess patient's health status for factors that can alter mechanisms of drug action (liver, renal, gastrointestinal, and cardiovascular function).
3. Devise a patient care plan to minimize risks and increase benefits of treatment, based upon where and how interactions are likely to occur.	Analyze what would change if mechanisms of drug action were altered by patient health factors, other drugs, or other therapies.
4. Evaluate effectiveness of patient care plan.	Monitor and document patient's response to drug therapy objectively (vital signs, clinical laboratory parameters, serum drug levels) and subjectively.
5. Devise alternative patient care plans if original plan does not aid in reaching ultimate goal of therapy.	Repeat steps 1 through 4. Consider additional nursing interventions. Consider increasing or decreasing drug dosages, using alternative drug forms or routes of administration, substituting drugs, discontinuing some drugs, or as a last resort, adding additional therapy to counteract drug side effects.

Distribution—Other drugs may take up important sites on proteins, freeing the drug for activity.

Metabolism—Other drugs may increase or decrease drug metabolism in the liver which, in turn, may increase or decrease the amount of active drug in the blood.

Excretion—Other drugs may alter how a drug or its active metabolites are excreted through the kidney.

3.   The pharmacodynamic phase: Other drugs may compete for receptor sites, which could impair the drug's activity, or influence normal physiologic function, which could inactivate the drug or make it more toxic.

A number of drugs may interact simultaneously at several different sites so that it may be difficult to attribute interaction to a single mechanism. For example, **aspirin** could interfere with the absorption, plasma protein binding, and active renal tubular secretion of other acidic drugs, and might also increase the toxicity of oral anticoagulants through effects on bleeding time, capillary fragility, platelet adhesiveness, intrinsic inhibition of clotting factor synthesis, and production of gastrointestinal erosions and ulcers, which might bleed.

Pharmaceutic Phase: Drug Incompatibilities

Incompatibilities result from undesirable physiochemical reactions most commonly occurring as acid-base reactions or solvent effects. By judicious admixing of parenteral drugs, this phenomenon can usually be avoided. There are two types of incompatibilities: visual and chemical.

Visual incompatibilities most often result from inadequate solubility and from acid-base reactions which produce poorly soluble, nonionized drug species or coprecipitates of oppositely charged drug ions. Also called physical incompatibilities, they are typified by precipitation, color change, evolution of gas, turbidity, or cloudiness. Concentration-dependent examples include **diazepam** (Valium) diluted in 5% dextrose in water (D_5W), **pentobarbital** (Nembutal) mixed with **meperidine** (Demerol), and **phenytoin sodium** (Dilantin) added to aqueous solutions (especially of acidic pH).

Chemical incompatibilities usually entail the degradation of drugs to inactive or toxic products. These degradation products may or may not be visible. Examples of chemical incompatibilities include **gentamicin** inactivation when mixed with **carbenicillin** and hydrolysis and precipitation of **tetracycline** when mixed in solutions containing large amounts of ascorbic acid.

Nurses should use care when mixing drugs and solutions. If there is doubt, a nurse should always consult a pharmacist, package insert, or current compatibility text for relevant information about potential incompatibilities. Changes in clarity or color, the formation of crystals, or sediment in solutions after drugs are added are signs that the nurse should seek orders for alternate solutions or medicines. The following general guidelines are helpful when adding drugs to solutions:

1.   Add one drug at a time, mix the solution thoroughly, and examine it visually before adding other drugs. If possible, avoid mixing more than two drugs in one intravenous solution.

2.   Some visual incompatibilities may require a certain concentration or amount of time to develop or appear. The former may be avoided by mixing the more concentrated additive solution first, then adding the more dilute solutions. Solutions should be used within the recommended time, and a new IV solution should be mixed and hung at least every 24 h.

3.   Chemical analogs or families of drugs react similarly, though not necessarily identically. For example, **lincomycin** and **clindamycin** would be expected to have similar chemical properties.

4.   Visual incompatibilities may be difficult to detect in colored solutions such as those containing B vitamins; therefore, additives that change the color of a clear solution should be added last.

Pharmacokinetic Phase

Drug Interaction at Sites of Absorption   A drug can be inactivated or blocked from absorption in the gastrointestinal tract after administration (see Table 6-4). Some drugs will not be absorbed due to chelation or binding when given with insoluble compounds such as **cholestyramine** (Questran), **kaolin**, or **charcoal**.

Alterations in gastrointestinal tract motility or acidity can slow or hasten drug absorption. **Anticholinergics, narcotics**, and **phenothiazines** delay gastric emptying time and delay the absorption of weakly basic drugs in the small intestines. However, acidic drugs may have increased absorption in the stomach. Conversely, drugs that increase gastric motility (e.g., **cholinomimetics**) will speed the absorption of basic drugs in the small intestines and decrease the absorption of acidic drugs in the stomach.

A drug inhibiting or decreasing stomach acidity might interfere with absorption of acid drugs such as **tetracycline**. Anticholinergics and histamine H_2 receptor antagonists (**ranitidine, cimetidine**), which inhibit gastric acid secretion, can theoretically affect absorption of weak acids and bases, such as **aspirin, digoxin**, and **quinidine**. It has also been theorized that cimetidine-induced reduction of gastric acid secretion may decrease the rate of inactivation of acid-labile drugs such as **penicillin**. Whether these mechanisms produce clinically significant alterations in serum drug levels is unknown.

Nursing care plans can include assessing for drug incompatibilities, scheduling meal and drug administration times to improve absorption, documenting gastrointestinal function by observing number and quality of stools or presence of nausea or vomiting, and offering interventions that can

TABLE 6-4 Drug-Drug Absorption Interactions

PRIMARY DRUG(S)/INTERACTING DRUG(S)	MECHANISMS OF ACTION AND EFFECT	NURSING ASSESSMENT AND INTERVENTION
Lincomycin/kaolin, pectin Tetracycline/antacids, iron	Prevents antibiotic absorption by binding; decreases drug plasma level and therapeutic effect	Assess for poor antibiotic response (increased temperature, wound drainage, increased white blood cell count). Separate doses by 2 h or more.
Tetracycline, levodopa/metoclopramide (Reglan)	Increases gastric motility; increases drug absorption in small intestine; increases drug level in blood	Document signs of patient improvement (resolving infection, improved motor functions in Parkinson's disease). Observe for changes in bowel function. Monitor for adverse levodopa effects (nausea, vomiting, dyskinesia), and decrease dose if they appear.
Digoxin/metoclopramide (Reglan)	Increases gastric motility; decreases drug absorption in stomach; lowers digoxin blood level	Monitor cardiac status, digoxin plasma levels. Increase digoxin dose if levels are subtherapeutic. Consider altering dosing times.
Quinidine, weak bases/atropine, phenothiazines, narcotics, antihistamines	Delays gastric emptying time; delays absorption in small intestine	Observe for delayed drug effect. Monitor cardiac status, quinidine plasma levels. Observe for changes in bowel function. Consider discontinuing interacting drug if necessary.
Digoxin/cimetidine	Decreases gastric acidity; slows absorption in stomach	Observe for delayed drug effect. Consider alternative routes for therapy. Monitor digoxin plasma levels, cardiac status. Change drug administration time.

prevent interactions. The nurse might suggest spacing dose schedules for drugs which interact in the intestinal tract. An alternative dosage route might be considered for one of the interacting drugs.

Drug Interaction at Sites of Distribution   The major mechanism of interaction in drug distribution occurs when there is competition for protein binding sites on plasma albumin (see Table 6-5). Acidic drugs have greater affinity for albumin and thus are more likely to compete for binding sites. This competition can increase availability of free drug and,

since only free drug is active, result in increased drug effect (see Fig. 6-2). For many drugs the increased free fraction is cleared more rapidly by the liver and kidneys, however.

The clinical significance of these types of interactions is dependent upon the magnitude of protein binding of the primary drug. For example, the anticoagulant **warfarin** (Coumadin) is highly bound, with approximately 2 percent free for action. If an additional 2 percent of **warfarin** is displaced from protein, twice as much free drug is available for action. Both the anti-inflammatory agents **phenylbutazone** (Butazolidin) and **sulindac** (Clinoril) have high affinity for protein binding. When they are added to therapy which includes

TABLE 6-5 Drug-Drug Distribution Interactions

PRIMARY DRUG/INTERACTING DRUG	MECHANISMS OF ACTION AND EFFECT	NURSING ASSESSMENT AND INTERVENTION
Warfarin/phenylbutazone* Warfarin/sulindac	Displaces drug from protein binding; increases warfarin free drug levels; causes hemorrhage	Observe for bleeding sites. Monitor prothrombin time. Decrease warfarin dose, based on prothrombin times.
Tolbutamide/phenylbutazone	Displaces drug from protein binding; increases tolbutamide free drug levels; causes hypoglycemia	Monitor blood glucose levels. Counteract hypoglycemia with IV glucose or PO sugar. Decrease tolbutamide dose or stop phenylbutyazone.
Methotrexate/sulfisoxazole	Displaces drug from protein binding; increases methotrexate toxicity; suppresses bone marrow	Monitor blood platelet and whole blood cell counts. Observe for altered bleeding tendencies, increased susceptibility to infection. Avoid concurrent use.

*See also metabolism interactions.

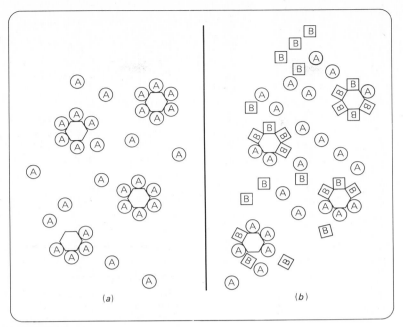

FIGURE 6-2

Schematic Representation of the Drug Interaction Due to Competition for Plasma Protein Binding Sites. (*a*) Drug A given alone is approximately 90 percent bound with 10 percent free (active drug). (*b*) The addition of drug B increases the unbound portion of drug A to 50 percent because drug B displaces drug A on the plasma protein and increases the availability of drug A to receptor sites. Metabolism and excretion of drug A may also be increased.

warfarin, the warfarin is displaced, increasing active drug and increasing the possibility of bleeding. If a drug has a wide therapeutic margin for safety, as **penicillin** does, displacement will have no significant effect on therapeutic response. If a drug is poorly bound to albumin, competition for binding sites will have little clinical significance.

Drugs do bind to protein binding sites throughout the body. Although the competition for sites other than those on albumin is not well-studied, the potential for alterations in drug pharmacokinetics at α_1-acid glycoprotein and tissue-binding sites does exist.

The nurse should monitor serum protein and albumin levels, especially if the patient is taking any drugs which are highly bound to protein (see Table 6-6) or when there is hepatic or renal impairment. If a patient has two or more drugs prescribed that are are highly bound to plasma protein (greater than 80 percent), the nurse should be alerted to the potential for drug interaction. Drug effect can be monitored by observing clinical parameters, serum levels of free drug, or tests reflecting drug action (e.g., prothrombin times in the case of **warfarin**). Standard observation of fluid balance and circulatory status, such as checking daily weight, edema, and vital signs, will alert the nurse to physical changes which will alter drug distribution and thus drug-drug distribution interactions.

Drug Interaction at Sites of Metabolism   Drug-drug interactions in drug metabolism result from the stimulation (induction) or inhibition by drugs of the drug-metabolizing enzymes, mainly in the liver. Many drugs, food substances, and environmental pollutants (e.g., DDT) are capable of altering their own metabolism and that of other drugs by stimulating or inhibiting microsomal enzymes, proteins associated with submicroscopic structures in the liver cell cytoplasm. Depending upon the dose and the drug, enzyme induction or inhibition usually develops over a period of several days to several weeks and persists for a similar period after discontinuation of the agent. If a drug changes the activity of one cytochrome P450 (microsomal) enzyme system, other drugs metabolized by that system will have altered pharmacokinetics (see Table 6-7). This can result in increased or decreased drug potency or longer or shorter duration of effect.

The clinical effects of induced or inhibited drug metab-

TABLE 6-6 Drugs That Are Highly Protein-Bound

Adjunctive agent in penicillin therapy
  Probenecid (Benemid)

Analgesics/antipyretics
  Aspirin
  Sodium salicylate

Anticoagulants
  Dicumarol
  Warfarin (Coumadin)

Antiepileptic agents
  Phenytoin (Dilantin)

Antihypertensive agents
  Diazoxide (Hyperstat IV)

Anti-inflammatory agents
  Ibuprofen (Motrin)
  Indomethacin (Indocin)
  Naproxen (Naprosyn)
  Phenylbutazone (Butazolidin)
  Sulindac (Clinoril)

Antineoplastic agents
  Methotrexate

Antiparkinsonian
  Bromocriptine

Antipsychotic
  Chlorpromazine (Thorazine)
  Haloperidol (Haldol)
  Thioridazine (Mellaril)

Cardiovascular agents
  Nifedipine (Procardia)
  Propranolol (Inderal)
  Verapamil (Calan, Isoptin)

Diuretics
  Chlorothiazide (Diuril)
  Ethacrynic acid (Edecrin)
  Furosemide (Lasix)
  Hydrochlorothiazide (HydroDIURIL, Esidrix)

Oral hypoglycemic agents
  Chlorpropamide (Diabinese)
  Tolbutamide (Orinase)

Lipid-lowering agents
  Clofibrate (Atromid-S)

Sedative/hypnotics
  Diazepam (Valium)
  Pentobarbital (Nembutal)
  Phenobarbital
  Secobarbital (Seconal)
  Thiopental (Pentothal)

olism depend upon whether the parent drug, metabolite, or both are active or inactive pharmacologically. Increased drug metabolism will lower blood levels of those drugs that are active in the parent state by altering those compounds to their less-active or inactive metabolites. The reverse is true if the metabolite is more active than the parent drug, such as in **phenylbutazone** conversion by the liver to oxyphenylbutazone (see Table 6-8).

A classic example of microsomal enzyme induction is the **phenobarbital-warfarin** combination. Patients given this combination will require larger doses of anticoagulant than is usually required to maintain a suitable state of anticoagulation, because **phenobarbital** induces the enzymes which metabolize **warfarin**. If the phenobarbital is discontinued upon hospital discharge without a decrease of the dose of anticoagulant, bleeding may occur. For drugs that have a low therapeutic index, such as **quinidine** and **warfarin**, this interaction has important clinical implications.

Inhibition of liver enzymes (usually causing a more-potent drug) is thought to occur by saturation of the available liver enzymes. **Cimetidine** (Tagamet) inhibits the microsomal oxidative enzyme system and increases blood levels of **warfarin, theophylline, propranolol** (Inderal), **phenytoin** (Dilantin), **carbamazepine** (Tegretol), **caffeine, diazepam** (Valium), and **chlordiazepoxide** (Librium).

Since alcohol use and abuse are widespread, the complex role that they play in drug interactions deserve discussion. Alcohol can both induce the liver enzymes and competitively inhibit metabolism of other drugs. The *acutely* intoxicated alcoholic with high blood alcohol levels will have potentiated effects from other drugs metabolized by the liver, since metabolism is decreased (inhibited). In the chronic, but *sober,* alcoholic there is decreased drug effect, since alcohol is an inducer of drug metabolism. This is why the rowdy inebriated person given **phenobarbital** for its sedative effect seems to sleep for days. As the alcohol blood level drops, and the patient awakes, large amounts of phenobarbital are needed to have any tranquilizing effect. Smoking tobacco or marijuana can also induce liver enzymes and interact with drugs in a clinically significant way. For example, smokers will require larger doses of **theophylline** to achieve therapeutic serum concentrations than will nonsmokers.

Adequate health history from patients regarding factors such as drinking and smoking habits and occupational exposures to chemicals can help identify potential interactions. Assessing prior drug effects (by asking at what dosage and how soon were previous drugs effective and with what combination of drugs) may point up susceptibility to alteration of liver enzyme function. Plasma drug levels can be com-

TABLE 6-7 Drugs That Alter Liver Metabolism

INDUCER	DRUGS WHOSE METABOLISM IS ENHANCED	INHIBITOR	DRUGS WHOSE METABOLISM IS INHIBITED
Barbiturates (e.g., phenobarbital)	Corticosteroids Doxycycline Griseofulvin Oral contraceptives Quinidine Warfarin	Cimetidine	Chlordiazepoxide Diazepam Flurazepam Phenytoin Quinidine Theophylline Warfarin
Carbamazepine	Doxycycline Warfarin	Disulfiram	Chlordiazepoxide Diazepam Phenytoin
Corticosteroids	Isoniazid		
Ethchlorvynol, glutethemide	Warfarin	Erythromycin	Carbamazepine Corticosteroids Theophylline
Griseofulvin	Warfarin		
Phenytoin	Corticosteroids Doxycycline Quinidine	Oral contraceptives	Carbamazepine Chlordiazepoxide Corticosteroids
Rifampin	Chlorpropamide Clofibrate Corticosteroids Diazepam Methadone Metoprolol Oral contraceptives Propranolol Quinidine Tolbutamide Warfarin		Diazepam Metoprolol Phenytoin Propranolol Theophylline
		Phenylbutazone, oxyphenbutazone	Phenytoin Tolbutamide Warfarin
		Sulfonamides	Phenytoin Warfarin

TABLE 6-8 Drug-Drug Metabolism Interactions

PRIMARY DRUG / INTERACTING DRUG	MECHANISMS OF ACTION AND EFFECT	NURSING ASSESSMENT AND INTERVENTION
Warfarin / phenylbutazone*	Inhibits metabolism; increases warfarin plasma levels; causes hemorrhage	Monitor prothrombin times. Decrease warfarin dose accordingly. Observe for sites of bleeding. Discontinue phenylbutazone if necessary.
Propranolol / cimetidine	Inhibits metabolism; decreases liver blood flow; increases blood levels of propranolol; increases cardiovascular effects	Monitor cardiac status. Monitor propranolol drug levels. Decrease propranolol as necessary. Discontinue cimetidine if clinically significant changes are occurring (bradycardia, CHF, atrioventricular block, GI upset).
Oral contraceptives / tetracycline	Alters enterohepatic circulation of steroids, including estrogens; decreases estrogen availability; decreases contraceptive effectiveness	Educate patients on alternative or supportive contraceptive methods while on tetracycline.

*See also distribution interactions.

pared with standard therapeutic ranges, and observations can be made for expected effects of a given dose. If the expected duration of drug effect is less or more than that reported in the literature, the nurse might suspect interactions at metabolic sites. If a patient has taken two known interacting drugs in the hospital, discharge preparation should include discontinuing one drug several days prior to the patient's going home, or maintaining the same doses of drugs upon discharge. In either case, *the nurse will ensure that the patient knows the signs of drug overdose or therapeutic failure and understands the importance of informing care providers of all drugs being taken, the need to keep appointments for reevaluations of drug therapy, and the dangers of discontinuing or adding any medication without consulting a health care provider.*

Drug Interaction at Sites of Excretion Potentials for interactions exist if drugs either alkalinize or acidify the urine (see Table 6-9). For example, **acetazolamide** (Diamox), **triamterene** (Dyrenium), **sodium bicarbonate**, and **sodium citrate** are all alkalinizing agents, while **ammonium chloride**, ammonium nitrate, **calcium chloride**, and salicylates (**aspirin**) are acidifying agents. This drug interaction potential can be used to therapeutic advantage; for example, a **phenobarbital** overdose can be partly treated through increased excretion of the drug by alkalinization of the urine. In general, if less than 20 percent of the active drug is normally excreted in the urine, the urinary excretion of the drug is not likely to be very sensitive to changes in urinary pH.

Competition for tubular secretion is another mechanism of drug interaction in the kidney. The classic example is the action of **probenecid**, which blocks tubular secretion of **pen-icillin**, creating the beneficial effects of more-sustained penicillin blood levels. Other drugs that interact in this way include **sulfonamide antibiotics, thiazide diuretics, chlorpropamide** (Diabinese), and **salicylates.**

Many drugs damage the glomerular membranes and alter excretion of drugs dependent upon this route of elimination (see Chap. 31). Impaired kidney function will result in increased serum blood levels, which can be clinically significant with drugs like **digoxin**, which are primarily renally excreted and have narrow therapeutic ranges. The adequacy of renal blood flow, based upon cardiac and vascular function, will determine how well the drug is delivered to the kidney for excretion.

Urinary pH testing should be performed when a pH-dependent drug interaction is suspected. When nephrotoxic drugs are given, serum levels can be monitored to prevent kidney damage. Kidney function can be assessed by presence of proteinuria, serum urea nitrogen, creatinine levels, and urine output (average 1.5 L/day). Assessment of cardiovascular function and patient weights will help determine if blood supply and circulation are adequate for the filtration process.

Pharmacodynamic Phase: Drug Interaction at Receptor Sites

Interactions can take place at receptor sites and cell membrane, creating either additive, synergistic, or antagonistic effects. Drugs are said to be *additive* if their effects, when the drugs are given together, are equal to the sum of their independent effects. If the effects of two drugs given concurrently are greater than the sum of their independent

TABLE 6-9 Drug-Drug Excretion Interactions

PRIMARY DRUG/INTERACTING DRUG(S)	MECHANISMS OF ACTION AND EFFECT	NURSING ASSESSMENT AND INTERVENTION
Aspirin/sodium bicarbonate	Alkalinizes urine; increases aspirin excretion; lowers blood levels of aspirin; has beneficial effect in severe salicylate toxicity	Observe for decreased therapeutic benefits from aspirin therapy unless treatment is for toxicity. Monitor urinary pH level.
Quinidine/mandelic acid	Acidifies urine; increases quinidine excretion; lowers blood levels of quinidine	Observe for decreased therapeutic effect of quinidine. Monitor cardiac status and quinidine blood levels. Increase quinidine dose or discontinue it; decrease dose of interacting drug. Monitor urine pH.
Digoxin/gentamicin, kanamycin	Damages or alters glomerular membranes (effect is caused by the aminoglycosides gentamicin and kanamycin); decreases excretion of digoxin; causes digoxin toxicity	Monitor cardiac status and digoxin blood levels. Monitor kidney function (blood chemistries, urine output). Monitor antibiotic level. Decrease digoxin dose as necessary. Possibly change to less-nephrotoxic antibiotic.
Lidocaine/propranolol	Competes for tubular secretion; decreases renal clearance of lidocaine; causes lidocaine toxicity	Monitor cardiac status. Monitor blood levels of lidocaine and propranolol. Decrease doses. Discontinue one drug and use alternative therapy.

effects, the drugs are considered to act *synergistically*. On the other other hand, two drugs are *antagonistic* if some effect of one is less when both are given than when one is taken alone. (See Chap. 5 for definitions of the types of antagonism.)

The effects of the combination of **antihistamines** and the antiarrhythmic **disopyramide** (Norpace), which both have anticholinergic effects, on parasympathetic function such as bladder contractility are additive. If an elderly man with prostatic enlargement were taking only disopyramide, he might experience urinary hesitancy, but if he added an over-the-counter antihistamine to treat cold symptoms, he could develop severe urinary retention. Some **penicillin** antibiotics are used with **aminoglycoside** antibiotics for their synergistic effects, resulting in far greater antibacterial action than when either is given alone. It is thought that penicillins damage the bacterial cell wall to increase the permeation of the aminoglycosides to their site of action.

An example of competitive antagonism which is used to therapeutic advantage is the treatment of narcotic overdose with the narcotic antagonist **naloxone** (Narcan), which competes for and blocks opiate receptors. Other pharmacodynamic interactions can lead to drug toxicity by acting at different receptors or altering a physiologic process related to drug action (see Table 6-10).

When drugs are added to a regimen, observations for enhanced or decreased physiologic effect can give the nurse clues to this type of drug-drug interaction. The most effective patient care plan is to monitor drug effect and duration through observation of clinical parameters specific to the drug's action. The nurse must suggest alternate drugs or cessation of therapy if severe ADRs occur.

Drug–Laboratory Test Interaction

The clinical laboratory plays an important role in both diagnostic and preventive medicine. With the increasing numbers of available medications and the potential of these drugs to interfere with laboratory test results, it is becoming increasingly difficult to evaluate laboratory test data without considering drug effects (see Table 6-11). There are basically two types of drug-laboratory interactions. The first is a change in the laboratory result that reflects a pharmacologic or toxicologic effect of a drug. Here, an *actual physiologic change* is produced by the drug in the parameter being measured. For example, **thiazide diuretics** cause hyperuricemia or hyperglycemia, and there are electrocardiographic changes in patients secondary to **digitalis** preparations. Another type of drug-laboratory interaction results from an *interference with the actual test procedure* and is usually more mechanical in nature. The drug or its metabolite becomes a contaminant. It may alter the components of body fluids or interact with the chemicals necessary for assay, creating error in results.

When unexpected or unanticipated laboratory results occur, the test should be repeated and/or the possibility of drug interference should be considered prior to changing patient drugs or care plans. If there is more than one method that can be used to perform the test, the method that is not affected should be used. The nurse can find resources for knowledge in this area from both pharmacists and the clinical laboratory specialists performing the tests.

Drug-Food Interaction

Though much has been published regarding drug interactions, there remains insufficient documentation of drug-food interactions and their clinical significance. Food can increase or decrease drug absorption and excretion (see Table 6-12). Some drugs are administered with foods to decrease the irritation of the gastrointestinal tract that the drugs may cause. Certain foods contain pharmacoactive substances capable of inducing enzymatic systems. Acid-labile drugs can be degraded in vitro in a weakly acidic vehicle, such as orange juice, as well as in the stomach.

Effects of Food on Drug Absorption Food affects absorption by influencing blood flow, solubility, gastric emptying time, and the physical characteristics of the gastrointestinal contents and epithelial lining. Probably one of the best-

TABLE 6-10 Drug-Drug Pharmacodynamic Interactions

PRIMARY DRUG / INTERACTING DRUG	MECHANISMS OF ACTION AND EFFECT	NURSING ASSESSMENT AND INTERVENTION
Digoxin / verapamil	Has additive effects on atrioventricular (AV) node of heart; prolongs QT interval on ECG	Monitor ECG for irregularities in cardiac rhythm. Monitor vital signs. Consider decreasing dose of verapamil or digoxin.
Propranolol / verapamil	Has additive effects on AV node of heart; prolongs QT interval on ECG; causes arrhythmias	Monitor ECG for irregularities in cardiac rhythm. Monitor vital signs. Decrease propranolol or verapamil doses.
Digoxin / chlorothiazide	Decreases potassium blood levels secondary to chlorothiazide; increases digoxin toxicity	Monitor serum electrolytes. Replace potassium if low. Monitor digoxin blood level. Monitor cardiac function. Decrease digoxin dose if necessary.

TABLE 6-11 A Few Examples of Effects of Common Drugs on Frequent Laboratory Tests

↑ = increased or positive results   x = pharmacologic effect of drug
↓ = decreased or negative results   * = drug interference with test

DRUG	BLOOD, SERUM, OR PLASMA TESTS												URINE TESTS				
	AMYLASE	BILIRUBIN	CHOLESTEROL	COOMBS' (DIRECT)	GLUCOSE	PHOSPHATASE (ALK)	POTASSIUM	PROTHROMBIN TIME	SGOT, SGPT[a]	THYROXINE	UREA NITROGEN	URIC ACID	CATECHOLAMINES	COLOR	GLUCOSE (BENEDICT'S)	PORPHYRINS	PROTEINS
Acetazolamide (Diamox)	x↑						x↓					x↑					*↑
Alcohol, ethyl	x↑	x↓	x↑		x↓			x↓	x↑			x↑	x↑	x↓		x↑	
Barbiturates	x↓	x↓				x↑		x↑								x↑	
Cephalosporins				*↑		x↑			x↑		x↑				*↑		
Chlorpropamide (Diabinese)		x↑	x↓	*↑	x↓	x↑			x↑	x↓						*↑	
Furosemide	x↑				x↑	x↑	x↓				x↑	x↑					
Indomethacin (Indocin)	x↑			*↑	x↓	x↑	x↑		x↑		x↑						
Oral contraceptives	x↑	x↑	x↑		x↑	x↑			x↑	x↑						x↑	
Phenytoin (Dilantin)		x↑↓			x↑	x↑			x↑	x↓				*↑			
Salicylates	x↓	x↑	x↓		x↑↓	x↑	x↓	x↑	x↑	x↑↓		x↑↓	x↓		*↑		*↑

[a]SGOT = serum glutamic oxaloacetic transaminase. SGPT = serum glutamic pyruvic transaminase.

TABLE 6-12 Drug-Food Interactions

DRUG	EFFECT OF FOOD	COMMENTS
Anti-infectives		
Erythromycin		
Base and stearate	Extent of absorption is decreased with food. Drug is unstable in acidic foods.	This is an example of where formulation and ionization influence interaction between drugs and food; it is probably best to administer drug on a fasting stomach, except for ethyl succinate salt.*
Enteric coated	Basic foods may cause premature dissolution in stomach, causing increased degradation and stomach irritation.	
Ethyl succinate	Extent of absorption is increased by food.	
Tetracycline	Administration with food decreases extent of absorption. Polyvalent ions (Ca^{2+}, Mg^{2+}, Fe^{2+}, Al^{3+}) present in milk, food, and antacids chelate most tetracyclines, decreasing solubility and net absorption. Iron salts have been shown to inhibit tetracycline absorption.	It is best to give drug on a fasting stomach with a full glass of water to decrease stomach irritation.*

Anti-inflammatory agents, nonsteroidal
    Phenylbutazone (Butazolidin)
    Ibuprofen (Motrin)
    Indomethacin (Indocin)
	Food helps decrease GI irritation caused by these drugs.	Administer with food.

Digoxin	Foods containing Ca^{2+} can bind digitalis glycosides, decreasing amount absorbed.	Avoid milk and antacids 1 h before and 2–3 h after digitalis dose.
Ferrous compounds	Food tends to decrease amount of irritation to GI tract caused by these compounds. However, elemental iron absorption is decreased 20%–40% when given with food.	It is probably best to administer drug with food only if patient has a problem with side effects, with decreased absorption to be taken into consideration.
Griseofulvin	Fatty meals tend to increase extent of absorption.	Higher blood levels will be achieved when drug is administered with meals.
Hydralazine (Apresoline)	Studies show that 2–3 times as much drug enters bloodstream when taken with food.	Clinical significance is not established, but smaller doses may be required if taken with food.
Levodopa	Food, by delaying stomach emptying, causes increased degradation in stomach, decreasing amount of drug available for absorption. Nausea and vomiting are common side effects that are decreased when drug is administered with a food. Food high in protein has been associated with poorer responses to drug; this may be due to competition with amino acids for neuromembrane transport. Vitamin B_6 in food tends to reverse effects of drug, possibly by decreasing levels of levodopa available for transport into central nervous system.	Not all patients are affected by vitamin B_6 and high-protein meals, but patient's diet should be reviewed for these possibilities if condition becomes refractory. Administer drug on a fasting stomach, in view of instability at low pH, unless nausea and vomiting are intolerable.*

Monoamine oxidase inhibitors
    Nialamide (Niamid)
    Pargyline (Eutonyl)
    Phenelzine (Nardil)
    Tranylcypromine (Parnate)
    Isocarboxazid (Marplan)
	Foods containing tyramine cause peripheral release of norepinephrine and can cause hypertensive crisis.	Patients should be advised to avoid foods with a high content of tyramine, which include aged foods.

Propranolol, metoprolol	Food given at time of administration tends to increase blood levels; this may be due to increased splanchnic blood flow during meals, decreasing first-pass effects.	Clinical significance is not established yet; however, it should be realized that consistency in meal timing and dosing can influence amount in body.

*A fasting stomach is defined as occurring 1 h before meals or 2–3 h after meals.

known drug-food interactions exists between **tetracycline** and milk products, where calcium ions chelate tetracycline into insoluble complexes that are not absorbed. Foods that affect gut pH have effects on the absorption of acidic or basic drugs that are similar to the effects of drugs that potentially alter gut pH.

Change in the rate of gastric emptying is probably the most important effect of food. Any substance in the stomach delays emptying and generally delays the rate of drug absorption. A good example of this occurs when certain **penicillin** antibiotics are administered with meals. Food delays gastric emptying, and a greater amount of the acid-labile antibiotic is degraded in the acidic stomach. There are instances where a delay in stomach emptying will increase the rate of absorption. **Ketoconazole**, a new antifungal agent, will be absorbed to a greater extent when taken shortly after a meal because of the drug's increased solubility in an acid medium.

Pharmacoactive Foods　One of the most publicized food-drug interactions occurs in patients using monoamine oxidase (MAO) inhibitors. These antidepression drugs inhibit enzymes responsible for the inactivation of catecholamines, particularly norepinephrine. If a patient on a MAO inhibitor ingests food containing tyramine (such as aged cheddar cheese and red wines), norepinephrine is displaced from nerve terminals and a potential hypertensive crisis can ensue.

The vitamin K content in leafy green vegetables can be responsible for reversal of oral anticoagulant therapy. **Warfarin** (Coumadin) acts as a competitive inhibitor of vitamin K–dependent clotting factor synthesis, and an increase in vitamin K can overcome drug action.

Effects of Food on Drug Elimination　By changing urine pH, foods can affect renal elimination of weakly acidic or basic drugs. Drug metabolism can also be affected by the induction of liver enzymes. Pesticides such as DDT and aldrin have been shown to induce these enzymes when ingestion of contaminated food occurs. Charcoal-broiled beef can also induce metabolizing enzymes and has been shown to decrease the half-life of **theophylline**, although the clinical significance of this has been questioned.

Effects of Food on GI-Irritating Drugs　Many drugs are irritating to gastrointestinal (GI) mucosa and cause nausea, vomiting, and diarrhea. To decrease or eliminate these discomforts, these drugs are usually administered with food, which tends to protect the epithelial lining of the gastric mucosa. Some drugs, such as salicylates, are known gastric irritants, and some preparations are enteric coated with a hard shell that is designed to resist dissolution in the acidic stomach and will dissolve only in the more neutral pH of the small intestine. Food and drugs that increase gastric pH, such as milk or antacids, may cause enteric coated drugs to dissolve in the stomach when administered concomitantly with these preparations.

Nursing Intervention in Drug-Food Interactions　Dietary management of a patient in conjunction with drug therapy has been a somewhat neglected area in general medical practice as well as in nursing care plans because of the scant information about drug-food interactions. However, dietary documentation, including what and when a patient eats, is an important nursing function related to drug therapy.

Nursing care plans can include dietary consultation if the patient is on many drugs or drugs known to interact with foods. This is especially important with elderly patients, who sometimes have unusual eating habits due to physical or social incapabilities (e.g., no teeth, low income, or poor home supervision). Special attention to food intake must be given to patients on antibiotics, since this group of drugs have better-known interactions with foods. Timing might be a problem with drug orders given as ac (before meals) or pc (after meals) when the patient's food is delayed because of npo (nothing by mouth) status for tests and examinations. In such instances, clarification of the medication order with the physician or consultation with a pharmacist will help determine proper drug and food administration times. Finally, discharge plans will include patient education on drug-food interactions where appropriate, with follow-up reinforcement at each outpatient visit.

NURSING PROCESS RELATED TO ADRs

Assessment

Aspects of the medication history particularly pertinent to prevention of adverse effects include: (1) a list of the patient's diagnoses, particularly those with implications for drug absorption, distribution, metabolism, and excretion, (2) a complete drug history including use of over-the-counter drugs, "culprit drugs" frequently implicated in ADRs (antibiotics, birth control pills, steroids, anticonvulsants, anticoagulants, antiarthritics, sedative-hypnotics), and social drugs (such as coffee, tea, tobacco, marijuana, alcohol), (3) a record of exposure to chemicals and pollutants, and (4) a description of prior ADRs.

Patients on drug therapy must also be closely monitored to detect ADRs. The monitoring can be performed by pharmacists, physicians, and/or nurses. Ideally, the system for monitoring ADRs should use an interdisciplinary approach.

Management

The implications for nursing action vary with the type of adverse reaction. Not all ADRs require the drug to be withheld or discontinued. However, the nurse is often the first person to identify ADRs, and the initial nursing intervention is extremely important to the ultimate outcome. If an event seems life-threatening or poses a risk to the well-being of the patient, the nurse *should* withhold the offending drug and notify the physician of the reaction. Even if the drug therapy is eventually reinstated, the nurse will have performed a function that meets professional, legal, and ethical standards.

If desired drug effects do not appear within a reasonable time period, or intolerable ADRs occur, the nurse can review the steps in drug and patient assessment for interventions that might have been overlooked. If conservative methods to increase or decrease drug action are not successful, alternative routes of drug administration, alternative drugs, or drug discontinuation could be considered through consultation with the physician. Other drug therapy might be added to decrease uncomfortable side effects, but the added potential for drug interactions must be weighed against the anticipated benefits.

Patient education of the risks for and symptoms of ADRs should be included in patient care plans. Patients should be encouraged to recognize and report suspected side effects. Nurses also should recognize that patients, as consumers, have a right to know about their medications, and nurses must provide this information. In addition, as patients become more aware of what the outcome of therapy should be, they will not allow the wrong medication or the improper dose to be administered, thus avoiding medication errors and other ADRs.

Evaluation

One of the major problems in controlling ADRs is recognizing their occurrence and evaluating their significance. Since patients are often on multiple drugs and there can be overlap between disease symptoms and symptoms of ADR, the process is difficult to evaluate. For example, infection is manifested by fever, but elevated temperatures can also occur with allergic drug responses. The accepted method of documenting a given sign or symptom as an ADR of a drug is to stop the drug and restart it after a "washout" period. However, this "drug challenge" is not always in the best interest of the patient when the symptom is serious (a suspected hepatotoxicity, for example) or causes significant patient discomfort. Many prescribers simply stop the drug and presume the symptoms or signs were drug-related if they subsequently subside.

Unfortunately, information regarding a drug's mechanisms of action or potential for ADRs is not available for all drugs. Duration of drug action and potentials for drug inter-actions are dependent upon highly variable factors. However, the nurse can weigh the probabilities of an interaction or adverse reaction of a particular drug by comparing it with drugs having similar actions, similar chemical compositions, or similar dispositions in the body.

Accurate description of the onset and duration of drug action after drug administration will help to assess drug effectiveness and nursing management in improving drug therapy. Documentation of drug action in relationship to drug dose and dosing schedules will not only identify effectiveness of therapy, but also may add to information on drugs and drug interactions under specific circumstances and clinical conditions. Drug treatment flow sheets allow such correlation of patient factors, drug administration, and drug effect. These flow sheets could include such information as laboratory data, drug plasma levels, vital signs, and psychologic and physiologic responses.

Finally, extending drug knowledge and applying it to the clinical setting will improve the way drugs are used. It is obvious that for one to know the effects of each and every available drug is an impossibility. It is possible, however, to know the effects and consequences of the drug that is just about to be given. Professional teamwork can provide a means for nurses, pharmacists, and physicians to share drug information. Bedside rounds, with patient consent and participation, can be an ideal learning approach. Multidisciplinary clinical conferences demonstrating drug effects in real patients with real problems can improve knowledge about drug therapy and ADRs.

CONCLUSION

Although all drugs have a potential for causing adverse effects, most ADRs are predictable and can be prevented. The nurse can contribute to safe drug use by assessing factors which might contribute to the development of ADRs, monitoring drug effects in all patients, and evaluating the outcomes of drug therapy. The nurse who is alert to the ever-present potential for ADRs in the clinical setting can avoid costly and dangerous adverse effects of drug therapy for patients.

REFERENCES

Bressler, R.: "Interactions Between Drugs," in P. B. Beeson and W. McDermott (eds.), *Cecil Textbook of Medicine,* 16th ed., Philadelphia: Saunders, 1982.

——, and J. Palmer: "Drug Interactions in the Aged," in W. E. Fann (ed.), *Drug Issues in Geropsychiatry,* Baltimore: Williams & Wilkins, 1974.

Broughton, L., and H. Rogers: "Decreased Systemic Clearance of Caffeine due to Cimetidine," *Br J Clin Pharmacol,* 12:155–159, 1981.

Carter, S.: "Potential Effect of Sulindac on Response of Prothrombin Time to Oral Anticoagulants," *Lancet* 2:698–699, 1979.

Davis, D. M. (ed.): *Textbook of Adverse Drug Reactions,* Oxford: Oxford University Press, 1977.

Dickerson, J.: "Adverse Reactions of New Drugs and What the Nurse Can Do About Them," *Nurses' Drug Alert,* 5:59–62, 1981.

Dukes, M. N. G. (ed.): *Meyler's Side Effects of Drugs,* 9th ed., Amsterdam: Excerpta Medica, 1980.

Gilman, A. G., L. S. Goodman, and A. Gilman (eds.): *Goodman and Gilman's The Pharmacological Basis of Therapeutics,* 6th ed., New York: Macmillan, 1980.

Graham, C., W. Turner, and J. Jones: "Lidocaine-Propranolol Interactions," *N Eng J Med,* 304:1301, 1981.

Hansten, P.: *Drug Interactions,* 4th ed., Philadelphia: Lea & Febiger, 1979.

Hoover, R., and J. F. Fraumeni: "Drug-induced Cancer," *Cancer,* 47:1071–1080, 1981.

Janz, D., and D. Schmidt: "Anti-epileptic Drugs and Failure of Oral Contraceptives," *Lancet* 1:1113, 1974.

Katcher, B. S., L. U. Young, and M. A. Koda-Kimble (eds.): *Applied Therapeutics: The Clinical Use of Drugs,* 3d ed., San Francisco: Applied Therapeutics, 1983.

Keller, N. S.: "Private Nursing Practice: Some Facilitators and Barriers in Health Care," in M. Leininger (ed.), *Barriers and Facilitators to Quality Health Care,* Philadelphia: Davis, 1975.

Lambert, M. L., Jr.: "Drug and Diet Interactions," *Am J Nurs,* 75:402–406, 1975.

Martin, E. W.: *Hazards of Medication,* 2d ed., Philadelphia: Lippincott, 1978.

Meyler, L., and A. Herxheimer (eds.), *Side Effects of Drugs,* Amsterdam: Excerpta Medica, 1976.

Miller, R. R., and D. J. Greenblatt (eds.): *Drug Effects in Hospitalized Patients,* New York: Wiley, 1976.

Newton, D. W.: "Physiochemical Determinants of Incompatibility and Instability in Injectable Drug Solutions and Admixtures," in *Handbook on Injectable Drugs,* Washington: American Society of Hospital Pharmacists, 1980.

Notelovitz, M., J. Tjapkes, and M. Ware: "Interactions between Estrogen and Dilantin in Menopausal Women," *N Engl J Med,* 304:788–789, 1981.

Petrie, J. C., et al.: "Awareness and Experience of General Practitioners of Selected Drug Interaction," *Br Med J,* 2:262–264, May 4, 1974.

Prescott, L. F.: "Clinically Important Drug Interactions," in G. S. Avery (ed.), *Drug Treatment,* Sydney: ADIS, 1976.

Resnekov L.: "Calcium Antagonistic Drugs: Myocardial Preservation and Reduced Vulnerability to Ventricular Fibrillation During CPR," *Crit Care Med,* 9:360–361, 1981.

Tobey, L. E., and T. R. Covington: "Antimicrobial Drug Interactions," *Am J Nurs,* 75:1470–1473, 1975.

Trinca, C., et al.: "The Drug Surveillance Program at the Arizona Medical Center," *Ariz Med,* 32:701–712, 1975.

Tweddel, A., et al.: "The Combination of Nifidipine and Propranolol in the Management of Patients with Angina Pectoris," *Br J Clin Pharmacol,* 12:229–233, 1981.

Wade, O. L., and L. Beeley: *Adverse Reactions to Drugs,* London: Heineman, 1976.

Yaw Twun-Barma, S., and G. Carruthers: "Quinidine-Rifampin Interactions," *N Engl J Med,* 304:1466–1469, 1981.

7

PHARMACOTHERAPEUTICS THROUGH THE LIFE SPAN*

BETTY JENNINGS
JOHN F. TOURVILLE
GINETTE A. PEPPER

Age is an important determinant of drug pharmacokinetics, the type and magnitude of adverse drug reactions, appropriate drug administration techniques, and the best approaches to patient education. However, it is the physical and psychologic development of an individual, rather than age per se, that influences drug response. This chapter addresses several important phases of development in which clinical pharmacology and therapeutics may differ from those in the young adult population (generally between 20 and 50 years of age), on whom most drug studies are done.

It is important to keep in mind that development is a continuous process and there are differences among persons assumed to be in the same developmental phase. In the newborn, renal function changes almost daily. Although anyone over 65 years is often identified as elderly, the physiology and psychology of a 65-year-old is very different from that of an 85-year-old. At each trimester of pregnancy the implications of drug therapy, for maternal response and teratogenesis, are profoundly different.

PREGNANCY AND LACTATION

LEARNING OBJECTIVES

Upon mastery of the contents of this section, the reader will be able to:

1. Describe how the physiology of pregnancy alters drug pharmacokinetics.
2. Explain the principles of placental transfer of drugs.

---

*Betty Jennings wrote the section on pregnancy and lactation. John F. Tourville contributed the section on infants and children. Ginette A. Pepper wrote the section on elderly adults.

3. Outline how fetal anatomy and physiology affects disposition of transplacentally acquired drugs.
4. Describe drug pharmacokinetics in human lactation.
5. List the variables that influence the effects of fetal drug exposure.
6. State nursing actions to minimize maternal, fetal, and breast-fed infant adverse drug effects.

In the presence of disease or complications of pregnancy, the pregnant woman's health may be dependent on drug use, yet the drugs affect two patients: the woman and her developing fetus, whose response to therapy cannot be directly observed and may not be fully measured until birth, during infancy, or even later in life. Likewise, the newborn must eliminate drugs acquired transplacentally during labor or birth. Drug use by a lactating woman may also have a deleterious effect on the infant.

PREGNANCY PHARMACOKINETICS

Maternal drug response during pregnancy and fetal drug exposure are dependent upon several factors:

1. The characteristics of the drug
2. The amount of drug administered to the pregnant woman
3. The effects of pregnancy-induced alterations in the physiology of absorption, distribution, and elimination of the drug in the mother
4. The amount of drug crossing the placenta, both from the mother to the fetus and vice versa
5. The possible role of drug metabolism by the placenta and fetal liver
6. The distribution and elimination of the drug by the fetus

Due to the potential for interaction between these variables, it is difficult to make simple predictions concerning dosage requirements and outcomes of drug use in pregnancy. In schematic form, Fig. 7-1 summarizes the pharmacokinetic processes in the maternal-placental-fetal system. The clinical significance of these processes can only be postulated in this chapter, while precise therapeutic implications remain to be elucidated by future research.

Maternal Physiology

Ingestion and Absorption

Nausea and vomiting may reduce drug ingestion and absorption, particularly during the first trimester of pregnancy. Gastric and intestinal tone and motility are generally believed to be decreased during pregnancy, because of the effect of progesterone. Hydrochloric acid secretion decreases during the first and second trimesters and increases during the third trimester. The most likely net effect of these changes would be a slower, yet enhanced, gut absorption with a delayed peak effect. Clincally, this would be important only when rapid onset was desirable.

Distribution

During normal pregnancy, plasma volume increases approximately 50 percent. Additionally, weight gain averages 10 to 12 kg over the entire gestation. Thus, once absorbed, a drug is diluted to a greater extent in the expanded plasma volume and increased body water and fat. Drug dosage requirements would be expected to be greater to achieve the same therapeutic effect than when the same woman was not pregnant, if this effect were not offset by other pharmacokinetic changes of pregnancy.

Protein Binding   Plasma expansion during pregnancy creates a physiologic hypoalbuminemia; the rate of albumin production is increased, but serum albumin concentration decreases because of plasma volume expansion. Further, many binding sites are occupied by hormones and other endogenous substances. The overall effect of decreased serum albumin concentration in pregnancy is to decrease the capacity for albumin binding of drugs and thus make more unbound, or free, drugs available for therapeutic or adverse effects and for placental transfer. As bound drug is inactive, the increased unbound portion of otherwise highly bound drugs may cause the pregnant woman to have an increased drug effect. Notable examples of drugs found in vitro to have increased unbound fractions during pregnancy include **diazepam**, **valproic acid**, **phenytoin**, **phenobarbital**, **lidocaine**, **meperidine**, **dexamethasone**, **propranolol**, **salicylic acid**, and **sulfisoxazole**. As free drug is also eliminated more rapidly in vivo, the steady state concentration of free drug is probably not altered, unless the unbound portion exceeds the body's capacity to eliminate the drug, as would occur in renal or liver disease.

Liver Metabolism

Blood flow to the liver is probably not decreased in pregnancy, but degradation of drugs by liver microsomal enzymes may be decreased. Stasis of bile in the liver is an effect of high estrogen levels in pregnancy, and drug clearance by biliary excretion would be delayed. Thus, physiologic changes of pregnancy in the liver may alter drug metabolism, but the extent cannot be quantified.

Excretion

Renal plasma flow increases 25 to 50 percent and glomerular filtration rate increases 50 percent in pregnancy secondary to increased cardiac output. These changes can increase the excretion of drugs by the kidney, especially of those drugs, such as the **penicillins**, **digoxin**, and **lithium carbonate**, which are excreted primarily unchanged in urine. In late pregnancy the weight of the uterus can decrease renal plasma flow in the supine position, resulting in prolonged effects of these drugs. This has implications for appropriate positioning of the laboring woman to facilitate drug elimination.

Placental Transfer

Placental Gate

Although the term *placental barrier* is still in use, increased knowledge has demonstrated that the placenta poses very little barrier between mother and fetus. In fact, the placental barrier at term is but a few cells thick and constitutes little mechanical barrier to drug transfer.

Drug Characteristics

Placental transfer of drugs is dependent upon the drug chemical properties of protein binding, molecular weight, ionization, and lipid solubility. The mechanism of placental drug transfer is primarily passive diffusion, so protein-bound drugs do not cross the placenta.

Molecular Weight   Substances with molecular weights less than 600 cross the placenta with ease, and most drugs have molecular weights of 250 to 500. However, this is not absolute, since some high-molecular-weight substances such as **gamma globulin** and **digoxin** cross the placenta and a few small molecules do not.

Ionization   Highly ionized substances do not cross the placenta readily. **Succinylcholine**, a highly ionized muscle relaxant commonly used during Cesarean birth, does not cross the placenta to any significant degree. Likewise, **heparin** undergoes little placental transfer.

Most drugs used in pregnancy are weak bases. Since fetal blood pH is around 7.3, compared with maternal blood pH of 7.44, such basic drugs tend to be "trapped" in the fetal blood. If administered in higher dosage ranges, even ionized

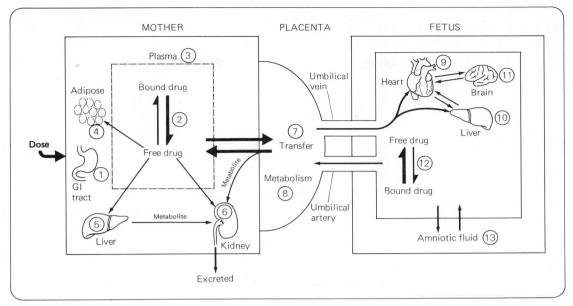

FIGURE 7-1

Drug Disposition in the Maternal-Placental-Fetal System. Numbers correspond to factors which potentially influence pharmacokinetics and drug effects on mother and fetus: (1) possible altered maternal absorption, (2) an increased maternal free drug fraction, (3) increased maternal plasma volume, (4) increased adipose secondary to maternal weight gain, (5) decreased maternal liver enzyme function, (6) increased maternal renal blood flow, (7) placental transfer of low-weight and lipid-soluble drugs (8) possible placental metabolism, (9) fetal circulation preferential to heart and brain, (10) low fetal liver enzyme activity, (11) an undeveloped fetal blood-brain barrier, (12) increased fetal free drug fraction, (13) recirculation of drugs excreted into amniotic fluid.

drugs can cross the placenta in significant amounts. For example, although **aspirin** is nearly 100 percent ionized at plasma pH, it crosses the placenta readily, because the nonionized portion is highly lipid-soluble.

Solubility Lipid-soluble substances cross the placenta easily. An unbound, nonionized drug of molecular weight less than 1000 is usually lipid-soluble and will rapidly penetrate the tissues which separate maternal and fetal circulations. Therefore, such drugs as **gaseous anesthetics, narcotics, ethanol,** and many of the drugs used in psychiatry will readily cross the placenta.

Placental Metabolism

The placenta has, at least to some extent, metabolic capacities. It is possible that certain drugs are available for placental transport only after transformation by the placenta. Likewise, the presence of certain drugs may induce or inhibit formation of placental enzymes necessary to its nutritive or elimination functions. The clinical significance of the biotransformation properties of the placenta requires further research, however.

Fetal Role in Transplacentally Acquired Drugs

The extent to which drug use by a pregnant woman affects her fetus depends on many factors. The concentration-time profile of the drug; fetal drug distribution, metabolism, and elimination; and age of the fetus all influence fetal drug exposure.

Concentration-Time Profile

The effects of a drug on the fetus are proportional to the concentration reaching fetal tissue and the duration of exposure. The maternal-placental-fetal system is dynamic, and changes occur throughout pregnancy that may alter pharmacokinetic processes and resultant drug exposure. Information about the concentration of drug to which the fetus is exposed at various times during pregnancy is somewhat limited, since most information comes from collecting blood samples from the mother and newborn at the time of birth.

Total drug exposure is a crucial factor influencing the intensity of the pharmacologic effect on the fetus. Drugs taken on a regular basis will most certainly reach equilibrium between mother and fetus. Most drugs taken regularly reach fetal levels which correspond to 50 to 100 percent of maternal serum concentrations, but some drugs are more concentrated in the fetus than in the mother. The only means of limiting fetal exposure to chronic maternal drug use is to use drugs which are lipid-insoluble and of large molecular weight.

Fetal Drug Distribution, Metabolism, and Elimination

Distribution of a drug in the fetus is a function of the unique fetal circulatory anatomy and results in a preferential circulation of blood and drug to the heart and brain, coincidently common sites of congenital anomalies. On the other hand, cardiac output is relatively greater in the fetus than in the adult, which serves to decrease the maternal-fetal concentration gradient and decrease total fetal exposure. Due to altered binding affinity, some drugs exhibit less protein binding in fetal plasma than in maternal plasma. Drugs demonstrating this effect include sulfonamides, barbiturates, phenytoin, and local anesthetics. These drugs would be more active in the fetus, increasing the risk of adverse drug effects. Finally, the fetal blood-brain barrier is poorly developed, which subjects the developing central nervous system to additional drug effects.

The capacity of the fetal liver for drug metabolism is less than in the adult, causing more pronounced and prolonged drug effects in the fetus. In addition, fetal circulation allows up to half of the blood from the umbilical vein to be directly circulated to the heart and brain without passing through the liver.

Fetal excretion of drug is primarily by diffusion of the drug back to the mother; thus, the mother metabolizes and excretes drugs for the fetus. Drugs metabolized by the fetus can be eliminated by the immature kidneys into amniotic fluid, but, as the fetus swallows amniotic fluid, drugs are recirculated.

Fetal Age

Gestational age of the fetus is important when effects of drug exposure on the fetus are considered (see the Teratogenicity section below). Drug transfer is probably greatest during late gestation for several reasons. There is increased uteroplacental blood flow because of the greater size and surface area of the placenta. The capillary endothelium becomes progressively thinner, thus reducing the distance between maternal and fetal blood. Breaks are more likely to occur as pregnancy advances. Fetal acid-base balance becomes progressively more acidotic, trapping ionized basic drugs. There is more free drug available because of increased maternal physiologic hypoalbuminemia. Of note is the fact that these processes create the possibility of greater drug levels existing at birth. Neonates, separated from their mothers' circulation and elimination capacity, are required to metabolize and excrete these drugs for themselves.

ADVERSE DRUG EFFECTS IN PREGNANCY

Fetal Effects

Society as a whole is concerned about use of drugs in pregnancy, as evidenced by the attention this topic receives in the public press. Difficulties avoiding harmful drug exposure in pregnancy arise from two problem areas: (1) incomplete information about specific effects of substances on the embryo and (2) application of available knowledge in a timely fashion to prevent adverse drug and substance effects on the fetus or embryo.

Incomplete Information

Knowledge of the effects of drugs in pregnancy is sometimes difficult to obtain. Much information comes from individual case studies, which serve to raise concern about a particular drug but do not prove causality. Epidemiologic studies are of two kinds. Case-control studies retrospectively compare abnormal babies with matched controls. Cohort studies compare groups of drug-exposed mothers with unexposed mothers. Problems identifying specific drug effects come from exposure of these women to many potentially harmful factors during their pregnancies and the necessity of large numbers of participants for analysis to afford statistical significance.

Animal studies are required in numerous species prior to release of a drug by the Food and Drug Administration. Drug testing in animals is of somewhat limited usefulness in pregnancy, as drugs may seem to be harmless in animals that are known teratogens to humans and vice versa. Certainly, teratogenicity in several species warrants concern and possible avoidance in human pregnancy.

Utilization of knowledge about drug use in pregnancy is further confounded by the fact that drug exposure alone often does not determine its effect on the fetus. Fetal susceptibility is determined by several factors including the drug, genetic makeup, maternal age, nutritional status, general health, and environmental pollutants.

Application of Available Knowledge

Some women, under medical care for chronic or acute health problems, become pregnant unknowingly and thus expose a developing human embryo to drugs best avoided in the first trimester. Improved contraception for some of these women could prevent this unnecessary drug exposure, as therapy could be altered or completed before a planned conception. Otherwise, women who are unable to avoid chronic drug therapy while attempting to conceive assume a known risk to the developing embryo.

A person's attitudes toward drugs and related substances affect drug exposure during human pregnancy. Some people do not consider cigarettes, caffeine, alcohol, various over-the-counter preparations, and "social drugs" (marijuana, cocaine, etc.) to be drugs. Increased public education is one

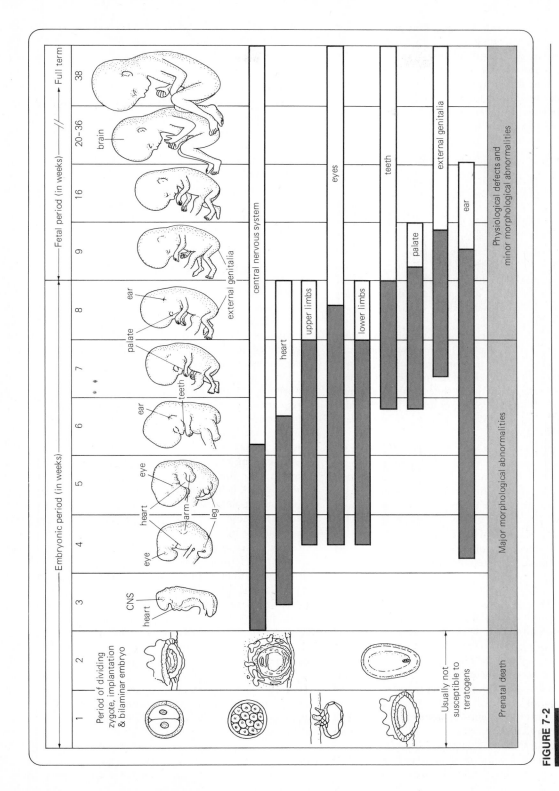

FIGURE 7-2

Schematic Illustration of the Sensitive or Critical Periods in Human Development. Shaded areas denote highly sensitive periods. Note that each organ or structure has a critical period during which its development may be deranged. (*From K. L. Moore: Before We Are Born, 2d ed., 1983. Courtesy W. B. Saunders Co.*)

means of assisting these women to become drug-free before conceiving and during pregnancy.

Another impediment to minimizing drug exposure in pregnancy is environmental pollution. Individuals may encounter harmful substances in the air they breathe, the water they drink, or the food they eat. Likewise, women's workplaces may be the sources of unwitting exposure. (See Chap. 49 and *Guidelines on Pregnancy and Work, 1977.*)

Teratogenicity

A *teratogen* is an agent toxic to cell differentiation which causes structural defects in the developing embryo. Drugs and related substances which cause intrauterine growth retardation or adverse biochemical and behavioral changes, as well as cancer, are also considered teratogens. The results of exposure to a specific substance depends on the gestational age of the embryo or fetus. Very early in gestation, an expected embryo might simply be aborted spontaneously because of adverse structural damage. Later during embryonic life, damage to various systems may occur, causing specific birth defects (see Fig. 7-2).

Thalidomide is an example of a drug which, when given to a mother between days 34 and 50 of gestation, has caused phocomelia (absence of the proximal portion of a limb). Later in pregnancy (after 8 weeks' gestation), structural damage will not occur but growth and functional development may be impaired. A number of drugs are to be avoided in the first trimester of pregnancy because of teratogenic effects. (See Table 7-1).

Later in pregnancy, drugs may still adversely affect the fetus. Hyperbilirubinemia with jaundice and even brain damage may be caused by competition for albumin binding sites between endogenous bilirubin and drugs such as **sulfonamides** and **aspirin**. Other examples are hemolytic anemia in infants with inherited glucose-6-phosphate dehydrogenase (G6PD) deficiency who receive drugs such as **sulfonamides** and **nitrofurantoin** and discoloration of teeth and enamel hypoplasia from **tetracyclines**.

Maternal Effects

Due to pharmacokinetic changes during pregnancy, a woman may be more or less sensitive to drug effects and need close monitoring for therapeutic and adverse effects. Although drug therapy may be necessary for maternal well-being during pregnancy, some drugs adversely affect uterine contractility. Beta-sympathomimetic drugs, commonly used to treat premature labor (see Chap. 46), may also be used to treat asthma; nonsteroidal anti-inflammatory drugs (see Chap. 26) may be used to treat arthritis. A side effect of both may be to prolong gestation, through smooth muscle relaxation and postaglandin inhibition respectively. **Magnesium sulfate**, used for treatment for preeclampsia, may sedate a woman and retard labor progress. Usually, to counteract any

drug effect which decreases uterine contractility, synthetic **oxytocin** (Pitocin) can be used to stimulate an effective labor pattern.

Fetal Therapeutics

Concern over drug use in pregnancy stems from the perspective that the fetus is a healthy individual and drug therapy is unnecessary, if not harmful. Therapeutic use of drugs during pregnancy for a compromised fetus is a new consideration. **Digoxin** has been given to the mother under carefully controlled circumstances to treat a fetus with heart failure. **Corticosteroids** have been used to stimulate fetal lung maturation when premature delivery seems inevitable. Further work in this new field may yield even greater application of the concept of fetal drug therapeutics.

NURSING PROCESS IMPLICATIONS

Education of the public about the risks of drugs and related substances is an area for nursing involvement. Opportunities for teaching women these facts before they conceive should be maximized. Annual health evaluations, women's organization meetings, and the classroom are settings where nurses may provide the public with this information.

Drug administration should include the principles of informed consent. The *Pregnant Patients' Bill of Rights and Pregnant Patients' Responsibilities* includes many principles of informed consent for pregnant women, and every health care provider who cares for pregnant or lactating women should be familiar with this document (see References). Administering drugs based on these principles can at least prevent some uninformed drug use by unconsenting individuals. The risk-benefit ratio must always be the basis for decision making about drug use during pregnancy. If a drug is necessary, those which have been used extensively in pregnancy and at least appear to be safe should be used, instead of new or experimental drugs. If possible, drug dosage should be determined by laboratory for blood levels of free drug, rather than by total drug concentration or usual drug dosage, particularly for those drugs considered possibly teratogenic. In practice the smallest effective dose should be used, since many teratogenic effects are probably dose-related. The nursing role includes the teaching of alternatives to drug use for common discomforts of pregnancy and concurrent, mild illnesses.

Drug administration in labor should be timed to minimize the magnitude of drug concentration in the infant at birth. Knowing the theoretical time interval between drug administration and peak drug concentration in the fetus for a specific drug helps to facilitate this critical timing.

Intravenous drug administration is often preferred during labor, as drug absorption is not a factor and smaller amounts are usually effective, compared with other routes of administration. When possible, intravenous injection of a

TABLE 7-1 Drugs with Significant Adverse Effects on the Fetus

DRUG	TRIMESTER	EFFECT
Aspirin, salicylates	Third	Prolonged labor; also possible salicylism and bleeding
Barbiturates	All	Neonatal dependence due to chronic use
Busulfan	All	Multiple congenital anomalies; growth retardation
Chloramphenicol	Third	Risk of "gray baby syndrome"
Chlorpropamide	All	Prolonged symptomatic neonatal hypoglycemia
Cortisone	First	Increased risk of cleft palate
Desipramine	Third	Withdrawal symptoms; breathlessness, tachypnea, tachycardia, difficult feeding
Diazepam	All	Neonatal dependence due to chronic use
Diethylstilbestrol	All	Vaginal adenosis; vaginal adenocarcinoma
Ethanol	All	High risk of fetal alcohol syndrome
Heroin	All	Neonatal dependence due to chronic use
Iodide	All	Congenital goiter; hypothyroidism
Kanamycin	All	Hearing impairment
Lithium	All	Cardiovascular malformations; hypotonia; hypoglycemia; nephrogenic diabetes
Methadone	All	Neonatal dependence due to chronic use
Methotrexate	First	Malformation of skull, face, and limbs
Methyltestosterone	Second and third	Masculinization of female fetus
Methylthiouracil	All	Hypothyroidism
Nitrofurantoin	Third	Hyperbilirubinemia and kernicterus
Norethindrone	All	Masculinization of female fetus
Phenytoin	All	Increased risk of cleft lip and palate
Propranolol	Third	Growth retardation; hypoglycemia; respiratory depression, bradycardia
Propylthiouracil	All	Congenital goiter
Sulfonamides	Third	Hyperbilirubinemia and kernicterus
Terbutaline	Third	Tachycardia; hypothermia; hypocalcemia, hypo- and hyperglycemia
Tetracycline	All	Discoloration of teeth; bone abnormalities
Thalidomide	First	Phocomelia in 20% of cases
Thiazides	Third	Thrombocytopenia; hypokalemia; hyponatremia; hypovolemia
Tolbutamide	All	Prolonged symptomatic neonatal hyperglycemia
Trimethadione	All	Multiple congenital anomalies
Warfarin	First Third	Hypoplastic nasal bridge; chondrodysplasia risk of bleeding (discontinue use 1 month before delivery)

Source: Compiled from M. S. Cohen, "Special Aspects of Perinatal and Pediatric Pharmacology," in B. G. Katzung (ed.), *Basic and Clinical Pharmacology,* Los Altos, CA: Lange Medical Publications, 1982; D. P. Hays: "Teratogenesis: A Review of the Basic Principles with a Discussion of Selected Agents," *Drug Intelligence and Clinical Pharmacy,* **15**(Part 1):444, 1981, **15**(Part 2):542, 1981, and **15**(Part 3):639, 1981; T. Tuchmann-Duplesis: "Embryonic Clinical Pharmacology," in G. S. Avery (ed.), *Drug Treatment,* Sydney: ADIS, 1980; R. M. Ward, S. Singh, and B. L. Mirkin: "Fetal Clinical Pharmacology," in G. S. Avery (ed.), *Drug Treatment,* Sydney: ADIS, 1980; and P. S. Weatherbee and J. R. Lodge: "Alcohol, Caffeine, and Nicotine Usage in Pregnancy," *U.S. Pharmacist* **6**(3):65, 1981.

drug with the onset of a contraction helps to reduce the amount of drug to the fetus. Equilibration occurs within the mother's bloodstream while the blood supply to the inter-villous space is shut off by the contraction, thus minimizing the bolus effect of intravenous injection. Conversely, pro-longed or repetitive intravenous infusion of a drug to the mother should be avoided, if possible, as this practice max-imizes fetal exposure to the drug.

Nursing responsibility for a woman during labor and birth includes care of the newborn. Being aware of the fetus's drug exposure allows the baby's needs to be ade-quately anticipated. Communicating drug history to the neonate's primary care provider also facilitates adequate observation and treatment in the critical first days of life.

General nursing responsibility relative to drug adminis-tration in pregnancy requires as complete an information base as possible about a drug's use in pregnancy. To facili-tate this understanding, the Food and Drug Administration has developed a categorization of the level of risk of drugs to the fetus (*FDA Drug Bulletin*, 1981).

Information of this type will assist care providers to be more knowledgeable about the use of drugs during preg-nancy and thus to obtain more fully informed consent from pregnant women prior to drug administration.

LACTATION PHARMACOKINETICS

Milk, produced by the alveolar cell, originates in maternal circulation. To get from maternal circulation to alveolus, substances must traverse the capillary endothelium, intersti-tial (extracellular) water, cell basement membrane, and cell plasma membrane.

The amount of drug or its metabolite which enters breast milk is determined by the same drug characteristics which influence all transport of drugs across membranes. Nonion-ized, lipid-soluble drugs of low molecular weight which are unbound to protein pass more easily and extensively into breast milk. Milk is more acidic than plasma. Weakly basic drugs will be more extensively ionized in breast milk, thus trapping ionized drug in breast milk.

Drug transport into milk can theoretically occur by sev-eral mechanisms. Milk proteins can serve as molecules for drug binding and transport into milk. Drugs and chemicals can bind to the outer lipoprotein membrane of milk fat globules or be trapped within the milk fat globule during fat formation. It is accepted that most drugs enter the breast milk by diffusion and that there is no evidence of back dif-fusion of a drug once it reaches the milk.

A neonate's exposure to a drug from breast-feeding depends on the concentration of the drug in the milk at the time of the feeding, the amount of milk consumed, the extent to which the drug is absorbed from the gastrointes-tinal tract, and the baby's ability to eliminate the drug. The dosage a baby receives depends on the milk/plasma concen-tration. If the concentration of the drug in the breast milk is known, the dose to the baby can be estimated. Table 7-2

TABLE 7-2 Percent of Maternal Drugs Appearing in Milk

DRUG	PERCENT OF MATERNAL DOSE
Cefazolin	0.075
Digoxin	0.07–0.14
Ethanol	1
Isoniazid	2.3
Nicotine	0.17
Prednisolone/prednisone	0.04–0.12
Propranolol	0.03–0.05
Salicylate	0.18–0.36
Sulfasalazine	0.16
Sulfone	2
Theophylline	4

Source: C. M. Berlin: *Obstetrics and Gynecology,* **58**(5 Sup-plement):17–23, 1981. Reprinted with permission from The Amer-ican College of Obstetricians and Gynecologists.

gives examples of the percent of maternal drug appearing in milk. The amount of drug in breast milk is seldom more than 1 to 2 percent of the maternal dose.

ADVERSE DRUG EFFECTS AND LACTATION

Determining whether to treat a breast-feeding woman with a particular drug or whether to advise cessation of breast-feeding during drug use is difficult. More information is available about drug use during lactation than during preg-nancy, as the process and outcome lend themselves more easily to observation and as milk/plasma concentrations can be determined. Long-term effects on suckling infants are more speculative; much information about drug effects dur-ing lactation comes from isolated case accounts. Continued, long-term, large studies are needed to more knowledgeably recommend drugs to be used during lactation.

The same problems exist during lactation as during preg-nancy concerning over-the-counter drug use, social and illicit drug use, and environmental pollutants. In fact, highly lipid-soluble environmental pollutants such as DDT and hal-ogenated hydrocarbons (PCB, vinyl chloride, dioxin) may be excreted through breast milk only. Education of women to avoid unnecessary drug use during lactation is indicated.

Effects on Infant

Table 7-3 summarizes specific information about commonly used medications, but there are several general consider-ations to be taken into account in decisions about drug administration in lactation and its potential effects on the infant: In utero exposure greatly exceeds that from breast-feeding. If gestation progressed concurrently with drug administration, it is unlikely that breast-feeding would be contraindicated because of exposure to the same drug. Long-term drug therapy is potentially more harmful than short-

TABLE 7-3 Commonly Used Drugs and Effects of Their Excretion into Breast Milk

DRUG	EFFECT ON INFANT	COMMENTS
Ampicillin	Minimal	There are no significant side effects. Occurrence of diarrhea or allergic sensitization is possible.
Aspirin	Minimal	Occasional doses are probably safe. High doses may produce significant concentration in breast milk.
Caffeine	Minimal	Caffeine intake in moderation is safe. Concentration in breast milk is about 1% of total dose taken by mother.
Chloral hydrate	Significant	Drug may cause drowsiness if infant is fed at peak concentration in milk.
Choramphenicol	Significant	Concentrations are too low to "cause gray baby syndrome." A possibility of bone marrow suppression does exist. Taking chloramphenicol while breast-feeding is not recommended.
Chlorothiazide	Minimal	No side effects have been reported.
Chlorpromazine	Minimal	Effect appears insignificant.
Codeine	Minimal	No side effects have been reported.
Diazepam	Significant	Drug will cause sedation in breast-fed infants. Accumulation can occur in newborns.
Dicumarol	Minimal	No adverse side effects have been reported. Nurse may wish to follow infant's prothrombin time.
Digoxin	Minimal	Insignificant quantities enter breast milk.
Ethanol	Moderate	Moderate ingestion by mother is unlikely to produce effects in infant. Large amounts consumed by mother can produce alcohol effects in infant.
Heroin	Significant	Drug enters breast milk and can prolong neonatal narcotic dependence.
Iodine (radioactive)	Significant	Drug enters milk in quantities sufficient to cause thyroid suppression in infant.
Isoniazid (INH)	Minimal	Milk concentrations equal maternal plasma concentrations. There is a possibility of pyridoxine deficiency developing in infant.
Kanamycin	Minimal	No adverse effects have been reported.
Lithium	Significant	Avoid breast-feeding.
Methadone	Significant	(See Heroin.) Under close physician supervision, breast-feeding can be continued. Signs of opiate withdrawal in infant may occur if mother stops taking methadone or stops breast-feeding abruptly.
Oral contraceptives	Minimal	They will suppress lactation in high doses.
Penicillin	Minimal	Very low concentrations are found in breast milk.
Phenobarbital	Moderate	Sedative-hypnotic doses can cause sedation in infant.
Phenytoin	Moderate	Amounts entering breast milk may be sufficient to cause side effects in infant.
Prednisone	Moderate	Low maternal doses are probably safe. Doses two or more times physiologic amounts should probably be avoided.
Propranolol	Minimal	Very small amounts enter breast milk.
Propylthiouracil, thiouracil	Significant	They can suppress thyroid function in infant.
Spironolactone	Minimal	Very small amounts enter breast milk.
Tetracycline	Moderate	There is a possibility of permanent staining of developing teeth in infant. Drug should be avoided during lactation.
Theophylline	Moderate	Drug can enter breast milk in moderate quantities but is not likely to produce significant effects.
Thyroxine	Minimal	No adverse effects have been reported from therapeutic doses.
Tolbutamide	Minimal	Low concentrations are found in breast milk.
Warfarin	Minimal	Very small quantities are found in breast milk.

Source: M. S. Cohen, "Special Aspects of Perinatal and Pediatric Pharmacology," in B. G. Katzung (ed.), *Basic and Clinical Pharmacology*, Los Altos, CA: Lange Medical Publications, 1982.

term therapy. Some drugs taken occasionally would be contraindicated if taken regularly over a long-term period.

If the drug is not absorbed orally, it is generally safe when delivered to the infant in the milk, although there may be local gastrointestinal effects. For example, if the lactating mother receives parenteral **kanamycin**, an aminoglycoside antibiotic which is not absorbed orally, the infant should not have any systemic effects but may experience altered gastrointestinal flora and resultant diarrhea.

Drugs which are given directly to infants for therapeutic reasons are logical choices for treating the lactating mother, because of the accumulated knowledge available about the drug's potential effects on the child. Generally, more caution is required when the estimated dose in the milk approaches a therapeutic quantity than when subtherapeutic amounts are involved, unless subtherapeutic doses of the drug could mask early signs of medical conditions in the infant.

Drugs commonly causing idiosyncratic or allergic reactions which are not dose-related should be avoided, if possible, since very small amounts of drug can sensitize the infant or even elicit a serious reaction. Similarly, alternatives should be sought for drugs with the potential for accumulation during prolonged therapy and those in which the effects are not easily recognizable in the infant. In all cases the least-toxic alternative for maternal therapy should be sought.

Maternal Effects

One concern about drug use during lactation is whether or not a drug might inhibit lactation. **Oral contraceptives** (combination pill), long-term use of **ergot derivatives**, and pharmacologic doses of **pyridoxine** (vitamin B_6) may serve as lactation inhibitors. Central nervous system depressants (**barbiturates, sedative-hypnotics, narcotics,** and **ethanol**) could interfere with the let-down reflex and impede successful lactation.

NURSING PROCESS IMPLICATIONS

Education of lactating women to avoid unnecessary drug use is indicated. Concurrently, education about treatment of various minor health problems with nonpharmacologic therapies can reduce reliance on drugs. Relaxation techniques for anxiety and insomnia; dietary modification for constipation; and fluids, rest, and room humidification for treatment of the common cold are examples of drug-free treatments of health problems likely to affect a lactating woman. When drugs are necessary, those known to be least noxious to the neonate should be selected.

To minimize the amount of drug an infant receives, the baby should be nursed after peak drug levels have subsided. This can be accomplished with most drugs by taking a drug just after breast-feeding and waiting as long as possible (e.g., 4 h) before breast-feeding the baby again. This principle is applicable to drugs taken in single doses or intermittently.

If there is doubt about a drug effect, the actual infant dosage can be measured. Maternal plasma, breast milk, and infant plasma can be collected and assayed. Although expensive, such steps can definitively determine an infant's actual drug exposure, and management can be more knowledgeably planned.

INFANTS AND CHILDREN

LEARNING OBJECTIVES

Upon mastery of the contents of this section, the reader will be able to:

1. Describe alterations in pharmacokinetics which occur in neonates and children, as compared with adults.

2. Identify five adverse drug reactions peculiar to infants or children and the appropriate interventions to prevent or minimize the reactions.

3. Compare five methods of dosage selection in the pediatric patient, and identify the best method for most pediatric patients.

4. Alter techniques or oral drug administration in keeping with a child's developmental stage.

5. List two reasons why an ambulatory pediatric patient might be underdosed.

6. Identify interventions appropriate to correcting underdosing problems.

The therapeutic administration of drugs in children differs from drug administration in adults in terms of selection of drugs, dosing, scheduling, techniques of administration, and therapeutic outcomes. Physiologic variations, which affect drug pharmacokinetics, and the child's growth and development, which affect administration techniques, are the basis for these differences.

In addition to these basic differences, children present special problems with regard to the legal and ethical factors governing drug research. Many drugs legally available for use in adults bear a warning in the product literature stating that because safety and efficacy have not been established for children, the drug should not be administered to them. Shirkey (1970) reported that more than 50 percent of drugs released for use in the United States since 1969 carried some type of warning to this effect. He reminds us that this makes children virtual "therapeutic orphans."

PEDIATRIC PHARMACOKINETICS

Most aspects of drug disposition in children (ages 1 to 12) are probably little different from those in adults. However, since physiologic processes change rapidly during infancy (the first year of life), and particularly during the first few weeks, a number of factors must be considered in selection of drug, dosage level, and dosage schedule for neonates (birth to 1 month), especially those born prematurely. Table 7-4 shows the pharmacokinetic differences in neonates, infants, and children, compared with adults.

Absorption

Absorption in neonates is usually slower than in older children, secondary to slower gastric emptying (two to three times longer), with irregular and unpredictable peristalsis. Examples of drugs more slowly absorbed by neonates are **phenytoin** (Dilantin), **phenobarbital**, and **acetaminophen** (Tylenol). The extent of absorption of drugs is usually not changed, except with drugs which are broken down by stomach acids. Thus, **penicillin** derivatives are better absorbed during the newborn period, since neonates have greatly reduced gastric acid production. Except during the first 2 days of life, when gastric acidity increases to high levels (pH of about 1), adult levels are not attained until about 3 years. Premature infants have very low gastric acidity. At about 6 to 8 months, oral absorption approaches the rate and extent seen in older children and adults.

Due to small muscle mass and frequently compromised perfusion, the sick premature infant may have irregular and unpredictable absorption from intramuscular injection sites. A sudden increase in perfusion can result in toxic blood levels of drugs such as the aminoglycoside antibiotics, so intravenous administration is the preferred parenteral route in these patients.

The rectal route of administration is sometimes used for acutely ill children who are unable or unwilling to swallow medications or who are in acute convulsions, when intravenous access is difficult. While rectal absorption is often slow and erratic, good results have been obtained using drugs in solution applied by a syringe with a specially designed blunt plastic tip (Boréus, 1982).

The skin and conjunctiva of the neonate, especially the premature, are quite permeable, and pharmacologic blood levels can result after topically administered drugs. **Hexachlorophene** is rapidly absorbed in small newborns, and percutaneous absorption of corticosteroids occurs when these drugs are used for eczema or diaper rash.

TABLE 7-4 Pharmacokinetic Parameters in Neonates, Infants, and Children, Compared with Adults

PARAMETER	NEONATES	INFANTS	CHILDREN
Absorption	↓	0	0
Protein binding	↓	0	0
Metabolism	↓↓↓	0	↑
Renal elimination	↓	0	0

0 = same as adult.
↓ = slightly decreased.
↓↓↓ = significantly decreased.
↑ = increased.

Distribution

Body Composition

A much higher percentage of the body mass of the full-term neonate is water (75 percent) in comparison to the adult (50 to 60 percent). Differences also exist between the full-term neonate and the premature infant (85 percent of body weight as water). Thus, in neonates those water-soluble drugs without extensive tissue bindings (e.g., **sulfonamides, penicillin, amoxicillin**) require higher doses relative to body weight to achieve the same plasma concentration. The total body fat content of the premature infant is 1 percent, compared with 15 percent in the full-term infant. Lipid-soluble drugs would tend to accumulate in smaller amounts in immature infants than in adults and older children, thus requiring lower doses relative to weight.

Plasma Protein Binding

Neonates have been shown to have decreased plasma protein binding, which means that more drug will be in the free form and, when the unbound portion of the drug exceeds the capacity to eliminate it, intoxication will occur at lower doses. The neonate also has a qualitatively different albumin, which has decreased binding potential and higher concentrations of bilirubin (secondary to the breakdown of fetal hemoglobin). Thus a potential for drug-induced displacement is created; drugs such as **sulfonamides** and **salicylates** may displace bilirubin and increase the risk of kernicterus (deposit of bilirubin in the central nervous system, which may cause brain damage).

Although an increased permeability of the blood-brain barrier in the neonate has been postulated, there are insufficient research data in humans to identify why neonates are more sensitive to the central nervous system effects of some drugs.

Metabolism

Both renal and hepatic factors contribute to the low clearance and prolonged half-life of many common drugs in neonates, as compared with older children and adults (see Table 7-5). Drug metabolism is altered in the neonate because of significantly decreased activity of liver enzymes, especially for phase II, or conjugation, reactions. However, the liver enzymes develop rapidly over the first month of life, necessitating frequent dosage adjustment during this time. Another consideration is whether, during the prenatal period, the mother took a drug such as **phenobarbital**, which induces early maturation of the microsomal enzymes. In this case normal neonatal doses may prove ineffective.

Older children tend to metabolize drugs faster, resulting in a shorter half-life. This has been documented for **propoxyphene** (Darvon), **diazoxide** (Hyperstat), **carbamazepine** (Tegretol), **ethosuximide** (Zarontin), **phenytoin** (Dilantin), **phenobarbital**, and **theophylline**. Children between 1 month and 2 years of age require higher doses of **digoxin** per unit

TABLE 7-5 Comparison of Plasma Half-Lives of Several Drugs in Neonates, Children, and Adults

DRUG	ROUTE OF ELIMINATION	HALF-LIFE, h		
		NEONATES	CHILDREN	ADULTS
Acetaminophen	Metabolized	2.2–5	3.1–3.4	1.9–2.2
Ampicillin	Renal, unchanged	2–4	1–1.3	1–1.3
Diazepam	Metabolized	25–100	18	15–25
Digoxin	Combined	60–107	36–37	30–40
Gentamicin	Renal, unchanged	6–8	2–3	2–3
Kanamycin	Renal, unchanged	6–18	2–4	2–4
Phenobarbital	Metabolized	100–500	50–65	64–140
Phenytoin	Metabolized	30–60	5	12–18
Theophylline	Metabolized	25–35	1.8–4	6–8

of body weight than older children and adults, possibly due to metabolic factors (Wettrell and Andersson, 1977). As more research is undertaken, other metabolized drugs may show similar characteristics. For the most part, then, drugs may be administered to children at the same dose intervals as for adults, but some agents which are metabolized may require higher doses with shorter dose intervals in order to offset the increased rate of metabolism in children.

Excretion

Glomerular filtration at birth is only 30 to 40 percent, and tubular secretion 20 to 30 percent, of adult values when adjusted for body surface area. Substantial improvement occurs in the first week of life, and glomerular filtration reaches adult levels by 6 to 12 months. Prolonged half-lives during the first weeks of life have been identified for such renally excreted drugs as the **penicillins, aminoglycosides,** and **digoxin.**

ADVERSE DRUG REACTIONS IN PEDIATRICS

Children respond to proper drug therapy in a manner similar to that of adults; however, they may have numerous peculiar adverse effects. In one published report, approximately 10 percent of 658 pediatric patients had at least one adverse reaction in an 8-month period (McKenzie et al., 1973). Others have found an incidence rate of approximately 56 percent in children on a specialty (hematology-oncology) floor where extremely toxic agents were administered (Collins et al., 1974). Whatever the incidence, children experience more peculiar adverse drug reactions than adults receiving the same drugs. Table 7-6 summarizes some of the reactions seen in pediatric patients. Changing physiologic systems, coinciding with varied pharmacologic effects, account for many of these unique reactions.

Tetracycline administration has been associated with dental staining and alterations in bone growth. Tetracycline forms a stable complex with calcium apatite, thereby alter-

ing normal bone and tooth growth. This reaction is apparently dose-related and appears to have the greatest incidence at a total dose of 3 g or in therapy which lasts longer than 10 days.

Chronic high-dose **corticosteroids** have resulted in severe growth retardation in infants and children. Steroids apparently inhibit normal epiphyseal maturation. This effect would naturally predominate in children, whose epiphyseal growth is active.

Although many adverse reactions may be explained in the light of coincidence of normal physiologic development with known pharmacologic activity, some reactions must be labeled idiosyncratic, including such reactions as the paradoxic hyperactivity caused by **phenobarbital**, increased intracranial pressure after **tetracycline** administration, and sudden death with **indomethacin** therapy.

NURSING PROCESS IMPLICATIONS

Dosage Selection

The selection of the proper dosage is one of the most crucial decisions made in pediatric drug therapy. Dosage modification formulas for children are filled with problems. Since it is the responsibility of the nurse to ascertain if the ordered drug dose is appropriate before it is administered, an understanding of the pitfalls of these formulas is crucial to safe nursing care.

One method of dosage selection is to administer the adult dosage to the child. Logic indicates that only in rare instances would this be the proper dosage; for most children the full adult dosage would be an overdose. But one instance in which the adult dosage is acceptable in children is the use of **mebendazole** in the treatment of enterobiasis: 100 mg is the accepted dosage for both adults and children.

An alternative method of dosage selection is to use a proportion of the average adult dosage. The two areas of possible error in this method are the definition of *average adult* and the determination of the proportion to be administered.

TABLE 7-6 Adverse Drug Reactions in Pediatrics

SYSTEM	REACTION	DRUG	RECOMMENDATIONS AND COMMENTS
Skeletal	Decreased bone growth	Corticosteroids	Avoid prolonged use. Infants may absorb topical agents enough to cause adrenal suppression.
	Weakened bone	Tetracycline	Avoid use in children under 8. Monitor for rickets and treat accordingly.
Central nervous	Sedation and impaired mentation	Chloral hydrate	Reactions have been seen in neonates with decreased metabolic capabilities.
		Hexachlorophene	In lab animals with high serum hexachlorophene levels, cystic spaces and cerebral edema have been seen. No human cases are known.
		Naphazoline	Avoid use.
		Tetrahydrozoline	Avoid use.
	Excitation	Phenobarbital	If phenobarbital level is high, decrease dose. If level is low, use another agent.
	Dystonias	Phenothiazines	Treat with diphenhydramine.
		Haloperidol	Drug may unmask Gilles de la Tourette's disease.
Dental	Staining	Tetracycline	Avoid use in children under 8.
		Iron	Effect is topical, due to liquid forms. Avoid contact with teeth.
	Gingival hyperplasia	Phenytoin	Practice good dental hygiene.
	Dental caries	Syrups and elixirs	Practice good dental hygiene. Choose sugar-free preparations.
Dermatologic	Diaper rash	Ampicillin	Rash is a frequent complication caused by a monilial overgrowth, possible with any broad-spectrum antibiotic.
	Maculopapular rash	Ampicillin	Occurs in 90% of all patients with mononucleosis and must be differentiated from a true allergy.
Hematopoietic	Hyperbilirubinemia	Novobiocin	Avoid use.
		Sulfonamide	Use with extreme caution.
		Vitamin K	Limit dosing to 1 mg.
	Increased calcium	Vitamin D (toxicity)	Do not exceed recommended dosing.
	Decreased calcium	Phenytoin, phenobarbital	Monitor for rickets.
	Peripheral vascular collapse	Chloramphenicol	Drug can cause "gray baby syndrome" in newborns. Use only when specifically indicated at 25 mg/kg/day.
Hepatic	Cirrhosis	Vitamin A	Effect is seen with toxic levels.
		Indomethacin	Effect may be seen at autopsy after sudden death.
Gastrointestinal	Diarrhea	Ampicillin	Diarrhea is a common sign of altered GI flora and may occur with any broad-spectrum antibiotic.
Miscellaneous	Hyperthermia, hyperventilation, excitation	Intoxication of aspirin anticholinergics phencyclidine	Determine exact cause of poisoning and treat accordingly.

The average adult dosage is just that—an average; it is the dosage to which *most* adults with adult illnesses respond. This is a dosage with a broad range of responses; it may be a safe range for adults but not for children. The determination of the proportion of the adult dosage to administer has led to the development of many rules based on weight, age, surface area, and even body water estimation.

Clark's Weight Rule   Clark's rule for children 2 years old and over, one of the oldest rules used, is based on the proportion of the child's weight to that of the adult.

$$\text{Child dose} = \frac{\text{Weight in pounds}}{150} \times \text{Adult dose}$$

The average adult weight used in this calculation is 150, but the average adult weight has increased over the decades. For example, the adult oral **erythromycin** dosage is 250 mg qid. Clark's rule would result in a dosage of 50 mg qid in an average 2-year-old child weighing 28 lb, or 13 kg. The actual recommended dose is 100 to 160 mg qid (7.5 to 12.5 mg/kg qid).

Age Rules   Two common dosage rules based on age are Young's and Fried's rules. *Young's rule* for children 2 years old or over calculates the approximate dosage for children as:

$$\text{Child dose} = \frac{\text{Age in years}}{\text{Age in years} + 12} \times \text{Adult dose}$$

Fried's rule for children less than 1 year of age calculates dosage as:

$$\text{Child dose} = \frac{\text{Age in months}}{150} \times \text{Adult dose}$$

Age is an even poorer basis than weight upon which to base dosage in children, since the physiologic characteristics of children at any given age vary greatly. The average 7-year-old child weighs 24.5 kg, with a range of 17 to 29 kg.

Body Surface Area   Dosages used on *surface area* (the best method available to date) have been calculated by such rules as the following:

$$\text{Approximate child's dose} = \frac{\text{Surface area of child's body}}{\text{Surface area of adult's body}} \times \text{Adult dose}$$

or

$$\text{Approximate child's dose} = \frac{\text{Surface area of child's body}}{1.73 \text{ m}^2} \times \text{Adult dose}$$

Surface area may be calculated by using a nomogram (see Fig. 7-3). The previously mentioned 2-year-old who weighs 13 kg is 87 cm tall and has a surface area of 0.57 m². The child's dose of erythromycin would be about 0.32 × adult dosage, or 80 mg qid, which is closer to the recommended dosage of 100 to 160 mg qid.

Body Water Formula   Dosage based on *body water estimation* has been suggested by Gill and Udea (1975). Their rationale is the fact that the child's body is made up of a greater percentage of water than the adult's (75 percent versus 60 percent). Any drug distributed in water would therefore have an altered concentration in younger children. This theory has sound scientific backing, but the formula is too cumbersome for clinical use, has not been tested in a broad spectrum of patients, and is again a function of "average adult dosage."

References   The problem is obvious: children cannot be dosed according to adult dosage recommendations. Dosages must be individualized for the child. At present, a compilation of these pediatric dosages can be found in current handbooks. Suggested pediatric dosage is given in terms of milligrams per kilogram of body weight or in milligrams per square meter of surface area. Both measurements have their pros and cons, but more importantly, both help give an average pediatric dose.

The ultimate method of dosage selection in children would be to measure the response desired. A dose-response curve is not available for most drugs, with such exceptions as a change in serum glucose as a result of insulin administration. The next best dosage-monitoring technique is to measure blood levels of drugs. This permits some individualization of dosage and should be mandatory in all pediatric patients on drugs with low therapeutic indices, such as **gentamicin, phenytoin, digoxin,** and **theophylline.**

Administration

The route and techniques of administration may have more of an effect on the outcome of therapy than all other considerations. If the child's bib or pajamas get more of the dose than the child or if the drug does not get to the site of action, all the time and effort involved in diagnosis, treatment, dosage determination, and pharmacokinetic individualization are lost.

Routes

Subcutaneous and intramuscular injections are often difficult in neonates and small children because of the small muscle size and the danger of nerve damage. Repeated injections may cause trauma, hematomas, or continued bleeding. These reactions, plus altered tissue perfusion, make drug absorption erratic in neonates.

Intravenous injections should be given slowly to avoid high peak drug levels. Drugs whose toxicity may be proportional to the peak concentrations (such as **gentamicin, amikacin,** and **phenytoin**) should be injected especially slowly in neonates. Intravenous administration of irritating drugs into scalp veins should be avoided, as permanent hair loss has been caused by extravasation. Older children tolerate intravenous and intramuscular injections in the same manner as adults.

Drugs, such as **aminophylline,** which require therapeutic blood levels within a narrow range may be ineffective when given as suppositories. Cases of intoxication following repeated rectal doses of drugs are due to erratic absorption. Children are also very aware of anything inserted into the rectum and may be upset by it. For the most part, rectal suppositories should be avoided unless the child is vomiting or has a fever. **Aspirin** or **acetaminophen** for fevers and **trimethobenzamide** (Tigan) for vomiting are effective when administered rectally. The buttocks should be held together manually or strapped with adhesive tape to prevent early evacuation of the suppository.

Topical therapy in the eyes, ears, or nose may be difficult to administer to children, as they move quickly. To prevent serious injury from a dropper, the hand which administers the medication into the eye, ear, or nose should rest firmly

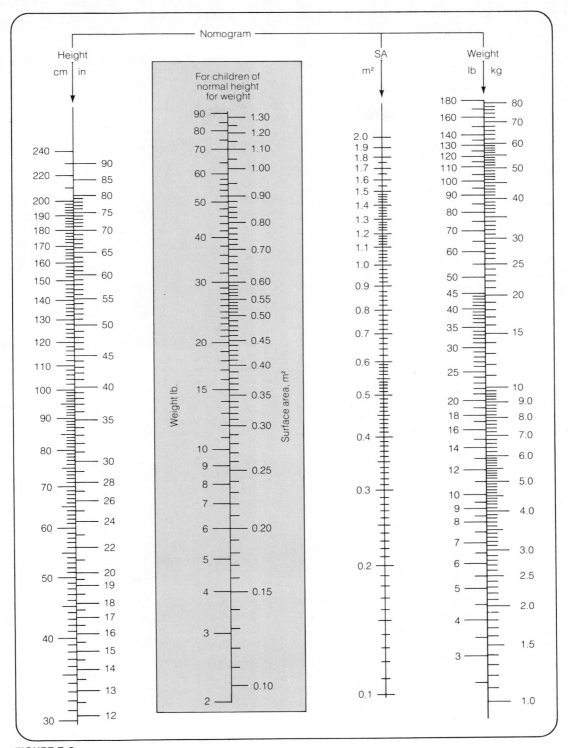

FIGURE 7-3

West Nomogram for Estimation of Surface Areas. The surface area is indicated at the point where a straight line connecting the height and weight intersects the surface area (SA) column and from the weight alone (enclosed area) if the patient is of roughly normal proportions. [*Nomogram modified from data of E. Boyd by C. D. West. From H. C. Shirkey: "Drug Therapy," in V. C. Vaughan and R. J. McKay (eds.): Nelson Textbook of Pediatrics, 10th ed., Philadelphia: W. B. Saunders, 1975.*]

on the child's head (see Fig. 7-4). Drops which are kept cold will be a shock to the child and should be warmed before administration. Results will be best if the entire dropper content is administered at once instead of by the "torture" method of 1 drop at a time.

Oral therapy is by far the most acceptable route for a child and in most situations will provide adequate therapy. An extra nursing challenge in oral administration to children is when and how to give an oral solid form, a chewable form, a liquid, or some other acceptable preparation. It has been shown that in some cases only 5 in 100 children receive the correct dose in the outpatient environment. Problems faced by the nurse include proper education of parents in administration techniques (the greatest problem arises from children spitting out the medication), standardizing the size of a teaspoon (household spoons vary in size from 2.5 to 7.2 mL), and reinforcement of the importance of following the directions exactly. Figure 7-5 shows various equipment used in administering drugs to children.

Techniques

Children in the 1- to 3-month age group move randomly yet have little head control. They must therefore be supported in a comfortable position, such as the feeding position, with their hands gently restrained. These babies usually do not retain all they take in, but they can suck, so a drug may best be given with a nipple; a syringe or dropper will be effective

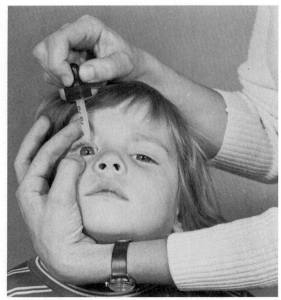

FIGURE 7-4

Proper Technique for the Instillation of Eye, Ear, or Nose Drops into a Child. Note that the hand holding the dropper rests firmly on the child's forehead so that if the head moves, the dropper will move with it. The other hand aids in holding he head steady and the eye open.

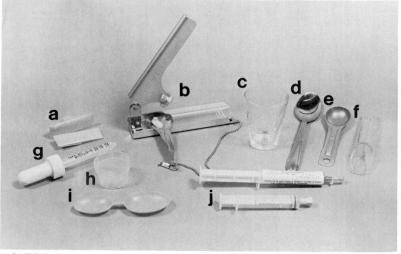

FIGURE 7-5

Equipment Used in Oral Administration of Medications to Children. (*a*) Powder papers. The exact dose amount is prepared by a pharmacist and placed in a paper. Preparation is time-consuming, and loss of the drug may occur. (*b*) Pill pulverizer. (*c*) Medicine cup. Highly inaccurate mode of dispensing oral liquids. (*d*) The household teaspoon. The size will vary from 2.5 to 7.2 mL. (*e*) Measuring teaspoon. Note sides of spoon; it is difficult to administer the entire dose. (*f, g, h, i*) Devices prepared by manufacturers for the administration of their products. (*j*) Pediatric oral syringes. Suspensions are prepared and exact amounts drawn up for easy administration.

if the medication is placed at the back of the mouth. The amount should be small enough and administration slow enough to avoid choking the child.

Children in the 3- to 12-month range are able to sit with support and even crawl. They have begun to finger-feed and even drink from a cup. These children must be carefully controlled while drugs are being administered, as they can resist with their entire bodies and put up an effective battle. By questioning the parent about normal feeding and medication habits, the nurse may learn that a child will take medications from a cup or may be used to taking them by some other technique. Great care should be taken to comfort the child, physically at first and verbally as a good reinforcement. Children at this age may remember uncomfortable experiences imposed during drug administration. The parent must be reminded that at this age children can start getting into mischief, so all drugs should be stored in a safe place.

By the age of 1 to 1½ years the child has usually advanced to independent (though messy) feeding, walking with support, and deliberate spitting. During this age period children begin to respond to commands, take part in daily routines, and become more independent and ambivalent. Drug administration at this age may be trying, and home feeding habits should be closely considered. Best results may come from having the child self-administer medications, aided by the use of familiar words for *drinking* or *swallowing,* which may be obtained from the parents. If the taste is bad (as with such preparations as **theophylline, potassium chloride,** and **prednisone,** the drug may be disguised. A small quantity of food or milk should be used for this purpose, as the child may not be able to eat a large amount. Before medications are mixed with food or beverages, drug-food interactions should be checked.

In the next year, chilren improve in walking, climbing, and seizing objects. They may run away or throw something in response to an offer of medications and, most importantly, may be able to get into any medications left nearby. By 2½ years of age they begin to be able to chew, take solid food, and respond to orders but become very independent. They take pride in their accomplishments. The clever nurse will be able to tell, at this point, whether a chewable tablet will go down more easily than a suspension. A firm approach, giving the child some alternatives, such as "How do you want to take this, on my lap or sitting in the chair?" will greatly facilitate drug administration. Involving the child with the routine will make the entire administration process easier.

The ages of 2½ to 3½ are times of increased proficiency. Children develop definite eating likes and dislikes, become ritualistic, and even develop fantasies. The tastes of medications may be disguised to fit their eating preferences. At this age children want to know "why" and want honesty from the people around. It is best to tell them why the drug is important (for example, "to make your throat better") and that it may taste bad but nonetheless is necessary. The nurse

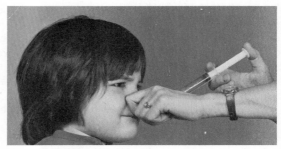

FIGURE 7-6

Poor Administration Technique. Never hold a child's nose to force swallowing of oral medications. Aspiration is a potential result of this practice.

should be *firm* but honest and should not "bargain" too long, as the stalemate will frustrate the child.

Up to the age of 6, children continue to refine motor movements and feeding abilities, and they become increasingly more independent. At this age they usually seek companionship and like to show their power to companions. The administration of medications will be easier if the nurse develops the friendship the child seeks and uses it to teach the child about the medication, its importance, and what it should do for the illness. At this age the child may be able to take a capsule but may be sensitive to loose teeth and obstacles to pill-taking which may be frustrating. A child's nose should never be held to force medication down, as this can easily result in aspiration of the drug (see Fig. 7-6).

From the age of 6 years to adulthood, the best technique is an honest but empathetic approach. Don't try to force medications because "the doctor said you should take this." These patients have developed their own attitudes toward their disease and toward the drug taken; they need to communicate these thoughts to the health professionals caring for them.

The best technique of oral drug administration may be hard to find, but by questioning both the parents and the child and by developing an armamentarium of innovative approaches, the task can be accomplished in even the most difficult patient.

ELDERLY ADULTS

LEARNING OBJECTIVES

Upon mastery of the contents of this section, the reader will be able to:

1. Describe how the normal physiology of aging alters drug pharmacokinetics and pharmacodynamics.

2. State modifications in drug dosage and schedule

appropriate to the pharmacokinetic and pharmacodynamic changes of aging.

3. Identify three adverse drug reactions that commonly occur in the elderly and the appropriate interventions to prevent or minimize the reactions.

4. List factors that might affect whether the elderly person takes a medication as prescribed.

5. Describe nursing interventions to assist the elderly in self-administration of medications.

The elderly are more heterogeneous in their responses to drugs than those in other age groups. Although "old age" is arbitrarily defined as commencing at 65 years, biologic aging begins early in life and proceeds at diverse rates in different organs and in different people. The secondary effects of aging, such as diseases common to the elderly and psychosocial adaptation processes, also contribute to this heterogeneity. Thus, statements about the effects of drug therapy in the elderly should be taken as broad generalizations, and treatment must be adapted according to individual patient response.

Clinicians have long recognized that older adults are more sensitive to drugs, experience prolonged drug effects, and have more adverse reactions, but only recently have researchers begun to systematically quantify these observations. Only a few drugs have been sufficiently studied in the elderly; therefore, much of the currently available information is theoretical or unsubstantiated. However, a rapid expansion of knowledge about drug effects in the elderly can be anticipated in the next few years.

Age-related changes in physiology can affect drug response by causing *pharmacokinetic* changes, which alter the concentration of a drug at the receptor site, or changes in *pharmacodynamics* and *capacity for organ response.* Figure 7-7 summarizes the changes in drug disposition common among the elderly.

GERIATRIC PHARMACOKINETICS

The half-lives of many drugs are prolonged in the elderly, as has been demonstrated for **diazepam** (Valium), **penicillin**, **digoxin, propranolol** (Inderal), **quinidine, kanamycin** (Kantrex), **acetaminophen** (Tylenol), **ethanol**, and others. While knowledge that a drug has a longer half-life in older patients alerts the nurse to extend the period of observation for drug effect, information about half-life alone does not give adequate information about how or whether the dosage level and administration schedule should be adjusted. This is because the half-life is determined both by *volume of distribution* and *rate of drug clearance,* either of which can be altered as a result of age-related physiologic changes. Only those increases in half-life associated with decreased clearance will necessitate dosage reduction. Therefore, the health care provider must be aware of how aging alters the absorption, distribution, metabolism, and excretion of various drugs.

Absorption

There are a number of age-related changes in the gastrointestinal tract that can be expected to affect oral drug absorption. Theoretically, the *decrease in gastric acid production* that occurs with age can limit the dissolution of some basic drugs, making them less absorbable when they reach the small intestine. Some tablets are formulated to disintegrate at a specific pH (e.g., enteric coated tablets), so decreased gastric acid can alter their dissolution. The increase in pH can be beneficial for drugs such as **penicillin**, which are broken down by stomach acid. Prodrugs, which must be hydrolyzed by stomach acid to an active form prior to absorption, can be affected by the lower gastric acidity. This is true for **clorazepate** (Tranxene), which is more slowly absorbed in the elderly.

In the small intestine of elderly persons there is a 30 percent *decrease in absorptive surface* (caused by atrophy of the villi) and *reduced motility.* Since most drugs are absorbed by passive diffusion, these changes theoretically can impair the absorption of drugs with low solubility or poor diffusibility, as has been shown for **digoxin**. Incomplete mixing can reduce the exposure of the soluble fraction to the mucosa, but this is offset because total contact time with the absorptive surface is increased. This increased contact time probably accounts for the greater extent of absorption noted in the elderly for drugs such as **cimetidine** (Tagamet) and **propranolol** (Inderal). The *intestinal blood flow of the elderly is reduced* to 50 to 60 percent of that in their younger counterparts, which also could adversely affect the absorption of poorly diffusible drugs, due to reduction of the concentration gradient between the intestine and the blood.

There are few studies of drug absorption in the elderly. Many drugs, such as **acetaminophen, phenylbutazone** (Butazolidin), **propoxyphene** (Darvon), and **aspirin**, have not demonstrated altered absorption with age. The few drugs which are associated with altered absorption in the elderly do not demonstrate any change in therapeutic effectiveness, so, apparently, normal aging alone does not significantly alter absorption. Other factors common to this age group that may cause significant alteration in absorption are gastrointestinal disease, altered dietary patterns, and concomitant drug therapy, especially with **anticholinergic** drugs (which delay gastric emptying) and **antacids** (which alter pH and form insoluble complexes with some drugs).

Distribution
Body Composition
Changes in size and body composition affect drug distribution in the elderly. As a group they are *smaller* in height, weight, and body surface area than younger adults; this alone warrants doses smaller than the usual adult doses for many elderly persons. *Body fat nearly doubles* with age, with a resultant decline in lean body mass. *Total body water declines* by 10 to 15 percent. Drugs such as **lithium** and **ethanol**, which are distributed in body water, have a smaller volume of distribution in the elderly. Conversely, with fat-

soluble drugs like **lidocaine, diazepam** (Valium), and many of the psychoactive drugs, the volume of distribution increases because of the larger reservoir of body fat. The half-lives of these drugs will be prolonged because the plasma concentration decays slowly.

Drugs distributed to body fat will require less-frequent dosing intervals in the elderly because of the slow decline in blood levels. There is no need to alter the total dose because of changes in volume of distribution, as the steady state plasma levels will not change. However, the time to achieve steady state is delayed if a loading dose is not given. The total loading dose required is greater, as the reservoir of body fat that must be filled is larger. Because of this it is often said that drugs such as diazepam "accumulate" in the elderly. What actually occurs is that the dose given to the smaller, elderly person is greater than that required to maintain the desired steady state blood levels, but the plasma concentration does not begin to rise into the toxic range until the total loading dose is given. This may take several days or weeks, during which the dose seems appropriate. Later, when the reservoir of body fat is filled, plasma concentration rises and the elderly person may become drowsy or confused as a result of overdosing.

Drugs distributed to body water require smaller loading doses in the elderly because of a smaller reservoir. Doses may need to be given more frequently to avoid wide fluctuations in blood levels.

Plasma Protein Binding

Since many drugs are bound to plasma proteins, the *decrease in albumin levels* of up to 20 percent which accompanies aging may alter drug distribution. Undernutrition, renal disease, and liver disease also decrease albumin binding capacity. The resultant increase in the free fraction of the drug can be expected to increase drug activity for most high-hepatic-clearance drugs (see Table 5-1). In the elderly, increased free fraction has been found as well for many renally excreted and low-hepatic-clearance drugs, including **warfarin, phenytoin, phenylbutazone, salicylates,** and **sulfadiazine,** probably because of age-related changes in elimination. This free fraction is also positively correlated with the number of drugs being taken, indicating that the elderly are at greater risk for drug interaction due to competition for albumin binding. Increased free drug levels mean greater drug response to a weight-adjusted dose, since only free drug is available for interaction with the receptor.

The protein alpha-1–acid glycoprotein is important to the plasma binding of many basic drugs such as **chlorpromazine** (Thorazine), **lidocaine,** and the tricyclic antidepressants. *Increased levels of α_1–acid glycoprotein* have been noted with aging. Although this is associated with enhanced drug binding, it is not of a magnitude to be of clinical significance. However, in chronic inflammatory states (e.g., cancer, arthritis) in which α_1–acid glycoprotein levels are further elevated, it is not known whether the increased binding has therapeutic significance.

There are several clinical implications of altered protein binding in the elderly. When interpreting drug blood levels, which are usually for total drug concentration (free and bound drug), allowance must be made for the increased free fraction of albumin-bound drugs, so lower total blood levels should be therapeutically effective. Dosages of highly albumin bound drugs should be decreased in the elderly:

1. For those drugs where hepatic clearance or renal excretion is also decreased in the elderly
2. For high-hepatic-clearance drugs (see Table 5-1), because the increased free fraction is not metabolized more rapidly
3. When the individual is on several drugs which are highly bound to plasma albumin

Careful observation for toxic effects or other adverse reactions is required whenever there is a change in drug regimen or the physiologic status of the elderly person, since body composition and drug binding may alter under these conditions.

Metabolism

Nutritional status, diet, pollutants, disease states, cigarette smoking, gender, genetic inheritance, and concomitant drug use contribute to an enormous interindividual variation in liver drug metabolizing function, making it difficult to quantify the effects of aging. There is a progressive decline in hepatic blood flow with age so that by age 60 it may be diminished by 40 to 50 percent. Most avidly metabolized (high-clearance) drugs, such as **propranolol,** are thus more slowly metabolized by the elderly.

The *size of the liver parenchyma as a percent of body weight also declines,* accompanied by a decrease in cytochrome P450 and other components of the microsomal enzyme system. This would be expected to decrease biotransformation of low-hepatic-clearance drugs, for which intrinsic enzyme activity is important. Evidence indicates that this is true for **amitriptyline** (Elavil), **imipramine** (Tofranil), **diazepam** (in men only), **chlordiazepoxide** (Librium), and **theophylline,** but not for **warfarin, lorazepam** (Ativan), **oxazepam** (Serax), or **isoniazid** (INH). Preliminary findings suggest that phase I oxidative metabolic pathways involving the *microsomal enzymes are somewhat impaired* in the elderly. In contrast the phase II conjugation reactions appear to remain relatively intact.

Elderly individuals seem to be *less prone to enzyme-inducing effects* of drugs and chemicals. Thus, older cigarette smokers metabolize drugs much more slowly than young smokers, at a rate comparable to their nonsmoking counterparts of a similar age. Effects of aging on first-pass metabolism are not clear, as both enhancement and impairment of bioavailability have been suggested.

Although there are insufficient data to make precise recommendations, it is advsied that with the elderly initial dosage levels of drugs metabolized by the microsomal enzymes

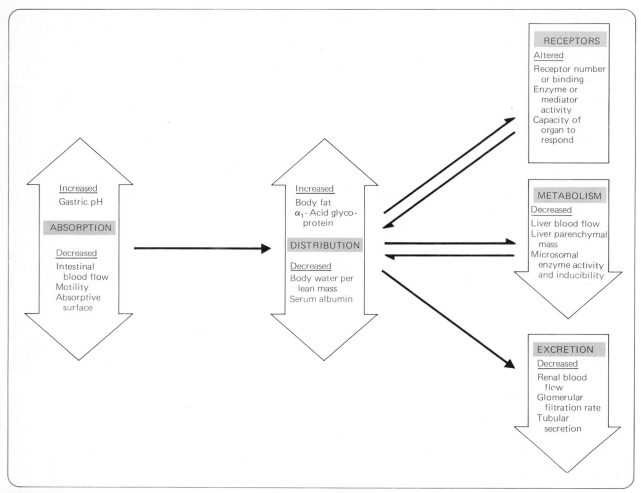

FIGURE 7-7

Summary of Pharmacokinetic and Pharmacodynamic Changes in the Elderly. Changes in absorption and distribution are complex, with increases in some parameters and decreases in others. Alteration in receptor sensitivity may result in increased or decreased response. Drug elimination is decreased due to declines in metabolism and excretion.

be reduced to one-half to two-thirds of the usual dosage for a younger adult. Those metabolized by nonoxidative pathways and phase II conjugation probably do not require dosage adjustment.

Excretion

There is a 50 percent *decline in renal function* between the ages of 20 and 70. Renal blood flow, glomerular filtration, and tubular secretion are all affected severely enough to require dosage reduction of those drugs whose major mode of elimination is through the kidney. These include **digoxin**, the **aminoglycoside antibiotics**, **procainamide** (Pronestyl), **nadolol** (Corgard), **clonidine** (Catapres), the **thiazide diuretics**, and the **penicillins**.

Because of the decline in endogenous creatinine formation secondary to reduced muscle mass with aging, the serum creatinine may give a deceptive impression of kidney function. The creatinine clearance can decrease significantly in the elderly while the serum creatinine remains within the normal range, so dosages of renally excreted drugs should be based upon an endogenous creatinine clearance test. Nomograms and dosage guidelines for a number of drugs have been developed based upon the creatinine clearance. If this test is not available or is impractical, the initial dosage for elderly persons should be based on the assumption of a 50 percent reduction in renal function and subsequently adjusted according to blood levels or clinical response.

PHARMACODYNAMICS AND ORGAN RESPONSE

In addition to altered pharmacokinetics, several factors may be responsible for the altered sensitivity of the elderly to some drugs. Changes in responsiveness may result from changes in receptor number or drug binding characteristics, alteration in the enzymes or mediators that translate the effect into the organ response, or changes in the capacity of the organ to respond.

The basis for the divergent pharmacodynamic responses of the elderly to most drugs is not well-studied. That the elderly are more sensitive to **diazepam** (Valium) and other benzodiazepines is well-established, but the mechanism is unknown. A change among the aged in beta-adrenoceptors has been implied from their decreased response to the sympathomimetic **isoproterenol** (Isuprel), but there is conflicting evidence regarding alteration in receptor number and binding. It is possible that there is less of the mediator adenosine 3′,5′-monophosphate (cyclic AMP), produced after β-stimulation in the elderly. The elderly are also more sensitive to the anticoagulant effects of **heparin** and **warfarin**, probably due to diminished capacity of the degenerated vessels to achieve mechanical hemostasis (intense vasospasm), although altered receptor activity may contribute to this effect.

Table 7-7 summarizes the pharmacokinetic and pharmacodynamic changes for selected drugs in the elderly.

ADVERSE DRUG REACTIONS IN GERIATRICS

The elderly have more chronic illnesses than other populations and take more prescription drugs. They frequently self-medicate with over-the-counter agents. As a result, the incidence of drug interactions and other adverse drug reactions is *two to seven times higher* in the elderly. Because of decreased compensatory capacity, adverse drug reactions are serious for the elderly and more often result in hospitalization. The signs of toxicity may manifest differently in the elderly or may be difficult to discriminate from symptoms of disease. Disease states also can make the elderly more susceptible to some adverse drug reactions. For example, ototoxicity (auditory nerve damage) is a more common result of **aminoglycoside antibotic** therapy when there is preexisting hearing impairment, a common finding in the elderly.

Risk factors for adverse drug reactions are being female, living alone, and being over 85 years old (referred to as "old old"). Those who are taking more than three drugs, who have renal impairment, and who have had previous adverse reactions are also more likely to develop an adverse drug

TABLE 7-7 Pharmacokinetic and Pharmacodynamic Changes with Common Drugs in the Elderly, Compared with Young Adults

DRUG	METABOLISM / EXCRETION	$t_{1/2}$	PLASMA PROTEIN BUILDING	V_d	CLEARANCE	RECEPTOR SENSITIVITY
Acetaminophen	Metabolized / 2% unchanged in urine	↑		0	↓	
Aminoglycosides	>95% unchanged in urine	↑	0	0	↓	
Amitriptyline*	Liver†	↑			↓	
Aspirin	Liver	↑	↓	0	↓	
Chlordiazepoxide	Liver†	↑	0	↑	↓	↑
Cimetidine	Liver / 60% unchanged in urine	↑		↓	↓	
Diazepam	Liver†	↑	0‡	↑	↓§	↑
Digoxin	Liver / 60–80% unchanged in urine	↑	0	↓	↓	0
Ethanol	Liver	0			↓	
Flurazepam	Liver†	↑		↑		↑
Lidocaine	Liver / 3% unchanged in urine	↑	0	↑	0	
Lithium	95% unchanged in urine	↑		↓	↓	
Lorazepam	Liver	0	0	0	0	↑
Meperidine	Liver	0	↓	0	0	↑‡
Oxazepam	Liver	0		0	0	↑
Penicillins	Primarily unchanged in urine	↑	0	↑	↓	
Procainamide	Liver / 50% unchanged in urine	↑			↓	
Propranolol	Liver	↑	0	0	↓	↓‡
Quinidine	Liver / 20% unchanged in urine	↑	0	0	↓	
Warfarin	Liver	0	↓	0	0	↑

0 = unchanged.   ↑ = increased.   ↓ = decreased.   Blank means no data available.   *Significantly higher blood levels following weight-adjusted dose.   †Active metabolites formed.   ‡Controversial finding.   §Men only, findings in women unchanged.

reaction. Common and troublesome adverse effects in the elderly include anticholinergic effects, dementia and depression, extrapyramidal symptoms, postural hypotension, and errors in drug self-administration. (See Chap. 6 for definition of adverse drug reaction.)

Anticholinergic Effects

Many drugs prescribed for the elderly or contained as ingredients in over-the-counter preparations (see Table 12-5) have anticholinergic action, which can cause discomfort and danger for the aged person. Anticholinergic effects are additive, and it is not uncommon for three agents with anticholinergic effects to be prescribed concomitantly for an elderly person. Anticholinergic effects include dry mouth, blurred vision, urinary hesitancy, constipation, ataxia, and confusion. Dry mouth impairs denture fit and can contribute to anorexia and poor nutritional status. For the man with prostatic hypertrophy, urinary retention can be life-threatening; urinary retention also contributes to incontinence in the elderly. Constipation leads to physical and psychologic discomfort in the individual raised to believe regular bowel function is crucial to good health, a common belief in the elderly. Ataxia predisposes to falls, and confusion is considered a symptom of dementia or depression. Anticholinergic effects can also impair temperature regulation and increase the risk of hyperthermia, precipitate an attack of acute angle-closure glaucoma in the predisposed individual, and increase the viscosity of respiratory secretions. The nursing process for these drug effects is considered in Chap. 12.

Dementia and Depression

The elderly often have decreased cognitive, as well as physical, reserve, so drugs can precipitate psychiatric disorders. Aging appears to be associated with altered levels of various neurotransmitters in the brain. For example, lower levels of the enzyme choline acetyltransferase, required for the production of acetylcholine, are found in the brains of elderly persons. Acetylcholine deficiency may be aggravated by the use of anticholinergic drugs, resulting in central anticholinergic syndrome, a type of reversible dementia. Digitalis toxicity can manifest as restlessness, agitation, and hallucinations, which are also typical of dementia. In fact 20 to 30 percent of reversible dementias in the elderly are secondary to drug effects. Endogenous and reactive depressions are common in the elderly, who are also highly susceptible to the depressant effects of centrally acting antihypertensive drugs, such as **methyldopa** (Aldomet) and **clonidine** (Catapres). Use of **reserpine** is discouraged in the elderly because of its tendency to cause gastric ulcers and depression. Antianxiety drugs and antipsychotics may also contribute to the development of depression.

Extrapyramidal Symptoms

Tremors and other abnormal movements are extrapyramidal symptoms, which often occur in elderly persons taking antipsychotic drugs. Decreased in brain neurotransmitters, such as dopamine and acetylcholine, probably contribute to the tendency of elderly persons to develop the symptoms. Parkinsonism (tremor and rigidity) usually appears early in treatment and can be controlled by anticholinergic drugs, which should not be used prophylactically because of their attendant risks. Tardive dyskinesia (abnormal movements in the area of the mouth and head) accompanies long-term antipsychotic therapy and may be irreversible.

Postural Hypotension

Impaired baroreceptor response and reduced peripheral venous tone in the elderly complicate the use of antihypertensives, diuretics, antipsychotics, and other drugs with hypotensive effects. When the older person goes rapidly from the lying to the standing position, a drop in blood pressure can occur, which may result in a fall, a fracture, even a stroke. The effect seems to be most pronounced at night, when many falls occur. Elderly persons should be taught to move slowly in stages from lying to standing and to seek assistance at night, especially when hospitalized.

Medication Errors

There are many reasons for the failure of elderly people to take a medication as intended by the prescriber (noncompliance). They may be unable to open the childproof container, to hear the instructions when the drug is prescribed, to read the small print on the label, or to swallow a capsule. Financial limitations may prevent them from having the prescription filled or cause them to take the drug less frequently than prescribed. They also may hoard old medications and lend or borrow medications among friends. Frequently, the labeling and the written and verbal directions about a medication are ambiguous or inadequate. Multiple medications and complex regimens are common. The elderly may see several specialists and have their prescriptions filled at several pharmacies, so it is not uncommon to find that they are taking two different brands of the same drug. Many elderly people feel that they are told too little about their diseases and their medications.

The current cohort of elderly typically hold a set of values and beliefs that affect medication taking. Independence is highly valued, and they are often reticent to "bother" the physician with questions or concerns, but then may ask the nurse or pharmacist. When they feel well, they are likely to discontinue medications because they don't understand that the drugs are still needed. The strength and importance of a medication is often judged by its size and color, and the elderly may not mention use of over-the-counter drugs, believing these are safe or "not drugs." From fear of being thought senile, many will not report and may even deny adverse drug effects like confusion, depression, or hallucinations.

NURSING PROCESS IMPLICATIONS

Assessment

The nurse must take careful medication histories from the elderly, including specific questions about when and how medications are taken, how they are stored, how nonprescription agents are used, financial status, what the patient knows about her or his disease and drugs, symptoms of adverse reactions, and values affecting medication-taking behaviors. Many older persons do not use the terms *medication* and *drug* as synonyms, reserving *drug* for very powerful or illicit substances, and may be offended if questioned about "drug use." Rather, the nurse should inquire about "medication use."

The drug regimen should be appraised for its appropriateness, for the individual elderly person (see Table 7-8). Dosages and dose intervals should be adjusted according to the age-related pharmacokinetics and pharmacodynamics of the drug as well as the weight, renal function, disease states, and drug sensitivity of the individual. Drug choice is also important. Agents with active metabolites and decreased clearance are often avoided in older people. For example, the half-lives of **diazepam** (Valium) and **flurazepam** (Dalmane)

TABLE 7-8 Summary of Geriatric Dosing Rules

General Guidelines

1. Geriatric patients will usually require one-third to one-half the dosage of drugs and less-frequent dosing.
2. Dosages should be started low and titrated upward until the desired therapeutic endpoint is reached.
3. Geriatric patients should be observed closely for changes in physiologic state that will alter drug requirements.

Specific Guidelines

1. Fat-soluble drugs have larger volumes of distribution, so they require larger loading doses, longer times to steady state, and less-frequent dosing.
2. Water-soluble drugs have smaller volumes of distribution in the elderly, so they require smaller loading doses and possibly more-frequent dosing to avoid wide fluctuations in blood levels.
3. Albumin-bound drugs probably require lower dosages if the elderly patient is on several highly albumin-bound drugs or if the drug is a high-hepatic-clearance drug.*
4. Drugs *oxidized* by the microsomal enzymes usually require lower doses.*
5. Drugs eliminated greater than 15–30% unchanged in the urine should have dosages reduced.*

---

*Dosing frequency may also be decreased.

are prolonged 2 to 4 times in the elderly, as are the half-lives of their active metabolites. **Oxazepam** (Serax) and **lorazepam** (Ativan) are metabolized by phase II conjugation reactions and have no active metabolites, and their pharmacokinetics do not appear to change with age. Therefore, oxazepam and lorazepam are considered the benzodiazepine drugs of choice for the elderly, although some clinicians regard the required frequent dosing as a disadvantage.

Many of the drugs elderly people take chronically can be safely discontinued. For example, about 75 percent of elderly persons in normal sinus rhythm on long-term **digoxin** therapy can have the drug withdrawn without problems and avoid the significant risk of digitalis toxicity, which is common in the elderly. All unnecessary drug use should be avoided.

Drug Administration

The most common general guideline regarding dosing in the elderly is to decrease the usual adult dose by one-half to one-third, but the best approach by far is to begin with a very low dose and titrate the dose slowly upward, according to patient response or blood level, until the preestablished goal is attained or adverse effects occur. The nurse is a vital team member in making the observations of patient response. Since dosage changes should not be made until steady state is attained (i.e., after 4 to 5 half-lives), the observations must be based on an assumption of prolonged half-life in the elderly. For the few drugs where this has been studied, information on half-life in the elderly is available in general drug references and in books and articles on drug therapy in the elderly.

Dosage Form and Packaging

Inadequate packaging and poor selection of dosage form contribute to noncompliance in the elderly. The directions on the container should be in dark, clear print and should give the name of the drug, its purpose, and specific instructions regarding when and how it is to be taken. A limited number of doses should be dispensed to the patient when a new agent is prescribed, to avoid expense and waste if the drug is ineffective or causes adverse effects. Patients who have difficulty opening childproof containers because of arthritis or poor hand grip strength should know that they can request other packaging, although this is dangerous if there are young children living in or visiting the household.

Solid oral dosage forms may be difficult for some elderly persons to swallow. Dividing tablets, even scored tablets, is difficult and inaccurate. Crushed tablets frequently yield particles that adhere to dentures and mouth structures. Liquid dosage forms, when available, are preferable because they are easy to swallow, most do not require dissolution, and they may be measured into small doses and dosage increments. However, those elderly persons with impaired dexterity or vision may have difficulty measuring liquid dosage forms. The abilities and preferences of the elderly person should be considered in selection of dosage form. Elderly persons often need to be instructed to take their medications with 8 oz of water to promote drug absorption and decrease the incidence of gastrointestinal adverse reactions.

Memory Aids

Simplified drug regimens with infrequent dosing and few medications are the best way to avoid omission and other medication errors. Yet optimum health and functioning of some elderly patients often require that they take several drugs and may require frequent dosing to avoid fluctuations in blood levels. Keeping the medications in a prominent place or associating medication administration with a routine daily activity is helpful for many elderly people. Written charts or calendars, where the drug can be checked off when it is taken, are useful to others (see Fig. 7-8). Color coding of the bottles with tape or felt tip pens, so that all medications administered at a certain time are marked in the same color, assists in assuring the proper number of dosings per day but does not assure correct dosage or number of pills per administration. Further, green and blue coding should be avoided, since yellowing of the lens with age makes the two colors difficult for many elderly to distinguish. The most controlled system is the use of special containers which have a compartment for each dose. The compartments can be filled in advance by the patient or a relative, friend, or visiting nurse. These containers are available commercially or can be improvised from an egg carton. A combination of several memory techniques can be used. It is often helpful for written instructions to include a description of the medication (color, size) and its purpose, as well as the name and dosing information.

Patient Education

The elderly have the same requirements for education regarding their disease and the medications (name, proper dosing, purpose, adverse effects, etc.) as any patient, but the need is magnified by the complexity of their drug regimen and the problems caused by age-related physical and psychosocial changes. The nurse should identify who is responsible

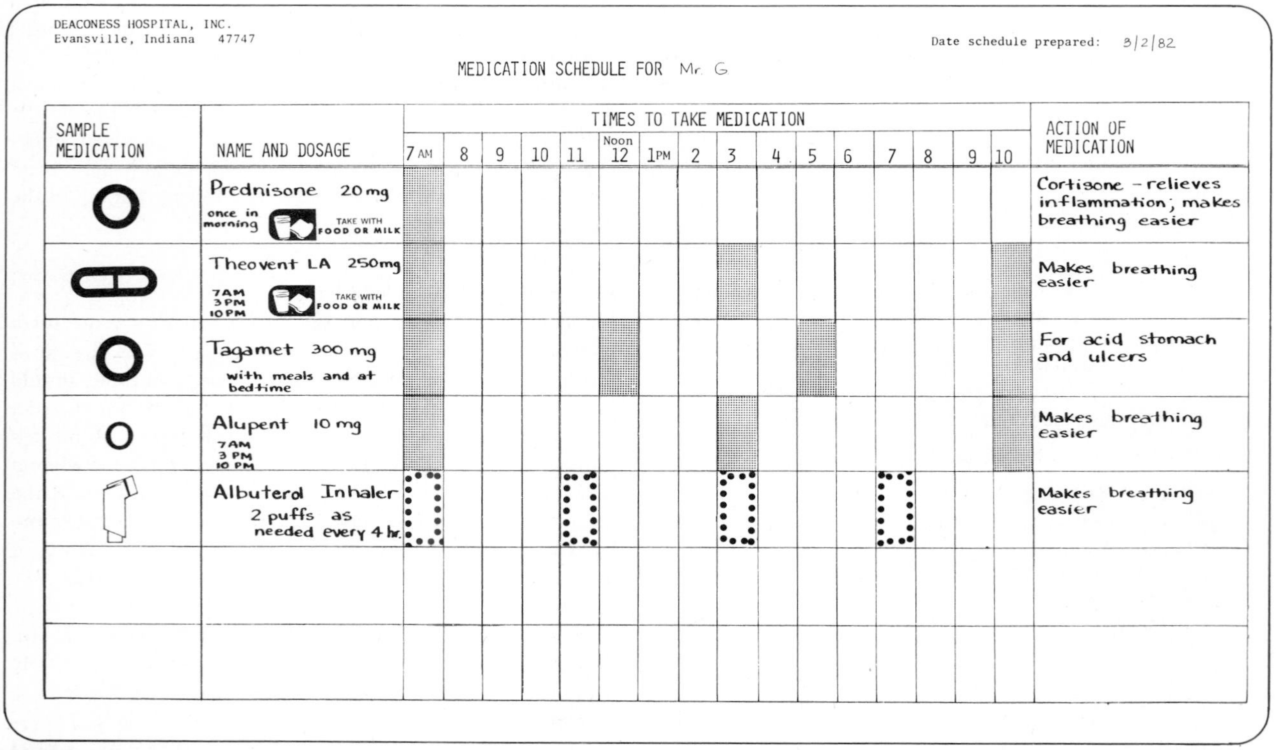

DEACONESS HOSPITAL, INC.
Evansville, Indiana 47747

Date schedule prepared: 3/2/82

MEDICATION SCHEDULE FOR Mr G

SAMPLE MEDICATION	NAME AND DOSAGE	7 AM	8	9	10	11	Noon 12	1 PM	2	3	4	5	6	7	8	9	10	ACTION OF MEDICATION
	Prednisone 20 mg once in morning TAKE WITH FOOD OR MILK																	Cortisone – relieves inflammation; makes breathing easier
	Theovent LA 250 mg 7 AM 3 PM 10 PM TAKE WITH FOOD OR MILK																	Makes breathing easier
	Tagamet 300 mg with meals and at bedtime																	For acid stomach and ulcers
	Alupent 10 mg 7 AM 3 PM 10 PM																	Makes breathing easier
	Albuterol Inhaler 2 puffs as needed every 4 hr.																	Makes breathing easier

FIGURE 7-8

Memory Aid. This medication administration record was planned with Mr. G. to suit his daily routine and usual requirements for PRN medication. The patient checks the shaded box when the drug is taken. Boxes outlined in dots indicate maximal frequency of the PRN drug. [*Source: P. S. Thompson and J. C. Willis: "Compliance Challenges in a Black Lung Clinic," Nurs Clin North Amer,* ***17****(3):513–521, 1982. Used by permission.*]

for administering or remembering the medications, if the elderly person is not *completely* independent in these activities, so all involved persons can be included in the education program. Instructions should be given both verbally and in large, legible print.

The best way to assure the patient can accurately self-administer his or her medications is to observe the actual procedure. Ability to read and comprehend the label instructions, to open the container, to select the correct dosage, and to swallow the dose should be assessed in the hospital or clinic when the drug is prescribed. Self-administration programs in the hospital provide opportunity for practice. The same brands that are to be used at home should be used in the hospital to familiarize the patient with the drugs' colors and sizes. The elderly patient should be taught how to store drugs and whether to take them with food, information which should be on the label. They should bring all medications with them to the clinic or when admitted to the hospital. They should also be told specifically what to do when they miss a dose or if an adverse reaction occurs.

Over-the-Counter Drugs

The elderly use a number of over-the-counter crugs, especially analgesics, laxatives, antacids, antidiarrheals, and cough and cold preparations. Part of the patient education program should concern the facts that these preparations are not entirely safe, may complicate or mask diseases common in aging, and have the potential to interact with prescription drugs. The patients should be encouraged to discuss these preparations with their pharmacists, nurses, or physicians. A pharmacy which keeps a record of what prescription drugs the patient is taking can help prevent overlapping and drug interactions between agents prescribed by several different specialists and with over-the-counter drugs.

Search for the Fountain of Youth

A number of vitamins, nutrients, hormones, enzymes, and other chemicals have been proposed at various times as the "cure" to aging or its effects. There is no convincing evidence to support claims that **vitamin E**, **hormones**, **procaine derivatives** (Gerovital, GH_3), **lecithin**, or other agents are effective in stopping or reversing aging. While often based on reputable theories of aging, the clinical research and rational therapeutic base for these agents is absent, and they have caused adverse effects. For example, it has been postulated that highly reactive oxygen-containing molecules contribute to cancer and aging. Superoxide dismutase, an enzyme that inactivates these molecules, is being proposed as an oral agent to prevent cancer and aging. Yet this drug is broken down in the stomach and does not reach the systemic circulation when given orally, and it has caused gastrointestinal distress. Health care providers must be able to provide the elderly with scientific appraisals of claims such as these, due to the cost and risk of ineffective agents.

CONCLUSION

This chapter has considered pharmacotherapeutics from a life-span developmental perspective. Clearly, age and other developmental states alter pharmacokinetics, susceptibility to adverse drug reactions, and nursing care approaches. Extremes of age (infancy and elderliness) are associated with decreased clearance, altered protein binding, and changes in distribution of many drugs, as well as other possible pharmacokinetic changes. During pregnancy and lactation the effects of maternal drugs on the child must be considered. Much more information is needed about the effects of development on the pharmacokinetics and pharmacodynamics of specific drugs and about the clinical implications of developmental changes for therapeutics.

REFERENCES

Pregnancy and Lactation

Beeley, L.: "Adverse Effects of Drugs in the First Trimester of Pregnancy," *Clin Obst Gynaecol*, 8:261–274, 1981.

———: "Drugs and Breast Feeding," *Clin Obstet Gynaecol*, 8:291–295, 1981.

Berkowitz, R. L., D. R. Coustan, T. K. Mochizuki: *Handbook for Prescribing Medications During Pregnancy*, Boston: Little, Brown, 1981.

Berlin, C. M.: "Pharmacologic Considerations of Drug Use in the Lactating Mother," *Obstet Gynecol*, 58 (Suppl. 5):17–23, 1981.

Bowes, W. A.: "The Effects of Medications on the Lactating Mother and her Infant," *Clin Obstet Gynecol*, 23:1073–1080, 1980.

Dickason, E. J.: "The Problem of Drug Use During Pregnancy," in E. J. Dickason, M. D. Schult and E. M. Morris (eds.), *Maternal and Infant Drugs and Nursing Intervention*, New York: McGraw-Hill, 1978.

Dilts, P. V.: "Placental Transfer," *Clin Obstet Gynecol*, 24:555–559, 1981.

FDA Drug Bulletin, 12:25, December 1981.

Guidelines on Pregnancy and Work, DHEW (NIOSH), Publication No. 78-118, Rockvllle, MD, U.S. Department of Health, Education, and Welfare, September 1977.

Levy, G.: "Pharmacokinetics of Fetal and Neonatal Exposure to Drugs," *Obstet Gynecol*, 58 (Suppl. 5):9–16, 1981.

Peterson, R. G., and W. A. Bowes: "Drugs, Toxins, and Environmental Agents in Breast Milk," in M. C. Neville and M. R. Neifert (eds.), *Lactation: Physiology, Nutrition and Breast Feeding*, New York: Plenum, 1983.

Pregnant Patients' Bill of Rights and Pregnant Patients' Responsibilities, Rochester, NY: International Childbirth Education Association, 1977.

Rayburn, W. R., and F. P. Zuspan: "Drug Use During Pregnancy," *Perinatal Press,* 4:115–117, 1980.

Infants and Children

Agurell, S., A. Berlin, H. Ferngren, and B. Hellstrom: "Plasma Levels of Diazepam after Parenteral and Rectal Administration in Children," *Epilepsia,* 16:277–283, 1975.

American Academy of Pediatrics Committee on Drugs: "Drug Tests in Children," *Pediatrics,* 43:463, 1969.

Bolme, P., et al.: "Pharmacokinetics of Theophylline in Young Children with Asthma: Comparison of Rectal Enema and Suppositories," *Eur J Clin Pharmacol,* 16:133–139, 1979.

Boréus, L. O.: *Principles of Pediatric Pharmacology,* New York: Churchill Livingstone, 1982.

Cohen, M. S.: "Special Aspects of Perinatal and Pediatric Pharmacology," in B. G. Katzung (ed.), *Basic and Clinical Pharmacology,* Los Altos, CA: Lange, 1982.

Collins, G. E., M. M. Clay, and J. M. Fallett: "A Prospective Study of the Epidemiology of Adverse Drug Reactions in Pediatric Hematology and Oncology Patients," *Am J Hosp Pharm,* 31:968–975, 1974.

Gill, M. A., and C. Udea: "Novel Method for the Determination of Pediatric Dosages," *Am J Hosp Pharm,* 33:389–392, 1975.

Mattar, M. E., J. Markello, and S. J. Yaffe: "Pharmaceutic Factors Affecting Pediatric Compliance," *Pediatrics,* 55:101–108, 1975.

McKenzie, M. W., R. B. Stewart, C. F. Weiss, and L. E. Cluff: "A Pharmacist-Based Study of the Epidemiology of Adverse Drug Reactions in Pediatric Medicine Patients," *Am J Hosp Pharm,* 30:898–903, 1973.

Mirkin, B. L.: "Pharmacodynamics and Drug Disposition in Pregnant Women," in K. L. Melmon and H. F. Morrelli (eds.), *Clinical Pharmacology: Basic Principles in Therapeutics,* New York: Macmillan, 1978.

Morselli, P. L.: "Clinical Pharmacokinetics in Neonates," *Clin Pharmacokinet,* 1:81–98, 1976.

Ormond, E. A. R., and C. Caulfield: "A Practical Guide to Giving Oral Medications to Young Children," *Am J Matern Child Nurs,* 1:320–325, 1976.

Shirkey, H. C.: *Pediatric Drug Handbook,* Philadelphia: Saunders, 1977.

———, "Therapeutic Orphans: Who Speaks for Children?" *J South Med Assoc,* 63:1361, 1970.

Tatro, D. S.: "Adverse Drug Reactions in Children," *Drug Intell Clin Pharm,* 7:109–113, 1973.

Wettrell, G., and K. E. Andersson: "Clinical Pharmacokinetics of Digoxin in Infants," *Clin Pharmacokinet,* 2:17–31, 1977.

Yaffe, S. J.: *Pediatric Pharmacology,* New York: Grune & Stratton, 1980.

Elderly Adults

Alford, D. M., and J. A. Moll: "Helping Elderly Patients in Ambulatory Settings Cope with Drug Therapy," *Nurs Clin North Am,* 17:275–282, 1982.

Anderson, W. F.: "Administration, Labeling, and General Principles of Drug Prescription in the Elderly," *Gerontol Clin,* 16:4–9, 1974.

Atkinson, L., I. Gibson, and J. Andrews: "An Investigation into the Ability of Elderly Patients Continuing to Take Prescribed Drugs After Discharge from the Hospital and Recommendations Concerning Improving the Situation," *Gerontology,* 24:225–234, 1978.

Bender, A. D.: "Pharmacodynamic Principles of Drug Therapy of the Aged," *J Am Geriatr Soc,* 22:296–303, 1974.

Blazer, D. G., C. F. Federspel, W. A. Ray, and W. Schaffner: "The Risk of Anticholinergic Toxicity in the Elderly: A Study of Prescribing Practices in Two Populations," *J Gerontol,* 38:31–5, 1983.

Boston Collaborative Drug Surveillance Program: "Clinical Depression of the Central Nervous Ssytem Due to Diazepam and Chlordiazepoxide in Relation to Cigarette Smoking and Age," *N Engl J Med,* 288:277–280, 1973.

Brown, M. M.: "Drug-Drug Interactions Among Residents in Homes for the Elderly," *Nurs Res,* 26:47–52, 1977.

Conrad, K. A., and R. Bressler (eds.): *Drug Therapy for the Elderly,* St. Louis: Mosby, 1982.

Davison, W.: "Neurological and Mental Disturbances Due to Drugs," *Age Ageing,* 7 (Suppl.):119–125, 1978.

Dellefield, K., and J. Miller: "Psychotropic Drugs and the Elderly Patient," *Nurs Clin North Am,* 17:303–318, 1982.

Divoll, M., B. Ameer, D. R. Abernethy, and D. J. Greenblatt: "Age Does Not Alter Acetaminophen Absorption," *J Am Geriatr Soc,* 30:240–244, 1982.

"Drugs and the Elderly," *Med Lett Drugs Ther,* 21:43–44, May 18, 1974.

Gerber, J. G.: "Drug Usage in the Elderly," in R. W. Schrier (ed.), *Clinical Internal Medicine in the Aged,* Philadelphia: Saunders, 1982.

Greenblatt, D. J., M. Divoll, S. K. Puri, I. Ho, M. A. Zinny, and R. I. Shader: "Reduced Single-Dose Clearance of Clobazem in Elderly Men Predicts Increased Multiple-Dose Accumulation," *Clin Pharmacokinet,* 8:83–89, 1983.

———, M. D. Allen, J. S. Harmatz, and R. I. Shader: "Diazepam Disposition Determinants," *Clin Pharmacol Ther,* 27:301–312, 1980.

Hollister, L. E.: "Prescribing Drugs for the Elderly Patient," in F. G. Ebaugh (ed.), *Management of Common Problems in Geriatric Medicine,* Reading, MA: Addison-Wesley, 1981.

Kaiko, R. F., S. L. Wallenstein, A. G. Rogers, P. Y. Grabinski, and R. W. Houde: "Narcotics in the Elderly," *Med Clin North Am,* 66:1079–1090, 1982.

Kiechel, J. R.: "Biotransformation of Drugs During Aging," *Gerontology,* 28 (Suppl. 1):101–112, 1982.

Kunze, M.: "Psychological Background of Noncompliance in Old Age," *Gerontology,* **28**(Suppl. 1):116–122, 1982.

Lamy, P. P.: *Prescribing for the Elderly,* Littleton, MA: PSG, 1980.

———: "Therapeutics and an Older Population: A Pharmacist's Perspective," *J Am Geriatr Soc,* **30**:53–55, 1982.

———: "Comparative Pharmacokinetic Changes and Drug Therapy in an Older Population," *J Am Geriatr Soc.* **30**:511–519, 1982.

———:"Over-the-Counter Medication: The Drug Interactions We Overlook," *J Am Geriatr Soc,* **30**:569–575, 1982.

LeSage, J.: "Drug Therapy in Long-Term Care Facilities," *Nurs Clin North Am,* **17**:331–340, 1982.

Ludin, D. V.: "Must Taking Medication be a Dilemma for the Independent Elderly?" *J Gerontol Nurs,* **4**:25–27, 1978.

———: "Medication-Taking Behavior and Compliance in the Elderly," in L. A. Pagliaro and A. M. Pagliaro (eds.), *Pharmacologic Aspects of Aging,* St. Louis: Mosby, 1983.

Meyer, B. R.: "Benzodiazepines in the Elderly," *Med Clin North Am,* **66**:1017–1036, 1982.

Oppeneer, J. E., and T. M. Vervoren: *Gerontological Pharmacology: A Resource for Health Practitioners,* St. Louis: Mosby, 1983.

Reidenberg, M. M.: "Drugs in the Eldery," *Med Clin North Am,* **66**:1073–1078, 1982.

Requarth, C. M.: "Medication Usage and Interaction in Long-Term Care Elderly," *J Gerontol Nurs,* **5**:33–37, 1979.

Salzman, C., R. I. Shader, J. Harmatz, and L. Robertson: "Psychopharmacologic Investigations in Elderly Volunteers: Effect of Diazepam in Males," *J Am Geriatr Soc,* **23**:451–457, 1975.

Schmucker, D. L.: "Age-Related Changes in Drug Disposition," *Pharmacol Rev,* **30**:445–456, 1979.

Schulz, P., K. Turner-Tamiyasu, G. Smith, K. M. Giacominci, and T. Blaschke: "Amitriptyline Disposition in Young and Elderly Normal Men," *Clin Pharmacol Ther,* **33**:360–365, 1983.

Shand, D. G.: "Biological Determinants of Altered Pharmacokinetics in the Elderly," *Gerontology,* **28** (Suppl. 1):8–17, 1982.

Vestal, R. E.: "Drug Use in the Elderly: A Review of Problems and Special Considerations," *Drugs,* **16**:358–382, 1982.

Vestal, R. F.: "Pharmacology and Aging," *J Am Geriatr Soc,* **30**:191–199, 1982.

Virtanen, F., J. Kanto, E. Iiasalo, E. U. M. Iiasalo, M. Salo, and S. Sjovall: "Pharmacokinetic Studies on Atropine with Special Reference to Age," *Acta Anaesthesiol Scand,* **26**:279–300, 1982.

Wallace, S., and B. Whiting: "Factors Affecting Drug Binding in Plasma of Elderly Patients," *Br J Clin Pharmacol,* **3**:327–330, 1976.

Wood, M., M. Blatman: "Drug Therapy in the Elderly," *Am Fam Physician,* **19**:143–152, 1979.

Wollner, L.: "Postural Hypotension in the Elderly," *Age Ageing,* **7** (Suppl.):112–114, 1978.

8

LEGAL AND ETHICAL CONSIDERATIONS IN PHARMACOTHERAPEUTICS*

MARY HARKNESS MAYERS
RITA J. PAYTON

While it is common to regard the legal and ethical aspects of an issue as similar or synonymous, the two perspectives are quite unique. Both involve application of rules or theories to decision making, but the source and substance of these principles are different for the ethical and legal viewpoints. What is legal may not be ethical, and ethical actions are not necessarily the legally sanctioned approaches.

Although neither the legal nor the ethical perspective offers an absolute prescription for all situations, these considerations constitute two components of nursing judgment. This chapter presents the legal and ethical bases for the role of the nurse in drug therapy.

LEGAL CONSIDERATIONS[1]

LEARNING OBJECTIVES

Upon mastery of the contents of this section, the reader will be able to:

1. List the state and federal laws which govern the administration of medications and devices and the general purpose and content of those laws.

2. Differentiate between codified, or legislature-passed, law and lawsuit, or court-written, law.

3. Identify the most important sources for determining legal standards of nursing care in drug administration.

4. Explain the function of standards, policies in manuals, and professional literature in assisting a legislature, judge, or jury in determining what the law should be.

5. Describe how the components of the nursing process assist in the logical application of legal guidelines to medication administration.

6. Differentiate informed consent as a fluid and variable process in administering medications from informed consent as a signed document.

Every time a nurse administers a medication, there arises a relationship between a pair of concepts. Those concepts are, first, the patient's personal *right* to competent and informed treatment and, second, the nurse's *responsibility* to give such care and treatment and nothing else. This right-responsibility relationship is the basis for describing the legal implications of the administration of medications by nurses. A nurse must know and understand the sources and theories of the responsibilities in administering medications, as well as the sources and theories of the patient's various rights. If an error or omission occurs and such knowledge is lacking, liability for negligence or intentional wrongdoing may ensue. The purpose of this section is to present and explain the various sources from which a nurse learns both the legal guidelines for pharmacotherapeutics and the basic theories of liability if the guidelines are not followed. A summary of the sources of law is presented in Table 8-1.

FEDERAL LAWS

The federal government controls drugs and devices chiefly in two ways. The first is general, whereby the government, under the Food, Drug, and Cosmetic Act, sets rigid standards for the development, research, manufacture, and sale of all drugs. In 1976 Congress added to this act the Medical Device Amendments, which govern the marketing of special equipment and devices used in medical care. The second

---

*The legal section was authored by M. H. Mayers; R. J. Payton wrote the section on ethical considerations.

[1]Previously published portions of this manuscript are used by permission of the publisher and author: M. H. Mayers, "Legal Guidelines," *Geriatric Nursing,* **2**(6):417–421, 1981. Copyright © 1981, American Journal of Nursing Company.

TABLE 8-1 Sources of Law Pertaining to the Nursing Role in Drug Therapy

SOURCE	REGULATORY OR ENFORCEMENT AGENCY	LAW OR PROVISION WITH EXAMPLES
		A. Codified Law

Federal government's United States code	Food and Drug Administration (Department of Health and Human Services)	Food, Drug, and Cosmetic Act of 1906 (amended 1938, 1962, 1972, 1976)
		  Establishes which drugs require prescriptions
		  Requires drugs to be safe and effective
		  Mandates proper manufacturing, labeling, shipping, and storing of drugs
		  Grants approval for use of an investigational new drug (IND)
		  Identifies therapeutically equivalent drugs
		  Governs development and marketing of medical devices

	Drug Enforcement Administration (Department of Justice)	Controlled Substances Act of 1970
		  Provides for five classes of controlled substances and their requisite use, handling, prescribing, and refill procedures (see Table 8-2)
		  Describes procedures necessary for registration for providers who prescribe, dispense, and administer controlled substances
		  Describes community mental health rehabilitation projects for drug abuse and addiction

State codes	Professional boards of the states	State practice acts
		  Define who can be licensed as a physician, nurse, or pharmacist
		  Define practice of those professional disciplines
		  Discipline practitioners for violations of act or for crimes of moral turpitude
		  (States also have food, drug, and cosmetic acts and controlled substances acts similar to federal ones.)

		B. Noncodified Law

Federal and state court decisions	Federal and state courts, boards, commissions, and agencies	Various doctrines adopted, such as patient's right
		  To have a professional relationship with a health care provider
		  To receive treatment and care commensurate with his or her needs
		  To give informed consent
		  To refuse treatment

		C. Quasi-Law *

Published guidelines, policies, and procedures	Joint Commission on Accreditation of Hospitals (JCAH)	Guidelines (see Table 8-3)
		  On preoperative medications (to be automatically cancelled at time of surgery)
		  On drugs to be added to intravenous solutions (only in a specific manner and under certain conditions)

	American Nurses Association American Medical Association American Pharmaceutical Association	Various promulgations and statements
		  Position papers
		  Codes of ethics
		  Joint practice publications

	Individual institutions	Policies and procedures
	Publications in textbooks and professional periodicals	Research, treatises, and articles

*Professional opinions and practices, which by virtue of their acceptance and adoption by practitioners respected and recognized as experts in their fields, would carry great weight in assisting judges, juries, and legislatures in determining the law on a particular point.

area specifically addressed by the federal government is the regulation of those drugs which have the potential to lead to abuse and therefore require strict handling; this authority is under the Controlled Substances Act.

Food, Drug, and Cosmetic Act

The Food and Drug Administration (FDA) has developed regulations which govern the purity, labeling, potency, safety, and effectiveness of drugs, cosmetics, and devices. It has complete jurisdiction to decide which drugs are considered safe for intended use and, therefore, which ones are allowed to be manufactured and sold to the general public. Of these, the FDA also determines which ones may be sold "over the counter" (OTC) and which ones will require a physician's supervision and therefore a physician's prescription. Elaborate and extensive mechanisms are in place to safeguard the approval process for new drugs (see Chap. 9).

Controlled Substances Act

The second area of federal jurisdiction falls under the Controlled Substances Act and involves those medications called "controlled substances," or "schedule drugs." The distribution and use of these medications—narcotics, depressants, stimulants, and hallucinogens—are rigidly controlled by very specific laws and regulations. The drugs can be dispensed and administered only if ordered by a physician who is registered with the federal Drug Enforcement Administration (DEA). Also, they can be delivered to and stored with only those physicians or registered institutions, such as hospitals and pharmacies. Whenever a nurse obtains and prepares a controlled substance for administration to a patient, a special control slip, individually numbered and labeled to indicate a specific type and amount of drug, must be completed to account for its proper use. The Controlled Substances Act divides the drugs into five classes according to the drugs' potential for being mishandled or misused (see Table 8-2). Some of the drugs on schedule I are not approved for medicinal use in the United States, although they may be so used in other countries.

Enforcement of the Controlled Substances Act is the responsibility of the DEA. According to the act, all registrants (who usually are physicians and pharmacists) must maintain and keep open to inspection complete, accurate records of all controlled substances received and disposed of; they must be able to show that safeguards are being maintained and that the drugs are not readily available to unauthorized persons or diverted to illegal uses. At minimum a locked storage cabinet with an alarm system is required. Also, virtually all hospitals require that the drugs available on nursing units be counted at the beginning and end of each nursing shift and that this count be compared to a "proof of use" sheet kept for each medication.

There are severe criminal penalties in the laws for violations of the Controlled Substances Act. The most frequent violations of the act are the illegal possession, use, or distribution of the drugs by physicians, pharmacists, and nurses. In addition to the criminal prosecution and penalty imposition (fine and/or imprisonment) by the state or federal attorney general, a practitioner in most states would lose, at least temporarily, his or her license to practice the profession. A nurse's responsibility in regard to these laws is not only to him- or herself and all patients, but also to other nurses, pharmacists, and physicians. Professional health care providers can be found to be conspirators to a crime if they have knowledge that controlled substances are being mishandled (not recorded or used properly), tampered with, or prescribed or administered in inordinate amounts, yet do not notify the proper hospital or government authorities.

STATE PRACTICE ACTS

States have three laws which describe who may prescribe, dispense, and administer medications or drugs to the general public. These three laws are the practice acts for nursing, medicine, and pharmacy.

The general practice acts for nursing as a rule do not specifically address medication administration. They do address in some manner the fact that the law sanctions the nurse to (1) follow the physicians' orders for the administration of

TABLE 8-2   Schedules of Controlled Drugs

SCHEDULE I	All nonresearch use is forbidden. Examples are heroin, LSD, marijuana, mescaline, peyote.
SCHEDULE II	No telephone prescriptions, no refills are allowed. Examples are opium, codeine, morphine, meperidine (Demerol), oxycodone (ingredient in Percodan, Tylox, Percocet), amphetamine, methylphenidate (Ritalin).
SCHEDULE III	Prescription must be rewritten after 6 months or five refills. Examples are benzphetamine (Didrex), butabarbital (Butisol), glutethimide (Doriden), Schedule II drugs in mixtures with noncontrolled drugs or suppository form.
SCHEDULE IV	Prescriptions must be rewritten after 6 months or five refills. Schedule IV differs from Schedule III in penalties for illegal possession. Examples are pentazocine (Talwin); propoxyphene (Darvon); diethylpropion (Tenuate); fenfluramine (Pondimin); benzodiazepines such as diazepam (Valium), lorazepam (Ativan), chlordiazepoxide (Librium); chloral hydrate; meprobamate (Miltown, Equanil), phenobarbital.
SCHEDULE V	Treat drugs like any other (nonnarcotic) prescribed drug. They may also be dispensed without prescription unless additional state restrictions apply. Examples are diphenoxylate (in restricted dosages and with atropine, as in Lomotil), restricted concentrations of codeine, dihydrocodeine, ethylmorphine.

medications and other treatments and (2) provides for the nursing care and teaching of patients.

Every state has promulgated a law defining the practice of pharmacy and regulating and licensing who may be a pharmacist. The practice of pharmacy is usually defined as preparing, compounding. dispensing, and retailing prescriptions, drugs, medicines, and chemicals. *Dispensing* is defined as labeling, delivering, or distributing drugs, usually in quantities of several doses, whereas *administration* is the apportionment of a single dose to a patient. Theoretically, any time a nurse removes a prescribed preparation from a pharmacy shelf or storage space in order to administer it, it is called dispensing and in almost every state is not authorized by law. Likewise, transfer of a medication to a new container for storage, and labeling or relabeling of containers are not authorized functions of the nurse.

The medical practice act usually provides that physicians may prescribe, dispense, and administer medications. These laws also generally contain a statement that no one else may administer medications *except* registered nurses or licensed practical nurses. Recently, legislatures in a few states have authorized qualified nurse practitioners to prescribe some medications within a protocol or under the supervision of a physician. Therefore, as far as the states are concerned, the control of diagnostic and therapeutic medications and devices is limited to a description of who may perform the three acts of prescribing, dispensing, and administering such substances and articles to the public.

The written laws of the states and federal government are among the formal promulgations adopted by legislatures for the health and welfare of all citizens. These basic laws are, however, broad or general measures. The two main sources of rules more specifically describing patients' rights and the nurse's concomitant responsibilities are (1) applicable case law (lawsuits for which decisions have been made and opinions have been written describing the decisions, also called common law and equal in force to codified law) and (2) guidelines for nursing found in publications of professional bodies, institutional policy and procedure manuals, textbooks, and periodicals.

STANDARDS OF CARE IN MEDICATION ADMINISTRATION

Case Law

Many lawsuits have been brought by patients against nurses or the nurses' employers because of errors or omissions related to the administration of or response to medications. From these cases—which are the most specific and important source of the applicable law for nurses—can be deduced four legal principles for proper drug administration:

1. The drug should be prepared according to a valid physician's order or protocol.
2. The drug should be administered correctly.

3. Consent to receive the drug should be informed.
4. Response to each drug should be assessed.

The following case discussions will serve to illustrate some of these principles.

Carrying out the physician's order exactly as it is written is one of the clearest responsibilities of the nurse. Not promptly noting and administering a stat order for **thioridazine** (Mellaril) was the source of a nurse's negligence in *Farrow v. Health Services Corporation* (604 P.2d 474, Utah, 1979). The patient received the thioridazine 2 h after it was ordered. Later that night he jumped from a window and died. The court said that the jury could decide the effect of this delay on the patient's death, that the nurse's testimony showed that a physician's order for medication to be administered stat means immediately, and that to give it at 10 P.M. after the 8 P.M. request did not comply with the order.

Correct administration of medications is always a legal responsibility of the nurse. Some of the most frequent errors occur when written physicians' orders can be correctly interpreted only by referring to previous orders or by having specialized knowledge, as in coronary care or pediatric nursing.

The "previous order" problem is illustrated by a 1961 case, *Larrimore v. Homeopathic Hospital Association* (176 A.2d 362, Super. Ct. Del., 1961). A nurse administered 30 mg of **pentolinium tartrate** (Ansolysen) intramuscularly to Mr. Larrimore, over his protest, after she had been off duty for 2 days. She checked only the most recent order, which read: "Reduce Ansolysen to 30 mg today." Three days earlier the nurse had given this patient Ansolysen 50 mg IM, per the then-current order. During her absence the route had been changed to oral. The nurse was held negligent for not validating her interpretation of the order and for not following the basic rule that any order that does not specify the route of administration is interpreted to mean oral administration.

Informed consent is required in any treatment situation, including drug therapy. Initially it is the prescriber's responsibility to discuss with the patient the purpose of the drug, its adverse effects, alternative treatment or drugs available, and risks if the drug is not used. The patient has the right, and must be given the opportunity, to question, postpone, or refuse the drug. The patient's consent need not be in writing.

Maintaining informed consent may be a troublesome matter. For example, certain antihypertensive drugs (e.g., reserpine) can cause severe depression. It is questionable whether the consent given by a patient who becomes depressed because of the drug remains complete and informed. Another problem is that a person may not be competent to grant or refuse consent. Legal competence is a relative concept, however, requiring various levels of apparent understanding for different purposes. Often a patient can give a clear, unequivocal response—either consent or refusal—during a lucid interval. Such a statement should be well-documented and respected. If a person is not competent, a close family member may be able to give consent or it may be necessary to have the court appoint a legal guardian. Once consent has been obtained, the nurse and physician are responsible for seeing that it continues to be informed and voluntary.

The last important responsibility of the nurse is noting and reporting the effects of the medication on the patient. These observations require that the nurse understand the condition of the patient which indicated the drug, what the expected outcome is, what adverse effects might occur, and the effects of drug reduction or withdrawl. This responsibility was highlighted in the case of *Weatherly v. New York* (441 N.Y.S.2d 319, Ct. Cl., 1981), concerning a patient who was receiving both **perphenazine** (Trilafon), an antipsychotic, and **amitriptyline hydrochloride** (Elavil), an antidepressant. After evaluating the patient's response and behavior for some time, the psychiatrist discontinued the perphenazine, which had been the "covering" medication allowing the antidepressant to be of greatest effect. During the next 5 days the patient became increasingly restless, confused, and ultimately quite terrified. A nurse and a nursing assistant were witnesses to these behaviors, but they did not notify the physician to explain what was occurring. At 7 A.M. one day the patient became extremely psychotic and jumped through a window, sustaining permanent injuries. In the lawsuit which was filed, the hospital and nursing staff were found liable for failing to exercise due care in monitoring and reporting the patient's condition after the cover drug was removed.

Professional Literature, Nursing Policies, and Procedure Manuals

Although they are not considered laws or regulations, the guidelines contained in reputable professional literature and references, in the manual of the Joint Commission on Accreditation of Hospitals (JCAH), and in written manuals developed by nursing departments of hospitals, clinics, and colleges are strongly persuasive about what the "law" should be in a nursing problem or situation. When administering medications, a nurse's decision to deviate from a written policy or procedure must be explained clearly and intelligently. "Following a doctor's order" is not sufficient reason for violation of an adopted guideline addressing the proper method of administering a medication, nor does it justify giving a dangerous dosage level or improper drug. The prescribing physician should always be notified of the conflict faced by the nurse, and either the order should be changed or the nurse should decline to administer the drug and should notify the pharmacist and nursing supervisor. Two examples of Joint Commission requirements are given in Table 8-3. One addresses the automatic cancellation of preoperative drug orders, and the other gives the requirements for adding drugs to intravenous solutions.

An example of a nurse's responsibility to adhere to a nursing policy and procedure manual's guideline is depicted

TABLE 8-3 Examples of Pharmacy Guidelines from the Joint Commission on Accreditation of Hospitals

Standard V

Written policies and procedures governing the safe administration of drugs and biologicals shall be developed by the medical staff in cooperation with the pharmaceutical department/service, the nursing service, and, as necessary, representatives of other disciplines.

Interpretation

Written policies and procedures governing the safe administration of drugs shall be reviewed at least annually, revised as necessary, and enforced. Such policies and procedures shall include, but not necessarily be limited to, the following:

There shall be an automatic cancellation of standing drug orders when a patient undergoes surgery. Automatic drug-stop orders shall otherwise be determined by the medical staff and stated in medical staff rules and regulations. There shall be a system to notify the responsible practitioner of the impending expiration of a drug order, so that the practitioner may determine whether the drug administration is to be continued or altered.

Cautionary measures for safe admixture of parenteral products shall be developed. Whenever drugs are added to intravenous solutions, a distinctive supplementary label shall be affixed to the container. The label shall indicate the patient's name and location; the name and amount of the drug(s) added; the name of the basic parenteral solution; the date and time of the addition; the date, time, and rate of administration; the name or identifying code of the individual who prepared the admixture; supplemental instructions; and the expiration date of the compounded solution.

Source: JCAH: *Accreditation Manual for Hospitals*, 1984.

in the case of a patient who is receiving the anticoagulant **warfarin sodium** (Coumadin). Standard medical practice dictates that prothrombin times shall be drawn and determined for all patients on warfarin. The written nursing procedure might provide: "If laboratory results for a patient's prothrombin time are greater than 2 times the control, it should be called to the attention of the physician." In this circumstance, for the nurse to either give the warfarin or withhold it but not call the doctor would violate the procedure and be an important ingredient in the accumulation of sufficient evidence to support a theory of negligence.

THE NURSING PROCESS

Since the nursing process is well accepted by the profession, its components describing the nurse's responsibilities would be used to frame legal analysis whenever there was a serious problem, resulting in a lawsuit, involving a nurse and the administration of medications. Some rights and responsibilities concerning medication administration are outlined with the nursing process in Table 8-4. Each of the previously described cases can be dissected into the responsibilities of

TABLE 8-4   Questions for Review in Using the Nursing Process to Ensure Safe Drug Administration

Assessment

Allergies?
Medications taken previously?
Drug-drug or drug-food interactions?
Kidney and liver status?
OTC or prescription drugs with patient?
Ability to swallow oral medications?

Management

Radiographic or other tests planned?
Extra teaching necessary?
Medications and laboratory test schedules?
Nothing-by-mouth status coming up?
Activity or visitors affected?
Relationship of medications to meals?
Generic or substitute?
Possibility of anaphylaxis?
Need for site rotation?
Is patient questioning drug?
Five rights: drug, route, dose, time, patient?
Does package or device appear tampered with?

Evaluation

Adverse effects?
Frequency of PRN administration?
Signs and symptoms of inadequate dosage or overdose?
Improvement being noted?

assessment, management, and *evaluation,* and in each case it can be determined where the nurse was derelict in fulfilling the particular duty concerning a certain medication and how that negligence caused harm or injury to the patient. The following cases also help to illustrate this legal analysis.

The importance of *assessment* is illustrated by the case of a nurse who cared for a postoperative patient who had a PRN narcotic order for pain (Oulton, 1982). The patient became very restless, and the nurse, interpreting this as pain, administered the narcotic. The patient went into respiratory arrest. Resuscitation was attempted but the patient remained comatose. The nurse was judged liable for failing to assess the patient properly—that is, recognize the signs of hypoxia in a postoperative patient.

Negligence in *management* is illustrated by the *Drewry* case (619 S.W.2d 397, Tenn. App., 1981). While receiving **calcium gluconate** intravenously, a patient called the nurse to complain about burning and swelling at the site. The nurse did nothing until the intravenous solution had been infused completely. Serious injury ensued, for which the nurse could have been completely responsible, since the tissue-sloughing properties of calcium gluconate should be known to anyone administering it.

Avoiding negligence in *evaluation* of patient response to a drug requires that the nurse recognize the most common adverse effects and signs of toxicity of drugs encountered in the particular specialty practiced. For example, in the 1977 *Dillon* case in California, a patient sued a physician and hospital because of deafness caused by excess administration of **kanamycin sulfate** (Kantrex) (#C-18319, Los Angeles Cty. Super. Ct., 1977). The court stated that the nurses should have recognized that the patient's hearing was deteriorating and should have alerted the doctor that the patient was receiving too much of the drug.

PRN Orders   The administration of "as needed" or "as necessary" (PRN) medications is a responsibility of nurses with implications for significant liability if the nursing process is not fulfilled properly. Such orders, whether given with one particular patient in mind or developed as part of a protocol or list of "standing" orders, represent a delegated prescribing function that is not to be taken lightly. A situation which illustrates the legal responsibilities of the nurse in following a PRN medication order is the following: A patient who was known to be an alcohol abuser was admitted after suffering smoke inhalation in a fire. She was placed on a ventilator with an endotracheal tube, and **chlordiazepoxide hydrochloride** (Librium) 50 mg IM every 4 h PRN for restlessness was ordered. The patient became very agitated and anxious, pulled out the endotracheal tube, and suffered serious injury from oxygen deprivation. The nurse was found negligent for not having administered the PRN chlordiazepoxide when serious signs of restlessness first appeared, although those signs of restlessness had been documented in the medical record.

There are three separate and distinct duties the nurse had in this case. The first is called awareness, or "mental mid-set." For any patient, the nurse must know in the beginning of her *assessment* that a PRN order exists, understand its purpose, and then continuously use assessment skills to be ready to pick up specific indications that the drug is needed. Second, the nurse must plan the best intervention and accurately administer the drug when indicated, which constitutes *management.* Third, after the drug is administered, it is the nurse's responsibility to *evaluate* whether the patient responds appropriately and, therefore, whether the PRN order is optimum (i.e., in strength and frequency of medication) in addressing the need. In this case, the nurse failed to relate the assessed data to the intended indications for the drug.

Summary of Legal Aspects

The sources of specific laws and regulations which govern health care in general, and the administration of drugs and devices in particular, are constantly changing. As knowledge about medicine and pharmacology expands, and as technologic innovations continue to be developed at a rapid rate, the laws and regulations will have to reflect higher and higher standards for nursing practice. However, the basic axiom in the law about patient care, which includes medication administration, will not be greatly affected. That axiom is:

> A registered nurse's duty owed to the patient is to exercise the requisite amount of care toward a patient that that particular patient's condition may require, and to protect the patient from dangers that may result from the patient's physical and mental incapacities, as well as from external circumstances peculiarly within the nurse's control. [*Daniel*, 415 So.2d 586, La. App., 1982]

ETHICAL CONSIDERATIONS

LEARNING OBJECTIVES

Upon mastery of the contents of this section, the reader will be able to:
1. Define an ethical dilemma.
2. Identify major ethical principles applicable in drug administration.
3. Identify problem areas in drug therapy which are potential sources of ethical dilemmas.

The term *ethics* refers to the right- and wrong-making characteristics of actions. Nurses are constantly in situations which require them to be concerned with ethical justification for their actions. An *ethical dilemma* occurs when there is a conflict between existing ethical principles in a given situation. The nurse has independent ethical responsibility for each nursing action. No one member of the health care team has greater or lesser responsibility for the ethics of actions which occur in the delivery of health care. Nurses' basic responsibilities in relationship to ethics include familiarity with ethical principles espoused by the profession and familiarity with some ethical decision-making process.

ETHICAL PRINCIPLES

Autonomy
Autonomy is also referred to as self-determination. Issues in patient self-determination often arise in relationship to drug therapy. Professional nursing strongly supports client autonomy. Client autonomy is reflected in behavior that is both authentic and independent. Self-determined behavior is reflected in the competent adult client's right to refuse medication regardless of the circumstances. The ability of an incompetent client to be autonomous may be limited.

Paternalism
Paternalism involves the use of coercion to gain client compliance with prescribed intervention patterns, including the taking of ordered drugs. Health care professionals tend to be highly paternalistic in our society. Paternalism is not necessarily an evil term. It is assumed that when nurses behave in a paternalistic fashion they do so out of concern for their client's health.

There are many forms of coercion. Most nurses would not agree with physically forcing medication down a patient's throat. However, even the statement "But you've got to take your pill—the doctor ordered it" can be perceived as coercive by many patients. Patients fear they will receive less than optimal care if they do not comply with prescribed therapy.

Truth Telling
Truth telling as a principle refers to being honest. Nurses can be less than honest with a client when they omit parts of the information the client needs in order to make an informed decision about whether or not to take a certain drug. Nurses practice information control, that is, the nonprovision of needed information to the client, more than they ever lie outright. Such unjustified information control violates the principles of truth telling just as much as the telling of an outright lie.

Respect for Property Rights
When a drug has been ordered for a patient and has been delivered from the pharmacy, the drug obviously belongs to the patient. Stealing of drugs by substitution of other substances is a direct violation of the principle of respect for property rights. Similarly, taking drugs or food from a patient's bedside stand without his or her consent violates this principle, even if it is done to protect the patient from harm or potential drug interaction.

DILEMMAS RELATED TO DRUG THERAPY

An *ethical dilemma* exists when, in a given situation, two or more ethical principles are in conflict. As you read the following problem areas which occur in relationship to drug therapy, identify the principles which are applicable in the situation. Remember that a list of absolute ethical rules does not exist, nor could one be generated or even prove useful over time. The individual nurse must establish priority of principles when principles are in conflict.

Answering a Patient's Questions about a Drug
Patients ask nurses many questions about the drugs they are taking. Some patients are simply interested in knowing the name of the drug; other patients want a detailed description of the purpose and side effects of the drug; and some patients want a comparison of the effectiveness and side effects of the drug that has been ordered with other drugs that are available. It is obvious that a nurse must be totally familiar with any drug that is being administered. In many clinical settings in which nurses practice, written or unwritten policies apply to what a nurse can tell a patient. But it is demeaning

to the nurse and less than honest to the patient if the nurse assumes a dumb "I don't know" attitude. The nurse should make every attempt to answer the patient's questions in an honest and straightforward manner.

Refusal or Noncompliance

Patients refuse to take prescribed medications for many reasons. They may be afraid of the drug, they may not believe in drug therapy, or they may be afraid the drug will make them sick. Nurses tend to react with disbelief and/or anger at overt refusal by a patient to take a prescribed drug. Nurses are sometimes afraid they will get into trouble if the patient does not take the drug. It really is important, therefore, to make efforts to understand why refusal is occurring. Many times the provision of additional information about the drug by the nurse will yield compliance in a noncoercive manner.

Dishonest measures such as disguising or hiding the drug in another substance are highly suspect. Verbal tactics which pressure the patient to comply may easily become coercive if they give rise to unreasonable fear within the patient. Patients in the institutional setting may comply out of fear, but once the patient is dismissed from the institutional setting, follow-through compliance in drug therapy will be greatly compromised.

Incompetent Patient

An incompetent patient is one who has not yet attained the age of reason, one who has temporarily lost the ability to behave in a rational fashion, or one who has permanently lost the ability to make rational decisions. Legal competency and ethical competency may not be the same. For example, some elderly persons who have been declared legally incompetent have been perceived by nurses as making very good sense in their refusal to enter another life-prolonging drug protocol.

In our society it is still assumed that parents will do what is best for their children. Therefore, for example, parental permission to use some coercion when administering injections to a 3-year-old is accepted. The administration of drugs to clients who are incompetent on a psychiatric basis involves many complex ethical dilemmas. Does the fact that a patient has a psychiatric diagnosis automatically make that patient incompetent to make any decisions regarding his or her treatment? Does the act of consent from a truly disturbed person mean anything? If a person is in a disturbed emotional state, is it assumed that she or he lacks rational decision-making powers all of the time? Each individual patient situation requires that the nurse examine ethical principles in a thoughtful manner.

Placebo Therapy

The very nature of placebo therapy involves deception. Before administering a placebo, the nurse should thoroughly understand the rationale for placebo therapy in the particular patient situation and should be in full agreement with the rationale. Placebo therapy overtly violates the principle of truth telling or honesty, and it is sometimes very difficult to honesty justify participation in administering placebos.

Experimentation

The development of new drugs requires human experimentation at some point. The nurse must explore the status of informed consent and be satisfied that all the provisions of informed consent have been attained before administering any experimental drug. The two-word phrase *informed consent* indicates two ingredients, each of which may give rise to ethical questions. First we must ask whether the patient's consent was obtained, and whether this consent was truly voluntary. Second, when consent has been established, we ask whether the patient was adequately informed beforehand. Informed consent is an ideal to which ethics seeks close approximation. The fact that a patient has signed a standard form in no way assures that truly informed consent has occurred. If a nurse is to participate in a drug experimentation protocol, the nurse should be aware of and in agreement with (1) the purpose of the experiment, (2) the methodology utilized in the experiment, and (3) the safeguards that have been established within the experimental design to protect the subject's rights.

The most common form of drug experimental design involves a double-blind study. Thus, the nurse will not know which patient is receiving which drug if, in fact, any drug at all. Nurses need to assume that all patients are receiving the experimental drug so that they can observe for both desirable and undesirable drug effects. An ethical informed consent from a subject related to a double-blind study would seem to require that the patient or subject be aware that not all subjects will receive the drug being tested and that, in fact, some patients will be receiving either alternate drugs or placebos. If all subjects are so informed, then valid informed consent can be achieved.

Impaired Nurse

The impaired nurse is a nurse who engages in substance abuse. It is not truly known whether there is a greater proportion of health care providers who become involved with substance abuse than the proportion in the population as a whole. However, there is no doubt that nurses, by virtue of their work setting and the responsibilities delegated to them, have relatively easy access to commonly abused drugs. It is ethically wrong to steal drugs from a patient's supply. One violates the patient's property rights in so doing. The nurse is also practicing extreme deception with the patient when, for instance, he or she substitutes normal saline for the **meperidine (Demerol)** in an injection.

Summary of Ethical Aspects

Ethical dilemmas are experienced frequently by nurses in relationship to their role in drug therapy. The nurse has individual ethical responsibility to examine the grounds of justification for all nursing actions, including the administration of drugs. The nurse must become familiar with ethical principles and learn to apply those principles in a rational manner. An ethical dilemma exists when two or more principles are in conflict in a given patient situation. The thoughtful nurse who is concerned with the ethical aspects of drug therapy will develop an ethical decision-making process which can be used consistently in all areas of the nursing role.

REFERENCES

Accreditation Manual for Hospitals 1984, Chicago: Joint Commission on Accreditation of Hospitals, 1984.

Armiger, B.: "Ethics of Nursing Research: Profile, Principles, Perspective," *Nurs Res,* 25:330–336, 1977.

Besch, L.: "Informed Consent: A Patient's Right," *Nurs Outlook,* 27:32–35, 1979.

Bok, S.: "The Ethics of Giving Placebos," *Sci Amer,* 231:17–23, 1974.

Bowie, R. B.: "Research Ethics for the Clinical Nurse," *AORN J,* 31:1016–1018, 1980.

Cazalas, M. W.: *Nursing and the Law,* 3d ed., Germantown, MD: Aspen, 1978.

Code for Nurses with Interpretive Statements, Kansas City: American Nurses' Association, 1976.

Cohen, S. N.: "Ethical and Legal Issues in Pediatric Drug Research," *Pediatr Pharmacol,* 1:25–29, 1980.

Controlled Substances Act, 21 U.S. Code 801, et. seq. 1970.

Daniel v. St. Francis Cabrini Hospital, 415 So. 2d 586 (La. App. 1982).

Davis, A. J.: "Pain Q3H . . . Ethical Issues," *Am J Nurs,* 80:974, 1980.

Dillon v. Hollywood Presbyterian Hospital, #C-18319, Los Angeles County Superior Court (Cal. 1977).

Drewry v. County of Obion, 619 S.W. 2d 397 (Tenn. App. 1981).

Dworkin, G.: "Paternalism," *The Monist,* 56:64–84, 1972.

———: "Autonomy and Behavior Control," *Hastings Cent Rep,* 6:23–28, 1976.

Farrow v. Health Services Corporation, 604 P. 2d 474 (Utah 1979).

Food, Drug and Cosmetic Act, 21 U.S. Code 201, et seq. 1906, 1938, 1962, 1976.

Human Rights Guidelines for Nurses in Clinical and Other Research, Kansas City: American Nurses' Association, 1975.

Larrimore v. Homeopathic Hospital Association, 176 A. 2d. 362 (Super. Ct. Del. 1961).

Levine, C.: "Depro-Provera and Contraceptive Risk: A Case Study of Values in Conflict," *Hastings Cent Rep,* 9:8–11, 1979.

Levine, R. J.: "Drug Testing in Prisons," *Prog Clin Biol Res,* 76:73–78, 1981.

Lewis, E. P.: "The Right to Inform," *Nurs Outlook,* 25:561, 1977.

Lipsett, M. B.: "On the Nature and Ethics of Phase I Clinical Trials of Cancer Chemotherapies," *JAMA,* 248:841–942, 1982.

Mayers, M. H.: "Legal Guidelines," *Geriatr Nurs,* 2:417–421, 1981.

Miller, B. L.: "Placebo Usage in Clinical Trials of Life-Saving Drugs," *Prog Clin Biol Res,* 38:263–274, 1980.

Murchison, I., T. S. Nichols, and R. Hanson: *Legal Accountability in the Nursing Process,* 2d ed., St. Louis: Mosby, 1982.

Oulton, R. (ed.): *Reciprocal News,* 5:2, 1982.

Payton, R. J.: "Information Control and Autonomy—Does the Nurse Have a Role?" *Nurs Clin North Amer,* 14:23–33, 1979.

Roginsky, M. S., and A. Handley: "Ethical Implications of Withdrawal of Experimental Drugs at Conclusion of Phase III Trials," *Clin Res,* 26:384–388, 1978.

Rollins, W. R.: "What Nurses Should Know About Administering 'New Drugs'" *Nursing Law and Ethics,* 1:1–2, 9–11, 1980.

Silber, T. J.: "Placebo Therapy: The Ethical Dimension," *JAMA,* 242:245–246, 1979.

Veatch, R. M.: "Drugs and Competing Drug Ethics," *Hastings Cent Stud,* 2:68–80, 1974.

Warren, D. G.: *Problems in Hospital Law,* 3d ed., Germantown, MD: Aspen, 1978.

Weatherly v. New York, 441 N.Y.S. 2d 319 (Ct. Cl. 1981).

9

NURSING IN RESEARCH AND CLINICAL TESTING OF DRUGS*

JUDITH UNDERWOOD GROTHE

LEARNING OBJECTIVES

Upon mastery of the contents of this chapter, the reader will be able to:

1. List the three sources of new drug products.
2. Describe the developmental program of a new drug, indicating the research activities in each stage.
3. Identify the nurse's role in the clinical testing of a new drug.
4. State criteria for evaluating a drug study.
5. Define the following terms: placebo control, double-blind, crossover, open-label, random assignment, matched pairs.

OVERVIEW OF DRUG DEVELOPMENT

From the time a potentially useful chemical is synthesized in the laboratory until the time it is available for use in the general population, some 10 years may elapse. During this time, hundreds of scientists and clinicians are involved in developing and testing this potentially useful agent. This step-by-step investigation of a new drug is called a *developmental program*.

Ongoing experiments in animals followed by testing on human subjects are paralleled by an in-depth scientific documentation process. At the conclusion of the entire testing process, animal and human data are presented to the Food and Drug Administration (FDA), Bureau of Drugs, for

review. Following extensive review of these data, which in itself may take years, a medicinal agent proven to be *safe* and *efficacious* for its specified clinical indications may be marketed. Only 1 in 10,000 potential drugs survives the entire development process and becomes available for clinical use.

Drug research proceeds according to a developmental program which permits decision making and data analysis at various stages. Table 9-1 places in a simplified sequence the events which may occur in the discovery and developmental process.

Isolation of Drug Materials

The first step in the system of drug development is the generation of drug materials to be tested. New drug products usually originate from one of three sources: (1) purification of chemical medicinals obtained from natural origins, such as digitalis from foxglove or quinine from cinchona bark, (2) identification and isolation of biologic chemicals which are determined to cause specific human responses, such as blood-clotting factors or hormones, or (3) modification by chemists who synthesize chemical agents, such as some of the recently developed antimicrobial drugs.

Once a potentially useful new chemical is isolated, several grams are purified for the next step, *preclinical research*.

Preclinical Research

Drugs must be tested in animals prior to their use with humans. The researcher tries to find several species of animal models in which the appropriate body system or function closely approximates the corresponding human systems or functions.

---

*Sections of this chapter were modified from the chapter "Clinical Testing" in the first edition, which was written by Marvin R. Frank.

143

TABLE 9-1 Steps in the Development of a New Drug

Potential new drug identified
  Exogenous chemical isolated
  Endogenous chemical purified
  Synthesized
Preclinical efficacy testing
  In vitro screening (test tube)
  In vivo screening (living organism)
Preclinical toxicity testing (animal)
  Acute toxicology (single dose)
  Subacute toxicology (lasting several weeks)
  Chronic toxicology (continuing for months or years)
  Teratology (potential to induce birth defects)
  Carcinogenicity (potential to induce cancer)
Clinical experimentation (human)
  Phase I (healthy human subjects; dosage range)
  Phase II (human subjects having disease; approx 100)
  Phase III (wider patient population; long-term data)
  Extended phase III–IV (longer-term data; postapproval)
Submission of new drug application to FDA
Pharmaceutical marketing

In Vitro and In Vivo Testing

Two types of preclinical tests are used to verify drug activity: in vitro and in vivo systems. An in vitro experiment is performed in an isolated test system, such as a test tube. An in vivo test is performed on living organisms.

Toxicity Screening

The second phase of preclinical study is *toxicity screening*. Animal toxicology is divided into acute, subacute, and chronic toxicity studies. An acute toxicity study consists of administering single doses of medication to observe and document the physiologic response. In subacute toxicity studies, the medication is given over a 2- to 3-week period. When the initial studies are completed, the medication is then tested for a prolonged period of time, sometimes continuing for years.

In addition, pathology studies should include teratology (potential to induce birth defects) experiments and may include carcinogenicity (potential to induce cancer) studies. The objectives of these studies are to identify abnormal changes in animal organs which are due to drug administration and to delineate the relatively safe therapeutic dose. A *control group* of animals, kept under similar conditions and receiving no drug, is compared with the experimental group.

Evaluation of Test Data

Information from animal tests is reviewed by experienced scientists, and a determination is made regarding the feasibility of testing the drug in human subjects, on the basis of its demonstrated toxicity and efficacy. When a decision to initiate human studies is made, one factor in the decision is an assessment of the seriousness of the disease to be treated as compared with the toxicity of the drug.

The *sponsor* (pharmaceutical company or independent researchers) will carefully document the results of all animal work performed. These data are combined with known information on the chemical features of the raw drug, as well as the manufacturing information on the formulated dosage and manufacturing controls designed to ensure a uniform product (quality control). This information is submitted to the FDA and is termed the *investigational new drug application,* or IND. If within 30 days of submission of the IND the FDA does not instruct the sponsor to postpone initiation of human studies, the clinical phase of drug development will begin.

Clinical Experimentation

Clinical experimentation may be divided into four phases, three of which occur prior to release of the drug for clinical use. Each phase has objectives which are designed to answer specific questions, and which generate data and information on a drug that will allow the scientists and clinicians involved in the research to assess the therapeutic value of the drug and estimate the risks attributable to the drug's use.

Phase I

The first group of human experiments with a new drug are called phase I studies. The objectives are to establish the human dosage range of the drug, based on how it is tolerated in *healthy* human subjects, and to determine the pharmacokinetics of the product.

If there are no demonstrated serious adverse drug effects, if the dosage range is well below that shown in chronic animal studies to induce pathology, and if the drug is eliminated in a reasonable time, phase II studies are initiated.

Phase II

The objective of phase II of human experimentation is to demonstrate the efficacy and relative safety of the drug in a group of subjects (usually no more than 100) having the *disease* for which the drug is intended. It is imperative that the clinical protocol, or plan, for these studies be a well-constructed document designed with the help of clinicians, statisticians, pharmacologists, pharmacists, nurses, and clinical research associates so that the data generated will answer the basic questions being posed and will evaluate questions relevant to clinical practice.

Clearly documented, statistically valid efficacy and safety must be established through well-designed studies in order to get FDA approval for drug release. It is therefore imperative that in the conduct of phase II and phase III studies a strong controlling input be exerted by the sponsor of the research, to ensure that the objectives of each phase of study are reached and that practitioners do not alter treatment methods.

If satisfactory efficacy and safety data are generated from phase II studies, phase III is initiated.

Phases III and IV

Phase III research encompasses all the objectives of phase II, but experience is sought for a wide patient population, and studies may be expanded to get long-term data if a chronic medication regimen is to be considered.

After all relevant data is compiled and analyzed, the sponsor submits a *new drug application* (NDA) to the FDA. Eventually a decision is made as to whether the drug will be approved (and released) or rejected or whether the NDA will be withdrawn and resubmitted at a later date, after research to answer specific questions generated by the FDA.

The final decision by the FDA may not, however, mark the termination of all research on the drug. Questions still must be answered regarding long-term use of the drug. This post-NDA approval research is sometimes referred to as phase IV.

DESIGN OF DRUG STUDIES

A controlled trial or drug study is a powerful tool in evaluating new and old drugs. To answer cause and effect questions, such as those about the safety and effectiveness of drugs or which of two treatments is better, an *experimental design* is required. By definition experimental designs are characterized by experimenter control over the administration of treatment; control groups, which may be untreated or treated with alternative methods; and random assignment of subjects to the treatment or control groups.

Several examples can help illustrate the principles of experimental designs. A retrospective study of the charts of all patients in a hospital during 1983 who had received a particular medication would be a *descriptive design,* or *nonexperimental design,* because there was no control group, random assignment, or experimenter manipulation of the treatment. Comparison of the mental status of those nursing-home patients receiving digoxin with those not receiving the drug is a *quasi-experimental design,* since there is a (nonequivalent) comparison group but no random assignment to treatment.

Such descriptive and quasi-experimental studies of intact groups do contribute to scientific knowledge but do not command the power of experimental designs to answer questions of cause. This is because too many factors which could potentially account for the observed findings are left uncontrolled. However, because of practical or ethical considerations, experimental designs may not always be possible. For example, while nonexperimental and quasi-experimental studies indicate an association or correlation in children between ingestion of aspirin during chicken pox or influenza infections and the subsequent development of Reye's syndrome, an experimental study to determine if aspirin causes Reye's syndrome in children with influenza would be unethical. Therefore, some clinical and scientific decisions are based on studies with nonexperimental or quasi-experimental designs. However, this is not desirable when experimental studies are feasible.

Problem Statement

In research the problem is usually stated as a question about the relationship between observable events. The observable phenomena are considered to be of three types: *independent variables, dependent variables,* and *intervening variables.* The researcher attempts to control as many intervening variables as possible so that the cause and effect relationship between the independent variable (the drug) and the dependent variables (the clinical responses) is clarified. In clinical drug studies *some* of the intervening variables likely to be of interest are age, sex, weight, disease states, size and color of the drug, diet, the social environment of the patient, and the mood of the patient and/or the physician. The important intervening variables will vary with the research question.

The *hypothesis* is a conjectural statement about the nature of the relationship between the identified variables. It is usually expressed in measurable terms, such as "Increasing serum **theophylline** concentrations will result in an increase in FEV_1 (a pulmonary function test) in asthmatic patients."

Control

Studies are designed to demonstrate the effect of the independent variable on the dependent variables. This is accomplished in experimental designs by dividing the subjects into two or more study groups. One group (*experimental group*), is exposed to the independent variable, while the other group(s) (*control groups*) are treated in the same manner except they are not exposed to the independent variable. If the groups are identical on all intervening variables and the hypothesis is true, the experimental group will show more change in the dependent variables than the control groups will. Control treatments in pharmacologic research consist of no drug; a different drug (an alternate active drug or a placebo); or the same drug in a different dose, route, or dosage schedule. A *placebo* is a substitute that is pharmacologically inert for the condition being treated. However, some proportion of the subjects will have a positive response to the placebo and others will experience adverse drug reactions to the placebo. Drugs are commonly compared with a placebo to ascertain if they cause more beneficial effects and/or more adverse effects than the pharmacologically "inert" placebo (see Chap. 5).

In studies involving diabetes mellitus, infections, or other diseases that may have severe morbidity or mortality if not treated, use of a placebo or untreated control group is ethically unacceptable. In these cases the control groups are treated with the best previously available forms of therapy.

Crossover Design   A study design frequently used in drug research is the *crossover design,* which involves several study periods for each subject. In the first period the experimental group receives the drug and the control group receives no treatment or the alternate form of treatment. After a wash-out period of no therapy in either group, the control group receives the drug and the experimental group receives the control form of therapy. Thus, in a crossover design the subject serves as his or her own control on some intervening variables.

Assignment to Treatment Group   The other goal of control in study designs is to eliminate the intervening variables as competing explanations for any change in the dependent variables. This is accomplished by making the experimental and control groups equal with respect to the intervening variables by *randomly assigning the subjects to treatment groups.* If the study sample is large enough, random assignment is the best way to achieve groups equal with respect to *known and unknown* intervening variables.

Sampling

Sampling involves obtaining information from a portion of a larger group. Researchers desire to generalize the findings from the sample to the larger group or *target population,* such as all patients with asthma, all women wanting to temporarily avoid pregnancy, or all patients with acute myelogenous leukemia. Generalization with relative confidence is possible when subjects are selected by *probability sampling* techniques. Probability sampling means that the subjects are randomly selected from a list of the entire target population. When the sample is randomly drawn only from a few clinics or hospitals, the findings can be confidently generalized only to patients in those particular settings. Generalization to the larger target population can be done only to the extent that the researchers can successfully argue that the actual population from which the sample was drawn is representative of the target population (e.g., same severity of disease, similar environments, diet, genetic influences).

Matched-Pair Design   If the investigator can identify the intervening variables which will affect the dependent variable, the sample subjects can be matched on these variables, such as age, sex, weight, and severity of disease. The matched members of the pairs are then randomly assigned to treatment groups, with one member in the experimental group and one in the control group. However, statistical problems that raise serious questions about the validity of the study occur if the matched pairs are not randomly assigned to treatment groups, as when patients in two hospital wards are matched on the intervening variables and then all those on one ward are given the experimental treatment while those on the other receive the control treatment.

Double-Blind Technique

One of the most influential intervening variables in drug studies relates to who knows the form of treatment the patient is receiving. While it is obvious that if the patient knows whether the substance is a placebo or a new drug, it might influence his or her response, it is less apparent that this knowledge might affect the prescriber's and investigator's attitudes toward the patient and clinical observations. Therefore, many studies are designed so that neither the prescribing physician nor the patient is aware of whether the experimental or control form of therapy is given to the patient. This is referred to as the *double-blind* technique. When an investigator other than the prescribing physician collects data, this observer is also unaware of the form of treatment the patient receives. (Some authors distinguish this procedure as the triple-blind technique.) In the double-blind methodology the pharmaceutical manufacturer, a pharmacist, a nurse, or another nonobserver maintains a code which identifies which form of treatment the patient is given. In most studies the research protocol specifies when the code should be broken (at the end of the study, when the patient has a severe adverse reaction, etc.).

A *single-blind* study is one in which only the subject is unaware of the form of treatment. An *open-label* study is one in which the observer, the prescribing physician, and the subject all know the form of treatment. Whenever possible the double-blind technique is the preferred method for drug investigation.

Measurement

The investigator must select the instruments to measure the dependent variables. Prior to the study it must be established that the instruments to be utilized are valid (measure what they are purported to measure), reliable (are consistent over time, circumstances, subjects), and sensitive (can identify clinically significant changes).

Interpretation of Data

The data that are generated from a study are evaluated using statistical methods. If probability sampling techniques were utilized, the statistical tests tell the researchers whether they should accept the hypothesis as tenable and how confident they can be that the change in the dependent variable was due to the effect of the independent variable rather than to chance alone. Some statistically significant findings are not clinically significant. For example, that a drug is shown in a study to cause a mean decrease of 2 mmHg in systolic blood pressure would not warrant its use clinically as an antihypertensive drug, although it is conceivable that the finding would be statistically significant in a large sample.

NURSING PROCESS IMPLICATIONS

Nurses are practicing in an area of rapidly expanding information on clinical pharmacology and therapeutics. In order for nurses to make decisions concerning the use of drugs, they must be able to critically evaluate the enormous amount of information generated about drugs (review articles, original research, manufacturer's promotional materials, etc.).

Patients ask nurses about alleged scientific claims for new or controversial forms of drug treatment, such as Laetrile for cancer and the so-called starch blockers for weight control. The nurse should explain to such patients whether the results of the studies were valid and why, stressing the importance of experimental designs, random assignment to treatment groups, placebo control, and double-blind provisions in drug studies.

In evaluating drug research, the nurse should ask the following questions:

1. Is the research question and/or hypothesis clearly stated?
2. Is the overall research design (experimental, quasi-experimental, or descriptive) appropriate to the research question?
3. Is there a control group, and were the subjects randomly assigned to treatment?
4. Are the measurement instruments used valid, reliable, and sensitive for the purposes for which they are used?
5. Was the double-blind technique used?
6. If the matched-pair design was used, were all the important intervening variables identified and used to match subjects?
7. Was the actual population from which the sample was drawn comparable to the target population (and to the population of interest to the nurse)?
8. Are the conclusions valid based on the data collected?
9. Are the findings clinically significant?

Nursing practice should not be chosen or altered based on a single study. The key to scientific method is reproducibility. If the same results are reproduced in several studies, then there is adequate support for changes in nursing practice.

Nurses as Drug Researchers

While it is the function of nurses in general to evaluate drug studies, a growing number of nurses are directly and primarily involved in drug research in various settings and capacities. Nurses do pharmacologic research in animal laboratories, medical schools, universities, and clinical settings, such as hospitals, nursing homes, community health agencies, physicians' offices, and clinics. Some conduct studies pertinent to elements of the nursing process in drug therapy, such as drug administration techniques and identification and management of adverse drug effects. Many work with interdisciplinary teams to study multifaceted questions. Overall, the nurse functions as a scientist, collaborator, and clinician-observer in drug research.

Nursing Role in the Development of New Drugs

The nurses most likely to be involved in the clinical experimentation phases of a drug development program are those in larger university hospital settings and those in clinics and physicians' offices where such research is conducted. Many institutions are now realizing the potentially key role of the nurse in a drug developmental program. Although all participants are part of a team effort, a nurse frequently functions as the *study coordinator,* who ensures communication between the sponsor, the physician, the institutional review board (IRB), the FDA, and the patient.

The participation of the nurse in a large university hospital setting usually involves data collection during the clinical experimentation phases, particularly phases II and III. In smaller institutions, clinics, and private physicians' offices, the nurse is often the initial contact of the sponsor. Although responsibilities may vary from institution to institution, nursing functions may include feasibility studies, protocol input, budget negotiation, attendance at institutional review board meetings, recruitment of potential subjects, screening of patients, assurance of informed consent, data gathering, and patient assessment. While these functions are discussed in this chapter specifically as they relate to nurses who are study coordinators in clinics, the descriptions can be generalized to other situations. Further, ethical considerations in research are an integral part of the nurse's responsibilities in all settings (see Chap. 8).

Feasibility Studies At the onset of clinical drug research, it is the nurse's responsibility to thoroughly read and evaluate the study design and protocol. Logistic questions that need to be answered are:

1. Is the patient population large enough to support this study?
2. Does the protocol provide sufficient safety measures to protect patients during the course of the study, i.e., complete physical examinations, laboratory tests, x-rays, electrocardiograms, etc.?
3. Is the equipment accessible? If not, will it be provided?
4. Are there any time limitations or conflicts between the actual patient visits required and the actual office hours of the clinic or institution?
5. Is adequate space available for storage of medications, case report forms, equipment, etc.?
6. Are enough physicians available, interested, and knowledgeable in the research to serve as coinvestigators and be on call in case medical problems arise?
7. What will be the nurse's role in the study?

Once these questions are answered, the nurse will collaborate with the physician and give a recommendation about whether or not it is feasible, or even wise, to initiate the study.

Protocol Input Many pharmaceutical companies are recognizing the importance of nursing input into the protocols. At the initial investigator's meetings of a multiclinic study, physicians and study coordinators are invited to participate in 1- or 2-day sessions designed to improve the study design and the protocol.

During the course of the study, unforeseen problems with the protocol may develop. It is the nurse's responsibility to communicate these to the primary investigator and/or physician and the pharmaceutical company. This nursing input will frequently result in an amendment to the protocol.

Budget Negotiation   Frequently, the nurse is involved in devising the budget necessary for the operation of the study. Cost effectiveness for the institution as well as the sponsor must be taken into consideration. Most protocols include a flow chart (see Table 9-2) that contains all the necessary office visits, clinical laboratory work, and special tests needed to be performed during the course of the study. These actual costs, as well as administrative costs (overhead), are included and submitted to the sponsor (pharmaceutical company, governmental agency, or grantor) for approval.

Advertising for and Screening Patients   A nurse in a large institution may not be involved in recruiting patients for research studies. However, in smaller institutions, this may be an added responsibility. The process of finding the appro-priate patients and screening them is perhaps one of the most crucial elements in determining the success of a study.

Every protocol has a list of inclusion-exclusion criteria for patients. These criteria must be *strictly* observed. Any deviation could render the research invalid and, more importantly, jeopardize the patients' health. Table 9-3 lists some of the more common criteria. Because of the strict adherence necessary, finding suitable candidates for research studies is a time-consuming, difficult process. Cost-effective recruitment can be obtained by advertising in small community newsletters, church newspapers, and other nonprofit organization newspapers, as well as radio and television commercials.

Screening patients involves obtaining accurate and detailed histories. The nurse's skill is essential in determining a patient's qualification to participate in the study.

Informed Consent   It is generally the responsibility of the physician or principal investigator and the drug sponsor to secure the investigational drug and alert the patient to the experimental process which will follow. The physician must explain to the patient the particular procedures which will be forthcoming and explain the risks, if any, associated with these procedures. This includes the risks of any tests used to

TABLE 9-2   Flow Chart for a Hypothetical Drug Study (Showing what data are collected at each patient contact)

	PRESTUDY	PLACEBO PHASE			ACTIVE-DRUG PHASE				POSTSTUDY
		DAY 1	DAY 8	DAY 16	DAY 24	DAY 32	DAY 40	DAY 48	
Complete physical examination	x	x							x
Brief office visit		x	x	x	x	x	x	x	
Laboratory work	x				x				x
Chest x-ray (if applicable)	x								
Electrocardiogram	x				x				x
Medication dispensed		x	x	x		x	x	x	
Blood pressure, height, weight	x	x	x	x	x	x	x	x	x
Adverse effects, concomitant drugs	x	x	x	x	x	x	x	x	x

TABLE 9-3 Inclusion-Exclusion Criteria for a Hypothetical Drug Research Protocol Involving an Experimental Antihypertensive Medication

Inclusions

1. Males and females between the ages of 18 and 70 years
2. Weights between 50 and 100 kg inclusively
3. Uncomplicated essential hypertension with systolic readings below 200 mmHg and diastolic readings between 90 and 120 mmHg
4. Patients receiving steroids or tranquilizers, only if the dose has been stable for the previous three months
5. Patients maintained on a sodium-restricted diet

Exclusions

1. Females with childbearing potential
2. Hypertension requiring surgical intervention
3. Severe target organ damage or diseases of any system including hepatic, renal, neurologic, or musculoskeletal
4. Coronary artery disease, a history of cardiac failure, or any other severe cardiac disease
5. Bronchial asthma, chronic bronchitis, emphysema

monitor the effects of the drug, as well as the risks of the drug itself. *Informed consent* implies that the patient has been informed to the fullest and has consented to the application of the procedure. Every person has the right to make the decision of whether or not he or she will participate in this type of medical practice and the right to withdraw at any time. It is the principal investigator's responsibility, in the case of the investigational drug, to obtain a *written* informed consent.

In many institutions today, it is the nurse's responsibility to write the informed consent statement, using the protocol and the rules and regulations of the FDA. The nurse *must* help in ensuring that consent is truly informed by eliciting and answering patients' questions and clarifying information that may be confusing to them.

Data Gathering The essence of a clinical investigational study is to compare the effectiveness of the drug in question to its toxicities. It is therefore essential that all information be recorded accurately and completely. It cannot be overemphasized that seemingly unrelated responses of the patient might be extremely significant and should always be documented. Many drugs that were originally being tested for one particular effect turned out to be marketed for a different indication. For example, **meprobamate** was originally being tested as a drug that would reduce muscle cramps, but under clinical investigation it was determined that patients using the drug were more relaxed and slept better. This type of information gathering is also necessary for drugs that have already been approved for one clinical use, since other effects of the drug might be later identified.

Patient Assessment All during the investigational study it is the responsibility of the nurse to assess the patient and observe and record the patient's own evaluation. Prompt reporting of adverse reactions to the physician and the sponsor is of the utmost importance whether it is a patient symptom, abnormal laboratory value, or other abnormal test result. In the event a patient dies, whether it is drug-related or not, it is the nurse's responsibility to notify the physician, the sponsor, institutional review board, and the FDA.

CONCLUSION

The complex developmental system for drug research has been designed to ensure that safe, effective medicines are available for the treatment of disease. At each stage of the investigative process, provision is made for decision making about the wisdom and feasibility of continuing the research. The nurse's role as a scientist, collaborator, and evaluator in drug research is required at all stages of the clinical investigation and is essential to the success of the study and the appropriate application of research to clinical practice.

REFERENCES

Anello, C.: "FDA Principles in Clinical Investigations," *Food and Drug Administration Papers,* 4:14–24, June 1970.

Associates of Clinical Pharmacology, P. O. Box 437, Furlong, PA 18925; 22 West Jefferson Street, Suite 301, Rockville, MD 20850.

Berkowitz, B. A.: "Drug Discovery and Evaluation," in B. G. Katzung (ed.), *Basic and Clinical Pharmacology,* Los Altos, CA: Lange, 1982.

Browers, J. Z., and G. P. Velo (eds.): *Drug Assessment Criteria and Methods,* New York: Elsevier/North Holland, 1979.

FDA Consumer, Superintendent of Documents, Government Printing Office, Washington, DC 20402.

Federal Register, "45 CFR Part 46 Final Regulations Amending Basic HHS Policy for the Protection of Human Research Subjects," vol. 46, no. 16, Jan. 26, 1981.

Jacox, A., and P. Prescott: "Determining a Study's Relevance for Clinical Practice," *Am J Nurs,* 78:1882–1889, 1978.

Levine, R. J.: *Ethics and Regulation of Clinical Research,* Baltimore-Munich: Urban & Schwarzenberg, 1981.

President's Commission for the Study of Ethical Problems in Medicine and Biomedical and Behavioral Research, Suite 555, 2000 K Street, N. W., Washington, DC 20006.

Public Responsibility in Medicine and Research, 15 Court Square, Suite 340, Boston, MA 02108.

Ross, W. S.: *The Life/Death Ratio: Benefits and Risks in Modern Medicine,* New York: Crowell, 1977.

Waife, S. O., and A. P. Shapiro, (eds.): *Clinical Evaluation of New Drugs,* New York: Hoebner-Harper, 1979.

Wardell, W. M.: "Drug Testing in Humans," in C. R. Craig and R. E. Stitzel (eds.), *Modern Pharmacology,* Boston: Little, Brown, 1982.

Williamson, Y. M.: *Research Methodology and Its Application to Nursing,* New York: Wiley, 1981.

UNIT III

NEURO-TRANSMISSION & THE AUTONOMIC NERVOUS SYSTEM

10

ANATOMY AND PHYSIOLOGY OF THE AUTONOMIC NERVOUS SYSTEM

ELEANOR H. BOYD
AMY M. KARCH

LEARNING OBJECTIVES

Upon mastery of the contents of this chapter, the reader will be able to:

1. List the sequence of events in transmission at the neuromuscular junction.

2. State the major ways in which transmission at an adrenergic synapse differs from transmission at a cholinergic synapse.

3. Explain the location of synapses in the somatic motor system and in the sympathetic and parasympathetic nervous systems.

4. Identify the neurotransmitter released at each of the above synapses.

5. List the effectors receiving sympathetic cholinergic innervation.

6. Define the terms *nicotinic* and *muscarinic* as they apply to receptors for acetylcholine.

7. State whether a given cholinergic synapse in the somatic motor, parasympathetic, or sympathetic nervous system is nicotinic or muscarinic.

8. Identify the adrenergic receptors in the heart, bronchi, and vasculature as α, β_1, or β_2.

9. List the effects of sympathetic and parasympathetic nerve impulses on various effectors.

10. Given a drug which mimics or blocks the effects of acetylcholine at nicotinic or muscarinic sites, predict the effects, if any, of the drug on the neuromuscular junction, autonomic ganglia, and effectors receiving cholinergic sympathetic and parasympathetic postganglionic innervation.

11. Given that a drug mimics or blocks the effects of sympathetic innervation of α, β_1, or β_2 receptors, predict the effects, if any, of the drug on the heart, bronchi, and blood pressure.

12. Give one example of the application of the anatomy and physiology of the autonomic nervous system to each step of the nursing process.

Many disease states involve the autonomic nervous system, and many disorders of the human body can be treated effectively by the use of drugs which mimic (these drugs are called *agonists*) or block (these drugs are called *antagonists*) the effects on organs produced by the autonomic nervous system. For example, the effective treatment of an acute attack of bronchial asthma sometimes includes the use of **isoproterenol hydrochloride** (Isuprel), a drug which dilates the bronchi, mimicking the effects of the sympathetic division of the autonomic nervous system. The effective treatment of sinus bradycardia sometimes includes the use of **atropine**, a drug which increases heart rate by blocking the effects of the parasympathetic division of the autonomic nervous system.

Understanding how autonomic drugs produce their desired, therapeutic effects, as well as learning what side effects to anticipate when these drugs are used, is greatly facilitated by knowledge of the anatomy and physiology of the autonomic nervous system. In the examples cited above, this knowledge would allow the health practitioner to anticipate that the asthmatic patient might experience palpitations after receiving isoproterenol, and to anticipate that the heart patient probably would complain about dryness of the mouth after receiving atropine.

It is the purpose of this chapter to provide the basic facts

153

essential to understanding the effects of the specific autonomic drugs. Using these basic facts, it should be possible for the nurse to figure out many of the effects of autonomic drugs with a minimum of rote memorization and to apply this knowledge in the clinical setting. In addition, it is appropriate to include in this section a discussion of the skeletal neuromuscular junction (*not* a part of the autonomic nervous system), both because it is likely to be a familiar example of synaptic transmission and because some autonomic drugs (the cholinesterase inhibitors) are used for their effects at both autonomic parasympathetic synapses and somatic neuromuscular junction.

FUNDAMENTALS OF NEUROANATOMY AND NEUROPHYSIOLOGY

The Neuron

The nervous system is composed of nerve cells, or *neurons,* and of glia and other cells and tissues which provide the nourishment, support, and protection which neurons require to function properly. It is the function of neurons to receive, to integrate, and to transmit information.

Neurons, like other mammalian cells, each have a nucleus, cytoplasm, mitochondria, granules, and other subcellular organelles enclosed by a cell membrane. Although the size and shape of neurons differ, all neurons have the same basic external features: a cell body, called the *soma,* and one or more *neuronal processes.* The neuronal processes are of two types, *axons* and *dendrites,* which are often highly branched (see Fig. 10-1).

Each neuron has one axon, which is specialized to carry information over distances to the site where the neuron makes a junction with another neuron; with an effector organ (*effector* means actor or doer), such as a smooth, striated, or cardiac muscle cell; or with a gland. These neurons, organs, or glands wlll be influenced by the information carried by the axon. Some neurons have axons which are quite short and transmit information only to cells near their own cell bodies. Other neurons, such as the spinal motor neurons which innervate the muscles of a foot or a toe in an adult human being, have longer axons, some longer than 1 m.

Each neuron typically has many dendrites. The dendrites and soma are the information-receiving sites of the neuron. The axon terminals of one neuron (called the *presynaptic* neuron) transmit information to the dendrites and the soma of another neuron (the *postsynaptic* neuron) at sites referred to as *junctions* or *synapses.* All the information received via synapses on the cell membrane of a postsynaptic neuron is integrated by this cell membrane.

The Nerve Action Potential

The axons of neurons are specialized to carry information in the form of electric signals called nerve impulses, or *action potentials.* An action potential is conducted without

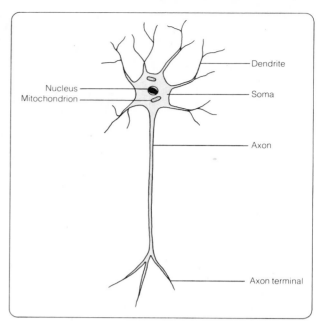

FIGURE 10-1

Diagram of a Typical Neuron.

loss of strength over the length of the axon from the region near the soma, where it is initiated, down into the finely branching axon terminals, which synapse with receiver areas on the cell membrane of another neuron or an effector cell.

Resting Membrane Potential

An electric potential, called the *membrane potential,* can be measured across the cell membrane between the cytoplasm or intracellular fluid of a neuron and the extracellular fluid surrounding the cell (see Fig. 10-2). The activity of neurons, as well as the activity of muscle or gland cells, is controlled by this membrane potential. At rest, the inside of the cell membrane is negatively charged and the outside of the cell membrane is positively charged. This potential, typically about 70 mV (or 70/1000 V) for a neuron, is the *resting membrane potential.*

The resting membrane potential of a cell is produced by the action of pumps in the cell membrane. These pumps are collectively referred to as the *sodium-potassium pump* or, more simply, the *sodium pump.* The sodium-potassium pump uses energy to push sodium ions out of the neuron at the same time that it is pulling potassium ions into the neurons. This allows sodium ions to be in low concentration and potassium ions to be in high concentration inside the cell. The situation is reversed in the extracellular fluid. In addition, the resting cell membrane is selectively permeable to potassium ions and is quite impermeable to sodium ions. Taken together, these facts allow biophysicists to account

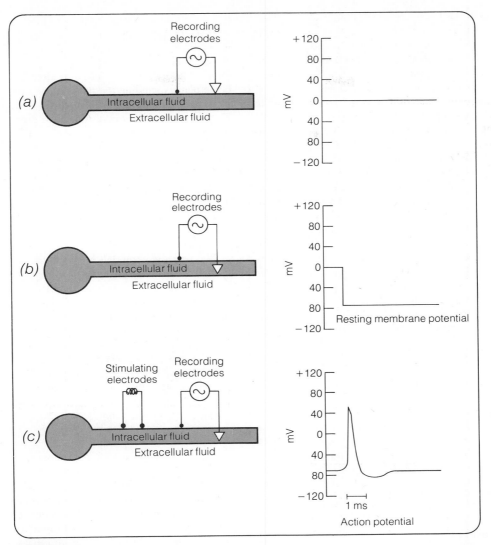

FIGURE 10-2

Membrane Potentials Recorded in a Neuron. In (a) both poles of the measuring device are in the extracellular fluid, and no potential difference is recorded between them. In (b), one of the poles, a glass micropipette electrode (with a tip about 1 μm in diameter), has penetrated the cell, and a potential difference of about 70 mV is recorded (the inside of the cell is negative with respect to the outside). In (c), a threshold stimulus has been applied to the nerve, and an action potential is generated and recorded; the membrane potential actually reverses polarity; then repolarization occurs.

for the measured values of resting membrane potential. Rather than understand membrane biophysics, it is more important for the nurse to remember that the membrane potential is important in controlling cellular activity, and to be aware that some foods that have a high potassium content, some drugs (cardiac glycosides and diuretics, for example), and some disease states (diarrhea and vomiting) can influence potassium levels and the membrane potential.

Threshold

When a neuron is stimulated, or excited, the membrane potential decreases locally at the site of the stimulus. The inside of the cell membrane becomes less negative with respect to the outside. This is usually referred to as *depolarization*. It is a characteristic of neuronal membranes that depolarization produces an increase in the permeability of the cell membrane to sodium ions. Sodium ions begin to flow into the cell from the extracellular fluid, where the concentration of sodium ions is high. This flow of positively charged sodium ions down their concentration gradient still further depolarizes the cell. When a critical level, called the *threshold membrane potential,* is reached, this process results in the generation of an action potential.

The action potential is a sudden, large, transient shift in membrane potential such that the inside of the cell actually becomes positively charged before normal polarity is restored (*repolarization*). Typically, in mammalian nerve, the entire depolarization-repolarization process constituting the action potential takes only about 1 ms (see Fig. 10-2). The depolarization phase of the action potential is accompanied by a further increase in membrane permeability to sodium ions. The membrane then becomes impermeable to sodium ions and more permeable to potassium ions. These factors terminate the depolarization phase of the action potential. The increase in permeability to potassium ions allows potassium to flow down its concentration gradient and out of the cell, thus restoring normal resting membrane potential and making the cell ready to fire another action potential. If repeated action potentials are fired, the sodium-potassium pump prevents sodium from building up inside the cell and prevents loss of intracellular potassium.

When a piece of membrane is brought to threshold and fires an action potential, this action potential sets up an electric field in the adjacent piece of cell membrane. The electric field acts as a stimulus to this adjacent membrane, which is brought to threshold, generates an action potential, and so on. In this way, the action potential is conducted without decrement along the length of the axon. Local anesthetics interfere with the conduction of action potentials. They block the conduction of sensory impulses responsible for pain perception by blocking the inflow of sodium ions needed to produce the action potential.

Synaptic Transmission

Sequence of Events in Synaptic Transmission

Electron microscopy has shown that a discrete space, called the *synaptic cleft,* intervenes between the terminals of most axons and the membranes of the neurons or effector cells with which they synapse. The electric signal (the action potential) in the presynaptic neuron cannot jump this high-resistance gap between the presynaptic and postsynaptic membranes. Instead, the arrival of the action potential in the axon terminal of the presynaptic neuron triggers the release of a chemical substance called a *neurotransmitter,* which has been stored in the axon terminal (see Fig. 10-3). This process requires the presence of calcium ions in the extracellular fluid. The neurotransmitter then diffuses across the snyaptic cleft and occupies special sites, called *receptors,* on the postsynaptic cell membrane.

The next step in the process of synaptic transmission differs somewhat, depending on the neurotransmitter released and the receptor. The interaction of a neurotransmitter with its receptor may be followed directly by an increase, or by a decrease, in the permeability of the membrane of the postsynaptic cell to one or more types of ion. Or the change in ionic permeability may occur only after a series of events has taken place, including the synthesis of a so-called secondary messenger (e.g., cyclic AMP or cyclic GMP) inside the cell. Elucidation of the series of molecular events following neurotransmitter-receptor interaction is the subject of much current research; our knowledge is still quite limited.

However the permeability change is brought about, it leads in turn to a small change in transmembrane potential, either a decrease (depolarization) or an increase (hyperpolarization). These small changes in membrane potential are called *synaptic potentials,* or, in the case of neuronal synapses with effectors, they are sometimes called *junctional potentials.*

Depolarizing potentials are excitatory in nature and may bring the membrane potential to the threshold for the generation of an action potential. Depolarizing synaptic potentials have several special names, depending on the site where they are generated. At the skeletal neuromuscular junction, they are called *end plate potentials;* at the synapse of one neuron with another, they are called *excitatory postsynaptic potentials* (EPSPs). Hyperpolarizing potentials are inhibitory. Hyperpolarizing synaptic potentials in neurons are referred to as *inhibitory postsynaptic potentials* (IPSPs). Another form of long-lasting neuronal inhibition, called *presynaptic inhibition,* has been known to exist in the central nervous system since the early 1960s but is still poorly understood.

Each neuron has many synapses on it, and its membrane potential at any moment reflects the summation of excitatory and inhibitory influences. If enough IPSPs are set up at the same time in a neuron, excitatory influences which otherwise would bring the neuron to threshold may be inadequate. This is one way by which the nervous system performs its function of integrating information.

The neurotransmitter is removed from the postsynaptic receptor by some combination of the following processes: diffusion, enzymatic inactivation, reuptake into the neuron which released it, or uptake into glial cells.

Although almost all known synaptic transmission in mammals involves a chemical neurotransmitter that diffuses across the gap between the adjacent cells, it should be noted that some synapses that operate electrically have recently been found in the mammalian brain; that is, adjacent cells are close enough together and the intercellular resistance is low enough that the neurons can communicate directly by electric, not chemical, means. (These synapses are all in brainstem nuclei; specifically, they are in Deiters nucleus, the mesencephalic nucleus of the fifth cranial nerve, and the inferior olive.) In addition, postganglionic parasympathetic neurons in the cardiac ganglion of a lower vertebrate also communicate electrically with one another. Because this type of synapse will probably remain a rarity, and because it

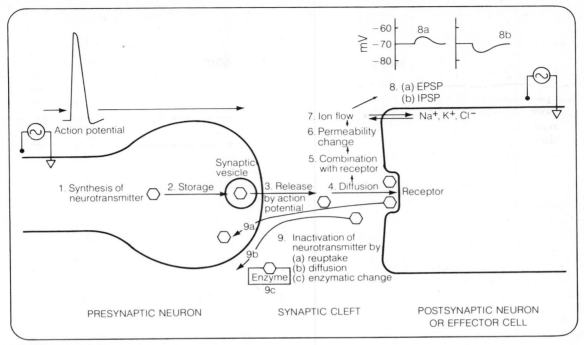

FIGURE 10-3

Sequence of Events in Synaptic Transmission. At some synapses, a more complex chain of biochemical events occurs in the postsynaptic cell: a "second messenger," such as cyclic AMP or cyclic GMP, is synthesized in a series of steps between events 5 and 6.

is not a likely site of action for autonomic drugs, it will not be discussed further.

Substances Identified as Neurotransmitters

To be accepted as a neurotransmitter at a given synapse, a candidate neurotransmitter substance must satisfy the following five criteria:

1. It must be synthesized in the presynaptic neuron.
2. It must be released from the terminals of this neuron.
3. When applied exogenously to the postsynaptic membrane, it must produce the same effects on the postsynaptic cell as the endogenously released neurotransmitter.
4. A specific mechanism must exist at the synapse for terminating the effects of the substance.
5. Drugs which increase or decrease the effectiveness of the endogenously released neurotransmitter must interact in the same way with the candidate neurotransmitter substance when it is applied exogenously.

In the mammalian autonomic nervous system two substances have been accepted as synaptic neurotransmitters: *acetylcholine* and *norepinephrine. Dopamine* may also have a modulating role in autonomic ganglia. In the mammalian

central nervous system, these three substances have been accepted as neurotransmitters, along with glycine, gamma aminobutyric acid (GABA), serotonin, and, perhaps, histamine and glutamate. The chemical structure of some of these neurotransmitters is shown in Fig. 10-4, along with the structure of epinephrine, which is released by the adrenal medulla. Dopamine, norepinephrine, and epinephrine have very similar structures and are often referred to as *catecholamines*. This is a chemical term which refers to the structure these substances have in common; that is, they are all 3,4-dihydroxyphenylethylamines.

Neuropeptides

Beginning in the 1970s researchers began finding some peptides in brain tissue that were previously unknown (endorphins and enkephalins, some of which have morphine-like analgesic activity) or were believed to occur only in other organ tissues (substance P, vasoactive intestinal polypeptide, cholecystokinin). Further investigation revealed that many of these peptides were not distributed uniformly in the brain; rather, they were localized in certain brain areas. Immunocytologic techniques allowed mapping of the locations of individual peptide-containing neurons in the brain, as well as in the spinal cord and autonomic nervous system.

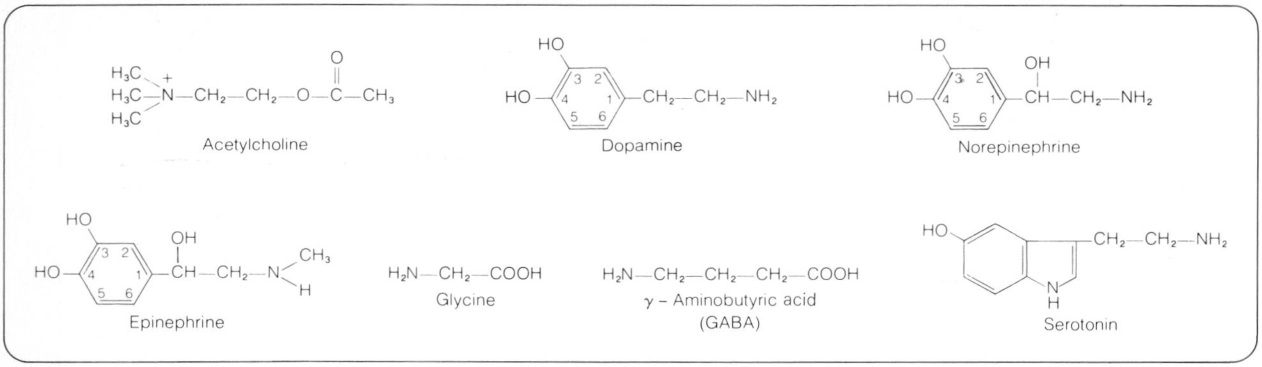

FIGURE 10-4

Chemical Structures of Some Neurotransmitters. Epinephrine, secreted by the adrenal medulla, is included to show its structural similarity to the neurotransmitters dopamine and norepinephrine; these three chemicals are all catecholamines.

Hormonal peptides such as adrenocorticotropin (ACTH), vasopressin, and oxytocin, previously believed to act only on remote target organs after release from the hypothalamus or pituitary into the circulation, were found in nerve terminals remote from the hypothalamus and pituitary, as were some peptides previously believed to have only an endocrine-regulating function within the hypothalamus and pituitary (luteinizing hormone-releasing hormone, LHRH; somatostatin; thyrotropin-releasing hormone, TRH). In addition, many of these peptides, when ejected in minute amounts from a micropipette brought near a neuron, were found to produce striking changes, either excitatory or inhibitory, in the neuron's activity. These are all indications that some of these peptides might have a physiologic role in the nervous system. What this role is, is unclear for most of the peptides, but, because they have a longer duration of action than neurotransmitters such as acetylcholine, and because some of them are found in the same neurons as one of the neurotransmitters mentioned above, it has been suggested that they modulate, in some way, the actions of neurotransmitters. They have been called *neuromodulators,* to distinguish them from neurotransmitters.

The role, if any, of these neuropeptides in mediating the therapeutic or adverse effects of any of our present drugs is entirely unknown. As more is learned about the role of these peptides in the body, in health and disease, it can be expected that new drugs will be developed to mimic their useful effects and to block their adverse effects.

THE AUTONOMIC NERVOUS SYSTEM

The autonomic nervous system acts to control and regulate the functioning of the heart, the smooth muscle in the walls of the respiratory and gastrointestinal tracts and elsewhere. It is sometimes called the *visceral nervous system.* Although some successful attempts have been made to train individuals to voluntarily control their own heart rates and blood pressures using biofeedback and psychologic conditioning techniques, we normally do *not* have voluntary control over the function of organs which are innervated by the autonomic nervous system. For this reason, the autonomic nervous system has been called the *involuntary nervous system.* This distinguishes it from the *voluntary,* or *somatic, motor system,* which innervates skeletal muscles and which we can control at will.

Autonomic Reflexes

The autonomic nervous system exerts continual, moment-to-moment control over heart rate, blood pressure, gastrointestinal tract motility, glandular secretions, and so on (see Table 10-1). It does this by reflexes. The control of systemic blood pressure by the baroreceptor reflex, originating in the carotid sinus, is illustrated in Fig. 10-5. This is only one of several baroreceptor reflexes that contribute to the control of systemic blood pressure. The anatomic substrate for autonomic reflexes consists of

1. Sensory receptors (in the example illustrated, the nerve endings in the carotid sinus).
2. Sensory nerves, or *afferent nerves* (the carotid sinus nerve, a branch of the glossopharyngeal nerve).
3. One or more areas of the central nervous system (the vasomotor center, the cardioaccelerator center, and the dorsal motor nucleus of the vagus nerve, all in the medulla, in the brainstem).
4. The motor nerves, or *efferent nerves* (the sympathetic nerves to blood vessels and the heart, and the parasympathetic nerves that innervate the sinoatrial node of the heart). Sensory receptors send information via afferent nerves into the central nervous system for integration with other information from many levels of the central nervous system. The central nervous system then instructs the effectors via efferent nerves.

Although some drugs and poisons affect the receptors involved in autonomic reflexes (for example, nicotine, in

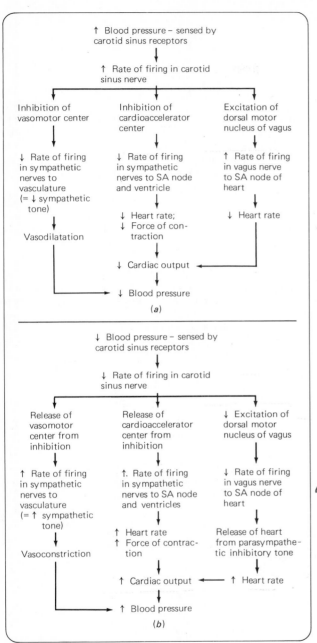

FIGURE 10-5

Baroreceptor Reflex. The carotid sinus baroreceptor reflex is an autonomic reflex that helps to control systemic blood pressure. Both increases (↑) in blood pressure (a) and decreases (↓) (b) are sensed by carotid sinus receptors and effector mechanisms are activated to maintain blood pressure within limits. Vasoconstricting drugs, such as phenylephrine and methoxamine, can increase blood pressure and set off the sequence of events shown in (a); when injected, both of these drugs cause reflex bradycardia. Vasodilating drugs, such as nitroglycerin and hydralazine, can decrease blood pressure and set off the sequence of events shown in (b); both of these drugs can cause reflex tachycardia.

tobacco, stimulates the carotid body) and some autonomic drugs probably act mostly in the central nervous system to produce their therapeutic effects [for example, the antihypertensive effects of α-**methyldopa** (Aldomet) and **propranolol** (Inderal) may be largely central], most autonomic drugs act as sites in the efferent pathways only. Subsequent discussion in this chapter is limited to autonomic efferent pathways.

Autonomic Efferents—Sympathetic and Parasympathetic Nervous Systems

Efferent pathways in the autonomic nervous system are classified as either sympathetic or parasympathetic. Most organs are innervated by both sympathetic and parasympathetic nerves. These two classes of autonomic nerve pathways differ in certain anatomic features and in function. If an organ receives both sympathetic and parasympathetic innervation, the effects of these nerves generally produce opposite and mutually antagonist effects (see Table 10-1). Only the salivary glands are possible exceptions to this statement; both sympathetic and parasympathetic nerve impulses stimulate salivary secretions, but the secretions are of different types. However, many effectors do *not* have both sympathetic and parasympathetic innervation.

Because the autonomic nervous system is often considered to consist only of these two classes of efferent pathways, these pathways are often referred to as the sympathetic and parasympathetic divisions of the autonomic nervous system, or simply the *sympathetic nervous system* and the *parasympathetic nervous system*.

The effects of the sympathetic nervous system on organs can be recalled if one associates them with a person in an emergency situation (the "flight or fight" syndrome). The effects of the parasympathetic nervous system are similar to the conditions in a person in a relaxed, after-dinner situation. Knowing these two fundamental principles allows the nurse to figure out many of the effector organ responses to sympathetic and parasympathetic nerve impulses and to drugs which mimic or interfere with the effects of these impulses. However, it is important to remember that, normally, both divisions of the autonomic nervous system are continually acting to maintain a constant internal environment, or homeostasis.

Comparison of the Somatic Motor, Sympathetic, and Parasympathetic Nervous Systems

In the somatic, or voluntary, motor system, the cell bodies of neurons which innervate skeletal muscle lie in the central nervous system in the ventral horn of the spinal cord, and the axons of these neurons proceed directly without interruption to synapse with the skeletal muscles which they innervate. This synapse is called the *neuromuscular junction*. Acetylcholine is the neurotransmitter. In contrast, in the autonomic nervous system, a *ganglion*, in which a synapse occurs, intervenes between the central nervous system and the effector organ innervated (see Fig. 10-6). The autonomic motor pathway is thus composed of two neurons in series, whereas the somatic motor pathway is composed of only one neuron.

The first neuron in the autonomic efferent pathway is called a *preganglionic neuron;* the second neuron is called a *postganglionic neuron.* The cell bodies of preganglionic neurons lie in the central nervous system, and the axons of these neurons synapse with postganglionic neurons whose cell bodies lie in autonomic ganglia outside the central nervous system. The neurotransmitter substance released by autonomic preganglionic neurons at this synapse with postganglionic neurons is acetylcholine. Actually, transmission in sympathetic ganglia has recently been shown to be more complex than this. Postganglionic neurons may synapse with one another. Furthermore, modulating interneurons in these ganglia release dopamine as a neurotransmitter onto postganglionic neurons. The physiologic significance of these dopaminergic interneurons is not clear, and their role, if any, in the therapeutic or adverse effects of drugs is also not known. Therefore, subsequent discussion will ignore these dopaminergic interneurons. The axons of postganglionic neurons synapse with the effector organs. The essential features of the somatic motor, sympathetic, and parasympathetic systems are illustrated in Fig. 10-6.

Cholinergic Synapses

The sequence of events in synaptic transmission is best understood at the neuromuscular junction in the somatic motor system, where acetylcholine is the neurotransmitter. Synapses, such as the mammalian neuromuscular junction, where acetylcholine is the neurotransmitter are referred to as *cholinergic* synapses. The term cholinergic is also applied to receptors for acetylcholine and to drugs mimicking the effects of acetylcholine.

The sequence of events in transmission at the neuromuscular junction is summarized in Fig. 10-7. Acetylcholine is synthesized in the neuron from two precursors, choline and acetyl coenzyme A, by the catalyzing action of the enzyme choline acetyltransferase. (*Enzymes* are intracellular protein molecules, which are needed to catalyze most cellular chemical reactions. Many enzymes, such as choline acetyltransferase, are specific for one chemical reaction.)

After it is synthesized, the acetylcholine is stored, probably in packets called *synaptic vesicles* which can be seen on electron micrographs of the nerve terminals. Conduction of the action potential into the fine axon terminals of the motor neuron causes some of this acetylcholine to be released from the nerve terminal. The released acetylcholine then diffuses across the cleft between the nerve cell membrane and the specialized area of skeletal muscle membrane in which receptors for acetylcholine are located. The occupation of receptor sites by acetylcholine causes a local increase in the permeability of the membrane to sodium and to potassium ions, and a depolarization, the end plate poten-

tial, occurs. Normally, the end plate potential rapidly brings the muscle to threshold, and a muscle action potential results, followed by contraction of the muscle fiber.

Some acetylcholine diffuses away from the synapse, but most acetylcholine is inactivated by the enzyme acetylcholinesterase, present at the synapse, which catalyzes the breakdown of acetylcholine to choline (which may be taken up and reused by the neuron) and acetic acid (which diffuses away into the circulation). A number of useful drugs, as well as some insecticides used in agriculture, act by inhibiting this enzyme and allowing the released acetylcholine to act more effectively and longer.

Acetylcholine is also the neurotransmitter at some synapses in the autonomic nervous system (at autonomic ganglia, at the synapses of all parasympathetic postganglionic neurons with their effector organs, and at the synapses of a few sympathetic postganglionic neurons with their effector organs). Although the sequence of events at all these synapses is similar to that shown in Fig. 10-7, it is important to recognize that acetylcholine does not affect all postsynaptic membranes in the same way, presumably because different ion permeability changes occur at different synapses. Although acetylcholine is an excitatory neurotransmitter at the neuromuscular junction and some other synapses, it is an inhibitory neurotransmitter elsewhere. For example, acetylcholine, released by parasympathetic postganglionic nerves to the heart, inhibits the spontaneous firing of the pacemaker cells in the sinoatrial node, thus decreasing heart rate.

Muscarinic and Nicotinic Cholinergic Receptors

Receptors for acetylcholine are not all the same. Some drugs specifically affect cholinergic receptors at the synapses of cholinergic postganglionic neurons with effectors, or at the synapses in autonomic ganglia, or at the skeletal neuromuscular junction. The receptors for acetylcholine on effector organs innervated by cholinergic postganglionic neurons are selectively blocked by drugs like **atropine.** These receptors are referred to as *muscarinic receptors,* because the alkaloid muscarine, a substance from a common species of poisonous mushroom (*Amanita muscaria*), mimics the effects of acetylcholine on these receptors. In contrast, the receptors for acetylcholine at autonomic ganglia and at the skeletal neuromuscular junction are not blocked by usual therapeutic doses of atropine, but are blocked by two different classes of drugs, ganglion blocking agents such as **trimethaphan camsylate** (Arfonad) and neuromuscular blocking agents such as **gallamine** (Flaxedil), respectively. Although drugs that block the receptors for acetylcholine at ganglia have little blocking effect at the neuromuscular junction and drugs that block the neuromuscular junction have little effect at ganglia, cholinergic receptors at both sites are referred to as *nicotinic receptors,* because the alkaloid nicotine mimics the effects of acetylcholine at both sites.

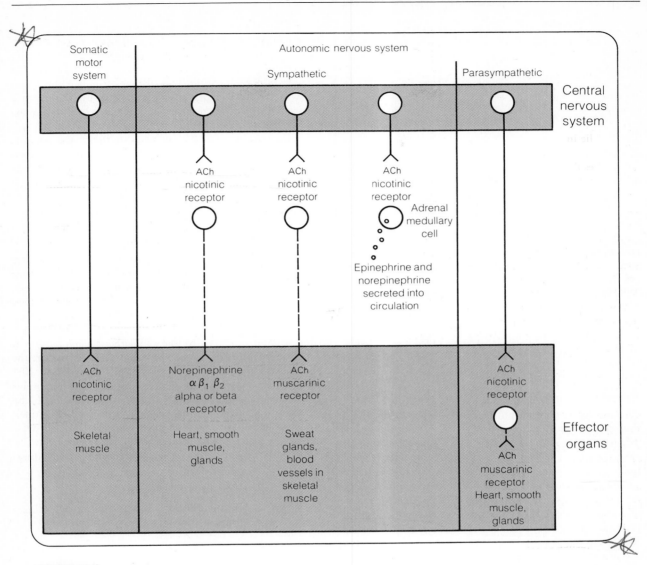

FIGURE 10-6

Diagram Comparing the Sympathetic, Parasympathetic, and Somatic Motor Systems. The central nervous system is represented by a box at the top of the diagram; effector organs are represented by a box at the bottom. In the somatic motor system, one neuron directly innervates skeletal muscle, releasing acetylcholine (ACh), which interacts with nicotinic receptors in skeletal muscle membrane. In the autonomic nervous system, preganglionic neurons (axons drawn as solid lines) synapse in autonomic ganglia with postganglionic neurons (axons drawn as dashed lines). Preganglionic neurons release acetylcholine, which interacts with nicotinic receptors in the membrane of postganglionic neurons or in adrenal medullary cells. Sympathetic postganglionic neurons characteristically have long axons. Most sympathetic postganglionic neurons release norepinephrine, which interacts with α or β receptors in the membrane of effectors. A few sympathetic postganglionic neurons and all parasympathetic postganglionic neurons release acetylcholine, which interacts with muscarinic receptors in the membrane of effectors. The adrenal medulla secretes epinephrine and norepinephrine, which are carried by the circulatory system to all parts of the body.

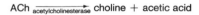

	1. Synthesis of neurotransmitter
Motor neuron	Choline + acetyl CoA $\xrightarrow[\text{acetylase}]{\text{choline}}$ acetylcholine
	2. Storage of acetylcholine in nerve terminal
	3. Action potential releases stored acetylcholine
Synaptic cleft	4. Acetylcholine diffuses across synaptic cleft
	5. Acetylcholine molecules occupy receptor sites in muscle membrane
	6. Membrane permeability to ions (Na^+, K^+) increases and ions flow across membrane
Skeletal muscle	7. End plate potential results
	8. Muscle membrane reaches threshold
	9. Action potential is generated
	10. Muscle cell contracts

FIGURE 10-7

Sequence of Events in Transmission at the Neuromuscular Junction. Action of acetylcholine is terminated by (1) destruction of the acetylcholine by the enzyme acetylcholinesterase

$$ACh \xrightarrow[\text{acetylcholinesterase}]{} \text{choline} + \text{acetic acid}$$

and (2) diffusion of the acetylcholine out of the synaptic cleft.

Adrenergic Synapses

Synapses where norepinephrine (also called noradrenaline) is the neurotransmitter are referred to as *adrenergic* synapses. The term adrenergic is also applied to drugs mimicking the effects of norepinephrine and to the receptors with which they interact. The sequence of events in transmission at an adrenergic synapse is summarized in Fig. 10-8. Norepinephrine is synthesized in neurons from the amino acid tyrosine in a series of steps. The synthesis of norepinephrine is more complex than the synthesis of acetylcholine and is more readily interfered with. Note that dopamine, which is itself a neurotransmitter at some synapses, is also a precursor in the synthesis of norepinephrine. After synthesis, norepinephrine, like acetylcholine, is stored in synaptic vesicles in the nerve terminal.

The nerve action potential causes the release of stored norepinephrine, which then diffuses across the synaptic cleft to occupy postsynaptic receptors, causing a change in the ionic permeability of the membrane and exciting or inhibiting the postsynaptic cell. Tyramine, found in certain foods, and some drugs, such as **amphetamine** and **ephedrine**, cause the release of stored norepinephrine, while another drug, **guanethidine** (Ismelin), depletes stored norepinephrine.

The effects of norepinephrine are terminated in a number of ways, but primarily by reuptake of the unchanged molecule into the presynaptic neuron from which it was released. Here, it may be reused, or it may be broken down by the enzyme momoamine oxidase (MAO). Several drugs [for example, **cocaine** and **imipramine** (Tofranil)] interfere with

the reuptake process. A number of drugs are MAO inhibitors, for example, **tranylcypromine** (Parnate), and allow norepinephrine to accumulate in the nerve terminals. The effects of norepinephrine may also be terminated by breakdown in the synaptic cleft (catalyzed by the enzyme catechol-*o*-methyltransferase, or COMT) or by diffusion out of the synaptic cleft.

Norepinephrine is the neurotransmitter at the synapses of most sympathetic postganglionic neurons with their effectors. Like acetylcholine, it has excitatory effects at some synapses and inhibitory effects at others. For example, it causes the smooth muscle in the walls of blood vessels to contract, but it causes bladder smooth muscle to relax.

α-Adrenergic and β-Adrenergic Receptors

Adrenergic receptors are not all the same. No single drug blocks all the effects of norepinephrine or all the effects of the adrenergic outflow of the sympathetic nervous system. That is, no single drug can block all adrenergic receptors. For many years, two receptor types, called alpha (α) and beta (β), have been postulated. Alpha receptors mediate the vasoconstriction produced by the sympathetic nervous system and some adrenergic drugs, whereas β receptors mediate the bronchodilation and the cardiac stimulation. Table 10-1 shows the type of receptor mediating the most important effector organ responses to sympathetic innervation. Alpha receptor–blocking drugs [e.g., **phentolamine** (Regitine)] block selectively the vasoconstriction produced by the sympathetic nervous system, but do not block the bronchodilation or cardiac stimulation. Beta receptor–blocking drugs

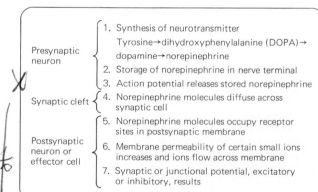

	1. Synthesis of neurotransmitter
Presynaptic neuron	Tyrosine→dihydroxyphenylalanine (DOPA)→ dopamine→norepinephrine
	2. Storage of norepinephrine in nerve terminal
	3. Action potential releases stored norepinephrine
Synaptic cleft	4. Norepinephrine molecules diffuse across synaptic cell
	5. Norepinephrine molecules occupy receptor sites in postsynaptic membrane
Postsynaptic neuron or effector cell	6. Membrane permeability of certain small ions increases and ions flow across membrane
	7. Synaptic or junctional potential, excitatory or inhibitory, results

FIGURE 10-8

Sequence of Events in Transmission at an Adrenergic Synapse. Action of norepinephrine is terminated by (1) reuptake of norepinephrine into the presynaptic neuron, where it is reused as a neurotransmitter or inactivated by the enzyme MAO, (2) inactivation of norepinephrine by the enzyme COMT, (3) diffusion of the norepinephrine out of the synaptic cleft.

[e.g., **propranolol** (Inderal)] block selectively the bronchodilation and cardiac stimulation, but do not block the vasoconstriction. Drugs that are agonists (sympathetic nervous system–mimicking drugs) also show selectivity. **Methoxamine** (Vasoxyl) produces vasoconstriction without bronchodilation or cardiac stimulation, and **isoproterenol** (Isuprel) produces bronchodilation and cardiac stimulation without vasoconstriction.

To the regret of students of pharmacology, drugs have recently become available with yet greater selectivity, and it has become necessary to divide both α and β receptors into two subgroups, called α_1 and α_2, and β_1 and β_2, respectively (see Table 10-1).

The subdivision of α receptors is very new. Although not all α receptors have been subtyped, most of the α receptors which have been known to pharmacologists for a long time are probably α_1 receptors. They occur postsynaptically on cells of effector organs. Alpha-1 receptors mediate the vasoconstriction described above as an effect of methoxamine. At present, the α_1 receptors appear far more important to a nurse's understanding of sympathomimetic and adrenergic blocking drugs than the α_2 receptors. The α_2 receptors are new to pharmacologists and usually occur presynaptically on adrenergic nerve terminals, where, it is hypothesized, they mediate a feedback inhibition of the release of norepinephrine. The significance of α_2 receptors in mediating therapeutic or adverse drug effects is still largely unknown, but it may contribute to our future understanding of observed drug effects and guide the development of new agents specific to one type of α receptor.

Both β_1 and β_2 receptors occur postsynaptically on the cells of effector organs, and both have clinical importance. The β_1 receptors mediate the cardiac stimulatory effects of the sympathetic nervous system and adrenergic drugs; the β_2 receptors mediate the bronchodilation and essentially all of the other β-receptor effects. Selective β_1 receptor blockers such as **metoprolol** (Lopressor) are useful in treating hypertension with less risk of precipitating asthma (a hazard when **propranolol**, a nonselective β_1 and β_2 blocker, is used for this purpose). Selective β_2 agonists such as **terbutaline** (Brethine, Bricanyl) are useful in treating asthma with less risk of causing cardiac stimulation and arrhythmias (a hazard when **isoproterenol**, a nonselective β_1 and β_2 agonist, is used).

The Sympathetic Nervous System

Anatomy

The sympathetic nervous system is sometimes referred to as the *thoracolumbar division of the autonomic nervous system* because the cell bodies of sympathetic preganglionic neurons lie in the thoracic and upper lumbar spinal cord. The axons of the preganglionic neurons leave the central nervous system in the ventral roots of the spinal nerves. Most sympathetic preganglionic neurons have short axons,

in comparison with parasympathetic preganglionic neurons (see Fig. 10-6). These axons synapse with postganglionic neurons in sympathetic chain ganglia, paired structures on either side of the spinal cord outside of the central nervous system, or in unpaired sympathetic ganglia in the abdomen. These postganglionic neurons send long axons to innervate effectors.

Some sympathetic preganglionic neurons also synapse on cells in the adrenal medulla, an organ which secretes epinephrine and norepinephrine into the bloodstream. The adrenal medulla is derived embryologically from the same type of tissue that gives rise to sympathetic ganglia, and adrenal medullary cells can be regarded as sympathetic postganglionic cells. The axon of a single sympathetic preganglionic neuron often branches extensively to synapse with many postganglionic neurons, an example of neuronal divergence. This anatomic relation in the sympathetic ganglia, as well as the release of epinephrine and norepinephrine into the circulation for distribution to the entire body, is the anatomic basis for the ability of the sympathetic nervous system to affect many organs and effectors simultaneously in an emergency.

Organs Innervated

The effectors innervated include the heart (sinoatrial node, specialized conduction tissue of the atria and ventricles, atrial and ventricular muscle), vasculature, bronchial smooth muscle, gastrointestinal smooth muscle and glands, detrusor muscle of the bladder, sphincters of the gastrointestinal and urinary tracts, sex organs, iris of the eye, salivary glands, liver, and sweat glands (see Table 10-1).

Neurotransmitters

All sympathetic *pre*ganglionic neurons, both those synapsing in ganglia and those synapsing with adrenal medullary cells, release acetylcholine as their neurotransmitter. The receptors for this acetylcholine on postganglionic neurons and on the adrenal medulla are one class of nicotinic receptors described earlier. Most sympathetic *post*ganglionic neurons release norepinephrine, but sympathetic postganglionic neurons innervating the sweat glands, and some blood vessels in skeletal muscle, release acetylcholine. These are referred to as *sympathetic cholinergic neurons*. The acetylcholine released by these neurons interacts with muscarinic receptors. Cells of the adrenal medulla release into the circulation a combination of epinephrine and norepinephrine, which is predominantly (80 percent) epinephrine in human beings.

Effector Organ Responses to Sympathetic Nerve Impulses

Table 10-1 summarizes the most important effects of impulses in the sympathetic nervous system on organs and lists the type of receptor mediating each effect.

It is relatively easy to figure out many of the effects of sympathetic stimulation if one associates the functions of the sympathetic nervous system with the physiologic changes which occur in an organism in an emergency situation. The rapidly beating, strongly contracting heart, that may even show an arrhythmia, and the copious outflow of sweat that often accompany a frightening or stressful situation are familiar to everyone and are the result of sympathetic stimulation. In addition, it is logical that in an emergency situation, when fight or flight may be necessary, the bronchi should be dilated to provide an optimum airway; the pupils should be dilated (*mydriasis*) to allow good visualiza-

TABLE 10-1 Effector Organ Responses to Autonomic Nerve Impulses

EFFECTOR	RESPONSE TO SYMPATHETIC NERVE IMPULSES	SYMPATHETIC RECEPTOR TYPE	RESPONSE TO PARASYMPATHETIC NERVE IMPULSES
Heart			
Sinoatrial node	Increased heart rate	β_1	Decreased heart rate
Atrioventricular node	Increased rate of conduction; increased irritability and arrhythmias	β_1	Decreased rate of conduction
His-Purkinje system	Increased irritability and arrhythmias	β_1	No innervation
Ventricular muscle	Increased force of contraction	β_1	No innervation
Smooth muscle in wall of			
Blood vessels*			
In skin, mucosa, and viscera	Contraction → vasoconstriction	α_1	No innervation
In skeletal muscle	Relaxation → vasodilation	Cholinergic, β_2†	No innervation
Bronchi	Relaxation → bronchodilation	β_2	Bronchoconstriction
Gastrointestinal tract	Relaxation → decreased motility	β_2	Increased motility
Bladder (detrusor muscle)	Relaxation	β_2	Contraction
Sphincters of gastrointestinal tract and urinary bladder	Contraction	α	Relaxation
Exocrine glands in gastrointestinal tract	Decreased secretion	?	Increased secretion
Eye			
Iris	Contraction of radial muscle → mydriasis (pupil dilates)	α	Contraction of sphincter muscle → miosis (pupil constricts)
Ciliary muscle‡	No innervation		Contraction → accommodation for near vision
Salivary glands	Viscous secretion	α	Copious watery secretion
Sweat glands	Increased sweating	Cholinergic	No innervation
Liver	Glycogenolysis → increased blood sugar	β_2	No innervation
Lacrimal and nasopharyngeal glands	No innervation		Increased secretion
Male sex organs	Emission	?	Erection

*Although investigators do not agree on many of the details of the autonomic innervation and regulation of blood vessels, there is general consensus regarding the effects of sympathetic impulses listed here, and sympathetic vasoconstrictor tone is vital to the maintenance of systemic blood pressure. It should be noted that parasympathetic cholinergic vasodilator nerves, and sympathetic vasodilator nerves to the coronary circulation, are sometimes described. If acetylcholine is injected, vasodilation and a fall in systemic blood pressure occur, but this does not mean that parasympathetic impulses cause vasodilation. Similarly, if epinephrine, which is secreted by the adrenal medulla in response to sympathetic impulses, is injected, coronary vasodilation can be observed (and complex vasodilation and vasoconstriction in other blood vessels), but local tissue metabolites and autoregulation are probably more important than the autonomic nervous system in regulating the coronary circulation. Vascular receptors for dopamine are important for the therapeutic response to that agent (Intropin) in shock but are of no demonstrated physiologic significance.

†The β_2 receptors in the blood vessels of skeletal muscle are not innervated and therefore do not respond directly to autonomic nerve impulses. However, they do respond to circulating epinephrine released from the adrenal medulla. Some sympathomimetic drugs cause vasodilatation mediated by these β_2 receptors.

‡The ciliary muscle controls the tension on the lens of the eye. Parasympathetic nerve impulses cause the ciliary muscle to contract, allow the lens to become more convex, and bring near objects to focus on the retina; when parasympathetic impulses are blocked, the lens assumes a shape in which far objects are focused on the retina and accommodation for near vision is lost.

tion of the threat; the blood pressure should be elevated by vasoconstriction of visceral and cutaneous blood vessels; and nutrients should be mobilized from the liver (*glycogenolysis*). Although defecation and urination are reactions sometimes observed in an organism in an emergency situation, the best evidence is that impulses in the sympathetic nervous system actually decrease the motility and secretions of the gastrointestinal tract, relax smooth muscle in the wall of the bladder, and contract the sphincters of the gastrointestinal and urinary tracts. Stress-induced urination and defecation are as yet not well understood in terms of the functioning of the autonomic nervous system.

In addition to the above effects, sympathetic impulses stimulate a scanty viscous secretion from the salivary glands and are responsible for male reproductive emission (ejaculation).

The Parasympathetic Nervous System

Anatomy

The parasympathetic nervous system is sometimes referred to as the *craniosacral division of the autonomic nervous system* because the cell bodies of parasympathetic preganglionic neurons lie in the brainstem (mesencephalon and medulla) and in the sacral spinal cord. The axons of the preganglioinic neurons leave the central nervous system in cranial nerves III, VII, IX, and X (the oculomotor, facial, glossopharyngeal, and vagus nerves, respectively) and in the ventral roots of the appropriate spinal nerves. In contrast to the axons of sympathetic preganglionic neurons, the axons of parasympathetic preganglionic neurons are characteristically long. Parasympathetic ganglia lie in or near the organ innervated by the postganglionic neurons whose cell bodies it contains. The axons of parasympathetic postganglionic neurons are thus very short. Generally, one preganglionic neuron synapses with only one postganglionic neuron. This one-to-one relation of pre- and postganglionic neurons is the anatomic basis for the discreteness of discharge and function observed in the parasympathetic nervous system.

Organs Innervated

The effectors innervated by the parasympathetic nervous system include the heart (sinoatrial and atrioventricular nodes and atrial muscle), bronchial smooth muscle and glands, gastrointestinal smooth muscle and glands, detrusor muscle of the bladder, sphincters of the gastrointestinal and urinary tracts, sex organs, iris and ciliary body of the eye, and salivary glands (see Table 10-1).

Neurotransmitters

Acetylcholine is the sole neurotransmitter released by the parasympathetic nervous system. It is released both by preganglionic neurons at their synapses in parasympathetic

ganglia with postganglionic neurons (nicotinic sites) and by postganglionic neurons at their synapses with effector organs (muscarinic sites). Although acetylcholine is the neurotransmitter at all parasympathetic synapses with effectors, it is important to remember that acetylcholine excites some cells and inhibits others. It will cause smooth muscle in the walls of the bronchi, gastrointestinal tract, and urinary bladder to contract, but it will cause smooth muscle in the sphincters of the gastrointestinal tract and urinary bladder to relax.

Effector Organ Responses to Parasympathetic Nerve Impulses

Table 10-1 summarizes the most important effects of parasympathetic stimulation on organs.

It is relatively easy to figure out many of these effects if one thinks of a person sitting quietly relaxed, after dinner, reading a book in a well-illuminated room. A person in such a situation would have a slow heart rate, an active and secreting gastrointestinal tract, small pupils (*miosis*), and an eye accommodated for near vision—all effects of parasympathetic stimulation. If one thinks of effects on other organs which are the opposite of those of sympathetic stimulation, one can figure out that parasympathetic impulses cause bronchoconstriction (and increased bronchial secretions), contraction of the detrusor muscle of the bladder, and relaxation of the sphincters of the gastrointestinal and urinary tracts.

In addition, impulses in the parasympathetic nervous system stimulate a copious and watery secretion from the salivary glands, stimulate secretion by lacrimal and nasopharyngeal glands, and are responsible for penile erection.

Sympathetic and Parasympathetic Tone

Some effectors are innervated by only one division of the autonomic nervous system. The vasculature, for example, receives no parasympathetic innervation. But it does receive sympathetic noradrenergic and cholinergic innervation. The adrenergic innervation plays an important role in controlling blood pressure. The vasculature is said to have *sympathetic tone*. There is, normally, ongoing, tonic impulse activity in sympathetic postganglionic adrenergic nerves, causing the release of norepinephrine, producing some degree of vasoconstriction, and maintaining blood pressure. Any drug (e.g., **phentolamine**) that interferes with the function of these nerves can remove sympathetic tone and lower blood pressure. The sweat glands also lack parasympathetic innervation and have sympathetic tone, which in their case is cholinergic (although circulating epinephrine stimulates some sweat glands).

Even when an effector or organ system receives dual innervation by both divisions of the autonomic nervous system, the effects of one division may predominate, and the effector is said to be under sympathetic or parasympathetic tone. The heart, gastrointestinal tract, and urinary bladder all usually have parasympathetic tone at rest. Any drug (e.g., **atropine**) which interferes with the function of the parasympathetic nervous system is therefore likely to increase heart rate, and may cause constipation and urinary retention.

THE NURSING PROCESS RELATED TO NEUROPHARMACOLOGY

An understanding of the autonomic nervous system should direct the activities of the nurse in each step of the nursing process with a wide variety of patients. An understanding of the functions of this system will be especially important when working with the patient taking any drug with autonomic activity. A quick review of the system's normal function will alert the nurse to what assessments to make, side effects and therapeutic effects to anticipate, and important teaching points to include when this normal function is altered in any way.

Assessment

When the patient is on an autonomic drug, presence of problems involving the cardiovascular system (myocardial infarction, congestive heart failure, hypertension, hypotension, arrhythmia), the respiratory system (asthma, obstructive lung disease), the urinary tract (prostatic hypertrophy, tumor), the gastrointestinal tract (obstruction, paralytic ileus), and the pressure of the eye (glaucoma) or in certain high-risk groups (elderly, depressed, diabetic) alert the nurse to assess for a drug-disease interaction that might contraindicate the drug or modify nursing management. A good data base for each of these systems is necessary for comparison with developments that occur during therapy. In the example of the patient who experiences palpitations while being treated with **isoproterenol** (Isuprel) for an acute asthma attack, the nurse would need to refer to charted objective data of the rate and rhythm of the heart before the drug therapy, to determine appropriate action.

Management and Evaluation

Due to the varied effects and uses of autonomic drugs, the goal-setting component of management is complicated, since it may be difficult to ascertain whether the desired therapeutic end has been reached. For example, the atropine effect of dry mouth is usually considered an adverse reaction to be minimized through dosage regulation and nursing intervention, but in Parkinson's disease this is one of the desired effects to control drooling. Many of the side effects of the autonomic drugs are predictable and can be alleviated or controlled by proper preventive and management plans. For example, for a patient placed on a cholinergic blocker who reports a history of constipation, immediate preventive action be taken (change in diet, increase in exercise, and adjustment of fluid intake) to avoid exacerbation of the problem.

Patient teaching is a vital component of the nursing care for patients receiving autonomic drugs. Using a concise educational approach, the nurse can prepare the patient for side effects and help the patient to cope effectively with them. The salient factors about the autonomic nervous system that underlie the therapeutic and adverse reactions can be simply explained to the patient: "You are probably most aware of the part of your nervous system which you can control voluntarily, but there is another part of the nervous system which is primarily nonvoluntary and controls your heart, blood pressure, sweating, salivation, digestion, and urination. The drug you are taking mimics the effect of this system by stimulating your heart, but some of the other effects may also be mimicked, and I would like to explain to you what to do if this occurs."

CONCLUSION

Many drugs used in varying clinical situations exert effects on the autonomic nervous system. In addition to the beneficial, therapeutic effects of these drugs, there are multiple undesirable but unavoidable effects which accompany their use. A knowledge of the anatomy and physiology of the autonomic nervous system enables the nurse to anticipate and monitor the actions of such drugs, which will be discussed in detail in the following chapters.

REFERENCES

Appenzeller, O.: *The Autonomic Nervous System: An Introduction to Basic and Clinical Concepts,* 3d ed., Amsterdam: North-Holland, 1982.

Bennett, M. R.: *Autonomic Neuromuscular Transmission,* London: Cambridge University Press, 1972.

Bloom, F. E.: "Neurohumoral Transmission and the Central Nervous System," in A. G. Gilman, L. S. Goodman, and A. Gilman (eds.), *Goodman and Gilman's The Pharmacological Basis of Therapeutics,* 6th ed., New York: Macmillan, 1980.

Cooper, J. R., F. E. Bloom, and R. H. Roth: *The Biochemical Basis of Neuropharmacology,* 4th ed., New York: Oxford University Press, 1982.

Johnson, R. H., and J. M. K. Spalding: *Disorders of the Autonomic Nervous System,* Philadelphia: Davis, 1974.

Kandel, E. R., and J. H. Schwartz: *Principles of Neural Science,* Amsterdam: Elsevier/North-Holland, 1981.

Koizumi, K., and C. McC. Brooks: "The Autonomic System and Its Role in Controlling Body Functions," in V. B. Mountcastle (ed.), *Medical Physiology,* 14th ed., St. Louis: Mosby, 1980.

Mayer, S. E.: "Neurohumoral Transmission and the Autonomic Nervous System," in A. G. Gilman, L. S. Goodman, and A. Gilman (eds.), *Goodman and Gilman's The Pharmacological Basis of Therapeutics,* 6th ed., New York: Macmillan, 1980.

Shepherd, G. M.: *Neurobiology,* New York: Oxford University Press, 1983.

11

DIRECT-ACTING PARASYMPATHO-MIMETIC DRUGS AND CHOLINESTERASE INHIBITORS

ELEANOR H. BOYD
AMY M. KARCH

LEARNING OBJECTIVES

Upon mastery of the contents of this chapter, the reader will be able to:

1. Describe the mechanism of action of the two classes of parasympathomimetic drugs.

2. Identify the clinical uses of bethanechol, carbachol, pilocarpine, physostigmine (Eserine), neostigmine, edrophonium, and isoflurophate (DFP).

3. Explain why the systemic administration of parasympathomimetic drugs usually produces side effects.

4. Give an example of one drug that is a specific antidote to and is useful in treating an adverse drug reaction to bethanechol.

5. Give an example of two different drugs that act by different mechanisms and are specific antidotes in organophosphorus poisoning.

6. State one nursing activity for each step of the nursing process applicable to patients using parasympathomimetic drugs for a given problem.

Drugs that mimic the effects of activation of the parasympathetic nervous system are called parasympathomimetic drugs. They are also sometimes called *cholinergic drugs,* or cholinergic agonists, because they produce effects in the body like those produced by acetylcholine when it is released from some cholinergic nerve terminals. Therapeutically useful parasympathomimetic drugs act by two differ-

ent mechanisms and are classified accordingly (see Fig. 11-1). Table 11-1 shows a more complete classification of the drugs described in this chapter and gives examples of important drugs in each class.

Direct-acting parasympathomimetic drugs interact with cholinergic receptors located on effector organs such as smooth muscle, glands, and the heart. These are the cholinergic receptors identified in Chap. 10 as *muscarinic* cholinergic receptors. They are innervated by parasympathetic postganglionic axons and by sympathetic cholinergic postganglionic axons.

Drugs in the second class of parasympathomimetic agents act indirectly. They inhibit the enzyme acetylcholinesterase, which catalyzes the breakdown of the acetylcholine released at synapses. Drugs in this class are referred to as inhibitors of acetylcholinesterase or, more simply, as *cholinesterase inhibitors,* or anticholinesterases. The inhibitors of acetylcholinesterase allow the acetylcholine released by nerve action potentials to accumulate at the synapses, where it is released. Endogenous acetylcholine therefore produces a greater effect of longer duration than it otherwise would. Cholinesterase inhibitors act at all cholinergic receptor sites to which they have access. This includes both muscarinic and nicotinic cholinergic sites in the peripheral nervous system. Some cholinesterase inhibitors can also act at cholinergic synapses in the central nervous system. Cholinesterase inhibitors produce therapeutically useful effects at muscarinic cholinergic synapses and at nicotinic cholinergic synapses at the neuromuscular junction. Both effects will be discussed in this chapter.

168

TABLE 11-1   Classification and Examples of Parasympathomimetic Agents

CLASS	EXAMPLES
Direct-acting parasympathomimetic drugs	
Synthetic esters of choline	Bethanechol, carbachol
Naturally occurring plant alkaloids	Pilocarpine
Cholinesterase inhibitors	
Reversible inhibitors	
Of moderately long duration	Neostigmine, physostigmine (esterine)
Of very brief duration	Edrophonium
Irreversible inhibitors (organophosphorus compounds)	
Drugs	Echothiophate, Isoflurophate (DFP)
Insecticides	Malathion, Parathion

REVIEW OF THE PARASYMPATHETIC NERVOUS SYSTEM NEUROPHYSIOLOGY

Many organs are innervated and influenced by the parasympathetic nervous system (see Table 10-1). For example, impulses in the parasympathetic nervous system cause salivation; stimulation (contraction) of the smooth muscle and relaxation of the sphincters of the gastrointestinal tract and urinary bladder; constriction of the bronchi and increased secretion from the mucus-secreting cells of the respiratory tract; slowing of the heart rate and slowing of the rate of conduction of the cardiac impulse through atrioventricular (AV) node; constriction of the pupil of the eye; accommodation of the eye for near vision; and secretion of tears.

Many of these parasympathetic effects would be uncomfortable and even life-threatening if they were not produced as part of a well-controlled and integrated autonomic reflex, acting with the help of the sympathetic nervous system to maintain homeostasis. For example, without the autonomic reflex, excessive stimulation of the gastrointestinal tract causes severe cramping and diarrhea, and bronchoconstriction or slowing of the heart can be fatal. However, when parasympathomimetic drugs are given, the parasympathomimetic effects produced are *not* part of a well-controlled reflex.

In addition, parasympathomimetic drugs act at cholinergic receptors besides those innervated by the parasympathetic nervous system. They act at *sympathetic* cholinergic receptors (see Chap. 10) to cause sweating. Of greater consequence, they act at sympathetic cholinergic receptors and at other cholinergic receptors in the vasculature to cause generalized vasodilatation and hypotension.

Cholinesterase inhibitors act at all of the above sites and at the neuromuscular junction. In low doses they cause skeletal muscle contractions; in high doses, paralysis.

Thus, these drugs can produce many potentially dangerous effects. Their safe and effective use requires knowledge of their potential adverse effects, and requires application of this knowledge in all steps of the nursing process. The clinical usefulness of these drugs is, in fact, limited by the diversity of the potentially serious adverse effects they can produce. Indications for their use have gradually declined as newer, more selective and more effective drugs have been found.

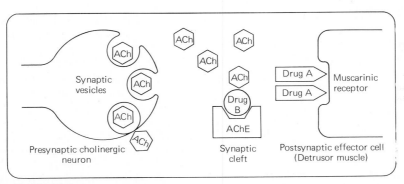

FIGURE 11-1

Schematic Representation of the Mechanisms of Parasympathomimetic Drugs in the Treatment of Urinary Retention. Drug A represents a direct-acting agent which elicits contraction of the bladder detrusor muscle by directly occupying the muscarinic receptor. Drug B represents an acetylcholinesterase (AChE) inhibitor, which prevents the breakdown of endogenous acetylcholine (ACh), increasing the availability of ACh to occupy the muscarinic receptors on the detrusor muscle.

CLINICAL USES OF DIRECT-ACTING PARASYMPATHOMIMETIC DRUGS AND CHOLINESTERASE INHIBITORS

When used judiciously, these drugs can effectively relieve gastrointestinal atony and urinary retention, can effectively treat some forms of glaucoma and prevent the ensuing blindness, and can restore neuromuscular function in some patients with myasthenia gravis. None of the drugs is used for all these indications; specific drugs and their uses are described in later sections.

Use in Treating Gastrointestinal Atony (Table 11-2)

The smooth muscle of the stomach and intestines can lose tone and motility after surgical manipulation of the viscera, after vagotomy, or after the administration of drugs like atropine (see Chap. 12), a drug often given as preoperative medication. Loss of tone by the smooth muscle of the stomach, called gastric atony, can delay gastric emptying; loss of tone by the smooth muscle of the intestines, called intestinal atony or paralytic ileus, can cause intense constipation, abdominal distention, and discomfort. Drugs with parasympathomimetic effects on the gastrointestinal tract are used to stimulate gastrointestinal smooth muscle and to relax sphincters, reducing gastric emptying time and restoring the normal peristaltic movements of the intestines.

Use in Treating Urinary Retention (Table 11-2)

Postoperative and postpartum urinary retention can be effectively treated by drugs with parasympathomimetic effects on the urinary bladder. These drugs cause the detrusor muscle of the bladder to contract and the sphincter and trigone to relax, thereby inducing urination. These drugs are also effective in treating neurogenic bladder.

TABLE 11-2 Drugs Used to Treat Gastrointestinal Atony and Urinary Retention

DRUG	DOSAGE AND ROUTE
Direct-acting parasympathomimetic drugs	
Bethanechol chloride (Myotonachol, Urecholine)	2.5–5 mg tid or qid subcutaneously; 10–30 mg tid or qid orally
Cholinesterase inhibitors	
Neostigmine bromide (Prostigmin Bromide)	15 mg orally
Neostigmine methylsulfate (Prostigmin Methylsulfate)	0.5–1.0 mg subcutaneously

TABLE 11-3 Drugs Used to Treat Some Forms of Glaucoma

Direct-acting parasympathomimetic drugs
  Carbachol
  Pilocarpine
Cholinesterase inhibitors
  Reversible inhibitors
    Demecarium (Humorsol)
    Physostigmine (Eserine)
  Irreversible inhibitors (organophosphorus compounds)
    Echothiophate iodide (Echodide, Phospholine)
    Isoflurophate (DFP, Floropryl)

Use in Treating Glaucoma (Table 11-3)

Parasympathomimetic drugs cause contraction of the sphincter muscle of the iris and contraction of the ciliary muscle (see Table 10-1). Secondary to these effects, in patients with some forms of glaucoma, the apertures of the canals of Schlemm may be more completely exposed, thereby permitting more normal drainage of aqueous humor, reducing intraocular pressure, and preventing permanent damage to the optic nerve. The reduction in intraocular pressure produced by these drugs when they are used to treat glaucoma may be partly due to the effects they have on the blood vessels of the eye and on the cells secreting the aqueous humor. To minimize side effects, drugs used to treat glaucoma are administered locally into the conjunctival sac of the eye in the form of ophthalmic preparations.

For a more detailed discussion of glaucoma and the use of these and other drugs in its treatment, see Chap. 39, "Ophthalmologic Disorders."

Use of Cholinesterase Inhibitors in Myasthenia Gravis (Table 11-4)

Myasthenia gravis is a progressive neuromuscular disorder, characterized by failure of transmission at the neuromuscular junction, with concomitant weakness and eventual paralysis of skeletal muscle. Drugs that inhibit acetylcholinesterase allow the molecules of acetylcholine released at the neuromuscular junction to have a longer time to interact with whatever cholinergic receptors are available. In patients with myasthenia, this results in a therapeutically useful facilitation of neuromuscular transmission. In fact, the improvement in strength of skeletal muscle contraction produced by a cholinesterase inhibitor is so characteristic of myasthenia that a very short acting cholinesterase inhibitor, **edrophonium**, is given for diagnostic purposes to patients suspected of having myasthenia.

However, it is a characteristic of nicotinic cholinergic receptors, including the cholinergic receptors at the neuromuscular junction, that too much acetylcholine *interferes*

TABLE 11-4 Cholinesterase Inhibitors Used for Treatment and Diagnosis of Myasthenia Gravis

Treatment

Neostigmine bromide (Prostigmin Bromide)
Neostigmine methylsulfate (Prostigmin Methylsulfate)
Pyridostigmine bromide (Mestinon)
Ambenonium chloride (Mytelase)

Diagnosis

Edrophonium chloride (Tensilon)

with transmission. It is sometimes difficult in myasthenic patients to adjust the maintenance dose of cholinesterase inhibitor properly to prevent the accumulation of too much acetylcholine. When too much acetylcholine accumulates, it can cause skeletal muscle weakness and paralysis that are very similar to those of the underlying disease. These drug-induced effects on skeletal muscle are part of a syndrome called *cholinergic crisis.* The edrophonium test used for diagnosing myasthenia is also useful in distinguishing cholinergic crisis from exacerbation of the disease. If edrophonium helps to overcome the muscle weakness, the dose of cholinesterase inhibitor should be increased; if edrophonium causes greater muscle weakness, the dose should be decreased.

For a more detailed description of myasthenia and the use of these and other drugs in its treatment, see Chap. 33, "Neurologic Disorders."

DIRECT-ACTING PARASYMPATHOMIMETIC DRUGS

Specific Drugs and Their Clinical Uses

These drugs are either synthetic esters of choline and chemically related to acetylcholine (see Fig. 11-2) or alkaloids, that is, naturally occurring nitrogen-containing substances found in plants. Acetylcholine itself is essentially never used clinically, because it is rapidly broken down by cholinesterases in the blood and tissues and because it lacks specificity, activating both muscarinic and nicotinic cholinergic receptors. (Ophthalmic preparations of acetylcholine are used, though rarely, to produce miosis of brief duration during eye surgery.) Muscarine, the mushroom alkaloid for which muscarinic receptors were named (see Chap. 10), is also not clinically useful because it lacks specificity.

Parasympathomimetic Esters of Choline

Research has led to the synthesis of several therapeutically useful drugs whose chemical structures, while resembling closely that of acetylcholine (see Fig. 11-2), confer on them the properties of stability (long duration of action) and greater specificity in their sites of action than acetylcholine.

Bethanechol Bethanechol (Urecholine, Myotonachol) is the drug of this group most likely to be given systemically. It is resistant to breakdown by cholinesterases and acts almost solely at muscarinic receptors, with some specificity for those muscarinic receptors located on smooth muscle of the gastrointestinal tract and urinary bladder. This means that at low doses it is more likely to produce parasympathomimetic effects on the gastrointestinal tract and urinary bladder than on other organs. It can be used systemically to relieve gastric and intestinal atony and urinary retention (see Table 11-2).

Molecules of bethanechol, like molecules of all parasympathomimetic choline esters, contain a quaternary (electrically charged) nitrogen atom (see Fig. 11-2). Bethanechol is therefore poorly absorbed after oral administration. When given orally, doses greater than those given subcutaneously are needed (see Table 11-2). Bethanechol is *never* given intravenously or intramuscularly, because it loses its specificity when given by those routes.

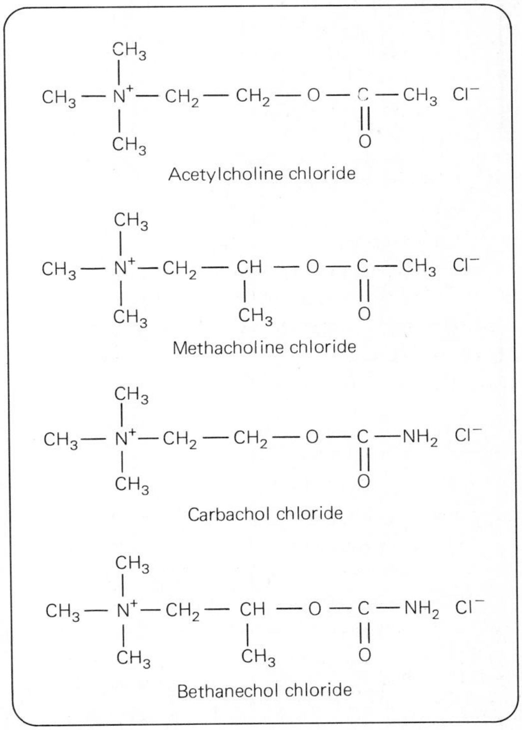

FIGURE 11-2

Chemical Structures of Acetylcholine and Synthetic Direct-Acting Parasympathomimetic Esters of Choline. Each of the agents shown is a quarternary ammonium compound (i.e., has a positively charged nitrogen atom), is absorbed poorly, and does not cross the blood-brain barrier in significant amounts.

Methacholine   Methacholine is somewhat resistant to breakdown by cholinesterase and is more specific in its sites of action than acetylcholine, affecting predominantly muscarinic receptors. However, methacholine lacks the specificity of bethanechol, and it produces profound and dangerous cardiovascular effects. It is used as a provocative test for obstructive airway disease, since it causes bronchoconstriction at low doses in susceptible individuals (see Chap. 27).

Carbachol   Carbachol (Carbacel, Isopto Carbachol) is resistant to cholinesterase, but it is not given systemically, because it is very nonspecific, acting at nicotinic as well as muscarinic receptors. When administered topically to the eye, carbachol is useful in treating certain forms of glaucoma (see Table 11-3).

Parasympathomimetic Alkaloids

Pilocarpine   Pilocarpine (Isopto Carpine, Pilocar) is an old drug, which was once used systemically when the induction of sweating (diaphoresis) was believed to be beneficial. Its use is now limited to local ophthalmic administration to treat glaucoma (see Table 11-3) or to overcome the effects of atropine and similar drugs used to facilitate examination of the eye.

Arecoline   Although pilocarpine is the only alkaloid used therapeutically as parasympathomimetic agent, arecoline, the active alkaloid in the betel nut, is used by the inhabitants of Papua New Guinea and other Pacific islands for the pleasurable effects it produces through the central nervous system. (Chewing the betel nut releases the arecoline.) Like pilocarpine, arecoline is an uncharged molecule and is both well-absorbed when ingested and capable of crossing the blood-brain barrier.

Adverse Effects of Direct-Acting Parasympathomimetic Drugs

Although the drugs used therapeutically are more specific in their effects than either acetylcholine or muscarine, they are still capable of affecting any organ having appropriate cholinergic receptors. In general, as with many modern drugs, their specificity decreases and the likelihood of unwanted and adverse effects increases as the dose is increased.

Most of the clinically important adverse effects produced by these drugs can be predicted from knowledge of the receptors with which they interact and from an understanding of the effects of activation of these receptors. Bethanechol will be discussed as a prototype drug because it is the drug in this group most likely to be given systemically, and therefore it is most likely to gain access to all potential sites of action. Methacholine, carbachol, and pilocarpine, in the rare instances when they are given systemically, or when they accidentally reach the systemic circulation after ophthalmic administration, can cause the same effects. The most important adverse effects of bethanechol are listed in Table 11-5.

Cardiovascular System

In doses used to treat paralytic ileus and urinary retention, bethanechol usually produces a slight fall in diastolic blood pressure that is accompanied by reflex tachycardia. Higher doses produce greater hypotension. The fall in blood pressure cannot be predicted from knowledge of the effects produced by activation of the parasympathetic nervous system. Parasympathetic nerve impulses *do not* produce vasodilatation, but parasympathomimetic drugs, interacting with muscarinic receptors, *do* cause dilatation of the entire vasculature. This effect of parasympathomimetic drugs was formerly used in the treatment of hypertension, but newer drugs lower blood pressure more effectively and specifically.

While the usual effect of bethanechol on the heart is

TABLE 11-5   Adverse Effects of Bethanechol*

ORGAN SYSTEM	EFFECT
Cardiovascular system	
Blood vessels	Vasodilatation and hypotension
Heart	Reflex tachycardia in therapeutic doses; sinus bradycardia at higher doses
	Various degrees of heart block
	Cardiac arrhythmias
Respiratory system	Bronchoconstriction
	Increased mucus secretion
	Wheezing and coughing
	Asthmatic attack
Gastrointestinal tract	Increased motility and increased peristalsis
	Intestinal cramps and diarrhea
	Increased gastric acid secretion
	Heartburn
	Nausea, vomiting
Urinary tract	Stimulation of detrusor muscle, which may cause discomfort in bladder region
Other organ systems	
Sweat glands	Sweating
Eye	Miosis and spasm of accommodation
	Lacrimation
	Headache in frontal region

*Atropine is a specific antidote.

reflex tachycardia, bethanechol may sometimes produce direct parasympathomimetic (vagomimetic) effects on the sinoatrial (SA) and atrioventricular (AV) nodes of the heart. These include sinus bradycardia, slowing of the conduction of the cardiac impulse through the AV node to the ventricles, and other degrees of heart block. Atrial or ventricular cardiac arrhythmias (i.e., the development of cardiac pacemakers outside the SA node) may also occur.

Respiratory System

Like the parasympathetic nervous system, bethanechol can stimulate tracheal and bronchial mucus-secreting cells, and it can cause bronchoconstriction. These effects can lead to coughing and wheezing.

Gastrointestinal Tract

Bethanechol is used therapeutically for its ability to stimulate gastrointestinal motility and tone. As a result of this effect, patients sometimes experience severe cramping, flatulence, and diarrhea. Secretions from salivary and digestive glands are also stimulated. The increased secretion of gastric hydrochloric acid can cause heartburn, nausea, and vomiting.

Urinary Tract

Bethanechol causes contraction of the detrusor muscle of the bladder, a therapeutically useful effect in patients with urinary retention, but the bladder contractions may cause lower abdominal discomfort.

Other Organ Systems

Patients receiving bethanechol may complain of feeling sweaty and flushed. Headache in the frontal region, possibly secondary to the effects on vision, is also a common complaint, especially after higher therapeutic doses. Patients may also have increased lacrimation (tearing).

Treatment of Adverse Effects Produced by Direct-Acting Parasympathomimetic Drugs

Atropine sulfate (see Chap. 12), a drug that *blocks* muscarinic cholinergic receptors, is a specific antidote to bethanechol and other direct-acting parasympathomimetic drugs. Whenever bethanechol is given by the subcutaneous route, **atropine sulfate** (0.5 to 1.0 mg, IM or IV) should be ready for injection. **Epinephrine** (see Chap. 13), a sympathomimetic drug, is also useful as a physiologic antagonist to the serious cardiovascular and respiratory effects of bethanechol. (See Chap. 48, "Emergency and Intensive Care," for the general principles of treating poisoning and adverse drug reactions.)

THE NURSING PROCESS RELATED TO DIRECT-ACTING PARASYMPATHOMIMETIC DRUGS

The basic nursing actions are the same for all patients receiving any of the direct-acting parasympathomimetics by a systemic route of administration. The particular patient problem, possible drug interactions, and the desired therapeutic effects must be considered for each individual patient, and the nursing approach should be altered accordingly.

Assessment

Past History The direct-acting parasympathomimetic drugs interact with the muscarinic cholinergic receptors to cause various predictable autonomic responses. Because these responses are no longer controlled and balanced by specific autonomic reflexes, they can be uncomfortable and even life-threatening in patients with particular compromised states.

The patient history should be taken to rule out any of the following problems, all of which are relative or absolute contraindications to use of the drugs:

Asthma or COPD Parasympathomimetics cause bronchoconstriction and increased mucus secretion in patients with asthma or other chronic respiratory diseases.

Bowel obstruction or recent bowel surgery Parasympathomimetics increase tone and motility of the gastrointestinal tract, which could lead to rupture in these patients.

Urinary bladder obstruction or recent bladder surgery Parasympathomimetics increase bladder muscle tone and contractions, which could cause intense pain or even rupture in these patients.

Peptic ulcer Parasympathomimetics increase gastrointestinal motility and acid production and could aggravate the ulcer.

Coronary insufficiency Parasympathomimetics have been shown to decrease blood flow to cardiac muscle, which could lead to angina or myocardial infarction.

Heart block Parasympathomimetics slow cardiac conduction through the atrioventricular node and decrease the normal rate of firing at the sinoatrial node; this can lead to escape rhythms and/or total block in these patients.

Hyperthyroidism Parasympathomimetics cause atrial fibrillation in these patients.

Physical Assessment Before giving any of these drugs, the nurse should assess the baseline functioning of all of the systems that are most affected by parasympathomimetics. This assessment includes blood pressure, apical and peripheral pulses (rate, rhythm, and character), heart sounds (by cardiac auscultation), respirations (rate, rhythm, character, and adventitious sounds), bowel sounds (rate and character), and urinary output (including assessment of bladder distention and tone).

Once a baseline assessment is established, the nurse will be able to detect changes in the patient that could indicate therapeutic or toxic effects of the drugs.

Management

The patient should be alerted to possible occurrence of common side effects such as flushing, nausea, diarrhea, urgency to void, flatulence, sweating, and headache. These side effects include many of the therapeutic uses of the drugs but are often seen as very uncomfortable by the patient, who should not be alarmed by them. Aspirin may help to relieve the headache. Immediate access to a bedpan or bedside commode will help to alleviate the anxiety produced by the feelings of urgency or the sudden diarrhea and cramping. A cool environment will help alleviate some of the discomfort associated with the flushing and diaphoresis. Atropine sulfate should always be available in case of severe side effects. The patient should be asked to report any feelings of light-headedness, faintness, excessive salivation, cramping, or pain. Any of these symptoms could indicate overdosage or excessive reaction to the drug.

Evaluation

The patient should be assessed for signs of therapeutic activity of the drug—voiding, increased bowel sounds, etc. A continual assessment of the patient for potential adverse side effects should be done. A decrease in heart rate or irregular heart rhythm; an increase in respiratory rate, wheezes, or rales; or abdominal rigidity and/or abdominal pain of any nature could indicate serious complications from the parasympathomimetic therapy, and the drug should be stopped and the physician notified immediately.

CHOLINESTERASE INHIBITORS

These drugs inhibit acetylcholinesterase and allow acetylcholine to accumulate and have a greater effect at the synapses, where it is released. Cholinesterase inhibitors can act at the muscarinic cholinergic sites where bethanechol acts, at the neuromuscular junctions, and at autonomic ganglia and the adrenal medulla. Some cholinesterase inhibitors also act at cholinergic synapses in the central nervous system.

Specific Drugs and Their Clinical Uses

These drugs are classed as either reversible or irreversible inhibitors of acetylcholinesterase (see Table 11-1), depending on their molecular mechanism of binding to acetylcholinesterase. The reversible inhibitors are themselves of two types, depending on their duration of action. **Edrophonium** has a very brief duration of action; the rest have moderately long durations of action. The irreversible inhibitors are organophorphorus molecules, originally synthesized as agents for chemical warfare. **Isoflurophate** and **echothiophate** are the only irreversible inhibitors used therapeutically. However, the irreversible inhibitors are used widely as pesticides. Many of them are readily absorbed through the intact skin and lungs, as well as orally, and in some agricultural communities exposure to and poisoning by these agents is not uncommon.

Reversible Cholinesterase Inhibitors

These drugs are used therapeutically for the same indications as the direct-acting parasympathomimetic drugs, i.e., to treat patients with paralytic ileus, urinary retention, and glaucoma. In addition, they are used for their effects at the neuromuscular junction to treat patients with myasthenia gravis.

Physostigmine Physostigmine (Isopto Eserine), is an alkaloid contained in the "ordeal bean," a seed of a west African plant, formerly used in witchcraft "trials by ordeal" in the parts of Africa where it grow. It is readily absorbed after oral administration and readily crosses the blood-brain barrier. Its major use now is in ophthalmic preparations to treat glaucoma. It can also be given systemically to treat both the central and the peripheral adverse effects of drugs like **atropine sulfate** and the **tricyclic antidepressants,** which block muscarinic cholinergic synapses. Physostigmine also is under investigation for treatment of memory impairment, as in senile dementia.

Demecarium Demecarium (Humorsol) is also used to treat glaucoma. Its duration of action is longer than that of physostigmine; therefore it is not administered as frequently. It is also relatively lacking in central nervous system effects, but its long-term use is associated with an unexplained high risk of cataract development.

Neostigmine Neostigmine (Prostigmin) contains a quaternary nitrogen atom and is therefore poorly absorbed after oral administration. It also penetrates the brain poorly and at therapeutic doses does not reach the central nervous system in concentrations sufficient to produce important effects. Neostigmine is given subcutaneously or orally, but to be effective orally, it must be given in higher doses than those effective subcutaneously.

Neostigmine has some specificity for muscarinic cholinergic synapses on cells of the gastrointestinal tract and urinary bladder. Its stimulatory effects on these organs can be used therapeutically to treat patients with paralytic ileus and urinary retention (see Table 11-2).

Neostigmine also has some specificity for the neuromuscular junction, where it both inhibits acetylcholinesterase and acts directly to stimulate skeletal muscle. It is used in the treatment of myasthenia gravis, as are two other cholinesterase inhibitors, *pyridostigmine* and *ambenonium* (see Table 11-4). Neostigmine is also sometimes used postoperatively by anesthesiologists to terminate the effects of tubocurarine and other competitive neuromuscular junction–blocking agents (see Chap. 16).

Edrophonium   Edrophonium (Tensilon), the cholinesterase inhibitor with very short duration of action, is unsuitable for therapeutic use in myasthenia, but, as described above, it is very useful in diagnostic procedures with myasthenic patients.

Irreversible Cholinesterase Inhibitors (Organophosphorus Compounds)

Echothiophate and Isoflurophate   Echothiophate (Echodide Phospholine Iodide) and isoflurophate (Floropryl) are the two therapeutically useful irreversible cholinesterase inhibitors. The latter drug is commonly referred to as DFP; the three letters are derived from its chemical name, di-isopropyl phosphorofluoridate. Echothiophate has the advantage of not penetrating the blood-brain barrier very readily.

Echothiophate and isoflurophate are used only in the form of ophthalmic preparations to treat glaucoma. They have a long duration of action, but, as with demecarium, their long-term use is associated with a high risk of cataract development. Their long duration of action reduces the frequency with which they must be administered, but also adds to the danger when inadvertent absorption into the systemic circulation occurs. These drugs bind irreversibly to acetylcholinesterase. This means that, unless an enzyme reactivator is given promptly (**pralidoxime**; see Treatment of Poisoning by Organophorphorus Compounds below), the action of these inhibitors is terminated only when the patient's nervous system has synthesized enough new molecules of acetylcholinesterase to restore normal synaptic function. Since enzymes are proteins, this may take several weeks.

Adverse Effects of Cholinesterase Inhibitors (Table 11-6)

After systemic administration or accidental systemic absorption of these drugs, they can produce adverse effects attributable to their actions at both muscarinic and nicotinic sites (the neuromuscular junction). Some cholinesterase inhibitors also act at central nervous system sites. The syndrome of serious toxic effects produced at these sites is called *cholinergic crisis.*

Cholinesterase inhibitors produce a spectrum of adverse effects at muscarinic receptors similar to that described for

bethanechol (see Table 11-5). Cholinesterase inhibitors also produce serious adverse effects at the neuromuscular junction. These include involuntary muscle contractions and eventual muscle weakness and paralysis. Loss of control of the respiratory muscles is a very serious consequence and, combined with bronchoconstriction and increased tracheobronchial secretions, is usually the primary cause of death in acute overdoses.

Those cholinesterase inhibitors that penetrate the blood-

TABLE 11-6   Adverse Effects of Cholinesterase Inhibitors*

ORGAN SYSTEM	EFFECT
Cardiovascular system	
Blood vessels	Vasodilatation and hypotension
Heart	Bradycardia
	Various degrees of heart block
	Cardiac arrhythmias
Respiratory system	Bronchoconstriction and increased mucus secretion
	Wheezing and coughing
	Asthmatic attack
	Paralysis of respiratory muscles
Gastrointestinal tract	Increased motility and increased peristalsis
	Intestinal cramps and diarrhea
	Increased gastric acid secretion
	Heartburn
	Nausea and vomiting
Urinary tract	Stimulation of detrusor muscle, which may cause discomfort in bladder region
Skeletal muscle	Stimulation of contractions, fasciculations
	Eventual muscle weakness and paralysis
Central nervous system	Confusion
	Slurred speech
	Loss of motor coordination
	Convulsions
	Coma
Other organ systems	
Sweat glands	Sweating
Eye	Miosis and spasm of accommodation
	Lacrimation
	Headache in frontal region

*Atropine is a specific antidote to muscarinic effects; pralidoxime should also be given when an organophosphorus compound has caused the adverse reaction, but pralidoxime is contraindicated when a reversible cholinesterase inhibitor such as physostigmine or neostigmine has caused the adverse reaction.

brain barrier (physostigmine and most of the organophorphorus agents) produce additional adverse effects attributable to their action in the brain. These include confusion, slurred speech, loss of motor coordination, and convulsions. Actions in the brain and at autonomic ganglia and the adrenal medulla also contribute to the adverse respiratory and cardiovascular effects.

Treatment of Adverse Effects Produced by Cholinesterase Inhibitors

Treatment of Poisoning by Reversible Cholinesterase Inhibitors

Atropine sulfate counteracts the effects of cholinesterase inhibitors at muscarinic receptors and in the central nervous system. Atropine should be given to treat an adverse reaction to any of the cholinesterase inhibitors. Atropine is not effective in counteracting the effects of cholinesterase inhibitors at the neuromuscular junction.

Treatment of Poisoning by Organophosphorus Compounds

Organophosphorus poisoning can occur as a result of the systemic absorption of echotiophate or isoflurophate or as a result of exposure to one of the organic phosphorus insecticides, such as parathion or malathion. When poisoning occurs as a result of handling or using an organophosphorus insecticide, it is important to realize that the patient's clothing may be a source of continued exposure. Since many of these insecticides are readily absorbed through the skin, as well as from the digestive and respiratory tracts, careful washing of the patient is also important. While the administration of specific antidotes (see below) is important, the general principles of treating poisoning (see Chap. 48) should not be forgotten. It may be necessary, for example, to give artificial respiration before an antidote can take effect.

Two drugs are useful as antidotes to organophosphorus agents: atropine and pralidoxime. **Atropine sulfate** should be given intravenously (IV) or intramuscularly (IM) in repeated doses (2 to 4 mg) at 10-min intervals to counteract the muscarinic and central nervous system effects. **Pralidoxime** (Protopam), often referred to as 2-PAM (a combination of letters derived from its chemical name), reactivates the molecules of acetylcholinesterase that are bound by the organophosphorus agents. Pralidoxime is ineffective and contraindicated in treating poisoning caused by the reversible cholinesterase inhibitors such as physostigmine or neostigmine. To be effective, pralidoxime (1 to 2 g, IV or IM) must be given promptly, before a process known as "aging" of the organophosphorus-acetylcholinesterase complex occurs. Pralidoxime does not penetrate the blood-brain barrier and therefore is not useful in overcoming the central nervous system effects of cholinesterase inhibition. Diacetyl oxime, a drug currently not available in the United States but available in other countries, is a reactivator of acetylcholinesterase that does reach the central nervous system.

THE NURSING PROCESS RELATED TO CHOLINESTERASE INHIBITORS

Patients who are receiving cholinesterase inhibitors need to be assessed and managed in much the same way as patients who are taking direct-acting parasympathomimetic drugs. The potentially serious side effects of these drugs require constant, acute evaluation of the patient's status, which must take into consideration the disease for which the patient is being treated, e.g., myasthenia gravis.

Assessment

Past History The cholinesterase inhibitors act to increase the effects of acetylcholine at muscarinic cholinergic sites (like the direct-acting parasympathomimetics), at the neuromuscular junction, at autonomic ganglia, and at the adrenal medulla. Because of their diverse actions, these drugs are potentially dangerous in some patients with particular compromised states.

Patients for whom the direct-acting parasympathomimetic drugs are contraindicated should also not receive cholinesterase inhibitors, for the same reasons. In addition, in patients with epilepsy or parkinsonism, cholinesterase inhibitors that cross the blood-brain barrier can aggravate either of these conditions.

The patient's occupation and living situation should be evaluated to determine if chronic exposure to organophosphorus insecticides is occurring. These insecticides are irreversible cholinesterase inhibitors and are readily absorbed through the skin and gastrointestinal and respiratory tracts. They can cause severe, but sometimes undiagnosed, toxicities in patients exposed to them.

Physical Assessment Before giving any of these drugs systemically, the nurse needs to establish baseline data for the patient similar to those obtained for patients on direct-acting parasympathomimetics. Other baseline data that are essential before administering cholinesterase inhibitors include muscular strength (handgrip, gait, resistance to passive movement of the limbs), visual acuity, pupil size and reactivity, and mental state (level of alertness, confusion, etc.).

Careful documentation of these baseline data will allow the nurse to detect changes in the patient that could signal toxicity from the drug or a lack of therapeutic effect.

Management

The patient should be monitored for changes in the baseline data that could indicate a toxic effect from the drug. The signs and symptoms of muscarinic toxicity, as well as the central and neuromuscular signs of cholinergic crisis, should be watched for. These include confusion, slurred speech, restlessness, fear, muscle cramps, twitching, weakness, and respiratory depression or arrest. In case a severe reaction should occur, atropine should be available, as well as pralidoxime if an organophosphorus drug is being given. Airway maintenance and respiratory support may be necessary in severe cases.

Patients with chronic glaucoma who are to self-administer ophthalmic preparations containing cholinesterase inhibitors need to be educated in the proper administration of the drug. It is important that pressure be maintained on the inner canthus of the eye during, and for a few seconds after, the administration of these drugs, to prevent their entering the nasolacrimal duct. If the opening of this duct is not occluded, the drug may reach the nose and throat, be swallowed, reach the systemic circulation, and cause serious systemic effects. The patient also needs to be made aware of the common side effects produced by these drugs, i.e., frontal headache, conjunctivitis, and eye pain, and should be assured that these usually abate within a few weeks. Aspirin may help relieve the headache; cool compresses on the eyes and the avoidance of bright light may also help to relieve the discomfort. The patient must also be aware that the eye drops should be clear solutions and should be kept sterile and that they may require special storage (which would be indicated on the bottle). The patient should be advised to discard the drug and get new medication if there is any doubt about the sterility of the solution. Many of these drugs can lead to lens opacities, and patients should be alerted to report any change in visual acuity.

Patients receiving cholinesterase inhibitors for the treatment of myasthenia gravis need intensive teaching about the signs and symptoms of therapeutic doses and toxic doses of the drug. A family member should also receive this education. The therapeutic dosages of the drug will change with the remissions and exacerbations of the myasthenia gravis, and the patient will need to learn to increase and decrease the dosage accordingly. The patient and his or her relative or friend should also have a list of what to watch for and when to call the physician, as well as instruction in the parenteral administration of the drug if swallowing becomes difficult.

Evaluation

The patient should be constantly assessed for evidence of the therapeutic effects of the drugs. The appearance of any of the toxic signs and symptoms should also be noted and reported immediately. A tolerance can develop to drugs used to treat chronic glaucoma, and the patient should receive periodic checks to determine if miosis is being maintained. Usually, stopping the drug for a short time will restore the patient's sensitivity to it. The patient may also have trouble seeing at night and should be evaluated for the development of problems with night vision and cautioned about nighttime activities, particularly driving.

The patient being treated for myasthenia gravis needs constant, ongoing evaluation of the disease and the warning signs of drug toxicity. The precariousness of the patient's physical condition should alert the nurse to be constantly prepared for emergency supportive treatment.

REFERENCES

Brimblecombe, R. W.: "Drug Actions on Cholinergic Systems," in P. B. Bradley (ed.), *Pharmacology Monographs,* Baltimore: University Park, 1974.

Holmstedt, B.: "Pharmacology of Organophosphorus Cholinesterase Inhibitors," *Pharmacol Rev,* 11:567–688, 1959.

Karczmar, A. G.: "Pharmacologic, Toxicologic, and Therapeutic Properties of Anticholinesterase Agents," *Physiol Pharmacol,* 3:163–322, 1967.

Koelle, G. B.: "Acetylcholine: Current Status in Physiology, Pharmacology and Medicine," *N Engl J Med,* **286**:1086, 1972.

Taylor, P.: "Cholinergic Agonists," in A. G. Gilman, L. S. Goodman, and A. Gilman (eds.), *Goodman and Gilman's The Pharmacological Basis of Therapeutics,* 6th ed., New York: Macmillan, 1980.

———: "Anticholinesterase Agents," in A. G. Gilman, L. S. Goodman, and A. Gilman (eds.), *Goodman and Gilman's The Pharmacological Basis of Therapeutics,* 6th ed., New York: Macmillan, 1980.

Volle, R. L.: "Pharmacology of the Autonomic Nervous System," *Annu Rev Pharmacol,* 3:129–152, 1963.

12

PARASYMPATHETIC BLOCKING DRUGS

ELEANOR H. BOYD
AMY M. KARCH

LEARNING OBJECTIVES

Upon mastery of the contents of this chapter, the reader will be able to:

1. Describe the mechanism by which atropine-like drugs act.

2. List the major effects of the atropine-like drugs on the following organ systems: salivary glands, gastrointestinal tract, heart, central nervous system, and eye.

3. Explain why atropine-like drugs are contraindicated in persons with glaucoma.

4. List five therapeutic uses for antimuscarinic drugs.

5. List two parameters for assessment of patients on parasympathetic blockers for each of the following: cardiovascular, gastrointestinal, and genitourinary systems; the eye; the exocrine glands.

6. List one approach to nursing management of patients on parasympathetic blockers for minimizing the adverse effects of the drugs on the following: cardiovascular, gastrointestinal, and genitourinary systems; the eye; the exocrine glands.

The drugs described in this chapter block the effects of the acetylcholine released at parasympathetic and at sympathetic cholinergic postganglionic synapses. Drugs of this group which penetrate the blood-brain barrier also block the effects of acetylcholine at some central nervous system cholinergic synapses. In addition, these drugs block the effects of direct-acting parasympathomimetic drugs and cholinesterase inhibitors.

Atropine is the prototype of the drugs discussed in this chapter, and the term *atropine-like drugs* is sometimes used to designate these drugs. The drugs in this group either are belladonna alkaloids (**atropine** and **scopolamine**) derived from belladonna plants or are synthetic or semisynthetic drugs. Chemically they are either tertiary amines or quaternary ammonium (containing a positively charged nitrogen atom) compounds.

These drugs are also called antimuscarinic drugs, parasympathetic blocking drugs, parasympatholytic drugs, anticholinergic drugs, or cholinergic blocking drugs. Each term indicates the site or mechanism of action of these drugs or the type of effect they produce.

MECHANISM OF ACTION

Atropine-like drugs act in a relatively specific manner at muscarinic cholinergic synapses to prevent the molecules of acetylcholine that are released at these synapses from combining with the muscarinic cholinergic receptors in the membranes of effector cells (see Fig. 12-1). Molecules of these drugs actually compete with molecules of acetylcholine for occupancy of cholinergic receptors. However, unlike acetylcholine, these drugs do not activate the cholinergic receptors; rather, they block the effects that normally would occur at muscarinic synapses in the presence of acetylcholine. This action is the basis for their being called *antimuscarinic drugs.*

Muscarinic cholinergic receptors occur at the synapses of parasympathetic postganglionic axons with autonomic effector cells. When these synapses are blocked, the effects of parasympathetic innervation are blocked. For this reason, these drugs are called parasympathetic blocking drugs or parasympatholytic drugs. These two terms do not completely describe the effects produced, because these drugs also block sympathetic cholinergic receptors. Recall that sympathetic cholinergic receptors mediate sweating as well as the dilatation of some blood vessels. Furthermore, the drugs of this group that cross the blood-brain barrier block cholinergic synapses in the central nervous system (CNS). Despite these limitations, the term *parasympathetic blocking drugs* will be used here because this chapter concentrates on describing the effects of the block of transmission of parasympathetic impulses to effector organs.

Besides blocking the effects of endogenous acetylcholine released from nerve terminals, these drugs block the effects of direct-acting parasympathomimetic drugs, such as betha-

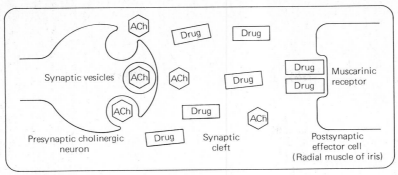

FIGURE 12-1

Schematic Representation of the Mechanism of Parasympathetic Blocking Drugs in Pupil Dilation. Drugs compete for the muscarinic receptor site with endogenous acetylcholine (ACh). Occupation of the receptor site on the radial muscle by the parasympathetic blocking drug results in pupil dilation.

nechol and pilocarpine, and they block the effect of cholinesterase inhibitors which are mediated by muscarinic receptors. Actually, these drugs block the effects of parasympathomimetic drugs more readily than they block the effects of endogenous acetylcholine, perhaps because it is more difficult for the drugs to reach some synaptic sites where acetylcholine is released.

The degree of receptor blockade depends on the dose. When acute toxicity is produced by an organophosphorus cholinesterase inhibitor, very high doses of atropine may be necessary to compete effectively with the many molecules of acetylcholine that have accumulated in the presence of the cholinesterase inhibitor. Atropine and other drugs of this group are *competitive blockers* of acetylcholine, bethanechol, etc.

Another frequently used term for this group of drugs is *anticholinergic drugs,* or *cholinergic blocking drugs.* These two terms are misleading because they imply that these drugs block indiscriminately *all* the effects of acetylcholine. This is not true. The tertiary amines in this group of drugs selectively block muscarinic cholinergic receptors. Low doses of those drugs that are quaternary ammonium compounds also selectively block muscarinic cholinergic receptors, but as the dose is increased, this selectivity is lost. Some of the effects produced by high doses of the quaternary ammonium compounds are attributable to blocking of nicotinic cholinergic receptors at autonomic ganglia. At toxic doses, the quaternary ammonium drugs in this group can also block the nicotinic cholinergic receptors at the neuromuscular junction.

CLINICAL USES OF PARASYMPATHETIC BLOCKING DRUGS

By blocking the influence of the parasympathetic nervous system on effector organs, these drugs leave unopposed the influences of the sympathetic nervous system, except for sweating, mediated by sympathetic cholinergic neurons, which is also blocked. Clinically, these drugs can thus cause a decrease in gastrointestinal secretions and motility, an increase in heart rate, a decrease in respiratory tract secretions, bronchodilatation, a decrease in tone of the urinary bladder, dilatation of the pupil of the eye and inability to focus on near objects, and a decrease in sweating.

These drugs are used clinically for their ability to block parasympathetic influences on the gastrointestinal tract, including the salivary glands; the heart; the eye; and the mucus-secreting and smooth muscle cells of the respiratory tract. Some of those with effects in the central nervous system also are useful in treating Parkinson's disease and in overcoming the toxic manifestations of cholinesterase inhibitors in the central, as well as the peripheral, nervous system. One drug, **scopolamine**, has clinically useful sedative properties and, in addition, has the ability to prevent motion sickness.

Use of parasympathetic blocking drugs is indicated for a variety of conditions:

To treat peptic ulcer and some states of spasticity and hypermotility of the gastrointestinal tract.

Sometimes to treat sinus bradycardia and to overcome a block of cardiac conduction at the atrioventricular (AV) node.

Preoperatively for their ability to decrease salivation and respiratory tract secretions, to counteract laryngospasm and dilate bronchi, and to block vagal influences on the heart which may be triggered by general anesthetics and some surgical procedures.

As ophthalmic preparations to dilate the pupil of the eye and paralyze accommodation for near vision during ophthalmologic examinations and in the treatment of certain eye disorders.

To treat Parkinson's disease.

To prevent motion sickness.

Atropine and **scopolamine** are each used for many of these indications, but none of these drugs is used for all the indications.

SPECIFIC DRUGS AND THEIR CLINICAL USES

Use as Antispasmodics in Treating Peptic Ulcer and Intestinal Spasticity and Hypermotility (Table 12-1)

The tone of the gastrointestinal tract is under parasympathetic control; thus, interfering with the transmission of parasympathetic nerve impulses to the gastrointestinal tract has been seen as logical therapy to decrease gastric secretion and to reduce intestinal spasticity and hypermotility in patients with peptic ulcer, spastic colon, and other conditions characterized by excessive peristalsis or increased intestinal tone.

These drugs have been widely used, often in conjunction with antacids, in treating peptic ulcer, but there is lack of unanimity as to their efficacy in promoting the healing of the ulcerated duodenal mucosa. Since the introduction of **cimetidine** (Tagamet), a histamine H_2 receptor–blocking agent that decreases gastric acid secretion, the use of para-

TABLE 12-1 Parasympathetic Blocking Drugs Used for Their Antispasmodic Effects on the Gastrointestinal Tract*

Tertiary amine compounds
 Atropine sulfate
 Belladonna extract
 Belladonna tincture
 Dicyclomine hydrochoride (Bentyl)
 Scopolamine (hyoscine) hydrobromide

Quaternary ammonium compounds
 Clidinium bromide (Quarzan)
 Glycopyrrolate (Robinul)
 Isopropamide iodide (Darbid)
 Mepenzolate bromide (Cantil)
 Methantheline bromide (Banthine)
 Propantheline bromide (Pro-Banthine)
 Tridihexethyl chloride (Pathilon)

*Many other antispasmodic drugs are marketed; this list represents a selected sample only.

sympathetic blocking agents in the management of peptic ulcer patients has declined. (See Chap. 30.)

These drugs are effective in controlling diarrhea produced by some drugs, such as **bethanechol** (see Chap. 11) and **guanethidine** (which interferes with the functioning of sympathetic postganglionic nerves and leaves unopposed the parasympathetic influences on the gastrointestinal tract). They are also effective in some neurogenic intestinal disorders. Their efficacy in controlling diarrhea associated with chronic inflammation or acute infection of the bowel is questionable.

One of the problems in the use of the parasympathetic blocking drugs for gastrointestinal disorders is that their gastrointestinal effects are produced only at relatively high doses, which also cause the side effects of dry mouth and blurred vision and also can cause urinary retention, constipation, tachycardia, etc. Because of these side effects, patient compliance in the use of these drugs is low. Many drugs have been synthesized in unsuccessful attempts to find one with specificity for the gastrointestinal tract.

When these drugs are given for gastrointestinal disorders, they are usually given orally, before meals and often also at bedtime. When the drugs are given to peptic ulcer patients, doses are given before meals for two reasons: to produce peak drug effects at the time of maximum meal-stimulated gastric acid secretion and to facilitate the absorption of the drug. The quaternary ammonium compounds (see Table 12-1) are poorly absorbed after oral administration, and they should always be given on an empty stomach to increase the amount absorbed. Doses are tailored as closely as possible to the individual patient, to achieve maximal therapeutic benefit with minimal side effects. It is especially easy to individualize the dosage of **belladonna tincture** because it is a liquid, instead of a fixed-dosage tablet, and it is usually measured out as drops, often put in fruit juice to increase palatability. Some of the drugs listed in Table 12-1 are available as sustained-release preparations, to minimize the number of doses the patient must remember to take, and some are available for parenteral administration. (See Chap. 30, "Disorders of the Alimentary Tract.")

Use in Treating and Preventing Sinus Bradycardia and Heart Block

Excessive vagal (parasympathetic) stimulation can cause sinus bradycardia accompanied by diminished cardiac output. When this occurs as the result of a hyperactive carotid sinus reflex (a baroreceptor reflex; see Fig. 10-5), or when it occurs initially following myocardial infarction, atropine is sometimes indicated. Administration of **atropine** after myocardial infarction is not without danger, because the ensuing tachycardia can increase myocardial ischemia and precipitate ventricular arrhythmias. Atropine can also be used to overcome AV nodal conduction block when it is due to excessive vagal tone, for example, after the administration of **digoxin** or other cardiac glycosides.

TABLE 12-2   Parasympathetic Blocking Drugs Used as Preanesthetic Medication

Atropine sulfate
Glycopyrrolate (Robinul)
Scopolamine (hyoscine) hydrobromide

Use as Preoperative or Preanesthetic Medication (Table 12-2)

Atropine, scopolamine, *or* **glycopyrrolate** is given prior to general anesthesia or surgery and intraoperatively to protect the heart from excessive vagal stimulation (bradycardia or AV nodal block); to decrease respiratory and salivary secretions, facilitating the maintenance of a clear airway; and to produce bronchodilatation and prevent laryngospasm. **Scopolamine** can produce sedation and amnesia, also useful in preoperative patients as well as with patients in labor. Glycopyrrolate is a quarternary ammonium agent, which does not readily cross the blood-brain barrier and thus causes negligible CNS effects. These drugs are also used intraoperatively for reversal of neuromuscular blocking drugs (see Chap. 47, "Surgery: Drugs Used in Perioperative Care").

Use in Ophthalmology (Table 12-3)

These drugs can be used, as ophthalmic preparations, to dilate the pupil of the eye to allow examination of the retina and head of the optic nerve. Their local ophthalmic use may precipitate an acute first attack of glaucoma in patients who, unknowingly, have narrow-angle glaucoma. Since glaucoma occurs primarily in persons over 40 years of age, risk of this occurring is reduced by measuring intraocular pressure in all patients over 40 years of age before the topical administration of parasympathetic blocking drugs into the eye.

TABLE 12-3   Ophthalmic Preparations of Parasympathetic Blocking Drugs Used for Diagnostic or Therapeutic Purposes

DRUG	CONCENTRATION	DURATION OF DETECTABLE OCULAR EFFECTS
Atropine sulfate solution (Atropisol)	0.5, 1, 2, or 3%	7–12 days
Cyclopentolate hydrochloride (Cyclogyl)	0.5, 1, or 2%	1 day
Homatropine hydrobromide ophthalmic solution	2 or 5%	1–3 days
Scopolamine (hyoscine) hydrobromide solution	0.25%	5–7 days
Tropicamide (Mydriacyl)	0.5 or 1.0%	< 6 h

These drugs are sometimes used therapeutically for certain inflammatory disorders of the iris. They are sometimes used alternately with miotics to break adhesions between the iris and lens.

Mydriasis produced by these drugs is accompanied at higher doses by cyloplegia (paralysis of accommodation for near vision), an effect mediated by their effects on the ciliary muscle/lens system. This effect is useful diagnostically in ophthalmologic exams and therapeutically in inflammatory eye disorders.

Atropine itself is of exceedingly long duration when administered locally in the eye (see Table 12-3); other drugs with shorter durations of action are often used diagnostically, or else a miotic, such as **pilocarpine** or **physostigmine**, is administered to terminate the drug effects (see Chap. 39, "Ophthalmologic Disorders").

Use in Treating Parkinson's Disease

Atropine was originally given to patients with Parkinson's disease to decrease salivation and to prevent the drooling that many of these patients experience as a result of impaired control of the buccal-lingual musculature. It was found to ameliorate some of the motor manifestations of this neurologic disease, especially the tremor. Despite the more recent therapeutic success of another drug, **levodopa,** in many patients with Parkinson's disease, several atropine-like drugs are still used in the management of Parkinson's disease patients. Some of these drugs are **benztropine mesylate** (Cogentin), **biperiden** (Akineton), **cycrimine hydrochloride** (Pagitane), **procyclidine hydrochloride** (Kemadrin), and **trihexyphenidyl hydrochloride** (Artane, Tremin). (See Chap. 33, "Neurologic Disorders.")

Use in Preventing Motion Sickness

Drugs are more effective in *preventing* than in treating motion sickness. **Scopolamine** (0.3 to 0.6 mg orally) has long been known to be effective in this regard. Although other drugs [**dimenhydrinate** (Dramamine), **cyclizine** (Marezine), **meclizine** (Bonine), etc.] have been used more often than scopolamine and are available as over-the-counter drugs without a physician's prescription, scopolamine has recently become the subject of renewed interest as a motion sickness preventative because of the introduction of a new and more convenient dosage form. A disposable drug-dispensing device, called Transderm-Scōp, applied to the skin behind the ear slowly releases scopolamine over a period of 3 days. The scopolamine is absorbed through the skin into the systemic circulation. (See Chap. 19, "Nausea and Vomiting.")

ADVERSE EFFECTS OF PARASYMPATHETIC BLOCKING DRUGS

Most of the adverse effects can be predicted if one knows the effects of parasympathetic influences on organ systems (see Table 10-1) and understands what happens when these influences are blocked. Another adverse effect occurs as the result of the blockade of the sympathetic cholinergic receptors that mediate sweating. The drugs that are tertiary amines also cause adverse effects attributable to their actions in the CNS, and high, toxic doses of the drugs that are quaternary ammonium compounds can block nicotinic receptors at autonomic ganglia and the neuromuscular junction.

Drugs in this group differ from most other modern drugs in that some unwanted side effects are produced by lower-than-therapeutic doses. For example, the muscarinic cholinergic receptors of the sweat and salivary glands are blocked by lower doses of these drugs than are the muscarinic cholinergic receptors of the gastric glands. (Receptors in the heart, eye, intestine, and urinary bladder are blocked by intermediate doses.) This means that therapeutic doses, administered systemically, will cause almost all patients to experience dry mouth and diminution of sweating.

The adverse effects of **atropine**, the prototype drug of this group, on various organ system are described below and summarized in Table 12-4. Poisoning by belladonna alkaloids occurs not only from the ingestion of pharmaceutical preparations, but, especially in children, from the ingestion of plant material, berries, etc., that contain these alkaloids. Further, many drugs from a wide variety of drug groups have atropine-like side effects (see Table 12-5).

Cardiovascular System

Low doses of atropine usually cause a slight *brady*cardia; higher doses cause a dose-dependent *tachy*cardia. Tachycardia is the expected effect of parasympathetic blockade; the bradycardia presumably results from a CNS effect. The degree of tachycardia depends on the degree of vagal tone normally exerting a braking action on heart rate; healthy young adults usually have the greatest degree of vagal tone on the heart and show the greatest increase in heart rate after atropine.

Usually no significant changes occur in blood pressure, although when atropine is given for sinus bradycardia or AV block, the improvement in cardiac output may lead to increased blood pressure.

Atropine blocks the vasodilatation and hypotension produced by parasympathomimetic drugs, but given alone, in therapeutic doses, it usually has no significant effects on the vasculature. This is as expected because the muscarinic cholinergic receptors in the vasculature are, for the most part, not innervated. Usually in toxic doses, and occasionally in therapeutic doses, atropine causes cutaneous vasodilatation in the blush area. The mechanism of this effect is not understood. Children given atropine as preanesthetic medication sometimes develop very red faces.

Respiratory System

Atropine blocks the respiratory tract secretions and bronchoconstriction produced by parasympathomimetic drugs, but given alone in the absence of bronchospastic disease, it

TABLE 12-4 Adverse Effects of Atropine*

ORGAN SYSTEM	EFFECT
Cardiovascular system	
Heart	Low doses: slight bradycardia
	High doses: tachycardia
Blood vessels	Vasodilatation in the blush area
Respiratory system	Decreased fluidity of respiratory tract secretion
Gastrointestinal tract	Dry mouth
	Constipation
Urinary tract	Urinary retention, especially in elderly males with prostate enlargement
Male reproductive system	Impotence
Visual system	Dilated pupils
	Photophobia
	Loss of accommodation for near vision
	Glaucoma attack
Sweat glands	Decreased sweating
	Dry skin
Central nervous system	Restlessness
	Excitement
	Delirium
	Coma
	Fever
Other effects	Headache

*Physostigmine is an antidote and should be administered to treat serious acute toxicity.

usually produces no effects on the respiratory system. The decreased fluidity of respiratory tract secretions caused by atropine may exacerbate the respiratory difficulties of patients with chronic obstructive pulmonary disease.

Gastrointestinal Tract

Often the gastrointestinal tract is the therapeutic target of atropine and other drugs of this group. Except when used as preanesthetic medication, the dry mouth is an undesired side effect, as is the constipation produced by higher doses.

Urinary Tract

Atropine can cause urinary retention and difficulty in urination, especially in elderly male patients, who may have some degree of prostatic enlargement.

Male Reproductive System

Block of parasympathetic influences on male sex organs can interfere with erection; ganglionic blockade, produced by

TABLE 12-5 Drugs with Atropine-like (Anticholinergic) Side Effects Due to Muscarinic Blockade

Antiarrhythmics

Disopyramide (Norpace)

Antidepressants

Maprotiline (Ludiomil)
Trazodone (Desyrel)
Tricyclic antidepressants (TCADs)
   Amitriptyline (Amitid, Amitril, Elavil, Endep)
   Amoxapine (Asendin)
   Desipramine (Norpramin, Pertofrane)
   Doxepin (Adapin, Sinequan)
   Imipramine (Janimine, Tofranil)
   Nortriptyline (Aventyl, Pamelor)
   Protriptyline (Vivactil)
   Trimipramine (Surmontil)

Antihistamine/Antivertigo/Antiemetic

Bromodiphenhydramine* (Ambodryl)
Brompheniramine* (Bromphen, Dimetane)
Chlorpheniramine (Chlor-Trimeton, Teldrin)
Cyclizine (Marezine)
Dimenhydrinate (Dramamine)
Cyproheptadine (Periactin)
Diphenhydramine* (Benadryl, Benylin)
Doxylamine (Decapryn)
Meclizine (Antivert, Bonine)
Promethazine (Anergan, Phenergan)
Pyrilamine*
Trimeprazine (Temaril)
Triprolidine* (Actidil)

Antiparkinsonians

Benztropin (Cogentin)
Biperiden (Akineton)
Cycrimine (Pagitane)
Procyclidine (Kemadrin)
Trihexyphenidyl (Artane, Tremin)

Antipsychotics†

Chlorprothixene (Taractan)
Molindone (Moban)
Phenothiazines
   Chlorpromazine (Thorazine)
   Mesoridazine (Serentil)
   Piperacetazine (Quide)
   Promazine (Sparine)
   Thoridazine (Mellaril)
   Triflupromazine (Vesprin)

Antispasmodics-Antiulcers

(See Table 12-1)

Skeletal Muscle Relaxants

Cyclobenzaprine (Flexeril)
Orphenadrine (Norflex)

*Available in over-the-counter preparations for cold and cough, either alone or in combination with other drugs.

†All antipsychotics have some atropine-like side effects, but those listed have moderate to marked effects.

the quaternary compounds, can also contribute to sexual dysfunction.

Visual System

Atropine given systemically in high therapeutic doses can cause mydriasis, loss of the pupillary light reflex, blurred vision, and inability to focus on near objects. When administered as eye drops or given systemically, it can raise intraocular pressure dangerously in patients with narrow-angle glaucoma.

Sweat Glands

Sweating is impaired even by low therapeutic doses of atropine. This may lead to an elevation of temperature, particularly in warm environments, where sweating is essential for dissipating body heat.

Central Nervous System

Atropine in high toxic doses causes restlessness, excitement, hallucinations, coma, and fever. Even **scopolamine**, which is used for its sedative properties at low doses, can cause excitement in high doses. Children may show marked fever after even therapeutic doses of atropine. The fever may be partly due to the effects of atropine in the CNS, as well as to the inhibition of sweating. The quaternary ammonium compounds do not penetrate the blood-brain barrier to a great enough extent to cause significant CNS effects. High doses of atropine often cause headache, but the mechanism may be visual changes, rather than CNS effects.

PHARMACOLOGIC TREATMENT OF ADVERSE REACTIONS

The slow intravenous administration of **physostigmine**, 1 to 4 mg, effectively counteracts most of the serious peripheral and central adverse effects of acute overdosage with atropine and other parasympathetic blocking drugs. Cool baths and alcohol sponges are useful in reducing the fever in children.

THE NURSING PROCESS RELATED TO PARASYMPATHETIC BLOCKING DRUGS

The parasympathetic blocking drugs have a diversity of uses, and thus many systemic side effects occur which may not be anticipated by the patient and which may be seen as quite uncomfortable. Because of these predictable problems, the nursing management of these patients becomes very important for assuring patient compliance with the medical regimen as well as for helping the patient to be as comfortable as possible. Those taking drugs with atropine-like side effects (see Table 12-5) require similar nursing care. This effect is additive if the patient is on several drugs with atropine-like side effects.

Assessment

Past History   Because the parasympathetic blocking drugs interrupt a wide range of autonomic reflexes, their use can produce responses that are uncomfortable or even life-threatening in patients with particular preestablished conditions. A careful patient history should be taken to rule out any of the following problems, all of which are specific contraindications to use of these drugs.

Coronary artery disease   Parasympathetic blockers cause an increase in heart rate, which, in patients with a compromised blood supply to the heart muscle, can lead to myocardial ischemia, angina, or ventricular irritability.

Chronic obstructive lung disease   Parasympathetic blockers cause a decrease in the fluidity of secretions in the respiratory tract, which can cause the development of mucous plugs and further compromise respiration in these patients. However, atropine is employed therapeutically for bronchodilatation in asthma and other chronic lung diseases.

Bowel obstruction or recent gastrointestinal surgery   Parasympathetic blockers decrease the tone and motility of the gastrointestinal tract, which could lead to paralytic ileus, severe impaction, or even intestinal rupture in these patients.

Urinary difficulty or prostatic hypertrophy   Parasympathetic blockers cause a decrease in urinary bladder tone, which can lead to urinary retention. This problem can be severe, especially in combination with prostatic hypertrophy.

Glaucoma   Parasympathetic blockers cause dilatation of the pupils of the eyes and can cause acute attacks of narrow-angle glaucoma.

Lactation   Parasympathetic blockers have been shown to suppress lactation and to pass into breast milk and should be avoided, if at all possible, in lactating mothers.

Physical Assessment   Before giving any of these drugs, the nurse should assess the baseline functioning of all of the systems that are most affected by the parasympathetic blockers. In this way, both therapeutic and toxic effects of the drugs can be carefully evaluated.

This assessment should include mental status (orientation, affect), apical pulse (rate, rhythm, character, presence of extra sounds), electrocardiogram (including assessment of conduction pattern and presence of blocks or extra beats), respirations (rate, rhythm, character, adventitious sounds), bowel sounds (rate and character), urinary output (including assessment of bladder distention, tone), eyes (pupil size, reactivity, and a check for glaucoma in all patients 40 years of age and older), and baseline temperature.

Management

Almost every effect of this group of drugs can be used therapeutically but can also be considered an adverse reaction when another effect is the desired one. Dry mouth (a desired effect when used preoperatively or with Parkinson's disease) is one of the most common and most unpleasant side effects of the parasympathetic blocking drugs. It can be so unpleasant to some people that they will discontinue the use of the drug to avoid the problem. The patient needs to be counseled to expect this problem, and several interventions can be used to help make the situation more tolerable: Meticulous oral hygiene is essential and will help rinse out dried secretions. Frequent, small sips of water (if not contraindicated by fluid restriction) will help moisten the mouth. Chewing sugarless gum or sucking on hard, sour, sugarless candy will help to stimulate some secretions, and the sugarless variety will help to protect the patient from tooth decay. Saliva substitutes (although expensive, several are available in over-the-counter form) will make chewing and swallowing easier. Lemon and glycerin swabs may be used for patients who are restricted from taking anything by mouth, but the long-range effect of these hypertonic solutions is often drier mucous membranes.

Constipation and/or abdominal distention are also frequent problems. Outpatients should be counseled to take preventive measures (high-roughage diet, lots of fluids, activity, and possibly laxatives); hospitalized patients should be observed for signs of constipation, and similar preventive measures should be taken.

Urinary retention can also be a problem, especially in patients who are predisposed to these problems (e.g., those with prostatic hypertrophy). The patient should be taught that this is an expected side effect and that careful attention should be paid to voiding. The patient should be asked to report any marked decrease in urinary output, feelings of abdominal fullness and pressure, or difficulty initiating a stream. If any of these occur, the drug will probably have to be stopped and the patient's status will have to be evaluated. The patient can also be advised always to urinate before taking each dose of the drug; at this time the drug effects should be at the lowest level, and the patient will then have an empty bladder before the drug effects reach their maximum.

Patients who receive parasympathetic blocking drugs prior to ophthalmic examinations may experience a prolonged period of dilatation of the pupil and photophobia. These patients can be advised to wear sunglasses when out of doors, to avoid bright lights indoors, and to be particularly careful when entering differing levels of light, as the loss of the normal pupillary reflex can cause pain and temporary blindness.

Patients who receive parasympathetic blocking drugs to decrease intestinal hypermotility should be advised to take the drug 30 to 60 min before meals, as food may stimulate intestinal motility and spasm.

Any patient who receives parasympathetic blocking

drugs has potential problems in the area of temperature control because of the loss of the ability to sweat. This can be most dangerous in young children or elderly adults, who already have marginal ability to regulate their temperature. Patients should always be cautioned to avoid extreme heat (several studies report the occurrence of heat strokes) and should be advised that they will be most comfortable in a cool environment. Patients who become pyrexic while on these drugs have to be managed very carefully, as sweating is one of the body's first defenses against fever.

Patients should also be cautioned that parasympathetic blocking drugs can cause dizziness, visual disturbances, and even sedation in some people. Because of this, safety can be a major problem. Outpatients should be advised against driving or operating dangerous machinery while on one of these drugs. Hospitalized patients should have safety precautions enforced and should receive periodic orientation to their environment. Elderly patients can develop *central anticholinergic syndrome,* a severe confusion reaction.

Another general point that should be incorporated into all patient teaching is to avoid the use of over-the-counter drugs unless it is first discussed with a health care provider. Many over-the-counter formulations contain atropine-like drugs, and the patient could inadvertently develop toxic levels of the drugs.

Evaluation

The patient should be evaluated for evidence of the therapeutic effect desired (pupillary dilatation, increased heart rate, dry mouth, etc.) and for the occurrence of any toxic or other side effects. The development of severe tachycardia, confusion, ataxia, restlessness, or hyperpyrexia could indicate severe toxicity; the drug should be stopped immediately, and the patient assessed appropriately. If any such drug is used during acute cardiac events, the patient should be on a cardiac monitor with constant evaluation of status and with appropriate emergency equipment available.

Patients should also be evaluated for any change in their response to other medications they may be taking. Atropine-like drugs delay gastric emptying and can therefore alter the degree of absorption of any drugs that are dissolved and absorbed in the gastrointestinal tract—e.g., digoxin, antibiotics.

Patients should also be evaluated for the occurrence of rash or contact dermatitis. These are signs of hypersensitivity to atropine-line drugs and are not uncommon. Dosage levels can often be adjusted to allow the patient to benefit from the drug without the toxic effects.

REFERENCES

Dukes, M. N. G.: *Meyler's Side Effects of Drugs,* 9th ed., Princeton: Excerpta Medica, 1980.

Nadel, J. A.: "The Place of Parasympathetic Drugs in the Management of Chronic Obstructive Airway Disease," *Postgrad Med,* 51(Suppl.):7–9, 1975.

Shader, R. I., and D. J. Greenblatt: "Belladonna Alkaloids and Synthetic Anticholinergics: Uses and Toxicity," in R. L. Shader (ed.), *Psychiatric Complications of Medical Drugs,* New York: Raven, 1972.

Volle, R. L.: "Pharmacology of the Autonomic Nervous System," *Ann Rev Pharmacol,* 3:129–152, 1963.

Weiner, N.: "Atropine, Scopolamine, and Related Antimuscarinic Drugs," in A. C. Gilman, L. S. Goodman, and A. Gilman (eds.), *Goodman and Gilman's The Pharmacological Basis of Therapeutics,* 6th ed., New York: Macmillan, 1980.

13

SYMPATHOMIMETIC DRUGS

ELEANOR H. BOYD
AMY M. KARCH

LEARNING OBJECTIVES

Upon mastery of the contents of this chapter, the reader will be able to:

1. List two therapeutically useful sympathomimetic effects mediated by alpha receptors, three therapeutically useful effects and one adverse effect mediated by beta-1 receptors, and two therapeutically useful effects mediated by beta-2 receptors.

2. Identify the types of adrenergic receptors at which epinephrine, norepinephrine, isoproterenol, dopamine, dobutamine, phenylephrine, methoxamine, terbutaline, and ephedrine act.

3. Explain why norepinephrine, phenylephrine, and methoxamine decrease heart rate, whereas epinephrine and isoproterenol increase it.

4. List the clinical indications for the use of each of the following: epinephrine, norepinephrine, phenylephrine, ritodrine, ephedrine, and dextroamphetamine.

5. List two nursing activities for each step of the nursing process for patients on sympathomimetic drugs.

6. Explain the importance of teaching patients about the use of over-the-counter preparations that contain sympathomimetic drugs.

Drugs that mimic the effects of the sympathetic nervous system are called *sympathomimetic drugs.* They are also called *adrenergic drugs* or *adrenergic agonists,* because they produce effects like those produced by the endogenous substances epinephrine (adrenaline) and norepinephrine (noradrenaline), which are released by sympathetic discharge.[1]

---

[1]Drugs such as **pilocarpine** and **bethanechol**, which mimic the effects of sympathetic cholinergic innervation, produce mainly parasympathomimetic effects. They are considered parasympathomimetic drugs and are described in Chap. 11.

Epinephrine and norepinephrine are themselves available as drugs and produce therapeutically useful effects when injected. Sympathomimetic drugs act by two different mechanisms (see Fig. 13-1) by a combination of these mechanisms:

1. Drugs such as epinephrine, norepinephrine, isoproterenol, and phenylephrine act *directly* on adrenergic receptors, to produce sympathomimetic effects.

2. Drugs such as amphetamine act indirectly, causing release of endogenous norepinephine from nerve terminals.

3. Drugs such as ephedrine act both directly on adrenergic receptors and by causing the release of norepinephrine.

Table 13-1 gives a classification of some of the most important sympathomimetic drugs.

REVIEW OF THE SYMPATHETIC NERVOUS SYSTEM AND ADRENERGIC RECEPTORS

The sympathetic nervous system innervates and influences many organs; in addition, epinephrine and norepinephrine, released into the systemic circulation from the adrenal medulla, influence all tissues to which they are distributed. The sympathetic nervous system acts quite discretely in the moment-to-moment control of the heart, viscera, glands, etc., but it acts by an intense and generalized discharge in emergencies (fright-fight-flight reactions).

Adrenergic receptors mediating these effects are of three types: alpha (α), beta-1 (β_1), and beta-2 (β_2) (see Chap. 10 and Table 10-1). Alpha receptors have recently been divided into two subtypes, α_1 and α_2 (see Chap. 10). The identification of α receptors as α_1 or α_2 is still incomplete, but most α_2 receptors appear to occur *pre*synaptically, while α_1 receptors appear to occur *post*synaptically and to be virtually synonymous with those receptors called, for many years, simply "α receptors." Since it is still unclear what role, of any, α_2 receptors play in producing the sympathomimetic drug

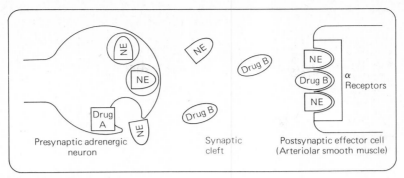

FIGURE 13-1

Schematic Representation of the Mechanisms of Alpha-Adrenergic Drugs on Arteriolar Tone. Drug A acts indirectly by releasing endogenous norepinephrine (NE) from presynaptic vesicles. Occupation of postsynaptic receptors by NE results in arteriolar constriction. Drug B is a direct-acting alpha agonist which produces arteriolar constriction by occupation of α sites. Similarly, drugs can act indirectly or directly (or both) to stimulate beta-1 and beta-2 (β_1 and β_2) receptors.

effects described in this chapter, the old terminology will be retained; that is, *α receptors* will indicate postsynaptic adrenergic receptors in the membranes of cells of effector organs.

The effects of sympathetic stimulation include the fol-

TABLE 13-1 Classification of Some Therapeutically Important Sympathomimetic Drugs

Direct-acting sympathomimetic drugs
  Catecholamines
    Epinephrine* (adrenaline)
    Norepinephrine* (noradrenaline)
    Dopamine*
    Isoproterenol
    Dobutamine
  Noncatecholamines
    Phenylephrine
    Methoxamine
    Albuterol (salbutamol)
    Isoetharine
    Metaproterenol
    Terbutaline
Indirect-acting sympathomimetic drugs
  Amphetamine
  Dextroamphetamine
  Methamphetamine
Sympathomimetic Drugs that Act Both Directly and Indirectly
  Ephedrine
  Mephentermine
  Metaraminol

---

*These catecholamines are endogenous substances as well as drugs.

lowing (the type of receptor mediating each effect is indicated in parentheses): increased heart rate (*positive chronotropic effect*: β_1 receptors), increased force of contraction of the ventricles (*positive inotropic effects*: β_1 receptors), increased rate of conduction of the cardiac impulse through the atrioventricular (AV) node (*positive dromotropic effect*: β_1 receptors), vasoconstriction (*α receptors*), bronchodilatation (β_2 receptors), dilatation of the pupils of the eye (mydriasis: *α receptors*), relaxation of the urinary bladder (β_2 receptors), contraction of intestinal and urinary bladder sphincters (*α receptors*), and glycogenolysis and other metabolic effects that make nutrients available (β receptors). Clinically important β_2 receptors also occur in the blood vessels of skeletal muscle and in the pregnant uterus. The β_2 receptors in the blood vessels in skeletal muscle are not innervated, but they mediate the vasodilatation caused by epinephrine and by some other sympathomimetic drugs. Beta-2 receptors in the pregnant uterus mediate uterine relaxation. Many β receptor effects are mediated by the "secondary messenger," cyclic adenosine monophosphate (cAMP).

Epinephrine and **norepinephrine** activate all types of adrenergic receptors, but the effects produced by these two agents are not identical; for example, epinephrine is a potent broncho- and vasodilator (both β_2 receptor effects); norepinephrine is only a weak broncho- and vasodilator, but it is a potent vasoconstrictor (*α receptor effect*). Some other sympathomimetic drugs have a greater degree of selectivity, interacting with only one type of adrenergic receptor and producing only a small part of the spectrum of sympathomimetic effects.

Sympathomimetic drugs are sometimes referred to by the type(s) of receptor with which they interact: *α (receptor) agonist, β_2 agonist, β_1 and β_2 agonist,* or *nonselective β*

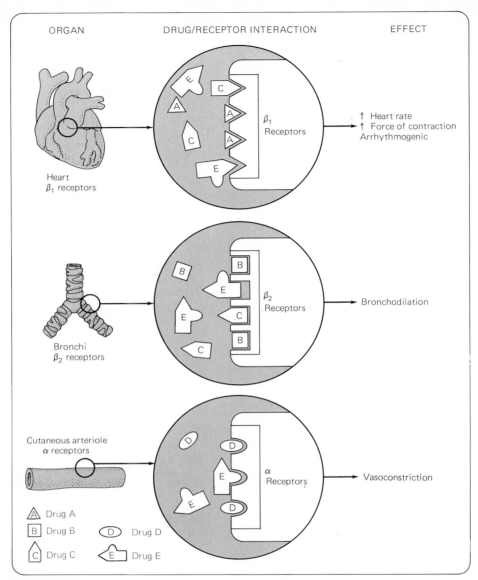

ORGAN   DRUG/RECEPTOR INTERACTION   EFFECT

Heart
β_1 receptors

β_1
Receptors

↑ Heart rate
↑ Force of contraction
Arrhythmogenic

Bronchi
β_2 receptors

β_2
Receptors

Bronchodilation

Cutaneous arteriole
α receptors

α
Receptors

Vasoconstriction

A Drug A
B Drug B   D Drug D
C Drug C   E Drug E

FIGURE 13-2

Schematic Representation of Receptor Selectivity of Adrenergic Drugs. Note that selectivity is only relative, and any so-called selective drug has some nonselective effects.

Drug A, a selective β_1 agonist (e.g., dobutamine), has cardiac inotropic and chronotropic effects.

Drug B is a selective β_2 agonist (e.g., terbutaline) resulting in bronchodilatation, vasodilatation, and other β_2-mediated effects.

Drug C is a nonselective β agonist (e.g., isoproterenol), active at β_1 and β_2 receptors, including cardiac, bronchial, and vascular β receptors.

Drug D is a relatively pure α agonist (e.g., phenylephrine) causing vasoconstriction.

Drug E can stimulate all adrenergic receptors (e.g., epinephrine), including α, β_1, and β_2 receptors.

188

agonist (see Fig. 13-2). The types of receptor with which the most important sympathomimetic drugs interact are described in the next section.

EFFECTS OF THE MOST IMPORTANT SYMPATHOMIMETIC DRUGS

Direct-Acting Sympathomimetic Drugs

Catecholamines

The term *catecholamine* indicates a particular chemical structure (see Chap. 10 and Fig. 10-4). It is of pharmacologic significance because sympathomimetic drugs that are catecholamines (epinephrine, norepinephrine, dopamine, isoprotenerol, and dobutamine) are rapidly inactivated in the intestines and liver by monoamine oxidase enzymes and by the enzyme catechol-o-methyltransferase (COMT). They are therefore ineffective by oral administration. Catecholamines also tend to have much shorter durations of action than noncatecholamines, and they do not cross the blood-brain barrier to an extent sufficient to produce therapeutically useful effects in the central nervous system.

Epinephrine (Adrenalin) Epinephrine, called *adrenaline* in Great Britain, is the prototype sympathomimetic drug to which other sympathomimetic drugs are most often compared. It acts at α, β_1, and β_2 receptors and can produce the full spectrum of sympathomimetic effects. Epinephrine has more clinical uses than any other sympathomimetic drug (see Tables 13-2 to 13-6). It produces therapeutically useful effects on the heart, blood vessels, bronchi, and eye; actions on β_1 receptors of the heart produce positive chronotropic, positive inotropic, and positive dromotropic effects, but actions at β_1 receptors also can cause cardiac arrhythmias.

In very low doses, epinephrine can cause a slight and transient decrease in blood pressure, an effect attributable to actions on the β_2 receptors that mediate dilatation of the blood vessels in skeletal muscle. In higher doses, the vasoconstrictor (α receptor) effect predominates, and blood pressure is increased. Epinephrine relaxes bronchial smooth muscle (β_2 receptor effect), produces mydriasis (α receptor effect), increases blood glucose and free fatty acids (β receptor effects), and decreases levels of circulating insulin (α receptor effect). Although it is difficult to demonstrate experimentally that injected epinephrine crosses the blood-brain barrier, it is well-documented clinically that patients receiving epinephrine experience anxiety, jitteriness, tremor, and headache, which are at least partly attributable to effects in the central nervous system, although they may in part be secondary to the cardiac and metabolic effects.

Norepinephrine (Levophed) Norepinephrine (*noradrenaline* in Great Britain and formerly called *levarterenol*) acts at α, β_1, and β_2 receptors, but its effects on β_2 receptors are very weak compared with those of epinephrine. It acts on α receptors to cause intense vasoconstriction that is unopposed by receptor vasodilator effects. The intense vasoconstriction causes an increase in mean blood pressure, which activates baroreceptor reflexes (see Fig. 10-5a) and leads to reflex bradycardia. This vagally mediated reflex bradycardia overcomes the direct effects of norepinephrine on the β_1 receptors of the sinoatrial (SA) node pacemaker. Although norepinephrine does not increase heart rate, it is important to remember that it *does* interact with cardiac β_1 receptors, and therefore, like epinephrine and other β_1 agonists, it can excite latent pacemaker cells and cause cardiac arrhythmias. It can cause the same untoward central nervous system symptoms (anxiety, headache, etc.) as epinephrine.

Dopamine Dopamine (Intropin) is a neurotransmitter in the central nervous system and is perhaps a neuromodulator in autonomic ganglia. So far as is known, its beneficial effects as a drug are unrelated to any of its neurotransmitter-neuromodulator roles. Dopamine acts at β_1 receptors of the heart to cause a positive inotropic effect and a slight increase in heart rate. It has some ability to release endogenous norepinephrine, and the released norepinephrine contributes to its cardiac effects. It also acts at α receptors to cause vasoconstriction, but in low doses it acts selectively on specific dopamine receptors in the renal and mesenteric vasculature to cause vasodilatation and to increase renal blood flow and glomerular filtration.

Isoproterenol Isoproterenol (Isuprel) is essentially a pure β receptor agonist. It acts at both β_1 and β_2 receptors. It has positive chronotropic, positive inotropic, and positive dromotropic effects on the heart; like epinephrine and norepinephrine, it has the disadvantage of causing cardiac arrhythmias. It causes vasodilatation and it relaxes bronchial smooth muscle (both β_2 receptor effects). It produces many of the same metabolic effects as epinephrine, but it is less likely to cause the central nervous system symptoms of anxiety, etc.

Dobutamine Dobutamine (Dobutrex) is essentially a pure β_1 receptor agonist. It has positive inotropic and positive dromotropic effects on the heart. It usually causes only a slight increase in heart rate, but it can cause cardiac arrhythmias. It has no important effects on the vasculature.

Noncatecholamines

These drugs are effective orally and have a longer duration of action than the catecholamines.

Phenylephrine Phenylephrine (Neo-Synephrine) is essentially a pure α receptor agonist. It causes vasoconstriction and increases blood pressure. The increased blood pressure causes reflex bradycardia (see Fig. 10-5a). It has minimal CNS effects.

Methoxamine   Methoxamine (Vasoxyl) is also essentially a pure α receptor agonist. Its effects are similar to those of phenylephrine.

Selective β_2 Agonists   **Albuterol** (Proventil, Ventolin), called *salbutamol* outside the United States, **isoetharine** (Bronkosol), **metaproterenol** (Alupent, Metaprel), and **terbutaline** (Brethine, Bricanyl) are used in the treatment of respiratory disease. They all relax bronchial smooth muscle and are less likely than isoproterenol or epinephrine to cause β_1 effects (tachycardia, palpitations, and cardiac arrhythmias). They can cause the same adverse central nervous system effects as epinephrine, i.e., anxiety, tremor, headache, etc. **Nylidrin** (Arlidin) and **isoxsuprine** (Vasodilan) are two other relatively selective β_2 agonists, possibly effective in treating peripheral vascular disease and cerebrovascular insufficiency. They can cause β_1 cardiac effects and CNS adverse effects.

Indirect-Acting Sympathomimetic Drugs

Amphetamines   These drugs have sympathomimetic effects but are used mostly for their effects in the central nervous system. **Amphetamine, dextroamphetamine,** and **methamphetamine** produce sympathomimetic effects in the periphery by releasing norepinephrine; thus, amphetamines produce α, β_1, and β_2 receptor effects. They are orally effective, and their effects last for several hours. They increase blood pressure and often produce reflex bradycardia; they can cause cardiac arrhythmias. They relax smooth muscle in the wall of the urinary bladder (β_2 receptor effect), and they cause contraction of the sphincter (α receptor effect), a combination of effects that may cause urinary retention and difficulty in urinating.

In the central nervous system, amphetamines also release norepinephrine, as well as dopamine, from nerve terminals. They may also have direct effects in the central nervous system. Amphetamines are potent stimulants of the central nervous system; they cause respiratory stimulation, insomnia, restlessness, tremor, agitation, depressed appetite, decreased sense of fatigue, elevation of mood, elation, and euphoria. Psychologic dependence develops with chronic use. In acute toxic doses or with the chronic use of high doses, they can cause psychosis with hallucinations and paranoia.

Anorexigenic Agents   Many sympathomimetic drugs are used only as appetite suppressants (anorexigenics) in the treatment of obese patients. These drugs still have the potential to cause the side effects already mentioned, since no drug has been found that is selective for the satiety center. Some of these drugs are listed in Table 13-7.

Sympathomimetic Drugs That Act Both Directly and Indirectly

The effects of these drugs are attributable in part to direct interaction with adrenergic receptors and in part to the release of norepinephrine. They produce effects mediated by α, β_1, and β_2 receptors.

Ephedrine   Ephedrine produces effects both in the periphery and in the central nervous system. It is orally effective and longer-acting than the catecholamines. It causes vasoconstriction, an increase in blood pressure, a positive inotropic effect on the heart, relaxation of bronchial smooth muscle, mydriasis, and central nervous system effects similar to those of amphetamine, but less intense. *Tachyphylaxis,* a rapid development of tolerance, occurs with respect to the peripheral effects of ephedrine and all indirect-acting drugs. Repeated doses produce fewer effects over time, presumably due to depletion of releasable stores of norepinephrine from nerve terminals.

Mephentermine and Metaraminol   Mephentermine (Wyamine) and metaraminol (Aramine) are vasoconstrictors that may cause reflex bradycardia. Their central nervous system effects are not prominent.

CLINICAL USES OF SYMPATHOMIMETIC DRUGS

These drugs produce therapeutically useful effects on the heart, blood vessels, bronchi, eye, pregnant uterus, and central nervous system. Table 13-2 summarizes the uses of sympathomimetic drugs. The use of an individual sympathomimetic drug is determined to a large extent by the type(s) of adrenergic receptor with which it interacts.

Clinical Uses of Cardiovascular Effects

Use in Treating Shock

Shock is a syndrome of circulatory insufficiency in which vital organs are inadequately perfused. Some sympathomimetic drugs may be helpful, as well as harmful, in treating shock.

In cases of shock where vasodilatation contributes significantly to the poor tissue perfusion, sympathomimetic drugs with α agonist vasoconstrictor activity may be useful. The pure α agonists, **phenylephrine** and **methoxamine**, are infused intravenously for this purpose, as are other sympathomimetic drugs with α agonist activity, such as **epinephrine, norepinephrine, mephentermine,** and **metaraminol**. All of these drugs are potent vasoconstrictors and have the disadvantage of *decreasing* blood *flow* to vital organs. The kidneys are especially at risk of sustaining irreversible damage when blood flow is compromised.

In actuality, the vasculature of patients in shock is often

TABLE 13-2 Miscellaneous Uses of Sympathomimetic Drugs

USE	DRUG
To treat shock and hypotension	(See Table 13-3)
To treat cardiac arrest	Epinephrine, isoproterenol
To treat heart failure	Dobutamine
To treat Stokes-Adams AV block and syncope	Ephedrine, epinephrine, hydroxyamphetamine (oral), isoproterenol (IV)
Symptomatic control of nasal congestion	(See Table 13-4)
Topical hemostasis	Epinephrine
To delay absorption of local anesthetics	Epinephrine
Bronchodilatation in COPD	(See Table 13-5)
To treat paroxysmal atrial tachycardia	Methoxamine, phenylephrine
To treat allergic reactions to drugs, venoms	Epinephrine
Topical application for ocular disorders	(See Table 13-6)
To treat vascular insufficiency	Isoxsuprine, nylidrin
To delay premature labor	Ritodrine (Yutopar)
For CNS effects	(See Table 13-7)

maximally constricted as a result of activation of baroreceptor reflexes by the shock syndrome. In such patients, vasoconstrictors would produce minimal increases in blood pressure and could further compromise blood flow. In these patients, α-*blocking* drugs or direct vasodilators such as **sodium nitroprusside** are sometimes used to overcome the vasoconstriction and restore blood flow to vital organs.

In cases of shock where decreased cardiac contractility and decreased cardiac output are contributing factors, sympathomimetic drugs that produce positive inotropic effects on the heart may be useful. These include **epinephrine, isoproterenol, dobutamine,** and **dopamine.** All of these drugs act on cardiac β_1 receptors to increase the force of ventricular contraction. Epinephrine and isoproterenol also increase heart rate. **Epinephrine** has the disadvantage, mentioned above, of decreasing renal blood flow. **Isoproterenol,** however, is a vasodilator (β_2 receptor effect) and thus usually increases renal blood flow in patients in shock. Both isoproterenol and epinephrine have the disadvantage of causing cardiac arrhythmias. By contrast, **dobutamine** acts quite selectively to increase the force of cardiac contraction, with minimal effects on other properties of the heart or on the vasculature. It is advocated for treating cardiogenic shock.

Dopamine increases cardiac contractility by an effect on cardiac β_1 receptors. It is less likely than epinephrine or isoproterenol to cause cardiac arrhythmias, and in low doses it has the added advantage of acting on dopamine receptors in the renal vasculature to increase renal blood flow. High doses of dopamine activate vascular α receptors, cause vasoconstriction, and decrease renal blood flow.

Table 13-3 summarizes the primary beneficial effects of these sympathomimetic drugs when they are used to treat shock. For a more detailed description of shock and its treatment, see Chap. 48, "Emergency and Intensive Care."

Use in Treating Hypotension

Hypotension, other than that associated with shock, can be caused by some general anesthetics, by an overdose of antihypertensive drugs, by some neurologic diseases such as

TABLE 13-3 Sympathomimetic Drugs Used to Treat Shock and Hypotension

DRUG	PRIMARY BENEFICIAL EFFECT IN SHOCK AND HYPOTENSION
Dobutamine (Dobutrex)	Positive inotropic effect, increased cardiac output, increased renal perfusion
Dopamine HCl (Dopastat, Intropin)	
Low dose	Positive inotropic effect, increased cardiac output, increased renal perfusion
High dose	Positive inotropic effect, increased cardiac output, vasoconstriction
Ephedrine sulfate	Positive inotropic effect, increased cardiac output, vasoconstriction
Epinephrine HCl (Adrenalin Chloride)	Positive inotropic effect, increased cardiac output, vasoconstriction
Isoproterenol HCl (Isuprel)	Positive inotropic effect, increased cardiac output, possible increased renal perfusion
Mephentermine sulfate (Wyamine Sulfate)	Positive inotropic effect, increased cardiac output, possible vasoconstriction or increased renal perfusion
Metaraminol bitartrate (Aramine)	Vasoconstriction
Methoxamine HCl (Vasoxyl)	Vasoconstriction
Norepinephrine bitartrate (Levophed)	Positive inotropic effect, increased cardiac output, vasoconstriction
Phenylephrine HCl (Neo-Synephrine)	Vasoconstriction

tabes dorsalis and syringomyelia, and by spinal anesthesia. The goal of spinal anesthesia is to block pain impulses entering the spinal cord in sensory fibers in the dorsal roots. The anesthetic may also block spinal cord outflow in the ventral roots. When thoracolumbar levels of the cord are involved, the sympathetic preganglionic outflow in the ventral roots may be blocked, sympathetic vasoconstrictor tone may be lost, and hypotension may result.

Sympathomimetic drugs are often used in restoring blood pressure. However, if the hypotension is caused by **cyclopropane** or by some of the halogenated hydrocarbon anesthetics (e.g., **halothane**), sympathomimetic drugs must be used with caution because of the likelihood of cardiac arrhythmias. **Ephedrine**, since it is orally effective, is often used to maintain blood pressure in patients with chronic neurologic disease. Either ephedrine or mephentermine is given intravenously to patients in whom spinal anesthesia has decreased blood pressure.

Use in Heart Block with Syncope and in Cardiac Arrest

In these cases, either **epinephrine** or **isoproterenol**, both of which have β_1 agonist activity, may be useful in restoring normal cardiac activity. The drugs are given intravenously in Stokes-Adams syndrome, and by intracardiac injection in cardiac arrest. In the syncope associated with Stokes-Adams syndrome, the block of conduction of the cardiac impulse through the AV node may be overcome by the positive dromotropic effect of the β_1 agonists. In cardiac arrest, the drugs may initiate cardiac pacemaker activity in cells of the SA node or in latent pacemaker cells.

Use in Treating Paroxysmal Atrial Tachycardia

Attacks of paroxysmal atrial tachycardia or nodal tachycardia are sometimes terminated by maneuvers that elicit intense vagal (parasympathetic) discharge to the heart. Two sympathomimetic drugs, **phenylephrine** and **methoxamine**, are sometimes given for this purpose. These drugs have negligible effects on cardiac β_1 receptors, but, by causing vasoconstriction and increasing blood pressure, they activate baroreceptor reflexes and increase the vagal (parasympathetic) discharge to the heart (see Fig. 10-5a).

Use as Nasal Decongestants (Table 13-4)

Sympathomimetic drugs with α agonist activity are used in the form of inhalers, as nasal sprays, as nose drops, and orally to produce constriction of blood vessels in the nasal mucosa and provide symtomatic relief from the nasal "stuffiness" that often accompanies the common cold, hay fever, allergic rhinitis, etc. Many of these preparations are available over the counter without a prescription. The nasal preparations of these drugs can cause rebound congestion, especially when they are used more frequently than recommended. (See Chap. 21, "Symptoms of 'Cold' and Allergy.")

TABLE 13-4 Some Sympathomimetic Drugs Used as Nasal Decongestants

Topical preparations (sprays, drops)
  Ephedrine HCl and sulfate (Efedron Nasal, Vatronol)
  Epinephrine HCl (Adrenalin Chloride)
  Naphazoline HCl (Privine)
  Oxymetazoline HCl (Afrin, Neo-Synephrine 12 Hour)
  Phenylephrine HCl (Alconefrin, Allerest Nasal, Neo-Synephrine)
  Tetrahydrozoline HCl (Tyzine)
  Xylometazoline HCl (Neo-Synephrine II Long Acting, Otrivin)
Nasal inhalers
  Desoxyephedrine (Vicks Inhaler)
  Propylhexedrine (Benzedrex)
Oral preparations
  Ephedrine sulfate
  Phenylephrine hydrochloride
  Phenylpropanolamine HCl (Propadrine)
  Pseudoephedrine HCl and sulfate (Sudafed)

Use to Produce Topical Hemostasis

Epinephrine, a potent constrictor of blood vessels in the mucosa, is used topically during nasolaryngeal surgery to reduce bleeding.

Use with Local Anesthetics

The vasoconstrictor properties of **epinephrine** are also used to limit the rate of absorption of local anesthetics that are infiltrated. Epinephrine is mixed with the local anesthetic before injection. By producing vasoconstriction at the injection site, epinephrine delays the absorption of the local anesthetic into the systemic circulation. This serves the dual purposes of prolonging the effect of the local anesthetic and reducing the likelihood of systemic toxicity from the local anesthetic. Epinephrine should *not* be mixed with solutions of local anesthetics to be injected into tissues whose circulation is supplied by end arteries, for example, the fingers, toes, earlobes, nose, and penis. The intense vasoconstriction produced in these tissues could cause necrosis or gangrene.

Use in Treating Vascular Insufficiency

Although efficacy has not been proved in controlled studies, **nylidrin** and **isoxsuprine** are used in conditions where local arteriolar dilatation may be of benefit. These drugs are used in cerebrovascular insufficiency, peripheral vascular disease (arteriosclerosis obliterans, thromboangiitis obliterans, and Raynaud's disease), frostbite, ischemic ulcer, and circulatory diseases of the inner ear.

Clinical Uses of Bronchodilator Effects

Use in COPD (Table 13-5)

Sympathomimetic drugs with activity as β_2 agonists are useful in treating chronic obstructive pulmonary disease

TABLE 13-5 Some Sympathomimetic Drugs Used as Bronchodilators in Treating Asthma and Other Bronchospastic Diseases

Albuterol* (salbutamol; Proventil, Ventolin)

Ephedrine sulfate

Epinephrine HCl (Adrenalin Chloride, Bronkaid Mist, Primatene Mist, Sus-Phrine, Vaponefrin)

Ethylnorepinephrine HCl (Bronkephrine)

Isoetharine HCl* (Bronkometer, Bronkosol)

Isoproterenol HCl (Aerolone, Isuprel, Norisodrine)

Metaproterenol sulfate* (Alupent, Metaprel)

Terbutaline sulfate* (Brethine, Bricanyl)

*Relatively selective β_2 sympathomimetic drug.

(COPD, i.e., asthma, emphysema, chronic bronchitis). The selective β_2 adrenergic agonists (**albuterol, isoetharine, metaproterenol**, and **terbutaline**) have been introduced. They are *relatively* selective for β_2 receptors and therefore cause fewer cardiac arrhythmias than the older agents, epinephrine and isoproterenol, but they are not totally devoid of β_1 cardiovascular effects. For a more detailed description of the use of these drugs and other drugs in the treatment of asthma and other bronchospastic diseases, see Chap. 27, "Respiratory Disorders."

Use in Treating Severe Allergic Reactions

Epinephrine is useful in treating severe allergic reactions to drugs, insect venoms, etc. These reactions can cause itching, urticaria (hives), bronchospasm, severe swelling of the tongue and lips, and edema of the glottis, which makes respiration difficult. Parenteral administration of epinephrine rapidly relieves these symptoms by combined vasoconstrictor (α) effects that reduce tissue edema and bronchodilator (β_2) effects.

Use of Ocular Effects (Table 13-6)

Sympathomimetic drugs with α agonist activity (**phenylephrine** and **hydroxyamphetamine**) are available as eye drops to dilate the pupil for ophthalmologic examination. Unlike parasympathetic blocking agents such as atropine, they produce mydriasis (pupil dilation) without cycloplegia (paralysis of accommodation). Sympathomimetic drugs are also used locally in the eye as decongestants to produce vasoconstriction and relieve the symptoms of minor eye irritation.

Paradoxically, sympathomimetic drugs are sometimes used to treat open-angle glaucoma, often in combination with a parasympathomimetic drug. It should be recalled that parasympathetic blocking drugs, which cause mydriasis, can precipitate glaucoma. It might be expected that since α agonists also cause mydriasis, they too could precipitate glaucoma. However, **epinephrine** and **phenylephrine** reduce intraocular pressure in open-angle glaucoma, probably by causing vasoconstriction, thereby reducing the rate of secretion of aqueous humor. For further discussion of the treatment of glaucoma, see Chap. 39, "Ophthalmologic Disorders."

Use in Preventing Premature Labor

Beta-2 receptors mediate relaxation of the uterus. The β_2 adrenergic agonist **ritodrine HCl** (Yutopar) is for delaying premature labor. Although the drug has some selectivity for β_2 receptors, it also can activate β_1 receptors. Maternal tachycardia and palpitations, and fetal tachycardia, have been reported. Ritodrine also causes changes in blood pressure and produces metabolic changes. When given with **corticosteroids** to patients in premature labor, ritodrine has caused maternal pulmonary edema. (See Chap. 46, "Women's Health Care.")

Uses of Central Nervous System Effects (Table 13-7)

Sympathomimetic drugs, such as ephedrine and amphetamine and some of its close chemical relatives, readily cross the blood-brain barrier; when used for their therapeutic effects in the periphery, they cause insomnia as an unwanted side effect. However, therapeutic use is made of this effect in treating narcolepsy, a syndrome characterized in part by inappropriate daytime lapses into sleep.

Amphetamine can also be used to offset the drowsiness produced by some antiepileptic drugs, such as **phenobarbital**; it is sometimes effective by itself in controlling the petit mal or absence types of epilepsy.

Paradoxically, dextroamphetamine and a related drug, **methylphenidate** (Ritalin), are useful in treating children with hyperkinetic syndromes (previously called minimal brain damage), whose restlessness and limited attention span interfere with their learning ability. Children maintained on

TABLE 13-6 Some Sympathomimetic Drugs Used as Ophthalmic Preparations

Dipivefrin HCl (Propine)

Ephedrine

Epinephrine bitartrate, borate, and HCl (Adrenalin Chloride, Epifrin, Epinal, Epitrate, Glaucon)

Hydroxyamphetamine HBr (Paredrine)

Naphazoline HCl (AK-Con Ophthalmic, Naphcon Forte Ophthalmic)

Phenylephrine HCl (Efricel, Neo-Synephrine)

Tetrahydrozoline HCl (Murine Plus Eye Drops, Visine)

TABLE 13-7   Some Sympathomimetic Drugs Used for Their Central Nervous System Effects*

	Uses					
	To Treat:			Adjunct in:		
DRUG	NARCOLEPSY	HYPERKINETIC SYNDROME	NOCTURNAL ENURESIS	EPILEPSY	PARKINSONISM	APPETITE SUPPRESSANT
Ephedrine	+		+			
Amphetamine sulfate (Benzedrine)	+		+			
Dextroamphetamine sulfate (Dexampex, Dexedrine)	+	+		+	+	+
Methamphetamine (Desoxyn, Methampex)	+					+
Methylphenidate HCl (Ritalin)	+	+				
Benzphetamine HCl (Didrex)						+
Chlorphentermine HCl (Pre-Sate)						+
Diethylpropion HCl (Tenuate, Tepanil)						+
Fenfluramine HCl (Pondimin)						+
Phentermine HCl (Ionamin, Wilpowr)						+
Phenylpropanolamine (Dexatrim, Diadex, Dietac, other over-the-counter preparations)						+

*For dosage and specific preparations of these drugs, see Chaps. 22, "Sleep Disturbances"; 33, "Neurologic Disorders"; and 25, "Nutritional Disorders."

these drugs can suffer growth retardation because the drugs suppress the appetite. (See Chapter 33, "Neurologic Disorders.")

Although controversial because of questionable efficacy and abuse potential, use is made of these appetite-suppressant properties of amphetamines in treating obese patients. Except for **fenfluramine** (Pondimin), all of the anorexigenic agents cause insomnia, jitteriness, etc.; in contrast, fenfluramine causes drowsiness. All of the drugs can produce peripheral sympathomimetic effects, especially on the cardiovascular system. (See Chap. 25, "Nutritional Disorders.")

Dextroamphetamine is also sometimes used to treat patients with Parkinson's disease who cannot tolerate more-effective drugs. It is not very effective, presumably because its beneficial effects depend on the release of dopamine from nigrostriatal neurons; dopamine is in very low concentrations in these neurons in parkinsonism patients.

Ephedrine and **amphetamine** are also used to treat patients with nocturnal enuresis; their effectiveness in these patients may be due to effects on both the central nervous system and the urinary bladder (β_2 receptors mediate relaxation) and its sphincter (α receptors mediate contraction).

ADVERSE EFFECTS OF SYMPATHOMIMETIC DRUGS AND THEIR TREATMENT

Table 13-8 summarizes the most common adverse effects of sympathomimetic drugs. Several considerations should be

kept in mind when this table is used. First, just as the clinical uses of an individual drug depend largely on the type(s) of adrenergic receptor with which it interacts, so too do the adverse effects. For example, many sympathomimetic drugs cause cardiac arrhythmias, but some, such as phenylephrine and methoxamine, which are essentially pure α agonists, are very much less likely to do so. On the other hand, it is important to remember that when a drug is described as having selectivity for a given type of receptor (e.g., when it is called a "selective agonist"), this means "relatively selective," and the drug may well produce adverse effects mediated by a type of receptor other than the one for which it shows selectivity. For example, the selective β_2 agonists used to treat asthma can and do produce tachycardia and cardiac arrhythmias, especially in sensitive patients, although the likelihood of their doing so is less than with epinephrine or isoproterenol. Finally, as with drugs in other classes, what is considered an adverse effect depends to some extent on the intended therapeutic effect in the individual patient. Insomnia is an unwanted side effect of ephedrine to the patient with chronic asthma, but the same basic drug is therapeutic to the patient with narcolepsy.

Most of the peripheral adverse effects of sympathomimetic drugs are effectively treated by dosage reduction or by the administration of the appropriate adrenergic blocking drug (see Chap. 14). For example, a cardiac arrhythmia produced by **isoproterenol** would be rationally and well treated by a β-blocking drug, such as **propranolol**, which is used as

TABLE 13-8 Adverse Effects of Sympathomimetic Drugs

ORGAN SYSTEM	EFFECT
Cardiovascular system	
Heart	Tachycardia*
	Palpitations*
	Cardiac arrhythmias*
	Angina*
Blood vessels	Hypertension,† possibly leading to
	Pulmonary edema
	Cerebrovascular accident
	After extravasation, local necrosis†
Urinary tract	Difficult and painful urination
	Urinary retention
Central nervous system	Anxiety
	Tremors
	Restlessness
	Headache
	Convulsions‡
	Insomnia‡
	Appetite suppression‡
	Hallucinations‡
	Psychosis‡
Other	Nausea
	Vomiting
	Sweating

*Effect most likely with drugs that have β_1 agonist activity.
†Effect most likely with drugs that have α agonist activity.
‡Effect most likely with amphetamines and anorexigenic agents.

an antiarrhythmic agent. If an α agonist such as **phenylephrine** were being infused intravenously and some of the drug leaked out of the vein, the tissue surrounding the intravenous injection site could be kept from becoming necrotic by infiltration of a solution of an α-blocking drug, such as **phentolamine**.

NURSING PROCESS RELATED TO SYMPATHOMIMETIC DRUGS

Sympathomimetic drugs produce life-saving effects in many acute situations; shock, severe asthma, etc. In these situations, many of the nursing implications relate to the constant monitoring and support of the vital functions of the cardiovascular, respiratory, nervous, and renal systems. The sympathomimetics are also used, however, for several chronic conditions, and they are available to patients in numerous over-the-counter preparations. In these situations, different nursing care considerations apply to the use of sympathomimetics.

Assessment

Past History The sympathomimetic drugs produce a wide range of autonomic effects. Normally, sympathetic effects are produced as a part of finely tuned autonomic reflexes, with sensory feedback and opposing parasympathetic influences. When produced by sympathomimetic drugs, without these balances and controls, these effects can be uncomfortable or even life-threatening in patients with particular pre-established conditions. A careful patient history should be taken and related to the spectrum of effects of the individual sympathomimetic drug, to ensure that the drug is not contraindicated in that particular patient. The following are relative or absolute contraindications to the use of some sympathomimetic drugs.

Coronary artery disease or angina Sympathomimetics cause an increase in heart rate, an increase in the force of myocardial contraction, and/or an increase in peripheral resistance (through vasoconstriction). Each of these increases the work load of the heart and can lead to angina, myocardial ischemia, or ventricular irritability in patients whose coronary circulation is compromised.

Cardiac arrhythmias Sympathomimetics can cause arrhythmias, especially in the patient whose heart is predisposed to arrhythmias, by activating latent pacemaker cells outside the SA node.

Diabetes mellitus Sympathomimetics with β agonist activity cause a change in metabolism which elevates serum glucose levels. This elevation of blood glucose can cause problems in diabetics, who already have difficulty in regulating blood glucose.

Hypertension Sympathomimetics cause an increase in systemic blood pressure, which could lead to stroke or myocardial infarction in patients with high blood pressure.

Glaucoma Sympathomimetics with α agonist activity cause dilatation of the pupils of the eyes and can cause acute attacks of narrow-angle glaucoma.

Urinary difficulty or prostatic hypertrophy Sympathomimetics with α agonist activity decrease bladder muscle tone; those with β agonist activity increase sphincter tone. Either of these effects can lead to urinary retention, especially in the presence of prostatic hypertrophy.

Seizures Those sympathomimetics that cross the blood-brain barrier can cause central nervous system stimulation with resultant tremors, anxiety, or convulsions; patients who have a history of seizures are especially prone to seizures after these drugs.

Mothers who are nursing should also avoid sympathomimetics, because they pass into breast milk and can affect the nursing infants.

Physical Assessment Before giving any of these drugs, the nurse should assess the baseline functioning of all of the systems that are most affected by the sympathomimetics. In this way, both therapeutic and toxic effects of the drugs can be accurately evaluated.

This assessment should include mental status (orientation, affect), neurologic status (pupils, tremors, muscle strength), blood pressure, apical pulse (rate, rhythm, character, presence of extra sounds), electrocardiogram (assessment for arrhythmias), respirations (rate, rhythm, character, adventitious sounds), and urinary output (bladder distention, tone).

Management

Solutions of catecholamines are unstable; a pink, red, brown, or black color indicates degradation of the drug. Only clear and colorless solutions should be administered.

Patients who receive sympathomimetics in an acute situation must be carefully monitored to assess the therapeutic action of the drug as well as to assess the occurrence of any toxic effects. The care of sites of IV infusion of α agonists has already been discussed; the patient also needs to be monitored for the occurrence of arrhymias, severe hypertension, flushing, restlessness, or cardiovascular collapse. Since a few milliliters of fluid can often make the difference between a therapeutic and a toxic level of the drug, the IV should be equipped with an infusion pump and the infusion rate must be watched carefully. Life support equipment, as well as appropriate aderenergic receptor blockers [**phenotolamine** (α blocker), **propranolol** (β blocker)], should be continuously available to counteract toxic effects.

Patients who are taking a sympathomimetic sublingually (isoproterenol) will need instruction on the proper procedure for taking the drug. The patient should be careful to avoid swallowing until the tablet has completely dissolved. The patient should be advised to change position slowly after taking the drug, to help minimize any postural hypotension that might occur.

Patients who are taking sympathomimetics through inhalers will need instruction on the particular inhalers they are using. Since there are several varieties of inhaler on the market, the patients will need to learn about the inhalers they are using and to learn that often inhalers cannot be interchanged. **Isoproterenol** inhalants may cause the saliva to turn pink; patients should be alerted to this and assured that it is not uncommon.

Sympathomimetic effects on the urinary bladder or sphincter sometimes lead to difficulty in urinating. Men with prostatic hypertrophy are especially vulnerable to this adverse reaction. If they have to take a sympathomimetic, these patients should be advised to monitor their urinary output and to void before taking each dose of medication, to ensure that the bladder is empty when the medication reaches its maximum effect.

All patients who are taking sympathomimetics should be taught the common side effects of the drugs. Restlessness, insomnia, tremulousness, flushing, sweating, palpitations, and loss of appetite are fairly common and uncomfortable reactions to some of these drugs. Assurance that these reactions are expected is beneficial to most patients. The patient should also be instructed to notify the nurse or physician if any of these occur, so dosage adjustment can be attempted, to alleviate these side effects.

Many over-the-counter (OTC) preparations contain sympathomimetics. They are found in cold capsules, nasal sprays, allergy medications, and diet pills. Patients who are taking prescribed sympathomimetics should be cautioned to avoid the use of OTC drugs unless they have discussed it with their physicians. Misuse of OTC preparations in combination with a prescribed sympathomimetic can lead to serious toxicity. Other patients also are at high risk for problems when using OTC drugs containing sympathomimetics. Patients with coronary artery disease, hypertension, diabetes, glaucoma, or history of stroke or cardiac arrhythmias should be cautioned about the use of such preparations. Since OTC drugs are often self-prescribed without an understanding of the ingredients they contain, this is a major problem in consumer education. Basic drug teaching plans should include reference to the potential dangers of specific OTC drugs. If patients are using nasal sprays to relieve nasal congestion, they should be instructed in the proper use of the sprays. Most of the sprays are designed to be used with the user's head in the upright position. Many people use the sprays with the head tilted backward; this can lead to systemic toxicity from the drug if the concentrated drops are absorbed from the mucous membrane. People also need to be taught that overuse of nasal decongestants can lead to rebound congestion.

Evaluation

The patient should be assessed for evidence of the therapeutic effect of the drug. If the patient is receiving the drug for an acute condition, frequent systemic assessment should be done of the patient's respiratory, cardiovascular, renal, and neurologic status. Other patients receiving sympathomimetics should receive period assessment to evaluate the effect of the sympathetic stimulation on their basic functioning.

Many drugs can interact dangerously with sympathomimetics. The patient's overall situation should be evaluated for the possible occurrence of any of these interactions.

Monoamine oxidase (MAO) inhibitors and **β adrenergic receptor blockers** can both potentiate the α sympathomimetic effects and lead to dangerous toxicity.

Tricyclic antidepressants, antihistamines, and **levothyroxine sodium** will all increase sympathomimetic activity.

When sympathomimetics are given with **general anesthetics, digitalis,** or other arrhythmogenic drugs, serious to fatal cardiac arrhythmias can occur. Sympathomimetic drug use should be stopped prior to surgery and should be reported to the anesthetist and prominently noted on the patient's chart.

Sympathomimetics decrease the effectiveness of many antihypertensive drugs (e.g., **guanethidine, reserpine**) and can cause a loss of blood pressure control. A patient who is regulated on an antihypertensive drug while taking a sympathomimetic should be told the importance of continuing to take both drugs. If only the sympathomimetic drug is stopped, the patient could experience severe hypotension.

It is important to remember that sympathomimetics are contained in many OTC preparations, and the drug-drug interactions discussed should be considered in evaluating unexpected effects of drug therapy.

REFERENCES

Goldberg, L. I.: "Dopamine: Clinical Uses of an Endogenous Catecholamine," *N Engl J Med,* **291**:707–710, 1974.

Hoffman, B. B., and R. J. Lefkowitz: "Alpha-Adrenergic Receptor Subtypes," *N Engl J Med,* **302**:1390–1393, 1980.

Kunos, G.: "Adrenoceptors," in R. George, R. O. Kien, and A. K. Cho (eds.), *Annual Review of Pharmacology and Toxicology,* Vol. 18, Annual Review, Palo Alto, CA, 1978.

Smith-Collins, A.: "Dobutamine: A New Inotropic Agent," *Nursing 80,* **10**:62–66, 1980.

Wiener, N.: "Norepinephrine, Epinephrine, and the Sympathomimetic Amines," in A. G. Gilman, L. S. Goodman, and A. Gilman (eds.), *Goodman and Gilman's The Pharmacological Basis of Therapeutics,* 6th ed., New York: Macmillan, 1980.

14

DRUGS INTERFERING WITH SYMPATHETIC NERVOUS SYSTEM FUNCTION

ELEANOR H. BOYD
AMY M. KARCH

LEARNING OBJECTIVES

Upon mastery of the contents of this chapter, the reader will be able to:

1. List three different sites at which sympatholytic drugs can act to interfere with sympathetic vasoconstrictor tone, and give an example of a drug acting at each site.

2. Differentiate between adrenergic receptor-blocking drugs and adrenergic neuron-blocking drugs.

3. Differentiate between the actions of alpha and beta adrenergic receptor blockers.

4. Explain the advantage of prazosin over phentolamine in treating hypertension.

5. Explain the advantage of metoprolol over propranolol in treating hypertension.

6. List six therapeutic uses of propranolol.

7. List the major adverse effects of nonselective alpha blockers.

8. List the major adverse effects of nonselective beta blockers.

9. List two nursing activities for each step of the nursing process for patients on sympatholytic drugs.

10. State three parameters that would be important in evaluating therapeutic effectiveness or adverse reactions in patients receiving sympatholytic drugs.

MECHANISMS OF ACTION

Drugs that interfere with sympathetic nervous system function do so in a variety of ways (see Figure 14-1), making description of these drugs more complicated than the description of parasympatholytic drugs, which act by only one mechanism: preventing molecules of the neurotransmitter acetylcholine from occupying and activating muscarinic cholinergic receptors in the cell membranes of effector organs.

Some *sympatholytic drugs* act by preventing molecules of the neurotransmitter norepinephrine from occupying and activating adrenergic receptors in the cell membranes of effector organs. These drugs are called *adrenergic receptor-blocking drugs*. For many years, these drugs were called simply "sympathetic blocking drugs" or "adrenergic blocking drugs." These terms are no longer adequate; they fail to distinguish between those drugs that block postsynaptic receptors and those that act in presynaptic adrenergic nerve terminals to interfere with the synthesis, storage, or release of norepinephrine.

Most adrenergic receptor-blocking drugs block either alpha or beta adrenergic receptors, but **labetalol** blocks *both* α and β receptors and is called an *alpha-beta blocker*. Drugs that block α receptors (e.g., **phentolamine**) are called *α-adrenergic receptor blockers*, or simply α *blockers*; drugs that block β receptors (e.g., **propranolol**) are called β *blockers*. Drugs are now available with yet greater selectivity; **prazosin** blocks α_1 receptors relatively selectively, and **metoprolol** blocks β_1 receptors with minimal effects on β_2 receptors. A goal of current pharmacologic research is to develop agents that have more selective receptor interactions. As more information is gathered on the adrenergic receptors in health and disease, clinicians should anticipate new α-specific compounds, as well as more selective β agents.

Adrenergic neuron-blocking drugs (**guanethidine, bret-**

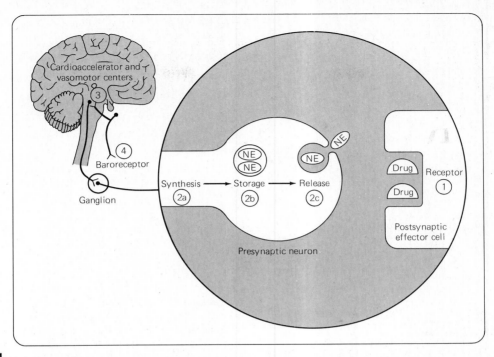

FIGURE 14-1

Mechanisms of Action of Sympatholytic Drugs. (1) Adrenergic receptor blockade of the postsynaptic receptor; (2) adrenergic neuron blockade by interference with (a) synthesis, (b) storage, and/or (c) release of norepinephrine (NE) from presynaptic neurons; (3) decrease of sympathetic outflow from the brain; and (4) activation of sensory endings in the baroreceptor to decrease sympathetic outflow from the brain. (The veratrum alkaloids, the only group of drugs to affect the baroreceptor site, were removed from the market by the manufacturer in 1984, making the fourth mechanism of action of historical interest only.) Receptor selectivity for adrenergic receptor blockade follows the same principles as for sympathetic agonists (see Fig. 13-2). β_2 selective blockers are currently marketed.

ylium, **reserpine,** and **metyrosine**) interfere with sympathetic nervous system function by interfering with the synthesis, storage, and/or release of norepinephrine from sympathetic postganglionic neurons. It is important to distinguish between adrenergic receptor- and adrenergic neuron-blocking drugs because these two groups of drugs produce different spectra of effects and they interact differently with drugs of other classes.

A third group of drugs (**methyldopa** and **clonidine**) act in the central nervous system to diminish sympathetic outflow from the brain, for example, from the vasomotor center and the cardioaccelerator center.

Drugs that block sympathetic ganglia also interfere with sympathetic nervous system function. These drugs, called ganglionic blockers, also block parasympathetic ganglia, although their sole therapeutic use is to interfere with sympathetic nervous system function. The ganglionic blockers are described in Chap. 15, "Ganglionic Blocking Drugs."

Table 14-1 gives a classification of some important sympatholytic drugs according to their sites and mechanisms of action.

CLINICAL USES OF SYMPATHOLYTIC DRUGS

Most of the *systemic* uses of sympatholytic drugs depend on their effects on the heart or on blood vessels. Sympatholytic drugs are used in the treatment of hypertension (see Table 14-2), cardiac arrhythmias (**propranolol** and **bretylium**), angina (**propranolol** and **nadolol**), peripheral vascular disease (**phentolamine** and **tolazoline**), and migraine headache (**propranolol**). They are used after myocardial infarction to limit infarct size (**metoprolol**) and to decrease the likelihood of reinfarction (**timolol** and **propranolol**). They are used to prepare patients for the surgical removal of the adrenal medullary tumor, pheochromocytoma, that secretes epinephrine and norepinephrine, and to control blood pressure and pre-

TABLE 14-1 Classification of Sympatholytic Drugs According to Sites and Mechanisms of Action

CLASSIFICATION	DRUGS
1. Adrenergic receptor blockers	
Alpha receptor blockers	
Competitive	
Nonselective α_1 and α_2 blockers*	Phentolamine HCl or mesylate (Regitine)
	Tolazoline (Priscoline)
Selective α_1 blockers	Prazosin HCl (Minipress)
Irreversible α_1 and α_2 blockers	Phenoxybenzamine HCl (Dibenzyline)
Beta receptor blockers (competitive)	
Nonselective β_1 and β_2 blockers	Propranolol HCl (Inderal)
	Oxprenolol (Trasicor)†
	Nadolol (Corgard)
	Timolol maleate (Blocadren, Timoptic)
	Pindolol (Visken)
Relatively selective β_1 blockers	Metoprolol tartrate (Lopressor)
	Atenolol (Tenormin)
Alpha-beta blocker	Labetalol (Trandate, Normodyne)
2. Adrenergic neuron blockers Impairing release and/or depletion of norepinephrine	Guanadrel (Hylorel)
	Guanethidine sulfate (Ismelin)
	Bretylium tosylate (Bretylol)
	Rauwolfia alkaloids, e.g., reserpine (Serpasil)
Impairing synthesis of catecholamines	Metyrosine (Demser)
3. Centrally acting depressants of sympathetic outflow	Clonidine (Catapres)
	Methyldopa (Aldomet)

*The ergot alkaloids—ergonovine, ergotamine, and ergotoxine—cause a reversible α blockade. However, clinically significant effects of the ergots—vasoconstriction in migraine, oxytocic effects in postpartum hemorrhage, and cognitive-acting effects in senile dementia—appear to result from other pharmacologic activity of the ergots.

†Approved by FDA in 1984 but not marketed.

vent cardiac arrhythmias in patients with inoperable pheochromocytoma (**phentolamine, phenoxybenzamine, propranolol,** and **metyrosine**). One drug, **timolol,** is used *topically* in the eye to treat open-angle glaucoma.

SPECIFIC SYMPATHOLYTIC DRUGS

Adrenergic Receptor-Blocking Drugs

These drugs act on either α or β receptors to prevent endogenous norepinephrine and epinephrine, and exogenous sym-

TABLE 14-2 Some Sympatholytic Drugs Used to Treat Hypertension*

Clonidine (Catapres)	Pindolol (Visken)
Guanadrel (Hylorel)	Prazosin (Minipress)
Guanethidine (Ismelin)	Propranolol (Inderal)
Methyldopa (Aldomet)	Reserpine (Serpasil)
Metoprolol (Lopressor)	Timolol (Blocadren)
Nadolol (Corgard)	

*For specific preparations and dosage, see Chap. 40, "High Blood Pressure."

pathomimetic drugs, from occupying and activating the receptors.

α Receptor Blockers

Phentolamine and Tolazoline Phentolamine (Regitine) and tolazoline (Priscoline) are competitive blockers of α_1 and α_2 receptors. By blocking α_1 receptors, they decrease sympathetic vasoconstrictor tone and decrease the effectiveness of drugs that activate α receptors. They are used in treating peripheral vascular disorders (e.g., Raynaud's disease), although their efficacy in these disorders is not established. Phentolamine is used to prevent necrosis when an α agonist drug (e.g., norepinephrine) leaks from an intravenous injection site. When vasoconstriction is present in shock, α blockers, such as these drugs, may be useful. The α receptor blockers were among the first drugs to be used to treat hypertension. They are now used to prevent or treat hypertensive crises in patients with pheochromocytoma. A disadvantage of these drugs is that they cause reflex tachycardia (see Fig. 10-5 and below). Newer drugs are more selective and efficacious in treating hypertension.

Prazosin Prazosin (Minipress) is a relatively selective α_1 blocker. Like phentolamine, it decreases sympathetic vasoconstrictor tone and reduces blood pressure. However, it is much less likely than phentolamine to cause reflex tachycardia. This difference makes prazosin one of the drugs used currently in treating hypertension. Understanding why prazosin is less likely than phentolamine to cause reflex tachycardia requires an understanding of α_2 receptors (one of the few instances to date where α_2 receptors currently have clinical importance). Alpha-2 receptors, located on the terminals of neurons that release norepinephrine, are believed to mediate feedback inhibition of further norepinephrine release. When α_2 receptors are blocked (e.g., by phentolamine), sympathetic nerve impulses can apparently release more norepinephrine than normal. How does this explain greater reflex tachycardia with phentolamine than with prazosin? Drugs such as phentolamine and prazosin block α_1 receptors, decrease blood pressure, and activate baroreceptor reflexes. This increases the rate of impulses in sympathetic cardioaccelerator nerves. Phentolamine, but not prazosin, blocks the α_2 receptors on the terminals of these cardioaccelerator nerves; thus, these nerves release more norepinephrine and produce more-intense reflex tachycardia when phentolamine has been given than when prazosin has been given. (See Fig. 14-2.)

Phenoxybenzamine   Phenoxybenzamine (Dibenzyline) blocks α receptors *irreversibly*. It thus has a very long duration of action. It is used in preventing hypertensive crises in patients with inoperable pheochromocytoma, and it is sometimes used in treating peripheral vascular disease.

β Receptor Blockers

Table 14-3 compares the β receptor blockers according to receptor type blocked, membrane-stabilizing activity, and intrinsic sympathomimetic activity (ISA). ISA means that the drug is a partial agonist at the adrenergic receptor. **Pindolol** and **oxprenolol**, the only β blockers demonstrating significant ISA, cause a smaller reduction in resting heart rate than the other β blockers and may cause less of the rebound phenomenon on withdrawal, but the clinical significance of these findings, if any, has not been adequately evaluated.

Nonspecific β Blockers

Propranolol (Inderal), **nadolol** (Corgard), **timolol** (Blocadren, Timoptic), **oxprenolol** (Trasicor), and **pindolol** (Visken) are all competitive blockers of both β_1 and β_2 receptors.

Propranolol is the oldest of these drugs and is approved for the greatest number of uses. All five drugs are used to treat hypertension. Part of their effectiveness in treating hypertension is attributable to their blockade of cardiac β_1 receptors and the resulting decrease in cardiac output, but other mechanisms of action are probably also involved. In some patients they may lower blood pressure by interfering with the release of renin; they may also act by actions (poorly understood) in the central nervous system.

Propranolol, which has significant membrane-stabilizing activity, is also used as an antiarrhythmic drug. Its effectiveness is probably dependent partly on its ability to block cardiac β_1 receptors and partly on its quinidine-like, local anesthetic, or membrane-stabilizing properties. **Oxprenolol** also has membrane-stabilizing activity but is not approved for antiarrhythmic use.

Propranolol and **nadolol** are used to treat angina. Angina is a syndrome in which cardiac oxygen demands exceed the ability of the coronary arteries to supply oxygen; myocardial ischemia and chest pain result. By blocking cardiac β_1 recep-

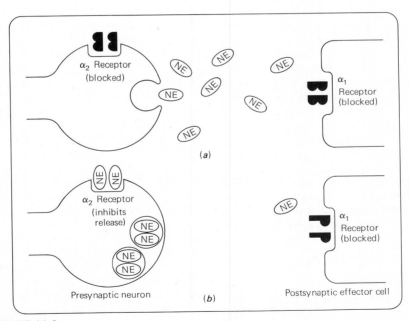

FIGURE 14-2

Schematic Representation of Blockade of α_1 and α_2 Adrenergic Receptors. (*a*) When a nonspecific α-blocking drug, such as phentolamine, blocks both α_1 and α_2 receptors, the following sequence occurs: decreased blood pressure → activation of baroreceptor reflexes → massive release of norepinephrine (NE) → intense reflex tachycardia. (*b*) With a specific α_1-blocking drug, such as prazosin, reflex tachycardia is absent or diminished because of negative feedback inhibition of NE release, which results when the α_2 receptor is free to be occupied by endogenous NE.

tors, these drugs decrease heart rate and decrease the force of ventricular contraction, thereby reducing cardiac oxygen demand. A vasodilator, such as nitroglycerin, and a β blocker are often given in combination to treat angina; they treat the angina by two different mechanisms, and the β blocker prevents the reflex tachycardia that the vasodilator might otherwise cause.

Propranolol is used in patients with pheochromocytoma to prevent tachycardia and cardiac arrhythmias. When propranolol is given to these patients, it is important to give an α blocker first, to prevent the reflex vasoconstriction and dangerous hypertension that could result from β blockade alone.

Timolol, metoprolol, and **propranolol** have been approved for use in patients whose condition has stabilized after myocardial infarction (MI). They have been found to decrease the likelihood of reinfarction and to decrease the mortality of post-MI patients. **Metoprolol** is used intravenously in the acute post-MI period to decrease the risk of sudden death.

Timolol is also used as an ophthalmic preparation (Timoptic) to treat open-angle glaucoma. Its mechanism of action in reducing intraocular pressure is not known.

Propranolol is also used prophylactically for migraine headaches. Many patients have found this drug effective in reducing the number of headaches they have; it appears to have a residual beneficial effect even after therapy is stopped. Both the mechanism of the beneficial effect and the mechanism of the residual effect are unexplained. Propranolol is not effective in *treating* migraine; it is effective only in preventing attacks. (A group of drugs, the ergot alkaloids, e.g., ergotamine and dihydroergotamine, are used both to treat and to prevent migraine. They have α adrenergic blocking activity, but they also cause vasoconstriction. Their mechanism of action in migraine is also unknown.)

Finally, **propranolol** has been found effective in decreasing the tremor and palpitations that often accompany both hyperthyroidism and anxiety. It prevents cardiac arrhythmias in hyperthyroid patients, whose hearts are especially sensitive to catecholamines. In patients with anxiety, it acts by unknown mechanisms to decrease the anxiety itself.

Because these drugs block β_2 receptors as well as β_1 receptors, they can cause wheezing and coughing in asthmatic and other chronic obstructive pulmonary disease (COPD) patients. Their cardiac depressant properties can lead to heart failure.

Cardioselective β_1 Blockers

Metoprolol (Lopressor) and **atenolol** (Tenormin) block β_1 receptors relatively selectively. They are thus less likely than the nonselective β blockers described above to cause bronchoconstriction. Both of these drugs are used to treat hypertension.

α and β Nonselective Blocker

Labetalol (Normodyne, Trandate) competitively inhibits both α and β receptors. It is used to treat hypertension. Labetalol has membrane-stabilizing properties but no intrinsic sympathomimetic activity. As a result of its nonselective blockade, it appears to cause less postural hypotension than pure α blockers and less bradycardia than pure β blockers.

Adrenergic Neuron-Blocking Drugs

These drugs are taken up into the sympathetic postganglionic neuron, where they interfere with one or more of the processes involved in the synthesis, storage, and release of norepinephrine from the nerve terminals.

Guanethidine and Guanadrel Guanethidine (Ismelin) and Guanadrel (Hylorel) initially impair the release of norepinephrine by nerve action potentials and then deplete the nerve terminal of norepinephrine by displacing it from storage granules. The displaced norepinephrine reaches the synaptic cleft and frequently causes transient sympathomimetic effects, such as increased blood pressure. With chronic therapy, guanethidine reduces blood pressure, its only clinical use. As expected, guanethidine decreases the sympathomimetic effects of indirect-acting sympathomimetic drugs (amphetamine, ephedrine), but neither guanethidine nor guanadrel decreases the central nervous system effects of these drugs because neither penetrates the blood-brain barrier to any significant extent.

Bretylium Bretylium (Bretylol) initially releases norepinephrine from sympathetic nerve terminals; therefore, like guanethidine, it may produce transient sympathomimetic effects. It then blocks the release of norepinephrine. Like guanethidine, it decreases the effectiveness of indirect-acting sympathomimetic drugs. It decreases blood pressure, but its main use is as an antiarrhythmic drug in ventricular fibrillation that has not responded to other therapy.

Reserpine Reserpine (Serpasil, others) is the prototype of the rauwolfia alkaloids, which deplete the brain and peripheral tissue of norepinephrine (and serotonin). Little norepinephrine is released from the nerve terminals by reserpine; therefore, unlike guanethidine and bretylium, reserpine produces little initial sympathomimetic effect. Reserpine

TABLE 14-3 Properties of β-Blocking Drugs

DRUG	ADRENERGIC RECEPTOR-BLOCKING ACTIVITY	INTRINSIC SYMPATHOMIMETIC ACTIVITY	MEMBRANE-STABILIZING ACTIVITY
Atenolol	β_1*	No	No
Metoprolol	β_1*	No	Slight
Nadolol	β_1, β_2	No	No
Oxprenolol	β_1, β_2	Yes	Yes
Pindolol	β_1, β_2	Yes	Slight
Propranolol	β_1, β_2	No	Yes
Timolol	β_1, β_2	No	No

*Blocks β_2 receptors at high doses.

has been used to treat hypertension and psychosis, but it is now rarely recommended for either indication. It produces many adverse effects attributable to actions in both the brain and the periphery.

Metyrosine   Metyrosine (Demser) is a new drug that inhibits the enzyme tyrosine hydroxylase, which converts the amino acid tyrosine to DOPA (see Fig. 10-8). It thus interferes with the synthesis of both norepinephrine and epinephrine (and dopamine). Its sole use is in the treatment of patients with pheochromocytoma.

Centrally Acting Depressants of Sympathetic Nervous System Outflow

Clonidine and Methyldopa   Clonidine (Catapres) and methyldopa (Aldomet) are both used to treat hypertension. The mechanism of action of these drugs is not known precisely, but evidence indicates that they act somehow in the brain to reduce sympathetic outflow to the cardiovascular system. Paradoxically, they are α adrenergic agonists; both drugs have been known to cause transient increases in blood pressure after an acute intravenous dose. Clonidine acts relatively selectively at α_2 receptors, as does the intraneuronal metabolite of methyldopa, α-methylnorepinephrine. The brainstem areas that control sympathetic outflow to the cardiovascular system are rich in norepinephrine-containing neurons and nerve terminals. These sites have been postulated to be the sites where these drugs act to reduce sympathetic outflow and blood pressure.

For further discussion of the uses of these drugs, as well as preparations available and dosage, see Chaps. 40, 43, and 45, on the cardiovascular disorders of high blood pressure, angina, and arrhythmias; Chap. 39, "Ophthalmologic Disorders"; and Chap. 33, "Neurologic Disorders."

ADVERSE EFFECTS OF SYMPATHOLYTIC DRUGS

Table 14-4 summarizes the most common adverse effects of sympatholytic drugs.

Many of these can be predicted from a knowledge of the mechanisms of action of the individual drugs, combined with an understanding of the normal physiologic functions that would be disrupted by these drugs' actions. For exam-

TABLE 14-4   Adverse Effects of Sympatholytic Drugs

ORGAN SYSTEM	EFFECT	SYMPATHOLYTIC DRUGS OR DRUG CLASSES CAUSING EFFECT
Cardiovascular	Bradycardia	β Blockers
	Decreased cardiac output	β Blockers
	Atrioventricular dissociation	β Blockers
	Cardiac arrhythmias	β Blockers
	Cardiac arrest	β Blockers
	Heart failure	β Blockers, guanethidine
	Reflex tachycardia	α Blockers
	Hypotension	α Blockers
	Postural hypotension	α Blockers, guanethidine, methyldopa
	Angina	α Blockers
Respiratory	Increased airway resistance	Nonselective β blockers*
	Bronchoconstriction	Nonselective β blockers*
	Asthmatic attack	Nonselective β blockers*
Digestive	Increased gastric acidity	α Blockers, reserpine
	Diarrhea	α Blockers, adrenergic neuron blockers, clonidine, methyldopa
Excretory	Sodium retention	α Blockers, β blockers, guanethidine, methyldopa, clonidine
Central nervous	Drowsiness	Phenoxybenzamine, reserpine, methyldopa, clonidine, metyrosine
	Depression, suicide	Phenoxybenzamine, propranolol, reserpine, methyldopa, clonidine
	Parkinsonism	Reserpine, methyldopa, metyrosine
	Hallucinations	Propranolol
	Insomnia	Propranolol
Other	Nasal congestion	α Blockers, adrenergic neuron blockers
	Male sexual dysfunction	Guanethidine, methyldopa, clonidine
	Sensitivity to insulin and blockade of hypoglycemic symptoms	β Blockers
	Drug fever and hepatic dysfunction	Methyldopa

*At higher doses, selective β_1 blockers will also cause these effects.

ple, drugs with β_1 receptor-blocking activity prevent impulses in sympathetic cardiac nerves from having their usual effects on the heart; therefore, they can cause bradycardia, decrease cardiac output, and even cause heart failure or cardiac arrest in sensitive patients. Some of these drugs cause sodium retention, which is at least partly secondary to cardiac depression and reduced renal blood flow. In diabetic patients and patients susceptible to attacks of hypoglycemia, **propranolol** increases insulin sensitivity (by blocking the β receptors that mediate glycogenolysis) and blocks the tachycardia that is a primary symptom of hypoglycemia. Drugs with β_2 receptor-blocking activity can increase airway resistance and cause breathing difficulty in sensitive patients. Many sympatholytic drugs, by interfering with sympathetic nervous system effects on the gastrointestinal tract, increase gastric acid secretion, increase intestinal motility, and cause diarrhea. These drugs can also interfere with male sexual function.

Some of the adverse effects are extensions of the desired therapeutic effects. For example, α receptor blockers and adrenergic neuron blockers, given to reduce the blood pressure of hypertensive patients, are likely to cause hypotension, especially *postural hypotension* (also called *orthostatic hypotension*) because they interfere with the reflex mechanisms (baroreceptor reflexes) that normally cause vasoconstriction when a person changes from a recumbent to a standing posture. Interference with normal vasoconstrictor tone causes another common adverse effect, nasal congestion.

Some sympatholytic drugs that penetrate the blood-brain barrier (**phenoxybenzamine, propranolol, reserpine, methyldopa, clonidine**) cause depression, possibly by interference with central neurotransmitter function, as well as other unwanted effects mediated by the central nervous system. The drug fever and hepatic dysfunction reported to result from **methyldopa** are apparently not related to the drug's sympatholytic actions.

NURSING PROCESS RELATED TO SYMPATHOLYTIC DRUGS

The varied mechanisms of action of the sympatholytic drugs and the wide range of specificities of these drugs make many aspects of the nursing care of patients on these drugs quite drug-specific. There are some general considerations, however, that should be incorporated into the nursing process for all patients on these drugs.

Assessment

Past History The sympatholytic drugs influence a wide range of autonomic effects. These effects are normally pro-

duced as a part of autonomic reflexes, with balances and controls. When the sympathetic reactions are blocked, normal controls and compensatory mechanisms no longer function. These effects can be uncomfortable or even life-threatening in patients with particular preestablished conditions. A careful patient history should be taken and related to the spectrum of effects of the individual sympatholytic drug. This can guide the nurse's teaching of the individual patient and can alert the nurse to the specific side effects the individual patient may experience. In addition, it can alert the nurse to the possibility that the particular sympatholytic drug may be contraindicated in that particular patient.

The following are relative or absolute contraindications to the use of some sympatholytic drugs.

Diabetes mellitus The nonselective β blockers increase insulin sensitivity by decreasing glycogenolysis. They also decrease the release of insulin in response to hyperglycemia. Thus, the dose of insulin or an oral hypoglycemic agent may need to be adjusted in the diabetic patient who is put on a β blocker. The β blockers also block all of the premonitory signs and symptoms of hypoglycemia (the sympathetic nervous system responses of increased heart rate, sweating, feelings of anxiety, etc.); therefore the patient will not have the usual warning signs, and blood glucose may fall dangerously low. If a β blocker must be given to a diabetic patient, atenolol is the one of choice, since it has few of these metabolic effects because of its receptor selectivity.

Chronic obstructive pulmonary disease The β blockers block bronchodilatation; this could be life-threatening in patients with obstructive or spastic bronchial diseases. Patients with seasonal asthma may also run into problems if bronchodilatation is blocked. Selective β_1 blockers are safer to use in these patients, but caution is still needed.

Congestive heart failure The compensatory mechanisms of the sympathetic nervous system protect the body in states of congestive heart failure. Blocking these reflex mechanisms can lead to severe cardiac failure and even death.

Angina or MI The reflex tachycardia caused by the α blockers can put increased demand on the heart muscle, resulting in angina in patients with compromised blood supply to the heart.

Physical Assessment Baseline functioning of the systems that would be most affected by interference with sympathetic nervous system function should be assessed before any of these drugs are given. In this way, the nurse will be able to accurately evaluate both the toxic and the therapeutic effects of the drugs.

This assessment should include mental status (orientation, affect), blood pressure (when supine, sitting, standing), apical pulse (rate, rhythm, presence of extra sounds), electrocardiogram (rate, pacing site, extra beats), respirations (rate, rhythm, character, adventitious sounds), and peripheral circulation (pulse, color, vascular filling). The policies of many institutions stipulate that *the apical pulse should be taken and recorded on the medication sheet prior to the administration of a β blocker.* In the presence of bradycardia (less than 50 to 60 beats/min) the drug is often withheld and the physician notified.

Management

Because of the wide spectrum of effects that these drugs have, patient teaching is a very important aspect of the management of patients on sympatholytics. Through careful teaching, the patient can learn to anticipate various side effects, learn ways to minimize discomfort, and be aware of when to notify the physician. Many of the sympatholytics cause CNS effects, such as dizziness, fatigue, nightmares, insomnia, mood changes, and especially depression. The patient should be alerted that they may occur. Often the dosage of the drug can be altered to alleviate some of these problems. Patients should be especially cautioned to avoid driving, or other tasks requiring alertness, while adjusting to the drug. **Prazosin** causes a "first dose effect" which frequently leads to severe postural hypotension and fainting. Patients starting on prazosin need to be extremely careful for the first 4 h after taking the drug; many people, therefore, would do best to start it at bedtime.

The loss of vasoconstrictor tone caused by these drugs frequently leads to nasal congestion or "stuffiness." This is a very annoying side effect that can be alleviated somewhat through the correct use of a saline nasal solution or nasal decongestant. Patients must be cautioned to avoid the use of oral over-the-counter cold, allergy, or cough medications, most of which contain sympathomimetics.

Patients must be taught not to discontinue taking their β-blocking drugs except with a physician's direction. Sudden stoppage of these drugs can cause a sympathetic rebound response, which can result in severe tachycardia, MI, or even death. The exact cause of this rebound is not clear, but patients should be tapered from their drugs over a 1- to 2-week period.

Patients should be taught to change position slowly, since many of these drugs have the effect of causing orthostatic hypotension. When rising from a supine position, the patient should sit first, with legs dangling, and then rise to standing with a support. A fine point the patient should remember is that rising from a squatting position (as in gardening or picking things up from the floor) could cause severe hypotension, as blood is trapped in the legs and autonomic reflexes are very slow. Hospitalized patients on sympatholytics should have safety precautions provided for them.

Male impotence is a side effect that is common with many of the sympatholytics (**propranolol, metoprolol, pindolol, guanethidine, clonidine, prazosin**). This side effect can be devastating to patients, and they will need support and understanding to deal with it.

Diabetics who must be given β-blocking drugs will need to have thorough teaching and will need to learn new ways to recognize hypoglycemia.

Propranolol and **metoprolol** should be taken with meals, to increase their absorption.

Patients should learn to recognize and report the signs and symptoms of congestive heart failure (difficulty breathing at night, shortness of breath with activity, swelling of the ankles or legs). They should also learn to take their pulses and blood pressures, if they are capable. Monitoring these parameters will involve them in their own care and alert them to toxic effects at an early stage so that corrective action can be taken.

Evaluation

The patient needs to be evaluated for therapeutic effectiveness of the drug. Blood pressure should be monitored frequently. Sitting and standing blood pressure readings should be done periodically to evaluate orthostatic changes. The patient should be monitored for signs of congestive heart failure—weight gain, intake-output disproportion, edema, rales, S_3—and corrective action should be taken immediately if any of these occur.

Over time, the nurse should be alert to behavioral changes in the patient. Bad dreams, hallucinations, or mood swings often precede the severe depression that can occur.

General anesthesia is contraindicated for these patients, since the blockage of their normal sympathetic response to stress prevents the compensatory mechanisms necessary to keep them alive during anesthesia. Patients should be tapered from the drugs before surgery. The patients' charts should clearly note the use of these drugs. If emergency surgery is required, **isoproterenol, nerepinephrine,** or **dopamine** can be given to reverse the effects of the sympatholytic drug. The patient must, however, be carefully monitored.

Overall, the patient should be evaluated for the possible occurrence of drug-drug interactions. Beta blockers are contraindicated with adrenergic-augmenting psychotropic drugs (such as **monoamine oxidase inhibitors** and **tricyclic antidepressants**). **Aminophylline** and β blockers are physiologically antagonistic, and the effectiveness of both is diminished. Propranolol plasma levels, and therefore propranolol effects, are increased in the presence of **chlorpromazine, cimetidine, furosemide,** and **hydralazine.** Any of the sympatholytics given with any catecholamine-depleting drugs (e.g., **reserpine**) can cause severe loss of sympathetic tone and cardiovascular collapse.

Each drug of this group should be checked individually for additional contraindications, side effects, or drug-drug interactions.

REFERENCES

Dukes, M. N. G.: *Meyler's Side Effects of Drugs Annual,* vol. 5, Princeton: Excerpta Medica, 1980.

Freshman, W. H.: *Clinical Pharmacology of the Beta Adrenergic Blocking Drugs,* New York: Appleton-Century-Crofts, 1980.

Kastrup, E. K. (ed.): *Facts and Comparisons,* Philadelphia: Lippincott, 1983.

Norwegian Multicenter Study Group: "Timolol-Induced Reduction in Mortality and Reinfarction in Patients Surviving Acute Myocardial Infarction," *N Engl J Med,* 304:801–804, 1981.

Wiener, N.: "Drugs That Inhibit Adrenergic Nerves and Block Adrenergic Receptors," in A. G. Gilman, L. S. Goodman, and A. Gilman (eds.), *Goodman and Gilman's The Pharmacological Basis of Therapeutics,* 6th ed., New York: Macmillan, 1980.

15

GANGLIONIC BLOCKING DRUGS

ELEANOR H. BOYD
AMY M. KARCH

LEARNING OBJECTIVES

Upon mastery of the contents of this chapter, the reader will be able to:

1. Explain why ganglionic blocking drugs are infrequently used therapeutically.

2. List three therapeutic uses of ganglionic blocking drugs.

3. List five adverse effects of ganglionic blocking drugs and a nursing intervention to mitigate each.

4. State one nursing activity for each step of the nursing process applicable to patients using ganglionic blocking drugs.

MECHANISMS OF ACTION OF GANGLIONIC DRUGS

Ganglionic Agonists

Acetylcholine is the neurotransmitter in all autonomic ganglia. Both sympathetic and parasympathetic preganglionic axons release acetylcholine, which stimulates postganglionic neurons and causes cells in the adrenal medulla to release epinephrine and norepinephrine into the circulation. Cholinergic receptors in ganglia and in the adrenal medulla are nicotinic (see Chap. 10). This means that the actions of acetylcholine on these receptors are like the actions of nicotine, the alkaloid contained in tobacco. Low doses of both acetylcholine and nicotine stimulate nicotinic receptors, but high doses of both block synaptic transmission. Nicotine and acetylcholine have no therapeutic usefulness as ganglionic drugs because of the great variety of effects they produce, representing parasympathomimetic and sympathomimetic actions at low doses, and parasympatholytic and sympatholytic actions at high doses.

Nicotine

Nicotine, which is self-administered by people who smoke tobacco, produces a variety of effects that are especially deleterious in patients with cardiovascular and peptic ulcer diseases. The predominant effects of the nicotine absorbed by smokers are increased heart rate and vasoconstriction (from stimulation of sympathetic ganglia and the release of adrenal catecholamines) and increased gastrointestinal motility and secretions (from stimulation of parasympathetic ganglia). The cardiovascular effects can increase blood pressure, aggravate peripheral vascular disease, increase cardiac work, and cause angina. Nicotine also acts at peripheral chemoreceptors and in the central nervous system. The chronic effects of nicotine and tobacco smoking are presented in greater detail in Chap. 49, "Community Health Nursing."

Ganglionic Blocking Drugs

The therapeutically useful drugs that act at autonomic ganglia *block* autonomic ganglia and are called *ganglionic blocking drugs*. They do not have acetylcholine- or nicotine-like effects on ganglionic transmission. They block transmission without causing initial stimulation. The block is of the competitive type; that is, these drugs combine with nicotine receptors in the ganglia and block the effects of acetylcholine released from preganglionic neurons. These drugs block both parasympathetic and sympathetic ganglia, as well as transmission of sympathetic preganglionic impulses to the cells of the adrenal medulla (see Fig. 15-1). Therefore, these drugs produce a great variety of effects; they affect virtually all aspects of autonomic function.

CLINICAL USES OF GANGLIONIC BLOCKING DRUGS

Because of their widespread actions, the ganglionic blocking drugs have very limited therapeutic usefulness. Their only therapeutically useful effect is reduction of blood pressure,

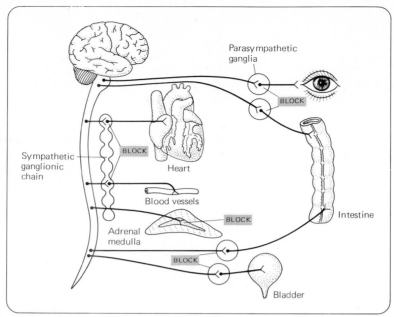

FIGURE 15-1

Sites of Ganglionic Blockade. Ganglionic blocking drugs block sympathetic and parasympathetic ganglia and sympathetic preganglionic transmission to the adrenal medulla, affecting numerous organs.

which occurs as a result of the blockade of transmission in sympathetic ganglia, which in turn blocks sympathetic vasoconstrictor tone. Blockade of the release of catecholamines from the adrenal medulla also contributes to the reduction of blood pressure. Ganglionic blocking drugs are used for initial blood pressure reduction with acute dissecting aortic aneurysms; they are also used in patients with autonomic hyperreflexia, a syndrome of excessive sympathetic discharge and high blood pressure that occurs mainly after upper spinal cord injuries. These drugs are also sometimes used to produce a controlled lowering of blood pressure to reduce the risk of hemorrhage during neurosurgery or cardiovascular surgery. Oral preparations are rarely used to treat severe essential hypertension and malignant hypertension.

SPECIFIC GANGLIONIC DRUGS

Hexamethonium is the prototype of ganglionic blocking drugs, but it is no longer used. In the United States, only **trimethaphan** and **mecamylamine** are approved ganglionic blocking drugs (see Table 15-1). Ganglionic blocking drugs still used in other parts of the world include **chlorisondamine, pempidine, pentolinium,** and **tetraethylammonium.**

Trimethaphan Camsylate   Trimethaphan camsylate (Arfonad) is available only for intravenous use. It is used for all the emergency situations described above, and during

surgery. It has a rapid onset of action but a short duration and must be infused continuously to maintain effectiveness. Tolerance may develop with prolonged use, because it can cause a sodium and water retention that negates the blood pressure–lowering effects of ganglionic blockade. Because of this, diuretics are sometimes added to the drug regimen, to prolong the efficacy of the drug.

Mecamylamine Hydrochloride   Mecamylamine hydrochloride (Inversine) is available for oral administration in tablet form. It is thus suitable for chronic administration in patients whose hypertension cannot be controlled by other antihypertensive drugs. This drug causes a very high incidence of orthostatic hypotension and constipation, which limits its usefulness.

TABLE 15-1   Ganglionic Blocking Drugs

DRUG	USUAL DOSAGE
Trimethaphan camsylate (Arfonad)	Intravenous drip of 0.3 to 6 mg/min, based on blood pressure response.
Mecamylamine hydrochloride (Inversine)	Beginning oral dosage of 2.5 mg twice daily; adjust as required to achieve desired blood pressure, but no more frequently than every 2 days. Average maintenance dose is 25 mg/day in three to four divided doses.

ADVERSE EFFECTS OF GANGLIONIC BLOCKING DRUGS

Ganglionic blocking drugs produce many adverse effects; essentially all of these are attributable to blockade of sympathetic or parasympathetic ganglia. The effect on an organ depends to a great extent on whether the sympathetic or the parasympathetic nervous system provides the dominant tone to that organ (see Chap. 10). The therapeutic effect of lowering blood pressure results from the reduction of sympathetic vasoconstrictor tone. Two very common adverse effects of these drugs, hypotension and orthostatic (or postural) hypotension, are extensions of this therapeutic effect.

The sympathetic nervous system also provides tone to the sweat glands (sympathetic cholinergic nerves). Blockade of sympathetic ganglia thus causes decreased sweating (*anhidrosis*).

The parasympathetic nervous system usually provides tone to the heart, the gastrointestinal tract, the urinary bladder, and the ciliary muscle and iris of the eye. Thus, ganglionic blocking drugs produce atropine-like effects on these organs.

Table 15-2 lists the most common adverse effects of ganglionic blocking drugs. The picture of an individual ("the hexamethonium man") who has been receiving a ganglionic blocking drug has been vividly portrayed by the British pharmacologist, Sir William Paton:

He is a pink complexioned person, except when he has stood in a queue for a long time, when he may get pale and faint. His handshake is warm and dry. He is a placid and relaxed companion; for instance he may laugh, but he can't cry because the tears cannot come. Your rudest story will not make him blush, and the most unpleasant circumstances will fail to make him turn pale. His collars and socks stay very clean and sweet. He wears corsets and may, if you meet him out, be rather fidgety (corsets to compress his splanchnic vascular pool, fidgety to keep the venous return going from his legs). He dislikes speaking much unless helped with something to moisten his dry mouth and throat. He is longsighted and easily blinded by bright light. The redness of his eyeballs may suggest irregular habits and in fact his head is rather weak. But he always behaves like a gentleman and never belches nor hiccups. He tends to get cold and keeps well wrapped up. But his health is good; he does not have chilblains and those diseases of modern civilization, hypertension and peptic ulcer, pass him by. He is thin because his appetite is modest; he never feels hunger pains and his stomach never rumbles. He gets rather constipated so that his intake of liquid paraffin is high. As old age comes on, he will suffer from retention of urine and impotence, but frequency, precipitancy, and strangury will not worry him. One is uncertain how he will end, but perhaps if he is not careful, by eating less and less and getting colder and colder, he will sink into a symptomless, hypoglycemic coma and die, as was proposed for the universe, a sort of entropy death. [*Scientific Basis of Medicine*][1]

TABLE 15-2   Adverse Effects of Ganglionic Blocking Drugs

ORGAN SYSTEM	EFFECT
Cardiovascular	
Heart	Increased heart rate (tachycardia)
Blood vessels	Vasodilatation
	Decreased blood pressure
	Orthostatic hypotension
Gastrointestinal	Decreased motility
	Decreased tone
	Constipation
	Paralytic ileus
Excretory (urinary bladder)	Urinary retention
Miscellaneous	
Salivary glands	Decreased production of saliva
	Dry mouth (xerostomia)
Sweat glands	Decreased production of sweat (anhidrosis)
Eye	Dilated pupils (mydriasis)
	Blurred vision (cycloplegia)
Male sexual function	Impotence

NURSING PROCESS RELATED TO GANGLIONIC BLOCKING DRUGS

The ganglionic stimulating/blocking agent nicotine is widely used in this country in the form of tobacco products, which introduce nicotine into the bloodstream. This practice has social, psychologic, and environmental implications beyond the physiologic response of the body. The role of the nurse in this arena of health teaching and preventive measures is covered in Chap. 49, "Community Health Nursing."

The only other use for the ganglionic blockers is in the treatment of severe hypertension or hypertensive emergencies. The side effects that the drugs produce include diverse responses of the autonomic nervous system, and nursing care should be directed at managing these responses.

[1]Used by permission of Professor Sir William Paton, CBE, FRS, and of the British Postgraduate Medical Federation.

Assessment

Past History A careful patient history should be taken, to rule out the presence of any preexisting condition that could be further compromised by the profound decrease in blood pressure caused by these drugs. Such conditions include coronary insufficiency, renal insufficiency, and cerebrovascular insufficiency.

Physical Assessment Baseline functioning of all of the systems affected by the ganglionic blocking agents should be assessed before these drugs are given. In the hypertensive emergency, these will be reevaluated constantly for any sign of toxic changes.

This assessment should include mental status (orientation), neurologic status (pupil reactivity, vision, handgrip) blood pressure (when supine, standing, sitting) electrocardiogram (rate, rhythm), respirations (rate, character, adventitious sounds), peripheral circulation (sensation, pulses, color, vascular filling), and gastrointestinal status (bowel sounds).

Management

Care of the patient in hypertensive crisis is covered in Chap. 40. Patients receiving chronic therapy with ganglionic blockers can anticipate many of the side effects exhibited by the "hexamethonium man." Nursing management should be directed at advising the patient to anticipate and deal with these effects. Since these effects are those of parasym-pathetic and sympathetic block, the measures described in Chaps. 12 and 14 for controlling adverse effects are appropriate for patients on ganglionic blocking drugs.

The loss of the ability to sweat can be a problem for the very young or for the older patient who has diminished ability to control body temperature and who relies on sweating to dissipate body heat. The patient should be advised to avoid extremes of temperature and should be monitored very closely if a fever develops.

The oral ganglionic blocker, mecamylamine, is readily absorbed. It should be taken after meals, to slow its absorption and provide a more constant blood level.

The patient must be taught never to discontinue the medication suddenly. Abrupt termination of the ganglionic blockade could result in a sudden return to the hypertensive level; stroke, myocardial infarction, or severe congestive heart failure could result.

Evaluation

The patient should receive ongoing evaluation for the therapeutic effectiveness of the drug. The patient should also be assessed for the occurrence of the anticipated adverse effects; dosage may need to be adjusted to minimize adverse reactions. Alcohol can potentiate the action of mecamylamine, and severe hypotension can result. Any sympathomimetic drug can decrease the therapeutic effects of the ganglionic blocking drugs while potentiating some of the adverse effects and should be avoided.

REFERENCES

Kastrup, E. K. (ed.): *Facts and Comparisons,* Philadelphia: Lippincott, 1983.

Paton, W. D. M.: "The Principles of Ganglionic Block," *Scientific Basis of Medicine,* vol. 2, London: Athlone Press, 1952–1953.

Salem, M. R.: "Therapeutic Uses of Ganglionic Blocking Drugs," *Int Anesthesiol Clin,* **16**:171, 1978.

Taylor, P.: "Ganglionic Stimulating and Blocking Agents," in A. G. Gilman, L. S. Goodman, and A. Gilman (eds.), *Goodman and Gilman's The Pharmacological Basis of Therapeutics,* 6th ed., New York: Macmillan, 1980.

Volle, R. L.: "Ganglionic Transmission," *Annu Rev Pharmacol,* **6**:135, 1969.

16

NEUROMUSCULAR JUNCTION BLOCKING DRUGS

ELEANOR H. BOYD
AMY M. KARCH

LEARNING OBJECTIVES

Upon mastery of the contents of this chapter, the reader will be able to:

1. Distinguish between neuromuscular junction blocking drugs, centrally acting skeletal muscle relaxants, and antispasmodics with respect to mechanisms of action, effects, and uses.

2. Describe the two different mechanisms by which neuromuscular junction blocking drugs act.

3. Predict the initial effect of administration of succinylcholine.

4. Given the name of a neuromuscular junction blocking drug, state whether a cholinesterase inhibitor would or would not be effective in reversing the drug's effects at the neuromuscular junction.

5. Describe three mechanisms by which tubocurarine can lower blood pressure.

6. List three parameters for assessing or evaluating patients in the preoperative and postoperative periods when they are using neuromuscular blocking agents.

MECHANISMS OF ACTION

Neuromuscular junction blocking drugs act by one of two mechanisms to produce paralysis and relaxation of skeletal muscles (see Fig. 16-1). One group of drugs, called *competitive blockers* or *nondepolarizing blockers,* compete with molecules of acetylcholine for cholinergic receptors at the neuromuscular junction. Competitive blockers occupy these receptors without initiating skeletal muscle contraction. They prevent the acetylcholine that is released by motor nerve terminals from occupying and activating the cholinergic receptors. Their neuromuscular junction blocking actions may be overcome by a cholinesterase inhibitor, such as **neostigmine** or **edrophonium.** Cholinesterase inhibitors prevent the enzymatic degradation of acetylcholine and thereby increase the amount of acetylcholine available to compete with the neuromuscular junction blockers.

The second group of neuromuscular junction blocking drugs, called *depolarizing blockers,* occupy cholinergic receptors at the neuromuscular junction, initially mimicking acetylcholine and causing skeletal muscle depolarization and contraction, and then blocking neuromuscular transmission. The mechanism of the neuromuscular block is not yet fully understood, but it differs from the block produced by the competitive, nondepolarizing, curare-like drugs in that it is *not* overcome by cholinesterase inhibitors.

Neuromuscular junction blocking drugs must not be confused with two other classes of drugs, namely, *centrally acting skeletal muscle relaxants*[1] and *antispasmodics.* Neuromuscular junction blockers act at the synaptic level to cause a flaccid paralysis of all skeletal muscles. The centrally acting skeletal muscle relaxants are used to treat skeletal muscle spasticity caused by injury (spinal cord transection) or disease (multiple sclerosis). They act at various sites in the brain and/or spinal cord to decrease impulses in motor nerves, causing reduced muscle spasm rather than skeletal muscle paralysis. (See Chap. 33, "Neurologic Disorders.") The antispasmodics are parasympathetic blocking drugs; they are essentially devoid of direct or indirect effects on

---

[1]The class of drugs called centrally acting skeletal muscle relaxants includes **baclofen** (Lioresal), **cyclobenzaprine** (Flexeril), the benzodiazepine **diazepam** (Valium), **carisoprodol** (Soma), **methocarbamol** (Robaxin), **orphenadrine** (Norflex), and other drugs. **Dantrolene** (Dantrium) is usually described with these drugs, although it acts *directly* on skeletal muscle, not in the central nervous system, to reduce skeletal muscle spasticity.

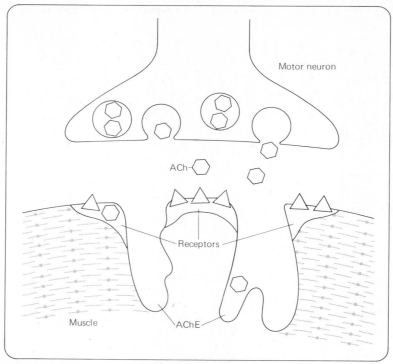

FIGURE 16-1

Mechanisms of Action of Neuromuscular Blockers. Schematic representation of the site of action of neuromuscular blocking drugs (△) at the myoneural junction. Nondepolarizing neuromuscular junction blocking drugs compete with endogenous acetylcholine (○) for receptor sites, to cause a flaccid paralysis, which can be reversed by acetylcholinesterase (AChE) inhibitors. Inhibition of AChE, located in invaginations of the motor end plate, increases the amount of acetylcholine competing with the drug and will reverse the paralysis. Depolarizing neuromuscular junction blocking drugs occupy the same sites noncompetitively and cause contraction of the muscle fibers.

skeletal muscle; they are used to treat spasms of gastrointestinal *smooth* muscle (see Chap. 12 and Table 12-1).

USES OF NEUROMUSCULAR JUNCTION BLOCKING DRUGS

These drugs are used mainly in conjunction with general anesthetic agents, in preparation for and during surgery. Some general anesthetics (e.g., **diethyl ether, cyclopropane,** and **enflurane** produce a significant degree of skeletal muscle relaxation by themselves, but others (e.g., **nitrous oxide, methoxyflurane,** and **thiopental** do not produce significant degrees of skeletal muscle relaxation, or they produce relaxation only at high concentrations which severely depress the cardiovascular and respiratory systems. Skeletal muscle relaxation is essential for many intraabdominal procedures and for the alignment of fractures and the repositioning of dislocations. Neuromuscular junction blocking drugs are given intravenously after the administration of the general anesthetic has begun and the patient has become uncon-

scious. A neuromuscular blocker may also be given to facilitate endotracheal intubation. The uses and dosages of these agents are discussed in Chap. 47, "Surgery: Drugs Used in Perioperative Care."

A short-acting neuromuscular blocker such as succinylcholine is sometimes given, along with a short-acting general anesthetic such as **thiopental**, prior to the administration of electroconvulsive therapy (ECT) to psychiatric patients. The therapeutic benefits of ECT do not depend on the grand mal convulsions that might otherwise occur, and by preventing the convulsions, **succinylcholine** also prevents fractures and other injuries.

Neuromuscular junction blockers are also used to prevent the severe and painful muscle contractions of tetanus or to prevent the convulsions caused by convulsant drugs such as **strychnine, pentylenetetrazol,** or **doxapram.** If untreated, the skeletal muscle contractions of tetanus, or those caused by convulsant drugs, may be not only painful but also life-threatening, since they can interfere with respiration and make artificial respiration ineffectual or impossible. When neuromuscular junction blockers are given in tetanus, the respiratory muscles (intercostal muscles and the diaphragm) are paralyzed and artificial respiration is essential to life. These patients are not anesthetized, and the neuromuscular junction blockers neither impair the patients' consciousness nor interfere with pain perception, but the patients are totally unable to respond by voice, eyes, or movements of any kind.

SPECIFIC NEUROMUSCULAR JUNCTION BLOCKING DRUGS

The drugs are listed, according to their mechanism of action, in Table 16-1. These drugs block rather selectively the nicotinic receptors at the neuromuscular junction, but some can also block, or stimulate, nicotinic receptors in autonomic ganglia.

The competitive blockers differ in several important ways from the depolarizing blockers; they differ in the initial effects they produce and in some of their interactions with other drugs. The treatment of patients who have received an overdose is also different for the two groups of drugs. Within the groups the individual competitive blockers and depolarizing blockers differ mainly in the adverse effects they produce and in their durations of action.

TABLE 16-1   Classification of Neuromuscular Junction Blocking Drugs According to Their Mechanism of Action

Competitive (nondepolarizing) blockers
  Curare derivatives
    Tubocurarine chloride
    Metocurine iodide (Metubine Iodide, a synthetic derivative)
  Synthetic drugs
    Gallamine triethiodide (Flaxedil)
    Pancuronium bromide (Pavulon)
    Atracurium besylate (Tracrium)†
    Vecuronium bromide (Norcuron)†
    Alcuronium chloride* (Alloferin)
    Fazadinium bromide*†

Depolarizing blockers
  Succinylcholine chloride (Anectine, Quelicin, Sucostrin, Sux-Cert)
  Decamethonium bromide (Syncurine)

Adjunct to succinylcholine
  Hexafluorenium bromide (Mylaxen; an inhibitor of plasma pseudocholinesterase and a weak competitive neuromuscular junction blocker)

*Not available in the United States.
†Significant portions of the drug are metabolized prior to elimination, so decreased renal function does not prolong recovery time.

Competitive, Nondepolarizing Neuromuscular Junction Blocking Drugs

These drugs cause an initial weakness of skeletal muscle that progresses rapidly to flaccid paralysis. Their neuromuscular junction blocking effects can be terminated by a cholinesterase inhibitor (**edrophonium** or **neostigmine**). Cholinesterase inhibitors (e. g., **physostigmine**) are sometimes administered when the duration of the neuromuscular block exceeds the duration of the surgery. The actions of **tubocurarine, metocurine iodide, gallamine,** and **pancuronium** are terminated largely by renal excretion, but nonrenal elimination is important for **atacurium** and **vecuronium**.

Tubocurarine   Tubocurarine chloride is a curare derivative. *Curare* is an arrow poison used for centuries by some South American Indians in hunting wild animals for food. An arrow tip inoculated with curare will paralyze and bring down the animals without making them unsafe to eat, since curare and the neuromuscular junction blocking drugs are ineffective orally.

Tubocurarine is one of the neuromuscular blockers that also causes some blockade of autonomic ganglia. Blockade of sympathetic ganglia and the adrenal medulla contributes to the lowering of blood pressure often produced by this drug. Secondary to the loss of skeletal muscle tone, pooling of blood in the legs may occur and can also contribute to hypotension.

Tubocurarine also releases histamine from mast cells. Histamine causes vasodilatation, which further lowers blood pressure. In addition, histamine can cause bronchoconstriction and stimulate bronchial and salivary secretions in sensitive individuals, such as those with a history of asthma. Tubocurarine is contraindicated in these patients for this reason.

Metocurine Iodide   Metocurine iodide (Metubine iodide) is a synthetic curare-like drug that causes less ganglionic blockade and less histamine release than tubocurarine. Like gallamine (see below), it is contraindicated in patients who are sensitive to iodine; both of these drugs are iodine salts.

Other Nondepolarizing Blockers   **Gallamine triethiodide** (Flaxedil) blocks vagal influences on the heart, thereby causing tachycardia and occasional cardiac arrhythmias. **Pancuronium bromide** (Pavulon) causes fewer autonomic side effects than some of the other competitive neuromuscular junction blocking drugs. **Atracurium besylate** (Tracrium) and **vecuronium bromide** (Norcuron) are intermediate-acting agents with a duration of action of one-third to one-half that of other nondepolarizing neuromuscular blockers at initially equipotent doses. Atracurium causes some histamine release, resulting in hypotension or bronchoconstriction in a small percentage of patients.

Depolarizing Neuromuscular Junction Blocking Drugs

These drugs differ from the competitive blockers in that they cause muscle fasciculations before they induce flaccid paralysis. These muscle contractions can be quite prominent, can release appreciable amounts of potassium into the circulation, and can sometimes cause muscle soreness postoperatively. The neuromuscular junction blocking effects of the depolarizing blockers are *not* overcome by cholinesterase inhibitors; cholinesterase inhibitors such as **neostigmine** and **edrophonium** should *not* be administered with these drugs, as they might increase the paralysis. Prolonged apnea produced by these drugs must be treated supportively by artificial respiration. Except for **succinylcholine** the effect of depolarizing blockers is terminated by renal excretion.

Succinylcholine Chloride Succinylcholine (Anectine) is a very short acting neuromuscular junction blocker. It is frequently used for brief surgical and diagnostic procedures. Its short duration of action is due to its rapid metabolism by pseudocholinesterases in the plasma and liver. Some patients show prolonged apnea after succinylcholine; many, but not all, of these patients have a genetically determined deficiency in the drug-metabolizing enzymes, or they have hepatic disease.

Hexafluorenium bromide (Mylaxen) is sometimes administered with succinlycholine to prevent the initial muscle fasciculations. Hexafluorenium is a weak competitive neuromuscular junction blocker. Hexafluorenium is also sometimes used to prolong the duration of action of succinylcholine; it inhibits selectively plasma pseudocholinesterase, thereby decreasing the rate at which succinylcholine is enzymatically degraded.

Succinylcholine can cause ganglionic stimulation, which, in turn, can cause hypertension and either tachycardia or bradycardia, depending on whether sympathetic or parasympathetic ganglia are more stimulated. Succinylcholine can release histamine, but this effect is less likely than with tubocurarine.

Decamethonium Bromide Decamethonium bromide (Syncurine) is rarely used now because it is long-acting. A competitive neuromuscular junction blocker, whose actions can be overcome by a cholinesterase inhibitor. is usually preferred when a long-acting blocker is needed.

NURSING PROCESS RELATED TO NEUROMUSCULAR JUNCTION BLOCKING DRUGS

The neuromuscular junction blocking drugs are administered by physicians or nurse anesthetists in acute care areas where ventilatory assistance and life support systems are readily available. Supportive nursing care is an essential aspect of the management of patients who receive these drugs.

Assessment

Past History A careful patient history should be taken, to rule out the presence of any preexisting condition which could be further compromised by the use of these drugs.

Chronic obstructive pulmonary diseases (COPD) Some neuromuscular junction blockers release histamine, which causes bronchoconstriction and increases bronchial secretions; these actions can cause severe exacerbations of disease in these patients.

Renal disease Since most of these drugs are excreted through the kidney, alteration in renal function can lead to prolonged and possibly life-threatening effects of the drug.

Physical Assessment A careful assessment of the patient's baseline functioning is essential for establishing the criteria necessary for monitoring patient care. The assessment should include neurologic status (cranial nerves, pupillary reflex), respirations (rate, rhythm, adventitious sounds), cardiovascular status (blood pressure, pulse rate, rhythm), and laboratory values (K^+ level, pH).

Management

Most of the nursing care of patients receiving neuromuscular junction blocking agents incorporates standard preoperative and postoperative procedures. Maintenance of respiration is a primary concern with these patients, and ventilatory support should be maintained until it is certain that the effects of the drugs have terminated. Relatives of those with known pseudocholinesterase deficiency will be tested prior to receiving succinylcholine, but screening the general population to determine who has this genetically determined condition is not practical, so all patients should be closely watched after receiving this drug for signs of prolonged paralysis.

Other patient conditions which lead to increased effectiveness of neuromuscular junction blocking agents include hypokalemia (secondary to thiazide diuretics, diarrhea, etc.); acidosis (secondary to ventilatory problems, diet, metabolic disorders); parenteral use of or irrigation of the surgical site with antibiotics (**aminoglycosides, bacitracin, polymyxin B, colistin,** and **tetracyclines**); and concurrent use of **quinine, quinidine, calcium** and **magnesium salts, propranolol, trimethaphan,** or certain inhalation anesthetics (**halothane, diethyl ether, methoxyflurane**). If a patient with any of the above conditions or drug histories is to receive a neuromuscular blocking agent, the condition should be documented and it should be clearly noted on the patient's chart or anesthesia flow chart. These patients will have to be monitored carefully for an extended period of time to assure that the effects of the drug have terminated.

Patients who are to receive a depolarizing agent should be alerted before the procedure that discomfort may be expected in the back, neck, and pharnyx because of the intense muscle contraction that may precede the paralysis. Massage, local heat, analgesics (e.g., aspirin), and proper positioning may help to relieve the discomfort.

It is very important to provide emotional and supportive care to patients, such as those with tetanus, who are receiving neuromuscular blocking agents without general anesthesia. These patients will need reassurance and pain control measures. As a patient advocate, the nurse will need to monitor what is said around these patients as well as to apprise the patients of procedures and activities to be done around them.

Evaluation

The patient will need to be constantly evaluated for evidence of the therapeutic effects of the drug. The flaccid muscle paralysis can be evaluated through peripheral and central neurologic examination. **Edrophonium** or **neostigmine** should be available for use in cases of severe and prolonged paralysis from the competitive blockers. The patient should also be evaluated for the need of supportive ventilation, suctioning, etc., until the full effects of the drug have terminated. Other side effects that can occur and should be watched for include arrhythmias and decreases in blood pressure, both of which may be severe and potentially life-threatening.

REFERENCES

Feldman, S.: *Muscle Relaxants,* New York: Elsevier/North-Holland, 1975.

Kastrup, E. K. (ed.): *Facts and Comparisons,* Philadelphia: Lippincott, 1983.

Taylor, P.: "Neuromuscular Blocking Agents," in A. G. Gilman, L. S. Goodman, and A. Gilman (eds.), *Goodman and Gilman's The Pharmacological Basis of Therapeutics,* 6th ed., New York: Macmillan, 1980.

Waud, B. E., and D. R. Waud: "Physiology and Pharmacology of Neuromuscular Blocking Agents," in R. L. Katz (ed.), *Muscle Relaxants,* Princeton: Excerpta Medica, 1975.

UNIT IV

CLINICAL PHARMACOLOGY & THERAPEUTICS OF COMMON MANIFESTATIONS OF DISEASES

PAIN*

ARTHUR G. LIPMAN
KATHLEEN MOONEY

LEARNING OBJECTIVES

Upon mastery of the content of this chapter, the student will be able to:

1. Define pain.
2. Explain the impact of pain theories on clinical practice.
3. Describe two major components of pain in terms of nociception, discrimination, affective-motivational influences, and cognitive aspects.
4. Explain the anatomy of referred pain and of affective influences on pain transmission.
5. Outline hypotheses about the functions of endorphins in pain perception.
6. Compare cutaneous, deep somatic, and visceral pain relative to origin, initiating mechanisms, effective analgesics, and likelihood of eliciting referred pain.
7. Differentiate acute and chronic pain syndromes on the basis of causes, endorphin response, dominant affect, and treatment.
8. Outline the assessment of pain, including both perceptive and reactive components.
9. Describe basic comfort measures for acute pain relief for children and adults.
10. Compare the effectiveness of aspirin to that of other analgesics and the nonsteroidal anti-inflammatory drugs.
11. Compare the mechanism and activity of nonsteroidal anti-inflammatory agents and acetaminophen.
12. Describe two components of an allergic reaction to aspirin.
13. Describe the clinical manifestations of acute and chronic salicylate intoxication and acute acetaminophen intoxication.
14. List five contraindications to the use of aspirin and the adverse effects of aspirin.
15. Describe the effect of dose and urine pH on aspirin pharmacokinetics.
16. State the indications for acetaminophen.
17. Describe the mechanism of action of narcotic analgesics.
18. Identify one nursing consideration when administering narcotics for each of the following systems: respiratory, gastrointestinal, cardiovascular, genitourinary, and neurologic.
19. Describe the reason for there being different oral-to-parenteral dose ratios for intermittently used (PRN) and regularly scheduled morphine sulfate.
20. Compare the agonist-antagonist analgesics to the pure agonist narcotics relative to efficacy and adverse effects.
21. Describe the efficacy of and precautions associated with propoxyphene.
22. Name the major narcotic antagonist drug.
23. Describe the pharmacologic and nonpharmacologic management of chronic pain.
24. Write a plan for evaluating pharmacologic management of pain.

Pain is one of the most common complaints for which patients seek professional health care. While pain has been the subject of treatises by philosophers, physiologists, and psychologists for thousands of years, discoveries as recent as the last 5 years have added much to our understanding. Yet much remains unknown. In spite of the fact that pain is a universal phenomenon, definitions of pain vary widely. The definition of pain adopted in 1979 by the International Association for the Study of Pain is "an unpleasant sensory and emotional experience associated with actual or potential tissue damage or described in terms of such damage." It is important to note that this definition includes both sensory and emotional components.

RELEVANCE OF PAIN THEORIES

Numerous theories about the cause, meaning, and purpose of pain have developed over the years and constitute a legacy

---

*The authors thank Brent Ekins for the section on salicylate and acetaminophen toxicity and Elvira Szigeti and Marti Sachse, who contributed the chapter on pain in the first edition.

to the health care provider. Although many of these theories are considered flawed or outmoded, certain components may affect health care providers' underlying assumptions about pain. It is important to identify one's assumptions about pain, to accept that unconscious assumptions may vary among people (both patients and providers), and to recognize that these assumptions can influence one's approach to a person in pain.

Even the derivation of the word *pain,* which comes from the Green *poine* and Latin *poene,* meaning penalty or punishment, reflects a theory of the purpose of pain. Many early civilizations (and some current religions) interpreted pain as a price paid for offense to a diety or moral principle. This assumption is seen in the health care provider who feels that people with sexually transmitted diseases or smokers with lung cancer "brought it on themselves."

Early thinkers defined pain entirely in affective terms. Aristotle described pain as an emotion, the opposite of pleasure. Epicuris, another Greek philosopher, described pain as the absence of pleasure. With the advent of modern science, however, the pendulum swung to regarding "real" pain as entirely a physical phenomenon.

In 1644, René Descartes explained pain in terms of the science of the seventeenth century (Fig. 17-1). In this *specificity theory of pain* Descartes suggested that for each unit of pain stimulus, one unit of pain is experienced. No allowance was made for psychologic influences on pain. Clinicians who classify pain as *either organic or psychogenic,* rather than on a continuum with varying influence of physical (organic) and emotional-cognitive (psychogenic) influence, are demonstrating an attitude congruent with this theory. Similarly, the statement to a patient, "You are requiring too much pain medicine for someone who is 3 days postop," reflects assumptions of a specificity theory of pain, i.e., that a specific injury results in a certain amount of pain.

Clinicians have long been aware that past pain experience, anxiety about pain, and beliefs about pain influence pain perception. To explain the role of these central control processes numerous *pattern-summation theories* were introduced during the nineteenth and twentieth centuries. The presumption with these theories is that continuous pain inputs over a period of time determine pain perception. The most recent of the pattern-summation theories, the *gate control theory,* published in 1965 by Melzack and Wall, proposes that a neural mechanism in the dorsal horns of the spinal column acts like a gate to pain impulses traveling from the periphery to the central nervous system where pain is perceived. The *ratio of impulses* from large inhibitory fibers and small facilatory fibers produce the painful experience. The large inhibitory fibers can be triggered by central or peripheral stimuli. According to this theory, rubbing an elbow after it is bumped decreases pain by stimulating the large fibers and increasing the proportion of inhibitory impulses. Pattern-summation theories have facilitated the introduction or acceptance of a wide variety of innovations in pain treatment, such as acupuncture, transcutaneous elec-

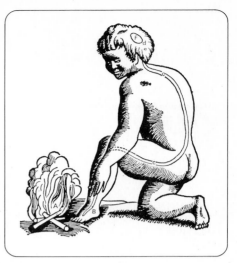

FIGURE 17-1

Descartes' (1644) Concept of the Pain Pathway. He writes: "If, for example, fire (A) comes near the foot (B), the minute particles of this fire, which as you know move with great velocity, have the power to set in motion the spot of the skin of the foot which they touch, and by this means pulling upon the delicate thread (cc) which is attached to the spot of the skin, they open up at the same instant the pore (de) against which the delicate thread ends, just as by pulling at one end of a rope one makes to strike at the same instant a bell which hangs at the other end." (*From F. Descartes:* L'homme, *Cambridge, England: Cambridge University Press, 1644.*)

trical nerve stimulation (TENS), and imagery, which are postulated to stimulate large inhibitory fibers through central or peripheral mechanisms.

A number of pain theories are currently under investigation, such as the endogenous opioid theory, the theories explaining limbic influences on pain, theories of acute and chronic pain, and others described below. As pain research continues, undoubtedly new theories will emerge and others wlll be refined, modified, or refuted. The nurse will need to scrutinize each for its validity and usefulness to clinical practice.

PSYCHOBIOLOGY OF PAIN

Components of Pain

Generally pain is conceptualized as having two broad components: a *perceptive* component and a *reactive* component. These components can be further subdivided into more specific functions. The perceptive component includes *nociception,* the detection and transmission of a painful stimulus to the thalamus, and *discrimination,* the conscious perception and recognition of the painful sensation. The reactive component involves the behavioral response to the pain and is under *affective-motivational* (emotional) and *cognitive* (interpretation; meaning) influences.

Research shows that people are much more similar relative to the perceptive component than they are in pain reaction. *Pain threshold* (the lowest intensity of stimulus that is perceived as painful) is nearly identical in all people, but how people rank a given painful stimulus with respect to intensity and tolerability is variable. However, the perceptive and reactive components are in reality parts of a holistic, indivisible process.

Pain Anatomy

Pain can be initiated by *mechanical* (cutting, pressure, shearing, tearing, distention, traction), *chemical* (endogenous pain chemicals, ischemia, or exogenous irritants), or *electrical* stimuli. These noxious stimuli are perceived primarily by free, undifferentiated, widely branched nerve endings (nociceptors). The nerve fibers for pain travel with other sensory, autonomic, and motor fibers through peripheral nerves and enter the spinal cord through the dorsal nerve routes, where two types of pain fibers arise: C fibers, which are small and unmyelinated, and A-delta fibers, which are large, myelinated, and transmit impulses much more rapidly. A-delta fibers carry acute, sharp pain, and C fibers primarily carry dull pain such as aching or burning. Pain fibers from the head enter the brainstem with the cranial nerves, rather than arriving through the spinal cord.

When pain fibers reach the dorsal horn of the gray matter of the spinal cord, most synapse with either (1) anterior horn (motor) cells to form primary reflex arcs, (2) second-order neurons which cross to the opposite side and ascend to the thalamus via the lateral spinothalamic tract, or (3) internuncial neurons, which then synapse with anterior horn cells or second-order neurons, although a few pain fibers ascend directly to the brainstem via dorsal tracts without synapsing with second-order neurons. In the thalamus conscious pain perception is thought to occur. At this site second-order neurons synapse with third-order neurons, which transmit information about the pain to the cerebral cortex where pain is recognized and interpreted.

Through an undefined mechanism activation of pain fibers initiates impulses which ascend via two secondary sensory tracts, the neospinothalamic tract, which carries messages relevant to localization and intensity of pain, and the paleospinothalamic tract, which has connections to the limbic system and underlies emotional and arousal components of pain. Descending pathways for pain regulation originate in the brainstem and synapse with internuncial neurons in the dorsal horn.

Segmental Innervation and Referred Pain

Due to the orderly way in which the pain fibers enter the spinal cord and brainstem, sensory innervation of the skin is *segmental* (see Fig. 17-2). Sensory fibers from the internal viscera and deep muscles enter the spinal cord with the cuta-

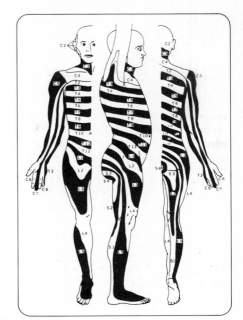

FIGURE 17-2

Sensory Dermatomes. Segmental innervation results in discrete areas of the skin representing the sensory domain of the spinal and cranial nerves. Visceral and deep musculoskeletal pain may be referred to the sensory dermatomes of the spinal nerves which innervate the painful internal organ. For example, the sensory pathways for the intrathoracic viscera are T1 to T4 and for the upper abdominal organs they are T6 to T8. Thus, disease of these organs are likely to be reflected as pain in the associated cutaneous segments. (*From G. M. Holmes:* Introduction to Clinical Neurology, *2nd ed., Baltimore: Williams & Wilkins, 1952. Used by permission.*)

neous nerves; pain from these deep structures often activates the pool of cutaneous sensory neurons which enter the cord at the same levels. This is the mechanism of *referred pain* and explains, for example, that cardiac pain in myocardial infarction is referred primarily to the substernum, left precordium, and left arm because the pain fibers from the heart enter the spine at the first four thoracic segments (T1 through T4). Some common sites of referred pain are shown in Table 17-1.

Pain Physiology and Biochemistry

Pain is thought to be initiated at nerve endings by the release of endogenous chemicals as a result of trauma, necrosis, ischemia, or inflammation. Bradykinin, histamine, potassium, and prostaglandins are among these implicated chemicals. The peripheral analgesic effect of **aspirin, acetaminophen**, and the **nonsteroidal anti-inflammatory drugs** is attributed to prostaglandin inhibition.

Strong, prolonged pain often stimulates muscle spasm or segmental reflexes (e.g., flexion of hips and knees in periton-

TABLE 17-1 Body Surface Areas Associated with Referred Visceral Pain

ORIGIN OF VISCERAL PAIN	LOCALIZATION OF PAIN ON BODY SURFACE
Appendix	Around umbilicus localizing in right lower quadrant of abdomen
Bladder	Lower abdomen directly over bladder
Esophagus	Pharynx, lower neck, arms, midline chest region
Gallbladder	Upper central portion of abdomen; lower right shoulder
Heart	Base of neck, shoulders, and upper chest; down arms (left side involvement more frequent than right)
Kidney and ureters	Regions of lower back over site of affected organ; anterior abdominal wall below and to the side of umbilicus
Stomach	Anterior surface of chest or upper abdomen
Uterus	Lower abdomen

Source: Reproduced with permission from W. K. Van Tyle, "Internal Analgesic Products," in *Handbook of Nonprescription Drugs,* 7th ed., Washington, D.C.: American Pharmaceutical Association, 1982.

itis) which serve to splint the diseased area, but may also contribute to further pain. Other responses to pain include avoidance, autonomic responses (blood pressure, pulse, pilomotor, etc.), and postural or gait adjustment.

Endogenous Opioids and Other Neuromodulators

For many years pharmacologists postulated that specific receptor sites for opioid narcotics must exist in the central nervous system for these drugs to act, and such stereospecific receptors were demonstrated in the 1970s. About the same time, endogenous opioids were isolated and generically termed *endorphins. Endorphin* is a contraction of the two words *endogenous and morphine.* Currently two groups of endogenous opioids are known: the endorphins (long-chain peptides) and the enkephalins (shorter-chain peptides). It has been postulated that the endorphins function in the substantia gelatinosa of the dorsal horn by modulating the release of substance P, the pain neurotransmitter at that site (see Fig. 17-3). The emotional component of pain relief may be associated with the endorphin-rich nuclei and opioid receptors found in and near the limbic system. Endorphins are also found in the periaqueductal region, and stimulation of this area causes release of endorphins into the cerebral spinal fluid, which impedes pain transmission.

There is evidence that endorphins play a role in the *pla-*

cebo effect in analgesia. Placebo analgesia is a phenomenon which occurs in about 35 percent of those with certain types of pain, including acute postoperative pain, dental pain, arthritic pain, angina, etc. **Naloxone**, a narcotic antagonist which works by blocking opioid receptors, will block placebo analgesia.

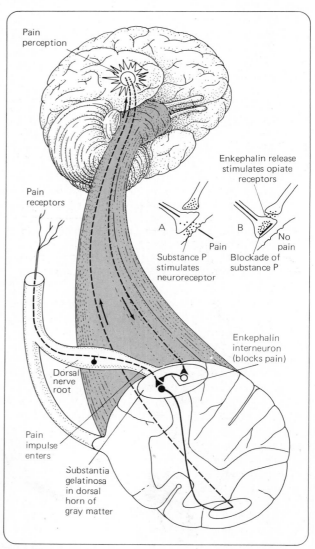

FIGURE 17-3

Current biochemical theory of pain stresses role of brain opiate receptors and endogenous opioids. Presence of specific binding sites in the limbic system and in substantia gelatinosa suggests that endogenous narcotics are active in both brain and spinal cord. Details (A and B) illustrate the hypothesis of how endogenous narcotics may operate to block pain perception. Intrinsic and extrinsic discrepancies in neurotransmissions are held to account for individual differences in psychophysiologic response to painful stimuli. (*From J. M. Luce, T. L. Thompson, C. J. Getto, and R. L. Byyny: "New Concepts of Chronic Pain and the Implications," Hospital Practice, 15(4):113, 1979.*)

Five different subtypes of opioid receptors have been postulated. Clinical effects have been suggested for three of these types of receptors (Table 17-2).

Pain Origins

The physiology and sensory experience varies with the origin of pain. Generally, pain may be experienced from alteration in three structural sites: *cutaneous* (skin and subcutaneous tissue), *deep somatic* (muscle and bone), and *visceral* (organ) sites.

Cutaneous pain is often localized, and the patient can point to it and indicate the specific painful areas. The severity of the pain is well-correlated with the degree of injury or damage. The pain may be characterized as tingling, prickling, stinging, as well as throbbing, burning, or sharp.

Deep somatic pain is generally more diffuse and is often described as dull, aching, or boring. The pain may be localized when highly pain sensitive tissues are involved, such as the periosteum of the bone, blood vessels, tendons, and ligaments. Deep somatic pain can be experienced as referred pain to the body surface resulting in cutaneous tenderness. Concurrent muscle contractions may heighten the pain perception. Ischemia and stretching in skeletal muscles, blood vessels, and periosteum of the bone can be highly painful. Deep somatic pain may fluctuate in severity depending on alteration in the stimulus or movement in the affected area.

Visceral pain is often difficult to localize, although over time it may become more localized. It is often described as vague, dull, aching, or burning. However, if it is due to an obstruction, as in the case of a bowel obstruction, it is cramping and rhythmic. Visceral pain also is often experienced as referred pain and may have trigger points located on the skin surface. Autonomic symptoms may be stimulated by visceral pain. The pain may increase in intensity if nothing is done to relieve it.

Milder musculoskeletal and cutaneous pain is frequently relieved by **aspirin**, **acetaminophen**, or **nonsteroidal anti-inflammatory drugs**. Visceral pain or musculoskeletal pain accompanied by muscle spasms less frequently respond to these nonnarcotic analgesics and often require **narcotic analgesics** or adjuvant drugs such as those which alter muscle tone.

PAIN PSYCHOSOCIOLOGY

Each individual's lifestyle, socialization process, cultural inheritance, support system, and past pain experiences may profoundly influence the manner in which pain is perceived. Pain perception is commonly increased by fatigue, anxiety, depression, and a feeling of isolation. Thus, the more chronic the pain, the more important past experience becomes. There are a number of stereotypes, some of which are based on research, about how people in certain cultural or ethnic groups respond to pain (e.g., the stoic Scandinavian or "old American," the vociferous Mediterranean). However, cultural stereotypes (whether research-based or not) do not apply to individuals; each person must be assessed as a unique being. Nurses must also be cognizant of their own culturally determined conceptions about the "proper" way for different individuals (e.g., men versus women, adults versus children) to respond to pain.

CLINICAL PAIN SYNDROMES

Pain is often described in terms of its temporal characteristics as acute or chronic pain. However, *acute pain* and *chronic pain* also differ in predominant causes and in anatomic, physiologic, biochemical, and psychosocial characteristics, as well as in duration.

Acute Pain

Acute pain, as typified by postoperative or immediate posttraumatic pain, is accompanied by anxiety and elicits an acute stress response. Since β endorphins are secreted from the pituitary with adrenocorticotropic hormone (ACTH), this response is adaptive in acute pain. Usually patients cope well with acute pain; it can easily be understood and rationalized as a body defense mechanism, a part of the healing process, or a parameter useful in monitoring clinical progress.

Severity of Acute Pain

Acute pain is commonly described as mild, moderate, or severe. Analgesic drugs are usually effective in all degrees of acute pain and can be taken as needed (PRN) to manage acute pain. **Aspirin** is the prototype drug for control of mild pain, aspirin or **aspirin plus codeine** for moderate pain, and **morphine** for severe pain (Fig. 17-4). **Acetaminophen** (Tylenol, others) appears to be as effective as aspirin in mild to moderate acute pain, and other opiates can achieve the analgesia of morphine.

TABLE 17-2   Clinical Effects of Opioid Receptors

μ	(mu)	Supraspinal analgesia
		Respiratory depression
		Euphoria
		Dependence
κ	(kappa)	Spinal analgesia
		Miosis
		Sedation
		Respiratory depression (?)
σ	(sigma)	Dysphoria
		Hallucinations
		Respiratory stimulation
		Vasomotor stimulation
δ	(delta)	Effects not yet clear
		Enkephalin binding site
ϵ	(epsilon)	Effects not yet clear
		β-endorphin binding site

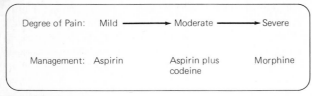

FIGURE 17-4

Acute Pain Continuum. The severity of acute pain can be correlated with drug therapy. The effectiveness of other drugs are compared to these prototype drugs for each type of acute pain.

Chronic Pain

Chronic pain is a continuous or recurring pain that is described as *intractable* if it is incapacitating and does not respond to usual treatments. Examples of chronic pain syndromes are *causalgia*, a severe burning pain in the distal extremity accompanied by trophic changes of skin and musculoskeletal structures; *phantom limb pain*, a tingling, burning, or itching perceived in an area that has been amputated; some *cancer pain*; severe *arthritis*; chronic *low back pain*; *tic douloureux*, a severe paroxysmal pain along the cutaneous distribution of the trigeminal nerve which may be initiated by stimulation of a "trigger point"; *migraine headaches*; and *thalamic pain syndrome*, a deep, severe, paroxysmal pain in the extremities of one side of the body.

Chronic pain has multiple dimensions (Fig. 17-5). It begins with the physical cause of the pain or event perceived as causing the pain. Stimuli which are normally innocuous or not painful can trigger pain in chronic pain syndromes. If the pain does not resolve, a psychologic dimension of anxiety followed by depression often presents after a few hours or days. As time passes without abatement of the pain, a social dimension is added which often presents as hostility. The pain becomes the central focus of the sufferer and changes in behavior occur. Communication patterns and interpersonal relations are disrupted.

Thus, a *chronic pain symptom complex* can be described with physical pain, anxiety, insomnia, and depression inextricably related (Fig. 17-6). Severity of chronic pain and the patient's mood vary together; one day the patient may experience only minor aches and another day the pain may be agonizing. Such changes do not often correlate with observable changes in the disease pattern or drug use. The biochemical relationship between depressive mood and pain may explain their correlation, however. Both pain and depression are associated with decreased cellular reuptake of serotonin and decreased levels of norepinephrine in the central nervous system. These neurotransmitters are involved in sensory-discriminatory and affective-motivational components of pain.

Aberrations in other biochemical and neuroanatomic functions occur in chronic pain. The endogenous pain control system does not appear to provide relief in chronic pain. The endorphins are released and do occupy the opioid recep-

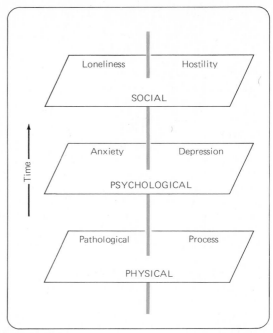

FIGURE 17-5

Dimensions of Severe, Chronic Pain. Chronic pain has physical, psychologic, and social ramifications. (*From A. G. Lipman: "Drug Therapy in Cancer Pain," Cancer Nursing, 2:39, 1980. Used by permission.*)

tors, but pain continues. Even surgical resection of the primary pain pathways or stimulation of the endorphin-rich periaqueductal gray matter does not relieve some chronic pain syndromes, further suggesting limbic system involvement in these pain states. Aberrant nerve regeneration may be another factor in some chronic pain syndromes.

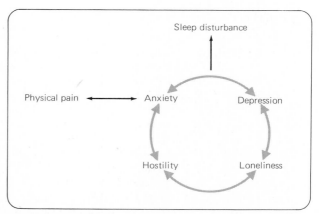

FIGURE 17-6

The symptom complex of severe, chronic pain. (*From A. G. Lipman: "Drug Therapy in Cancer Pain," Cancer Nursing, 2:39, 1980. Used by permission.*)

ASSESSMENT OF PAIN

Comprehensive assessment of pain must involve both the perceptive and the reactive components of pain. The nursing diagnosis of pain is made simply and entirely on the basis of an individual's statement that pain exists, but assessment must result in an analysis of the *cause* and *manifestations* of the pain. When it is possible to determine cause of pain, nursing or medical interventions may be initiated to resolve the pain by addressing the cause. Analysis of the manifestations of pain aids in determining appropriate symptomatic treatment, so nursing diagnosis is directed at determining *acuity or chronicity, origin* (visceral, cutaneous, deep somatic, or specific organ, such as the heart in angina), *severity* (mild, moderate, severe), and *psychosocial response* (affect, coping, meaningful interpersonal interactions, etc.).

Assessing Pain Perception

The nurse elicits a description of the pain characteristics (sensory experience) from the patient. A variety of descriptors are explored. The wording of questions asked about pain are crucial in determining the quality of information derived. The nurse should question the patient in both a nonjudgmental and nonleading manner. An adequate description of pain characteristics can be determined by assessing the following seven specific areas: type and quality, location, onset, duration, progression and severity, aggravating factors, and relief techniques. Some questions which can be utilized to assess these characteristics and the function of the data derived are shown in Table 17-3.

Chronic pain is often more difficult for patients to describe than acute pain. Other symptoms and adverse effects of drugs may exacerbate pain. For example, dry mouth or constipation from narcotics and anticholinergics can increase pain or stimuli which elicit the pain. Drugs also can induce mood changes which affect pain perception.

Much of patients' communication about pain is figurative or nonverbal. They frequently underreport pain, so observation is an important part of assessment. This is particularly true for children, who do not respond with the adult terminology we use in assessing pain and may not know how to make their pain relief needs known. In addition, children may try to hide pain because they fear the injection of pain medication. For the most valid assessments nurses can observe patients when they are not aware of this observation. Clues that a person is experiencing pain include splinting, guarding, rigid or tense posture, limping, or other pain-expressive behaviors. Sleep patterns, ability to accomplish activities of daily living, and alertness are useful parameters in assessing pain. Parents may be able to point out atypical behavior indicating their child is in pain.

Observation can also help the nurse to identify relief mechanisms. If the patient has less pain when distracted by conversation or activity or after the visit from a favorite grandchild, these can be built into the pain management strategies.

Assessing Pain Response

In assessing pain perception, data about pain response are collected simultaneously by observing facial expression, body posture, word selection, and tone of voice. The health care provider should ask about previous pain experiences in self or others, social interaction, family or job stress, social support, and specific coping mechanisms (Table 17-3).

The nurse must strive to understand the unique meaning of pain to the patient. The pain may signal weakness, dependency, or loss of control. The patient may fear rejection by loved ones, the medical team, or others. Patients may be worried about loss of job, income, and status or believe the pain is a form of punishment. They may fear dying or feel lonely and isolated. It may have been possible to deny or ignore the disease causing pain in nonpainful stages, but the constant nature or intensity of the pain may continually remind patients that they have a serious or incurable illness, which leads to increased anxiety and pain perception.

Pain questionnaires and rating scales have been developed to evaluate patients' comfort. Visual analog scales are instruments which allow patients to mark on a descriptive anchored line their current perceptions of pain (Fig. 17-7). A well-known and research-validated scale is the McGill-Melzack Pain Questionnaire, which actually assesses both the perceptive and reactive components of pain. Such tools give a reliable technique to assess pain and evaluate efficacy of pain relief measures.

Physiologic Response

Physiologic response to pain occurs through stimulation of the autonomic nervous system which commonly accompanies visceral pain. Although stimulation usually activates a sympathetic response, a combined sympathetic and parasympathetic response may occur. If the sympathetic portion of the autonomic nervous system responds, typically the patient's pupils will be dilated; respiration, heart rate, and blood pressure will increase; perspiration may be evident; and urinary output as well as gastrointestinal peristalsis will decrease. If the parasympathetic portion of the autonomic nervous system is stimulated, pupils will constrict, heart rate and blood pressure will lower, and gastrointestinal peristalsis will increase.

Autonomic responses are less evident in long-term chronic pain. The body cannot continually support an autonomic response. Therefore adaptation occurs and physiologic alterations are less pronounced. This does not mean that the patient no longer experiences the pain. The pain is just as intense, but the physiologic response that the nurse can measure through pulse, respiration, and blood pressure has been modified.

ACUTE PAIN MANAGEMENT

Pain is a symptom. When the cause of pain can be identified and is treatable, pain should be managed as a manifestation of the disease rather than as a discrete condition. Surgical, medical, or drug treatment other than analgesics may be more appropriate than analgesics alone for many specific causes of pain. For example, pain is a common concomitant of inflammatory processes of bones and joints; if analgesics which do not reduce the inflammation are used, a relatively painless destruction of joints can occur. For pain with a large psychogenic component, analgesic intervention is rarely indicated and may contribute to the pain problem. In such cases, psychosocial interventions should be initiated.

The nurse, in conjunction with other health team members and the patient, identifies the strategy for pain relief. The strategy is generally multimodal, that is, it includes more than simply administering prescribed analgesics, and it considers all aspects of the particular patient's pain experience including physical, psychological, social, cultural, and spiritual factors. In dealing with acute pain of short duration, primary attention is to physical relief of pain, and drugs combined with basic comfort measures are generally

TABLE 17-3 Assessment of Pain

DESCRIPTOR	QUESTIONS TO ASK*	RATIONALE/ANALYSIS
General	Do you have discomfort? Tell me about your pain/discomfort.	Some people will admit to "discomfort" but will deny pain. Begin description with an open-ended question.
Type or quality	Is the pain dull or sharp, aching, burning, radiating, pulsating, cramping, intermittent, or steady?	Differentiate visceral or deep somatic origin or specific organ source.
Location/radiation	Where does it hurt? Point to it. Does the pain seem to go anywhere else? Where?	Determine cause, presence of pain. Pointing is more accurate as it does not require anatomic vocabulary.
Onset/aggravating factors	When did (does) the pain occur? What were you doing? Was the occurrence sudden or gradual? What makes the pain start or become worse (position, foods—which ones, heat/cold, tension/worry, exercise)?	Ascertain acuity or chronicity. Onset and aggravating factors are the most useful in diagnosing cause. Try to reproduce pain on examination.
Duration	How long have you had this pain? Has it been intermittent or steady? Have you ever had this pain before? When?	Determine acuity or chronicity.
Progression/severity	What have you had to do differently because of this pain? Does it help? When is the pain worse? Is the pain worse now than when it started? On a scale of 0–10, with 10 being the worst pain you can imagine and 0 being no pain, what number describes this pain?	May use visual analog scale to assess severity. These are important questions to ascertain reactivity as well.
Relief mechanisms	What relieves the pain (rest/sleep, exercise, diet, aspirin or other medication, heat/ice)?	Establish cause and management plan. Data about previous analgesia should be specific as to drugs, dosage, scheduling.
Past experience	Have you ever before known anyone with this kind of pain? Compare this pain to other pain you have known.	Pain experiences in self or others influence expectations and sensory experience.
Meaning	Do you know what might be causing your pain? Why did you seek medical help for this pain?	Fear of the cause of pain is important in pain response.
Affective response	Which of the following words describe your mood: jittery, blue, calm, depressed, unconcerned, nervous, hopeless, uptight, energyless, angry, lonely, frightened.	Detection of anxiety and depression by asking for yes/no to each adjective.
Coping/social support	How are you getting along with your family, coworkers, friends? Who helps you do the things which your condition prevents you from doing? Who can you talk to about your pain and your feelings? When you have a problem or a dilemma, what methods work best for solving it?	Identify coping mechanisms that have worked in the past, sources of social support, secondary gains in pain experience.

*The patient, family member, caretaker, or significant other can be the source(s) of this information.

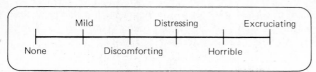

FIGURE 17-7

Visual Analog Scale for Rating Pain with Behavioral Anchor Description.

effective. Chronic pain requires additional strategies, such as psychosocial, physical, and surgical modalities.

Basic Comfort Measures

A number of nursing techniques may provide pain relief or promote the effects of analgesics. Failure to attend to these basic comfort measures will increase the dosage of analgesic required and may totally compromise drug efficacy.

Proper positioning and rest are two major principles of basic comfort. For pain relief this indicates (1) rest of the entire organism, (2) rest of the painful part, (3) elevation of the painful part when possible, (4) management of the environment (e.g., control of sensory overload or sensory deprivation), and (5) support of painful part (e.g., elastic bandage wraps, slings, braces). Local heat, cold, or local massage is often comforting as well, if not otherwise contraindicated. Strain on muscles and joints can occur when a painful part is guarded or positioned without regard for total body alignment.

Distraction may be a very useful technique. Reading to the patient, listening to a favorite musical selection on portable headsets, or a visit from a loved one may assist in sustaining other pain relief measures. Comfort and relaxation techniques such as a back rub or a hot bath may also be beneficial. Families may wish to participate in providing these forms of pain relief.

Other interventions may be directed at psychological, social, or spiritual aspects of pain. An opportunity to air one's concerns, a visit by a chaplain or a spiritual advisor, or an opportunity to resolve minor family misunderstandings or situational worries (e.g., a pet at home alone) may contribute significantly to the patient's comfort in acute pain situations. Prior knowledge of the sensations to be anticipated following a diagnostic or surgical procedure significantly reduces reported pain and analgesic requirements. Therefore preoperative or preprocedural patient education is an important nursing consideration.

The manner in which an analgesic is administered is often as important as the analgesic in relieving pain. The verbal and nonverbal messages the patient receives about the nurses' confidence in the medication is a crucial factor in outcome. In addition, when analgesia is required, it will be more effective if it is given before pain becomes too severe and the emotional component of anxiety reaches overwhelming levels.

With children the nurse is often placed in the paradoxical position of trying to relieve pain by injection of medications, which the child perceives as an intolerable physical assault. If possible, subcutaneous or intramuscular injections should be avoided in children. If the child has an intravenous line in place, the medication may be administered intravenously. Preferred routes for analgesia administration are oral or rectal. Children should not be allowed to become so uncomfortable that they must remain in pain for long periods of time waiting for analgesics to reach maximum effectiveness. A child who is experiencing pain needs expressive outlets. Play therapy programs have an important role in assisting the child to deal with painful experiences. Explanations to children should be based on their developmental level and ability to understand the information. A child, as well as an adult, deserves an explanation of the way and reason for pain medication administration and the expected lag between administration and pain relief. The nurse should be realistic and honest with the child, never promising a painless procedure or total pain relief if that is not possible. Finally, the nurse should remember the value of comfort techniques, cuddling, and distraction with a favorite toy as powerful adjuncts to analgesic administration.

Analgesic Drug Therapy

Analgesia is the diminution of pain perception without loss of consciousness. It may involve the alteration of the physical or emotional component of pain, or both. Drugs other than analgesics (e.g., skeletal muscle relaxants, local anesthetics, anxiolytics) are also used to promote this effect.

The objective of pain management is to make the individual reasonably comfortable without markedly impairing central nervous system function. Analgesics provide only symptomatic relief; they do not correct the underlying disorder which is causing or contributing to the pain. There is risk of analgesics masking pain, fever, inflammation, or other symptoms while the disease progresses. In acute pain, it is therefore advantageous for patients to take as little drug as necessary for them to be reasonably comfortable. Dosing on an as needed (PRN) schedule is usually appropriate. If the prescriber believes that the acute pain stimulus will be active for a limited time (e.g., 3 days), it may be reasonable for the drug to be given on a regularly scheduled basis for part of that time (e.g., 2 of the 3 days) and then given on a PRN schedule.

Analgesics are commonly classified as *nonnarcotics* and *narcotics*. Nonnarcotic analgesics work primarily in the periphery to lessen the transmission of pain impulses to the spinal column. Narcotic analgesics work primarily to lessen pain perception through occupation of the opioid receptor sites in the central nervous system, including those anatomic areas involved with both sensory perception and emotional response.

Most pain can be managed by **aspirin** (or **acetaminophen**). If aspirin or combinations of aspirin with nonnarcotic analgesics are insufficient, a second level of analgesia can be accomplished through combinations of **aspirin with codeine, oxycodone,** or **pentazocine.** When such combinations do not provide sufficient analgesia, **morphine** or another opiate should be considered. The combination of morphine with aspirin or another nonnarcotic agent will often permit the use of a lower dose of morphine than would be necessary were the opiate used alone.

Nonnarcotic Analgesics

Nonnarcotic analgesics are the nonsalicylate nonsteroidal anti-inflammatory drugs (NSAIDs), aspirin and other salicylates, and acetaminophen. Several salicylates have been used in the past, but aspirin is the most important and commonly used drug in this group today. Aspirin is actually an NSAID but is often discussed separately.

Aspirin and Other Salicylates Aspirin (ASA, acetylsalicylic acid) is unsurpassed by other nonnarcotic drugs. Research in cancer patients with mild to moderate pain shows aspirin to be an equivalent or better pain reliever than six other nonnarcotic analgesics, codeine, and one psychotropic agent (Moertel and others, 1972). Further, as shown in Table 17-4, only combinations of aspirin with codeine, oxycodone, and pentazocine were shown to be more effective than aspirin alone (Moertel and others, 1974). Since

TABLE 17-4　Relative Therapeutic Effects of Oral Analgesics*

ANALGESIC COMPOSITION	COMPARABLE TRADE NAME†	MEAN PERCENT PAIN RELIEF	MORE EFFECTIVE THAN PLACEBO	MORE EFFECTIVE THAN ASPIRIN, 650 mg
Codeine sulfate, 65 mg + aspirin, 650 mg	Emcodeine #4[a] Empirin w/Codeine no. 3[b]	63	Yes	Yes
Oxycodone, 9.76 mg + aspirin, 650 mg	Percodan[b]	63	Yes	Yes
Pentazocine hydrochloride, 25 mg + aspirin, 650 mg	Talwin compound[b]	59	Yes	Yes
Aspirin, 650 mg	Numerous	56	Yes	—
Propoxyphene napsylate, 100 mg + aspirin, 650 mg	Darvon-N w/ASA[a]	55	Yes	No
Pentazocine, 50 mg	Talwin	54	Yes	No
Promazine hydrochloride, 25 mg + aspirin, 650 mg	Sparine[c]	51	Yes	No
Acetaminophen, 650 mg	Tylenol, Panadol, others	50	Yes	No
Pentobarbital sodium, 32 mg + aspirin, 650 mg	Nembutal[c]	50	Yes	No
Phenacetin‡		48	Yes	No
Caffeine, 65 mg + aspirin, 650 mg		48	Yes	No
Ethoheptazine citrate, 75 mg + aspirin, 650 mg	Zactarin‡	48	Yes	No
Mefenamic acid, 250 mg	Ponstel	47	Yes	No
Codeine, 65 mg		46	Yes	No
Propoxyphene, 65 mg	Darvon, Dolene, others	43	No	No
Ethoheptazine, 75 mg	Zactane‡	38	No	No
Promazine, 25 mg	Sparine	37	No	No
Placebo		33	—	No

*Sources of data are Moertel and others (1972) and Moertel and others (1974).
†Precise composition of various trade names will vary. Doses of listed products approximately equivalent to:
　[a]One tablet of product listed plus 325 mg aspirin.
　[b]Two tablets of product listed.
　[c]One tablet or capsule of product listed plus 650 mg aspirin.
‡No longer available commercially in the U.S.A.

aspirin works peripherally and these narcotics work centrally, the two appear to have a complementary action.

Aspirin, like other salicylates, is an analgesic, antipyretic, and anti-inflammatory agent. Salicylates reduce platelet adhesiveness. Aspirin does this irreversibly by acetylating the platelets. Therefore, aspirin is of potential usefulness as an anticoagulant in a variety of thromboembolic disorders (Chap. 42, "Thromboembolic Disorders").

Many patients do not believe that aspirin is a particularly effective analgesic because of its common availability and nonprescription status. This is not an appropriate belief, and nurses should inform patients that aspirin is indeed a drug of choice in mild to moderate pain. However, aspirin is contraindicated for patients taking oral anticoagulants, with bleeding disorders, with peptic ulcer disease, who are pregnant and near term, and who are allergic to the drug, as well as in children with influenza or chickenpox. Acetaminophen is the alternative of choice for simple analgesia and antipyresis. If anti-inflammatory activity is needed, a nonsteroidal anti-inflammatory drug should be considered.

Mechanism of action   Salicylates and other NSAIDs work primarily by inhibiting the synthesis of prostaglandins. This is accomplished through the inhibition of prostaglandin synthetase, the enzyme necessary for the production of these chemicals. Prostaglandin E is a necessary part of the biochemical transmission of pain impulses from the periphery to the spinal cord. These drugs also have a slight effect on pain perception in the hypothalamus.

Pharmacokinetics   Oral salicylates are rapidly absorbed, primarily from the small intestine and to some extent from the stomach. While absorption normally occurs within 30 min, the presence of food will delay stomach emptying and absorption. Peak plasma concentrations are reached in approximately 2 h. Timed-release preparations and enteric-coated tablets are expensive, give delayed and often erratic absorption, and are inadvisable for analgesic use due to delayed onset of action. Rectal absorption is often incomplete, so the rectal suppository is not a preferred means of administration and should be used only when oral administration is not feasible.

After absorption aspirin is rapidly distributed throughout the body tissues, with 50 to 90 percent of the salicylate bound to serum protein. Aspirin is rapidly hydrolyzed to salicylic acid in plasma and tissue. Because this is a rapid process, aspirin plasma half-life is only 20 min, whereas the salicylic acid half-life is 3 to 6 h in low doses and 15 to 30 h in large doses because of the liver's limited capacity for biotransformation of salicylic acid to its water-soluble form for excretion. Thus, while aspirin is pharmacologically active, it owes most of its activity to its hydrolyzed form, salicylic acid, which is metabolized mainly in the liver. Ten percent of salicylic acid is excreted unchanged, but this is highly variable, depending on the pH of the urine (5 percent at low pH to 85 percent at high pH).

Adverse reactions   The major untoward effect of aspirin is gastric intolerance. This can usually be minimized by the patient taking the aspirin with a full glass of water. When aspirin is used chronically or by patients who are predisposed to gastric ulceration, it may be ulcerogenic. Aspirin may exacerbate bleeding disorders.

Because aspirin is highly serum protein-bound, there is a high risk of interaction with other drugs which are highly serum protein-bound. These include **anticoagulants, anticonvulsants,** and **oral antidiabetic agents.** Aspirin blocks uric acid excretion in analgesic doses. Therefore, it may precipitate or exacerbate gout in hyperuricemic patients. Most other adverse effects of aspirin are seen primarily in chronic salicylism or acute toxicity states.

Aspirin allergy presents most commonly as asthma-like bronchospasms or as rash, but anaphylaxis has occurred. Aspirin allergy is more common in asthmatics, but less than 20 percent of asthmatics are intolerant to aspirin. Gastrointestinal upset is not indicative of allergy. Patients who report aspirin allergy which was manifested as gastric upset should be advised that they are probably not allergic to the drug. When patients are unable to tolerate aspirin, acetaminophen is the usual alternative of choice. However, acetaminophen provides no anti-inflammatory activity. Therefore, if an anti-inflammatory drug is indicated, other nonsteroidal anti-inflammatory drugs should be considered.

In 1982, an association between aspirin use by children with chickenpox or influenza and the occurrence of Reye's syndrome was documented. Reye's syndrome is a rare, acute, life-threatening encephalopathy occurring mostly in children under 16 years of age who are recovering from viral infections (see Chap. 18, "Alterations in Body Temperature," for further discussion).

Salicylate intoxication   A dose of aspirin greater than 150 mg/kg of body weight is considered toxic. The common signs and symptoms of salicylate intoxication include nausea and vomiting, tinnitus, hyperventilation, and abdominal pain. Infants often do not exhibit hyperventilation. These symptoms are all consistent with a mild intoxication. Moderate or severe intoxication may include these and other symptoms including fever, acid-base imbalance, disorientation, diaphoresis, convulsions, coagulopathies (bleeding), and hypoglycemia. The areas of assessment that should be evaluated include the state of hydration, neurologic status, vital signs, acid-base balance, electrolytes, renal function, urine output, and the hematologic status. It is important to determine if the intoxication represents a single ingestion and the time of ingestion. A blood salicylate level in the range of 50 mg/dL at 6 h indicates mild intoxication, whereas the same blood level at 24 h indicates moderate to serious intoxication. If the intoxication is chronic, i.e., aspirin has been taken in too large a dose for a long period of time or in a normal dose too frequently, blood levels are less useful in determining the severity of a poisoning. Therapy of salicylate intoxication is directed at removal of the drug using emesis or gastric lavage followed by at least 50 g of activated charcoal in an adult or 20 to 25 g in a child as a water slury. Catharsis should be induced with up to three doses of an osmotic or saline cathartic given at 1- to 2-h intervals until a charcoal-laden stool is seen. Of importance is the state of hydration in such a patient. Catharsis may not be possible in the dehydrated patient until the hydration is accomplished with fluid replacements as well as electrolyte replacements. Any indication of developing acidosis should be managed aggressively and potassium losses replaced. Forced alkaline diuresis, as with sodium bicarbonate and diuretics, is effective in accelerating the elimination of the absorbed salicylate. Adequate urine flow of 3 to 6 mL/kg of body weight per hour should be obtained and the pH of the urine should be at least 7. If the blood level remains high and major manifestations cannot be controlled, dialysis or hemoperfusion should be employed to remove the salicylate. Criteria for initiation of these procedures include severe intoxication unresponsive to conservative measures, a serum salicylate level greater than 150 mg/dL, a major serum half-life of greater than 15 h, failure to alkalinize the urine with the appropriate bicarbonate therapy, and renal or hepatic failure.

Patient education   Many combination products containing aspirin are commercially available. These combinations are no more effective than the equivalent dose of the total ingredients as aspirin alone. Combinations of **aspirin with phenacetin and caffeine** (APC) have been removed from the market since the combination of phenacetin with aspirin used chronically may lead to nephrotoxicity. Additionally, no advantage of adding **caffeine** to aspirin has been demonstrated. Advertisements for many combination products intimate that the combinations are more effective than aspirin alone. Studies have demonstrated such agents to be more effective than aspirin only when the aspirin-equivalent of the combinations exceeds the dose of plain aspirin to which the combinations have been compared. For example, Anacin tablets each contain 400 mg of aspirin, but three 325-mg aspirin tablets contains 975 mg of aspirin, which is more than the 800 mg in two Anacin tablets. Further, three aspirin tablets may be less expensive than two Anacin tablets.

Since aspirin is unstable in solution, no liquid aspirin is commercially available. Many consumers are unaware that such common products as Anacin, Bufferin, Excedrin, Midol, Pabalate, Vanquish, Empirin, Ascriptin, Alka-Seltzer, Coricidin, Triaminicin, Dristan, Quiet World, etc., contain salicylates and should be taught to read product labels. If aspirin is contraindicated for an individual, the patient should inform the family pharmacist so that prescriptions containing aspirin will not be dispensed.

Until recent years, aspirin was the major drug implicated in pediatric poisonings. The federal requirements for packaging of salicylates in containers with child-resistant closures resulted in a dramatic decrease in aspirin poisonings. Such containers have frequently been criticized in the lay and professional press as causing difficulty for elderly and arthritic patients. This can occur, and therefore federal regulations permit one package size of each product to be marketed in a traditional container. Nurses should emphasize to patients the importance of using safety containers, especially when there are young children in the home. Many poisonings occur when children are visiting in homes where no children live. Therefore, use of child-resistant containers should be encouraged.

For pain which will resolve readily, patients should be advised to take their analgesics, including salicylates, only as needed. However, many patients suffer pain needlessly due to their belief that it is bad to take drugs even when they are indicated. Therefore, nurses should ascertain patients' beliefs about drug use and provide counseling accordingly. Patients should be advised of the risks of both acute and chronic salicylate toxicity. Patients should be advised to stop taking the salicylates and contact their physicians if there are any signs of bleeding. Nurses should describe such problems as hematemesis, epistaxis, melena, ecchymosis, and hematuria in language which patients can understand. Patients should also be advised that if they experience wheezing, rash or hives, tinnitus, dizziness, or severe stomach upset, they should stop taking the drug and contact their physicians. It is important for patients to take aspirin with a full glass of water if they experience gastrointestinal upset. This will aid dissolution and thus minimize gastric upset. Additionally, patients may take the drug with food if gastric upset continues.

Most people need not use more expensive "buffered" aspirin, e.g., Bufferin, Ascriptin. These dosage forms contain very small amounts of antacid, which results in mild alkalinization of the immediate environment of the tablet during dissolution. This pH change accelerates ionization, thus minimizing the risk of undissolved particles of aspirin directly contacting and irritating the gastric mucosa. For most patients, a full glass of water is equally effective in minimizing gastric upset.

Patients should be advised that on occasion salicylates have caused a slight green or brown tint to the urine. This is usually not noticeable unless the patient is dehydrated and the urine is highly concentrated. The patient should also be advised that direct application of aspirin to a tooth or irritated mucosa can cause severe chemical irritation and will not aid in pain relief.

Any aspirin exposed to heat and humidity will degrade. Aspirin with a very strong vinegar odor or excessive loose powder in the bottom of the bottle is unstable and will produce less clinical effect. It may also cause more gastritis than a fresh drug. To help ensure that fresh drug is being used, nurses should advise patients to purchase amounts of aspirin that will normally be used within a year. Bottles should be tightly capped between uses and protected from environmental extremes of moisture and heat. Therefore, many bathroom medicine cabinets are not ideal places to store aspirin.

Other salicylates   Several other salicylates have been developed. They are useful for patients unable to tolerate aspirin. **Sodium salicylate** is the most common of these. It is generally considered somewhat less effective than aspirin but can be used by some patients who are allergic to aspirin. **Choline salicylate** (Arthropan) is available in an oral liquid dosage form. This allows patients unable to swallow aspirin tablets to take a salicylate orally. **Diflunisal** (Dolobid) is a salicylic acid analog which also possesses uricosuric activity. Side effects associated with the use of diflunisal are similar to those occurring with other salicylates. It may cause less gastrointestinal upset and has a longer half-life than aspirin. **Magnesium salicylate** is sodium free but should not be used in renal failure.

Dosage and preparations **Aspirin** is available in a wide variety of oral dosage forms and strengths and as rectal suppositories. The average analgesic dosage range is 60 to 100 mg/kg/24 h divided into five to six doses for children (see Table 18-6) and 325 to 975 mg every 4 h for adults. When adult dosages are written in number of tablets, the nurse should clarify with the prescriber which strength should be used.

The average dosage range of **sodium salicylate** is the same as for **aspirin**. **Choline salicylate** (Arthropan) is available as an 870 mg per 5 mL oral liquid. The 5-mL dose is equilvalent to 650 mg of aspirin.

Magnesium salicylate (Doan's pills, Magan, others) is administered in doses of 500 to 600 mg three or four times daily. **Diflunisal** (Dolobid) is normally dosed only every 12 h. It is available as 250- and 500-mg tablets. The average adult loading dose is 1 g followed by 500 mg every 12 h.

Acetaminophen Acetaminophen, which is marketed under numerous trade names such as Tylenol, Datril, and Panadol, is the second most popular and important nonprescription analgesic in the United States. It is equipotent with aspirin as a simple analgesic. It is also comparable as an antipyretic. However, acetaminophen has little anti-inflammatory activity. Therefore, it may not be effective in inflammatory painful states such as rheumatoid arthritis. If acetaminophen or another analgesic which is not an anti-inflammatory agent were used in such conditions, painless destruction of the joint could occur.

Mechanism of action The mechanism of action of acetaminophen is unclear. It appears to act as a central prostaglandin synthetase inhibitor but its peripheral actions are unclear. Acetaminophen is the alternative of choice to aspirin in patients who cannot tolerate aspirin and in whom a simple analgesic without anti-inflammatory activity is indicated.

Pharmacokinetics Absorption of acetaminophen from the gastrointestinal tract is rapid and nearly complete, with plasma concentrations peaking in ½ to 2 h. The gastric emptying time influences the rate of absorption, so the patient who has eaten immediately before taking the drug or who is taking drugs with anticholinergic effects may experience some delay in onset of analgesia. Half-life is approximately 1 to 3 h. Distribution of acetaminophen is uniform throughout the body fluids; however, binding to plasma proteins is variable and is clinically important only in acute intoxication. Metabolism of acetaminophen occurs by hepatic microsomal enzymes; the major metabolites have no bio-

logic activity and are excreted in the urine. The minor metabolites are further detoxified by hepatic glutathione and excreted. In overdoses glutathione may be exhausted, leaving these minor metabolites free to bind with hepatocellular macromolecules, causing liver necrosis. Only a small percentiage of acetaminophen is excreted unchanged in the urine.

Adverse effects Acetaminophen is not associated with the gastrointestinal irritation and ulcerogenesis that may be seen with aspirin. Acetaminophen does not appreciably potentiate oral anticoagulants or affect uric acid excretion or mental processes. In therapeutic doses, acetaminophen is relatively nontoxic, but in large doses it can be extremely toxic. The adverse reactions associated with the drug at normal doses are primarily due to a relatively rare hypersensitivity reaction.

Acetaminophen intoxication This drug produces few adverse effects as compared to aspirin, but large overdoses can be life-threatening. A dose greater than 110 mg/kg of body weight (7.5 g in an adult) may be toxic. Following large overdose, immediate symptoms may include only mild nausea and vomiting or anxiety. The assessment of the severity of the poisoning is best determinined by an acetaminophen blood level and comparison of the level to a standard nomogram. A patient who has taken an overdose of acetaminophen must be aggressively evaluated as soon as possible after detection. Gastric lavage or emesis with activated charcoal and cathartics should be withheld unless other toxic drugs have been taken or activated charcoal is indicated. A blood sample should be drawn at least 4 h after ingestion and the value plotted on available nomograms. This will enable prognostic evaluation of the severity of possible outcome of the poisoning. Blood levels of greater than 300 μg/mL at 4 h usually indicate hepatotoxicity. Patients with blood levels of less than 120 μg/mL invariably have no evidence of liver damage.

If the serum level exceeds the nomogram line for safety or if the acetaminophen level will not be available prior to 16 h following ingestion, oral **acetylcysteine** (Mucomyst) is administered as an initial oral dose of 140 mg/kg followed by 17 doses of 70 mg every 4 h. The benefit of this agent has been demonstrated up to 16 h post ingestion with decreasing effectiveness after that period of time.

Dosage and preparations Dosage for acetaminophen is usually 325 to 975 mg q4 h to a maximum daily dose of 2.6 g for adults. Dosage for children under 3 years is 60 mg, for those 3 to 6 years, 60 to 120 mg, and for those 6 to 12 years, 120 to 240 mg (see Table 18-6). The children's dosages can be repeated every 3 to 4 h up to four times daily. Children's chewable tablets and liquids are commercially available. *It is important to note that the concentration of drug per unit volume in the pediatric drops and the pediatric liquid vary.* See Chap. 18 for further discussion of children's preparations.

Patient education Acetaminophen, like other analgesics, should be used only when necessary. If pain persists for more than 10 days, the patient should seek medical advice. Acetaminophen should be stored in tight, light-resistant containers. Nurses should emphasize the danger of massive overdose. There is a common misconception that acetaminophen is more safe than aspirin. While this may be true in marginal overdose situations, massive overdose of acetaminophen is potentially fatal.

Generally, acetaminophen is more expensive than aspirin. It has no advantage over aspirin in patients who can tolerate aspirin. Tylenol is the most widely known brand of the drug. Numerous other brands and generic dosage forms are available, as well as combinations containing acetaminophen (Table 17-7).

It is important to note that following a severe acetaminophen overdose, symptoms may be absent for several hours. Therefore, if an individual is suspected of having ingested a large amount of acetaminophen, that individual should be brought to medical attention immediately. The drug should be kept out of reach of children. Nurses should stress to patients the maximum daily dose.

Nonsteroidal Anti-Inflammatory Drugs   In recent years, several nonsalicylate, nonsteroidal anti-inflammatory drugs (NSAIDs) have been developed. These drugs are generally equianalgesic to aspirin and have similar anti-inflammatory activity. Some may be more effective than aspirin in dysmenorrhea. In other indications, no clinical advantage has been generally demonstrated. They are primarily used in treating arthritic diseases.

Establishing which agent may be more effective than another in a given patient is generally accomplished clinically. If a patient does not respond to one of the drugs within 2 weeks of initiating therapy, another may be tried. Sometimes, one agent is effective in patients resistant to other drugs in the group. Some of the newer NSAIDs are useful in patients who do not respond to older NSAIDs, but also some of the newer drugs may cause more gastrointestinal and other side effects. Some NSAIDs may be preferred to others due to longer durations of action necessitating less frequent dosing or better patient tolerance. Many patients who are unable to tolerate aspirin due to gastric side effects can tolerate NSAIDs. The NSAIDs are many times more expensive than aspirin and most are prescription drugs. These agents are discussed in detail in Chap. 26, "Immune and Inflammatory Disorders." **Mefenamic acid** (Ponstel) is an NSAID used primarily for acute analgesia due to the serious diarrhea it may cause with chronic use. **Ibuprofen** (Advil, Nuprin) is available as a nonprescription analgesic.

Narcotic Analgesics

The term *narcotic* is traditionally used to describe those analgesics which are derived from or are chemically analogous to the active alkaloids of the opium poppy. Opium is the exudate of the poppy plant *Papaver somniferum*. When the exudate is extracted and dried, it is called powdered

opium. The powdered opium contains numerous alkaloids such as **morphine, codeine, and papaverine**. Morphine and codeine have analgesic effects, while papaverine has a smooth muscle–relaxant effect. In addition to the natural opiates, there are a number of synthetic opiates. Analgesics which act centrally by occupying opiate receptor sites can be divided into the pure agonist and the partial agonist (agonist-antagonist) narcotics. All of the narcotic agonists except **propoxyphene** (Darvon, others) are effective for moderate to severe pain.

Narcotic Agonists   The pure narcotic agonists are listed in Table 17-5. These agents are indicated for treatment of severe pain. Postoperative pain and severe pain resulting from carcinoma, myocardial infarction, and major trauma require the analgesic potency afforded by the narcotics and may not be responsive to nonnarcotic analgesics. Members of this class of agents are also used as preanesthesia agents, in neuroleptanesthesia (**fentanyl**), in management of narcotic dependence (**methadone**), as antitussives (**codeine**), and antidiarrheals (**paregoric**).

Mechanism of action   The narcotic analgesics act through occupation of the opiate receptors in the central nervous system. Narcotic analgesics alter the release from afferent (sensory) neurons sensitive to noxious stimuli of several neurotransmitters, including norepinephrine, serotonin, dopamine, and other catecholamines. The effects of the narcotic include analgesia, drowsiness, mood changes, mental clouding, decreased sensitivity of the respiratory center to carbon dioxide, and stimulation of the chemoreceptor trigger zone associated with vomiting. Some patients say they feel euphoric and that the worry, tension, and anxiety associated with the pain disappears. Patients may still perceive pain, but their emotions about it are altered. Peripheral effects include decreased sensitivity of α-adrenergic receptors resulting in hypotension, inhibited peristalsis which may cause constipation, and increased bladder sphincter tone.

Pharmacokinetics   Many of these agents undergo a significant first pass effect when administered orally, but this decreases with chronic regular dosing. All are metabolized by the liver with inactive metabolites excreted in the urine. Their pharmacokinetics are compared in Table 17-5.

Adverse effects   The major adverse effects of narcotic agonists are listed in Table 17-6. In addition, hypersensitivity reactions such as urticaria, although rare, have been reported. Patients who experience allergic reactions to morphine or other natural alkaloids may not experience reactions to synthetic opiates such as **methadone** or **meperidine**.

Elderly and debilitated patients and others known to be particularly sensitive to CNS depressants should be dosed carefully. Cardiovascular, pulmonary, and hepatic disease, hypothyroidism, bronchial asthma, Addison's disease, toxic psychosis, severe CNS depression, and coma are other conditions in which narcotics should be used with extreme caution.

TABLE 17-5 Narcotic Agonist Analgesics

DRUG	TRADE NAME	Equianalgesic Dose (mg)[1]			ONSET (min)/ PEAK (h)	DURATION (h)	HALF-LIFE (h)	DEPENDENCE POTENTIAL	GI EFFECTS[2]
		IV	IM/SQ	PO					
Morphine		4	10	60 [3]	20/0.5–1.5	4–6[4]	2–3	Moderate	Marked
Alphaprodine	Nisentil	20	45	—	2–30/1–2	1–2[5]	2	Moderate	Slight
Codeine		—	—	—	15–30/1.5	4–6[4]	3–4	Slight	Slight
Fentanyl	Sublimaze	0.1	0.1	—	10/0.5	1–2[5]	2–6	Moderate	Moderate
Hydromorphone	Dilaudid	2	2	7.5	20/1	4–5[4]	2–4	Slight	Moderate
Levorphanol	Levo-Dromoran	2	2	2–3	60/2	4–8[6]	—	Slight	Moderate
Meperidine	Demerol, others	50–75	75–100	150+	10/1	2–4[7]	4–8	Moderate	Slight
Methadone	Dolophine	—	10	12.5+	15/1.5	4–6[8]	24	Moderate	Slight
Oxycodone	Percodan (contains ASA)	—	—	—	30/1–2	4–6[4]	—	Moderate	Moderate
Oxymorphone	Numorphan	0.5	1.0	6	5–10/1	3–6[4]	—	Marked	Marked

[1]Comparable to 10 mg morphine IM. There are no equianalgesic doses for codeine and oxycodone (see text).
[2]Nausea, vomiting, constipation.
[3]Equivalent oral dose based on PRN administration is 60 mg, but on regular schedule it is 15–25 mg (see text).
[4]Dosed every 4–6 h.   [7]Dosed every 2½–3½ h.
[5]Dosed every 1–2 h.   [8]Dosed every 3–4 h.
[6]Dosed every 6–8 h.

TABLE 17-6 Effects of Narcotics on Various Systems and Areas of the Body

SYSTEM OR AREA	EFFECTS
Consciousness	Drowsiness, euphoria, sleep, mental clouding
Eye	Miosis (constriction of pupil)
Respiratory	Rate and depth of respiration depressed
Cough reflex	Depression of cough reflex
Medulla	Possible nausea and vomiting
Pituitary	Stimulates release of antidiuretic hormone, which decreases urinary output
Gastrointestinal	Slows peristalsis; delays emptying of stomach; decreases gastric, pancreatic, and biliary secretions; causes constipation and anorexia
Gallbladder and common bile duct	Spasm of biliary tract
Genitourinary	Difficulty in voiding

Before administering the narcotic analgesic the nurse should check the vital signs. In the presence of *severe* hypotension relative to the patient's baseline readings, or if severe dehydration or hypovolemia is present, it is unwise to give large analgesic doses, since narcotics lower the blood pressure. After administration of a narcotic, the patients should avoid rapidly assuming the upright position, as they may experience postural hypotension.

Respiratory depression is a potential danger associated with narcotics, particularly those administered parenterally. The nurse should therefore analyze the rate and character of respiration before a narcotic is administered and give the drug cautiously if the patient shows respiratory depression, i.e., shallow respirations, respiratory rate of 10 or less per minute, or a decrease of 8 or more respirations per minute from baseline resting rates. Monitoring of the patient's respiration is important in such cases. Narcotics should be administered judiciously to those with chronic obstructive lung conditions, as complete respiratory suppression can occur, especially if the patient is also receiving oxygen at a rate of more than 3 L/min. A patient with impaired gaseous exchange in the lungs should be observed carefully for signs of hypoxia (restlessness, irritability, cyanosis, hypotension) when narcotics are given. Patients receiving narcotics should be encouraged to exercise, turn, cough, and breathe deeply. This is particularly important since the cough center may be depressed by the narcotic. However, excessive fear of analgesia-induced respiratory depression should not prevent adequate pain treatment. Since the respiratory center is low in the central nervous system and central nervous system depression proceeds from higher centers to lower centers, it is improbable that narcotics will cause respiratory depression in the absence of clouded thinking and obtundation in a patient with otherwise normal respiratory function.

Nausea and vomiting may occur after the initial narcotic dose, after several doses, or not at all. Since ambulation enhances stimulation of the central vomiting center, the patient should be cautioned to remain quiet or an antiemetic should be administered.

For most patients in pain a change in the level of consciousness may be beneficial, but such changes should be carefully evaluated and reported if severe. While the patient with cardiovascular problems or recovering from surgery needs sleep and rest, narcotics are contraindicated for the patient with a head injury or increased intracranial pressure, as they may mask important neurologic changes or actually increase intracranial pressure. Safety is important in the patient receiving narcotics; side rails should be used and the patient cautioned to remain in bed if there are changes in mental status, especially alterations in judgment, or if there is unsteadiness.

Intake and output of patients taking narcotics must be accurately measured, since these drugs not only increase the secretion of antidiuretic hormone (ADH) but can decrease the effectiveness of bladder function. Difficulty in voiding after surgery may be in part attributable to narcotics. Nursing measures such as having the male patient stand to void, providing the sound of running water, or encouraging the patient to relax are usually all that is necessary. In some cases, however, medications are given or the patient is catheterized.

During therapy with narcotic analgesics, accurate assessment of bowel function is important, since narcotics can impair intestinal peristalsis, leading to constipation and even paralytic ileus. Frequency of stools and number and character of bowel sounds are checked. To maintain optimal bowel function, adequate exercise, fluids, and dietary roughage are important. Occasionally the patient will require a laxative in spite of these preventive measures.

Many antitussives contain a narcotic, most often codeine. These agents retain the properties of narcotics and may cause the same adverse effects. Since most antitussives are taken in the home, teaching is important. Teaching should include the necessity of keeping medication out of the reach of children; avoidance of driving, etc., since narcotics may impair judgment; and the danger of simultaneously taking alcohol or any other drug that depresses the central nervous system.

The patient who experiences some of the side effects of narcotics caused by the dilatation of cutaneous blood vessels, such as flushed skin, sweating, and unusual warmth to the head, neck, and thorax, may need to be reassured that nothing is wrong. A change of bed and pajamas or a cool cloth to the forehead may be needed to make the patient more comfortable.

Narcotic abuse Tolerance to and dependence on narcotic analgesics are important considerations in the use of these agents for analgesia. *Tolerance,* exemplified by the need for increasing doses for the same effect, and *dependence,* a state which involves withdrawal symptoms when the drug is discontinued, both involve physiologic changes in the body. Drug abuse behavior, including drug-seeking and drug-taking patterns, may be associated with tolerance and dependence.

These undesirable effects occur in persons using the drugs for recreational purposes and in persons taking the drugs in the absence of physical pain. Patients with physical pain seldom develop treatment-induced dependence from which they cannot be easily withdrawn once the pain resolves. Additionally, tolerance is not an important clinical problem in patients with severe, chronic pain due to physical causes.

Tolerance to the respiratory-depressant, analgesic, sedative, emetic, and euphoric effects of the narcotics develops, but users still exhibit miosis and complain of constipation. The lethal dose is greatly altered with the development of tolerance. Tolerance occurs among the opioids regardless of chemical dissimilarities. Tolerance disappears with withdrawal, a factor accounting for fatal overdose when addicts take prewithdrawal doses after a period of abstinence.

Many clinicians harbor excessive fears of dependence and toxicity from narcotic analgesics. Recent clinical and epidemiologic studies have demonstrated that these fears are often unfounded. Investigators from the Boston Collaborative Drug Surveillance Program reported that dependence occurred in only 4 of 11,882 patients who did not have prior drug abuse histories and who received at least one narcotic preparation for medical indications. Fear of inducing dependence should not prevent health professionals from using narcotics in sufficient doses at frequent enough time intervals to provide effective analgesia (see Fig. 17-8).

Drug interactions **Phenothiazines, monoamine oxidase inhibitors,** and **tricyclic antidepressants** enhance the depressant effects (respiratory, sedative, and hypotensive) of the analgesics. **General anesthetics, antipsychotics, antianxiety agents,** and **sedative-hypnotics** may also enhance their depressant effects. Dosages of narcotics should be decreased, often by 25 to 50 percent, when they are given concurrent with phenothiazines such as **prochlorperazine** (Compazine) or **promethazine** (Phenergan).

Dosage and administration The patient may have orders for several different analgesics, e.g., a potent parenteral narcotic, a less potent narcotic such as **oxycodone** compound, and a nonnarcotic analgesic. Further, the nurse may have the options of selecting a dosage within a range

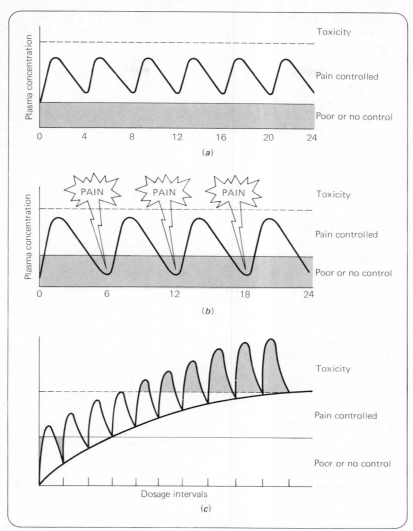

FIGURE 17-8

(*a*) Appropriate narcotic analgesic plasma profile obtained with regularly scheduled (every 4 h) doses. (*b*) Plasma profile for inappropriate dosing (too infrequent) resulting in intermittent pain. (*c*) Plasma profile of accumulation of narcotic due to too-frequent dosing.

ordered by the physician and of using another agent, such as an antianxiety drug or phenothiazine, along with the analgesic. In many situations these drugs are ordered on a PRN basis. Obviously, the nurse can select the most beneficial method of management only after a thorough assessment of the patient's immediate pain experience.

Severity of pain is not the only criterion upon which the nurse should base the selection of a narcotic analgesic, since narcotics affect a variety of organ systems (Table 17-6) and the nurse will want to avoid compounding other problems with adverse effects of the analgesic. If the narcotic analgesic effect is required because of severity of the pain, however,

the nurse can often initiate measures to prevent or minimize these adverse effects.

In elderly patients, analgesics are frequently eliminated from the body more slowly than in younger patients. Therefore, lower doses may be necessary. In all patients, titration to response is the key to successful analgesic therapy. When patients are receiving relatively high doses, but their sensoriums are clear and their vital signs are within the normal range, additional drug should be administered if the pain is not yet relieved. Alternatively, if patients are receiving seemingly low doses, but their central nervous system functions appear to be depressed by the drug, the doses should be lowered. In children the narcotics approved for use in moderate to severe pain, pediatric dentistry, and/or preoperative preparation are **meperidine** (Demerol), 0.5 to 1 mg/kg intramuscularly or subcutaneously; **alphaprodine** (Nisentil), 0.3 to 0.6 mg/kg by the submucosal route for dental procedures; and **codeine**, 0.5 mg/kg or 15 mg/m² by oral, intramuscular, or subcutaneous routes. Other narcotics may be used, but their safety and efficacy in children is not well-documented.

Most narcotic analgesics provide equal analgesia when administered at equianalgesic (equal pain relief) doses and appropriate time intervals (see Table 17-5). The exceptions are **codeine** and **oxycodone**, which appear to have multiphasic dose-response curves (Fig. 17-9). Other narcotic analgesics appear to have a relatively straight line dose-response curve. Therefore, as the dose of **morphine, methadone,** or most other narcotic analgesics increases, the analgesia produced increased proportionally. However, with **codeine** and **oxycodone** a ceiling effect appears to occur; further dose increments provide decreasing amounts of additional analgesia. This change has been observed to occur at doses exceeding 30 to 60 mg of **codeine** q3–4h, or two **oxycodone** **compound** tablets (e.g., Percodan, Percocet, Tylox) q3–4h.

As a result of this multiphasic dose-response curve, **codeine** and **oxycodone** are used for mild to moderate pain, often in combination with **aspirin** or **acetaminophen** (see

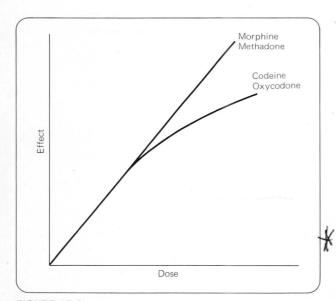

FIGURE 17-9

Relative Dose-Response Curves. Increasing the dose of methadone and morphine increases the response, while increasing doses of oxycodone and codeine reach a plateau or ceiling effect. (*From A. G. Lipman: ''Pain Management in Clinical Pharmacy and Therapeutics,''* in *E. T. Herfindal and J. R. Hirschman* (eds.), Clinical Pharmacology and Therapeutics, *3rd ed.*, Baltimore: Williams & Wilkins, 1983.)

Table 17-7). **Codeine** is dosed for analgesia at 15 to 60 mg q4–6h. **Oxycodone** is given in doses averaging 5 mg q4–6h.

The other narcotics are given in doses approximately equianalgesic to 5 to 10 mg of **morphine** intramuscularly. Dosages may be repeated as needed at intervals appropriate to the half-life and duration of action of the specific drug. Table 17-5 lists these dosages and dosing intervals.

The oral-to-parenteral dose ratio of **morphine** (and other narcotics) is much lower if the drug is given on a regularly scheduled basis rather than on an intermittent basis. This appears to be due to an altered first pass effect. When the morphine is taken orally, it is absorbed into the portal circulation and is distributed to the liver before it reaches the central nervous system. In the liver, much of the morphine is metabolized. Thus, a six times higher dose is needed orally as opposed to parenterally when the drug is given intermittently. If, however, the morphine serum level is maintained with regularly scheduled dosing, the liver metabolism sites may become saturated. In such cases, much of the drug will proceed to the central nervous system without being metabolized. Therefore, with regularly scheduled doses, the oral-to-parenteral dose ratio for morphine diminishes to 1.5 to 2.5 to 1. This first pass effect is not nearly as noticeable with other narcotic analgesics.

The initial dosing interval for **morphine** is normally 4 h. Once relative analgesia is accomplished, patients can frequently maintain pain relief with a dose every 6 h. The initial dose interval for **methadone** (Dolophine) or **levorphanol** (Levo-Dromoran) is normally every 6 h. This time interval can often be extended to every 8 h once pain relief is accomplished. Some patients report maintenance of pain relief with every 10- to 12-h dosing of the longer-acting analgesics. The longer-acting drugs are more convenient for patients and staff. Additionally, they allow greater ease in maintaining analgesia without the necessity to interrupt sleep for nighttime doses. Another important advantage is that fewer daily doses result in fewer reminders to the patients of their pain. The major additional risk of the longer-acting drugs is accumulation toxicity (see Fig. 17-8c). Such accumulation frequently occurs gradually, and clinical signs may not be observed for 5 to 10 days. The risk of accumulation is low if the drug is administered no more often than every 6 h. **Meperidine** (Demerol) has a relatively short duration of action and requires dosing every 2½ to 3½ h to maintain adequate analgesia.

Propoxyphene (Darvon, Others) Propoxyphene is a congener of methadone and is as available as both the hydrochloride (Darvon, Dolene, Doxaphene, others) and napsylate salts (Darvon-N). The latter and combinations thereof are more expensive than generic propoxyphene HCl. No clinical advantage of the napsylate over the hydrochloride salt has been demonstrated. Several studies have demonstrated lesser or equal potency of propoxyphene as compared with aspirin or codeine. Others have suggested that a dose of 120 mg of propoxyphene hydrochloride may be equivalent to 60 mg of codeine. However, that dose of propoxyphene approaches gastric intolerance levels. The drug provides no anti-inflammatory or antipyretic activity.

Mechanism of action The analgesic activity of propoxyphene is produced by direct action on the opiate receptors of the central nervous system (CNS). In doses equianalgesic to codeine propoxyphene produces central nervous system effects similar to the opiates, as well as nausea, dizziness, and lightheadedness. Persons taking propoxyphene may experience tremulousness, restlessness, and mild euphoria associated with a CNS-stimulant effect.

Pharmacokinetics The napsylate salt (Darvon-N) is less soluble than the hydrochloride, but no differences in absorption, metabolism, or effects between the two salts have been shown in humans. Peak plasma concentration differences between the two salts are small, and both peak at about 2 h. Half-life is approximately 3½ h. Doses given every 6 h require approximately 2 days to reach steady plasma levels. The drug is metabolized in the liver, and the metabolites are excreted in the urine. Combination of **propoxyphene** with **aspirin** (Darvon compound, SK-65 compound, etc.) or **acetaminophen** (Darvocet-N, Dolacet, Wygesic) provides greater analgesia than propoxyphene alone.

Adverse effects Adverse drug reactions from propoxyphene include gastrointestinal complaints (nausea, vomiting, heartburn, and constipation), dizziness, skin rash, dysphoria, and minor visual disturbances.

Overdosage with propoxyphene can be fatal, especially in

TABLE 17-7 Content of Some Combination Analgesics

TRADE NAME	ASPIRIN	ACETAMINOPHEN	NARCOTIC	OTHER
Excedrin	250 mg	250 mg		Caffeine, 65 mg
Equagesic	250 mg			Meprobamate, 200 mg
Excedrin PM		500 mg		Diphenhydramine, 38 mg
Fiorinal	325 mg			Caffeine, 40 mg; Butalbital, 50 mg
Trigesic	230 mg	125 mg		Caffeine, 30 mg
Vanquish Caplets	227 mg	194 mg		Caffeine, 33 mg; magnesium hydroxide, 50 mg; aluminum hydroxide, 50 mg
Bufferin	325 mg			Magnesium carbonate, 97.2 mg; aluminum glycinate, 48.6 mg
Ascriptin	325 mg			Magnesium hydroxide, 76 mg; aluminum hydroxide, 75 mg
Alka-Seltzer	325 mg			Sodium bicarbonate, 1.9 g; citric acid, 1 g
Tylenol with codeine no. 3		300 mg	Codeine, 30 mg	
Tylenol with codeine no. 4		300 mg	Codeine, 60 mg	
Phenaphen with codeine no. 4		300 mg	Codeine, 60 mg	
ASA and codeine compound	380 mg		Codeine, 30 mg	Caffeine, 30 mg
Fiorinal with codeine	325 mg		Codeine, 30 mg	Caffeine, 40 mg; Butalbital, 50 mg
Darvon compound-65	389 mg		Propoxyphene HCl, 65 mg	Caffeine, 32.4 mg
Darvocet-N 100		650 mg	Propoxyphene napsylate, 100 mg	
B & O Supprettes no. 15A			Opium, 30 mg	Belladonna, 16.2 mg
Tylox capsules		500 mg	Oxycodone, 4.88 mg	
Percodan	325 mg		Oxycodone, 4.88 mg	
Percodan-Demi	325 mg		Oxycodone, 2.44 mg	

young children. Blood levels are not good indications of prognosis, as low levels have been associated with death, while persons with high levels have survived. The clinical picture of overdosage, which may occur as early as ½ h after ingestion, is similar to overdosage with a narcotic and includes nausea, vomiting, drowsiness, stupor, miosis, respiratory depression, and cyanosis. Hypotension, seizures, coma, neurogenic pulmonary edema, cardiac bundle branch block, and cardiovascular collapse can also occur.

Propoxyphene is a controlled substance because of its abuse potential. Misuse seems to occur because the CNS-stimulant effect is pleasurable to some people. Misuse is often seen when the drug is used in drug-abuse treatment programs.

Drug interactions with propoxyphene are rare. The CNS-depressant effect may be additive with other drugs having similar effects. Alcohol in particular should be avoided, since overdoses and death have been associated with alcohol ingestion.

Dosage   Due to the differences in the weight of the salts, 65 mg of the hydrochloride is equal to 100 mg of the napsylate. Recommended dosages are **propoxyphene hydrochloride** 65 mg and **propoxyphene napsylate** 100 mg. Dosage may be repeated every 4 h but should not exceed six doses per day.

Patient education   It is important that patients not exceed the prescribed dose of propoxyphene. Should they do so, the risk of central nervous system depression and gastric upset increases greatly. Patients should be advised that the drug frequently causes drowsiness or sedation, especially early in therapy. Therefore, patients should exercise caution about driving or other activities requiring alertness. Gastrointestinal distress can be decreased by taking the drug with food or milk. Dizziness can often be counteracted by the patient lying down following the dose. Patients should be advised of the interaction between this agent and alcohol or other sedating drugs.

Although the published studies on propoxyphene in which it is compared with aspirin and other analgesics are not very positive, nurses should be positive when administering this drug. Many patients report excellent analgesia with propoxyphene. It is not clear whether this effect is pharmacologic or a mixture of pharmacologic activity and psychologic expectations.

Agonist-Antagonist Analgesics   Three analgesics categorized as narcotic agonist-antagonist drugs are available in the United States. The first of these is **pentazocine** (Talwin), which is available in both oral and parenteral dosage forms. **Nalbuphine** (Nubain) and **butorphanol** (Stadol) are available only in parenteral dosage forms.

Mechanism of action   These agents are partial agonists (see Chap. 5) and when given alone they provide effective analgesia, but antagonize narcotic analgesics if given concurrently. Thus, use of these agents in patients who currently have narcotic analgesics in their system may result in acute withdrawal from the narcotics or sudden loss of all analgesia. The agonist-antagonist analgesics provide analgesia which is equivalent to codeine according to some studies and equivalent to morphine according to others. However, these drugs offer little clinical advantage over other analgesics. The risk of dependence due to these agents is less than with morphine and other narcotics. The agonist-antagonist analgesics are controlled substances, like all other narcotics.

Pharmacokinetics   Pentazocine undergoes significant first pass effect. Its oral bioavailability is 20 percent. All of the agonist-antagonist analgesics are metabolized in the liver with less than 5 percent excreted in unchanged form by the kidneys. The pharmacokinetics of these agents is outlined in Table 17-8.

Adverse effects   Adverse reactions most commonly associated with these agents are sedation, sweating, dizziness, lightheadedness, and nausea. There appears to be a higher incidence of dysphoria, hallucinations, and vasomotor and respiratory stimulation with these agents than with narcotics. This may be due to preferential binding of the agonist-antagonist agents to sigma opioid receptors in the central nervous system. These adverse effects are more noticeable with chronic use and in elderly patients. Similar to the opiates, agonist-antagonist analgesics also produce sedation and respiratory depression.

Dose   The recommended dose of **pentazocine** by the oral route is 50 mg, while for subcutaneous or intramuscular

TABLE 17-8   Narcotic Agonist-Antagonist Analgesics

DRUG	TRADE NAME	USUAL ROUTE*	ONSET (min)	PEAK (h)	DURATION (h)	HALF-LIFE (h)	USUAL DOSAGE (mg)†
Pentazocine	Talwin	PO IM	15–30	½–1 2–3	3	2–3	50–100 30
Butorphanol	Stadol	IM	5–10	½–1	3–4	2–4	1–4
Nalbuphine	Nubain	IM, SQ	15	1	3–6	5	10–20

*Can be given IV or SQ as well. IV onset at 2–3 min and peak at 10–30 min. Dosages (IV): pentazocine, 30 mg; butorphanol, 0.5–2 mg; and nalbuphine, 10 mg.

†Dosage may be repeated every 3–4 h.

injection it is 30 mg. The usual adult recommended dose of **nalbuphine** is 20 mg q3–4h. The usual recommended adult dose of **butorphanol** is 2 mg with a dose range of 1 to 4 mg q3–4h. These drugs are not advised for analgesia in children.

Narcotic Antagonists

Because the opiate analgesics act through occupation of the opiate receptors, specific antagonists which have a high affinity for the receptors but which do not produce pharmacologic activity can antagonize the opiate drugs. **Naloxone** (Narcan) is the drug of choice for this purpose. A single intravenous injection of 0.4 to 2 mg of naloxone in an adult or 0.1 to 0.2 mg/kg in children can reverse a narcotic-induced coma in a very brief time. Patients who have received narcotic antagonists must be carefully monitored because the antagonists are often shorter-acting than the opiates. Therefore, the patients may relapse into respiratory depression and coma unless an additional dose of the antagonist is administered when indicated.

Centrally Acting Nonnarcotic

Methotrimeprazine (Levoprome) is an analgesic which works in the central nervous system but does not occupy opiate receptors. Structurally related to the phenothiazines, methotrimeprazine produces analgesia comparable to that of morphine but is accompanied by marked sedation. It is indicated in obstetric analgesia, preanesthesia, and management of moderate to severe pain where respiratory depression is undesirable. Like phenothiazines (see Chap. 34) it causes hypotension, anticholinergic effects, and extrapyramidal (movement disorder) effects. With CNS depressants and hypotensive drugs, it has additive effects. The usual dosage of methotrimeprazine (Levoprome) is 10 to 20 mg IM q4–6h (range 5 to 40 mg); smaller doses are indicated for the elderly.

CHRONIC PAIN MANAGEMENT

Chronic pain ranges from intermittent and bothersome to intractable and agonizing. Unlike acute pain, it is often not possible, or even helpful, to rationalize chronic pain, as it is pain which has outlived its usefulness. Rather, coping with the pain must become incorporated into the individual's lifestyle. Coping strategies include nonpharmacologic techniques to alter the sensory and reactive components and judicious use of analgesics.

Nonpharmacologic Therapy

Behavior therapies are aimed at cognitive and motivational-affective factors of pain reaction. Electroanalgesia, acupuncture, surgery, and similar therapies are directed toward decreasing the noxious stimuli that reach the brain.

Behavior Therapy

Psychotherapy, including relaxation techniques, hypnosis, and conditioning are major treatments for many chronic pain patients. Operant conditioning is a very useful modality when secondary gain is a factor. Secondary gain occurs when patients receive attention in response to complaints of pain. The desire for such attention may result in patients continuing to complain after the physical pain is no longer present, resulting in a chronic pain syndrome. Operant conditioning is the process through which behavior is changed or influenced by manipulation of consequences (positive or negative reinforcement). Such behavior modification is generally reserved for patients whose chronic pain is not associated with physical disorders which normally cause severe pain or when pain cannot be eliminated. Behavior modification requires active participation of the patients and their support group.

Electromyographic biofeedback allows patients to learn when they are becoming tense and thus to relax. Biofeedback machines provide a visual or an audio signal when muscle tension increases. Biofeedback is particularly useful in teaching patients autonomic and somatic control because it provides immediate feedback of their muscular tension levels. It is most useful in treating tension headaches, neck pain, and other pain syndromes which are associated with high levels of muscle tension.

Imagery is a technique in which patients are taught to use their imaginations as a therapeutic tool. This may include focusing on pleasant sensory experiences and memories to draw attention away from the pain or conjuring images of containment and dissociation from the pain. For example, a child might be told to imagine putting the pain in a balloon and letting it float away above the bed.

Electroanalgesia

The phenomenon of pain relief by electrical stimulation is purposed to be explained by the gate-control theory, that is, the electrical current blocks pain transmission. Two types of electroanalgesia are used clinically. *Trancutaneous electrical nerve stimulation (TENS)* uses low-intensity high-frequency electrical stimulation to the painful area or its segmental nerve. Endorphins apparently are not involved in this phenomenon, as it is not blocked by **naloxone**. *Acupuncture analgesia* in which there is low-frequency, high-intensity electrical stimulation or manual twirling of the needle appears most effective in acute pain. It may be mediated by the endogenous opioids.

Other Nonpharmacologic Modalities

Acupressure, physical therapy, palliative irradiation (for bony metastases of cancer), and surgical disruption of pain pathways are other methods used in chronic pain. Anesthesiology procedures are being utilized increasingly in the management of chronic pain problems. These local injection procedures include both reversible blocks with local anesthetic and irreversible (neurolytic) nerve blocks with phenol or absolute alcohol. They have been used successfully in causalgias, reflex sympathetic dystrophy syndromes, drug-induced vasospasm, and abdominal visceral disease. Myofascial trigger points are small, circumscribed areas of focal hyperirritability, possibly associated with sympathetic pain pathways. **Local anesthetics** injected into the trigger point may provide relief for several days to weeks, even though the drugs would normally be expected to act for only a few hours. With surgical and blockade procedures pain often returns as alternate pain pathways develop over time.

Pharmacologic Therapy

Mild to intermittent chronic pain due to diseases such as rheumatoid arthritis is commonly managed with aspirin or other analgesics. Appropriate exercise, rest, and diet are essential parts of the management of such pain problems. However, when severe, chronic pain results in the symptom complex of a chronic pain syndrome (physical pain, anxiety, depression, and insomnia), a coordinated management approach is required. Attempts to treat each symptom in the complex separately often result in undesirable drug side effects for which further drugs are prescribed. This approach may lead to a vicious cycle of multiple drug use and escalating drug-induced symptoms. The physical pain and anxiety should be addressed as the initial target symptoms. Interruptions of the pain-anxiety axis may result in diminution of the other symptoms. Specific drug therapy for the insomnia and depression is required only if these do not resolve once appropriate analgesic therapy is introduced.

Anxiety and Pain

Commonly, the major cause of anxiety is the continual recurrence of the pain. Chronic pain consists of current pain, remembered pain, and anticipated pain. Even when current pain is controlled, anxiety is induced by pain memory which elicits anticipated pain. While narcotic analgesics alone or in combination with an NSAID are the drugs indicated to treat chronic pain with physical causation, the dosing should be *regularly scheduled rather than PRN* if the anxiety about pain recurrence is to be reduced. If the patient waits for the pain to recur before taking the next dose, increased anxiety about the recurrence of pain will increase pain perception and necessitate a higher analgesic dose. After patients experience several days of relative freedom from pain, their anticipation about pain recurrence commonly diminishes and their anxiety decreases. As a result, pain perception is lessened and the patients' analgesic requirements also decrease.

Various antianxiety agents have been used to treat the anxiety component of the symptom complex. However, research shows no clear benefit from **phenothiazines, benzodiazepines,** or **hydroxyzine** (Vistaril) as adjuncts to regularly scheduled analgesia.

In the management of acute pain, narcotic doses are often started at a low level and titrated upward until an effective dose is reached. This approach is strongly discouraged in the management of severe, chronic pain, since patients will usually experience greatly increased anxiety if they are given doses of narcotic analgesics which do not provide pain relief. Therefore, it is preferable for the initial dose to be in the effective range. For most chronic pain patients, a small overdose is preferable to a small underdose. Once initial pain relief is established with regularly scheduled doses, the dose of narcotic can frequently be lowered. Dose decrements should only take place after the drug has reached steady-state serum levels (four to five half-lives). Reasonable dose reductions are 20 percent of the total daily dose every 2 days for **morphine** or every 3 days for **methadone.** When narcotic analgesics are used continually, it is reasonable to attempt dosage reduction every 1 to 2 weeks.

A patient who is dozing off due to the narcotic is likely to be receiving excessive amounts of the drug. Since total elimination of pain often results in clouded thinking, a reasonable objective may be to lower the pain to a level the patient can tolerate. If an adequate serum level of narcotic is not maintained, the patient may alternate between pain and obtundation. In such cases, lower doses should be administered on a more frequent schedule. If a patient continues to experience severe, chronic pain while receiving regularly scheduled doses which are highly sedating, other causes of anxiety may be the principal problem, and psychologic consultation may be indicated.

When pain increases, dosage should be titrated upward with increments implemented at each dosing interval. The difference between a serum narcotic level which produces little or no analgesia and one which produces effective analgesia may be small, so reasonable increments are 20 to 25 percent of the previous dose added at the next dose.

The single advantage of parenteral over oral doses of narcotics is a more rapid effect. If the drugs are given on a regularly scheduled basis patients can nearly always receive their drugs orally as long as they are receiving nutrition orally. A number of oral dosage forms are available for use in chronic pain, although lower bioavailability means oral doses are often higher than parenteral doses (see Table 17-5). If patients cannot take drugs orally, rectal administration may be considered. Intramuscular or subcutaneous administration is sometimes necessary. Intravenous administration of analgesics is necessary in only 5 to 10 percent of chronic pain patients. When intravenous administration is required, infusion pumps should be used, as roller clamps provide inconsistent dosing and may result in insufficient analgesia or overdose.

Depression

The depressive component of the chronic pain symptom complex requires antidepressant medications in 10 to 15 percent of the cases. These may be the same patients who have a genetic predisposition to depression, but most patients' depression has been linked to the pain and anxiety. Side effects of the antidepressant drugs have generally presented greater risk than benefit in most pain patients. Antidepressant drugs have been demonstrated to be useful in certain specific pain states including trigeminal neuralgia and postherpetic neuralgia. In such neurologic problems, the effect of the antidepressant agents on neurohumoral transmitter levels in the central nervous system may result in direct analgesic activity.

Insomnia

Chronic pain patients frequently experience insomnia due to the pain and depression of the chronic pain symptom complex. Therefore, once some relative analgesia is accomplished, it is common for patients to sleep. This is often in response to their sleep deficit; not necessarily an indication of a narcotic drug overdose. If patients' respiratory rate and other clinical monitoring parameters are relatively normal while they are sleeping following a dose of narcotic, nurses should not assume that the dose is excessive. Generally, hypnotic drugs are not indicated for insomnia secondary to chronic pain. Resolution of the pain problem results in more normal sleep patterns.

Special Analgesia Techniques

Hospice programs provide support and analgesia management to terminally ill patients and their families. Another innovation, pain clinics, uses a multidisciplinary approach in the diagnosis of pain etiology and in chronic pain management. These organizations have been instrumental in the development of some of the new narcotic dosing systems: epidural analgesia, patient-controlled analgesia, and analgesic cocktails.

Epidural Analgesia Epidural analgesia in patients with intractable, chronic pain is used as an alternative to intravenous therapy. Epidural analgesia may be administered through a variety of specialized catheters and reservoir systems which deliver the narcotic directly into the epidural space in the spinal cord. Doses of as little as 1 to 4 mg of **morphine** q12–14h by this route often provide excellent analgesia with minimal clouding of the sensorium.

Patient-Controlled Analgesia Patient-controlled analgesia, also termed *demand analgesia,* is a system whereby a specific dose of narcotic is delivered through an indwelling intravenous catheter when the patient pushes a button. The syringe pump can deliver the drug no more frequently than the preset interval. Because pain intensity has some diurnal variation, this method more closely conforms to the patient's daily variation in needs than do regularly scheduled doses. Although principally used to date for acute postoperative pain, advantages noted are more normal sleep patterns, patient acceptance and preference, and a decreased risk of

tolerance and dependence since patients [...] their dosages.

Analgesic Cocktails A number of "co[...] analgesia in a hydroalcoholic base, such as the [...] cocktail (heroin or morphine with cocaine in alcohol and water with flavoring), have been used in chronic pain. Controlled studies show that some of the ingredients in these mixtures do little more than increase the risk of drug interaction. Cocaine offers no additional analgesia over narcotics alone, but does produce dysphoria in some patients. Heroin, not a legal drug in the United States, is no more effective than morphine as an analgesic. Alcohol is undesirable for patients whose digestive tracts are irritated by disease, chemotherapy, or irradiation and may actually increase pain in some cancer patients. Therefore (according to a personal communication) even Drs. Saunders and Twycross, the two leaders in the British hospice movement who popularized the Bromptom cocktail, now recommend aqueous morphine as their analgesic of choice.

EVALUATION OF PAIN TREATMENT

Once the pain treatment plan has been initiated, the nurse evaluates the effectiveness of the plan. Because nurses are the health team members who spend the greatest amount of time with the patients, nurses are able to collect the most comprehensive data on the patient's responses to the treatment plan. The nurse follows up after each administration of an analgesic and elicits and records the degree, onset, and duration of pain relief. The nurse also observes the effectiveness of nonpharmacologic strategies. Patients' subjective feedback provides the major evaluation data that nurses receive.

Chronic pain patients are often open to suggestions. Therefore, nurses should ask about pain in positive ways, e.g., "Are you comfortable?", rather than negative ways, e.g., "Are you still experiencing pain?" Nurses should also note restlessness, anxiety, and the autonomic signs of depression. Patients' vital signs will often diminish once pain control is obtained.

The pain treatment plan cannot be appropriately altered unless the nurse collects and documents accurate accounts of drug and other treatment administration and patient response. When the patient no longer experiences adequate pain relief, the nurse should facilitate a revision in the current treatment plan. It is important to include the patients in all changes so that they continue to feel the interest, support, and responsiveness of the health care team to their unique pain experience.

Nurses and other health professionals who counsel pain patients have good reason to be optimistic about available pain management modalities. This optimism should be shared with patients. Both health professionals and the public subscribe to many misconceptions about pain and analgesics, especially narcotics. Patient education may be necessary to convince some patients to take their regularly scheduled analgesics before the pain returns. New technology, including infusion pumps, patient-controlled analgesia devices, and equipment needed for the new routes of administration directly into the central nervous system all offer promise of being useful in managing some patients' pain. Because of their close interaction with patients, nurses can be most influential in the management of pain.

CASE STUDY

Mrs. C.G. is a 72-year-old woman with infiltrating ductal cancer of the left breast. She had a radical mastectomy 6 years ago. Since that time she has had progressive and extensive metastatic disease. She has received multiple courses of chemotherapy and hormonal therapy to which she is no longer responding. She, her family, and her physician have determined that further curative treatments are no longer appropriate.

Mrs. C.G. lives at home with her 73-year-old husband, who has been in relatively poor health with diabetes and coronary heart disease. They have three grown children, two daughters and a son, all of whom are married. They have two grandchildren. Both Mrs. C.G. and her husband have previously been active in a Protestant community church, but due to their illnesses they have not actively participated in the last year. She now presents with diffuse, dull, continuous abdominal pain and pain in her right femur which has not been adequately controlled by acetaminophen with codeine.

Assessment

Mrs. C.G. has been taking acetaminophen 650 mg with codeine 65 mg approximately four times a day but not during the night. She reports that the pain is rarely relieved. She spends most of her day on the couch, dozing when possible. She says she often has difficulty sleeping at night. Mrs. C.G. describes the abdominal pain as aching and gnawing, covering her entire abdomen. It has been worse in the morning but fluctuates depending on the day. No change of position seems to help. The right femur pain is intense and easily localized. It is excruciating to have pressure placed on the site. She reports that the only time she has really felt well in spite of the pain has been on the several occasions that her children have brought Sunday dinner to her home. She particularly enjoys talking about her two grandchildren who are 7 and 10 years old. She comments that as much as she had dreaded this, she guessed she would have to have pain "shots."

Mrs. C.G. is realistic about her limited life expectancy. It is somewhat difficult for her to talk about this with her family although they also know. She confides that the pain has really interfered with any enjoyment left in life. She is also worried about what will become of her husband, whom she describes as needing a lot of supervision of his health and diet. When asked what would make this time more meaningful, Mrs. C.G. said she needed sufficient pain relief so that she could spend more time with her family and to feel comfortable that everything would be all right with her family in the future.

Management

The goals for Mrs. C.G. included adequate pain relief and improved interactions and quality of time with her family. In order to obtain adequate pain relief both physical and psychosocial interventions were required.

The right femur pain was caused by bony metastasis. Short-term, low-dose radiation therapy was given to the right femur. Such radiation is often appropriate pain relief intervention for localized bone metastasis. An anti-inflammatory analgesic would be more appropriate for residual bone pain than a narcotic alone.

Mrs. C.G. was started on an analgesic program. Oral morphine sulfate 25 mg in liquid form, was administered every 4 h around the clock. Over the course of the following week, the dose was reduced to 20 mg every 6 h. This dose offered adequate pain relief without significant sedation. Before the narcotic analgesic program was begin, the plan was explained to Mrs. C.G. and her family. The rationale for titrating the dose, dosing schedule around the clock, using the oral route for medication, and fears of addiction and tolerance were addressed. They were also told that if she should experience further pain once the drug and dose were established, an appropriate adjustment would be made so that pain control would be maintained throughout the course of her illness. An order for ibuprofen (Motrin) 400 mg every 4 h if bone pain returned, was also written. This drug was not needed. A bulky diet, frequent oral liquids, and a bulk laxative (Metamucil) were recommended to control constipation which resulted from narcotic administration and decreased food intake and activity.

A family meeting was held to discuss Mrs. C.G.'s illness and plans for the future. The two daughters, who were not employed, offered to alternate staying with their parents during the day so that meals could be prepared and Mrs. C.G.'s husband could receive help in taking his medication. On Saturdays the son volunteered to help with errands and jobs around the house. They agreed to look into the cost and availability of a night nurse in case one was needed in the future. Sunday family dinners at Mrs. C.G.'s home were planned on a regular basis.

A referral was also made to the local home care Hospice Program for continuing follow-up and support. Mrs. C.G. had expressed some regret over missing her participation in their community church. A contact was made with the minister of the church informing him of the family's medical needs and desire for continuing spiritual support.

Evaluation

Mrs. C.G. received immediate and permanent pain relief from the right femur pain after the radiation treatments were completed. She also reported that her other pain was quite adequately relieved with the 20 mg of morphine every 6 h. She commented that the pain was not totally gone, but it didn't seem to bother her anymore. She did not report nausea as a side effect. However, constipation was an intermittent problem which required bulky diet, oral liquids, and an oral peristaltic stimulant type of laxative.

Mrs. C.G. reported that she felt somewhat weaker each week, but she was enjoying her time with her family. She was relieved that her husband was getting the support he needed from their children. She stated that the hospice staff were extremely helpful and she slept easier knowing there was someone they could call if a problem developed in the night. Mrs. C.G. said the hospice staff were helping her family to make realistic plans for the ongoing care of her husband after her death which, as difficult as it was to talk about, made her feel relieved. The minister, who visited regularly, also helped her and her husband deal with their impending separation. With the relief of her pain, Mrs. C.G. reported that she was once again sleeping well. Therefore, no sleeping medication was needed.

REFERENCES

Adams, R. D., and J. B. Martin: "Acute and Chronic Pain: Pathophysiology and Management," in R. G. Petersdorf et al. (eds.), *Harrison's Principles of Internal Medicine*, 10th ed., New York, McGraw-Hill, 1983.

Boss, B. J., and J. W. Goloskov: "Pain," in S. M. Lewis and I. C. Collier (eds.), *Medical Surgical Nursing: Assessment and Management of Clinical Problems*, New York: McGraw-Hill, 1983.

Churcher, M. D.: "Pain and the Autonomic Nervous System," *Recent Progress in Anesthesiology and Resuscitation,* Amsterdam: Excerpta Medica, 1975, pp. 59–62.

Clarke, I. M. C.: "Amitryptyline and Perphenazine in Chronic Pain," *Anesthesia*, **36**:210, 1981.

Jacox, Ada K.: *Pain: A Source Book for Nurses and Other Health Professionals*, Boston: Little, Brown, 1977.

Kaiko, R. F., S. L. Wallenstin, A. G. Rogers, P. Y. Grabinski, and R. W. House: "Analgesic and Mood effects of Heroin and Morphine in Cancer Patients with Postoperative Pain," *N Eng J Med*, **304**:1501, 1981.

Kastrup, E. K., et al. (eds.): *Facts and Comparisons*, St. Louis: J. B. Lippincott, 1984.

Koch-Weser, J.: "Drug Therapy—Acetaminophen," *N Engl J Med*, **295** (23): 1297–1300, 1976.

Lipman, A. G.: "Drug Therapy in Cancer Pain," *Cancer Nursing*, **2**:: 39, 1980.

Magora, F., L. Aldjemoff, J. Tannebaum, and A. Magora: "Treatment of Pain by Transcutaneous Electrical Stimulation," *Acta Anesthesia Scand*, **22**: 289, 1978.

Maher, R. M.: "Cancer Pain in Relation to Nursing Care," *Nursing Times*, **75**: 344–349, 1975.

Markes, R. M., and E. J. Sachar: "Undertreatment of Medical Inpatients Narcotic Analgesics," *Ann Intern Med*, **78**: 173, 1973.

McCaffrey, M.: *Nursing Management of the Patient with Pain*, 2nd ed., Philadelphia: J. B. Lippincott, 1971.

Melzack, R., B. M. Mount, and R. Gordon: "The Brompton Mixture Versus Morphine Solution Given Orally: Effects on Pain," *Can Med Assoc J*, **120**: 435, 1971.

Melzack, R. and P. D. Wall: "Pain Mechanisms: A New Theory," *Science*, **150**: 971, 1965.

——: *The Challenge of Pain*, New York: Basic Books, 1983.

Merskey, H.: "Pain Terms: A List with Definitions and Notes on Usage," *Pain*, **6**: 249, 1979.

——: "Assessment of Pain," *Physiotherapy*, **60** (4): 96–98, 1974.

Merskey, J.: "The Perception and Measurement of Pain," *J Psychosomatic Res*, **17**: 251–255, 1973.

Miller, R. R., A. Feingold, and J. Paxinos: "Propoxyphene Hydrochloride: A Critical Review," *J Am Med Assoc*, **213**: 996, 1970.

Moertel, C. G., D. L. Ahmann, W. F. Taylor, and N. Schwartz: "Relief of Pain by Oral Medications," *J Am Med Assoc*, **229**: 55, 1974.

——: "A Comparative Evaluation of Marketed Analgesic Drugs," *N Eng J Med*, **286**: 813, 1972.

"Pain and Suffering: A Special Supplement," *Am J Nursing*, **74** (3): 491–520.

Painter, J. R., J. L. Seres, and R. I. Newman: "Assessing Benefits of the Pain Center," *Pain*, **8**: 101, 1980.

Poletti, C. E., A. M. Cohen, D. P. Todd, R. G. Ojemann, W. H. Sweet, and N. G. Zervas: "Cancer Pain Relieved by Long-Term Epidural Morphine with Permanent Indwelling Systems for Self-Administration," *J Neurosurgery*, **55**: 581, 1981.

Porter, J., and J. Jick: "Addiction Rare in Patients Treated with Narcotics" (letter), *N Eng J Med*, **302**: 123, 1980.

Revler, J. B., D. E. Girard, and D. F. Nardone: "The Chronic Pain Syndrome: Misconceptions and Management," *Ann Intern Med,* **93**: 588, 1980.

Robbie, D. C. "Control of Pain by Drugs," *Physiotherapy,* **60** (5): 128–130, 1974.

Skinner, B. F.: *Science and Human Behavior,* New York: Macmillan, 1953.

Snyder, S. H. "Opiate Receptors in the Brain," *N Engl J Med,* **297** (5): 266–271, 1977.

———: "Opiate Receptors and Internal Opiates," *Sci Am,* **236**: 44, 1977.

Tamsen, A., P. Hartvig, and M. Holmdahl: "Patient Con-trolled Analgesic Therapy in the Early Postoperative Period," *Acta Anesthesia Scand,* **23**: 462, 1974.

Turk, D. C., D. H. Meichanbaum, and W. H. Berman: "Application of Biofeedback for Regulation of Pain: A Critical Review," *Psychol Bull,* **86**: 1322, 1979.

Twycross, R.: "Value of Cocaine in Opiate-Containing Elix-irs" (letter) *Brit Med J,* **2**: 1348, 1977.

Ulett, G. A.: "Acupuncture Treatments for Pain Relief," *J Am Med Assoc,* **245**: 768, 1981.

Wyant, G. M.: "Chronic Pain Syndrome and Their Treat-ment, II. Trigger Points," *Can Anaesthesia Soc J,* **26**: 216, 1979.

18

ALTERATIONS IN BODY TEMPERATURE

ANNE G. DAVIS
MARY A. MURPHY

LEARNING OBJECTIVES

Upon mastery of the content of this chapter, the reader will be able to:

1. Describe normal and abnormal thermoregulation.
2. Define hypothermia and the various types of hypothermia.
3. List drugs which can alter temperature regulation.
4. List five types of fever.
5. Describe the cause, symptoms, and treatment of malignant hyperthermia.
6. Describe the assessment of fever with reference to the methods of taking a temperature and a history, performing a physical examination, and appropriate follow-up.
7. Formulate a plan for the management of a fever specifically defining the objectives of management and citing examples of both nonpharmacologic and pharmacologic modalities.
8. Compare and contrast the two main drugs chosen for fever management with emphasis on their pharmacokinetic, pharmacodynamic, and adverse effect characteristics.

The body temperature in healthy human beings is normally maintained within a very narrow range despite variations in the environmental conditions or the amount of physical exercise. Although a "normal" body temperature is hard to define, oral temperatures above 37.2°C (99°F) in a person at bed rest would signify fever and probably would be indicative of systemic disease. The lower range of "normal" in healthy persons is 35.8°C (96.5°F). Some individuals consistently maintain slightly elevated temperatures at rest, and most people have temperature fluctuations throughout the day. A few clinicians and researchers contend that elevations in body temperature are beneficial and should not be suppressed. In addition to being a good indicator of systemic disease, there may be added benefit to the infected host by enhancement of the activity of the host defense system. The body also diverts circulating iron into the liver and spleen during fever, thus denying microbes this source of a vital nutrient. Most clinicians, however, believe that the discomfort and potential complications (e.g., seizures in young children) outweigh any potential benefits and will treat fever.

PHYSIOLOGY OF THERMOREGULATION

The neural control for integrating sensations of temperature changes is located in the hypothalamus (specifically, the preoptic anterior hypothalamus, which has also been named the thermoregulatory center). Specialized neurons located within the hypothalamus and spinal cord act as sensors to respond to internal and external environmental temperatures. When deviations from normothermia are sensed, the body responds by dissipating heat through flushing and sweating or by conservation and production of heat through vasoconstriction and shivering.

A *pyrogen* is defined as a fever-producing substance. Foreign substances such as viruses, bacteria, antigen-antibody complexes, and endotoxins serve as sources of *exogenous pyrogens*. These agents or their by-products are pyrogenic in the human body, and upon introduction to the circulation they initiate a series of reactions that result in fever. First, phagocytic leukocytes, such as monocytes, eosinophils, neutrophils, and Kupffer cells, are stimulated to produce *endogenous pyrogen*. This endogenous pyrogen in turn circulates to the thermoregulatory center within the hypothalamus and stimulates the thermosensitive neurons to produce fever. Several mediators within the hypothalamus are suspected of facilitating the process, such as prostaglandins (E_1 series), cyclic AMP, and monoamines, like serotonin. These mediators cause the thermoregulatory center to "reset"; the higher temperature is sensed as being the new normal body temperature, and heat is produced by shivering, vasoconstriction of the periphery, and sensations of cold causing the affected person to seek additional clothing.

245

Once the offending agent has been effectively removed or destroyed, the body again resets its temperature control to a lower level, and the person will register the prior normal resting body temperature. Although the exact mechanism for this is still unclear, it is felt that the central nervous system in some way inactivates the endogenous pyrogen and/or that the kidneys filter the endogenous pyrogen from the circulation.

HYPOTHERMIA

Hypothermia is defined as any core body temperature below 35°C (95°F). An individual will lose consciousness when the body temperature falls below 26.7°C (80°F). An incubator thermometer or thermocouple must be used to document temperatures below 35°C (95°F) because clinical thermometers will not register the lower numbers. Hypothermia is defined as being generalized or localized (Table 18-1).

Assessment

Hypothermia can be a symptom of acute illness or the result of environmental exposure. Clinical symptoms of hypothermia vary according to magnitude of temperature depression, humidity and wind chill factor, length of exposure, amount of body exposed, rate of rewarming, and degree of damage. Generalized accidental hypothermia causes the individual to appear cold and pale. There may be uncontrollable shivering (which is ineffective in producing core heat), and with time this may progress to stiffness of muscles, miotic pupils, slow, shallow respirations, bradycardia, hypotension, edema, metabolic acidosis, ventricular fibrillations, unconsciousness, and death. Hypothermia associated with an acute illness will present with some of the same symptoms as generalized accidental hypothermia, but with no history of environmental exposure. These patients may arrive at the hospital comatose.

Localized hypothermia begins with a feeling of numbness and loss of sensation. The skin is initially white, followed by erythema and edema. If exposure is not curtailed,

frostbite will result, manifested by formation of blisters and bullae, necrosis of tissue, and eventual gangrene.

Elderly people are particularly vulnerable to hypothermia and may become hypothermic even with household temperatures set in the range of 60 to 70°F. Although research data are lacking, clinicians cannot overlook the possible role of drugs in producing hypothermia. Some **nonsteroidal anti-inflammatory drugs** (including **aspirin**), **alcohol**, and **vasodilators** prescribed to treat hypertension or peripheral vascular disease, might lower the body temperature or predispose the elderly to hypothermia in cool environments.

Management

Immediate care for hypothermia is passive rewarming. Wet, cold clothing should be removed and warm, dry clothing wrapped around the victim or affected part. Additionally warm drinks should be given if the patient is conscious, and isometric exercises should be performed if the patient is able. Then the victim should be transferred to a hospital for active rewarming, which can include a warm-water bath (37 to 41°C, or 100 to 105°F) of the victim or affected part, wraps in heating pads, warmed intravenous fluids, warm gastric lavage, warm peritoneal lavage, inhalation of warmed gases (oxygen). If the patient is unconscious, resuscitation procedures should be vigorous and prolonged, since young healthy victims have been known to survive the most severe conditions.

Evaluation

Hypothermia is a serious condition requiring careful monitoring for acidosis (blood gases), volume depletion (blood pressure, central venous pressure, urine output), arrhythmias (pulse, ECG monitor), and temperature changes during treatment. The nurse should be aware that even though the periphery has been rewarmed, arrhythmias and even ventricular fibrillation which are refractory to drugs and electroconversion can occur if the myocardium has not been sufficiently rewarmed. Respiratory status (respiratory rate and character, lung sounds) are also monitored, as these patients are prone to pneumonia.

Monitoring of the affected part in local hypothermia requires evaluation of pulses, motion, sensation, lesions, and signs of infection. Local hypothermia may result in residual symptoms of pain, excess sweating, numbness, and discoloration, especially in the winter and following exposure to cold.

HYPERTHERMIA

Hyperthermia is a core body temperature above 41.1°C (106°F) and is generally associated with environmental conditions. Hyperthermia is classified according to degrees; mild, moderate, and severe (Table 18-2). *Malignant hyperthermia* is an inheritable form of severe hyperthermia that is characterized by a rapid increase in body temperature (39

TABLE 18-1   Types of Hypothermia

Generalized

Accidental environmental exposure

Acute illness: congestive heart failure, diabetes, acute respiratory failure

Generalized immersion

Localized

Frostnip: distal parts of the body

Frostbite: vascular and tissue injury

Immersion foot: damaged nerve and muscle tissue

TABLE 18-2   Types of Hyperthermia

Mild Hyperthermia

Heat cramps
Stroker's cramps

Moderate Hyperthermia

Heat exhaustion
Heat prostration
Heat collapse

Severe Hyperthermia

Heat stroke
Heat pyrexia
Sunstroke
Malignant hyperthermia

42°C, or 102 to 107°F) upon stimulation by inhalational anesthetics or muscle relaxants (see examples in Table 18-3).

Assessment

Clinical symptoms of hyperthermia vary according to the severity. *Heat cramps* can develop in individuals who are in good physical condition and have recently finished strenuous physical exercise. Body temperature may not be elevated; however, the patient will complain of excessive perspiration followed by painful spasms of the voluntary muscles, especially in the legs.

When the cardiovascular system fails to respond to high environmental temperatures and profuse sweating causes excessive extracellular volume depletion, the result is *heat exhaustion.* Other symptoms include sudden onset of weakness, dizziness, headache, muscle cramps, anorexia, nausea and vomiting, diarrhea, clammy skin, mydriasis, hypotension, oliguria, tachycardia, and fluctuations in body temperature. Rest in a cool environment generates a quick recovery.

Heat stroke is more commonly seen in elderly people with an underlying chronic illness (arteriosclerosis, diabetes mellitus, alcoholism). Direct sun exposure is not necessary, but high humidity (over 60 to 75 percent) is required for the "sweat fatigue" to develop. Antipsychotics, diuretics, and drugs with anticholinergic effects (see Table 12-5) retard

TABLE 18-3   Drugs That Cause Malignant Hyperthermia

Anesthetics	Lidocaine
General	Muscle relaxants
Local	Pancuronium
Atropine	Phencyclidine
Bupivacaine	Salicylate overdose
Enflurane	Suxamethonium chloride
Fenfluramine	Tocopherol
Halothane	Tubocurarine

sweating and may predispose to hyperthermia. Generally the victim will sweat profusely, cease sweating, and then develop symptoms: unconsciousness, headache, vertigo, nausea, visual disturbances, faintness, abdominal cramping, confusion, breathing difficulties, hypertension, and hypotonia followed by lethargy, stupor, coma, and death. The skin will be hot, flushed, and dry, and the body temperature may register over 41.1°C (106°F).

A thorough drug history will aid in detection of prior episodes of malignant hyperthermia in the patient or a close relative. Agents listed in Table 18-3 should be avoided or used with caution in these individuals. Patients who manifest symptoms of malignant hyperthermia will experience less relaxation during induction of anesthesia, and muscle fasciculations, hot skin, tachycardia, muscle rigidity, hypotension, and cyanosis during surgery. Death can occur from metabolic disorders and acute renal failure.

Management

Management of hyperthermia must be prompt and extensive with the more severe types. Heat cramps generally require only rest in a cool environment, loosening of clothing, and water replacement. Salt tablets, salt water (¼ tsp of salt to 1 pint of water), or a balanced electrolyte solution like Gatorade may be given. Heat exhaustion requires the same measures with the possible addition of intravenous replacement of fluids. Heat stroke victims require total immersion in an ice-water bath. Following the bath, the victim is placed in an air-conditioned, cool room and massaged to increase heat loss. Sedation is not recommended, but phenothiazine compounds (**prochlorperazine, promethazine, chlorpromazine**), to reduce shivering, intravenous fluids, and heparinized blood may be necessary.

Malignant hyperthermia is a medical emergency. Treatment consists of interrupting surgery, discontinuing all anesthetics, cooling the patient with ice, and administering 100% oxygen along with **sodium bicarbonate** to combat metabolic acidosis. Hyperkalemia can be treated with generous amounts of fluids and **furosemide** (Lasix). The drug of choice for malignant hyperthermia is **dantrolene sodium** (Dantrium; see Chap. 33) by rapid intravenous infusion. This muscle relaxant should be given initially in a dose of 1 mg/kg and continued until the patient's symptoms abate or until a maximum cumulative dose of 10 mg/kg has been reached. **Procainamide** (Pronestyl; see Chap. 45) in a dose of 0.5 to 1 mg/kg/min will combat arrhythmias.

Evaluation

Treatment of severe hyperthermia requires constant monitoring of the rectal temperature during therapy. Baths may be discontinued when the temperature falls below 38.3°C (101°F), but the rectal temperature is still monitored in case there is febrile rebound. These patients should be observed for the complications of hyperthermia. Central venous pressure and renal output are monitored for dehydration, congestive heart failure, and acute renal failure. Respiratory status is also evaluated, since aspiration, airway obstruction, and respiratory insufficiency can occur. If phenothiazines are used to decrease shivering, it should be remembered that these agents can themselves contribute to the hyperthermic reactions.

FEVER

The "normal" oral body temperature is 37°C (98.6°F), the "normal" rectal temperature is 37.6°C (99.6°F), and the "normal" axillary temperature is 36.5°C (97.6°F), but body temperature may vary several tenths of a degree among individuals. Temperatures that are measured rectally will read 1°F higher and axillary temperatures will read 1°F lower than oral temperatures. Normal temperatures can be altered by time of day, ovulation, excitement, stress, diet, environment, or humidity. *Fever* is an elevation of core body temperature over 37.8°C (100°F) orally or 38.4° (101°F) rectally. Several descriptive patterns that may help in determining the etiology of fever are shown in Table 18-4.

Etiology

Acute short-term fevers are often caused by bacterial or viral infections and are frequently self-limiting, but long-term fevers may be difficult to diagnose. There are many diseases that cause prolonged fever in humans. Examples of these are granulomatous infections (tuberculosis, fungi), pyogenic infections (liver abcess, cholecystitis), bacterial endocarditis, bacteremias, neoplasms, connective tissue disease (rheumatic fever, systemic lupus erythematosis, rheumatoid arthritis), multiple pulmonary emboli, thyroiditis, and drug fever.

Drug Fever

A febrile reaction precipitated directly or indirectly by the administration of a medication is considered a *drug fever*. Many drugs have been implicated as causes of drug fever, which constitutes 3 to 5 percent of all adverse drug reactions (Table 18-5). Several mechanisms for this disorder exist, including contamination of the preparation with pyrogenic foreign substances, drugs which act as pyrogens, local inflammation and tissue injury after administration, and hereditable biochemical defects (e.g., glucose 6-phosphate dehydrogenase deficiency) which predispose the patient to adverse drug reactions. However, the most common is an immunologic reaction; frequently allergic manifestations (rash, urticaria, eosinophilia) are a part of the symptomatology of drug fever. The patient with drug fever may show a remittent temperature elevation, an intermittent pattern of

---

TABLE 18-4 Definitions of Fever Syndromes

Intermittent fever: The temperature falls to normal each day.

Remittent fever: The temperature falls each day but does not return to normal.

Sustained fever: There is persistent elevation of temperature without diurnal variation.

Relapsing fever: Short febrile periods occur between days of normal temperature.

Fever of unknown origin (FUO): Occurrence of prolonged, unexplained fever; different patterns may exist.

TABLE 18-5 Drugs Reported to Cause Drug Fever

Allopurinol	Cocaine*	Isoniazid	Procarbazine
Amphetamine	Colchicine	Levamisole	Propylthiouracil
Amphotericin B	Corticosteroids	Lithium	Prostaglandins
Anesthetics	Cytarabine	Mercurials	Quinidine*
Antihistamines*	Diazoxide	Methyldopa*	Quinine
Asparaginase*	Dicyclomine	Mithramycin	Reserpine
Atropine*	Digitalis†	Nialamide	Rifampin
Azathioprine	Folic acid	Nitrofurantoin	Salicylates*
Barbiturates*	Glutethimide	Novobiocin*	Streptokinase
Benzatropine	Haloperidol	Para-aminosalicylic	Streptomycin
Bleomycin*	Heparin	acid*	Sulfonamides*
Carbachol	Hydralazine	Penicillins*	Tetracyclines†
Cephalosporins	Ibuprofen	Penicillamine	Thioridazine
Chlorambucil	Imipramine	Pentazocine	Thiouracil
Chloramphenicol†	Immunizations	Phenolphthalein	Tolmetin
Chloroquine	Insulins†	Phenothiazines	Trimeprazine
Chlorpromazine	Interferon	Phenytoin*	Tuberculin PPD
Cimetidine	Iodides	Potassium iodide	Vancomycin
Clofibrate	Iron dextran	Procainamide*	Warfarin

*Most commonly.   †Very rarely.

elevation, or the fever may appear at fixed time intervals following the drug's administration. Upon discontinuation of the drug therapy, the fever should abate within 48 h, provided delayed metabolism and excretion or tissue injury are not present.

The diagnosis of drug fever caused by hypersensitivity is often missed, but should be suspected when the patient appears well when febrile and lacks the tachycardia, chills, headache, and myalgia that generally accompany temperature elevations. Rarely, drug fever may also manifest a symptom pattern similar to a septic process. Drug fever from allergy characteristically occurs on the seventh to tenth day of therapy but may appear within hours if the patient has been previously exposed to the drug. When hypersensitivity fever is suspected, all nonessential medications should be discontinued. If the fever abates, drugs are sequentially rechallenged to identify the responsible agent. If the patient is taking a drug commonly implicated in causing drug fever, this agent is discontinued first. Substitution of a chemically unrelated compound (e.g., **erythromycin** for **penicillin**) allows for continuation of the identification process. Corticosteroids (e.g., **prednisone**) may be used to suppress the fever if continued therapy with the causal agent is deemed essential, but **antihistamines** and **desensitization** programs are ineffective.

Assessment

Taking a Temperature

Temperatures can be taken with glass thermometers, electronic thermometers, or Clinitemp fever detectors (black, flexible strips of plastic with heat-sensitive crystals). Thermometers are calibrated in Fahrenheit (°F) or Celsius (°C) degrees, as shown in Fig. 18-1. The choice of a thermometer depends on the patient's age and condition. Patients who mouth-breathe, have oral problems, are confused, or may bite the thermometer should have temperatures taken rectally.

Whatever type of thermometer is selected, proper use and timing is crucial. A glass thermometer must be vigorously shaken to contain all the mercury below the 95°F mark before insertion. The glass rectal thermometer must stay in place for 4 min to obtain an accurate reading, but when the room temperature is 72°F or more, the time may be reduced to 2 to 3 min. Temperatures can be taken at the axilla, but they are generally considered unreliable, and the thermometer must be held in place for 5 to 10 min. Oral temperatures are taken for 3 to 5 min, although some researchers feel 8 min is required in a room of 65 to 75°F to obtain a stabilized oral temperature. The advantage of an electronic thermometer is that it registers the correct temperature almost immediately.

Diurnal and Variable Rhythms

Although most thermometers would indicate that 37°C (98.6°F) is a "normal" tem-

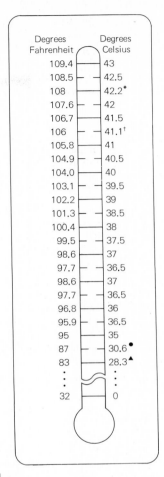

FIGURE 18-1

Schematic representation of a thermometer showing temperature conversions and extremes of body temperature. To convert Fahrenheit to Celsius: °C = ⅝ (°F − 32). Physiologic effects of dysthermia: *brain damage; †convulsions; ●loss of consciousness; ▲ventricular fibrillation.

perature, body temperature is variable and dynamic. Some healthy persons may register a temperature as low as 35.8°C (96.5°F). Temperature readings will also vary depending on environmental changes, physical exercise, and type of clothing. Circadian (diurnal) variations in temperature occur in healthy people with low temperature readings in the morning upon waking, rising slowly throughout the day with a peak effect between 6 P.M. and 10 P.M., and then declining until the minimum levels are reached at 2 A.M. to 4 A.M. The febrile patterns of humans will also mimic this diurnal pattern. The female reproductive cycle, with temperature elevation at midcycle ovulation, is another source of rhythmic variation.

Body temperature in children is more variable than in adults. Children experience transient elevations of temperature with only slight physical exertion. Adults who exercise in excess, such as marathon runners, may show severe elevations in temperature as high as 41°C (105.8°F). The body can compensate for such alterations through subcutaneous vasodilatation, hyperventilation, and sweating. Should these homeostatic mechanisms not be operational, hyperthermia may result.

Ascertaining the Cause of Fever

Fever is one of the distinguishing characteristics of many diseases, such as meningitis, otitis, urinary tract infection, and pneumonia. The history should contain some basic questions: patient's age, onset of fever, similar episodes in the past, gradual or sudden onset, total duration of fever, character of the fever, any aggravating factors (recent exposures, drugs, immunizations), any treatment used with this fever or prior fevers, course of this fever, and the effect of the fever on daily activities. Also included are questions concerning chronic or acute conditions that might precipitate a fever, such as cardiac disease, diabetes, tuberculosis, mononucleosis, pneumonia, asthma, and ulcers. Notation is made of associated symptoms such as shivering, chills, change in weight, night sweats, and environmental history that may indicate exposure to diseases or working conditions that precipitated the fever.

The physical examination should begin with a general observation. The patient who looks "good" (walks in, sits comfortably, talks without strain) and has a fever is less worrisome initially than the child who looks toxic (slumped in mother's arms and immobile during the entire history), has a dull look across the face, and has a fever. McCarthy et al. (1981) identified eight observational variables on which to base clinical judgment when assessing febrile children: playfulness, alertness, consolability, motor ability, eating, color, respiration, and hydration.

Depending on the information gathered during the history and how the patient looks, the physical examination may be either a brief check of the troubled, localized area or a complete physical examination looking for additional clues to identification of the reason for the fever. Any question of fever origin should precipitate the full physical examination.

If the history and physical examination define the problem, no diagnostic testing may be necessary. If there is some doubt about fever origin, the simplest, least invasive procedures such as white blood cell counts, urinalysis, throat cultures, and x-rays are performed before invasive, costly tests are done. The patient may have to be hospitalized for more extensive work-ups.

Management

Nonpharmacologic Management

A patient with a fever caused by a specific condition such as infectious disease should receive treatment for that condi-

tion in order to eliminate the fever. A febrile patient with no associated symptoms can be treated to be made comfortable. It is best to begin with simple procedures for eliminating the fever while allowing time for the development of more specific symptoms. No treatment for simple fevers is preferred, since many fevers appear and disappear without intervention. This is especially common in children. A patient who is uncomfortably warm may be sponged or submerged in *lukewarm* water (96 to 100°F) for 15 to 20 min to reduce the feeling of warmth. Cold-water or alcohol sponging should not be performed because this causes too much discomfort, will not reduce the fever, and may increase temperature in the extremities. The patient should be dressed in minimal clothing with a light blanket on the bed, because overdressing can increase a fever. Encouragement of extra fluids such as water, tea, juice, ginger ale, balanced electrolyte solutions (Gatorade, Pedialyte), and light broth are helpful. If the patient is feeling nauseated, the fluids can be given in small sips, or as ice chips and popsicles.

A fever of 24-h duration with no other major symptoms may be treated with sponge bathing, fluids, and antipyretics. The exception to this management is the infant under 6 weeks of age who may have a fever as the only symptom of a major illness (sepsis or meningitis). Infants may be hospitalized if the fever is over 100°F for a day.

Pharmacologic Management

Medications that have been used as antipyretics include salicylates [**aspirin** (ASA, Anacin, Bufferin, others)], aminophenols [**acetaminophen** (Tylenol, Datril, Tempra, Anacin 3, others)], nonsteroidal anti-inflammatory drugs [**indomethacin** (Indocin), **ibuprofen** (Motrin, Rufen, Nuprin, Advil], and corticosteroids (**prednisone**, others). The mechanism of fever reduction for all of these drugs is inhibition of prostaglandin synthesis. Additionally, corticosteroids reduce the amount of pyrogen produced by monocytes. Corticosteroids and the nonsteroidal anti-inflammatory drugs are not often used for antipyresis, due to their potential for causing serious adverse effects.

Aspirin and Acetaminophen   Aspirin and acetaminophen are by far the most commonly used antipyretics and are considered the antipyretic drugs of choice. Aspirin has analgesic, antipyretic, antiplatelet, and anti-inflammatory activity. Acetaminophen has only analgesic and antipyretic properties. The pharmacology of these agents and their use in analgesia is discussed in Chap. 17, while the anti-inflammatory and antiplatelet uses of aspirin are discussed in Chaps. 26 and 42, respectively.

Aspirin and acetaminophen are very similar in their efficacy as antipyretics, although one study (Steele et al., 1972) indicates that acetaminophen may act more rapidly. In this comparison of aspirin and acetaminophen in children the reduction in temperature from 39.5°C (105°F) to 38.4°C (101°F) occurred in 3 h with aspirin and in 1½ h with acetaminophen. Thus, since there is little difference in effectiveness, the selection of aspirin or acetaminophen for antipyresis in an individual patient is dependent upon pharmacokinetic and adverse effect differences.

Pharmacokinetics   Although aspirin undergoes significant hydrolysis to salicylic acid during absorption, salicylic acid is an active antipyretic, so there is little effective difference in absorption between aspirin and acetaminophen. Metabolism of both **acetaminophen** and aspirin occurs in the liver. The metabolites of acetaminophen are pharmacologically inactive, but one metabolite is highly reactive. In the usual therapeutic dosage range, this minor metabolite is rapidly inactivated by conjugation. However, in large doses (single doses greater than 5 g), as in suicide attempts, the capacity of liver enzymes to inactivate the compound is overwhelmed, and this metabolite then reacts with tissues in vital organs such as liver and kidney, causing significant damage.

Aspirin is totally converted to salicylic acid during and after absorption. Salicylic acid is then metabolized in the liver to several metabolites, only one of which is active (gentisic acid). The metabolic pathway for salicylic acid has limited capacity (zero-order kinetics; see Chaps. 5 and 26), and thus may cause toxicity at high doses. Thus, serum salicylate concentrations are monitored in patients receiving chronic salicylates and may be considered for patients who routinely take "around-the-clock" aspirin therapy during febrile episodes. Blood salicylate levels of 100 μg/mL are considered therapeutic for analgesia, antiplatelet effects, and antipyresis, while much higher levels (150 to 300 μg/mL) are required for anti-inflammatory effects.

Adverse effects   Rarely are adverse effects seen with **acetaminophen** when recommended doses are not exceeded, although hypersensitivity reactions do occur. In overdose liver damage can result. **Phenacetin**, a compound chemically related to acetaminophen, causes renal papillary necrosis when used chronically, and since acetaminophen is a metabolite of phenacetin, some researchers suggest that this may also be a problem with chronic acetaminophen use.

Adverse effects of **aspirin** at recommended doses do occur more commonly. There is evidence in both adults and children that a conscientious patient or relative can cause salicylism by use of this drug routinely in recommended doses for fever. *Salicylism* is the term used to describe toxicity from salicylates, and it may result from acute overdosage or chronic use. The major manifestations are acid-base and electrolyte disturbances, dehydration, hyperpyrexia, and hyperglycemia. Patient complaints include tinnitus, hearing loss (may be permanent with chronic use), headache, dizziness, sweating, thirst, hyperventilation, and nausea and vomiting. Individuals who are dehydrated prior to using aspirin are more susceptible to salicylism. This could easily occur with fever syndromes.

Even in doses that do not reach toxic plasma levels, aspirin can cause considerable gastrointestinal discomfort and can actually aggravate a preexisting ulcer. Because of the antiplatelet effects of aspirin, some surgeons will want to know when their prospective patients last received aspirin and may request bleeding times to monitor residual effects. Recent research (Ferraris and Swanson, 1983) indicates the risk of perioperative blood loss due to preoperative aspirin use is less than was once thought. There is a correlation between the administration of aspirin to children and adolescents during illness from influenza or chicken pox and the subsequent development of Reye's syndrome, a severe neurologic disorder. Aspirin also causes hypersensitivity reactions, especially in those with nasal polyps or atopy (hay fever, asthma, allergies).

Although both aspirin and acetaminophen probably increase the hypoprothrombinemic effects of oral anticoagulants, acetaminophen is the antipyretic of choice in patients taking anticoagulants, since aspirin affects coagulation through several mechanisms in these patients. Oral contraceptives increase the metabolism of acetaminophen by 20 to 30 percent, so the recommended dosage may be less effective in women taking both drugs. Aspirin is involved in many drug interactions, increasing the ulcerogenic potential and gastric irritation of corticosteroids and nonsteroidal anti-inflammatory drugs. Drugs which alter urine pH will affect the excretion of salicylates.

Dosage and administration   Current dosing recommendations for both acetaminophen and aspirin are very similar (Table 18-6). The pediatric patient may receive 10 to 15 mg/kg/dose of either drug every 4 to 6 h without exceeding five doses in 24 h. Adult doses for antipyresis with aspirin or acetaminophen are 325 to 600 mg/dose given every 4 h as necessary without exceeding 2.6 g/day. Adults also also should be cautioned about using high doses of either drug chronically without proper instruction and monitoring by a physician. With sustained temperature elevations, the patient will be more comfortable if the antipyretic is given regularly, rather than only after the temperature becomes elevated.

TABLE 18-6   Antipyretic Doses of Aspirin and Acetaminophen by Age*

AGE	ASPIRIN (mg)†	ACETAMINOPHEN (mg)
0–3 months	33–65	40
4–11 months	81	80
12–24 months	120 or 130	120
2–3 years	162	160
4–5 years	243	240
6–8 years	324	320
9–10 years	405	400
11–12 years	486	480
Adults	648	650

*Dose may be repeated four to five times daily at 4- to 6-h intervals.

†Aspirin for children is available in 65-mg and 81-mg tablets (33 mg = one-half of a 65-mg tablet; 40 mg = one-half of an 81-mg tablet; 120 mg = one and one-half 81-mg tablets).

Both agents should be taken with adequate fluid (120 mL in children and 240 mL in adults). The gastric irritation caused by aspirin will be further diminished if the drug is given with food or milk. When liquid forms of acetaminophen are used, the nurse and patient or relative should be aware that the liquid forms of the drug are available in several concentrations, such as 120 mg/5 mL elixir (Pedric, Valadol, PeeDee Dose, others), 160 mg/5 mL elixir (Tempra, Tylenol, Aceta, Bayapap, others), 325 mg/5 mL elixir (Dolanex), 165 mg/5 mL elixir (Tylenol Extra Strength), 100 mg/mL solution (acetaminophen or APAP Drops, Tylenol Drops, Tempra Drops, others), and 120 mg/2.5 mL solution (Liquiprin drops). Therefore, when liquid dosages are prescribed, the concentration or entire trade name (Tylenol drops versus Tylenol elixir), as well as an accurate method of measurement (device provided by the manufacturer, dosing syringe, pediatric dosing spoon; see Chap. 7), *must be specified*. Because only acetaminophen is available in a liquid form and due to the risks of salicylism, Reye's syndrome, and gastric irritation with aspirin, acetaminophen is the generally preferred antipyretic for children.

Both aspirin and acetaminophen are available in several strengths of various solid dosage forms (e.g., tablets, capsules, chewable tablets, suppositories). Therefore, it is equally important with solid dosage forms to ascertain the dosage the patient has on hand or to suggest the strength to purchase if the drug order is by number of dosage units (e.g., "Take two aspirin"), rather than by milligrams.

Upon the advice of a physician, pediatric patients may require both aspirin and acetaminophen together for fever control, as this may provide a more prolonged effect, although it will not lower the temperature below that which can be achieved by using either agent alone. Some clinicians, however, will avoid concurrent use of aspirin and acetaminophen due to the dangers associated with aspirin and the currently unsubstantiated hypothesis that chronic use of this combination may increase the risk of renal papillary necrosis.

Evaluation

The temperature should be retaken 2 to 3 h after the antipyretic is administered and the patient evaluated for comfort level. The goal of antipyretic therapy is not necessarily to return the temperature to normal, but to decrease it to a level where the patient is comfortable and the risk of febrile complications (e.g., convulsions in children) is minimized. Patients on aspirin should be evaluated for gastric irritation. Reye's syndrome begins with vomiting and lethargy, progressing to delirium and coma, so the nurse should monitor for these symptoms in those under 18 who have received aspirin. It is also important to evaluate the parent's knowledge of the possible hazards of the administration of aspirin to children (since fever may appear before it is possible to identify the condition as influenza or chicken pox) and of the signs of Reye's syndrome. Nurses should ensure that patients, especially parents of growing children whose dosage requirments change over time, know the correct antipyretic dosages and have them in written form for reference.

CASE STUDY

J.B. is an 18-month-old toddler seen in his pediatrician's office for a fever. His mother reports that he has had a fever of 40°C (104°F) for 3 days and she is worried about the possibility of convulsions.

The history reveals J.B.'s fever began 3 days ago. It begins to rise in the morning and reaches a peak around 4 or 5 o'clock in the afternoon. Mrs. B. reports that it was 103°F the first day, 105°F the second day, and 104°F on the third day. He feels hot to touch and is a little irritable in the evening, but otherwise J.B. has had no symptoms of illness and has been eating and drinking as usual. J.B. does not have diarrhea or constipation and his sleep has been normal. He was exposed to chicken pox 5 days ago at the babysitter's. Mother has been treating the fever with acetaminophen (Tylenol) 80 mg q6–8h and extra fluids.

On examination J.B. has a rectal temperature of 104°F and feels warm to the touch. He does not look toxic and is seen playing with some toys on and off his mother's lap and wandering around the examining room. Further examination reveals a warm flushed skin, slight puffiness of the upper eyelids, gray tympanic membranes with all landmarks visible, a slightly injected pharynx, and some small cervical nodes. The heart, chest, abdomen, and genitalia were all found to be normal along with a neurologic exam reported as grossly intact. His present weight is 11.3 kg.

Assessment

This is a healthy-looking toddler with a negative history and physical examination who probably has roseola infantum. The differential should also include urinary tract infection, streptococcal pharyngitis, otitis media, flu syndrome, drug fever, meningitis, neoplasia, tuberculosis, Rocky Mountain spotted fever, and rheumatic fever.

Management

Laboratory tests for throat culture, urinalysis, and white blood cell count were sent. Mother was given instructions on the time course for roseola, that is, to expect 3 to 4 days of high fever followed by 8 to 24 h of a skin rash. She was asked to give 1 tsp of Tylenol elixir (160 mg/5 mL) every 4 to 6 h to J.B. when needed for temperature control and to try sponge bathing as needed along with encouraging fluid intake. Mrs. B. was instructed to return J.B. to the office if the fever did not subside and/or if the skin rash did not appear. The importance of using the measuring cup provided by the manufacturer or a pediatric dosing spoon when measuring liquid medications was explained to Mrs. B.

Evaluation

All the diseases listed in the differential have fever as an early symptom. The laboratory work-up will probably be negative, and the child will go on to develop a fine macular rash over the upper trunk. In the event the rash does not appear and the elevation in temperature persists, the child should be reexamined to rule out other diagnoses. While the prescribed dose exceeds age-related recommendations, acetaminophen in a dose of 10 to 15 mg/kg given every 4 to 6 h is appropriate for an 18-month-old child provided not more than five doses are given in 24 h, especially when the fever has not responded to lower doses. The mother should bring J.B. back or call the clinic if the fever is not decreased below 101°F (38.3°C) within 3 h of the dose.

REFERENCES

Abbey, J. C., et al.: "How Long is That Thermometer Accurate?" *Am J Nurs,* **78**:1375–1376, 1978.

Bernheim, H. S., L. H. Block, and E. Atkins: "Fever: Pathogenesis, Pathophysiology, and Purpose," *Ann Intern Med,* **91**:261–270, 1979.

Cone, Jr., T. E.: "Diagnosis and Treatment: Children with Fevers," *Pediatrics,* **43**:290–293, 1969.

DeLapp, D.: "Accidental Hypothermia," *Am J Nurs,* **83**:62–67, 1983.

Dinarello, C. A., and S. M. Wolff: "Pathogenesis of Fever in Man," *N Engl J Med,* **298**:607–612, 1978.

Dube, S., and S. Pierog (eds.): *Immediate Care of the Sick and Injured Child,* St. Louis: Mosby, 1978.

Ferraris, V. A., and E. Swanson: "Aspirin Usage and Perioperative Blood Loss in Patients Undergoing Unexpected Operations," *Surg Gynecol Obstetr,* **156**:439–442, 1983.

Goldfrank, L., and H. Osborn: "Heat Stroke: Dx and Rx," *Health Pract Physician Assist,* **2**:12–16, 1978.

——, and R. Kirstein: "Emergency Management of Hypothermia," *Health Pract Physician Assist,* **2**:20–21, 37, 1978.

Green, M., and R. Haggerty (eds.): *Ambulatory Pediatrics II,* Philadelphia: Saunders, 1977.

Greene, J. W., C. Hara, S. O'Connor, W. A. Altemeier: "Management of Febrile Outpatient Neonates," *Clin Pediatr,* **20**:375–380, 1981.

Hasaday, J. D.: "Drug Fever," *Drug Ther,* **10**:78–80, 1980.

Hayes, A. H.: "Therapeutic Implications of Drug Interactions with Acetaminophen and Aspirin," *Arch Intern Med,* **141**:301–304, 1981.

Hoekelman, R. A., S. Blatman, P. A. Brunell, S. B. Friedman, and H. Seidel: *Principles of Pediatrics: Health Care of the Young,* New York: McGraw-Hill, 1978, pp. 275–279.

Illingworth, R. S.: *Common Symptoms of Disease in Children,* Oxford: Blackwell Scientific, 1982.

Jarvis, M.: "Vital Signs: How to Take Them More Accurately . . . and Understand Them More Fully," *Nursing,* **6**:31–37, 1976.

Kluger, J.: "Special Article: Fever," *Pediatrics,* **66**:720–724, 1980.

Levy, G.: "Comparative Pharmacokinetics of Aspirin and Acetaminophen," *Arch Intern Med,* **141**:279–281, 1981.

Lipsky, B. A., and J. V. Hirschmann: "Drug Fever," *JAMA,* **245**:851–854, 1981.

Lovejoy, F. H.: "Aspirin and Acetaminophen: A Comparative View of Their Antipyretic and Analgesic Activity," *Pediatrics,* **62**:904–909, 1978.

McCarthy, P. L., C. A. Stashwick, J. F. Jekel, et al.: "Further Definition of History and Observation Variables in Assessing Febrile Children," *Pediatrics,* **67**:687–693, 1981.

——, J. F. Jekel, C. A. Stashwick, S. Z. Spiesel, and T. F. Dolan: "History and Observation Varibles in Assessing Febrile Children," *Pediatrics,* **65**:1090–1095, 1980.

Moffet, H. L.: *Pediatric Infectious Diseases,* 2d ed., Philadelphia: Lippincott, 1981.

Nichols, G.: "Taking Adult Temperatures: Rectal Measurements," *Am J Nurs,* **72**:1092–1093, 1972.

——, and D. Kucha: "Taking Adult Temperatures: Oral Measurements," *Am J Nurs,* **72**:1091–1092, 1972.

Peterson, R. G., and B. H. Rumack: "Age as a Variable in Acetaminophen Overdose," *Arch Intern Med,* **141**:390–393, 1981.

Reynolds, J.: "How to Take a Temperature," *Pediatr Nurs,* **4**:67–68, 1978.

Robinson, L., K. E. Roper, and R. G. Fischer: "Nursing Considerations in the Use of Non-prescription Analgesic-Antipyretics: Aspirin and Acetaminophen," *Pediatr Nurs,* **3**:18–24, 1977.

Rumack, B. H.: "Aspirin and Acetaminophen: A Comparative View for the Pediatric Patient with Particular Regard to Toxicity, Both in Therapeutic Dose and in Overdose," *Pediatrics,* **62**:943–946, 1978.

Schmitt, B. D.: "Fever Phobia—Misconceptions of Parents About Fevers," *Am J Dis Child,* **134:**176–181, 1980.

Shaver, J. F.: "The Basic Mechanisms of Fever: Considerations for Therapy," *Nurse Pract,* **7:**15–19, 1982.

Steele, R. W., P. T. Tanaka, R. P. Lara, and J. W. Bass: "Evaluation of Sponging and of Oral Antipyretic Therapy to Reduce Fever," *J Pediatr,* **77:**824–829, 1970.

———, F. S. H. Young, J. W. Bass, et al.: "Oral Antipyretic Therapy: Evaluation of Aspirin-Acetaminophen Combination," *Am J Dis Child,* **123:**204–206, 1972.

Stern, R. C.: "Pathophysiologic Basis for Symptomatic Treatment of Fever," *Pediatrics,* **59:**92–98, 1977.

Wasson, J. B., T. Walsh, R. Tompkins, and H. Sox: *The Common Symptom Guide,* New York: McGraw-Hill, 1975.

Young, E. J., V. Fainstein, and D. M. Musher: "Drug-Induced Fever: Cases Seen in the Evaluation of Unexplained Fever in a General Hospital Population," *Rev Infect Dis,* **4:**69–77, 1982.

19

NAUSEA AND VOMITING

RUTH MERRYMAN
BRENDA FONT CLARKE

LEARNING OBJECTIVES

Upon mastery of the contents of this chapter, the reader shall be able to

1. Differentiate among the following terms: *nausea, vomiting, retching,* and *regurgitation.*
2. Describe the physiologic regulation of nausea and vomiting.
3. List four drug classes that are commonly associated with nausea and vomiting.
4. Describe three signs and symptoms which differentiate the causes of nausea and vomiting.
5. List three complications of vomiting.
6. Explain the nonpharmacologic treatment of nausea and vomiting.
7. Name three types of antiemetics and give examples of each.
8. Describe the mechanism of action of antihistamines in motion sickness.
9. List the major side effects of the antihistamines.
10. Explain the mechanism of action of the scopolamine transdermal therapeutic system.
11. Describe the considerations in selecting an approach to management of nausea and vomiting in pregnancy.
12. List three causes of vomiting in the pediatric patient.
13. Discuss the use of antihistamines in the treatment of motion sickness.
14. Give the dose, route of administration, and common adverse effects of the following antiemetics: prochlorperazine, benzquinamide, trimethobenzamide, and metoclopramide.

Nausea and vomiting may be symptoms of a disease process or a response to stimuli such as drugs, radiation, or motion. The underlying cause should be sought and corrected if possible; the etiology may suggest which measures are optimal for symptomatic treatment. Some nausea and vomiting is mild and self-limiting and does not require drug therapy. In other situations, untreated vomiting may delay or interrupt wound healing after surgery or may cause fluid and electrolyte loss, perpetuating the symptoms of nausea and vomiting.

PHYSIOLOGY OF NAUSEA AND VOMITING

Nausea and vomiting are a physiologic response to noxious stimuli. *Nausea* is a feeling, usually referred to the throat or epigastrium, of an imminent desire to vomit. Autonomic changes often accompany the feeling of nausea, including skin pallor, anorexia, diaphoresis (increased perspiration), salivation, and occasional hypotension associated with bradycardia (vasovagal syndrome). Nausea is produced by excitation of an area in the medulla which is either closely associated with or actually part of the vomiting center. Nausea can be caused by irritative impulses from the gastrointestinal tract, by impulses which originate in the brain and which are associated with motion sickness, or by impulses originating from the cortex to initiate vomiting.

Vomiting is a forceful oral expulsion of upper gastrointestinal tract contents. Physiologically, vomiting is the means by which the upper gastrointestinal tract expels its contents when it becomes excessively irritated, overexcited, or overdistended. Since vomiting can occur without being preceded by the sensation of nausea, it appears that only certain parts of the vomiting center are associated with producing the sensation of nausea.

When the gastric mucosa of the upper gastrointestinal tract becomes irritated, impulses are relayed to the vomiting center via visceral afferent pathways. From the *vomiting center,* impulses travel efferent pathways along the phrenic nerve (to the diaphragm), the spinal nerves (to the abdominal

*The editors thank Robert A. Kerr and Joan M. Stanley, who contributed the chapter on this subject in the first edition.

musculature), and the visceral efferent nerves (to the stomach and esophagus). These efferent impulses then produce the act of vomiting (Fig. 19-1).

Some stimuli to vomiting do not traverse the afferent pathways to the vomiting center but rather act directly on an area in the brain called the *chemoreceptor trigger zone* (*CTZ*). The CTZ is located in a V-shaped band of tissue called the area postrema on the lateral walls of the fourth ventricle. This area is highly permeable to a variety of substances, which seems to account for its ability to be directly stimulated. By directly acting on the CTZ, drugs (like apomorphine), nauseating smells, and motion all can cause vomiting. Some antiemetic drugs prevent or alleviate vomiting by directly acting on the CTZ and are therefore able to block drug-induced vomiting; however, such an approach will not alleviate vomiting caused by gastrointestinal distention or irritation.

PATHOPHYSIOLOGY OF NAUSEA AND VOMITING

The exact mechanisms by which pathologic states induce vomiting are not well-understood. However, it is apparent that there is an eventual stimulus in the vomiting center or chemoreceptor trigger zone leading to the efferent impulses which produce the act of vomiting. The following paragraphs discuss pathophysiologic causes of vomiting.

Central Nervous System

Emotional reactions to major life events, neurosis, and psychosis can be associated with nausea and vomiting, probably via direct action on the central nervous system. Pain, shock, and vascular changes such as those resulting in migraine headaches can also induce vomiting. Increased intracranial pressure caused by brain swelling secondary to inflammation, neoplasm, concussion, intracranial hemorrhage, and acute hydrocephalus may lead to projectile vomiting, which is often not associated with nausea.

Drug-Induced Response

Most drugs are capable of causing nausea or vomiting. Drug-induced vomiting may be secondary to direct action on the CTZ or vomiting center [as with **apomorphine**, the digitalis glycosides (**digoxin** and **digitoxin**), **narcotic analgesics**, or **cancer chemotherapeutic** agents] or to direct irritating effects on the gastrointestinal mucosa (as with **alcohol**, **aspirin** and other **nonsteroidal anti-inflammatory agents**, and **antibiotics**).

Physiologic Response

Acute febrile illnesses (acute infections), especially in young children, are frequently accompanied by vomiting as well as diarrhea. Accumulation of endogenous chemicals apparently leads to noxious stimuli to the vomiting center or CTZ; this can be seen in viral hepatitis, renal failure (leading to uremia), and diabetic ketoacidosis.

Endocrine Changes

Endocrine deficiencies can cause vomiting probably secondary to biochemical changes and effects on the hypothalamus and medullary centers. Diabetic acidosis, adrenal insufficiency, adrenal crisis, hyperthyroidism, and the hormonal changes of pregnancy can induce vomiting by sending stimuli up the afferent nerve pathways to the vomiting center.

Visceral Abnormalities

Organic diseases of the stomach and upper small intestine can cause vomiting by sending stimuli up the afferent nerve pathways to the vomiting center. Such visceral abnormalities include peptic ulcer disease, malignant neoplasm, obstruction, acute appendicitis, pancreatitis, cholecystitis, viral hepatitis, gastroenteritis, and any peritoneal irritation. Radiation therapy and chronic severe pain can also cause vomiting.

Deficiency States

Vomiting can be associated with fasting and starvation with hypovitaminosis.

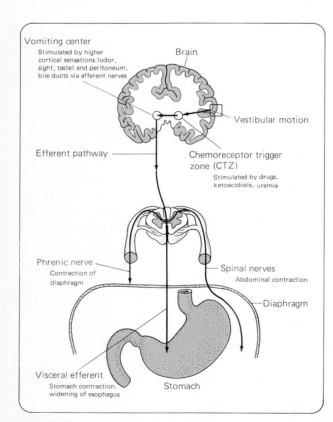

FIGURE 19-1

Neural and Chemical Mechanisms of Vomiting.

Vestibular Disturbances

Motion sickness resulting from movements of the head, neck, and eye muscles stimulates the cholinergic synapses of the vestibular nuclei leading to stimulation of the CTZ and the vomiting center. Other labyrinthine diseases such as otitis media and Ménière's disease can produce the same vestibular stimuli.

Psychogenic Causes

Vomiting may be self-induced, as seen in anorexia nervosa and bulimia (binge/purge syndrome). Vomiting may also be a mental association or anticipatory response as seen in patients receiving cancer chemotherapy.

Cardiac Abnormalities

Nausea and vomiting have been associated with acute myocardial infarction, congestive heart failure, and hypertensive crisis.

Ocular Abnormalities

Nausea or vomiting may occur in patients with uncontrolled glaucoma. Nausea is often seen when errors occur in refractive lens prescriptions.

The characteristics of nausea and vomiting and associated pathophysiologic conditions are summarized in Table 19-1.

TABLE 19-1 Characteristics of Vomiting and Pathologic Conditions

CHARACTERISTICS OF VOMITING	CONDITION TO CONSIDER
Occurs immediately after eating	Functional or organic processes in the stomach
Occurs 1 h or more after eating	Gastric motility disturbance, gastric atony, pyloric obstruction
Digested food in vomitus 12–48 h after eating	Pyloroduodenal obstruction
Frequent prolonged vomiting	Fluid and electrolyte depletion; acid-base imbalance
Large amount of food containing bile in vomitus	Obstruction below ampulla of Vater
Bloody and/or coffee-ground appearance of vomitus	Acute or chronic gastrointestinal bleeding
Fecal odor to vomitus	Intestinal obstruction, peritonitis, gastrocolonic fistula
Projectile vomiting	Increased intracranial pressure, pyloric stenosis in small children

ASSESSMENT AND CLINICAL FINDINGS

Assessment should be directed toward determining if the symptom represents a medical emergency, a manifestation of another medical problem, or a physiologic alteration which needs to be corrected. Patient variables which may alter the therapeutic approach must be defined.

History

The patient may present with nausea and vomiting as the chief complaint, which may be a manifestation of an underlying pathologic condition. Often the nurse must initially clarify what the patient means by the terms *nausea* and *vomiting*. Nausea usually precedes vomiting. The term *vomiting* should be differentiated from (1) *regurgitation*, which is the bringing up of material into the esophagus without nausea and without participation of the gastric musculature; (2) *retching*, which is an attempt to vomit characterized by labored, rhythmic respiratory activity which frequently precedes the act of vomiting but does not actually result in expulsion of gastric contents; and (3) *coughing*, which often results in retching and the passing of sputum rather than vomitus.

There are many characteristics which may differentiate the causes of nausea and vomiting. The nurse should follow a pattern of systematic questioning which will elicit a comprehensive history of nausea and vomiting from the patient. Questioning should include all aspects of the patient's symptomatology.

Time

The time of day may be indicative of the underlying pathology. The hormonal changes of pregnancy frequently induce either early morning or evening nausea and vomiting; vomiting may be the presenting complaint in a woman who is unaware of her pregnancy. Vomiting shortly after eating may be indicative of gastritis or pylorospasm. Nausea and vomiting in the cancer patient may correlate with the times of chemotherapy administration or may be due to other causes including progressive disease.

Severity

This feature of nausea and vomiting is generally described by having patients tell how the nausea and/or vomiting affects their normal activity. Aspiration pneumonitis may be seen in patients with decreased epiglottis reflexes either post anesthesia, after excessive alcohol ingestion, or after trauma. Gastric acid aspirated into the lungs can produce a life-threatening pneumonitis. Wound disruption may occur if forceful vomiting follows soon after surgery.

Quantity and Character

The specifics concerning the character and quantity of the vomitus itself are important in differentiating the underlying cause. It is difficult for many people to estimate the amount of vomitus. Comparison to familiar measurements such as a tablespoonful, a cup, or a quart may help the patient accurately quantify the amount. Excessive vomiting may result in metabolic complications—hypokalemia, hyponatremia, and hypochloremic alkalosis. In addition, dehydration and renal failure may further compound the metabolic problems.

A description of the vomitus by the patient must include the consistency, color, texture, odor, and contents. The consistency and contents are helpful in determining the source of the vomitus. Mucus may be from postnasal drip, rhinorrhea, or chronic inflammation of the gastric mucosa. If particles of food are present in the vomitus, the degree of digestion of these particles should be described as well as the length of time that has passed since ingestion. If large particles of food are vomited immediately after eating, it may indicate only a functional disorder such as improper chewing of food. If vomiting is associated with large amounts of belching, the problem may be due to swallowing of air (aerophagia). Bile will be present in all vomitus if the vomiting has been persistent.

The presence of blood and whether it is bright red or dark must be assessed and quantified. Blood in the vomitus may signify esophogeal, gastric, or duodenal bleeding. Blood that is bright red is usually fresh, secondary to ulceration in the mouth, esophagus, stomach, or duodenum. Blood exposed to gastric juice is often coffee-ground in appearance, as the blood is changed to hematin by gastric acid. The patient must distinguish between the vomiting of gross blood (hematemesis) and the coughing up of blood (hemoptysis). Blood in the vomitus may frighten the patient and thus heighten anxiety, which in turn can lead to an overexaggeration of the amount of blood that is actually lost.

The final element in the description of the vomitus is the odor. Hydrochloric acid has a definite, penetrating odor. The absence of an odor of hydrochloric acid may indicate that the material vomited has come from above the level of the stomach or that there is a decrease in acid production. A smell of putrefaction (like rotten eggs) may indicate gastric stasis if accompanied by a history of foul belching. A putrid or fecal odor may indicate lower bowel obstruction or fistula.

Duration

This line of questioning should include the onset and frequency of the symptom. The frequency of a symptom should be defined as closely as possible as times per minute, hour, day, week, or month. Prolonged vomiting is often found in conjunction with ethanol abuse and may cause a rupture in the cardioesophogeal junction (Mallory-Weiss syndrome) and life-threatening blood loss. Dental decay has been caused by chronic vomiting.

Influencing Factors

The patient should be asked what factors seem to precipitate the nausea and/or vomiting or to make it worse, and what

factors seem to relieve the nausea and/or vomiting either partially or totally. This information is important since the patient may not associate the nausea and/or vomiting with any specific events or realize the importance of associated factors and may therefore not volunteer the information.

Factors which should be considered are any change in food patterns, use of irritants such as alcohol or nicotine, prescribed medications, over-the-counter medications, any change in physical activities, emotional events, and/or recent trauma. Vomiting is often self-induced by those with anorexia nervosa to rid themselves of the food they were compelled to eat; antiemetics should not be the primary treatment.

Another factor to consider is a recent family history of vomiting. This may indicate either the ingestion of a toxin or an infectious illness. Because the vomiting threshold varies from person to person, the absence of a family history does not necessarily exclude either the ingestion of a toxin or an infectious illness as a cause of the nausea and vomiting. Similarly, allergies may affect some family members and not others, so it is important to question the patient regarding a possible allergy to food, animals, etc.

Generally a patient will very quickly determine consciously or subconsciously what exacerbates the symptoms. Position change or movement of the head and neck may exacerbate the symptoms if caused by vestibular disease. Food ingestion may relieve or increase the symptoms. Specific types of foods, such as carbohydrates, may relieve symptoms during pregnancy. Often, a person may have tried numerous home remedies or nonprescription drugs, which may or may not have alleviated the symptoms, prior to seeking health care.

Associated Symptoms

Symptoms may occur in body regions not directly involved with the nausea and/or vomiting. Abdominal pain accompanies vomiting in many gastrointestinal diseases. Rapid, dramatic weight loss may indicate intestinal obstruction, though women with anorexia nervosa or bulimia may also have difficulty maintaining body weight.

Vomiting associated with headaches may indicate acute glaucoma; with vertigo, it may suggest middle ear pathology; with jaundice, it suggests liver disease; with urinary symptoms, it suggests renal disease; and with chest pain, it may indicate acute myocardial infarction.

A change in bowel habits may occur with nausea and/or vomiting. Vomiting may be accompanied by diarrhea in gastroenteritis and by constipation in an obstruction.

The Pediatric Patient

Self-limiting gastroenteritis is a frequent cause of nausea and vomiting in children. In infants, fluids represent a larger percentage of body weight than in older children. Infants should be observed for signs of excess fluid loss or electrolyte imbalance and referred immediately to a physician if signs of dehydration are present. In the neonatal period, vomiting may be due to a congenital obstruction of the intestine or bile ducts. Later causes are pyloric stenosis, intussusception, volvulus, and strangulated umbilical or inguinal hernias. Treatment of the cause of the obstruction will abate the vomiting.

Postoperative Nausea and Vomiting

Anesthetic agents and narcotic agents sensitize the vestibular apparatus, the organ of balance. Due to this sensitization, rough handling during transportation from the operating room to the recovery room and frequent changes of position are frequent causes of nausea and vomiting during the posttanesthetic recovery phase. The vomiting center may be stimulated directly by chemical materials in the blood such as **morphine** and **meperidine**. Cerebral anoxia is another mechanism which stimulates the vomiting center during the immediate postanesthetic recovery period. Nausea has been found to be significantly related to pain in the postoperative period. The dosages of any analgesics should be sufficient to reduce pain and relieve nausea. The use of **naloxone** to reverse narcotic anesthetic agents during surgery will usually stimulate nausea and vomiting in the immediate postanesthetic recovery period.

Physical Examination

After completing the patient history, an examination of the abdomen is essential. Care must be taken during the examination not to exacerbate the symptoms excessively. Pulsations, protruberances, asymmetry, and general shape of the abdomen should be noted. Auscultation of the bowel sounds should precede any physical examination of the abdomen; the tenderness in turn interferes with the motility of the bowel. This will change the frequency and character of the bowel sounds. Peristaltic sounds occur anywhere from 2 to 3 times a minute to a maximum of 10 to 15 times a minute depending upon the stage of the digestive process at the time of the examination.

The absence and distribution of bowel sounds are important in isolating an obstruction. Abdominal arterial bruits may indicate vascular problems. Light and deep palpation should be performed in order to note any tenderness, organomegaly, or abnormal masses or fullness. Rectal examination may be helpful in distinguishing acute appendicitis in the patient who presents with nausea and/or vomiting. A stool specimen should be examined for fresh blood.

General patient assessment measures are summarized in Table 19-2.

MANAGEMENT

Clinical Pharmacology and Therapeutics

Therapeutic measures can be directed at the underlying pathologic condition or cause, or they can be directed at

TABLE 19-2   General Patient Assessment Measures

1. General appearance
   a. Does the patient look acutely ill?
   b. Skin color and turgor
   c. Sweating
2. Vital signs: Pulse, temperature, blood pressure (supine, sitting, standing)
3. What does the patient mean by "vomiting"? Differentiate between vomiting, regurgitation, retching, coughing.
4. When did vomiting start?
5. What time of day does vomiting occur?
6. What was the patient doing at the time?
7. What are the precipitating factors?
8. What are the associated symptoms?
9. How long has the vomiting been going on?
10. What is the frequency of the vomiting?
11. What is the appearance of the vomitus?
12. What is the amount of vomitus?
13. What are the temporal relations between vomiting and eating?
14. Physical examination of the abdomen

relieving the act of vomiting. Vomiting is a symptom and should not be treated with antiemetic measures until the reason for the vomiting has been assessed. Antiemetic therapy may not only eliminate vomiting as a diagnostic symptom but may also mask other diagnostic findings. However, if the disease process cannot be rapidly reversed, symptomatic measures may be taken to alleviate the nausea and vomiting.

Nonpharmacologic Management

Often nausea and vomiting may be relieved by simple measures other than drug treatment.

Diet

Small quantities of oral fluids may be given, such as gelatin, weak tea, carbonated beverages, or Gatorade (a commercially available fluid and electrolyte replacement) as tolerated. If vomiting is prolonged, parenteral fluids and electrolyte solutions may be indicated to maintain homeostasis. Oral solids should be begun with small servings of dry, bland foods such as crackers or dry toast and progressed until the patient can tolerate a normal diet. Frequent small feedings in place of normal or large meals will prevent the possibility of gastrointestinal distention.

Pharmacologic Management

The drugs, dosage forms, and regimens used to treat nausea and vomiting are summarized in Table 19-3. Drugs used for the prophylaxis of nausea and vomiting should be administered prior to the patient's exposure to the causative agents (motion or travel, cancer chemotherapy).

TABLE 19-3 Antiemetic Drugs and Regimens

DRUG	BRAND NAME	DOSAGE FORMS	ADULT DOSE	PEDIATRIC DOSE
Phosphorylated carbohydrate solutions	Emetrol, Especol, Nausetrol	Liquid	15–30 mL at 15-min intervals until vomiting stops.	5–10 mL at 15 min intervals until vomiting stops.
ANTIHISTAMINES				
Cyclizine	Marezine	Tablet Injection	50 mg taken 30 min before travel. May be repeated every 4–6 h. Do not exceed 200 mg/day. 50 mg q4–6h	1 mg/kg q8h.
Meclizine	Bonine, Antivert	Tablet	25–50 mg taken 1 h before travel. May be repeated every 24 h for duration of travel.	Safety not established in children.
Dimenhydrinate	Dramamine, Marmine, Motion-Aid	Tablet, liquid, injection	PO or IM: 50 mg q4–6h.	1.25 mg/kg four times a day. Maximum daily dose of 300 mg.
Diphenhydramine	Benadryl, Benahist, Nordryl, Phen-Amin, many others	Capsule, elixir, injection	PO: 25–50 mg taken 30 min prior to travel; repeat before meals and at bedtime. IV or IM: 10–50 mg	1.25 mg/kg four times a day. Maximum daily dose of 300 mg.
Buclizine	Bucladin-S Softtab	Tablet	50 mg taken at least 30 min prior to travel. Maximum daily dose is 150 mg.	Dosage not established.
PHENOTHIAZINES				
Chlorpromazine	Thorazine	Tablet, suppository, liquid, injection	PO: 10–25 mg q4–6h; may be increased if needed. PR: 50–100 mg q6–8h if needed. IM: 25 mg. If no hypotension occurs, then 25–50 mg q3–4h if needed.	2 mg/kg/24 h in four to six doses.
Prochlorperazine	Compazine	Tablet, suppository, liquid, injection	PO: 5–10 mg q3–4h. PR: 25 mg twice daily. IM: 5–10 mg q3–4h. Do not exceed IM dose of 40 mg/day.	PO or PR: 0.4 mg/kg/24 h in two or three doses. Not recommended for children under 10 kg.
Promethazine	Phenergan	Tablet, syrup, suppository, injection	12.5–25 mg q4–6h.	0.25 mg/kg q4–6h.
Triethylperazine	Torecan	Tablet, suppository, injection	10–30 mg daily in divided doses.	Dose not established in children.

TABLE 19-3   Antiemetic Drugs and Regimens (*Continued*)

DRUG	BRAND NAME	DOSAGE FORMS	ADULT DOSE	PEDIATRIC DOSE
MISCELLANEOUS DRUGS				
Benzquinamide	Emete-Con	Injection	IM: 50 mg (0.5–1 mg/ kg); may be repeated in 1 h with subsequent doses q3–4h. IV: 25 mg (0.2–0.4 mg/ kg) slowly.	Not recommended for use in children.
Trimethobenzamide	Tigan, Tegamide	Capsule, suppository, injection	PO or PR: 250 mg three to four times/day. IM: 200 mg three to four times/day.	100–200 mg three to four times daily.
Scopolamine transdermal therapeutic system	Transderm-Scop	Patch	One system postauricularly every 3 days if needed.	Dose not established in children.
Metoclopramide	Reglan	Tablet, injection	1–2 mg/kg diluted in 50 mL of IV fluid. Begin 30 min prior to chemotherapy. Repeat q2h for two doses, then q3h for three doses.	Age 6 to 14: 2.5 to 5 mg. Under 6: 0.1 mg/kg.

Phosphorylated Carbohydrate Solutions

These preparations consist of phosphoric acid and hyperosmolar concentrations of various carbohydrates. The products provide for the symptomatic relief of uncomplicated nausea and vomiting. The mechanism of action is probably that of a direct effect on the wall of the gastrointestinal tract by reduction of smooth muscle contraction. The effectiveness of these drugs is in a direct proportion to the amount administered. Phosphorylated carbohydrate solutions should not be diluted before administration. Patients should be cautioned to avoid taking oral fluids immediately before and at least 15 min after the dose. An osmotic diarrhea may occur when these drugs are taken in excessive amounts. Diabetics should avoid these products because of the carbohydrate concentration.

Antihistamines

Antihistamines are effective in the treatment of motion sickness but offer little protection against other causes of nausea and vomiting, including cancer chemotherapy. The antiemetic effect is probably due to the central nervous system depressant and anticholinergic properties of these drugs. Motion sickness appears to be a result of stimulation of the labyrinthine system and transmission of this stimulus through cholinergic and adrenergic fibers to the vestibular network located near the vomiting center. With strong stimulation, impulses radiate outward through the adjacent cholinergic-mediated reticular system to the vomiting center. Thus, the inhibition of the cholinergic-mediated spread of impulses from the vestibular nucleus to the vomiting center provides for the effectiveness of antihistamines in motion sickness. The pharmacology of the antihistamines is discussed in detail in Chap. 21.

In order to be the most effective, these drugs should be administered at least 30 to 60 min prior to exposure to the motion or to beginning travel. These agents are used as a prophylactic measure; responses to drug or motion and susceptibility to motion sickness may vary with the patient's age, previous exposure to drug or motion, severity, and duration of the motion. If one antihistamine is ineffective, another should be tried.

Until 1983, an estimated 10 to 25 percent of pregnant women in the United States received prescriptions for the antihistamine combination Bendectin (**doxylamine/pyridoxine**). This was usually prescribed for nausea and vomiting during the first trimester of pregnancy. There was considerable public interest surrounding this drug after a highly publicized case of a child with birth defects whose mother had taken Bendectin during gestation appeared in the news media. In 1983, the manufacturer voluntarily removed the product from the market in the United States.

Phenothiazines

The phenothiazines are best utilized in the control of nausea and vomiting of short duration since the incidence of adverse effects increases with prolonged use. These drugs should not be used prophylactically due to potential adverse effects. The pharmacology of the phenothiazines is discussed in detail in Chap. 34. In usual therapeutic doses, the phenothiazines prevent vomiting by action on the CTZ and the vomiting center. They are effective in uremia, gastroenteritis, radiation sickness, cancer, and postoperative nausea and vomiting. Phenothiazines are also capable of suppressing nausea and vomiting due to other drugs such as those used in cancer chemotherapy, estrogens, and narcotic analgesics. The most commonly seen adverse effects in the antiemetic doses are mild to moderate drowsiness. The phenothiazines used as antiemetics also have the highest incidence of extrapyramidal symptoms. **Chlorpromazine** (Thorazine) and **promazine** (Sparine) are the most likely to produce a parkinson-like syndrome (tremors, rigidity, akinesia, pill-rolling). **Prochlorperazine** (Compazine) and **trifluoperazine** (Vesprin) are most likely to cause dyskinetic reactions involving the muscles of the face and neck, perioral spasms with or without tongue protrusion, tics, alteration of the mandibular joint function, oculogyric crisis, and difficulty in speech and swallowing. Symptoms usually subside in a few hours. If symptoms persist, the dosage should be lowered or the drug discontinued. Extrapyramidal symptoms may be relieved with **diphenhydramine** (Benadryl) or **benztropine** (Cogentin) (see Chap. 34). It is important to note that the phenothiazines when used alone or in combination with other drugs such as anesthetics, narcotic analgesics, or preoperative medications may cause hypotension, respiratory depression, and extrapyramidal effects, and may increase the actual postanesthesia recovery time.

Miscellaneous Antiemetic Agents

Benzquinamide (Emete-Con) Benzquinamide is used parenterally for the prevention and treatment of nausea and vomiting associated with anesthesia and surgery. The drug has been used investigationally in the treatment of cancer chemotherapy–induced vomiting. Benzquinamide is believed to exert a depressant effect on the CTZ. The drug is rapidly absorbed following oral, intramuscular, or rectal administration. The antiemetic effect usually occurs within 15 min of administration with a duration of action of 3 to 4 h. At therapeutic concentrations, the drug is approximately 60 percent protein-bound. It has not been established whether the drug crosses the blood-brain barrier and the placenta, or appears in breast milk. The drug is metabolized by the liver, and the inactive metabolites are excreted in the urine. The most common side effects are drowsiness and sedation. Intravenous administration of benzquinamide has been associated with a sudden increase in blood pressure and transient arrhythmias; therefore, it is preferable to administer the drug by the oral, intramuscular, or rectal routes.

Trimethobenzamide (Tigan, Spengan) Trimethobenzamide is structurally related to the antihistamines. This drug is less effective as an antiemetic than the phenothiazines but is comparatively free of the toxicity associated with the phenothiazines. Severe nausea and vomiting should not be treated with trimethobenzamide alone. Limited studies indicate that trimethobenzamide may be useful in the control of nausea and vomiting associated with postoperative proce-

dures and radiation therapy. The drug appears to have antiemetic activity in 10 to 40 min with a duration of action of 3 to 4 h. After intramuscular administration, the onset of action is 15 to 35 min and the duration of action is 2 to 3 h. From 50 to 75 percent of the drug is metabolized in the liver. The remaining drug is excreted unchanged in the urine. Side effects with this drug occur infrequently and seldom require discontinuation of the drug. Parkinson-like syndromes and skin sensitivity have been reported. Pain, stinging, burning, redness, and swelling may occur at the injection site. This may be remedied by injecting the drug into the dorsogluteal site and avoiding the escape of solution along the needle track. Local irritation has also been reported with rectal administration. Rectal suppositories contain benzocaine and should not be administered to patients with a benzocaine allergy.

Scopolamine Scopolamine is one of the most effective drugs used for motion sickness. Scopolamine is an anticholinergic agent and acts primarily by reducing the excitability of the labyrinthine receptors and by depressing the conduction in the vestibular-cerebellar pathway. It is especially effective in the prevention of motion sickness. When administered orally or intramuscularly, it has frequently been associated with adverse effects including drowsiness, dry mouth, blurred vision, and, with high doses, mental confusion and hallucinations.

A transdermal therapeutic system has been developed that releases small amounts of scopolamine for a 3-day period. The transdermal system is a thin film with a matrix containing 1.5 mg of scopolamine. An initial priming dose of scopolamine is released from the system's adhesive layer. This brings the blood concentrations to a therapeutic level. The system is placed behind the ear several hours before the antiemetic effect is required. A dose of 0.5 mg of scopolamine will be delivered over the 3-day period that the system is left in place. The delivery system should be replaced every 3 days if continued therapy is required.

Metoclopramide (Reglan) Metoclopramide stimulates motility of the upper gastrointestinal tract without stimulating the gastric, biliary, or pancreatic secretions. Its mode of action is unclear. The onset of pharmacologic action of metoclopramide is 1 to 3 min following intravenous administration. Eighty-five percent of the drug appears in the urine within 72 h of administration; approximately one-half of the drug is eliminated in the unchanged form. Extrapyramidal effects are the most common side effects. If an extrapyramidal reaction occurs, it can be reversed with an intramuscular or intravenous dose of **diphenhydramine** (Benadryl).

Investigational Agents
Several drugs have been used investigationally for the management of chemotherapy-induced nausea and vomiting.

Haloperiodol and Droperidol Both haloperidol (Haldol) and droperidol (Inapsine) possess antiemetic potential. Droperidol has been used to control postoperative and obstetrical nausea and vomiting. These drugs appear to block afferent nerve transmissions to the CTZ. Haloperidol and droperidol have been useful in suppressing vomiting in patients refractory to treatment with either the phenothiazines or benzquinamide. The most common side effects are sedation and occasional dystonic reactions.

Corticosteroids The observation that patients treated for Hodgkin's disease with regimens that included *prednisone* seemed to have less nausea and vomiting due to chemotherapy led to the trial of corticosteroids for antiemetic therapy. The proposed mechanism of action of steroids in chemotherapy-induced nausea and vomiting is conjectural. To date, **methylprednisolone** and **dexamethasone** have been used with varying degrees of success.

Cannabinoids **Delta-9-tetrahydrocannabinol** (THC) and its chemical congeners **nabilone** and **levonantradol** have been studied. The optimal dose or route of administration which is effective for nausea and vomiting without producing the psychotropic "high" has not been established. It is believed that the congeners of THC may show more promise for practical clinical use.

EVALUATION

Evaluation of the management of nausea and vomiting begins with the patient's subjective statement on the effectiveness of the approach and, if possible, observation of any emesis that occurs. Intake and output measurements should be kept until the vomiting is well-controlled as well as observation for fluid and electrolyte imbalances.

Anticholinergic side effects are common to most antiemetics, and so the patient should be observed for drowsiness, constipation, dry mouth, urinary retention (especially in elderly males), and blurred vision.

CASE STUDY

B.R., a 25-year-old married woman, brought her second child, age 2 months, to the clinic for well-child care. She asked the family nurse practitioner if there were any special precautions which should be taken for the baby during the 1000-mile airplane flight the family was taking the following week. The nurse explained that babies usually travel well by airplane if they have a bottle to suck, or are nursing during ascent and descent in order to equalize the ear pressures. B.R. thanked the nurse and remarked that she wished there was something that simple that could prevent the airsickness that was a severe problem for B.R. herself.

Assessment

The nurse further explored with B.R. what she meant by "airsickness." B.R. explained that each time she had flown in her life she had been nauseated and vomited whatever was in her stomach; when she did not eat the day of the flight, she only retched for the entire trip. This problem occurred only during air travel and amusement park rides, which she had learned to avoid. B.R. had no history of allergies or glaucoma and had not had relief from any of the over-the-counter antiemetic agents.

Management

The nurse referred B.R. to the family practice physician. B.R. returned with a prescription for the scopolamine transdermal delivery system (Transderm-Scop). The nurse counseled B.R. to apply the unit at least 4 h before beginning travel. B.R. should select a hairless area of skin behind one ear and be sure that the area was clean and dry. She should remove the backing from the unit, being careful not to touch the adhesive surface and apply the adhesive side to the clean dry area behind the ear so that the tan-colored side is showing. A gentle but firm pressure should be used.

B.R. could leave the unit in place for up to 3 days if necessary. The nurse also explained to B.R. that she must wash her hands carefully after applying the unit to remove any scopolamine. B.R. should keep the area as dry as possible; however, limited contact with water such as in swimming or bathing would not affect the system.

Evaluation

The next month when B.R. brought the child for her checkup, the nurse inquired about the airplane flight and whether B.R. or the baby had experienced any difficulties. The patient stated that the child had slept throughout the flight, and she had been able to control the vomiting and retching with the scopolamine transdermal delivery system applied before each flight, although she had continued to feel a little "queasy" on landings.

REFERENCES

Barbezat, G. O.: "The Vomiting Patient: The Rational Approach," *Drugs,* **22**:246–253, 1981.

Beland, J. L., and J. Y. Passos, *Clinical Nursing: Pathophysiological and Psychosocial Approaches,* 4th ed., New York: Macmillan, 1981.

Berry-Opersteny, D., and K. B. Heusinkveld: "Prophylactic Antiemetics for Chemotherapy-Associated Nausea and Vomiting," *Cancer Nurs,* **6**:117–123, 1983.

Biggs, J. S. G.: "Treatment of Gastrointestinal Disorders of Pregnancy," *Drugs,* **19**:70–76, 1980.

Bouchier, I. A., and J. S. Morris: *Clinical Skills: A System of Clinical Examination,* 2d ed., Philadelphia: Saunders, 1982.

Cirrillo, V. J., and K. F. Tmepero: "Pharmacology and Therapeutic Use of Antihistamines," *Am J Hosp Pharm,* **33**:1200–1207, 1976.

Claggert, M. S.: "Anorexia Nervosa: A Behavioral Approach," *Am J Nurs,* **80**:1468–1472, 1980.

Cordero, J. F., G. P. Oakley, F. Greenberg, and J. M. Levy: "Is Bendectin a Teratogen?" *JAMA,* **245**:2307–2310, 1981.

Drain, C. B., and S. B. Shipley: *The Recovery Room,* Philadelphia: Saunders, 1979.

Frytak, S., and C. G. Moertel: "Management of Nausea and Vomiting in the Cancer Patient," *JAMA,* **245**:393–396, 1981.

Holme, K. A.: "Binge Eating and Vomiting: A Survey of a College Population," *Psychol Med,* **11**:697–706, 1981.

Huff, P. S.: "Safety of Drug Therapy for Nausea and Vomiting of Pregnancy," *J Fam Pract,* **11**:969–970, 1980.

Isselbacher, K. J.: "Anorexia, Nausea, and Vomiting," in Peteresdorf, R. G. et al. (eds.), *Harrison's Principles of Internal Medicine,* 10th ed., New York: McGraw-Hill, 1983.

Jick, H., C. B. Holmes, J. R. Hunter, S. Madson, and A. Stergachis: "First Trimester Drug Use and Congenital Disorders," *JAMA,* **246**:343–346, 1981.

Johnson, P. E.: "Nausea and Vomiting," in Katcher, B. S., L. Y. Young, and M. A. Koda-Kimble (eds.), *Applied Therapeutics: The Clinical Use of Drugs,* 3d ed., San Francisco: Applied Therapeutics, 1983.

Luckman, J., and K. C. Sorenson: *Medical Surgical Nursing: A Psychosocial Approach,* Philadelphia: Saunders, 1980.

Marlow, D. R.: *Textbook of Pediatric Nursing,* 5th ed., Philadelphia: Saunders, 1977.

McCauley, M. E., J. W. Royal, J. E. Shaw, and L. G. Schmitt: "Effect of Transdermal Administered Scopolamine in Preventing Motion Sickness," *Aviat Space Environ Med,* **50**:1108–1111, 1979.

Odera, G. M., and S. West: "Emetic and Antiemetic Products," in Laitin, S. C. (ed.), *The Handbook of Non-Prescription Drugs,* 6th ed., Washington: American Pharmaceutical Association, 1982.

Schwinghammer, T.: "Antiemetics: Choosing from Alternatives," *Hosp Formul,* **21**:139–143, 1980.

USP Dispensing Information, vol. I and II, 2d ed., Rockville, Md.: United States Pharmacoepeial Convention, 1983.

Wood, C. D.: "Antimotion Sickness and Antiemetic Drugs," *Drugs,* **17**:471–532, 1979.

Wyman, J. B.: "The Vomiting Patient," *Am Fam Physician,* **21**:139–142, 1980.

20

CONSTIPATION AND DIARRHEA

JOHN M. HOOPES
KATHLEEN SIMONS PIGGOTT
ANN E. GUNNETT

LEARNING OBJECTIVES

Upon mastery of the content of this chapter the reader will be able to:

1. Explain why it is difficult to define the terms constipation and diarrhea.

2. Describe at least two complications or sequelae of constipation and of diarrhea.

3. Outline the assessment of patients with constipation and with diarrhea.

4. State the therapeutic objectives in the management of constipation and of diarrhea.

5. Describe the types of patients at risk of developing constipation.

6. Indicate which class of laxatives has the most physiologic action.

7. Describe three nonpharmacologic management modalities for constipation and three for diarrhea.

8. Describe two types of enemas and give an indication for each.

9. Give at least three drugs that can cause constipation and three that can cause diarrhea.

10. List four classes of laxatives and give at least two examples of each.

11. List three classes of antidiarrheal agents and give at least one example of each.

12. State the mechanism of action and adverse effects of each class of laxative.

13. State the mechanism of action and adverse effects of each class of antidiarrheal agent.

14. Write patient education plans for the patient using (1) a laxative and (2) an antidiarrheal agent.

As a society, we have a tendency to be overly concerned with our bowel habits. The overuse of laxatives, both prescription and nonprescription, is a major health problem. Sales of over-the-counter laxatives were in excess of $337 million in 1980, and in the institutional setting laxatives are the second most prescribed drug. The apprehension that surrounds constipation usually far exceeds its significance. In reality, there are only a few indications for the use of laxatives, and more often it is a responsibility of the nurse to try to assist the patient in breaking the laxative habit.

Diarrheal illnesses are very common, short-lived, and usually without complications. However, to certain patients (i.e., infants, children, and the elderly), the loss of fluid and electrolytes can be devastating. Appropriate management of the original problem can prevent these unfortunate sequelae, and nurses traditionally have played a prominent part in the care of these patients. Although antidiarrheal preparations are not abused to as great an extent as laxatives, they are often misused.

PHYSIOLOGY OF NORMAL STOOL FORMATION

The process of absorption and digestion of a meal and the resultant stool formation requires normal flow of digestive enzymes, proper pH regulation, and normal somatic and smooth muscle activity. This function is regulated by gastrointestinal hormones and the autonomic and enteric nervous systems. Fats, carbohydrates, and proteins each have digestive processes that if inadequate or overwhelmed will alter stool formation. When large amounts of unabsorbed fatty acids, mono- or disaccharides, amino acids, or bile salts reach the terminal ileum and colon, their osmotic action and stimulant properties will alter stool formation.

Within the gastrointestinal tract large amounts of water and electrolytes are processed. It is estimated that of the total 9 L of fluid in the gastrointestinal tract daily (2 L consumed and 7 L of secretion), only 100 to 200 mL is excreted in the stool. An appreciation of the relative concentration of each ion at different levels of the intestines is important since loss of fluid from a specific area is associated with a particular electrolyte loss. In the upper intestinal tract the fluid is high in sodium and chloride and relatively acid, whereas lower intestinal contents are predominantly potassium and bicarbonate. The gastrointestinal contents are still fluid in the ascending colon. It is not until reaching the transverse and descending colon that the contents become semisolid. The product of the absorption process is feces, which are 75% water and 25% solid material, predominantly bacteria. Since water continues to be absorbed from the rectum while the stool remains there, the longer the stool remains there, the harder it will become.

Motility

Smooth muscle activity of the bowel is of three types. Isolated segmental contractions are responsible for the mixing functions in the small intestine. Propulsive movements are a result of coordinated segmental contractions (peristaltic movement) in the small intestine. Finally, the colon is capable of quickly shortening its length resulting in special "mass movements." Peristaltic contractions occur regularly, while "mass movements" occur only three to four times a day. These mass movements are usually associated with food entering the stomach (gastrocolic reflex).

Primary control of motility is through enteric nerve fibers composed of two groups of nerve structures called Auerbach's and Meissner's plexuses. The enteric nerves provide coordination of bowel motility which is facilitated by parasympathetic input and inhibited by sympathetic input. Sphincter tone is reflexly mediated through the enteric nervous system.

Various neurotransmitters are active in controlling bowel motility. Acetylcholine and norepinephrine are the transmitters for the postganglionic parasympathetic and sympathetic nerves, respectively. In addition, noncholinergic-nonadrenergic neurotransmitters which are either inhibitory or excitatory have been identified. Serotonin, substance P, gastrin, cholecystokinin, and thyrotropin-releasing hormone are excitatory in action. Purines, somatostatin, opium derivatives, vasoactive intestinal polypeptide (VIP), γ-aminobutyric acid (GABA), glucagon, and secretin are inhibitory.

Defecation Reflex

When feces move into the rectum by mass movement, the rectum is distended, causing a series of responses known as the defecation reflex. The muscles of the descending and sigmoid colons contract, the internal and external sphincters relax, and defecation takes place. The defecation reflex can be controlled voluntarily until the proper time for defecation. The defecation reflex diminishes over time if it is voluntarily delayed too long. Reflexes can be initiated by contracting the abdominal muscles, forcing feces into the rectum. However, these reflexes are not usually as effective as those initiated by the mass movement.

CONSTIPATION

There is no consensus as to the definition of constipation. Since it is a symptom, it is subject to interpretation by the patient. The patient's attitudes regarding regularity or consistency of the stool may be influenced by social and psychologic factors.

A working definition of constipation may be the condition causing the patient to complain of infrequent stool production or the passage of dry, hard stools. Another definition is the functional impairment of the colon in producing properly formed stools at regular intervals. In both these definitions there is a large degree of flexibility and subjective interpretation of the terms.

Pathophysiology

Causes of constipation are listed in Table 20-1. One of the major factors contributing to constipation is not allowing

TABLE 20-1 Etiology of Constipation

Behavioral
Low dietary fiber
Delayed defecation reflex
Lack of exercise
Stress

Psychosomatic
Depression
Psychosis
Anxiety

Neurologic
Segmental cord lesion
Strokes
Multiple sclerosis

Lesions of the Bowel
Diverticulosis
Irritable bowel
Obstruction (appendicitis, tumors, hernia)
Systemic sclerosis
Inflammatory bowel disease
Rectal prolapse
Hirschsprung's disease

Endocrine and Metabolic
Hypothyroidism
Hypercalcemia
Porphyria
Diabetes mellitus
Uremia
Hypokalemia
Panhypopituitarism

Miscellaneous
Immobility
Pregnancy
Aging
Anal lesions

the normal physiologic defecation reflex to proceed. Stress may also lead to constipation. Another primary cause of constipation is a diet low in fiber and/or fluids. The use of laxatives on a regular basis tends to lead to chronic constipation by evacuating the rectum and parts of the colon. This results in physiologic delay in stool formation that in turn is interpreted by the patient as constipation. Thus, the patient enters a cyclic behavioral pattern of using laxatives to cause evacuation of the bowel; and once the dependence on the use of laxatives is established, the behavior is very difficult to change.

Neurologic impairments of the GI tract (e.g., Hirschprung's disease) and spinal cord injuries which alter the stimulation of the internal and external sphincters of the rectal colon will inhibit passage of stool, as will any pathophysiologic process which slows peristalsis. Examples of such processes include hypothyroidism and hypokalemia.

The use of drugs (Table 20-2) which slow peristalsis will contribute to constipation. Examples of these drugs are the anticholinergics, such as **atropine** and **scopolamine**, which are used preoperatively to decrease salivary and bronchial secretions, to decrease gastric acid secretion in peptic ulcer disease, and to inhibit nausea and vomiting. **Tricyclic antidepressants, MAO inhibitors, antipsychotics,** and **antiparkinsonian** drugs used in the treatment of mental illness have anticholinergic effects.

Opiates and opiate derivatives (e.g., morphine, codeine, and meperidine) are used in the treatment of pain, but will also decrease peristaltic activity. Drugs which contain aluminum (e.g., antacids and phosphate binders) and iron will

TABLE 20-2   Drugs That Induce Constipation

Narcotic analgesics
Anesthetic agents
Antacids (calcium and aluminum compounds)
Anticholinergics
Anticonvulsants
Antidepressive agents
Barium sulfate
Bismuth
Diuretics
Drugs for parkinsonism
Ganglionic blockers
Hematinics (especially iron)
Hypotensives
MAO inhibitors
Metallic intoxication (arsenic, lead, mercury, phosphorus)
Muscle paralyzers
Opiates
Psychotherapeutic drugs
Laxative addiction

Source: Adapted with permission from J. S. Fordtran and M. Sleisenger, eds.: *Gastrointestinal Disease,* Philadelphia: W. B. Saunders, 1978.

cause the stool to become harder, contributing to constipation.

Immobility is a leading cause of constipation in the hospitalized patient. The weakened abdominal and perineal muscles and decreased gastric motility of the bedridden patient lead to an alteration in the ability to maintain a normal pattern of defecation. The patient required to use a bedpan for defecation may, because of embarrassment at a lack of privacy or concern with the odor, suppress the urge to defecate for a period of days.

Clinical Sequelae and Complications

Constipation is seldom complicated by serious sequelae. Patients may complain of incomplete emptying of the rectum, bloating, malaise, headache, lower abdominal discomfort, and other general disorders. The association of these symptoms with constipation is inferred from observation and from the fact that the symptoms are promptly relieved by enemas or laxatives, reinforcing laxative misuse.

There are, however, a few potentially serious problems that may result from constipation. Constipation may be a major contributor to sudden death in patients with organic heart disease. Straining initiates a *Valsalva maneuver* that serves to compromise coronary circulation and cerebral blood flow. Intrathoracic and intracerebral pressure has been found to be further increased during straining when the patient is constipated. Thus, measures to reduce the risk of constipation in patients with a myocardial infarction, eye surgery, or potentially increased intracranial pressure must be implemented. In these cases a stool softener such as **docusate** (e.g., Colace) is usually prescribed.

There may be gastrointestinal complications. Gas and fecal accumulation may distend the colon, resulting in megacolon. Hemorrhoids can be exacerbated by constipation and can in turn contribute to the problem. Impaction is probably the most frequently encountered result of constipation. Impaction may take the form of hard, round fecal masses called *scybala* or a soft fecal mass called a *pultaceous impaction.* They are most frequently found in the rectum (98 percent) or in the sigmoid, transverse, or ascending colon (1.6 percent) or in the ileum (0.4 percent). Not infrequently impaction may result in diarrhea with fecal incontinence.

The feeling of "fullness" or "bloatedness" associated with constipation is of concern in terms of a patient's nutritional status. The anorexia which is often associated with constipation may lead to a decrease in nutritional intake, causing a negative nitrogen balance and compromising healing.

Assessment

A careful history is necessary first to establish the meaning of the patient's complaint. Deliberate questioning about the frequency of bowel movements, nature of the stool, symptoms associated with defecation, use of drugs, diet, level of exercise, social history, and a review of gastrointestinal systems with special note of recent changes are absolutely necessary. The frequent contribution of drug therapy to constipation is often overlooked. At admission to the hospital, data about patient's normal bowel habits should be collected so that a plan of care can focus on reinforcing factors which contribute to functional bowel habits and identify areas in which patient reeducation may be beneficial.

A thorough abdominal examination for bowel sounds, distention, masses, organomegaly, and tenderness is required in addition to inspection of the anus, rectum, and stool. Important laboratory data include a complete blood cell count (CBC), in particular the hematocrit or hemoglobin to detect chronic gastrointestinal blood loss. The stool should be tested for occult blood.

Management

Therapeutic Objectives

The wide variation in bowel frequency among normal persons needs to be emphasized. There is no *absolute normal* for the frequency of movements. Rather, the frequency of movements is determined by what is appropriate for the individual.

Therapeutic objectives in the management of constipation are as follows:

1. Relief and/or prevention of impaction
2. Removal of aggravating factors (social, psychologic, drugs)
3. Correction of primary disease processes
4. Restoration of appropriate frequency of bowel movements
5. Improvement of consistency of the stool so that it can be passed without difficulty

Nonpharmacologic Management

Nursing measures related to the prevention or nonpharmacologic management of constipation focus primarily on the patient's diet, exercise patterns, and bowel habits. These measures are safer than the use of drugs and are more likely to encourage health-promoting behaviors on the part of the patient.

Diet It has long been appreciated that increasing dietary fiber content may be helpful in treating constipation. Recent evidence suggests that low fiber content of Western industrialized countries is associated with constipation. It has been established that the addition of *bran* to the diet shortens transit time and helps prevent constipation. The use of bran is extremely safe. However, large amounts may cause gas with flatulence and distention. Bran should not be consumed dry. Liberal amounts of fluid are advised to aid in proper bulk formation.

An intake of 2 g of bran daily should significantly improve function. Dietary fiber in the form of carbohydrates (cellulose, polysaccharides, hemicellulose, and pectins) and noncarbohydrates act by entrapping water. The stool is made softer, bulkier, and heavier. Hence, peristalsis is made more effective, and the stool is easier to pass.

The effectiveness of a food to impart these characteristics to the stool is directly proportional to its fiber content and particle size. Fiber from wheat and corn bran is more effective than that from fruit, vegetables, oats, or rice, because it is more concentrated. Coarse bran (raw milled bran) is superior to fine bran (processed) because of its larger particle size. In addition to wheat and corn bran, carrots, apples, oranges, and brussels sprouts have substantial water-holding capacities.

Other foods that will soften the stool are listed in Table 20-3.

Exercise Regular exercise can be expected to aid the treatment of constipation. For most patients this is best achieved by encouraging some activity after meals, especially after breakfast, in order to help form appropriate bowel habits by establishing regularity in the daily schedule for this function. In the hospital, ambulation or even range-of-motion exercise can often obviate the need for medication to treat constipation or gaseous abdominal distention.

Bowel Habits Institution of proper bowel habits may be the most rewarding area of therapy but is often difficult. One needs to begin by urging the patient to set a time of day for bowel movements and to give this function a priority. Delaying response to the urge to defecate must be discouraged, and the reasons for delaying it should be examined. Other elementary problems may be encountered and should not be overlooked because of their simplicity. For example, the use of a bedside commode can eliminate the need to use a bedpan, while devices to raise the height of the toilet enhance the comfort of the arthritic patient or the patient in a cast.

In the hospital, the nursing staff should assist patients to achieve their usual bowel patterns. This may involve allowing the patient to sip a cup of coffee or tea or read a magazine; every effort should be made to avoid rushing the patient and to provide adequate privacy.

Odor control is of utmost importance for the patient who must use a bedpan. Emptying the pan immediately after its use and attaching a nonperfumed air deodorizer near the bedside will eliminate some of the embarrassment felt by the patient.

Pharmacologic Management

Pharmacologic approaches to constipation include laxatives and cathartics, suppositories, and enemas. Commonly used products and dosages are shown on Table 20-4.

Laxatives and Cathartics The term *laxative* and *cathartic* are often used interchangeably, but they refer to a difference in the intensity of the action produced. Laxative action will produce a soft, formed stool, while cathartics produce a more watery evacuation. Laxatives and cathartics are classified as contact (stimulant) cathartics, saline cathartics, bulk-forming laxatives, and emollient laxatives.

Very little difference has been demonstrated among agents within each class. Generally, an individual drug has the same basic clinical and pharmacologic uses and limitations as the other members of its class.

Contact (Stimulant) Cathartics   Contact or stimulant cathartics have been classified in three subgroups: castor oil, anthraquinone, and diphenylmethane derivatives. They dif-

fer in location and latency of onset, but the mechanism of action and adverse effects are similar.

Mechanism of action   It is thought that a contact cathartic stimulates peristalsis by irritating the mucosa, by stimulating the nerve plexus, or by a direct action on the smooth muscle. An alternative mechanism of action may be that these agents cause the secretion of fluid and electrolytes into the lumen of the intestines and that motor activity of the intestines is modified by the increase in mass in the lumen. Castor oil affects the lumen of the small intestine, while the diphenylmethane and anthraquinone cathartics effect the large intestine. The intensity of the response of the stimulant cathartics varies with the dose, but interpatient variation

TABLE 20-3   Foods Used to Soften the Stool

FOOD GROUP	FOODS RECOMMENDED	FOODS WITH NEUTRAL OR LITTLE EFFECT ON STOOLS
Beverage	A large intake of mild beverages	Water, coffee, tea
Breads	Whole-wheat bread, crackers, muffins, and quick breads; bran breads and muffins	Bread, crackers, and cakes that are not whole grain
Cereals	Natural whole-grain cereals: barley, bran, whole wheat	All others
Desserts	All products containing seeds, nuts, coconut, fruit, and fruit pulp	Cakes, cookies, etc., with low-fat and low-whole-grain content and moderate- to low-sugar content
Eggs	Fried and scrambled eggs; omelets	Egg white; eggs cooked in other ways
Fats and oils	All	
Fruits and juices	All fruits except bananas; prune juice and fresh fruits are especially good	Limited serving of citrus; if diet is low in vitamin C, use supplementary prescription.
Meat, fish, poultry, and cheese	Fatty fish, e.g., salmon, tuna; marbled or fatty beef; fatty poultry, e.g., goose and duck; pork; yellow or white cheese with high fat; processed meats; poor-quality (fatty) hamburger	Beef, chicken, lamb, turkey, liver.
Potatoes and substitutes	Hominy grits, whole grains, or wild rice	Potatoes, macaroni, noodles, spaghetti.
Sugar and sweets	Sweets containing nuts and whole fruit, marmalade, molasses, jams	
Soups	All soups with fat	
Vegetables	Fresh and raw vegetables	All cooked vegetables. May be some variation with some individuals.
Miscellaneous	Salt, catsup, chili, peanut butter, coconut, garlic, horseradish, nuts, olives, pickles, relish, popcorn, and herbs	

Source: Modified from Chapman, W., Hill, M., and D. B. Shortleff. Management of the Neurogenic Bowel and Bladder. Oak Brook, Ill.: Eterna, 1979.

may vary four- to eightfold. Therefore, a dose in one patient may be ineffective, while the same dose in another patient may produce an exaggerated response.

Adverse effects All the contact cathartics have been known to cause griping, intestinal cramps, increased secretions, and excessive fluid evacuation. The patient who abuses contact cathartics is at risk for developing hypokalemia. Such cathartics should therefore be used judiciously if the patient is receiving **digoxin** or **potassium-depleting diuretics** or if the patient is at risk for developing cardiac arrythmias.

With immobilized or debilitated patients or when a serious pathologic bowel or neuromuscular condition exists, strong stimulation cathartics are sometimes required. Their use is always attended with some risk, and even the most benign agents may have serious consequences.

Castor oil Castor oil is a bland oil, but in the presence of the lipase of the small intestine it is hydrolyzed to ricinoleic acid. It is the ricinoleic acid that produces the cathartic effect. Castor oil acts by irritating and increasing fluid secretion from the small bowel, producing a prompt and thorough evacuation. It is recommended only for use in special procedures like certain radiologic examinations. As castor oil will achieve its effect in 2 to 6 h, it is not recommended to be taken at bedtime. It is advisable to give it in well-iced fruit juice to increase palatability. Because castor oil may precipitate abortion it should not be used by pregnant women. It is excreted in the milk of nursing mothers.

Diphenylmethane cathartics The two primary types of diphenylmethane cathartic are phenolphthalein and bisacodyl.

Phenolphthalein is available in any variety of over-the-counter preparations. Its site of action is on the colon, and since its onset of action is usually not less than 6 h, it can therefore be taken at bedtime. Phenolphthalein in an alkaline environment will turn pink. Thus if a patient uses a soapsuds enema and then uses phenolphthalein, the stool will be pink. The major problem with overdoses of phenolphthalein is that it causes fluid and electrolyte imbalances; however, allergic reactions and death have also been reported.

Bisacodyl (Dulcolax) is unique among the stimulant cathartics in that it is available both in an oral dosage form and as a suppository. Adverse effects of the oral drug include cramping and excessive cathartic effect. Bisacodyl is available as a 5-mg enteric coated tablet which should not be crushed, chewed, or taken with milk or an antacid. The onset of action for the oral tablets is 6 to 12 h.

Anthraquinone cathartics The major anthraquinone preparations are **senna**, **cascara sagrada**, and **danthron**. Their effects are limited to the large intestine and seldom occur before 6 h after oral administration, and sometimes their action can be delayed for 24 h.

Adverse reactions to the anthraquinones include excessive catharsis and melanosis coli, which has been observed in patients using these drugs over prolonged periods. *Melan-*

osis coli is a benign pigmentation and reversible over several months. Anthraquinones also will discolor the urine, and patients should be warned of this. See Table 20-4 for the various preparations of senna, cascara sagrada, and danthron.

The agents within this class have had little comparison, and for the purpose of management of constipation no difference between them can be expected. Choice is based on safety and convenience, and on this basis senna has advantages, although cascara is also a reasonable choice. However, senna is the only one of this class found to be safe in pregnant women and nursing mothers.

Saline Cathartics The saline cathartics include several magnesium, sodium, and potassium salts. The most popular of these agents are **magnesium hydroxide** (milk of magnesia) and **sodium phosphate** (Phospha-Soda).

Mechanism of action These agents are incompletely absorbed, increasing osmolality of the intestinal lumen; they cause water to be retained in the intestinal lumen, which leads to an increase in peristalsis. Transit time is reduced, and the feces are delivered in a semifluid state. Since the onset of action is ½ to 3 h, these cathartics should not be given at bedtime.

Adverse effects The adverse effects of the saline cathartics are due to the absorption of the ions into the systemic circulation which may produce toxicity. This may be a particular problem with the magnesium salts, since 20 percent of the ion may be absorbed. In a patient with normal renal function, this is not a problem, since they are capable of excreting the ion, but in patients in renal failure, these agents are contraindicated, since magnesium intoxication may result. Symptoms of magnesium intoxication include hypotension, respiratory depression, and loss of deep tendon reflexes. Sodium cathartics are contraindicated in cases of congestive heart failure. When a solution is administered that is strongly hypertonic (like the saline cathartics), it will draw water from the circulation in order to become isoosmotic. Therefore, to avoid fluid imbalance, saline cathartics should be administered with plenty of water (e.g., 1 L water over 6 h).

Preparation and dosage For preparations and dosage of saline cathartics see Table 20-4.

Bulk-Forming Laxatives The bulk-forming laxatives include a variety of natural and semisynthetic polysaccharides and cellulose derivatives, represented by **psyllium**, **methylcellulose** (MC), and **carboxymethylcellulose** (CMC).

The mechanism of action is through substances which dissolve and swell in water, producing an emollient gel or viscous solution that serves to hydrate the feces, promoting peristalsis and defecation. Its effect is evident in 12 to 24 h, but the full therapeutic effect may not be evident until the third or fourth day. For some patients, an increase in dietary bulk is also recommended instead of the use of bulk-forming agents. These agents are devoid of systemic adverse effects. Flatulence may develop but can be relieved by increasing the

TABLE 20-4   Classification and Properties of Drugs to Treat Constipation

AGENT	DOSAGE FORM	TRADE NAMES	ADULT DOSE	PEDIATRIC DOSE	SITE OF ACTION*	APPROXIMATE TIME REQUIRED FOR ACTION (h)
Contact Cathartics						
Castor oil	Liquid	Emulsoil, Neolid, Purge	15–30 mL	<2 yr: 1–5 mL 2–12 yr: 5–15 mL	Small intestines	2–6
Phenolphthalein	Tablets/liquid	Ex-Lax, Correctol, Phenolax, Feen-a-Mint	30–195 mg	<2 yr: Avoid 2–6 yr: 15–30 mg >6 yr: 30–60 mg	Colon	6–8
Bisacodyl	Tablets	Cenalax, Deficol, Dulcolax	10–15 mg	>6 yr: 5–10 mg	Colon	6–10
Senna	Tablets	Senexan, Senekot, Senolax	2 tablets	>60 lbs: 1 tablet	Colon	6–10
	Granules	Senekot, Black-Draught	¼–1 tsp†	See label†		
	Syrup	Casafru, Senekot	5–15 mL†	See label†		
	Liquid/powder	X-Prep	Preradiologic: 75 mL or 22.5 g	⅛–½ adult dose		
Cascara sagrada	Tablets		325–650 mg	Avoid	Colon	6–8
	Aromatic fluid extract		5 mL	¼–½ adult dose		
	Fluid extract		1 mL	¼–½ adult dose		
Danthron	Solid/liquid	Modane, Dorbane	37.5–150 mg	<12 yr: Avoid	Colon	8
Saline Cathartics						
Magnesium hydroxide (milk of magnesia, M.O.M.)	Liquid	Phillips Milk of Magnesia, others	15–30 mL	0.5 mL/kg/dose	Small and large intestines	0.5–3
Magnesium citrate (citrate of magnesia)	Liquid	Citroma, Citro-Nesia	240 mL	5 mL/kg/dose	Small and large intestines	0.5–3
Magnesium sulfate (Epsom salts)	Powder		15 g	0.25 g/kg/dose	Small and large intestines	0.5–3
Sodium phosphate and sodium biphosphate	Liquid	Phospho-Soda	20–40 mL	5–15 mL	Small and large intestines	0.5–3
Bulk-Forming Laxatives						
Methylcellulose	Powder/liquid	Cologel, Maltsuprex	1–2 tbsp once or twice daily	½–2 tbsp daily	Small and large intestines	12–72
Psyllium	Flakes/granules	Mucilose, Siblin	1–2 tsp with fluid twice daily	See label.	Small and large intestines	12–72
	Powder	Metamucil, Perdiem, Hydrocil	1 rounded tsp one to three times daily	>6 yr: 1 level tsp daily		

TABLE 20-4 Classification and Properties of Drugs to Treat Constipation (*Continued*)

AGENT	DOSAGE FORM	TRADE NAMES	ADULT DOSE	PEDIATRIC DOSE	SITE OF ACTION*	APPROXIMATE TIME REQUIRED FOR ACTION (h)
Emollient Laxatives and Stool Softeners						
Mineral oil	Liquid	Nujol, Agoral, Petrogalar	5–30 mL	5–10 mL	Colon	6–8
Docusate sodium (dioctyl sodium sulfosuccinate, DSS)	Tablets/ capsules/ liquid	Colace, Doxinate, Comfolax, Colax	50–240 mg	<3 yrs: 10–40 mg 3–6 yrs: 20–60 mg 6–12 yrs: 40–120 mg	Small and large intestine	12–72
Docusate calcium (dioctyl calcium sulfosuccinate)	Capsules	Surfak, Surfac, Pro-Cal-Sof	240 mg	50–150 mg	Small and large intestine	12–72
Docusate potassium	Capsules	Dialose, Kasof	100–300 mg	Avoid	Small and large intestine	12–72
Polaxamer 188	Capsules	Alaxin	480 mg	240–480 mg	Small and large intestine	12–72
Suppositories and Enemas						
Bisacodyl	Suppository	Dulcolax, Cenalax, Theralax	10 mg	5 mg	Colon	0.5–1
Senna	Suppository	Senokot	One	One-half	Colon	0.5–2
CO_2-releasing	Suppository	Ceo-Two	One	Avoid	Colon	0.5–2
Glycerin	Suppository/ rectal liquid	Fleet Babylax	One	1 or 4 mL liquid	Colon	0.5–2
Sodium phosphate and sodium biphospate	Enema	Fleet	118 mL	60 mL	Colon	0.5–2
Bisacodyl	Enema	Fleet Bisacodyl, Clysodrast	One package	Avoid	Colon	0.5–1
Docusate potassium and benzocaine	Enema	Therevac	3.9 g	Avoid	Colon	0.5–8
Mineral oil	Enema	Fleet Mineral Oil	120 mL	30–60 mL	Colon	0.5–8
Miscellaneous and Combinations						
Polycarbophil	Tablets	Mitrolan	1 g four times daily	3–6 yr: 500 mg twice daily 6–12 yr: 500 mg tid	Small and large intestine	12–72
Lactulose	Syrup	Chronolac	15–60 mL	Avoid	Small and large intestine	24–48
Docusate plus casanthranol	Capsules/ tablets/ liquids	Peri-Colace, Diothron, Stimulax, Dialose-Plus	1–2 tablets or capsules; 7.5–30 mL†	See label†	Small and large intestine and colon	8–24
Docusate plus danthron	Capsules/ tablets	Unilax, Modane Plus, Doxidan, Dorbantyl	1–2 tablets or capsules; 7.5–30 mL†	See label†	Small and large intestine and colon	8–24

*All agents except the bulk laxatives are absorbed to some extent.
†Varies by preparation; follow label directions.

patient's fluid intake. Intestinal obstruction has been reported with these agents, and impaction has occurred when there was a pathologic intestinal condition. Esophageal obstruction has occurred when the patient took the preparation dry. It is therefore recommended that the patient take all bulk-forming agents with several glasses of water. The choice of the various bulk-forming agents is based mainly on patient preference, since there is no significant clinical advantage of one preparation over the other.

The initial dose for methylcellulose and carboxymethylcellulose is 1 g, and for psyllium it is 5 g. Doses are then increased according to response and may be divided into twice daily doses (see Table 20-4). Adequate fluid intake must be maintained, and patients should be instructed to swallow immediately upon mixing and to follow each dose with at least one full (8-oz) glass of water.

Emollient Laxatives and Stool Softeners **Mineral oil** is the most common emollient laxative. It is only slightly absorbed, and it exerts its effect probably by retarding the reabsorption of water, thus softening the stool and by coating the intestinal lining, making passage of stool less difficult. Mineral oil has many potential serious adverse effects, and its use is *not recommended*. The **docusates** (dioctyl sulfosuccinates; DSS or DOSS) lower the surface tension of stool allowing it to be penetrated by intestinal fluids. Preparations are **docusate calcium** (Surfak) and **docusate sodium** (Colace). For dosages see Table 20-4.

Adverse effects Significant interference with absorption of essential fat-soluble vitamins like vitamin A, D, E, and K is one of the major adverse effects of **mineral oil**. It is contraindicated in the pregnant woman because it may lower the level of vitamin K in the fetus, causing a predisposition to bleeding. Mineral oil is absorbed and deposited in intestinal mucosa, mesenteric lymph nodes, liver, and spleen, where foreign body reactions are elicited. It may leak through the anal sphincter causing soiling and even pruritus. Wound healing can be delayed, and it is also reported to interfere with defecation by decreasing sensation in the rectum. Finally, mineral oil can be aspirated into the lungs, causing lipoid pneumonia. The onset of this reaction can be insidious and is a danger in aged, recumbent, or dysphagic patients or those suffering from hiatal hernia. The public is not generally knowledgeable of the risks with mineral oil, and it is the obligation of all health care professionals to discourage its use.

In therapeutic doses, the **docusates** rarely have adverse effects. Large doses may cause vomiting and diarrhea.

Miscellaneous Preparations **Lactulose** (Cephulac) is a semisynthetic disaccharide that is not hydrolyzed by intestinal enzymes. It is used for its laxative action and in the treatment of portal encephalopathy in patients with chronic liver disease. The laxative effect of lactulose comes about because water and electrolytes are retained in the lumen of the intestine, causing an osmotic effect. Lactulose is metabolized to lactate and other organic acids which lowers the luminal pH; the exact effect of the pH reduction on motility is still unknown.

The adverse effects of lactulose include flatulence, cramps, abdominal discomfort, and nausea and vomiting, which are most common when the drug is initiated. Excessive diarrhea can lead to fluid and electrolyte problems and should be avoided. Lactulose may be countraindicated in patients who have diabetis mellitus and should be avoided in patients who need a galactose-free diet. The usual laxative dose is 10 to 15 mL (7 to 10 g) in a single or divided dose. The response to the laxative effect may require several days, and if no response is seen, the dose may be increased.

Combination Preparations Combination products are widely available. Except for barium enema "preps," there is very little to indicate any particular advantage with these over other methods or single agents. Most combinations are unnecessary, irrational, and generally expensive.

Suppositories **Glycerin** suppositories are a popular drug for relief of constipation in infants and adults. Their site of action is on the lower bowel, and their efficacy is questionable in the presence of hard stools.

Bisacody (Dulcolax) 10-mg suppositories stimulate the bowel mucosa and initiate a reflex peristalsis. They are safe for use by pregnant women and nursing mothers because the bisacodyl is not absorbed sytemically. The suppositories may produce a mild burning sensation in the rectum. They work in 15 to 60 min. Bisacodyl suppositories are frequently used for bowel training in neurologically impaired patients. Approximately 30 min after the suppository is inserted, the patient is assisted to the commode or bedpan. Often this is scheduled after a meal to take advantage of mass movements. Gentle digital stimulation while the patient performs the Valsalva maneuver may be required to initiate peristalsis. A course of bowel training should be tried prior to the use of suppositories, oral stimulant laxatives, or enemas since many patients can achieve bowel training without pharmacologic intervention.

Enemas Enemas are useful when rectal and lower bowel evacuation is indicated in preparation for radiologic exams, endoscopy, and surgery. Enemas may be used to treat impaction and to maintain a regular bowel program for neurologically impaired individuals. A variety of enema solutions are available, but not all are safe to use on a regular basis.

The **normal saline-solution** enema is the safest, most effective, and well-tolerated type. Large volumes may be used to effectively cleanse the rectum and sigmoid colon. Administered properly, this is achieved with little mucosal irritation or alteration in fluid or electrolyte balance.

Oil-retention enemas administered in small volumes may be used effectively for softening impacted feces. Removal of impaction is facilitated if this is followed by a normal saline solution enema after 4 to 6 h. A large impaction may need to be removed digitally by insertion of a well-lubricated, gloved finger into the rectum. The nurse's fingernail should be cut short, and removal of the feces should be done slowly and gently.

During digital removal of impacted feces, the patient must be observed carefully for signs of discomfort and changes in vital signs. The process may need to be stopped and resumed at intervals during the day.

Some patients may find retaining a **mineral oil enema** difficult. Applying a cotton ball to the anus and taping the buttocks together gently will help such patients to retain the enema. If this is done, the nurse must assess the response of the patient's skin to the tape.

Disposable, **hypertonic saline solution enemas** (e.g., Fleet) usually contain mixtures of sodium phosphates and sodium citrates. They have the advantage of being convenient for self-administration, and they are disposable. While they act by drawing water into the lumen of the bowel, the quantities involved generally cause insignificant problems with fluid and electrolyte imbalance.

Hypotonic enema solutions such as tap water should be avoided if at all possible. The low osmolality of the tap water in proportion to the osmolality of the mesenteric blood supply will cause a shift of water from the bowel to the plasma resulting in water intoxication.

Strong stimulant enemas such as soap and peroxide should also be avoided. They pose threats to the mucosa and offer no significant advantage over other enemas. In addition, administration is associated with severe discomfort and may cause rapid depletion of body water and electrolytes.

Patient Education

The nurse should elicit the patient's beliefs regarding "normal" bowel patterns. It is important that the nurse not attempt to force the patient to accept changes in patterns that have evolved over along period of time.

Patients must be informed in basic, explicit terms about bowel physiology and the important role various factors play in the pathogenesis of constipation. Patients must receive unbiased information regarding what is a "normal" bowel pattern and the wide range of variation about this norm. They must be carefully instructed as to what changes to expect in bowel movements during treatment and when. Patients should be encouraged to avoid laxatives except those prescribed. Nonpharmacologic means of achieving bowel patterns acceptable to the patient are preferred over pharmacologic means.

The role of laxatives in aggravating constipation and their side effects must be impressed upon all patients. These drugs are much abused and overused. The wide variety and quantity of products on the market testify to their popularity among the general public, but their use should be limited to situations in which nonpharmacologic interventions are either too slow or inappropriate.

Evaluation

In an outpatient setting the subjective statements of the patient relative to number and character of stools are the main method of evaluation, although the nurse should also judge whether patient education has altered attitudes and knowledge regarding normal bowel functioning and patterns of laxative use. For some conditions it may be necessary to obtain stool specimens for analysis.

In most inpatient settings a routine evaluation and recording of the patient's bowel movements has been established in order to identify deviations which often occur in this population due to drugs, immobility, diet modifications, stress, and disease. Patients who are at risk for constipation due to these conditions or who are receiving treatment for constipation should receive a more in-depth analysis than mere determination of presence or absence of a bowel movement each day. To be noted are actual frequency of stools; consistency; related factors such as diet, fluids, and exercise; actual observation of the stools; and adverse effects specific to the laxative used.

DIARRHEA

Pathophysiology

The term diarrhea comes from the Greek, meaning "to flow through." There is no standard definition of diarrhea; the term is used to refer to the passage of feces, which may be liquid or semiformed, with increased frequency. Diarrhea results when there is reduced bowel tone, decreased segmental contractions, or increased mass movements in the colon.

The clinical significance of the diarrhea is based not only on that of the underlying etiologic factor (see Table 20-5) but also on fluid and electrolyte losses which may accompany increased fecal output. Frequently, diarrhea is acute, self-limiting, and only a minor inconvenience. In the infant, the child, or the debilitated adult, however, diarrhea can cause a significant upset in fluid and electrolyte, acid-base, and nutritional homeostasis.

Clinical Sequelae and Complications

The infant, the child and the debilitated adult is at risk for altered homeostasis secondary to diarrhea. Because intestinal fluids are rich in water, sodium, potassium, and bicarbonate, the individual with diarrhea may develop minor to severe dehydration. The loss of bicarbonate places the patient at risk for developing metabolic acidosis.

In situations of chronic diarrhea, e.g., malabsorption syndromes, the patient is at risk for developing nutritional deficiencies. The type of nutritional deficiency is dependent upon the area of bowel affected.

A transient lactose intolerance may develop secondary to the loss of intestinal disaccharidase enzymes. Disaccharidase enzymes (lactose, sucrase, maltase, and isomaltase) are secreted by the epithelial cells lining the intestinal mucosa. These epithelial cells are sheared off by the diarrheal pro-

TABLE 20-5 Diarrhea and Its Treatment

TYPE	HISTORY	SYMPTOMS	USUAL DURATION	TREATMENT	PROGNOSIS
Acute:					
Salmonella	Recent ingestion of contaminated food; affects all age groups	Sudden onset of abdominal cramps, watery diarrhea, nausea, vomiting, fever; onset of symptoms usually within 12–24 h after ingestion; infects perineal ileum and cecum	1–5 days	Symptomatic; bed rest, fluid, and electrolyte replacement; antibiotics (ampicillin if susceptible; chloramphenicol in life-threatening cases for 3–5 days)	Usually self-limiting
Shigella	Affects all age groups	Sudden onset of abdominal cramps, diarrhea containing shreds of mucus and specks of blood, tenesmus (frequently), fever; infects small bowel (early) and colon (later)	4–7 days	Symptomatic; bed rest, fluid, glucose, electrolyte replacement; antibiotics (ampicillin if susceptible)	Usually self-limiting
Escherichia coli	Affects children under 2 and the elderly in an overcrowded environment (e.g., hospital nursery or nursing home)	Abdominal cramps, fever, tenesmus; infects mostly small bowel	7–21 days	Fluid, glucose electrolyte replacement	Severe if not treated
Staphylococcus	Recent food ingestion	Sudden onset (1–2 h) of nausea, vomiting, diarrhea	6–12 h	Supportive; fluid replacement	Self-limiting
Viral, infantile	Predilection for children and infants; usually occurs in summer and autumn; very contagious	Abrupt onset of profuse, watery diarrhea, slight fever; frequent vomiting; upper respiratory symptoms	1–21 days	Symptomatic and supportive	Usually self-limiting
Traveler's diarrhea (caused by *Escherichia coli, Salmonella, Shigella, Giardia lamblia*)	Travel outside normal locus	Sudden onset of nausea, abdominal cramps, tenesmus, fever, prostration	5 days (onset is 6 days)	Symptomatic and supportive	Usually self-limiting
Drug-induced	Broad-spectrum antibiotics, autonomic drugs, laxative, nitrofurantoin, antacids, antineoplastics, antituberculins, ferrous sulfate, colchicine, nonsteroidal antiinflammatory drugs, digoxin	Sudden onset of rectal urgency, abdominal cramps	Variable	Discontinue or change drug; vancomycin	Usually self-limiting; however, can be fatal
Chronic	History of repeated episodes; poor health history	Weight loss, anorexia, mucus and/or blood in feces	Weeks to years	Depends on etiology	Severe if not treated

Source: Copyright 1982 by the American Pharmaceutical Association. *Handbook of Nonprescription Drugs,* 7th ed., Reprinted with permission of the American Pharmaceutical Association.

cess, but regenerate once the diarrhea is resolved. Diarrhea can also be produced by foods in the patient's diet. Food allergy, eating foods high in roughage, and food poisoning (food toxins) can all produce diarrhea. Food intolerance and diarrhea are associated with disaccharidase deficiency (lactase deficiency). These enzymes are reduced in intestinal disorders such as infectious diarrhea, congenital disaccharidase deficiency, and gastrointestinal allergy. The disaccharides ingested in the diet are not metabolized and pool in the lumen of the intestine, where they produce osmotic and pH changes.

Assessment

The assessment process can be broken down into three components: history, physical examination, and examination of the stool. Relevant historical factors include the time of onset; factors associated with the onset, e.g., travel, food, concurrent illnesses, and association with others who have similar symptoms; and symptoms experienced by the patient. Significant symptoms include fevers, chilling, cramping, abdominal pain, nausea, and vomiting.

The physical examination includes auscultation of bowel tones, percussion and palpation for masses and tenderness, including rebound tenderness, and assessment of hydration status. Laboratory tests to rule out infection include a white blood cell count, differential, and erythrocyte sedimentation rate.

Examination of the stool will help to identify etiologic factors. The stool should be examined for blood, mucus, and pus, and a sample should be sent to the lab for culture and sensitivity if the patient is febrile, if symptoms are severe, or if symptoms do not subside within 48 h. Evaluating the stool for reducing substances will determine the presence of simple sugars, indicating malabsorption. Presence of fat in the stool is also indicative of malabsorption.

Sigmoidoscopy will determine presence of mucosal changes associated with ulcerative colitis and may be necessary to locate carcinoma. Radiopaque examination of the bowel may be useful in diagnosing changes associated with inflammatory bowel disease and carcinoma.

Management

Therapeutic Objectives

The objectives in the therapy of diarrhea are:

1. Prevention and treatment of fluid and electrolyte imbalance, if present.
2. Treatment of specific etiologic processes.
3. Relief of associated symptoms such as cramping and tenesmus (spasmodic contractions of sphincter with persistent desire and straining to empty bowel).
4. Prevention of perianal irritation.
5. Decrease in frequency of unformed stools to patient's normal frequency.

Nonpharmacologic Management

An essential component of the therapy of diarrhea consists of modifications in the patient's patterns of behavior. Any dietary substance that can potentially irritate the bowel further should be avoided (see Table 20-6). Clear liquids followed by gradual progression to the regular diet will decrease bowel stimuli. Milk products should be avoided and should be deleted from the diet for several days after resolution of the problem. Low-fat diets have been advocated for patients with steatorrhea. Glucose and electrolyte solutions orally have been recommended, because glucose facilitates absorption of electrolytes and water in the small intestine. The recommended solution contains, per liter, sodium chloride, 3.5 g; sodium bicarbonate, 2.5 g; potassium chloride, 1.5 g; and glucose, 20 g. This solution would have an osmolarity of approximately 320 mosmol/L, and the patient should be allowed to drink it freely. Solutions of commercial products like Gatorade and liquid Jell-O have been recommended. They are, however, very low in electrolytes and are not recommended if the patient has a sodium or potassium deficit. Pedialyte and Lytren are two examples of commercially prepared electrolyte preparations that are recommended for infants.

Replacement of fluid and electrolyte losses can be critical. Patients with severe vomiting or altered level of consciousness (confused or comatose) will not be able to ingest sufficient liquids to meet their metabolic needs. During replacement therapy patients with problems predisposing to fluid and electrolyte imbalance or susceptible to fluid overload must be monitored carefully. For example, patients with chronic renal failure and patients with congestive heart failure may be at risk for fluid overload.

Oral fluids are the treatment of choice to prevent fluid and electrolyte imbalance, where oral fluid intake is not limited. However, if oral fluids in sufficient amounts to meet the patient's needs cannot be ingested or if severe imbalance is present, parenteral fluids will be necessary. The oral fluids of choice are the glucose and electrolyte solutions discussed previously. The patient should be allowed to drink freely unless oral intake exacerbates the symptoms.

Because exercise will increase stool formation in diarrhea, rest is recommended. The activity level should be adapted to the severity of the diarrhea and fluid and electrolyte loss as well as other problems. The presence of frequent bowel movements of fluid content will be irritating to the perianal mucosa. Good hygiene is essential to prevent excoriation. Washing with a gentle soap and water following each bowel movement may be necessary, especially if the individual's skin is excoriated. Emollients (vitamin A and D ointment, white petrolatum) may be used to protect the skin.

Pharmacologic Management

The treatment of diarrhea whenever possible should be directed at the underlying problem. Patients with *lactose intolerance* can purchase **lactase enzyme** at health food stores or pharmacies and pretreat each quart of milk with 4 to 10 drops of the liquid (LactAid) or the contents of 1–2 capsules (Lactrase). Alternatively, 1 or 2 capsules can be ingested with the dairy products, or sprinkled over the food.

There is a wide variety of preparations that are commercially available to treat the symptoms of diarrhea but the **opiates** are considered the most effective. Other preparations that are used include the **anticholinergics, polycarbophil,** and other adsorbents.

Opiates   The antidiarrheal effects of opiates are due to their morphine content. **Morphine** increases nonpropulsive and decreases propulsive contractions while the tone of the sphincters is increased, slowing transit time in the small and large bowel.

Adverse effects   In the normal doses used for their antidiarrheal effects the opiates have little dependency potential. However, if these preparations are used chronically and in doses larger than those recommended, the dependency risk exists. The use of these preparations in cases of diarrhea caused by shigellosis should be avoided because resolution of the infection is delayed. Other effects may include sedation, drowsiness, and cramping.

Dosage and preparations   The most common preparations are **tincture of opium** (laudanum, deodorized tincture of opium); **camphorated tincture of opium** (paregoric); **opium powder; diphenoxylate,** a synthetic opiate, with **atropine sulfate** (Lomotil); **loperamide** (Imodium), also a synthetic opiate; **codeine;** and **morphine.** Opium is commonly used in doses of 15 to 20 mg, which is equivalent to 1.5 to

TABLE 20-6   Foods Used to Harden the Stool

FOOD GROUP	FOODS RECOMMENDED	FOODS WITH NEUTRAL OR LITTLE EFFECT ON STOOL
Beverages	2% milk (fat-free), carbonated beverage, Kool-Aid	Relatively low intake of water; coffee, tea, buttermilk
Breads	Melba toast, rusk, zweiback, or crackers with low-fat and whole-grain content	
Cereals	Cooked, refined wheat, corn, rice cereals, strained oatmeal, prepared cereals made from refined corn or rice	
Desserts	Ice milk, arrowroot, plain sugar, cookies and cakes low in fat, plain desserts, Jell-O or gelatin pudding with skim or 2% milk or with strained fruit juices	
Eggs	Hard-cooked, poached	Egg white
Fats and oils	Not recommended; attempt to reduce intake to absolute minimum	
Fruit and fruit juices	Canned fruits, tender raw fruits without skins (only to tolerance)	Strained fruit juices including one serving citrus juice daily
Meat, fish	Lean meats*	Chicken, turkey, lean fish, lean beef, veal, and pork
Cheese	Dry cottage cheese, skim milk cheese, natural or plain yogurt (unpasteurized)	
Sugars and sweets	Plain candy, honey, jelly, sugar and syrup	
Vegetables	Tender, cooked vegetables with little fiber; grated raw vegetables	Tomato juice, soft-leaf lettuce
Miscellaneous	Dilute vinegar	Mild spices in moderation; white sauce and gravy in moderation

*Avoid marbled or fatty cuts and cheap hamburger.
Source: Modified from Chapman, W., Hill, M. and D. B. Shurtleff. Management of the Neurogenic Bowel and Bladder. Oak Brook, Ill.: Eterna, 1979.

2.0 mg of morphine. See Table 20-7 for doses of the opiate antidiarrheals.

Laudanum and paregoric Laudanum (tincture of opium) and paregoric (camphorated tincture of opium) preparations are administered after each loose stool not to exceed four doses per day. Laudanum contains 25 times more morphine than paregoric, and package labels should be checked closely so that confusion between the two doses does not occur. Both laudanum and paregoric are given in combination with an adsorbant such as pectin or bismuth subsalicylate. Paregoric is sometimes used to treat infants of mothers addicted to narcotics.

Diphenoxylate Diphenoxylate (Lomotil and others) is a synthetic opiate closely related to **meperidine** (Demerol). Its only recognized use is in combination with atropine sulfate for treatment of diarrhea. At high doses (40 to 60 mg) Lomotil may produce morphine-like symptoms of euphoria and dependence. In therapeutic doses, Lomotil is safe for adults but should be used with caution in children. It is contraindicated in children under 2 years of age. In cases of overdose, **naloxone hydrochloride** (Narcan) should be used to counteract respiratory depression. Diphenoxylate should be used with caution in pregnant women and is not recommended for use by nursing mothers.

Loperamide (Imodium) Loperamide is a synthetic antidiarrheal drug which is used in the treatment of acute nonspecific diarrhea and chronic diarrhea associated with inflammatory bowel disease and to reduce the volume of discharge from ileostomies. Loperamide is as effective an inhibitor of gastrointestinal motility as diphenoxylate, codeine, or morphine without causing their morphine-like effects even in high doses.

Pharmacokinetics of loperamide shows that the stomach absorption is low; only about 10 percent of the drug is recovered from the urine, and 42 percent is excreted in the feces. The half-life of loperamide that has been *absorbed* is approximately 7 to 14 h.

As with most other antidiarrheal preparations, constipa-

tion is the most frequent adverse effect of loperamide, although drowsiness, dizziness, abdominal discomfort, nausea, vomiting, tiredness, skin rash, and dry mouth have all been reported. Overdoses with loperamide can cause central nervous system (CNS) depression, and the treatment should be with gastric lavage and the administration of activated charcoal. If CNS depression occurs, it may be treated with repeated doses of the narcotic antagonist **naloxone hydrochloride** (Narcan). There is inconclusive data for the safety of loperamide for children, pregnant women, or nursing mothers.

Adsorbents The adsorbents are the most frequently used over-the-counter antidiarrheal preparations. Their action is to adsorb quantities of water and electrolytes as well nutrients and other material. The most common agents used are **activated charcoal, aluminum hydroxides, attapulgite** (magnesium aluminum silicate), **bismuth subsalicylate** and **bismuth subnitrate, kaolin, pectin,** and **magnesium trisilicate.** Although these products have been used for years, their effectiveness in the treatment of diarrhea has not been proved or at best have been shown to be only marginally effective.

Adverse effects Since these agents are relatively nonabsorbed, adverse effects are rare. In some cases giving these agents in conjunction with drugs might decrease the absorption of the drug, but drug absorption is inhibited in the presence of diarrhea to begin with.

Dosage and preparation **Kaolin** and **pectin** mixture is given usually after each loose bowel movement (Table 20-8). **Bismuth subnitrate** should not be used, since it may form nitrite ion which may be absorbed, causing hypotension and methemoglobinemia. With the use of bismuth salts the stool becomes darker. **Bismuth subsalicylate** may be effective in the treatment and prevention of traveler's diarrhea.

Anticholinergic Drugs The anticholinergic agents have a limited role in the treatment of diarrhea. They act by inhibiting parasympathetic activity of the intestinal tract, which decreases intestinal motility. The objective of their use should be to decrease cramping when associated with diarrhea rather than to treat the diarrhea.

Adverse effects When given in doses to produce antispasmotic activity, anticholinergic agents have effects on other organs: cardiovascular system, urogenital tract, salivary glands, and eye. Thus, these agents have all the contraindications associated with the use of any anticholinergic preparation (see Chap. 12).

Dosage and preparations These agents are effective only when given in doses equivalent to 0.6 to 1 mg of **atropine sulfate.** The amount of atropine in over-the-counter preparations (Table 20-8) and Lomotil is subtherapeutic for its antispasmotic effect. A commonly used preparation is **belladonna tincture,** 0.3 mg/mL of alkaloids given alone or

TABLE 20-7 Narcotic Medications Used to Treat Diarrhea

DRUG	TRADE NAME	ADULT DOSE	PEDIATRIC DOSE
Opiates			
Laudanum		0.3–1.0 mL	
Paregoric		5–10 mL	2–4 mL/m²
Diphenoxylate with atropine sulfate	Lomotil, others	2.5–5 mg	2 mg tid, 2–5 years 2 mg qid, 5–8 years 2 mg 5 times daily, 8–12 years
Loperamide	Imodium	2–4 mg	Not recommended, <12 years

in combination with other products. The most common combination preparation is Donnagel.

Miscellaneous Lactobacillus preparations (Lactinex, Bacid, yogurt) are in theory used to help return the normal intestinal flora of gastrointestinal tract. Antibiotics are known to alter the normal intestinal flora, and it sometimes is recommended that these preparations be taken as adjunct therapy. Milk containing higher concentrations of *Lactobacillus acidophilus* is available in supermarkets. Capsules should be taken with at least 4 oz of milk or tomato juice. Granules can be sprinkled on foods.

Polycarbophil Polycarbophil (Mitrolan) has the ability to bind free water; it can absorb 60 times its weight in water and is effective in treating diarrhea. Paradoxically, it is also effective in treating constipation by preventing the stool from becoming hard and dry. It has few adverse effects since it is nonabsorbed and relatively nontoxic.

Patient Education

The use of over-the-counter and prescription medications for the treatment of diarrhea is recommended only after the etiology of the diarrhea is determined. Various types of diarrhea secondary to bacterial infections are often treated with antibiotics, in which case the patient should be taught proper self-administration of the antibiotics.

Diarrhea secondary to infectious and parasitic agents can be highly contagious. Teaching proper hand-washing techniques is essential. The need for appropriate hand-washing should be emphasized in the education of both patients and health care providers.

Replacement of fluids is an important adjunct to the management of diarrhea. The recommended amount of fluid is based upon the patient's age, weight, and degree of fluid losses. Types of replacement fluids are discussed in Chap. 24. Small amounts taken frequently are better tolerated than large amounts taken at greater intervals. Parents of infants

TABLE 20-8 Antidiarrheal Products

PRODUCT	DOSAGE FORMS	OPIATES	ADSORBENTS	OTHER ACTIVE INGREDIENTS	INACTIVE INGREDIENTS
Bacid	Capsule			Carboxymethyl cellulose sodium, 100 mg *Lactobacillus, acidophilus* 500 million U	
Donnagel	Suspension		Kaolin, 200 mg/mL Pectin, 4.76 mg/mL	Hyoscyamine sulfate, 0.0035 mg/mL Atropine sulfate 0.0006 mg/mL Hyoscine hydrobromide 0.0002 mg/mL	Alcohol, 3.8% Sodium benzoate, 2 mg/mL
Donnagel-PG	Suspension	Powdered opium, 0.8 mg/mL	Kaolin, 200 mg/mL Pectin, 4.76 mg/mL	Hyosycamine sulfate, 0.0035 mg/mL Atropine sulfate, 0.0006 mg/mL Hyoscine hydrobromide, 0.0002 mg/mL	Alcohol, 5% Sodium benzoate, 2 mg/mL
Kaolin Pectin	Suspension		Kaolin 190 mg/mL Pectin, 4.34 mg/mL	Carboxymethyl cellulose sodium, 0.4%	Glycerin, 1.75% lime mint flavor saccharin Sodium, 0.025%
Kaopectate concentrate	Suspension		Kaolin, 290 mg/mL Pectin, 6.47 mg/mL		
Lactinex	Tablet Granules			*Lactobacillus acidophilus, L. bulgaricus*	
Pepto-Bismol	Tablet		Bismuth subsalicylate, 300 mg/tablet		
	Liquid		Bismuth subsalicylate, 525 mg/30 mL		

Source: Modified from American Pharmaceutical Association: *Handbook of Nonprescription Drugs,* 7th ed., reprinted with permission.

and small children, especially, need to be given explicit guidelines for home management of diarrhea as well as indications for when medical intervention is indicated.

Dietary adjustments should be made when the diarrhea is associated with specific food tolerances. The patient with celiac disease, for instance, should refrain from foods which contain gluten, while the patient with a lactose intolerance or lactase deficiency needs to avoid milk products or use lactase enzyme as previously discussed. Teaching the patient to read product labels on commercially prepared foods and providing the patient with recipes that avoid implicated foods will enhance patient compliance with dietary restrictions.

When the diarrhea is secondary to a chronic malabsorptive disorder, the patient often requires nutritional supplements such as **vitamins** and **minerals.** Pancreatic enzymes are indicated in cystic fibrosis. Diarrhea which occurs secondary to the irritation of bile salts in the bowel is common in patients with biliary tract disease. **Cholestyramine** is often indicated in this situation.

In general, patients with diarrheal episodes which last longer than 48 h or which cause significant fluid losses should be encouraged to seek medical evaluation. Infants, children, and debilitated adults are at particular risk, and questionable episodes of diarrhea should always be brought to medical attention.

Evaluation

To monitor the achievement of the therapeutic objectives, the appropriate indices of effect are identified. Estimates of fluid intake in comparison with fluid loss (vomiting, urinary loss, diaphoresis, diarrhea) should be made. If fever is present, it will increase fluid needs. Specific etiologic processes should be monitored, for example by use of stool cultures. Objective data should be obtained where possible, for example by examination of perianal mucosa. Stool consistency and frequency also need to be evaluated.

CASE STUDY

Q.F., a 63-year-old widow, was admitted to the orthopedic unit for an internal fixation of a fractured left hip. On Q.F.'s tenth postoperative day Ms. P., the team leader, returned to the unit after a vacation to find that the patient was recovering well from the surgery, had begun gait training in physical therapy, and had been on a regular diet for 7 days.

Assessment

In reviewing the patient's drug orders, Ms. P. was surprised to note that not only were there orders for Colace, 100 mg at bedtime; Metamucil, 2 tsp bid PRN; soapsuds enema PRN; and paregoric, 10 mL q3–4h PRN, but each had been administered at least once in the previous 48 h. Review of the medical orders and nurses' notes revealed how Q.F. had come to have this "regimen": The physician routinely ordered Colace after this surgical procedure. On the second postoperative day, Q.F. had begun to worry about constipation even though she had advanced only to a full liquid diet, and the physician ordered the Metamucil at the patient's request, since she had used this drug routinely at home. On the fifth postoperative day, Q.F. had developed "diarrhea," and the evening nurse had phoned the physician, received the paregoric order, and withheld the Colace for two nights. Two days later the patient had complained of being constipated and "feeling of fullness," requesting an enema, as had been her habit at least once weekly before hospitalization. The nurse's aide who had administered the enema on the physician's order indicated that the patient

had insisted on two successive enemas. The record showed that the next day she had received the Metamucil again.

Interview of the patient revealed that she thought that "normal" bowel habits were essential to health, and that one well-formed stool daily was the only "normal" pattern she recognized. Any deviation from this was termed "diarrhea" or "constipation" and promptly treated.

Q.F. had high blood pressure and had developed secondary congestive heart failure 2 years previously, which had resolved with medication. The hypertension was presently controlled by 50 mg of hydrochlorothiazide daily.

Ms. P.'s nursing diagnosis for Q.F. was chronic laxative abuse, coupled with misuse of antidiarrheals, creating a "seesaw" pattern in bowel habits. The cause of the condition was misinformation, and it was made more dangerous by the patient's cardiac condition.

Management

Ms. P. contacted Q.F.'s physician and presented the data about the problem and her analysis. The physician agreed that the situation was highly undesirable and supported the program suggested by Ms. P. for discontinuation of all medication and enemas, for patient education, and for use of behavioral means to achieve optimum bowel functions.

The variation of elimination patterns that are considered normal, the cause and dangers of laxative abuse, and the role of diet, exercise, and fluids in control of elimination were presented by Ms. P. The nurse met with the patient and dietitian to plan a high-bulk diet. The patient was extremely reluctant to change her normal habits and agreed to forgo the laxatives only with maximal encouragement and support from the physician and nursing staff. Fluid intake and activity, both of which were encouraged, and number and character of stools were recorded meticulously.

Evaluation

During hospitalization it was possible to control bowel elimination adequately with behavioral means, although the patient's elimination pattern was every second day. However, long-term follow-up by the physician revealed that Q.F.'s basic attitudes were apparently unchanged, for she resumed her former habit of laxative abuse within 2 months of returning home.

REFERENCES

Alvear, D. T., et al.: "Constipation in Infants and Children: Personal Observations and Management," *Enterostomal Ther*, 10:14–18, January–February 1983.

Aman, R. A.: "Treating the Patient, Not the Constipation," *Am J Nurs*, 80:1634–1635, January 1980.

American Hospital Formulary Service, Bethesda, MD: American Society of Hospital Pharmacists, 1982.

Angel, J. E.: *Physician's Desk Reference*, 37th ed., Oradell, NJ: Medical Economics, 1983.

Bertholf, C. B.: "Protocol: Acute Diarrhea," *Nurse Pract*, 3:17–20, May–June 1978.

Chapman, W., M. Hill, and D. B. Shurtleff: *Management of the Neurogenic Bowel and Bladder*, Oak Brook, IL: Eterna, 1979.

Chow, M. P., et al.: *Handbook of Pediatric Primary Care*, New York: Wiley, 1979.

DeGennaro, M. D., et al.: "Antidepressant Drug Therapy," *Am J Nurs*, 81:1304–1310, July 1981.

Evans, D. W.: "Practical Advice about a Delicate Pediatric Problem," *RN*, 41:51–52, August 1978.

Gerald, M. C.: *Pharmacology: An Introduction to Drugs*, Englewood Cliffs, NJ: Prentice-Hall, 1981.

Gilman, A. G., L. S. Goodman, and A. Gilman (eds.): *Goodman and Gilman's The Pharmacological Basis of Therapeutics*, 6th ed., New York: Macmillan 1980.

Groer, M. E., and M. E. Shekleton: *Basic Pathophysiology: A Conceptual Approach*, St. Louis: Mosby, 1979.

Handbook of Nonprescription Drugs, 7th ed. Washington: American Pharmaceutical Association, 1982.

Iseminger, M., et al.: "Bran Works," *Geriatr Nurs*, 3:402–404, November–December, 1982.

Ling, L., et al.: "Dietary Treatment of Diarrhea and Constipation in Infants and Children," *Issues Compr Pediatr Nurs*, 3:17–28, October 1978.

McGrath, B. J.: "Fluids, Electrolytes and Replacement Therapy in Pediatric Nursing," *Am J Maternal Child Nurs*, 5:58–62, January–February 1980.

Miller, M. J.: *Pathophysiology: Principles of Disease*, Philadelphia: Saunders 1983.

Obrien, M. T., and P. J. Pallett: "Bowel Training for Stroke Patients," *Nursing 79*, 9:54, July 1979 (Abstract).

Quinn, R. J.: "Bowel Program after Spinal Fracture," *Nursing*, 10:106, April 1980.

Vigliarolo, D.: "Managing Bowel Incontinence in Children with Meningo-Myelocele," *Am J Nurs*, 80:105–107, January 1980.

21

SYMPTOMS OF "COLD" AND ALLERGY*

VAUGHN C. CULBERTSON
BEVERLY A. BURTON

LEARNING OBJECTIVES

Upon mastery of the content of this chapter the reader will be able to:

1. Describe the causes and symptomatology of the common cold, allergic rhinitis, and influenza.

2. Outline the assessment of the patient with symptoms of rhinorrhea, nasal congestion, cough, and pharyngitis.

3. Explain histamine release and the effects of H_1 and H_2 receptors.

4. State the major pharmacologic and adverse effects of antihistamines, nasal decongestants, antitussives, and expectorants.

5. Describe the precautions of nasal decongestants in patients with ischemic heart disease, thyroid disease, diabetes mellitus, and hypertension.

6. Explain the etiology of the drug-induced rebound phenomena produced by topical nasal decongestants.

7. Describe the indications for adverse effects of topical nasal steroids in the treatment of nasal congestion.

8. Outline recommendations to patients for rational management of sneezing, rhinitis, nasal congestion, and pharyngitis due to the common cold.

9. Outline recommendations to patients for rational management of sneezing, rhinitis, nasal congestion, and conjunctival itching due to allergy.

10. Write teaching plans for patients receiving antihistamines, systemic and topical nasal decongestants, and antitussives.

11. Describe the evaluation of the treatment of common cold and allergic rhinitis.

*The editors thank Thomas H. Wiser and Thomasine D. Guberski, who contributed the chapter on this subject in the first edition.

A variety of pathologic conditions—the common cold, influenza, allergic rhinitis, vasomotor rhinitis, rhinitis medicamentosa—can produce symptoms of nasal congestion, nasal discharge, cough, sore throat, fever, headache, and general malaise. Although the treatment is symptomatic, it is important to differentiate the cause of the symptoms.

PATHOLOGY

The Common Cold

Success in treating the common cold, like other viral infections of the respiratory tract, has proved to be elusive. Most adults have two to four colds per year; children may have up to twelve per year. The common cold has been described as the most expensive illness in the United States. The American public spends between $500 million and $700 million annually on cold and cough preparations, more than on any other kind of over-the-counter products. These figures do not include monies spent on prescription medications such as antihistamines, antitussives, and antibiotics. Aside from the vast amount of money the public spends on treating the symptoms of common cold, the disease accounts for a large amount of time lost from work and school.

Transmission of the common cold usually occurs through airborne respiratory droplets. After a 1- to 4-day incubation period, clinical manifestations occur. Contrary to what many believe, fatigue or exposure to drafts do not increase one's susceptibility to colds.

Symptoms vary from one patient to another, but generally include pharyngitis, nasal congestion, rhinorrhea, headache, malaise, lethargy, and possibly fever, chills, and cough. The classic symptom of the common cold is nasal discharge which usually begins as a clear, watery, and profuse discharge; later it becomes mucopurulent, yellow-green, and thick. Generally, major signs of the cold diminish after 3 days. However, a residual stuffed-up feeling and cough, usually dry, may persist for 1 or 2 weeks.

Any one of over 100 viruses may be responsible for the

infection, and there are no explicit diagnostic tests to isolate specific organisms. White blood count and differential are within normal limits during the common cold. Consequently, diagnosis rests on typically mild, localized upper respiratory symptoms.

Physical examination of the patient reveals erythematous, edematous nasal mucosa (as opposed to pale, boggy mucosa in hay fever). Further findings may include mildly erythematous pharynx, mild conjunctivitis, and occasionally low-grade fever. The remainder of the physical examination is normal. Infants may present with elevated fever as well as erythematous tympanic membranes.

Treatment is aimed at purely relieving symptoms and promoting patient comfort as there is no known cure for the common cold. Bed rest or a reduction in activity is a logical response to the lethargy and malaise that accompany a cold. Liberal fluid intake is necessary to liquefy secretions and maintain adequate hydration. Management may include a variety of over-the-counter products and prescription medications which are directed at treating one or more symptoms.

Patients may also use a variety of home remedies which may have some psychologic and social value but very little scientific basis. Home remedies that have been used include chicken soup, a combination of boiled wine and aspirin, or a mixture of hot tea, sugar, and the patient's favorite alcoholic beverage (e.g., the "hot toddy"). These home remedies may have a strong placebo effect and should not be rejected as a form of therapy since they may be more effective than some of the advertised treatments.

Many patients request antibiotics for treating their cold. The nurse plays an important role in emphasizing to patients that antibiotics are not effective for viral infection. The routine use of antibiotics is indicated only in patients at risk of developing a secondary bacterial infection [e.g., chronic obstructive pulmonary disease (COPD), recurrent sinusitis].

Patients should be made aware of which symptoms would indicate a condition more complicated than the common cold. Clues to a more serious condition include a temperature elevation over 100°F (37.8°C), a general feeling of increased illness (malaise, anorexia, tachycardia), tonsillar exudate, tender lymph glands and severely erythematous pharynx.

Vitamin C and the Common Cold

The claims for the value of vitamin C in treatment of the common cold, in doses of up to 15 g, have emanated from Dr. Linus Pauling (*Vitamin C and the Common Cold*). The benefits at this time are still debatable, and the theory of its effects, if any, is not well understood. When used in large doses, the potential for adverse effects is present; however these are uncommon. Adverse effects include diarrhea, urinary acidification (modifies the pharmacokinetic pattern of some drugs), possible precipitation of urate or oxalate stones in the urinary tract, and interference with laboratory tests.

As with most megavitamin therapy, the issues are extremely controversial. In some cases, it is judged that vitamin C actually prevents the development of a cold, while in others it is thought that the vitamin may at least shorten the duration.

Allergic Rhinitis

Although the first onset of allergic rhinitis is greatest in children and young adults, it may begin at almost any age. Symptoms usually decrease with age. A family history of allergic disease is common. Allergic rhinitis is a reaction of the nasal mucosa manifested by nasal edema, sneezing, itching, rhinorrhea, and nasal congestion resulting from allergy to a specific antigen. The allergy may be due to antigen-like pollen which exists only during certain seasons (hay fever or seasonal) or to others which are present all year long (perennial). Hay fever varies with the geography, the type of local vegetation, and the time of year that the plants pollinate. Allergies may also be caused by a variety of antigens like household dust or animal dander. When the antigen (allergen) is inhaled, it comes in contact with the sensitized mucosa, and antigen-antibody reactions occur, causing nasal congestion, increase in watery secretions, and itching which leads to sneezing. Many think this reaction is mediated by chemicals such as histamine and the leukotrienes.

Rhinorrhea associated with allergic rhinitis is typically a watery, thin discharge that may be quite profuse and continuous. The nasal congestion of allergic rhinitis is due to swollen turbinates, and, if severe, may cause headaches or earaches. Commonly there is associated conjunctival itching and lacrimation. Patients with eye symptoms may complain of photophobia and tired eyes.

The most valuable tool in the diagnosis of allergic rhinitis is a carefully taken history with specific attention to details of occurrence of symptoms. The history should include when the symptoms first began and the intervals between exacerbation. Patients with seasonal allergic rhinitis (hay fever) tend to exhibit more severe symptoms on windy days due to an increase in pollen in the air. On rainy days when pollen is cleared from the air, many patients will notice a decrease in symptoms. Patients with perennial allergic rhinitis may have continuous symptoms because of the continual presence of the allergen (dust or dander) in their environment. The presence of exacerbations occurring certain times of the year is important to the differentiation between seasonal and perennial allergic rhinitis. The treatment is similar with both types.

Treatment of allergic rhinitis involves avoiding the allergen if possible, altering the immune response by injecting allergen extracts (immunotherapy), and treating the symptoms.

Symptomatic treatment of allergic rhinitis is aimed at achieving relief with a minimum of side effects (e.g., drowsiness). Since the principal mediator of the allergic rhinitis reaction is histamine, use of antihistamines is beneficial.

Immunotherapy

To alter an immune response to an antigenic material, the patient is treated with the antigenic material so that specific blocking antibodies to the antigen may be produced. These antibodies react with naturally occurring antigen blocking their interaction with endogenous antibodies and preventing the inflammatory antigen-antibody reaction. Therapy begins by skin testing to identify specific antigens. Next, trial therapy aimed at avoidance of the offending antigen (i.e., environmental control) and aggressive therapy with medication to treat the symptoms is initiated. If unsuccessful, immunotherapy may be added to the regimen. Small doses of the offending antigen(s) are injected subcutaneously at approximately 2-week intervals. The dose is gradually increased until severe adverse local or systemic reactions to the injected allergen occur or until satisfactory relief of symptoms is achieved. Although extremely beneficial to some patients, therapy is expensive and inconvenient often involving several years of injections; results are inconsistent; and there is always the risk of serious adverse reactions, including anaphylaxis. Thus, immunotherapy is indicated only for a selected population whose symptoms cannot be controlled by more conventional therapeutic measures.

Influenza

Influenza is an acute contagious viral infection which is marked by fever, prostration, and benign outcome. The accompanying headache, myalgia, and weakness may be more severe than the respiratory symptoms of influenza. Respiratory symptoms include a spasmodic, nonproductive cough, sore throat, nasal congestion, and rhinorrhea which is usually less prominent than other symptoms.

Treatment of influenza is directed at relieving the symptoms and includes aspirin or acetaminophen for fever and myalgia, liberal fluid intake, and cough suppressant if needed. Routine use of antibiotics is indicated only in patients who risk developing a secondary bacterial infection (e.g., elderly, severe asthmatics, patients with COPD, patients with an altered immune response).

ASSESSMENT

In assessing the patient with symptoms of rhinitis, nasal congestion, pharyngitis, malaise, and cough, it is important to differentiate the cause of the symptoms. In addition to the common cold, allergic rhinitis, and influenza, causes can also include impending exacerbation of asthma, prodromal symptoms of measles, or more serious disorders such as streptococcal pharyngitis or pneumonia.

A history of the onset and duration of symptoms including a detailed description of malaise, fever, nasal discomfort and discharge, sneezing, cough, sputum, and sore throat should be elicited from the patient. Physical assessment emphasizes examination of ears, nose, throat, cervical lymph node, and thorax as well as general appearance (see Table 21-1). A review of systems should also be done so that symptoms indicative of more serious conditions are not overlooked.

MANAGEMENT OF SYMPTOMS

Rhinorrhea (Nasal Discharge)

In allergic rhinitis and the common cold, histamine, along with other chemical mediators, is released and initiates the

TABLE 21-1 Differential Diagnosis of Allergies, Colds, and Influenza

	APPEARANCE OF NARES	NASAL DISCHARGE	PHARYNX	COUGH	CHEST AUSCULTATION	PERTINENT LAB FINDINGS
Common cold	External nares reddened; internal nares red and swollen	Mucopurulent	Mild to moderate erythema without exudates	Usually dry, scanty, accompanied by substernal aching	Usually clear	Usually none, possibly mild leukocytosis
Allergic rhinitis	Enlarged nasal turbinates, pale, boggy and swollen mucosa; possible nasal polyps	Profuse, continuous thin, watery, clear	May be mildly erythematous due to postpharyngeal secretions	Nonproductive from irritation of post-pharyngeal secretions	Usually clear	Eosinophilia
Influenza	Noncontributory	Noncontributory	Dull, red; faucial pillar slightly edematous	Brief, spasmodic, nonproductive	Rhonchi and occasional scattered rales	Generally none

inflammatory response producing rhinorrhea. Although it is common to both, the contribution histamine makes varies due to differences in the mechanism of release and the amount released.

Antihistamines are considered rational therapy for prevention and attenuation of allergic rhinitis. However, their value in the treatment of the common cold and influenza is controversial and lacks scientific basis. Understanding the role of histamine and the mechanism of action of antihistamines will allow the practitioner to advise patients to use these agents more effectively.

Histamine

Histamine is present in nearly all body tissues and biologic fluids, but is more prominent in the skin and gastrointestinal mucosa. Mast cells store endogenous histamine and release it into tissue in response to a variety of stimuli (i.e., physical or chemical injury, infection, antigen-antibody reaction). In allergic disorders (e.g., allergic rhinitis, anaphylaxis, and hypersensitivity), interaction of antibody-coated mast cells with allergen (i.e., antigen) results in cell lysis and histamine release.

The physiologic action of histamine can be classified on the basis of its receptor activity in much the same way adrenergic receptors are classified. Two types of histamine receptors have been identified, H_1 and H_2. Stimulation of H_1 receptors results in constriction of extravascular smooth muscle, while the most important effect of H_2 stimulation is induction of exocrine gland secretion. Some effects, most notably vascular dilation, are mediated by a combination of H_1 and H_2 receptors.

The dominant pharmacologic action of histamine involves three organ systems: the cardiovascular system, extravascular smooth muscle, and exocrine glands.

Capillary vasodilation results from a direct action of histamine on blood vessels. This may decrease systemic blood pressure and, in large doses, can produce shock. A second vascular effect, an increase in capillary permeability, results in transudation of fluid and protein into the extracellular space and in edema formation. These actions are thought to be important determinants of the classic "triple response" phenomena following intradermal injection of histamine (i.e., erythema, flare, and wheal). Furthermore, these vascular effects on cerebral vessels may account for the so-called histamine headache.

Histamine activates H_1 receptors in nonvascular smooth muscle, primarily in the gastrointestinal tract, causing constriction. Bronchial smooth muscle is less prominently affected in normal individuals, but severe bronchoconstriction may be induced in patients with bronchial asthma or other specific pulmonary diseases.

Histamine dramatically increases gastric acid secretion and may evoke large volumes of high-acidity gastric juice. **Betazole** (Histalog), a histamine isomer with preferential effects on gastric acid secretion, is utilized diagnostically for this purpose. Other exocrine glands are not significantly affected.

The importance of histamine as a mediator of the inflammatory response is well documented. However, histamine is not the only chemical mediator released, and, in emergency situations (i.e., anaphylaxis), antihistamines are not the first drugs of choice.

Antihistamines

Some antihistamines are listed in Table 21-2. These agents are active at H_1 receptors.

Mechanism of Action   Antihistamines do not affect the release of histamine; instead they compete with histamine for the receptor site thus preventing its pharmacologic response. This type of receptor blockade, termed competitive antagonism, reflects the ability of increasing doses of histamine to overcome antihistaminic activity. Most antihistamines block H_1 receptors and are frequently used to treat rhinorrhea, while agents like **cimetidine** (Tagamet) and **rantidine** (Zantac) block H_2 receptors. The actions of the H_1 blockers include histamine antagonism and muscarinic blockade.

Histamine antagonism results in inhibition of most of the smooth muscle responses to histamine, including those of the GI tract, bronchi, and vasculature. However, antigen-antibody induced bronchospasm is only weakly antagonized, and the vascular dilatory effects are only partially reversed owing to the participation of H_2 receptors in this response. Antihistamines effectively antagonize histamine-induced increases in capillary permeability and edema formation. Flare and itch reactions following endogenous histamine release are also suppressed.

Central nervous system effects are also quite prominent with antihistamines. Most commonly, they depress the central nervous system causing drowsiness but, occasionally, they may produce CNS stimulation resulting in restlessness, nervousness, and inability to sleep.

Most antihistamines have some anticholinergic (antimuscarinic) property which accounts for dryness of mouth and decrease in other secretions. These effects may be the mechanism by which antihistamines reduce rhinorrhea. In addition, central anticholinergic properties of some H_1 blockers may be at least partially responsible for their usefulness in preventing motion sickness and emesis.

Pharmacokinetics   Specific pharmacokinetic information is lacking for most antihistamines. In general they are rapidly absorbed following oral and parenteral administration. Onset of action begins within 15 to 30 min and is usually fully developed in 1 or 2 h. Duration of action as judged by suppression of wheal-and-flare reaction is several days for most antihistamines and can be up to 4 days for **hydroxyzine** (Atarax).

Furthermore, several antihistamines, including **chlor-**

TABLE 21-2 Antihistamines

| GENERIC NAME | BRAND NAME | Dosage (Maximum Dose per 24 h) | | | COMMENTS |
		ADULTS	CHILDREN, 6 TO <12 YEARS	CHILDREN, 2 TO <6 YEARS	
		Ethanolamines			
Diphenhydramine hydrochloride*	Benadryl, Nordryl, Valdrene, Diphen	25–50 mg q4–6h (300 mg)	12.5–25 mg q4–6h (37.5 mg)	6.25 mg q4–6h	Prominent sedation and anticholinergic effects; commonly used in urticaria, pruritus, and anaphylaxis; effective antitussive; available as OTC products
Carbinoxamine maleate†	Clistin	4–8 mg q6–8h	4 mg q6–8h	2 mg q6–8h	Sedation infrequent
Dimenhydrinate*	Dramamine	50–100 mg q4h	25–50 mg q8h		Used for motion sickness
		Ethylenediamines			
Tripelennamine hydrochloride†	Pelamine, PBZ	25–50 mg q4–6h (600 mg)	5 mg/kg/24 h in divided doses 4–6 times per day (300 mg)	5 mg/kg/24 h, 4–6 doses	
Pyrilamine maleate*		25–50 mg q6–8h (100 mg)	12.5–25 mg q6–8h (100 mg)	6.25 mg–25 mg q6–8h (50 mg)	
		Alkylamines			
Triprolidine hydrochloride†	Actidil	2.5 mg q8–12h	1.25 mg q8–12h	0.6 mg q8–12h	
Brompheniramine maleate*	Dimetane Bromphen	4 mg q4–6h (24 mg)	2 mg q4–6h (12 mg)	1 mg q4–6h (6 mg)	Congenital malformations in humans; in many OTC products
Chlorpheniramine maleate*	Chlor-Trimeton, Teldrin, Aller-Chlor	4 mg q4–6h (12 mg)	2 mg q4–6h (6 mg)	1 mg q4–6h (6 mg)	Available as OTC product
		Phenothiazines			
Promethazine†	Phenergan	12.5 mg–25 mg q6–8h	6.25–12.5 mg q6–8h		Prominent sedative effect
		Piperazines			
Hydroxyzine hydrochloride†	Atarax	25–75 mg q6–8h (300 mg)	12.5–25 mg q6–8h (150 mg)	50 mg/daily in 3 or 4 doses	May be drug of choice for allergic rhinitis
Hydroxyzine pamoate†	Vistaril	See above	See above	See above	
Cyclizine*	Marezine	50 mg 30 min prior to travel (200 mg)	25 mg (100 mg)	Not established	Used for motion sickness
Meclizine*	Antivert	25–50 mg	Not established	Not established	Used for motion sickness
		Miscellaneous			
Cyproheptadine†	Periactin	4 mg q8h (32 mg)	4 mg q8–12h (16 mg)	2 mg q6–8h (12 mg)	Used for pruritus

*Over-the-counter drug.
†By prescription only.
Source: Adapted from The American Pharmaceutical Association: *Handbook of Nonprescription Drugs,* 7th ed., Washington, D.C.: The American Pharmaceutical Association, 1982.

pheniramine (Chlor-Trimeton) and **brompheniramine** (Dimetane), are eliminated from the serum slowly (i.e., half-lives of 30 to 36 h). This suggests that administering these agents four times a day may be unnecessary, although it is the recommended dosage interval.

Adverse Effects Although adverse effects are similar for all antihistamines, the incidence and severity varies with the individual drug. Minor adverse effects often disappear with continual therapy, or may be relieved by a decrease in dosage or change of antihistamine. Serious toxicity (e.g., ataxia, stupor, coma, excitement, hyperthermia, and convulsions) can result from large overdoses but is extremely rare with therapeutic doses.

The most common adverse effect accompanying antihistamine therapy is sedation. This ranges from mild drowsiness to deep sleep and occurs in 25 to 50 percent of all patients treated. By administering most of the daily dosage at bedtime, this effect may be used to some benefit. Some patients, especially children, may react with paradoxical excitement manifested by nervousness, restlessness, tremors, insomnia, palpitations, and, rarely, convulsions. Other CNS effects include dizziness, lassitude, and disturbed coordination.

Gastrointestinal complaints are the next most commonly reported adverse effects. The complaints include nausea, vomiting, diarrhea, constipation, and anorexia; they may be alleviated by administering the drug with food or milk. Skin rash (i.e., contact dermatitis) may occur during systemic therapy, but is most common following topical application. Cross-sensitivity with some local anesthetics may occur, but systemic hypersensitivity reactions are rare. Anticholinergic properties may lead to dry mouth, blurred vision, urinary retention (especially in elderly male patients), and constipation.

Several antihistamines (e.g., meclizine) are teratogenic in animals. Because safe use in pregnancy has not been established in humans, it is generally recommended that these agents be avoided.

Preparations A vast array of preparations is available for treating symptoms of cold and allergy. Many of these preparations are single-entity products, while others are a combination of ingredients ("shotgun" approach). Single-entity products are preferred, since many of the multiple-entity preparations have irrational combinations and include drugs that the patient might not need.

Diphenhydramine (Benadryl) is probably the best known of all the antihistamines because of its widespread use for disorders other than cough and cold. However, its comparatively greater sedative and anticholinergic properties increase the likelihood of side effects and limit its usefulness, particularly in daytime. The usual adult oral dose is 25 to 50 mg qid.

The alkylamine class of antihistamines, which includes **pheniramine**, **chlorpheniramine** (Chlor-Trimeton), **brom-**

pheniramine (Dimetane), and **triprolidine** (Actidil), have less tendency to produce sedation and are probably better agents for daytime therapy. Consequently, these drugs are common ingredients in over-the-counter cough and cold preparations (see Tables 21-2, 21-7, and 21-9).

Hydroxyzine is available as a hydrochloride salt (Atarax) and a pamoate salt (Vistaril). A recent, controlled clinical trial documented the superiority of hydroxyzine over **chlorpheniramine** and placebo in the prophylaxis of allergic rhinitis. Prior to pollen season, an adult oral dose of 25 mg is given at bedtime and gradually increased at 2- or 3-day intervals to a maximum of 150 mg/day. Gradual dose titration allows tolerance to sedative effects to develop while H_1 receptor blockade is cultivated. Treatment is maintained throughout the pollen season.

A newly developed investigational phenothiazine derivative, **terferadene**, has shown promising results. It compares favorably with traditional antihistamines, but sedation and other CNS side effects have been minimal.

Patient Education Patients should be advised that drowsiness, dizziness, disturbance of coordination, dry mouth and throat, blurred vision, nausea, constipation, and, occasionally, urinary retention are all potential side effects of antihistamines. Hypersensitivity reaction, although rare, indicates a need for discontinuance of the drug and notification of the primary care provider.

The sedative property of antihistamines must be emphasized to the patient. Although the degree of drowsiness and slowing of reflexes varies with the antihistamine used, none is entirely free of this effect. If a person's job or other activities requires a high degree of mental alertness or a short reaction time (e.g., driving a motor vehicle and working with hazardous machinery or tools), any antihistamine must be used cautiously. Patients may need help in scheduling the best times for taking these medications. Children should avoid activities (such as climbing) which could result in injury.

In addition, patients should be advised that antihistamines may potentiate effects of alcohol and other CNS depressants, including hypnotics, sedatives, narcotics, tranquilizers, and analgesics. If concurrent administration of these agents is necessary, caution must be exercised because of the increased possibility of drowsiness. Many over-the-counter medications contain alcohol, and patients should be warned to avoid this hidden source. (See alcohol content of OTC products in Tables 21-7 and 21-9.)

If a patient experiences adverse or irritating effects or an unsatisfactory clinical response from one antihistamine, an antihistamine from a different chemical class may provide a more favorable response with fewer side effects.

Nasal Congestion

Dilation of nasal blood vessels with transudation of fluid into submucosal tissue produces swelling of the turbinates and narrowing of the nasal cavities. Symptoms are treated with topical or systemically administered sympathomimetic amines or topical corticosteroids.

Nasal Decongestants

Mechanism of Action The sympathomimetic amines, whether administered topically to the nasal mucosa or orally, stimulate α-adrenergic receptors, produce vascular smooth muscle constriction of the arterioles within the nasal mucosa, and thus decrease blood flow to shrink engorged mucous membranes. This relieves nasal stuffiness and helps the patient breathe. Although not well documented, some degree of tolerance (i.e., tachyphylaxis) may develop after chronic use.

Adverse Effects Sympathomimetic amines frequently produce symptoms of CNS stimulation consisting of nervousness, insomnia, and irritability after systemic administration. Less common adverse effects are caused by the sympathomimetic action of these drugs on the cardiovascular and endocrine systems. However, vasoconstriction is not limited to the nasal mucosa and occurs in other vascular beds as well.

In normotensive individuals, compensatory cardiovascular reflexes prevent any clinically significant increase in blood pressure. However, hypertensive patients should be cautioned about a potential increase in blood pressure, although there is probably little harm with short-term use (e.g., cold management). Similarly, individuals with ischemic heart disease or thyroid disease may experience an exacerbation of symptoms.

Sympathomimetics can pharmacologically increase blood glucose and possibly worsen diabetic control. Since hyperglycemia is principally a β_2-adrenergic response, the effects of nasal decongestants on blood glucose control, if any, are probably modest.

With frequent use, topical decongestants can produce a *rebound nasal congestion* (rhinitis medicamentosa). This is caused by intense local vasoconstriction and irritation, which later may produce rebound vasodilation and severe engorgement as the drug effect subsides. An endless cycle is created since the drug is being used to treat symptoms the drug itself is producing. A drug history will reveal whether the patient is using it too frequently. If the patient is abusing the topical decongestant, an oral nasal decongestant and/or routine saline washes can be recommended. Recently, the use of **intranasal coticosteroids** was found to be effective therapy for rhinitis medicamentosa. These products are discussed in more detail under topical nasal decongestant preparations. Use of topical nasal decongestants in excess of recommended daily dosage may result in dry nasal mucosa and loss of ciliary action.

Topical Preparations and Administration A variety of topical and oral preparations are available (see Tables 21-3 and 21-4). **Phenylephrine** (NeoSynephrine), used in concentrations of 0.125 to 1.0% qid, is one of the most effective nonprescription nasal decongestants, but may cause prominent nasal irritation. **Naphazoline** (Privine) is more potent than phenylephrine, and when absorbed systemically, can produce CNS depression rather than stimulation. It should not be given to children. It is administered as a 0.05% solu-

TABLE 21-3   Systemic Nasal Decongestants

DRUG	SINGLE-ENTITY PRODUCT	PREPARATIONS AVAILABLE	Dosage (Maximum Dose/24 h) *			COMMENTS
			ADULTS	CHILDREN, 6 TO <12 YEARS	CHILDREN, 2 TO <6 YEARS†	
Phenylephrine	None; see combination products listed in Table 21-7		10 mg q4h (60 mg)	5 mg q4h (30 mg)	2.5 mg q4h (15 mg)	Poor bioavailability; usually present in subtherapeutic dosage
Phenylpropanolomine	Propadrine Propagest	25 and 50 mg capsules; 20 mg/5mL elixir (16% alcohol)	25 mg q4h (150 mg)	12.5 mg q4h (75 mg)	6.25 mg q4h (37.5 mg)	
Pseudoephedrine	Sudafed, Novafed	30- and 60-mg tablets; timed-release, 60 and 120 mg; liquid, 30 mg/5 mL	60 mg q6h (240 mg)	30 mg q6h (120 mg)	15 mg q6h (60 mg)	Short duration of action (3 h); sustained-release preparations now available

*The FDA advisory review panel on nonprescription cold, cough, allergy, bronchodilator, and antihistamine products has recommended these ingredients as safe and effective (category 1) at the dosages specified.

†There is no recommended dosage for children under 2 years of age except under the advice and supervision of a physician.

Source: Adapted from The American Pharmaceutical Association: *Handbook of Nonprescription Drugs,* 7th ed., Washington, DC: The American Pharmaceutical Association, 1982.

tion, one to three drops every 4 or 5 h. Preparations of **xylometazoline** (Otrivin) and **oxymetazoline** (Afrin) are longer-acting and should be used only twice a day. Other agents include the sympathomimetic amines **levodeoxyephedrine** and **propylhexedrine**. Clear-cut differences of these OTC preparations have not been demonstrated.

Oral Preparations Oral agents have a slower onset of action but a more prolonged effect and have not been associated with rebound congestion.

Ephedrine is more effective as a bronchodilator and should not be recommended for nasal decongestion. Its main adverse effect is CNS stimulation which may cause

nervousness, anxiety, and palpitations. Some commercial preparations may contain a CNS depressant to counteract this effect.

Pseudoephedrine (Sudafed) has less vasoconstrictor and CNS stimulation effect than ephedrine. The adult dose is 30 to 60 mg tid or qid. (the 30-mg tablet is sold over-the-counter). For children between 2 to 5 years, doses are 15 mg tid or qid as an elixir (30 mg/5 mL). Its peak action occurs in 4 h. Because its duration of action is only 3 or 4 hours, several new sustained-action preparations have been marketed. These products can be administered twice daily for effective relief of nasal congestion.

Phenylpropanolamine (Propadrine) is similar to ephed-

TABLE 21-4 Topical Nasal Decongestants*

DRUG AND CONCENTRATION	SINGLE-ENTITY PRODUCTS	Dosage, Number of Daily Applicaitons			COMMENTS
		ADULTS, DROPS OR SPRAYS	CHILDREN 6 TO <12 YEARS, DROPS OR SPRAYS	CHILDREN 2 TO <6 YEARS†	
Ephedrine, 1.0% (various salts)	Epnedsol-1%	2–3 (≥4 h)	1–2 (≥4 h)	—	Also available in 0.5 and 3% solutions
Naphazoline hydrochloride, 0.05%	Privine drops and spray	1–2 (≥6 h)	Not recommended (refer to 0.025%)	—	May produce CNS depression following systemic absorption
Oxymetazoline hydrochloride, 0.05%	Afrin drops and spray Bayfrin, Duration	2–3 (morning and evening)	Same as for adults	Not recommended (refer to 0.025%)	Long duration of action
0.025%	—	—	—	2–3 (morning and evening)	
Phenylephrine hydrochloride, 0.5%	NeoSynephrine drops	2–3 (≥4 h)	Not recommended (refer to 0.25%)	Not recommended (refer to 0.125%)	Also available as 1% solution and 0.5% jelly
0.025%	Nasal spray, in 0.25% and 0.5% only	Same as 0.5%	2–3 (≥4 h)	Not recommended (refer to 0.125%)	
0.125%	—	—	—	2–3 drops (≥4 h)	
Xylometazoline hydrochloride, 0.1%	Otrivin drops and spray	2–3 (8–10 h)	Not recommended (refer to 0.05%)	Not recommended (refer to 0.05%)	Long duration of action
0.05%	—	—	2–3 (8–10 h)	2–3 (8–10 h)	

*The FDA advisory review panel on cold, cough, allergy, bronchodilator, and antiasthmatic products has recommended these ingredients as safe and effective (category I) at the dosages specified. Only drops should be used in children 2 to <6 years, since the spray is difficult to use in the small nostril. These products should not be used in patients with chronic rhinitis because of the risk of rhinitis medicamentosa.

†For children under 6 there is no recommended dosage of ephedrine, naphazoline, or oxymetazoline except under the advice and supervision of a physician.

Source: Adapted from The American Pharmaceutical Association: *Handbook of Nonprescription Drugs*, 7th ed., Washington, DC: The American Pharmaceutical Association, 1982.

rine but more active as a vasoconstrictor and less active as a bronchodilator and CNS stimulant. The oral dose is 25 to 50 mg tid. Its peak action occurs in 3 h.

Phenylephrine is a frequent ingredient in combination cough and cold products. Unfortunately, it has poor bioavailability, and its efficacy is questionable.

Use of systemic nasal decongestants, with or without antihistamines, for the treatment of middle ear infection and/or effusion is controversial. Since nasal congestion frequently accompanies this condition, systemic decongestants are frequently utilized in an attempt to reduce eustachian tube congestion and to facilitate drainage. Little objective evidence is available to support any benefit from reduced symptomalogy or shorter recovery, however.

Patient Education Administering topical decongestants properly is essential to promote drug effectiveness and to prevent the negative effects caused by systemic absorption of the drug. The patient should be instructed that rebound congestion, which may occur if the patient uses the drug too often or too much, be explained. Rebound congestion becomes part of a vicious cycle as it leads to more frequent use of the agent that causes it.

Nasal sprays are designed so that one squeeze of the plastic container delivers the required dose. The nasal spray is administered with the patient in the upright position by squeezing once into each nostril and waiting 3 to 5 min before blowing the nose. A second dose may be administered if necessary to clear congestion.

To administer nasal drops, the patient should be supine and should remain in that position for approximately 5 min after the drug is administered. To ensure more uniform absorption of the medication, the head may be turned from side to side while the patient is reclining. After topical application, patients may experience discomfort such as burning, sneezing, and dryness. Nasal sprays are probably more convenient for adults and older children while nasal drops are more effective for children under 6 years of age.

Topical solutions can quickly become contaminated with use and may serve as reservoirs of bacterial and fungal infections. To minimize contamination, it is essential that no more than one person use the same dropper or spray.

In addition to using topical solutions, the patient may find it helpful to apply heat to frontal and maxillary sinus areas. This encourages drainage and relieves pain and pressure. Patients with hypertension, hyperthyroidism, diabetes mellitus or ischemic heart disease should use oral decongestants with caution, if at all. Also, sympathomimetic amines are contraindicated in patients receiving monoamine oxidase inhibitors. These adverse interactions are not likely to occur with topically applied agents.

Intranasal Corticosteroids

In severe cases refractory to other drug therapy, it may be necessary to add a corticosteroid nasal spray such as dexa-methasone (Decadron Turbinaire), beclomethasone (Beconase or Vancenase), or Flunisolide (Nasalide).

Mechanism of Action The mode of action of these agents in treating nasal congestion remains unknown, but a reduction of histamine-containing cells in the epithelium and decreased release of leukotrienes is thought to be of importance. These agents have potent glucocorticoid activity with weak mineralcorticoid activity. The topical administration of these agents produces anti-inflammatory and vasoconstrictor effects.

Pharmacokinetics When administered intranasally, these agents are readily absorbed. It is not known whether the absorption site is the gastrointestinal tract, the nasal membranes, the respiratory tract, or a combination of all three sites. The distribution and elimination characteristics of these agents following intranasal administration have not been well described.

Adverse Effects Sneezing, burning, and nasal irritation are all common adverse effects of intranasal corticosteroids and usually decrease over time. These adverse effects on the nasal membranes may be due to irritation from the propellant. If local adverse effects are severe, it may be necessary to switch to a different intranasal corticosteroid. These agents may also cause nasal dryness, nasal bleeding with hemorrhagic crusting, and nasal mucosal ulcerations.

The overgrowth of the yeast *Candida albicans,* which is common when the drugs are inhaled into the lungs, occurs much less frequently when the drugs are administered intranasally. Adrenal suppression usually does not occur when these drugs are employed in the recommended doses. However, adrenal suppression can occur when larger doses are employed and when these agents are used in conjunction with other corticosteroids.

Dosage When used to treat nasal congestion the inhaled dose of beclomethasone diproprionate (Vancenase, Beconase) is 1 or 2 sprays (42 to 84 μg) three to four times daily. Flunisolide (Nasalide) yields 25 μg per metered spray, and dexamethasone sodium phosphate (Decadron Turbinaire) delivers 100 μg per metered spray. The usual dosage of both of these agents is two sprays in each nostril two or three times daily.

Patient Education Patient education is extremely important for optimal therapeutic effect of topical corticosteroids. Compliance may be facilitated by emphasizing that improvement does not occur immediately and will require continuous therapy. Since sprays are ineffective during periods of severe obstruction, patients should be instructed to administer these agents only in a patent (open) nostril, even if it necessitates postponing a dose for several hours. It is also important, particularly with pressurized aerosols, to point the nozzle straight backward and avoid pointing it directly at the nasal septum. This is helpful in preventing the anterior nasal dryness and hemorrhagic crusting mentioned previously.

Cromolyn Sodium

Cromolyn sodium (Nasalcrom) is a 4% liquid nasal spray intended for the prevention and treatment of allergic rhinitis. The mechanism of action is thought to be prevention of the antigen-stimulated release of mediators. The nasal solution for most patients is well tolerated although transient nasal stinging, burning or irritation, and sneezing can occur. The cromolyn is delivered through a patient-activated pump which releases 5.2 mg of cromolyn per actuation. Prior to administration of the Nasalcrom, it is recommended that the patient clear the nasal passages with either a decongestant and or with nasal saline washes. The usual dose is one spray in each nostril three to six times a day. Since it has a prophylactic action, it is recommended that the medication be continued even when symptoms are not present.

Cough

The cough reflex, like the sneeze reflex, is a protective mechanism designed to remove inhaled foreign bodies, secretions, and cellular debris from the respiratory tract. Successful operation of the cough reflex results in sputum production and a productive cough. Patients may need to learn that this type of cough is beneficial and should not be suppressed. However, in many cases, the cough can be uncomfortable and unnecessary. A dry, nonproductive cough may further irritate the respiratory tract and perpetuate the cough.

Expectorants

Expectorants are administered orally to increase the flow of respiratory secretions and to aid expectoration. For an expectorant to work properly, there must be normal ciliary function, normal viscosity of mucus, a patent airway, appropriately humidified air, and an intact cough reflex. Failure of any one of these functions will result in ineffective expectoration.

Mechanism of Action Most expectorants are thought to work by thinning hyperviscous mucus. **Ammonium chloride** and **ammonium carbonate** are still common expectorants in many cold preparations. They may function by breaking down complex proteins in sputum and by an osmotic effect, resulting in attraction of water from cells and blood vessels. Confirmation of these effects has been demonstrated in animals using high doses, but human studies have failed to support this effect.

Iodides have long been used for their mucolytic and expectorant effects. A commonly used saturated solution of potassium iodide directly stimulates lacrimal, salivary, and mucous glands. **Terpin hydrate** and **guaifenesin** (glyceryl

guiacolate) also seem to act by a similar mechanism. Guaifenesin is absorbed by the stomach and then taken up by the bronchial glands where it stimulates secretion. Unfortunately, this occurs only with large, almost nauseating doses of the drug. A controlled trial has failed to show any beneficial effects.

Another drug occasionally used in expectorant products is **syrup of ipecac**. As with most agents in this class, effects in animal studies have not been demonstrated in humans. It has been postulated that ipecac aids expectoration by stimulating vagal afferent nerves in the gastric mucosa. This could produce cholinergic stimulation of bronchial glands and an increase in respiratory tract secretion.

Adequate hydration and fluid intake is important since water comprises 95% of tracheobronchial secretions. This, presumably, aids expectoration by thinning hyperviscous sputum and improving mucokinesis. Humidifying inspired air is also frequently employed for this effect. Although cool air vaporizers have been recommended on the premise that they do no harm, recent evidence suggests this may not be true. Disadvantages of aerosol therapy include frequent contamination of the aerosol generator with microorganisms, an increase in airway resistance, and patient discomfort from being damp and chilled.

In summary, using expectorants to aid productive cough is controversial since clinical evidence has not proved their efficacy. The most effective treatment remains simple maintenance of a liberal fluid intake.

Adverse Effects Most expectorants have few adverse effects and are usually limited to gastrointestinal upset. Ammonium chloride may be toxic in large doses and should not be used by patients with renal or hepatic failure or chronic heart disease.

Preparations Many expectorant preparations are marketed as combination products containing antihistamines, antitussives, and other ingredients (see Table 21-7). These are irrational combinations for treating productive cough since antihistamines may dry up respiratory secretions, and antitussives would prevent effective expectoration by inhibiting the cough reflex. Therefore, it is best to use single-entity products. The most frequently used expectorant is **guaifenesin** in doses of 100 mg every 3 or 4 h (see Table 21-5).

Antitussives

Cough suppressants (antitussives) are indicated when the patient presents with a bothersome, dry nonproductive cough. These agents act by either depressing the cough center in the medulla or by suppressing sensory or motor nerve fibers in the respiratory tract. Both narcotic and nonnarcotic drugs are available.

Nonnarcotic Preparations Dextromethorphan is considered by many to be the antitussive of choice because of its safety and efficacy. Gastrointestinal upset and drowsiness are mild infrequent complaints, and it produces no dependency liability or respiratory depression. Antitussive effects of dextromethorphan are comparable to equal doses of codeine although, at upper dosage limits, codeine may have slightly greater activity. Previous hypersensitivity constitutes the only contraindication to its use.

The antihistamine agent **diphenhydramine** is also an FDA-approved nonnarcotic antitussive. Most evidence supports a central mechanism of action, but a possible peripheral effect has also been suggested. Doses of 25 to 50 mg are effective in reducing both the intensity and frequency of pathologic cough due to upper respiratory infection or chronic bronchial disease. Because of its prominent sedative action, diphenhydramine may be more suited for use as a nighttime cough suppressant. (See antihistamines for adverse effects.)

Benzonatate (Tessalon Perles) is a local anesthetic structurally related to procaine. It is believed to act by anesthetizing peripheral stretch receptors in the respiratory tract, thereby suppressing the cough reflex at its source. Release of benzonatate by chewing the perle causes local anesthesia of the oral mucosa, an effect which has been used clinically prior to endoscopic procedures to prevent gagging (and coughing) in addition to cough suppression. Hypersensitiv-ity reactions to **procaine** or related compounds contraindi-cates the use of benzonatate. Side effects are minor and generally involve gastrointestinal complaints. The usual adult dose is 100 mg three times daily.

Narcotic Preparations   Most narcotics (e.g., **morphine** and its congeners) possess antitussive properties. **Codeine** is the most commonly used narcotic antitussive for several reasons. First, it has low dependency liability, and when used in recommended doses for short periods, has no danger of psychologic or physical dependence. Abuse of codeine-containing cough products does occur, however, and chronic use is rarely justified. Second, following oral administration, it is equal in antitussive efficacy to morphine with approximately one-fourth the respiratory depressant effects.

Common adverse effects of codeine are gastrointestinal distress, drowsiness, lightheadedness, and constipation. It may also have a drying effect on respiratory mucosa. Hypersensitivity reactions, usually involving skin rash and pruritus, are not common but are potentially serious. Because of possible cross-sensitivity, patients with a true hypersensitivity reaction to morphine or related congeners should probably not use a codeine-containing antitussive preparation. The adult antitussive dose is 15 to 30 mg administered orally every 4 h as needed.

TABLE 21-5   Expectorants

DRUG*	Dosage (Maximum Dose per 24 h)			
	ADULTS	CHILDREN, 6 TO <12 YEARS	CHILDREN, 2 TO <6 YEARS	COMMENTS
Ammonium chloride	300 mg q2–4h	150 mg q2–4h	75 mg q2–4h	Avoid in renal, hepatic, and cardiac disease
Guaifenesin	200–400 mg q4h (2400 mg)	50–100 mg q4h (600 mg)	50 mg q4h (300 mg)	Available as single-entity product (Robitussin 100 mg/5 mL)
Syrup of ipecac	0.5–1.0 mL (of syrup containing not less than 123 mg and not more than 157 mg of total ether-soluble alkaloids of ipecac per 100 mL) 3 or 4 times per day	0.25–0.5 mL (of syrup containing not less than 123 mg and not more than 157 mg of total ether-soluble alkaloids of ipecac/100 mL) 3 or 4 times per day	Not recommended	
Terpin hydrate	200 mg q4h (1200 mg)	100 mg (of terpin hydrate alone or in a nonalcoholic mixture) q4h	50 mg (of terpin hydrate alone or in a nonalcoholic mixture) q4h (300 mg)	High alcoholic content of elixir precludes use in children under 12

*The FDA advisory review panel on nonprescription cold, cough, allergy, bronchodilator, and antiasthmatic products has concluded that the available data are insufficient to permit classification of these ingredients (category III).

Source: Adapted from The American Pharmaceutical Association: *Handbook of Nonprescription Drugs,* 7th ed., Washington, DC: The American Pharmaceutical Association, 1982.

Preparations Numerous antitussive products are available. As with other preparations, irrational combination of antitussives and other cough and cold ingredients makes rational selection of the appropriate product difficult. **Dextromethorphen** and **diphenhydramine** have the added advantage of being nonprescription products. Antitussive drugs and selected commercial products are listed in Table 21-6.

Patient Education In addition to information about cough suppressants, patients need to know other ways to alleviate the discomfort of an irritating cough. Liberal fluid intake, unless otherwise contraindicated, is essential. Deep breathing exercises, postural drainage, elevating the head of the bed or using several pillows, limiting or cessation of smoking, and maintaining adequate humidity in the environment are helpful in reducing irritation of cough. Hard candy or lozenges, tea with lemon, sips of honey, or carbonated beverages may also provide a soothing effect on pharyngeal mucosa. Diabetics must be cautioned about the sugar content when considering these home remedies and when selecting over-the-counter products. Some sugar-free (SF) products are listed in Table 21-7.

Patients receiving iodides for any length of time should be alerted to stop medication and contact their primary care provider if symptoms of iodism appear. These symptoms include brassy taste, burning sensation in the mouth, sneezing, irritation of the eyes, gastric distress, fever, and (often) severe headache.

Sore Throat (Pharyngitis)

Sore throat is more commonly seen with the common cold than with allergic rhinitis, although with allergic rhinitis continuous mouth breathing may produce pharyngitis. Many other factors may lead to a sore throat, including other diseases ("strep" throat, influenza) or the use of tobacco and alcohol. The symptomatic relief of the soreness may be obtained by using lozenges (see Table 21-8) or mouthwashes. The so-called benefit of these preparations is attributed to the inclusion of antibacterial compounds (phenols, alcohols, quatenary ammonium compounds, volatile oils, oxygenating agents, and iodine-containing products) and local anesthetics (benzocaine, phenol, benzyl alcohol). The problem with antibacterial agents is that since most infections are viral, there is no proof that changing the bacterial flora of the oral cavity will have any therapeutic benefit. The use of the local anesthetics can produce some

TABLE 21-6 Antitussives

DRUG*	SINGLE-ENTITY PRODUCTS	PREPARATIONS AVAILABLE	Dosage (Maximum Dose per 24 h)			COMMENTS
			ADULTS	CHILDREN, 6 TO <12 YEARS	CHILDREN, 2 TO <6 YEARS*	
Codeine	Various	15-, 30-, and 60-mg tablets	10–30 mg q4–6h (120 mg)	5–10 mg q4–6h (60 mg)	2.5–5 mg q4–6h (30 mg)	With antitussive doses, respiratory depression and dependence liability are insignificant in otherwise healthy individuals; avoid in patients with chronic pulmonary disease and history of drug abuse or concurrent use of other CNS depressants.
Dextromethorphan	Pertussin 8-Hour, Romilar Chewable Tablets for Children, Hold	30 mg/20 mL, 7.5 mg/tablet	10–20 mg q4h or 30 mg q6–8h (120 mg)	5–10 mg q4h or 15 mg q6–8h (60 mg)	2.5–5 mg q4h or 7.5 mg q6–8h (30 mg)	Adverse effects are mild and infrequent; available in numerous OTC cough and cold products.
Diphenhydramine hydrochloride	Benylin Cough Syrup	12.5 mg/mL	25 mg q4h (150 mg)	12.5 mg q4h (75 mg)	6.25 mg q4h (37.5 mg)	Sedation and anticholinergic effects prominent; may be useful as nighttime cough suppressant.

*The FDA advisory review panel on nonprescription cold, cough, allergy, bronchodilator, and antiasthmatic products has recommended all these ingredients as safe and effective (category I).

Source: Adapted from The American Pharmaceutical Association: *Handbook of Nonprescription Drugs,* 7th ed., Washington, DC: The American Pharmaceutical Association, 1982.

TABLE 21-7 Selected Antitussive and Expectorant Preparations

BRAND NAME	ANTITUSSIVE	EXPECTORANT	SYMPATHOMIMETIC	ANTIHISTAMINE
Cheracol (3%)*	Codeine phosphate 10 mg/5 mL	Guaifenesin 100 mg/5 mL		
Cheracol D (4.75%)	Dextromethorphan hydrobromide, 9.86 mg/5 mL	Guaifenesin 100 mg/5 mL		
Chlor-Trimeton expectorant (1%)		Ammonium chloride, 100 mg/5 mL Guaifenesin, 50 mg/5 mL	Phenylephrine hydrochloride, 10 mg/5 mL	Chlorpheniramine maleate, 2 mg/5 mL
Coricidin Cough Formula (N/A)†	Dextromethorphan hydrobromide, 10 mg/5mL	Guaifenesin, 50 mg/5 mL	Phenylpropanolamine hydrochloride, 12.5 mg/5 mL	
Dorcol Pediatric (5%)	Dextromethorphan hydrobromide, 5.0 mg/5 mL	Guaifenesin, 50 mg/5 mL	Phenylpropanolamine hydrochloride, 6.25 mg/5 mL	
Dristan (2%)	Dextromethorphan hydrobromide, 7.5 mg/5 mL	Guaifenesin 30 mg/5 mL	Phenylephrine hydrochloride, 5 mg/5 mL	Chlorpheniramine maleate, 1 mg/5 mL
Halls Decongestant Cough Formula (22%)	Dextromethorphan hydrobromide, 15 mg/10 mL		Phenylpropanolamine hydrochloride, 37.5 mg/10 mL	
Histadyl EC (5% SF)‡	Codeine phosphate, 10 mg/5 mL	Ammonium chloride, 110 mg/5 mL	Ephedrine hydrochloride, 5 mg/5 mL	Chlorpheniramine maleate, 2 mg/5 ml
Entex capsules		Guaifenesin, 200 mg	Phenylpropanolamine hydrochloride, 45 mg, and phenylephrine hydrochloride, 5 mg	
Novahistine DMX (5%)	Dextromethorphan hydrobromide, 10 mg/5 mL	Guaifenesin, 100 mg/5 mL	Pseudoephedrine hydrochloride, 30 mg/5 mL	
Novahistine expectorant (7.5%)	Codeine phosphate, 10 mg/5 mL	Guaifenesin, 100 mg/5 mL	Pseudoephedrine hydrochloride, 30 mg/5 mL	
Ornacol capsules and liquid (5%, SF)‡	Dextromethorphan hydrobromide, 30 mg/capsule, 15 mg/5 mL		Phenylpropanolamine hydrochloride, 25 mg per capsule, 12.5 mg/5 mL	
Romilar III (20%)	Dextromethorphan hydrobromide, 5 mg/5 mL		Phenylpropanolamine hydrochloride, 12.5 mg/5 mL	
Triaminic Expectorant (5%)		Guaifenesin, 100 mg/5 mL	Phenylpropanolamine hydrochloride, 12.5 mg/5 mL	
Triaminic expectorant with codeine (5%)	Codeine phosphate, 10 mg/5 mL	Guaifenesin, 100 mg/5 mL	Phenylpropanolamine hydrochloride, 12.5 mg/5 mL	

TABLE 21-7 Selected Antitussive and Expectorant Preparations (*Continued*)

BRAND NAME	ANTITUSSIVE	EXPECTORANT	SYMPATHOMIMETIC	ANTIHISTAMINE
Triaminicol (N/A)	Dextromethorphan hydrobromide, 10 mg/5 mL		Phenylpropanolamine hydrochloride, 12.5 mg/5 mL	Chlorpheniramine maleate, 2.0 mg/ 5 mL
Vicks Cough Syrup (5%)	Dextromethorphan hydrobromide, 3.5 mg/5 mL	Guaifenesin, 25 mg/5 mL		

* % denotes percentage alcohol content.
† N/A denotes nonalcoholic.
‡ SF denotes sugar free preparations.
Source: Adapted from The American Pharmaceutical Association: *Handbook of Nonprescription Drugs,* 7th ed., Washington, DC: The American Pharmaceutical Association, 1982.

comfort due to the fact that it may desensitize the nerve endings. However, in most cases, these agents are present in subtherapeutic concentrations. **Benzocaine** is effective in concentrations of 5% to 20%, **phenol** in 0.5% to 1.5%, and **benzyl alcohol** near 10%. The best judge of the effectiveness of the product is the patient since the placebo effect must not be excluded. Hard candies or cough drops may have a soothing effect on the sore throat and may be just as effective.

EVALUATION

Temporary relief of symptoms or the discomfort they cause is the basis of evaluation. The duration of the relief from symptoms should also be considered. A cold persisting for more than 10 days requires reassessment of the patient for complications or misdiagnosis. If symptoms rapidly recur after medication, a rebound effect (as with the sympathom-

imetic drops) may be taking place, or tolerance (as with antihistamine) may have developed. Drowsiness, excitement, gastrointestinal distress, and other side effects should also be evaluated to ascertain if the benefit of symptomatic relief outweighs the discomfort, inconvenience, or potential dangers posed by the side effects.

SUMMARY

Treatment of the common cold remains largely symptomatic, (see Table 21-9). Antihistamines are frequently incorporated into cold preparations and may reduce nasal rhinorrhea by a weak anticholinergic effect. Effectiveness in preventing or relieving symptoms of the common cold, however, have not been conclusively demonstrated in well-controlled clinical trials. Although considered fairly innocuous drugs, sedation is a common adverse effect which may be hazardous during daytime use. Therefore, the common

TABLE 21-8 Lozenge Products

PRODUCT	ANESTHETIC	ANTIBACTERIAL AGENTS	OTHER INGREDIENTS
Cepacol		Cetylpyridinium chloride 1:1500	Benzyl alcohol 0.3%, sucrose
Cepacol Troches	Benzocaine, 10 mg	Cetylpyridinium chloride 1:1500	Sucrose 1 g
Cherry Chloraseptic		Phenol-sodium phenolate (total phenol, 1.4%); these ingredients are also anesthetic	
Chloraseptic Cough Control		Phenol-sodium phenolate (total phenol, 32.5 mg); these ingredients are also anesthetic	Dextromethorphan hydrobromide, 10 mg
Sucrets		Hexylresorcinol, 2.4 mg	
Vicks Throat Lozenges	Benzocaine, 5 mg	Cetylpyridinium chloride, 1.66 mg	Menthol, camphor, eucalyptus oil

Source: Adapted from the American Pharmaceutical Association: *Handbook of Nonprescription Drugs,* 7th ed. Washington, DC: The American Pharmaceutical Association, 1982.

practice of recommending antihistamines to placate symptomatic patients is not acceptable without first considering the risks involved.

Antihistamine use in allergic rhinitis is considered more rational since histamine is thought to play a more important role in the pathogenesis of symptoms. Treatment must be initiated prior to the onset of the allergy season; this timing allows the patient to gradually develop a tolerance to the sedative effects. Antihistamines effectively prevent or suppress the symptoms of sneezing, rhinorrhea, nasal pruritus, and conjunctivitis, and are considered the treatment of choice for individuals in which elimination of the allergen cannot be accomplished.

Nasal congestion, a frequent complaint in both the common cold and allergic rhinitis, generally responds to systemically administered sympathomimetic agents. Topical preparations are useful in cases of severe congestion but should be used only in recommended doses for a short period of time (3 days or less) to avoid the rebound syndrome of rhinitis medicamentosa. They decrease engorgement and congestion by α-adrenergic vasoconstriction of nasal blood vessels.

TABLE 21-9 Combination Cold and Allergy Products

PRODUCT	DOSAGE FORM	SYMPATHOMIMETIC AGENTS	ANTIHISTAMINE	ANALGESIC	OTHER INGREDIENTS
Alka-Seltzer Plus	Effervescent tablet	Phenylpropanolamine bitartrate, 24.08 mg	Chlorpheniramine maleate, 2.0 mg	Aspirin, 324 mg	
Congesprin Children's Cold Tablets	Tablet	Phenylephrine hydrochloride, 1.25 mg		Acetaminophen, 81 mg	
Chlor-Trimeton Decongestant	Tablet	Pseudoephedrine sulfate 60 mg	Chlorpheniramine maleate, 4 mg		
Contac	Time capsule	Phenylpropanolamine hydrochloride, 75 mg	Chlorpheniramine maleate, 8 mg		
Coricidin	Tablet		Chlorpheniramine maleate, 2 mg	Aspirin, 325 mg	
Coricidin "D"	Tablet	Phenylpropanolamine hydrochloride, 12.5 mg	Chlorpheniramine maleate, 2 mg	Aspirin, 325 mg	
Co Tylenol Cold Formula	Tablet capsule	Pseudoephedrine hydrochloride, 30 mg	Chlorpheniramine maleate, 2 mg	Acetaminophen, 325 mg	Dextromethorphan hydrobromide, 15 mg
Dimetane Decongestant	Tablet/ liquid	Phenylephrine hydrochloride 10 mg (tablet), 1 mg/mL (liquid)	Brompheniramine maleate 4 mg (tablet), 0.4 mg/ mL (liquid)		Alcohol, 2.3% (liquid)
Dristan Advanced Formula	Tablet	Phenylpropanolamine hydrochloride, 12.5 mg	Chlorpheniramine maleate, 2 mg	Acetaminophen, 325 mg	
Novahistine Elixir	Syrup	Phenylephrine hydrochloride, 1.0 mg/mL	Chlorpheniramine maleate, 0.4 mg/mL		Alcohol, 5%
NyQuil	Liquid	Pseudoephedrine hydrochloride, 20 mg/mL	Doxylamine succinate 0.25 mg/ mL	Acetaminophen, 20 mg/mL	Alcohol 25% Dextromethorphan, 0.5 mg/mL
Sine-Aid	Tablet	Pseudoephedrine hydrochloride, 30 mg		Acetaminophen, 325 mg	

Source: Adapted from the American Pharmaceutical Association: *Handbook of Nonprescription Drugs,* 7th ed., Washington, DC: The American Pharmaceutical Association, 1982.

Antitussives work primarily through depression of the medullary cough center and should only be employed for suppression of a dry, nonproductive cough. Dextromethorphan is preferred for cough due to colds because its minimal toxicity affords safe use in children and avoids the more bothersome and potentially serious toxicity of narcotic antitussives.

There is little, if any, conclusive evidence to support the therapeutic benefit of expectorants. Furthermore, the common practice of combining an antitussive and expectorant in cough and cold preparations is irrational since effective expectoration requires an intact cough reflex. Maintenance of a liberal oral fluid intake is probably the treatment of choice.

The use of antibacterial agents like penicillin and tetracycline for the treatment of viral pharyngitis is irrational and should be avoided, even though many patients demand these agents. It must be remembered that much of the public's information—or misinformation—is gained through advertising, and the nurse should try to educate the patient about these symptoms and the value of prudent drug therapy.

CASE STUDY

R.S., a 21-year-old geology student reported to the student health clinic complaining of a runny nose, nasal congestion, and a general feeling of malaise.

Assessment

R.S.'s symptoms had begun 2 days previously with a mild sore throat. He felt feverish at that time, although he had not taken his temperature. The day before, he had developed a clear, watery, profuse nasal discharge. Now this discharge was thick and yellow-green, and he had a dry, hacking cough. R.S. denied ever having had allergies and stated there was no family history of allergies. He denied symptoms of conjunctival itching, lacrimation, photophobia, headache, or earache. Review of systems was noncontributory. The physical exam revealed vital signs: blood pressure 126/84, pulse 80 and regular, respiratory rate 20, temperature 99°F. There was mild conjunctivitis bilaterally. External auditory canals were clear with no bulging or retraction of tympanic membranes. External nares were reddened. Nasal mucosa was erythematous and edematous with mucopurulent nasal discharge. No nasal polyps were present. Pharynx was mildly erythematous without exudate. Sinuses were nontender with palpation. There was no cervical lymphadenopathy. His chest was clear to percussion and auscultation. Remainder of the physical exam was entirely normal. Complete blood count with differential showed only a mild leukocytosis with normal eosinophil count.

After assessing R.S.'s symptoms, physical findings, and laboratory data, the nurse felt he had a common cold as opposed to allergic rhinitis, influenza, or a more serious condition.

Management

The nurse gave R.S. an explanation of the exam. He was told that there is no cure for the common cold, but that symptoms should subside in approximately 7 days. He was told why antibiotics and antihistamines are irrational treatment for the common cold and was advised that the best treatment for him would be aimed at relieving symptoms and promoting his comfort.

The nurse advised R.S. to reduce his activity, get plenty of sleep at night, take a liberal amount of fluids and aspirin or acetaminophen to relieve his myalgia and feeling of feverishness. For the pharyngitis, the nurse recommended that R.S. suck on hard candies or throat lozenges or that he drink tea with lemon or carbonated beverages. Since R.S. gave no history of diabetes, hypertension, cardiac, or thyroid problems and review of these systems was normal, a sympathomimetic amine nasal spray was recommended for the rhinitis and nasal congestion. The nurse gave careful instructions to R.S. for administering these topical decongestants as well as an explanation of how to avoid the phenomenon of rebound congestion.

R.S. was told what symptoms would develop if he had a more serious condition. He was advised to return to the student health clinic if the cold had not resolved in a week or if new symptoms should appear.

Evaluation

R.S. did not return to clinic until a month later when he came for a flu immunization. He said that the cold had lasted five more days and that the symptomatic treatment had kept him "fairly comfortable" for the duration of the cold.

REFERENCES

Boyd, E. M.: "Antitussives, Antiemetics, and Dermatomucosal Agents," in J. R. Dipalma, (ed.), *Drill's Pharmacology in Medicine,* 4th ed., New York: McGraw-Hill, 1971.

Bryant, B. G., and J. F. Cormier: "Cold and Allergy Products," in *Handbook of Nonprescription Drugs,* 7th ed., Washington, DC: American Pharmaceutical Association, 1982.

Capel, L.: "Rhinitis and Its Management," in *Nurs Mirror,* **145:**20–21, 1977.

Coulehan, J. L.: "Ascorbic Acid and the Common Cold—Reviewing the Evidence," *Postgrad Med,* **66:**153–160, 1979.

Douglas, W. W.: "Histamine and 5-Hydroxytryptamine (Serotonin) and Their Antagonists," in A. G. Gilman, L. S. Goodman, and A. Gilman (eds.), *The Pharmacological Basis of Therapeutics,* 6th ed., New York: Macmillan, 1982.

Hendeles, L., M. Weinberger, and L. Wong: "Medical Management of Noninfectious Rhinitis," *Am J Hosp Pharm,* **37:**1496–1504, 1980.

Hirsh, S., P. F. Viernes, and R. C. Kory: "The Expectorant Effect of Glycerol Guaiacolate in Patients with Chronic Bronchitis," *Chest,* **63:**9–14, 1973.

Hoole, A., R. Greenberg, and C. G. Pickard, Jr. (eds.): "Allergic Rhinitis," "Upper Respiratory Infection (Common Cold)," in *Patient Care Guidelines for Nurse Practitioners,* 2d ed., Boston: Little, Brown, 1982.

Howard, Jr., J. C., T. R. Kantner, L. S. Lilienfield, et al.: "Effectiveness of Antihistamines in the Symptomatic Management of the Common Cold," *JAMA,* **242:**2414–2417, 1979.

Hutchinson, R.: "The Common Cold Primer," *Nursing 79,* **9:**57–61, 1979.

Iveson, J.: "Allergies, Silent Suffers," *Nurs Mirror,* **151:**38–39, 1980.

Levy, M. L., G. D. Ericson, and L. K. Pickering: "Infections of the Upper Respiratory Tract," *Med Clin North Am,* **67:**153–171, 1983.

Mygind, N.: "Topical Steroid Treatment for Allergic Rhinitis and Allied Conditions," *Clin Otolaryngol,* **7:**343–352, 1982.

Proctor, D. F., and K. G. Adams: "Physiology and Pharmacology of Nasal Function and Mucus Secretion," *Pharm Ther,* **2:**493–509, 1976.

Roth, F. E., and L. Tabachnick: "Histamine and Antihistamines," in J. R. Dipalma, (ed.), *Drill's Pharmacology in Medicine,* 4th ed., New York: McGraw-Hill, 1971.

Schoaf, L., L. Hendeles, and M. Weinberger: "Suppression of Seasonal Allergic Rhinitis Symptoms with Daily Hydroxyzine," *J Allergy Clin Immunol,* **63:**129–133, 1979.

Schumacher, L.: "Common Cold," *Nursing 82,* **12:**78–79, 1982.

Weiner, N.: "Norepinephrine, Epinephrine, and the Sympathomimetic Amines," in A. G. Gilman, L. S. Goodman, and A. Gilman (eds.), *Goodman and Gilman's The Pharmacological Basis of Therapeutics,* 6th ed., New York: Macmillan, 1980.

West, S., B. Brandon, P. Stolley, et al.: "A Review of Antihistamines and the Common Cold," *Pediatrics* **56:**100–106, 1975.

Zanjanian, M. H.: "Expectorants and Antitussive Agents: Are They Helpful?" *Ann Allergy,* **44:**290–295, 1980.

22

SLEEP DISTURBANCES*

RICHARD J. MARTIN
PATRICIA K. BRANNIN

LEARNING OBJECTIVES

Upon mastery of the contents of this chapter the reader will be able to:

1. Describe the two major categories of sleep.
2. Describe normal sleep in terms of various sleep stages.
3. Describe the differences in normal sleep as a function of age.
4. Outline the behavioral manifestations of insomnia and the indications for spirometric and polysomnographic examination of patients with insomnia.
5. List at least three causes of insomnia.
6. Describe the types of respiratory disorders that can occur during sleep and the possible treatment modalities.
7. Name at least three nondrug therapies for insomnia.
8. List the specific drugs for therapy of five different sleep disorders.
9. Describe the long- and short-term efficacy of various hypnotic agents.
10. Describe the effects of various hypnotic agents on REM sleep.
11. Define REM rebound.
12. List three drug interactions of hypnotic agents.
13. List five pertinent questions about sleep pattern, sleep, and hypnotic medications that can be asked in assessing the patient.
14. Write a teaching plan for patients on hypnotic agents.
15. Name the class of hypnotic drugs which appears to offer the fewest disadvantages in the treatment of insomnia.
16. State the common adverse effects of hypnotic drugs.
17. Identify nursing measures to minimize the adverse effects of hypnotic drugs.
18. Explain why hypnotics should be given on an empty stomach.
19. Describe the evaluation of interventions to improve sleep.

Sleep is a complex condition that is only slightly understood. Approximately one-third of our lives is spent in a state of sleep, the components of which are both passive and active. Sleep is necessary to help prepare the individual for the waking period.

Recent research has brought significant advances to our knowledge of normal sleep and sleep disorders, thereby resulting in improvement in the therapy of sleep disorders. In this chapter, normal sleep, sleep disorders, and their therapies will be discussed, with special emphasis on insomnia and *hypnotic* agents (drugs used to induce sleep).

NORMAL SLEEP

Sleep consists of two categories: rapid eye movement (REM) sleep and nonrapid eye movement (NREM) sleep. NREM sleep is further divided into sleep stages 1, 2, 3, and 4.

Normal sleep consists of sequences of NREM and REM sleep. In normal young adults, there are periods of stage 1 and 2 sleep followed by periods of stages 3 and 4 sleep. After 70 to 100 min of NREM sleep, the first episode of REM sleep occurs. This sequence then repeats itself between four and six times throughout the night at approximately 90-min intervals. The total amount of time spent in REM sleep is approximately 20 to 25 percent of the total sleep time. The length of the REM periods increases as sleep progresses. The adult experiences short periodic episodes of wakefulness. This pattern is largely the same in children, except that there are fewer periods of wakefulness and a longer duration of

*The authors thank John J. Fordice and Debbie Walder, who contributed the chapter on this subject in the first edition.

stages 3 and 4 sleep. In the elderly, there is a decrease in stage 4 sleep (and to some extent stage 3) and an increase in the frequency and duration of wakeful periods, resulting in a marked increase in the total time awake.

The amount of time spent sleeping in a 24-h period varies with age: the infant spends some 20 h/day sleeping; a child, up to 10 or 12 h; and most adults, an average of 7 or 8 h/day. Elderly patients have more fragmented sleep and as a result may spend more time in bed and nap more during the day. Among the elderly, however, there is generally a preference for sleep at night.

Although the exact requirements for the different stages of sleep are not known, it is known that persons who are deprived of sleep in general or of any specific stage of sleep do not feel as well subjectively or perform as well objectively as those who are not sleep-deprived. Those deprived of sleep experience a variety of unpleasant symptoms including fatigue, irritability, and inability to concentrate. Illusions and hallucinations may intrude into consciousness as well. Performance of motor tasks deteriorates, and the incentive to work diminishes. One may see certain neurologic signs such as nystagmus, slight tremor of the hands, ptosis, expressionless face, and difficulty in speaking. Persons deprived of REM sleep show hyperactivity, emotional lability, and impulsive behavior.

Research with subjects undergoing prolonged sleep deprivation indicates that for complete recovery these subjects require more sleep than was lost. Selective deprivation of stage 4 or REM sleep results in an excessive amount of sleep in those stages on the first several nights of undisturbed sleep. General sleep deprivation results in excessive stage 4 sleep during the first night, while the second night is characterized by excessive amounts of REM sleep, or *REM rebound*. These findings have suggested to many investigators that there is a specific need for each stage of sleep, though investigation into this hypothesis has been unrewarding thus far.

After prolonged use of hypnotic drugs (which can result in REM deprivation), REM rebound frequently associated with nightmares, insomnia, and severely disturbed sleep can occur when the drug is stopped. Patients experiencing REM rebound or *rebound insomnia* frequently revert to drug use to suppress the unpleasant symptoms.

SLEEP DISORDERS

Although there is considerable overlap among categories, sleep disorders are classified into four groups.

Insomnia Difficulty initiating and maintaining sleep.

Hypersomnia Excessive somnolence including narcolepsy.

Disorders of the sleep-wake cycle such as jet lag, work shift change, and persistent phase-shift change.

Parasomnias including sleepwalking, night terrors, and enuresis.

Sleep-induced respiratory disorders (sleep apnea syndrome and alveolar hypoventilation syndrome) can cause both insomnia and hypersomnia. Because they respond to pharmacologic intervention and are important to nursing care, insomnia and sleep apnea syndrome will be the focus of this discussion. Less common sleep disorders are outlined in Table 22-1.

Insomnia

Insomnia is the most frequently encountered sleep disorder. It is present in 5 to 10 percent of healthy young adults, in at least 20 percent of patients in general hospitals, and in up to 80 percent or more of psychiatric patients. The prevalence of insomnia increases with age and is higher in women than in men.

Insomnia is present when persons have difficulty falling asleep, when they are unable to sleep as well as they would like, and when this inability to sleep affects their psychologic well-being or their ability to function. The insomnia may manifest itself as inability or difficulty in falling asleep, inability or difficulty staying asleep, or awakening too early in the morning. These variations of insomnia may occur by themselves or in combination.

Care must be taken not to rely only upon the patient's statement that insomnia is present. Sometimes patients who think they have insomnia fall asleep after a normal length of time and have a normal sleep pattern. In addition, the term insomnia is used by patients who really have the *sleep apnea syndrome* and are actually hypersomnolent. The term *insomnia,* unfortunately, is used indiscriminately and should be corroborated by a good history and/or polysomnographic testing (a sleep study).

Causes of Insomnia

Environmental Factors Noise, bright light, unfamiliar surroundings, climatic conditions, and the condition of the bed may play a role in the etiology of insomnia. City dwellers who live on a busy street may be awakened by street noise, but it is actually an unfamiliar sound that awakens people, as they tend to adapt to consistent noise. Sunlight can interfere with sleep, particularly in those who sleep during the day because of nighttime vocational demands. A hospitalized patient is in unfamiliar surroundings and will hear strange noises, both of which may cause temporary sleep problems. Bright lights in an intensive care unit or the hall lights in a hospital ward may also interfere with sleep. The temperature and humidity of the room may affect sleep; even the "best sleepers" may have difficulty sleeping on an extremely warm and humid evening. A mattresss that is too soft or one that has lumps in it may also contribute to difficulties in sleeping.

Drug-Induced Insomnia Ingestion of substances containing CNS-stimulating compounds may also interfere with sleep. Coffee, tea, and cola beverages contain caffeine, which can keep some individuals awake if ingested just prior to sleep (Table 22-2). Drugs such as **methylphenidate** (Ritalin), **dextroamphetamine** (Dexedrine), and analgesic compounds containing **caffeine** (e.g., Anacin, Empirin compounds, etc.) can also prevent people from sleeping. Ingestion of a diuretic at bedtime may interfere with sleep because of the need to urinate during the night. Alcoholic beverages can facilitate falling asleep but may then cause multiple arousals throughout the night.

Physical and Psychiatric Conditions Any medical disorder associated with pain or physical discomfort can produce insomnia. Arthritis, athletic injuries, headache, and other painful or uncomfortable disorders can cause insomnia on a short- or long-term basis. Paroxysmal nocturnal dyspnea in congestive heart failure is also associated with insomnia. In fact, insomnia may be a presenting symptom in congestive heart failure.

Cerebral arteriosclerosis and CNS neoplasia have been associated with insomnia. In addition, thyrotoxicosis, Cushing's syndrome, fever, and normal pregnancy (in the last trimester) have been reported to be associated with insomnia.

It is of considerable importance to remember that respiratory disorders can worsen dramatically during sleep causing the symptom of insomnia. The two most common respiratory diseases that have been most extensively studied are asthma and chronic obstructive pulmonary disease. Patients with these diseases may awaken during the night, due to wheezing, coughing, shortness of breath, hypoxemia, and hypercapnia. Commonly these patients state that they are merely having trouble sleeping unless specific questions are asked or pulmonary function testing is performed during the night. In these patients, the symptom of difficulty in sleeping should not be taken lightly, and further information should be sought as mortality is the highest from midnight to 6 A.M. in these patients.

Psychologic factors are important considerations in the etiology of insomnia. It is thought that "high pressure" living can cause insomnia. Young adults who are poor sleepers

TABLE 22-1 Less Common Sleep Disorders

DISORDER	DESCRIPTION	TREATMENT
Somnambulism (sleepwalking)	Most common in male children with family history; high incidence of enuresis. Episodes vary, usually lasting several minutes, with total amnesia for episodes. Occur during NREM, especially stages 3 and 4. Child and adolescent somnambulists show little evidence of pathology; adults often schizophrenic, neurotic.	Safety measures: Lock doors, remove dangerous objects, provide ground floor room. Children will outgrow the disorder; adults should be referred for psychiatric treatment. Suppressants of stage 4 sleep (diazepam) have shown little efficacy.
Night terrors and nightmares	Night terrors characterized by intense anxiety, autonomic discharge, vocalization, and little recall; occur more frequently in children, usually during stage 3 or 4 sleep. Nightmares are frightening; occur at all ages during REM sleep. Particularly evident during REM rebound after withdrawal of hypnotics. Night terrors and nightmares in children usually transient and situational, but sometimes associated with psychologic disorders.	Children tend to outgrow the disorder; adults should be referred for psychiatric help. Suppressants of stage 4 sleep (diazepam) have been effective in adults.
Narcolepsy	Characterized by irresistible sleep attacks of less than 15 min. Associated with cataplexy (loss of muscle tone) and hallucinations. Frequently occur after meals. Patients awaken refreshed with refractory period of 1–5 h. Disorder usually appears before age 30. Association with psychologic disorders questionable.	Relatives, friends, employers may misinterpret symptoms and so should be told of disorder. Amphetamine or other CNS stimulants effective, but depress REM sleep. Tricyclic antidepressant (imipramine) effective for auxiliary symptoms but not sleep attacks. Patients with narcolepsy not controlled by drugs should avoid driving or operating machinery.

TABLE 22-2 Caffeine Concentration in Common Beverages and in Prescripton and Nonprescription Drugs

BEVERAGE	CAFFEINE, mg/serving
Coffee	
Instant	86–99
Brewed	100–150
Decaffeinated	2–4
Tea	55–80
Cocoa	50
Cola (12 ounces)	35–55

OVER-THE-COUNTER DRUGS	CAFFEINE, mg/tablet
Anacin (aspirin compound)	32
Coricidin	32
Empirin compound	32
Excedrin	65
Cold preparations, average	40
Anorexan*	100
Dexatrim*	200

PRESCRIPTION MEDICATION	CAFFEINE, mg/tablet
A.S.A. & Codeine Compound	32
Cafergot	100
Fiorinal	40

*Federal regulations require the phasing-out of caffeine from diet aids containing phenylpropanolamine. Consumers should read the labels during the transitional period to ascertain caffeine content.

and are without obvious organic or psychiatric disorders have been found to have minor psychologic disorders predisposing them to chronic feelings of inadequacy and tension. The symptom complexes of the major psychiatric illnesses, schizophrenia, depression, and mania include insomnia. The nonspecific psychologic stress or anxiety associated with catastrophic medical illnesses (e.g., cancer) can also cause insomnia.

Sleep Apnea Syndrome

Specific questions related to the *sleep apnea syndrome* (SAS) can help to identify these individuals. The signs and symptoms of SAS can be seen in Table 22-3. The hallmark of SAS is daytime hypersomnolence. This excessive sleepiness can be potentially lethal because of the increased possibility of industrial and automotive accidents. In addition, because of the severe sleep apnea hypoxia that occurs, patients are at a greater risk of developing pulmonary hypertension, heart failure, and erythrocytosis. When the apneic episode is broken, the patient may be aroused or may awaken. In this case the patient will complain of "insomnia."

Three types of apneas can occur. An *upper airway obstruction* occurs when the tongue and other posterior pharyngeal structures lose their muscular tone and occlude the tracheal opening. Respiratory effort is still made, but because of the obstruction there is no airflow. A *central*

apnea occurs when the brain stops sending impulses to the respiratory muscles to initiate airflow, and as a result no effort is made to breathe. A *mixed apnea* is a combination of a central apnea and an upper airway obstruction; i.e., during an episode there is a lack of respiratory effort followed by increasing attempts.

Alveolar hypoventilation syndrome occurs when airflow continues but at a consistently reduced rate. This sleep-induced respiratory disorder clinically presents exactly the same as the sleep apnea syndrome.

ASSESSMENT

Each patient has unique sleep patterns and habits which can be identified by questioning the patient or a family member. A sleep assessment should include the following questions:

How long do you sleep?

What is your usual bedtime and arising time?

What is your routine at bedtime or awakening (e.g., bath, beverages, activities)?

What is your normal sleep environment?

Do you take naps during the day? If so, what is the number and length of the naps?

Do you have values and beliefs related to sleep needs?

Do you have a sleep problem?

If the patient admits to a sleep problem, the following information should be obtained.

How long has the problem existed?

Does this problem occur every night?

Is the problem initiating sleep, staying asleep, or awakening early?

TABLE 22-3 Sleep Apnea Syndrome

Daytime hypersomnolence
Restless sleep ("insomnia")
Loud snoring
Sexual impotency
Intellectual and personality changes
Morning headaches
Systemic hypertension
Pulmonary hypertension
Right heart failure
Congestive heart failure
Erythrocytosis
Nocturnal (apnea) arrythmias

Can you associate a cause with your sleep problem?

Does your sleep problem interfere with your job or daily routine?

Do you drink alcohol or caffeine beverages such as coffee, tea, or cola? (Table 22-2). How much? What time of day do you drink them?

Are you taking sleeping tablets, tranquilizers, or any other medications? If so, what do you take, and when and how often do you take them? Have you brought any of these products to the hospital with you?

The patient's subjective statement is the primary source of information for identification of a sleep disturbance, although behavioral manifestations such as irritability, difficulty in concentrating, episodes of disorientation and misperception, and feelings of persecution may be cues that indicate a need to assess for sleep problems. In some settings, such as intensive care, sleep deprivation is almost inevitable. Whenever the patient must be awakened frequently, the risk of stage 4 and REM deprivation is increased. Identification of environmental, organic, and emotional factors that contribute to sleep disturbances is the basic purpose of assessment in the hospitalized or ambulatory patient.

When pulmonary disease is present, questions may be asked about the patient's breathing status during the night and if respiratory treatments are taken. Simple bedside spirometry (forced vital capacity and forced expiratory volume in one second) both at bedtime and when an awakening occurs may be beneficial in documenting the decrement in lung function. A check of arterial blood gas may be helpful to document any severe hypoxemia or hypercapnia that develops.

If any of the symptoms or signs that are listed in Table 22-3 are present, then a polysomnographic evaluation is necessary to document which type of apnea or if hypoventilation is present and to what degree. Observation by the nursing staff is beneficial in determining whether irregular breathing occurs; however, a formal study is always necessary for specific diagnosis.

MANAGEMENT

The treatment of insomnia should start with the alleviation of environmental, psychiatric, or medical problems which may contribute to the difficulty in sleeping. For insomnia patients who have serious problems not aided significantly by modifying the environment or treating organic and psychiatric conditions, hypnotic drugs should be considered for symptomatic relief.

If the patient has brought sleep medication to the hospital, such medications should be sent home or kept in the pharmacy until discharge. If the patient has taken prescribed hypotics at home, the physician should be informed, since abrupt withdrawal can cause adverse effects of REM rebound and/or withdrawal symptoms.

Nonpharmacologic Management

There are several nonpharmacologic measures that can be taken to help relieve insomnia which are preferable to drug therapy. The patient should arise at a specific early hour each morning regardless of the previous night's sleep, minimize naps during the day, and avoid caffeine-containing beverages and nonprescription stimulant and cold preparations.

The patient should avoid heavy meals for several hours before bedtime and should perform light exercise such as a leisurely swim or walk before bedtime. Strenuous exercise should be avoided before bedtime. Patients should schedule a specific time for going to bed and learn to relax by participating in activities such as taking a warm bath, reading, watching TV, or listening to restful music. Environmental factors which might disturb sleep such as noise, light, temperature, an uncomfortable mattress, or poor ventilation should be minimized. Some patients find that drinking milk beverages at bedtime aid in sleeping.

Eliminating unnecessary noise (e.g., loud talking or laughing by hospital staff and banging of equipment) and reducing the number of times sleep is interrupted to give medications or perform treatments will help minimize the hospitalized patient's sleep difficulties and improve the quality of sleep. Hospitalization causes a transient insomnia which can be treated appropriately with short-term use of hypnotics at bedtime. The hospitalized patient should be able to expect a darkened, tidy, well-ventilated sleep environment that is kept at a comfortable temperature and free from noxious noises and odors.

Psychiatric problems associated with sleep disorders should be adequately diagnosed and treated in an attempt to alleviate sleeping problems. Although insomnia patients are frequently emotionally disturbed, they rarely seek or are referred for psychiatric treatment. Insomnia patients tend to reject the possibility of psychopathology as the root of their sleep problems and instead focus on somatic problems. The prognosis of this group of patients can be greatly improved if they are referred for psychiatric treatment.

While it is helpful to follow the patient's normal bedtime routine as closely as possible during hospitalization, some changes undoubtedly will be necessary. The nurse can discuss with the patient these deviations from the usual routine and can help to plan alternatives. As anxiety over insomnia can aggravate the problem, the patient should be assured that these symptoms are not unusual when there is change in the environment and that they usually disappear in a few days.

Anxiety may cause many sleep disturbances in the hospital. The hospital is an unknown to most people, and the hospitalized patient, who is often apprehensive about test results and procedures, looks back at night on a day of mysterious experiences. The opportunity to ask questions (and getting adequate answers) and an accepting atmosphere for expressing fear and anxiety are vital to a patient's comfort and rest.

Treating the Medical Causes of Insomnia

Insomnia resulting from painful medical conditions can be treated by relieving the pain that interferes with sleep. Non-pain-producing medical conditions, such as congestive heart failure, thyrotoxicosis, and Cushing's syndrome, should be treated appropriately. "Insomnia" caused by respiratory problems is not only more difficult to treat but if not diagnosed correctly and treated appropriately may result in significant morbidity and/or mortality. In patients who have asthma or chronic obstructive pulmonary disease with nocturnal symptoms, several modalities must be checked and treated. Therapeutic levels of bronchodilator (long-acting theophylline and inhaled β-agonist at bedtime) must be present throughout the night. At times a postural drainage treatment can be beneficial in patients who have copious secretions. If noctural hypoxia is present, oxygen should be used. Also common in this group of patients is gastroesophageal reflux which not only gives "heart burn" but can worsen pulmonary function. **Cimetidine** and/or **antacids** at bedtime and elevation of the head of the bed by blocks will help overcome this problem.

The sleep apnea syndrome (SAS) can be treated in several ways. Central apneas and hypoventilation respond to respiratory stimulants (these are not total body stimulants) such as the carbonic anhydrase inhibitors (**dichlorphenamide** and **acetazolamide**; see Chaps. 27 and 39), **progesterone**, or supplemental low-flow oxygen can be instituted. Upper airway obstruction and mixed apneas are always improved by tracheostomy, but unless life-threatening arrhythmias during sleep are present, nonsurgical procedures are undertaken first. **Protriptyline**, a tricyclic antidepressant, alleviates upper airway obstruction, and though its mechanism of action is unknown at this time it is successful in about 20 percent of the patients. About 80 percent of these patients with SAS are grossly obese, and weight loss can also be beneficial, though it is extremely difficult for these patients to lose weight and keep it off. Unfortunately, some patients have lost as much as 150 lb (70 kg) with no improvement in their condition. Supplemental oxygen has also been shown to be beneficial in a subset of obstructive apnea patients. A new method for treatment is to give continuous positive airway pressure (CPAP) through the nose, thereby producing a "pneumatic splint" in the oropharynx and maintaining a patent airway.

Pharmacologic Management— Hypnotic Agents

Hypnotic agents (see Table 22-4) frequently alleviate insomnia. It is important to recognize that hypnotic doses of the majority of these agents interfere in varying degrees with REM sleep. The difference between sedatives and hypnotics is the dose. The rationale for prescribing hypnotic agents for a particular patient should be based upon the following considerations:

1. Degree of insomnia.
2. Type of work.

3. History of pulmonary insufficiency.
4. Suicidal tendencies.
5. History of drug or substance abuse.
6. Age.
7. Associated illness.
8. History of noncompliance with medications.
9. Anticipated length of therapy.

Lastly, the withdrawal of the majority of hypnotic drugs may result in restlessness or abnormal sleep.

Therapeutic Objective

The objective of the hypnotic agent is to induce and maintain sleep, making it as much like natural sleep as possible. The patient should awaken in the morning with no residual effects from the hypnotic agent. It is therefore preferable that the hypnotic agent be rapidly absorbed after oral administration and then rapidly eliminated.

Efficacy

The majority of individuals with insomnia do not require long-term treatment. Carefully monitored therapy of short duration appears to be associated with minimal hazards. When a hypnotic agent is introduced into the therapeutic regimen, a schedule to attempt to discontinue the drug periodically should be developed to assess the necessity of and/or efficacy of treatment.

Most hypnotics have been proved to be effective in inducing and maintaining sleep when used for short periods of time. When used in adequate doses and only occasionally, these drugs consistently reduce the time of onset of sleep, prolong the duration of sleep, and reduce the number of nocturnal wakings. With the exception of morning hangover (which most hypnotic drugs produce), the patient usually awakens feeling well-rested and refreshed.

Adverse Effects

All hypnotic drugs may produce *morning hangover*, residual drowsiness or heavy-headedness after a bedtime dose. Up to 15 percent of hospitalized patients who have taken a hypnotic drug complain of hangover. Patients who do not experience hangover may experience impairment of reaction time, incoordination, impaired motor function, or diminished intellectual performance the day after taking a sleeping pill.

Virtually all of these hypnotic drugs are subject to *abuse*. Many of them are widely abused (e.g., **barbiturates**, **glutethimide**, and **methaqualone**), and all these drugs are capable of producing dependence in persons using them. **Chloral hydrate** and related compounds are less frequently abused, and they are less likely to be implicated in cases of intentional overdose than are other agents. **Flurazepam** and the other benzodiazapines appear to be the least hazardous hypnotic drugs available in terms of abuse and dependence potential.

It appears that all hypnotic agents have the potential to suppress REM sleep, depending upon the dose, but the usual therapeutic doses of flurazepam and chloral hydrate do not suppress REM sleep. Therapeutic doses of **barbiturates, glutethimide**, and **methyprylon** all suppress REM sleep.

Drug Interactions Clinically significant drug interactions with hypnotic agents are mediated by three mechanisms; enzyme induction, protein-binding displacement, and potentiating CNS-depressant effects.

Barbiturates and **glutethimide** cause clinically significant stimulation of drug-metabolizing hepatic microsomal enzymes. The pharmacologic activity of other drugs which are metabolized by this enzyme system is thus diminished when barbiturates or glutethimide are coadministered. This interaction has been well documented with oral anticoagulants. The dose of the oral anticoagulant would have to be raised in a person who is started on a barbiturate or glutethimide regimen. The greatest danger, however, is when a patient is left on the anticoagulant but the barbiturate is discontinued: excessive bleeding may occur. Enzyme induction with **methaqualone** and **ethchlorvynol** has been suggested in some reports. **Flurazepam** does not cause clinically significant enzyme induction.

Chloral hydrate is metabolized to trichloroethanol and then to trichloroacetic acid (TCA). Since TCA is strongly protein-bound, it can displace other drugs from protein-binding sites. This results in a transient increase in the free, unbound, pharmacologically active drug in the serum and consequently causes an increase in the action of the drug. Thus, when the anticoagulant warfarin is used, the addition of chloral hydrate could cause potential bleeding problems. However, since TCA also induces microsomal enzymes, it may neutralize the protein displacement effect. The concurrent use of **chloral hydrate** and **warfarin** should be avoided. Other drugs that are highly protein-bound and could potentially interact with chloral hydrate and related compounds are **phenytoin** (Dilantin), **phenylbutazone** (Butazolidin), and **imipramine** (Tofranil); however, to date no clinically significant interactions have been reported. The other hypnotic drugs do not cause protein-binding displacement.

All hypnotics are CNS depressants and can potentiate the effects of any other CNS depressant, including narcotics, antipsychotic agents, antidepressants, anticonvulsants, antihistamines, and alcohol. Deaths have resulted from the combined use of barbiturates and alcohol. In addition, alcohol induces the action of the hepatic enzymes and enhances the metabolism of drugs, including other hypnotics. These agents potentiate apneas during sleep and are contraindicated in these patients.

Drug Administration Nurses should generally avoid simultaneous administration of hypnotics and other CNS depressants (i.e., narcotics, sedatives, anxiolytics, "tranquilizers," antipsychotics). For example, if the patient has orders for **diazepam** (Valium), 5 mg qid, and **flurazepam** (Dalmane), 30 mg at bedtime, doses of both medications would probably be scheduled for 9 P.M. (depending on hospital routine). The patient who is also having pain could also receive a narcotic analgesic, such as **meperidine** (Demerol), 75 mg IM, at nearly the same time, and CNS depression could result, especially in an elderly patient.

It would be unsound to make a rule that two CNS depressants should never be given simultaneously, but usually they should be given *only* if there are definite indications, based upon thorough assessment of the patient. For example, if on the previous night the patient had received pain medication at 8 P.M., a hypnotic at 9:30 P.M., pain medication again at 11 P.M., a repeat dose of the hypnotic drug at 1:30 A.M., and pain medication again at 4 A.M., and if the patient had obviously slept poorly and shown no signs of CNS depression or impaired liver or renal function, the simultaneous administration of the hypnotic and narcotic analgesic could be indicated to ensure a better night's sleep that next night.

Another decision the nurse must often make when there is a "may repeat" order is whether to readminister the hypnotic dose later in the night when the patient awakens. Generally, nonpharmacologic measures such as positioning, listening to the patient, straightening the bed, a warm noncaffeine drink, offering the bedpan or assistance to the bathroom, or giving a back rub will allow the patient to return to sleep. The nurse should express confidence, verbally and nonverbally, that the patient will get back to sleep without further medication. If these measures are not effective, the hypnotic should be administered only when its effect will be diminished by morning, as indicated by the onset, peak, and half-life of the drug's activity. Consideration should be given to other drug therapy or activities scheduled for the next morning (such as a preprocedural medication containing a CNS depressant ordered for 7 A.M.). Only if the benefits demonstrably outweigh the risks should a lactating mother receive a hypnotic, even if she is not to nurse the chld during that night. When a patient is scheduled for surgery the next day, specific approval of the anesthesiologist is necessary before administering a hypnotic.

Benzodiazepines

All benzodiazepines can be used as sedative-hypnotic agents. The benzodiazepine with the fastest onset of action and the shortest duration of effect is the hypnotic agent of choice.

Mechanism of Action Benzodiazepines are well known for their ability to suppress anxiety and produce sedation and sleep. In addition, they decrease the discomfort secondary to muscle spasms, control seizures, and counteract spasticity.

There are both peripheral and CNS benzodiazepine-binding sites (receptor sites). The greatest number of these receptor sites is in the central nervous system. The affinity of a specific benzodiazepine for such receptor sites approximately corresponds to its pharmacologic potency. The binding process is the initial step which leads to the reported net effect of benzodiazepines to augment the inhibitory properties of the neurotransmitter γ-aminobutyric acid (GABA).

Pharmacokinetics The pharmacokinetic properties of the benzodiazpines can best be appreciated by the range of elimination half-life and pathway of metabolism. This group of hypnotic agents is metabolized by the liver via one of two pathways—oxidation or conjugation. The majority of benzodiazapines are biotransformed by oxidation, which is mediated by hepatic microsomal enzymes. The other metabolic pathway is conjugation, which results in the direct conjugation of benzodiazepines to glucuronic acid, producing water-soluble glucuronide metabolites that are excreted in the urine. It should be noted that although oxidation is the common metabolic pathway, it is influenced by many factors such as normal aging, cirrhosis, and simultaneous administration of other pharmacologic agents which are enzyme inhibitors (i.e., **cimetidine, alcohol**, and **isoniazid**).

Preparations In reality, any of the benzodiazepine derivatives may be prescribed for the treatment of insomnia. Selection of a specific benzodiazepine will depend upon the age, condition, and tolerance of the patient and drug availability. The most common problem with insomnia is the inability to fall asleep. Therefore, the absorption rate of the benzodiazepine is a critical issue. The three available hypnotics specifically for insomnia are **flurazepam** (most rapidly absorbed), **triazolam** and **lorazepam** (intermediate absorption rates), and **temazepam** (slower absorption rate). **Lorazepam** (Ativan) is also indicated as an anxiety agent and is discussed in Chap. 34.

Flurazepam hydrochloride (Dalmane) Flurazepam is both pharmacologically and chemically similar to the other benzodiazepines. It significantly decreases sleep-induction time, the numbers of awakenings, and the time spent awake, and it subsequently increases the duration of sleep.

Flurazepam is the most rapidly absorbed benzodiazepine. Adequate hypnotic effects begin an average of 17 min after oral administration and last from 4 to 8 h. Effectiveness of the drug is reportedly maintained up to 4 weeks (if taken daily). The elimination half-life is long, averaging 74 to 160 h. As a result of this slow elimination, the drug may be given every other day, and the probability of rebound insomnia is minimal.

Accumulation of the metabolites may result in drowsiness and impairment of daytime functioning. Vertigo and ataxia may occur. Paradoxical reactions such as nervousness, irritability, and euphoria have also been reported. Like other hypnotic agents, it may result in drug dependence.

Triazolam (Halcion) Triazolam has the shortest half-life of the hypnotic benzodiazepines (2.5 h), which makes it well suited for sedative-hypnotic therapy. It produces the CNS depression typical of benzodiazepines, presumably by interaction with benzodiazepine receptors at the neurotransmitter γ-aminobutyric acid (GABA) synapses. Both sleep induction and noctural awakening time are decreased. Neither rebound insomnia upon abrupt withdrawal nor drug tolerance has been reported.

Triazolam is rapidly and completely absorbed after oral administration, which results in a rapid onset of action. The time elapsed to peak concentration is about 1.25 h. Because this agent is metabolized to pharmacologically inactive metabolites with short elimination half-lives, CNS depression is of short duration. Recommended dosage for the geriatric or debilitated population is decreased from the usual average dosage by 50 percent until the individual response is determined.

Triazolam adverse effects are similar to all currently available benzodiazepines, with the dose-dependent production of ataxia, euphoria, fatigue, lack of coordination, and drowsiness. However, recommended dosages reportedly produce only slight residual effects the following morning.

Temazepam (Restoril) Temazepam is a metabolic derivative of the benzodiazepine diazepam. It is metabolized by conjugation, so old age or coadministration with enzyme inhibitors such as **cimetidine** is minimally significant. This agent appears not to affect the induction of sleep but rather decreases the frequency of awakening with resultant prolonged total duration of sleep.

Absorption of temazepam is relatively slow, producing peak plasma concentrations within 2.5 h after administration. The elimination half-life is approximately 9 to 12 h.

Side effects have reportedly consisted of gastrointestinal distress, hangover, headache, morning drowsiness, unpleasant dreams or nightmares, vertigo, depression, and confusion. Doses of 40 mg or more could produce respiratory distress. With doses of 15 mg, daytime skills should not be impaired—except in some elderly patients.

Barbiturates

Mechanism of Action Barbiturates have been used extensively as hypnotics, sedatives, and anticonvulsants, but the introduction of newer agents has diminished their use as hypnotics and sedatives. The newer agents, in particular the **benzodiazepines**, have fewer adverse effects, including a lower potential for causing suicide and somewhat lower incidence of physical dependence.

Barbiturates are nonspecific CNS depressants. They are similar to the benzodiazepines in that they facilitate neurotransmission in the central nervous system, but their sites of action are less selective. In normal hypnotic doses they induce sleep, while in lower doses they induce sedation and have been used as a daytime sedative.

Pharmacokinetics The barbiturates are well absorbed with both oral and intramuscular administration. Onset of action is correlated directly with duration of action, which in turn is primarily dependent upon drug distribution. Distribution is indirectly related to brain and plasma binding as well as lipid solubility. The elimination half-life is relatively long, (from 25 h for **amobarbital** to 79 h for **phenobarbital** and 100 h for **butabarbital**), and morning hangover is a frequent complaint. Most barbiturates are metabolized in the liver, and in the presence of liver disease their excretion will be delayed, producing an excessive hypnotic effect. It appears there is a normal elimination pattern even in the presence of renal failure (with the exception of **amobarbitol**). Barbiturates are rapidly and extensively distributed to all body tissues. They pass the placental barrier and can depress the neonatal respiration and central nervous system. These agents appear in breast milk, but in insignificant amounts.

Adverse Effects   Morning "hangover" is a frequent occurrence. Lethargy and drowsiness in individuals who are sensitive (i.e., those with severe liver disease and the elderly) is common. Symptoms of organic brain disorders may develop, especially in the elderly. The opposite effect of sedation may occur with the development of excitement. Significant respiratory depression may occur in patients with pulmonary insufficiency. It is of utmost importance to be cognizant of the fact that barbiturates continue to be one of the major causes of fatal drug poisoning.

Preparations   Barbiturates are marketed in a wide variety of preparations and are available in various dosage forms (see Table 22-4).

Miscellaneous Hypnotic Agents

Chloral Hydrate   Chloral hydrate is one of the oldest hypnotic agents, although it is not used as frequently as it once was. Its clinical effects are due to its metabolite, trichlorethanol, although chloral hydrate does have some hypnotic effect itself. Chloral hydrate has a rapid onset of action accompanied by a short half-life following a rapid absorption and conversion in the liver to trichlorethanol and ultimately to trichloroacetic acid. Because of the rapid onset of action and short half-life, the drug is especially useful in patients who have difficulty falling asleep. In comparison to the benzodiazepine the benefit-risk ratio is probably not as good. However, it may be the agent of choice among the nonbenzodiazepine hypnotics.

Chloral hydrate has an unpleasant taste; it is irritating and may produce nausea, vomiting, flatulence, and epigastric distress. Central nervous system effects include lightheadedness, malaise, ataxia, and nightmares. Allergic reactions have also been reported. Chloral hydrate should not be

TABLE 22-4   Hypnotic Drugs

GENERIC NAME	TRADE NAME	DOSAGE RANGE, mg (hs)	ADVERSE EFFECTS
Benzodiazepines			
Flurazepam	Dalmane	15–30	Drowsiness, confusion, ataxia, hangover, hypotension, tolerance, physical dependence, blood dyscrasias, jaundice
Triazolam	Halcion	0.125–0.5	Drowsiness, headache, dizziness, nervousness, lightheadedness, coordination disorders, and ataxia
Temazepam	Restoril	15–30	Drowsiness, dizziness, lethargy, confusion, euphoria
Lorazepam	Ativan	2–4	Drowsiness, lethargy, confusion, dizziness
Barbiturates			
Pentobarbital	Nembutal	100–200	Hangover, ataxia, gastric irritation, tolerance, physical dependence, rashes, respiratory depression, hypotension
Secobarbital	Seconal	100–200	
Amobarbital	Amytal	50–200	
Phenobarbital	Luminal	100–200	
Butabarbital	Butisol	100	
Secobarbital/amobarbital	Tuinal	50–100	
Chloral Hydrate and Derivatives			
Chloral hydrate	Noctec, Somnos	500–1500	Hangover, ataxia, gastric irritation, tolerance, physical dependence, excitement
Triclofos sodium	Triclos	750–1500	
Miscellaneous			
Glutethimide	Doriden	500–1000	Rashes, hangover, ataxia, tolerance, physical dependence, exfoliative dermatitis, hypotension, paradoxic excitement
Methyprylon	Noludar	200–400	Hangover, dizziness, ataxia, hypotension, tolerance, physical dependence, GI disturbances, paradoxic excitement, rashes, blood dyscrasias
Ethchlorvynol	Placidyl	500–750	Hangover, ataxia, hypotension, vomiting, blurred vision, urticaria, paradoxic excitement, tolerance, physical dependence, toxic amblyopia, prolonged hypnosis

given to patients with hepatic, renal, or severe cardiac disease.

Chloral hydrate (Noctec) is available in soft capsules. It is best taken with a full glass of water or milk to prevent gastric irritation. It can also be administered rectally as a retention enema (in olive oil) or as a suppository (Aquachlor), but rectal absorption is erratic. The preparation **triclofos** (Triclos) contains chloral hydrate in the form of a prodrug which then releases the chloral hydrate.

Paraldehyde Paraldehyde is a rapidly acting (10 to 15 min) hypnotic agent. It has often been used to treat the tremulousness associated with alcohol withdrawal. Paraldehyde has a burning, disagreeable taste, a pungent odor, and an irritating effect on the mucous membranes, making its use during nausea, vomiting, or gastritis undesirable. The drug is 70 to 80 percent metabolized by the liver, and 11 to 28 percent is excreted via the lungs. It should not be given in the presence of liver disease but may be given in the presence of renal disease.

It is administered orally in doses of 5 to 10 mL or rectally as a retention enema. Orally it is given over crushed ice or with orange juice or milk to help mask the taste and decrease gastric irritation. A fresh preparation of paraldehyde must be used and the old preparation should be discarded after it has been open for 24 h. The solution should be discarded if it is not clear or if it smells like acetic acid (vinegar). When administered rectally, it is given in a concentration of one part drug to two parts oil. Intramuscular injection of paraldehyde can be hazardous owing to local tissue irritation, nerve damage, and possible circulatory collapse.

Carbamates **Ethinamate** (Valmid) has a rapid onset of action and a short duration. Its effect on REM sleep is unknown, and it is inactivated by the liver. Adverse effects include nausea and vomiting and, infrequently, rash. The hypnotic dose is 0.5 to 1 g at bedtime. It offers no advantage over the other hypnotics.

Bromides Bromides were once used to produce sedation, as anticonvulsants and, to some extent, as hypnotics. They have a low therapeutic index and therefore should not be used clinically as hypnotics. **Acetylcarbromal** (Paxarel, Sedamyl) is the only agent of this type currently marketed.

Meprobamate (Miltown and Equanil) Meprobamate can be used as a sedative in doses of 400 mg; its hypnotic dose is 800 mg. It offers no advantage over the benzodiazepines. Adverse effects of meprobamate include excessive drowsiness, ataxia, allergic reaction, and (rarely) blood dyscrasias.

Ethchlorvynol (Placidyl) Ethchlorvynol, in addition to its sedative-hypnotic properties, also has anticonvulsant and muscle relaxant properties. Adverse effects include a disagreeable aftertaste, dizziness, nausea and vomiting, hypo-

tension, and facial numbness. It commonly produces morning-after hangover. It may produce an idiosyncratic reaction which causes stimulation and giddiness. Hypnotic doses are 500 mg at bedtime. It offers no advantage over other hypnotic agents.

Glutethimide (Doriden) The action of glutethimide is similar to that of the barbiturates, but it has no real advantage over them. Absorption from the gastrointestinal tract may be erratic. The drug is metabolized in the liver where it is conjugated and then excreted. It is also capable of inducing liver enzymes. Adverse effects can include hangover, excitement, blurred vision, gastrointestinal irritation, and skin rash. It is contraindicated in porphyria. The dose is 500 mg at bedtime.

Tricyclic Antidepressants Tricyclic antidepressants are not primary drugs for the treatment of sleep disorders with the exception of **imipramine** in the treatment of auxiliary symptoms in narcolepsy and **protriptyline** for sleep apnea. Tricyclic antidepressants are indicated for the treatment of depression. Patients who are being treated for depression frequently experience sleep problems and may take advantage of the sedative effects of these drugs by using once-daily, bedtime doses. The sedation produced by these drugs frequently promotes restful sleep and thus may eliminate the need for a hypnotic drug (see Chap. 34, "Psychiatric Disorders").

Over-the-Counter Drugs Over-the-counter (OTC) products are usually a combination of antihistamines (diphenhydramine, doxylamine succinate, or pyrilamine maleate) and may contain analgesic agents (see Table 22-5).

Antihistamines like **diphenhydramine**, **hydroxyzine**, and **promethazine** have secondary pharmacologic properties that cause central nervous system depression; they have been promoted as "safer" hypnotics, although there is no evidence that this claim is true. Furthermore, antihistamines have anticholinergic properties that may cause problems in elderly patients, and they also suppress REM sleep. **Diphenhydramine** (Benadryl, Nytol, Compoz, etc.) is effective and used clinically to induce sleep in doses of 50 to 100 mg at bedtime.

The amino acid L-tryptophan (Tryptacin, Trofan) is sold as a nutritional supplement. It is not currently marketed as a single-entity preparation as a sleep aid. It has been used in the treatment of insomnia in doses of 1 to 5 g at bedtime.

Patient Education

The following key points should be included in the education of patients taking hypnotic agents:

The patient should inform all health professionals about *all* medications and alcohol usage—including nonprescription drugs. In general, alcohol should be avoided during treatment with hypnotics.

TABLE 22-5 Nonprescription Sleep Aids

PRODUCT	ANTIHISTAMINE
Compoz tablets	Diphenhydramine, 50 mg
Nervine	Pyrilamine maleate, 25 mg
Nytol with DPH	Diphenhydramine, 25 mg
Quiet Tabs	Pyrilamine maleate, 25 mg
Quiet World tablets*	Pyrilamine maleate, 25 mg
Sedacaps	Pyrilamine maleate, 25 mg
Sleep-Eze 3	Diphenhydramine, 50 mg
Sominex	Pyrilamine maleate, 25 mg
Sominex Formula 2	Diphenhydramine, 25 mg
Somnicaps	Pyrilamine maleate, 25 mg
Tranquil capsules	Pyrilamine maleate, 25 mg
Unisom	Doxylamine succinate, 25 mg

*Also contains aspirin 227.5 mg and acetominophen 162.5 mg.

The patient should inform health care providers if she is planning to become pregnant, if she is already pregnant, or if she becomes pregnant while taking the medicine.

The patient should inform the health care providers if she is nursing an infant.

The patient should avoid driving a car or operating heavy equipment until he or she has experienced the effects of the medication.

The patient should take only the prescribed dose of medication.

The patient should inform the health care provider if he or she experiences an increase in sleep problems (rebound insomnia) on the first few nights after discontinuing the drug.

Care should be taken to avoid allowing the patient to become too dependent on the use of sleep medication. Patients who are receiving a "sleeping pill" may not need detailed information as to the drug's mechanism of action, but there is other important information of which the patient should be aware. Both hospitalized and ambulatory patients should be informed of the possibility of morning hangover with these drugs and their effects on intellectual performance and motor behavior. This is especially important in ambulatory patients who are likely to be driving a car or operating machinery in the morning.

Because of the additive effects of alcohol and other central nervous system depressants when used in combination with hypnotic agents, patients should be advised to avoid these preparations when hypnotics are prescribed.

Patients should be instructed in ways to avoid multiple doses of hypnotic agents. Patients who awaken after the first dose of a hypnotic agent may be very confused and forget they have taken the first dose and take a second dose. To avoid overdosing, patients should be instructed not to keep the bottle of sleeping pills at the bedside. Delayed onset of action if hypnotics are taken with food may cause the patient to take a second dose because it may seem that the first dose "didn't work." This could result in excessive and prolonged CNS depression. Antacids may interfere with hypnotic drug absorption. Therefore, sleeping medications should be given on an empty stomach with a glass of water after such activities as taking a shower or brushing teeth are completed.

EVALUATION

While notoriously unreliable, the patient's subjective statements must be the basis for evaluation of sleep. Often the night nurse will observe patients hourly and find them apparently sleeping, while these same patients will report that they never even dozed all night. Signs of sleep deprivation may validate the presence of a sleep disturbance, but the signs are not necessarily present even if the patient has significant insomnia. As a result, the evaluation of approaches planned to improve sleep can be difficult with both inpatients and outpatients.

The problem of evaluating sleep is further complicated by the fact that the nurse who implements the plan can rarely actually observe its effects because the shift usually ends before evaluation can be accomplished. Other nurses may fail to evaluate drugs they have not administered. Therefore, nurses on all shifts must be aware of the patient's sleep status and communicate the necessary data to other nurses so that a coordinated and effective approach may be taken.

Each morning, data should be collected from patients who are on hypnotics about the presence of hangover symptoms, the patient's subjective evaluation of the night's sleep, the presence of REM rebound or vivid dreams, and daytime drowsiness. The nurse caring for the patient at night may note CNS depression (difficult arousal, decreased rate and depth of respiration, and decreased blood pressure), signs of ataxia (stumbling or falling), paradoxic excitement, or gastrointestinal distress. These problems should be communicated to the prescriber and/or the nurse who prepares the patient for sleep so that drug therapy can be modified accordingly. The nurse who finds an effective nonpharmacologic approach for a particular patient should make sure that it is written on the patient's care plan. If observation of apneic or irregular breathing is found, further medical investigation may be necessary.

CONCLUSION

Sleep disorders of various types are important problems, insomnia being the most frequently encountered. Sleep disorders other than insomnia are usually related to specific psychologic, environmental, or medical causes, and may require specific therapy. Rational treatment of insomnia begins with a thorough search for underlying causes.

Hypnotic drugs are indicated only in selected cases of insomnia. Older hypnotic drugs (barbiturates, meprobamate, etc.) are seen to be effective for short-term treatment but are ineffective over extended periods. In addition, the older drugs interfere with various sleep stages and can produce dependence; they are dangerous when taken in suicide attempts. There appear to be few good reasons to prescribe these older drugs.

Benzodiazepines (flurazepam, triazolam, temazepam, lorazepam) seem to be the agents of choice in most cases of temporary insomnia. Flurazepam may be effective with an every-other-night dosing schedule due to its prolonged effect.

CASE STUDY

G. F., a 52-year-old corporate executive, was admitted to a general hospital for treatment of hypertension, congestive heart failure, a painful left knee, and obesity, and to rule out gout, gastric ulcers, and arteriosclerotic heart disease. The physician's orders included flurazepam (Dalmane) 15 mg at bedtime PRN for sleep and hydrochlorothiazide (HydroDiuril) 50 mg stat and 50 mg bid.

Assessment

When the admission history was taken, the patient denied using any medications except aspirin for joint pain. However, he normally consumed 10 to 15 cups of coffee daily. Upon specific questioning about medications used for sleep, he recalled using antihistamines approximately three times per month to help him sleep. Normally he slept 6 to 10 h each night, making up on the weekend for sleep missed during the week. He often slept in a king-size bed alone since his wife worked nights. He used one pillow and one electric blanket. The room was darkened, soundproof, and kept at 62°F both summer and winter. Normally he went to bed between 10 P.M. and midnight after showering and reading while he had a final cup of coffee. He would awaken at 6 A.M., dress, and drive to work without breakfast in order to avoid the traffic. He would drink several cups of coffee in the cafeteria before going to his office at 7:30 A.M. G. F. admitted that he slept poorly if one of his children was not home, when he was out of town on business, and on Sunday nights due to "worry over business problems" anticipated for the next week. He would seldom wake up once he went to sleep.

The nurse noted that G. F. seemed very anxious as he sat rigidly on the edge of the chair. His wife confirmed this, stating that G. F. was firmly convinced that no one at his age entering the hospital ever left alive.

G. F. was in a private room at the end of the hall. The nurse anticipated that due to his past history of periodic situational insomnia, initial stat dose of diuretic administered at 7 P.M., painful knee, and high anxiety level, G. F. would probably have sleep problems in the hospital and a hypnotic would be appropriate.

Management

G. F. was offered flurazepam (Dalmane) 15 mg on the first night, but he refused it, citing fear of addiction. The nurse explained that flurazepam was considered useful during the initial period of hospitalization, since the change in environment commonly caused sleep disorders, and that it had a very low addiction potential when used for a short period of time. However, G. F. still insisted that he did not want the medication.

The nurse encouraged G. F. to shower at night and furnished him with a hot cup of decaffinated coffee at bedtime. Because of his usual excessive coffee intake, it was unlikely that caffeine would keep him awake; it was more likely that he would have difficulty waking up and staying awake during the day without his accustomed intake. As a result, he might sleep during the day, making it more difficult to fall asleep at night. However, in light of the potential cardiac and ulcer problems, the nurse elected to serve a decaffeinated coffee. The air conditioning was turned to its coolest setting, but the temperature never went below 70°F. G. F. was given a single pillow and blanket and offered a back rub, which he also refused.

On subsequent days, diuretics were scheduled for A.M. and 3 P.M. to allow their effect to abate before bedtime. Care was taken to explain each test and its results to G. F. and to encourage him to ask questions and express his feelings about hospitalization. Heart disease and ulcers were ruled out, but gouty arthritis and hiatal hernia were diagnosed and treatment was instituted.

When the nurse discovered that G. F. had refused the back rub because he did not want to bother the nursing staff, the purpose of back rubs was explained, and on the second through sixth nights he accepted both the Dalmane and the back rub. On the seventh night he refused the Dalmane since he expected to be discharged in 2 days and felt he could sleep without it. The nurse supported him in this decision.

Evaluation

G. F. found the bed too hard and too small, the unit too noisy, and the room too hot for sleeping. Although the effects of the diuretic seemed to end around 11 P.M., he slept very little the first night. Since he was scheduled for numerous tests the next day, there was no opportunity for napping. On subsequent nights he slept well without any hangover or residual drowsiness. His anxiety level decreased markedly as his condition improved and problems were ruled out.

REFERENCES

Briemer, D.: "Clinical Pharmacokinetics of Hypnotics," *Clin Pharmacokinet,* **2:**93–109, 1977.

Bunker, M. L., et al.: "Caffeine Content of Common Beverages," *J Am Diet Assoc,* **74:**28–32, January 1979.

Drug Evaluations, 5th ed., Chicago: American Medical Association, 1983.

Greenblatt, D. J., and R. R. Miller: "Rational Use of Psychotropic Drugs: I. Hypnotics," *Am J Hosp Pharm,* **31:**990–995, 1974.

—— and R. I. Shader: "The Clinical Choice of Sedative-Hypnotics," *Ann Intern Med,* **77:**91–100, 1972.

—— and ——: *Benzodiazepines in Clinical Practice,* New York: Raven, 1974.

—— and ——: "Psychotropic Drugs in the General Hospital," in R. I. Shader (ed.), *Manual of Psychiatric Therapies: Practical Psychiatry and Psychopharmacology,* Boston: Little, Brown, 1975, chap. 1.

—— et al.: "Clinical Pharmacokinetics of the Newer Benzodiazepines," *Clinical Pharmacokinetics,* **8:**233–252, May–June 1983.

—— et al.: "Current Status of Benzodiazepines," *New Engl J Med,* **309:**354–358, pt. 1, Aug. 11, 1983.

—— et al.: "Current Status of Benzodiazepines," *The New England Journal of Medicine,* **309:**410–416, pt. 2, Aug. 18, 1983.

Guilleminault, C., J. van den Hoed, and M. M. Mitler: "Clinical Overview of the Sleep Apnea Syndrome," in C. Guilleminault and W. C. Dement (eds.), *Sleep Apnea Syndromes,* New York: Liss, 1978, pp. 1–12.

Handbook of Nonprescription Drugs, 7th ed., Washington, DC: American Pharmaceutical Association, 1982.

Johns, M. W.: "Sleep and Hypnotic Drugs," *Drugs,* **9:**448–478, 1975.

Kales, A.: "Psychophysiological Studies of Insomnia," *Ann Intern Med,* **71:**625–629, 1969.

——: "The Evaluation and Treatment of Sleep Disorders: Pharmacological and Psychological Studies," in M. Chase (ed.), *The Sleeping Brain,* Los Angeles: UCLA Brain Information Service/Brain Research Institute, 1972, pp. 447–491.

——, E. O. Bixler, and T. L. Tan: "Chronic Hypnotic Use: Ineffectiveness, Drug Withdrawal Insomnia and Hypnotic Drug Dependence," *JAMA,* **227:**513–518, 1974.

—— and J. D. Kales: "Recent Advances in the Diagnosis and Treatment of Sleep Disorders," in G. Usdin (ed.), *The Relevance of Sleep Research to Clinical Practice,* New York: Brunner/Mazel, 1972, pp. 61–94.

—— and ——: "Sleep Disorders: Recent Findings in the Diagnosis and Treatment of Disturbed Sleep," *N Engl J Med,* **290:**487–498, Feb. 28, 1974.

Koch-Weser, J., and E. M. Sellers: "Drug Interactions with Coumarin Anticoagulants," *N Engl J Med,* **285:**487–498, 547–558, 1971.

Lasagna, L.: "Hypnotic Drugs," *N Engl J Med,* **287:**1182–1184, Dec. 7, 1973.

Martin, R. J., M. H. Sanders, B. A. Gray, and B. Pennock: "Acute and Long-Term Ventilatory Effects of Hyperoxia in the Adult Sleep Apnea Syndrome," *Am Rev Respir Dis,* **125:**175–180, 1982.

Miller, R. R., D. V. DeYoung, and J. Paxinos: "Hypnotic Drugs," *Postgrad Med J,* **46:**314–317, 1970.

Mitchell, P. H.: *Concepts Basic to Nursing,* 2d ed., New York: McGraw-Hill, 1977.

Morgan, A. J.: "Minor Tranquilizers, Hypnotics, and Sedatives," *Am J Nurs,* **73:**1220–1222, July 1973.

Olson, E., et al.: "Recognition, General Considerations, and

Techniques in the Management of Drug Intoxication," *Heart and Lung,* **12**:110–130, March 1983.

Oswald, I. D., L. F. Dunleavy, and J. A. Strong: "Hyperthyroidism and the Sleeping Brain," *Hormones,* **3**:278–281, 1972.

———, and R. G. Priest: "Five Weeks to Escape the Sleeping Pill Habit," *Br Med J,* **2**:1093–1099, 1965.

Parish, P. E.: "The Prescribing of Psychotropic Drugs in General Practice," *J. R. Coll Gen Practitioners,* **21**(Suppl.):1–77, 1971.

Reynolds, J. (ed.): *Martindale's The Extra Pharmacopoeia,* 28th ed., London: Pharmaceutical, 1982.

Sellers, E. M., and J. Koch-Wiser: "Potentiation of Warfarin-Induced Hypoprothrombinemia by Chloral Hydrate," *N Engl J Med,* **283**:827–831, 1970.

Shapiro, S., D. Stone, G. P. Lewis, and H. Jick: "Clinical Effects of Hypnotics: II. An Epidemiologic Study," *JAMA,* **209**:2016–2020, 1969.

Sharpless, S.: "Hypnotics and Sedatives," in L. S. Goodman and A. Gilman (eds.), *Goodman and Gilman's The Pharmacological Basis of Therapeutics,* 6th ed., New York: Macmillan, 1983.

Traver, G.: *Respiratory Nursing, The Science and the Art,* New York: Wiley, 1982.

UCLA Interdepartmental Confercne: "Drug Dependency: Investigations of Stimulants and Depressants," *Ann Intern Med,* **70**:591–614, 1969.

Way, W. L., and A. J. Trevor: "Sedative-Hypnotics," *Anesthesiology,* **34**:170–182, 1971.

Westerholm, B.: "Consumption of Psychotropic Drugs in Sweden," *Act Nerv Super,* **15**:156–157, 1973.

23

EDEMA

MARTHA H. STONER

LEARNING OBJECTIVES

Upon mastery of the contents of this chapter, the reader will be able to:

1. Explain the mechanisms that preserve normal tissue water balance, including colloid osmotic pressure and capillary hydrostatic pressure.

2. Define edema.

3. Identify the conditions where edema may be present.

4. Describe the methods used to assess and monitor edematous patients.

5. Explain the nonpharmacologic management of edema.

6. Name four types of diuretics which might be used to treat edema.

7. Relate the site of action of the diuretics to their therapeutic and adverse effects.

8. State the mechanism of action of the thiazide and loop diuretics and of spironolactone.

9. List the adverse effects of each group of diuretics used to treat edema.

10. Explain the nursing process for hypokalemia, hyperkalemia, hyponatemia, hypovolemia, hyperglycemia, hypercalcemia, and hyperuricemia associated with diuretic therapy.

11. Outline a plan of education for the patient taking diuretics.

Edema, the retention of excess fluid in interstitial spaces, is not a primary disease process; it is an indicator of underlying pathologic conditions. Edema is a physical sign important in detecting and monitoring both local and systemic disorders influencing fluid balance. Acute inflammatory reactions such as allergic conditions and obstruction of lymphatic channels following radical mastectomy are examples of *local processes* frequently accompanied by edema. Congestive heart failure, nephrotic syndrome, and hepatic cirrhosis are *systemic conditions* which produce edema. Management of the underlying condition is essential, but monitoring of edema as an accessible parameter of the manifestation of a pathologic process may prevent unnecessary damage to involved organ systems and increase the patient's potential for rehabilitation.

ETIOLOGY

The primary etiology of edema is an imbalance in the distribution of water due to a shift of fluid from the plasma to the interstitial space. The resultant expansion of the interstitial space is evidenced as tissue swelling, or edema. Edema occurs when there is disruption of the regulating forces controlling the exchange of fluid across vessel walls (Fig. 23-1). Two major forces, capillary hydrostatic pressure and plasma colloidal osmotic pressure, regulate fluid distribution at the tissue level.

Capillary Hydrostatic Pressure

Capillary hydrostatic pressure is the force created by the fluid within the capillaries. An elevation of the hydrostatic pressure forces fluid out of the capillary into the tissue spaces, resulting in increased interstitial fluid pressure and edema. Increased capillary hydrostatic pressure accompanies any condition that causes an increase in venous pressure or arteriolar dilation. Underlying conditions influencing hydrostatic pressure include local allergic reactions, hypertension, congestive heart disease, primary and secondary hyperaldosteronism, and thrombophlebitis. Certain drugs (Table 23-1) cause edema by increasing sodium and water retention, resulting in increased hydrostatic pressure.

Plasma Colloidal Osmotic Pressure

Plasma colloidal osmotic pressure (oncotic pressure) is the force exerted by plasma proteins in the vascular space. Colloidal pressure is that developed when two solutions of different concentrations of the same solute are separated by a membrane permeable only to the solvent. If plasma colloidal osmotic pressure is low, fluid is not drawn from the interstitial space into the capillaries. Rather, capillary hydrostatic pressure overrides the osmotic pressure, and fluid is pushed out of the capillaries into tissue spaces. The most common cause of decreased colloidal osmotic pressure is hypoproteinemia associated with burns, liver and kidney diseases, malabsorption of amino acids, and starvation.

313

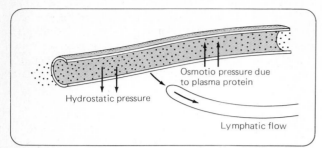

FIGURE 23-1

Factors Involved in Fluid Balance between Blood Vessels and Tissues. Hydrostatic pressure tends to push fluid into the interstitial spaces. This is largely balanced by the osmotic pressure exerted by plasma protein (dots) which ordinarily do not pass through vessel walls. The fluid which does pass into the interstices drains via the lymphatics. (*Adapted from G. D. Abrams: "Response of the Body to Injury," in S. A. Price and L. M. Wilson (eds.),* Pathophysiology: Clinical Concepts of Disease Processes, *2d ed., New York: McGraw-Hill, 1982. Used by permission.*)

ASSESSMENT OF EDEMA

The practitioner can elicit subjective data about edema by asking the client to respond to a set of descriptors (Table 23-2). The presence of edema can be detected and monitored during physical examination. Measurement of weight provides objective data useful in monitoring edema. To be accurate, weights should be measured at the same time of day under similar conditions such as with the same amount of clothing, and after emptying the bladder. Taking and recording pulse and blood pressure measurements provides information useful in evaluating fluid status (e.g., a bounding pulse and elevated blood pressure may indicate excess fluid volume). Palpation over bony surfaces, especially in dependent areas, such as the tibia and the sacrum, determines the amount of edema present based on the depth of indentation (pitting) when pressure is applied. Shiny, pale skin which appears tight also indicates the presence of edema.

Additional assessments of edema include auscultation of the lungs for rales and pleural friction rub, palpation of the chest wall for diminished tactile fremitus, inspection of neck veins for distention, and percussion of the abdomen for the presence of ascites. Neurologic signs (level of consciousness, pupil response, and motor and sensory function) are significant in assessing edema within the cranial vault. Laboratory assessment of serum albumin for hypoalbuminemia and serum electrolytes will help to elucidate the cause of systemic edema.

MANAGEMENT OF EDEMA

Nonpharmacologic Management

Treatment of edema is directed toward the cause of the edema with the goal of correcting the maldistribution of fluid. Nonpharmacologic management of edema such as restriction of sodium and water intake may be adequate to control edema. A high-protein diet may be used in edematous conditions associated with hypoproteinemia. Wearing supportive stockings, restricting physical activity, and elevating extremities are examples of nonpharmacologic methods used to mobilize fluid in the treatment of edema. Edema of pregnancy is generally due to hormonal changes and mechanical obstruction of venous return caused by the posi-

TABLE 23-1   Drugs That May Cause Edema by Expanding Plasma Volume

DRUG	COMMENT
Steroids	
Glucocorticoids	Agents with strong mineralcorticoid activity (e.g., hydrocortisone) are more likely to cause edema than those with weak mineralocorticoid activity (e.g., prednisone).
Estrogens	Includes oral contraceptives.
Androgens	May occur with or without congestive heart failure, especially with long-term use.
Progestins	Includes oral contraceptives.
Antihypertensives	
Diazoxide	May occur with repeat injection and compromise antihypertensive effects, especially in patients with low cardiac reserve.
Sympatholytics, such as guanethidine (Ismelin), methyldopa (Aldomet), reserpine, prazocin (Minipres), minoxidil (Lonetin)	Cause sodium and water retention as a compensatory response. Usually require concurrent diuretic therapy.
Antiarthritis Drugs	
Nonsteroidal anti-inflammatory drugs, especially indomethacin (Indocin), zomepriac (Zomax), phenylbutazone (Butazoladin)	Cause sodium and water retention, especially in higher doses.
Salicylates	In anti-inflammatory doses may increase sodium and water retention.
Miscellaneous	
Osmotic diuretics (mannitol, urea, etc.)	Volume overload may occur if administered too rapidly.
Glycerrhyzic acid	Component of licorice which has mineralocorticoid effect.

TABLE 23-2 Descriptors Used to Elicit Subjective Data about Edema*

Time Sequence

Onset/commenced
Duration of episodes
Frequency of episodes
Number of episodes

Time Relationships

Precipitated by
Continuous or intermittent
Associated with other events or conditions
Time of day noted

Characteristics

Anatomic location
Bilateral/unilateral
Intensity/degree
Quantity/severity at worst

Course

Getting better/relieved by
Getting worse/not relieved or made worse by
Unchanging
Response to therapy

---

*Interviewer should phrase questions for each descriptor to fit the patient's understanding and symptoms (e.g., When did you first notice the swelling/weight gain?)

tion of the fetus; nonpharmacologic methods of treatment (rest and elevation of extremities) are the only management indicated for simple edema of pregnancy, as drugs may be dangerous to both mother and fetus. Localized edema may be relieved by drainage, as in removal of ascitic fluid by paracentesis and drainage of excess cerebral spinal fluid by spinal or ventricular tap.

Pharmacologic Management

Goals of pharmacologic therapy of edema are to decrease hydrostatic pressure by increasing renal excretion of sodium and water and/or to increase colloidal osmotic pressure. Diuretics are the drug group used to decrease hydrostatic pressure. Colloids, such as albumin, can be given intravenously to increase colloidal osmotic pressure (see Chap. 24).

Diuretics

The six groups of diuretics are: carbonic anhydrase inhibitors, mercurial diuretics, osmotic diuretics, thiazide diuretics, loop diuretics, and the potassium-sparing diuretics. The *carbonic anhydrase inhibitors* (e.g., **acetazolamide**) are primarily used in the treatment of glaucoma and for their effects on acid-base balance (e.g., urinary alkalinization, acute mountain sickness, and sleep apnea). The pharmacology of these agents is discussed in Chap. 39.

Mercurial diuretics are available but are primarily of historical interest. They are seldom used because they require parental administration, while newer effective agents can be given orally.

Osmotic diuretics are used to increase water excretion in preference to sodium excretion (e.g., to maintain urine volume when renal hemodynamics are compromised, to decrease intracranial and intraocular pressure). **Mannitol, urea,** and **glycerol** are examples of osmotic diuretics (see Chap. 39).

Drugs with mild diuretic action contained in *over-the-counter preparations* promoted for the treatment of water retention ("bloating") and symptoms associated with menstruation (e.g., Fluidex, Aqua-Ban, Pamprin, Midol), include **caffeine** and **pamabrom**. The thiazide diuretics, loop diuretics, and potassium-sparing agents are the prescription drugs most commonly employed for edematous conditions, although these drugs are also indicated in the treatment of hypertension (Chap. 40) and to reduce preload and afterload in cardiac conditions (Chaps. 43 and 44).

Mechanism and Sites of Diuretic Action Diuretics increase urine output through prevention of the reabsorption of water from the kidney tubules. This is accomplished by increasing the osmotic pressure of the tubular fluid, usually as a result of decreased reabsorption of electrolytes (e.g., sodium, chloride, bicarbonate). This causes excretion of large amounts of dilute urine. The magnitude and type of drug effects of diuretics depend upon where in the kidney tubule the drug effect is exerted and the normal tubular functions of the sites of drug action. (See Fig. 23-2.)

Once the plasma is filtered through the glomerulus, it sequentially passes through the proximal convoluted tubule, the loop of Henle, the distal convoluted tubule, and the collecting duct. As the tubular filtrate travels through the nephron, substances are *reabsorbed* from the filtrate or *secreted* into the filtrate at various points in order to maintain chemical homeostasis in the body. In the *proximal tubule* much bicarbonate is reabsorbed under the influence of the enzyme, carbonic anhydrase. Diuretics which are sulfonamide derivatives (**carbonic anhydrase inhibitors, thiazides, furosemide, bumetanide**) are all antagonists to carbonic anhydrase and may affect acid-base status by action in the proximal tubule. In addition, organic acids such as uric acid are actively secreted in the proximal tubule, and competition (between diuretics and uric acid) for the carriers at this site can raise serum uric acid levels and precipitate gout in the susceptible person.

The *loop of Henle,* particularly the thick ascending limb, is the site of massive Na^+ and Cl^- reabsorption, as well as reabsorption of divalent cations (Mg^{2+}, Ca^{2+}). Only the *loop diuretics* are active at this site, which accounts for their potent diuretic effects, as well as their tendency to deplete calcium and magnesium.

The early *distal convoluted tubule* has receptors for parathormone and is a site of active Ca^{2+} reabsorption, as well as the reabsorption of Na^+ and Cl^- ions. Acting at this site, the thiazides and related diuretics cause moderate diuresis, as well as retention of calcium.

In the *terminal distal tubule* and *collecting duct,* sodium can be reabsorbed in exchange for potassium. Diuretics with

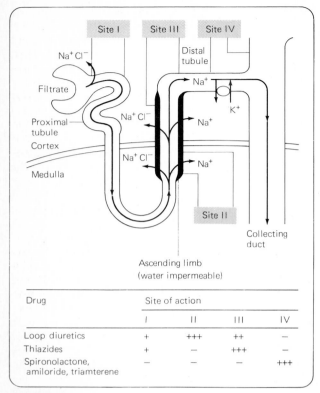

FIGURE 23-2

Sites of Action of Diuretics. I. Proximal tubule. II. Ascending Henle's loop. III. Early distal tubule. IV. Terminal distal tubule and collecting duct. (*Adapted from D. L. Davies and G. B. Wilson: "Diuretics, Mechanism of Action and Clinical Application," Drugs, 9:181, 1975. Used by permission.*)

sites of action prior to the collecting tubule (e.g., **thiazides, loop agents**) cause *kaluresis* (potassium depletion through the urine), because the filtrate reaching the duct is high in sodium which is exchanged for potassium. On the other hand, diuretics active at this site (**amiloride, spironolactone,** and **triamterene**) are considered *potassium-sparing diuretics,* since they retard potassium excretion. Receptors for aldosterone are present at this site and antidiuretic hormone (ADH) is active at the collecting duct. Spironolactone is an antagonist for aldosterone, and thus is useful in treating hyperaldosteronism. **Lithium carbonate** can cause nephrogenic diabetes insipidus by inhibiting antidiuretic hormone action at the collecting duct.

Thiazides and Related Diuretics   By chemical composition these drugs (Table 23-3) are all sulfonamides, and so cross-allergy can occur between these agents and the sulfonamide antibiotics or sulfonylurea oral antidiabetic agents. Although not thiazides, **quinethazone** (Hydromox), **metolazone** (Diulo, Zaroxolyn), **chlorthalidone** (Hygroton, Thali-

tone), and **indapamide** (Lozol) are structurally and pharmacologically similar to the thiazides.

Mechanism of action   The thiazides produce diuresis by inhibiting the reabsorption of sodium, chloride, and water in the early distal tubule. Being sulfonamide diuretics, these agents also inhibit carbonic anhydrase in the proximal tubule. Increased potassium excretion, decreased uric acid excretion, and calcium retention are other actions of these drugs. The mechanism of the antihypertensive action of these drugs is thought to involve more than diuresis, and the thiazides may exert a direct vasodilator effect on the vascular wall.

Pharmacokinetics   The onset of action of the thiazides and related diuretics is approximately 2 h, except for **hydroflumethiazide** (Diucardin, Saluron), **bendroflumethiazide** (Naturetin), and **metolazone** (Diulo, Zaroxolyn) which begin to exert their effects in 1 h, and **cyclothiazide** (Anhydron, Fluidil) in which the onset of action may be delayed up to 6 h. Cardiac failure may impair absorption, but food appears to increase the absorption of several thiazides. The long duration of action of **chlorthalidone** is attributed to its slow absorption.

The onset and duration of action of the thiazides and related diuretics is shown in Table 23-3, although renal impairment and congestive heart failure can prolong the elimination half-life and effects of these drugs. Most are eliminated primarily by renal excretion in unchanged form, although **bendroflumethiazide** and **indapamide** are eliminated up to two-thirds or more by nonrenal routes (hepatic metabolism).

Adverse effects   The most common, major adverse effects of thiazide and related diuretic therapy are *volume and electrolyte* disturbances. *Hypovolemia* or volume depletion usually occurs shortly after therapy is initiated and is of particular importance in elderly individuals. Careful monitoring of weight, blood pressure, and pulse to detect fluid loss, postural hypotension, and tachycardia are necessary. Symptoms such as dizziness, weakness, and thirst should also be evaluated as indicators of hypovolemia. Dehydration may result if hypovolemia is extreme.

Electrolyte disturbances found in patients taking thiazides and related diuretics include hyponatremia and hypokalemia. Hyponatremia is rare but can be life-threatening in elderly individuals.

Hypokalemia (a serum potassium level of less than 3.5 meq/L) is a common adverse effect of thiazides. Serum potassium levels are an effective and generally available method for monitoring potassium balance. In asymptomatic patients, serum potassium should be measured before therapy begins, after 1 month of therapy, and every 3 to 6 months thereafter. Symptomatic patients (e.g., those reporting generalized weakness, fatigue, bilateral calf pain or cramps, palpitations, dizziness, or nausea) and individuals at risk (e.g., those receiving digitalis glycosides or corticosteroids, those with dietary intake low in potassium or excessive in salt, or those with documented history of hypokalemia) require more frequent monitoring and will need potassium replacement therapy (see Chap. 24). Potassium replacement can be in the form of increased dietary intake of potassium (e.g., bananas, oranges), but replacement requires large amounts of these foods which are generally high in calories. Dietary approaches are, therefore, not a practical alternative to supplementation with potassium salts. However, high-potassium diets are advocated by some clinicians in the prevention of hypokalemia in asymptomatic and low-risk patients taking thiazides. Concomitant use of a potassium-sparing diuretic (e.g., **spironolactone, triamterene,** or **amiloride**) may be an appropriate alternative to potassium replacement therapy.

Hyperuricemia (serum uric acid greater than 7 mg/dL) is another common adverse effect of thiazide therapy. Baseline serum uric acid levels should be obtained before and repeated 1 to 2 months after thiazide therapy is initiated. A history of gout does not preclude the use of thiazides, but individuals with gout may require prophylactic therapy with antigout drugs to avoid complications.

Hyperglycemia (an increase in blood glucose) is an adverse effect of thiazide therapy in elderly people and individuals who have or are predisposed to diabetes mellitus. The mechanism of the hyperglycemia is poorly understood, but may be associated with the hypokalemic effects of thiazide agents. Diabetics and people at risk for diabetes should be routinely questioned regarding symptoms of diabetes, and urine and blood glucose should be monitored periodically.

Thiazides also cause hypercalcemia and dermatologic

reactions. The nursing process for the adverse effects of thiazide diuretics is described in Table 23-4.

Drug interactions   Thiazides and related diuretics may *potentiate* the response to certain drugs (e.g., antihypertensives, including ganglionic blockers or peripheral adrenergic blockers; tubocurarine; quinidine). Decreased potassium levels and increased calcium levels caused by thiazides increase the risk of digitalis toxicity in those taking the digitalis glycosides. Because thiazides reduce the renal clearance of lithium, producing a high risk of toxicity, these two drugs should generally not be prescribed concomitantly. However, thiazides are used to treat lithium-induced nephrogenic diabetes insipidus. **Thiazide** therapy may *decrease* the action of drugs such as norepinephrine and antidiabetic agents. **Sulfonamide** antibiotics potentiate the diuretic effect of thiazides by displacing them from protein binding sites, while **indomethacin** may antagonize the hypotensive effect of thiazide diuretics.

Adverse effects of thiazides may be aggravated by drug interactions. For example, hypokalemia is more likely to develop in patients receiving both thiazides and **corticosteroids** or **ACTH**. Hypercalcemia is more common when thiazides are combined with **calcium carbonate.**

Dosage and administration   Usual doses of the **thiazides** and related diuretics are shown in Table 23-3. Dosage should be individualized and usually begins in the lower ranges and is titrated upward according to therapeutic response. Once diuresis has occurred and the patient has attained "dry weight" (weight prior to onset of edema), a

TABLE 23-3   Thiazides and Related Diuretics

DRUG	TRADE NAMES (EXAMPLES)	PEAK, h	DURATION, h	Usual Adult Oral Dosage,* mg INITIAL	MAINTENANCE	USUAL MAINTENANCE FREQUENCY
Bendroflumethiazide	Naturetin	6–12	18–24	20	2.5–5	qd
Benzthiazide	Aquatag, Exna, others	4–6	12–18	50–200	50–150	qd
Chlorothiazide	Diuril	4	6–12	500–1000	500–1000‡	qd or bid
Chlorthalidone†	Hygroton	2	48–72	50–100	50–200	qd or qod
Cyclothiazide	Anhydron, Fluidil	7–12	18–24		1–2	qd or qod
Hydrochlorothiazide	Esidrex, HydroDiuril, Oretic, others	4	6–12	25–200	25–100§	qd or bid
Hydroflumethiazide	Diucardin, Saluron	2–4	6–12	50	25–200	qd or bid
Indapamide†	Lozol	1–2	12–24		2.5–5	qd
Methyclothiazide	Aquatensen, Enduron	6	24		2.5–10	qd
Metolazone†	Diulo, Zaroxolyn	2	12–24		5–20	qd
Polythiazide	Renese	6	36		1–4	qd
Quinethazone†	Hydromox	6	18–24	50–100	50–200	qd
Trichlormethiazide	Metahydrin, Naqua	6	24		1–4	qd

*Dosages given are for treatment of edema. Doses to treat hypertension may differ.

†A sulfonamide, but not a thiazide. Actions are similar to thiazides.

‡Intravenous form and oral suspension available. Oral pediatric doses are generally 10 mg/lb/day in two doses, but infants under 6 months may require 15 mg/lb/day. Intravenous administration not recommended for infants and children. Should not be given by IM or SC routes.

§Oral pediatric doses are generally 1 mg/lb/day in two doses, but infants under 6 months may require 1.5 mg/lb/day.

TABLE 23-4 Adverse Effects of Diuretics

DRUG	ADVERSE EFFECT	INCIDENCE	ASSESSMENT	MANAGEMENT	EVALUATION
Thiazide	Hypokalemia	8–40%, depending on dose and product	Take serum K^+ level. Ask about bilateral calf pain, paresthesia of extremities, palpitations, and generalized muscle weakness. Hypokalemia is more common in patients with salt intake greater than 5 g/day, congestive heart failure, ascites, diarrhea, and cirrhosis. Serum level less than 3.5 meq/L.	Usually 40–60 meq qd and recommend decrease in sodium chloride intake. May use salt substitute containing potassium chloride. Spironolactone 50–100 mg daily or triamterene 100 mg daily. Teach patient to identify symptoms of hypokalemia and food containing potassium.	Serum potassium and disappearance of symptoms. K^+ levels at beginning, 1 month after start, then every 3–6 months PRN.
	Hyperglycemia	Mostly in patients with existing diabetes or chemically undetected diabetes. Onset may be 1 to 4 weeks or longer.	Patient should have fasting blood glucose test, but may be reserved for patients with diabetes or suspected prediabetes. Patient should be questioned about symptoms: polyuria, polydipsia, polyphagia.	In diabetics, usually control by increasing dose of insulin (reg.) 3–5 units daily. Increase dose of oral diabetic agent to maximum, or use more dietary control.	Check fasting blood glucose at start, 1 month, then every 3–6 months until disappearance of symptoms.
	Hyperuricemia	Hyperuricemic serum levels greater than 7.0 mg/dL occur in 65–75% of patients in treatment (normal untreated 25–35%). Incidence of clinical gout not well established.	Check serum uric acid levels. Question about joint pains or stiffness. Should treat if serum level goes to 9 mg/dL. Make two uric acid determinations before asymptomatic treatment is begun.	Change to spironolactone or add allopurinol (200–300 mg qd). Acute attack treated with colchicine 0.6 mg qh until relief of pain or adverse effects (maximum 12 tablets).	Serum uric acid levels.
	Hypercalcemia	Rare. Mechanism is a decrease in calcium excretion and some suppression of parathyroid hormone secretion.	Most common in patients with chronic renal disease, hyperparathyroidism, vitamin D–treated hypoparathyroidism, or metabolic bone disease.	May return to normal without discontinuing drug or can switch to furosemide.	Measure calcium levels before and during therapy in high-risk patients.

Drug	Reaction	Incidence/Comments	Signs/Symptoms	Management	Outcome
	Dermatologic reaction	Rare; includes necrotizing vasculitis, photosensitivity; allergic in nature and not dose-related.		May disappear in time or may try chlorthalidone or loop diuretics.	
Furosemide, ethacrynic acid, and bumetanide	Hypokalemia	More common than with hydrochlorothiazide.	See thiazide.		
	Hyperglycemia	Less common than with thiazide.	See thiazide.		
	Hyperuricemia	Same as for thiazide.	See thiazide.		
	Hypovolemia	Most common with intensive IV therapy and in elderly.	Dry mouth, thirst, weakness, lethargy, hypotension, oliguria, and tachycardia may be noted.	Decrease dose or change to another diuretic. Correct any accompanying electrolyte imbalance.	Disappearance of symptoms. Return to normal electrolytes.
Spironolactone	Hyperkalemia	Rare with doses of 100–200 mg/day. Approximately 3% in horpitalized patients with normal renal function and not receiving K^+ supplement. If K^+ is added or patient is azotemic, incidence is 42%.	Serum potassium levels. ECG (tall T waves, low-amplitude P waves, and atrial asystole) before muscle weakness and flaccid paralysis. Assess renal function and concurrent drug administration.	Discontinue spironolactone or potassium supplement in accordance with assessment of cause of hyperkalemia. Combination with thiazides may prevent.	ECG and potassium levels.
	Gynecomastia	Actual incidence unknown. Problem may be patient-specific and dose-related.	Breast exam for tenderness, enlargement, and lumpiness. Onset 1–20 months. Other drugs such as methyldopa and digitalis may also be a cause.	Reduce dose. Discontinue drug. Switch to triamterene or amiloride.	Disappearance of symptoms.
	Amenorrhea	Not well established. More common with prior menstrual problems.	Accurate history.	Use another diuretic.	Return to normal menses.
Triamterene, amiloride	Hyperkalemia	About 10% with amiloride. Rare with triamterene.	See spironolactone.		

lower maintenance dosage is usually given; doses given every other day or 3 to 5 days/week may be adequate and minimize adverse effects. A "ceiling effect" probably occurs with these agents, and doses in excess of those recommended do not produce additional therapeutic response. For example, initial evidence indicates that **chlorothiazide** may be no more effective in doses of 500 mg than in doses of 250 mg, although increased response may be obtained by multiple daily doses of the lower dosage. These drugs may cause gastrointestinal irritation and should not be taken on an empty stomach; they should be taken early in the day since they cause urination that may interfere with sleep.

Loop Diuretics The loop diuretics (Table 23-5), or *high ceiling diuretics,* include three potent diuretics: **bumetamide** (Bumex), **furosemide** (Lasix), and **ethacrynic acid** (Edecrin). Since response to these drugs apparently increases as the dose is increased, it is the adverse effects rather than a response ceiling that usually limits dosages. Like the thiazides, furosemide and bumetanide are sulfonamides, but ethacrynic acid is not.

Mechanism of action The loop diuretics inhibit Na, Cl, and water reabsorption in the thick ascending limb of the loop of Henle, as well as in the proximal and distal tubules. They also decrease excretion of uric acid, increase calcium excretion, and increase sodium elimination. Thus, the thiazides and the loop diuretics have *opposing effects on serum calcium,* but both are considered *potassium-wasting,* and they cause the *retention of uric acid* and *elevate serum glucose* levels. Loop diuretics can increase urine flow even in the presence of renal insufficiency. The diuresis elicited by loop diuretics is profound and may occur more rapidly than fluid can be mobilized from the tissues, resulting in low cardiac output or even circulatory collapse. As a result of their powerful effects, loop diuretics are indicated in acute pulmonary edema, edema refractory to thiazides, hypercalcemia, nephrosis, hypertension, and acute renal failure.

Pharmacokinetics All three drugs are rapidly absorbed and excreted primarily unchanged by the kidneys. Bioavailability with **furosemide** is 65 percent and 90 to 100 percent with **ethacrynic acid** and **bumetanide**. The loop diuretics are greater than 90 percent plasma protein-bound. Onset of action is within minutes after intravenous injection and occurs 30 to 60 min after oral administration. The peak and duration of oral dosage forms is shown in Table 23-5. Peak action occurs 15 to 30 min after intravenous injection and

persists 2 to 4 h. Metabolites of ethacrynic acid, furosemide, and bumetanide have been identified, but it is not known if they have any diuretic action.

Adverse effects Because the mechanism of action of loop diuretics is similar to thiazide diuretics, they share the similar adverse effects of hypokalemia, hyperglycemia, and hyperuricemia. The extension of the site of action to the loop of Henle makes these more potent diuretics and increases the potential for more extreme adverse effects due to excessive diuresis (Table 23-4). The patient should be weighed periodically to assess the amount of diuresis and thus avoid the possibility of electrolyte and fluid imbalance. Serum electrolyte measures (Na^+, K^+, Ca^{2+}, Mg^{2+}) need to be performed periodically to monitor possible imbalances. Signs of excessive diuresis such as dry mouth, thirst, anorexia, orthostatic hypotension, weakness, lethargy, drowsiness, restlessness, numbness, muscle cramps, pain or fatigue, nausea or vomiting, irregular or rapid heart rate, and decreased urine volume must be monitored. Loop diuretics have also been associated with tinnitus and irreversible hearing loss, as well as hypocalcemia. Ethacrynic acid should be discontinued immediately if profuse diarrhea occurs soon after therapy is initiated.

Drug interactions Loop diuretics, like thiazides, potentiate the effects of **antihypertensive medications,** including ganglionic or peripheral adrenergic blocking drugs. Hypokalemia associated with diuresis is increased by **corticosteroid** or **ACTH** and may precipitate **digitalis** toxicity in patients taking digitalis drugs. Furosemide may alter the effects of **theophylline, metolazone,** and **succinylcholine.** It may also decrease the effect of **norepinephrine** and **tubocurarine.** Salicylate toxicity has occurred in patients taking high doses of **salicylates** with furosemide.

Adverse effects of loop diuretics may be aggravated by drug interactions. For example, concomitant administration of parental loop diuretics and **aminoglycoside antibiotics** should be done cautiously because of the increased potential for ototoxicity. Orthostatic hypotension associated with loop diuretic therapy may be worsened by consumption of **alcohol, barbiturates,** or **narcotics.** Concurrent intravenous administration of furosemide with **gentamicin** may enhance the nephrotoxicity associated with gentamicin. **Indomethacin** and other nonsteroidal anti-inflammatory drugs may reduce the antihypertensive effect of furosemide. Absorption of furosemide may be reduced by **phenytoin. Oral anticoagulant** requirement to maintain a desired prothrombin time

TABLE 23-5 Loop Diuretics Used in Edema

NAME	TRADE NAME	$t_{1/2}$, min	PEAK, min	DURATION, h	USUAL DAILY DOSAGE (PO)
Bumetanide	Bumex	60–90	60–120	4	0.5–2 mg
Ethacrynic acid	Edecrin	60	120	6–8	50–100 mg
Furosemide	Lasix	50	60–120	6–8	*Adult:* 20–80 mg *Child:* 1–2 mg/kg (IV)

may be decreased for patients taking **ethacrynic acid**. **Lithium** should not be taken with loop diuretics.

Dosage and administration   These drugs are available as tablets and parenteral solutions; **furosemide** is also supplied as an oral suspension. **Furosemide** and **bumetanide** can be given intravenously or intramuscularly, but **ethacrynic acid** is too irritating to be injected into intramuscular or subcutaneous tissue. Intravenous boluses should be given slowly (over 1 or 2 min or longer). Continuous infusions of **furosemide** should not exceed a rate of 4 mg/min. Oral dosage may be given with milk or meals if gastrointestinal upset occurs.

Dosage should be individualized based on patient response. After diuresis is established, lower or intermittent maintenance doses may be adequate. **Ethacrynic acid** and **bumetanide** are not currently recommended for use by children. Dosage early in the day will minimize sleep disturbances from the need to urinate.

Potassium-Sparing Diuretics

Spironolactone   Spironolactone (Aldactone) is a *potassium-sparing diuretic* indicated in the diagnosis and treatment of primary aldosteronism, in essential hypertension, in edematous conditions, particularly those accompanied by secondary hyperaldosteronism (e.g., congestive heart failure, cirrhosis of the liver), and to prevent and treat hypokalemia.

Mechanism of action   Spironolactone is a competitive pharmacologic antagonist to aldosterone in the terminal distal tubule and collecting duct. Therefore, it increases the excretion of sodium and water, while retaining potassium. Spironolactone also interferes with testosterone synthesis, permitting a relative overactivity of estrogen. This may account for its endocrine effects.

Pharmacokinetics   Spironolactone is well-absorbed and rapidly converted to the apparently inactive metabolite, canrenone, which has complex, biphasic elimination. Spironolactone and canrenone are highly bound to plasma proteins. They are eliminated primarily by the kidneys, but also in the bile. The onset, duration, and magnitude of action of spironolactone is determined by levels of aldosterone secretion.

Adverse effects   Spironolactone may produce symptoms of cramping, diarrhea, lethargy, confusion, headache, and ataxia. Gynecomastia, irregular menses, amenorrhea or postmenopausal bleeding, and male impotency (an inability to achieve or maintain erection) may occur in patients taking spironolactone. Hyperkalemia is a potentially dangerous effect of spironolactone therapy.

Drug interactions   The risk of *hyperkalemia* makes potassium supplementation—either through medication (potassium replacement or use of other potassium-sparing diuretics) or changes in diet—dangerous in patients taking any potassium-sparing diuretic. This retention of potassium may reduce the cardiac effects of **digitalis glycosides**. **Oral anticoagulants** may be less effective because of the spirono-

lactone-induced concentration of clotting factors. Spironolactone and other potassium-sparing diuretics reduce the vascular responsiveness to **norepinephrine**, but may potentiate the effects of **antihypertensives**.

Dosage and administration   Generally it requires several days of therapy to achieve full therapeutic effect of spironolactone. It is available only as tablets which may be given as a single or divided dose (see Table 23-6).

Triamterene. *Mechanism of action*   The exact mechanism whereby triamterene inhibits sodium reabsorption in the terminal distal tubule and collecting duct is unknown, but it is not through competitive antagonism of aldosterone. It exerts only a mild to moderate diuretic activity, due to the fact that it is active only in the terminal portions of the nephron.

Pharmacokinetics   Triamterene is 30 to 70 percent absorbed orally. Its onset of action is 2 to 4 h after oral administration, and its duration is 7 to 9 h. Triamterene is primarily metabolized in the liver, but a small amount is excreted unchanged in the urine. Little is known about the activity and elimination of its metabolites.

Adverse effects   Triamterene has been associated with relatively minor adverse effects such as weakness, headache, dry mouth, rash, photosensitivity, and gastrointestinal disturbances. Patients with a history of renal calculi may be at increased risk for stone formation while receiving triamterene. Similarly, individuals predisposed to gouty arthritis who are taking triamterene may have increased serum uric acid levels. Drug interactions with triamterene are the same as those related to spironolactone.

Dosage and administration   Dosage should be individualized to patient response. Usual doses are shown in Table 23-6, but are lower when another diuretic is taken concurrently.

Amiloride. *Mechanism of action*   Amiloride is an antikaluretic (*potassium-sparing*) diuretic whose site of action is the collecting duct. It is useful as an adjunct to potassium-depleting diuretics in treating edema, congestive heart failure, and hypertension. Its mechanism of action is unknown, but it is not an aldosterone antagonist.

TABLE 23-6   Potassium-Sparing Diuretics

NAME	TRADE NAME	USUAL DOSE*	USUAL FREQUENCY
Amiloride	Midamor	5–10 mg	qd
Spironolactone	Aldactone	*Adult:* 25–200 mg *Child:* 3.3 mg/kg	qd
Triamterene	Dyrenium	100–200 mg Maximum: 300 mg/day	bid, after meals

*Usually lower if taken concurrently with thiazide diuretic.

Pharmacokinetics Onset of action of amiloride is 2 h with a peak 6 to 10 h after administration and a duration of about 24 h. Amiloride is not metabolized; it is excreted unchanged, 50 percent in the urine and 40 percent in the feces.

Adverse effects Few significant adverse effects have been reported by patients taking amiloride. Like the other potassium-sparing diuretics, amiloride may cause *hyperkalemia.* Other adverse effects probably related to amiloride include nausea, anoxia, abdominal pain, flatulence, and mild skin rash. Drug interactions for amiloride are the same as those listed for spironolactone.

Dosage and administration Amiloride can be taken with food if it causes gastrointestinal upset. Dosage should be individually adjusted to the patient's response (Table 23-6). Maintenance therapy may be intermittent (every other day or 4 to 5 times weekly).

Combination Diuretic Therapy In cases of refractory edema, a thiazide and a loop diuretic may be given concurrently. These two groups have additive effects, but some of their adverse effects are off-setting or not overlapping. In addition, thiazides and potassium-sparing diuretics are given concurrently for their complimentary effects on potassium elimination. Several agents are available in fixed combinations (see Table 23-7). Adverse effects of combination diuretics are a summation of the adverse effects of the components. When potassium-sparing and potassium-wasting diuretics are combined, the serum potassium is usually maintained in normal ranges; although either hyperkalemia or hypokalemia can occur with this combination, potassium depletion is more common. A problem with fixed combinations is that adjustment of the dosage of a single component is not possible.

TABLE 23-7 Combination Diuretics

TRADE NAMES	THIAZIDE	POTASSIUM-SPARING AGENT	USUAL DOSE
Alazide, Aldactazide, Spironazide, Spirozide	Hydrochloro-thiazide, 25 mg	Spironolac-tone, 25 mg	2–4 qd
Dyazide	Hydrochloro-thiazide, 25 mg	Triamterene, 25 mg	1–2 qd after meals
Moduretic	Hydrochloro-thiazide, 50 mg	Amiloride, 5 mg	1–2 qd after meals

Patient Education

Patient education is an integral part of the treatment plan for edematous patients. The patient and family members must be provided information to increase their understanding of the pathologic process underlying the formation of edema. This, together with knowledge about the factors that contribute to fluid retention, encourages clients to be informed, active participants in their treatment program. Patients can become responsible for monitoring their fluid status by weighing themselves and taking their blood pressure daily. Thorough, accurate instructions regarding medications, fluid restrictions, sodium restrictions, and other dietary changes must be provided initially and periodically. Assessment of patient's knowledge and understanding of the treatment regimen is an essential ingredient of a patient education plan. Patients may call diuretics "water pills," but should be taught instead to use the generic name and know the purpose and dosage of their drugs.

EVALUATION

With any therapy instituted to treat edema, it is important to evaluate the effect of the regimen. On each visit, the nurse should elicit from the patient any history of dyspnea on exertion or orthopnea. The extent of dependent edema should be evaluated by observation and palpation over bony prominences and, if appropriate, measurement of the abdomen, thighs, and calves. Other parameters to assess edematous patients include weight, serial blood pressure readings to evaluate for postural variations, inspection of jugular veins for distention, auscultation of the heart for extra heart sounds and of the lungs for rales, and examination of the abdomen for ascites and masses. Laboratory studies such as serum electrolytes, blood urea nitrogen, uric acid creatinine, and urinalysis should be performed periodically (e.g., every 3 to 6 months) and/or in response to symptoms, to monitor any underlying pathology and to evaluate the effectiveness of the treatment program.

Evaluation of the edematous client includes an assessment of adherence to concomitant therapies such as dietary restriction of sodium, avoidance of prolonged standing or sitting with legs in a dependent position, and wearing of support stockings. In addition, it is also important to evaluate for possible adverse effects of any diuretics being taken by the patient. The nurse should inquire about symptoms such as calf muscle pain, generalized muscle weakness, palpitations, polyuria, polydipsia, polyphagia, and joint pain. If these symptoms of adverse effects occur, laboratory analysis (particularly for serum potassium and hyperglycemia) should be done.

CASE STUDY

B. S., a 42-year-old white rancher, lives on an isolated western ranch with his wife and four school-aged daughters. He had been vigorously healthy all of his adult life with the exception of two episodes of acute pyelonephritis with proteinuria during the past 2 years. The most recent episode was 6 months prior to this clinic visit.

B. S. had no family history of urinary disease or diabetes. The episodes of pyelonephritis were treated with ampicillin, 500 mg orally every 6 h for 10 days; acetaminophen, 650 mg as needed for fever; increased fluid intake; restricted sodium diet, and rest.

B. S. came to clinic because the swelling of his feet had progressively gotten worse over the past month. As he had been instructed, B. S. brought a 24-h urine sample with him to the clinic. He reported that the sample had been refrigerated and then transported in an ice chest cooler. He was wearing slippers because he was unable to wear his boots following the 4-h drive to the clinic. B. S. reported that he had persistent headache the past 3 or 4 days.

Assessment

B. S. was in no apparent distress and was breathing without obvious effort. His weight was 86 kg (189 lb), up 6 kg (13 lb) from 6 months ago. Blood pressure in the right arm while seated was 150/88, a slight increase since last visit (144/82). A new finding, pitting edema (+++), was present in the feet and ankles and the posterior tibial and dorsalis pedis pulses were weak bilaterally. In addition, slight edema of the eyelids was noted. Diagnostic test findings which were within normal limits included chest x-ray, ECG, and fasting blood sugar. Other results of blood analysis were normal except for: potassium 6.1 meq/L (3.5–5.5 meq/L); sodium 130 meq/L (136–145 meq/L); albumin 3.0 g/dL (3.5–5 g/dL); creatinine 2.5 mg/dL (0.7–1.5 mg/dL). A 24-h analysis of urine revealed proteinuria 3 g/day (0.1 g/day) and creatinine clearance 65 mL/mm (70–130 mL/min).

The nurse's diagnosis was disturbance of fluid and electrolyte balance with progressive edema associated with a medical diagnosis of nephrotic syndrome.

Management

The goal of therapy was to decrease edema and correct the electrolyte imbalance. B. S. was placed on fluid restriction (1000–1500 mL/day) for 3 days, after which a return to normal fluid intake was expected. Other prescription included 100 g/day protein (high-protein) diet and 1 g/day sodium (low-sodium). Temporary bed rest was recommended. Medications prescribed were prednisone 40 mg/day for 10 days and chlorothiazide 500 mg bid. Instructions were given to taper the prednisone dose over four additional days to avoid adverse effects from adrenal suppression.

The nurse advised B. S. to avoid prolonged periods of sitting or standing and to elevate his feet and legs frequently during the day. B. S. was instructed regarding the purposes for the prescribed treatment and medications.

The nurse provided him with information about what to expect from the treatment regimen, including any adverse effects of the prescribed medications. The nurse emphasized the symptoms of hypokalemia, because B. S. was at high risk of potassium depletion since he was taking both a corticosteroid and a thiazide diuretic. No potassium supplement was required at this time due to his elevated potassium level. He was told that the chlorothiazide would cause him to urinate and was instructed to take the doses with breakfast and lunch to avoid sleep disruption.

B. S. was informed that further diagnostic studies would be scheduled for future visits when they became appropriate or necessary. He was given an appointment to return to the clinic in 3 weeks.

Evaluation

On his return to the clinic, B. S. reported that he had had no headaches since 2 or 3 days after his last appointment. He said that he had taken the chlorothiazide as prescribed even though he was sometimes inconvenienced by the need to urinate frequently. No obvious edema of the eyelids was noted, and the edema of his feet was markedly decreased (+ pitting). His blood pressure had returned to 144/82 and pedal pulses were easily palpated. His weight had decreased by 4 kg. All serum electrolytes were within normal limits.

In response to questioning, B. S. reported that he had not experienced any symptoms of adverse effects of chlorothiazide therapy (e.g., calf muscle pain, generalized weakness, palpitations, joint pain, or stiffness). He said that he had followed the advice to take frequent rest periods during which he elevated his feet. B. S. indicated that he understood his condition by explaining that his salt-restricted diet and chlorothiazide therapy were associated with his increased urinary output and decreased dependent edema. He was able to describe the purposes of his therapy and identified the symptoms of adverse effects of the medication.

Because B. S. attained the desired goal of the therapeutic regimen without apparent adverse effects, the prescriber decided to keep him on chlorothiazide and the sodium restriction. The chlorothiazide was to be taken weekdays only (Monday through Friday) to avoid adverse effects.

Continuation of conservative measures (e.g., rest periods) was encouraged. His prognosis included the expectation of repeated episodes of acute nephrotic syndrome. Prednisone would be prescribed as needed in response to worsening of symptoms. B. S. would be monitored in clinic every 3 months unless his condition should warrant more frequent evaluations.

REFERENCES

Brater, D. C., and S. O. Thier: "Renal Disorders," in K. L. Melmon and H. F. Morelli (eds.): *Clinical Pharmacology: Basic Principles in Therapeutics,* New York: Macmillan, 1978.

Culbertson, V.: "Hypertension: 3. Assessment and Monitoring of the Hypertensive Patient," in M. Malone (ed.): *A Continuing Education Series in Pharmacy,* Stockton, CA: Cal Central Press, Accepted for publication in 1984.

Drug Information for the Health Care Provider, 1983 USPDI, Kingsport, TN: Kingsport, 1983.

"Indapamide for Hypertension and Edema," *Facts and Comparison Newsletter,* **26:** 47–48, 1983.

Isselbacher, K. J., R. Adams, E. Braunwald, R. Petersdorf, and J. Wilson (eds.): *Harrison's Principles of Internal Medicine,* 10th ed., New York: McGraw-Hill, 1983.

Kastrup, E. K. (ed.): *Facts and Comparisons,* Philadelphia: Lippincott, 1983.

Lawson, D., W. Tilstone, J. Gray, et al.: "Effect of Furosemide on the Pharmacokinetics of Gentamicin in Patients," *J Clin Pharmacol,* **22:**254–258, 1982.

Licht, J. H., R. J. Hale, B. Pugh, et al.: "Diuretic Regimens in Essential Hypertension: A Comparison of Hypokalemic Effects, BP Control, and Cost," *Arch Int Med,* **143:**1694–1699, 1983.

Mudge, G. H.: "Diuretics and Other Agents Employed in the Mobilization of Edema Fluid," in A. G. Gilman, L. S. Goodman, and A. Gilman (eds.): *Goodman and Gilman's Pharmacological Basis of Therapeutics,* 6th ed., New York: Macmillan, 1980.

Price, S. A., and L. M. Wilson: *Pathophysiology: Clinical Concepts of Disease Processes,* 2d ed., New York: McGraw-Hill, 1982.

Riddiough, M. A.: "Preventing, Detecting, and Management of Adverse Reactions in Antihypertensive Agents in the Ambulant Patient With Essential Hypertension," *Am J Hosp Pharm,* **34:**405–478, May 1977.

Stillwell, S. B.: "The Edematous Client: Causes, Physical Assessment and Treatment," *Nurse Pract,* **8:**21–27, 41, 1983.

Treseler, K. M.: *Clinical Laboratory Tests: Significance and Implications for Nursing,* Englewood Cliffs, NJ: Prentice-Hall, 1982.

Warnock, D. G.: "Diuretics," in B. G. Katzung (ed.), *Basic and Clinical Pharmacology,* Los Altos, CA: Lange, 1982.

Wright, N., and J. S. Rolson: "Renal Diseases," in G. S. Avery (ed.), *Drug Treatment: Principles and Practice of Clinical Pharmacology and Therapeutics,* 2d ed., New York: ADIS, 1980.

24

FLUID, ELECTROLYTE, AND ACID-BASE IMBALANCES

ANITA G. LORENZO
LEIGH K. KASZYK

LEARNING OBJECTIVES

Upon mastery of the contents of this chapter, the reader will be able to:

1. State the four main goals of management of fluid and electrolyte disorders.
2. Describe the functions of sodium, potassium, plasma proteins, and hydrostatic pressure in maintaining normal fluid balance.
3. List the most common causes of hypovolemia and hypervolemia.
4. Describe the assessment of fluid balance status.
5. Explain the principles of selection of dose, rate, route, and type of solution to treat hypovolemia.
6. Distinguish dextrose solutions, crystalloids, and colloids according to uses and precautions.
7. Explain the terms *isotonic, hypertonic,* and *hypotonic,* giving examples of intravenous (IV) solutions with each property.
8. Explain the hazards of too-rapid removal of fluid excess.
9. Relate sodium and water physiology to osmolality balance.
10. Relate the physiologic function of potassium to the clinical findings in potassium imbalance.
11. List drugs which can cause hypokalemia and methods to prevent this effect.
12. Describe the factors that determine the dose, rate, and route of potassium replacement therapy.
13. State the precautions in administration of oral and parenteral potassium therapy.
14. Describe three methods to treat hyperkalemia.
15. Explain the precautions in administration of oral and parenteral calcium, phosphate, and magnesium replacement.
16. List drugs which can affect calcium balance and the mechanisms of these effects.
17. Explain the mechanism of antacids when used to treat hyperphosphatemia.
18. Explain how the elemental calcium content of an oral calcium supplement is calculated.
19. Describe the indications for intravenous sodium bicarbonate, tromethamine, sodium lactate, ammonium chloride, and hydrochloric acid solutions in acid-base imbalances.
20. Describe the nursing process related to fluid and electrolyte imbalances.

Common to many diseases and symptoms (e.g., vomiting, diarrhea, fever, hyperventilation) are aberrations in fluid and electrolyte balance. (See Fig. 24-1.) Furthermore, therapeutic modalities can cause fluid and electrolyte loss; overzealous or poorly monitored therapy may result in excesses of fluid or electrolytes. Nurses must be aware of patients who are at risk for fluid and electrolyte imbalances and implement measures to *prevent the occurrence* of those imbalances. When a disorder of fluid or electrolyte imbalance occurs, a primary goal is to treat or *remove the cause.* If this does not correct the imbalance or if the imbalance results in serious physiologic complications, direct measures are instituted to *restore normal fluid and electrolyte levels and/or to counteract the physiologic complications.* The clinical pharmacology and therapeutics and nursing process related to disorders in fluid, potassium, polyvalent ion (calcium, phosphate, and magnesium), and acid-base balance are described in this chapter.

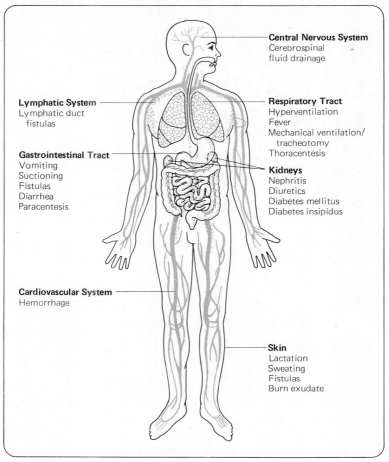

FIGURE 24-1

Routes of Abnormal Body Fluid and Electrolyte Losses. (*Adapted from Parenteral Products Division, Fundamentals of Body Water and Electrolytes. Reproduced with permission from Travenol Laboratories, Inc., copyright 1981, Travenol Laboratories, Inc. All rights reserved.*)

FLUID BALANCE

Normal Physiology

Distribution

Since there is virtually no water in neutral fat, total body water (TBW) constitutes 60 percent of the adult's body weight but varies with gender, age, and body fat. Obese individuals or adults over 60 years of age have only 45 to 50 percent of body weight present as water, whereas infants or emaciated patients may have 70 to 75 percent of body weight present as water.

Total body water is distributed into two major compartments, the extracellular fluid (ECF) and the intracellular fluid (ICF), as shown in Fig. 24-2. In an adult, the ECF is 15 percent of body weight, or approximately 12 L, and the ICF is 45 percent of body weight, or approximately 30 L. The extracellular fluid can be further divided into two compartments containing the interstitial fluid (environment around cells) and the plasma (intravascular fluid). Water found in dense connective tissues, bone, and epithelial secretions such as intraocular or synovial fluids is also part of the extracellular compartment.

Osmolality

The distribution of water into various body compartments is controlled primarily by osmotic forces. The osmotic activity of a compartment of fluid depends upon the number of particles per kilogram of water, or *osmolality,* which is expressed in units of milliosmoles per kilogram of water (mosmol/kg H_2O, or mosmol/L). Since water can move across the cell membrane that divides the extracellular fluid from intracellular fluid, the distribution of water between

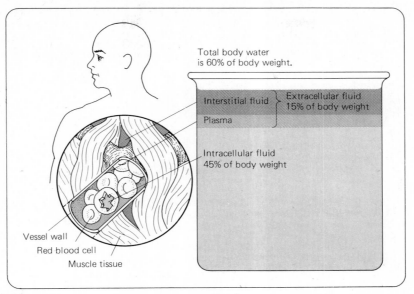

FIGURE 24-2

Body Fluid Compartments. (*Adapted from Parenteral Products Division, Fundamentals of Body Water and Electrolytes. Reproduced with permission from Travenol Laboratories, Inc., copyright 1981, Travenol Laboratories, Inc. All rights reserved.*)

the two compartments is determined by their osmolality. Sodium is the major contributor to the osmality of the ECF, although potassium plays this role in the ICF. If the osmolality of the compartment changes, water will move to restore osmotic equilibrium across the cell membrane.

The normal measured *plasma osmolality* (posmol) is 275 to 290 mosmol/L. Although urea is a solute in plasma, it can freely diffuse across cell membranes and does not act as an effective osmole to hold water in the extracellular space. Therefore, the effective posmol is less than the measured values and ranges between 270 and 285 mosmol/L. Only under abnormal circumstances does plasma glucose or urea become an important contributor to the plasma osmolality. Because of the close relation between the plasma sodium concentration and plasma osmolality, usually *hypo*natremia reflects *hypo*osmolality and *hyper*natremia represents *hyper*osmolality.

Sodium does not play an important role in the movement of water between capillary and interstitial spaces, because the concentration of sodium normally is the same in these two compartments (135 to 145 meq/L). The major osmotically active particles inside the capillaries are the plasma proteins (colloids), because such proteins cannot move across the capillary membrane. The plasma colloid osmotic pressure is also called the *oncotic pressure*. The pressure exerted by the plasma proteins pulls fluid into the capillaries from the interstitial fluid, thereby increasing the plasma volume. A counterbalancing force of blood perfusion pressure from the heart, termed *hydrostatic pressure,* pushes fluid out of the capillaries into the interstitial space. Opposing

forces exert counterbalancing effects at the arterial and venous end of the capillary to prevent the abnormal movement of fluids between compartments (Fig. 24-3); edema may result when these forces are not balanced (see Chap.23).

Regulation

Water homeostasis in the body is determined by a balance between intake and output. Normal daily water requirements for healthy adults and children are 1500 to 2000 mL per square meter (m^2) of body surface area. This daily intake of water may come from ingested liquids or foods, endogenous water production from metabolic processes, or parenteral fluids. In order to maintain a balance, a corresponding amount of water is lost from the body every day. The four major routes of fluid output include the kidney (60 percent), skin (20 percent), lung (15 percent), and intestine (5 percent). The daily fluid balance in an adult is outlined below.

INTAKE, mL		OUTPUT, mL	
Ingested	500–1700	Lung, skin	850–1200
Solids	800–1000	Intestine	50– 200
Endogenous	200– 300	Kidney	600–1600

Regulation of water homeostasis in the body is controlled by physiologic responses to changes in plasma osmolality and volume as shown in Fig. 24-4. Because of the close relation between plasma osmolality and plasma sodium concentration, the two are regulated by similar mechanisms. As plasma osmolality decreases (hypoosmolality) because of

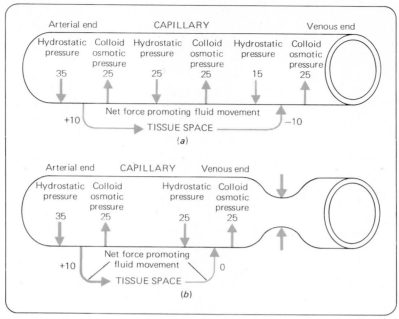

FIGURE 24-3

Mechanism of Edema in Vascular Occlusion. (*a*) Normal fluid movement across the capillary membrane. (*b*) Abnormal fluid distribution in edematous states. [*From P. J. Cannon and D. W. Seldin, "Physiology and Pharmacology of Edema," in M. H. Maxwell et al.* (eds.), The Patient with Edema. *Reprinted with the permission of the copyright holder, Hoechst-Roussel Pharmaceuticals, Inc., Somerville, NJ, 1976.*]

excess water in the body, hypothalamic osmoreceptors are stimulated. The central thirst mechanism and antidiuretic hormone (ADH or vasopressin) secretion are both suppressed. The decreased thirst drive retards fluid intake. Normally, ADH increases the permeability of the renal collecting duct cells to water, allowing reabsorption of large amounts of water filtered in the kidney. The absence of ADH prevents the reabsorption of renal water and increases urine output. The three other routes of water loss (lung, skin, and intestine) maintain relatively constant outputs.

Losses of fluid in the body, resulting in increased osmolality (hyperosmolality) and hypovolemia, trigger several physiologic regulatory processes. ADH is liberated to increase renal water absorption, the central thirst mechanism is stimulated, there are a decrease in glomerular filtration and an increase in proximal tubular reabsorption, and aldosterone is liberated by the adrenal cortex in the face of ECF losses. Aldosterone acts on the distal tubule to increase sodium reabsorption and therefore increase water retention. All these processes work to increase ECF volume and decrease plasma osmolality.

Hypovolemia

Etiology

A decrease in body fluid volume, termed *hypovolemia* or dehydration, may be due to derangements in the physiologic

regulation of water balance. Therefore, excess output via any of the four water elimination routes (intestines, kidneys, lungs, or skin) without compensatory increased intake will result in hypovolemia, but gastrointestinal and renal losses are most frequent. The common finding in many dehydrated patients is the loss of gastrointestinal tract fluid by vomiting, nasogastric suction, diarrhea, fistulas, surgical drains, or bleeding. Renal losses may be due to diuretics, hyperglycemia, diabetes insipidus, or hypoaldosteronism. Other causes of hypovolemia include increased skin and lung water losses when patients have a fever or burns. Sequestration of fluid into a space away from the ECF and ICF, termed *third space losses,* may result in hypovolemia. Potential third space losses occur in patients with peritonitis, pancreatitis, crush injuries, and intestinal obstruction and after abdominal surgery. Finally, patients who are comatose or nonambulatory, as well as young children who cannot ask for water, may become dehydrated.

Assessment

The manifestations of hypovolemia are a result of fluid deficits in the extracellular compartment as well as the various electrolyte and acid-base disorders that may accompany the deficits. Hypovolemia results in increased thirst, dry mucous membranes, postural dizziness, decreased skin turgor, weight loss, and lethargy. Hypovolemia will manifest as

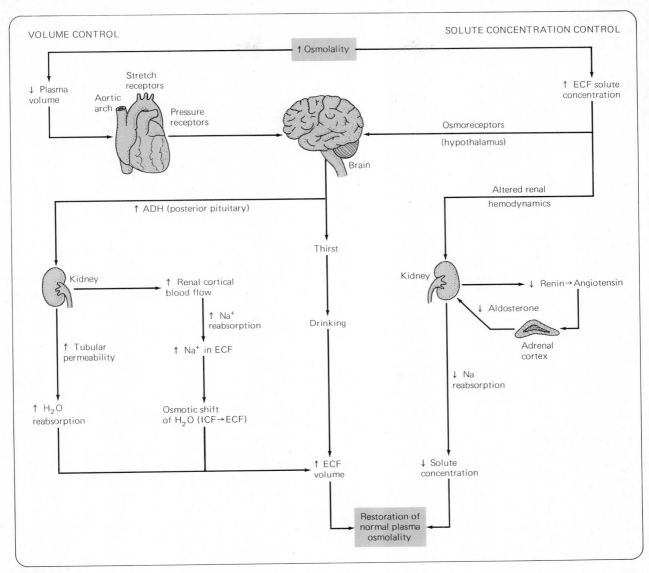

FIGURE 24-4

Regulation of Plasma Osmolality. Under normal conditions plasma osmolality is a function of volume and number of osmotically active particles (solute concentration). Volume is sensed by stretch receptors and pressure receptors in the aortic arch and elsewhere. Volume is controlled by the effects of antidiuretic hormone (ADH) from the posterior pituitary on renal blood flow distribution and renal tubular permeability. Osmotic shifts of the ICF to the ECF also affect plasma volume. Solute concentration of ECF is largely regulated through the renin-angiotensin-aldosterone axis, which controls sodium (Na⁺) reabsorption at the kidney. (*After Weil and Bailie, 1977.*)

shock when tissue perfusion becomes severely compromised. Tachycardia, hypotension, and coma may ensue. Laboratory values that become deranged in hypovolemia include high urine and serum osmolality (750 to 1400 mosmol/L and 280 to 295 mosmol/L, respectively), a blood urea nitrogen to serum creatinine ratio greater than 10 to 15, low urine output (< 20 to 40 mL/h), and concentrated hematocrit. Plasma sodium may be unchanged, decreased, or increased, depending upon the concentration of sodium in the fluids lost from the body and the sodium content of any fluids administered or ingested.

The classification of hypovolemia may be based upon degree of weight loss or symptomatology. Mild deficits are seen with loss of 5 percent of body weight (50 mL/kg) in infants and loss of 3 percent of body weight (30 mL/kg) in older children and adults. Similar estimates can be made to determine moderate (10 percent or 100 mL/kg, infant; 6 percent or 60 mL/kg, adult) and severe (15 percent or 150 mL/kg, infant; 9 percent or 90 mL/kg, adult) deficits.

Management

Prevention of hypovolemia involves identification of those patients at risk (i.e., those whose fluid output exceeds or potentially exceeds intake) and assurance that daily intake approximates output. Nonedematous patients with normal renal function should be encouraged to drink *at least* 3 to 5 glassfuls (750 to 1250 mL) of fluid daily, especially if taking diuretics. Confused or activity-restricted people require access to palatable fluids and reminders to drink. Those not eating solid foods will need to acquire the 800 to 1000 mL normally derived from the diet through other sources. Elevated temperature and hyperventilation increase insensible losses and must be considered in planning fluid requirments.

The goal of therapy in patients with hypovolemia is to reverse the symptoms and signs of fluid deficit while minimizing the risk of fluid overload. Elimination of any etiologic factors, if possible, should be a primary objective of treatment. This may be a change in drug regimens, such as discontinuing or decreasing doses of diuretics, or treatment of an infectious diarrheal illness in order to limit gastrointestinal losses. In some cases, the precipitating event cannot be remedied immediately, as in the example of a patient with third space losses after trauma to the abdominal viscera or a patient with a chronic, draining gastrointestinal fistula. In these cases, the excess losses of fluid should be estimated and replaced on a daily basis. Sometimes the clinician has the opportunity to actually measure the amount and electrolyte concentration of the fluid loss. For example, the drainage from a patient with gastric outlet obstruction and nasogastric suction may be collected and measured. If it contains 35 meq/L of sodium, 10 meq/L of potassium, and 45 meq/L of chloride, then *a solution of similar composition* should be administered at a rate equal to the output.

In order to correct the hypovolemia, the total body deficit plus maintenance fluid requirement must be administered concomitantly. Daily fluid *maintenance* requirements are 1500 mL/m^2 in children and adults. Replacement of fluid *deficits* requires careful planning of the dose, rate, route, and composition of the solution for administration.

Dose The degree of dehydration (mild, moderate, or severe) gives an initial estimation of the replacement dose. However, patients lose fluid and sodium in varying ratios, and there are no formulas that will provide exact replacement of both deficits for *every* patient. The best method is to estimate the replacement dose as shown in Table 24-1 and then to evaluate the adequacy of this initial replacement dose by the degree of reversal of clinical manifestations of hypovolemia, using both physical signs and laboratory values.

Rate The rate of volume replacement also depends upon the severity of the patient's signs and symptoms. A patient in shock with urine output less than 0.5 mL/kg/h, mental status changes, systolic blood pressure less than 90 mmHg, central venous pressure less than 5 mmHg, cardiac index less than 2.2 L/min/m^2, tachycardia, hypoxemia, and collapsed peripheral veins requires immediate resuscitation with volume. Parenteral fluids at a rate of 350 to 500 mL/m^2/h should be administered. The patient's requirements should be reassessed in 2 h and the rate of infusion may be decreased to 3000 mL/m^2/day when the vital signs stabilize. Less severe volume deficits require administration of fluids at a lower rate. Once the patient becomes asymptomatic, the remaining volume deficit can be gradually replaced over the next 2 to 5 days.

Route The enteral route is the preferred route of administration of water in order to minimize complications secondary to intravenous catheters. The exceptions are patients who cannot tolerate or should not be administered enteral fluids. Any patient with severe hypovolemia or hypovolemic shock should have immediate resuscitation with parenteral fluids, preferably with a central venous catheter.

Composition of Solution The composition of the replacement solution depends upon the plasma osmolality, serum electrolytes, and acid-base balance, as well as the etiology, type, and degree of fluid loss (refer to Table 24-1). In general, patients with mild deficits should be administered solutions containing 30 to 80 meq/L of NaCl (0.2 to 0.45% NaCl) with 5% dextrose and maintenance amounts of potassium. Patients with moderate to severe deficits require varying concentrations of NaCl in the replacement solution, depending upon the plasma osmolality. *Hyperosmolality states necessitate hypotonic solutions* containing 30 to 80 meq/L of NaCl, and *hypoosmolality states need isotonic to hypertonic solutions* containing 140 to 500 meq/L of NaCl (see the following section, Osmolality Imbalances).

For patients in hypovolemic shock, controversy surrounds the appropriate type of replacement fluids. There is actually a role for both electrolyte solutions (crystalloids) and plasma expanders (colloids). The only type of solution that is not appropriate is free water or pure dextrose in water. Initial volume replacement with a crystalloid solution is adequate and preferred. Plasma expanders are confined to the vascular space and will not replace interstitial deficits. In addition, patients who have lost large amounts of sodium and colloidal solutions may not adequately replenish these losses. The primary indications for colloid solutions are clinical situations where protein is lost, e.g., for burn patients requiring albumin replacement and bleeding patients requiring blood or blood component replacement.

Associated Disorders Patients may also experience problems associated with the hypovolemia. *Hypoxemia* requires oxygen administration and, if severe, mechanical ventilation. *Electrolyte deficits,* determined by serum electrolytes, can be corrected by replacement doses added to the sodium chloride solution. Unless the patient is symptomatic, the correction of electrolyte deficits is secondary to restoration of adequate volume. Potassium doses are usually withheld until the establishment of adequate urine output (see section on potassium therapy). *Metabolic and/or respiratory acidosis* are common and will usually reverse with establishment of adequate tissue and lung perfusion. Sodium bicarbonate should not be administered unless the arterial pH falls below 7.2 units (see section on acidemia therapy). *Oliguria* will also usually reverse with adequate volume repletion and kidney perfusion. Intravenous diuretics such as **mannitol** and **furosemide** (Lasix) may be administered to increase renal perfusion but have not been shown to prevent acute tubular necrosis and renal failure due to inadequate perfusion in hypovolemia.

Evaluation

With adequate fluid volume replacement the indicators of dehydration, including urine output, weight, skin turgor, serum urea nitrogen, central venous pressure, and blood pressure, return to normal ranges. One sensitive and non-invasive parameter to monitor is the *urine sodium concentration.* A urine sodium value that has increased to greater than 15 meq/L during fluid therapy indicates adequate replacement, because sodium excretion is liberalized once normal volumes are attained.

Adverse Effects Table 24-2 illustrates that adverse effects of parenteral fluid therapy relate to (1) contaminants, (2) immunlogic/allergic responses of the recipient, and (3) method of administration. Minimizing the hazards associated with administration is a particularly important nursing responsibility. One category is those hazards associated with intravenous cannulation, such as thrombophlebitis, infection, air embolism, and particle thrombosis. The second category includes fluid overload caused by excessive speed of infusion.

Careful observation for fluid overload is maintained during fluid therapy, particularly in patients with congestive heart failure, renal insufficiency, cirrhosis, or malnutrition. Fluid overload is indicated by weight gain, basilar rales, dependent edema, venous distention, and increased blood pressure.

TABLE 24-1 Therapy of Hypovolemia and Dysnatremia*

VOLUME DEFICIT	REPLACEMENT RATE AND DOSE	ADMINSTRATION ROUTE†	NaCl SOLUTION,‡ meq/L (g/dL)
None	1500 mL/m²/day	Enteral	30–40 (0.20)
Mild	2000 mL/m²/day	Enteral (preferred)	
With hyponatremia			70–80 (0.45)
With normonatremia			30–40 (0.20)
With hypernatremia			30–40 (0.20)
Moderate	2500 mL/m²/day	Enteral (preferred)	
With hyponatremia			140–150 (0.90)
With normonatremia			70–80 (0.45)
With hypernatremia			30–40 (0.20)
Severe	3000 mL/m²/day	Intravenous (preferred)	
With hyponatremia			500 (3.00)
With normonatremia			140–150 (0.90)
With hypernatremia			70–80 (0.45)
Shock§	350–500 mL/m²/h for 2 h, then 3000 mL/m²/day	Intravenous (only)	140–150 (0.90)

*The dysnatremias (hyponatremia and hypernatremia) represent the osmolality disorders (hypoosmolality and hyperosmolality) except in rare cases such as hyperglycemic states inducing hyponatremia and hyperosmolality.

†Intravenous route is used whenever the patient can not tolerate or should not be administered fluids via the enteral route.

‡Dextrose (5 to 10%) and other electrolytes may be added to the NaCl solution if needed. Strength of sodium chloride solution expressed in milliequivalents per liter and (grams per 100 milliliters). 0.90 NaCl commonly referred to as normal saline; 0.45 NaCl as half normal saline; 0.20 NaCl as one-fourth normal saline.

§Initial volume replacement with a NaCl solution (crystalloid) is adequate and preferred; however, whole blood or components (colloid) should also be transfused if there is significant blood or protein loss.

TABLE 24-2 Adverse Effects of Parenteral Fluid Therapy

CAUSE	REACTION	CLINICAL MANIFESTATIONS	FACTORS INCREASING SUSCEPTIBILITY	TO PREVENT OR MINIMIZE REACTION
Elements contained in the fluid	Pyrogenic, embolic, vasomotor	Rise in temperature, severe chills, cyanosis, circulatory collapse	Febrile diseases, liver diseases, hypoproteinemia	Use only sterile, pyrogen-free solutions and apparatus
	Posttransfusion hepatitis	Homologous serum jaundice		Use pasteurized blood fractions
Method of administration	Speed reactions	Circulatory overload, cardiac failure	Cardiac decompensation	Avoid too rapid administration
	Embolic	Air embolism		Replace air in tubing with solution before injecting. Stop injection with 2 or 3 mL still remaining in receptacle
	Thrombotic	Trauma to walls of vein	Poor nutritive state, low serum protein level	Avoid constant use of same vein
	Tissue necrosis	Edema		Reduce fluid volume. Be sure needle remains constant in vein
Specific incompatibility of recipient	Hemolytic	Chills, nausea and vomiting, lumbar pain, abdominal cramps, oliguria	Blood group incompatibility, Rh type incompatibility, hemolytic anemia	Administer cross-matched blood
	Allergic	Urticaria, angioneurotic edema, asthma	Recipient sensitivity to allergens in donor plasma	Interrupt infusion at first sign of reaction

Source: *Parenteral Solutions Handbook,* Berkeley, CA: Cutter Medical, Division of Miles Laboratories, Inc., 1979. Used by permission.

Available IV Solutions

Intravenous solutions can be classified as sources of free water and calories, crystalloids, and colloids. Agents used for total parenteral nutrition are discussed in Chap. 25. Dextrose (glucose) solutions are the most common sources of free water and calories. *Crystalloids* are ionic solutions, whereas *colloids* consist of large molecules (such as proteins or sugar polymers) dispersed in liquids.

Sources of Free Water and Calories Dextrose solutions (Table 24-3) are available in concentrations of 2.5, 5, 10, 20, 40, 50, 60, and 70 g per 100 mL (2½%, 5%, 10%, 20%, 40%, 50%, 60%, and 70% solutions, respectively). When the sugar in the solution is metabolized, free water is available to the body. Five percent dextrose solutions (abbreviated D_5W for 5% dextrose in water) are isotonic. Since 1 L of D_5W supplies only 170 calories, hypertonic solutions that supply more calories in less fluid volume are marketed. Solutions greater than 10% should be administered by central venous catheter, as they are irritating to peripheral veins. Glycosuria will result if dextrose is administered at rates greater than 0.5 g

dextrose/kg per hour and requires monitoring of blood and urine glucose levels. Electrolytes can be added to dextrose solutions, and D_5W is a common vehicle for the administration of intravenous medications.

Crystalloids Sodium chloride solutions (saline) comprise the basic crystalloid solutions (Table 24-3). Saline solutions approximately equal to the sodium chloride concentration of blood (0.9%) are isotonic and are termed **normal saline** (NS). Hypertonic solutions of 3 and 5% sodium chloride are available; hypotonic solutions of 0.45% sodium chloride are termed "half normal saline," or ½ NS. Combined saline and dextrose solutions are marketed, for example, 5% dextrose in 0.2% sodium chloride (D_5W¼ NS).

More than 100 different crystalloid solutions are marketed in the United States. *Polyionic products* (e.g., **lactated Ringer's**) are claimed to contain "balanced" mixtures of electrolytes; however, there are no proven advantages to using these solutions. A combination of dextrose and sodium chloride with potassium and other electrolytes added according to the individual patient requirements is

TABLE 24-3 Crystalloid Solutions and Sources of Free Water*

SOLUTION TYPES (EXAMPLES)	PRIMARY INDICATIONS	DEXTROSE, g/L	Electrolytes, meq/L						OSMOLALITY, mosmol/L	Cal/L
			Na$^+$	K$^+$	Cl$^-$	Ca^{2+}	Mg^{2+}	LACTATE		
Dextrose solutions	Free water, calorie source									
D$_5$W		50							253	170
D$_{10}$W		100							505	340
D$_{50}$W		500							2526	1700
Saline solutions	Volume deficits, hyponatremia									
0.45% sodium chloride (½ NS)			77		77				154	
0.9% sodium chloride (NS)			154		154				308	
3% normal saline			513		513				1026	
Dextrose/saline solution	Volume deficits									
Dextrose 5% in 0.2% sodium chloride (D$_5$W ¼ NS)		50	34		34				324	170
Dextrose 5% in 0.45% sodium chloride (D$_5$W ½ NS)		50	154		154				561	170
Dextrose 10% in 0.45% sodium chloride (D$_{10}$W ½ NS)		100	77		77				660	340
Potassium solutions	Maintenance fluid, replacement fluid									
Dextrose 5% in 0.2% sodium chloride, 15% potassium chloride		50	34	20	54				360	170
Dextrose 5% in a 0.45% sodium chloride, 15% potassium chloride		50	77	20	97				445	170
Dextrose 5% in 0.45% sodium chloride, 20 meq potassium chloride		50	77	20	97				445	170
Polyionic solutions	Maintenance fluids, replacement fluids									
Ringer's injection			147	4	156	5			309	
Lactated Ringer's injection			130	4	109	3		28	272	
Lytren†		75	30	25	25	4	4			255
Pedialyte†		50	30	25	30	4	4			70

*Pure water is never given intravenously, as it would cause hemolysis.
†Lytren and Pedialyte are polyionic solutions for enteral administration.

preferable to these fixed combinations. *Multiple-electrolyte products* for oral use (Lytren, Pedialyte) are also available (Table 24-3).

Colloids Colloids (Table 24-4) are termed *plasma expanders* because they function physiologically like plasma proteins in maintaining oncotic pressure and blood volume. Human plasma is the source for several colloidal solutions (**albumin** and **plasma protein fraction**), and others are large polysaccharide chains (**dextran** and **hetastarch**).

Plasma protein fraction contains albumin and globulins. Both albumin and plasma protein fraction can cause hypotension if administered at rates greater than 10 mL/min.

Blood pressure should be monitored during the infusion, and the rate should be slowed or discontinued if hypotension occurs. Allergic or pyrogenic reactions, manifested mainly by fever and chills, can occur and require discontinuation of the infusion. Because of the increased protein load, patients with renal or hepatic failure should be monitored carefully if albumin or plasma protein fraction is administered.

Anaphylaxis or milder hypersensitivity reactions also occur with hetastarch and dextran, although they are significantly less common with low molecular weight dextran (Dextran 40) than with high molecular weight dextran (Dextran 70). These agents retard coagulation, and dextran 40 is used in doses of 500 to 1000 mL/day to prevent thrombosis following surgery. Patients receiving multiple infusions of hetastarch or dextran should be observed for bleeding.

Hypervolemia and Edema

Excess fluid circulating in the intravascular space is termed *hypervolemia* and can result from too-rapid administration of fluid. However, the most common state of excess fluid is an expansion of the interstitial fluid volume, known as *edema* (see Chap. 23, "Edema"). The primary etiology of edema is not an imbalance in the regulation of input versus output of water, but an imbalance of the distribution of water. Fluid overload is only life-threatening if *pulmonary edema* is present. Pulmonary edema necessitates immediate therapy, as discussed in Chap. 43. In other fluid excess states removal of excess fluid should proceed very slowly, since fluid is initially lost from the intravascular space. Fluid from the interstitial space then equilibrates with the intravascular space. There is a net movement of fluid out of the interstitial space to be excreted in the urine. However, the equilibration process can take place no faster than about 2 to 3 L in 24 h for peripheral edema and 0.5 L in 24 h for ascitic fluid (peritoneal cavity). Removal of fluid at faster rates results in intravascular volume depletion and all the manifestations and risks of hypovolemia.

Osmolality Imbalances

Hypervolemia and hypovolemia are imbalances of *fluid volume,* whereas hypoosmolality and hyperosmolality are imbalances of the *concentration of solutes* in the fluid. Because sodium is the major osmotically active solute in the ECF, in most cases hyperosmolality represents hypernatremia and hypoosmolality represents hyponatremia.

Etiology

Hypoosmolality

Although hyponatremia (hypoosmolality) theoretically could be caused by pure sodium loss, this condition does not occur. The common etiology in hypoosmolal syndromes is either water retention or net sodium loss. Administration of diuretics, loss of volume (burns, vomiting), as well as dysfunction of kidneys and adrenals are the most frequent causes. Another mechanism for abnormal water retention and hyponatremia is the *syndrome of inappropriate antidiuretic hormone secretion* (SIADH). Neurologic disorders (meningitis, tumors); certain drugs (**chlorpropamide, vincristine, cyclophosphamide, carbamazepine, vasopressin, and oxytocin**); pulmonary disorders (tuberculosis, oat-cell carcinoma); and postoperative stress may all cause SIADH and hypoosmolality.

In a few conditions, hyponatremia and hypoosmolality *do not* occur concurrently. Severe hyperlipidemia (lipid clearance disorders), severe hyperproteinemia (multiple myeloma), or isotonic glycine flushes (following transurethral resections of prostate) may displace plasma sodium and cause a pseudohyponatremia with normal osmolality. Another exception is diabetic ketoacidosis (DKA), in which the plasma glucose is increased because of insulin insufficiency, but the plasma sodium is decreased as a result of a combination of vomiting and polyuria accompanied by a salt-free water intake. When a patient in DKA exhibits extremely elevated plasma glucose levels (950 mg/100 mL), low plasma sodium levels and symptoms of *hyper*osmolality, the hyperosmolality and the hyperglycemia, rather than the serum sodium value, are treated.

Hyperosmolality A common factor in most hypernatremia (hyperosmolality) states is water loss. A less frequent cause is sodium excess as with administration of hypertonic

TABLE 24-4 Colloid Solutions

GENERIC NAME (BRAND)	SOLUTION COMPOSITION*	CONCENTRATION, % OR g/dL	INITIAL IV DOSE, mL/kg	ADVERSE EFFECTS
Normal serum albumin (Albuminar, Buminate, others)	Human albumin Human albumin	5 25	5.0 0.3	Hypotension, allergy
Dextran (Gentran, Rheomacrodex, Macrodex, others)	Dextran 40 Dextran 70, 75	10 6	20 20	Alter coagulation, hypersensitivity
Hetastarch (Hespan)	Hydroxyethyl-starch	6	20	Alter coagulation, anaphylaxis
Plasma protein fraction (Plasmanate, Plasmatein, others)	Plasma proteins	5	5.0	Hypotension, allergy

*All solutions contain approximately 150 meq/L of sodium chloride (0.9% NaCl).

sodium chloride solutions or improperly diluted infant formulas. Water deficits leading to hyperosmolality include insensible loss (burns, sweating); renal loss (diabetes insipidus, osmotic diuresis); and hypothalamic dysfunction (hypodipsia). Diabetes insipidus is divided into two clinical categories. Complete or partial failure of ADH secretion is called central diabetes insipidus (CDI), and failure of ADH effect on the kidney tubule is called nephrogenic diabetes insipidus (NDI). Neurologic disorders (meningitis, tumors) and trauma may cause CDI. NDI may be a result of acute and chronic renal failure, sickle cell anemia, hypercalcemia, hypokalemia, or administration of **diuretics**, **lithium**, or **demeclocycline**.

Assessment

The *signs and symptoms of hypoosmolality* (hyponatremia) are due to the movement of water from an area of low osmolality (extracellular fluid) to an area of high osmolality (intracellular fluid). The cellular overhydration results in the symptoms of nausea, malaise, headache, and lethargy. Seizures and coma can occur with plasma sodium concentrations less than 100 meq/L or with rapid drops in the plasma sodium concentration.

Symptomatic hypernatremia (hyperosmolality) virtually never occurs if there are an intact thirst mechanism and free access to water. Patients with diabetes insipidus will complain of polydipsia and polyuria, which are due to their desire to drink water triggered by the hypernatremia (hyperosmolality). The *signs and symptoms of hyperosmolality* are due to the movement of water from the area of low osmolality (intracellular fluid) to an area of high osmolality (extracellular fluid). The cellular dehydration results in dry, sticky mucous membranes, rubbery tissue turgor; and the neurologic symptoms of lethargy, muscle weakness, hyperreflexia, seizures, and coma. The presence of symptoms is related both to the absolute degree of hyperosmolality and to the rate of rise in the effective plasma osmolality.

Before any therapy is initiated for osmolality disorders, the patient must have an adequate assessment of the severity of the osmolality disturbance. The serum electrolytes, plasma and urine osmolality, mental status, vital signs, input and output, and physical exam should be performed and recorded as a baseline.

Management

The goal of therapy in patients with osmolality imbalances is reversal of the signs and symptoms of neurologic dysfunction, not necessarily normalization of the serum sodium value. A patient with hypoosmolality may have volume depletion (hypovolemia) with net sodium loss or volume expansion (edema) without sodium loss. Hyperosmolality cases may have net volume depletion (hypovolemia), with or without sodium loss, or volume expansion (edema) with sodium gain. Therapy depends upon the fluid, osmolality,

and sodium balance as well as the underlying disease state and is administered as described previously in the section on hypovolemia (Table 24-1) and Chap. 23. Additional therapy for specific disorders of osmolality is outlined in Table 24-5.

Evaluation

Rapid correction of osmolality imbalances can result in cerebral edema, seizures, and death. Meticulous attention to the intake and output of both sodium and water is required during therapy. Serum electrolytes, vital signs, and mental status must be monitored frequently.

POTASSIUM BALANCE

Normal Physiology

Distribution

Potassium is a vital cation for the normal function of the human cell. Ninety-eight percent of the potassium in the body is located in the intracellular compartment. The large amount of potassium in the intracellular compartment maintains an osmotic pressure to help keep fluid inside the cell. The difference between the concentration of potassium in the intracellular compartment and that in the extracellular compartment is maintained by an active metabolic pump. Potassium is maintained at a relatively constant value of 160 meq/L in the ICF. The concentration of the ECF is measured in the serum, and normal values range from 3.5 to 5.0 meq/L.

Function

The ratio of the intracellular fluid to the extracellular fluid potassium concentration ($ICF-K^+ : ECF-K^+$) is the principal determinant of cell membrane potential in excitable tissue such as cardiac and skeletal muscle. Since the concentration of potassium in the ECF is so much lower than the concentration inside the cell, small changes in the ECF potassium, as reflected by serum potassium values, can significantly alter this ratio. A high or low serum potassium value will increase or decrease cell excitability, respectively. Muscle weakness and/or cardiac dysrhythmias may result in either case.

Regulation

The homeostasis of potassium in the body is influenced by the distribution between ECF and ICF, as well as the balance between intake and output. Acid-base disorders and cellular metabolism may affect the serum potassium concentration. As the hydronium ion (H_3O^+) moves into the cell in metabolic acidosis, potassium is shifted into the ECF, resulting in higher serum potassium values. Decreases in serum potassium values occur with metabolic alkalosis. Potassium moves into the cell during the metabolic processes of gly-

TABLE 24-5 Management of Osmolality Imbalances

DISORDER OR CAUSE	IMBALANCE	MANAGEMENT
Hypoosmolality States		
Vomiting, fistula, diuretics, burns	Water and sodium deficit (sodium loss > water)	Treat hypovolemia
Heart failure, cirrhosis, nephrotic syndrome, renal failure	Excess water and sodium (water gain > sodium)	Treat edema
Adrenal insufficiency	Excess water; sodium deficit	Mineralocorticoid replacement
Syndrome of inappropriate ADH secretion (SIADH)	Excess water	Restrict fluids 3% NaCl plus furosemide Lithium, demeclocycline
Hyperosmolality States		
Fever, burns	Water and sodium deficit (water loss > sodium)	Treat hypovolemia
Central diabetes insipidus (CDI)	Water deficit	Fluids Desmopressin (DDAVP) Diuretics Carbamazepine, chlorpropamide, clofibrate (for partial CDI only)
Nephrogenic diabetes insipidus (NDI)	Water deficit	Fluids Diuretics
Hypothalamic dysfunction	Water deficit	Forced fluids Chlorpropamide (Diabinese)
Sodium overload	Excess sodium and water (sodium gain > water)	Diuretics Dialysis

cogen formation and protein synthesis. Insulin promotes the entry of potassium into skeletal muscle and hepatic cells. In contrast, breakdown of cells during trauma or other conditions results in release of potassium into the ECF. The primary route of elimination from the body is through secretion of potassium into the distal tubular lumen of nephrons. When stimulated by a low serum sodium, low blood volume, or high plasma potassium concentration, aldosterone acts on the distal tubule to increase the secretion of potassium.

Hypokalemia

Etiology

A decrease in the serum potassium, termed *hypokalemia*, may be due to derangements in the physiologic regulation of this electrolyte. Therefore, serum potassium may be abnormally low because of changes in the distribution between ICF and ECF or the balance between intake and output. Potassium may shift into the cell in patients developing metabolic alkalosis secondary to nasogastric suction or receiving large glucose loads as in hyperalimentation. Potassium entry may also occur during anemia therapy because of increased red blood cell production. Patients may lose excess potassium in the urine when treated with loop and **thiazide diuretics, corticosteroids** (e.g., **prednisone**), **carbenicillin**, high sodium diets, or low magnesium intakes. Vomiting, diarrhea, fistulas, ostomies, and drains or tubes may all cause losses of potassium from the gastrointestinal tract.

Assessment

Patients with hypokalemia may experience skeletal muscle dysfunction with muscle weakness or leg cramps and gastrointestinal smooth muscle dysfunction with constipation or abdominal distention. Common signs of hypokalemia include electrocardiogram changes such as inverted T waves and renal impairment noted by polyuria. Severe hypokalemia may cause respiratory muscle paralysis, paralytic ileus, and cardiac dysrhythmias. It is important to remember that patients can have low serum potassium values and be asymptomatic, especially if the hypokalemia developed over a long period of time. Before any therapy is initiated, the patient must have an adequate assessment of the severity of the hypokalemia. Monitoring of the electrocardiogram, respiratory muscle function, skeletal muscle function, gastrointestinal tract function, and serum potassium (including an initial and repeat level to rule out laboratory error) should be performed.

Management

Prevention of hypokalemia in patients who have excessive losses, such as those taking potassium depleting diuretics (**thiazides** and related diuretics, **furosemide**, and so on) or **corticosteroids**, may be accomplished by teaching the patient to consume a diet high in potassium and low in sodium (Table 24-6). It should be pointed out to patients that most high potassium food is also high in calories, and this aspect must be considered in menu planning. Since low potassium predisposes patients taking digitalis glycosides (e.g., **digoxin**) to dangerous toxicity, many clinicians institute prophylactic oral potassium supplements for patients taking potassium-depleting diuretics and digitalis drugs concurrently and for those with prior history of drug-induced hypokalemia. An alternative to potassium supplements is the addition of a potassium-sparing diuretic, such as **spironolactone** (Aldac-

tone), **amiloride hydrochloride** (Midamor), or **triamterene** (Dyrenium) to the patients' drug therapy regimen (see Chap. 23).

The goal of therapy in patients with hypokalemia is reversal of the symptoms and signs of neuromuscular dysfunction, which is not necessarily synonymous with normalization of the serum potassium value. Elimination of any etiologic factors, if possible, is the primary objective. Patients may need to have changes in drug regimens, such as converting to a corticosteroid with minimal mineralocorticoid activity (e.e., **triamcinolone, dexamethasone**). Treatment of an infectious diarrheal illness may limit gastrointestinal losses. At other times, the precipitating event cannot be remedied immediately, as in the example of a patient with continual drainage of a small bowel fistula. In these cases, the excess losses of potassium should be estimated or mea-

TABLE 24-6   Potassium, Sodium, and Calorie Content of Selected Foods

FOOD	AMOUNT*	POTASSIUM, meq	SODIUM, meq	CAL	FOOD	AMOUNT*	POTASSIUM, meq	SODIUM, meq	CAL
Vegetables					*Fruits*				
Asparagus	½ cup	4.7	—	15	Apple	1 small	2.3	—	70
Beans					Apricots				
Dried, cooked	½ cup	10.0	—	55–75	Canned	½ cup	6.0	—	110
Lima	½ cup	9.5	—	130	Dried	4 halves	5.0	—	39
Bean sprouts	½ cup	4.0	—	17	Fresh	3 small	8.0	—	55
Beet greens	½ cup	8.5	3.0	13	Avocado	⅛	4.6	—	46
Broccoli	½ cup	7.0	—	20	Banana	1 small	9.6	—	100
Cabbage, raw	1 cup	6.0	0.9	15	Cantaloupe	½ small	13.0	—	60
Carrots, raw	1 cup	8.8	2.0	20	Figs, dried	1	2.5	—	60
Celery, raw	1 cup	9.0	5.4	15	Peach	1 medium	6.2	—	35
Collards	½ cup	6.0	0.8	28	Strawberries	1 cup	6.3	—	55
Green beans					Raisins	1½ tbsp	4.3	—	40
Fresh/frozen	½ cup	4.0	—	15	Rhubarb	½ cup	6.5	—	193
Canned	½ cup	2.5	10.0	23	Watermelon	½ slice	5.0	—	58
Mustard greens	½ cup	5.5	0.8	18					
Peas					*Meat*				
Dried, cooked	½ cup	6.8	1.5	145	Beef	3 oz	8.4	2.4	245
Canned	½ cup	1.2	10.0	84	Chicken	3 oz	9.0	3.0	115
Fresh	½ cup	2.5	—	58	Frankfurters	1	3.0	24.0	170
Potatoes					Liver	3 oz	9.6	7.2	195
Baked, white	½ cup	13.0	—	90	Pork	3 oz	9.0	2.7	310
Boiled, white	½ cup	7.3	—	80	Veal	3 oz	11.4	3.0	185
Spinach	½ cup	8.5	—	20	Tuna				
Tomatoes	½ cup	6.5	—	40	Fresh	¼ cup	2.3	0.6	100
Squash					Canned	¼ cup	2.6	4.6	170
Winter, baked	½ cup	12.0	—	65					
Winter, boiled	½ cup	6.5	—		*Miscellaneous*				
Milk					Peanut butter	2 tbsp	4.5	7.8	190
Whole	1 cup	8.8	5.2	160	Cheese				
Buttermilk	1 cup	8.5	13.6	90	American	1 slice	0.6	9.1	105
Skim	1 cup	8.8	5.2	90	Cottage	¼ cup	1.1	5.0	65
Powdered, skim	¼ cup	13.5	6.9	61	Egg	1	1.8	2.7	74

*Approximate.

sured and replaced on a daily basis. Assessment of potassium loss may involve both measurement of total volume of drainage and laboratory determination of potassium concentration in samples of drainage.

In order to correct the hypokalemia, the total body deficit and maintenance needs of potassium must be administered concomitantly. Daily maintenance requirements are 50 meq/m² in children and adults. Generally, potassium deficits are corrected by administration of potassium salts, but mild deficits may be treated with the potassium-sparing diuretic **spironolactone** (Aldactone, others) in doses of 25 to 100 mg daily (see Chap. 23). Replacement of the potassium deficit requires careful planning of the dose, rate, and route for administration.

Dose The dose of potassium required to replace the deficit depends upon total body losses of potassium in *both the ICF and the ECF.* The serum potassium values (ECF-K) do not correlate with the total amount of body losses. For example, the serum potassium concentration may only have decreased from 4 meq/L to 2 meq/L, but total body deficit may be 400 meq of potassium. Once enough potassium has been administered to render the patient asymptomatic, then the rest of the deficit can be replaced very slowly over the next 5 to 7 days.

Rate The rate of potassium replacement depends upon the severity of the patient's signs and symptoms. A patient with flaccid paralysis should receive intravenous potassium at a rate of up to 0.5 meq/kg over 60 min, whereas an asymptomatic patient should receive oral potassium at a rate of 20 to 40 meq/m² per day divided into two to four doses.

Route The route of administration depends on the severity of symptoms and the availability of enteral versus parenteral access. A patient with severe symptoms or a patient who cannot tolerate oral feedings needs intravenous potassium. Potassium may be administered peripherally or centrally, but the concentration of potassium should never exceed 80 meq in a liter bottle of intravenous solution to be given peripherally, since the potential for the entire dose of potassium to be infused into the patient in a very short period of time is always present. Such an event could result in rapid reversal of the hypokalemia to hyperkalemia with a resultant fatal dysrhythmia. Potassium may be given mixed in more concentrated solutions, if given via a central vein by using an infusion pump and continuous electrocardiographic monitoring.

Evaluation

Monitoring for efficacy and toxicity of potassium therapy is crucial. Whenever a patient is being given potassium by rapid intravenous infusion, continuous electrocardiographic monitoring is essential. The patient's serum potassium should be monitored hourly in this instance. Patients receiving oral potassium therapy require less vigorous monitoring, which includes observation for return of normal muscle function (bowel sounds, improved muscle tone), as well as serum potassium determinations. If the patient's fluid and electrolyte intake and output are stable, the serum potassium may not have to be monitored except once a month.

Adverse Effects Overtreatment causes hyperkalemia, manifested by oliguria, abdominal cramps, diarrhea, and electrocardiogram (ECG) changes of peaked T waves and arrhythmias. Before potassium is administered, adequate urinary output should be established to decrease the risk of hyperkalemia. During intravenous infusion the vein should be observed for phlebitis and the blood pressure monitored, as too-rapid infusion may cause vasodilation. Oral forms of potassium can cause gastrointestinal (GI) irritation, especially if administered with inadequate liquids. Enteric-coated and other slow release forms can cause bleeding or ulceration of the gastrointestinal tract, so the nurse should note abdominal pain; distention; black, tarry stools; and decreased hemotocrit levels.

Preparations and Administration

Potassium is available in several salts, including chloride, acetate, phosphate, gluconate, and combinations of several salts. In hypokalemic patients, whether administered intravenously or orally, potassium chloride is the salt of choice, because patients with potassium depletion often have concomitant metabolic alkalosis and hypochloremia, and the hypokalemia will not correct until the chloride is also replaced. In rare instances when hypokalemia is present with metabolic acidosis, potassium acetate can be used to correct both imbalances.

Parenteral Preparations Parenteral potassium is available in a variety of premixed solutions, containing 20 meq/L of potassium or less (Table 24-3). These are utilized for maintenance of a normal serum potassium in patients without oral intake. In treatment of severe hypokalemia the solution may have concentrations greater than 40 meq/L. Potassium salts are also available in highly concentrated solutions, packaged in vials of 10 to 50 mL. These concentrated solutions are *never* to be administered to the patient without prior dilution with a bulk parenteral solution. The undiluted concentrates contain as much as 3000 meq/L, and a very small dose could be fatal.

An excessive volume or rapid rate of infusion may cause hyperkalemia with resulting cardiac arrest due to the high serum concentrations of potassium. Parental potassium may be administered by central or peripheral veins. Intramuscular or subcutaneous administration is not recommended because of significant pain and irritation of these tissues. Nurses should consult with a hospital pharmacist or appropriate written reference on drug incompatibilities before adding any drug, including potassium, to an intravenous solution. Three rules are essential to remember when administering intravenous potassium:

1. Do not administer more than 80 meq of potassium per liter of solution.
2. Do not administer more than 10 meq/h.
3. Never break the above two rules without close monitoring of the patient's ECG and frequent serum potassium levels.

Oral Preparations It is always preferable to give potassium orally in order to prevent the potential complications of intravenous therapy. Potassium may be given as a liquid, effervescent tablets and granules, powder, or slow release tablets and capsules (Table 24-7). Liquids, granules, powders, and effervescent tablets must always be well diluted (in 240 mL) in some form of beverage, orange juice being the

most common type of dilutant as it has a high potassium content (5.7 meq K^+/120 mL). The usual regime for mild to moderate hypokalemia is 20 to 40 meq/m^2 per day given once or twice a day. Oral potassium preparations are irritating to the stomach mucosa; therefore, they should be administered with or after meals.

The salty taste of liquid oral potassium supplements makes them unpalatable to some patients. Inclusion of the liquid potassium supplement in a gelatin dessert or frozen juice bar sometimes allows patients to tolerate the taste and to avoid more expensive dosage forms. To prepare the gelatin form, the daily dosage of the potassium supplement is included as part of the liquid when the commercial gelatin (e.g., Jell-O) or homemade recipe is prepared. After the gelatin sets, it is cut into portions, one for each dose. Frozen juice bars can be similarly prepared.

TABLE 24-7 Oral Potassium Preparations

TRADE NAME	POTASSIUM CONTENT*	SALT
Liquids		
Kaochlor 10%, Kay Ciel, Klorvess 10% liquid	20 meq/15 mL	Chloride
Kaon Cl-20, Klor-Con 20%, Potachlor 20%	40 meq/15 mL	Chloride
Kaon, K-G elixir, Bayon	20 meq/15 mL	Gluconate
Bi-K, Twin-K, Duo-K	20 meq/15 mL	Combinations
Trikates, Tri-K	45 meq/15 mL	Combinations
Powder and Granules		
Kay Ciel, K-Lor, Klorvess (effervescent)	20 meq/unit	Chloride
Klor-Con/25, K-Lyte/Cl	25 meq/unit	Chloride
Capsules and Tablets		
Kaochlor-Eff, Klorvess, K-Lyte/Cl (effervescents)	20, 25, 50 meq/tab	Chloride or combinations
Potassium Cl (enteric coated)	4, 13.4 meq/tab	Chloride
Micro-K Extencaps (controlled release)	8 meq/cap	Chloride
Kaon Cl-10, Slow-K, Klotrix (wax matrix)	6.7, 8.0, 10 meq/tab	Chloride
K-Forte Regular, Osto-K (chewable with vitamin C)	1.0 meq/tab	Combinations
Kao-Nor, Kaon (plain)	2.5, 5 meq/tab	Gluconate

*Not all products are available in all strengths listed. Consult label or package insert for each product.

Hyperkalemia

Etiology

An increase in the serum potassium, termed *hyperkalemia* (>5.0 meq/L), may be due to derangements in the physiologic regulation of this electrolyte. Therefore, serum potassium may be abnormally high because of changes in the distribution between ICF and ECF, as well as the balance between intake and output. Potassium may shift out of the cells in patients with metabolic acidosis and insulin deficiency as in diabetic ketoacidosis. These patients may have high serum potassium concentrations even though total body stores of potassium are depleted. Excess potassium is released into the serum from cells when there are tissue damage and breakdown secondary to trauma or chemotherapy-induced cytotoxicity. Spurious elevations of serum potassium concentration can be observed when mechanical trauma during blood collection causes hemolysis of red blood cells, an example being the heel stick in infants.

There are three major clinical conditions in which the output of urinary potassium is inadequate: renal failure, ineffective or decreased aldosterone secretion, and volume depletion. *Any patient who has diminished renal function (whatever the cause may be) must be monitored for hyperkalemia.* Salt substitutes and drugs containing large amounts of potassium must be used with caution in order to prevent hyperkalemia. Ineffective or decreased aldosterone level prevents normal excretion of potassium in the urine. Potassium-sparing diuretics such as **spironolactone, triamterene,** and **amiloride hydrochloride** act upon the same site in the distal tubule as aldosterone to diminish potassium excretion. Serum potassium levels must be monitored in patients taking these diuretics to prevent hyperkalemia, especially if renal dysfunction is also present.

Hyperkalemia can be caused by excessive intake of potassium, in addition to the mechanisms of cellular shifts and decreased output mentioned above. Clinical examples of excessive intakes of potassium include the administration of stored blood that contains potassium released from red cells, intravenous solutions of potassium that are infused very quickly, and drugs that contain large amounts of potassium, such as some penicillins. Whatever the source of the potassium, excessive intakes are potentially fatal in the presence of renal failure.

Assessment

The cardiac conduction problems produced by hyperkalemia may result in ventricular fibrillation of asystole. These dysrhythmias are the potentially life threatening effects of hyperkalemia. Early changes of hyperkalemia that can be anticipated by monitoring the electrocardiogram include peaked T waves and a shortened QT interval; eventually the QRS complex widens. Severe hyperkalemia, serum concentrations greater than 8.0 meq/L, prevents repolarization of muscle cells, leading to muscle weakness and paralysis. An adequate assessment of the severity of the hyperkalemia includes the electrocardiogram, muscle function, and serum potassium (a repeat level).

Management

The goal of therapy in patients with hyperkalemia is reversal of the symptoms and signs of cardiac and neuromuscular dysfunction, not merely the normalization of the serum potassium value. Elimination of any etiologic factors, if possible, is the primary objective of therapy. Patients may need to have changes in drug regimens, such as converting to a diuretic that allows excretion of potassium instead of a potassium-sparing diuretic. They may require elimination of oral and intravenous potassium intake and repletion of volume status. At other times, the precipitating event can not be remedied, as in the example of a patient with renal failure. In these cases, dietary and intravenous intake of potassium must be minimized.

Treatment of hyperkalemia depends upon the severity of the patient's signs and symptoms. A patient with muscle weakness, ECG changes, or serum levels greater than 8 meq/L requires immediate therapy. **Calcium gluconate**, 5.0 to 10.0 mL of a 10% solution, is administered by intravenous push over 2 to 3 min in order to protect excitable membranes against the effects of hyperkalemia. The onset of action is within minutes but the duration of effect is transient (1 to 2 h). Calcium gluconate is preferred to calcium chloride because it has a much lower osmolality and does not cause thrombophlebitis or hyperosmolality. The next step is the intravenous administration of 100 to 200 mL of a **20% solution of glucose** ($D_{20}W$) containing 20 to 30 units of **regular insulin**, which helps to move potassium from the serum into the cells. **Sodium bicarbonate** (50 meq) may also be given intravenously to drive potassium into the cells, particularly if metabolic acidosis is present. The effects of glucose plus insulin and sodium bicarbonate therapy have a rapid onset and may last for hours. However, the underlying etiology of the hyperkalemia must still be corrected.

For patients with mild or absent signs and symptoms of hyperkalemia, treatment may be less aggressive. Diuretics such as **furosemide** will increase potassium excretion if renal function is adequate. Cation-exchange resins (**sodium polystyrene sulfonate**; Kayexalate) may be administered as oral or rectal solutions. Although both of these modalities actually eliminate potassium from the body, the onset of action is slow. In special cases, such as acute renal failure with trauma and chronic renal failure with anuria, peritonial dialysis and hemodialysis are used to remove potassium from the body.

Evaluation

In severe hyperkalemia the ECG should be monitored constantly, since there is danger of dysrhythmias as long as the serum potassium level is elevated. The nurse should observe for decreased peaking of the T waves and lengthening of the QT interval as the patient improves. Serum potassium and muscle strength are monitored every 1–2 h. When calcium gluconate, glucose-insulin infusions, and sodium bicarbonate are used to lower the serum potassium or to protect excitable tissues, the serum calcium, glucose, and pH should also be monitored. Since these drugs provide only temporary benefit, monitoring continues even after the patient begins to improve. Development of confusion, muscle weakness, and ECG changes (flattening or inversion of the T waves and prominent U waves) may indicate hypokalemia resulting from overtreatment. It is also important to evaluate urine output and other indicators of renal function. When the patient is taking oral therapy to reduce the serum potassium, such as diuretics or an ion exchange resin, it is important to remember that there will be a lag between the initiation of therapy and the achievement of the desired therapeutic endpoint because these agents work relatively slowly.

Sodium Polystyrene Sulfonate (Kayexalate)

Sodium polystyrene sulfonate is an ion exchange resin which takes up potassium and liberates sodium as it passes through the large intestine. The effectiveness of this agent in treating hyperkalemia is highly variable. The agent is not absorbed and is eliminated in the feces.

Adverse Effects Sodium polystyrene sulfate should be used with caution in edema and congestive heart falure where increased sodium loads may be harmful. Since other cations may be depleted, calcium and magnesium as well as potassium serum levels must be monitored. Gastric irritation, nausea, vomiting, and constipation may occur. The drug is usually mixed with 10 to 20 mL of 70% sorbitol to reduce constipation and fecal impaction.

Dosage and Administration   Adult dosage is 15 to 60 g daily, divided into doses of 15 g (approximately 4 level tsp of the powder). Rectal administration requires 30 to 60 min retention of the enema, preceded and followed by a cleansing enema with a sodium-free solution. Good skin care is indicated since diarrhea may result from the sorbitol.

POLYVALENT ION BALANCE

Normal Physiology

Distribution

Calcium, phosphate, and magnesium are polyvalent ions that play important roles in normal body function. These ions are stored in the bone with only a very small percentage of the total found in the extracellular fluid. Of the portion in the serum, only about 50 percent is in the active, ionized form, and the rest is either protein-bound or complexed. Normal serum concentrations of the polyvalent ions range from 8.5 to 10.5 mg/dL for calcium, 3.0 to 4.5 mg/dL for phosphorus, and 1.8 to 3.0 mg/dL for magnesium.

Function

Calcium, phosphate, and magnesium are integral elements of normal bone structure and physiology. All three ions are involved in metabolic and enzyme systems such as the blood clotting cascade (calcium) and red blood cell oxygen delivery (phosphate). Of major importance are the roles of magnesium and calcium in regulation of neuromuscular and cardiac excitability.

Regulation

The polyvalent ions calcium, phosphate, and magnesium have similar regulatory mechanisms in the body. Normal serum concentrations and body stores are maintained by three mechanisms: gastrointestinal or intravenous intake, exchange between extracellular fluid and bone, and renal excretion. The homeostases of these ions are interrelated and under hormonal control. *Parathyroid hormone, vitamin D,* and *calcitonin* act on the intestine, bone, and kidney to maintain a normal balance, as outlined in Table 24-8. Serum levels of calcium and phosphate are reciprocal, so as levels of one rise, the levels of the other decline. Normal daily requirements of the polyvalent ions are age-dependent and range from 800 to 1200 mg/day for calcium and phosphorus, and 150 to 450 mg/day for magnesium (see Chap. 25).

Deficits of Polyvalent ions

Hypocalcemia

Etiology   Hypocalcemia may occur because of a sudden increase in deposition of calcium in bone or soft tissue. Various conditions, including hypoparathyroidism following neck or thyroid surgery, the development of hyperphosphatemia, or the osteoblastic metastases of certain types of tumors, may cause hypocalcemia. Massive transfusions or plasma exchange may result in transient but symptomatic hypocalcemia. **Furosemide** (Lasix) and other loop diuretics increase calcium excretion. Other drug-induced causes of hypocalcemia are excessive **corticosteroid** or **calcitonin** supplementation, malabsorption of vitamin D caused by **mineral oil**, and impaired activation of vitamin D caused by **anticonvulsants**. Factitious hypocalcemia occurs in hypoalbuminemia (total serum calcium low with normal levels of ionized calcium). Hyperventilation and alkalosis will transiently lower ionized calcium without any effect on total serum calcium.

Assessment   Patients with rapid development of hypocalcemia experience neuromuscular and cardiac abnormalities, including parasthesias, seizures, tetany, hypotension, and prolonged QT intervals on electrocardiogram. Chronic hypocalcemia is manifested by mental confusion, skin

TABLE 24-8   Hormonal Regulation of Polyvalent Ions*

	PARATHYROID HORMONE	VITAMIN D	CALCITONIN
Bone	↑Bone resorption	↑Bone resorption	↓Bone resorption
Kidney	↑P; ↓Ca and Mg excretion	↓P and Ca excretion	↑P, Ca, and Mg excretion
Intestine	↑P, Ca, and Mg absorption	↑P, Ca, and Mg absorption	↓P, Ca, and Mg absorption
Hypercalcemia, hypophosphatemia, hypermagnesemia	↓Secretion	↓Production	↑Secretion
Hypocalcemia, hyperphosphatemia, hypomagnesemia	↑Secretion	↑Production	↓Secretion

*Polyvalent ions: phosphate (HPO_4^{3-}), calcium (Ca^{2+}), magnesium (Mg^{2+}).

changes, and cataracts. Assessment for these clinical signs and serum calcium, phosphate, and magnesium levels should be done prior to therapy. Calcium therapy is contraindicated if the patient has renal stones.

Management Calcium is available for *parenteral administration* as the chloride, gluconate, levulinate, and gluceptate salts. The amount of calcium present in 1 g of the product will vary, depending upon the salt form (Table 24-9). Parenteral administration is indicated only for patients having symptomatic hypocalcemia or requiring intravenous fluids. Other uses of parenteral calcium include treatment of hypermagnesemia, hyperkalemia, and cardiac emergencies. The drug may be given via central or peripheral veins, but calcium injection is very irritating, and injection into tissues must be avoided. For symptomatic hypocalcemia calcium should be administered by slow intravenous push not to exceed 1 meq/min or by infusion in an IV solution. The total dose of calcium administered is the amount necessary to reverse life-threatening symptoms. An initial dose is 3 meq per square meter of body surface area with monitoring of patient symptoms, ECG, and serum calcium. If response to parenteral calcium is not adequate, 4 to 5 g of **magnesium** (8 to 10 mL of 50% solution) added to the intravenous infusion and infused over 4 to 24 h may promote serum calcium response. Seizure precautions are instituted for hypocalcemic patients, and treatment of the cause of hypocalcemia is initiated, if possible. For example, **thiazide diuretics** which spare calcium can replace **loop diuretics** or hyperphosphatemia can be reversed.

Oral calcium, available as numerous salts (Table 24-9), is used to correct asymptomatic hypocalcemia and in the chronic treatment of senile osteoporosis (Chap. 46), hypoparathyroidism (Chap. 36), and rickets (Chap. 25). Vitamin D is used in rickets and may also be required in long term therapy for other disorders related to calcium balance, provided hyperphosphatemia is reversed prior to therapy (see Chap. 25). If renal function is not impaired, a magnesium-containing antacid can be used to offset the constipation and oversecretion of stomach acid that may be stimulated by calcium supplements.

Patients will need education on the importance and methods of taking the calcium supplements in spite of poor palatability and GI adverse effects (see Table 24-9). They should be warned to consult their health care provider prior to changing calcium supplements, as the elemental calcium content will vary depending upon the salt in the product. For example, a daily dosage of 1.5 g elemental calcium would require sixteen 1000-mg tablets of **calcium gluconate**, but only three 1.25-g tablets of **calcium carbonate** (Os-Cal 500). The elemental calcium is determined by multiplying the percentage of elemental calcium by weight of the salt (Table 24-9) times the weight of the dosage unit. Therefore, 325-mg tablets of calcium lactate contain 42.25 mg calcium (13% × 325 mg).

Evaluation As the hypocalcemia resolves, the symptoms and signs of nerve and muscle irritability, such as tingling fingers and perioral area, muscle cramps, positive Trousseau's sign (carpopedal spasm when blood pressure cuff is applied for 3 min to upper arm), Chvostek's sign (twitching of facial muscles when area below temple is tapped), and ECG changes disappear. The total serum calcium returns to normal range (8 to 10 mg/100 mL when corrected for pH and hypoalbuminemia or ionized calcium of 2.3 to 2.8 meq/L). With chronic therapy urine calcium losses should not exceed 4 mg/kg/day. *Overtreatment* can cause hypercalcemia manifested by flaccid muscles, flank pain (kidney stones), nausea and vomiting, weight loss, polyuria, polydipsia, stupor, headache, and tachycardia.

The nurse should also evaluate possible *drug interactions* which can occur with calcium salts. Patients on digitalis glycosides (**digoxin**) may experience enhanced effects or toxicity, and there may be a decreased response to calcium channel blockers (e.g., **verapamil**). The absorption of **tetracyclines**, except **doxycycline**, is impaired by concomitant ingestion of calcium. **Corticosteroids** may impair calcium absorption from the bowel.

Hypophosphatemia

Etiology and Assessment Hypophosphatemia may develop as a result of cell catabolism in starvation since phosphate is the major intracellular anion. A common cause of low serum phosphate is decreased intake or absorption. Patients may not be given adequate phosphate supplementation during intravenous therapy or may be prescribed aluminum antacids, which bind phosphate in the gut and prevent absorption. Patients with hyperparathyroidism, diabetic ketoacidosis, acute alcoholism, or total parenteral nutrition may have decreased serum phosphate due to increased movement into tissues. Phosphate may also be lost in excessive amounts through renal excretion as in renal tubular acidosis. Acute hypophosphatemia is a life-threatening situation. Patients may experience hemolysis, rhabdomyolysis, and tissue hypoxia. The assessment of hypophosphatemia includes adequate monitoring of patient symptoms, serum phosphate, and serum calcium values.

Management and Evaluation If possible, correction of the underlying cause such as discontinuing **aluminum antacids**, is the initial step in management. Intravenous phosphate is indicated only for patients having symptomatic hypophosphatemia or requiring intravenous fluids. **Parenteral phosphate** is available as the sodium or potassium salt in concentrations of 3 millimoles/mL (Table 24-9). It is to be administered only through central or peripheral veins after dilution in a large volume of fluid because of the high osmolality. The dose and rate of administration depend upon the serum determinations. Chronic hypophosphatemia may be treated with **oral phosphorus** preparations (Table 24-10) available as the potassium and/or sodium salt. Oral phosphorus is hyperosmolar and may cause severe diarrhea, which may be prevented by beginning supplementation at low doses and gradually increasing to fully efficacious doses. The oral phosphates should be diluted with water to decrease the osmolality and increase gastrointestinal toler-ance. With the administration of intravenous phosphate, the concomitant sodium or potassium load must be considered, especially in patients with congestive heart failure and renal failure. In addition, intravenous phosphates have greater risk than oral phosphates for tissue calcification, renal cortical necrosis, and fatal shock.

In patients with renal dysfunction special care must be

TABLE 24-9 Calcium Preparations

INGREDIENT(S)	TRADE NAME(S)	Elemental Calcium Content		COMMENTS
		% BY WEIGHT	meq	
Parenteral				
Calcium chloride (10%)		27	1.36/mL	Calcium salts are irritating to tissues in proportion to concentration; avoid extravasation. Should be given IV no faster than 1 meq/min; calcium chloride should not be given by IM route.
Calcium gluconate (10%)	Kalcinate	9	0.45/mL	
Calcium gluceptate (22%)		8.2	0.9/mL	
Combination Parenterals				
Calcium glycerophosphate 1%/calcium levulinate 1.5%	Cal-Nor	—	0.19/mL	Patient may complain of calcium taste, "hot flushes," or tingling on injection. Not compatible with bicarbonate. IV tubing should be flushed with saline between infusions containing incompatible drugs.
Calcium glycerophosphate 0.5%/ calcium lactate 0.5%	Calphosan	—	0.08/mL	
Oral Products				
Calcium carbonate (tablets, powder, liquid)	Os-Cal 500 Tablets, Equilet, Tums, Chooz, Alka-2 Chewable Antacid Tablets, Titralac	40	20/g	Usual oral doses in 1 mg elemental calcium vary according to indications, usually divided into four doses: Dietary supplement: 1.0–1.5 g/day Hypoparathyroidism: 1.5–3.0 g/day Osteoporosis: 1.0–1.5 g/day
Calcium gluconate (tablets, powder)		9	4.5/g	
Calcium glubionate (syrup: 115 mg Ca^{2+}/5 mL)	Neo-Calglucon Syrup	6.5	3.3/g	Oral absorption of calcium is reduced by foods containing oxalic acid (spinach, rhubarb), phytic acid (bran and whole grains), and phosphorus (dairy products, cola beverages).
Calcium lactate (tablets, powder)		13	6.5/g	
Dibasic calcium phosphate dihydrate (tablets, powder)		23	11.5/g	
Calcium/magnesium carbonate (dolomite)		22	5.4/g	Tablets should be chewed thoroughly. Powders are sprinkled on food or mixed in warm liquid; cool water may then be added to improve palatability. Taking carbonate products with meals may limit belching caused by carbon dioxide release.
Calcium/magnesium (from oyster shell flour)	Elecal	280 mg/tablet		
Calcium carbonate/sodium fluoride	Florical	145.6 mg/capsule		Some natural sources of calcium (e.g., dolomite, oyster shells) have been found to be contaminated with lead, arsenic, and other trace metals. These preparations also vary in calcium content, depending upon source.

TABLE 24-10 Phosphate Supplements

INGREDIENT(S)	TRADE NAME(S)	PHOSPHATE CONTENT*	CATION CONTENT*	USUAL DOSE
		Parenteral (IV)		
Potassium phosphate		3 mM	4.4 meq K	See text
Sodium phosphate		3 mM	4.4 meq Na	See text
		Oral		
Dibasic sodium and potassium phosphate/monobasic sodium and potassium phosphate	Neutra-Phos Powder and Capsules	3 mM	7.1 meq Na, 7.1 meq K	1 capsule mixed with 75 mL H_2O qid†
Dibasic and monobasic potassium phosphate	Neutra-Phos-K Powder and Capsules	8 mM	14.2 meq K	As above†
Dibasic sodium phosphate/sodium acid phosphate monohydrate/potassium acid phosphate	K-Phos Neutral Tablets	8 mM	12.6 meq Na, 1.5 meq K	1 tablet qid with glassful H_2O

*Content per mL for parenterals and per dose unit (e.g., tablet, capsule) for oral forms. Milligram equivalents of phosphate: 3 mM = 93 mg, 8 mM = 250 mg.

†Also available as powder. One bottle (67.5 g) is mixed with water to make 1 gal of solution; dose is 75 mL qid.

taken to avoid iatrogenic hyperphosphatemia. Therapy should be evaluated by serum phosphate levels, as the initial clinical manifestations of hyperphosphatemia are nonspecific: weakness, flaccid muscles, paresthesias, mental confusion, hypotension, dysrhthmias, and signs of hypocalcemia.

Hypomagnesemia

Etiology and Assessment Serum magnesium levels less than 1.8 mg/dL or 1.5 meq/L, termed *hypomagnesemia,* may develop as the result of decreased intake or increased output. Patients with gastrointestinal dysfunction who may have reduced intake or absorption of magnesium include those having extensive bowel resections, chronic diarrhea, postoperative status, bowel fistulas, malabsorption syndromes, inflammatory bowel disease, alcoholic cirrhosis, and prolonged magnesium-free diets/fluids. Multiple factors may induce renal losses of magnesium and resultant hypomagnesemia. Renal diseases (renal tubular acidosis, chronic renal failure, and acute tubular necrosis), endocrine disorders (hyperparathyroidism and hyperaldosteronism), and drug therapy (**diuretics**, **aminoglycosides**, and *cis*-**platinum**) may all cause excess renal wasting of magnesium. Muscle tremors, hyperactive deep tendon reflexes, disorientation, positive Chvostek's sign, cardiac dysrhythmias, and seizures may be exhibited in hypomagnesemia. Prior to magnesium therapy, urine output of at least 100 mL/4 h must be established.

Management The underlying cause of hypomagnesemia should be eliminated if possible. Severely symptomatic

patients may be given magnesium, 0.5 to 1.0 meq/kg diluted with 5% dextrose or sodium chloride solution, in a slow infusion over 3 to 4 h. Then, 0.5 meq/kg may be given every 24 h in divided doses either by intramuscular (IM) or intravenous route until the serum magnesium normalizes. **Magnesium sulfate** is available in several strengths for parenteral administration (Table 24-11). These solutions must never be administered intravenously undiluted or at rates greater than 1 meq/min. The patient's symptoms, ECG, and serum magnesium should be monitored. When patients are unable to tolerate enteral feedings, parenteral fluids should contain a maintenance magnesium dose of 0.25 to 0.5 meq/kg/day to prevent hypomagnesemia.

Oral magnesium supplements are employed in patients

TABLE 24-11 Magnesium Supplements

INGREDIENT(S)	TRADE NAME	MAGNESIUM CONTENT
	Parenteral	
Magnesium sulfate		
10%		0.8 meq/mL
12.5%		1.0 meq/mL
50%		4.0 meq/mL
	Oral	
Magnesium gluconate	Almora Magonate	4.4 meq/g (2.2 meq/tablet)
Magnesium-protein complex	Mg-PLUS	11 meq/tablet

who can tolerate enteral dosing. These preparations may be used for treatment of asymptomatic hypomagnesemia or prevention of hypomagnesemia in patients with excessive losses. The dose is 0.25 to 0.5 meq/kg/day administered in four divided doses. Oral magnesium is available as the chloride, citrate, gluconate, hydroxide, or sulfate salt in solution, tablet, and powder preparations. Oral magnesium may cause diarrhea if used in large doses.

Evaluation Special care must be taken in any patient with renal dysfunction to prevent hypermagnesemia, which is manifested by lethargy, respiratory depression, and depressed deep tendon reflexes. Vital signs, especially respirations, should be monitored every 15 min during an infusion containing therapeutic levels of magnesium and for at least 1 h afterward.

Excesses of Polyvalent Ions

Hypercalcemia

Etiology and Assessment Serum calcium levels greater than 6.0 meq/L (11.0 mg/dL) in the presence of a normal serum albumin and arterial pH is termed *hypercalcemia*. This condition is most commonly caused by increased bone resorption in patients with hyperparathyroidism, tumor metastasis, immobilization, hematologic neoplasms, and vitamin A or D intoxication. Increased calcium intake or absorption, an example being the milk-alkali syndrome due to **calcium antacids**, may also result in hypercalcemia. Less frequent etiologies include decreased bone formation, as in hypothyroidism, and decreased renal excretion, as with **thiazide diuretic** usage. Acute hypercalcemia is manifested by nausea and vomiting; polyuria, nocturia, and polydipsia; as well as confusion, stupor, and coma. Prolonged hypercalcemia will result in chronic renal insufficiency, nephrocalcinosis, and metastatic tissue calcification.

The baseline assessment in hypercalcemia includes patient symptoms and serum calcium, phosphate, pH, and albumin levels. The presence of disease states which complicate fluid administration (renal or cardiac insufficiency) should also be noted.

Management and Evaluation The therapeutic approach to hypercalcemia depends upon the cause of the abnormality, the patient's signs and symptoms, and the serum calcium level. Table 24-12 outlines the treatment modalities used or being investigated.

Central nervous system changes, serum calcium levels in excess of 12.0 mg/100 mL, or arrhythmias require immediate treatment. Because of its speed, efficacy, and safety, the preferred method to reduce serum calcium is an intravenous **saline infusion** (0.9 or 0.45%) at 200 to 500 mL/h or more to achieve diuresis in excess of 150 mL/h. The naturesis caused by this infusion is accompanied by urinary calcium

loss but requires close monitoring of fluid balance (auscultation of lungs, evaluation for third heart sound, central venous pressure) and of serum electrolytes and urinary output.

Loop diuretics, which promote renal calcium wasting as well as diuresis, may be added to the fluid therapy. **Furosemide** (Lasix), 20 to 100 mg every 1 to 2 h, requires monitoring for dehydration, hypotension, hyperglycemia, or auditory damage. However, the duration of effect of saline infusions and diuretics is only 4 to 6 h.

A number of other agents have been used to treat acute hypercalcemia. The bone resorption-inhibiting hormone **calcitonin**, available from salmon (Calcimar) or pig (investi-

TABLE 24-12 Management of Hypercalcemia

THERAPY	DOSING REGIMEN*	ADVERSE EFFECTS
Hydration	3000 mL/m²/day (0.9% NaCl) IV	Fluid overload
Furosemide	1 mg/kg q1–2h IVP	Potassium and fluid depletion
Sodium sulfate†	3000 mL (0.12 *M*) over 12 h IV	Sodium and fluid overload
Phosphate, IV†	100 m*M*/day IV	Hypocalcemia, tetany
Phosphate, oral	1.0–3.0 g/day PO	Severe diarrhea
Diphosphonates clodronate‡	3200 mg/day PO	Diarrhea
EDTA†	1.5 g/m³ over 3–4 h IV	Hypocalcemia, cardiac arrest
Plicamycin	25 µg/kg q24–48h IVP	Thrombocytopenia, renal damage
Calcitonin	2–8 MRC units/kg q6–12h IM, SQ	Headache, flushing, allergies
Glucocorticoids	Prednisone, 30–60 mg/day or its equivalent, PO or IV	Fluid retention, immune suppression
Indomethacin‡	300–600 mg/day PO	Gastrointestinal upset, ulcers, headache
Dialysis	Peritoneal or hemodialysis	Related to procedure

*Administration routes: intravenous infusion (IV), intravenous push (IVP), oral (PO), intramuscular (IM), subcutaneous (SQ).

†Because of the severe adverse effects compared to the potential benefits of these agents and the availability of alternative therapy, these agents are not currently recommended.

‡Investigational use only.

§Formerly called mithramycin.

gational) sources, has a rapid onset and duration of up to 24 h (see Chap. 36). **Intravenous phosphates** (Table 24-10) and **ethylenediaminetetraacetic acid** (EDTA) (chelating agent; see Chap. 48) are rarely used, because of severe adverse effects. **Plicamycin** (Mithracin) and **diphosphonates**, such as **etidronate disodium** (Didronel), are most commonly used in hypercalcemia due to malignancy. Plicamycin is very effective in preventing bone resorption by inhibiting osteoclasts but is associated with severe side effects (see Chap. 37). **Etidronate** and **dichloromethylene diphosphonate**, investigational oral agents for hypercalcemia, are accompanied by relatively few adverse effects. **Corticosteroids** have low efficacy except in hypercalcemia secondary to tumors or due to excessive gastrointestinal absorption of calcium (hypervitaminosis D, sarcoidosis) and require 3 to 6 days prior to onset of action because of their mechanism of slowing osteoclast activity. **Mineralocorticoids** (**fludrocortisone** or **DOCA**), which increase tubular reabsorption of sodium at the expense of calcium and other cation excretion, have a rapid onset but are rarely used because of the massive edema obligate with therapy. **Indomethacin** (Indocin) and other nonsteroidal anti-inflammatory drugs inhibit prostaglandins which have parathormone-like activity and have an onset of hypocalcemia activity of approximately 3 days. **Indomethacin** and **aspirin** are being investigated for use in parathormone-secreting tumors and hyperparathyroidism not amenable to surgery.

Hypercalcemia due to a nonreversible etiology requires chronic therapy. Oral **phosphates** (Table 24-10) are given in doses of 1.0 to 3.0 g/day, but their usefulness is usually limited by diarrhea.

Hyperphosphatemia

Renal failure, whether acute or chronic, is the most common cause of *hyperphosphatemia*, in which serum phosphate values are greater than 5 to 6 mg/dL. Other etiologies include hypoparathyroidism and release of phosphate from cells after chemotherapy. Hyperphosphatemia may result in metastatic calcification and should be treated. **Aluminum hydroxide antacids** are effective in binding phosphate in the gut prior to absorption. The dose is titrated to the serum phosphate value. The usual starting regimen is 500 mg four times a day administered as capsules, tablets, or suspension (see Chap. 30).

Hypermagnesemia

Serum level of magnesium greater than 2.5 meq/L (3.0 mg/dL), termed *hypermagnesemia*, is not a common electrolyte abnormality. This condition may be caused by reduced renal elimination or increased intake. Hypermagnesemia has been reported in patients poisoned by **Epsom salt** and in those with renal failure treated with magnesium-containing antacids or enemas. Clinical manifestations include depressed neuromuscular function, hypotension, nausea, and prolonged QT interval. The only treatment is elimination of the underlying cause. In renal failure patients, dialysis may be

necessary to eliminate the magnesium load. Acutely, a 10-mL dose of **calcium gluconate** 10% solution administered by slow intravenous push (IVP) may prevent cardiac dysrhythmias.

ACID-BASE BALANCE

Normal Physiology

The ECF hydronium ion (H_3O^+; hydrated hydrogen ion) concentration is maintained within narrow limits. The range is 38 to 42 meq/L, which corresponds to an arterial pH of 7.38 to 7.42. Any significant deviation will lead to profound disruption of homeostasis. There are three major mechanisms whereby the body compensates for derangements in the acid-base balance.

1. The ECF contains weak acids and their anions, which buffer the addition of strong acid or base and resist pH changes.
2. The excretion of bicarbonate ion, which is controlled by the kidney.
3. The lungs are able to increase expiration of carbon dioxide to compensate for acid loads.

Acid-Base Imbalances

Definitions

States where blood pH is above 7.42 or below 7.38 units are defined as *alkalemia* and *acidemia*, respectively. There are four primary types of clinical disorders leading to these abnormal acid-base states. Alkalemia may be caused by an increase in serum bicarbonate ion (HCO_3^-) called *metabolic alkalosis* or by a decrease in arterial carbon dioxide concentration (P_{CO2}) called *respiratory alkalosis*. Acidemia may be caused by a decrease in serum bicarbonate ion called *metabolic acidosis* or by an increase in arterial carbon dioxide concentration called *respiratory acidosis*. All of the preceding disorders have acute and chronic forms, occurring alone or in combination. Clinical states with a combination of imbalances are called *mixed acid-base disorders*.

Etiology

The common etiologies of these disorders are outlined in Table 24-13. In general, conditions leading to GI or renal losses of bicarbonate and those increasing acid production or ingestion will result in *metabolic acidosis*. Renal failure, diabetic ketoacidosis, and salicylate overdose are examples. *Respiratory acidosis* is commonly caused by acute and chronic forms of obstructive airway diseases such as asthma and emphysema. The net loss of hydronium ions or precursors in the extracellular fluid (ECF) can result in *metabolic alkalosis*. A greater loss of chloride ions than bicarbonate ions leads to metabolic alkalosis. Examples include diuretic therapy and nasogastric drainage. *Respiratory alkalosis* is an uncommon primary imbalance but can be caused by increased elimination of carbon dioxide in the lungs. Conditions stimulating respiration such as head trauma, fever, and mechanical hyperventilation result in respiratory alkalosis.

Assessment

The clinical manifestations of acid-base disorders are varied. Patients with acidemia will have an arterial pH less than 7.38 units and deep, rapid respirations. Prolonged acidemia can result in decreased myocardial contractility and periph-

eral vascular resistance. The patient may become hypotensive and comatose, develop refractory ventricular fibrillation, and die. The arterial P_{CO_2} and serum bicarbonate are both decreased in primary metabolic acidosis but are increased in primary respiratory acidosis.

The clinical manifestations of alkalemia are dominated by the underlying disease state. Patients may exhibit neuromuscular irritability, including hyperactive deep tendon reflexes or tetany. Laboratory findings include an arterial pH greater than 7.42 with a decreased arterial P_{CO_2} in both metabolic and respiratory alkalosis. An increased serum bicarbonate value is present in metabolic alkalosis, although the opposite is true for respiratory alkalosis.

TABLE 24-13   Acid-Base Imbalances

	Metabolic Imbalance		Respiratory Imbalance	
Mechanism	Acidosis results from loss of fixed base and/or accumulation of organic or fixed acids. Compensation occurs by the blowing off of CO_2 if respiratory mechanism is normal.	Due usually to excessive K^+ loss, loss of acid or, rarely, alkali ingestion. Compensation occurs by CO_2 retention.	Acidosis is due to retention of CO_2 resulting from improper ventilation. Compensation occurs with saving of fixed base by renal synthesis of NH_4.	Alkalosis due to excessive blowing off of CO_2. Compensation occurs by renal excretion of fixed base.
Diseases or Causes	Renal loss (failure), diabetic acidosis, loss of base from GI tract, other causes.	Urinary K^+ loss without replacement, gastric vomiting, or, rarely, alkali ingestion.	Any disease interfering with proper respiration: pneumonia, emphysema, congestive failure, asthma, poorly functioning respirator.	Hyperventilation; voluntary, psychological, or overuse of respiratory aids (e.g., respirator).
Treatment	Remove excessive anions and replace fixed base by the use of fluids and electrolytes (if diminished). Correction of $H.HCO_3$ results from respiratory retention of CO_2.	Replace K^+ deficit (large doses of K^+ are often necessary) and any Na^+ deficit indicated by using Cl^- salt. May use NH_4Cl but with caution.	Treat underlying disease and attempt to improve ventilation. Base is rarely used. Correction will result when disease resolves or is corrected and excess CO_2 is blown off.	Hold breath; rebreathe into paper bag; breathe 5% CO_2–O_2; correct respiratory appliance. Correction will occur. Fixed base will return to normal by body's retention of base.

SOURCE: M. J. Chatton, S. Margen, and H. Brainerd, *Handbook of Medical Treatment*, Los Altos, CA: Lange Medical Publications, 1964. Used by permission.

Management

Acidemia Management of patients with acidemia is correction of the underlying cause or exacerbating condition (see Table 24-14). Oxygen therapy is appropriate for processes inducing respiratory acidosis.

For respiratory or metabolic acidosis, **sodium bicarbonate** ($NaHCO_3$) therapy is only administered for severe acidemia states where the arterial pH is less than 7.2 or the serum bicarbonate concentration is less than 15 meq/L. The dose of sodium bicarbonate depends upon the patient's weight and the degree of acidemia. The lower the serum bicarbonate concentration, the more sodium bicarbonate required. The serum bicarbonate value should not be restored above 15 meq/L, in order to prevent iatrogenic metabolic alkalosis and sodium overload. Sodium bicarbonate is available in an 8.4% solution for parenteral administration. The solution contains 1 meq/mL of sodium and 1 meq/mL of bicarbonate. The osmolality of the solution is very high and should be diluted one to one with sterile water for pediatric patients. The usual dose is 1 meq/kg body weight for children and adults, given by slow IVP (1 to 2 meq/kg/min).

Tromethamine (Tham Solution) is an organic buffer available as a 0.3 M solution (300 meq/L) for parenteral administration. The only advantage of tromethamine over sodium bicarbonate is that it is sodium-free. The solution is useful in neonates who can not tolerate large sodium loads. Tromethamine is associated with several adverse effects

including transient hypoglycemia, respiratory depression, and local vasospasm on extravasation.

Solutions containing precursors of bicarbonate such as **sodium lactate** and **sodium acetate** are also available for parenteral administration. These solutions should never be used for the acute therapy of acidemia because the conversion of the precursors to bicarbonate can be delayed, especially in the presence of tissue hypoxia. These solutions do have a place in the therapy of chronic metabolic acidosis associated with hyperchloremia. In this condition, lactate or acetate salts should be used instead of chloride salts for parenteral fluids.

Alkalemia Volume and chloride depletion are crucial to the generation and maintenance of metabolic alkalosis. The kidney will preserve ECF volume by reabsorbing sodium bicarbonate even in the face of alkalemia. The kidney will also preserve electroneutrality by reabsorbing sodium with bicarbonate ion instead of the deficient chloride ion even in the face of alkalemia. Therefore, volume and chloride replacements are vital for the correction of metabolic alkalosis. For patients with large losses of gastric fluid, hydrogen ion, and chloride ion as with nasogastric drainage, **cimetidine** (Tagamet) may be administered to inhibit hydrochloric acid secretion and prevent metabolic alkalosis. Other therapy available for use in metabolic alkalosis includes direct replacement of hydrogen and chloride ions with **hydrochloric acid, ammonium chloride,** or **arginine hydrochloride.** Of the three agents, hydrochloric acid is associated with the least side effects and may be used in renal or hepatic failure, although the other two drugs may not. A 0.15 N hydrochloric acid solution (sterile, pyrogen-free) is isotonic and may be given as an intravenous infusion. The dose is that amount sufficient to replace one-half of the chloride deficit in the first 24 h. A reevaluation of fluid, electrolyte, and acid-base balance after that time will help determine further replacement requirements. Ongoing losses of volume and chloride must be replaced at least every 8 h. Hemodialysis or peritoneal dialysis is also effective for correction of severe metabolic alkalosis.

Respiratory alkalosis requires correction of the underlying disorder. Often these situations are self-limiting, as in the case of fever, anxiety, head trauma, or salicylate overdose. The only therapy available for severe respiratory alkalosis is ventilatory manipulation, including mechanical ventilation (decreased minute ventilation or increased dead space), use of rebreathing masks, and inhalation of 3% **carbon dioxide.**

Evaluation

Arterial blood gas determinations and serum electrolytes are monitored to assure adequate therapy and to avoid overtreatment. Rapid IV administration or extravasation of the agents can result in pain, and tissue damage. Signs of fluid excess and respiratory function should also be evaluated regularly during therapy.

TABLE 24-14 Commercially Available Drugs Used in Acid-Base Imbalances

DRUG	Content %	Content meq/mL*	INDICATIONS
Sodium bicarbonate	4.0	0.48	Metabolic acidosis in renal disease, uncontrolled diabetes, cardiac arrest, shock, etc.; urinary alkalinization
	4.2	0.5	
	5.0	0.595	
	7.5	0.892	
	8.4	1.0	
Sodium lactate	1.9	0.167	Chronic metabolic acidosis with hypochloremia. Converted to bicarbonate in liver, so contraindicated in severe hepatic disease
	28.0	2.5	
	44.8	4.0	
Sodium acetate	16.4	2.0	
Tromethamine (Tham)	3.6	0.3	Acute metabolic acidosis in cardiopulmonary bypass, cardiac arrest. Renally excreted. Sodium-free
Ammonium chloride	2.14	0.4	Hypochloremic metabolic alkalosis not accompanied by severe hepatic disease
	26.75	5.0	

*Milliequivalents of cation and anion per mL.

CASE STUDY

B.J., a 63-year-old married women was admitted to the hospital for severe vomiting of 3 days' duration. One year prior to this admission, B.J. had undergone colon resection for a carcinoma. No evidence of metastatis of the low-grade tumor was noted at that time. Admitting diagnosis was bowel obstruction of unknown cause.

Assessment

B.J. appeared anxious and severely ill to the admitting nurse. Vital signs were blood pressure, 86/64; temperature, 101.5°F; pulse, 102; respirations, 16 (shallow). Admission weight was 132 lb; she stated that her weight the week before she became ill was 138 lb. Her last stool was 5 days before admission. She had been voiding small amounts of concentrated urine and had been able to tolerate only a few sips of chicken broth and room-temperature lemon-lime soda in spite of extreme thirst. The patient was able to void 50 mL, which was tested for specific gravity (1.041) and then sent to the laboratory for urinalysis.

B.J. was alert and oriented, although she was restless and anxious. Diminished patellar and Achilles reflexes, flabby muscles, and absence of bowel sounds were noted. Her skin lacked turgor, her mucous membranes were sticky, and her tongue was furrowed.

Laboratory tests revealed hematocrit, 50% (37–47); BUN, 24 mg/dL (10–20); Na^+, 136 meq/L (135–145); K^+, 3.2 meq/L (3.5–5.0); Cl^-, 90 meq/L (98–100); Ca^{2+}, 8.8 mg/dL (8.5–10.5); Mg^{2+}, 1.2 meq/L (1.5–2.5); HPO_4^{3-}, 4.0 mg/dL (3.0–4.5). Blood gases showed pH, 7.48 (7.38–7.42); P_{CO_2}, 50 mmHg (35–45); P_{O_2}, 78 mmHg (95–100); HCO_3^-, 36 meq/L (22–26). (Numbers in parentheses are normal ranges.)

From analysis of the data, the nurse noted multiple fluid and electrolyte imbalances: hypovolemia, hypokalemia, hypochloremia, hypomagnesemia, and metabolic alkalosis. Other problems were anxiety about the cause of the obstruction and moderate abdominal pain.

Orders included barium enema in the morning; nasogastric (NG) tube for low intermittent suction; meperidine hydrochloride, 50 mg IM every 3 to 4 h as necessary for pain; IV orders of 3000 mL of 0.9% sodium chloride solution with 20 meq/L of KCl at 300 mL/h, followed by 2000 mL of 5% dextrose in 0.45% sodium chloride with 40 meq/L of KCL and 8 meq/L of magnesium sulfate at a rate of 150 mL/h; and oxygen, 2 to 4 L/min.

Noting that the patient would receive a large amount of fluid in 24 h, the nurse assessed the order based on the replacement guidelines for patients with severe hypovolemia and normoatremia; 3000 mL/m² of body surface area should be infused in 24 h. B.J.'s body surface area was about 1.7 m², so the approximately 5 L of fluid she would receive in the next 24 h was correct. Since the patient had voided, indicating her kidneys were functioning, the potassium in the solution could be given safely, although the nurse would continue to observe output.

Management

Oxygen by nasal prongs at 2 L/min was initiated for borderline hypoxemia secondary to compensation for the alkalosis. The NG tube was inserted and IV therapy started. Until the patient's blood pressure increased, the nurse was reluctant to administer the narcotic analgesic, which could further lower the blood pressure of this volume-depleted patient, who potentially could develop shock. However, the pain was controlled by comfort measures and positioning.

B.J. continued to complain of thirst and asked for a drink or ice chips. Since replacement of water without electrolytes can increase imbalance, the nurse requested an order to allow the patient to such ice chips made out of electrolyte solution.

The nurses' time spent with the patient and family to allow them to ask questions and to discuss their fears. Although the patient had previously had barium enemas, the procedure was reviewed with her.

Ongoing assessment for signs and symptoms of imbalance of electrolytes and fluids included observing daily weight, intake, and output (including nasogastric drainage, which should be replaced on a volume-for-volume basis); checking vital signs every 4 h, performing neurologic assessment; and monitoring urine specific gravity, arterial blood gases, and serum electrolytes.

Evaluation

During the barium enema, a volvulus of the colon was discovered, but distention of the bowel by the barium caused it to be released. However, the paralytic ileus was not corrected for 3 days, and the nasogastric suction and intravenous maintenance was continued until the return of bowel sounds. No evidence of tumor was found.

REFERENCES

Arruda, J. A. L. (ed.): "Symposium on Acid-Base Balance," *Semin Nephrol,* **1**:211–289, 1981.

Brass, E. P., and W. L. Thompson: "Drug-Induced Electrolyte Abnormalities," *Drugs,* **24**:207–228, 1982.

Brenner, B. M. (ed.): "Symposium on Disorders of Extracellular Volume and Composition," *Am J Med,* **72**:273–374, pt. 1; 473–550, pt. 2, 1982.

Burgess, A.: *The Nurse's Guide to Fluid and Electrolyte Balance,* 2d ed., New York: McGraw-Hill, 1979.

Carroll, H. J., and M. S. Oh: *Water, Electrolyte, and Acid-Base Metabolism,* Philadelphia: Lippincott, 1978.

Catchpole, M.: "Electrolytes, Their Physiological Action and Interactions: A Review," *Am Assoc Nurs Anesth J,* **50**:476–481, 1982.

Cohen, J. J., and J. P. Kassirer: *Acid-Base,* Boston: Little, Brown, 1982.

Cunningham, S. G.: "Fluid and Electrolyte Disturbances Associated with Cancer and Its Treatment," *Nurs Clin North Am,* **17**:579–593, Dec. 1982.

Cutter Medical: *Parenteral Solutions Handbook,* Berkeley, Calif.: Cutter Laboratories, 1978.

Finberg, L., R. E. Kravath, and A. R. Fleischman: *Water and Electrolytes in Pediatrics,* Philadelphia: Saunders, 1982.

Flenley, D. C.: "Blood Gas and Acid-Base Interpretation," *Basics of RD,* **10**:1–6, 1981.

Flever, L.: "Understanding the Electrolyte Maze," *Am J Nurs,* **80**:1591–1595, September 1980.

Guyton, A. C.: "The Body Fluids and Kidneys," in *Textbook of Medical Physiology,* 6th ed., Philadelphia, Saunders, 1981.

Juliani, L. M.: "Precautions to Take with Dextrose and Hypotonic Saline," *RN,* **44**:66–69, 1981.

———: "Electrolyte Solutions: Monitor, Monitor, Monitor," *RN,* **44**:48–49, 1981.

Kaehny, W. D.: "Pathogenesis and Management of Respiratory and Mixed Acid-Base Disorders," in R. W. Schrier (ed.), *Renal and Electrolyte Disorders,* Boston: Little, Brown, 1980.

———, and P. A. Gabow: "Pathogenesis and Management of Metabolic Acidosis and Alkalosis," in R. W. Schrier (ed.), *Renal and Electrolyte Disorders,* Boston: Little, Brown, 1980.

Kastrup, E. K. (ed.): *Facts and Comparisons,* Philadelphia: Lippincott, 1983.

Kee, J. L.: *Fluids and Electrolytes with Clinical Applications,* New York: Wiley, 1971.

Krause, M. V., and L. K. Mahan: *Food, Nutrition and Diet Therapy,* Philadelphia, Saunders, 1979.

Levinsky, N. G.: "Fluid and Electrolytes," in R. G. Petersdorf, et al. (eds.), *Harrison's Principles of Internal Medicine,* 10th ed., New York: McGraw-Hill, 1983.

Luckmann, J., and K. C. Sorenson: *Medical-Surgical Nursing, A Psychophysiologic Approach,* 2d ed., Philadelphia: Saunders, 1980.

Maxwell, M. H., and C. R. Kleeman: *Clinical Disorders of Fluid and Electrolyte Metabolism,* New York: McGraw-Hill, 1980.

Metheny, N.: "Preoperative Fluid Balance Assessment," *AORN J,* **33**:51–56, 1981.

Monitoring Fluid and Electrolytes Precisely: Nursing 78 Skillbook Series, Springhouse, PA.: Springhouse Intermed, 1978.

Rando, J. T.: "Fluid and Electrolyte Management of the Adult Surgical Patient," *Am Assoc Nurs Anesth J,* **50**:49–54, 1982.

Robinson, C. H.: *Normal and Therapeutic Nutrition,* 14th ed., New York: Macmillan, 1972.

Rose, B. D.: *Clinical Physiology of Acid-Base and Electrolyte Disorders,* New York: McGraw-Hill, 1977.

Schwartz, A. B., and H. Lyons: *Acid-Base and Electrolyte Balance,* New York: Grune & Stratton, 1977.

Skorecki, K. L., and B. M. Brenner: "Body Fluid Homeostasis in Man," *Am J Med,* **70**:77–88, 1981.

Soltis, B.: "Fluid and Electrolyte Imbalance," in W. J. Phipps, B. C. Long, and N. F. Woods (eds.), *Medical-Surgical Nursing Concepts and Clinical Practice,* 2d ed., St. Louis: Mosby, 1983.

Stroot, V. R., C. A. Lee, and C. A. Schapper: *Fluids and Electrolytes: A Practical Approach,* Philadelphia: Davis, 1974.

Stukler-Schlag, M. R.: "Pre and Post Operative Fluids and Electrolytes: Nursing Assessment and Interventions," *Today's OR Nurse,* **4**:11–5, 66–67, September 1982.

Yu, P. Y. K., et al.: "Symposium on Fluid Balance in the Newborn Infant," *Clin Perinatol,* **9**:451–658, 1982.

Weil, W. B., and M. D. Bailie: *Fluid and Electrolyte Metabolism in Infants and Children,* New York: Grune & Stratton, 1977.

UNIT V

CLINICAL PHARMACOLOGY & THERAPEUTICS OF COMMON DISORDERS

25

NUTRITIONAL DISORDERS*

MARGARET BALL
LYNNE JOHNSON PHILLIPS

LEARNING OBJECTIVES

Upon mastery of the contents of this chapter, the reader will be able to:

1. Differentiate between U.S. RDA and RDA estimates of nutrient requirements.

2. Indicate the name of the related deficiency state, at least one important dietary or environmental source, uses other than dietary supplementation, and the signs of overdosage (where applicable) for each of the following vitamins: vitamin A, ascorbic acid, vitamin D, thiamine, vitamin K, and pyridoxine.

3. List at least four essential minerals or elements.

4. Compare breast milk and infant milk formulas by constituents.

5. List the major types of therapeutic and standard infant formulas and describe the sources of protein, fat, and carbohydrate.

6. Indicate when vitamin and mineral supplements should be prescribed in infancy, pregnancy, and lactation.

7. Indicate the site of action and drug family of the amphetamine and nonamphetamine anorectic drugs.

8. List the adverse effects of the anorectic drugs.

9. Indicate the efficacy of the following drugs in the treatment of obesity: human chorionic gonadotropin, thyroid hormones, amphetamines, starch blockers, fad diets.

10. Explain patient education associated with anorectics use in obesity.

11. State the components of a nutritional assessment.

12. List the three major types of enteral formulations and their distinguishing characteristics.

13. List advantages and disadvantages associated with five routes of enteral product administration via tubes.

14. Describe the pertinent nursing care for the patient on enteral therapy.

15. Define the term *total parenteral nutrition* (TPN) and list the indications and advantages of this approach.

16. List the constituents of a total parenteral solution.

17. Explain the advantages of parenteral fat emulsions in parenteral hyperalimentation.

18. Differentiate between the nutritional support therapies of partial parenteral nutrition (PPN) and total parenteral nutrition (TPN).

19. List the key components of central access catheter care.

20. List the adverse effects of TPN.

DIETARY REQUIREMENTS

Of the substances required for human metabolism, all but 40 can be manufactured by the body. It is essential that these 40 be provided in the diet. The requirements for these essential nutrients vary widely from person to person and are influenced by differences in activity, growth, drug use (Table 25-1), and other physiologic circumstances.

Estimates of daily requirements known as the *Recommended Daily Allowances (RDA)* have been summarized and published by the National Research Council (Table 25-2). The Recommended Daily Allowances are the levels of intake of essential nutrients considered, in the judgment of the NRC Food and Nutrition Board and on the basis of available scientific knowledge, to be adequate to meet the nutritional needs of practically all healthy persons. Persons consuming less than the RDA are not necessarily malnourished.

The Food and Drug Administration (FDA) has proposed a set of standards, *the United States Recommended Daily*

---

*The editors thank Harold Silverman, Pharm. D., who wrote portions of the chapter on this subject in the first edition.

TABLE 25-1 Selected Drug-Nutrient Interactions

DRUG	NUTRIENT	EFFECT ON NUTRIENTS	DRUG	NUTRIENT	EFFECT ON NUTRIENTS
Aspirin	Folic acid	↓Serum levels; altered transport	Corticosteroids	Vitamin D	↑Metabolism ↑Requirement
	Vitamin C	↑Urinary excretion		Vitamin B₆	↑Requirement
	Thiamin	↑Urinary excretion		Vitamin C	↑Requirement
	Vitamin K	↑Urinary excretion			↑Urinary excretion
	Iron	May cause blood loss		Calcium	↓Absorption
Anticonvulsants	Folic acid	↓Serum levels			↑Urinary excretion
	Vitamin B₆	↓Serum levels		Phosphorus	↓Absorption
	Vitamin B₁₂	↓Serum levels		Zinc	↑Urinary excretion
	Vitamin D	↓Conversion to active forms			↓Serum levels
				Glucose	↑Serum levels
	Vitamin K	↑Requirement		Triglycerides	↑Serum levels
Tetracycline	Fat	↓Absorption		Cholesterol	↑Serum levels
	Amino acids	↓Absorption		Nitrogen	↑Urinary excretion
	Calcium	↓Absorption	Hydralazine	Vitamin B₆	↑Urinary excretion
	Iron	↓Absorption	Laxatives		
	Magnesium	↓Absorption	Cathartics	Vitamin D	↓Absorption
	Zinc	↓Absorption		Calcium	↓Absorption
	Niacin	↑Urinary excretion	Mineral oil	Fat-soluble vitamins	↓Absorption
	Riboflavin	↑Urinary excretion			
	Folacin	↑Urinary excretion		Calcium	↓Absorption
	Vitamin C	↑Urinary excretion		Phosphates	↓Absorption
Antitubercular drugs					
Cycloserine	Vitamin B₆	Vitamin B₆ antagonist	Levodopa	Amino acids	↑Requirement
	Protein	↓Synthesis		Vitamin B₆	↑Requirement
Isoniazid (INH)	Vitamin B₆	Vitamin B₆ antagonist ↑Urinary excretion		Vitamin C	↑Requirement
		Causes deficiency	Oral contraceptives	Vitamin B₆	↑Requirement ↓Blood levels
	Niacin	Causes deficiency		Riboflavin	↑Requirement, ↓Blood levels
	Vitamin B₁₂	↓Absorption ↓Serum levels		Folic acid	↓Absorption, ↓Blood levels
Cholesterol-Lowering Agents				Vitamin B₁₂	↓Blood levels
Cholestyramine	Fat-soluble vitamins	↓Absorption		Vitamin C	↓Blood levels
				Vitamin A	↑Blood levels
	Folic acid	↓Absorption		Calcium	↑Absorption
	Iron	↓Absorption		Iron	↑Serum levels
	Vitamin B₁₂	↓Absorption ↓Blood levels		Copper	↑Serum levels
	Calcium	↑Urinary excretion ↓Blood levels	Penicillamine	Vitamin B₆	↑Requirement ↑Urinary excretion
Clofibrate	Vitamin B₁₂	↓Absorption		Zinc	↑Urinary excretion
	Iron	↓Absorption		Iron	↑Urinary excretion
	Intake	Alters taste; causes nausea and GI irritation		Copper	↑Urinary excretion Alters taste; causes anorexia, nausea, vomiting
Colchicine	Fat	↓Absorption			
	Nitrogen	↓Absorption			
	Folic acid	↓Absorption			
	Vitamin B₁₂	↓Absorption			

Source: Adapted by permission from *Understanding Normal and Clinical Nutrition* by Eleanor Noss Whitney and Corinne Balog Cataldo, Copyright © 1983 by West Publishing Company. All rights reserved.

Allowances (*U.S. RDA*), for use in food labeling for nutrient content. They replace the Minimum Daily Requirements (MDR) formerly used by the FDA for labeling. These standards are derived from the RDA but are based on broad age groups, rather than on the larger number of age/sex groups for which the RDA are established. As nutrient information on food labels increases, the U.S. RDA will be the reference standard for content values listed.

Since the RDA are intended to maintain 95 percent of the population adequately, we will consider them briefly.

Energy

Caloric requirements vary widely with age, size, sex, and degree of activity. The recommendation for average males 23 to 50 years of age is 2700 kcal daily; that for average females in the same age group is 2000 kcal daily. Pregnancy requires the addition of 300 kcal/day and lactation 500 kcal/day. Energy may be obtained from dietary carbohydrates, fats, and proteins.

Proteins

Protein is essential in the daily diet because it is composed of many essential amino acids. Food proteins contain various combinations of the 20 naturally occurring amino acids, 9 of which are essential for human beings. Histidine is required for infants, but its essentiality for adults has not been clearly established. Amino acids recovered from the dietary protein are either used in the synthesis of body protein or catabolized for energy. The average male (70 kg) requires 56 g of protein and the average female 44 g.

Vitamins

Vitamins may be broadly defined as chemical substances essential for certain ongoing metabolic processes and not synthesized within the body. These essential nutrients generally act as coenzymes or hormones and may normally be obtained from a nutritious diet. Situations may arise, however, in which the level of one or more of the vitamins falls below acceptable levels. In these cases, generally brought about by specific dietary deficiencies or drug interactions, supplementation with additional vitamins may be indicated.

A list of oral and parenteral multivitamin preparations is given in Table 25-3. The nurse should check the compatibility of vitamins with solutions and other drugs whenever they are added to intravenous solutions.

Vitamin A

Vitamin A is a fat-soluble substances produced in the body from carotene, a material found in the deep-yellow and dark-green vegetable foods (milk, butter, fortified margarine, eggs, liver, and kidney). Vitamin A is essential for normal healthy skin, eyes, and hair and, in general, for the maintenance of all epithelial structures.

Vitamin A deficiencies result in anatomic abnormalities of the eye called *xerophthalmia*, which involves drying of corneal secretions and eventual corneal damage. Moderate vitamin A deficiencies result in an inability to see in subdued light and a decrease in vision immediately following exposure to bright light. Nonocular manifestations of vitamin A deficiency are generally obscured by the signs and symptoms of general malnutrition or the existence of some other condition which precludes effective absorption of vitamin A.

The therapy of vitamin A deficiency is 50,000 international units (IU)/day for 1 to 2 weeks. [Currently, vitamin A amounts may be stated in retinal equivalents (RE) in some references.] Also, the entire diet should be reviewed, since other deficiencies are likely. Unless blindness has already occurred, treatment of vitamin A deficiency results in corneal healing. However, any scar tissue present will cause limitation of vision. Topical vitamin A and **isotretinoin** (13-*cis*-retinoic acid; Accutane), a derivative of vitamin A, are used in the treatment of cystic acne (see Chap. 38).

Overdosage Hypervitaminosis A results from the ingestion of large doses of vitamin A (as much as 500,000 IU/day) for long periods. In infants, signs of acute intoxication are drowsiness, vomiting, and bulging of the fontanels from increased intracranial pressure. Chronic overdosage produces failure to gain weight, loss of hair, coarseness of hair texture, liver enlargement, and bone pain. In adults, vitamin A overdosage produces headache, blurred vision or diplopia (double vision), nausea, and vomiting. Bone pain and changes similar to those occurring in children also occur. Additionally, peeling of the skin, neuritis, fissures and sores at the corners of the mouth, hair loss, coarseness of skin texture, and local areas of hyperpigmentation are common. The prognosis for both children and adults is good once vitamin A ingestion is stopped.

Vitamin D

The name *vitamin D* is commonly used to describe several related fat-soluble substances which function as hormones in conjunction with parathyroid hormone and calcitonin to regulate calcium homeostasis. Vitamin D promotes calcium absorption in the intestine, increases bone resorption, and decreases calcium excretion by the kidney. It also affects magnesium metabolism. Deficiency of vitamin D leads to *rickets* in children and *osteomalacia* in adults. The metabolism of natural vitamin D and its synthetic analog, **dihydrotachysterol** (DHT) (Hytakerol), is shown in Fig. 25-1. **Cacifediol** (Calderol) has weak pharmacologic activity and must be converted by the kidneys to calcitriol, the active form of natural vitamin D. Therefore **calcitriol** (Rocaltrol) is the preferred natural vitamin D supplement in those with renal failure. **Dihydrotachysterol** (Hytakerol) must be activated by the liver but has a more rapid onset of action and shorter duration of effect than the natural vitamin D forms.

TABLE 25-2   Recommended Daily Dietary Allowances,[1] Revised 1980
Designed for the maintenance of good nutrition of practically all healthy people in the United States

	AGE, years	Weight kg	Weight lb	Height cm	Height in	PROTEIN, g	VITAMIN A, μg RE[2]	VITAMIN D, μg[3]	VITAMIN E, mg α-TE[4]	VITAMIN C, mg	THIAMIN, mg
							Fat-Soluble Vitamins				
Infants	0.0–0.5	6	13	60	24	kg × 2.2	420	10	3	35	0.3
	0.5–1.0	9	20	71	28	kg × 2.0	400	10	4	35	0.5
Children	1–3	13	29	90	35	23	400	10	5	45	0.7
	4–6	20	44	112	44	30	500	10	6	45	0.9
	7–10	28	62	132	52	34	700	10	7	45	1.2
Males	11–14	45	99	157	62	45	1000	10	8	50	1.4
	15–18	66	145	176	69	56	1000	10	10	60	1.4
	19–22	70	154	177	70	56	1000	7.5	10	60	1.5
	23–50	70	154	178	70	56	1000	5	10	60	1.4
	51+	70	154	178	70	56	1000	5	10	60	1.2
Females	11–14	46	101	157	62	46	800	10	8	50	1.1
	15–18	55	120	163	64	46	800	10	8	60	1.1
	19–22	55	120	163	64	44	800	7.5	8	60	1.1
	23–50	55	120	163	64	44	800	5	8	60	1.0
	51+	55	120	163	64	44	800	5	8	60	1.0
Pregnant						+30	+200	+5	+2	+20	+0.4
Lactating						+20	+400	+5	+3	+40	+0.5

Source: Food and Nutrition Board, National Academy of Sciences—National Research Council

[1]The allowances are intended to provide for individual variations among most normal persons as they live in the United States under usual environmental stresses. Diets should be based on a variety of common foods in order to provide other nutrients for which human requirements have been less well defined. See text for detailed discussion of allowances and of nutrients not tabulated.

[2]Retinol equivalents. 1 RE = 1 μg retinol or 6 μg β-carotene. See text for calculation of vitamin A activity of diets as retinol equivalents.

[3]As cholecalciferol. 10 μg cholecalciferol = 400 IU of vitamin D.

[4]α-tocopherol equivalents. 1 mg d-α-tocopherol = 1 α-TE. See text for variation in allowances and calculation of vitamin E activity of the diet as α-tocopherol equivalents.

Vitamin D is present in liver, butter fat, egg yolk, and fatty fish. Human milk and cow's milk also contain somewhat limited amounts. In many countries, including the United States, milk, margarine, butter, and other foods are fortified with vitamin D. Rickets can be prevented in infants by supplementation with 400 units (U) per day for the first 2 years of life. Premature infants require considerably larger doses as a supplement, because they have no vitamin D stores. Persons with dark skins may also require supplementation. The available forms of vitamin D and recommended doses are listed in Table 25-4.

Overdosage   Hypervitaminosis D results from the ingestion of excessive amounts of the vitamin. The clinical features of hypervitaminosis D are associated with hypercalcemia. Patients experience weakness, lethargy, anorexia, nausea and vomiting, excessive weight loss, excessive thirst and urination, irritability, and depression. Laboratory findings in hypervitaminosis D include hypercalcemia, hyperphosphatemia or hypophosphatemia, and decreased alkaline phosphatase. Renal damage from calcium deposits in the kidney follows the development of these findings. Calcium deposits may also be found in skin, heart, lung, pancreas, stomach, and other soft tissue. This disorder is treated by discontinuation of the vitamin D supplementation and treatment for hypercalcemia (see Chap. 24).

Vitamin E

Vitamin E is a fat-soluble substance which is a mixture of naturally occurring tocopherols. Food sources rich in vitamin E include vegetable oils, margarine, shortening, wheat germ, egg yolk, milk, liver, and leafy vegetables. Although vitamin E is known to affect certain biochemical pathways, its deficiency produces few effects in human beings. Plasma vitamin E concentration in the newborn infant is about one-third that of adults, and that of the low-birth-weight infant

Water-Soluble Vitamins					Minerals					
RIBO-FLAVIN, mg	NIACIN, mg NE[5]	VITAMIN B_6, mg	FOLACIN[6], μg	VITAMIN B_{12}, μg	CALCIUM, mg	PHOS-PHORUS, mg	MAG-NESIUM, mg	IRON, mg	ZINC, mg	IODINE, μg
0.4	6	0.3	30	0.5[7]	360	240	50	10	3	40
0.6	8	0.6	45	1.5	540	360	70	15	5	50
0.8	9	0.9	100	2.0	800	800	150	15	10	70
1.0	11	1.3	200	2.5	800	800	200	10	10	90
1.4	16	1.6	300	3.0	800	800	250	10	10	120
1.6	18	1.8	400	3.0	1200	1200	350	18	15	150
1.7	18	2.0	400	3.0	1200	1200	400	18	15	150
1.7	19	2.2	400	3.0	800	800	350	10	15	150
1.6	18	2.2	400	3.0	800	800	350	10	15	150
1.4	16	2.2	400	3.0	800	800	350	10	15	150
1.3	15	1.8	400	3.0	1200	1200	300	18	15	150
1.3	14	2.0	400	3.0	1200	1200	300	18	15	150
1.3	14	2.0	400	3.0	800	800	300	18	15	150
1.2	13	2.0	400	3.0	800	800	300	18	15	150
1.2	13	2.0	400	3.0	800	800	300	10	15	150
+0.3	+2	+0.6	+400	+1.0	+400	+400	+150	—[8]	+5	+25
+0.5	+5	+0.5	+100	+1.0	+400	+400	+150	—[8]	+10	+50

[6]The folacin allowances refer to dietary sources as determined by *Lactobacillus casei* assay after treatment with enzymes (conjugases) to make polyglutamyl forms of the vitamin available to the test organism.

[7]The recommended dietary allowance for vitamin B_{12} in infants is based on average concentration of the vitamin in human milk. The allowances after weaning are based on energy intake (as recommended by the American Academy of Pediatrics) and consideration of other factors, such as intestinal absorption; see text.

[8]The increased requirement during pregnancy cannot be met by the iron content of habitual American diets nor by the existing iron stores of many women; therefore the use of 30–60 mg of supplemental iron is recommended. Iron needs during lactation are not substantially different from those of nonpregnant women, but continued supplementation of the mother for 2–3 months after parturition is advisable in order to replenish stores depleted by pregnancy.

is even lower. Malnourished infants have been known to develop an anemia responsive to vitamin E.

Laboratory animals have exhibited a variety of other effects attributable to vitamin E deficiency, but these have not been reported in human beings.

Vitamin K

Vitamin K is a fat-soluble substance essential for blood clotting becuase of its role in prothrombin production. Vitamin K deficiency occurs only in the newborn infant, before the intestinal flora and diet begin to supply the vitamin, so infants are given parenteral vitamin K as a single IM dose of 0.5 to 2 mg. Vitamin K supplementation in doses of 2 to 25 mg may also be necessary in the presence of overdosage with one of the oral anticoagulant drugs, for which it is a specific antidote, and after oral antibiotic therapy, which sterilizes the gut and diminishes the natural supply of the vitamin produced by the action of intestinal flora on green leafy vegetables. Available vitamin K preparations are listed in Table 25-5.

Thiamin

Thiamin, or vitamin B_1, is a water-soluble substance found in whole-grain and enriched breads, cereals, and flour and in organ meats, other meats, poultry, fish, legumes, nuts, milk, and green vegetables. Thiamin functions as a coenzyme in a number of different metabolic transformation reactions, the most important of which is carbohydrate metabolism. The thiamin requirement is related to metabolic rate and is greatest when carbohydrate is the chief energy source. A mineral intake of 1 mg of thiamin per day is recommended for adults to maintain body stores when caloric intake is restricted. There is an increase in the RDA for both pregnancy and lactation.

Thiamin deficiency brings on the condition known as *beriberi*, consisting of neurologic involvement, heart failure,

TABLE 25-3 Selected Multiple Vitamin Preparations

PRODUCT	VITAMIN A, IU	VITAMIN D, IU	VITAMIN E, IU	ASCORBIC ACID (C), mg	THIAMIN (B₁), mg	RIBOFLAVIN (B₂), mg	NIACIN, mg	FLUORIDE, mg
Abdee Baby Drops (per 0.6 mL)	5,000	400		50	1.0	1.2	10	
Cod liver oil concentrate capsules	10,000	400						
Flintstones Chewable	2,500	400	15	60	1.05	1.2	13.5	
Geritol liquid					5.0	5.0	100	
Larobec†				500	15	15	100	
MVI-12 injection*† (per 5 mL)	3,300	200	10	100	3	3.6	40	
Materna 1-60 tablets†	8,000	400	30	100	3	3.4	20	250
Myadec	10,000	400	30	250	10.0	10.0	100	
Natalins Rx tablets†	8,000	400	30	90	2.5	3	20	
One-A-Day	5,000	400	15	60	1.5	1.7	20	
One-A-Day Vitamins Plus Minerals	5,000	400	15	50	1.5	1.7	20	
Pancebrin Injection (per mL)*†	5,000	500	1.1	30	5	1	10	
Poly-Vi-Sol drops (per 0.6 mL)	1,500	400	5	35	0.5	0.6	8	
Poly-Vi-Sol with Iron drops (per 0.6 mL)*	1,500	400	5	35	0.5	0.6	8	
Solu-B*† (per mL)					5	5	125	
Solu-B with Ascorbic Acid (per 5 mL)*†				500	10	10	250	
Stuart Prenatal	8,000	400	30	60	1.7	2.0	20	
Theragran	10,000	400	15	200	10.3	10.0	100	
Tri-Vi-Sol Drops	1,500	400		35				
Tri-Vi-Sol with Iron Drops	1,500	400		35				
Unicap	5,000	400	15	60	1.5	1.7	20	
Unicap Chewable	5,000	400	15	60	1.5	1.7	20	
Vi-Daylin/F Drops (per mL)	1,500	400	5	35	0.5	0.6	8	0.25

*For parenteral use; check compatibility with solutions and other drugs.

†Requires a prescription.

PYRIDOXINE HYDROCHLORIDE (B_6), mg	CYANOCO-BALAMIN (B_{12}), μg	FOLIC ACID, μg	PANTO-THENIC ACID, μg	IRON, mg	CALCIUM, mg	PHOSPHO-RUS, mg	MAGNE-SIUM, mg	OTHER INGREDIENTS
1.0			5.0					
1.0	4.5	0.3						
1.0	3.0		4.0	100				Methionine, 75 mg/oz Choline bitartrate, 100 mg
	5	500	18					
4			15					
4	12	1000		60	250			Cu, I, Mg, Docusate sodium
5.0	6.0	400	20	20			100	Cu, Zn, Mn, I
10	8	1000	15	60	200			Cu, I, Mg, Zn Biotin
2.0	6.0	400						
2.0	6.0	400	10.0	18	100	100	100	Zn, Cu, I
1.5			1.5					
0.4								
0.4				10				
2.5			25					
5			50		500			
4.0	8.0	800		60	200		100	Iodine
4.1	5.0	21.4						
				10				
2.0	6.0	400						
2.0	6.0	400						
0.4	2							

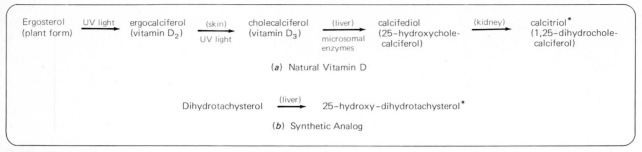

FIGURE 25-1

Metabolism of Vitamin D. (*a*) Natural vitamin D can be derived from a plant sterol and activated in a series of steps in the skin, liver, and kidneys. (*b*) The synthetic analog dihydrotachysterol is activated in the liver. *Calcitriol, or 1,25-dihydrocholecalciferol (1,25[OH]$_2$-D$_3$), and 25-hydroxy-dihydrotachysterol are the physiologically active forms of vitamin D.

and/or edema. Thiamin deficiency most commonly occurs in economically deprived countries in the Far East but can also result from poor dietary habits, as in the alcoholic patient (so-called occidental beriberi). In such patients thiamin deficiency leads to weakness of the myocardial muscles, heart failure, and a mild peripheral neuritis. Treatment should begin with up to 60 mg/day **thiamin hydrochloride** (Betalin S, Bewon, Biamine), although 15 mg of thiamin is usually sufficient to treat beriberi without cardiac involvement. Oriental beriberi responds much more gradually to thiamin administration, since the deficiency has been severe

enough to cause damage to structural elements of the myocardium.

Riboflavin (Vitamin B$_2$)

Riboflavin is found in eggs, enriched bread and cereals, leafy green vegetables, lean meats, liver, dried yeast, and milk. Dietary deficiency of riboflavin has been associated with loss of visual acuity (rare), mild lesions of the lips (cheilosis), and a scrotal seborrheic dermatitis. The diagnosis of riboflavin deficiency is usually associated with a dietary history showing deficient intake and the appearance of dermatologic

TABLE 25-4   Vitamin D Supplementation

PREPARATION	TRADE NAME	DOSE (DAILY)	CAUTIONS
Ergocalciferol (vitamin D$_2$)	Drisdol, Calciferol, Deltalin	Rickets prophylaxis: 400 IU Rickets treatment: 1000–4000 IU Hypoparathyroidism: 50,000 IU (as much as 200,000 IU daily may be required in some cases)	Usually accompanied by calcium supplement. Therapeutic goal is to return serum calcium to normal concentration (8 mg/dL) while minimizing urinary calcium loss (4 mg/kg/day) and restoring bone mass.
Calcifediol	Calderol	50–125 μg daily or every other day	Evaluate response to starting dose at 2- to 4-week intervals. Reduce calcium and vitamin D supplements as normal serum calcium is approached.
Calcitriol (1,25-dihydroxycholecalciferol)	Rocaltrol	0.25 μg (as much as 1 μg daily may be required)	Mineral oil may decrease absorption. Cholestyramine, barbiturates, and phenytoin may decrease utilization of vitamin D. Thiazide diuretics may potentiate the hypercalcemic effect.
Dihydrotachysterol (DHT)	Hytakerol	Initial dose: 0.75–2.5 mg Maintenance: 0.2–1 mg	Signs and symptoms of overdosage include symptomatic hypercalcemia, profuse sweating, nephrotoxicity, anemia, headache. Normal serum vitamin D: 50–135 IU/dL. Analogs not requiring kidney hydroxylation are preferred in renal disease (calcitriol, dihydrotachysterol).

*Table prepared by Celeste Martin Marx, Pharm.D.

symptoms. The recommended allowances call for an increase for pregnancy and lactation. Low urinary riboflavin levels have been reported by several investigators in women taking oral contraceptives. The data are insufficient to suggest an increased allowance.

Pyridoxine (Vitamin B₆)

Pyridoxine is found in wheat germ, vegetables, dried yeast, meat, and whole-grain cereals. It is found in such a wide variety of foods that dietary deficiency is rare. Experimental B_6 deficiency produces cachexia, scaling of the skin, and microcytic hypochromic anemia. Convulsive seizures may be seen, especially in babies.

Some drugs such as **isoniazid** and **hydralazine** (Apresoline), exert an anti-vitamin B_6 effect, thereby increasing the dietary requirement for pyridoxine. This is particularly true of patients who are slow acetylators (genetically determined; see Chap. 5), pregnant, diabetic, elderly, or who have liver disease. Polyneuritis may appear as a consequence of this effect but is easily treated with 25 to 50 mg/day of pyridoxine. Prophylactic therapy with **pyridoxine** (Hexa-Betalin, Beesix, others) is customarily given to patients receiving isoniazid to prevent the development of vitamin B_6 deficiency.

Ironically, pyridoxine ingestion can cause the inactivation of **levodopa**, used to treat Parkinson's disease. For this reason patients receiving levodopa therapy are warned to avoid pyridoxine supplementation in their diets unless taking a combined **levodopa-carbidopa** preparation (e.g., Sinemet) (see Chap. 33, "Neurologic Disorders").

High doses of vitamin B_6 have been used therapeutically. Normally given in doses of up to 2 mg, it may be used in daily doses of up to 500 mg. In vitamin B_6-dependent infantile convulsions, 10 to 25 mg/day has been shown to be effective. In vitamin B_6–responsive anemia, 10 mg/day has proved adequate. In cystathioninuria, a metabolic disorder with no known clinical manifestations, daily doses of up to 400 mg have been employed. In xanthuremic aciduria, a metabolic disorder which is considered a potential cause of mental retardation, up to 10 mg/day has been used. Homocystinuria, a metabolic disease which maybe a cause of arterial and venous thromboses and mental retardation, has been treated with up to 500 mg/day. The vitamin has been used in the treatment of nausea and vomiting in pregnancy and following radiation. There is an increase in the recommended allowance for pregnancy and lactation. Women on estrogen-progesterone oral contraceptives are reported to require additional B_6. Abnormal tryptophan metabolism is also cited in recent studies as contributing to an increased vitamin B_6 requirement.

Niacin

Nicotinic acid, or niacin, another component of the vitamin B complex, is found in whole grains and enriched breads, flours, and cereals and in lean meats, liver, fish, dried yeast, nuts, legumes, coffee, and eggs. Niacin serves as part of coenzymes involved in a variety of functions. Specifically, it is part of nicotinamide adenine dinucleotide (NAD) and nicotinamide adenine dinucleotide phosphate (NADP), two coenzymes involved in many enzymatic reactions of intermediary metabolism. Liver microsomal enzymes containing NADP play an important role in the metabolism of many drugs, and niacin deficiency may alter drug disposition. Niacin deficiency leads to the development of *pellagra,* a disease characterized by skin lesions, alimentary tract lesions, and neurologic signs. Allowances for niacin are commonly related to energy expenditure.

Pellagra is most often seen in females of childbearing age and is associated with dietary deficiency of nicotinic acid. In

TABLE 25-5 Vitamin K Supplementation

PREPARATION	TRADE NAME	DOSAGE FORMS	CAUTIONS
Phytonadione	Mephyton AquaMEPHYTON	Tablets Injection	IV injection of AquaMEPHYTON has resulted in deaths, apparently from anaphylaxis. IV injection should be avoided whenever possible and should not exceed 1 mg/min.
	Konakion	IM injection only	IM injection should be given deep into muscle. In infants the anteriolateral thigh or deltoid sites are recommended.
Menadione (vitamin K_3)		Tablets	Use of mineral oil with oral forms may restrict absorption.
Menadiol sodium diphosphate (vitamin K_4)	Synkayvite	Injection, tablets	Repeat dosage may be required after 6–8 h in anticoagulant-induced hypoprothrombinemia.
			Menadione and menadiol sodium diphosphate are contraindicated in infants and during late pregnancy.

the United States, where primary pellagra is not often seen, secondary causes of pellagra, such as malabsorptive syndromes and alcoholism, are an important consideration.

Severe illness with pellagra must be treated as an emergency, with primary efforts aimed at correction of fluid and electrolyte imbalance and replacement of **niacin** (Nicobid, Diacin, Nicolar, others) with up to 300 mg/day. **Niacinamide,** or nicotinic acid amide, produces the beneficial effects of niacin without some of the unpleasant side effects.

Niacin has been used in the treatment of schizophrenia, and as a peripheral vasodilator, although its efficacy in these conditions remains to be established. It is also used in hyperlipidemia (see Chap. 41).

Pantothenic Acid

Pantothenic acid deficiency may contribute to the disease states seen with other nutrient deficiencies or with severe malabsorption. Natural pantothenic acid deficiency has not been seen in human beings but has been well documented in animals, where it produces dermatitis, adrenal degeneration, and central nervous system symptoms. Pantothenic acid is found in eggs, nuts, broccoli, liver, yeast, and egg yolk. It plays an important role in the metabolism of carbohydrates and fats and the formation of acetylcholine through its role in forming coenzyme A.

Cyanocobolamin (Vitamin B$_{12}$)

Found generally in liver, kidney, milk, saltwater fish, oysters, lean meat, and foods of animal origin, vitamin B$_{12}$ is a cofactor in synthesis of the nuclear material of red blood cells. Nutritional deficiency of vitamin B$_{12}$ resulting from inadequate dietary intake is rare. It is most likely the result of a strict vegetatian diet devoid of animal protein foods. Pregnant women and young children in strict vegetarian diets may need oral supplementation with **cyanocobolamin** (Redisol, Kalbovite). B$_{12}$ deficiency is treated with 15 to 30 μg of B$_{12}$ parenterally q2h for three or four doses; thereafter, 25 μg supplementation may be given once a week. The administration of larger doses of B$_{12}$ is not advantageous, since the percentage excreted increases with the size of the dose.

Vitamin B$_{12}$ deficiency leads to the development of *pernicious anemia,* a disorder characterized by megaloblastic anemia, lack of normal gastric juice, and neurologic damage. The deficiency arises from inability of the gastric fundus to secrete intrinsic factor, without which vitamin B$_{12}$ cannot be absorbed. Pernicious anemia requires lifelong parenteral supplementation (see Chap. 36).

Folic Acid

The term *folic acid,* or *folacin,* refers to a group of substances widely distributed in green leafy vegetables, yeast, liver, and meats. This vitamin acts with B$_{12}$ in the transfer of single carbon units essential for hemopoiesis and mucosal proliferation. Folate deficiency leads to the development of *megaloblastic anemia* (see Chap. 36). There is an increased need for folic acid during pregnancy and lactation. Stressful situations such as disease and excess alcohol consumption increase the requirement for folacin. Doses greater than 0.1 mg daily may obscure pernicious anemia, correcting the hematologic signs while permitting progression of the associated neurologic damage, which is irreversible.

Ascorbic Acid (Vitamin C)

Ascorbic acid deficiency is responsible for the disease known as *scurvy.* Scurvy shows three primary manifestations in the adult: swollen gums with loss of teeth, skin lesions, and pain and weakness in the lower extremities. As the disease progresses, the skin lesions become more conspicuous and hemorrhages occur. In children the most characteristic changes are found in the skeleton, where bone formation is abnormal. Dietary sources of vitamin C include citrus fruit, tomatoes, berries, melons, broccoli, cabbage, sweet potatoes, chili peppers, and green peppers.

After the age of 6 months, infants may be treated by the administration of orange juice. Adults are treated with 500 mg/day of vitamin C. Once therapy has begun, the effects of scurvy begin to recede within 2 to 3 days. Bone formation begins to correct itself within that period of time, and hemorrhages disappear.

Ascorbic acid is also used to acidify the urine and alter the excretion of some drugs. Doses of 4 to 12 g daily are required for this effect. The drug is given in divided doses around the clock and the pH of the urine is monitored.

Megavitamin Therapy

Many persons, including some health professionals, believe that massive doses of vitamins either as single entities such as vitamin C or vitamin E or as combinations of vitamins, minerals, and trace elements are effective in preventing and treating diseases. The concept of megavitamin therapy is extremely controversial, with a lack of good clinical studies to support or refute the theories. It is obvious that there is need for well-controlled clinical studies in this area. Nurses should understand that their patients may strongly believe in megavitamin therapy, and if it is causing the patient no harm the possible placebo effect should not be discounted.

Recently there has been controversy over the use of massive doses of ascorbic acid as therapy for the common cold, to reduce its frequency and severity. Several large-scale studies have shown little or no effect of ascorbic acid on the common cold, despite the fact that a large number of anecdotal reports attest to its efficacy. Excessive intakes of ascorbic acid have been reported to lower serum cholesterol in some individuals, but not in others.

All health professionals who are teaching health care should be aware of the unfavorable effects of overuse of vitamin C. Large doses of ascorbic acid can produce "rebound scurvy." There is evidence that megadoses of vitamin C can produce adverse effects on growing bones, and they interfere with laboratory tests by causing a false positive on the reduction tests for sugar in the urine (e.g., Clinitest) and a false negative on some tests for occult blood in the stool and on enzyme tests for sugar in the urine (e.g., Chemstrip uG, Diastix, Tes-Tape). Large amounts may reverse the anticoagulant activity activity of warfarin and precipitate crises in sickle-cell anemia. Megadoses of vitamin C may also induce uterine bleeding in pregnant women and have been reported to terminate pregnancy, presumably by increasing the production of estrogen. Massive doses destroy substantial amounts of vitamin B_{12} in food; there have been recent reports of vitamin B_{12} deficiency in patients taking megadoses of ascorbic acid. Other reported adverse effects of excessive intakes of ascorbic acid include absorption of excessive amounts of food iron, impaired bactericidal activity of leukocytes, precipitation of calcium oxalate renal stones, and altered drug excretion.

Minerals and Elements

Calcium

Since only 40 percent of dietary calcium is absorbed, 800 mg is required to replace the 300 mg in obligatory losses each day in adults. In the United States, 75 to 85 percent of calcium intake is derived from milk and dairy products. In those who are still growing or in pregnant or lactating women, up to 1200 mg may be required daily. If a supplement is indicated, calcium lactate and calcium gluconate are preferred to the other calcium salts, particularly the phosphate salts, because of their increased solubility (see Table 24-9 for list of calcium supplements). It is especially important for those still growing to accumulate sufficient bone mass, because the amount accumulated in the growing years is steadily depleted thereafter. Furthermore, the appearance of subsequent disorders involving demineralization may be a function of this starting mass.

Phosphorus

Phosphorus is closely related to calcium. Both minerals function in bone building and both are regulated metabolically by the parathyroid hormone. Phosphorus is involved in a great variety of chemical reactions in the body and is an important anion within the cell. It is recommended that in infancy the calcium/phosphorus ratio in the diet be 1.5:1, decreasing to 1:1 at one year of age. Phosphorus preparations are shown in Table 24-10.

Iodine

Iodine is an essential part of the thyroid hormones. Pregnant and lactating females require increased iodine. Natural sources vary widely, depending on the iodine content of the soil. Iodized salt is the main dietary source of iodine.

Iron

Iron is an indispensable element which is often found in inadequate amounts in the human diet. Iron intoxication can occur, especially when high iron intake is coupled with a low-protein diet. (See Chap. 48 for symptoms and treatment of iron toxicity.) Since only 10 percent of dietary iron is absorbed and absorption varies with the source of the iron, the exact amount of iron absorbed is often uncertain. Supplemental iron is necessary during pregnancy and lactation, since the requirement cannot be met by ordinary diets. In the growth periods of infancy and adolescence, particular attention should be paid to iron intake. The healthy adult male loses approximately 1 mg/day and the menstruating female loses an *additional* 0.5 mg to 1.4 mg/day. An average of 6 mg of elemental iron is available in each 1000 kcal in a mixed diet. Dietary sources and a discussion of iron therapy can be found in Chap. 36.

Magnesium

Magnesium is important as a cofactor for many body enzymes. The required amount is readily found in most American diets; approximately 120 mg is usually ingested with each 1000 kcal. Magnesium is found abundantly in vegetable food sources. Magnesium deficiency produces a nonspecific set of neurologic, muscular, and gastrointestinal problems related to calcium and potassium losses.

Copper

Deficiency of copper, an essential element in the diet, is thought to be quite rare. The usual daily requirement is easily obtained in the human diet. Copper is necessary to the function of several enzymes.

Zinc

Zinc has recently been identified as an important dietary element because of its effects on wound healing, taste sensation, appetite, growth, immune function, and other phenomena. Animal meats and seafoods are better sources of available zinc than vegetables. Zinc can cause gastrointestinal irritation, and large doses (> 2 g) cause emesis. Bran and dairy products impair zinc absorption.

Miscellaneous Elements

Certain other elements (sodium, chloride, potassium) are found in the diet in such plentiful quantities that no special supplementation is normally necessary. Fluoride, although not essential, has useful therapeutic applications in small supplementary doses. Other trace elements (chromium, cobalt, manganese, molybdenum, nickel, tin, vanadium, silicon, selenium) are known to produce specific effects. The required amounts of these elements are quite small, and they are generally found in sufficient quantities in the average diet.

Food Additives

Food additives have been defined by the FDA as substances that are directly added to food and become part of it or substances that may affect food without becoming part of it. Because of the banning of some food additives by the FDA, the public has become suspicious of these substances. Many feel that the so-called natural foods offer more safety. However, merely being "natural" does not assure safety. Consider the toxicity of natural tobacco, some forms of mushrooms, and certain molds which grow on crops. On the other hand, it cannot be overlooked that the use of food additives, like the use of many drugs, is not without adverse effects. There is no question that the use of many food additives is unnecessary, but many others such as antioxidant, antimold, and antibacterial agents are necessary to the safety and availability of food.

In addition to the threat of cancer induced by food additives, a wide variety of other disorders are attributed to these agents. Some have claimed that many behavioral and learning disabilities are due to artificial food flavors and colors in foods, but the evidence is not conclusive.

The nurse may be asked about the safety of these agents. By the same criteria used throughout this text to evaluate other pharmacologic agents, the nurse can recommend that products that serve no real purpose except to color or add taste can easily be avoided, just as many of the preservatives can be avoided. It is obvious, however, that more conclusive data are necessary in this area, and until they are available this is a matter of personal decision.

Patient Education Related to Dietary Supplements

Because of escalation of the vitamin and mineral enrichment of foodstuffs, such as breakfast cereals, and proliferation of businesses specializing in vitamin supplements, many people have come to believe that nearly every malady is preventable or curable by the proper vitamin. No matter what their personal views on the value of vitamin supplementation, nurses' educative role requires screening the various claims for vitamin therapy by analyzing the validity of the research and disseminating the information objectively to the public and to patients. Not uncommonly, people self-prescribe or overindulge in vitamin food supplements hoping for a cure of some malady and therefore do not seek medical assistance in time for optimal treatment. When patients are taking professionally prescribed or self-prescribed vitamin supplements, the nurse should teach them about the potential dangers and proper use. The teaching should include warnings that the use of vitamins is not a substitute for seeking competent diagnosis and treatment; that excessive amounts of some agents can interfere with laboratory tests; that disease can be masked by vitamins; that hypervitaminosis can occur; and that vitamins, like all drugs, should be kept out of the reach of children. Further, patients should know that vitamins lose potency relatively rapidly, so they should be kept in tightly closed containers and checked for expiration dates. The nurse should warn patients to avoid mineral oil as a laxative, since it can interfere with the absorption of fat-soluble vitamins (A, D, E, and K).

INFANT NUTRITION

Although breastfeeding is recommended for most infants, there are factors which would limit its use. Aside from maternal illness, employment, or preference for bottle feeding, breastfeeding may not be possible when therapeutic infant formulas are needed.

Standard Infant Formulas

The standard infant formula contains approximately 20 kcal/oz of protein derived from cows' milk, mainly casein. Most preparations use a vegetable oil such as corn or soy oil to supply fat content. Carbohydrates supply 40 percent of the calories of the typical commercial infant formulas. This source may be lactose, sucrose, or corn syrup. Excess disaccharides can produce diarrhea in the child. A list of formulas is given in Table 25-6.

There are three basic types of standard formulas: ready-to-feed, concentrated liquid, and concentrated powder. The concentrated formulas and powders require the addition of water to make the proper formula. The parent must be able to follow the directions, since diarrhea or more serious reactions can occur if an excessively concentrated preparation is administered. The nurse should ensure that the manufacturer's directions are explained to and understood by the parents, and that they are able to prepare the formula with proper aseptic technique.

Therapeutic Formulas

Milk Allergy It is estimated that 1 percent of the infant population is allergic to the protein in cows' milk. In most of the therapeutic formulas used in cases of cows' milk allergy a substitute protein source is used. These formulas include a water-soluble soy (Isomil, Soyalac, Pro-Sobee, Nursoy), enzymatic hydrolysates of casein (Nutramigen, Pregestimil), or a meat-based formula derived from beef heart.

Fat Restriction Conditions such as cystic fibrosis, celiac disease and other malabsorption disorders may require the use of infant formulas containing triglycerides with medium chain-length triglycerides (MCT). These include Pregestimil (2.8 g MCT/dL) and Portagen (3.1 g MCT/100 mg mix).

Carbohydrate Deficiency Premature infants require more calories and are less able to utilize them. Formulas that are used include Enfamil Premature Formula and Similac PM 60/40. Disaccharidase deficiency may occur as a congenital defect or secondary to cystic fibrosis or celiac disease. In these cases, RCF Liquid, which has no carbohydrates, is employed. Later a formula lacking the specific disaccharide may be given (e.g., Isomil SF).

Phenylketonuria When phenylketones accumulate in infants unable to metabolize phenylalanine to tyrosine because of an inborn error of metabolism, they cause an alteration in brain development and produce mental retardation. In these cases a formula which has no phenylalanine is indicated. Since phenylalanine is an essential amino acid it must be provided in the diet, but only in a limited amount. To limit amounts of phenylalanine a formula which uses whey proteins (e.g., SMA Iron Fortified) is often preferred to one which uses casein as the source of the protein (e.g., Lofenalac).

Vomiting and Diarrhea In severe gastrointestinal upset with vomiting and diarrhea, the infant may be unable to tolerate milk products and may become depleted of electrolytes. Electrolyte solutions (e.g., Pedialyte) may restore fluid balance until the child again can tolerate the usual formula. However, since there are only 20 kcal/dL of this formula and it contains no protein, fat, or vitamins, it can be used only for a limited amount of time.

MALNUTRITION

Malnutrition is often thought to reflect a shortage of proper nutrients only. However, malnutrition can be as much a reflection of overnutrition as of undernutrition. In the underdeveloped areas of the world and in the underprivileged areas of the technically developed countries, the problems of too little food, lack of choice and variety in available foods, poor judgment in food selection due to lack of information, and poor methods of preparation all contribute to the development of nutritional deficiencies. In technically developed areas, malnutrition occurs as a result of misguided or misinformed selection of foods or the consumption of highly refined and processed foods, which can result in dietary imbalance and nutritional deficiency. Additionally, disease or associated medical interventions can cause malnutrition. Overnutrition, manifested as obesity, is the major form of malnutrition in developed countries such as the United States, but adult malnutrition has significant implications for nursing practice.

Determining Nutritional Status

There have been many advances over the past 10 years in the identification of patients who may have macronutrient deficiencies or may be at risk of developing such. The methodology of nutritional assessment in the determination of clinical outcome is still under development. Therefore, health professionals will encounter many variations of assessment parameters in different institutions and different parts of the country. Frequently, it is the dietitian who performs the nutritional assessment and, if appropriate, ongoing assessments; however, the nurse should be familiar with the components of this assessment and its interpretations in order to form a more appropriate nursing nutritional care plan.

Effective nutritional assessment can often identify and more accurately define malnutrition in its early stages so that effective nutritional therapeutics can aid the clinical management. This is true whether the patient is overnourished or undernourished.

Nutrition History

An important tool in the assessment of nutritional status is the nutrition history which reviews food consumption and eating habits. Two common methods of obtaining this information are the 24-h recall and the diet dairy.

In the *24-h recall method* the patient lists the food and amounts eaten in the previous 24 h. From these data the interviewer can estimate protein, carbohydrate, fat, and calorie intake. The disadvantages of this methodology are that the patient may not remember dietary intake very accurately and that 24 h may not be very representative of this individual's normal diet. Of course, if the patient is in an institution, it is easier to obtain accurate information.

The other method of obtaining a diet history, a *diet dairy,* requires that the patient record all of the foods eaten for 3 to 7 days. The time of food intake and the amounts eaten are recorded. Both weekdays and weekends should be included during the history, as food consumption may vary. Additionally, a listing of physical activity for each day may provide helpful data for examining caloric expenditure.

Since many people know what they should eat although they may not actually eat correctly, care must be taken during the diet history interview to assume a nonjudgmental attitude and to avoid leading questions, so that the information will be as accurate as possible. The interviewer should, of course, precede the discussion with an explanation of why the information is collected.

All of the data must then be analyzed for adequacy in type and amount of nutrients according to the patient's age, sex, and activity level. Additionally, economic status, general health practices, and psychologic and sociocultural factors, can affect nutritional status.

Somatic Protein Measurements

Weight and Height Charts indicating the desirable ranges of weight according to height, sex, and body frame size are readily available. The health care practitioner should make accurate measurements rather than relying on a patient's recall. For patients unable to stand unassisted, a chair, litter, or sling type scale may be used. In order to enhance the accuracy of serial measurements, the patient should ideally be weighed each time with the same precalibrated scale, wearing an equal amount of clothing, and at the same time

TABLE 25-6 Normal and Therapeutic Infant Formulas Compared to Breast Milk

PRODUCT	Calories per 30 mL	Calories per 100 mL	PROTEIN, g/100 mL	FAT, g/100 mL	CARBO-HYDRATE, g/100 mL	SODIUM, meq/100 mL	POTASSIUM, meq/100 mL	CHLORIDE, mg/100 mL	CALCIUM, mg/100 mL	PHOSPHORUS, mg/100 mL
Breast milk	22	75	1.1	4.5	6.8	0.7	1.3	1.1	33.6	16.0
Cow's milk: whole, fortified	21	69	3.5	3.5	4.9	2.5	3.6	2.7	120.0	96.0
Enfamil	20	68	1.5	3.7	7.0	1.0	1.7	1.4	53.0	44.0
Evaporated milk: diluted 1:1, fortified	21	69	3.5	4.0	4.9	2.8	3.9	3.2	134.6	102.5
Goat's milk, fresh	21	69	3.6	4.0	4.6	1.4	4.6	4.5	128.0	104.9
Similac	20	68	1.55	3.6	7.23	1.1	2.0	1.5	51.0	39.0
Similac with Iron	20	68	1.55	3.6	7.23	1.1	2.0	1.5	51.0	39.0
SMA Iron-Fortified	20	68	1.5	3.6	7.2	0.65	1.4	1.0	44.0	33.0
Isomil	20	68	2.0	3.6	6.80	1.3	1.8	1.5	70.0	50.0
Meat Base Formula (1:1 dilution)	20	68	2.7	3.5	6.4	1.2	1.4	1.4	102	68.0
Nutramigen	20	68	2.2	2.6	8.8	1.6	2.0	1.7	63	48
ProSobee	20	68	2	3.6	6.9	1.3	2.1	1.6	63	50
Pedialyte	6	20	None	None	5.0	3.0	2.0	3.0	8.0	None
Portagen	20	68	2.4	3.2	7.8	1.4	2.2	1.6	63	48
Pregestimil	20	68	1.9	2.7	9.1	1.4	1.9	1.6	63	42
Lofenalac	20	68	2.3	2.7	8.8	1.4	1.8	1.3	63	48

Source: Copyright 1982 by the American Pharmaceutical Association, *Handbook of Nonprescription Drugs*, 7th ed. Reprinted with permission of the American Pharmaceutical Association.

each day. When the patient is unable to stand, height can be measured from heel to top of the head by using a flexible tape measure, while the patient lies flat in bed with arms folded across the chest. In addition to comparing the patient's current weight with a desirable weight, the examiner should record changes in weight over the recent past, especially any history of sudden weight gain or of weight loss.

Body Frame Size Estimation of body frame size is necessary to use the height and weight charts. *Elbow breadth* (distance between the medial and lateral epicondyles of the humerus) has replaced wrist circumference as the most reliable measurement for estmating body frame size. This measurement is compared to norms for medium-framed persons by sex and age (Table 25-7). Measurements greater than the norm indicate a large frame, and those smaller than the norm indicate a small frame.

Skin Fold Measurements Skin fold measurements are one means of estimating body fat content of subcutaneous tissue. Although various areas of the body can be used to obtain this measurement (e.g., biceps, subscapular, abdominal), the triceps skin fold (TSF) is most commonly used. The TSF measurement, performed by pinching a lengthwise double fold of skin and fat between the thumb and forefinger about 1 cm above the midpoint of the arm is used to determine midarm circumference (MAC) [see the section Mid Upper Arm Circumference (MAMC)], with the patient's arm hanging freely. A caliper is then applied to the pinched portion of skin and fat and its thickness is measured in millimeters (Fig. 25-2). This measurement is then compared to age and sex standards (Table 25-8).

Indications for Further Assessment At this point it may be determined that no further nutritional assessment is needed and that no recommendations for support and/or changes of dietary habits are currently appropriate. However, the group of patients considered high risk for nutritional deficits and requiring further nutritional assessment include those with recent loss of 7 to 10 percent of body weight, recent surgery or chemotherapy, recent illness lasting more than 3 weeks, serum albumin less than 3.5 g/dL, lymphocyte count less than 1500/mm^3, disorders of GI tract, burns, trauma, or can-

IRON, mg/100 mL	TYPE OF CARBOHYDRATE	SOURCE OF PROTEIN	TYPE OF FAT	VIT. A, IU/L	VIT. D, IU/L	THIAMINE, mg/L	NIACIN EQUIVALENT, mg/L	ASCORBIC ACID, mg/L
0.15	Lactose	Human milk	Human milk fat	2400	5	0.16	3.5	8
0.05	Lactose	Cow's milk	Butterfat	1850	400	0.29	1.0	10
0.05	Lactose	Cow's milk	Butterfat	1850	400	0.20	1.0	7
0.15	Lactose	Cow's milk	Soy, coconut oils	1690	420	0.53	8.5	55
1.3	Lactose	Cow's milk	Soy, coconut oils	1690	420	0.53	8.5	55
0.15	Lactose	Cow's milk	Soy, coconut oils	2500	400	0.65	7.0	55
1.3	Lactose	Demineralized whey	Safflower oil (blend), soy, coconut oils	2640	423	0.71	10.1	58
1.2	Sucrose, corn syrup	Soy protein	Soy, coconut oils	2500	400	0.40	9.0	55
1.37	Sucrose, modified tapioca, starch	Beef heart	Sesame, beef fat	1808	407	0.60	4.1	61
1.3	Sucrose, modified tapioca, starch	Hydrolyzed casein	Corn oil	1690	420	0.53	8.5	55
1.3	Corn syrup solids	Soy isolate	Soy oil, coconut oil	2100	420	0.53	8.5	55
None	Dextrose	None	None	None	None	None	None	None
1.3	Corn syrup solids, sucrose	Casein	Corn, MCT oils	5300	530	1.1	13.7	55
1.3	Corn syrup solids, modified tapioca starch	Hydrolyzed casein	Corn, MCT oils	2100	420	0.53	8.5	55
1.3	Corn syrup, modified tapioca starch	Hydrolyzed casein	Corn oil	1690	420	0.53	8.5	55

TABLE 25-7   Norms for Elbow Breadth of Medium-Framed People*

HEIGHT, in†	ELBOW BREADTH, in‡
Men	
62–63	2½–2⅞
64–67	2⅝–2⅞
68–71	2¾–3
72–75	2¾–3⅛
76	2⅞–3¼
Women	
58–63	2¼–2½
64–71	2⅜–2⅝
72	2½–2¾

*For estimating body frame size.
†In shoes, 1-in heels.
‡Distance between median and lateral epicondyles of humerus. Measurements smaller than norms indicate small frame. Measurements larger than norms indicate large frame.
Source: Metropolitan Life Insurance Company, 1983.

cer (Tuckerman, 1983). These patients require a complete nutritional assessment (nitrogen balance, MAMC, CHI, immune function, visceral protein stores, etc.; see below) and analysis of the need for nutritional therapy. For the overweight person further assessment should include history, physical examination, and further laboratory testing as necessary to rule out endocrine, cardiac, psychiatric, renal, or hepatic causes of weight gain.

Mid Upper Arm Muscle Circumference (MAMC) The MAMC measurement reflects muscle mass and protein-calorie adequacy of dietary intake. It is computed by determining the midarm circumference (MAC) minus the circumference of the skin fold thickness (see Fig. 25-3). Decreased arm circumference occurs with both acute and chronic wasting. MAC is measured at the midpoint of the upper arm, and the computed MAMC is compared to standards for age and sex (Table 25-8).

Creatinine-Height Index (CHI) The creatinine height index is an indirect measurement of muscle mass depletion. A 24-h urine collection is assayed for total creatinine excre-

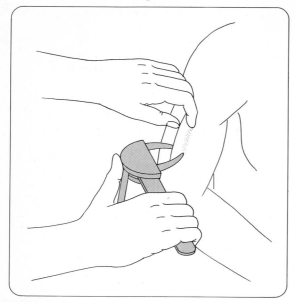

FIGURE 25-2

Use of Skin Calipers. Triceps skinfold thickness is measured 1 cm above the midpoint between the acromion process of the scapula and the olecranon process of the ulna.

tion. The CHI is expressed as a percentage and compares the actual milligrams of creatinine excreted for the 24-h period with the predicted creatinine excretion based on height (from Table 25-8).

$$\text{CHI} = \frac{\text{Measured urinary creatinine} \times 100}{\text{Ideal urinary creatinine}}$$

An average of three serial 24-h urine collections will give the most accurate results. A limitation of the CHI is that body frame size and musculature and changes in creatinine excretion that occur with age are not taken into account by established norms.

Nitrogen Balance

Nitrogen balance is examined to evaluate the adequacy of calorie and protein intake. Nitrogen loss is determined from a 24-h urine collection, and nitrogen gain is ascertained by recording the grams of protein intake during the same 24-h period. Nitrogen loss is subtracted from the nitrogen gain; the result provides a positive or negative nitrogen balance number, according to the following formula, which assumes 2.5 g to be the approximate sum of urinary nonurea nitrogen, fecal loss, and integumental loss (Rudman and Bleier, 1983):

$$\begin{aligned}\frac{\text{Nitrogen balance}}{\text{number}} &= \frac{\text{Daily protein intake (g)}}{6.25} \\ &- [\text{24-h urine urea nitrogen (g)} + 2.5\ \text{g}]\end{aligned}$$

The clinical significance of this obtained value is that repair of significant protein deficits can only occur if the nitrogen balance is significantly positive, e.g., +4 to +6. This means the nitrogen intake, in the form of protein, needs to be greater than the nitrogen losses the patient is experiencing. If the obtained nitrogen balance number is 0 or near 0, this result indicates that no change in the patient's nutritional status is likely to occur; if no deficits exist, the goal of therapy becomes to maintain this 0 nitrogen balance. A large negative nitrogen balance number indicates that the

TABLE 25-8 Standards for Nutritional Status Parameters*

| AGE, yr | Triceps Skin Fold, mm† | | | | | | Midarm Muscle Circumference, cm‡ | | | | | | Ideal Creatinine§, mg/24 h/cm | | |
| | Standard | | 80% Standard | | 60% Standard | | Standard | | 80% Standard | | 60% Standard | | | | |
	M	F	M	F	M	F	M	F	M	F	M	F	HEIGHT	M	F
0.5	10.0	10.0	8.0	8.0	6.0	6.0	11.4	11.2	9.1	9.0	6.8	6.7	150	—	5.68
1	10.3	10.2	8.2	8.2	6.2	6.1	12.7	12.4	10.2	9.9	7.6	7.4	160	8.28	5.93
2	10.0	10.1	8.0	8.1	6.0	6.1	13.1	12.8	10.5	10.2	7.9	7.7	165	8.40	6.09
5	9.1	9.4	7.3	7.5	5.5	5.7	14.1	13.9	11.3	11.1	8.5	8.3	170	8.62	6.32
10	8.2	10.4	6.6	8.3	4.9	6.2	17.1	16.6	13.7	13.3	10.3	10.0	175	8.86	6.51
15	6.3	11.4	5.0	9.1	3.8	6.8	23.0	20.8	18.4	16.6	13.8	12.5	180	9.11	6.69
Adult	12.5	16.5	10.0	13.2	7.5	9.9	25.3	23.2	20.2	18.6	15.2	13.9	185	9.38	—

*Triceps skin fold (TSF) and midarm muscle circumference (MAMC) given by sex (M = male; F = female) and age; ideal weight creatinine by sex and height. (Condensed from C. E. Butterworth and C. L. Blackburn: "Hospital Malnutrition and How to Assess the Nutritional Status of a Patient," *Nutrition Today*, **10**:8, 1975. Reproduced with permission of *Nutrition Today* magazine, P.O. Box 1829, Annapolis, Maryland, 21404. Consult the original source for a more complete breakdown of age and height standards.)

†See Fig. 25-2 for method of measurement.

‡See Fig. 25-3 for method of calculation.

§Derived by multiplying ideal weight for height by creatinine coefficient (23 mg/kg for males; 18 mg/kg for females) and dividing by height in cm. Creatinine height index (CHI) is expressed as the percentage of this ideal creatinine which is actually excreted in a 24-h urine collection.

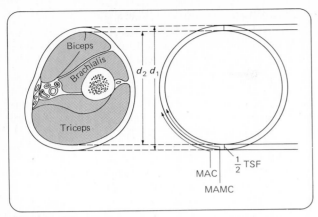

FIGURE 25-3

Measurement and Computation of Mid Upper Arm Muscle Circumference (MAMC). Midarm circumference (MAC) is measured in centimeters with a tape measure, and triceps skinfold is measured in centimeters as described in Fig. 25-2. Mid upper arm muscle circumference (MAMC) is calculated as follows;

$$MAMC = \pi d_2$$
$$= \pi[d_1 - (d_1 - d_2)]$$
$$= \pi d_1 - \pi(d_1 - d_2)$$
$$= MAC - \pi TSF$$

where d_1 = arm diameter
          d_2 = muscle diameter
          TSF = $2 \times$ subcutaneous fat = $d_1 - d_2$
and   MAC = πd_1 .

(*Adapted from C. E. Butterworth and G. L. Blackburn: "Hospital Malnutrition and How to Assess the Nutritional Status of a Patient," Nutrition Today, 10:8, 1975. Reproduced with permission of* Nutrition Today *magazine, P.O. Box 1829, Annapolis, MD 21404.*)

patient has an existing and continuing protein deficit, a finding which supports a conclusion of inadequate nutrition and/or needed nutritional support.

Immune Functions

Cell-Mediated Immunity   Body defenses are affected by numerous factors, one of which is malnutrition. Patients with suspected malnutrition are skin tested via intradermal injection to measure their cutaneous hypersensitivity to known antigens, to provide information about the adequacy of the cellular immune system. Common antigens used include mumps, candida, and purified protein derivative (PPD). The skin tests are read at 24 and 48 h. Normal response is a wheal of at least 15 mm in diameter. A result of 10 to 15 mm indicates a mild immune deficiency; between 5 to 10 mm, moderate deficiency; and less than 5 mm, a severe immune incompetency. If an immune deficiency is ascertained from skin testing, the causative factor

may be malnutrition. Some controversy exists about the reliability of this test because of other existing factors, such as surgery, anesthesia, sepsis, chemotherapy, and radiotherapy, which also affect immunocompetence. Thus, skin testing is only one of the many indices used to determine nutritional status.

Lymphocyte Count   Another immunocompetence study is the determination of total lymphycyte count:

TLC = Lymphocytes (%)
$$\times \text{ White blood cell count (WBC)}$$

A count of less than 1500/mm³ is suggestive of impaired immunocompetence.

The immune function tests discussed here are used not so much to determine the presence of malnutrition but to determine the scope of effects of that state. Other tests discussed in this section are more definitive for the detection of malnutrition.

Visceral Protein Measurements

Visceral or nonmuscle protein levels are measured by serum laboratory tests. The most commonly measured proteins are albumin and transferrin. Serum albumin has a long half-life of approximately 21 days and therefore changes slowly with poor dietary protein intake. Transferrin, which has a much shorter half-life of 8 to 10 days, reflects dietary protein changes more acutely. However, hydration level and the presence of stress or trauma may significantly alter the valves of both of these proteins, thus detracting from their nutritional significance.

Prealbumin, another visceral protein, has an extremely short half-life of 1 to 2 days and is therefore a sensitive indicator of visceral protein status. However, the serum concentration of prealbumin also changes acutely with minor stress and therefore can be a misleading nutritional indicator.

Physical Examination

Physical exam of the patient with malnutrition or the potential for malnutrition is important. Special emphasis is given to those body areas which most commonly reflect nutritional deficiencies: skin, hair, eyes, and mouth. Glands and the nervous system are less commonly affected. Physical signs of nutritional deficiencies occur only after significant body nutrient depletion. While a patient is acutely ill, the commonly affected body systems should be assessed at least weekly for nutrient deficiency (e.g., rashes, lesions, texture changes) and the results recorded.

Compiling Data

The compilation of all the above data is generally summarized in some standard format which varies from institution to institution. The degree of nutritional depletion is measured and evaluated by a series of tests. No single test is used to determine any degree of impairment or to establish goals for nutritional repletion. Figure 25-4 demonstrates an example of a nutritional assessment profile.

OBESITY

When caloric intake exceeds the energy requirements of the body for physical activity and growth, the result is the accumulation of adipose tissue. If this continues for a prolonged period, obesity results. Obesity is a serious health hazard, increasing the risks of diseases (such as diabetes mellitus, coronary atherosclerosis, hypertension, respiratory difficulties); increasing surgical risk; complicating pregnancy; and causing growth disturbances in the adolescent. Weight reduction will generally result in the normalization of the risks.

Clinical Pharmacology and Therapeutics

Three modalities for treatment of overnutrition are education, diet adjustment, and medication. A major role of the nurse, working with the dietitian and other health professionals, is education. Probably the most complex of the educational goals are those related to motivation, a major determinant of patient compliance. For some patients, presentation of the benefits or risks to overall health and longevity will induce adequate motivation, although for others this type of approach may even have negative effects. Any time the nurse is dealing with lifelong patterns and values in an area that has important social and psychologic implications, such as eating habits, it is not enough simply to tell the patient to do something. The most effective approaches are active involvement of the patient and/or family in planning and implementation, coupled with sincere interest and concern by the nurse and frequent follow-up.

ANERGIC/METABOLIC PROFILE*

PATIENT _____ ROOM _____ DATE _____

| | | DEFICIT | | | |
PARAMETERS	VALUE	SEVERE	MOD	MILD	ADEQUATE
MARASMUS — SOMATIC PROTEINS					
WEIGHT/HEIGHT					
TRICEPS SKINFOLD (mm)					
ARM MUSCLE CIRCUMFERENCE (cm)					
CREATININE/HEIGHT INDEX					
KWASHIORKOR — VISCERAL PROTEINS					
ALBUMIN					
TRANSFERRIN					
TOTAL LYMPHOCYTE COUNT					
CELL—MEDIATED IMMUNITY					

NITROGEN IN (g/day) _____

NITROGEN OUT (g/day) _____

NITROGEN BALANCE (g/day) _____

NUTRITIONAL STATUS	DEGREE
☐ ADEQUATE	☐ NONE
☐ MARASMUS	☐ MILD
☐ KWASHIORKOR	☐ MODERATE
☐ MARASMUS-KWASHIORKOR MIX	☐ SEVERE

STANDARDS	SEVERE	MODERATE	MILD
SOMATIC PROTEINS - % DEFICIT	> 30%	> 15-30%	> 5-15%
ALBUMIN (g/dl)	< 2.5	< 3.0-2.5	< 3.5-3.0
TRANSFERRIN (mg/dL)	< 160	< 180-160	< 200-180
LYMPHOCYTE COUNT (No/mm^3)	< 900	< 1500-900	< 1800-1500
CELL—MEDIATED IMMUNITY (mm)	< 5-0	< 10-5	< 15-10

*Adapted from Metabolic Support Service, St. Mary of Nazareth Hospital, Chicago, Ill.

FIGURE 25-4

Example of a Nutritional Assessment Profile. (*Used through courtesy of Abbott Laboratories from* Contemporary Parenteral Nutrition, *1980.*)

Many people would like to think that the answer to obesity or overnutrition lies in a pill or injection. However, anorectic drugs are ineffective without concomitant diet modification, and the amphetamines and nonamphetamine anorectics usually lose efficacy with prolonged use. Furthermore, anorectics, hormones, and fad diets in the treatment of obesity can be very dangerous. Diet, exercise, and modification of behavior remain the major determinants of weight loss.

Amphetamines

The amphetamine and nonamphetamine anorectics are *sympathomimetic agents* used to suppress appetite to help patients tolerate low-calorie diets. Many physicians do not prescribe these agents because of their low efficacy and safety and their potential for abuse (see Chap. 49). Amphetamines are also used in narcolepsy and attention deficit disorder in children (see Chap. 33).

Mechanism of Action   Amphetamines have central nervous system (CNS) stimulant activity. They are thought to exert their anorectic activity in the lateral hypothalamic feeding center, but the precise mechanism is not known. Amphetamines also have weak α- and β-adrenergic stimulating ability.

Pharmacokinetics   Amphetamines are *basic* (alkaline) drugs which are rapidly absorbed from the small intestine and widely distributed throughout the body. Therapeutic blood levels are between 5 and 10 μg/dL. Amphetamines are metabolized by the liver, but the portion excreted unchanged in the urine and the half-life depend upon the urinary pH. Urine at a pH less than 5.6 results in a half-life of about 7 h; for every one-unit increase in urine pH, the half-life is extended by 7 h.

Adverse Effects   A number of disease states require cautious use of amphetamines: hypertension, hyperthyroidism, cardiovascular disease, prior drug abuse, and agitation. Possible teratogenic effects have occurred when pregnant women have used amphetamines. Allergic reactions also occur.

Cardiac effects (tachycardia, palpitations, increased blood pressure) and CNS stimulation (restlessness, irritability, insomnia, tremor, euphoria) are the most common adverse effects. Dry mouth, diarrhea, constipation, and unpleasant taste also occur. High doses may cause sexual dysfunction and reversible increases in serum thyroxine levels. Although tolerance and tachyphylaxis to the anorectic effect occur, the dosage should *not* be increased when loss of effect occurs.

Drug Interactions   Hypertensive crisis may occur if amphetamines are taken within 14 days of administration of **monoamine-oxidase (MAO) inhibitors. Insulin** requirements may be altered by amphetamines. Effects of **guanethidine** (Ismelin) and other antihypertensives may be decreased by amphetamines. The various amphetamine preparations are shown in Table 25-9.

Nonamphetamine Anorectics

Like the amphetamine anorexiogenic drugs discussed above, the nonamphetamines are *indirect-acting sympathomimetics*. All except **mazindol** (Mazanor, Sanorex), **phenmetrazine** (Preludin), and **phendimetrazine** (Metra, Trimstat, others) are analogs of amphetamine and thus have similar effects (Table 25-9). **Fenfluramine** (Pondimin) is unique in that it causes CNS depression by depleting serotonin in the brain.

Mechanism of Action   The precise mechanism of these drugs is not known. They are thought to have a direct stimulant effect on the satiety center in the hypothalamus and limbic regions.

Pharmacokinetics   Nonamphetamine anorectics are well absorbed and distributed throughout the body. Most agents exert their effects for 4 to 6 h, although this period is longer (8 to 18 h) for **mazindol, fenfluramine,** and sustained-released dosage forms. These drugs are metabolized by the liver, and only fenfluramine has pH-dependent renal excretion.

Adverse Effects   The contraindications, precautions, adverse effects, and drug interactions of the nonamphetamine anorectics are similar to the amphetamines (see the section on amphetamines), although the potential for abuse is slightly less. **Fenfluramine** may cause CNS depression, drowsiness, impotence, and withdrawal symptoms (ataxia, tremor, confusion). It should not be used with other CNS depressants or by alcoholics who may have psychotic reactions. Fenfluramine potentiates rather than antagonizes the effects of antihypertensive drugs, may increase the risk of cardiac arrest during surgery, and has hypoglycemic activity. **Mazindol** also has hypoglycemic activity and may potentiate the pressor effects of catecholamines. **Diethylpropion hydrochloride** is associated with increased seizure activity in epileptics.

Nonprescription Anorectics

The most common ingredient in over-the-counter diet aids is the sympathomimetic **phenylpropanolamine,** which is also commonly used as a decongestant in cold preparations. Phenylpropanolamine shows many of the same adverse effects and drug interactions as the amphetamine and nonamphetamine anorectics (see the section on nonamphetamine anorectics), such as blood pressure elevation, palpitations, tachycardia, restlessness, seizures, and insomnia, but it also is associated with renal failure accompanied by muscle lysis (rhabdomyolysis) and hypertensive episodes when administered with **propranolol** (Inderal) or **indomethacin** (Indocin). Vitamins and minerals are other ingredients in these preparations (e.g., Vita-Slim, Dexatrim Plus Vitamins, Trendex, Appedrine), as are grapefruit extract and mild diuretics (Fluidex Plus).

Benzocaine, a local anesthetic, decreases taste perception, which is thought to be an important factor in overeating. Methylcellulose or other bulk producers may be included to give the sensation of fullness. Examples of nonprescription diet aids are shown in Table 25-9.

Patient Education Related to Anorectics

A crucial aspect of nursing care for the patient taking anorectics, whether self-medication with nonprescription drugs

or prescribed agents, is education. These agents are adjuncts in weight loss and are effective only if combined with dietary modification and exercise. Anorectics should not be used longer than 8 to 12 weeks, and the prescribed or labeled dosage and frequency should not be exceeded. The prescription drugs are controlled substances (see Chap. 8) because of their abuse potential.

Since these drugs may cause insomnia, they should be taken early in the day. Sustained-release forms should be taken 10 to 14 h before bedtime and should not be chewed, crushed, or opened. These drugs are usually taken on an empty stomach ½ to 1 h before meals, although **mazindol** may be taken with meals if gastrointestinal irritation occurs.

Patients should be aware of the adverse effects of the prescribed agent. They should know to inform a health care

TABLE 25-9 Amphetamines and Other Anorectic Agents

GENERIC NAME	TRADE NAME	DOSAGE FORMS	USUAL ANORECTIC DOSE*
Amphetamines			
Amphetamine sulfate		Tablets	5–30 mg daily in divided doses before meals
Dextroamphetamine sulfate	Dexedrine, Dexampex, Fendex, others	Tablets, capsules, elixir, sustained release capsules (spansules)	As above; spansules taken once daily, in morning
Methamphetamine HCl (desoxyephedrine HCl)	Desoxyn, Methampex	Tablets, long-acting tablets	5 mg before meals tid, or 10–15 mg in morning
Amphetamine mixtures (mixtures of salts of various amphetamines)	Biphetamine, Delcobese, Obetrol	Long-acting tablets or capsules	5–20 mg total amphetamines daily
Nonamphetamine Anorectics			
Benzphetamine HCl	Didrex	Tablets	25–50 mg one to three times daily
Diethylpropion HCl	Tenuate, Tepanil, others	Tablets, sustained release tablets	25 mg tid before meals or 75 mg in the morning
Fenfluramine HCl	Pondimin	Tablets	20–40 mg tid before meals
Mazindol	Sanorex, Mazanor	Tablets	1 mg tid one before meals or 2 mg before lunch
Phendimetrazine tartrate	Adipost, Trimcaps, others	Tablets, capsules, sustained release capsules	35 mg two to three times daily before meals or 105 mg in the morning
Phenmetrazine HCl	Preludin	Tablets, sustained release tablets	25 mg two to three times daily before meals or 50–75 mg once daily
Phentermine HCl	Tora, Phentrol, Fastin, others	Tablets, capsules, timed release capsules	8 mg tid before meals or 15–37.5 mg once daily
Nonprescription Anorectics			
Phenylpropanolamine	Control, Dexatrim Caffeine Free, Acutrim, others	Tablets, capsules, timed release capsules	25 mg tid before meals or 75 mg in morning
Benzocaine	Ayds, Slim-Line	Candy, gum	5–15 mg tid before meals

*Once-daily dosages are for sustained release forms.

professional if palpitations, chest pain, nervousness, dizziness, severe constipation, or other severe gastrointestinal effects occur.

Other Agents Used in Obesity

Hormones   Various hormones have been used in the treatment of obesity. **Human chorionic gonadotropin** (HCG) has been studied in this regard, but studies to date have not substantiated efficacy. The applicability of HCG as a therapeutic entity in the treatment of obesity is still unproved, and the possibility of adverse endocrinologic reactions from it should be kept in mind (see Chap. 46).

Progesterone has been used to improve the pulmonary function of obese patients. Many of these patients exhibit a form of alveolar hypoventilation called the *Pickwickian syndrome* (see Chap. 22). They exhibit somnolence, twitching, cyanosis, periodic respiration, secondary polycythemia, and right ventricular hypertrophy and failure.

Thyroid hormones have been used for many years as adjuncts to weight loss therapy. There is no doubt that thyroid hormone will produce reductions in body weight, if given in adequate doses and durations of therapy. These reductions are transitory, however, and are limited to the period when the thyroid hormone is being administered. Patients tend to regain all weight lost after therapy has been terminated, because of larger appetites than before therapy and decreased level of activity from muscle fatigue and weakness. Furthermore, weight lost by this method tends to be lean body mass and not adipose tissue.

Chronic therapy with thyroid hormones for the purpose of weight reduction is associated with cardiovascular symptoms, including palpitations and sweating, loss of urinary calcium and nitrogen, and development of osteoporosis. Therapy with thyroid hormones should be considered only in obese patients in whom hypothyroidism can be documented. In these cases, the hormone should be given only in doses sufficient for physiologic replacement. A combination that has proved lethal is a digitalis glycoside (**digoxin**), a thyroid preparation, and **dextroamphetamine**.

Starch Blockers   Starch blockers are substances which supposedly prevent the normal digestion of starch by blocking the action of the enzyme amylase. Research has shown no demonstrable effect on the absorption of starch calories. Users of starch blockers have reported symptoms including nausea, vomiting, diarrhea, and abdominal pain (bloating and gas).

Ultra-Low Calorie Diets   There were numerous deaths in 1977 due to the use of liquid protein diets. Very-low-calorie diets (including powdered instant mix formulas and premixed liquid preparations) pose a significant health hazard to dieters not under continuous medical supervision by a physician knowledgeable in the metabolism and nutrition of such diets, including appropriate laboratory evaluation at regular intervals. No one should be on a very-low-calorie diet (less than 800 kcal) without close and continuous medical supervision throughout the dieting and refeeding period.

UNDERNUTRITION

Categories of adult macronutrient malnutrition can be classified as kwashiorkor, marasmus, and marasmus-kwashiorkor. *Kwashiorkor* is defined by visceral protein deficiency (serum albumin, transferrin, and prealbumin). Persons with this type of deficiency often appear well nourished and are in many cases obese. However, because the visceral protein stores are inadequate and cellular immune functions are depressed, these patients are at a risk of morbidity and mortality due to their malnutrition.

Marasmus is defined by gradual wasting of body fat and skeletal muscle mass in the presence of preservation of visceral protein stores and immunocompetence. These persons are typically underweight, appear emaciated, and are at a relatively low risk of nutritionally related morbidity and mortality. However, they have minimal nutritional reserves and tolerate repeated or prolonged stress poorly.

Marasmus-kwashiorkor is a combination of all of the deficiencies listed: skeletal muscle wasting, depletion of fat stores, serum visceral protein concentrations below normal, and immunologic incompetence. These persons appear cachectic and typically suffer acute catabolic stress and starvation secondary to chronic illness. This is the group of malnourished patients who have the highest risk of serious morbidity and mortality without intensive nutritional intervention.

Clinical Pharmacology and Therapeutics

Current studies are beginning to establish the relation between the assessed nutritional status and patient prognosis, both in terms of complication rate and morbidity and mortality. However, the techniques discussed for nutritional assessment have only recently been used in the selection of patients who require nutritional support. Published data for normal ranges for all age groups, especially 40 years and older, are incomplete and of questionable accuracy. Therefore, data obtained from a nutritional assessment must be carefully interpreted and utilized as supportive, rather than definitive, information in patient selection for nutritional support.

Indications for Nutritional Support

Increasing numbers of patients receive enteral or parenteral nutritional support because of the recognized relation between sound nutritional status and recovery. Further, the realization of the depleting effects of stress and illness on nutrient stores has resulted in use of nutritional therapy in patients who are currently nutritionally sound but who are candidates for nutritional depletion. Decisions about the use of nutritional support therapy are based upon a review of dietary adequacy, somatic and visceral protein parameters, nitrogen balance, immune competence, and potential for stress and nutrient depletion. Patients requiring nutritional support can be separated into five categories:

1. Nonhypermetabolic
2. Slight deficit and/or slightly hypermetabolic
3. Hypermetabolic
4. Severely malnourished
5. Chronic inability to maintain nutrition

Nonhypermetabolic *Nonhypermetabolic* patients are nutritionally sound, but their disease state or surgery can result in protein deficiency if preventative therapy is not initiated. Typically, this group includes stroke, cancer chemotherapy patients, some surgical patients, and any other patient who is not experiencing a high degree of stress or infection. The goal of therapy for these patients is to maintain their current nutritional level; thus, a nitrogen balance of 0 to −2 is acceptable. If the nitrogen balance becomes significantly less than −2 or the visceral protein markers begin a downward trend, protein sparing nutritional support, in the form of nonprotein calories, is indicated.

Slight Deficit Patients with *slight deficits* are nutritionally sound or may have mild to moderate deficits and/or are slightly hypermetabolic (nitrogen balance of −2 to −5). Often these patients may have been in the first category, nonhypermetabolic, but protein sparing nutritional support has not prevented a declining patient trend. At this point, these patients require more calories than can be obtained by normal protein sparing methods but do not require central vein hyperalimentation. The logical choice in this situation is partial parenteral nutrition, which can repair minor deficits and prevent severe nutritional deficits.

Hypermetabolic *Hypermetabolic* patients require intensive nutritional support even though they are nutritionally sound. By definition of *hypermetabolism,* nutritional and metabolic needs are at levels so great that they cannot be met by normal means. These demands are often twice those of a healthy person; their caloric demands can reach 5000 to 6000 kcal and 24 to 36 g of nitrogen per day. These patients include most victims of major burns, trauma, and infection. The goal of therapy becomes maintenance of current sound nutritional status and achievement of a zero nitrogen balance. These needs can only be met with central vein hyperalimentation. Maintenance of a zero nitrogen balance requires that adequate nonprotein and protein be provided to repair injury and to preserve existing protein compartments. The status of those protein stores affect the ability of the patient to withstand stress; the hypermetabolic patient is in a state of severe stress and of tremendous nutritional need.

Severely Malnourished *Severely malnourished* patients are those who have abnormal results in all the nutritional parameters previously discussed. Moderate to severe malnutrition has been demonstrated in up to 20 percent of hospitalized patients. The therapeutic goal of repairing protein deficits requires the achievement of a +4 to +6 nitrogen balance. The only clinical means to achieve this balance is via central vein hyperalimentation.

Chronic Inability to Maintain Nutrition There is a growing population of patients who for numerous reasons (e.g., chronic vomiting, cancer, ulcerative colitis) cannot adequately meet nutritional needs by standard means. These individuals have no need to be hospitalized and can live normal lives. However, they need some form of daily nutritional support that they or their family can manage at home, independent of health care professionals.

Approaches to Nutritional Therapy

Nutritional support is always necessary when the patient's oral intake is inadequate to meet nutritional requirements and therapeutic goals. The two methods for administration of nutrients to achieve repair of nutritional deficits or for maintenance of body cell mass are into the gastrointestinal tract (*enteral*) or into the venous system (*parenteral*). The enteric route, whether oral or tube feeding techniques are used, is *always* preferred whenever it is possible. If this approach fails or is not feasible, parenteral nutrition is necessary.

Nutritional support should be an integral part of the patient's total therapy, not an incidental treatment. Based upon a thorough assessment and carefully identified goals, nutritional therapy is a component of total nursing care in a variety of settings from the acute care hospital to the extended care facility, the long-term rehabilitation center, the clinic or health care office, and even in the home!

Enteral Nutrition

Enteral nutrition requires that the patient have a minimal level of function of the gastrointestinal tract (approximately 3 ft of functioning jejunum) and that the degree of repletion and/or maintenance required can be met by enteral products. Potential contraindications to enteral therapy include upper gastrointestinal hemorrhaging, gastrointestinal obstruction or malabsorption, paralytic ileus, fistulas, recent gastrointestinal surgery, or severe vomiting.

The enteral route for nutritional support encompasses a wide range of techniques and products. Some patients may simply need a nutritional supplement to their orally consumed diet, but some require total nourishment with an enteral product via a tube which allows access to a distal portion of the gastrointestinal tract.

Nutrient Sources

Because patients' nutritional needs and gastrointestinal tract function are variable, numerous innovations in enteral products have occurred. Enteral feeding products are no longer synonomous with hospital blenderized diets which have undefined nutrient levels. The products available differ from each other in many ways. Some are dehydrated and require reconstitution; others are ready-to-use liquids.

Some products are complete nutritional formulas, whereas others are only nutritional supplements. The formulas may contain protein, fat, and/or carbohydrates, which can be derived from a variety of sources, a fact that produces significant product differences. Additionally, the complexity of nutrients may vary. For example, the nitrogen substrate of a formula may be whole protein, peptides of various sizes, or amino acids. Other product differences include the characteristics of digestibility; caloric density; caloric distribution across carbohydrates, fats, and proteins; viscosity; pH, osmolarity; amount of residue; taste; palatability; and flavoring.

Many of these product differences have clinical significance. For example, taste and palatability, which greatly affect patient compliance if the oral route is being used, have little significance if an enteral feeding tube is being used. Viscosity may have an impact on the gauge of tube used and high viscosity may require an infusion pump. High osmolarity may encourage the dumping syndrome, especially if the formula is delivered too fast, another indication for use of an infusion pump. Some fats such as medium chain triglycerides may be tolerated better than others in patients with whole fat intolerance. Products which contain lactose may not be tolerated in patients who have a lactose deficiency and lactose intolerance. Fecal formation is influenced by the amount of residue. In patients who require fluid restriction, the desirable product is one which has a high caloric density per volume of fluid. Thus, the choice of enteral product must be based on knowledge of the constituents and characteristics of various products, correlated with an understanding of the patient's individual needs.

Classification of Enteral Formulas

A majority of enteral products can be classified as one of three basic types of mixtures, polymeric, elemental, and modular. (See Table 25-10.)

Polymeric *Polymeric* solutions, composed of protein, carbohydrate, and fat of a high-molecular-weight form, are the most inexpensive of the enteral formulas, have a low osmolarity, and are based on milk proteins. These diets tend to be more palatable than others because the fat component contributes a greater percentage of the total calories than with other diets. These preparations are complete with respect to vitamins and minerals and are isoosmolar. Most average a ratio of 1 kcal/mL, and there are some products available

that offer 2 kcal/mL and are useful for the patient who requires fluid and/or sodium restriction. These enteral solutions are used to supplement inadequate caloric intake or to provide complete nutrition; because of palatability, they can be tolerated for long periods of time if necessary. They require normal digestive ability, and some products are lactose free for patients who have a lactose intolerance. The primary disadvantage of polymeric formulas is the fixed nutrient composition, which is a drawback for only a small group of patients.

Elemental *Elemental* solutions are low in residue and are composed of a predigested and easily absorbed protein source (hydrolyzed protein, dipeptides and tripeptides, and/or crystalline amino acids), a carbohydrate source that requires little amylase activity (glucose, sucrose, dextrin, and oligosaccharides), and a small amount of fat in the form of essential fatty acids. All essential minerals and vitamins are included. However, these formulas do have several disadvantages. Most are unpalatable and are therefore not very suitable for oral use, although flavoring somewhat alleviates this problem. They are also hyperosmolar, and therefore can cause cramping and an osmotic diarrhea if infused too rapidly. However, these formulas remain the product of choice for patients who have impaired digestive and absorptive capability and require feeding in a simple, readily available "elemental" form.

Modular Modular formulas are individual modules of protein, carbohydrate, and fat; vitamin and mineral modules are still in the research and development stage. Until the latter modules are on the market, a complete nutritional formula can be attained by adding these vitamins, minerals, and trace elements to the core modules. The core modules can also be added to polymeric formulas in order to change the protein, carbohydrate, and/or fat content of the original formula.

Indications

Table 25-11 relates the appropriate use of enteral formula types to disease states.

Routes of Administration

If a patient is unable to take an enteral product orally, tube feedings can be administered by the following routes: nasogastric, nasoduodenal, nasojejunal, esophagostomy, gastrostomy, and jejunostomy. The latter three routes require surgical access to a portion of the gastrointestinal tract but are useful for long-term therapy because the tube is removed or covered between feedings.

The complications of nasopharyngitis, rhinitis, otitis media, parotitis, and stricture of the gastroesophageal sphincter previously associated with large-bore (e.g., 16 French) stiff nasointestinal tubes have been largely elimi-

TABLE 25-10 Examples of Enteral Formulas

| TYPES | EXAMPLE | Osmolality | | DAILY VOLUME FOR 100% RDA, mL | Protein | | Carbohydrate | |
		mosm/kg	kcal/mL or g		g/1000 kcal	SOURCE	g/1000 kcal	SOURCE
Elemental	Vivonex HN	810	1.00	3000	46	Amino acids	210	Glucose oligosaccharides
	Vital	460	1.00	1500	42	Peptides from whey, soy, meat, + 9 amino acids	188	Corn syrup, sucrose
	Travasorb HN	560	1.00	2000	45	Peptides from lactalbumin	175	Glucose oligosaccharides
Polymeric	Sustacal	625	1.00	1080	60	Casein, soy	138	Sucrose, corn syrup
	Ensure	450	1.06	1900	35	Casein, soy	135	Corn syrup, sucrose
	Isocal	300	1.06	1900	32	Casein, soy	125	Glucose oligosaccharides
	Portagen	354	1.00	2525	36	Casein	117	Corn syrup, sucrose
	Compleat B	300	1.07	1500	40	Beef, casein	133	Cereal, vegetable, fruit
	Ensure Plus	600	1.50	1920	37	Casein, soy	133	Corn syrup, sucrose
	Magnacal	590	2.00	1000	35	Casein	125	Maltodextrin, sucrose
Modular	Polycose	850	2.00	NA	0	NA	250	Glucose polymers
	Casec	NA*	3.70	NA	230	Casein	0	NA
	MCT oil	NA	7.70	NA	0	NA	0	NA
	Product 80056	NA	4.90	NA	0	NA	146	Corn syrup, tapioca
Altered amino acids	Hepatic-Aid	1158	1.65	NA	26	Amino acids	175	Maltodextrin, sucrose
	Amin-aid	1095	1.95	NA	10	Amino acids	187	Maltodextrin, sucrose

*NA = not applicable.

Source: J. C. Bleier and D. Rudman: "Diet Therapy," in R. G. Petersdorf et al. (eds.), *Harrison's Principles of Internal Medicine*, 10th ed., McGraw-Hill, New York, 1983. Used by permission.

nated or minimized. The newer feeding tubes used are flexible, generally an 8 French size, and many have a mercury weighted tip or stylet which aids in the insertion. The disadvantage of these tubes is that they can easily be removed by the disoriented or uncooperative patient.

Feeding tubes that deliver enteral formula to the stomach (nasogastric, esophagostomy, gastrostomy) take advantage of the bacteriocidal effects of gastric acid and allow the digestive process to begin in the stomach. They permit the stomach to empty its contents at a controlled rate, thereby decreasing the risk of dumping syndrome, and reduce problems associated with bacterial contamination of the formula. Jejunal feeding results in less nausea, vomiting, and bloating, but formulas must be easily digestible, isoosmolar, and prepared, stored, and delivered with least risk of bacterial contamination. Skin excoriation and peritonitis are risks with gastrostomy and jejunostomy.

Adverse Effects

The adverse effects of enteral hyperalimentation and appropriate management are outlined in Table 25-12.

Dosage and Administration

Regardless of type of enteral feeding tube used, the general principle is always to use the smallest tube through which

g/1000 kcal	Fat SOURCE	Ca, mg/1000 kcal	P, mg/1000 kcal	Na, mg/1000 kcal	K, mg/1000 kcal	MICRONUTRIENTS
<1	Safflower oil	333	333	529	1173	Yes
11	55% safflower oil 45% MCT oil	667	667	383	1167	Yes
13	MCT oil Sunflower oil	500	500	920	1170	Yes
23	Soy oil	1000	920	920	2060	Yes
35	Corn oil	511	511	708	1179	Yes
42	80% soy oil 20% MCT oil	600	500	500	1250	Yes
48	86% MCT oil 12% corn oil	936	707	468	1248	Yes
34	Beef, corn oil	625	875	625	1313	Yes
35	Corn oil	422	422	704	1267	Yes
40	Soy oil	500	500	500	625	Yes
0	NA	150	30	290	100	No
5	Milk	4312	2156	408	0	No
120	92% MCT oil	0	0	0	0	No
46	Corn oil	1102	606	147	688	Yes
22	Soy oil	0	0	0	0	No
24	Soy oil	0	0	173	0	No

the formula will run. In general, more viscous preparations require a size 10 French tube, although thinner formulas will easily flow through a 6 to 8 size French tube. If a smaller tube is desired for a viscous formula, the use of an enteral pump will aid in solution delivery.

When to begin the enteral infusion and the rate of administration are dependent upon the patient's overall condition and nutrient tolerance. A jejunal feeding may be started immediately postoperatively, despite expected postoperative ileus because the jejunum is still able to absorb sufficient water, electrolytes, and organic substrates. However, some prescribers prefer to wait until 24 h after surgery to begin jejunal feedings.

If the enteral solution is being delivered nasoenterically,

the formula should infuse over a period of 18 to 24 h each day. Use of an infusion pump permits continuous, even flow; prevents abdominal cramping; and avoids occlusion of the tube by a viscous solution. The concentration and flow rate of the formula should be increased slowly, beginning with a one-half to one-quarter-strength solution (especially with hyperosmolar elemental diets) at a rate of 25 mL/h and increasing to full strength and an optimal flow rate over 3 to 4 days.

Bolus or intermittent feedings by tube are not common in current practice because of problems with gastric reflux and the chance of aspiration when a large volume of enteral formula is delivered at one time. Additionally, it is thought that the absorption of nutrients is much greater with a con-

TABLE 25-11 Disease States, Nutritional Sensitivities, and Appropriate Selection of Enteral Solution

DISEASE STATES	Nutritional Sensitivity								Enteral Formula		
	LACTOSE	FAT MALABSORPTION	PROTEIN MALABSORPTION	PROTEIN ENCEPHALOPATHY OR UREMIA	SODIUM	POTASSIUM	RESIDUE	FLUID VOLUME	POLYMERIC	ELEMENTAL	MODULAR
Medical											
Anorexia									+		
Inflammatory bowel disease	+	+	+							+	
Chronic pancreatitis		+	+				+			+	
Short bowel syndrome	+	+	+				+			+	
Cancer											
Anorexia									+		
Partial esophageal obstruction									+		
Radiation enteritis	+	+	+				+			+	
Cirrhosis											
Ascites				+	+†			+	+(HCD)		+
Encephalopathy				+							+
Cardiac cachexia		±	±		+†			+	+(HCD)		+
Pulmonary cachexia					±			±	+		+
Renal insufficiency				+	+	+		+	+		+
Surgical											
Major injury											
Head trauma		+							+		
Long bone fracture			±						+		
Bowel resection*							+	+			
Bowel obstruction							+				
Fistulas										+	
Severe burn							±	+	+(HP, HCD)	+(HP)	

Abbreviations: HCD = high caloric density; HP = high protein.

*Symptoms and treatment vary with extent of resection.

†High dosages of diuretics and secondary hyperaldosteronism may increase potassium requirement.

Source: S. B. Heymsfield, J. Horow, and D. H. Lawson: *Developments in Digestive Diseases*, Philadelphia: Lea and Febiger, 1980. Reprinted with permission.

TABLE 25-12 Complications of Enteral Hyperalimentation and Their Management

TYPE OF COMPLICATION	FREQUENCY, %	MANAGEMENT
Mechanical		
Tube lumen clogged by solution	Infrequent (<10)	Flush with water; replace tube if unsuccessful
Pulmonary aspiration of stomach contents	Rare (<1)	Unlikely with head of bed elevated; discontinue if aspiration occurs
Esophageal erosion	Rare (<1)	Discontinue tube
Stomal erosion	2	Discontinue tube
Wound infection	2	Treat with antibiotics
Herniation through interostomy site	Rare (<1)	
Tube dislodgement:		
Nasoenteral	10–20	Replace tube
Gastrostomy	Rare (<1)	Replace tube
Jejunostomy	Rare (<1)	Use intravenous nutritional support
Gastrointestinal Symptoms		
Vomiting and bloating	10–15	Reduce flow rate and give 10 mg metoclopromide; add peripheral hyperalimentation if needed
Diarrhea and cramping	10–20	Reduce flow; dilute solution; consider different type solution; add antidiarrheal drug
Metabolic, Fluid, and Electrolyte Abnormalities		
Hyperglycemia and glucosuria	10–15	Reduce flow; administer insulin
Hyperosmolar coma	Rare (<1)	Discontinue therapy
Edema	20–25	Usually none; may reduce Na content or slow hyperalimentation rate; rarely use diuretics
Volume overload in uremia	10	Dialyze more frequently
Congestive heart failure	1–5	Slow hyperalimentation; administer diuretics and digoxin
Hypernatremia, hypercalcemia	<5	Adjust electrolyte content of hyperalimentation
Essential fatty acid deficiency	Common	Linoleic acid supplement orally or intralipid intravenously

Source: J. C. Bleier and D. Rudman: "Diet Therapy," in R. G. Petersdorf et al. (eds.) *Harrison's Principles of Internal Medicine,* 10th ed., McGraw-Hill, 1983. Used by permission.

stant, even rate and that the problems of dumping syndrome are decreased when the patient receives a constant infusion of formula.

The mechanical and technical aspects of enteral care are beyond the scope of this book but can be found in standard fundamental or medical-surgical nursing texts. Table 25-13 summarizes pertinent observations for the patient receiving enteral therapy.

Parenteral Nutrition

Some patients require intensive metabolic support which can only be met by parenteral (intravenous) solutions. (See Table 25-14.) Malnutrition can develop very rapidly, causing these patients to tolerate the stress of illness poorly. Wound healing is impaired, and susceptibility to infection and other complications is heightened. Thus, early detection of malnutrition and correction of this state can often prevent a prolonged and/or catastrophic hospital course.

Total parenteral nutrition (TPN), or *parenteral hyperalimentation*, refers to the administration of markedly hypertonic solutions into a central vein (to avoid peripheral vein irritation). Patients who do not require intensive nutritional support may receive *partial parenteral nutrition* (PPN) either alone or concurrently with enteral nutrition.

Total Parenteral Nutrition (TPN)

Since TPN is often the patient's sole means of nourishment, it is imperative that the nutrients administered closely approximate those of a balanced oral diet. To achieve this, parenteral solutions should contain protein (amino acids), carbohydrates, fats, electrolytes, and micronutrients.

Protein (Nitrogen) Sources More recently developed nitrogen sources for parenteral solutions are crystalline amino acids which are composed of essential and nonessential L-amino acids (Aminosyn, Travasol, Freamine, Veinamine). The L (*levo*) form is preferable to the D (*dextro*) form because the former can be readily metabolized whereas the latter is largely excreted. These amino acids are used to replete and spare protein stores. These commercial solutions

TABLE 25-13 Monitoring of the Patient on Enteral Nutritional Therapy

When initiating a new or intermittent feeding	Check the placement (NG tube). Check amount of residual (if 150 mL, consider possible reasons for delayed gastric emptying).*
Every ½ h	Check gravity drip rates when applicable.*
Every hour	Check pump drip rate when applicable.*
Every 2–4 h of continuous feeding	Check residual.*
Every 4 h	Check vital signs, including blood pressure, temperature, pulse, and respiration.
	Check sugar and acetone in urine (in nondiabetic patient, can be discontinued after 48 h if consistently negative).
	Refill feeding container.
	Check ice, when applicable.
Every 8 h	Check intake and output.
	Check specific gravity of urine.
	Charting
Every day	Weigh patient.
	Change feeding bag and tubing.
	Check electrolyes, blood urea nitrogen, and blood glucose daily until stabilized.
Every 3–4 days	Change irrigation set.
Every 7–10 days	SMA-12 and SMA-6 (blood chemistries)
	Complete blood count
	Make nutritional assessment.
PRN	Observe patient for any untoward responses to tube feeding (nausea, vomiting, diarrhea, others).
	Check tube placement (NG).
	Check nitrogen balance.
	Clean feeding equipment.

*Applicable only when tubes are employed

Source: Modified from *Monitoring Summary and Checklist, Tube Feedings: Clinical Applications,* June, 1980. Reprinted with permission of Ross Laboratories.

come in concentrations ranging from 3.5% to 10%. In addition, products for the uremic patient which contain only minimal requirements of the eight essential amino acids (Aminosyn-RF, Nephramine) are available.

Calorie Sources—Glucose   It is critical to remember that the energy requirements of ill persons are increased; it has been estimated that hospitalized patients require 20 percent more calories above their resting energy needs in order to perform limited physical activity. Other investigators have recommended that caloric intake be increased 50 percent over resting energy needs in order to achieve positive nitrogen balance.

The primary caloric sources in parenteral solutions are glucose and fats. Generally, 50% dextrose (500 mL), a markedly hypertonic solution, is used, mixed with an equal volume of amino acid solution (typically 7 or 8.5%); the resultant dextrose concentration is 25%. The final volume of 1 L

TABLE 25-14   Indications for Parenteral Nutrition

Impaired digestive function due to
Bowel inflammation or obstruction
Intractable diarrhea
Ulcerative colitis
Crohn's disease, especially with enterocutaneous fistulae
Mouth, throat, and stomach carcinoma
Malabsorption syndrome
Short bowel syndrome
Pancreatitis
Peritonitis
Chronic vomiting

Iatrogenic nutritional or growth disturbance
Adrenocorticosteroid therapy
Chemotherapy
GI surgery
Radiotherapy

Malnutrition secondary to
Alcoholism
Anorexia
Cancer
Connective tissue disorders
Hepatic failure
Renal failure

Hypercatabolic states
Postsurgery
Sepsis
Severe burns
Trauma

Source: G. L. Blackburn, E. M. Copeland III, and G. B. Rankin: "Aggressive Parenteral Nutrition; Feeding the Malnourished Patient," *Patient Care,* **15**(1):55, January 30, 1981. Adapted with permission. Copyright © 1981, Patient Care Communications, Inc., Darien, CT. All rights reserved.

(1000 mL) provides 850 nonprotein calories and 150 protein calories. For example, a highly hypermetabolic patient, as seen in severe burns, may require 5 L of TPN per day, which would provide 4250 nonprotein calories. A comparable volume of 5% dextrose would provide only 850 cal. Thus, caloric density is a significant feature of TPN solutions.

Calorie Sources—Fats (Lipids)   Fat, in the form of a 10 or 20% safflower (Liposyn) or soybean oil (Intralipid, Travamulsion) emulsion offers a great advantage for patients requiring substantial nutritional repletion. Since the caloric value of fat is more than twice that of carbohydrate sources (9 kcal/g vs. 3.4 kcal/g), the addition of **intravenous fat emulsions** to TPN regimens can greatly increase caloric load without a concomitant increase in fluid volume. A 10% emulsion provides about 555 kcal/500 mL, and a 20% concentration approximately 1000 kcal/500 mL. However, the general guideline is that intravenous fats should not compose more than 40 to 60 percent of the total calories per day. Carbohydrate calories are needed to satisfy the glucose requirements of the brain and to prevent gluconeogenesis (from an inadequate glucose supply). Regardless of the caloric requirement, the amount provided in fat should not exceed 2.5 g/kg of body weight for adults; for the pediatric patient the upper limit is 4 g/kg.

The recognition of *essential fatty acid depletion* (EFAD) with prolonged nutritional programs devoid of fat has prompted clinicians to regard fat emulsion as an indispensable part of a TPN regimen, so fats serve two purposes in parenteral nutrition, calorie source and source of essential fatty acids.

Vitamins, Electrolytes, and Trace Elements   All vitamins can be supplied parenterally by commercially available multiple-vitamin preparations which contain water-soluble forms of vitamins A, D, and E, along with the B group vitamins and ascorbic acid. These commercial preparations do not have vitamin K, which must be added separately. It must be mentioned that further research is needed to determine more accurately the requirements for parenteral vitamins and the effects of severe stress, trauma, infection, malnutrition, and intravenous use of protein and large amounts of carbohydrates on those requirements.

Electrolytes must be added to TPN solutions to provide maintenance requirements, as well as to replace antecedent and/or ongoing, abnormal losses. The physician makes the determination of electrolyte requirements on the basis of laboratory and clinical evaluations. Some commercially available amino acid solutions have electrolyte content, which may be sufficient to meet patient requirements, or they may be supplemented by the use of additives.

Trace elements include such substances as copper, zinc, magnesium, and chromium. There is documentation on the daily dietary allowances for trace elements; however, trace element requirements for parenteral use have not been established with any certainty. Commercially prepared solutions of trace elements are added to TPN solutions.

Insulin When patients are receiving highly concentrated dextrose solutions, they often require exogenous insulin administration to maintain serum glucose levels within normal ranges, particularly early in therapy. Insulin given subcutaneously or intramuscularly can cause large fluctuations in serum glucose; therefore, the appropriate insulin dosage may be added directly to the TPN solution. All TPN patients require frequent urinary testing for glucosuria to determine the need for and to guide the appropriate dosage of insulin.

Heparin Heparin is frequently added to TPN solutions to prevent clotting in the subclavian catheter and to enhance the clearance of administered fat particles. The dosage of 1 U/mL of TPN solution is sufficient to prevent catheter clotting; 1 to 2 U/mL of fat emulsion is recommended to enhance clearance of fat particles. Heparin can be added to either the TPN solution or the fat emulsion, but never to both when they are infusing concurrently.

Partial Parenteral Nutrition

Partial parenteral nutrition (PPN) was developed in order to provide an easier means of administering nutritional prophylaxis, that is, prevention of nutritional depletion in hospitalized patients that might inhibit recovery or develop into more serious malnourishment. It is intended as short-term therapy to supply a limited amount of nutrients, not the full nutritional requirements, to the nonstressed or marginally malnourished patient for whom TPN is really not indicated. Because PPN is indicated for patients who need replacement of protein losses as they occur or in whom oral intake is contraindicated, the gastrointestinal (GI) surgical patient is an excellent candidate. Such patients include those undergoing gastric or colonic resection or pancreatic or hepatic surgery. Other candidates include those in intensive care units who may experience severe but short-term stress. However, if nutritional support becomes necessary for more than 10 to 12 days, then TPN is indicated. Three basic therapeutic regimens may be used for PPN:

1. Nitrogen source with carbohydrate solution
2. Nitrogen source, carbohydrate solution, and lipid emulsion
3. Nitrogen source alone (controversial)

Protein (Nitrogen) Sources The same crystalline amino acid solutions is discussed in the section on TPN are used for PPN; however, generally, the lesser-concentration (3.5 and 5.5%) solutions of amino acids are used.

Calorie Sources—Glucose PPN is administered via peripheral routes. This means of infusion is easier to establish and is not associated with the potential complications of the central venous route used with TPN. However, the peripheral route has a distinct limitation; hypertonic solutions cannot be infused because of the associated problems of vein irritation, sclerosis, and phlebitis. Therefore, less-concentrated solutions of dextrose, i.e., 10% dextrose, must be employed as a calorie source. For example, when 500 mL of 10% dextrose is combined with an equal volume of 5.5% amino acid solution, the final dextrose concentration becomes 5%, yielding 170 nonprotein kcal/L and 4.63 g nitrogen/L. This results in a nonprotein calorie to nitrogen ratio of approximately 37:1, contrasted to the typical ratio of TPN solutions at 180:1. Any attempt to increase the PPN ratio will require increasing the dextrose concentration, which will increase the potential for vein irritation and subsequent multiple intravenous recannulations.

Calorie Sources—Fats If more calories are desired in PPN regimens, the use of intravenous fats is recommended. As discussed with TPN, these emulsions provide 1.1 kcal/mL and can augment nonprotein calorie needs. The peripheral administration route can be used because these solutions are isotonic; thus vein irritation is unlikely.

Vitamins and Electrolytes Other nutrients required for successful PPN include vitamins and electrolytes. These are added to the solutions, as in TPN, and are individualized according to patient needs.

Vascular Access and Management

The administration of TPN solutions requires the cannulation of the central venous circulation, most commonly the superior vena cava, via the subclavian vein. As previously mentioned, this procedure is necessary because of the hyperosmolar nature of these solutions. There are numerous commercially available catheters today, most of which are made of silicone elastomer, which has surface characteristics which impede thrombus formation.

Historically, patients who require long-term nutritional support, on an inpatient or outpatient basis, undergo a surgical procedure to place a Hickman or Broviac catheter. These catheters have a large-bore, 1.6-mm and 1.0-mm inside diameter, respectively, with one or two dacron cuffs used to anchor them in place subcutaneously. The external end of the catheter is threaded and comes with a male luer lock cap. These catheters are able to stay in place for at least a year with meticulous care to prevent infection.

A newer technique being used now in some institutions employs a Centrasil or Intrasil catheter system. The subclavian vein is cannulated to obtain access to the superior vena cava, as in the traditional subclavian catheter placement technique; however, this product affords the opportunity to perform a catheter exchange over a guide wire without the need for a second needle cannulation of the vessel.

Complications seen with subclavian vein catheterization include air embolism, catheter embolism, penumothorax, arterial puncture, improper tip location, subclavian vein thrombosis, and infection. It is generally accepted that catheter insertion by practitioners with extensive experience in placement of subclavian catheters significantly reduces complication rates. Complication rates related to insertion are currently 1 percent or less.

Patients who are receiving TPN are predisposed to infection because they are often catabolic, have concomitant infections for which they may be receiving broad-spectrum antibiotics (and perhaps corticosteroids), and have a foreign body in the vascular system. The TPN solutions are potentially rich substrates for bacterial growth because of their high dextrose content. Thus, proper aseptic techniques in caring for the catheter site and IV tubing are critical. Failure of asepsis greatly increases infection complications. Guidelines for TPN catheter care are listed in Table 25-15.

Adverse Effects

Any therapeutic regimen has associated risks which can be decreased by careful monitoring. Complications associated with PPN have generally been fewer and less serious than those identified with centrally administered TPN, which involves use of the central route and intensive metabolic support. However, the goals and benefits of TPN that cannot be achieved with PPN justify the greater risks.

Sepsis Sepsis is a critical complication of TPN which is often procedure-related. Contamination of the TPN solution can occur from solution preparation (which should be done in pharmacies under laminar flow hoods—not at the nursing station), catheter placement, connection of the IV tubing, catheter site care, contamination of the administration set and/or solution container, or inappropriate manipulation of the system (e.g., administering blood products or withdrawing blood samples).

In the beginning years of TPN (early 1970s), rates of contamination and septicemia were unacceptably high and con-

---

TABLE 25-15 Guidelines for Catheter Care for TPN

1. Intravenous administration sets should be changed at least every 24 h. In some institutions tubing is changed with each new bottle.

2. When the tubing is changed at the catheter the patient should be lying down, and the health practitioner should request the patient to perform the Valsalva maneuver if at all possible. These two techniques help to prevent air embolus. The patient who has a Hickman or Broviac catheter *must* have the catheter *clamped* whenever opening it to air. These are different from the subclavian catheter because the lumen is much larger, thus making air embolism more likely.

3. A bottle of TPN should not infuse any more than 24 h because of the increased possibility of bacterial growth. Some institutions have guidelines limiting the duration of infusion of a single TPN bottle to 12–18 h. Prior to administration, solutions should be kept refrigerated at 39°F (4°C).

4. Stopcocks, anywhere in the line, are not advised, as these are potential sites for bacterial growth.

5. No piggyback infusions should be administered through the TPN line because of increased chance of contaminating the solutions. Additionally, there are serious questions about the stability of many drugs when admixed with TPN solutions.

6. Blood sampling from the catheter is not recommended unless there is no other vascular access. Blood is a rich culture medium, and unless scrupulous technique is used, the potential for infection is great.

7. Dressings over the catheter site should be changed aseptically and routinely and should always be dry and intact. Procedures for dressing changes vary with the institution and physician. Generally, the skin is defatted with acetone (which also destroys bacterial cell walls) and then cleaned with povidone-iodine solution (**Betadine**). The catheter is also painted with povidone-iodine. The use of acetone around the Hickman/Broviac catheter requires careful application, as it breaks down the integrity of the catheter. For this reason, many institutions do not allow the use of acetone with the Hickman/Broviac catheters. Finally povidone-iodine ointment is applied at the insertion site. Antibiotic ointments have less toxicity to both bacteria and fungi and increase the fungal colonizations of the catheter. Finally, a gauze dressing or clear adhesive dressing (e.g., Op-site, Tegaderm) is applied and must be totally occlusive. Gauze dressings are generally changed three times per week, whereas the newer clear dressing may be left on up to 7 days if they remain occlusive.

stituted a significant patient risk. However, with realization that most of the sepsis was of an iatrogenic origin, meticulous protocols to dictate virtually every aspect of the TPN regimen, combined with a heightened awareness of the absolute necessity of aseptic technique, resulted in a marked reduction of contamination and sepsis. Current sepsis rates average 3 to 7 percent when meticulous technique is used. Most septicemias are fungal; however, gram-positive and to a lesser extent gram-negative bacteria may also cause sepsis. The most common fungal agent involved in sepsis is *Candida,* which grows well in the hypertonic, somewhat acidic solution of TPN.

Consideration should be given to the use of in-line filters to decrease the risk of infection secondary to contaminated solutions. The 0.22-μm filter is most typically used and will block fungi and virtually all bacteria from reaching the patient; this filter also requires the use of a pump to maintain flow rate. It can also trap small amounts of air in the solution as it infuses. Of course, this micropore filter is of no use for bacterial/fungal contamination that occurs below the filter. Additionally, if lipid emulsions are being administered with the TPN solution, they have to be "piggybacked" or "Y-connected" below the filter, so the fat particles will not clog the filter. It must be noted that many institutions do not use filters, under the premise that sepsis is prevented by properly prepared solutions, proper care of the TPN catheter, and good metabolic management.

Osmotic Diuresis Osmotic diuresis occurs when the patient's renal threshold for glucosuria is exceeded, leading to an increased water loss and dehydration. Ongoing evaluation of the patient's urinary and serum glucose will allow prompt identification of osmotic diuresis, and appropriate measures can correct this situation before serious sequelae (dehydration, hyperglycemia, nonketotic coma) develop. If the patient has a glucosuria of ¾ percent (+2), it can be lowered by decreasing the rate of TPN administration. If glucosuria has reached levels of 1 percent or 2 percent or more (+3 or +4), insulin administration is required.

Other Metabolic Complications Other metabolic complications include hyperammonemia, hyperchloremic metabolic acidosis, hypoglycemia, hypokalemia, hypomagnesemia, hyponatremia, hypophosphatemia, and prerenal azotemia. All of these can be avoided or arrested by alert biochemical and clinical monitoring, as outlined in Table 25-16.

Dosage and Administration

All patients except those with fluid intolerance should start out their TPN regimen by receiving 2000 mL of solution over 24 h. This is well within the ranges for normal water metabolism and carbohydrate utilization. After the first 24 h

the volume may be increased in increments of 1000 mL/day (averages 2400 to 3000 mL/24 h). If glucose intolerance exists, regular insulin should be added to the solutions rather than gradually increasing the glucose loads in hopes of avoiding the use of insulin. Patients who have normal pancreatic function will tolerate rapid increases of carbohydrate infusion. Patients who have deficient pancreatic function or insulin resistance may require more than a week before carbohydrate tolerance improves, if it does at all, and during this time significant nutritional losses may occur (Grant, 1980).

It is very important that TPN solutions be infused at a steady rate. Large changes in the rate ($\pm$15 percent or more) can cause significant hypoglycemia or hyperglycemia and, if great, coma, convulsions, or even death. If the solution administration is off schedule, the flow rate should not be increased or decreased to compensate for the off schedule. Instead, the flow rate should be adjusted to the correct hourly rate and continued at this rate thereafter. The concern over a constant rate dictates the use of an infusion pump, which eliminates the guesswork and variables of infusion therapy. Additionally, use of a pump prolongs catheter life by preventing occlusion of the catheter tip by a clot or fibrin sheath.

Home Nutritional Therapy

There are people who cannot sustain life without frequent hospital admissions for dehydration, malnourishment, and electrolyte deficiency unless they receive nutritional therapy chronically. These include patients with GI problems, such as inflammatory bowel disease, fistulas, obstruction, malabsorption, and radiation enteritis, as well as those with multiple-system trauma, burns, renal failure, hepatic disease, stroke or comatose patients, and those with cancer. The patients and their families are taught how to care for their IV catheters, pumps, and solutions and how to monitor any signs of complications. Generally, they infuse "cyclically," that is, over 12 h, usually while asleep at night, rather than over 24 h as is done in the hospital. This affords them the time to participate in family and community affairs and perhaps even employment. In many communities, nutritional support companies have appeared, assuming the responsibility for supplying and delivering the required solutions and ancillary supplies needed and bearing all financial risks in seeking third-party reimbursement.

Psychosocial Responses to TPN

Total parenteral nutrition is a relatively new therapy which is increasing in inpatient and long-term home use. As with many lifesaving therapies such as hemodialysis, TPN may be associated with numerous psychologic problems.

A 1-year study examined the psychosocial responses of 59

TABLE 25-16   Complications of TPN

COMPLICATIONS	POSSIBLE PREVENTIVE MEASURES
Problems related to catheter misplacement	
Pneumothorax, hemothorax, hydrothorax, chylothorax Puncture of subclavian artery Catheter embolism Hydromediastinum or hemomediastinum Brachial plexus injury Myocardial perforation	Confirm catheter site in superior vena cava by an x-ray film before starting infusion
Air embolism	Ask patient to hold breath on inspiration during placement of catheter and when bottles and tubing are being changed.
Infections	
Septicemias and fungal septicemias; septic thrombosis or thrombophlebitis	Use strict aseptic technique during catheter insertion and maintenance, while changing the tubing and filter, and during storage of TPN solution (store at 4°C).
Metabolic problems	Ensure accurate metabolic assessment before initiation of infusion, appropriate total dose, accurate infusion rate, careful monitoring of hematologic variables.
Glucose	
Hyperglycemia, hyperosmolar coma	Gradually increase (over 48 h) the concentration of dextrose administered.
Hypoglycemia	Gradually decrease dextrose concentration before TPN is discontinued.
Calcium-phosphorus	
Hypercalcemia, hypophosphatemia, hypercalciuria	Monitor serum electrolytes.
Amino acids	
Hyperammonemia, azotemia, hyperchloremic acidosis	Monitor serum electrolytes, BUN, cognitive function.
Miscellaneous	
Essential fatty acid deficiency (clinical or biochemical or both)	Provide intravenous fat emulsion, with cyclical administration of carbohydrate calories, oral or cutaneous administration of safflower oil, administration of linoleic acid.
Trace element deficiencies (zinc)	Provide adequate amounts of trace metals in IV formula.*
Skin abnormalities; elevations in serum SGOT and alkaline phosphatase levels	Consider lipid infusions to reduce need for hypertonic dextrose.

*Patients with excessive GI losses of trace elements, particularly zinc, may need more than maintenance therapy.
Source: Contemporary Parenteral Nutrition, Central Vein, 1982. Used through courtesy of Abbott Laboratories.

patients after they were placed in TPN. The researchers were able to identify three general patterns dependent upon the medical or surgical diagnosis and duration of TPN therapy (Malcolm et al., 1980).

Acute illness with brief TPN for 1 to 4 weeks had minimal psychosocial effects. Patients and their families did not appear to react to TPN as a specific treatment modality.

The pattern of *convalescence with intermediate-term TPN* included patients who were beginning oral intake although TPN was continued for another 1 to 12 weeks in order to improve anabolic effects. In this group of patients

and families minor psychosocial reactions developed, taking the form of anxiety and apprehension about the importance of TPN and the cost of this therapy. Very few patients (fewer than 5 percent) developed more severe psychiatric syndromes in the absence of cerebral insufficiency. At this stage family reactions played little part in the adjustment to TPN therapy.

Chronic illness with long-term TPN subjected patients to long-term stresses and alterations in lifestyles, vocational roles, and personal identities. These changes generally began about the time home training for self-care started. Family

TABLE 25-17   Evaluation of TPN Therapy

VARIABLES TO BE MONITORED	Suggested Frequency	
	FIRST WEEK	LATER
I. Energy Balance		
Weight	Daily	Daily
II. Metabolic Variables		
1. Blood measurements:		
Plasma electrolytes (Na^+, K^+, Cl^-)	Daily	2 times weekly
Blood urea nitrogen	3 times weekly	2 times weekly
Plasma osmolarity	Daily	2 times weekly
Plasma total calcium and inorganic phosphorus	3 times weekly	Weekly
Blood glucose	Daily	2 times weekly
Plasma transaminases	3 times weekly	Weekly
Plasma alkaline phosphatase	Weekly	Weekly
Plasma total protein and fractions	2 times weekly	Weekly
Blood acid-base status	Daily	Daily
Hemoglobin and hematocrit	Weekly	Weekly
Platelet count and WBC	Weekly	Weekly
Ammonia	2 times weekly	Daily
Magnesium	2 times weekly	As needed
2. Urine measurements:		
Glucose	4–6 times daily	4 times daily
Specific gravity or osmolarity	2–4 times daily	Daily
3. General measurements:		
Volume of infusate	Daily	Daily
Oral intake (if any)	Daily	Daily
Urinary output	Daily	Daily
III. Prevention and Detection of Infection		
1. Clinical observations (activity, temperature, symptoms)	Daily	Daily
2. WBC and differential	As indicated	Weekly
3. Cultures	As indicated	Weekly
IV. Nutritional Assessment		
1. Anergic / metabolic profile	Initially	Weekly
2. Nitrogen balance	2 times weekly	2 times weekly
V. Lipid Utilization (tolerance)		
Triglycerides	Daily	Weekly
Cholesterol	Daily	Weekly
Fat clearance	Daily	Weekly

Source: Contemporary Parenteral Nutrition, Central Vein, 1982. Used through courtesy of Abbott Laboratories.

members and patients assumed roles that were difficult to deny or avoid. Issues of dependency, negative body image, control, and ambivalence to caretakers began to surface. Patients developed concerns and perhaps phobic behaviors based on rational or irrational fears related to their TPN therapy. Complications requiring further hospitalizations and causing news fears arose. Questions about cost and longevity were a constant source of worry. A few developed delusional thinking. Chronic TPN programs are in their infancy, and there are no data on morbidity and mortality or on long-term psychosocial adaptation.

Evaluation of Nutritional Therapy

Evaluating nutritional support interventions involves appraisal of the changes or maintenance of nutritional status by somatic protein measurements, nitrogen balance, immune function, visceral protein measurement, and weight. The monitoring of specific adverse effects of enteral and parenteral therapy is outlined in Table 25-13 and Table 25-17, respectively. For long-term therapy the psychosocial response of the patient and family must be considered.

CASE STUDY

C.C., a 21-year-old female college student, had been diagnosed 5 months previously as having ulcerative colitis. She was admitted to the hospital for treatment of severe diarrhea of 4 days' duration, weakness, and a 10-kg (22-lb) weight loss over the preceding 3 months.

Assessment

C.C. reported to the nurse that she had been experiencing anorexia, nausea, and four to five watery stools daily for the last 2 months and that the stools had increased in number to more than eight per day and had become grossly bloody over the last 4 days. Admission vital signs included height, 170 cm (57 in); weight, 48 kg (105 lb); temperature, 36.6°C; pulse, 106/min; respirations, 16/min; blood pressure (right arm, lying), 102/62 without evidence of orthostatic changes. On physical examination she appeared as a pale, thin, slightly anxious white female with pain on palpation, guarding of the left lower abdominal quadrant, and marked excoriation of the perianal area. Other physical findings were noncontributory. Relevant laboratory values included hemoglobin, 9 g/dL; hematocrit, 30%; lymphocytes, 2000/mm³; albumin, 4.2 g/dL; total protein, 7.0 g/dL; plasma urea nitrogen, 14.0 g/dL; creatinine, 0.9 g/dL; sodium, 138 meq/L; potassium, 3.0 meq/L; chloride, 106 meq/L; and bicarbonate, 22 meq/L.

The nurse recognized that not only was C.C. anemic and hypokalemic, but also she was at significant risk for (or already experiencing) a macronutrient deficiency state. The nurse proposed to the patient's physician that she be seen by the Nutritional Support Team for thorough assessment and consideration for nutritional support therapy.

The dietitian, clinical nurse specialist, physician, and clinical pharmacist of the Nutritional Support Team gathered the following additional laboratory data: 24-h urinary creatinine excretion, 850 mg (5 mg/cm height); prothrombin time, 11.1 s; partial thromboplastin time, 35 s; total iron binding capacity (TIBC), 220 µg/dL (indicator of transferrin levels; normal: 25 to 400 µg/dL); 24-h urinary urea excretion, 6.3 g. The patient's mid upper arm circumference (MAC) was 19 cm, her triceps skin fold thickness (TSF) was 11.5 mm, and her elbow breadth was 5.5 cm (about 2½ in). Delayed hypersensitivity skin reaction to mumps and *Candida* was 12 mm and 10 mm, respectively, at 24 h and 10 mm for both sites at 48 h. She tolerated food poorly because of anorexia, nausea, and exacerbation of diarrhea by oral intake. Therefore, during the assessment she was placed on enteral formula, which was tolerated somewhat better. Her protein intake was estimated at less than 30 g/day.

The following parameters were computed; TSF, 70 percent of standard (from Table 25-8); medium body frame (from Table 25-7), indicating she was about 80 percent of the ideal weight for her height (60 kg; from height-weight tables); creatinine height index (CHI), 80 percent (actual creatinine excretion divided by ideal value from Table 25-8); MAMC, 80 percent of standard (computed to be 18.6 cm by formula in Fig. 25-3 and compared with data in Table 25-8); and a nitrogen balance of −4 (computed by formula in narrative of this chapter). The diagnosis of the team was that C.C. did not demonstrate visceral protein depletion as evidenced by normal (or marginally low) serum albumin, TIBC, total protein, lymphocyte count, delayed hypersensitivity, and coagulation tests. However, she did exhibit marasmus (depletion of peripheral fat and somatic muscle mass), as indicated by the below-standard TSF, MAMC, and CHI. A nitrogen balance of −4 suggested she had a moderate deficit, and partial parenteral nutritional support was recommended to supplement the enteral intake. The approximate daily fluid, nonprotein calories, and protein requirements for C.C. (based on weight of 48 kg) were 2500 mL, 1920 kcal, and 58 g, respectively.

Management

Medications ordered or C.C. were prednisolone sodium phosphate 30 mg IV bid (to treat the acute ulcerative colitis); loperamide hydrochloride (Imodium) 2 mg after each stool; and iron dextran (Feostat) 50 mg IV daily × 3, administered by the physician (to replenish iron stores). A combined enteral-parenteral approach to nutritional therapy was ordered, with an elemental enteral solution (Vivonex-HN), 300 mL qid, and protein carbohydrate peripheral parenteral nutrition (2 L daily of a solution of 500 mL of a 5.5% amino acid solution with 500 mL of 20% dextrose solution). Electrolytes were added to each infusion; Na, 30 meq/L; K, 40 meq/L; PO₄ 13 mM/L; Mg, 10 meq/L; Ca, 7 meq/L; Cl, 15 meq/L. Potassium supplementation was extremely important because the patient was hypokalemic and because corticosteroids have potassium-depleting effects. Chloride supplementation was initially less than maintenance levels because of the slight hyperchloremia at admission. Vitamins and trace minerals were added to one bottle daily, since the enteral formula did not meet her entire RDA.

The patient was provided with warm, damp washcloths for cleansing after each stool and given a petrolatum-based ointment to protect the perianal area. Nurses measured stool volume for fluid content and recorded this as part of the patient's output, which was considered in planning composition of the nutritional therapy the next day.

Enteral feedings were presented in a visually pleasing manner, were kept iced, and, when possible, the nurses joined C.C. while she "ate." Enteral feedings were diluted or accompanied with water to avoid diarrhea and cramping. Intake of formula and fluid was meticuously recorded.

Evaluation

C.C. was weighed and electrolytes and blood glucose were evaluated daily. Tests for glucosuria and urine specific gravity were performed several times daily. Biweekly tests for nitrogen balance, magnesium levels, total protein, and plasma urea were done.

Nurses observed C.C. carefully for signs of intestinal perforation (loss of bowel sounds, pain) and megacolon (pain, abdominal enlargement), which may be exacerbated by the corticosteroid and antidiarrheal drug therapy. The peripheral vein access site was observed for signs of infection. As C.C. improved, corticosteroid dosages were tapered and switched to the oral route. Plans were made for the gradual switch to entirely enteral supplementation and oral feeding.

REFERENCES

American Council of Science and Health, September–October, 1982.

Bo-Linn, G., et al.: "Starch Blockers—Their Effect on Calorie Absorption from a High-Starch Meal," *N Engl J Med*, **307**:1413–1416, Dec. 2, 1982.

Butterworth, C. E., and G. L. Blackburn: "Hospital Nutrition and How to Assess the Nutritional Status of a Patient," *Nutr Today*, **10**:8, 1975.

Chernoff, R.: "Nutritional Support: Formulas and Delivery of Enteral Feeding," *J Diet Assoc*, **79**:426, 1981.

Contemporary Parenteral Nutrition—Central Vein, North Chicago: Abbott Laboratories, 1982.

Crosby, W.: "Who Needs Iron?" *N Engl J Med*, **297**:427–431, Aug. 25, 1977.

Facts and Comparisons, St. Louis: Facts and Comparisons, Inc., 1984.

Forlaw, L., et al.: *Introduction to Nutritional and Physical Assessment of the Adult Patient for the Nurse*, Rockville, MD: Aspen Systems, Inc., 1983.

Fundamentals of Nutritional Support, Deerfield, IL: Travenol Laboratories, 1981.

Grant, J. P.: *Handbook of Total Parenteral Nutrition*, Philadelphia: Saunders, 1980.

Guthrie, H.: *Introductory Nutrition*, 5th ed., St. Louis: Mosby, 1983.

Handbook of Nonprescription Drugs, 7th ed., Washington: American Pharmaceutical Association, 1982.

Heymsfield, S. B., et al.: "Enteral Hyperalimentation," in J. E. Berk (ed.), *Developments in Digestive Diseases*, Philadelphia: Lea & Febiger, 1980.

Jubes, T. H.: "Food Additives," *N Engl J Med*, **297**:427–431, Aug. 25, 1977.

Lasagna, L.: "Attitudes toward Appetite Suppressants," *JAMA*, **225**:44–48, July 2, 1974.

Malcolm, R., et al.: "Psychosocial Aspects of Total Parenteral Nutrition," *Psychosomatics*, **21**:115, 1980.

McSweeney, G. W.: "Parenteral Nutrition," in B. S. Katcher, et al. (eds.), *Applied Therapeutics*, 3d ed., San Francisco: Applied Therapeutics, 1983.

Press release, American Society of Bariatric Physicians, Oct. 22, 1981.

Recommended Dietary Allowances, 9th ed., National Academy of Sciences, 1980.

Rivlin, R. S.: "Therapy of Obesity with Hormones," *N Engl J Med*, **297**:1158–1161, Nov. 24, 1977.

Rudman, D., and J. C. Bleier: "Assessment of Nutritional Status," in R. G. Petersdorf et al. (eds.), *Harrison's Principles of Internal Medicine*, 10th ed., New York: McGraw-Hill, 1983.

Tube Feedings: Clinical Application, Columbus, OH: Ross Laboratories, 1980.

Tuckerman, M. M., and S. J. Turco: *Human Nutrition*, Philadelphia: Lea & Febiger, 1983.

Ulmer, D. D.: "Trace Elements," *N Engl J Med*, **297**:318–321, Aug. 11, 1977.

Van Itallie, T. B., and M. Yang: "Diet and Weight Loss," *N Engl J Med*, **297**:1158–1161, Nov. 24, 1977.

Williams, S. R.: *Nutrition and Diet Therapy*, 4th ed., St. Louis: Mosby, 1981.

Whitney, E. N., and C. B. Cataldo: *Understanding Normal and Clinical Nutrition*, St. Paul: West, 1983.

26

IMMUNE AND INFLAMMATORY DISORDERS

MICHAEL A. CARTER
RONALD P. EVENS
RALPH E. SMALL

LEARNING OBJECTIVES

Upon mastery of the contents of this chapter the reader will be able to:

1. Compare and contrast immune and inflammatory responses.

2. State the major components of the humoral immune system and cell-mediated immunity.

3. Differentiate the mechanisms of action of nonsteroidal anti-inflammatory drugs, disease-modifying drugs, and antigout drugs in terms of their effects on the immune system and inflammation response.

4. Give at least five examples of nonsteroidal anti-inflammatory drugs.

5. List the effects of and indications for nonsteroidal anti-inflammatory drugs.

6. Relate the pharmacokinetics of nonsteroidal anti-inflammatory drugs to their dosage schedule and clinically significant drug interactions.

7. Compare the efficacy and safety of aspirin to the other nonsteroidal anti-inflammatory drugs in the treatment of arthritis.

8. List four major adverse effects of the nonsteroidal anti-inflammatory drugs as a group.

9. List adverse effects particularly prevalent with (a) indomethacin, (b) phenylbutazone, and (c) meclofenamate, compared with other nonsteroidal anti-inflammatory drugs.

10. Describe parameters useful for monitoring for the therapeutic effects of nonsteroidal anti-inflammatory drugs, disease modifying drugs, and antigout drugs.

11. Differentiate the goals of therapy with nonsteroidal anti-inflammatory drugs from those of therapy with disease modifying drugs.

12. List five groups of disease modifying drugs and give examples of specific drugs from each group.

13. Describe the temporal aspects of the onset of action of disease modifying drugs.

14. Explain the mechanism of anti-inflammatory or immune suppressive action of gold compounds, antimalarials, penicillamine, and the immune suppressive agents.

15. Identify disease modifying drug(s) and nursing process commonly associated with the following adverse effects: gastric distress, skin rash, hair loss, blood dyscrasias, ocular disturbance, bladder damage, and reproductive problems.

16. Relate the pharmacokinetics and adverse effects of disease modifying drugs to clinically significant drug interactions and dosing regimen.

17. List the adverse effects of chronic corticosteroid therapy.

18. List four categories of drugs used for gout therapy.

19. Describe the mechanism of action, adverse effects, and nursing process for allopurinol, the uricosurics, and colchicine in gout.

20. Relate the pharmacokinetics and adverse effects of antigout drugs to clinically significant drug interactions and dosing regimen.

21. Relate the pathogenesis of the following immune and inflammatory disorders to their control by drug therapy: bursitis and tenosynovitis, degenerative joint disease, rheumatoid arthritis, systemic lupus erythematosis.

The body's defense against assault by foreign material, such as microorganisms and particles, includes immune and inflammatory processes. The *immune process* is a response mounted by the body to neutralize, destroy, or eliminate specific foreign materials (antigens). *Inflammation* occurs whenever cells or tissues of the body are injured or killed. It is a vascular reaction in which fluid, chemical mediators, and cells are delivered to the interstitial tissue site of injury or necrosis. The inflammatory reaction is the same regardless of the cause of tissue disruption or previous occurrence of the same injury. However, the immune response is specific for a particular antigen and requires an initial exposure before it can be initiated. Immune responses can trigger the inflammatory reaction but at a rate more rapid than would have otherwise occurred.

Immune and inflammatory diseases include bursitis and tenosynovitis, gouty arthritis, osteoarthritis, rheumatoid arthritis, and systemic lupus erythematosus. The primary tissue under attack in these autoimmune and trauma diseases is connective tissue, particularly in the joints of the body but also in other areas such as skin. The diseases are generally progressive, with cumulative tissue damage over time. The chronic progressive course is often punctuated with periods of acute exacerbations and spontaneous remissions. Joint destruction is a potential result of these diseases, which afflict at least 20 million people in the United States alone. Women make up about two-thirds of these patients. Arthritic diseases are much more common in older people (tenfold higher incidence for those over 45 than for those below); however, they cause disease in all ages. Drug therapy involves over 35 different drugs used alone and in combinations. The annual health care costs including drug therapy, physical therapy, hospitalization, and assistive devices is calculated in the billions of dollars.

IMMUNE SYSTEM

The *immune system* comprises several components: white blood cells (e.g., lymphocytes, monocytes, macrophages, and neutrophils); proteins (e.g., antibodies); and chemical mediators (e.g., complement and lymphokines). Anatomically, the immune system involves the *lymphatic* and *reticuloendothelial* (RE) *systems,* which are the two related organ systems that house and participate in the immune processes. The lymphatic system contains lymph fluid (extracellular fluid), lymph nodes and ducts, a capillary system, and lymphocytes. Its function is drainage and cleansing of foreign material from the extracellular fluid of all cells. Lymphocytes circulate between the blood and the lymphatic system. The RE system involves phagocytic white blood cells (monocytes and macrophages) and lymphocytes and is located in the spleen, lymph nodes, bone marrow, and liver. The roles of the RE system are phagocytosis of foreign material, preliminary processing of antigens for lymphocytes, and enhancing lymphocyte activity.

The immune system is divided into two distinct functional units, that is, *humoral immunity* and *cell-mediated immunity.* In response to foreign material in the body (an antigen), lymphocytes and macrophages can be activated in either or both arms of the immune system. *Humoral immunity* (HI) involves B lymphocytes which produce antibodies

that remove or destroy antigens by utilizing the chemical mediator complement and macrophages. *Cell-mediated immunity* (CMI) is an immunologic reaction to specific antigens and is mediated by cells, rather than by protein antibodies. These cells are *T lymphocytes* that become specialized in their function and remove or destroy antigens directly or by invoking the assistance of phagocytic macrophages and neutrophils. Figure 26-1 schematically depicts the immune system, showing the cellular changes and their sequence. The immune disorders, such as rheumatoid arthritis and systemic lupus erythematosus, involve malfunction of the immune systems. Normal tissues are recognized as or become antigens, and the products of the immune system (antibodies and lymphocytes) attack normal connective tissue.

Cell-Mediated Immunity

The T lymphocytes of the CMI system originate in the bone marrow, but the *thymus gland* is the primary site for their storage and development. T lymphocytes are found in the RE system, and they also continuously circulate between the bloodstream and lymphatic system. Following antigen invasion, macrophages carry antigens from tissues to the lymphocytes and facilitate the interaction of antigens with T lymphocytes in the RE system. T lymphocytes contain receptors to a single antigen on their cell surface, which is called *clonal restriction.* Thus one clone of T lymphocytes reacts with only one antigen. Through this interaction, T lymphocytes are then stimulated to undergo maturation, proliferation, and differentiation into five types of effector T cells. *T delayed hypersensitivity cells* promote an inflammatory reaction against antigens by releasing inflammatory mediators, lymphokines. *T amplifier cells* enhance the responsiveness of other immunocompetent cells. *T cytotoxic cells* are directed against specific target cells and kill them. *T helper cells* interface with the humoral immune system and enhance antibody production. *T suppressor cells* also influence antibody production, but in an opposite, counterbalancing fashion to T helper cells.

Humoral Immunity

Lymphocytes also form the basis of the humoral immune system (HI), but are a different type (B lymphocytes) than in the CMI system (T lymphocytes). B lymphocytes are coated with surface immunoglobulins that impart specificity for the reaction of a single B lymphocyte to a single antigen (*clonal specificity*). B lymphocytes are activated by two factors, that is, the antigen and an antigen-specific T helper cell. This activation is also assisted by the macrophage, which serves as a carrier of the antigen. After the interaction between the antigen and B lymphocyte, the B lymphocytes differentiate into plasma cells and eventually produce specific *antibodies* against the specific antigen. The antibodies stimulate the *complement system,* which is a cascade of factors that participate in inflammatory reactions. Complement factors

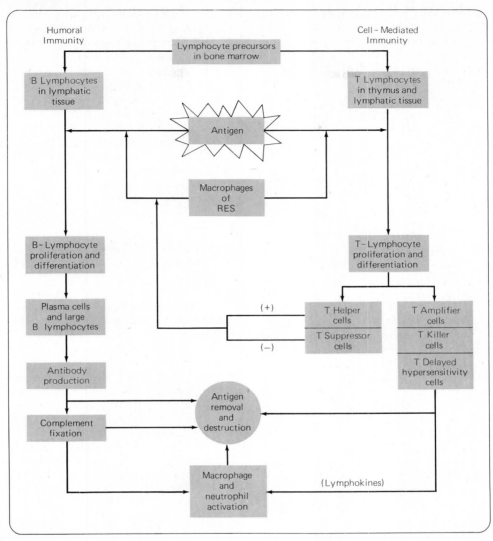

FIGURE 26-1

The Immune System, Showing Humoral Immunity and Cell-Mediated Immunity. Introduction of an antigen into the body causes differentiation and proliferation of lymphocytes characteristic of each division. B lymphocytes in the humoral system develop into plasma cells which secrete antibodies. Antibodies are immunoglobulins specific to one antigen and bind to antigens, leading to their removal and destruction. T lymphocytes in the cell-mediated immune system differentiate into five subtypes, which directly attack the antigen and mediate the function of B lymphocytes.

stimulate proteolysis, chemotaxis, and phagocytosis by leukocytes; cytolysis of cells; edema; anaphylaxis; vascular congestion; and pain. Figure 26-1 summarizes these humoral immune changes.

Antibodies of the HI system are multichain proteins composed of four polypeptides with an amino acid sequence specific for a single antigen. Each clone of plasma cells produces a different antibody for a different antigen. Antibodies possess two antigen binding sites permitting cross-linking and clumping (agglutination) of antigens for their removal. Also, antibodies stimulate phagocytic cells and activate com-

plement to help eliminate foreign materials (antigens) from the body. Four major classes of antibodies or immunoglobulins are produced: IgA, IgE, IgG, and IgM. Table 26-1 indicates their location and roles. A fifth class (IgD) is found, but its role is yet to be delineated.

INFLAMMATION

The *inflammation* process is a defense mechanism of the body to localize, destroy, and remove foreign particles and damaged cells. During an inflammatory episode, the patient

TABLE 26-1   Immunoglobulins of the Immune System

TYPE	LOCATION	FUNCTION
IgA	Body secretions (tears, saliva, sweat, mucus)	Complement activation
		Antigen removal and destruction in body lumens
IgE	Tissue bound	Primary immunoglobulin in immediate hypersensitivity reactions
		Sensitization of mast cells for anaphylaxis (edema and bronchoconstriction)
		Cytophilic binding to cell
		No complement activation
IgG	Serum	Primary immunoglobulin in systemic immune response
		Complement activation
		Recruitment of phagocytic cells
		Neutralization of toxins and viruses
		Placental transfer; fetal and neonatal protection
IgM	Serum	Early immunoglobulin in systemic immune response
		Agglutination of foreign particles (most active Ig)
		Blood group differentiation
		Complement fixation

has the classic signs and symptoms of pain and edema, often accompanied by redness and heat. This dynamic process is a result of a complicated cascade of events, indicated by acute stimuli such as trauma (tissue disruption) or foreign substance invasion. It involves a myriad of chemical and cellular reactions and leads to tissue disruption and/or antigen removal and destruction, resulting in tissue repair and/or fibrosis.

Figure 26-2 summarizes the chronic inflammation process for connective tissue diseases, such as arthritis. This simplified diagram shows four basic components of inflammation: stimuli, chemical mediators, cellular reactions, and tissue disruption and repair. Each agent listed under the four components of inflammation in Fig. 26-2 is identified by its effects on, or reactions involved in, the process.

In *chronic inflammatory diseases,* an unknown foreign substance or trauma initiates the inflammation process in a patient who is generally predisposed by several factors. These factors include chronic trauma over a period of years to the connective tissue, genetic predisposition, abnormal connective tissue synthesis, or aging tissue with compro-

mised repair processes. These antigenic changes in normal tissue lead to cellular changes in lymphocytes and macrophages and stimulate their release of chemical mediators. Both chemicals and cells dynamically interact to stimulate and amplify each other and are directed against normal connective tissue, especially in the joints and skin. *Chemical reactions* induce many systemic changes: production of inflammatory mediators such as complement, kinins, prostaglandins, and many others; attraction and stimulation of phagocytic neutrophils and monocytes; vascular congestion; and tissue edema, pain, and destruction. *Cellular reactions* include phagocytosis, release of chemical mediators, and tissue destruction. The result of the two types of reactions is destruction of synovial and osseous tissues that is progressive in nature with inadequate repair and fibrosis.

Prostaglandins and Related Mediators

Prostaglandins are a group of biologically active lipids produced in many organs and having broad regulatory activity in the body. These mediators and a number of related substances (e.g., leukotrienes, thromboxanes) are synthesized from the same precursors in a cascade of reactions (see Fig. 26-3) and are called *eicosanoids* as a group. The nine groups of prostaglandins identified to date are arbitrarily assigned letter designations *A* to *I* (i.e., PGA, PGB, PGC, PGD, PGE, PGF, PGG, PGH, PGI). They are further identified by subscripts which describe the chemical structure (e.g., $PGF_{2\alpha}$, PGF_{β}, PGE_2). Similar designations have been devised for the two groups of *thromboxanes* (e.g., TXA_2, TXB_3) and the five groups of *leukotrienes* (e.g., LTA, LTB_3, LTC_5, LTD_4, LTE). The *hydroperoxyeicosatetraenoic acids* (HPETEs) and *hydroxyeicosatetraenoic acids* (HETEs) are identified according to their chemical structure by a numerical prefix (e.g., 12-HPETE, 12-HETE).

Physiologic Function   In addition to their functions as chemical mediators in the inflammatory process, the prostaglandins and related substances regulate smooth muscle in blood vessels, gastrointestinal tract, respiratory system, and reproductive tract; protect the gastrointestinal mucosa; regulate renal blood flow and distribution; maintain a patent ductus arteriosus in the fetus; and control platelet function. Because the prostaglandins and other eicosanoids are rapidly inactivated in the organs in which they are synthesized and in the systemic circulation, they are involved in fine regulation of basic cell functions. Further, their actions are *cell-specific;* that is, they may be different or even opposing in various cells. For example, a single prostaglandin, PGE_2, has the following effects: it relaxes arterial smooth muscle; contracts or relaxes uterine smooth muscle, depending on the concentration present; relaxes the bronchi; stimulates renin release in the kidney; activates the thermoregulatory center in the hypothalmus to induce fever; and in the GI tract contracts longitudinal smooth muscle but relaxes the circular smooth muscle.

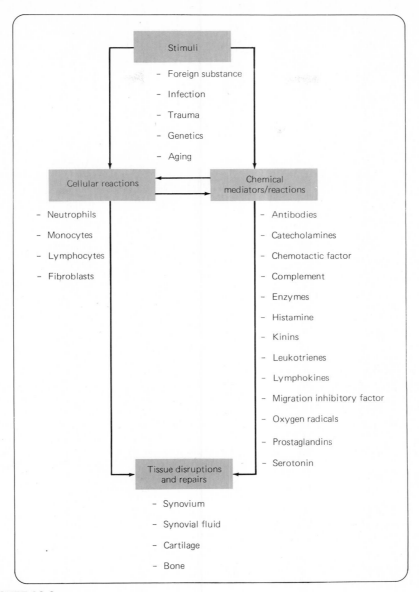

FIGURE 26-2

The Chronic Inflammation Process. Arthritic diseases are characterized by a chronic inflammatory process. Several proposed stimuli elicit the release and production of chemical mediators and promote cellular reactions. Inflammatory cells can produce more chemical mediators and reactions, and chemical mediators can stimulate further cellular reactions. The result of the chemical and cellular reactions during the chronic inflammatory process is a gradual disruption of synovial tissues (synovial lining, cartilage, and bone).

Clinical Implications The diverse and widespread effects of the prostaglandins and other eicosanoids complicate the therapeutic use of these substances and of agents which inhibit formation of endogenous prostaglandins and thromboxanes, as adverse effects often accompany the desired action. Prostaglandins are employed clinically as abortifacients and for induction of labor (see Chap. 46). **Alprostadil,** or PGE_1, (Prostin VR Pediatric) is approved for presurgical use in maintaining the patency of the ductus arteriosus in neonates with certain congenital heart defects. Prostaglandins have been investigated as therapeutic agents in bronchoconstrictive pulmonary disease (PGE_2) and peripheral vascular disease (PGE_1 and PGI_2, or prostacyclin).

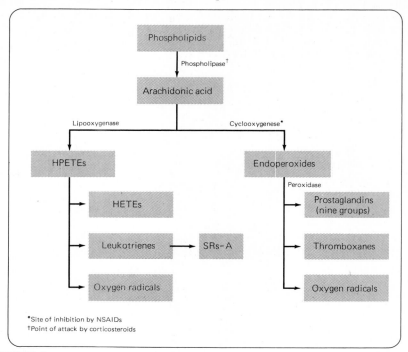

FIGURE 26-3

Prostaglandin Synthesis and the Sites of Action of Anti-inflammatory Drugs. Prostaglandins and related eicosanoids, such as thromboxanes, leukotrienes, and oxygen radicals, are synthesized in a cascade of reactions starting from the phospholipids in cellular membranes. Arachidonic acid is the systemically found free fatty acid that is the parent compound for all these prostaglandin-related compounds. Enzymes mediate the production of these inflammatory mediators and are susceptible to blockade by anti-inflammatory drugs. (HPETEs = hydroperoxyeicosatretraneoic acids, HETEs = hydroxyeicosanoid acids; SRS-A = slow-reacting substance of anaphylaxis).

Therapeutic *inhibition of endogenous synthesis* of prostaglandins and other eicosanoids has been used in dysmenorrhea (Chap. 46) and to inhibit platelet function in clotting disorders (Chap. 42), induce closure of the ductus arteriosus in premature infants, and reduce fever (Chap. 18), as well as in the treatment of inflammatory and immune diseases discussed in this chapter. The nonsteroidal anti-inflammatory drugs and corticosteroids constitute the available inhibitors of the synthesis of prostaglandins and other eicosanoids (Fig. 26-3). Doubtless there will be numerous future developments in the therapeutic use of prostaglandins and their inhibitors.

DRUGS THAT MODIFY IMMUNE OR INFLAMMATORY PROCESSES

Drug treatment for immune and inflammatory rheumatic disorders, along with physical therapy, controls the clinical manifestations of the diseases and possibly slows or halts disease progression. However, the drugs do not cure the diseases or eradicate the underlying etiology (often unknown).

Therefore, the general goals of therapy with these drugs are threefold:

1. Amelioration of the signs and symptoms of the inflammatory and immunologic diseases.

2. Maintenance of function of the joints and adjoining muscles.

3. Prevention of deformities.

The list of drugs efficacious for inflammatory diseases is lengthy. These anti-inflammatory drugs will be discussed in three sections: nonsteroidal anti-inflammatory drugs (NSAIDs), the disease-modifying antirheumatic drugs (DMARDs), and the antigout drugs. (See Table 26-2).

Nonsteroidal Anti-Inflammatory Drugs (NSAIDs)

Twenty individual drugs constitute the class of nonsteroidal anti-inflammatory therapeutic agents. They can be subdivided into six chemical classes, including salicylates, pyrazolones, propionic acids, oxicams, indoles and indenes, and anthranylic acids. General principles of therapy common to all NSAIDs will be discussed first, followed by discussion of each class of compounds.

Mechanism of Action

Although their chemical structures are somewhat diverse, the pharmacology of all the NSAIDs is very similar. The NSAIDs as a class of drugs reduce inflammation by interrupting the cascade of production of inflammatory mediators. Specifically, their mechanism of action is an inhibition of the enzyme (cyclooxygenase or prostaglandin synthetase) responsible for the conversion of the endogenous systemic fatty acid, arachidonic acid, to prostaglandins, thromboxanes, and oxygen radicals. Thus, these drugs have been called "prostaglandin inhibitors." Figure 26-3 shows the site of action of NSAIDs in inflammation. Major mediators are removed from the inflammation process, but others remain active to cause some inflammation.

Indications

The goal of treatment of rheumatic disorders with NSAIDs is control of *synovitis* (joint inflammation). NSAIDs are the drugs of first choice in treating rheumatic diseases because of their efficacy and low toxicity. Their efficacy is good to excellent in mild to moderate disease, with over 50 percent of the patients experiencing full resolution or at least a major reduction in severity of pain and inflammation. Monitoring success of therapy is a subjective process employing various symptoms and signs of disease. However, scaled assessments are available to quantify the process and improve discrimination for the degree of relief (e.g., ring size assessment employs a series of rings to measure degree of inflammation in the joints of the fingers). Also, use of a group of symptoms will enhance documentation of response (e.g., degree of pain or pain relief, ring size, range of motion of joints, grip strength, and many others).

In comparing the efficacy among these drugs, **aspirin** is the standard of effectiveness, and all other NSAIDs are considered equally effective to aspirin at appropriate doses of each drug. Cost is always a salient factor in deciding the drug of choice. Aspirin is by far the least expensive NSAID. It should be remembered that a *placebo* effect is pronounced in these diseases, with up to one-third of the patients having a response to placebo therapy. Individual patients will respond better to one NSAID versus another, even though their overall efficacy is not different. Therefore, when one

TABLE 26-2   Anti-Inflammatory Drugs

Anthranylic acids*	Oxicams*
Mefenamic acid (Ponstel)	Piroxicam (Feldene)
Meclofenamate (Meclomen)	Penicillamine (Cuprimine)†
Antimalarial agents†	Propionic acids*
Chloroquine (Aralen)	Benoxaprofen (Oraflex)§
Hydroxychloroquine (Plaquenil)	Fenbufen (Cinopal)‡
Quinacrine (Atabrine)	Fenoprofen (Nalfon)
Corticosteroids, oral	Ibuprofen (Motrin, Rufen)
Methylprednisolone (Medrol)	Naproxen (Naprosyn, Anaprox)
Prednisolone (Delta-Cortef)	Zomepirac (Zomax)§
Prednisone (Deltasone)	Pyrazolones*
Corticosteroids, intraarticular	Oxyphenbutazone (Tandaeril)
Betamethasone acetate (Celestone Soluspan)	Phenylbutazone (Butazolidin)
Predinisolone tebutate (Hydeltra T.B.A.)	Salicylates*
Triamcinolone hexacetonide (Aristospan)	Aspirin, plain
Gold salts†	buffered (Ascriptin, Bufferin)
Auranofin (Ridaura)‡	enteric coated (Ecotrin, Easprin)
Aurothioglucose (Solganol)	sustained release (Zorprin)
Gold sodium thiomalate (Myochrysine)	Choline salicylate (Arthropan)
Immunosuppressive agents†	Diflunisal (Dolobid)
Azathioprine (Imuran)	Magnesium salicylate (Magan)
Cyclophosphamide (Cytoxan)	Salsalate (Disalcid)
Methotrexate	Salicylamide (Uromide)
Indole/indenes*	Sodium salicylate (Uracel 5)
Indomethacin (Indocin)	Sodium thiosalicylate (Asproject, Thiocyl)
Sulindac (Clinoril)	
Tolmetin (Tolectin)	

*Nonsteroidal anti-inflammatory agents.
†Disease-modifying anti-inflammatory agents.
‡Investigational agents.
§Drug was withdrawn from market because of side effects.

drug fails at full doses, another from a different chemical class (see Table 26-2) is used. The onset of anti-inflammatory response is 1 to 2 weeks. Some patients with more severe inflammation can require up to 3 to 4 weeks for a full response. Pain and fever caused by arthritis or other conditions can also be relieved by NSAIDs. However, the response is more rapid, often within a few hours to days. Acute painful states that respond to NSAIDs include headache, dysmenorrhea, and muscle pain (Chap. 17).

Pharmacokinetics

All NSAIDs are well absorbed upon oral administration. Concurrent consumption of food or antiacids with NSAIDs will reduce absorption by as much as 25 to 30 percent, but no failure of therapy due to this interaction has been established. NSAIDs are cleared from the body by hepatic metabolism, usually by a conjugation reaction; the metabolites are excreted by the kidney. The plasma half-life varies from 2 h for **fenoprofen** to more than 100 h for **piroxicam**. (See Table

26-3). All NSAIDs are highly bound to plasma proteins (90 to 98 percent). NSAIDs distribute well from plasma into synovial fluid. The levels in synovial fluid are about half those in plasma, peak at a later time, and persist for several hours longer.

Adverse Effects

NSAIDs have very similar adverse effects on the gastrointestinal, pulmonary, cutaneous, gynecologic, cardiovascular, and renal system. Prostaglandins are mediators of tissue functions in all tissues. Therefore, many adverse effects common to all NSAIDs are hypothesized to be related to *inhibition of prostaglandin synthesis*. However, some major differences do exist, as characterized in the individual drug presentations that follow.

Gastric distress is a common dose-related complaint associated with NSAIDs and is reported by patients as nausea, epigastric discomfort, gastric distention, or vomiting at incidence rates of 5 to 20 percent. NSAIDs possess a direct

TABLE 26-3 Nonsteroidal Anti-Inflammatory Agents: Doses and Pharmacokinetics

	DOSAGE FORM	HALF-LIFE, h	DOSAGE RANGE, g/day	NUMBER OF DOSES PER DAY
Aspirin	Tablets	3 or 18*	4–6	4–6
	Sustained release tablets			2–3
Choline salicylate (Arthropan)	Oral liquid	3 or 18*	4–6	3–4
Diflunisal (Dolobid)	Tablets	10–12	0.5–0.75	2
Fenbufen (Cinopal)	Capsules	10–12	0.8–1.2	2
Fenoprofen (Nalfon)	Tablets	2–3	1.2–3.6	3–4
Ibuprofen (Motrin, Rufen)	Tablets	2–4	1.2–3.6	3–4
Indomethacin (Indocin)	Capsules	2–10	0.075–0.15	3–4
	Sustained release			1–2
Magnesium salicylate (Magan)	Tablets	3 or 18*	4–6	3–4
Meclofenamate (Meclomen)	Capsule	2–3	0.3–0.4	3–4
Mefenamic acid (Ponstel)	Capsules	4–6	0.75–1.0	3–4
Naproxen (Naprosyn, Anaprox)	Tablets	12–15	0.5–0.75	2
Oxyphenbutazone (Tandaeril)	Tablets	75	0.2–0.4	3–4
Phenylbutazone (Butazolidin)	Tablets	30–175	0.2–0.4	3–4
Piroxicam (Feldene)	Capsules	14–158	0.02–0.04	1–2
Salsalate (Disalcid)	Tablets, capsules	3 or 18*	4–6	3–4
Sodium magnesium salicylate (Trilisate)	Tablets, liquid	3 or 18*	4–6	3–4
Sulindac (Clinoril)	Tablets	7 or 18†	0.2–0.4	2
Tolmetin (Tolectin)	Capsules	1	1.2–2.0	3–4

*Salicylates have a long half-life at the high antirheumatic doses. At low doses (1–2 g/day), the half-life is about 3 h.

†Sulindac is the parent drug with a 7-h half-life; its active metabolite has an 18-h half-life.

irritative action to gastric lining. Also, prostaglandins provide a cytoprotective effect for gastric mucosa, which is compromised with NSAID use. NSAIDs can produce occult blood loss, and acute gastrointestinal bleeding is possible. Patients with peptic ulcer disease should be given NSAIDs with caution.

Allergic reactions are produced by salicylates, particularly in asthma patients, and present either as acute bronchospasm or as a cutaneous urticarial reaction. Cross-reactivity occurs almost universally among the NSAIDs. Patients with a history of aspirin hypersensitivity should be given NSAIDS with caution if at all. NSAIDs cause various skin rashes. In addition to allergic urticarial rashes, nonallergic maculopapular or other nonspecific rashes have been associated with each NSAID.

NSAIDs have *reproductive system* adverse effects. During childbirth, prostaglandins play a key role as a mediator or uterine contraction. NSAIDs potentially can interfere with uterine contractions and should be avoided during the third trimester of pregnancy. The fetus has a patent ductus arteriosus (PDA), which is needed for proper fetal shunting of blood from the pulmonary artery to the aorta. Prostaglandins are key mediators in maintaining the PDA, and NSAIDs can disturb this special fetal circulation. The chance of premature closure of PDA necessitates avoidance of NSAIDs or at least downward dosage adjustment in late pregnancy.

Salt and water retention is produced by NSAIDs in some patients because of prostaglandin inhibition resulting in reduction in renal blood flow, glomerular filtration, and salt and water excretion. Cardiac and renal patients are at the highest risk of these fluid/electrolyte problems. *Hepatic damage* is an uncommon reaction associated with NSAIDs. Liver enzymes can increase, but these changes do not produce clinical hepatitis and usually do not alter drug utilization. **Aspirin** carries the highest risk of hepatic damage. *Platelet function* is inhibited by NSAIDs. Aggregation of platelets is compromised, prolonging bleeding time and predisposing patients to easy bruising. **Aspirin** causes the most problems, and all other NSAIDs are much less toxic to platelets.

Highly protein bound drugs potentially will interact with NSAIDs. They displace each other from these binding sites, increase the amount of free drug in the blood, and produce greater pharmacologic effects and even toxicity. Such drugs include anticoagulants (e.g., **warfarin**), oral hypoglycemic agents (e.g., **tolbutamide**), sulfonamides, and hydantoin anticonvulsants (e.g., **phenytoin**).

Dosage and Administration

Doses of NSAIDs are generally higher for inflammation control than for pain relief or antipyresis. (See Table 26-3.) The severity of pain and inflammation will influence the dosing level. The dose should not be fixed at one level but should be adjusted to the pattern of changing disease activity over time. The dosing frequency is adapted to the half-life of the NSAID. **Fenoprofen** is dosed three to four times a day because its half-life is 2 to 3 h, and **diflunisal** is dosed twice daily because of a 10- to 12-h half-life. Also, the occurrence of gastric distress with NSAID ingestion can alter the dosing scheme. A change from a twice-daily dose to lower and more frequent doses often can reduce gastric irritation.

The duration of therapy follows the chronic nature of the disease. Drugs are continued during apparently quiescent periods to maintain disease control. However, arthritic disease sometimes will have periods of disease remission that do not require treatment. Acute traumatic arthritis (e.g., acute tenosynovitis) obviously is only treated for the expected short duration of problem, often a few days.

Salicylates

Aspirin is the drug of first choice in most arthritic disorders, as long as the patient can tolerate its adverse effects. Seven salicylates (see Table 26-2) and five dosage forms of aspirin (plain, buffered, effervescent/buffered, enteric coated, and sustained release tablets) have been developed to improve the efficacy and reduce toxicity of salicylates.

Pharmacokinetics   A plasma salicylate level of 15 to 30 mg/dL is considered necessary for anti-inflammatory activity. The half-life of salicylates changes with the dosage, as noted in Table 26-3. Salicylates are metabolized by six pathways in the liver; the contribution of each pathway changes with the dose. Because two pathways are saturable, metabolism slows and plasma half-life increases with higher doses. See Chap. 17 for further pharmacokinetic information.

Adverse Effects   Aspirin is the most gastrotoxic NSAID, causing gastric distress and occult blood loss at a frequency and degree of severity which is at least twofold higher than that of the other salicylates and other NSAIDs. Aspirin also causes tinnitus at the higher anti-inflammatory blood levels and reversible hearing loss. If hearing problems occur, blood levels of salicylate should be drawn to evaluate aspirin's involvement. Chronic aspirin abuse, particularly in combination products containing phenacetin, can cause chronic interstitial nephritis. Hepatotoxicity is relatively common in children with rheumatic diseases, such as rheumatic fever, who are receiving aspirin. Overdosage with aspirin produces metabolic acidosis then alkalosis. Further elaboration of salicylate side effects is found in Chap. 17.

Dosage and Administration   The doses and dosing frequencies for all the salicylate derivatives are found in Table 26-3. The standard dosage range for anti-inflammatory effects is 3 to 6 g of salicylate. Although **aspirin** has an 18-h half-life at the above dosage range, gastric side effects necessitate that the large daily dose be divided into 3 to 4 doses/day. However, enteric coated tablets reduce gastric problems and can be given in larger doses and less frequently, for instance, 2 to 3 doses/day. **Diflunisal** (Dolobid) is a salicylate derivative with an extended half-life permitting twice-daily dosing. Also, a sustained release formulation (Zorprin), which can be given 2 to 3 times/day, is available.

Pyrazolones

Phenylbutazone (Butazolidin, Azolid) and **oxyphenbutazone** (Tandaeril, Oxalid) are two available pyrazolones, which are NSAIDs possessing anti-inflammatory, analgesic, antipyretic, and uricosuric effects. Their indications are acute gout, rheumatoid arthritis, degenerative joint disease, and bursitis/tenosynovitis. Because of serious adverse effects, rational use requires careful patient selection, close supervision, and discontinuation of therapy if no favorable response occurs after a 1-week trial.

Pharmacokinetics   Phenylbutazone is metabolized in the liver to the active drug oxyphenbutazone. Although the half-life is quite long (see Table 26-3), gastric side effects limit dosing to 3 to 4 times a day. The long half-life can lead to accumulation of the drugs in the body with chronic dosing.

Adverse Effects   In addition to the potential reactions common to all NSAIDs, such as gastric distress, allergic reactions, skin rashes, and gynecologic effects, phenylbutazone and oxyphenbutazone tend to produce sodium and water retention in about 10 percent of the patients. Expansion of the circulatory volume can lead to congestive heart failure, pulmonary edema, and elevated blood pressure. Dosage reduction and sodium restriction can reverse these effects.

Hematologic abnormalities, especially agranulocytosis, are the major adverse effects limiting pyrazolone usage. Although the reaction is uncommon (0.15 percent incidence or less), fatalities have occurred in patients treated with phenylbutazone. The reaction is insidious and variable in onset (days to weeks) and is not dose-related. Other hematologic disorders include leukopenia, thrombocytopenia, pancytopenia, and hemolytic anemia. Because of these blood dyscrasias, clinicians recommend blood cell counts to be performed at intervals of 2 to 4 weeks during chronic therapy.

The protein binding in the blood is very high for these drugs, about 98 percent; therefore, drug interactions will occur as a result of competition at albumin binding sites. Potentiation of activity is possible for anticoagulants, oral hypoglycemic agents, and sulfonamides.

Dosage and Administration   Doses for arthritis are found in Table 26-3. Phenylbutazone has been used also for acute gout attacks. A loading dose of 100 to 200 mg is given three times a day for 2 to 3 days; the dose is then tapered rapidly over a few days. Side effects can limit this use, and these drugs are taken usually with food or milk to minimize the adverse gastric effects. Elderly patients are at greater risk of toxicity and should be monitored more closely.

Propionic Acid Derivatives

The currently marketed propionic acid derivative drugs include **fenoprofen** (Nalfon), **ibuprofen** (Motrin, Rufen), and **naproxen** (Anaprox, Naprosyn). **Ibuprofen** is also available without prescription as Advil and Nuprin. **Fenbufen** (Cinopal) is an investigational drug, and **benoxaprofen** (Oraflex) and **zomepirac** (Zomax) were removed from the market in 1983 by the manufacturers. These NSAIDs are all equal in anti-inflammatory and analgesic activities to salicylates. They all can be used to treat bursitis and tenosynovitis, acute gouty arthritis, osteoarthritis, and rheumatoid arthritis when a NSAID is indicated, even though each drug does not have a Food and Drug Administration (FDA) approved indication for each disease. **Ibuprofen**, **fenoprofen**, and **naproxen** have been used successfully for acute gout attacks.

Adverse Effects   This group of NSAIDs can all cause gastric distress, allergic reactions, salt and water retention, skin rashes, gynecologic effects, and fetal changes. The propionic acid derivatives are all superior to aspirin in causing less frequent and less severe gastrointestinal reactions. They can be used in salicylate-intolerant patients, but they still can cause gastric reactions, including reported severe gastric bleeding in rare cases.

Two types of nephrotoxicity occur with propionic acid derivatives. Nephrotic syndrome with proteinuria is an uncommon reaction. **Fenoprofen** has caused this problem most frequently, but **zomepirac**, **ibuprofen**, and **naproxen** have been implicated. The reaction is reversible with cessation of the drug. Sodium and water retention related to elevated prostaglandin levels and changes in kidney renin levels occurs with the propionic acid derivatives. It is reversible when the drug is discontinued.

Dosage and Administration   The dosage ranges for chronic arthritis therapy are found in Table 26-3. The only significant difference among these six NSAIDs is the *dosing frequency* (number of doses per day), which is based primarily on the different half-lives. Although the half-lives vary from 3 to 30 h, each of the propionic acid drugs is similarly highly protein bound and metabolized in the liver.

Acute gout can be treated with high doses of these drugs for a couple of days followed by rapid dosage tapering. Therapy usually continues for only 1 week. This indication is not approved by the FDA.

Piroxicam

Piroxicam (Feldene) is equal in efficacy to aspirin and other NSAIDs for arthritic diseases. However, the dosage schedule is once a day because it has the longest half-life among the NSAIDs (about 40 h). Although piroxicam is a different chemical class (oxicams) from the other NSAIDs, its liver metabolism, high protein binding, and adverse effects (gastric, liver, skin, kidney, uterus, and lungs) are similar to the other nonsalicylate NSAIDs.

Indole and Indenes

Indomethacin (Indocin, Indocin SR), sulindac (Clinoril), and tolmetin (Tolectin, Tolectin DS) are indicated in the treatment of all the arthritis diseases. Indomethacin is also used for gouty arthritis to stop an acute attack. It is effective in over 80 percent of these cases. Investigationally, indomethacin (0.3 to 0.6 mg/kg/24 h) is used as the medical treatment alternative to surgery for closure of a persistent patent ductus arteriosus in premature infants.

Pharmacokinetics Sulindac is a prodrug, which has a dual half-life. The parent compound is inactive, with a half-life of about 7 h. The active sulfide metabolite has a longer half-life of 18 h and is further metabolized to an inactive sulfone derivative. Indomethacin and tolmetin are metabolized to inactive compounds, which are excreted into the urine by the kidney. Indomethacin undergoes some enterohepatic recirculation.

Adverse Effects Indomethacin frequently causes gastrointestinal and especially central nervous system (CNS) reactions. These adverse reactions are dose-related. Frontal headaches are the most prominent adverse effects, occurring in about 25 percent of the patients and often accompanied by throbbing. Faintness and dizziness are observed in about 15 percent of patients. Other CNS manifestations include insomnia, nightmares, hallucinations, confusion, drowsiness, depression, and psychosis. Sulindac and tolmetin also cause dizziness, drowsiness, tiredness, and headache, but much less frequently.

Gastrointestinal reactions are more common with indomethacin than other NSAIDs: nausea (over 10 percent), diarrhea (10 percent), abdominal pain (3 percent), and ulcers (2 percent). Occult blood loss occurs less often than with aspirin. Sulindac and tolmetin cause these same adverse effects, but they are less severe and less common.

Other reactions include salt and water retention, skin rashes, allergic reactions, and possible uterine effects with all three of these NSAIDs; dry mouth with sulindac; and rare bone marrow depression with indomethacin (leukopenia in children, agranulocytosis, aplastic anemia, and thrombocytopenic purpura). Tolmetin has caused increased high blood pressure in hypertensive patients.

Dosage and Administration See Table 26-3 for standard doses for chronic arthritis. For acute attacks of gout, a loading dose technique is employed for indomethacin over a few days. The dose is 75 mg, then 25 to 50 mg every 6 h for 1 to 2 days, and then 25 to 50 mg every 8 h. The rate of dosage decrease depends on the response of gout to therapy. With

indomethacin and sulindac dosing at bedtime is commonly used to control nocturnal pain. Also, an extra nighttime dose boosts blood levels during the night so that more drug is available in the morning to control excessive morning stiffness. Indomethacin sustained-release (SR) is a 75-mg capsule containing polymer coated pellets of indomethacin, designed for immediate release of 25 mg, followed by prolonged release of 50 mg of indomethacin. A twice-daily regimen is possible with indomethacin SR instead of the usual 3 to 4 times/day schedule. These drugs should be taken with meals or a full glass of milk to reduce gastric distress.

Anthranylic Acids

The efficacy and pharmacokinetics of meclofenamate (Meclomen) and mefenamic acid (Ponstel) are similar to those of other NSAIDs. However, their clinical utility is significantly hindered by the frequent gastrointestinal and neurologic adverse effects. Diarrhea is quite common with mefenamic acid (10 to 15 percent incidence) and meclofenamate (greater than 40 percent). Up to 90 percent of patients receiving meclofenamate experience nausea, dyspepsia, diarrhea, or flatulence. These adverse effects are considered so severe that about one-third of the patients will stop the drug.

Mefenamic acid commonly causes dyspepsia (33 percent). Mefenamic acid also produces headache, dizziness, and drowsiness. Other adverse effects common to all NSAIDs can occur, such as allergic reactions and others. Mefenamic acid is approved for the treatment of pain and dysmenorrhea, given on an every-6-h schedule. Meclofenamate is approved for use in rheumatoid and osteoarthritis.

NURSING PROCESS RELATED TO NSAIDs

Assessment

Prior to the commencement of therapy with NSAIDs, baseline masurements of the patient's signs and symptoms are performed and recorded. Severity of pain, degree and pattern of stiffness, and impairment of activities of daily living are obtained by history. A goniometer is used to measure joint range of motion.

Careful questioning and examination will help to identify patients for whom NSAIDs are contraindicated or who will require special considerations and monitoring. Such conditions include the following.

NSAID sensitivity Because of cross-sensitivity among NSAIDs, extreme caution should be taken if the patient has previously experienced urticaria, difficulty in breathing, rhinitis, or angioedema after taking any NSAIDs. Aspirin sensitivity is more common in people with asthma or nasal polyps. Parenteral salicylates (i.e., injectable sodium salicylate) are avoided in patients with asthma.

Hemorrhagic states: hypoprothrombinemia; hemophilia; bleeding ulcers; anemia NSAIDs may complicate hemorrhagic disorders because they inhibit platelet aggregation and cause prolonged bleeding times and gastrointestinal blood loss. **Aspirin** has the most sustained and marked effects on platelet function; many clinicians will discontinue aspirin therapy 1 week prior to surgery, but other clinicians do not believe this precaution is necessary. Prior to therapy with **phenylbutazone** a complete blood count is indicated.

Elderly The elderly have more frequent adverse effects from NSAIDs than other patients. An even more thorough assessment is indicated prior to initiation of therapy for patients over 60 years of age.

Pregnancy and lactation NSAIDs are contraindicated particularly during the last trimester of pregnancy because of possible adverse effects in the fetus or newborn and inhibition of uterine contractility. Women who must take these drugs chronically probably should not nurse their infants.

Cardiovascular disease; fluid retention states; congestive heart failure NSAIDs may cause problems for patients with limited cardiac reserve since these drugs can cause retention of sodium and water. The effects of diuretics and antihypertensive medications may be physiologically antagonized by these effects of NSAIDs. A baseline weight and blood pressure should be recorded in the patient's record.

Impaired hepatic function In the presence of impaired hepatic function, NSAIDs may promote hepatocellular damage. Lupus and pediatric arthritic patients are at highest risk of liver malfunction. Baseline and regularly repeated liver function tests are indicated when there is a history of hepatic dysfunction. Hepatic disease may affect the pharmacokinetics of NSAIDs by altering drug metabolism and albumin binding, thereby increasing the drug effects. Protein binding may also be altered by malnutrition, renal disease, or rheumatoid arthritis with a resulting increase in free, active drug.

Peptic ulcer; gastritis; GI bleeding NSAIDs require cautious administration to patients with upper gastrointestinal disease since deaths have occurred in patients with peptic ulcers or GI bleeding while they were taking NSAIDs. **Indomethacin, phenylbutazone,** and **aspirin** should not be used by patients with active peptic ulcers.

Impaired renal function The incidence of adverse renal effects is higher in patients with preexisting renal impairment. These patients require baseline tests of renal function (urinalysis, urea nitrogen, creatinine clearance) and regular follow-up. Although only 20 percent or fewer of these drugs are usually excreted unchanged in the urine, severely impaired renal function could result in elevated plasma levels of NSAIDs.

Depression; chronic headaches; psychotic symptoms Patients with a history of headache or psychiatric disturbances may be more prone to the dose-related neuropsychiatric adverse effects of **indomethacin** and other indoles. These include headache, unpleasant cerebral sensations, nightmares, and psychotic disturbances.

Therapy with oral anticoagulants; oral antidiabetic agents; thiazide diuretics; β-adrenergic blockers Concurrent therapy with NSAIDs and drugs which are highly bound to plasma protein may result in increased effects of the interacting drugs. The sodium and water retention of NSAIDs may counteract the effects of diuretics and antihypertensive drugs.

Management

Nonpharmacologic therapy, patient education, and psychosocial support are important to the management of the conditions for which NSAIDs are prescribed (see following discussions of diseases), particularly since NSAIDs do not affect the cause or the course of the disease. Selecting the simplest dosing regimen possible and assisting the patient to control adverse effects may encourage compliance to this chronic therapy. Cost should not be overlooked, however, and **aspirin** remains an effective and relatively inexpensive form of therapy in spite of the fact that three to six doses may be required daily. Since aspirin is such a common drug, patients may doubt its value in their disease. Therefore, the nurse must educate the patient in the efficacy of aspirin and emphasize that its value as an anti-inflammatory drug requires different dosage patterns than does its use for analgesia and antipyresis.

Gastrointestinal adverse effects of NSAIDs are minimized by multiple daily dosing, taking the drug with food or a full glass of milk, and using the smallest effective dose. Although absorption may be altered, NSAIDs can be taken with antacids, but use of sodium bicarbonate as the antacid should be avoided. Patients who develop peptic ulcer disease while taking NSAIDs may continue the drug while the ulcer is treated with **cimetidine** (Tagamet) or **ranitidine** (Zantac). Close follow-up is important in these cases to assure that healing is taking place.

Drowsiness is an occasional CNS adverse effect of NSAIDS and may constitute a safety hazard, especially early in the course of treatment. The patient should be instructed to avoid driving or hazardous activities until it can be ascertained whether this effect occurs. Taking the drug at bedtime may decrease this hazard, as well as rendering any headaches which occur less troublesome. Use of analgesic doses of **acetaminophen** (Tylenol, Datril, and others) may be useful in controlling headache. Aspirin should be avoided because it may interact with the other NSAIDs and increase adverse effects. Switching to another NSAID may be necessary if symptoms continue.

Patients should be instructed to contact their care provider if they develop severe epigastric or abdominal pain, edema or weight gain, unusual bruising or bleeding, black stools, rash, pruritis, tinnitus, or persistent headache. The importance of returning for the evaluation of drug effect and adverse effects also requires emphasis.

Evaluation

Subjective appraisal of the patient's pain and joint activity, as well as objective tests of inflammation and function, should be made to determine the efficacy of these drugs. To evaluate adverse effects, the clinician should gather subjective data by review of all systems, with emphasis on the GI system (epigastric or abdominal pain, black stools, jaundice, anorexia, mouth sores); CNS (drowsiness, insomnia, dizziness, headache, paresthesias, tremors, fatigue, confusion, mental clouding); cardiovascular system (weight gain, edema, dyspnea, chest pain); dermatologic system (rash); and the special senses (blurred vision, photophobia, scotoma, tinnitus, hearing loss, ear pain).

Objective information collected at each patient evaluation includes observation for gastric irritation or ulceration (stool for occult blood periodically and whenever there are GI complaints); fluid retention (weight gain, increased blood pressure, palpation for edema); hematologic or allergic response (check skin for rash, petechiae, bruising, blood counts for signs of bleeding); hepatic involvement (jaundice, periodic liver function tests); visual changes (eye examinations periodically and whenever there are visual complaints); and auditory effects (audiometric evaluation for those with symptoms). Further, those taking **phenylbutazone** and **oxyphenbutazone** should have regular hematologic laboratory evaluations.

Disease-Modifying Antirheumatic Drugs (DMARDs)

When the NSAIDs do not control immune-mediated arthritic disease to a sufficient degree, other drugs can directly influence the disease process, although they are more toxic. The *disease-modifying antirheumatic drugs* (DMARDs) are listed in Table 26-4, including antimalarials, gold compounds, immunosuppressive agents, and penicillamine. Corticosteroids are not disease-modifying drugs but are discussed in this section because of their efficacy in symptom control and their incidence of serious adverse effects with chronic use. Non-immune-mediated disorders such as degenerative joint disease do not respond to these drugs.

Indications

The goals of treatment with DMARDs are twofold:

1. Control of clinical manifestations.
2. Arrest or slowing of disease progression.

In addition to symptoms, other monitoring parameters are useful for the DMARDs to assess pathologic changes in the diseases (e.g., x-ray; immunologic tests such as C-reactive protein, latex fixation, and rheumatoid factor; and joint or bone biopsy). About two-thirds or more of the patients who can tolerate the side effects are expected to respond to DMARDs with disease control. This high rate of efficacy occurs even in patients with moderate to severe arthritis. The onset of response to DMARD therapy is delayed and gradual. Often 3 to 6 months of therapy is required before any significant improvement in the disease occurs. Maximum response in some patients occurs after 1 year of treatment. During the initial latency period for the DMARD's onset of effects, NSAIDs are continued for pain and inflammation. Also, NSAIDs are often continued throughout DMARD therapy because they produce some degree of control.

The sequence of DMARD use is listed in Fig. 26-4 for rheumatoid arthritis. Table 26-4 contains the dosage ranges and the number of daily doses for each DMARD.

Adverse Effects

Table 26-5 lists and compares the adverse effects of the DMARDs. The major adverse effects involve the skin, GI system, blood cells, and kidney. Because of the scope and severity of the side effects of DMARD therapy, thorough patient assessment for other concurrent diseases must be performed prior to initiation of these drugs to avoid exacerbation of these diseases.

TABLE 26-4 Doses of Disease-Modifying Antirheumatic Drugs

DRUG	DOSAGE FORM	DOSAGE RANGE, mg	DOSES/DAY
Auranofin (Ridaura)	Tablet	3–9	2
Aurothioglucose (Solganal)	Injection	50	(Weekly)
Azathioprine (Imuran)	Tablet	75–150	1–2
Chloroquine (Aralen)	Tablet	250–375	1
Cyclophosphamide (Cytoxan)	Tablet	75–150	1–2
Gold sodium thiomalate (Myochrysine)	Injection	50	(Weekly)
Hydroxychloroquine (Plaquenil)	Tablet	200–400	1–3
Methotrexate	Tablet	5–20	(Weekly)
Penicillamine (Cuprimine)	Capsule	250–1250	1–4
Quinacrine (Atabrine)	Tablet	100–150	1

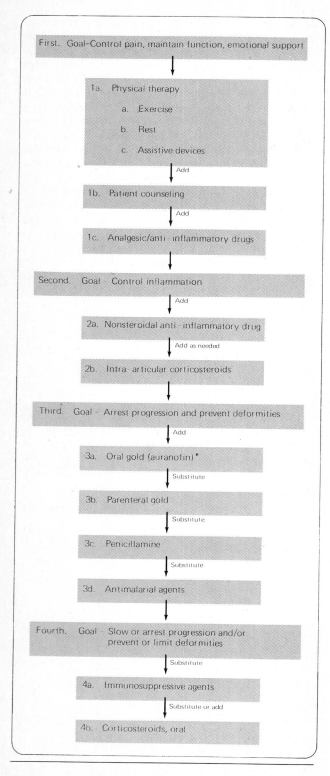

First. Goal-Control pain, maintain function, emotional support

1a. Physical therapy

   a. Exercise

   b. Rest

   c. Assistive devices

Add

1b. Patient counseling

Add

1c. Analgesic/anti-inflammatory drugs

Second. Goal - Control inflammation

Add

2a. Nonsteroidal anti-inflammatory drug

Add as needed

2b. Intra-articular corticosteroids

Third. Goal - Arrest progression and prevent deformities

Add

3a. Oral gold (auranofin)*

Substitute

3b. Parenteral gold

Substitute

3c. Penicillamine

Substitute

3d. Antimalarial agents

Fourth. Goal - Slow or arrest progression and/or prevent or limit deformities

Substitute

4a. Immunosuppressive agents

Substitute or add

4b. Corticosteroids, oral

*Oral gold is investigational.

Gold Compounds

The use of gold as an antirheumatic drug is called *chrysotherapy*. This class of drugs includes two parenteral preparations, **aurothioglucose** (Solganal) in an oil base and **gold sodium thiomalate** (Myochrysine) in an aqueous vehicle, and an investigational oral preparation, **auranofin** (Ridaura). Parenteral gold therapy is highly efficacious in treating rheumatoid arthritis, with about 75 percent of patients responding and remission in 20 to 25 percent. Both clinical and pathologic improvements are observed with gold therapy. Response is more likely in a patient with active polyarticular involvement in earlier stages of the disease. If joint deformities already exist, response will be compromised. Treatment is continued indefinitely, even during apparent quiescent periods. The response usually is delayed for 3 to 6 months, and some patients will continue to improve into the second year of treatment. **Auranofin** has the advantage of oral dosing with similar efficacy and less severe toxicity, although the scope of adverse effects is about the same.

Mechanism of Action   No specific mechanism has been identified to explain fully the influence of gold on rheumatoid arthritis. Parenteral gold salts possess anti-inflammatory and probably immunoregulatory properties. The phagocytic activity of monocytes and polymorphonuclear leukocytes are inhibited. Lysosomal enzyme and prostaglandin actions are suppressed. Lymphocyte stimulation is reduced. Gold is hypothesized to react with collagen, increasing cross-linkages to create a more stable molecule with more resistance to inflammation. Also, gold may retard the formation of disulfide bonds and abnormal proteins such as rheumatoid factor. In addition, normal immunoglobulins that are turned into antigens in rheumatoid arthritis may be restructured back to normal by a catalytic action of gold. Among the many mechanisms proposed for gold's beneficial effects on arthritis, no one or composite of them has been definitively established.

    Auranofin (Ridaura) is a new salt form of gold for oral use currently under investigation. Its pharmacologic actions are similar but broader in scope and degree than the parenteral salt forms of gold. Both humoral and cell-mediated

FIGURE 26-4

Rheumatoid Arthritis: Steps in Therapy. Therapy employs four steps to manage arthritis and incorporates several therapeutic alternatives at each step. The first step includes physical therapy, patient and family counseling, and administration of anti-inflammatory drugs. This step constitutes the basic chronic therapy that is continued throughout the arthritic patient's lifetime of disease. As the disease worsens, additional treatments are added to this basic program. The drug choices in steps three and four of therapy are added and substituted for each other, depending on disease activity, drug effectiveness, and drug toxicity.

immune systems are suppressed with auranofin, as evidenced by reductions in antibody-induced cell lysis, cytotoxicity, and agglutination and also by suppression of lymphocyte stimulation, transformation, and activity. Anti-inflammatory actions are also more consistent with reductions in chemotaxis, phagocytosis, lysosomal enzyme release, oxygen radical production, and aggregation of leukocytes.

Pharmacokinetics Parenteral and oral gold differ in the pharmacokinetic properties of absorption, serum concentration, extent of distribution, and excretory pattern. About 25 percent of an oral dose of **auranofin** is absorbed. Only 1 percent of **gold sodium thiomalate** (a parenteral drug) is absorbed with oral use. Serum concentrations differ greatly in levels, but persistence in the blood and tissues is common for both oral and parenteral gold. A 50-mg intramuscular dose produces a peak level of 700 μg/mL, and a 50-mg monthly dose achieves a serum level range of 75 to 125 μg/mL. A 2-mg and 6-mg dose of **auranofin** for 12 weeks achieves serum levels of 30 and 80 μg/mL, respectively.

Tissue distribution is significant with gold. In the blood, red blood cells account for a major percentage of the gold concentration (16 percent, parenteral; 25 to 50 percent, oral). Synovial fluid levels are about 50 percent of serum levels. Gold is found in skin, liver, spleen, eyes, and kidney at much higher concentrations than blood for parenteral gold and at about equal levels for auranofin. The plasma half-lives for gold are 5 days for parenteral and 20 days for oral forms. However, gold is retained in tissues for months; 25 percent of parenteral gold remains in tissues at 8 months and only 15 percent of oral gold at 10 days. Excretion of parenteral gold is 70 percent by the kidneys and 30 percent in the feces, whereas oral gold is 5 percent and 95 percent, respectively.

Adverse Effects The frequency (8.4 to 62 percent) and severity of gold toxicity limits its clinical utility (see Table 26-5). Serious reactions occur approximately 4.5 percent of the time. The incidence of toxic reactions is unrelated to the plasma levels of gold but may possibly be dependent on the total body content. The most common toxic effects are those involving the skin and buccal mucosa (20 to 30 percent) and vary from simple erythematous scales to severe exfoliative dermatitis. Pruritis is almost always present with the rash. Gold dermatitis may be a *nitritoid* reaction (vasomotor skin changes) observed with the parenteral aqueous salt form, **gold sodium thiomalate**. Gold is also toxic to the kidney and may cause proteinuria (17 percent); however, there are only a few documented cases of irreversible toxic nephropathy.

Of all the adverse effects the most dangerous are the blood dyscrasias, as these may prove fatal. Thrombocytopenia, leukopenia, agranulocytosis, and aplastic anemia may all occur. White blood cell counts, platelet counts, and urinalysis should be assessed by the nurse before each injection. Ophthalmic reactions are possible, including discoloration of iris (chrysiasis), cataracts, corneal ulceration, and retinopathy. If toxic symptoms progress, the gold will have to be discontinued and other forms of therapy instituted. Auranofin produces the same scope of reactions, but gastrointestinal reactions are more frequent, especially diarrhea (a 40 percent incidence), and skin reactions are less common. Blood dyscrasias may be less frequent.

Dosage and Administration Parenteral gold is given intramuscularly on a weekly basis. A 10-mg test dose is given first to determine patient tolerance to gold. A 25-mg dose is then used for 1 to 2 weeks. If the patient tolerates this dose, it is increased to 50 mg for 3 to 6 months to induce a response.

TABLE 26-5 Adverse Effects of Disease-Modifying Drugs*

	GOLD	PENICILLAMINE	CHLOROQUINE	AZATHIOPRINE	CYCLOPHOSPHAMIDE	METHOTREXATE
Gastric distress	+	++	++	+++	+++	+++
Stomatitis	++	+	+	+++	++	+++
Metallic taste	+	++	0	0	0	0
Hepatotoxicity	+	0	+	++	0	++++
Skin rash	+++	+++	++	++	+	++
Alopecia	0	0	0	+	++++	++
Leukopenia	++	+	0	++++	++++	++
Thrombocytopenia	+	++	0	+++	+++	++
Anemia	0	0	0	+	+	++
Proteinuria	++	++	+	+	+	0
Nephrotic syndrome	+	+	0	0	0	0
Bladder damage	0	0	0	0	+++	0
Ocular disturbance	+	0	+++	0	0	0
Neurologic problems	+	+	++	0	0	+
Fertility disruption	0	0	0	++++	++++	+++
Teratogenesis	0	0	0	++++	++++	++++

*Scale for incidence of adverse effects: 0: none reported; +: seldom; ++: occasional; +++: common; ++++: frequent.

A total dose of 500 mg to 1 g is given over this period. Once a maximum response is achieved, the 50-mg dose is given at wider intervals during maintenance therapy. A biweekly up to a monthly schedule is employed as long as disease control is sustained. Auranofin is given in a daily oral dose of 2 to 6 mg.

Penicillamine

Penicillamine (Cuprimine) is indicated for rheumatoid arthritis, poisonings with heavy metals (e.g., lead and iron), and Wilson's disease (abnormal metabolism of copper). Penicillamine's efficacy is similar to that of parenteral gold in the percentage and rate of disease control of arthritis.

Mechanism of Action Although penicillamine is a chelating agent, binding with heavy metals, its mechanism related to arthritis is unknown. However, immunosuppressive effects are observed, e.g., interference in B and T lymphocyte functions, decrease in antibody response to antigens, decrease in circulating immunoglobulins, and altered complement activity.

Pharmacokinetics Penicillamine is absorbed well after oral use with a peak level within 1 to 2 h, although food will significantly reduce its absorption. In the blood, it is bound to albumin and excreted rapidly through the kidney (about 90 percent in 6 to 7 h). Because it chelates minerals, such as iron, drug interactions will occur with multivitamins containing minerals and iron tablets.

Adverse Effects The scope of adverse effects is similar to that of gold. Previously, the overall incidence (50 to 60 percent) was considered to be higher than with gold salts, but the lower doses used currently should reduce this frequency. The adverse effects are reversible with discontinuation of treatment. Skin rashes are common (2 to 40 percent incidence). An early rash is pruritic and maculopapular within 1 month of treatment; a scaly rash occurs later. A loss of taste is found in 10 to 20 percent of patients, sometimes accompanied by nausea, vomiting, dyspepsia, or stomatitis. Thrombocytopenia occurs in 10 to 20 percent of the patients, but sudden leukopenia is less common (fewer than 5 percent). Nephrotoxicity manifests as proteinuria at a 2 to 15 percent incidence. Proteins in the urine can exceed 2 g every 24 h. Rare reactions include myasthenia gravis, polymyositis, Goodpasture's syndrome, and systemic lupus erythematosus. **Penicillamine** should not be administered with gold, because the gold will be chelated by penicillamine and removed from the body.

Dosage and Administration The dosing scheme is characterized as "start low, go slow" to minimize side effects (see Table 26-4). A starting dose is 125 to 250 mg, with increments at 1- to 3-month intervals. Most patients will respond to doses at or below 750 mg/day.

Antimalarial Drugs

Antimalarial antirheumatic drugs include **chloroquine** (Aralen), **hydroxychloroquine** (Plaquenil), and **quinacrine** (Atabrine). The response rate and onset of response for chloroquine and hydroxychloroquine for rheumatoid arthritis are delayed, as they are in the other DMARDs. Antimalarials frequently are used along with NSAIDs to treat SLE. Quinacrine is used only for SLE.

Mechanism of Action Chloroquine has been shown to stabilize lysosomal membranes, suppress lymphocytes, inhibit chemotaxis, inhibit DNA polymerase, and inhibit disulfide bonds. These effects would be beneficial in arthritis, but a specific mechanism has not been identified. The other two antimalarial drugs probably have the same actions.

Pharmacokinetics Oral absorption is good with **chloroquine**, and it is concentrated highly in tissues. Pigmented tissues contain the highest amounts; melanin binds the antimalarials, especially in the eyes. Excretion is very slow through the kidneys. **Hydroxychloroquine** and **quinacrine** possess the same properties.

Adverse Effects Table 26-5 lists the adverse effects of antimalarial drugs. Ocular reactions are the major problem limiting the use of these drugs for arthritis. These drugs concentrate in the eye 100-fold higher than in the blood. Visual disturbance occurs commonly (15 to 50 percent), with diplopia and loss of accommodation. Corneal opacities also occur. Retinopathy gradually increases during therapy with blurred vision, night blindness, and scotoma; blindness is the result if therapy is not stopped. Routine ophthalmologic exams are recommended. Neurologic side effects include headache, dizziness, and myopathy. Gastric reactions are nausea and diarrhea. Skin effects include hyperpigmentation and lichenoid rash, with exfoliative dermatitis possible.

Dosage and Administration The dosage forms, dosage range, and the number of doses/day are found in Table 26-4. Therapy continues for up to a total cumulative dose of 600 g; then the drug is stopped to prevent an excessive increase in ocular side effects. Some clinicians will treat a patient for several months, stop treatment temporarily for a week, and then resume antimalarials. This regimen is used in an attempt to prevent toxicity.

Immunosuppressive Agents

Azathioprine (Imuran), **cyclophosphamide** (Cytoxan), and **methotrexate** are cytotoxic drugs. Chapter 37 describes the pharmacology of methotrexate and cyclophosphamide (pharmacokinetics, adverse effects, etc.). Azathioprine is discussed in Chap. 31. As immunosuppressants, they produce decreased lymphocyte and antibody responses which are pathologic features of rheumatoid arthritis. **Azathioprine** and **cyclophosphamide** can produce partial or complete remissions in 70 to 100 percent of the patients with moderate to severe rheumatoid arthritis. **Methotrexate** is an investigational drug in the treatment of psoriatic arthritis and rheumatoid arthritis with a response rate of about 75 percent. Onset of disease control is gradual, as noted for DMARDs in general.

The six criteria for use of immunosuppressive agents in arthritis are life-threatening or crippling disease, conventional treatment failure, reversible synovitis, absence of preexisting infection or blood cell problems, and capability for close patient monitoring. Corticosteroid-dependent arthritis patients often can be tapered off their steroids when these agents are used. Table 26-4 contains the dosage forms, dosage ranges, and number of doses per day. Table 26-5 lists the potential adverse effects observed with immunosuppressive agents.

Corticosteroids

Five indications are recognized as appropriate for corticosteroid use in immune and inflammatory disease. First, chronic oral therapy is employed for recalcitrant patients who fail to respond to NSAIDs and DMARDs. Second, the oral corticosteroids are useful during the initial period required for onset of DMARD action. Third, intraarticular injections are indicated for acute exacerbation of synovitis in single joints in which mobility is impaired significantly. Response is rapid, with inflammation control within a few days for oral therapy and within 24 h for intraarticular dosing. Fourth, occasionally **adrenocorticotropic hormone** (**ACTH**) injection is used for gouty arthritis when standard therapy fails. Fifth, high-dose oral corticosteroids, e.g., 20 to 70 mg/day of prednisone, are used for short periods for a severe attack of the systemic rheumatic disorders, rheumatoid arthritis, and SLE.

Mechanism of Action Both anti-inflammatory and immunosuppressive properties are associated with the corticosteroids. Inflammation is reduced by blockade of prostaglandin formation (see Fig. 26-3), inhibition of leukocyte and monocyte chemotaxis and phagocytosis, stabilization of lysosomal enzymes, and prevention of changes in capillary membranes. Immunosuppression is caused by decreased reticuloendothelial processing of antigens and altered functions of lymphocytes, including decreases in blastogenesis, mediator release, proliferation, and cytotoxicity. Therefore, synovitis of rheumatoid arthritis and bursitis is controlled by corticosteroids. See Chap. 35 for more information on the pharmacology of corticosteroids.

Adverse Effects Table 26-6 lists 25 adverse effects associated with chronic (at least several months) corticosteroid use at pharmacologic doses. All organ systems can be disturbed by corticosteroids. Close patient monitoring is essential to identify and manage these many iatrogenic problems. The nursing process relevant to these often serious adverse effects is presented in Chap. 35.

Dosage and Administration Oral therapy is kept at the lowest doses which will control target symptoms (e.g., 10 to 12 mg/day of **prednisone**) to minimize side effects during chronic corticosteroid use, even though higher doses would be more effective. The dose is given daily in the morning for **prednisone** or **prednisolone**, providing coverage over a full 24 h and simulating normal physiologic steroid secre-

TABLE 26-6 Adverse Effects of Chronic Corticosteroid Therapy

Cardiovascular and renal	*Neurologic*
Sodium retention	Euphoria
Fluid retention	Dependence
Potassium wasting	Depression
	Psychosis
Endocrine	
Adrenal suppression*	*Ophthalmic*
Fat redistribution	Cataracts
Hyperglycemia	Ocular hypertension (glaucoma)
Hyperlipidemia	
Menstrual irregularity	*Skin*
	Acne
Musculoskeletal	Bruisability
Bone fractures	Hirsutism
Growth retardation	Petichiae
Muscle wasting	
Osteoporosis	*Miscellaneous*
	Infection
	Weight gain
	Gastric distress
	Wound healing problems

*Life-threatening adrenal insufficiency may occur if these drugs are discontinued abruptly. Dosage should be tapered.

tion patterns. Every-other-day dosing has been used to minimize adrenal suppression but will not control symptoms in all patients.

The doses of intraarticular steroids are adjusted to the joint size (e.g., phalanges, 0.1 mL; wrist, 0.5 mL; knee, 1.0 mL). The drugs are in suspension formulations which afford prolonged duration of action (2 to 4 weeks) with a single injection. Table 26-2 lists three such corticosteroid injectable suspensions. Injections should be given no more often than at 4- to 8-week intervals to minimize local joint destruction. Their administration requires meticulous injection technique to avoid local toxicity. The injection process requires local anesthetic application to reduce pain during corticosteroid injection into an inflamed joint, aseptic technique to avoid infecting synovial fluid, withdrawal of excess fluid to relieve pain and increase drug concentration, and flushing of the needle with saline to avoid accidental depositing of crystals from the needle tip into tissues while withdrawing the needle. The joint given a corticosteroid injection should have reduced activity for about 24 to 48 h, to avoid joint damage from prematurely excessive mobilization.

NURSING PROCESS RELATED TO DMARDs

Assessment

The disease-modifying antirheumatic drugs represent a diverse group of agents. Excluding the corticosteroids, the characteristic that links these drugs is their ability to modify the course of the immune-mediated rheumatic diseases. In addition, these drugs are usually used for extended periods of time, e.g., 1 year to life, and are likely to produce adverse effects gradually over this period. Baseline measurement of the patient's signs and symptoms are focused upon those body systems in which the intended action of the drug is directed, as well as upon those systems in which adverse effects are likely to occur:

Renal A history of renal insufficiency or abnormality is an important consideration in penicillamine therapy, since renal function is crucial to its elimination. Most of the DMARDs can cause bladder or renal adverse effects (e.g., hematuria, proteinuria, nephrotic syndrome), so a baseline urinalysis precedes therapy.

Hematologic The incidence of blood dyscrasias (i.e., leukopenia, anemia, thrombocytopenia) with these drugs indicates a CBC prior to therapy. American blacks or individuals of Mediterranean ancestry may be tested prior to **chloroquine** (or other antimalarial drug) therapy for deficiency of glucose-6-phosphate dehydrogenase (G6PD), since acute hemolysis can result from this drug in persons with this genetic disorder.

Dermatologic Inspection of the skin prior to therapy will aid identification of skin rash attributable to a drug.

Reproductive Pregnancy or lactation generally contraindicates DMARDs, which may cause fetal abnormalities or harm to the breast-fed infant. The initial assessment should include a reproductive history, including current contraception practices.

Other systems Any patient who is elderly or has uncontrolled endocrine, hepatic, or cardiovascular disease (e.g., diabetes mellitus, severe hypertension, congestive heart failure) has a higher risk of severe adverse reaction to the DMARDs, especially to parenteral gold. Patients allergic to drugs related to the DMARD prescribed (e.g., the penicillin-sensitive person who is to receive penicillamine) should receive the related DMARD with extreme caution, if at all. A thorough eye examination, including acuity, visual field, color discrimination, and ophthalmoscopic examination, should be performed prior to antimalarial (e.g., chloroquine) therapy.

Management

DMARDs are frequently combined with other forms of drug therapy in the treatment of patients with immune-mediated disorders. This means that multiple-dosing patterns may be used and the patient may be confused about the purpose of each type of drug. Also, the patient may be required to adhere to a DMARD schedule for a number of months before any noticeable change is seen in symptoms. An intense education program that focuses upon the actions, adverse effects, and drug interactions of these agents is necessary.

Some of the adverse effects may be difficult to prevent since DMARDs are given for such long periods. These adverse effects are balanced against the therapeutic effects to determine whether the drugs should be continued. Chills, fever, bruising, bleeding, or sore throat are signs of blood dyscrasias that may occur with the DMARDs; patients should be encouraged to report these to their care provider as soon as they notice them. Rashes, gastric distress, diarrhea, jaundice, and stomatitis (inflammation of the mouth) are other signs which should be reported if they occur during DMARD therapy. Patients must also be educated in the identification of adverse effects of the specific DMARD which they are taking (e.g., ocular effects with **chloroquine**, fertility disruption with **cyclophosphamide**, hepatotoxicity with **methotrexate**).

Although **penicillamine** must be taken on an empty stomach, gastric distress may be diminished if other DMARDs are taken with food. Increased dietary pyridoxine (found in grains, meat, molasses) or supplementation (25 mg/day) may be required with penicillamine, since the requirement for this vitamin is increased by penicillamine.

Evaluation

The modification of the disease process will usually produce gradual changes in the patient's signs and symptoms. During each visit, the patient's subjective changes are evaluated and a thorough review of systems, with a particular focus upon those systems likely to demonstrate adverse effects of the DMARD, is made.

Since the individual DMARDs are so different, the nurse needs to be familiar with each drug in order to know which systems to examine, but many DMARDs cause hematologic or renal toxicities. Complete blood counts should be performed routinely and whenever the patient complains of fatigue, sore throat, bruising, fever, or other signs of anemia, leukopenia, or thrombocytopenia. Urinalysis performed routinely with particular attention to proteinuria or hematuria will facilitate early identification of renal or bladder adverse effects. Patients on combined antiarthritis therapy are often at increased risk of adverse effects due to overlapping toxicities (e.g., phenylbutazone, an NSAID, and the DMARDs both may cause blood dyscrasias).

The nursing process for the corticosteroids, which are quite different from the other DMARDs, is discussed in Chap. 35. The nursing process for the antimalarials is further discussed in Chap. 29, and that for the immunosuppressants is in Chaps. 31 and 37.

Antigout Drugs

Four distinct classes of drugs are employed for gout therapy: *allopurinal, uricosuric drugs* (probenecid and sulfinpyrazone), *colchicine,* and *NSAIDs.* The goals of therapy are cessation of acute attacks, control of inflammation, and reduction of systemic uric acid. The clinical signs and symptoms of gout can be controlled with drug therapy in almost all patients.

Mechanism of Action

Gout is an inflammatory and metabolic disease involving the joints and other soft tissues. Uric acid is the normal catabolic product of purine nucleic acids, but it deposits in tissues and incites an inflammatory reaction in a gouty patient. The mechanisms of action of the antigout drugs are shown in Fig. 26-5, as are the physiology of the production of uric acid and the pathologic changes in gout. Various antigout drugs work by blocking the formation of uric acid from its precursors (xanthine and hypoxanthine) by inhibiting the enzyme xanthine oxidase, enhancing the excretion of uric acid by blocking renal tubular reabsorption, or reducing inflammation.

Dosage and Administration

Therapy for acute gouty arthritis is aggressive short-term high-dose therapy with colchicine or NSAIDs. Loading doses are used for 1 to 2 days to stop the acute attack. then the dose is tapered over a few days to maintenance levels.

Chronic inflammation is treated with NSAIDs (see previous discussion). **Colchicine** is used prophylactically at low doses to prevent acute attacks. Hyperuricemia is treated with allopurinal and/or uricosuric drugs. Table 26-7 contains the doses for acute and chronic treatment of gout.

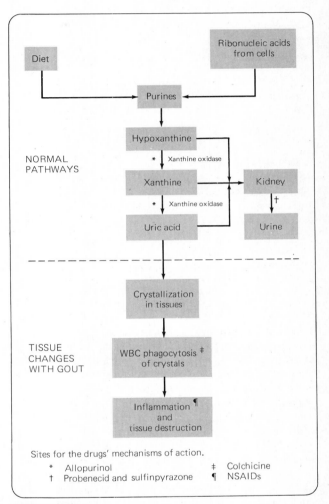

FIGURE 26-5

Gout Pathogenesis and Sites of Drug Action. Uric acid is the metabolic product of nuclear ribonucleic acids and normally is excreted completely by the kidney into the urine. In gout, excess systemic uric acid is deposited in tissues and elicits a chronic destructive inflammatory process. Antigout drugs inhibit the pathogenesis of gout at four distinct sites of action. Allopurinol blocks uric acid formation by inhibiting the enzyme xanthine oxidase. Probenecid and sulfinpyrazone increase uric acid excretion in the kidney by blocking renal reabsorption. Colchicine interrupts inflammation by suppressing WBC activity. NSAIDs reduce inflammation by blocking the formation of inflammatory chemical mediators.

TABLE 26-7 Antigout Drugs: Doses

DRUG	CHRONIC THERAPY DAILY DOSAGE RANGE, mg	ACUTE THERAPY LOADING DOSES, mg
Allopurinol (Zyloprim)	200–400	—
Colchicine (Various)	0.5–1.2*	4–8
Probenecid (Benemid)	500–1000*	—
Sulfinpyrazone (Anturane)	200–800*	—
NSAIDs		
Fenoprofen (Nalfon)	1200–2400*	2400†
Ibuprofen (Motrin, Rufen)	1200–3600*	3600†
Indomethacin (Indocin)	75–150*	100–200
Naproxen (Naprosyn, Anaprox)	500–750*	750
Phenylbutazone (Butazoladin)	200–300*	600–800
Sulindac (Clinoril)	200–400*	300–400

*Divide into two to four doses.

†The maximum doses of these two NSAIDs have not been determined.

Allopurinol

Allopurinol (Zyloprim) is indicated in the treatment of primary gout and gout secondary to other disease states which cause hyperuricemia. Allopurinol is sometimes used in combination with uricosuric drugs to lower uric acid levels. Allopurinol is preferable to uricosuric drugs in the treatment of patients with a history of stone formation, excessive production of uric acid, or renal disease. Serum uric acid is reduced within 24 to 48 h after starting allopurinol, and peak effect occurs in 1 to 2 weeks. Control of gouty attacks is achieved in 60 to 100 percent of allopurinol patients within a few months. Initiation of allopurinol can precipitate an acute attack of gout in about 10 percent of patients; therefore, colchicine may be used prophylactically and concomitantly for a few months. Allopurinol is used indefinitely, since drug cessation often leads to acute attacks of gout.

Allopurinol is also used to prevent acute uric acid nephropathy during cancer therapy with antineoplastic agents. These drugs are used to destroy rapidly proliferating cells (cancer cells) in the body. This destruction of cells results in an increase in purines, which are metabolized in the body to uric acid. The uric acid may be presented to the kidney in sufficiently elevated concentrations to result in precipitation in the tubules, resulting in renal failure. Allopurinol is utilized to block the formation of this excess uric acid.

Mechanism of Action Figure 26-5 shows that the enzyme xanthine oxidase is primarily responsible for the final metabolic conversion of purines into uric acid, which is then excreted by the kidney. Allopurinol's blockade of this enzyme reduces uric acid levels in the blood and prevents uric acid from achieving a saturation point for crystallization. Purines then are excreted as uric acid precursors (xanthine and hypoxanthine) in addition to uric acid.

Pharmacokinetics Allopurinol is rapidly metabolized in the body to oxypurinol, which has a half-life of 30 h. This metabolite is active to a lesser degree as a xanthine oxidase inhibitor. Renal clearance of oxypurinol is slower than that of allopurinol, and it is this metabolite which is responsible for the extended action of that drug.

Adverse Effects The most common side effect of allopurinol is a pruritic maculopapular skin rash, possibly accompanied by fever. Dermatitis of various intensities has also occurred. Alopecia has been produced. Cases of life-threatening toxic epidermal necrolysis and exfoliative dermatitis have been observed. The milder skin reactions seem to be dose-related and may disappear if therapy is stopped and then resumed at a lower dosage. However, because of the fatal skin reactions, any rash requires close followup.

Other side effects include nausea and vomiting, anorexia, abdominal pain, and diarrhea. Some patients may exhibit an idiosyncratic or hypersensitivity reaction to the drug, e.g., vasculitis. Some cases of hepatoxicity have been reported in patients taking allopurinol. For this reason, liver function tests should be done before and during therapy. Rarely leukopenia and thrombocytopenia have been reported with allopurinol.

Dosage and Administration Single daily doses are used because of the extended half-life of the active metabolite. Initial doses are 100 mg/day with upward titration to 300 mg. Recalcitrant patients may require up to 1 g/day. Dosage adjustments are made according to serum uric acid levels, with a therapeutic goal of a level of 6 mg/dL or less. Since allopurinol and oxypurinol are excreted by the kidney, a creatinine clearance of only 10 to 50 mL/min will require a dose of 200 mg/day. If the clearance is less than 10 mL/min, the dose should be reduced to 100 mg/day or less.

Colchicine

Colchicine is the drug of choice in the treatment of acute gouty arthritis. Ninety percent of patients with gout will respond favorably if this treatment is started within hours after the attack begins. Initiation of therapy in later stages will increase the possibility of treatment failure. Colchicine is indicated also as prophylactic therapy for patients with recurrent acute attacks of gout and as a preventive measure during the first few months of allopurinol or uricosuric therapy. Tolerance does not develop, and no loss of efficacy has been observed after repeated use of the drug.

Mechanism of Action   The drug is thought to work by decreasing the inflammatory response to deposited urate crystals by inhibiting leukocyte migration and phagocytosis. A lactic acidosis is produced by leukocytes as they attack the urate deposits, and this results in a further increase in urate deposition. The interruption of this cycle by colchicine results in a decrease in the inflammatory response. The drug enters the leukocytes and can be detected in these cells up to 9 days after administration. Colchicine binds to microtubular proteins in the leukocytes, causing disaggregation and inhibiting cell function.

Pharmacokinetics   The drug is absorbed rapidly and then is avidly taken up into tissue, such that the plasma half-life is very short, only 20-30 min. Colchicine is partially metabolized in the liver. Biliary excretion is the major route of elimination from the body for both the drug and its metabolites, all of which undergo enterohepatic cycling.

Adverse Effects   Gastrointestinal toxicity, especially diarrhea, occurs in 25 to 80 percent of patients receiving acute therapy. Since the drug is given every hour in acute attacks, a buildup of unchanged drug is presented to the GI tract, both as recycled and newly administered colchicine. When this accumulation reaches toxic concentrations in the GI tract, the patient experiences symptoms of nausea, vomiting, diarrhea, hyperperistalsis, and abdominal cramping. These manifestations of gastrointestinal toxicity may not be seen with intravenous administration, since the amount of unchanged drug reaching the intestine after administration is not supplemented by additional, oral doses. With chronic administration, gastrointestinal reactions are much less common. The danger of bone marrow depression is serious but rare, resulting in agranulocytosis, thrombocytopenia, leukopenia, and aplastic anemia. Loss of body and scalp hair, rashes, myopathy, anuria, renal damage, and hematuria also have been reported.

Colchicine should be used cautiously for elderly or debilitated patients and patients with serious renal, GI, or cardiac disorders, as these groups have a tendency toward accumulating the drug. If toxicity does occur, dialysis is of no value, and therapy is directed at correcting the dehydration, electrolyte imbalances, acidosis, and shock.

Dosage and Administration   For acute gout, colchicine is administered until pain is relieved (usually 12 to 24 h) or signs of gastrointestinal toxicity (diarrhea) appear. When administered orally, colchicine should be given as an initial dose of 1.0 to 1.2 mg followed by 0.5 to 0.6 mg every hour. The maximum total dose is 8 mg.

Parenteral colchicine can be used for acute gout in order to achieve a more rapid response with less GI toxicity. A 1- to 2-mg dose is given slowly (at least 2 to 5 min) in an established intravenous line over several minutes. The dose can be repeated one or two times at 6- to 12-h intervals. Parenteral administration must avoid any extravasation into tissue as this will result in serious necrosis. An excessive rate of infusion will cause sclerosis of veins.

Uricosuric Agents

Probenecid (Benemid) and **sulfinpyrazone** (Anturane) belong to the antigout class of drugs called *uricosuric agents* because they promote urate excretion. Clinical improvement and sustained reduction in serum uric acid occur in 75 percent or more of patients with gout or hyperuricemia treated with either of these two drugs. Some patients will have control of uric acid levels but still experience acute attacks. During initiation of treatment, fluxes in uric acid lead to acute gouty attacks, requiring prophylactic colchicine for a few months. These drugs are not effective when the patient is in renal failure. Sulfinpyrazone also decreases platelet aggregation and is used prophylactically to prevent thrombus formation in thromboembolic disease, such as transient cerebral ischemic attacks and myocardial infarction. **Probenecid** is also used to prolong the effects of certain **penicillins** and **cephalosporins** because it interferes with their elimination by tubular secretion.

Mechanism of Action   Uric acid is excreted from the body almost exclusively via the kidney (see Fig. 26-5). It is first filtered by the glomerulus, reabsorbed proximally, and finally secreted distally. The reabsorption and secretion phases are active processes, so that if interference with the carriers involved occurs either by competition with uric acid for their binding sites or by deactivation of the carrier itself, there will be a significant change in the amount of uric acid excreted from the body. As a result, interference with the reabsorption process results in a significant increase in uric acid excretion even though secretory carriers are also blocked. A number of drugs, predominantly organic acids, interfere with the tubular reabsorption of uric acid in the kidney and enhance urate excretion, but **probenecid** and **sulfinpyrazone** are the two organic acids utilized specifically for their uricosuric effect.

Pharmacokinetics   Following oral administration, sulfinpyrazone and probenecid are almost completely absorbed, attaining a peak level in 1 to 4 h. Protein binding is high for both drugs (90 percent for probenecid and 98 percent for sulfinpyrazone). Elimination is via glomerular filtration and then reabsorption from the tubule. The drugs are then metabolized in the liver and excreted slowly by the kidney as glucuronide conjugates and other metabolites. The half-lives are 6 to 12 h for probenecid and 2 to 4 h for sulfinpyrazone.

Adverse Effects   Probenecid is usually well tolerated; however, side effects may include headache and GI disturbances, such as anorexia, nausea, vomiting, diarrhea, constipation, and abdominal discomfort. The disturbances are usually dose-related, and reduction in dosage may overcome them. Skin rashes, anaphylactic reactions, and drug fever may be manifestations of hypersensitivity, but they do not occur often. Flushing, dizziness, and anemia have also been reported. Sulfinpyrazone also produces GI reactions and hypersensitivity skin rashes.

The possibility of renal stone formation exists during the initial stages of therapy. Alkalinization of the urine and maintenance of urinary volume with hydration will decrease the possibility of this occurrence.

Dosage and Administration   Therapy is initiated at low doses (0.5 to 1 g probenecid and 200 to 200 mg sulfinpyrazone) in order to minimize abnormal fluxes in uric acid and secondary acute attacks of gout. Doses are gradually increased over several weeks (see Table 26-7).

Nonsteroidal Anti-Inflammatory Drugs

Fenoprofen, ibuprofen, indomethacin, naproxen, phenylbutazone, and **sulindac** are all effective in controlling the inflammation in acute and chronic gout when a patient cannot tolerate the adverse effects of colchicine or allopurinol. Their response rate is almost as high as the above two conventional treatments. Table 26-7 contains the doses for chronic and acute treatment. Acute gout is treated with a loading dose for 1 to 2 days, as noted in the table, with dosage tapering over a few days after the response of the gout to NSAIDs.

Salicylates in Gout   Salicylates have been used in the treatment of both acute and chronic gout. They increase the urinary excretion of urates by competing for active transport sites in the tubule, but this action is dose-related. In low doses (1 to 2 g/day), salicylates may decrease urate excretion by blocking tubular secretion, producing a rise in serum urate levels. In doses above 5 g/day both tubular secretion and tubular reabsorption are blocked, increasing the excretion of urates and resulting in a lower plasma urate level. Salicylates in large doses are seldom used in the treatment of gout, as they are not well tolerated, especially by the elderly. The salicylate effect is enhanced in an alkaline urine, and both uric acid and salicylate excretion are increased.

Salicylates, at any dosage level, inactivate the effect of uricosuric drugs and can cause urate retention. The mechanism of this interaction is not known, although it is thought that salicylates block the receptor sites in the renal tubule. Salicylates should be avoided in gouty arthritis.

NURSING PROCESS RELATED TO ANTIGOUT DRUGS

Assessment

Baseline information gathered prior to antigout drug therapy includes an assessment of all drugs currently being taken, a careful history of any hypersensitivities, serum uric acid level, and a creatinine clearance. If a uricosuric is being considered, the patient should be questioned concerning a history of uric acid kidney stones and blood dyscrasias. Additional conditions that require special considerations include the following.

Renal impairment   Since uricosurics increase the kidney's excretion of uric acid, adequate renal function is necessary for these drugs to function. In addition, the dosage of allopurinol will need to be adjusted downward in decreased renal functioning.

Elderly   The elderly may have decreased renal and GI functioning and these can alter the absorption and excretion of the drugs and uric acid.

Management

A major management activity is to assure that the patient maintains an adequate intake of fluids to produce approximately 2 L of urine per day. This procedure will increase the excretion of uric acid and will dilute the uric acid in the urine in an effort to prevent the formation of kidney stones. Patients should be cautioned from beginning other drug therapy without informing their care provider that they are taking chronic antigout drug therapy. Alkaline urine, which results from drinking citrus fruit juices, for example, promotes uric acid secretion and inhibits urate stone formation.

Evaluation

The drug therapy is evaluated by decreases in serum uric acid and by the absence of acute gouty attacks. If any tophi were present before beginning therapy, they should be decreasing in size and should disappear over time. The patient is evaluated for adverse drug effects that are renal (the development of renal stones, decreased creatine clearance); dermatologic (rash, alopecia, urticaria, purpura); gastrointestinal (nausea, vomiting, diarrhea); and hematologic (anemia, bone marrow depression, and agranulocytosis).

SPECIFIC IMMUNE AND INFLAMMATORY DISORDERS

Nonarticular Rheumatism: Bursitis and Tenosynovitis

Nonarticular rheumatism is a group of disorders having the common characteristics of musculoskeletal pain and stiffness. Two similar problems within this category are bursitis and tenosynovitis. These problems both involve inflammation of synovium of unilateral, isolated joints. *Bursae* are closed synovial sacs located at friction sites throughout the body. Inflammation of these sacs can be caused by excessive frictional forces or by direct trauma. *Tenosynovitis* is an inflammation of the synovial lining of the fibrous tube through which a tendon moves. This inflammation is also caused by excessive friction or trauma.

Clinical Findings

The most common clinical findings in bursitis and tenosynovitis are pain with movements of the afflicted joint, tenderness, and swelling. There may also be redness over the affected site. There are no specific laboratory tests that are useful in the assessment of these problems. Nursing assessment includes determining from the patient's history of daily activities the type of increased friction or trauma that caused the bursitis or tenosynovitis. Activities that are rapid, repetitive, and stressful to limited parts of the body, such as scrubbing floors, raking leaves, or playing tennis, are likely causes. The locations of pain, tenderness, swelling, increased warmth, and redness are noted on examination.

Clinical Pharmacology and Therapeutics

Treatment includes physical therapy, rest, analgesic, and anti-inflammatory drugs. Splinting and padding will give the afflicted area rest and protection. Joints in the lower extremities should be relieved of weight bearing with rest and assistive devices. Thermotherapy with warm moist heat will provide analgesic and anti-inflammatory actions.

NSAIDs are used for acute and chronic bursitis and tenosynovitis. Doses are adjusted to the severity of the pain and the presence of inflammation. Very painful joints with compromised mobility warrant short courses of opiate analgesia for only a few doses. Intraarticular corticosteroids are indicated if NSAIDs do not decrease the inflammation within 3 or 4 days. Some specially trained nurses may perform this procedure. The dosage and administration guidelines for these drugs are found earlier in this chapter.

The patient will need to learn the principles of protection of the tendons and bursae in order to prevent a recurrence of these problems. These principles include avoiding rapid, repeated actions that cause excessive friction to the tendons or bursae and altering activities of daily living that cause direct trauma to these areas.

Monitoring and Prognosis

Both bursitis and tenosynovitis are acute, self-limiting disorders. The patient's adherence to the drug regime and the physical therapy recommendations are evaluated especially if improvement does not occur within 3 or 4 days. Improvement is demonstrated by decreased pain, tenderness, swelling, and redness, as well as by increased range of motion in the affected area. These disorders tend to recur since they are related to the person's daily living habits that cause excessive friction and/or trauma to the bursae or tendons.

CASE STUDY

R.J. is a 24-year-old male who was recently employed at a factory assembling small engine components. After being at work for eight days Mr. J. visited the occupational health nurse with a complaint of acute pain on top of his right hand. He believed the pain was brought on by his activities at work.

Assessment

Mr. J. cannot recall having ever had a problem like this in the past. Since the onset of this problem he has been using "some" aspirin, which he says decreased the pain slightly. The pain is severe enough to disturb his sleep at night and is limiting his ability to perform on the job. On physical examination, the nurse noted a warm enlarged boggy area on the dorsum of the Mr. J.'s right hand around the extensor tendons of the third through fifth fingers. Flexion and extension of the wrist were limited to approximately 5°. There were no other significant physical findings. The nurse assessed the problem as tenosynovitis of the extensor tendinous area of the right hand secondary to increased friction from repetitive motion.

Management

The specific goals established for Mr. J. were to decrease the pain in his right hand, decrease the inflammation of the

tendinous sheath, and to alter the activities at work that were causing the problem. An immediate application of a cold pack was performed in the clinic for 30 min. Mr. J. was instructed to take aspirin, 3.9 g/day (three 325-mg tablets qid), with meals. The nurse worked with the line supervisor to reassign Mr. J. to an activity that did not require repeated flexion and extension of his wrist.

The nurse explained the inflammatory process to Mr. J. and explained the role of aspirin in altering the inflammatory response. Patient education sheets explaining the inflammatory process were provided to Mr. J. A patient education handout concerning the side effects and drug interactions of aspirin was given to Mr. J.

Evaluation

Mr. J. was seen in the nurse's office two days later. At this time he had a marked decrease in the swelling and an increase in the range of motion for both flexion and extension of the right wrist. He had been assigned new assembly activities as a part of his work and was no longer causing trauma to the affected area.

Degenerative Joint Disease

Degenerative joint disease (DJD), including osteoarthritis and hypertrophic arthritis, is an arthritic disorder of movable joints, characterized by deterioration and abrasion of articular cartilage and formation of new bone at the articular surface. The exact cause of DJD is unknown but appears to have some relation to the biomechanics of the joint. Type II collagen, which makes up the articular cartilage, begins to lose its compressibility secondary to proteoglycan malfunction.

DJD is more common in women than in men and is found primarily in people over the age of 45. This problem was once thought to be a normal consequence of the aging process since the incidence of its occurrence increases with age. In younger people the same joint changes can be documented secondary to cartilage damage from joint injury, infection, or congenital deformities.

Although degenerative joint disease involves primarily biochemical and biomechanical changes within the joint, synovitis frequently accompanies the problem. Therefore, medications that offer analgesic and anti-inflammatory effects may be useful in the treatment of this disorder.

Clinical Findings

DJD involves the weight-bearing joints, including the cervical and lumbar spine, the hips, and the knees, as well as the distal and proximal interphalangeal joints of the hands. The most common symptom is an aching pain in the joint, especially with movement and weight bearing. The individual may have stiffness after resting, but this generally goes away with motion. Morning stiffness, if present, usually lasts only a few minutes. Muscle spasms or pressure on the nerves in the region of the joint may also be a major source of pain. The physical signs seen with DJD include a restricted range of motion, local tenderness, bony enlargements around the joint, small effusions, and crepitation.

Since DJD is a local, arthritic disorder, there are no specific blood tests for the illness. X-ray changes may become evident as the disorder progresses. There will be narrowing of the joint space and increased density of subchondral bone. Bone spurs may be seen at the joint margin, and cystic changes of various sizes are sometimes seen. The extent of the change in the joints noted with x-ray may not be related, however, to the presence of symptoms. Nursing assessment for the patient with DJD includes an assessment of the nature of the person's pain and current techniques used for pain control, the limitations in joint range of motion and the problems these cause in performing activities of daily living, and any undue stresses placed on affected joints by such factors as work pattern and excessive body weight. A thorough medication history that includes all prescribed and over-the-counter drugs, dosages, frequency, duration of use, adverse effects, and allergies is required to analyze potential drug interactions and adverse effects for which the patient may be at risk.

Clinical Pharmacology and Therapeutics

The goals of therapy are to disrupt the progression of the illness and control pain so that the patient may perform activities of daily living. In order to accomplish these goals, management programs include active physical therapy, including the application of heat and cold, and appropriate exercise; drug treatment with analgesics and anti-inflammatory agents; and surgical procedures designed to correct joint malalignment, debridement of loose bodies, and partial or total joint replacement.

In degenerative joint disease NSAIDs are used for analgesia and for control of synovitis. Disease-modifying anti-rheumatic drugs are not used in the treatment of DJD. Because of the chronic nature of DJD, patient education is directed at establishing new patterns of living. A therapeutic exercise and rest program is developed with the consultation of physical and occupational therapists to maintain joint functioning and to reduce joint trauma. The patient will need to understand the illness and the principles of management, as well as the purposes, actions, adverse effects, and potential drug interactions of the prescribed drug regimen. Patient education should also include assistance in identifying adaptive devices to maintain activities of daily living and methods of pain control, including NSAIDs, other analgesics, and the application of hot and cold packs.

Monitoring and Prognosis

DJD generally progresses very slowly in an individual. The major problems encountered are pain upon use of the joint and increasing instability with weight bearing. If exercise and drug regimens fail to provide pain relief and appropriate range of motion, surgical procedures that replace the joints can offer both. Joint replacement is a fairly new procedure, with the majority of the success being in the area of hip joint replacement. Long-term evaluation studies of total prosthesis for knees, finger joints, and other joints are still underway. If the joint replacement procedure is unsuccessful, it may be necessary to fuse the joint permanently in order to provide pain relief and stability.

Nursing evaluation of therapy for DJD has three components. The patient's abilities to perform activities of daily living are evaluated to determine any changes as a response to therapy or to indicate a need to provide additional therapy. The patient's success in the management of pain is evaluated to determine whether changes are needed. Finally, the occurrence of adverse effects of any of the medications is evaluated to determine whether alterations in the drug therapy regimen are necessary.

CASE STUDY

B.B. is a 61-year-old female employed as a waitress who was presented to the nurse practitioner in the Arthritis Clinic with a chief complaint of increased pain in both knees.

Assessment

Ms. B. began to experience progressive limitation of activities over the past 4 years and within the last 3 months had begun to have difficulty maintaining her usual level of work. Her medication history showed that she had taken aspirin therapy in a sporadic pattern over the past several years and that when it did not "cure" her problem she discontinued its use. The aspirin had caused epigastric discomfort and ringing in her ears, which also led to the sporadic drug use. Six years ago a course of indomethacin (Indocin) 25 mg tid with food, provided "some" pain relief but caused headaches and nightmares. She was then changed to ibuprofen (Motrin), 300 mg, which she reports that she takes "off and on" primarily for pain relief. She does not want to take "too many" pills for fear that she might become "hooked" on these drugs.

Ms. B. is the primary source of income for a family that consists of herself, her disabled husband, and a grandchild. She has worked as a waitress in the same restaurant for the past 6 years, and this is the only type of work for which she believes she is prepared.

On physical examination the nurse practitioner noted nontender, bony enlargements of the distal interphalangeal joints of the first and second fingers of the right hand and first, second, and third fingers of the left hand. Elbows, soulders, cervical spine, and lumbar spine showed no abnormalities. The right hip had a 5° flexion contracture, and the left hip was normal. The right knee had a mild effusion, lacked 10° of full extension, and had laxity of the medial collateral ligament. The left knee had no effusion, lacked 5° of full extension, and also demonstrated instability of the medial collaterial ligament. The patient was 35 percent over her desirable weight. There was no evidence of cardiac or gastrointestinal disease.

Ms. B's complete blood count was normal with erythrocyte sedimendation rate of 12 mm/h (normal, 0 to 20 mm/h). X-ray studies indicated normal hip joints and uniform narrowing of the medial joint space of both knees with extensive osteophyte formation and increased subchondral bone density. The nurse practitioner assessed the problem as osteoarthritis of both knees, resulting in impairment of normal activities of daily living.

Management

The goals established for Ms. B. were to assist her with the management of pain, to decrease the further progression of the illness, and to assist her with the management of activities of daily living. A patient education program was designed to assist Ms. B. with the understanding of her illness and the medications that were to be used in its treatment. The anti-inflammatory and analgesic properties of NSAIDs were discussed, as were the side effects and drug interaction. Ms. B. was enrolled in a weight reduction program offered by a local civic group to assist in reducing her weight to within normal range. She was enrolled in a patient club provided by the local chapter of the Arthritis Foundation to provide her with a support group to assist in the management of her illness. A therapeutic exercise program was designed to strengthen her muscle groups around her knee and to increase the range of motion to her knees.

Drug therapy consisted of aspirin, 3.9 g/day (three 325-mg tablets qid), with a full glass of water and meals.

Evaluation

Ms. B. was instructed to return to clinic in 2 weeks, followed by a monthly appointment for the next 6 months. The aspirin dosage of 3.9 g/day maintained a salicylate blood level of about 20 mg/dL, which is in the therapeutic range. However, Ms. B. complained of epigastric discomfort and frequent and easy bruising (a new problem). A stool guaiac test established occult blood loss. Because of aspirin-induced side effects, NSAID therapy was changed from aspirin to sulindac (Clinoril), 200-mg tablet bid. A return to the clinic in 2 weeks showed relief of pain, minimal gastric complaints, and cessation of bruising.

At 6 months following the initial appointment, Ms. B. had less swelling and improved range of motion in both knees. She had reduced her weight by 38 lb. She reported that she had been able to alter activities of daily living and her job to reduce the amount of stress placed on her knees. Most of the practical hints in this area had been provided as a part of her patient club and from materials on DJD provided by the Arthritis Foundation.

Rheumatoid Arthritis

Rheumatoid arthritis is a chronic, systemic, inflammatory disorder of unknown etiology. This disorder can produce pain, stiffness, and deformities of the joints, in addition to the systemic manifestations that can affect the hematologic, pulmonary, neurologic, and cardiovascular systems. Rheumatoid arthritis belongs to a complex group of autoimmune disorders, and the symptoms are manifested primarily in the diarthrodial joints and related structures. The onset of 70 percent of the cases occurs between the ages of 30 and 70 with a peak onset between the ages of 40 and 50 years. Women are affected two to three times more frequently than men. Rheumatoid arthritis occurs more seriously in children under 16 years of age and is defined as *juvenile rheumatoid arthritis (JRA)*. The pathogenesis of rheumatoid arthritis is outlined in Fig. 26-2 and associated discussion.

Synovitis is the most characteristic of changes seen in the joint. The normal synovial lining becomes vascular and edematous. A layer of pannus, or granulation tissue, made of proliferating fibroblasts, blood vessels, and chronic inflammatory cells forms. The pannus continues to grow and to cover the entire articular cartilage, leading to marked destruction of the cartilage and subchondral bone.

Clinical Findings

There are a large number of clinical features and laboratory studies specifically useful in diagnosing rheumatoid arthritis. The disease undergoes an insidious onset and usually follows a slow, progressive course characterized by periods of remission and exacerbation. The most common symptom is morning stiffness lasting more than 1 h. Affected joints are warm, swollen, tender, and red. The synovium will be palpable and boggy around the joint. Joint range of motion is generally limited, especially with extension. The patient will frequently experience symptoms of fatigue, anorexia, weight loss, crepitus, and characteristic joint deformities.

The complete blood count will frequently indicate a mild to moderate normocytic, normochronic anemia and a mild leukocytosis. The erythrocyte sedimentation rate can be markedly increased, and antinuclear antibodies may be positive with a very high titer. Specific macroglobulins known as *rheumatoid factors* are found in about 75 percent of the patients with rheumatoid arthritis. Serum iron may be decreased, although total iron binding is normal secondary to ineffective erythropoiesis.

Synovial fluid analysis is usually performed to help confirm the diagnosis. This analysis will show a white, translucent to opaque fluid with low viscosity. There will be a fair to poor mucin clot and often a spontaneous clot. The fluid will have an elevated white blood count of 3000 to 50,000, and greater than 70 percent will be polymorphonuclear leukocytes.

X-rays for the diagnosis of rheumatoid arthritis are not useful in the early course of the disease since only soft tissue swelling is present. Joint deformities come from fibrous or bony ankylosis. Cartilage and bone destruction are characteristic radiologic findings in the later stages of rheumatoid arthritis.

In the early stages an accurate diagnosis is often difficult to determine. Individuals with rheumatoid arthritis have symptoms for a number of years before a characteristic pattern of the disorder emerges and laboratory and x-ray findings confirm the diagnosis. Nursing assessment includes a complete history of symptoms such as length of morning stiffness; frequency, distribution, and time of joint pain; fatigue; and weight loss. All joints are examined for range of motion, swelling, tenderness, and color. This information is noted in the patient's record. The patient's ability to perform activities of daily living is also recorded, along with the patient's family's understanding of the illness. Evidence of nonrheumatologic tissue involvement is also identified since rheumatoid arthritis is a systemic multiorgan illness. An analysis of the current medication regime, including dose, frequency, duration of use, adverse effects, and allergies, is important for subsequent drug management. Over-the-counter preparations, as well as products not approved for the treatment of rheumatoid arthritis, should be included in this analysis.

Clinical Pharmacology and Therapeutics

There is no known cure for rheumatoid arthritis. The basic program of treatment includes education of the patient, family, and society; application of heat and cold to the affected joints; prescription of therapeutic exercises; systemic, joint, and emotional rest; salicylates to tolerance; and a well-balanced diet and drug therapy.

Figure 26-4 shows the steps in the treatment of rheumatoid arthritis. The rate of progression through these steps depends on the severity of the patient's pain and inflammation, the degree of disability caused by the inflammation, and the responsiveness of the disease to therapy. The general principles included in the discussions of the NSAIDs and DMARDs apply most directly to the rheumatoid arthritis patient.

Together with the treatment team, the nurse develops a patient and family education program that focuses upon the cause and treatment of the illness and the role of the complex medical regimen in the total treatment program. The patient and family are taught to apply heat and/or cold packs to the affected joints. A therapeutic exercise program is designed with the goal of maintaining the range of motion of the joints and muscle strength while minimizing deformities. The exercise program is paced with a program of rest to assure that the patient and the joints are not overexerted. The use of adaptive and assistive devices can enable the patient to remain functional in activities of daily living. Both the patient and family can be helped by the special programs offered by the Arthritis Foundation, whose national offices are located at 3400 Peachtree Road NE, Atlanta, Georgia 30326. Local chapters are located throughout the United States and Canada.

Monitoring and Prognosis

The natural course of rheumatoid arthritis is variable. Some patients experience spontaneous remission, others have a progressive steady deterioration leading to death. The most common course is one of remissions and exacerbations with a gradual decline in functional capability secondary to joint destruction.

The course of the disease and the efficacy of the drug therapy can be monitored by evaluating the erythrocyte sedimentation rate, duration of stiffness each morning, time of onset of fatigue after awakening, changes in grip strength, frequency of awakening at night with pain, and number of tender and painful joints. Evaluation for the adverse effects of medications must be thorough and systematic in order to distinguish these effects from the signs and symptoms of the disease process. In addition, many patients are on multiple-drug regimens, and drug interactions can occur.

CASE STUDY

S.C. is a 45-year-old mother of three who is employed as a secretary to a vice president of an oil company in a large metropolitan city. Over the past year she has noticed that it has become increasingly difficult to arise and get to her office on time. She has experienced pain in her hands, which she has attributed to fluctuating work loads involving increased typing. Ms. C's symptoms have been frequent and severe enough that she has visited her physician twice in the last 6 months. She was told that she was likely going through menopause and that she should not worry about these symptoms.

Assessment

After watching a television program on arthritis, Ms. C. visited the company nurse and explained her symptoms. The company nurse referred her to a rheumatologist for evaluation. Ms. C. had recalled that she had experienced a number of diffuse joint complaints since the age of 20. These complaints disappeared during each of her pregnancies and for a short period afterward. Upon close questioning she was able to report a slow onset of generalized fatigue which she had attributed to increasing age. There was no significant family history of arthritis or other systemic inflammatory disorders.

On physical examination Ms. C. had swollen and tender proximal interphalangeal and metacarpal-interphalangeal joints in both hands, tender metatarsal-interphalangeal joints in both feet, and slight tenderness in both knee joints. All other joint exams were essentially negative at this time.

Diagnostic studies showed a mild normochronic, normocytic anemia; erythrocyte sedimentation rate of 40 mm/h (normal, 0 to 20 mm/h); and positive rheumatoid factor and antinuclear antibodies (ANA). X-ray studies revealed only soft tissue swelling on the joints of the hands and feet and no abnormal changes in other joints. The rheumatologist tentatively diagnosed Ms. C. as having rheumatoid arthritis.

Management

The rheumatologist, clinical nurse specialist, and clinical pharmacist designed a program of treatment for Ms. C. that included an educational program for herself and her family; referral to a physical therapist for the program of therapeutic exercise and application of heat and cold; a medication regime of aspirin, 5.2 g/daily (four 325-mg tablets qid) with meals, and a well-balanced diet.

Ms. C. had discussed her illness with individuals at work. One of her coworkers had a sister who had a similar illness and reported that she had been "cured" by an arthritis clinic in Mexico. Ms. C. asked her rheumatologist and clinical specialist about this form of cure. They informed her that generally the treatment in these programs was corticosteroids. Ms. C. was told that at some point she might need both intraarticular and systemic corticosteroids but that these were not indicated at this time since the adverse effects were greater than the beneficial effects. Ms. C. was advised of the widespread marketing of unproven treatment methods for arthritis. Specifically, she was instructed that there are over 120 forms of arthritis and no one treatment can "cure" or treat all forms. She was encouraged to feel free to discuss with her health care providers all forms of treatment prior to beginning them. She was provided materials available from the Arthritis Foundation and was enrolled in a patient support group of other individuals who have rheumatoid arthritis.

Evaluation

Ms. C. was able to remain at work and convinced her employer to trade her typewriter for a word processor which required much less stress on her hand joints. She discovered that enteric coated aspirin provided less gastric irritation than regular aspirin. She found that she needed to alter her dose to between 4 and 6 g/day in order to manage her pain and decrease her morning stiffness.

At her return visit at 6 months she reported that she was beginning to come to grips with the fact that she had a lifelong illness for which there was no cure. She reported that she had moved through being angry over her diagnosis and in many ways was comforted to know that her illness was not "in her head." However, she had not experienced a period of remission in her illness and was currently being evaluated for penicillamine therapy, rather than parenteral gold, because she was afraid of injections. The initial dose was only 125 mg in order to minimize side effects. Ms. C. was informed of the very slow onset of beneficial effects produced by penicillamine and told to continue her enteric coated aspirin indefinitely for pain and stiffness. Over 4 months, her penicillamine dose was raised to 750 mg/day, one 250-mg capsule tid, and the swelling and tenderness in her hands and knees were almost fully cleared. During this period, a dry rash attributed to penicillamine appeared on her extremities, but because of disease control, the drug was continued. The rash cleared spontaneously over several weeks.

At her physician's visit 6 months after initiation of penicillamine, urinalysis revealed 2+ proteinuria, which was felt to be caused by penicillamine. The dose was reduced to 500 mg/day, and a follow-up urinalysis at 1 month showed trace protein.

Ms. C. is now receiving her aspirin and penicillamine with good disease control. Morning stiffness is reduced to 30 min, pain and swelling usually only occur with excess physical activity, and her productivity at work is improving.

Systemic Lupus Erythematosus

Systemic lupus erythematosus (SLE) is a chronic inflammatory and immunologic disorder of unknown etiology. The disorder is found primarily in females, in a ratio of seven to one over males; blacks have a higher incidence than other racial groups. The disorder may affect multiple organ systems and produce a remarkably diverse number of symptoms. The disorder may progress in a large number of ways, including acute, fulminating disease or slowly progressive disease with long periods of remission.

SLE belongs to a group of systemic autoimmune collagen diseases that includes progressive systemic sclerosis (scleroderma), rheumatoid arthritis, dermatomyositis, and polyarteritis nodosa. These disorders have a number of overlapping symptoms and laboratory findings, and similar drugs are used in their treatment.

Although the etiology of SLE is unknown, much is known about the mechanisms of tissue damage that occurs in this disorder. Circulating complexes of antinuclear antibodies and their antigens are thought to be responsible for the major pathologic changes seen in SLE. A fixation of complement at the site follows the deposition of the antigen-antibody complexes. This occurrence leads to activation of the complement system and the inflammatory process.

An unusual finding in SLE is that the individual may have an increase in symptoms following exposure to sunlight. Ultraviolet-irradiated deoxyribonucleic acid (DNA) is extremely antigenic. One explanation given for the relation of sunlight exposure to the development of symptoms is that the ultraviolet light waves induce antigenicity of the skin DNA.

Drug-Induced Systemic Lupus Erythematosus

Hydralazine (Apresoline) and **procainamide** (Pronestyl) are able to induce a syndrome that is very similar to SLE in certain individuals. This syndrome includes most of the symptoms of SLE, including positive tests for ANA, but renal and central nervous system involvement do not occur. The SLE symptoms begin to disappear within a few weeks of the discontinuation of these drugs. The positive ANA test reverts to negative after several months. A number of other drugs are capable of producing a positive ANA. These include **penicillamine, isoniazid, chlorpromazine,** and anticonvulsants such as **barbiturates, phenytoin, ethosuximide, methsuximide,** and **primidone.** Drugs which may cause an exacerbation of SLE in a patient who is in a remission of SLE include **sulfonamides, penicillins,** and **oral contraceptives.**

Clinical Findings

Over 90 percent of the individuals with SLE will have complaints of arthralgia and arthritis as early manifestations of this disorder. There can also be profound weakness and generalized muscle tenderness reflecting myositis. Some of the common manifestations also seen in SLE are fever, fatigue, malaise, anorexia, and weight loss. The characteristic cutaneous feature is a facial eruption described as a "butterfly" erythematous rash over the bridge of the nose.

Another form of rash which may occur with or without SLE is discoid lupus erythematosus. These lesions may be present anywhere on the body but mainly occur as a chronic keratotic scaling with atrophy, telangiectasia, and keratotic plugging on the face, arms, neck, and scalp. These lesions may eventually lead to permanent scarring. Individuals with discoid lupus may also have short broken hairs above the forehead known as "lupus hairs." Once this stage has occurred, a rapid loss of large amounts of scalp hair (alopecia) may occur.

Involvment of the mucous membranes may occur as oral, nasopharyngeal, or vaginal ulceration. These ulcerations, in combination with effects on the GI tract, can lead to the development of anorexia, nausea, vomiting, diarrhea, or abdominal pains. Raynaud's phenomenon may cause severe vasoconstriction and necrosis of the fingtertips. A nontender, diffuse, or local lymph node enlargement is frequently seen in SLE.

The most serious complications of the disorder involve the heart, kidney, and the central nervous system. Renal complications (lupus nephritis) have been detected in 50 percent of all individuals with SLE. These complications may advance to renal failure. SLE can lead to the development of organic neurologic problems, which may consist if convulsive disorders, abnormalities in the cranial nerves, changes in mental function, psychosis, depression, and chorea.

There may be a variety of changes in hematologic and immunologic laboratory tests. Some of these tests are nonspecific, and others are specifically seen in SLE. As with other autoimmune disorders, there is frequently an alteration in the complete blood count. A normocytic, normochronic anemia and leukopenia are frequently seen. Occasionally there is a mild thrombocytopenia. The erythrocyte sedimentation rate can be elevated, indicating an inflammatory process. Immunologic abnormalities that are the most useful in evaluating this disorder are ANA cells and occasionally lupus erythematosus (LE) cells.

Nursing assessment of the person with SLE is multifaceted and includes physical and psychosocial elements. A complete physical assessment provides a baseline by which to identify subtle changes in the multiple organ systems affected by the illness. The psychosocial impact of this disorder upon patients and their families is crucial. Since the drug regimen is often complex and changes frequently, the nurse assesses the treatment for sufficient dosage, frequency, adverse effects, and compliance. All medications taken by the patient, not just those used to treat the illness, are assessed for possible contraindications in this complex disease. Since SLE can affect the kidney with devastating results, frequent urinalysis is conducted to detect the presence of hematuria and proteinuria.

Clinical Pharmacology and Therapeutics

SLE is treated with NSAIDs, DMARDs (usually antimalarials or immunosuppressive agents), and corticosteroids. The specific complications will influence treatment. NSAIDs are used to control the articular inflammation in a fashion similar to their action in rheumatoid arthritis. **Aspirin** is falling into disuse as a NSAID alternative because it produces the highest incidence of hepatotoxicity, and some SLE patients have hepatic involvement. In addition, SLE patients are at higher risk of the cutaneous, hepatic, and renal adverse effects of NSAIDs. If the NSAIDs are inadequate to control the symptoms of disease, antimalarials may be effective and usually are the next drugs of choice. Initial antimalarial doses are high to achieve a remission. Clearance of skin lesions offers a monitoring parameter to use in dosage adjustment.

Acute exacerbations of SLE of rheumatologic and especially nonrheumatologic involvement, e.g., interstitial nephritis, are treated with high-dose oral corticosteroids (e.g., 0.5 to 1.5 mg/kg/day of **prednisone**) for short periods, depending on disease response (a few days to 3 months). This dosage is reduced to maintenance dosage levels (7.5 to 10 mg/day) gradually over several weeks. In patients with severe disease and inadequate response to corticosteroids, immunosuppressive drugs are employed at doses noted previously. A major component of the nursing management of the patient with SLE is an educational program for the patient and the family focusing upon the complex and multifaceted treatment regime. Avoidance of exposure to the sun is very important; patients are advised to use umbrellas, hats, and long-sleeved shirts. Compliance with these measures may be problematic in teenagers with SLE. The patient should use a sunscreen with a sun protection factor (SPF) of 15 (see Chap. 38) and reapply the sunscreen after swimming or heavy exercise. The patient should receive a list of drugs that should be avoided because of their potential for exacerbating SLE. Special programs and information are available to patients and their families from the Lupus Foundation. Local chapters are located in most states.

Monitoring and Prognosis

The prognosis in SLE is variable, depending upon the severity of the symptoms, the organs involved in the disorder, and the length of time remissions may be maintained. Since there is no specific cure for SLE, prognosis is based upon how well the symptoms are managed. Evaluation of the effectiveness of therapy will depend upon the organ systems involved. Adverse effects of drugs must be distinguished from exacerbations or extensions of the disease into other organ systems. Changes in mental status should be evaluated to determine whether they are caused by increased central nervous system involvement due to the illness or are side effects of the corticosteroid drug therapy or depressive reactions to the illness and the requisite psychosocial adaptation. Urinalysis for proteinuria and hematuria is used to monitor for increased renal involvement, which may require alterations in drug regimens. The effectiveness of measures to protect the skin from the sun should also be evaluated.

Gout

Gout is a term used for a group of approximately nine metabolic disorders that are characterized by an elevated serum uric acid concentration (hyperuricemia). Ninety-five percent of the individuals who develop gout are men, and the peak incidence is in the fifth decade of life. The problem develops when crystals of monosodium urate monohydrate form in the joints and surrounding tissues. These needlelike crystals are responsible for the acute inflammatory reaction that produces the severe pain commonly associated with a gouty attack. These crystal deposits can cause extensive joint and soft tissue damage if left untreated. Figure 26-5 shows the physiologic changes associated with uric acid.

There are four stages in the clinical progression of gout. The first stage is asymptomatic hyperuricemia during which the individual has no symptoms other than an elevated serum uric acid. Only 5 percent of these individuals go on to develop an acute gouty attack. The second stage is acute gouty arthritis in which there is a sudden onset of exquisitely painful swelling and tenderness, usually of the great toe metatarsophalangeal joint. The third stage, the intercritical period, follows the acute gouty attack. During this period the individual is asymptomatic and may remain so for months to up to 10 years. Most individuals, however, have a repeat gouty attack in less than 1 year if they are untreated.

The fourth stage is the chronic gouty arthritis stage in which the urate pool continues to expand, resulting in the development of tophi.

Drug-Induced Gout

A number of drugs can elevate the serum uric acid level by blocking tubular secretion of uric acid by the kidneys. This action can cause an acute gouty attack in the individual with gout. The drugs include the **thiazide** and **loop diuretics, levodopa, ethambutol, aspirin** in low doses (1 to 2 g/day; see above), **diazoxide, acetazolamide,** and **alcohol.**

Clinical Findings

The individual with gout will generally seek medical attention during an acute attack. There is usually only one distal, lower-extremity joint involved. The joint will be warm, red, and so tender that palpation will not be possible.

The basic laboratory test utilized to diagnosis gout is a serum uric acid level. Serum levels reflect both the rate of metabolism and renal excretion of uric acid. Normal serum levels are less than 7 mg/dL for males and less than 6 mg/dL for females.

Nursing assessment during an acute gouty attack includes obtaining a history of precipitating factors such as changes in medication, alcohol intake, or diet. A medication history including all current drugs as well as drug sensitivities is an important baseline. The patient's joints are assessed, noting the location, color, and tenderness of those joints involved with the acute attack. In chronic gout, the nurse assesses the current medication regime for dosage, frequency, drug interactions, and adverse effects.

Clinical Pharmacology and Therapeutics

The treatment of an acute gouty attack is different from the treatment of chronic gout. During an acute attack, **NSAIDs** or **colchicine** may be given in high doses or in loading doses to reduce the acute inflammation of the joint. The nurse carefully observes for adverse effects of these drugs during this time. The involved joint(s) should be protected from injury and elevated to reduce swelling. The nurse also evaluates any decreases in pain, swelling, or tenderness in the affected joint.

Chronic gout is treated with **allopurinol** or uricosuric agents to lower systemic uric acid levels. If the patient is taking a uricosuric agent, the nurse evaluates for decreased creatinine clearance by the kidneys which would result in diminished drug effect. Fluid intake for patients taking an uricosuric agent should be at least 1500 mL/day to promote the excretion of uric acid. An educational program describing the cause of the disorder, the medication regimen used in its treatment, the potential drug interactions between prescribed and over-the-counter drugs, and the role of alcohol and diet in precipating acute attacks is developed.

Monitoring and Prognosis

The prognosis for gout can be very favorable. Drug therapy is usually successful in lowering the serum urate level. The individual can remain essentially free of acute gouty attacks with maintenance therapy. Some of the damage done to the joint during the acute gouty attack can be reversed; however, if joint destruction is extensive, degenerative joint disease can occur.

REFERENCES

Adams, S. S., and J. W. Buckler: "Ibuprofen and Flurbiprofen," *Clin Rheum Dis,* 5:359–380, 1979.

Brown-Skeers, V.: "How the Nurse Practitioner Manages the Rheumatoid Arthritis Patient," *Nursing 79,* 9:26–35, 1979.

——: "Rheumatoid Arthritis," *Crit Care Update,* 10:21–25, 1983.

Buckananan, W. W., P. J. Rooney, and J. A. N. Rennie: "Aspirin and the Salicylates," *Clin Rheu Dis,* 5:499–540, 1979.

Buckingham, R. B.: "Bursitis and Tendonitis," *Compr Ther,* 7:52–57, 1981.

Bunch, T. W., and J. D. O'Duffy: "Clinical Pharmacology. 6. Disease-Modifying Drugs for Progressive Rheumatoid Arthritis," *Mayo Clin Proc,* 55:161–179, 1980.

Dahl, S. L., and J. R. Ward: "Pharmacology, Clinical Efficacy, and Adverse Effects of Piroxicam, A New Nonster-oidal Anti-Inflammatory Agent," *Pharmacotherapy,* 2:80–90, 1982.

Davis, J. D., H. B. Muss, and R. A. Turner: "Cytotoxic Agents in the Treatment of Rheumatoid Arthritis," *South Med J,* 71:58–64, 1978.

Dickerson, G., and T. Gorman: "Adult Arthritis: The Assessment," *Am J Nurs,* 83:262–265, 1983.

Ehrlich, G. E.: "Tolmetin Sodium: Meeting the Clinical Challenge," *Clin Rheum Dis,* 5:481–498, 1979.

Gall, E. P.: "Hyperuricemia and Gout," *Postgrad Med,* 65:163–168, 1979.

Garcia, C.: "Gold Therapy in Arthritis Treatment," *Nurse Pract,* 6:35–38, 1981.

Gray, R. G., J. Tenenbaum, and N. L. Gottlieb: "Local Corticosteroid Injection Treatment in Rheumatic Disorders," *Seminars Arthritis Rheum,* 10:231–254, 1981.

Harmon, C. E., and J. P. Portanova: "Drug-Induced Lupus:

Clinical and Serological Studies," *Clin Rheu Dis,* 8:121–135, 1982.

Hughes, G. R. V.: "The Treatment of SLE: The Case for Conservative Management," *Clin Rheum Dis,* 8:299–313, 1982.

Huskisson, E. C.: "Classification of Anti-rheumatic Drugs," *Clin Rheum Dis,* 5:353–358, 1979.

——: "Routine Drug Treatment of Rheumatoid Arthritis and Other Rheumatic Diseases," *Clin Rheum Dis,* 5:697–706, 1979.

Katz, W. A.: *Rheumatic Diseases,* Philadelphia: Lippincott, 1977.

Koerner, M. and G. Dickerson: "Adult Arthritis: A Look at Some of Its Forms," *Am J Nurs,* 83:255–262, 1983.

Lyle, W. H.: "Penicillamine," *Clin Rheum Dis,* 5:569–602, 1979.

Mangani, R. J.: "Drug Therapy Reviews: Pathogenesis and Clinical Management of Hyperuricemia and Gout," *Am J Hosp Pharm,* 36:497–504, 1979.

Mooney, N.: "Coping with Chronic Pain in Rheumatoid Arthritis: Patient Behaviors and Nursing Interventions," *Rehabil Nurs,* 8:20–21, 24–25, 1983.

Morishima, M.: "Diagnosis of Arthritis," *Nurse Pract,* 5:49, 1980.

Moskowitz, R. W.: "Management of Osteoarthritis," *Hosp Pract,* 14:75–87, 1979.

Porter, S., M. Johnson, and C. Foran: "Adult Arthritis: Hand Splints," *Am J Nurs,* 83:276–278, 1983.

Rhymer, A. R.: "Sulindac," *Clin Rheum Dis,* 5:553–568, 1979.

——, and D. C. Gengos: "Indomethacin," *Clin Rheum Dis,* 5:541–552, 1979.

Ridolfo, A. S., R. Nickander, and W. M. Mikulashek: "Fenoprofen and Benoxaprofen," *Clin Rheum Dis,* 5:393–410. 1979.

Rodnan, G. P., and H. R. Schumacher (eds.): *Primer on the Rheumatic Diseases,* 8th ed., Atlanta: Arthritis Foundation, 1983.

Rothermich, N. O.: "Chrysotherapy in Rheumatoid Arthritis," *Clinics Rheum Dis,* 5:631–640, 1979.

Sack, K. E.: "Arthritis: Specifics on Long-Term Management," *Geriatrics,* 35:32–37, pt. 1, 1980.

Simkin, P. A.: "Tendonitis and Bursitis of the Shoulder," *Postgrad Med,* 73:177–190, 1983.

Simpson, C.: "Adult Arthritis: Heat, Cold, or Both?" *Amer J Nurs,* 83:270–273, 1983.

——, and G. Dickinson: "Adult Arthritis: Exercise," *Amer J Nurs,* 83:273–275, 1983.

Singleton, Jr., P. T.: "Salsalate: 'Its Role in the Management of Rheumatic Disease'" *Clin Ther,* 3:80–102, 1980.

Sisco, D.: "Systemic Lupus Erythematosus and Resultant Renal Failure," *Nephrol Nurse,* 4:48–49, 1979.

Spiegel, T. M., and J. Weiss: "Anti-inflammatory Agents in Arthritis," *Comp Ther,* 7:18–23, 1981.

Spruck, M.: "Gold Therapy for Rheumatoid Arthritis," *Am J Nurs,* 79:1246–1248, 1979.

Strand, C., and S. Clark, "Adult Arthritis: Drugs and Remedies," *Am J Nurs,* 83:266–270, 1983.

Strodthoff, C.: "Pathophysiology of Rheumatoid Arthritis," *Nurse Pract,* 7:32–35, 1982.

Swezey, R. L.: *Arthritis: Rational Therapy and Rehabilitation,* Philadelphia: Saunders, 1978.

Talbot, J. H.: "Drug Treatment of Gout," *Clin Rheum Dis,* 5:657–672, 1979.

Todd, B.: "For Arthritis—Plain Aspirin or an Aspirin Alternative?" *Geratr Nurs,* 3:191–192, 1982.

Torbett, M. P., and J. Ervin: "The Patient with Systemic Lupus Erythematosus," *Am J Nurs,* 77:1299–1302, 1977.

Waterson, M.: "Exercises to Help Manage Your Rheumatoid Arthritis," *Nursing 79,* 9:32–33, 1979.

Wright, V.: "Rheumatoid Arthritis: 5. Surgical Treatment," *Nurs Times,* 73:1955–1958, 1977.

27

RESPIRATORY DISORDERS

MATTHEW B. WIENER
ROSEMARY A. SIMKINS

LEARNING OBJECTIVES

Upon mastery of the contents of this chapter, the reader will be able to:

1. Describe the role of cyclic nucleotides, prostaglandins, beta-receptors, mast cells, and mucus production in the etiology of respiratory diseases.

2. Compare the chronic obstructive lung diseases, asthma, chronic bronchitis, and emphysema, as to clinical manifestation, assessment, and management.

3. List five factors that can induce bronchoconstriction.

4. Explain the rationale for using bronchodilators in the treatment of cystic fibrosis and bronchiectasis.

5. Describe the therapy of hypersensitivity pneumonitis.

6. Discuss the therapeutic interventions for the treatment of acute mountain sickness (AMS).

7. Give three therapeutic goals in the therapy of respiratory diseases.

8. Differentiate which of the following drugs can cause bronchodilation: theophylline, metaproterenol, atropine sulfate, prednisone, cromolyn sodium, and beclomethasone.

9. Differentiate which of the following drugs can produce changes in pulmonary function tests: theophylline, terbutaline, cromolyn sodium, and prednisone.

10. List three classes of drugs that can be used to treat exercise-induced bronchoconstriction (EIB). Describe how and when they should be administered.

11. Describe the mechanism of action, pharmacokinetics, adverse effects, and dosing for bronchodilating drugs: xanthine preparations, sympathomimetic agents, and parasympathetic blocking drugs.

12. Explain the value of monitoring theophylline levels and give four factors that can increase or decrease these levels.

13. Discuss the advantages of using sustained-release theophylline preparations in the therapy of chronic lung diseases.

14. List three routes of administration of the sympathomimetic agents and the advantage of each route.

15. Explain the technique involved in using a respiratory treatment employing a metered dose inhaler (MDI), a nebulizer with either a hand-bulb nebulizer or a compressor, and the MDI with a tube spacer (Aerochamber).

16. Describe three conditions in which cromolyn sodium will be beneficial.

17. Give an indication for the use of cromolyn sodium in the nose and eye.

18. Describe the onset of action and three pharmacologic effects of corticosteroids in the treatment of lung diseases.

19. Compare the dosing of corticosteroids in the treatment of acute and chronic respiratory disorders.

20. Describe the administration of oxygen and two possible adverse effects with its therapy.

21. List four antimicrobial agents that can be used in the treatment of upper respiratory infections based on clinical impression.

22. Explain the role of troleandomycin when used with methylprednisolone in the therapy of asthma.

23. List three drugs that can be used as mucokinetic agents.

24. Describe three therapeutic interventions for excessive mucus production.

25. Describe the role of the nurse, including assessment, management, and evaluation, in caring for patients' respiratory disorders.

26. Write the pharmacologic aspects of a nursing care plan for the patient with a respiratory disorder.

This chapter will discuss respiratory disorders, with the main focus on the clinical pharmacology and therapeutics of the chronic obstructive lung diseases. The therapy of chronic obstructive lung diseases and most other respiratory diseases uses similar agents (bronchodilators, corticosteroids, oxygen, and others). The main differences when treating these diseases are their responses to therapy. Asthma is considered more reversible and therefore more responsive to therapy, whereas chronic bronchitis and emphysema are considered more irreversible and less responsive to pharmacologic therapy. Restrictive lung diseases are also less responsive to drug therapy.

Our understanding of the pathophysiology of the numerous respiratory disorders is limited, and therefore specific therapeutic intervention has not been developed. In most cases the therapy of respiratory diseases is based on preventing the problem (avoiding antigens, employing immunotherapy, stopping smoking) or reversing the symptoms of the disorders. Once the cellular alterations are better understood, therapeutic intervention can become more specific and possibly more effective.

ANATOMY AND PHYSIOLOGY OF THE RESPIRATORY TRACT

The main function of the respiratory tract is to provide gas exchange between the atmosphere and the blood. Oxygen is carried to the alveoli during inspiration, and the carbon dioxide is removed from the lungs by expiration. Ventilation is performed by the respiratory and cardiac muscles. The respiratory tract is divided into upper and lower respiratory airways. The upper airway conducts, cleans, warms, and humidifies air, so it is suited for gas exchange in the distal air spaces. The structures of the upper airways are the nose, mouth, nasopharynges and oropharynges, and larynx. The structures of the lower respiratory tract include the trachea, bronchi, bronchioles, alveolar ducts, and alveolar sac. The most important structures in the respiratory system in terms of drug therapy are the smooth muscles, the ciliated epithelium lining the airways, the bronchial glands, and the mast cells.

Physiology of the Lung

Cyclic Nucleotides

The cyclic nucleotides [cyclic adenosine monophosphate (AMP) and cyclic guanosine monophosphate (GMP)] are involved in the autonomic control of bronchial smooth muscle and the release of mediators from the mast cells. By increasing cyclic AMP or by decreasing cyclic GMP bronchial smooth muscle will be relaxed and mediator release from the mast cells prevented. The cyclic nucleotides are also thought to interact with calcium to produce their effects on smooth muscle and mast cells (see Fig. 27-1).

Bronchial Smooth Muscle

Smooth muscle is present from the trachea to the alveolar ducts and is under the control of the autonomic nervous system. The innervation of the respiratory tract by the parasympathetic (vagal) nervous system has been established, but direct innervation by the sympathetic nervous system is lacking. However, there are β receptors (mostly β_2) in the bronchial smooth muscle, which upon stimulation cause bronchial smooth muscle relaxation. One theory (Szentivanyi, 1968) for the pathophysiology of asthma postulates a lack or a partial blockade of the β receptors.

The Mast Cell

The mast cells are distributed throughout the respiratory tract from the nasopharynx to the bronchial lumen. The sensitized mast cell can release a series of mediators in response to antigens. The principal mediators which cause respiratory problems are histamine, SRS-A (leukotrienes C_4 and D_4) ECF-A, prostaglandin D_2, platelet-activating factor (PAF), and others. The *degranulation* (release of mediators) of mast cells is a major factor in allergic asthma, and a great deal of pharmacologic research is directed at altering the mast cell response.

Prostaglandins

The prostaglandin E series has been shown to have a bronchodilating effect, and the prostaglandin F series is a potent bronchoconstricting compound. There is also a theory that relates the development of asthma to an imbalance in the two different prostaglandin series. Currently, prostaglandin E is not used therapeutically because upon inhalation it has a marked irritating effect on the pharynx and trachea and its duration of action is short.

Sputum

Sputum or phlegm is an abnormal, viscous, excretory product of the diseased respiratory tract. The healthy respiratory tract is bathed with secretions that are carried upward toward the pharynx and then removed without the person's awareness. Mucus is produced in the lungs by submucosal glands (goblet cells) in the bronchi. Sputum production is associated with various respiratory disorders and is treated with nondrug therapy (postural drainage, hydration) and drug therapy (acetylcysteine, alcohol).

RESPIRATORY DISEASES

Diseases of the Upper Airways

Disorders of the upper respiratory tract affect the nose, nasopharynx, paranasal sinuses, and the larynx. These disorders are extremely common and are more of an annoyance than a life-threatening problem. Examples of upper respiratory

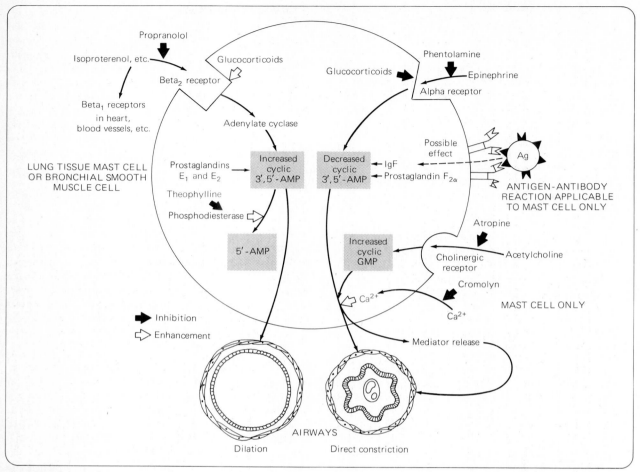

FIGURE 27-1

Representation of the Pharmacologic Action of Drugs Used in the Treatment of Respiratory Disease. Bronchodilation can occur from stimulation of the β_2 receptors, inhibition of phosphodiesterase, blockade of the cholinergic receptors. Cromolyn sodium prevents the influx of calcium and stabilizes mast cells and prevents mediator release. Corticosteroids may increase the numbers of β_2 receptors. *(Modified from R. G. Townley: Pharmacologic Blocks to Mediator Release: Clinical Applications, Adv Asthma Allergy, 2:7, 1975).*

tract diseases include sinusitis (both acute and chronic), allergic rhinitis and vasomotor rhinitis, and acute pharyngitis (see Chapters 21 and 28 for therapy). Upper respiratory tract problems (acute sinusitis) may cause exacerbation of lower airway diseases (asthma). In those cases the upper airways diseases should be aggressively treated. Vocal cord problems may present symptoms similar to those of asthma but will usually be unresponsive to pharmacologic therapy. Paradoxical vocal cord function can be successfully treated with speech therapy.

Diseases of the Bronchi and Bronchioles

It is estimated that more than 16 million people in North America suffer from some form of chronic airflow limitation. Asthma, chronic bronchitis, emphysema, bronchiec-

tasis, and cystic fibrosis all have as a common feature the resistance to airflow.

Asthma

It is estimated that asthma (literally meaning "difficult breathing") affects over 7 million people in the United States. It is the most frequent cause of school absences in children exceeding all other chronic disorders. Asthma is characterized by increased responsiveness of the airways (airway hyperreactivity) to various stimuli (see Table 27-1). The airway narrowing is reversible with bronchodilating drugs, or it may reverse spontaneously. Asthma is characterized by recurrent, paroxysmal attacks of cough; chest tightness; and difficulty in breathing. This is often accompanied by wheezing. Excessive sputum production is often present and the sputum is difficult to expectorate.

TABLE 27-1   Some Factors That Can Stimulate Bronchoconstriction

Allergens
  House dust, inhaled pollen, mold spores, dust mites, pet dander
Specific irritants
  Odors and chemical fumes, air pollution, cold air, tobacco smoke, perfumes, gastric reflux
Nonspecific irritants
  Infections (viral or bacterial); exercise; emotions (stress, anxiety, fatigue)
Foods
  Nuts, seafood, milk, eggs
Drugs
  Aspirin, NSAIDs, tartrazine, propranolol, methacholine, indomethacin, narcotics
Occupational exposure
  Toluene diiocynate, wood dust, textile dust (byssinosis)
Coexistent conditions
  Upper respiratory diseases, hyperthyroidism vagal reflexes

Status asthmaticus represents a life-threatening medical emergency. Status asthmaticus is severe asthma that is not responsive to bronchodilating drugs. Therapy of status asthmaticus includes oxygen, fluid, aminophylline (IV), β-adrenergic agonist (depending on the number of previous treatments), corticosteroids (IV), and possibly mechanical ventilation.

Chronic Bronchitis

It is estimated that over 7 million individuals have chronic bronchitis. Chronic bronchitis is characterized by chronic cough with excessive sputum production that is not due to a known cause such as tuberculosis or bronchiectasis. The cough and mucus production are present on most days for at least 3 months of the year for two successive years. Chronic bronchitis rarely occurs in the pure form. Most commonly it occurs along with emphysema or, in some cases, asthma. In chronic bronchitis there is an increase in size and function of the mucus-secreting cells along with a decreased ability to remove the mucus. Factors suspected to cause these changes include cigarette smoking (the single most important factor), occupational exposure, infections, air pollution, and postnasal drainage.

Emphysema

Emphysema (literally meaning "overinflation") is characterized by an increase beyond the normal size of air spaces distal to the terminal nonrespiratory bronchioles accompanied by destructive changes in the alveolar walls. Advances in understanding the pathogenesis of emphysema have been made. Emphysema has been associated with the severe deficiency of α-1-antitrypsin. This has lead to the concept that emphysema is due to an imbalance of protease (elastase), which is capable of destroying alveolar tissue, and the antiprotease effects of α-1-antitrypsin (Fig. 27-2). Research efforts are directed at developing compounds which have antiprotease activity. Emphysema is thought to develop when the airways are continuously inflamed, leading to the

development of a complete or partial obstruction. The most frequent cause of the inflammation is cigarette smoking. The inflammation also leads to the release of protease from the neutrophils and this results in more lung tissue damage. It is also thought that cigarette smoking may also alter the function of antiproteases.

Bronchiectasis

Bronchiectasis is a disease characterized by a permanent abnormal dilation of the bronchioles, bronchi, or both. The majority of the cases of bronchiectasis develop after atelectasis. When there is a narrowing of the bronchial lumen, bronchiectasis can occur distal to the narrowing. Since bacterial infections are frequently associated with bronchiectasis, antibiotics are used in prevention and in treatment.

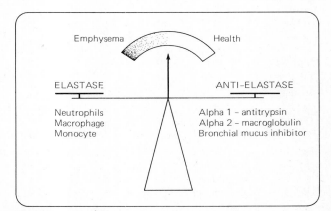

FIGURE 27-2

The health of the lung tissue is dependent on the balance between proteases (elastase) and antiproteases (antielastase). Emphysema may develop because of an increase in activity of elastase or a decrease in antielastase activity. *(Reprinted with permission from R. M. Cherniack and Cherniack: Respiration in Health and Disease, 3d ed., Philadelphia: Saunders, 1983.)*

Additional therapies include postural drainage, bronchodilators for those patients who are responsive, and bronchial lavage when other therapies have failed.

Cystic Fibrosis

Cystic fibrosis is an inherited disease that involves the exocrine glands and possibly other organs. The majority of the morbidity and mortality involves the respiratory tract. Problems associated with cystic fibrosis occur because of obstruction caused by excessive secretions in the respiratory tract, sweat glands, small intestines, pancreas, and the bile ducts. These hypersecretions and decreased clearance of the respiratory secretions lead to airway obstruction. The stagnant mucus also becomes an excellent medium for microorganisms. The management of the pulmonary problems associated with cystic fibrosis include antimicrobial agents, postural drainage, and bronchodilators if there is evidence of a response.

Diseases of the Parenchyma

The normal healthy lung avoids damage even though it is continuously exposed to the environment and foreign substances. If the normal protective mechanisms (cough reflex, mucociliary, and immunologic systems) of the lungs are altered, infection can develop in the lung parenchyma. The aspiration of irritating substances such as mineral oil can lead to the inflammation of the lung parenchyma, causing a lipid pneumonia. The inhalation of various toxic substances (cadmium, beryllium, mercury) may produce inflammation which will allow the spread of microorganisms and/or the development of interstitial fibrosis.

Extrinsic allergic alveolitis (hypersensitivity pneumonitis) is an allergic inflammation of the lung parenchyma in a sensitized susceptible individual following the inhalation of an antigen (Table 27-2). Treatment is usually avoidance of the antigen, and in some cases corticosteroids can be used. Drugs that can produce pulmonary disease are listed in Table 27-3.

Pulmonary Vascular Diseases

Primary (Idiopathic) Pulmonary Hypertension

The blood pressure in the pulmonary artery of a healthy adult is approximately 23 over 8 mmHg (systolic over diastolic) with a mean pressure of 14 mmHg. Pulmonary hypertension occurs when the systolic pressure is greater than 30 mmHg and the diastolic pressure is greater than 15 mmHg. Chronic elevation of the pulmonary blood pressure will ultimately lead to right-side heart failure. The therapy of pulmonary hypertension may include digoxin, pulmonary vasodilators, (see Table 27-4), anticoagulants, and/or oxygen.

TABLE 27-2 Selected Examples of Hypersensitivity Pneumonitis

DISEASE	ANTIGEN	SOURCE OF ANTIGEN
Farmer's lung	Thermophilic actinomycetes, *Aspergillus* sp.	Contaminated hay, grain, silage
Bird fancier's, breeder's or handler's lung	Parakeet, pigeon, dove, chicken, turkey proteins	Avian droppings
Humidifier or air-conditioner lung	Thermophilic actinomycetes, *Aureobasidium pullulans*, ameba, other	Contaminated water in humidification aerosols, vaporizers, sprays
Woodworker's lung	Wood dust; Alternaria	Oak, cedar, mahogany dusts; pine and spruce pulp
Sauna taker's lung	*A. pullulans*, other	Contaminated sauna steam
Bagassosis	Thermophilic actinomycetes	Contaminated bagasse (sugar cane)
Malt worker's lung	*Aspergillus fumigatus, A. clavatus*	Moldy barley
Mushroom worker's lung	Thermophilic actinomycetes, other	Mushroom compost
Sequoiosis	Pullularia, *Graphium* sp.	Redwood sawdust
Maple bark stripper's disease	*Cryptostroma corticale*	Maple bark
Coffee worker's lung	Coffee bean dust	Coffee beans
Miller's lung	*Sitophilus granarius* (wheat weevil)	Infested wheat flour
Bathtub refinisher's lung	Toluene diisocyanate (TDI)	Porcelain surfacing catalyst
Chemical worker's lung	Toluene diisocyanate (TDI), methylene diisocyanate (MDI), phthallic anhydride, vinyl chloride, other	Polyurethane foam and insulation, synthetic rubber manufacturing, meat wrapping and labeling, other

Source: H. B. Richardson: ''Extrinsic Allergic Alveolitis,'' in R. C. Cherniack (ed.), *Current Therapy of Respiratory Disease, 1984–1985*, Philadelphia: B. C. Decker; St. Louis: C. V. Mosby, 1984.

TABLE 27-3 Drug-Induced Pulmonary Disorders

DRUG	PULMONARY EFFECTS AND THERAPY*
Chemotherapeutic Bisulfan (Myleran) Cyclophosphamide (Cytoxan) Bleomycin Nitosoureas (BCNU, CCNU, etc.) Chlorambucil (Leukran) Mitromycin Melphalan (Alkeran) Methotrexate Procarbazine Hydroxyurea Cytosine arabinoside (Ara-C) Azathioprine (Imuran)	Usually presents as diffuse pulmonary infiltrates, fever, and occasionally as hypoxemia. Treatment is to stop the drug prior to fibrosis. In some cases, prednisone is indicated.
Anti-infectives Nitrofurantoin	Acute bronchospasm, acute alveolar damage, and chronic diffuse interstitial pneumonitis fibrosis.
Azulfidine	Pneumonitis, in some cases progressing to irreversible fibrosis
Sulfonamides, INH, PCN, TCN	Pulmonary infiltrates with eosinophilia syndrome
Aminoglycosides	Neuromuscular blockade
Anti-inflammatory Drugs Corticosteroids	Mediastinal lipomatosis; no treatment is necessary.
Salicylates	Bronchospasm, pulmonary infiltrate with eosinophilia, noncardiac pulmonary edema, or respiratory alkalosis through hyperventilation
Gold	Interstitial fibrosis
Penicillamine	Bronchiolitis obliterans
Analgesics Methadone, propoxyphene, and heroin	Noncardiac pulmonary edema
Inhaled Agents General	Any inhaled agent can produce irritating bronchitis. Treatment is to avoid the drug; pretreatment with beta agonists.
Oxygen	High doses for a few days can produce adult respiratory distress syndrome.
Miscellaneous INH, hydralazine, phenytoin procanamide, penicillamine, and others	SLE with pleuropulmonary reactions
Methylsergide (Sansert)	Pleural thickening
Oral contraceptives	Pulmonary embolism
Hydrochlorthiazide	Noncardiac pulmonary edema
Amiodarone	Acute interstitial pneumonitis

*The drug should be discontinued or avoided whenever possible.

Source: Modified from R. C. Rosenow: "Drug-Induced Lung Disease," in R. M. Cherniack (ed.), *Current Therapy of Respiratory Disease 1984–1985,* Philadelphia: B. C. Decker; St Louis: C. V. Mosby, 1984.

TABLE 27-4 Pulmonary Vasodilators Used in Pulmonary Hypertension

DRUG	ACUTE DOSE	CHRONIC DOSE
Hydralazine	10–20 mg IV	50–150 mg PO q6h
Diazoxide	45–600 mg into PA	—
Nitoprusside	6 µg/kg/min IV	—
Nifedipine	10–40 mg PO	20 mg PO q26h
Verapamil	5–10 mg IV	80–120 mg PO q8h
Diltiazem	—	30 mg PO q8h
Phentolamine	1–10 mg IV	—
Prazocin	2–5 mg PO	5 mg PO q8h
Isoproterenol	3 µg/min into PA	—
	0.5–5 µg/min IV	
Captopril	—	25–150 mg PO q8h

PA = Pulmonary artery.
Source: Modified from D. S. Lukas: "Primary Pulmonary Hypertension," in R. M. Cherniack (ed.), *Current Therapy of Respiratory Disease 1984–1985,* Philadelphia: B. C. Decker; St. Louis: C. V. Mosby, 1984.

Pulmonary Thromboembolitic Disorders

Pulmonary embolism and infarction are leading causes of illness and death in many clinical centers. In many cases this condition is only established at post mortem examination. For a complete discussion of the therapy of thromboembolic disorders see Chap. 42.

Acute Mountain Sickness (AMS)

When unacclimatized people ascend high enough and fast enough almost all will experience the syndrome of AMS. The AMS is due in part to hypobaric hypoxia. This syndrome may occur in individuals ascending to a moderate altitude (8000 to 14,000 ft), as well as those ascending to high altitude (14,000 to 18,000 ft). Patients may present the following signs and symptoms: headaches, insomnia, anorexia, nausea, dizziness, vomiting, oliguria, cough, ataxia, cyanosis, and dyspnea. The therapy of AMS is to descend to a lower altitude. Other therapeutic measures that have been used include oxygen, **acetazolamide** (see Chaps. 22 and 23), and **dexamethasone**. The easiest form of therapy is prevention by allowing for acclimatization prior to ascending to higher elevations.

Respiratory Failure

Respiratory failure occurs when the gas exchange is impaired or inadequate so that hypoxia and/or hypercapnia develop. Respiratory failure can occur with adult respiratory distress syndrome, interstitial lung diseases, chronic obstructive lung diseases, and acute respiratory disorders. The management of acute respiratory failure includes oxygen therapy, reduction in the work of breathing, and the reduction of airway obstruction. Acute exacerbations of respiratory failure are often caused by infections. These should be treated with the appropriate antibiotics. Mechanical ventilation of the patient may be necessary.

CLINICAL FINDINGS

The primary symptoms of pulmonary disease are excessive nasal secretions, cough, expectoration of sputum, expectoration of blood, shortness of breath, wheezing, cyanosis, and chest pain. Signs associated with respiratory disease are alterations in lung sounds, lung size, chest distensibility, clubbing of fingers and toes, and poor growth in children.

The patient's history should include personal habits (alcohol consumption, smoking history); hobbies and pets; age of residence; flora; and occupation. Family history should assess α-1-antitrypsin deficiency, cystic fibrosis, allergies, and tuberculosis. Medical history should include the occurrence of wheezing and shortness of breath associated with beta blocking agents, aspirin, tartrazine, foods, drink, and so on. After completing the physical examination and taking the history, a chest x-ray may give additional information on pulmonary lesions. However, in many conditions the chest x-ray is not helpful.

Laboratory assessment of respiratory diseases includes bacteriologic, cytologic, and chemical examination of abnormal secretions; sweat test; histologic examination of tissues; skin testing; bronchoprovocation testing; pulmonary function testing; and immunologic work-ups. Bronchoprovocation testing can assess airway reactivity with the inhalation of histamine or methacholine. Exercise testing can also be used as a bronchoprovocation test. If occupational asthma is suspected, inhalation of the antigen (toluene diiocyanate, wood dust, flour) can be diagnostic.

Pulmonary function testing can assess respiratory function as well as monitor the patient's response to therapy. Measurements of ventilation are useful in differentiating restrictive diseases (usually normal flow rates but decreased volumes) from obstructive diseases (decreased flow rates with usually increased lung volume). Spirometry is a simple test that will give information on the flow-resistive properties of the lungs. Spirometry will give the forced expiratory volume in 1 s (FEV_1) and forced expiratory capacity (FVC) and components of vital capacity. The peak flow meter is a useful tool that the patient can use to evaluate the disease. The peak flow meter is hand-held and measures flow rates in liters per minute. The body plethysmograph (body box) is a more complicated piece of equipment that will give information on thoracic gas volumes, airway resistance, and specific conductance. A disadvantage of spirometry and the peak flow meter is that both tests require the patient to give a good effort. The body plethysmograph depends less on the efforts of the patient (see Fig. 27-3).

CLINICAL PHARMACOLOGY AND THERAPEUTICS

The principal drugs used in the treatment of chronic obstructive lung diseases include bronchodilators (xanthine

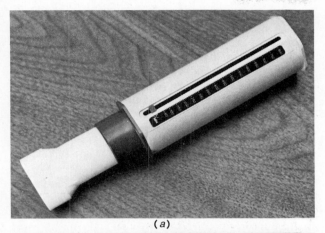

(a)

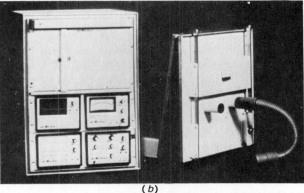

(b)

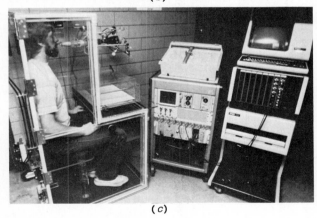

(c)

FIGURE 27-3

Pulmonary Function Testing. (*a*) An example of a peak flow meter; (*b*) spirometry; (*c*) body plethysmograph (body box).

symptoms for many respiratory diseases are very similar, therapy will be similar.

Therapeutic Goals

Therapeutic goals for patients with respiratory disorders are

1. To improve pulmonary function measurements.
2. To increase exercise performance.
3. To improve arterial blood gases.
4. To increase the patient's understanding of the disease, thus maintaining the highest quality of life possible.

The pulmonary function test ideally should be between 80 and 120 percent of predicted, or the best that the patient can perform. Arterial blood gases should indicate normoxyia and no alkalemia or acidemia. Goals for exercise performance can include climbing stairs, performing activities of daily living, and participating in activities with peers. The goal of patient education is to help the patient to develop a lifestyle appropriate to the disease and to live as fulfilling a life as possible. This may include complying with drug therapy, dealing with acute exacerbations, learning methods to decrease the working of breathing, and learning pulmonary hygiene.

Nondrug Therapy

"Every time I pet Aunt Sally's cat I start to wheeze and my nose runs." For many patients, respiratory problems can be associated with a food, an animal, a time of the year, and other events. In these cases the easiest form of therapy is to avoid the precipitating event. This may require changes in the patient's lifestyle. If possible, drug therapy may be avoided. Immunotherapy (allergy shots) has proved to be effective in some conditions (bee stings, ragweed allergy, and others) in controlling allergic symptoms and reducing respiratory problems.

Additional nondrug therapeutic intervention may include weight reduction, smoking cessation, psychologic counseling, routine aerobic exercise, and others, all of which may decrease the patient's need for medication.

Bronchodilators

Bronchodilator drugs are compounds that have an antibronchoconstrictor effect (reverse bronchoconstriction). By this definition drugs such as the xanthine derivatives (**theophylline**); sympathomimetic agents (beta adrenergic receptor agonists, **epinephrine**, and related compounds); and parasympatholytic agents (**atropine**) will relax bronchial smooth muscles and can be considered bronchodilators. **Cromolyn sodium** and **corticosteroids** will not relax bronchial smooth muscle and are not considered bronchodilators. However, corticosteroids may produce bronchodilation indicated by clinical improvement and increase in pulmonary functions.

Some of the compounds used to treat respiratory diseases

derivatives, sympathomimetic agents, and anticholinergic agents); corticosteroid; cromolyn sodium; oxygen; antimicrobials; mucokinetic agents; and corticosteroid sparing agents (these are agents added to the treatment program to reduce the effective dose of corticosteroids). Most of this discussion will be appropriate for the treatment of asthma, since it responds best to therapy. However, since signs and have been used for many years. The Chinese used Ma Huang more than 5000 years ago. Its active ingredient is **ephedrine**. Until 1900 the most effective therapy was various atropine-line drugs, which were smoked, injected, or taken orally. In 1936 **aminophylline** (theophylline ethylenediamine) was first used for the treatment of acute asthma. Aminophylline or theophylline is still used intravenously for acute treatment of asthma, but its role in the chronic therapy of asthma may vary. Physicians in the United States use it extensively in clinical practice and in many cases consider theophylline as the first drug to be introduced. Physicians in Australia and the United Kingdom use other agents more extensively, most notably cromolyn sodium. The selection of initial drug may vary with geographic location, experience of the prescribers, and clinical status of the patient.

The goal of drug therapy in the management of respiratory diseases is to minimize the use of corticosteroids by maximizing the use of bronchodilators and other drugs.

Xanthines

Methylxanthines, which include theophylline (aminophylline is the salt theophylline ethylenediamine; the active component of aminophylline is theophylline), theobromine and caffeine, all occur naturally. Caffeine is contained in tea, colas and coffee; recently (Becker, 1984) it has been reported to improve pulmonary functions as well as having a CNS stimulant effect. Theobromine is found in cocoa and chocolate and is not used therapeutically. Theophylline and its derivatives are the main drugs used in the treatment of respiratory disease.

Mechanism of Action   Theophylline, caffeine, and to a lesser extent theobromine all cause stimulation of the central nervous system, produce diuresis in the kidneys, stimulate cardiac muscle, and relax smooth muscle (bronchial smooth muscle, lower esophageal sphincter). Methylxanthines also inhibit the secretion of mast cell mediators and possibly other sources of inflammation, while increasing gastric secretions. Because methylxanthines also stimulate medullary respiratory centers they are useful in the treatment of Cheyne-Stokes respiration and apnea of preterm infants.

The cellular mechanism of action of theophylline has often been explained as inhibiting phosphodiesterase and producing an increase in cyclic AMP (cAMP) (see Fig. 27-1). However, this does not adequately explain its mechanism of action, and other theories postulate inhibition of translocation of intracellular calcium, blockage of adenosine receptors, inhibition of prostaglandin synthesis, and alterations in metabolism of catecholamines.

Pharmacokinetics   Serum theophylline levels have been correlated with bronchodilating effects and adverse effects. The goal of therapy with theophylline is to have a serum concentration between 5 and 20 μg/mL. Serum theophylline concentrations above 20 μg/mL have been associated with a greater incidence of adverse effects. Concentrations between 5 and 20 μg/mL have been associated with most therapeutic effects. On rare occasions patients require theophylline concentrations above 20 μg/mL.

The absorption of theophylline has classically been described as rapid and complete when given orally (liquid, short-acting tablets, or sustained-release preparations). Food and antacids have a negligible influence. Recent studies (Rogers et al., in press; Dederich et al. 1981) have demonstrated that an additional factor in altering theophylline levels is the absorption of the drug. The fluctuations have been shown with the short-acting preparations, as well as the sustained-release formulations. Variations in absorption of theophylline produce swings in theophylline levels during the same dosage interval at the same dose. These variations in serum theophylline levels make dosage adjustments based on theophylline levels more difficult. The effects of variations in the serum theophylline levels must be interpreted in terms of the clinical status of the patient.

Problems in the absorption of theophylline may be due to the effects of food, gastrointestinal physiology, or dosage formulation. The significance of variations in the absorption of theophylline preparation needs to be evaluated further.

Theophylline is distributed to all the compartments of the body. It also crosses the placenta and into breast milk. The distribution of theophylline into breast milk and the fetus is not an absolute contraindication for breast feeding or pregnancy. Theophylline is approximately 50 to 65 percent bound to plasma proteins.

The serum half-life for theophylline ranges from 3 to 12.8 h (average 3 to 7 h) in otherwise healthy nonsmoking adults; from 1.5 to 9.5 h in children, and from 15 to 58 h in premature infants. The rate of theophylline clearance shows wide variations based on the age of the patient, concurrent drug therapy, and other diseases (see Table 27-5). The elimination of theophylline usually follows first-order kinetics,

TABLE 27-5   Factors That May Require Alteration in Theophylline Dosage

Increase in Theophylline Dosage

Younger children (2–16 years)
Smokers of cigarettes and marijuana
Diets that are high in protein and low in carbohydrate
Diets that include large amounts of charcoal-broiled beef
Concurrent treatment with phenobarbital, phenytoin, or carbamazepine

Decrease in Theophylline Dosage

Premature neonate with apnea
Elderly patients
Patients with cardiac disease: heart failure, cor pulmonale, or acute pulmonary edema
Patients with hepatic disease: cirrhosis or hepatic insufficiency
Some infections
Concurrent therapy that includes one of the following drugs: troleandomycin, erythromycin, cimetidine, ranitidine (possible), and allopurinol

but dose-dependent kinetics have been reported. Variations in theophylline clearance in some patients follow a circadian rhythm.

Theophylline is metabolized in the liver with only about 10 percent of the drug being excreted unchanged in the urine. The principal metabolites of theophylline are 1,3-dimethyluric acid, 1-methyluric acid, and 3-methylxanthine. It is thought that only 3-methylxanthine has some bronchodilating effect.

Adverse Effects   The adverse effects associated with theophylline include gastrointestinal upset manifested by anorexia, nausea, vomiting, and abdominal discomfort. Central nervous system effects include nervousness, headache, insomnia, irritability, and the severe toxicity of convulsions and coma (usually associated with levels above 40 μg/mL). Cardiovascular effects seen include tachycardia, and with very high levels, hypotension or arrhythmias have been reported.

The treatments of high theophylline levels include liquid charcoal, magnesium sulfate, and discontinuation of all theophylline preparations. When very high levels are encountered charcoal hemoperfusion is indicated.

Preparations   The short-acting theophylline preparations (which include uncoated tablets, oral liquids, and IV solutions; see Table 27-6) usually have the disadvantage of requiring multiple daily doses associated with poor patient compliance. The short-acting preparations for many patients are still useful. The use of sustained-release theophylline preparations has increased in clinical practice since they avoid the problem of frequent dosing in patients who are rapid eliminators of theophylline and improve patient compliance. The variability in absorption of theophylline preparations and the difference in theophylline release systems in the various sustained-release products make these products noninterchangeable.

Theophylline should not be given as a suppository because of slow and erratic absorption. The IM route should also be avoided because of the pain associated with the injection. Aminophylline and a theophylline solution can be given for IV use. **Choline theophyinate**, oxtriphylline (Choledyl) is a partially enteric coated formulation of theophylline which in theory reduces gastric upset by releasing the theophylline in the small intestines. This is of little value since the gastric upset is usually centrally mediated on the basis of serum theophylline concentrations and not local irritation.

Anhydrous theophylline concentration of various drugs is listed in Table 27-7. It is important to remember that the amount of theophylline in the various formulations of aminophylline varies with the manufacture. The IV preparation of aminophylline (G. D. Searle) contains 80 percent theophylline, and Somophyllin (Fisons) contains 85 percent theophylline. **Dyphylline** (Lufyllin) is a xanthine derivative but has no clinical advantage over other theophylline prepara-

tions. Since it has the disadvantage that one is not able to monitor the levels of dyphylline, dyphylline therefore should not be used.

Dosage   The dosage of theophylline should be based on serum theophylline concentrations or the clinical status of the patient. The general principles of dosing theophylline are as follows.

Acute treatment   If immediate bronchodilation is needed, it is best achieved by giving a loading dose intravenously. A loading dose of 6 mg/kg of aminophylline (4.8 mg/kg of theophylline) can be given slowly over 20 to 30 min. This dosage assumes that the patient is not using any theophylline preparation. If the patient is already taking a

TABLE 27-6   Theophylline Preparations

Short-Acting Preparations

Uncoated Tablets
  Slo-phyllin
  Aminophylline
  Theophyl Chewable
  Theolaire

Oral Liquids
  Somophyllin
  Slo-phyllin GG Syrup

Intravenous Solutions*
  Aminophylline
  Theophylline

Rectal Solution
  Somophyllin Rectal Solution

Sustained-Release Preparations

Sustained-Release Tablets
  Aminodur Dura-Tabs
  Choledyl SA
  Constant-T
  LaBid
  Quibron-T/SR Dividose
  Respbid
  Sustaire
  Theo-dur
  Theolair-SR

Sustained-Release Bead-Filled Capsules
  Bronkodyl S-R
  Ellixophyllin SR
  Slo-bid Gyrocaps
  Somophyllin-CRT
  Theo-bid Duracaps
  Theo-dur sprinkles
  Theovent

24-Hour Preparations
  Theo-24
  Uniphyl

TABLE 27-7 Theophylline Content of Common Xanthine Preparations

GENERIC NAME	CHEMICAL NAME	ANHYDROUS THEOPHYLLINE CONTENT, %
Aminophylline USP	Theophylline ethylenediamine	78–86
Oxtriphylline	Choline theophyllinate	65
Theophylline calcium salicylate	—	48
Theophylline monoethanolamine	—	75
Theophylline monohydrate NF	—	90
Theophylline sodium glycinate	—	50

theophylline preparation it may only be necessary to give the maintenance dose intravenously or to give an adjusted loading dose (it is expected that a loading dose of 0.5 mg/kg of theophylline will increase the serum theophylline concentration by $1\mu g/mL$). A rapidly absorbed preparation of theophylline can also be used in the treatment of acute bronchospasm. Again, if the patient is not using theophylline a loading dose of 6 mg/kg can be administered. The dosage for the treatment of acute bronchospasms for oral and IV therapy is listed in Table 27-8.

Chronic therapy Patients can be maintained on a short-acting theophylline preparation, which usually requires four daily doses. Sustained-release preparations require less frequent dosing and can be given every 8, 12, or 24 h. Patients can usually be maintained on theophylline doses of 12 to 24 mg/kg/day (Table 27-9). However, therapy must be individualized. If there is no clinical need to achieve a theophylline level rapidly, it is best to titrate the patient's dose of theophylline upward slowly. When theophylline is titrated slowly, adverse effects are less severe and the clinical response can be more closely evaluated.

Patient Education Patients should be instructed on the most common adverse effects associated with theophylline therapy. If these effects occur, they should be reported to the prescribers since they may indicate toxicity. Patients should also be instructed in the importance of using theophylline on a maintenance basis and what to do when a dose is missed. Maintenance doses of theophylline may also help to prevent exercise-induced bronchoconstriction (EIB). The use of theophylline may not preclude the need for pretreat-

ment with other drugs in the treatment of EIB. Patients should also understand the value of theophylline concentrations in monitoring their therapy.

Theophylline may be taken with food or antacids if the patient feels it minimizes gastrointestinal problems. For faster absorption it should be taken with a full glass of water and on an empty stomach. The sustained-released tablets should not be chewed and must be taken whole. The sustained-release bead-filled capsules can be emptied on food (still should not be chewed) for patients who have difficulty in swallowing tablets or capsules.

Sympathomimetic Agents (Adrenergic Receptor Agonists)
Epinephrine was first introduced in 1910 as a bronchodilator. In 1941 **isoproterenol** was the first pure β-adrenergic agonist drug introduced: it has no α-adrenergic stimulating properties. Its disadvantage is that it is not orally active since it is metabolized in the gastrointestinal tract. In 1961 **metaproterenol** was marketed; because it has the advantages of selectivity for β_2-adrenergic receptors, longer duration of action than previously available products, and resistance to catechol-O-methyltransferase (COMT) it can be given orally. Since the introduction of metaproterenol numerous other selective β_2 agonists have been marketed, with more to follow. It is hoped that the newer preparations will be more selective for β_2 receptors and have a quicker onset and longer duration of action, with fewer adverse effects.

Adrenergic receptor agonists increase cAMP (see Fig. 27-1) to produce bronchodilation and inhibit mast cell degranulation. In addition, they cause vasodilation and increases in ciliary motility.

TABLE 27-8 Approximate Dosage of Intravenous Aminophylline for Treatment of Acute Bronchospasm*

GROUP	MAINTENANCE DOSE, per h
Children 6 months to 9 years	1.0 mg/kg
Children 9–16 and young adult smoker	0.8 mg/kg
Otherwise healthy nonsmoking adult	0.5 mg/kg
Older patients with cor pulmonale	0.3 mg/kg
Patients with CHF or liver disease	0.1–1.2 mg/kg

*IV aminophylline (G.D. Searle) contains approximately 80 percent theophylline. Therefore 1 mg of aminophylline contains approximately 0.8 mg of theophylline.

TABLE 27-9 Maximum Recommended Maintenance Dosage of Theophylline*

GROUP	DAILY THEOPHYLLINE DOSAGE†
Children to 9 years	24 mg/kg
Children 9–12 years	20 mg/kg
Patient 12–16 years	18 mg/kg
Patients 16 years and older	13 mg/kg

*Larger doses can be given but must be based on serum theophylline concentrations.

†Dosages are expressed as anhydrous theophylline.

There is little information available on the correlation between serum concentrations of β agonists and pharmacologic activity. However, it has been shown that when the β agonists are given by inhalation there is an increase in pulmonary function before there is a detectable serum concentration of the drug.

Routes of Administration   β Agonists can be administered parenterally (usually by subcutaneous injection for acute problems), orally, or by inhalation. The inhalation route is usually preferred because it delivers the drug directly to the receptors in the lungs, and therefore a smaller dose is required. Parenteral and oral therapy require systemic delivery of the drug, which is usually associated with a greater incidence of adverse effects.

The usefulness of oral and parenteral β-receptor agonists is limited by their adverse effects. The patient's susceptibility to tremors and palpitations will limit the dose if the drug is used at all. When these drugs are used orally it is best to start with low doses and slowly titrate upward. The adverse effects for many patients diminish with continuous therapy.

Since a therapeutic response can usually be achieved with inhaled medications, the use of oral β agonists still has a limited value. Very small children and patients who have difficulty in administering a nebulizer or meter dose inhaler will require oral therapy. Oral administration of the medication may have the advantage of producing bronchodilation in the small airways that may not be reached by an inhaled treatment. Inhaled bronchodilators can affect the small airways, but this response is dependent on the patient's administration technique. The use of both oral and inhaled β agonists for maintenance therapy is a controversial practice, and for the majority of patients should be avoided.

Selection of β-Adrenergic Agonists   Large interpatient variation with the β-agonist drugs and the difficulties encountered in establishing well-controlled clinical trials cause the selection of a β-agonist to be based on the clinical response of the individual patient. The β-agonists are said to have variations in their onset of action and the duration of action, but the clinical significance of this finding is questionable (see Table 27-10). β-agonist response can be evaluated by administering the medication and then measuring pulmonary functions (usually spirometry) over time (time-response curves). The cost of medication as well as the taste of the drug may play a role in the selection of the drug.

TABLE 27-10   Sympathomimetic Bronchodilators

DRUG	TRADE NAME	COMMENTS
Selective β₂ Agonists		
Albuterol	Proventil, Ventolin	Slow onset of action and longer duration; available as tablets and MDI*
Metaproterenol	Alupent, Metaprel	Rapid onset with a slightly shorter duration of action; available as a tablet, syrup, MDI, solution for inhalation
Terbutaline	Brethine, Bricanyl, Brethaire	Slow onset of action with a long duration; available as a tablet, injectable, and MDI
Isoetharine hydrochloride	Bronkosol, Beta-2	Rapid onset and short duration; solution for inhalation
Isoetharine mestylate	Bronkometer	MDI
Fenoterol	Berotec	Not on the market; has a long duration of action
Rimiterol		Not on the market; has a short duration of action; intended for IV use
Nonselective β₂ Agonists		
Isoproterenol	Isuprel	Has significant cardiac effect and a short duration of action; available as a solution for inhalation and MDI
α and β Receptor Agonists		
Epinephrine	Adrenalin	Short duration of action; available as SC injection and for inhalation
Epinephrine Aqueous Suspension	Sus-Phrine	Long-acting epinephrine
Ephedrine	Numerous	Available as a syrup and capsules; numerous adverse effects

*MDI = Metered dose inhaler.

In treatment of patients with severe respiratory diseases it is usually preferred to administer the beta-agonists (for chronic therapy) by a nebulizer which is either powered by a compressor or a hand-bulb. (The nebulizer is a device which suspends particles of liquid medication in a gas stream. In contrast the metered dose inhaler (MDI) suspends particles in a volatile propellant.) It is believed that the nebulizer gives a better response to the medication, although the newer techniques to administer the MDI may improve response. Isoetharine and metaproterenol are available as solution and are the selective β_2 agonist that are most often prescribed for nebulization. When it is difficult to take a nebulized treatment, the metered dose inhaler can be substituted.

Epinephrine   Epinephrine is still the drug of choice in the treatment of anaphylactic reactions since it causes both alpha and beta effects. The newer, more selective β_2 agonists have replaced its use in the therapy of chronic obstructive lung diseases. It is still useful in the treatment of acute bronchoconstriction when it is given subcutaneously. The alternative to epinephrine is the subcutaneous administration of terbutaline. Epinephrine can not be given orally, but it can be administered by inhalation. Many of the over-the-counter asthma preparations contain epinephrine as the active principle (see Table 27-11).

Ephedrine   Ephedrine has been replaced with the newer, more selective β-agonists, which have fewer side effects and

TABLE 27-11   Asthma Product Table

PRODUCT	DOSAGE FORM	EPHEDRINE	EPINEPHRINE	THEOPHYLLINE	OTHER INGREDIENTS
Amodrine	Tablet	25 mg (as racemic hydrochloride)			Aminophylline, 100 mg Phenobarbital, 8 mg
AsthmaNefrin	Inhalant solution		2.25% (epinephrine base as racemic hydrochloride)		Chlorobutanol, 0.5%
Bronitin Mist	Inhalant		7.0 mg/mL (as bitartrate)		Freon propellant
Bronkaid	Tablet	24 mg (as sulfate)		100 mg (anhydrous)	Guaifenesin, 100 mg Magnesium trisilicate, 74.52 mg
Bronkaid Mist	Inhalant		0.5%		Ascorbic acid, 0.07% Alcohol, 34% Hydrochloric and nitric acid buffers
Bronkotabs	Tablet	24 mg (as sulfate)		100 mg	Guaifenesin, 100 mg Phenobarbital, 8 mg
Primatene M	Tablet	24 mg (as hydrochloride)		130 mg	Pyrilamine maleate, 16 mg
Primatene Mist	Inhalant		5.5 mg/mL		Alcohol, 34% Freon propellant
Primatene P	Tablet	24 mg (as hydrochloride)		130 mg	Phenobarbital, 8 mg
Tedral	Tablet Elixir Suspension	24 mg/tablet 1.2 mg/mL (elixir) 2.4 mg/mL (suspension) (all as hydrochloride)		130 mg/tablet (anhydrous) 6.5 mg/mL (elixir) 13 mg/mL (suspension)	Phenobarbital, 8 mg/tablet 0.4 mg/mL (elixir) 0.8 mg/mL (suspension)
Vaponefrin Solution	Inhalant		2.25% (epinephrine base as racemic hydrochloride)		Chlorobutanol, 0.5%
Verquad	Tablet Suspension	24 mg/tablet 2.4 mg/mL (both as hydrochloride)		130 mg/tablet 13 mg/mL (both as calcium salicylate)	Guaifenesin, 100 mg/tablet or 10 mg/mL Phenobarbital, 8 mg/tablet or 0.8 mg/mL

Source: Adapted from The American Pharmaceutical Association, *Handbook of Nonprescription Drugs,* Washington, D.C.: American Pharmaceutical Association, 1982.

greater bronchodilating effects. It is still found in many over-the-counter preparations (Bronkaid, Tedral). The usual oral dose is 25–50 mg every 3–4 h.

Isoproterenol Isoproterenol affects both β receptors, causing marked cardiac effects. As with the other β-receptor agonists, some patients respond better to therapy with isoproterenol than the other agents and it should be used for those patients. It has been used intravenously in the treatment of severe asthmatic attacks but is usually given by inhalation either as a metered dose inhaler or as a solution for nebulization.

Isoetharine Isoetharine was the first drug introduced that had selective β_2-agonist activity. It is administered by inhalation in a metered dose inhaler (Bronkometer) or as a solution for nebulization (Bronkosol, Beta-2). It has a rapid onset of action (15 min) with a short duration (2 h).

Metaproterenol Metaproterenol can be given orally, intravenously (only for investigational use), or by inhalation. Metaproterenol (Alupent, Metaprel) is similar to isoproterenol in degree of bronchodilating effect but has fewer cardiovascular effects. It has a shorter duration of action than the newer selective β agonists but a rapid onset of action.

Newer Selective β_2-Adrenergic Receptor Agonists The number of drugs introduced that are selective β_2 agonists is steadily increasing. All drugs in this classification can be given by inhalation or orally. They all have longer duration of actions and do not cause direct cardiac stimulation. The major adverse effects associated with their use are tremors and tachycardia. The tremors are due to a direct stimulation of β_2 receptors in the skeletal muscles. The β_2 stimulation of blood vessels supplying the skeletal muscle also results in decreased peripheral resistance causing a reflex tachycardia. The agents in this group include **albuterol** (Ventolin, Proventil); **terbutaline** (Brethine, Brincanyl, Brethaire); **fenterol** (Berotec); **carbuterol** and others.

Adverse Effects Many of the side effects associated with the β agonists can be explained by the action of the drugs on the sympathetic nervous system (see Chap. 13). The major adverse effects of this class of agents include nervousness, palpitations, agitation, hand tremors, and loss of sleep.

Many of the adverse effects diminish with time. It also has been suggested that the bronchodilating effect of these agents may also decrease with continued use. Tolerance with these agents has been difficult to establish, but it is believed to occur. Its clinical significance still needs to be established.

Corticosteroids are thought to increase the number of beta-receptors and therefore enhance the β-adrenergic bronchodilating response. Patients on corticosteroids and β-adrenergic agents avoid the problem of tolerance (see Fig. 27-1).

Hypoxemia has been described as a complication in the administration of β agonists, atropine, and theophylline. The decrease in arterial oxygen tension can occur because there is a drug-induced increase in pulmonary blood flow to areas that are poorly ventilated because of bronchoconstriction. This will further aggravate the ventilation-perfusion imbalance. This effect can be prevented by administering oxygen along with the drugs.

Deaths have been associated with excessive use of the aerosol form of β-adrenergic agonists, in particular **isoproterenol**. In the years 1961 to 1966 there was an increase in deaths of asthma patients in the United Kingdom. This increase was loosely associated with an increase in the use of inhaled isoproterenol. The deaths may have been related to either an idiosyncratic reaction to isoproterenol or to an increase in cardiac irritability caused by the Freon propellant. A cause and effect relationship between the increased deaths and the use of metered dosed inhaler has not been positively established, but many practitioners still limit the patient's use of aerosol medications.

One group of chemicals known to produce asthma is sulfiting preservatives (metabisulfite, bisulfite, and sulfur dioxide). These agents are present in many of the solutions used for inhalation (**isoetharine, metaproterenol, and isoproterenol**) and for injection (**epinephrine**). In most cases the bronchodilating effects of the β agonists outweigh the bronchoconstricting effects of the sulfiting agents. If a patient is known to be sensitive to the sulfiting agents it is best to avoid their use. The metered dose inhalers (since they are usually powders) and the unit dose preparations of metaproterenol do not contain any sulfiting agents.

Dosage The inhalation of the β agonist allows a degree of flexibility in dosing. Patients who are only mildly obstructed may require only one inhalation of medication once or twice a day, although patients who are severely obstructed may require larger and more frequent doses. Patients using inhaled β-adrenergic agonists to prevent exercise-induced bronchoconstriction can administer it 15 to 20 min prior to the exercise. The usual dosage of inhaled beta agonist solution should be the least number of inhalations of the least concentrated solution that will produce the therapeutic effects. The solutions for nebulization may be inhaled undiluted but in most cases are diluted with either fresh tap water or normal saline. The inhaled solutions that can be nebulized include 1% (1:100) **epinephrine hydrochloride** (Adrenalin), 2.25% **racemic epinephrine** (S-2, Vaponephrin), 0.1–1% **isoetharine hydrochloride** (B-2, Bronkosol), 0.25–1% **isoproterenol hydrochloride** (Isuprel) and 5% **metaproterenol sulfate** (Alupent, Metaprel). The selective beta agonists **metaproterenol sulfate** and **isoetharine hydrochloride** are the preferred agents. Metaproterenol is commonly inhaled after mixing 0.3 mL of metaproterenol sulfate with 2.2 mL of normal saline. Isoetharine hydrochloride can be administered by a nebulizer after mixing 0.5 mL of the 1% solution with 1.5 mL of normal saline. Alternatively, both isoetharine and metaproterenol can be given by a hand-bulb nebulizer as an undiluted solution. The dosage and preparation should be changed based on the clinical response of the patient.

The metered dose inhalers are in most cases a more convenient method to administer inhaled beta agonists, but many clinicians prefer the inhaled solution for the more difficult patient. The usual dosage of inhaled beta agonist given by MDI is one to four inhalations (puffs) q4–6h. As with the inhaled solutions, the least number of sprays is preferred. Examples of beta agonists that can be given by MDI include **epinephrine** (160–270 μg per metered spray (Primatene, Bronkaid), **isoetharine mesylate** (0.340 mg per metered spray, Bronkometer), **metaproterenol sulfate** (0.65 mg per metered spray), **isproterenol sulfate (80 μg per metered spray, Isuprel), albuterol sulfate** (90 μg per metered spray), and terbutaline sulfate (0.25 mg per metered spray, Brethaire).

Metaproterenol, terbutaline, and **albuterol** are given orally in doses of 10 to 20 mg, 2.5 to 5 mg, and 2 to 4 mg three or four times a day, respectively.

Patient Education: Method of Administration It is essential that the patient inhale the medication properly, since the effectiveness of the drug is dependent on the method of administration. Even when proper technique is used only about 10 percent of the drug actually reaches the lung. Most of the medication is deposited in the back of the mouth, exhaled, or left in the delivery system. Of the portion of the drug swallowed, only about 50 percent is eventually absorbed. Factors that improve the deposition of the drug into the tracheobronchial tree are (1) small droplets of the medication and (2) a slow deep inspiration. It is therefore recommended that when the solution is administered by a hand-bulb nebulizer or compressor, a tube (smooth surfaced) be attached to the end of the nebulizer. When the metered dose inhaler is used, certain products (Inspir-Care, Aero Chamber) can be attached to a metered dose inhaler that will select the appropriate particle size and improve patient technique (see Fig. 27-4).

Independent of the method of administration (nebulizer or MDI), the basic technique is as follows:

1. The patient exhales slowly, and places the mouthpiece between the lips.
2. The drug delivery system is actuated.
3. The patient slowly inhales to TLC (total lung capacity).
4. At the end of the full inspiration the patient should hold his or her breath for 6 to 10 s and then exhale it slowly through pursed lips.

If another dose is given the patient should wait 5 to 10 min to allow the first treatment to have an effect. Many patients find the use of a hand-bulb nebulizer to be tiring and prefer to use a compressor. When a compressor is used a Y-connector allows the patient to control the delivery of the medication. If the patient is not able to take a deep inspiration or cannot coordinate the administration technique, a simple face mask or a positive-pressure breathing machine (IPBB) can be used. When used long term, the IPBB machine is no more effective than other methods of administration. Whatever method of administration is used, the technique of administration is most important.

Parasympatholytic Agents
Atropine sulfate is the prototype agent used in the treatment of respiratory diseases. The quaternary ammonium compounds **SCH 1000 iprotropium** (Atrovent) (still an investigational agent in the United States), and **atropine methylnitrate** have also been used in the treatment of respiratory disorders.

Mechanism of Action Parasympatholytic drugs competitively antagonize the muscarinic actions of acetylcholine (see Fig. 27-1). The muscarinic receptors are located on the smooth muscle of the bronchi, the gastrointestinal tract, various secretory glands (sweat and bronchial glands), the heart, and in the eyes. The parasympatholytic drugs lack selectivity, and there is a clinical need for an agent that affects primarily the receptors in the respiratory tract. Effects produced in respiratory disorders are relaxation of the bronchial smooth muscle, decreased release of mediators from mast cells, and blockage of the efferent end of the vagal irritant receptor reflex.

Pharmacokinetics Atropine is well absorbed when taken by mouth; most of the drug is excreted in the urine within 2 h, with up to 50 percent excreted as unchanged atropine. The metabolites of atropine have not been well described.

The quaternary ammonium compounds **atropine methylnitrate** and **ipratropium bromide** are poorly absorbed orally and do not cross the blood brain barrier. Approximately 45 percent of ipratropium is excreted unchanged in the urine when the drug is given by inhalation.

Adverse Effects The adverse effects of **atropine sulfate** and the related drugs can be attributed to their effects on the autonomic nervous system (see Chap. 12). Adverse effects include dry mouth, blurred vision, urinary retention, inhibition of sweating, and tachycardia. The most annoying effect to the patient is dry mouth. This may be prevented by reducing the dose.

Dosage **Atropine sulfate** solution for inhalation can be compounded from the dry powder in a concentration of 2 mg/mL or 4 mg/mL. It is also commercially available in a unit dose package that contains 1 mg. The usual adult dose is 0.025 mg/kg given two to four times a day by inhalation. **Iprotropium** is available in a metered dose inhaler that delivers 20 μg per actuation. The usual dose is one to two puffs (20–40 μg) two to four times a day.

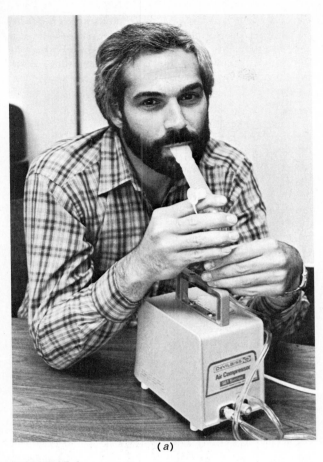

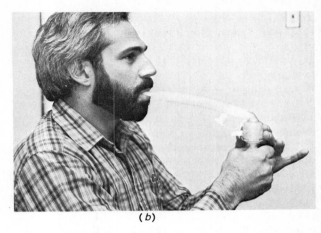

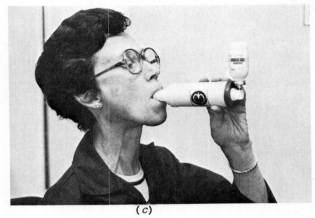

FIGURE 27-4

Methods of Administering Inhaled Respiratory Treatments. (*a*) Solutions can be administered by inhalation with a nebulizer powered by a compressor; (*b*) solution can be administered with a hand-bulb nebulizer; and (*c*) metered dose inhaler using an Aerochamber by Monaghan.

Clinical Efficacy   **Atropine sulfate** can be a bronchodilating drug in the treatment of chronic obstructive lung disease. When the therapeutic goals can not be reached with theophylline or β-adrenergic agonist, atropine should be tried. As for all the other bronchodilators, its effects should be carefully evaluated. It is rational to use the three different types of bronchodilators in the same patient if a response can be demonstrated. The three types of bronchodilators all have different mechanisms of action.

Cromolyn Sodium

Cromolyn sodium is used *only* in the prophylactic treatment of bronchial asthma and is not effective in the management of other respiratory diseases. The problems associated with the use of cromolyn include the following: many patients do not respond to cromolyn and it is difficult to predict which patients will respond; there may be a long lag time before the drug is effective; and it is not absorbed orally. This has

led researchers to try to develop similar compounds that would be orally active and more effective.

Mechanism of Action

Cromolyn sodium has no bronchodilator or anti-inflammatory properties. It is believed to inhibit the release of mediators from the mast cells (see Fig. 27-1). Cromolyn is suspected of blocking the calcium channel and producing a "membrane stabilization" effect. If calcium is prevented from entering the mast cells degranulation is prevented and mediator release is inhibited. Attempts have also been made to explain cromolyn action on the basis of its anticholinergic effect. The exact mechanism of action is still unknown.

Pharmacokinetics

Cromolyn is poorly absorbed from the gastrointestinal tract (about 1 percent of the drug is absorbed). When inhaled, less than 10 percent of the dose reaches the lungs. The majority of the drug is excreted by the gastrointestinal tract. The portion that is inhaled into the lungs is absorbed and then excreted in the urine and bile. After inhalation the drug is rapidly absorbed, then excreted unchanged in the urine and bile. The half-life of cromolyn is about 90 min.

Indications

Cromolyn on a maintenance basis is useful in the prophylaxis of asthma and other allergic conditions. It is not effective in the treatment of chronic bronchitis or emphysema, nor is it effective in the treatment of acute asthma. Cromolyn or the inhaled β agonists can be used in the treatment of exercise-induced bronchoconstriction (EIB). When given to treat EIB, it is given as a single dose 15 to 20 min prior to exercise. In refractory cases of EIB, cromolyn and a β_2 agonist can be used together. Cromolyn is also available as a nasal solution (Nasalcrom) for the treatment of allergic rhinitis and as a ophthalmologic solution (Opticrom; not on the U.S. market) for the treatment of seasonal allergic conjunctivitis and vernal keratoconjunctivitis. It has been administered orally in the treatment of food allergy and chronic inflammatory diseases.

Cromolyn has proved to be most effective in younger patients who are corticosteroid-dependent and have extrinsic asthma (antigen-induced). A trial (6 to 8 weeks) of cromolyn is frequently indicated in patients who are not easily controlled by bronchodilators.

Adverse Effects

The main problems associated with the use of cromolyn powder are bronchospasm and pharyngeal irritation. This may be avoided or lessened by using an inhaled bronchodilator prior to the use of cromolyn, and then following the cromolyn powder with a glass of water. The introduction of cromolyn solution has reduced the problems associated with the inhalation of the powder, but the treatment requires a large volume for inhalation (2 mL) so administration is time-consuming. Cromolyn has also been associated with eosinophilic pneumonia, pulmonary granulomatosis, anaphylaxis, and other problems, but these adverse effects are uncommon.

Dosage

The usual dose for cromolyn by inhalation is 20 mg (one capsule or one ampul) given four times a day. Patients who are unstable may require more frequent dosing in the beginning of therapy. Later, the dosage schedule can be reduced. In other cases the dosage schedule may be reduced to twice a day.

Patient Education: Method of Administration

It is important that the proper inhalation technique be followed (see previous section). When the cromolyn powder is used the spinhaler should be properly maintained. If the cromolyn causes pharyngeal irritation, sucking on candies or following the treatment with a glass of water may reduce the irritation. The patient should be told that this medication is not used in the treatment of an acute asthma attack (it may not be necessary to stop the drug) and that it may take up to 6 to 8 weeks to determine whether it is effective.

Corticosteroids

Corticosteroids are used to treat the acute exacerbation of respiratory diseases and as maintenance therapy. Corticosteroids are extremely effective in the treatment of respiratory disorders, but their adverse effects limit their usefulness. A more complete discussion of corticosteroids is presented in the chapter on endocrine disorders (Chap. 35).

The exact mechanism of action by which the corticosteroids exert their action on the lungs is still not completely known. The steroids' effects in respiratory disease may relate to (1) inhibition of mediator release from mast cells, (2) suppression of inflammation, and (3) synergism of corticosteroids and β agonist.

Dosing of Corticosteroids

Acute Exacerbations (Status Asthmaticus)   In the treatment of acute exacerbations the goal is to give enough corticosteroids to reverse the airway obstruction. An exact dosage appropriate for all patients cannot be given, since the dose-response relationship in the therapy of asthma has not been established. **Hydrocortisone**, 200 mg, or **methylprednisolone**, 40 mg, given IV every 4 to 6 h is a frequent starting dose. Larger doses can be used since the adverse effects of high-dose short-term corticosteroid therapy are usually fewer than the problems associated with the disease. The steroid dosage selected is dependent on the clinical status of the patient and the experiences of the medical staff.

When the acute problem is over, the patient can be rapidly or slowly tapered to their maintenance doses. If the tapering is too rapid the patient will develop respiratory problems; to prevent this, many practitioners always reduce the steroid dosage slowly.

Chronic Therapy   In contrast to the acute management of respiratory problems the chronic use of corticosteroids requires minimizing the dose and maximizing the dosage interval as much as possible. In chronic therapy the beneficial effects may have to be reduced to avoid the toxicities associated chronic steroid therapy. The preferred maintenance regimen is to avoid using steroids. If steroids are required, a short course of therapy (boost) followed by a period of time without any steroids is the next best regime. If steroids are required more often, an every-other-day program is preferred to daily administration of steroids. When every-other-day or daily steroids are used a single early morning dose is employed. Multiple daily doses of corticosteroids should be reserved for the treatment of acute exacerbations and not for chronic therapy.

Preparations   **Prednisone**, **prednisolone**, and **methylprednisolone** are the most common drugs used for oral maintenance therapy. Their duration of action allows alternate-day dosing and has minimum salt and water retention properties. Prednisone should be the first drug tried since it is inexpensive and is available in numerous tablet strengths. Prednisolone is the active metabolite of prednisone, but it has the disadvantage of offering only a few tablet strengths, therefore making dosage adjustments more difficult. Methylprednisolone has the disadvantage of being expensive; however, some patients respond better to it.

Patient Education   An important component in the treatment of respiratory disorders is self-care. Patients with moderate to severe asthma should be able to recognize when their respiratory disease is not responding to the usual maintenance regime. The early aggressive treatment of the acute problem may avoid hospitalization. In many cases this aggressive treatment may require the patient to take a steroid boost (high-dose corticosteroid therapy for a short period of time). Therapy is always initiated under the supervision of the medical team, but patients should be taught how and when to take steroids. After the short course of high-dose corticosteroid therapy the maintenance program should be resumed.

Patients frequently get upset with the adverse effects steroids have on their body and mind when taken chronically. Their desire to avoid these problems may cause patients to discontinue therapy abruptly. Patients who have been on steroids for a long period of time must be reminded to have their dosage reduced slowly.

Topical Inhaled Steroid Preparations

Beclomethasone diproprionate (Vanceril and Beclovent) and **triamcinolone acetonide** (Azmacort) are topically active corticosteroids that are given by inhalation. The topical corticosteroids can be used to reduce or eliminate the need for systemic corticosteroids. This is advantageous since beclomethasone and triamcinolone don't produce the adverse effects of the oral corticosteroids. Topical steroid preparations are not recommended for the treatment of the acute attack. Care should be observed when switching patients from oral to inhaled corticosteroids so as not to cause acute adrenal insufficiency. The patient may also experience withdrawal side effects during the switching from system to topical steroids. *Candida albicans* or *Aspergillus niger* infections can occur in the mouth and pharnyx during beclomethasone and triamcinolone therapy. This may require antifungal treatment or stopping of the medication. The problem of infection may be reduced by rinsing the mouth out with mouthwash after an inhaled treatment. Patients should use their inhaled topical steroids after an inhaled bronchodilator treatment. Beclomethasone is usually administered in doses of two to four puffs four times a day. The usual dosage of triamcinolone is two inhalations three to four times a day. Various dosing schedules, including an alternate-day program, have been used.

Miscellaneous Agents

Oxygen Therapy

Hypoxemia (low oxygen in the blood) is the single most important factor contributing to respiratory mortality during acute respiratory failure. The goal of oxygen therapy is to increase the amount of oxygen carried by the blood to as close to normal as possible (Pa_{O_2} 70–100 mmHg at sea level, varying among patients).

There are numerous methods of administering oxygen, including nasal cannulas (prongs), face masks, hoods, face tents, and T-tube systems. Each system has its own particular advantages and disadvantages. The adverse effects of the drying of secretions associated with oxygen therapy can be avoided if the oxygen is well humidified. High concentrations (greater than 60 percent) of oxygen may eliminate nitrogen normally present in the alveoli. This may lead to atelectasis. High concentrations of oxygen for more than 48 to 72 h may cause oxygen toxicity. Oxygen supports combustion and when compressed in a tank may act as a projectile if not properly vented. Patients using home oxygen must be aware of hazards and measures to ensure safety. Rules for home oxygen use include the following:

1.   Secure the oxygen tank either to a wall or in a special stand.
2.   When initially "tapping" a tank ensure that the regulator is turned off and opened gradually.
3.   Ensure there is no smoking where oxygen is stored or used.
4.   Keep all tanks away from heat sources and electrical devices.
5.   Check all oxygen equipment regularly and report any faulty equipment to supplier immediately.

Liquid oxygen and oxygen concentrators are excellent alternatives for home oxygen therapy.

Antimicrobials

The basic principles of antimicrobial therapy are presented in Chaps. 28 and 29. The use of antimicrobials in treatment of chronic obstructive lung diseases is often based on clinical impression and history. A patient with asthma and a history of severe respiratory problems (hospitalization or visits to the ER) associated with upper respiratory infections may have antimicrobials started without a culture and sensitivity testing. In other patients the development of abnormal sputum (change in color or viscosity) or the symptoms of sinusitis indicates the need for antimicrobial therapy. The antimicrobials most frequently used orally in the treatment of respiratory disorders are **ampicillin, amoxicillin, tetracycline, erythromycin,** and **trimethoprim-sulfmethoxazole.**

Mucokinetic Agents

Mucokinetic agents are used to aid in the loosening and liquefaction of sputum and to improve expectoration. Although the efficacy of these agents is controversial, they are used in cases where the problem of sputum production is severe. Adequate hydration is still the most effective treatment. Mucokinetic agents can be administered orally or by inhalation (see Table 27-12).

Troleandomycin (TAO)

TAO is a macrolid antibiotic which is not used clinically to treat infections. TAO is used in the treatment of severe recalcitrant asthma that has not been responsive to other therapies. When used in the treatment of asthma it is considered a steroid-sparing agent. TAO must be used with the steroid methylprednosolone. Traditionally, TAO therapy is started by using multiple daily doses (loading dose) then tapered to the maintenance dose of 250 mg once a day or every other day. The mechanism of action of TAO is still not completely understood. One theory is that it decreases the clearance of the methylprednisolone and that a lower dose reflects only a decrease in the elimination of the steroid. Another theory states that it has a steroid-sparing effect unrelated to the methylprednisolone. Whatever the mechanism of action is, some patients show a marked clinical improvement and a lowering of their steroid dosage when placed on the combination of TAO and methylprednisolone. Prior to initiating therapy liver function tests must be obtained since the use of TAO may be limited by alteration in liver functions.

Agents That Affect Respiration

The clinical role of respiratory stimulants is limited (Table 27-13). The clinical preference is to use mechanical methods rather than drugs to stimulate respiration. The analeptic respiratory stimulants were once used in the treatment of overdose of narcotic and other central nervous depressant. These agents have a short duration of action with numerous adverse effects. Narcotic overdoses are now treated with the narcotic antagonists. Hormones such as **medroxyprogesterone** (Depo-Provera) are used in the treatment of certain respiratory disorders including hypoventilation associated with obesity (Pickwickian syndrome). Adrenergic agents have been used in the treatment of alveolar hypoventilation. Carbonic anhydrase inhibitors cause a metabolic acidosis which has a stimulant effect on the respiratory center.

TABLE 27-12 Inhaled Mucokinetic Agents

DRUG	COMMENT
Water	In most cases should be given orally; can be given via a nebulizer for individual therapy; also can be given via a room humidifier or a hot shower.
Saline solution	Normal saline is well tolerated. Hypotonic saline (0.45%) can be given by ultrasonic nebulization. Hypertonic saline is most effective in stimulating productive cough.
Propylene glycol	Is a hygroscopic drug (absorbs water). In some cases 1–2 mL of a 2% solution is inhaled.
Acetylcysteine (Mucomyst)	1–2 mL of either a 10 or 20% solution can be inhaled 3–4 times a day. It is stable for only 96 once the bottle is opened.
Deoxyribonuclease (Dornase), trypsin, chymotrypsin,	Infrequently used; expensive, toxic, relatively ineffective.
Sodium bicarbonate	Acts as a surfactant when inhaled as a 2% solution; 1.4% solution is almost isotonic. Also used in 5 and 7% concentrations.
Ethanol	Has been inhaled as a mucokinetic agent. The usual dose is 1–2 mL of a 30–50% solution given by inhalation.

TABLE 27-13 Respiratory Stimulants

Analeptics

Bemegride (Megride)
Doxapram (Doxapram)
Nikethamide (Coramine)
Pentylenetetazole (Metrazole)

Hormones

Medroxyprogesterone (Provera)
Progesterone
Estrogens

Methylxanthines

Caffeine
Theophylline

Adrenergic Agents

Dextroamphetamine (Dexedrine)
Methylphenidate (Ritalin)
Levarternol (Levophed)

Carbonic Anhydrase Inhibitors

Acetazolamide (Diamox)
Dichlorphenamide (Daranide)

Narcotic Antagonist

Naloxone (Narcan)
Levallorphan (Lorfan)

A more common problem is that drugs that depress respiration may be taken purposefully or accidentally. Patients who have preexisting respiratory disorders are particularly sensitive to the effects of respiratory depressants. The respiratory depressants include narcotics (antitussives), sedative-hypnotics, tranquilizers, and antidepressants.

NURSING PROCESS RELATED TO OBSTRUCTIVE LUNG DISEASE

Assessment

Clinical signs of obstructive lung disease, as discussed earlier, include cough, sputum production, changes in chest x-ray, and pulmonary function tests. Frequently, the nurse may detect signs of respiratory problems in patients who present with other medical problems. Since lung disease affects many systems and can complicate various therapeutic modalities such as anesthetics, oxygen, and drug therapy, the nurse must carry out a thorough pulmonary assessment during the earliest contact with the patient. Nursing diagnoses frequently identified in the patient with pulmonary problems include ineffective breathing patterns, ineffective airway clearance, airway irritability, poor nutrition, poor hydration, decreased activity tolerance, depression, sleep disturbances, cognitive deficits, and impaired sexuality.

As dehydration and electrolyte imbalance may accompany acute episodes, clinical and laboratory assessment of fluid and electrolyte balance are imperative initially and throughout treatment. Some imbalances may occur as results of treatment or may not be initially evident, for example, the hypokalemia that appears after respiratory acidosis is corrected.

Blood gas analysis during an acute episode may indicate hypoxemia and metabolic and respiratory acidosis. The best indicator of respiratory failure is the slope of the arterial curve. Hypoxemia and hypercapnia are often manifested by anxiety, mental confusion, and restlessness, although an exhausted patient may not exhibit these signs. Frequent mental status assessment during an acute episode is imperative.

Serial pulmonary function tests are an invaluable tool to detect and monitor pulmonary status. Spirometry, flow-volume loops, body plethysmograph, and peak flow meters provide means for the medical team to objectively assess changes in respiratory status.

Management

The goals of nursing care during the acute phase are to reduce hypoxemia, promote pulmonary hygiene, improve pulmonary functions, and relieve patient and family anxiety. It is desirable during the interim period between acute episodes to ensure that the patient is able to maintain the highest level of health and functioning and to identify early signs of deterioration and take appropriate steps to avoid acute problems, if possible.

Administration of oxygen and decreasing the demand for oxygen by promoting rest are methods of reducing hypoxia. The objective is usually to raise the arterial oxygen pressure above 50 mmHg, without elevation of the arterial carbon dioxide level due to respiratory depression. The blood gas measurements and the signs of CO_2 narcosis (lethargy, confusion, respiratory depression, difficult arousal) must be monitored. Oxygen should be administered continuously and not intermittently to the patient with hypoxia, as the Pa_{O_2} may drop dangerously low if oxygen is withdrawn abruptly for ambulation to the bathroom, eating, and so on. This may necessitate the use of portable oxygen tanks or extensions on the oxygen line.

The use of bronchodilators such as sympathomimetic or theophylline to relieve bronchospasm will also be helpful to reverse hypoxia. If the arterial pH drops below 7.2, the sympathomimetic bronchodilators will be ineffective. Constant IV infusion of aminophylline and/or isoproterenol requires constant ECG monitoring being cognizant of cardiac arrhythmias, tachycardia, vital signs, and arterial blood gas measurements. Pulse rate parameters should be delineated by the physician. Observation of mental changes, excitation, or exhaustion may necessitate modification of the use of these agents.

The upright position (high Fowler's with arm resting on a table) promotes respiratory excursion. Patients also must be taught proper methods of pursed-lip exhalation and breathing exercises when well and be encouraged and coached in their performance during acute episodes.

Pulmonary hygiene includes adequate hydration, coughing and deep breathing (with interspersed rest periods and postural drainage), clapping, and vibration (if not otherwise contraindicated). Postural drainage, clapping, and vibration should be performed after the bronchodilator is administered to prevent the bronchospasms that can result from these procedures.

Proper use of the nebulizer is an important part of patient education. Although the use of space tubes and air chambers seems to improve delivery of aerosols in patients with coordination problems, it is not generally better than employing good technique. Patient education is the key to interim management. The patient should know the names, dosage, frequency, actions, and adverse effects of drugs to be taken at home. Young children should be actively involved in their own care and be given increasing responsibility for own medications as they develop. Since the effects of bronchodilators can be cumulative or harmful to the respiratory tract, patients should be aware of the maximum number of doses that may be used each day.

Calm, competent, quick performance of necessary activities by the nurse serves to decrease anxiety. Appropriate use of touch, as during breathing exercises, can also be reassuring. All patients should be able to identify their own triggers, how to avoid triggers when possible, and, when it is not, how to recognize and treat early signs of respiratory distress.

Education programs must also stress when to call the physician. Symptoms requiring outside intervention are specific for each patient but might include changes in sputum production, increasing respiratory distress, chest tightness and pain, unusual fatigue, and ankle swelling. Anytime subcutaneous epinephrine is given at home the physician should be notified.

Dehydration is a frequent effect of increased respiratory work. Hydration is best achieved with oral fluids to maintain urine specific gravity between 1.005 and 1.015 in an otherwise healthy individual. Patients with cor pulmonale, kidney disease, and so on, need closer monitoring. Other factors influencing patient success include cessation of smoking and increasing physical activity; swimming, aerobic exercises and jogging are excellent physical exercises. The obese patient should be taught appropriate and safe diet regimes. Group support such as the Weight Watchers program has proved to be one of the most successful approaches to weight control.

Family education in addition to patient education is a nursing responsibility. Chronic illness of any member affects the whole family. Lack of knowledge, fear of the unknown, changes in lifestyle, and financial drain increase stress levels of all those affected. Family discord, divorce, depression, and patient isolation often result. Integration of family members into the education process and into the patient's care may decrease fear with knowledge of how to cope effectively with an acute episode of respiratory distress. If inappropriate coping or depression persist, family and individual therapy is often helpful.

Evaluation

Outcome criteria for ineffective breathing patterns may include improvement in dyspnea, fatigue, and Pa_{CO_2} and Pa_{O_2}. The patient should be able to demonstrate breathing exercises and relaxation techniques. Ineffective airway clearance outcome criteria most likely will include changes in chest x-ray; wheezes and rales; improvement in hypoxia and hypercapnea; demonstrated knowledge of adequate hydration; and so on. Evaluation of nursing care is the essential component if care of the patient with respiratory disease is to be successful.

CASE STUDY

P.K. is a 62-year-old married house painter. Recently he had noticed exertional dyspnea. He had rarely sought health care in the past but had now come to the clinic complaining of a "bad chest cold" with severe shortness of breath.

Significant history included a 40-year habit of smoking two packs of cigarettes a day. He admitted to a smoker's cough with sputum production in the morning and evening. Among the positive findings on examination were bilateral inspiratory and expiratory rhonchi; easily expectorated sputum in which D. pneumoniae was later identified: Pa_{O_2} of 50 mmHg and Pa_{CO_2} of 50 mmHg on room air; increased anteroposterior diameter of the chest wall and depressed diaphragm on chest x-ray; FEV_1 60 percent of forced vital capacity (normal, 75 to 85 percent); heart rate 100/min, respirations 22, and oral temperature 100°F; and hematocrit reading 50 percent.

Ampicillin was started orally at a dose of 500 mg q6h for 3 days and then reduced to 250 mg q6h for an additional 4 days. The physician advised the patient to discontinue smoking. Referral was made to the respiratory nurse specialist for patient education and follow-up of chronic bronchitis.

Assessment

The nurse met with P.K. and his wife briefly. In view of the physician's findings, the nurse determined that the patient was too ill for any in-depth teaching at that time, so only essential instruction was done. The nurse explained that the ampicillin should be taken with a full glass of water and that concurrent ingestion of food could inhibit the absorption of the drug and reviewed the dosage schedule. The patient was encouraged by the nurse to reduce his smoking, with an explanation that cigarettes are a leading cause of chronic bronchitis but that damage could be halted or even reversed if he quit smoking. Mr. and Mrs. K. agreed to meet with the nurse in 2 weeks at his return appointment and were instructed to call the nurse if he did not improve steadily or if they had any questions.

At the next appointment, the patient's pulmonary function studies had improved but were still consistent with airway obstruction; his vital signs were normal; his Pa_{O_2} had increased to 60 mmHg. The nurse noted rare inspiratory and expiratory rhonchi and wheezes on auscultation. The patient reported that he had decreased his smoking to one pack of cigarettes per day. His weight was 85 kg, 15 kg over his optimal weight, which constituted an excess burden to his heart and lungs.

Because of the importance of preventing mucus impaction due to impaired mucociliary clearance, a bronchodilator, isoetherine (Bronkosol) 0.05 mL bid, was ordered by the physician. He was also started on a sustained-release theophylline (Theodur) 300 mg bid.

Management

The patient was given the choice of administering the bronchodilator by hand bulb or pump-driven nebulizer after a demonstration of each by the nurse. He chose the latter and was instructed to use 0.5 mL of isoetherine and 0.5 mL of water followed by 5 min of inhaling nebulized water. The patient first carried out self-administration of the drug at the clinic with the nurse watching. Coughing exercises produced large amounts of yellow sputum, which impressed the patient with the value of the drug and exercises. Mr. and Mrs. K. were told to contact the nurse if he experienced severe headache, nausea, palpitations, or tremor, which the drug occasionally caused. The importance of further decreasing smoking was stressed.

The nurse instructed Mr. and Mrs. K. in a reducing diet. Along with this plan the patient was encouraged to walk three or four times a day, gradually increasing the distance. This would in time improve his exercise tolerance and decrease his dyspnea.

Proper breathing could also alleviate dyspnea. The patient was instructed to sit in a comfortable supported position, take a relaxed slow breath, and tense the abdominal muscles and purse his lips while slowly exhaling (without force). This form of breathing was to be utilized at the onset of dyspnea or anxiety. By being provided with a method to alleviate the dyspnea, he would be better able to control his anxiety, thus breaking the cycle of dyspnea leading to anxiety causing increased dyspnea, etc.

Even though Mr. and Mrs. K. seemed to understand all the nurse's instructions, these were reinforced with a simple illustrated manual that would serve as a reference at home.

Evaluation

At a return appointment in 2 weeks, the couple demonstrated good retention of instructions. Even though the patient had not lost any weight, he had further reduced his smoking to three-quarters of a pack. His theophylline concentration was 12 μg/mL, which is in the therapeutic range. The nurse reinforced the previous teaching and commended him on his progress. On auscultation the nurse noted improved breath sounds, and the patient reported increased exercise tolerance and no signs of adverse effects.

The patient would be seen at the clinic every 3 months and understood that he was to come immediately if he developed a change in pulmonary symptoms.

REFERENCES

Guidelines for Nursing Care of the Pulmonary Patient, Los Angeles: California Thoracic Society, 1984.

"Manual on the Standardization of Care of the Severely Asthmatic Care, American Academy of Pediatrics," *J Asthma Res,* 13:1976.

Bauer, L. A., M. Gibaldi, and R. E. Vestal: "Influences of Pharmacokinetic Diurnal Variation on Bioavailability Estimates," *Clin Pharmacokinet* 9:184–187, 1984.

Becker, A. B., K. J. Simons, C. A. Gillespie, and F. R. Simons: "The Bronchodilator Effects and Pharmacokinetics of Caffeine in Asthma," *N Engl J Med,* 310:743–746, 1984.

Boushey, H. A., and W. Gold: "Anticholinergic Drugs," in E. Middleton, C. E. Reed, and E. F. Ellis (eds.), *Allergy Principles and Practice,* St. Louis: Mosby, 1983.

Cherniack, R. M.: *Current Therapy of Respiratory Disease 1984–1985,* Philadelphia: B. C. Decker; St. Louis: C. V. Mosby; 1984.

Cherniack, R. M., and L. Cherniack: *Respiration in Health and Disease,* 3d ed., Philadelphia: Saunders, 1983.

D'Agonstino, J. S.: "Set Your Mind at Ease on Oxygen Toxicity," *Nursing 83,* 13:54–56, 1983.

Dederich, R. A., S. J. Szefler, and E. R. Green: "Intrasubject Variation in Sustained-Release Theophylline Absorption," *J Allergy Clin Immunol,* 67:465–471, 1981.

Ellmyer, P.: "A Guide to Your Patient's Safe Home Use of Oxygen," *Nursing 82,* 12:55–57, 1982.

Eriksson, N. E., K. Haglind, and K. C. Hindinger: "A New Inhalation Technique for Freon Aerosols: Terbutaline Aerosol with a Tube Extension: A 2 Day Crossover Comparison with Salbutamol Aerosol," *Allergy,* 35:617–622, 1980.

Gordon, M.: *Manual of Nursing Diagnosis,* New York: McGraw-Hill, 1982.

Hendeles, L., and M. Weinberger: "Theophylline," in E. Middleton, C. E. Reed, and E. F. Ellis (eds.), *Allergy Principles and Practice,* St. Louis: Mosby, 1983.

Hendeles, L., M. Weinberger, and G. Johnson: "Theophylline," in W. E. Evens, J. J. Schentag, and W. J. Juskeo (eds.), *Applied Pharmacokinetics, Principles of Therapeutic Drug Monitoring,* San Francisco: Applied Therapeutics, 1980.

Johnson, H. G.: "Cromoglycate and Other Inhibitors of Mediator Release," in E. Middleton, C. E. Reed, and E. F. Ellis (eds.), *Allergy Principles and Practice,* St. Louis: Mosby, 1983.

King, C.: "Examining the Thorax and Respiratory System," *RN,* 45:54–63, 1982.

Mascia, A.: "Rehabilitation of the Child with Chronic Asthma," in J. A. Downey and L. L. Niels (eds.) *The Child with Disabling Illness,* New York: Raven, 1982.

Mitenko, P. A., and R. I. Ogilvie: "Rational Intravenous Doses of Theophylline," *N Engl J Med,* 289:600–603, 1973.

Morris, H.: "Pharmacology of Corticosteroids in Asthma," in E. Middleton, C. E. Reed, and E. F. Ellis (eds.), *Allergy Principles and Practice,* St. Louis: Mosby, 1983.

Paterson, J. W., A. J. Woolcock, and G. M. Shenfield: *Am Rev Respir Dis,* **120**:1149–1179, 1979.

Powell, J. R., and L. Hak: "Asthma Products," in *Handbook of Nonprescription Drugs,* 7th ed., Washington, DC: American Pharmaceutical Association, 1982.

Rall, T. W.: "Central Nervous System Stimulants, The Xanthines," in A. G. Gilman, L. S. Goodman, and A. Gilman (eds.), *Goodman and Gilman's The Pharmacological Basis of Therapeutics,* 6th ed., New York: Macmillan, 1980.

Rogers, R. J., S. J. Szefler, M. B. Wiener, and A. Kalisker: "Inconsistent Absorption from a Sustained-Release Theophylline Preparation during Continuous Therapy in Asthmatic Children," *J Pediatrics* (in press).

Sjoberg, E. L.: "Nursing Diagnosis and the COPD Patient," *Am J Nurs,* **83**:244–248, 1983.

Szentivanyi, A.: "The Beta Adrenergic Theory of Atopic Abnormality in Bronchial Asthma," *J Allergy Clin Immunol,* **42**:203–232, 1968.

Venter, J. C., C. M. Fraser, H. S. Nelson, and E. Middleton: "Adrenergic Agents," in E. Middleton, C. E. Reed, and E. F. Ellis (eds.), *Allergy Principles and Practice,* St. Louis: Mosby, 1983.

Westra, B.: "Assessment under Pressure: When Your Patient Says I Can't Breath," *Nursing 84,* **14**:34–39, 1984.

Ziment, I.: *Respiratory Pharmacology and Therapeutics,* Philadelphia: Saunders, 1978.

28

INFECTIOUS DISORDERS I: GENERAL PRINCIPLES OF ANTIMICROBIAL THERAPY AND ACUTE BACTERIAL INFECTIONS*

SHELDON LEFKOWITZ
SANDE JONES
CATHERINE JOHNSON

GENERAL PRINCIPLES OF ANTIMICROBIAL THERAPY

LEARNING OBJECTIVES

Upon mastery of this section of this chapter, the reader will be able to:

1. Describe the two basic principles used in the selection of an antimicrobial agent.

2. Describe the differences between the disc diffusion and tube dilution tests for determining antimicrobial sensitivity.

3. List four host factors used in selecting an antimicrobial agent for the treatment of an infectious disease.

4. Define and give examples of broad-spectrum and narrow-spectrum antimicrobials.

5. Define and give examples of bactericidal and bacteriostatic antimicrobial agents.

6. List four possible mechanisms of action for antimicrobial agents and give an example for each.

7. Name three antimicrobials that cannot be given orally.

8. Give two indications for using antimicrobials intravenously.

9. Describe two methods to avoid IV incompatibilities of antimicrobials.

10. List three mechanisms by which microorganisms can become resistant to antimicrobials.

11. Give two techniques that will prevent the development of resistance.

12. Give three indications for antimicrobial prophylaxis.

13. Describe the problems associated with noncompliance to antimicrobial therapy and the nurse's role in assuring compliance.

14. Discuss the role of the nurse in the assessment, management, and evaluation of infectious disease.

With the introduction of **sulfanilamide** (a sulfonamide) in 1936, a new era began in the treatment of infectious diseases. In 1941 **penicillin** was introduced as the first antimicrobial agent which could be mass produced in quantities large enough to reach a wide patient population. In the years since then, numerous antimicrobial agents which have dramati-

*The editors thank Arthur Lipman and Susan Molde, who contributed the chapter on infectious disease in the first edition.

cally improved the outlook for the treatment of infectious diseases have been introduced. However, the widespread use of these new "wonder drugs" has brought about its own set of new problems. Aside from their adverse side effects, these drugs have become a widely misused tool in medicine. This misuse has led to the emergence of drug-resistant pathogens. This, in turn, has led to the development of still more antimicrobial agents, as well as improved methods for monitoring drug concentrations and better methods for isolating and identifying the pathogenic organisms themselves.

Antibiosis is the process in which a substance from one living organism destroys or inhibits the growth of another type of organism. Although antibiotics were originally produced from bacteria, fungi, and other microorganisms, some of the new drugs broadly classified as antibiotics have been totally or partially synthesized. This has increased their production while greatly lowering their cost.

To be useful in chemotherapy a chemical must not only inhibit microbial growth; it must also have few harmful side effects in the host. Such drugs are said to have a *favorable therapeutic index.* Potentially toxic chemicals can also be used if care is taken to identify persons at risk for the toxicity before administering the drug.

The information on infectious diseases will be presented in two chapters. The first covers the therapeutic principles of treatment, the basic clinical pharmacology and therapeutics of the drugs, and a discussion of the treatment of some bacterial infections. The second chapter (29) covers the treatment of nonbacterial infections, including mycobacterial, fungal, protozoal, and viral infections.

SELECTION OF ANTIMICROBIAL AGENTS

The cornerstone of treatment for an infected patient is the isolation and identification of the microorganism involved, then determining the antimicrobial agents to which it is susceptible. However, because of the time lag involved in this process (often about 48 h), the initial treatment must frequently be based entirely on clinical impression (history, physical examination, microscopic examination and rapid laboratory tests), although specimens should always be obtained for culture before antimicrobial therapy is started. Assuming the site of the infection and the circumstances under which it developed are known, an educated guess can be made about the likely pathogens. Then antimicrobial therapy can be started with agents that cover the suspected microorganisms (Table 28-1).

The patterns of antibiotic resistance for an organism can vary dramatically in different parts of the world, and this must be taken into consideration when choosing the antibiotic used for initial treatment. For example, regional differences in the organisms causing gram-negative endocarditis in drug abusers exist in the United States. Even within a single hospital the antibiotic susceptibility of a microor-

ganism can change abruptly. This can be seen in the spread of methicillin-resistant *Staphylococcus aureus* in American hospitals. Other factors which should be taken into consideration when deciding on an initial course of therapy are the relative cost of the antibiotics, patient allergies, and the possible effects on organ functions.

The value of simple laboratory examinations in choosing antibiotics cannot be overemphasized. Gram-stained material from an infection site may help identify pathogens and focus antibiotic therapy. When a culture from a single site yields several organisms, a Gram's stain can help determine the most likely pathogen. An acid-fast smear test can also be very useful for diagnosis.

Once the list of possible pathogens has been narrowed down, initial therapy can be started. This initial therapy will naturally be open to revision when the organism(s) are positively identified and sensitivity tests performed.

Sensitivity Tests

Two different sensitivity tests can be used to determine the in vitro sensitivity of microorganisms to antimicrobial agents. They are the disc diffusion method and the tube dilution method.

The *disc diffusion* technique uses an agar-filled petri dish that has been streaked with the organism. Small filter paper discs containing known amounts of antimicrobial agents are placed on the agar and allowed to diffuse into it for 18–24 h in an incubator. If the organism is sensitive to the antibiotic, an area of no growth (called a *zone of inhibition*) will occur around the discs. The larger this zone of inhibition, the more sensitive the organism is to the drug. The test is easy to perform, relatively inexpensive, and provides some quantitative information on the susceptibility of an organism to a drug. The antibiotics tested are often classified as sensitive, resistant, or intermediate sensitivity to the drug tested.

The *tube dilution* method uses known dilutions of the antibiotic in a liquid or solid medium that is inoculated with the organism. After incubation the lowest concentration of the drug that inhibits growth is known as the *minimum inhibitory concentration (MIC).* The lowest concentration that sterilizes the medium is called the *minimum bactericidal concentration (MBC).* The MBC is used only in special clinical situations when exact measurement is needed. Some laboratories report MIC while others translate this information into the categories of sensitive or resistant.

Host Factors

The clinical status of the host (the patient) determines when the antibiotic therapy is started, how it is administered, and which drug is chosen. If the patient is stable, the therapy can be delayed until laboratory tests are completed. Patients with

TABLE 28-1 Antimicrobial Drugs of Choice

INFECTING ORGANISM	DRUG OF FIRST CHOICE	ALTERNATIVE DRUGS
Gram-Positive Cocci		
Staphylococcus aureus or S. epidermidis[*]		
Non-penicillinase-producing	Penicillin G or V[1]	A cephalosporin[2,3]; vancomycin; clindamycin
Penicillinase-producing	A penicillinase-resistant penicillin[4]	A cephalosporin[2,3]; vancomycin, clindamycin
Methicillin-resistant[5]	Vancomycin, with or without rifampin[6] and/or gentamicin	Trimethoprim-sulfamethoxazole[6]
Streptococcus pyogenes (Group A) and Groups C and G	Penicillin G or V[1]	An erythromycin[7]; a cephalosporin[2,3], vancomycin[6]
Streptococcus, Group B	Penicillin G or ampicillin	A cephalosporin[2,3]; vancomycin; an erythromycin[6]
Streptococcus, viridans group[8]	Penicillin G with or without streptomycin	A cephalosporin[2,3]; vancomycin[6]
Streptococcus, enterococcus group		
Endocarditis[8] or other severe infection	Ampicillin or penicillin G with gentamicin or streptomycin	Vancomycin[6] with gentamicin or streptomycin
Uncomplicated urinary tract infection[9]	Ampicillin or amoxicillin	Nitrofurantoin
Streptococcus, anaerobic (peptostreptococcus)	Penicillin G	Clindamycin; chloramphenicol[6,11]; a cephalosporin[2,3]; an erythromycin[6]
Streptococcus pneumoniae (pneumococcus)	Penicillin G or V[1,12]	An erythromycin[7,12], a cephalosporin[2,3], chloramphenicol[6,11,12], vancomycin[6]
Gram-Negative Cocci		
Neisseria gonorrhoeae[13] (gonococcus)	Amoxicillin followed by a tetracycline[10] or penicillin G	A tetracycline; ampicillin; spectinomycin; cefoxitin,[2] cefuroxime,[2] cefotaxime,[2] or ceftizoxime[2]
Neisseria meningitidis[14] (meningococcus)	Penicillin G	Chloramphenicol[6,11]; cefuroxime[2]; cefotaxime[2]; a sulfonamide[15]
Gram-Positive Bacilli		
Bacillus anthracis (anthrax)	Penicillin G	An erythromycin[6]; a tetracycline[10]
Clostridium perfringens (welchii)[16]	Penicillin G	Chloramphenicol[6,11], clindamycin[6]; metronidazole; a tetracycline[10]
Clostridium tetani[17]	Penicillin G	A tetracycline[10]
Clostridium difficile	Vancomycin	Metronidazole; bacitracin[6]
Corynebacterium diphtheriae[18]	An erythromycin	Penicillin G

445

TABLE 28-1 Antimicrobial Drugs of Choice (*Continued*)

INFECTING ORGANISM	DRUG OF FIRST CHOICE	ALTERNATIVE DRUGS
Enteric Gram-Negative Bacilli		
Bacteroides		
Oropharyngeal strains	Penicillin G[6,19]	Clindamycin; cefoxitin[2]; metronidazole
Gastrointestinal strains[20]	Clindamycin or metronidazole	Cefoxitin[2], chloramphenicol[6,11]; mezlocillin, ticarcillin, or piperacillin
Enterobacter	Gentamicin,[21] tobramycin,[21] or netilmicin[21]	Amikacin[21]; cefotaxime[2] or ceftizoxime[2]; carbenicillin, ticarcillin, mezlocillin, piperacillin, or azlocillin; trimethoprim-sulfamethoxazole; chloramphenicol[6,11]
Escherichia coli[22]	Gentamicin,[23] tobramycin,[23] or netilmicin[23]	Amikacin[23]; ampicillin; carbenicillin, ticarcillin, mezlocillin, piperacillin, or azlocillin; a cephalosporin[2,3]; trimethoprim-sulfamethoxazole; a tetracycline[10], chloramphenicol[6,11]
Klebsiella pneumoniae[22]	Gentamicin,[24] tobramycin,[24] or netilmicin[24]	Amikacin[24]; a cephalosporin[2,3], trimethoprim-sulfamethoxazole; a tetracycline[10], chloramphenicol[6,11]; mezlocillin or piperacillin
Proteus mirabilis[22]	Ampicillin[25]	A cephalosporin[2,3], gentamicin, tobramycin, or netilmicin; amikacin; carbenicillin, ticarcillin, mezlocillin, piperacillin, or azlocillin; trimethoprim-sulfamethoxazole; chloramphenicol[6,11]
Proteus, * indole-positive (including *Providencia rettgeri, Morganella morganii, and Proteus vulgaris*)	Gentamicin,[21] tobramycin,[21] or netilmicin[21]	Amikacin[21]; cefotaxime[2] or ceftizoxime[2]; carbenicillin, ticarcillin, mezlocillin, piperacillin, or azlocillin; trimethoprim-sulfamethoxazole; a tetracycline[6,10], chloramphenicol[6,11]; cefoxitin[2]
Salmonella typhi[26]	Chloramphenicol[11]	Ampicillin; amoxicillin[6], trimethoprim-sulfamethoxazole
Other *Salmonella*[27]	Ampicillin or amoxicillin[6]	Chloramphenicol[11]; trimethoprim-sulfamethoxazole
Serratia *	Gentamicin[21] or amikacin[21]	Cefotaxime[2] or ceftizoxime[2]; trimethoprim-sulfamethoxazole[6]; carbenicillin,[6] ticarcillin,[6] mezlocillin,[6] or piperacillin,[6] or azlocillin, cefoxitin[2,6]
Shigella *	Trimethoprim-sulfamethoxazole	chloramphenicol[6,11]; a tetracycline[10], ampicillin
Other Gram-Negative Bacilli		
Acinetobacter (Mima, Herellea) *	Tobramycin,[6,28] gentamicin,[6,28] or netilmicin[6,28]	Amikacin[28], kanamycin; carbenicillin,[6] ticarcillin,[6] mezlocillin,[6] piperacillin,[6] or azlocillin,[6] trimethoprim-sulfamethoxazole[6]; minocycline[10], doxycycline[10]
Bordetella pertussis (whooping cough)	An erythromycin	Trimethoprim-sulfamethoxazole,[6] ampicillin[6]
Brucella (brucellosis) *	A tetracycline[10] with or without streptomycin	Chloramphenicol[6,11] with or without streptomycin; trimethoprim-sulfamethozazole[6]
Francisella tularensis (tularemia) *	Streptomycin, gentamicin,[6] tobramycin,[6] or amikacin[6]	A tetracycline[10], chloramphenicol[6,11]
Fusobacterium *	Penicillin G	Metronidazole; clindamycin[6], chloramphenicol[6,11]
Gardnerella (Haemophilus) *vaginalis*[13]	Metronidazole[6]	Ampicillin[6]

Haemophilus ducreyi (chancroid)	Trimethoprim-sulfamethoxazole[6] or an erythromycin[6]	A tetracycline[10]; streptomycin
Haemophilus influenzae		
Meningitis, epiglottitis, arthritis, and other serious infections	Chloramphenicol plus ampicillin initially[29]	Cefuroxime[2]; cefotaxime[2]; trimethoprim-sulfamethoxazole[6]
Other infections	Ampicillin or amoxicillin	Trimethoprim-sulfamethoxazole; cefuroxime[2]; a sulfonamide; cefaclor[2]; cefamandole,[2] cefotaxime[2]; ceftizoxime[2]; a tetracycline[10]
Legionella micdadei (*L. pittsburgensis*)	An erythromycin[6] with or without rifampin[6,30]	
Legionella pneumophila	An erythromycin with or without rifampin[6,30]	
Leptotrichia buccalis (Vincent's infection)	Penicillin G	A tetracycline[6,10]; clindamycin[6]
Pseudomonas aeruginosa		
Urinary tract infection	Carbenicillin or ticarcillin	Piperacillin, mezlocillin, or azlocillin; gentamicin; tobramycin; netilmicin; amikacin; a polymyxin
Other infections[31]	Tobramycin, gentamicin, or netilmicin with carbenicillin, ticarcillin, mezlocillin, piperacillin, or azlocillin	Amikacin with carbenicillin, ticarcillin, mezlocillin, piperacillin, or azlocillin; cefoperazone[2,3]
Pseudomonas pseudomallei (melioidosis)	Trimethoprim-sulfamethoxazole[6]	A tetracycline[6,10] with or without chloramphenicol[11,32]; chloramphenicol[11] plus kanamycin, gentamicin or tobramycin; a sulfonamide[6]
Pseudomonas cepacia	Trimethoprim-sulfamethoxazole[6]	Chloramphenicol[6,11]
Spirillum minus (rat bite fever)	Penicillin G	A tetracycline[6,10]; streptomycin
Streptobacillus moniliformis (rat bite fever; Haverhill fever)	Penicillin G	A tetracycline[6,10]; streptomycin
	Acid-Fast Bacilli	
Vibrio cholerae (cholera)[33]	A tetracycline[10]	Trimethoprim-sulfamethoxazole[6]
Yersinia pestis (plague)	Streptomycin	A tetracycline[10]; chloramphenicol[6,11]; gentamicin[6]
Mycobacterium tuberculosis[34]	Isoniazid with rifampin[35]	Ethambutol; streptomycin[11]; pyrazinamide; para-aminosalicylic acid (PAS); cycloserine[11]; ethionamide[11]; kanamycin[6,11]; capreomycin[11];
Mycobacterium kansasii[34]	Isoniazid[6] with rifampin[6] with or without ethambuto[6]	Streptomycin[11]; ethionamide[6,11]; cycloserine[6,11]
Mycobacterium avium-intracellulare-scrofulaceum complex[34]	Isoniazid,[16] rifampin,[6] ethambutol,[6] and streptomycin[11]	Clofazime[36]; capreomycin[6,11]; ethionamide[6,11]; cycloserine[6,11]; ansemicin[36]; thienamycin[36], amikacin[6]
Mycobacterium fortuitum[34]	Amikacin[6,11] and doxycycline[6]	Rifampin[6], an erythromycin[6]
Mycobacterium leprae (leprosy)	Dapsone[11] with rifampin[6] with or without clofazimine[36]	Acedapsone[11,36]; ethionamide[11]; prothionamide[36]

447

TABLE 28-1 Antimicrobial Drugs of Choice (*Continued*)

INFECTING ORGANISM	DRUG OF FIRST CHOICE	ALTERNATIVE DRUGS
	Actinomycetes	
Actionmyces israelii (actinomycosis)	Penicillin G	A tetracycline[10]
Nocardia	Trisulfapyramidines	Trimethoprim-sulfamethoxazole[6]; minocycline,[6] trisulfapyrimidines with minocycline,[6] ampicillin,[6] or erythromycin[6]; amikacin[6,11]; cycloserine[6,11]
	Chlamydiae	
Chlamydia psittaci (psittacosis; ornithosis)	A tetracycline[10]	Chloramphenicol[11]
Chlamydia trachomatis[13]		
(Pneumonia)	An erythromycin[6]	A sulfonamide; a tetracycline[10]
(Urethritis or pelvic inflammatory disease)	A tetracycline[10] or an erythromycin[6]	Sulfisoxazole[6]
	Mycoplasma	
Mycoplasma pneumoniae	An erythromycin or a tetracycline[10]	
Ureaplasma urealyticum	An erythromycin[6]	A tetracycline[6,10]
	Rickettsia	
Rocky Mountain spotted fever, endemic typhus (murine), tick bite fever, trench fever, typhus, scrub typhus, Q fever	A tetracycline[10]	Chloramphenicol[11]
	Spirochetes	
Leptospira	Penicillin G[6]	A tetracycline[6,10]
Treponema pallidum (syphilis)	Penicillin G[1]	A tetracycline[10], an erythromycin
Treponema pertenue (yaws)	Penicillin G[6]	A tetracycline[10]
	Viruses	
Herpes simplex (keratitis)	Trifluridine (topical)	Vidarabine (topical); idozuridine (topical)
(Genital)	Acyclovir	
(Encephalitis)	Vidarabine	Acyclovir[6]
(Neonatal)	Vidarabine	Acyclovir[6]
(Disseminated, adult)	Acyclovir	Vidarabine[6]
Influenza A	Amantadine	
Varicella zoster	Vidarabine[6] or acyclovir[6]	

*Resistance may be a problem, and susceptibility tests should be performed.

[1]Penicillin V is preferred for oral treatment of infections caused by non-penicillinase-producing staphylococci and other gram-positive cocci but is ineffective for gonorrhea. For initial therapy of severe infections, crystalline penicillin G, administered parenterally, is first choice. For somewhat longer action in less severe infections due to Group A streptococci; pneumococci, gonococci, or *Treponema pallidum*, procaine penicillin G, an intramuscular formulation, is administered once or twice daily. Benzathine penicillin G, a slowly absorbed intramuscular preparation, is usually given in a single monthly injection for prophylaxis of rheumatic fever, once for treatment of Group A streptococcal pharyngitis, and once or more for treatment of syphilis.

[2]The cephalosporins have been used as alternatives to penicillins in patients allergic to penicillins, but such patients may also have allergic reactions to cephalosporins.

[3]For parenteral treatment of staphylococcal infections, a "first-generation" cephalosporin such as cephalothin, cephapirin, cephradine, or cefazolin can be used; for staphylococcal endocarditis, some Medical Letter consultants prefer cephalothin or cephapirin. For oral therapy, cephalexin or cephradine can be used. The "second-generation" cephalosporins cefamandole, cefuroxime, and cefoxitin and the "third-generation" cephalosporins cefotaxime, cefoperazone, and ceftizoxime have greater activity against enteric gram-negative bacilli, and cefoxitin is active against many strains of Bacteroides fragilis. Moxalactam, another "third-generation" cephalosporin, has been associated with serious, sometimes fatal, bleeding disorders, and some Medical Letter consultants now advise against its use; in any case, it should not be used to treat infections caused by gram-positive organisms. With the exception of cefoperazone, the activity of all currently available (February 1984) cephalosporins against Pseudomonas aeruginosa is poor or inconsistent.

[4]For oral use against penicillinase-producing staphylococci, cloxacillin or dicloxacillin is preferred; for severe infections, a parenteral formulation of methicillin, nafcillin, or oxacillin should be used. Neither ampicillin, amoxicillin, bacampicillin, cyclacillin, hetacillin, carbenicillin, ticarcillin, mezlocillin, azlocillin, nor piperacillin is effective against penicillinase-producing staphylococci.

[5]Occasional strains of coagulase-positive staphylococci and many strains of coagulase-negative staphylococci are resistant to penicillinase-resistant penicillins; these strains are also resistant to cephalosporins.

[6]Not approved for this indication by the U.S. Food and Drug Administration.

[7]Occasional strains of Group A streptococci and pneumococci may be resistant to erythromycins.

[8]In endocarditis, disc sensitivity testing may not provide adequate information; dilution tests for susceptibility should be used to assess bactericidal as well as inhibitory end points. Peak bactericidal activity of the serum against the patient's own organism should be present at a serum dilution of at least 1:8.

[9]Routine antimicrobial susceptibility tests may be misleading. Because of high urine concentrations, ampicillin may be effective in urinary tract infections, even when the organism is reported to be "resistant."

[10]Tetracycline hydrochloride is preferred for most indications. Doxycycline is recommended for uremic patients with infections outside the urinary tract for which a tetracycline is indicated. Tetracyclines are generally not recommended for pregnant women, infants, or children eight years old or younger.

[11]Because of the frequency of serious adverse effects, this drug should be used only for severe infections when less hazardous drugs are ineffective.

[12]In patients allergic to penicillin, an erythromycin is preferred for respiratory infections, and chloramphenicol is recommended for meningitis. Rare strains of Streptococcus pneumoniae may be resistant to penicillin; these strains are susceptible to vancomycin.

[13]For more details, see Table 28-21.

[14]Rifampin is recommended for prophylaxis in close contacts of patients infected by sulfonamide-resistant organisms. Minocycline may also be effective for such prophylaxis but frequently causes vomiting and vertigo. An oral sulfonamide is recommended for prophylaxis in close contacts of patients known to be infected by sulfonamide-sensitive organisms.

[15]Sulfonamide-resistant strains are frequent in the United States and sulfonamides should be used only when susceptibility is established by susceptibility tests.

[16]Debridement is primary. Large doses of penicillin G are required. Hyperbaric oxygen therapy may be a useful adjunct to surgical debridement in management of the spreading, necrotic type.

[17]For prophylaxis, a tetanus toxoid booster and, for some patients, tetanus immune globulin (human) are required.

[18]Antitoxin is primary; antimicrobials are used only to halt further toxin production and to prevent the carrier state.

[19]The proportion of penicillin-resistant Bacteroides species from the oropharynx has been increasing recently; for patients seriously ill with infections due to these organisms, or where response to penicillin is delayed, clindamycin is preferred.

[20]When infection is in the central nervous system, either intravenous metronidazole or chloramphenicol is recommended.

[21]In severely ill patients Medical Letter consultants would add carbenicillin, ticarcillin, meelocillin, piperacillin, or azlocillin (but see footnote 31) or cefotaxime or ceftizoxime.

[22]For an acute, uncomplicated urinary tract infection, before the infecting organism is known, the drug of first choice is one of the oral soluble sulfonamides, such as sulfisoxazole, or (for E. coli or Proteus mirabilis) ampicillin or amoxicillin, or (for Klebsiella) a cephalosporin. Trimethoprim or trimethoprim-sulfamethoxazole may also be useful for treatment of urinary tract infections caused by susceptible organisms.

[23]In severely ill patients Medical Letter consultants would add ampicillin, carbenicillin, ticarcillin, mezlocillin, piperacillin, azlocillin, or a cephalosporin, but see footnote 31.

[24]In severely ill patients Medical Letter consultants would add a cephalosporin.

[25]Large doses (6 grams or more daily) are usually necessary for systemic infections. In severely ill patients, some Medical Letter consultants would add gentamicin, tobramycin, netilmicin, or amikacin.

[26]Ampicillin or amoxicillin may be effective in milder cases. Ampicillin is the drug of choice for S. typhi carriers.

[27]Most cases of Salmonella gastroenteritis subside spontaneously without antimicrobial therapy.

[28]In severe infections some Medical Letter consultants would add carbenicillin, ticarcillin, mezlocillin, piperacillin, or azlocillin, but see footnote 31.

449

Footnotes to Table 28-1 (*Cont.*)

[29]Some strains of *H. influenzae* are resistant to ampicillin and rare strains are resistant to chloramphenicol. Chloramphenicol (100 mg/kg/day IV) plus ampicillin can be used initially for treatment of meningitis in children more than one month old until the organism is identified and its antimicrobial susceptibility is determined. Ampicillin is preferred by some *Medical Letter* consultants for treatment of organisms known to be susceptible.

[30]Rifampin should be added only for patients who do not respond to erythromycin alone.

[31]Neither gentamicin, tobramycin, netilmicin, nor amikacin should be mixed in the same bottle with carbenicillin, ticarcillin, mezlocillin, piperacillin, or azlocillin for intravenous administration. In high concentration or in patients with renal failure carbenicillin or ticarcillin may inactivate the aminoglycosides.

[32]Seriously ill patients should be treated with both tetracycline and chloramphenicol.

[33]Antibiotic therapy is an adjunct to and not a substitute for prompt fluid and electrolyte replacement.

[34]Susceptibility tests should be performed by appropriate reference laboratories, but antituberculosis drugs may be effective *in vivo* even when *in vitro* tests show resistance. Some isolates may require vigorous chemotherapy using multiple drugs.

[35]Rifampin should be used concurrently with other drugs to prevent emergence of resistance. It is always included in treatment regimens for isoniazid-resistant organisms and is generally used together with isoniazid in the treatment of cavitary and far-advanced pulmonary tuberculosis as well as for extrapulmonary tuberculosis.

[36]An investigational drug in the United States.

Source: Modified from *Medical Letter on Drugs and Therapeutics* **26**:19–26, Mar. 2, 1984.

serious infections usually need higher and more predictable blood levels, which indicate the use of IV therapy. In less severe infections intramuscular (IM) or oral therapy can be used.

Allergy   Anyone can have an allergic reaction to an antibiotic, but patients with a history of allergic disorders (asthma, hives, hayfever, eczema) are at higher risk for severe, even life-threatening allergic reactions to antibiotics. **Penicillin** and its derivatives and the **sulfonamides** are the most well known causes of antibiotic allergies, especially with parenteral administration. In some situations the risk of developing an allergic reaction must be weighed against possible therapeutic benefits.

Patients may assume that they have an allergy because of pain they've experienced with injections or a gastrointestinal (GI) upset associated with the drug. However, some people who claim allergy have been reported to tolerate the drug without any reaction when inadvertently reexposed to it. Other patients who have successfully used the drug in the past may have an allergic reaction on subsequent exposure. Desensitization (giving progressively larger doses of the drug) has been successful, but it is a complex procedure that carries a significant risk and should be tried only when no alternative drug is available.

Age   The patient's age is an important consideration in any antimicrobial therapy, since the pharmacokinetics of the drug will change with age. The very young and the very old are most likely to have unusual responses. The renal function of a child is not mature until 1 year of age. Kidney function in elderly patients is also frequently diminished. Liver enzymes in the newborn are less able to metabolize **chloramphenicol** which may accumulate and cause gray baby syndrome. **Sulfonamides** displace bilirubin from binding sites on albumin, resulting in kernicterus in the newborn. The functioning of the immune system also tends to be altered in the very old and very young.

Pregnancy   Most antimicrobials cross the placenta and can accumulate in significant concentrations in the fetus, but this risk must be weighed against the benefits to the mother. The following drugs carry the most risk: chloramphenicol, tetracycline, sulfonamide, streptomycin, and the plasmocides (chloroquine and quinine). Chloramphenicol and sulfonamide may be toxic because the liver enzymes of the fetus may not be able to excrete the drugs. Streptomycin and other aminoglycosides have been associated with 8th cranial nerve damage. The plasmocides chloroquine (in large doses) and quinine have been associated with abortion and fetal abnormalities.

Breast Feeding   The following drugs should be avoided during breast feeding: **amantadine hydrochloride, tetracyclines,** and **chloramphenicol.** Breast feeding does not necessarily contraindicate the use of other antimicrobial agents, but the infant should be carefully monitored for any problems. **Aminoglycosides** are very polar compounds, so they pass into the breast milk poorly. **Cephalosporins** and **penicillins** pass into the breast milk in small amounts, so that allergic reactions and alterations in GI flora may occur. **Sulfonamides** pass into the milk in sufficient concentrations that they may cause problems in the infant, although they are not absolutely contraindicated.

Immunity   Antimicrobial drugs may only halt the growth of an organism, leaving it up to the host's normal immunity to actually eradicate the infection. If the patient is immunodeficient, the eradication of the infection will be diminished. Immunodeficiency can be caused by a congenital condition, splenectomy, diabetes mellitus, surgery, burns, or massive antimicrobial therapy. Immunodeficient patients may have unusual infections [e.g., autoimmune deficiency syndrome (AIDS) patients may have *Pneumocystis carinii*].

Diabetes Mellitus   The absorption of intramuscular drugs may be lower in diabetes patients, and peak blood levels of penicillin G may be lower. When higher blood levels are needed, IV injections should be used.

Renal Disease   There are two main problems which arise when antibiotics are given to patients with renal disease. The first is that any drugs which are normally excreted through the kidneys may quickly reach toxic levels unless the doses are adjusted to take the impaired kidney function into account. The second problem is that several classes of antibiotics (most notably the aminoglycosides) are nephrotoxic and may exacerbate any preexisting nephropathy. Because of this, only drugs with minimal nephrotoxic effects should be used in patients with any renal disease.

When nephrotoxic drugs must be used in renally impaired patients, kidney function should be monitored. Dosage should start as it would for normal patients, but subsequent doses must be reduced or the time between doses increased (see Chap. 31). Adjustments can be made according to either creatinine clearance, blood urea nitrogen (BUN) levels, or serum creatinine levels. Of these three indicators, creatinine clearance is the most reliable (see Fig. 28-1). Serum assays are also very helpful in maintaining the proper levels of the drugs in the blood. Most nephrotoxic reactions are reversible if they are recognized in time.

In practice, the proper approach to determining the correct dose is to measure the drug's disappearance from the blood over time. This allows an accurate match between the dose and the patient's loss of renal excretory capacity. If the drug is eliminated mainly by the kidneys, conventional measurement of renal function should allow estimation of the dose reduction needed to compensate for the decreased kidney function.

Liver Disease   Many antimicrobial drugs are partially metabolized and eliminated by the hepatobiliary system,

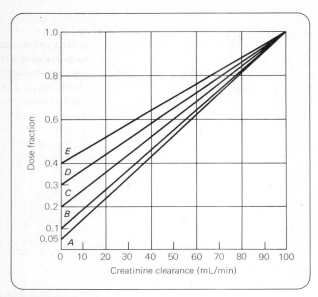

FIGURE 28-1

Dose Fraction as a Function of Creatinine Clearance. Lines *A* to *E* are dosing lines appropriate for different antibiotics based on the dose fraction for anephric patients. (*R. J. Anderson and R. W. Schrier: Clinical Use of Drugs in Patients with Kidney and Liver Disease, Philadelphia: Saunders, 1981.*)

including ampicillin, cephalosporins, clindamycin, linco-mycin hydrochloride monohydrate, erythromycins, and tet-racyclines. Care should be taken when administering these drugs to patients with liver disease. Very little is known about the disease's effects on clearance of the drugs.

CHEMOTHERAPEUTIC AGENTS

Antibiotics can be classified by their mechanism of action or by their spectrum of activity. Tetracycline and chloram-phenicol are examples of broad- or extended-spectrum anti-biotics because they are active against both gram-positive and gram-negative bacteria. Penicillin G is active primarily against gram-positive bacteria, so it is classified as a narrow-spectrum antibiotic. Modification of the parent compound

can extend the range of a narrow-spectrum antibiotic (e.g., amoxicillin and ampicillin are both derivatives of penicillin, but are broader-spectrum antimicrobials).

Mechanism of Action
Antimicrobial drugs work by one or more of the following processes (see Table 28-2):

1.   They inhibit formation of the cell wall, which leads to cell lysis or loss of function.
2.   They cause the loss of cell components by changing the permeability of the cell membrane.
3.   They cause reversible effects in protein synthesis by altering ribosomal activity.
4.   They bind to the 30S ribosomal subunit, which causes nonreversible alterations in protein synthesis.
5.   They affect nucleic acid metabolism.
6.   They block essential metabolic steps in the organism (antimetabolites).

Drugs which inhibit the growth of the pathogen are called *bacteriostatic;* drugs which kill the pathogen are called *bactericidal.* Assignment of a drug to these categories is determined both by the action of the drug and the con-centration used. For example, low concentrations of a par-ticular drug may be bacteriostatic, whereas high concentra-tions of the same drug may be bactericidal.

Pharmacokinetics
Oral therapy is the preferred method of administration if the patient is able to tolerate it and can reach sufficient serum and tissue drug levels. Three groups of antimicrobials can-not be given orally because of poor GI absorption. They are (1) the aminoglycosides, (2) the polymyxins, and (3) the polyenes (**amphotericin B** and **nystatin**). Acid lability accounts for the lack of effectiveness of **methicillin sodium** and **carbenicillin disodium** given orally. On the other hand, **penicillin G** is only slightly affected by gastric acidity, and many preparations are buffered for better absorption. Intra-venous (IV) therapy produces higher blood levels and more rapid increases in levels than either intramuscular (IM) or oral administration.

Distribution of antibiotics follows the same principles as other drugs. After absorption nearly all antimicrobials are

TABLE 28-2   Mechanism of Action of Antimicrobial Agents

ALTERATION IN CELL WALL	CELL MEMBRANE	REVERSIBLE INHIBITION OF PROTEIN SYNTHESIS	IRREVERSIBLE INHIBITION OF PROTEIN SYNTHESIS	ALTERS NUCLEIC ACID METABOLISM	ANTIMETABOLITES
Penicillin	Polymyxin	Chloramphenicol	Aminoglycosides	Rifampin	Trimethoprim
Cephalosporins	Amphotericin B	Tetracyclines			Sulfonamides
Cycloserine	Nystatin	Erthyromycin			
Bacitracin	Colistin	Lincomycin			
Vancomycin		Clindamycin			

protein bound, mostly to albumin. **Chloramphenicol** is distributed into the central nervous system (CNS), but **ampicillin**, **cephalosporins**, and **penicillin** are not, except in cases of meningitis and similar diseases in which membrane permeability increases. Effective drug concentrations can be reached in the fetus with **ampicillin**, **methicillin**, **penicillin** (**penicillin G**), **tetracyclines**, **chloramphenicol**, **streptomycin**, **cephalosporins**, **sulfonamides**, and **isoniazid** (**INH**). Because of the toxicity of aminoglycosides, tetracyclines, and chloramphenicol to the fetus, other antimicrobials, such as cephalosporins and penicillins, should be used during pregnancy. Since therapeutic concentrations are reached in the synovial fluid, intraarticular injections are usually unnecessary.

Some of the means by which antimicrobials are removed are excretion through the kidneys, inactivation by the liver, and secretion into the bile. Renal excretion of the active drug accounts for the elimination of penicillins, cephalosporins, aminoglycosides, trimethoprim, chloroquine, 5-fluorocytosine, sulfonamides, nitrofurantoin, and most tetracyclines except minocycline; these are excreted primarily in bile and feces.

Drugs which are excreted or metabolized by the liver include chloramphenicol, rifampin, INH, erythromycin, and lincomycin. As mentioned earlier, liver disease may impair the ability of the liver to handle these drugs, and dosage adjustment may be necessary.

Adverse Effects

Toxicities of antimicrobial agents are presented in Table 28-3.

TABLE 28-3   Selected Toxicities of Antimicrobial Drugs

SYSTEM	DRUGS
Renal	
Decreased GFR	Aminoglycosides, polymyxins, amphotericin B, cephaloridine
Nephritis	Penicillins, sulfonamides
Renal tubular acidosis	Amphotericin B
Electrolyte disturbances	Carbenicillin; tetracycline worsens uremic state
Hematologic	
Anemia-hypoliferative	Chloramphenicol, amphotericin B, 5-FC
Hemolytic	G6PD deficiency—sulfonamides, nitrofurantoin, chloramphenicol, primaquine
Hypersensitivity	Penicillins, cephalosporins, sulfonamides
Neutropenia	Chloramphenicol, 5-FC, others through hypersensitivity
Thrombocytopenia	Chloramphenicol, rifampin, 5-FC, others through hypersensitivity
Optic	Ethambutol
Auditory	Aminoglycosides, vancomycin
Vestibular	Aminoglycosides
CNS and peripheral nervous system	INH, tetracycline, penicillins, polymyxins, nitrofurantoin
GI	Entercolitis—all broad-spectrum drugs and clindamycin
Hepatic	Oxacillin, tetracycline, INH, rifampin
Pulmonary	Nitrofurantoin
Cutaneous	Hypersensitivity (all drugs); phototoxicity (tetracycline); Stevens-Johnson syndrome (sulfonamides and others)
Musculoskeletal	Serum sickness (all drugs, particularly penicillins, cephalosporins, and sulfonamides); bone development (tetracycline)
Cardiovascular	Sodium overload (carbenicillin)
Dental	Tooth staining under age 7 (tetracycline)

Source: R. K. Root and W. J. Hierholzer, "Infectious Disease in Clinical Pharmacology," in *Clinical Pharmacology: Basic Principles in Therapeutics*, 2nd ed., K. L. Melmon and H. F. Morrelli, eds., New York: Macmillan, 1978.

Idiosyncratic Reactions Idiosyncratic reactions are unrelated to either the immune system or to a known pharmacologic property of the drug. For example, **sulfonamides** may cause acute hemolysis in people who are genetically deficient in the enzyme glucose-6-phosphate dehydrogenase (G6PD). Another example is the development of a peripheral neuropathy after **INH** therapy in people who are genetically slow acetylators of isoniazid.

Gastrointestinal Effects Oral antimicrobial drugs can cause nausea anorexia, vomiting, and diarrhea although these symptoms are usually minor. Many antimicrobials can cause GI upset when given orally in high doses or for more than a few days. This upset is usually dose-related and can be attributed to chemical irritation of the GI mucosa and/or disturbances in the normal gut flora (which occur when an unabsorbed drug inhibits floral growth in the colon). Chemical irritation can be minimized by diluting the drug in the stomach with a glass of fluid or a small amount of food. Dairy foods should not be taken with tetracyclines. Stomatitis and glossitis can be associated with broad-spectrum antibiotics (such as tetracycline), but these symptoms will usually subside if the drug is discontinued. Occasionally treatment with an antifungal agent (such as nystatin) may be necessary.

Diarrhea is the most common GI complication. It is generally caused by changes in the gut flora.

Hepatotoxicity Antimicrobial agents can cause a variety of hepatotoxicities, which are classified according to the type of lesion (see Chap. 32).

Isoniazid (INH) can cause hepatitis syndrome. Preliminary symptoms are fatigue, weakness, anorexia, malaise, and/or fever. If these symptoms appear, the drug should be immediately discontinued. Preexisting liver disease or mild transaminase elevation does not contraindicate INH therapy.

Erythromycin estolate (Ilosone Oral Preparations) has been associated with a few cases of obstructive jaundice (hepatocanalicular hepatotoxicity). If this occurs, the estolate can be discontinued in favor of the free base or stearate. **Troleandomycin** can also occasionally cause obstructive jaundice and alterations in liver enzymes. **Tetracycline**-induced fatty infiltrates can occur with IV doses larger than 2 g. This is commonly associated with the use of tetracycline during pregnancy.

Central Nervous System (CNS) Effects CNS toxicities are encountered less frequently than other adverse effects. **Penicillin G** encephalopathy is characterized by CNS stimulation and manifested by delirium or coma with intense myoclonic and generalized seizures. It is usually associated with doses greater than 60 million U/day (IV) and is often preceded by cerebral disease and accompanied by renal failure. Patients given procaine penicillin G intramuscularly have complained of visual and auditory disturbances, although this reaction is rare (1 in 400). Tetracycline can (only rarely) cause an increase in intracranial pressure.

Neuromuscular blockade, skeletal muscle weakness, and respiratory depression are all associated with the **aminoglycosides** and **polymyxins**. These side effects can be rapidly reversed by discontinuing the drug and administering **calcium chloride** (1 g IV).

Superinfections Many antibiotics alter the normal flora in the body. Sometimes when the drug-sensitive flora are removed, an overgrowth of a different and drug-resistant flora occurs, causing a *superinfection* (an infection by a secondary pathogen). These superinfections are most often seen in patients less than 2 years or more than 50 years of age. Superinfections rarely occur when a drug is given for less than a week. Broad-spectrum antibiotics such as ampicillin and tetracycline increase the risk of superinfections because of their greater suppression of normal flora. *Pseudomonas* colitis, a superinfection caused by an overgrowth of *clostridium difficile* in patients on broad-spectrum antibiotics (ampicillin, tetracycline, chloramphenicol, and clindamycin) causes a severe diarrhea that may be life-threatening but is usually reversed with **vancomycin**.

Hematologic Complications Hematologic complications occur infrequently. When they do they are associated with a high incidence of sickness and death. Chloramphenicol can cause fatal aplastic anemia (1 case in 40,000) and simple "iron deficiency" anemia. It is not yet known how to predict which patients are susceptible, so careful use is necessary. Hemolytic anemia associated with a glucose-6-phosphate dehydrogenase (G6PD) deficiency can occur with sulfonamides, nitrofurantoin, nalidixic acid, or chloramphenicol.

Intravenous Incompatibilities Intravenous therapy can be seriously compromised by improperly reconstituting the drugs, mixing the drugs with other incompatible drugs, and storing the solutions too long. Any of these problems can cause degradation of the drugs (Table 28-4).

In vitro incompatibility of many drugs precludes their being mixed together before administration. Additives such as vitamins and multiple electrolytes may also be incompatible. When multiple drugs are used, they should ideally be mixed in the same solution unless they are chemically incompatible. In actual practice it may not be practical to determine compatibility for more than two drugs, in which case they should be mixed separately to avoid problems. Blood should never be mixed with IV drugs, since its in vitro compatibility is unpredictable.

Drug Interactions Antimicrobials interact by a variety of mechanisms with other drugs and foods. These interactions may result in loss of antimicrobial efficacy, increased or decreased efficacy of the interacting drug, or increased drug toxicity. A few examples of drug interactions are shown in Table 28-5. The clinical significance of these reactions will vary.

TABLE 28-4 Selected Antibiotics Incompatible in IV Solutions

ANTIBIOTIC	INTERFERING AGENT	REMARKS
Amphotericin B	Antihistamines	Incompatible
	Vitamins	Incompatible
	Amikacin sulfate	Physically incompatible; immediate precipitate
	Sodium chloride 0.9%	Physically incompatible
	Calcium salts	Haze develops over 3 h
	Carbenicillin disodium	Haze develops over 3 h
	Procaine HCl, lidocaine HCl	Precipitation of amphotericin B
	Penicillin G (K^+ and Na^+)	Physically incompatible
	Potassium chloride	Physically incompatible
Ampicillin	Dextrose in water	Ampicillin decomposition increases with increase in dextrose concentration
	Chlorpromazine HCl	Immediate precipitate
	Dopamine HCl	36% ampicillin decomposition in 6 h at 23–25°C
	Clindamycin	Physically incompatible
Cefamandole (Mandol)	Calcium gluconate	Incompatible
	All aminoglycoside antibiotics, e.g., gentamicin, tobramycin	Haze or precipitate within 4 h
	Solutions containing magnesium	Incompatible
Cefazolin (Kefzol, Ancef)	Amikacin, kanamycin	Turbidity observed at 24 h
	Calcium gluconate	Incompatible
	Erythromycin gluceptats	Incompatible
	Tetracycline HCl	Incompatible
	Cimetidine HCl	Immediate precipitate
	Lidocaine HCl	Formation of precipitate
Clindamycin (Cleocin)	Aminophylline	Physically incompatible
	Ampicillin	Physically incompatible
	Magnesium sulfate	Physically incompatible
	Phenytoin Na^+ (Dilantin)	Physically incompatible
Oxacillin (Prostaphlin, Bactocill)	Gentamicin sulfate	Incompatible
	Tetracycline	Physically incompatible
Penicillin G potassium	Aminophylline	Increases decomposition of penicillin
	Amphotericin B	Haze develops over 3 h
		Physically incompatible
	Dopamine HCl	14% penicillin decomposition in 24 h
	Sodium bicarbonate	Penicillin decomposition
	Tetracycline	pH outside stability range for penicillin
	Thiopental sodium	Physically incompatible
Tetracycline	Carbenicillin	Haze develops over 3 h
	Cefazolin	
	Erythromycin	Physically incompatible
	All penicillinase-resistant antimicrobials, e.g., oxacillin	Physically incompatible

455

TABLE 28-5 Drug Interactions Involving Antimicrobial Agents

DRUG	INTERACTING DRUG OR FOOD	EFFECT
Tetracyclines	Dairy products, iron antacids	Chelation of TCN; decreased absorption
Penicillins, cephalosporins	Probenecid	Decreased tubular secretion of the antimicrobials; increased half-life. This is often used clinically.
Broad-spectrum antimicrobials (except rifampin)	Oral anticoagulants	Enhanced anticoagulant effect, presumably due to decreased vitamin K synthesis by bacterial flora
Aminoglycosides	Nephrotoxic drugs or ototoxic drugs	Increased nephrotoxicity and ototoxicity
	Neuromuscular blockers	Prolonged muscular paralysis
Chloramphenicol	Phenytoin, oral anticoagulants, oral antidiabetic drugs	Decreased metabolism with increased risk of interacting drug
Erythromycin	Theophylline, carbamazepine	Decreased metabolism with increased risk of toxicity with interacting drug
Rifampin	Beta blockers, oral contraceptives, oral antidiabetic drugs, quinidine	Increased metabolism with decreased efficacy of interacting drug

Resistance to Antimicrobial Agents

Pathogens are tested in vitro to determine their sensitivity to particular drugs. Microorganisms have various means of surviving antibiotics, so their sensitivity will vary from organism to organism, from drug to drug, and from one geographic location to another.

A population of pathogens can become resistant to a drug after therapy has started, through the process of selection. This occurs because the sensitive organisms in the population are killed off by the drug, leaving the resistant organisms to multiply. Pathogen populations can also overcome the effects of drugs through genetic changes passed on from generation to generation. These changes can occur via mutation, transduction, transformation, or conjugation. Whatever the method of genetic change, the basic mechanism is related to

1. Elaboration of drug-metabolizing enzymes such as β-lactamase (penicillinase, cephalosporinase) or acetylating enzymes
2. Changes in the bacteria's permeability to the drug
3. Increased amounts of internal antagonists to the drug's action
4. Changes in the binding between the sites of the drug's action and the drug itself

Therapy with a combination of drugs may slow down or prevent the pathogen's development of resistance. For example, the tubercle bacillus rapidly develops resistance to a single drug such as INH, but using rifampin in combination with INH delays the development of resistance.

Duration of Therapy

If the course of antibiotic therapy is too short, it invites a relapse of the original pathogen and fosters the rise of drug-resistant pathogens. If the course is too long, the patient runs the risk of superinfection and drug toxicity. Generally antibiotic therapy should be continued until all evidence of infection (including fever, leukocytosis, and positive cultures) has been absent for 48 to 72 h. Frequently the drug suppresses the obvious symptoms of infection within 3 to 4 days of starting therapy, and the patient stops taking the drug (noncompliance). Patients who do this run the risk of a relapse several days later. The best way to prevent noncompliance is to explain the reasons for completing the therapy course to the patient.

A secondary complication of noncompliance is that patients may have several doses of the drug left in the medicine cabinet and be tempted to take these left-over drugs the next time they feel ill even when they are contraindicated for the new illness. Even if the drug is not dangerous there will nearly always be an insufficient number of doses for proper treatment, so the risk of relapse and the rise of drug-resistant pathogens exists.

As mentioned above, the prolonged use of antibiotic drugs, particularly broad-spectrum drugs, brings with it the risk of superinfections. Recurring fever in a patient receiving antimicrobial therapy may indicate a superinfection, drug fever, or incorrect original diagnosis. This usually requires discontinuing the drug and reevaluating the patient. Some superinfections can be managed by simply stopping the use of the drug. Duration of therapy for specific infections is discussed in the final section of this chapter and in Chap. 29.

Combination Therapy

When drugs are used in combination, their modes of action are important considerations because they can either counteract or enhance each other. The combined use of a bacteriostatic drug with a bactericidal drug can impair the bactericidal effect. For example, tetracyclines at low doses are bacteriostatic; they inhibit protein synthesis and growth of the microorganism. Penicillin, on the other hand, is bactericidal; it affects cell wall synthesis and is efficacious only if the bacteria are actively growing. When these two drugs are combined, the tetracycline slows down the growth of the bacteria to the point that the penicillin no longer kills it.

An example of two drugs which enhance each other's effects is the combination of **trimethoprim** with **sulfamethoxazole** (a sulfonamide). Both of these drugs inhibit folic acid production by acting sequentially on the folic acid biosynthetic pathway, thereby increasing the inhibitory effect on bacterial growth. Generally, combination therapy is indicated in infections caused by multiple pathogens, to prevent the emergence of resistant strains, and when two drugs have additive or synergistic effects.

Clavulanic acid is a compound that has little antibacterial effect, but it inhibits the enzyme β-lactamase. When combined with amoxicillin, penicillins, or cephalosporin, it can prevent the breakdown of the antibiotic by inhibiting the enzyme β-lactamase.

Antimicrobial Prophylaxis

The indications for prophylactic use of antibiotics are these: immunocompromised patients, those with chronic disease in which prevention of bacterial infections is especially important (e.g., chronic obstructive lung disease), those having certain types of surgery, and prophylaxis of endocarditis. The beneficial effects of using antibiotics prophylactically must always be weighed against the possible risks, including adverse effects of the drugs themselves, development of drug resistance, and superinfections.

When antibiotics are used prophylactically for surgery they should be administered just prior to the operation. A second dose may be required if the operation is delayed or the procedure is prolonged. Generally postsurgical antibiotic therapy is unnecessary except in cases of ruptured viscus or traumatic wounds (see Table 28-6).

NURSING PROCESS RELATED TO ANTIMICROBIAL DRUGS

Assessment

Patients are given antibiotics for a wide variety of diseases. Before starting drug therapy the nurse should know:

1. Why the patient is receiving the drug
2. Which drug the patient is receiving
3. What the route of administration will be
4. What factors might complicate or contraindicate the use of the drug

Knowing the answers to these questions not only helps in treatment but also defines the need for patient education in each case.

Some of the factors which determine the effectiveness of drug therapy are the nature of the pathogen, its sensitivity to the drugs used, the state of the patient's natural defense mechanisms, and the patient's age, medical history, kidney and liver functions, and compliance.

First, baseline values should be determined. Vital signs, pertinent laboratory results (e.g., CBC with differential, urinalysis, BUN, creatinine and sedimentation rate); appearance of sputum, urine, or stool (color, odor, amount); appearance of wounds, lesions, or incisions (size, color, odor, description of drainage, swelling, erythema); signs of organ or tissue dysfunction; symptoms of pressure; and pain should all be noted. The nurse should also make neurologic and audiometric assessments, especially if the patient will be receiving aminoglycosides. All this will help in identifying and treating adverse reactions. From these examinations or by other means, the nurse should determine whether the patient is immunodeficient or immunosuppressed. If so, the particular requirements for dealing with a compromised patient should be analyzed. For example, the patient who is using corticosteroids will probably need to have her corticosteroid dose increased to help overcome the stress of infection. The infected diabetic may need to have his insulin dosage adjusted and change his method of urine testing, since some antibiotics give a false-positive result with Benedict's solution and Clinitest.

An allergy history is extremely important since antibiotics can cause allergic reactions, and cross-sensitivities exist between many antibiotics. Patients should describe any problems they have had with medications including over-the-counter drugs and preparations used for eye, skin, or dental problems. Before receiving the first dose of any antibiotic, especially penicillin, patients should be asked again whether they have ever taken that specific drug before and, if so, whether they noticed any unusual reactions. Patients who cannot remember what antibiotic they have taken may be reminded by looking at a picture chart of the various preparations (such as those found in the *Physician's Desk Reference*). Patients who have histories of multiple allergies and drug reactions (especially to drugs related to the one prescribed) will need a rigorous clinical assessment for allergic reactions.

Since determining the infecting organism is crucial to proper treatment the nurse should check to see whether cultures need to be taken before starting treatment. It may be necessary to take throat, nose, ear, or vaginal swabs, or to obtain specimens of sputum, urine, stool, or blood. These samples should be taken as soon as possible. Since the point of taking these samples is to look for microorganisms, contamination of the specimen must be avoided.

TABLE 28-6 Prevention of Wound Infections and Sepsis in Surgical Patients

NATURE OF OPERATION	LIKELY PATHOGENS	RECOMMENDED DRUGS AND ADULT DOSAGE BEFORE SURGERY†
	Clean	
Cardiovascular Prosthetic valve and other open-heart surgery	*Staphylococcus epidermidis, S. aureus, Corynebacterium* sp. enteric gram-negative bacilli, fungi	Cefazolin, 1 g IM/IV *or* Vancomycin, 1 g IV
Arterial reconstructive surgery involving the abdominal aorta, a prosthesis, or a groin incision	*S. aureus, S. epidermidis,* enteric gram-negative bacilli	Cefazolin, 1 g IM/IV
Orthopedic Total joint replacement, internal fixation of proximal femoral fracture	*S. aureus, S. epidermidis*	Cefazolin, 1 g IM/IV *or* Vancomycin, 1 g IV
	Clean-Contaminated	
Head and neck (entering oral cavity or pharynx)	*S. aureus,* streptococci, oral anaerobes	Cefazolin, 1 g IM/IV *or* Aqueous penicillin G, 1 million U IV
Gastroduodenal	Enteric gram-negative bacilli, gram-positive cocci	*High risk or gastric bypass only:* Cefazolin, 1 g IM/IV
Biliary tract	Enteric gram-negative bacilli, group D streptococcus, *Clostridium*	*High risk only:* Cefazolin, 1 g IM/IV
Colorectal	Enteric gram-negative bacilli, anaerobic bacteria, group D streptococci	*Oral:* Neomycin plus erythromycin base, 1 g of each at 1 P.M., 2 P.M., and 11 P.M. the day before the operation *Parenteral:* Cefoxitin, 1 g IV *or* Clindamycin, 600 mg IV, plus gentamicin or tobramycin, 1.5 mg/kg IM/IV
Appendectomy	Enteric gram-negative bacilli, anaerobic bacteria	Cefoxitin, 1 g IV
Vaginal or abdominal hysterectomy	Enteric gram-negative bacilli, anaerobes, group B and D streptococci	Cefazolin, 1 g IM/IV
Cesarean section	Same as for hysterectomy	*High risk only:* Cefazolin, 1 g IV after cord clamping
Abortion	Same as for hysterectomy	*First trimester in patients with previous pelvic inflammatory disease:* Aqueous penicillin G, 1 million U IV *Second trimester:* Cefazolin, 1 g IM/IV
	Dirty	
Ruptured viscus	Enteric gram-negative bacilli, anaerobes, group D streptococci	Clindamycin, 600 mg IV q6h, plus gentamicin or tobramycin, 1.5 mg/kg q8h IM/IV *or* Cefoxitin, 1 g q4–8h IV, with or without gentamicin or tobramycin, 1.5 mg/kg q8h IM/IV
Traumatic wound	*S. aureus,* group A streptococcus, *Clostridium, Pasteurella multicoda**	Cefazolin, 1 g q4–8h IM/IV

*With dog or cat bites.   †Parenteral prophylactic antimicrobials for clean and clean-contaminated surgery can be given as a single dose just before the operation. For prolonged operations, additional intraoperative doses should be given q4–8h for the duration of the procedure. For dirty surgery therapy should usually be continued for 5–10 days.

Source: Medical Letter on Drugs and Therapeutics, vol. 25, Dec. 23, 1983.

Whenever caring for patients the nurse must keep an open mind and be alert for those patients who can be considered high risks for infection. For example, the nurse should be aware that any patient receiving invasive therapy (insertion of a Foley catheter, peripheral IV, intraarterial or central venous catheter, temporary pacemaker) is at risk for gram-negative septicemia or septic shock. Nurses must know and watch for the early warnings of complications so that proper treatment can be started.

Management

Nursing management in antimicrobial therapy includes actual administration of the drug and patient education.

Before administering the antibiotic the nurse should

1. Recheck the physician's order.
2. Be sure the medication is indicated for the patient's infection by checking culture and sensitivity reports.
3. Verify that the dosage is correct for the patient's age, renal and hepatic function, and site of infection.

The nurse must know what medications the patient is currently taking and watch for pharmacologically antagonistic combinations: either drugs which counteract each other or drugs which have the potential for increased toxicity. The nurse must be familiar with the drug's action and potential adverse effects and must explain these to the patient. Particular emphasis should be given to symptoms the patient should watch for.

Anaphylactic shock is sudden, acute, and potentially fatal. Whoever is administering the drug must be prepared to treat it. It usually begins with diffuse flushing, itching, and a feeling of warmth. Hives may appear on the patient's face and chest. Upper respiratory edema is characterized by massive facial angioedema and respiratory difficulty which is manifested by wheezing and shortness of breath. The patient may become anxious, have a choking sensation, and feel chest tightness and pain. If this continues, respiratory and/or circulatory failure will result, ending in coma and death. Outpatients who have received parenteral antibiotics should wait at the clinic for at least 20 min after the dose and be monitored for adverse effects.

The nurse responsible for drug preparation should consult and follow the package insert or institutional protocol. In institutions that have IV admixture programs the IV antibiotic will be prepared in the pharmacy under a laminar flow hood, and the drug will be delivered to the nursing unit. The nurse should then check the label against the medication order before administering the IV.

It is important to include all the IV fluid administered on the patient's intake and output record, especially for a patient whose fluid intake is restricted, such as a chronic dialysis patient or a patient with increased intracranial pressure.

Nurses should know the indications for both the general categories of antibiotics and the specific antibiotics they are dealing with. Any special measures required for a specific patient should be written into the patient's care plan and medical record.

Patients with endocrine or renal problems may need to have their electrolytes monitored since some antibiotics contain large amounts of sodium and potassium. Patients using antibiotics that are metabolized in the liver (chloramphenicol, clindamycin, erythromycin, and some tetracyclines) may need liver function studies such as serum glutamic oxaloacetic transaminase (SGOT), serum glutamic pyruvic transaminase (SGPT), bilirubin, and alkaline phosphatase. Patients taking drugs that are excreted by the kidneys (aminoglycosides, cephalosporins, most penicillins, and some tetracyclines) may need their BUN, urine output, specific gravity, creatinine clearance, and serum creatinine levels monitored. Patients with altered renal or liver function may need to have the antibiotic dosage decreased or may need to be given a different antibiotic. When patients are being typed and cross-matched for transfusions it is important that the blood bank know which antibiotic they are taking, since some may cause a false positive on the Coombs' test. Since some antibiotics affect the hematopoietic system the nurse must know the early signs of blood dyscrasias and watch lab results for these. Any patients using aminoglycosides should be tested frequently for signs of toxicity in the 8th cranial nerve, such as tinnitus, dizziness, and hearing loss.

Proper administration of the drug maximizes its effectiveness and decreases its adverse effects. Many antibiotics cause gastric irritation. These drugs (e.g., sulfonamides) can be given with a full glass of water to decrease the irritation. Food can also have an effect on absorption. Some drugs, such as some oral **penicillins** and **erythromycin** should be taken on an empty stomach (1 h before eating or 2 to 3 h after). Others, such as the oral cephalosporins, should be taken with meals to minimize gastric irritation. Giving antibiotics such as clindamycin and erythromycin via IV or IM injection can be painful, cause phlebitis (IV), or sterile abscess (IM). Unless contraindicated by concurrent conditions (such as fluid restrictions), IV drugs should be diluted with 50 to 100 mL of fluid to prevent irritation of the vein wall. Changing IV sites every 48 h will not only lessen the irritation but will also help prevent a superinfection at the injection site. Scrupulous care when using central venous lines and Hickman catheters will help to prevent septicemia. For large IM injections the site should be changed frequently and the injection given into a large muscle mass. Massaging the muscle for a full 2 min after injection will improve absorption of the drug.

Scheduling drug administration should not be done without considering the patient's other needs. Blood levels are most consistent when the drugs are given at regular doses throughout the entire day. In severe infections, when using IV administration of drugs with a very short half-life, the injections are usually given around the clock at evenly spaced intervals. However, there are times when the patient's uninterrupted sleep is more important than an absolutely consistent blood level. In these cases the drug should be spread out only over waking hours. If the drug can be taken with food, patients on self-medication can take the pill with each meal and at bed time. This is an easily remembered routine which helps patient compliance.

Patient education is a very important part of management, since noncompliance is a major cause of therapeutic failure. Patients taking oral antibiotics need specific instructions on food-drug interactions. It cannot be overemphasized that the drug should be taken as long as ordered, and that dosage should not be changed without asking the clinician. Often patients will stop their antibiotic when their symptoms cease but before the infection is completely eradicated. This can only lead to relapse or drug resistance, and the patient should be told this. When antibiotics are administered to children, the drugs should not be stopped when the fever or sore throat is relieved. It should also be explained that unused antibiotics, should there be any, are to be discarded and never used for a subsequent illness. Self-diagnosis and medication with leftover drugs can lead to serious health consequences. Patients who are being discharged with Hickman catheters need detailed instructions on the care of the catheter from the nurse prior to the anticipated discharge so that discharge is not delayed.

Besides explaining the disease and the action of the antibiotic against it, the nurse must help the patient and others who might be involved to understand how the disease is spread and what they can do to break the chain of infection (see Table 28-7). Part of this process is to identify other people who may have been exposed to the disease. The nurse

TABLE 28-7   The Infectious Process in Acute Communicable Diseases

These six factors must be present in sequential order for the spread of a communicable disease. Breaking any link in this chain will stop the disease spread.

1. *Causative Agent*   The invading organism
2. *Reservoir*   A place for the invading organism to live and multiply; may be human, animal, or nonanimal
3. *Mode of Escape*   From the reservoir; may be various body systems, open lesions, or mechanical, such as an animal bite
4. *Mode of Transmission*   A way of reaching the host; may be direct or indirect contact
5. *Mode of Entry*   For the organism to enter the human body
6. *Susceptible Host*   Whether person becomes ill after the organism enters the body depends on organism, degree of exposure, duration of exposure, and person's general physical, emotional, and mental state

must exercise particular sensitivity in cases of sexually transmitted disease (STD). It is crucial that the nurse use a calm, supportive, nonjudgmental attitude. Criticism or sarcasm by the interviewer is most unprofessional and may result in the patient's failure to list all sexual contacts. These unreported contacts will then become "silent victims" perpetuating the spread of these diseases.

Other important aspects of patient education include detailed information about how and when to take the drug, especially for the patient being discharged with a Hickman catheter in place. Each patient should be told the importance of starting medication as soon as possible. It is very important to explain the signs of adverse drug reactions and ineffectiveness, as well as what to do if these happen. All patients should receive information on correct storage and handling of their medication.

Since prevention is a key underlying principle, patients and their families need to be told how to minimize the spread of disease through proper hand washing and disposing of contaminated waste (tissues, dressings, and so on). Those close to the patient need to understand how the disease is spread to help prevent reinfection. Sometimes environmental disinfection must be explained (see Chap. 38). In all this the clinician should serve as a role model for proper technique.

Evaluation

In addition to administering the drugs and educating the patient, the nurse is responsible for seeing whether the drug is effective. The usual signs of improvement are a decrease in fever and pulse rate, a decrease in white blood cell or colony count, a decrease in the amount of sputum or wound drainage, or an increase in urinary output. Other, more general signs include an increased sense of well-being, an increase in appetite, and decreased complaints of pain.

The nurse must always be alert for drug resistance if the infection becomes less responsive to therapy and/or the patient's condition worsens. Signs of new infections must also be watched for. Injection sites or the sites of indwelling catheters are especially susceptible to secondary infections and superinfections. Other sites commonly involved are the mouth, GI tract, and vagina. New infections can be manifested by diarrhea, change in stool character, stomatitis or glossitis, and vaginal discharge.

The nurse should continue to watch for adverse effects and, for patients on self-medication, compliance with the regimen. In an institutional setting the nurse needs to check automatic stop dates for drugs and to discuss with the physician whether the drug should be continued, discontinued, or changed.

CLINICAL PHARMACOLOGY AND THERAPEUTICS OF ANTIBACTERIAL DRUGS

LEARNING OBJECTIVES

Upon mastery of this section of this chapter, the reader will be able to:

1. List four adverse reactions of penicillins.
2. Describe the assessment of penicillin allergy.
3. Compare penicillin G, penicillin V, ampicillin, carbenicillin, dicloxacillin, and piperacillin with respect to antimicrobial spectrum, penicillinase sensitivity, and acid stability.
4. Describe the differences between the first-, second-, and third-generation cephalosporins giving an example of each and an indication for its use.
5. List three adverse effects of the cephalosporins.
6. Give three indications for erythromycin therapy.
7. Give an indication and an adverse effect of clindamycin.
8. Compare tetracycline, doxycycline, and minocycline as to spectrum of activity and dosage.
9. Give three adverse effects of the tetracyclines.
10. List three examples of aminoglycosides.
11. List the major indications and adverse effects of the aminoglycosides.

PENICILLINS

The penicillins and their derivatives are antibiotic derivatives, all sharing the same *basic* chemical structure. Penicillin G (benzylpenicillin) was the first penicillin used in humans. Newer penicillins were developed by first adding precursors to the penicillin G fermentation tanks and later by adding semisynthetic side chains to the penicillanic acid nucleus. Penicillins are generally divided into three groups: penicillin G and penicillin V, the penicillinase-resistant penicillins, and the broad-spectrum penicillins.

Mechanism of Action

Penicillins are bactericidal drugs that act by interfering with the synthesis of bacterial cell wall mucopeptide. This interference causes increased internal osmotic pressure and results in rupture of the cell. The drugs act during cell division and do not affect nondividing cells. Therefore, bacteriostatic antibiotics such as chloramphenicol that prevent cell division may impair or negate the activity of penicillins. However, the clinical significance of this interaction may be questionable in many situations.

Spectrum of Activity

Penicillin G is the drug of choice for susceptible organisms in nonallergic patients. It is effective in vitro against the majority of gram-positive and gram-negative cocci. Most common pathogenic streptococci (excluding group D streptococci-enterococci) are highly sensitive. Most *Staphylococcus aureus* strains are now resistant, however, because of their ability to produce the enzyme penicillinase. Penicillin G remains the drug of choice for both gonococci and *Treponema pallidum* (the causative organism of syphilis). Some gram-negative bacilli, notably *Proteus mirabilis*, are sensitive to high doses of penicillin G, but other drugs are generally preferred for clinical use against infections caused by gram-negative organisms. The penicillinase-resistant penicillins are indicated *only* when the organism is penicillinase-producing. No advantage is gained by using these agents or broad-spectrum penicillins for organisms sensitive to penicillin G or penicillin V.

Pharmacokinetics

About one-third of an oral dose of penicillin G is absorbed; therefore, an oral dose must be four to five times greater than a parenteral dose to achieve similar serum concentrations.

Following IM or subcutaneous injection, aqueous penicillin G produces peak plasma levels within 1 to 3 h. This level falls rapidly, resulting in the need for injections every 4 to 6 h if the serum level is to be maintained. Procaine penicillin G is therefore usually preferred for IM injection because it provides more consistent steady-state levels.

Penicillin G is widely distributed throughout the body. Significant amounts of the drug appear in most body tissues. The drug does not enter the cerebrospinal fluid (CSF) except when the meninges are inflamed. In acute meningitis, levels are attained in the CSF, but therapeutic levels are not predictable. Penicillins are excreted primarily unchanged by the kidneys, largely by tubular secretion. **Probenecid** (Benemid) is excreted through the same route and competes with penicillins for secretion sites. Therefore, serum levels of penicillins can be raised 50 to 100 percent by concurrent administration of probenecid. The half-life of penicillin G is normally about 30 min but may be increased 20-fold in patients with renal disease. Table 28-8 outlines the pharmacokinetic parameters for many of the available penicillins.

Adverse Effects

Their low incidence of toxicity and cost make penicillins the drugs of choice for the treatment of susceptible organisms in nonallergic patients (Table 28-9). The most frequent adverse effects to penicillins are hypersensitivity reactions that occur in 0.7 to 10 percent of patients. The variation in the incidence is dependent on method of reporting, route of administration, and particular penicillin or derivative. The

TABLE 28-8 Pharmacokinetic Parameters of Selected Penicillins

DRUG	SERUM $t_{1/2}$ (h) N	SERUM $t_{1/2}$ (h) R	PEAK SERUM CONCENTRATION ($\mu g/ml$)	% ORAL ABSORPTION	PROTEIN, % PROTEIN-BOUND
Ampicillin 500 mg	1–1.5	10–20	2–6	30–70	15–25
Amoxicillin 500 mg PO	7–1.4	10–20	4–12	74–92	20–25
Carbenicillin 1g IV	1–1.5	10–20	10–40		—
Cloxacillin 500 mg PO	0.5	0.8	7–15	50	94
Dicloxacillin 250 mg PO	0.7	1–2	5–9	74	96
Oxacillin 500 mg IM	0.5	0.5–1.0	11	33	90
Methacillin 1 g IM	0.5	4	12	—	—
Nafcillin 500 mg PO	0.5–1	1.2	7	50	90
Penicillin G 500 mg	0.5	7–10	0.5–2.7	33	30–60
Penicillin G procaine 300,000	—*		0.9		—
Penicillin G benzathine			30 ng/mL†		
Penicillin VK 500 mg			3.0–13.5‡	60	80
Ticarcillin	1–1.5	10–20			

N = normal renal function; R = decreased renal function.
*Slowly released following IM injection.
†Levels are produced for 21–28 days.
‡Penicillin V levels two to five times greater than penicillin G.

allergic reaction can range from as mild as a rash to a life-threatening anaphylaxis (overall incidence 0.05 percent). The more serious reactions usually occur after IV administration but reactions can occur after oral or even intradermal skin testing. Fever or eosinophilia may be the only presenting sign of penicillin allergy. Other uncommon hypersensitivity reactions include the development of a positive Coombs' test and hemolytic anemia or hematologic reactions such as thrombocytopenia, thrombocytopenic purpura, leukopenia, and agranulocytosis. These reactions are usually reversible when the drug is stopped.

The cause of the penicillin allergy has been attributed to penicillin and its degradation products, mainly penicillenic or penicilloic acid. These antigenic determinants are classified as major and minor determinants. The classification is based on frequency of occurrence rather than the type of allergic reaction it may produce. The *major determinants* are involved in accelerated or delayed urticarial reactions and other dermatologic reactions and consist mainly of penicilloyl polylysine (PPL). The immediate reactions are caused by the *minor determinants,* which include penicillin G, penicilloic acid, and α-benzylpenicilloylamine.

Patients who have a positive history for penicillin allergy can be skin-tested. **PPL** (Pre-Pen) and **minor determinants mixture** (MDM) are the most useful screening methods for patients with a history of immediate reactions. A scratch test with the material is performed; if the test is positive, no further testing is needed. If the test is negative, intradermal testing is then done. Pre-Pen is commercially available, but minor determinants are not marketed commercially. An alternative to employing minor determinants is using an old solution of aqueous penicillin G along with the Pre-Pen.

The GI effects of oral preparations of penicillin include nausea, vomiting, epigastric distress, black hairy tongue, and diarrhea for oral preparations. Pseudomembranous colitis has also been reported with oral penicillins, especially with ampicillin, amoxicillin, and other broad-spectrum agents.

Penicillin can be irritating to the central and peripheral nervous system. Neurologic toxicity is associated with large doses of penicillin G (greater than 20 million U/day, or 10 g of carbenicillin) in patients with decreased renal function. The patients may exhibit hallucinations, hyperreflexia, seizures, and impaired sensorium.

Acute interstitial nephritis appears to be a hypersensitivity reaction that has been reported with methicillin, parenteral ampicillin, nafcillin, penicillin G, and oral oxacillin.

Electrolyte imbalance is a possibility with rapid IV administration of carbenicillin disodium, ticarcillin disodium, or potassium or sodium penicillin.

Bacterial Resistance Penicillin, penicillin derivatives, and cephalosporin antibiotics (all antibiotics which contain a β-lactam ring) can be enzymatically inactivated by penicillinases (β-lactamases). β-Lactamases are produced by staphylococci and by some *Bacteroides* and *Bacillus* species. Some bacteria remain resistant to penicillin because the antibiotic cannot penetrate the cell wall.

Preparations: Penicillin G and Penicillin V

Penicillin G Penicillin G (benzylpenicillin) is available in oral and parenteral dosage forms (see Table 28-10). The oral drug is slightly acid-labile (destroyed by gastric acid). Therefore, penicillin V, which is acid-stable, is preferred for oral use. Topical use of penicillin is discouraged because of questionable efficacy and a high potential for sensitization.

TABLE 28-9 Adverse Reactions to Some of the Penicillins

Shared by all Penicillins

Allergic reactions, rarely anaphylactic

Skin rashes

Diarrhea

Neuromuscular irritability, including seizures with large doses of renal failure

Hematologic changes such as neutropenia, anemia (at times hemolytic)

Drug-induced fever

Nephropathy, as component of serum sickness type reaction

Commonly Associated with the Following Individual Drugs

Ampicillin
Skin rash
Diarrhea
Pseudomembranous colitis

Azlocillin
Chest pain with rapid infusion

Carbenicillin
Hypokalemic alkalosis, sodium overload
Platelet dysfunction (high dose)

Methicillin
Interstitial nephritis
Anemia, neutropenia, granulocytopenia

Mezlocillin
Bleeding abnormalities (high doses)

Nafcillin
Thrombophlebitis
Elevated serum glutamic oxalacetic transaminase
Bleeding disorders (high doses)

Oxacillin
Elevated serum glutamic oxalacetic transaminase
Granulocytopenia

Pipercillin
Bleeding disorders (high doses)

Potassium penicillin G
Hyperkalemia and arrhythmias with IV doses given rapidly

Procaine penicillin G
Neurologic reactions and abnormal behavior with high doses

Ticarcillin
Bleeding disorders (high doses)

Aqueous penicillin G is highly irritating to soft tissues and provides a short duration of activity when administered intramuscularly. Two salts of penicillin G, procaine and benzathine, are used for IM administration. Vessels have been occluded by inadvertent IV injection of these salts.

Procaine penicillin G (Duracillin, Wycillin) is a viscous, white, opaque fluid which provides consistent therapeutic penicillin G serum levels for 12 h. The injection is nonirritating, partly because of the mild local anesthetic effect of the procaine. This is usually the IM dosage form of choice.

Benzathine penicillin G (Bicillin L-A) is a viscous, white, opaque fluid which provides low serum levels of penicillin G for up to 21 to 28 days. It is useful for periodic injections in the treatment or prevention of infection due to organisms that are sensitive to very low serum levels of penicillin (streptococcal prophylaxis in patients with rheumatic heart disease).

Combinations of the two salts (benzathine penicillin and procaine penicillin) are available in equal parts (Bicillin C-R injection) and three parts benzathine to one part procaine (Bicillin C-R 900/300). These dosage forms provide high initial levels with sustained lower levels for up to 10 days. They may be useful in single-dose therapy of streptococcal infection but do not provide sufficient serum levels for most other infections.

Penicillin V Penicillin V potassium (phenoxymethyl penicillin) possesses an antibacterial spectrum that is identical and pharmacologic properties that are very similar to penicillin G. Penicillin V is significantly more acid-stable, with better absorption following oral administration. When administered in equal oral doses, penicillin V produces serum levels two to five times those of penicillin G. However, penicillin V is available only in an oral dosage form.

Dosage Penicillin doses have been expressed in units rather than by weight since early penicillins were impure, and equal weights of drug did not necessarily produce equal biologic effects. One milligram of pure penicillin G sodium equals 1667 U. The conversion varies with other salts because of the varying weights of the salts. Thus, pure penicillin G doses are traditionally expressed in units. Doses of other penicillin dosage forms are usually expressed in milligrams, and doses of the newer penicillins are always expressed by weight. The common clinical conversion is 400,000 U of penicillin G equals 250 mg.

Oral adult doses of penicillin G or V are in the range of 250 to 500 mg three or four times a day. Oral pediatric doses of penicillin V are commonly 25,000 to 100,000 U/kg/day, divided into four doses.

Intravenous adult doses of aqueous penicillin G are between 1.2 and 24 million U/day, divided into four to six doses. Intramuscular adult doses of procaine penicillin G range from 300,000 to 1.2 million U q12h. Pediatric doses of penicillin G injection are usually between 25,000 and 250,000 U/kg/day, divided into four doses.

Preparations: Penicillinase-Resistant Penicillins
When penicillin was first used clinically, the majority of staphylococci were sensitive to penicillin G. Within a decade, however, resistance began to develop. The majority of

TABLE 28-10 Classification of Penicillins

GENERIC NAME	TRADE NAME	ADULT DOSAGE*
Natural		
Penicillin G	Pentide	Oral: 25,000–90,000 U/kg in 3–6 divided doses IV: Infused at a rate of 5000–100,000 U/h or, in severe infection, 20–80 million U/day in divided doses or as constant infusion
Penicillin G procaine	Wycillin, Duracillin	300,000–1.2 million U q48–72h
Penicillin G benzathine	Bicillin LA, Permapen	600,000–1.2 million U, usually q15–30 days
Penicillin G benzathine with procaine		
Phenoxymethyl penicillin (penicillin V potassium)	Pen-Vee K, V-Cillin K, Veetids	125–500 mg, 4–6 times daily; infants, 50 mg/kg/day
Semisynthetic Penicillinase-Resistant		
Methicillin	Staphcillin	IM or IV: 1 g q4–6 h; may give double or more IV dose in severe infections
Oxacillin	Bactocill, Prostaphlin	Oral: 500 mg q4–6 h; may double in severe infections IM or IV: 250–500 mg q4–6 h; may double in severe infections
Cloxacillin	Tegopen	Oral: 250–500 mg every 6 h; may double in severe infections
Nafcillin	Unipen	Oral: 250 mg to 1 g q4–6h IM: 500 mg q4–6h IV: 500 mg 1 g q4h
Dicloxacillin	Dynapen, Pathocil	Oral: 250–500 mg q6h; may double in severe infections
Broad-Spectrum Penicillins		
Ampicillin	Polycillin (many)	Oral: 250–500 mg q6h IM or IV: 0.25 g–2 g q6h to a maximum of 8–14 g/day
Amoxicillin	Larotid, Amoxil	Oral: 250–500 mg q8h to a maximum of 6 g/day
Carbenicillin indanyl sodium	Geocillin	Oral: For urinary tract infections only; 50–65 mg/kg/day in 4 doses
Carbenicillin disodium	Geopen, Pyopen	IM: 50–500 mg/kg/day in 4 doses; larger doses given IV IV: 50–500 mg/kg/day in 4–6 doses; maximal adult dose about 36 g
Ticarcillin	Ticar	IM: 50–100 mg/kg/day in 3–4 doses IV: 200–300 mg/kg/day in 4–6 doses; maximal adult dose about 24 g
Mezlocillin	Mezlin	IM: 1–2 g q6h IV: 200–300 mg/kg/day in 4–6 doses; maximal adult dose about 24 g
Azlocillin	Azlin	IM: 1–2 g q6h IV: 200–300 mg/kg/day in 4–6 doses; maximal adult dose about 24 g
Pipracillin	Pipracil	IM: 1–2 g q6h IV: 200–300 mg/kg/day in 4–6 doses; maximal adult dose about 24 g

*High dosage may be given for severe infections.

staphylococci are now penicillin G–resistant because of their ability to produce penicillinase. **Methicillin** (Staphcillin) was the first penicillin analog developed which was resistant to penicillinase. The drug is available for parenteral use only, and, although it is still effective, newer and more potent penicillinase-resistant penicillins are available (see Table 28-10). The isoxazole penicillins include **oxacillin** (Prostaphlin, Bactocill), **cloxacillin** (Tegopen), and **dicloxacillin** (Dynapen, Pathocil, Veracillin). They are the drugs of choice for treating infections due to penicillinase-producing staphylococci. Until bacteriology proves otherwise, one must assume that most staphylococci are now penicillinase producers. However, staphylococcal infections of the oral cavity are commonly sensitive to penicillin G or V.

Oxacillin and nafcillin are effective parenteral drugs for staphylococcal infections. They are administered in doses of 2 to 12 g/day divided into four to six doses. Dicloxacillin is the oral drug of choice because of its better absorption and lower minimum inhibitory concentration (MIC) for staphylococci as compared with the other drugs. This drug is administered in doses of 2 to 4 g/day in four doses.

Oral dicloxacillin doses for children (weighing <40 kg) are 12.5 mg/kg/day in four doses. Young children may object to the taste of dicloxacillin suspension; in this case the nurse should ask the prescriber to substitute oxacillin.

The penicillinase-resistant penicillins should not be used to treat infections due to penicillin G–sensitive organisms. These drugs do include the penicillin G spectrum but are less effective. Mixed infections due to both penicillinase-producing staphylococci and penicillin G–sensitive organisms can often be treated with a penicillinase-resistant penicillin alone.

Staphylococcal strains resistant to all of the penicillinase-resistant penicillins have been reported. These organisms, called *methicillin-resistant staphylococci*, develop resistance by mechanisms other than penicillinase production. **Vancomycin** may be indicated in infections due to these organisms.

Preparations: Broad-Spectrum Penicillins

Ampicillin   Ampicillin is a semisynthetic broad-spectrum penicillin that is acid-stable and penicillinase-sensitive. Its antimicrobial spectrum includes many gram-positive and gram-negative bacteria. It is not as effective against penicillin G–sensitive gram-positive cocci as penicillin G. When ampicillin was introduced, most *Escherichia coli, Haemophilus influenzae, Neisseria gonorrhea,* and *Proteus mirabilis* strains were sensitive. Today, organisms resistant to ampicillin are becoming more common.

Ampicillin is well absorbed following oral administration, but peak serum levels are higher when it is taken on an empty stomach. Oral doses produce peak levels in 2 h; IM doses peak at about 1 h. Adult doses are 2 to 4 g/day orally and 2 to 12 g/day parenterally, each divided into four

doses. Pediatric oral doses are 50 to 100 mg/kg/day, and parenteral doses range from 100 to 200 mg/kg/day, also divided into four doses. Meningitis should be treated more aggressively with more frequent IV dosing.

Amoxicillin   Amoxicillin (Amoxil, Larotid) is an analog of ampicillin similar in spectrum and pharmacologic characteristics. It is less effective than ampicillin against *Shigella.* It is available for oral use only and is better absorbed than ampicillin. Amoxicillin causes less diarrhea and may therefore be advantageous for patients who suffer severe GI upset from ampicillin. Amoxicillin is given three times a day, as compared to ampicillin's four times a day. The one less dose per day in both the adult and pediatric age groups may improve compliance. Otherwise it offers little advantage and is usually more expensive than ampicillin. Amoxicillin is available in combination with potassium clavulate (Augmentin). Potassium clavulate inhibits the enzyme β-lactamase and effectively expands the amoxicillin spectrum to include organisms that produce β-lactamase.

Carbenicillin   Carbenicillin (Geopen, Pyopen) is a semisynthetic penicillin which in large, parenteral doses is effective against severe gram-negative pathogens, including indole-positive *Proteus* and *Pseudomonas aeruginosa;* this drug has fallen into disuse in favor of other agents. The drug is penicillinase-sensitive. Carbenicillin is administered intravenously for severe systemic infections in a dose of 25 to 40 g/day in four divided doses. The pediatric dose is 100 to 500 mg/kg/day in four divided doses. Carbenicillin injection is a disodium salt containing approximately 5 meq of sodium per gram. **Carbenicillin indanyl sodium** (Geocillin) is an oral drug used exclusively in the treatment of urinary tract infections. The adult dose is 500 to 1000 mg orally qid. The pediatric dose is 50 to 65 mg/kg/day of carbenicillin indanyl in four divided doses.

Ticarcillin   Ticarcillin (Ticar) is given intramuscularly or intravenously since it is not absorbed orally. When used in the treatment of *Pseudomonas* infections, it requires high serum levels (60 µg/mL or greater) to be effective. The low toxicity associated with ticarcillin usually allows for the high levels to be achieved.

Ticarcillin is bactericidal and is active against both gram-positive and gram-negative organisms. It may be synergistic when used with **gentamicin sulfate** or **tobramycin sulfate** in the treatment of *Pseudomonas* infections.

It is given intravenously for serious infections in doses of 200 to 300 mg/kg/day (18 to 24 g/day) in three to eight divided doses. The dose for complicated urinary tract infections is 150 to 200 mg/kg/day given in four to six divided doses. When given by IM injection the dose should not exceed 2 g per injection. The pediatric dosage ranges from 75 to 100 mg/kg given IV every 8 h.

Azlocillin Azlocillin (Azlin) has a spectrum of activity similar to those of mezlocillin sodium and piperacillin. It is less active than the latter agents against most *Enterobacteriaceae* and anaerobes but is more active against *Pseudomonas aeruginosa.* Its primary use is in *Pseudomonas* infections, generally in combination with an aminoglycoside for severe infections.

Adverse reactions are similar to those seen in carbenicillin and mezlocillin (Table 28-9). The sodium content is 2.17 mg/g. The adult IV dosage for serious infections is 200 to 300 mg/kg/ day or 4 g q4h in life-threatening infections. Dosage should be decreased in renal impairment, with a dose of 30 g q12h if the patient is anuric.

Mezlocillin Mezlocillin (Mezlin) has a spectrum of activity similar to that of carbenicillin, but it is more active against *Streptococcus faecalis* (like ampicillin), indole-positive *Proteus, Klebsiella, Enterobacter* and *Serratia.* Its activity against *Pseudomonas aeruginosa* is greater than that of carbenicillin, but similar to that of ticaricillin. Adverse reactions are similar to those for azlocillin and carbenicillin. The sodium content is 1.85 meq/g.

Dosage for adults is 200 to 300 mg/kg/day in 4- to 6-g divided doses; in renal failure the dose is reduced to 2 to 3 g q4–6h.

Piperacillin Piperacillin (Pipracil) has a spectrum of activity similar to carbenicillins, except that it is more active against *Streptococcus faecalis* (like ampicillin) and many gram-negative bacteria, including *Pseudomonas aeruginosa, Klebsiella, Enterobacter* and *Bacteroides fragilis.* The emergence of resistant organisms during therapy has occurred when piperacillin was used alone in treatment of *Pseudomonas aeruginosa* infections. Adverse reactions are similar to those for carbenicillin, although a lower sodium content (2 meq/g) may reduce the risk of sodium overload. The adult IV dosage for serious infections is 200 to 300 mg/kg/day in equally divided doses q4–6h. Dosage must be reduced in cases of renal impairment.

CEPHALOSPORINS

The cephalosporins are semisynthetic antibiotic derivatives. They are similar to penicillins both chemically and in their mechanism of action. The drugs are significantly less sensitive to β-lactamase enzymes than are the penicillins. Organisms producing high levels of penicillinase and/or cephalosporinase may be resistant to cephalosporins. Cephalosporins are used as alternatives to penicillin in penicillin-allergic patients, but deaths due to acute cephalosporin allergic reaction have occurred in individuals with histories of penicillin allergy.

Spectrum of Activity

The cephalosporin antibiotics are classified into first-, second-, and third-generation antibiotics. The cephamycins are also classified with the cephalosporins because of their similar spectrum of activity. The first-generation cephalosporins are usually active against the gram-positive organisms, including *Staphylococcus aureus, Staphylococcus epidermidis,* group A and B hemolytic streptococci, and *Streptococcus pneumoniae.* The gram-negative organisms are somewhat more resistant, but cephalosporins may be active against *E. coli, K. pneumoniae, P. mirabilis,* and *Shigella.* The second-generation cephalosporins have a broader spectrum of activity, including most strains of *H. influenzae, Enterobacter, Neisseria* and all the strains susceptible to first-generation cephalosporins. The third-generation cephalosporins usually have less activity toward the gram-positive organisms but have a broader spectrum of activity toward gram-negative organisms.

The cephalosporins are among the most frequently overused antibiotics. Sensitive *Klebsiella* are among the only organisms for which the cephalosporins are considered the drug of choice. The cephalosporins can be considered a primary drug when toxicity and bacterial resistance indicate their use.

Pharmacokinetics

Cefamandole nafate, cefazolin sodium, cefotaxime sodium, and **cephalothin sodium** are not absorbed from the GI tract. **Cefaclor, cefadroxil monohydrate, cephalexin,** and **cephadrine** can be given orally. The cephalosporins are widely distributed in the body to pleural and synovial sites and into bones. They are poorly distributed into the CSF even when the meninges are inflamed. Oral probenecid will slow the renal excretion of the cephalosporins. The pharmacokinetic parameters are listed in Table 28-11.

Adverse Effects

Allergic reactions have occurred in about 5 percent of the patients receiving cephalosporins. Anaphylaxis has occurred (rarely), with the most common adverse reactions being rashes (maculopapular, morbilliform, and erythematous); fever; serum sickness; urticaria; pruritus; eosinophilia; and joint pain.

Approximately 3 percent of the patients receiving cephalosporins have a positive direct or indirect Coombs' test. Other hematologic effects include rare transient neutropenia, thrombocythemia, thrombocytopenia, and leukopenia.

The renal problems with cephalosporins include a mild transient increase in BUN and serum creatinine. A few cases of nephrotoxicity have been reported with **cephalothin, cephalexin,** and **cefazolin.** Liver problems include mild transient increase in SGOT, SGPT, and alkaline phosphatase which reverses when the drug is stopped.

TABLE 28-11 Pharmacokinetic Parameters of Selected Cephalosporins

DRUG	SERUM $t_{1/2}$ (h)		PEAK SERUM* CONC. ($\mu g/mL$)	PROTEIN BINDING (%)
	N	R		
Cefaclor	1	2.5	25†	25
Cefadroxil	1–2	15–20	28–33‡	90
Cefamandole	1	11–18	20–35	70
Cefazolin	1.5–2	20–70	50–75	85–95
Cefoperazone	2	—	75	90
Cefotaxime	1	1.5–3	20	30
Cefoxitin	1	20	23	85–90
Ceftizoxime	1.7	24–36	35	28
Cefuroxime	1	—	40	33
Cephalexin	1	20–40	35§	5–15
Cephalothin	0.5	2–3	15–20	60–70
Moxalactam	2–3	20–40	30–50	50

N = normal renal function; R = renal dysfunction.
*The peak concentration is based on 1-g injection given IM.
†Oral administration of a 500-mg dose gives peak levels of 23–25 $\mu g/mL$.
‡Oral administration of a 500-mg dose gives peak levels of 15–16 $\mu g/mL$.
§Oral administration of a 500-mg dose gives peak level of 32–39 $\mu g/mL$.

Pain is associated with the IM administration of all cephalosporins (especially **cephalothin**). Infusion phlebitis occurs in 30 to 50 percent of the patients receiving IV cephalosporins.

The intrathecal use of cephalosporins has been associated with CNS toxicities, including hallucinations, seizures, and nystagmus.

Preparations: First-Generation Cephalosporins

The dosages and preparations of cephalosporins are given in Table 28-12.

Cephalothin Cephalothin (Keflin) appears to be the cephalosporin most resistant to β-lactamase. It is available only in the injectable form and most commonly administered in doses of 2 to 12 g/day (four to six divided doses) in adults. The pediatric dose is 60 to 100 mg/kg/day, administered in four to six doses. Higher doses carry greater risks of nephrotoxicity.

Cephaloridine Cephaloridine (Loridine) is seldom used today because it produces nephrotoxicity. Intramuscularly, it is the best-tolerated cephalosporin, producing peak levels within 30 min. Although this drug produces the highest CSF levels of the cephalosporins, it is generally not useful in meningitis because of its toxicities.

Cefazolin Cefazolin (Ancef, Kefzol) is better tolerated after IM injection than cephalothin and produces higher serum levels. Approximately 500 mg every 8 h of cefazolin is equal to 1 g of cephalothin every 6 h.

Cephapirin Cephapirin (Cefadyl) is pharmacologically similar to cephalothin. It is better tolerated on IM injection, although cephalothin may be more resistant to β-lactamase.

Cephalexin Cephalexin (Keflex) is an acid-stable oral cephalosporin that is well absorbed from the GI tract. Peak serum levels are reached in 1 h. The drug is excreted primarily unchanged in the urine. It is useful in treating systemic or urinary tract infections. The adult dose is 1 to 4 g/day, given in four divided doses. The pediatric dose is 25 to 50 mg/kg/day, given in four divided doses. Cephalexin and oral cepharadine appear to be clinically interchangeable.

Cefadroxil Cefadroxil (Duricef) is acid-stable and is rapidly and almost completely absorbed from the GI tract. The absorption of cefadroxil is not delayed in the presence of food. The other oral cephalosporins have their absorption delayed in the presence of food. The serum half-life of cefadroxil is 63 to 119 min in adults with normal renal function. Cefadroxil is excreted unchanged in the urine. More than 90 percent of a single 500-mg or 1-g oral dose is excreted within 8 h in adults with normal renal function. The usual daily oral adult dosage for the treatment of urinary tract infections is 1 to 2 g, given in one or two divided doses. For the treatment of skin and skin structure infection, the usual daily adult dosage is 1 g in one or two divided doses. For group A β-hemolytic streptococcal pharyngitis, the usual adult dosage is 1 g, given in two divided doses. In patients with impaired renal function, doses and/or frequency of administration must be modified in response to the degree of impairment.

TABLE 28-12 Cephalosporins

DRUG	TRADE NAME	ADULT DOSAGE*
First-Generation		
Cephalothin	Keflin	IV: 500 mg to 1 g q4–6h IM: not recommended
Cephaloridine	Loridine	IM: 500 mg to 1 g q6–8h
Cefazolin	Ancef, Kefzol	IM or IV: 250 mg to 1 g q6–12h
Cephapirin	Cefadyl	IM or IV: 500 mg to 1 g q4–6h
Cephalexin	Keflex	Oral: 250–500 q6h
Cephaloglycine	Kafocin	Oral: 250–500 mg q6h
Cefadroxil	Duricef	Oral: 500 mg to 1 g q12–24h
Cephradine	Velosef, Anspor	Oral: 250 mg to 1 g q6h IM or IV: 500 mg to 1 g q4–6h
Cefuroxime	Zinacef	*Adult:* 75–100 g q8h *Child:* 50–100 mg/kg/day
Second-Generation		
Cefaclor	Ceclor	Oral: 250–500 q6–8h
Cefamandole	Mandol	IM or IV: 500 mg to 1 g q4–8h
Cefoxitin (Cephamycin)	Mefoxin	IV: 1–2 g q6–8h
Third-Generation		
Cefotaxime	Claforan	IM or IV: 1–2 g q6–8h
Cefoperazone	Cefobid	IM or IV: 1–2 g q8–12h
Moxalactam	Moxam	IM or IV: 1–2 g q8–12h
Ceftizoxime	Cefizox	1–2 g q8h

*Higher dosages may be given for severe infections.

Cephradine Cephradine (Anspor, Velosef) possesses characteristics very similar to those of cefazolin. This drug is also available in oral dosage forms that are pharmacologically very similar to cephalexin (Keflex).

Preparations: Second-Generation Cephalosporins

Cefaclor Cefaclor (Ceclor) is a semisynthetic cephalosporin antibiotic. It is acid-stable and is well absorbed from the GI tract. The serum half-life of cefaclor is 25 to 60 min in adults with normal renal function. The drug is excreted unchanged in the urine. Approximately 50 to 85 percent of a single oral dose is excreted within 8 h in adults with normal renal function. Cefaclor is indicated in the treatment of the following infections:

1. Otitis media caused by *S. pneumoniae, H. influenzae, Staphylococcus,* and *S. pyogenes.*
2. Respiratory tract infections including pneumonia due to *S. pneumoniae, H. influenzae,* and *S. pyogenes.*
3. Infections in the upper respiratory tract, skin, and urinary tract.

Adult dosage is 250 to 500 mg, given orally every 8 h. Larger doses have been used to treat severe infections. In children the usual dose is 20 mg/kg/day, given in divided doses every 8 h.

Cefamandole Nafate Cefamandole nafate (Mandol) is not absorbed orally and must be given parenterally. It is hydrolyzed in the plasma to cefamandole, which has the majority of the antibacterial activity. Cefamandole has greater resistance to β-lactamase than the second-generation cephalosporins. It also has improved activity compared to first-generation cephalosporins against gram-negative bacteria, including *H. influenzae* (including ampicillin-resistant strains), *E. coli, Proteus,* and many *Enterobacter.* The adult dose of 500 mg to 1 g every 4 to 8 h can be increased in patients with serious infections, not to exceed 12 g/day. The usual pediatric dose is 50 to 100 mg/kg, given in divided doses every 4 to 8 h. Dosage must be adjusted in renal diseases. The adult dosage is 500 mg to 1 g every 4 to 6 h, to a maximum of 12 g/day, given IM or IV.

Cefoxitin Cefoxitin (Mefoxin) has greater gram-negative activity than first-generation cephalosporins (e.g., cefazolin), especially against *B. fragilis* and other anaerobic organisms, generally because of the greater β-lactamase resistance of cefoxitin. Gram-positive activity is equivalent to or less than cefazolin's. Adverse reactions are similar to those of other cephalosporins except that cefoxitin is very painful on IM injection. The adult IV dosage is 1 to 2 g every 6 to 8 h, to a maximum of 12 g/day.

Cefuroxime Cefuroxime (Zinacef) is a second-generation cephalosporin which has similar activity to cefamandoles. It is not orally bioavailable and therefore must be given IM or IV. The serum half-life is 60 to 120 min and it should be given every 6 to 8 h. Cefuroxime is widely distributed to most body tissues and penetrates the inflamed meninges, making it useful in the treatment of bacterial meningitis (it is the only second-generation cephalosporin to be approved to treat bacterial meningitis). It is excreted unchanged in the urine. The usual adult dose is between 0.75 and 1.0 g every 8 h. In severe cases of meningitis 1.5 g may be required every 6 h. In infants and children 3 years of age and older, a dose of 50 to 100 mg/kg/day is recommended.

Preparations: Third-Generation Cephalosporins

Cefotaxime Cefotaxime (Claforan) can be distinguished from previous agents by markedly increased activity against a variety of gram-negative organisms, including some potentially useful activity (similar to ticarcillin's) against *Pseudomonas aeruginosa*. Gram-positive activity is inferior to that of cefazolin. Adverse effects are similar to other cephalosporins. Most strains of *Clostridium difficile* are resistant, and cases of pseudomembranous colitis have been observed. The usual adult IV dosage is 1 to 2 g every 6 to 8 h, to a maximum of 12 g/day.

Cefoperazone Cefoperazone (Cefobid) is a third-generation cephalosporin similar to cefotaxime and moxalactam. However, its activity against *Pseudomonas aeruginosa* is superior, inhibiting 50 percent of strains at 5 to 6.2 μg/mL. The pharmacokinetics of cefoperazone have not been studied completely, but it appears to undergo very significant biliary elimination, producing biliary concentration exceeding 1 mg/mL. Only 15 to 30 percent of the drug is excreted in the urine. The half-life of the drug is 2 h. The pharmacokinetic properties allow cefoperazone to be given every 12 h. Early studies have reported frequent diarrhea, perhaps related to biliary elimination, and a disulfiram-like reaction (flushing and nausea when alcohol is consumed). The adult IV and IM dose is 1 to 2 g every 8 to 12 h, and adverse reactions are similar to those for other cephalosporins.

Moxalactam Moxalactam (Moxam) shares most pharmacologic properties with cephalosporins. It closely resembles cefotaxime in its spectrum and activity, although moxalactam's activity against streptococci and staphylococci is inferior and its activity against anaerobic organisms is superior. It is not significantly metabolized and is primarily eliminated unchanged in the urine, with a half-life of 2 to 3 h. Early trials suggest that it may provide effective CSF con-

centrations for the treatment of meningitis. Adverse reactions are similar to reactions of cephalosporins, although several cases of thrombocytosis, enterococcal superinfection, agranulocytosis, and colitis have been reported. A vitamin K-responsive hypoprothrombinemia and bleeding have occurred, as has a disulfiram-like interaction with alcohol. The usual dosage (IM or IV) for adults is 2 to 6 g/day, to a maximum of 12 g/day in two to three divided doses.

Ceftizoxime Sodium Ceftizoxime sodium (Cefizox) is indicated for serious infections caused by susceptible organisms. It has a high degree of resistance to β-lactamase. It is similar to the other third-generation cephalosporins in that it also lacks oral bioavailability and must be given IV or IM. Ceftizoxamine has a serum half-life of about 2 h and is excreted unchanged in the kidneys. Dosage should be reduced in patients with decreased renal function. The most common adverse effects are GI disturbances (nausea, vomiting, diarrhea), rash, and pruritis. The usual adult dose is 1 to 2 g every 8 to 12 h; higher doses can be given in more serious infections.

MACROLIDE ANTIBIOTICS

The macrolide antibiotics are so named because they contain a large lactone ring. Erythromycin is the only true macrolide that is used clinically. Troleandomycin (TAO) is a semisynthetic macrolide that is less effective and more toxic (hepatotoxic) than erythromycin and is used as an adjunctive therapy in respiratory disease (see Chap. 27).

Erythromycin

Erythromycin is available as erythromycin base, plus three salts for oral use, one salt for IM use, and two salts for IV use (Table 28-13). The salts provide stability and other formulation advantages, but the free erythromycin base is the biologically active form.

Mechanism of Action

Erythromycin inhibits protein synthesis by binding to the 50S subunit of the ribosomes of sensitive microorganisms. The drug does not act on the cell wall and is therefore effective against some cell-wall-deficient organisms. Erythromycin is usually bacteriostatic, although high concentrations may be bactericidal.

Spectrum of Activity

Erythromycins have a bacterial spectrum of activity that is larger than that of penicillin G. They are most effective against gram-positive cocci (staphylococci and streptococci) and bacilli. Their gram-negative activity includes cocci (*Neisseria*) and bacilli (*H. influenzae*, *Legionella pneumophila*, *Pasteurella*, and *Brucella*). Erythromycins also inhibit

TABLE 28-13 Erythromycins

FORM	TRADE NAME	DOSAGE*
Erythromycin base	E-mycin, Ilotycin, Eryc	*Adults:* 250–500 mg PO q6h to a maximum of 4 g/day *Pediatric:* 30–50 mg/kg/day PO in four divided doses
Erythromycin estolate	Ilosone	*Adults:* 250–500 mg PO q6h to a maximum of 4 g/day
Erythromycin ethylsuccinate	E.E.S., Pediamycin	*Orally:* 400 mg q6h to a maximum of 4 g/day†
Erythromycin glucceptate	Ilotycin	*Adults:* IV: 15–20 mg/kg/day in four divided doses *Pediatrics:* Same dose†
Erythromycin lactobionate	Erythrocin, Lactobionate IV	Same as glucceptate†
Erythromycin stearate	Erythrocin, Bristamycin	*Adults:* 250–500 mg PO q6h *Pediatric:* 30–50 mg/kg/day PO in four divided doses

*Higher dosages may be given for severe infections.
†Dosage is expressed in terms of erythromycin.

some strains of *Mycoplasma pneumoniae, Rickettsia, Treponema, Entamoeba histolytica,* and atypical mycobacteria.

Clinical Use

The major clinical uses of erythromycin are as alternatives to penicillin in penicillin-allergic patients, particularly in streptococcal, staphylococcal, and pneumococcal infections. It is also useful prophylactically in penicillin-allergic patients with rheumatic heart disease. Erythromycin is a first-line agent in respiratory and otic infections due to *Mycoplasma pneumoniae.* It is effective in eradicating the diptheria carrier state. Erythromycin has been used in the treatment of Legionnaires' disease. Erythromycin is also useful as a second-line drug in a variety of other infections.

Pharmacokinetics

Orally administered erythromycin is absorbed from the small intestine but is acid-labile. Erythromycin-base tablets (E-Mycin, Ilotycin, Eryce, others) are therefore enteric-coated. **Erythromycin stearate** tablets (Bristamycin, Erythrocin Stearate, others) provide more consistent levels than many enteric-coated base tablets (stearate tablets are generally film-coated). **Erythromycin estolate** capsules (Ilosone) provide the highest, most consistent serum levels, but this advantage must be weighed against the known hepatotoxicity of this preparation. Erythromycin estolate oral suspension (Ilosone) is also available.

Oral erythromycin dosage forms produce peak plasma levels in 1 to 4 h (levels of 0.1 to 2 μg/mL). The drugs are best absorbed when taken on an empty stomach. The serum half-life of erythromycin is 1.5 to 2 h. In patients with renal

disease the half-life increases to 6 h. This feature is usually not clinically important. Body tissue levels, except in the CNS, usually exceed serum levels. The drug diffuses into cerebrospinal, peritoneal, and pleural fluids. Less than 5 percent of orally administered erythromycin is excreted unchanged in the urine. The drug is largely metabolized in the liver and excreted into the bile feces. Erythromycin crosses the placenta, giving fetal concentrations of 5 to 20 percent of the maternal serum concentrations.

Adverse Effects

Erythromycin is associated with a low incidence of adverse effects. GI upset following oral drug is the most frequent complaint. Hypersensitivity reactions of fever and rash occur rarely. Significant toxicity is seen only with erythromycin estolate, which can produce cholestatic hepatitis. The syndrome generally occurs after 1 to 3 weeks of treatment and produces nausea, vomiting, and abdominal cramps similar to those of acute cholecystitis. These symptoms are resolved upon discontinuation of the drug. IM injections of erythromycin cause severe, lasting pain. IV infusions cause a high incidence of phlebitis and have been associated with reversible hearing loss. Superinfection is also a potential problem.

Dosage

The oral adult dose is 1 to 2 g/day, divided into four doses for all forms except the ethylsuccinate. The IV dose is 1 to 4 g/day, divided into four doses. Oral and parenteral pediatric doses are 30 to 50 mg/kg/day, divided into four doses.

Preparations

Erythromycin ethylsuccinate is available in both tablets (E.E.S. 400) and oral suspension (Erythromycin Ethylsuccinate Suspension, Pediamycin). This ester salt is absorbed as is and must be enzymatically cleaved in the serum to free erythromycin in order to be effective. This gradual process results in only about 60 percent of the drug's being biologically active at any given time. Therefore, 400 mg of the ethylsuccinate is needed to produce the in vivo activity of 250 mg of the base, stearate, or estolate.

The IM dosage form is erythromycin ethylsuccinate (Erythrocin Ethylsuccinate-IM). IV erythromycin is available as the glucceptate (Ilotycin Glucceptate Intra Venous) and the erythromycin lactobionate (Erythrocin Lactobionate—I.V.) (see Table 28-13).

CLINDAMYCIN AND LINCOMYCIN

Clindamycin (Cleocin) and lincomycin (Lincocin) have similar spectra of activity, but clindamycin is more effective against those sensitive organisms (see spectrum of activity). It also has been associated with less toxicity, and therefore it is more frequently used clinically. This discussion emphasizes clindamycin.

Mechanism of Action

Clindamycin and lincomycin act in the same manner as erythromycin, chloramphenicol, and troleandomycin by binding with the 50S subunit of the ribosomes of sensitive organisms and inhibiting protein synthesis. They both are bacteriostatic in low concentrations and may be bactericidal in higher concentrations.

Spectrum of Activity

Clindamycin is active against most aerobic gram-positive organisms, including staphylococci, streptococci (except *S. faecalis*), and pneumococci. Clindamycin and lincomycin are active against anaerobic and microaerophilic gram-positive and gram-negative organisms. The MIC for many organisms is 0.1 to 4.0 μg/mL.

Pharmacokinetics

Clindamycin palmitate hydrochloride and clindamycin phosphate are well absorbed from the GI tract, but prior to absorption they must be hydrolyzed to clindamycin. Following a 150-mg dose of clindamycin, peak plasma levels are 1.9 to 3.9 μg/mL 45 to 60 min after the dose. Clindamycin is well distributed throughout the body, with good levels in bone and synovial fluid but poor levels in the CSF even when the meninges are inflamed. It is approximately 93 percent protein-bound. It is largely liver-metabolized, and the metabolites are excreted in the urine and bile. Approximately 10 percent of each dose is excreted in the urine unchanged. The normal half-life of clindamycin is 2 to 3 h.

Clinical Use

The main use of clindamycin is in the treatment of serious infections of the respiratory tract, skin, soft tissue, septicemia, and intraabdominal and other sites that are due to anaerobic organisms. A major use is in the treatment of *Bacteroides fragilis*.

Adverse Effects

Untoward effects of clindamycin and lincomycin are similar, the most serious being pseudomembranous colitis. Skin rash occurs in about 10 percent of patients, and Stevens-Johnson syndrome has occurred. IV use may produce thrombophlebitis. Because of the potential for severe GI toxicity, clindamycin should not be used when less toxic drugs are active against the pathogen.

The most common adverse effect is diarrhea, occurring in about 20 percent of patients receiving the drug. It may begin after a few days of therapy or days to weeks after the drug is discontinued. This diarrhea can be severe. Pseudomembranous colitis has occurred and has caused fatalities. Oral administration has also produced stomatitis, nausea, vomiting, skin rashes, and vaginitis. Parenteral use has produced reversible neutropenia, leukopenia, and thrombopenia.

Dosage

The usual adult dosage of clindamycin is 150 to 450 mg every 6 h. The usual pediatric dose is 8 to 25 mg/kg in three or four divided doses. The usual adult dose IM or IV is 600 mg to 2.7 g daily in two to four divided doses. An IV infusion can be given in a dose of 10 mg/min for 30 min, followed by an infusion rate of 0.75 mg/min. This should give a clindamycin level of 4 to 5 μg/mL (see Table 28-14).

TETRACYCLINES

Tetracyclines are broad-spectrum bacteriostatic agents, and all have similar pharmacologic and antimicrobial spectrum characteristics. Cross-resistance usually exists among tetracyclines, with the exception of **minocycline**, which may be effective against strains of staphylococci that are resistant to other tetracyclines.

Mechanism of Action

Tetracyclines act by binding to the 30S ribosomal subunit, thus inhibiting protein synthesis. This is the basis of the drug's bacteriostatic action. It affects only rapidly multiplying organisms. Higher concentrations of drug are needed to affect susceptible gram-negative organisms than are required for susceptible gram-positive organisms. Higher concentrations may be bactericidal.

Spectrum of Activity

The tetracyclines are classified as broad-spectrum antibiotics with activity against many gram-positive and gram-negative

TABLE 28-14   Clindamycin Dosage Forms

DRUG	TRADE NAME	DOSAGE
Clindamycin hydrochloride	Cleocin	*Adult:* Orally: 150–450 mg q6h
Clindamycin palmitate HCl	Cleocin Pediatric	IM or IV: 600 mg–2.7 g/day in 2–4 divided doses to a maximum of 4.8
Clindamycin phosphate	Cleocin Phosphate	g/day; single IM dose greater than 600 mg is not recommended.
		Note: Infuse no faster than 30 mg/min.
		Pediatric: Oral: Child over 10 kg: 8–25 mg/kg/day in 3–4 divided doses
		Child under 10 kg: Give no less than 37.5 mg q8h.
		IM or IV (over 1 month): 15–40 mg/kg/day in 3–4 divided doses (not less than 300 mg/day in severe infection regardless of weight)

organisms, and *Rickettsia, Chlamydia, Mycoplasma,* and spirochetes. Although the tetracyclines are active in vitro against many aerobic gram-positive cocci, they should not be used to treat staphylococcus, group A β-hemolytic streptococcus, or *Streptococcus pneumoniae* infections because of their resistance to tetracyclines. Patients with severe staphylococcal infections should not use tetracycline because a bactericidal antimicrobial is preferred.

Pharmacokinetics

Tetracyclines are readily but incompletely absorbed from the GI tract. Divalent and trivalent cations (aluminum, calcium, iron, and magnesium found in antacids, hematinics, iron preparations, and dairy foods) all chelate tetracyclines in the gut and can significantly reduce GI absorption. Drugs and foods should not be taken within 2 h of a dose of oral tetracycline. Sodium bicarbonate also decreases GI absorption of tetracyclines.

Differences exist in the absorption of various tetracyclines. Oxytetracycline and tetracycline are least well absorbed. Peak serum levels following a single oral dose occur in 2 to 4 h, and therapeutic levels persist for 6 to 12 h. Demeclocycline and methacycline are only 60 to 80 percent absorbed when given on an empty stomach but produce therapeutic plasma levels for 24 h. Doxycycline and minocycline are well absorbed, even when taken with food, producing peak plasma levels in 2 h; therapeutic levels are maintained for 24 h. Except for doxycycline and minocycline, which should be taken with food, tetracyclines should be taken on an empty stomach (1 h before or 2 h after meals).

The various tetracyclines differ in their degrees of serum protein binding, but these differences are not generally clinically significant (see Table 28-15). Patients with liver disease or bile-duct obstruction may have decreased clearance of tetracyclines. The half-life of tetracyclines increases when given to patients with decreased renal function. Doxycycline and minocycline are excreted primarily by nonrenal routes, and their half-life does not change. Liver dysfunction or bile duct obstruction may significantly increase the duration of tetracycline levels. The drugs are well distributed throughout body tissues, cross the placenta, and are found in human milk. CSF levels are about one-fourth those of serum levels.

Adverse Effects

The adverse effects of the tetracyclines have led to the use of newer agents in other drug classes to treat infections for which tetracyclines were once commonly used. Sensitization can occur, and angioedema and anaphylaxis may occur with the oral drug. Hives, rashes, and exfoliative dermatitis may occur with any tetracycline.

Gastrointestinal discomfort is common and dose-related. Gastritis, nausea and vomiting, and diarrhea may occur from chemical irritation. Superinfection may also produce diarrhea. Intramuscular administration produces poor absorption and great discomfort; intravenous use is associated with a high incidence of phlebitis. Fatty infiltration of the liver was initially observed with IV doses of more than 2 g/day of tetracycline hydrochloride in pregnant women. Although pregnancy introduces greater risk of hepatoxicity, this effect may occur with high doses of any tetracycline by parenteral or oral routes in any patient with impaired excretory capability. Intravenous doxycycline is associated with less hepatotoxicity because it is mainly excreted with the bile. Fatty liver secondary to tetracycline toxicity carries a significant risk of mortality.

Tetracyclines are teratogenic and may cause irreversible tooth mottling in children as a result of the drugs' high affinity for calcium. The metabolic effects include increased catabolism and disturbances in nitrogen balance. Tetracyclines may delay blood coagulation. Administration to infants has produced increased intracranial pressure. Dizziness, ataxia, and nausea have been reported among a significant number of patients taking minocycline, and photosensitization has been reported with demeclocycline. Outdated or degraded tetracycline has produced a severe nephropathy similar to Fanconi syndrome and lupus-like skin lesions. Tetracyclines have been shown to exacerbate preexisting nephropathy. Thus, with the possible exception of doxycycline and minocycline, tetracyclines are contraindicated in patients with renal dysfunction. Long-term tetracycline use may produce changes in blood elements and thrombocytopenic purpura.

Nonabsorbed tetracycline passes into the intestinal contents. Gut flora are significantly changed within 48 h after oral tetracycline therapy is initiated. Changes in stool color, odor, and consistency are common. Gastrointestinal cramp-

TABLE 28-15 Pharmacokinetic Parameters of Tetracyclines

DRUG	PERCENT BOUND TO SERUM PROTEIN	SERUM HALF-LIFE (h)	PREDOMINANT ROUTE OF EXCRETION
Demeclocycline	36–91	10–17	Renal
Doxycycline	25–93	14–24	Biliary
Methacycline	75–90	7–15	Renal
Minocycline	55–88	11–26	Liver
Oxytetracycline	10–40	6–10	Renal
Tetracycline	20–67	6–12	Renal

ing and diarrhea may occur. Flora return to normal within a few days of cessation of therapy. However, superinfection may result from tetracycline-resistant organisms. Fatal superinfections due to coagulase-positive staphylococci have been reported.

Clinical Use

The tetracyclines are active in vitro against many urinary pathogens and are safe, inexpensive, and effective therapy for most cases of uncomplicated lower urinary tract infections caused by susceptible microorganisms in adults. Because the tetracyclines are less active in vitro in an alkaline medium, effectiveness may be enhanced if the pH of the urine is maintained in the acidic range during the treatment of urinary tract infections. The tetracyclines should not be used for the treatment of acute pyelonephritis unless use of other antimicrobial agents, such as the aminoglycosides or semisynthetic penicillins, is contraindicated. Currently, the tetracyclines are the agents of choice for the treatment of urethritis caused by *Chlamydia* and *ureaplasma urealyticum*. Doxycycline is effective therapy for chlamydia cervicithis and pelvic inflammatory disease (PID).

Tetracycline or erythromycin is considered the agent of choice for the treatment of *Mycoplasma pneumoniae* infections. Combination therapy with a tetracycline and streptomycin is the most effective treatment for brucellosis. The tetracyclines can be used for the treatment of syphilis and gonorrhea in patients who are allergic to penicillin, although tetracycline-resistant gonococcus strains have been reported. Tetracycline is also effective treatment for rickettsial infections and other uncommon infections.

Doxycycline is effective prophylactic therapy for traveler's diarrhea caused by toxicogenic strains of *Escherichia coli*. The tetracyclines are effective in the treatment of patients with cholera. The tetracyclines should not be used as prophylaxis for subacute bacterial endocarditis or recurrent acute rheumatic fever.

Tetracyclines may be alternated with ampicillin and other broad-spectrum antimicrobial agents for long-term, intermittent, suppressive therapy in patients with chronic bronchopulmonary infections. The tetracyclines are effective in the treatment of acne; they presumably act by decreasing the fatty acid content of sebum. Low-dose tetracycline (250 mg twice daily) is effective therapy for this condition. Minocycline is reportedly effective in the treatment of nocardia infections. Although rifampin is the agent of choice for meningococcal carriers, minocycline may be used alternatively if use of rifampin is contraindicated.

Dosage

The oral adult dose of tetracyclines varies both with the drug and the disease being treated. Tetracycline and oxytetracycline are normally administered in doses of 1 to 2 g/day as four divided doses. The oral dose of demeclocycline and methacycline is 600 mg/day, in two to four divided doses per day. The oral dose of doxycycline and minocycline is 100 mg once or twice a day. The parenteral dose of tetracycline, oxytetracycline, and chlortetracycline is 0.75 to 1 g/day, divided into two to four intravenous doses. IM use is discouraged because of pain on injection and poor absorption. Doxycycline and minocycline injections are administered as 100 to 200 mg/day, in one or two divided doses. Tetracyclines are generally not recommended for pediatric use. In children the oral dose of tetracycline is 20 to 40 mg/kg/day as four divided doses, and the parenteral dose is 10 to 20 g/kg/day in two divided doses. Table 28-16 lists the available tetracycline preparations.

AMINOGLYCOSIDES

The aminoglycoside antibiotics are frequently used in the treatment of life-threatening gram-negative bacterial infections. They are synergistic with the penicillins, cephalosporins, and clindamycin; therefore, in the critically ill patient

TABLE 28-16 Tetracyclines

DRUG	TRADE NAME	DOSAGE
Tetracycline HCl	Achromycin, Sumycin	*Adult:* Orally 250–500 g q6–12h IV: 250–500 mg every 6–12h to a maximum of 2 g/day Pediatric (over 8 years of age): 25–50 mg/kg daily in four divided doses
Demeclocycline	Declomycin	*Adult:* Oral: 600 mg/day in 2–4 divided doses
Doxycycline	Vibramycin	*Adult:* Oral: 100 mg q12h for 1 day, then 50–100 mg/day IV: 200 mg in 1–2 divided doses for 1 day, then 100–200 mg/day
Methacycline	Rondomycin	*Adult:* Oral: 300 mg q12h
Minocycline	Minocin	*Adult:* Oral or IV: 200 mg initially, then 100 mg q12h
Oxytetracycline	Terramycin, others	*Adult:* Oral: 250–500 mg q6h IM: 100–250 mg q12h IV: 250–500 mg q6–12h to a maximum of 2 g/day

combination therapy is frequently used. The main disadvantage of using aminoglycosides is their low therapeutic index and the adverse effects of ototoxicity and nephrotoxicity. Neomycin is the most active of the aminoglycosides and also the most toxic, and streptomycin is the least active and least toxic. Gentamicin, kanamycin, tobramycin, amikacin, and netilmycin all have intermediate activity and toxicity (see Table 28-17).

Mechanism of Action

All aminoglycosides are bactericidal, since they inhibit protein synthesis through their effect on the 30S subunit of the ribosomes of susceptible organisms. Bacterial resistance is acquired slowly, except with streptomycin. Cross-resistance among aminoglycosides is common.

Spectrum of Activity

The spectrum of activity of the various aminoglycoside antibiotics will vary with the individual drug and the organisms being treated. In general the aminoglycosides are active against numerous aerobic gram-negative and some gram-positive bacteria. Aminoglycosides are inactive against anaerobic bacteria. The gram-negative organisms are most susceptible to amikacin, gentamicin, netilmicin, and tobramycin, with resistance being more common with kanamycin. Other susceptible gram-negative organisms include *Enterobacter, E. coli, Klebsiella, Proteus* (indole-positive and indole-negative), *Pseudomonas, Salmonella, Serratia,* and *Shigella*. Streptomycin is active against numerous strains of mycobacteria, including *Mycobacterium tuberculosis*.

Pharmacokinetics

Aminoglycosides are poorly absorbed after oral administration and therefore must be given parenterally (IM or IV). After parenteral administration they are excreted almost entirely by the kidney and are only minimally bound to plasma proteins (except streptomycin, which is 35 percent protein-bound). After an IV dose the drug is rapidly distributed to highly perfused organs and to extracellular water. The elimination of the half-life aminoglycosides in patients with normal renal function is 2 to 4 h. Aminoglycosides are excreted unchanged in the urine by glomerular filtration and some tubular reabsorption. Dosages should be adjusted for those with renal impairment (Table 28-18).

TABLE 28-17 Aminoglycosides

DRUG	ROUTE	DOSAGE (NORMAL RENAL FUNCTION)	SPECTRUM	COMMENTS
Amikacin	IV or IM	*Adult*: 15 mg/kg/day in divided doses q8–12h *Children*: 7.5 mg/kg q12h	Similar to gentamicin but active against many isolates of *Proteus, Pseudomonas,* and *Serratia* resistant to gentamicin and tobramycin	A semisynthetic derivative of kanamycin that is resistant to many bacterial enzymes which degrade gentamicin and tobramycin
Gentamicin	IV or IM	*Adult*; 3–5 mg/kg/day in divided doses q8h *Children*: 6–7.5 mg/kg/day in divided doses q8h	Most aerobic gram-negative bacteria sensitive	Resistance is still uncommon among gram-negative aerobes but is increasing. Some strains of *Proteus, Klebsiella, Serratia,* and *P. aeruginosa* are resistant.
Kanamycin	IV or IM	*Adults and Children*: 15 mg/kg/day in divided doses q6–12h maximum (1.5 g/day)	Most *Pseudomonas* are resistant. Some *E. coli* and *Klebsiella* are resistant	
Netilmicin	IV or IM	3.5 mg/kg/day in divided doses q8h	Similar to gentamicin	Less active than gentamicin against *P. aeruginosa;* data suggest it may be less nephrotoxic and ototoxic than gentamicin.
Neomycin	Oral	2–8 g/day in 2–4 divided doses	Activity between kanamycin and gentamicin	
Streptomycin	IM	15 mg/kg/day in divided doses q12h (maximum 2 g/day)	Many gram-negative bacilli are resistant.	The only aminoglycoside with demonstrated activity against *Mycobacterium tuberculosis*
Tobramycin	IV or IM	*Adults and Children*: 3–5 mg/kg/day in divided doses q8h	Similar to gentamicin	Although most strains of *Pseudomonas* are sensitive to tobramycin and gentamicin, tobramycin is inhibitory at one-third the concentration of gentamicin; *Serratia* may be less sensitive to tobramycin than to gentamicin.

TABLE 28-18 Aminoglycoside Dosing for Adults with Renal Impairment*

1. Select loading dose in mg/kg (based on estimated ideal body weight) to provide peak serum concentrations in range listed below for desired aminoglycoside.

AMINOGLYCOSIDE	USUAL LOADING DOSES	EXPECTED PEAK SERUM CONCENTRATIONS
Tobramycin, Gentamicin	1.5–2.0 mg/kg	4–10 µg/mL
Amikacin, Kanamycin	5.0–7.5 mg/kg	15–30 µg/mL

2. Select maintenance dose (as percentage of chosen loading dose) to continue peak serum concentrations indicated above according to desired dosing interval and the patient's corrected creatinine clearance [C(c)cr].

$$C(c)cr \text{ male} = 140 - age/serum \ creatinine$$
$$C(c)cr \text{ female} = 0.85 \times C(c)cr \text{ male}$$

C(c)cr (mL/min)	HALF-LIFE† (h)	8 h	12 h	24 h
90	3.1	84%	—	—
80	3.4	80	91%	—
70	3.9	76	88	—
60	4.5	71	84	—
50	5.3	65	79	—
40	6.5	57	72	92%
30	8.4	48	63	86
25	9.9	43	57	81
20	11.9	37	50	75
17	13.6	33	46	70
15	15.1	31	42	67
12	17.9	27	37	61
10‡	20.4	24	34	56
7	25.9	19	28	47
5	31.5	16	23	41
2	46.8	11	16	30
0	69.3	8	11	21

*Do not use in hemodialysis or peritoneal dialysis patients or in children.

†Alternatively one-half of the chosen loading dose may be given at an interval approximately equal to the estimated half-life.

‡Dosing for patients with C(c)cr ≤ 10 mL/min should be assisted by measured serum concentrations.

Source: Modified from F. A. Sarubbi, Jr., and J. H. Hull: "Amikacin Serum Concentrations: Prediction of Levels and Dosage Guidelines," *Ann Intern Med*, **89:**612–618, 1978. *American Hospital Formulary Service Drug Information 84*, Bethesda, MD: American Society of Hospital Pharmacists, 1984.

The aminoglycosides have a low therapeutic index, and the monitoring of serum levels is indicated. The peak level (approximately 30 min after an IV infusion or 1 h after an IM dose) should be in the range of 4 to 12 µg/mL for gentamicin, tobramycin, and netilmicin and 12 to 36 µg/mL for amikacin and kanamycin. The development of toxicities is more frequent when the peak serum concentrations are above 12 µg/mL for gentamicin and tobramycin, above 16 µg/mL for netilmicin, and above 35 µg/mL for amikacin and kanamycin. As with all other pharmacokinetic parameters, the drug concentrations must be correlated with the clinical status of the patient.

Adverse Effects

The most serious adverse effects of the aminoglycosides are ototoxicity and nephrotoxicity. Patients who are dehydrated, receiving other ototoxic and nephrotoxic drugs, elderly, or having renal problems are at a higher risk of developing aminoglycoside toxicities. The vestibular problems associated with aminoglycosides (8th cranial nerve damage) are usually reversible when the drug is stopped. The hearing loss associated with aminoglycosides may be permanent. Audiometric testing is needed to detect hearing loss because the loss of high-frequency hearing occurs prior to clinical hearing loss. Nephrotoxicity is usually reversible when the drug is discontinued.

The aminoglycosides can also cause neuromuscular blockade resulting in respiratory paralysis and may enhance the neuromuscular blockade produced by skeletal muscle relaxants. Other CNS effects include headaches, lethargy, tremors, peripheral neuritis, and encephalopathy.

Preparations and Dosage

Streptomycin Streptomycin is not used as a single agent because of the rapid development of organism resistance. It is used in the treatment of plague at dosages of 4 g/day for the first 2 days then 2 g/day for the next 7 days. It is also used to treat tularemia in a dosage of 1 to 2 g/day for 7 to 10 days. Streptomycin is used in combination with penicillin (the combination is synergistic and both are bactericidal) to treat bacterial endocarditis. The dosage of streptomycin is still used during the early stage of tuberculosis chemotherapy.

Dosages of streptomycin greater than 2 g/day should not be given for longer than 2 weeks because of its toxicity, but dosages of 1 g/day can be given for 30 to 90 days without toxicity.

Neomycin Neomycin (Mycifradin, Neobiotic) is rarely given parenterally because of its toxicity. However, it is sometimes used in the treatment of hepatic coma and topically as an antibacterial agent (this use should be limited because of the dangers of sensitization).

Kanamycin   The major use of kanamycin (Kantrex) is in the treatment of infections due to gram-negative bacilli (except *Salmonella typhosa* and *Pseudomonas*). The usual dose is 15 mg/kg/day, in doses given every 6 to 12 h (not to exceed 1.5 g/day). Pain at the injection site occurs frequently with kanamycin. It can also be given IV (very slowly) in a diluted solution. It is used to suppress gut flora in doses of 3 to 4 g/day given orally as four divided doses in adults and 50 mg/kg/day as four to six doses in children.

Gentamicin   Gentamicin (Garamycin) has a broader spectrum than kanamycin but should be reserved for gram-negative infection caused by *Proteus* or *Pseudomonas* bacilli. It is the most widely used of all aminoglycosides, but its usefulness has been reduced because a growing number of gram-negative bacilli have become resistant to its effects. Gentamicin and carbenicillin are clearly synergistic in treating *Pseudomonas* infection, but they cannot be mixed in the same bottle. The bacterial spectrum of gentamicin includes *Pseudomonas aeruginosa* and *Serratia,* and it is also effective in treating gram-negative bacilli that have become resistant to other agents, for example, *E. coli* and *Klebsiella*. Additionally, nearly all strains of *Staphylococcus aureus* are sensitive to gentamicin.

The usual dosage of gentamicin is between 1 and 5 mg/kg/day, producing blood levels of 4 to 10 mg/L (4 to 10 μg/mL). Peak blood levels are achieved in about 1 h and last for 6 to 8 h. When treating urinary tract infections, dosages of 0.5 to 1.0 mg/kg/day are effective because of the high concentration of drug in the urine.

Tobramycin   Tobramycin (Nebcin) is thought to have an increased concentration in bronchial secretion, which may make it more useful in pulmonary infections than the other aminoglycosides. In vitro testing also suggests that tobramycin is more effective against *Pseudomonas aeruginosa,* although the clinical significance of this finding is still unclear.

Amikacin   Amikacin (Amikin) shows activity against organisms that are resistant to gentamicin, for example, *Serratia,* indole-positive *Proteus,* and others. The dosage of amikacin is 15 mg/kg/day, and its role in the institution should be restricted to use against organisms resistant to gentamicin.

Netilmicin   Netilmicin (Netromycin) is an aminoglycoside antibiotic that is effective against a broad range of gram-negative and gram-positive organisms. Development of newer aminoglycoside antibiotics occurs because of the emergence of aminoglycoside-resistant organisms. Bacterial resistance to aminoglycosides is due to enzymatic inactivation. Netilimicin is pharmacologically, pharmacokinetically, and microbiologically similar to other aminoglycosides. However, it is effective against gentamicin-resistant bacteria and can be mixed in the IV bottle with **carbenicillin** or **ticarcil-**

lin. Additionally, it has been suggested that netilmicin may have less ototoxicity and nephrotoxicity.

Ototoxicity and nephrotoxicity remain the major limitations to long-term netilmicin therapy. Decreased renal function and concomitant use of nephrotoxic or ototoxic drugs increase the incidence of these side effects. The adult dose is 6 mg/kg/day IV or IM in three equally divided doses every 8 h.

CHLORAMPHENICOL

Mechanism of Action

Chloramphenicol is bacteriostatic since it inhibits the protein synthesis by binding to 50S ribosomal subunits. It may also be bactericidal in higher concentrations. The salts of chloramphenicol palmitate and sodium succinate must be hydrolyzed to chloramphenicol in vivo to be active.

Spectrum of Activity

The spectrum of activity of chloramphenicol includes most gram-positive and gram-negative organisms, *Rickettesia, Mycloplasma,* and *Chlamydia*. The resistance to chloramphenicol especially among some gram-negative organisms (*Salmonella* and *E. coli*) is increasing.

Pharmacokinetics

Chloramphenicol is rapidly absorbed after oral administration. Peak levels are attained within 2 h. It is well distributed throughout the body and reaches the CSF. Chloramphenicol is found in bile, crosses the placenta, and reaches the breast milk. The drug is metabolized primarily in the liver, is excreted by the kidneys, and has a half-life of 1.5 to 3.5 h (normal renal and liver function). Less than 10 percent is excreted as active drug. Severe liver disease significantly delays clearance of the drug from the plasma. Intramuscular administration is contraindicated because of extremely poor and erratic absorption from the injection site.

Adverse Effects

Hypersensitivity reactions producing cutaneous or respiratory manifestations are rare. Idiosyncratic bone marrow toxicity due to hypersensitivity is the most serious toxic effect of chloramphenicol. Life-threatening pancytopenia, agranulocytosis, or thrombocytopenia occurs in from 1 in 40,000 to 1 in 60,000 patients receiving the drug orally. Seventy percent of these occurrences are fatal pancytopenia. Toxicity may occur after the course of therapy is completed. It is not dose-related, and discontinuation of the drug does not reverse the effect. This idiosyncratic toxicity is not to be confused with the mild, dose-related, reversible anemia that is frequently seen with chloramphenicol therapy.

Nausea, vomiting, unpleasant taste, and diarrhea are associated with oral therapy. Serious superinfections can occur. Chloramphenicol is extremely toxic in neonates because of the inability of the immature liver to conjugate the drug to inactive metabolites, resulting in inadequate excretion. This "gray syndrome" usually occurs 2 to 9 days after initiation of therapy and is dose-related. The syndrome progresses rapidly. Infants are in distress within 24 h, and 40 percent of those affected die.

Clinical Use

The use of chloramphenicol is limited to those infections in which the drug is shown to be effective by sensitivity tests and for which no less toxic drug is adequate. Typhoid fever is a major indication for chloramphenicol. Some *Salmonella typhosa* strains have become resistant to the drug, however. Chloramphenicol is useful in meningitis and epiglotitis caused by ampicillin-resistant *Haemophilus influenzae*. The drug is also effective against most rickettsiae and anaerobic bacteria.

Chloramphenicol, as the ophthalmic solution and ointment, is the drug of choice for many ocular infections, since these dosage forms are effective, have a broad antimicrobial spectrum, and are relatively nontoxic.

Dosage

Chloramphenicol is administered to adults as 30 to 50 mg/kg/day in four divided doses parenterally and orally as 30 to 100 mg/kg/day in four divided doses. The pediatric dose is 50 mg/kg/day in four divided doses parenterally and 50 to 100 mg/kg/day in four divided doses orally. Neonatal doses are 25 mg/kg/day (up to 1 week) and 50 mg/kg/day (1 to 4 weeks), both as four divided doses. Chloramphenicol doses must be decreased in patients with hepatic impairment. Decreased kidney function does not necessitate dosage adjustments, since the excretory delay principally affects inactive metabolites of the drug.

MISCELLANEOUS ANTIMICROBIALS

Peptide Antibiotics

The polymyxins and bacitracin are similar in that they all contain peptide linkages and are elaborated by bacilli and principally used as topical agents.

Polymyxins

Mechanism of Action **Polymixin B sulfate** (Aerosporin Powder) and **polymyxin E** (colistin, Coly-Mycin) are bactericidal surface-acting agents that disrupt the cell walls of susceptible organisms. Their spectra are similar, encompassing primarily gram-negaive organisms. Colistin is more potent than polymyxin B against *Pseudomonas, Salmonella, Shigella,* and the *E. coli* group.

Pharmacokinetics These drugs are not absorbed after oral administration. Colistin has been used orally for enteric infections. Polymyxins do not enter the CSF and are slowly excreted by the kidneys. Impaired renal function necessitates decreased doses. Polymyxin B is poorly absorbed in topical administration but is useful in treating local infections because of its low potential for producing hypersensitivity. Pain with IM administration is great, and infusion phlebitis is common with IV use. Intrathecal injection of the polymyxins causes meningeal irritation and adverse CNS effects.

Adverse Effects Untoward reactions seen with polymyxins include flushing, dizziness, paresthesias, diplopia, weakness, clouding of the sensorium, nephropathy, and dyspnea. Superinfections may also occur. The drugs may cause neuromuscular blockade, producing respiratory paralysis.

Clinical Use Polymyxins are useful systemic agents only for rare infections that are not sensitive to less toxic drugs. The drugs are most useful topically, and are preferable to topical aminoglycosides (especially neomycin) for application to skin and mucous membranes infected with gram-negative organisms.

Bacitracin

Bacitracin is a cell wall synthesis antagonist effective against a variety of gram-positive organisms and a few gram-negative bacteria. It is not absorbed after oral administration and is rarely used parenterally because of its great nephrotoxicity.

Topical bacitracin rarely causes hypersensitivity reactions and is the topical antibiotic of choice for susceptible gram-positive organisms. It is also useful when applied topically in ophthalmological infections due to susceptible organisms. Combinations of bacitracin and polymyxin B (Polysporin, Polycin) provide broad-spectrum topical antibiotic therapy without the risk of hypersensitization found with the three-drug combination of neosporin, bacitracin, and polymyxin B (Neosporin, Mycitracin, NeoPolycin).

Spectinomycin

Spectinomycin (Trobicin) is a bacteriostatic antibiotic that is effective against several gram-negative pathogens in vitro but is clinically useful only in the treatment of acute genital and rectal gonorrhea as a second-line drug for use in penicillin-allergic patients. It is also useful in patients with penicillinase-producing gonorrhea. When it is given as a single dose the adverse effects are uncommon. Severe toxic reactions such as ototoxicity and nephrotoxicity have not been reported. Adverse effects include urticaria, fever, chill, nausea, vomiting, insomnia, and dizziness. The dose is a single 2-g IM injection for both males and females. Although spectinomycin is excreted as active drug in the urine, no dosage adjustment is necessary in renal impairment since the single-dose regimen precludes accumulation of toxic levels. The drug does not eradicate established or incubating syphilis.

Vancomycin

Vancomycin (Vancocin) is an antibiotic that inhibits bacterial cell wall synthesis in many strains of staphylococci and streptococci. In combination with streptomycin or gentamicin the drug is effective against most, but not all, staphylococci.

The drug is poorly absorbed after oral administration but is used orally to treat staphylococcal enteritis and to prevent that condition in immunosuppressed patients with high enteric colony counts. The drug is primarily excreted unchanged in the urine, and dosage must be reduced in impaired renal function.

Vancomycin can produce hypersensitivity reactions, which include macular skin rashes and anaphylaxis. It can cause marked infusion phlebitis with IV administration. Ototoxicity and nephrotoxicity can be severe. The drug should be avoided whenever possible in patients concurrently receiving other nephrotoxic agents. Vancomycin can be given orally to treat colitis caused by toxin-producing bacteria *Clostridium difficile* and *Staphylococcus aureus*.

Vancomycin is indicated in methicillin-resistant staphylococcal infections, that is, diseases due to staphylococci that are resistant to penicillinase-resistant penicillins. Vancomycin is also useful in patients with staphylococcal disease who cannot tolerate safer agents. The usual adult IV or oral dosage of vancomycin is 500 mg q6h or 1 g q12h.

SULFONAMIDES AND TRIMETHOPRIM

Mechanism of Action

Sulfonamides are usually classified as bacteriostatic in their action. All sulfonamides interfere with the bacteria's ability to utilize para-aminobenzoic acid (PABA), which is needed to produce folic acid essential for some bacteria's growth. Only bacteria that synthesize their own folic acid will be affected by sulfonamides or trimethoprim. Sulfonamides competitively inhibit dihydrofolic acid synthetase, which is needed for the conversion of PABA to folic acid.

Trimethoprim is another antagonist anti-infective which can act synergistically with the sulfonamides. Trimethoprim inhibits the folic acid pathway by preventing the conversion of dihydofolic acid to tetrahydrofolic acid, the metabolically active form of folic acid. Trimethoprim acts at a different stage of the folic acid synthesis; it can be combined with sulfamethoxazole [**co-trimoxazole** (Bactrim, Septra)]. This can be given orally or by injection.

Spectrum of Activity

Sulfonamides were originally very effective against a wide spectrum of gram-positive and gram-negative bacteria, but their usefulness has decreased with the development of resistant bacteria. Sulfonamides are active in vitro against gram-positive bacteria, including staphylococci, streptococci, *Clostridium tetani, Bacillus anthracis,* and others. Their activity toward gram-negative organisms may include *Enterobacter, E. coli, Klebsiella, Proteus mirabilis, P. vulgaris, Salmonella,* and *Shigella.*

Pharmacokinetics

Sulfonamides (with the exception of sulfapyrimidine and sulfasalazine which are only slightly absorbed) are well absorbed. The following are rapidly absorbed with peak concentrations in 2 to 4 h: **sulfacytine, sulfamerazine, sulfmethazine, sulfamethizole,** and **sulfisoxazole. Sulfadiazine, sulfamethoxazole,** and **sulfapyridine** are absorbed at a slower rate, with a peak level in 3 to 7 h.

The absorbed sulfonamides are widely distributed throughout the body. **Sulfisoxazole** appears to be the only sulfonamide to be distributed only extracellularly. Sulfonamides readily cross the placenta, and concentrations may be half of those achieved in the maternal blood concentration. The sulfonamides vary in the degree of protein binding: sulfacytine, sulfamethizole, and sulfisoxazole are reported to be 85 to 90 percent protein bound.

The sulfonamides are acetylated by enzymes in the liver. The metabolites do not have antibacterial activity and are excreted by the kidneys. Those that are not absorbed are excreted in the feces.

Adverse Effects

Sulfonamides have been implicated in a variety of adverse reactions. These reactions occur in about 5 percent of the patients receiving the drug. Many of the adverse effects reverse upon stopping of the drug. The hypersensitivity reaction appears to be the most common, and the frequency of the reaction appears to increase with increasing dose. There appears to be cross-sensitivity between the anti-infective sulfonamides, some diuretics such as acetazolamide and thiazide diuretics, and the sulfonylurea antidiabetic agents. Numerous dermatologic reactions have been reported, including a mild pruritic rash, exfoliative dermatitis, and erythema multiforme of the Stevens-Johnson type. Because sulfonamides can also cause photosensitivity reactions, patients should be cautioned about spending long periods of time in the sun. A serum sickness reaction characterized by headache, fever, hives, bronchospasm, and conjunctivitis may occur.

Crystalluria and hematuria were once significant problems but are now uncommon with the newer more soluble sulfonamides. Alkalinization of the urine is usually not necessary if the urine output is kept at a minimum of 1500 mL/day. Toxic nephrosis has occurred rarely. Acute hemolytic anemia may occur in patients who are deficient in the enzyme glucose-6-phosphate dehydrogenase (G6PD).

Sulfonamides are generally contraindicated in patients under 2 months of age because of the potential problem of kernicterus.

Clinical Use

Sulfonamides are used in the treatment of uncomplicated urinary tract infections, most of which are caused by sulfonamide-sensitive *E. coli*. Sulfonamides are also the first-line drugs in the treatment of infections due to nocardiosis. In some cases the treatment of nocardiosis will include a second antibiotic (**minocycline**, **ampicillin**, **erythromycin**, or **cycloserine**). Sulfadiazine, sulfisoxazole, and sulfamethoxazole have been used in the treatment of toxoplasmosis.

The combination of **sulfamethoxazole-trimethoprim** (Septra, Bactrim) has produced an oral effective drug for the treatment of recurrent urinary tract infections and respiratory infections, including *Pneumocystis carinii*.

Sulfapyridine is the drug of choice for the treatment of dermatitis herpetiformis (Duhring's disease). This is the only current indication for sulfapyridine.

Preparations

Trisulfapyrimidines include sulfadiazine, sulfamerazine, and sulfamethazine (Sulfaloid, Triple Sulfa). The combination of three different sulfonamides was originally formulated to prevent the development of crystalluria. The newer, more soluble sulfonamides have reduced the problem of crystalluria. The main use of the triple-sulfonamide preparations is in the treatment of intravaginal bacterial infections. Sulfacetamide is the most commonly used ophthalmologic preparation. **Mafenide acetate** (Sulfamylon Acetate Cream) and **silver sulfadiazine** (Silvadene) are used topically in the treatment of burn patients to aid in the prevention of infections.

The oral sulfonamide preparations, including **sulfisoxazole** (Gantrisin); **sulfamethoxazole** (Gantanol); and **sulfamethizole** (Thiosulfil, Urifon), are usually administered in doses of 2 to 4 g/day in two to four divided doses. The pediatric dosage is usually 20 to 40 mg/kg/day as four divided doses. The parenteral preparation of sulfisoxazole (Gantrisin 400 mg/mL) is given in a dose of 100 mg/kg/day, divided into three or four doses.

The combination of 400 mg of sulfamethoxazole with 80 mg trimethoprim, known as *co-trimoxazole* (Bactrim, Septra), has the advantage of requiring only a twice-daily dosage. The dosage is either one or two tablets every 12 h. There are double-strength tablets which contain 800 mg of sulfamethoxazole and 160 mg of trimethoprim (Bactrim DS, Septra DS). It is also available as parenteral preparations which contain 16 mg/mL trimethoprim and 80 mg/mL sulfamethoxazole. Co-trimoxazole indications include urinary tract infections, otitis media, enteritis, pneumocystis infections, bronchitis, nocardiosis, and others. Trimethoprim (Proloprim, Trimpex) is available as a single-entity product for the treatment of urinary tract infections. The dosage is 100 to 200 mg twice a day.

NURSING PROCESS RELATED TO ANTIBACTERIALS

The nursing process related to the penicillins, cephalosporins, erythromycin, clindamycin, tetracyclines, and sulfonamides is summarized in Table 28-19.

THERAPY OF COMMON ACUTE INFECTIOUS DISORDERS

LEARNING OBJECTIVES

Upon mastery of this section of this chapter, the reader will be able to:

1. Give the principal drug and an alternative agent used in the treatment of the following organisms that can cause pneumonias: pneumococcus, *Haemophilus influenzae*, *Legionella pneumophila*, and *Klebsiella pneumoniae*.

2. Discuss the treatment of viral pneumonias.

3. Give the most likely causal organism and an antibiotic that would be effective in treating bacterial meningitis in adults and in children.

4. Indicate which antibiotics should be given intrathecally in the treatment of bacterial meningitis.

5. Give an example of an antibiotic that can be given to prevent meningococcal meningitis.

6. List two treatment programs that can be utilized to prevent the development of infectious endocarditis in patients undergoing dental procedures.

7. Give two drugs that can be used in the treatment of endocarditis due to *Candida albicans.*

8. Give two therapeutic regimens that can be used in the treatment of the following sexually transmitted diseases: urethritis gonorrhea, pelvic inflammatory disease, early primary syphilis, and chancroid.

9. Give two treatment regimens for the acute management of an uncomplicated urinary tract infection.

10. Give two advantages to a single-dose treatment of urinary tract infection.

11. Discuss the nursing assessment, management, and evaluation associated with the treatment of pneumonia, meningitis, endocarditis, urinary tract infections, and sexually transmitted diseases.

PNEUMONIAS

Pneumonia is an inflammatory process in lung parenchyma most commonly caused by infection. Among conditions that predispose to pneumonia are viral respiratory diseases, malnutrition, exposure to cold, noxious gases, alcohol intoxication, depression of cerebral function by drugs, and cardiac failure.

Approximately half of the acute pneumonias are of bacterial origin; other principal causes are viruses and mycoplasma. Early identification of the infectious agent is essential for the proper treatment of pneumonia.

A careful history will often help to differentiate bacterial from viral infections and also identify noninfectious diseases

TABLE 28-19 Nursing Process Related to Antibacterial Drugs

ASSESSMENT	MANAGEMENT	EVALUATION
	Penicillins	
Contraindicated in patients with history of allergic reaction. Assess for asthma or sensitivity to cephalosporins or multiple allergens. With infants under 3 months of age, check mother's allergy history. When giving procaine penicillin, also check for procaine sensitivity.	Patient should be monitored for first 30 min after administration. Penicillin G binds to food, is poorly absorbed in acid media, so give no food for 1 h before or 2 h after the drug. Advise patients not to take with caffeine, citrus fruit, cola drinks, fruit juices, pickles, tomatoes, and vinegar. Monitor electrolytes, renal, hepatic, and hematopoietic function; IV and IM administration may cause localized tissue irritation; give deep IM into gluteal muscle. Dilute well when giving IV, and change infusion site every 48 h. IM procaine penicillin, if given IV, may cause emboli and toxic mental and cardiac symptoms.	Common adverse reactions: rash, dermatitis, fever, joint pain, itching. Emergency treatment of anaphylactic shock consists of epinephrine IV or SQ, airway management, oxygen, steroids, vasopressors, and cardiopulmonary resuscitation. Advise allergic patients to wear Medi-alert tags. Hyperkalemia and hypernatremia may result if giving large IV doses of sodium and potassium salts. May give false-positive Coombs' test. May give false-positive urine glucose with Benedict's test, and false-positive urine protein. Mezlocillin, azlocillin, and carbenicillin sometimes cause bleeding manifestations, with abnormalities of coagulation tests, so prothrombin time should be monitored.
	Cephalosporins	
Check for hypersensitivity to penicillins; use with caution in patients with history of drug allergies and renal or liver impairment. Use with caution with patients on furosemide, ethacrynic acid, colistin, or aminoglycosides.	Oral cephalosporins (Keflex, Duricef, Anspor, Velosef) may be given with food although absorption may be delayed. Patients on parenteral feedings may show vitamin K deficiencies, resulting in coagulation abnormalities, corrected by supplemental doses of vitamin K. Give deep IM injections; sterile abscesses occur if given SQ. Monitor output and check for casts, RBCs, or protein in urine. Check on renal function studies. Large IV doses of Keflin may cause thrombophlebitis; the addition of 10–25 mg of hydrocortisone to IV solutions containing 4–6 g of Keflin may reduce the incidence of phlebitis. Warn patients against taking alcohol concurrently. IM doses of Keflin may cause pain, induration, tenderness, and temperature elevation after repeated injections. Velosef for Infusion should not be mixed with Lactated Ringer's Injection.	Adverse effects: diarrhea, nausea, and vomiting, abdominal discomfort, oral candidiasis (thrush). Hypersensitivity reactions may include rash, urticaria, angioedema, drug fever, and anaphylaxis. Prolonged use may result in overgrowth of nonsusceptible organisms. May give false-positive Coombs' test, false-positive urine glucose with Benedict's or Clinitest, false-positive for urine protein, and increase of urine steroids with 17-ketosteroid test. Large doses may cause nephrotoxicity, with dose-related acute tubular necrosis.

showing signs and symptoms of pneumonia. A sudden onset of symptoms, including fever, chills, cough, and frequent chest pain, suggests bacterial infection. Viral pneumonia is more often gradual in onset, with malaise and low-grade fever without chills, and is more likely to follow an upper respiratory infection. Elderly patients, especially those with chronic obstructive pulmonary disease and other chronic illnesses, may have bacterial pneumonias without typical symptoms. A generalized, nonspecific deterioration of the patient's previous condition can mark the onset of a pulmonary infection and usually requires more aggressive management.

TABLE 28-19 Nursing Process Related to Antibacterial Drugs (*Cont.*)

ASSESSMENT	MANAGEMENT	EVALUATION
	Tetracyclines	
Use caution in impaired renal or liver function, pregnancy, postpartum and lactation. Incompatible with cephalothin; may be toxic with sulfonamides; inhibits bacterial action of penicillins. Should not be given to children under 8; may cause permanent tooth discoloration.	Check expiration date carefully; expired products may cause Fanconi syndrome. Do not expose to extreme humidity, heat, or light. Do not give with food, milk, or dairy products, or antacids with aluminum, calcium, or magnesium. Advise patients to avoid calcium-rich foods (almonds, buttermilk, cheese, cream, ice cream, milk, pizza, waffles, yogurt); do not give concurrently with iron or sodium bicarbonate. Minocycline and doxycycline may be taken with milk products. Monitor I&O, especially with demeclocycline, which promotes water excretion by inhibiting ADH. Alert patients to photosensitive skin reactions; prolonged exposure to sun should be avoided. Monitor BUN. If pruritis ani, advise patient to cleanse anal area carefully after each bowel movement. Administer drug 1 h before or 2 h after meals except minocycline and doxycycline.	Common adverse effects: minor GI disturbances, rash, local irritation at injection site, and anogenital lesions. May alter urine tests to show increase in catecholamines and false-positive with Clinitest or Benedict's. Pruritis ani may result from contamination with breakdown products. Products of degradation may cause adverse effects on kidney function; may show decrease in blood ammonia from destruction of gut bacteria or an increase from drug-induced liver damage; have an antianabolic effect; reduce protein synthesis, resulting in increased BUN.
	Aminoglycosides	
Use with caution in impaired liver or renal function; with anticoagulants, diuretics, cephalothins, skeletal muscle relaxants, and general anesthesia.	Have patient report any tinnitus (early symptom of hearing loss). Check for early signs of vestibular toxicity: headache, nausea, vomiting, vertigo, nystagmus, dizziness, and loss of balance. Patients who are hypocalcemic or have had IV muscle relaxants and/or general anesthesia must be watched for muscle weakness, apnea, or respiratory paralysis. Monitor patients on anticoagulants for bleeding problems. Advise patient that drug is potentiated by alcohol. Monitor I&O, and observe urine for oliguria or casts. Monitor for rise in BUN, NPN, serum creatinine, and decrease in creatinine clearance levels. Do not mix with other medications.	Patients treated with aminoglycosides need to be observed closely because of the potential nephrotoxicity and neurotoxicity associated with their use. Watch for decreased renal function and disturbances of the eighth cranial nerve. Adverse effects: numbness, skin tingling, muscle twitching, and convulsions; alters the following lab tests: increase seen in SGOT, SGPT, LDH, and bilirubin; decrease seen in calcium, sodium, potassium, and CBC. Neuromuscular blockade can be reversed with calcium salts.

Gram-Positive Organisms

Gram-positive cocci include *Streptococcus pneumoniae* (pneumococcus), *Staphylococcus aureus*, and *Streptococcus pyogenes* (group A β-hemolytic streptococci). Pneumococcus accounts for 60 to 80 percent of the community-acquired bacterial pneumonias. *Staphylococcus aureus* accounts for 2 percent of the community-acquired infections and 10 to 20 percent of the hospital-acquired infections. *Streptococcus pyogenes* is a relatively rare pulmonary pathogen. Most patients with pneumonias can be treated as outpatients. Those who are seriously ill and require IV therapy should be hospitalized. Supportive care for the patient

TABLE 28-19   Nursing Process Related to Antibacterial Drugs (*Cont.*)

ASSESSMENT	MANAGEMENT	EVALUATION
	Chloramphenicol	
Potent drug that should not be used for trivial infections or as a prophylactic antibiotic. Use with caution in patients who are pregnant, have impaired liver or hepatic function, or who are presently on medication that might cause bone marrow depression.	Advise patients of need for hospitalization during therapy to monitor for bone marrow depression; monitor blood studies for appearance of reticulocytopenia, leukopenia, thrombocytopenia, or anemia. Observe infants for "Gray syndrome": abdominal distention with or without emesis, progressive pallid cyanosis, vasomotor collapse, with irregular respirations, followed by death a few hours after onset of symptoms. Chloramphenicol sodium succinate for injection must be given IV and is ineffective if given IM.	Serious and fatal blood dyscrasias have occurred after administration of this drug, also aplastic anemia later terminated in leukemia. Adverse effects include nausea and vomiting, stomatitis, glossitis, and diarrhea. Drug should be stopped if otic or peripheral neuritis occurs. "Gray syndrome" toxicity with infants can be fatal and can occur if the mother received the drug during delivery.
	Sulfonamides	
Assess for prior allergy to sulfonamides. Contraindicated in pregnancy and lactation, severe hepatitis, glomerular nephritis, and uremia. Use with caution in patients with impaired renal or hepatic function, severe allergy, bronchial asthma, concurrent use of anticoagulants or antidiabetic sulfonylurea drugs. Assess patients who will receive Bactrim for sensitivity to trimethoprim and for folate deficiency.	Observe for early indications of blood disorders: sore throat, fever, pallor, purpura or jaundice. Monitor CBC and urinalysis; maintain a fluid intake of at least 2500 mL/day to have an output of at least 1000 mL/day to prevent crystalluria and stone formation. Observe for bleeding abnormalities with patients on oral anticoagulants. Elderly patients concurrently taking thiazide diuretics should be monitored for thrombopenia with purpura. Monitor patients who are deficient in the enzyme glucose-6-phosphate dehydrogenase for acute hemolytic anemia. Monitor blood sugar; if given concurrently with tolbutamide, may cause severe hypoglycemia.	Adverse reactions include blood dyscrasias, rash, skin eruptions, nausea, diarrhea, tachycardia, and palpitations. Sulfonamides may cause kernicterus in children. Kidney damage and urinary complications such as urolithiasis, oliguria, hematuria, renal colic, obstruction anuria, and nitrogen retention may occur after sulfapyridine, sulfathiazole, and sulfamerazine administration.

with pneumonia includes clearing of secretion; oxygenation; antipyretics; fluids, administration of electrolytes and antitussives; and treatment of other complications.

Pneumococcal Pneumonia

Penicillin G is the drug of choice for pneumococcal pneumonias. It is given initially in dosages ranging from 600,000 U of procaine penicillin G IM every 12 h for moderate illness to 1 million U of aqueous penicillin G, given every 4 h rapidly as an IV infusion in severe cases. Only after there has been a definite response to treatment should oral penicillin V, 250 to 500 mg every 4 to 6 h, be considered. All pneumococci are susceptible to penicillin at present,

although some strains require higher dosages to be effective. Some strains are resistant to **tetracyclines** and **erythromycin**. If a patient is allergic to **penicillin**, alternative agents that can be used include **erythromycin, tetracycline,** and **cephalosporin** (**cephalexin** 500 mg q6h orally or 1 g of **cefazolin** IV q6h).

Pneumococcal polysaccharide vaccine (Pneumovax) has been shown to be effective in preventing pneumococcal bacteremia and contains the 23 serotypes associated with 70 percent of the pneumococcal infections. It is currently recommended for high-risk patients over the age of 2 years with chronic obstructive lung disease, congestive heart failure, sickle cell anemia, asplenia, diabetis mellitus, alcoholism, nephrotic syndrome, or chronic immunosuppression,

TABLE 28-19 Nursing Process Related to Antibacterial Drugs (*Cont.*)

ASSESSMENT	MANAGEMENT	EVALUATION
	Clindamycin	
Use with caution in patients with history of GI disease, particularly colitis. Elderly patients with severe illness may not tolerate diarrhea. Erythromycin and clindamycin are antagonistic and should not be given together. Use with caution in patients with impaired liver and kidney function.	Give IV no faster than 30 mg/min; too rapid IV administration may cause hypotension and cardiac arrest. Oral form should be taken with a full glass of water to avoid esophageal irritation. Patients should be advised that the oral form is partially excreted in saliva and may cause a bitter taste. Monitor patients for colitis characterized by severe persistent diarrhea, abdominal cramps, and passage of blood and mucus. Monitor renal function studies.	Clindamycin therapy has been associated with potentially fatal pseudomembranous colitis; vancomycin has been found to be effective in the treatment of antibiotic-associated colitis produced by *Clostridium difficile*. Antiperistaltic agents should not be given to treat severe diarrhea since they may prolong or worsen the condition. Adverse effects include abdominal pain, nausea, vomiting, diarrhea, jaundice, transient neutropenia, and eosinophilia. High doses may cause increase in liver enzymes and serum bilirubin and may enhance the action of neuromuscular blocking agents.
	Erythromycins	
Contraindicated in patients with known sensitivity. Use with caution in patients with impaired liver function, and if concurrent with theophylline administration.	Allow only water 1–2 h before and after administering. Acidic fruit or juice or carbonated beverages may decompose the drug prematurely (exceptions are enteric-coated erythromycin base and erythromycin ethylsuccinate). For full effect, children's chewable tablets (EES) should be fully chewed. IV erythromycin is irritating and should not be given IVP; buffers such as sodium bicarbonate (Neut) may be added to the IV solution. Observe for manifestations of malaise, nausea, vomiting, abdominal colic, fever, and severe abdominal pain. If due to Ilosone administration, symptoms will disappear when drug stopped. Patients on theophylline must be observed for toxicity.	Hepatic dysfunction with or without jaundice has occurred with erythromycin estolate administration, so monitor patient's hepatic function. Adverse reactions may be GI and are dose-related; reversible hearing loss associated with high doses of IV erythromycin have been reported rarely. Theophylline dosage may have to be reduced to avoid theophylline toxicity.

and for all persons over age 50. The vaccine should not be used in children under the age of 2 years or in pregnant women.

Streptococcal Pneumonia

Pneumonia due to hemolytic streptococci usually follows a viral infection of the respiratory tract, especially influenza or measles, or it develops in persons with underlying pulmonary disease. The patients are usually severely toxic; cyanotic pleural effusion develops frequently and early and progresses to empyema in one-third of untreated patients.

Penicillin G is the drug of choice with treatment of streptococcal pneumonia. It is given initially in dosages ranging from 600,000 U of procaine penicillin IM every 12 h for moderate illness to 1 million U of aqueous penicillin G given IV every 4 h in severe cases. Alternate forms of therapy include **erythromycin, tetracycline,** or a **cephalosporin.**

Staphylococcal Pneumonia

Pneumonia caused by *Staphylococcus aureus* occurs as a sequela to viral infections of the respiratory tract (e.g., influenza) in debilitated (e.g., postsurgical) patients or hospitalized infants, especially after antimicrobial drug administration.

Initial therapy (based on sputum smear) consists of nafcillin sodium, 6 to 12 g/day or vancomycin, 2 g/day, given IV in divided doses. If the staphylococcus proves to be penicillin-sensitive, aqueous penicillin G, 10 to 60 million

U/day in divided doses IV is the drug of choice. Drugs should be continued for several weeks. Supportive measures and treatment of complications are essential.

Gram-Negative Bacilli

Klebsiella Pneumonia

Klebsella pneumoniae occurs as a member of the normal bacterial flora of the respiratory tract or gut of 5 to 20 percent of the population. Pneumonia due to this organism occurs mainly in persons over 40 years of age with a history of alcoholism, malnutrition, or debilitating diseases. Klebsiella pneumoniae also occurs as a superinfection in persons hospitalized for serious disease, including other types of pneumonia treated with antimicrobial drugs.

Immediate antimicrobial treatment is essential. A cephalosporin such as **cefotaxime** (Claforan), 1 to 2 g, is injected IV as a bolus every 4 h. **Tobramycin** or **gentamicin**, 5 to 8 mg/kg/day, may be given in addition. Antimicrobial treatment may have to be continued for more than 2 weeks to avoid relapses. General supportive treatment of the patient is essential.

Haemophilus Influenzae Pneumonia

Haemophilus influenzae pneumonia is a rare form of primary bacterial pneumonia. In adults, it has occurred in the presence of cardiac disease and chronic lung disease. Treatment is with **ampicillin**, 1 to 1.5 g PO every 6 h or 150 mg/kg/day IV, may be used unless penicillinase-producing Haemophilus is present. An alternative treatment is chloramphenicol, 500 mg PO or IV every 6 h. **Trimethoprim-sulfamethoxazole** (Bactrim and Septra) has been used in antibiotic-resistant Haemophilus pneumoniae.

Legionella Pneumonia

Legionella pneumophila is a poorly staining gram-negative bacterium that has biochemically distinct characteristics. During severe outbreaks, the mortality rate has been 10 percent in those with legionella pneumonia. Death is attributed to respiratory or renal failure or shock, with disseminated intravascular coagulation.

The treatment of choice is **erythromycin**, 0.5 to 1 g IV or PO every 6 h for 2 to 3 weeks. This usually results in improvement in 2 to 3 days. **Rifampin**, 10 to 20 mg/kg/day, has been suggested for those patients who fail to respond to erythromycin.

Mixed Bacterial Pneumonias

Mixed bacterial pneumonias include those in which culture and smear reveal several organisms, not one of which can clearly be identified as the causative agent. These pneumonias usually appear as complications of anesthesia, surgery, aspiration, trauma, or various chronic illnesses (cardiac failure, advanced carcinoma, uremia). They are common complications of chronic pulmonary diseases such as bronchiectasis (dilation of the small bronchial tubes) and emphysema.

Mixed bacterial pneumonias must be differentiated from tuberculosis, carcinoma, and other specific mycotic, bacterial, and viral pulmonary infections. Unless a probably significant etiologic agent can be identified, **amoxicillin**, 500 mg PO q8h or **cefoxitin** intravenously, as a 1-g bolus every 4 h should be given as initial therapy. This will be modified according to clinical and laboratory results.

Aspiration Pneumonia

Aspiration pneumonia is an especially severe type of pneumonia, often with a high mortality rate. It results from the aspiration of gastric contents in addition to aspiration of upper respiratory flora in secretions. Pulmonary injury is due in large part to the low pH (<2.5) of gastric secretions.

Removal of aspirated material by catheter suction or bronchoscopy may be attempted, but this procedure usually fails to remove all aspirate completely.

Some aspiration pneumonias have no bacterial component, but in many other pneumonias, mixed bacterial flora are involved. Antimicrobial drugs directed against the latter (e.g., **penicillin G** plus an **aminoglycoside** or an appropriate cephalosporin) are sometimes administered without waiting for evidence of progressive pulmonary infection. Appropriate change in therapy can occur after laboratory and clinical evidence of microbial infection.

Mycoplasmal Pneumonia

Mycoplasmal pneumonia is a frequent cause of nonbacterial pneumonia. It is usually endemic and occurs throughout the year. Mycoplasmal and viral pneumonias present similar clinical features. In mild and moderate cases of mycoplasmal pneumonia treatment is not indicated. Severe cases may be treated with **tetracycline** or **erythromycin**, 0.5 g PO q4–6h.

Viral Pneumonia

Viruses account for over 90 percent of acute respiratory diseases among all age groups, ranging from the common cold to diffuse pneumonia. They affect children under the age of 6 years most commonly. In children the most frequent organism is respiratory syncytial virus. In the adult population type A influenza is the most common pathogen. In most cases no antibiotic therapy is indicated. In severe infections and in debilitated patients antibiotics may be used to prevent secondary bacterial infections. **Amantadine hydrochloride** (Symmetrel) has also been used to treat some influenza A infections.

CASE STUDY

S.G. is an 85-year-old white male who was admitted to the hospital for repair of a fractured left hip. He had previously been hospitalized for a possible myocardial infarction (MI) with recurrent chest pains. He has a past history of diabetes with a questionable history of chronic bronchitis.

In the 2 weeks post surgery for the repair of his hip, S.G. was experiencing episodes of wheezing and shortness of breath. He developed a sore throat and a cough with production of yellow sputum. The wheezing was characterized by inspiratory stridor. A loading dose of aminophylline was given, followed by an infusion of aminophylline. Methylprednisolone was also given intravenously. His chest x-ray showed left lower lobe infiltrates. He became febrile and his blood gas showed arterial P_{O_2} of 46 mmHg on room air. S.G.'s respiratory status continued to deteriorate to acute respiratory failure. He was then transferred to the intensive care unit.

Assessment

In the intensive care unit S.G. was endotracheally intubated with ventilator support. He appeared to be an elderly, well-nourished male, awake and oriented. There was no evidence of cyanosis or clubbing and once intubated was in no acute distress. His electrocardiogram showed atrial fibrillation with a control rate of 80. His blood pressure was 110/70, respiration 14. He was febrile with a temperature of 103.6°F, and his lungs on examination had scattered rales. His chest x-ray showed bilateral alveolar infiltrates, and he was diagnosed as having an aspiration pneumonia. Cultures were taken by a bronchoscopy and sent to the laboratory for sensitivity tests.

Management

The culture showed numerous gram-negative bacilli, with *Pseudomonas aeruginosa* which was sensitive to tobramycin and ticarcillin. S.G. was started on tobramycin, 80 mg IV q8h, and ticarcillin, 2 g IV q6h. Aminophylline and methylprednisolone were also continued.

Evaluation

After 1 week on the antibiotics S.G. was afebrile with a temperature of 100°F, and his chest x-ray was clear. He was extubated, placed on supplemental oxygen, and transferred out of intensive care. The antibiotic regimen was continued for 12 days. The aminophylline was also discontinued, and the methylprednisolone was slowly tapered. At the time of discharge he was given an outpatient follow-up appointment.

BACTERIAL MENINGITIS

Bacterial meningitis is a medical emergency. It has a mortality rate of 10 to 20 percent. The earlier the treatment is started during an episode of meningitis, the better the prognosis. Nonspecific symptoms such as headache, vomiting, lethargy, or irritability may be the earliest indications of meningitis. A high index of suspicion and a clinician's willingness to do a lumbar puncture when the diagnosis of meningitis is considered are essential for its early detection and treatment.

Once the diagnosis of meningitis is made, the choice of antibiotic therapy is one of the most important decisions the clinician will make. Antibiotic therapy of meningitis is largely affected by the physiology of the blood-brain barrier. The blood-brain barrier excludes many antibiotics (e.g., cephalothin) from the CSF. Others (for instance, aminoglycosides) need to be instilled directly into the CSF. Bactericidal levels of antibiotics must be obtained in the CSF to ensure a successful outcome.

The causes of bacterial meningitis vary with the age of the patient, as follows: (1) *Streptococcus pneumoniae* cause 30 to 50 percent of the cases in adults and only 10 to 20 percent in children; (2) *Haemophilis influenzae* is responsible for 35 to 45 percent of the cases in children (6 months to 5 years) but only 1 to 3 percent of the adults; (3) *Neisseria meningitidis* causes 10 to 30 percent of the adult cases and 30 to 40 percent of those in children (up to the age of 15); (4) gram-negative bacilli and group B streptococcus are the main organisms in neonates.

Clinical Pharmacology and Therapeutics

The antibiotics generally used in the treatment of meningitis include the penicillins, aminoglycosides, chloramphenicol, and cephalosporins (cefotaxime and moxalactam).

The initial antibiotic therapy should be based on CSF gram stain and the clinical setting, and should be modified when the CSF culture and sensitivity are available. Before sensitivities are obtained, *Haemophilus influenzae* meningitis should be treated with chloramphenicol and ampicillin, since many strains are now ampicillin-resistant, and a few are chloramphenicol-resistant. When the sensitivity results are available, the effective antibiotic may be continued alone. Moxalactam and cefotaxime also appear to be effective against *Haemophilus influenzae* and may be used as alternative therapy for strains that are resistant to both ampicillin and chloramphenicol (see Table 28-20).

Antibiotics should be continued in the recommended doses for 5 to 7 days after the patient is afebrile for a total

TABLE 28-20   Therapy of Specific Meningitis Infections

ORGANISM	THERAPY
Streptococcus pneumoniae	Penicillin G or chloramphenicol
Neisseria meningitidis	Penicillin G or chloramphenicol; prophylaxis with rifampin or minocycline
Haemophilus influenzae	Ampicillin, chloramphenicol, co-trimoxazole, moxalactam
Staphylococcus aureus	Nafcillin or oxacillin
Staphylococcus epidermidis	Vancomycin with or without rifampin
Gram-negative bacillary meningitis	Moxalactam or cefotaxime
Listeria monocytogenes	Ampicillin or penicillin G with aminoglycosides

of at least 10 days of therapy. Neonatal meningitis requires treatment for a minimum of 3 weeks. Meningitis due to gram-negative rods or staphylococci generally requires 3 to 6 weeks of therapy.

All patients with meningitis should be hospitalized throughout the duration of their antibiotic treatment. As with all seriously ill patients, vital signs should be monitored frequently. Mental status changes should be noted. Patients should be monitored for seizures, which may be due to hyponatremia, subdural effusion, fever, or brain abscess. These causes should be sought and treated. IV **diazepam** will control seizures in some patients. Alternative drugs in the acute situation include **phenobarbital** and **phenytoin** (Dilantin).

Persons who are intimate contacts of patients with meningococcal meningitis are at an increased risk of meningitis. They can be treated with **rifampin**, 600 mg twice a day for 2 days. **Minocycline**, 100 mg twice a day for 5 days, may also be used.

INFECTIVE ENDOCARDITIS

Infective endocarditis implies the presence of microorganisms (bacteria, fungi, chlamydiae, and so on) in the heart valves or endocardium. Traditionally, endocarditis was called "acute" or "subacute," but developments of the past decade make it more desirable to group endocarditis according to the causative microorganism. The traditional subacute infective endocarditis has an insidious onset, with slow deterioration, anemia, valve damage leading to heart failure, cachexia, and death. It is superimposed mainly on preexisting congenital, rheumatic, or calcific abnormalities of the heart valves. Bacteremia frequently occurs after dental procedures and endoscopic or other manipulations of the

respiratory, urinary or GI tract. *Streptococcus viridans* (50 percent) and *Streptococcus faecalis* (10 percent) are among the most common causative agents, but virtually any microorganism can cause endocarditis.

The traditional acute infective endocarditis is a rapidly progressive, destructive infection of the normal, abnormal, or prosthetic valves, usually developing in the course of intense bacteremia, IV narcotic abuse, surgery on infected tissues, urologic procedures, or infection of a prosthesis. Acute infective endocarditis can be caused by *Staphylococcus aureus*, pneumococcus, group A streptococcus, and others.

Clinical Pharmacology and Therapeutics

Prevention   Some cases of endocarditis arise after dental procedures or surgery of the oropharynx or genitourinary tract. Patients with known cardiac abnormalities who are to have any of these procedures should have prior treatment in one of the following ways (dosages are for adults):

1.   600,000 U procaine penicillin mixed with 1 million U aqueous crystalline **penicillin** IM 60 min before the procedure, then penicillin VK, 500 mg q6h for eight doses.

2.   **Penicillin** VK, 2 g PO 1 h prior to the procedure and then 500 mg PO q6h for eight doses.

3.   In case of **penicillin** sensitivity or allergy, erythromycin, 1 g PO 2 h before the procedure and then 500 mg PO q6h for eight doses can be given.

4.   For genitourinary instrumentation or surgery, give gentamicin, 5 mg/kg/day in addition to medication listed in 1.

5.   For GI surgery, give **cefazolin**, 1 g IM 1 h before and 4, 12, and 18 h after the procedure.

Treatment   The most important consideration in the treatment of infective endocarditis is keeping a bactericidal concentration of antibiotics in contact with the infecting organism, which is often localized in a vascular tissue or in vegetation. Penicillins, because of their high degree of bactericidal activity against many bacteria that produce endocarditis and their low toxicity, are by far the most useful drugs. Synergistic combinations of antibiotics have proved valuable at times.

Specific antimicrobial regimens are as follows:

1.   Endocarditis due to *Streptococcus viridans (S. salivarius, S. mutans, S. sanguis, S. bovis)*: penicillin G, 5 to 10 million U daily (in divided doses given as a bolus q4h into an intravenous infusion) continued for 3 to 4 weeks. Enhanced bactericidal action is obtained if an aminoglycoside (e.g., gentamicin, 3 to 5 mg/kg/day IM) is added during the first 10 to 14 days of treatment. Doses will vary because of resistant organisms.

2. Endocarditis due to *Streptococcus fecalis:* The *S. fecalis* causes 5 to 10 percent of cases of spontaneously arising endocarditis and occasionally also follows abuse of IV drugs. Treatment requires simultaneous use of penicillin and an aminoglycoside. Penicillin G, 20 to 40 million U, or ampicillin, 6 to 12 g/day, is given in divided doses as bolus injections q2–4h into an IV infusion. An aminoglycoside (gentamicin, 5 mg/kg/day) is injected IM q8–12h.

3. Endocarditis due to staphylococcus (*Staphylococcus aureaus, S. epidermidis*): If the infecting staphylococci are not penicillinase producers, **penicillin G**, 10 to 20 million U in divided doses (as an IV bolus), is the treatment of choice. If the staphylococci produce penicillinase, **nafcillin** (penicillinase-resistant) 8 to 12 g daily, given as a bolus q2h into an IV infusion, is the drug of choice.

4. Endocarditis due to gram-negative bacteremia: The susceptibility of these organisms to antimicrobial drugs varies so greatly that effective treatment must be based on laboratory tests. Therapy usually consists of an aminoglycoside in combination with a penicillin or cephalosporin.

5. Endocarditis due to yeast and fungi: This type rarely arises spontaneously but is seen with increasing frequency in abusers of IV drugs, after cardiac surgery, or in immunosuppressed individuals. *Candida albicans, Candida parapsilosis,* and *Torulopus glabrata* are among the organisms encountered commonly. The drugs most active against yeast and fungi are amphotericin B (0.4 to 1 mg/kg/day IV) and **flucytosine** (150 mg/kg/day orally). However, these drugs will rarely eradicate fungal endocarditis.

6. Prosthetic valve endocarditis: This may occur early within days after insertion of a valve, when it is usually caused by staphylococci, gram-negative enteric bacteria, or *Candida.* Treatment is aimed at the infecting organism.

7. Culture-negative endocarditis: With a clinical picture suggestive of infective endocarditis but with persistently negative blood cultures, empiric treatment with penicillin G, 20 to 50 million U/day IV, plus an aminoglycoside (e.g., gentamicin, 5 mg/kg/day IM) can continue for 4 weeks. There should be significant improvement in some manifestations of the disease within 1 week. If there is not, a therapeutic trial with other drugs may be warranted.

CASE STUDY

T.P. is a 44-year-old black male who was admitted to the hospital, presenting symptoms of intermittent fever, weakness, malaise, and alternating chills and sweats.

Assessment

Upon obtaining the patient's history, the admitting nurse found that T.P. had a history of rheumatic fever as a child. He also had had a substantial weight loss over the past few months and complained that he never had any energy and was "tired all the time." On physical examination, T.P. appeared thin, pale, and anemic-looking, with enlarged lymph nodes. His heart rate was slightly increased at 110, blood pressure was 100/60, and temperature was 101.4°F. Moderate clubbing of the fingers was evidenced, and some petechial hemorrhage was found on the skin. Blood and throat cultures were taken, as well as routine laboratory tests.

Management

Once T.P. was admitted to the hospital he was placed on strict bed rest. The cultures grew *Streptococcus viridans.* Echocardiogram showed some valvular damage due to vegetation present on the mitral valve. A diagnosis of subacute bacterial endocarditis was made. T.P. was not allergic to penicillin so he was started on aqueous crystalline penicillin G, 2 million U IV every 6 h. The penicillin was to be continued for the next 6 weeks.

Evaluation

T.P. was discharged to home care after 6 weeks with instructions on limited activity, diet, and medication. Plans were made for further cardiologic evaluation of his impaired cardiac function for possible need for valvular replacement surgery.

SEXUALLY TRANSMITTED DISEASES (STDs)

Diseases that can be transmitted by sexual contact (venereal) include not only gonorrhea, syphilis, chancroid, lymphogranuloma venereum, and granuloma inguinale but a new generation of diseases which includes pediculosis pubis, venereal warts, herpes simplex, and others. A major problem in the therapy of STD is the failure to treat the sexual partners of patients with STDs. In the United States, local health departments will work with patients and local medical people to treat and contact sexual partners for many of the STDs. The treatment of STDs is presented in Table 28-21.

Gonorrhea

Gonorrhea is the most reported STD in the United States and the most commonly reported communicable disease. Uncomplicated infections of the urethra and cervix with *Neisseria gonorrhoeae* can be treated with a single dose of amoxicillin and probenecid, followed up with tetracycline.

TABLE 28-21 Treatment of Sexually Transmitted Diseases

TYPE OR STAGE	DRUGS OF CHOICE	DOSAGE	ALTERNATIVES
Gonorrhea			
Urethritis or cervicitis	Amoxicillin *plus* probenecid *followed by* Tetracycline HCl*	3 g PO once plus 1 g PO once. 500 mg PO qid × 7 days	Penicillin G procaine 4.8 million U IM† once *plus* probenecid 1 g PO once Spectinomycin 2 g IM once. Cefoxitin 2 g or cefuroxime 1.5 g IM once *plus* probenecid 1 g PO once. Cefotaxime 1 g IM once.
Anal			
Women	As for urethritis or cervicitis	See above.	See above.
Men	Penicillin G procaine *plus* probenecid	As for urethritis	Spectinomycin 2 g IM once
Pharyngeal	Tetracycline HCl* *or* Penicillin G procaine *plus* probenecid	As for urethritis As for urethritis	Trimethoprim-sulfamethoxazole 9 tablets‡ daily × 5 days
Ophthalmia (adults)	Penicillin G crystalline *plus* saline irrigation	10 million U IV daily × 5 days	Cefoxitin 1 g or cefotaxime 500 mg IV qid × 5 days *plus* saline irrigation
Bacteremia and arthritis	Penicillin G crystalline *followed by* Amoxicillin	10 million U IV daily × 3 days 500 mg PO qid × 4 days	Tetracycline 500 mg oral qid* × 7 days Spectinomycin 2 g IM bid × 3 days Erythromycin 500 mg oral qid × 7 days Cefotaxime 500 mg or cefoxitin 1 g IV qid × 7 days
Meningitis	Penicillin G crystalline	At least 10 million U IV daily for at least 10 days	Cefotaxime 2 g IV q4h for at least 10 days
Endocarditis	Penicillin G crystalline	At least 10 million U IV daily for at least 3–4 weeks	Chloramphenicol 4–6 g/day for at least 10 days
Neonatal			
Ophthalmia	Penicillin G crystalline *plus* saline irrigation	50,000 U/kg/day IV in 2 doses × 7 days	
Arthritis and septicemia	Penicillin G crystalline	75,000–100,000 U/kg/day IV in 4 doses × 7 days	
Meningitis	Penicillin G crystalline	100,000 U/kg/day IV in 3 or 4 doses for at least 10 days	
Children (under 45 kg)			
Urogenital, anal and pharyngeal	Amoxicillin *plus* probenecid *or* Penicillin G procaine *plus* probenecid	50 mg/kg oral once 25 mg/kg (max. 1 g) once 100,000 U/kg IM once 25 mg/kg (max. 1 g) once	Spectinomycin 40 mg/kg IM once Tetracycline (over 8 years old) 10 mg/kg PO qid × 5 days
Arthritis	Penicillin G crystalline	150,000 U/kg/day IV × 7 days	Cefoxitin 100 mg/kg/day or cefotaxime 50 mg/kg/day IV in divided doses × 7 days Tetracycline (over 8 years old) 10 mg/kg PO qid × 7 days Erythromycin 50 mg/kg/day PO in 4 divided doses × 7 days
Meningitis	Penicillin G crystalline	250,000 U/kg/day IV in 6 divided doses for at least 10 days	Cefotaxime 200 mg/kg/day IV for at least 10 days Chloramphenicol 100 mg/kg/day IV for at least 10 days

Condition	Drug	Dosage
Chlamydia trachomatis		
Urethritis or cervicitis	Tetracycline HCl*	500 mg PO qid × 7 days
	or	
	Erythromycin	500 mg PO qid × 7 days
Proctitis	Tetracycline* or erythromycin	500 mg PO qid for 7 days
Neonatal		
Ophthalmia	Erythromycin	12.5 mg/kg PO or IV qid × 14 days
Pneumonia	Erythromycin	10 mg/kg PO or IV qid × 14 days
Lymphogranuloma venereum	Tetracycline* or erythromycin	500 mg PO qid × 21 days
Pelvic inflammatory disease		
Outpatients	Cefoxitin	2 g IM once
	plus probenecid	1 g PO once
	followed by doxycycline	100 mg PO bid × 10 days
Hospitalized patients	Cefoxitin *plus* doxycycline	2 g IV qid
	followed by doxycycline	100 mg IV bid until/improvement
		100 mg PO bid to complete 10 days
Epididymitis	Amoxicillin *plus*	3 g PO once
	probenecid *followed by*	1 g PO once
	Tetracycline HCl*	500 mg qid × 10 days
Syphilis		
Early (Primary, secondary, or latent less than 1 year)	Penicillin G benzathine	2.4 million U IM once
Late (more than one year's duration, cardiovascular)	Penicillin G benzathine	2.4 million U IM weekly × 3
Neurosyphilis	Penicillin G crystalline	2–4 million U IV q4h × 10 days
	or	
	Penicillin G procaine	2.4 million U IM daily plus probenecid PO 500 mg qid, both × 10 days
	or	
	Penicillin G benzathine	2.4 million U IM weekly × 3
Congenital syphilis		
CSF normal	Penicillin G benzathine	50,000 U/kg IM once
CSF abnormal	Penicillin G crystalline	25,000 U/kg IM or IV bid for at least 10 days
	or	
	Penicillin G procaine	50,000 U/kg IM daily for at least 10 days
Chancroid	Trimethoprim-sulfamethoxazole	Two tablets‡ bid × 5 days
	or	
	Erythromycin	500 mg PO qid × 7 days

Additional therapy notes:

- Sulfisoxazole 500 mg PO qid × 10 days
- Sulfisoxazole 100 mg/kg/day PO or IV in divided doses (for children more than 4 weeks old)
- Tetracycline HCl 500 mg PO qid × 10 days
- Doxycycline 100 mg IV bid *plus* metronidazole 1 g IV bid until improvement *followed by* doxycycline 100 mg oral bid *plus* metronidazole 1 g oral bid to complete 10 days
- *Chlamydia* only:
  Erythromycin 500 mg qid × 10 days
  Gonococci only: Amoxicillin 500 mg tid × 10 days
- Tetracycline 500 mg PO qid × 15 days
  Erythromycin 500 mg PO qid × 15 days
- Tetracycline 500 mg PO qid × 30 days
  Erythromycin 500 mg PO qid × 30 days
- Tetracycline 500 mg PO qid × 30 days
  Erythromycin 500 mg PO qid × 30 days

*Or doxycycline 100 mg PO bid.   †Divided into two injections at one visit.   ‡Each tablet contains 80 mg trimethoprim and 400 mg sulfamethoxazole.

Source: The Medical Letter on Drugs and Therapeutics, **26:**5–10, Jan. 20, 1984.

If compliance with the oral therapy is expected to be a problem treatment with procaine penicillin G plus probenecid can be implemented. The penicillinase-producing strains of *N. gonorrhoeae* (PPNG) should be treated with spectinomycin or a cephalosporin (cefotaxime or cefoxitin).

Syphilis

Syphilis is a complex infectious disease caused by *Treponema pallidum*, a spirochete. Parenteral penicillin G is still the drug of choice for the treatment of syphilis. Treatment may be associated with the Jarisch-Herxheimer reaction, which is attributed to the sudden massive destruction of spirochetes and is manifested by fever and aggravation of the existing clinical picture. Therapy should be continued unless the symptoms become severe or life-threatening.

CASE STUDY

A 19-year-old woman came to the venereal disease clinic complaining of frequent, urgent, and painful urination. This problem began suddenly about 12 h after she had sexual intercourse.

Assessment

The patient's medical history and physical examination were unremarkable. However, the patient had noted a small amount of vaginal discharge for several months. Because the discharge was not profuse, pruritic, or malodorous, the patient was unconcerned. Her only medication was birth control pills (Ovral).

The pelvic examination was within normal limits except for a small amount of white discharge from the cervical os. Samples of the discharge were taken for microscopic examination and gonococcal culture. The Gram's stain and wet mount showed no trichomonads or yeasts but did show numerous gram-positive rods (lactobacilli) and a few gram-negative rods.

Microscopic examination of the urine sediment showed increased red and white blood cells, numerous bacteria, and a few epithelial cells. A "clean catch" urine specimen was sent to the laboratory for culture. The presumptive diagnosis was acute uncomplicated cystitis, probably due to *E. coli*, and a vaginal discharge of uncertain etiology.

Management

The patient was given a prescription for trimethoprim-sulfamethoxazole double-strength (Bactrim DS or Septra DS) and instructed to take three tablets all at once. She was instructed to drink plenty of fluids, including orange and grapefruit juices. She was asked to call the clinic within 48 h to obtain the results of the other cultures and if she developed rash, fever, chills, or flank pain.

The urine culture grew out more that 10^5 bacteria/mL of *E. coli*, and the cervical culture showed a few *Neisseria gonorrhoeae*. The patient was contacted and asked to return to the clinic. She was informed of the culture results and questioned about her sexual practices and partners. She was given 1 g of probenecid orally and 30 min later 4.8 million U or procaine penicillin intramuscularly. A serologic test for syphilis was also taken. The patient was advised against sexual intercourse until after her next clinic appointment 6 days later. Arrangements were made to have her sexual partners treated, and a venereal disease case report for gonorrhea was completed and sent to the local health department.

Evaluation

On the return appointment a repeat urine culture and another culture from the endocervical canal were taken. Minimal discharge was present. She agreed to call the clinic 48 h later for the results of her second culture and VDRL. All follow-up tests proved to be negative, and she was discharged from the clinic.

URINARY TRACT INFECTIONS

Acute infection of the urinary tract can be divided into those which affect the lower tract (urethritis, cystitis, and prostatitis) and those which affect the upper tract (acute pyelonephritis). Active urinary tract infections (UTIs) are characterized by more than 100,000 (10^5) bacteria per milliliter collected from a clean catch urine sample. Patients who are symptomatic may have a UTI with less bacteriuria (10^2 to 10^4). The term *relapse* implies recurrence of infection with the same organism; *reinfection* implies infection with a different organism.

Acute UTIs affect up to 20 percent of adult women during their lives. Males rarely develop acute UTIs before the age of 45 unless they have anatomic abnormalities.

Virtually any microorganism can produce a UTI, but the

most common are the gram-negative bacilli. Up to 90 percent of all community-acquired UTIs are caused by *E. coli;* other common organism include *Enterobacter, Klebsiella, Serratia, Pseudomonas,* and *Proteus.* The latter organisms are more common in recurrent infections or patients with structural abnormalities.

Clinical Pharmacology and Therapeutics

Acute Urinary Tract Infections
The treatment of an acute uncomplicated UTI most often will respond to a 7- to 10-day course of a **sulfonamide, nitrofurantoin, ampicillin, nalidixic acid,** or **tetracycline,** since most of these infections are due to *E. coli* and most strains are still sensitive to the drugs. A single-dose therapy has been effective, using 3.5 g of ampicillin, 3.0 g of amoxicillin, and three to four tablets of double-strength trimethoprim-sulfamethoxazole (Bactrim DS, Septra DS) (see Table 28-22). Single-dose therapy has the advantages of improved patient compliance and lower expense. **Phenazopyridine** (Pyridium) has analgesic or local anesthetic effect (it has no antibacterial action) on the urinary tract and can be given alone or in combination with various sulfonamides [**sulfamethoxazole** (Azo Gantanol)]. It is taken to relieve symptoms of the urinary tract infection. The drug is best used as a single-entity product since therapy is usually only needed for the first 2 days.

The treatment of recurrent infections is based on the results of culture and susceptibility tests. The drug is then given for 10 to 14 days in doses sufficient to produce high urinary levels. If a patient does not respond, a 12- to 20-week trial of trimethoprim-sulfamethoxazole or ampicillin may be tried.

Chronic Urinary Tract Infections
Urine cultures are the guide to therapy and are repeated before, during, and after therapy. Treatment may consist of surgical correction of the anatomic abnormalities, usually performed in conjunction with therapy for the UTI.

If the same organism is isolated from at least two sequential urine cultures, antimicrobial drug sensitivity tests should be performed. From the group of drugs to which the organism is susceptible, in vitro, the least toxic is selected and given daily for 4 weeks. Repeated examination of urine after

TABLE 28-22 Overview of Outpatient Antimicrobial Therapy for Lower Urinary Tract Infections

INDICATION	ANTIMICROBIAL AGENT (ORAL ADMINISTRATION)	DOSE	INTERVAL	DURATION
Acute bacterial cystitis	Trimethoprim-sulfamethoxazole, double-strength tablet*	3 tablets	Single dose	—
	Amoxicillin, 500-mg capsule	6 capsules	Single dose	—
	Sulfisoxazole, 500-mg tablet	4 tablets	Single dose	—
	Trimethoprim, 100-mg tablet	1 tablet	Every 12 h	7 days
	Macrodantin, 100-mg capsule	1 capsule	Every 6 h	7 days
	Nalidixic acid, 500-mg caplet	2 caplets	Every 6 h	7 days
Acute urethral syndrome Initial therapy	Trimethoprim-sulfamethoxazole, double-strength tablet*	3 tablets	Single dose	—
	Amoxicillin, 500-mg capsule	6 capsules	Single dose	—
After failure	Doxycycline, 100-mg capsule	1 capsule	Every 12 h	10 days
Asymptomatic bacteriuria during pregnancy	Amoxicillin, 250-mg capsule	1 capsule	Every 6 h	7 days
	Cephradine, 250-mg capsule	1 capsule	Every 6 h	7 days
Prophylaxis against recurrent bacteriuria	Trimethoprim-sulfamethoxazole, single-strength tablet†	½ tablet	Every evening	6 months
	Trimethoprim, 100-mg tablet	½ tablet	Every evening	6 months

*Each double-strength tablet consists of 160 mg of trimethoprim and 800 mg of sulfamethoxazole.
†Each single-strength tablet consists of 80 mg of trimethoprim and 400 mg of sulfamethoxazole.
Source: T. E. Keys and R. F. Edson, "Antimicrobial Agents in Urinary Tract Infections," *Mayo Clin Proc,* **58:** 166,1983.

TABLE 28-23 Antibacterial Agents Used Principally for Urinary Tract Infections

DRUG	ACTIVITY SPECTRUM AND CHARACTERISTICS	DOSAGE	ROUTE	SIDE EFFECTS
Sulfonamides Sulfisoxazole (Gantrisin), sulfamethizole (Thiosulfil), sulfamethoxazole (Gantanol), trimethoprim-sulfamethoxazole [Bactrim & Septra]	Short-acting sulfonamides are best because of high urinary concentration and good solubility at acid pH; more active in alkaline urine; especially effective against E. coli and P. mirabilis; many strains of Klebsiella, Aerobacter, Proteus, and Pseudomonas are resistant.	Varies with drug (see text)	Oral	Allergic reactions; skin rash, drug fever, pruritus, photosensitization; periarteritis nodosa, S.L.E., Stevens-Johnson syndrome, serum sickness syndrome, myocarditis; neurotoxicity (psychosis, neuritis); hepatotoxicity; blood dyscrasias, usually agranulocytosis; crystalluria; nausea and vomiting, headache, dizziness, lassitude, mental depression, acidosis, sulfhemoglobin; hemolytic anemia in G6PD-deficient individuals; possible teratogenic effects; should not be used in newborn infants or in pregnant women near term.
Nitrofurantoin (Furadantin, Macrodantin)	Many gram-positive and gram-negative organisms; as relates to urinary tract, nitrofurantoin is effective against likely pathogens except Pseudomonas and some Klebsiella, Enterobacter, and Proteus species, high urinary concentration (ineffective in renal failure); increased activity in acid urine; action much reduced at pH 8 or over.	100 mg q6h, 5–7 mg/kg	Oral, IV	Nausea and vomiting, hypersensitivity, peripheral neuropathy, pulmonary infiltrate, intrahepatic cholestasis, hemolytic anemia in G6PD deficiency; contraindicated in renal failure; should not be used in infants less than 1 month of age.
Methenamine mandelate (Mandelamine), methenamine hippurate (Hiprex, Urex)	Combination effect against most organisms in vitro; methenamine has no action per se but in acid medium is slowly decomposed with liberation of formaldehyde; mandelic acid also requires acid pH; effective only when acid urine (preferably at or below pH 5) can be maintained; limited place in therapy; should not be used in tissue infection (pyelonephritis).	0.5–1 g q6h	Oral	Nausea and vomiting; contraindicated in renal failure because it leads to acidosis; should not be used with sulfonamides.
Nalidixic acid (NegGram)	Gram-negative urinary tract pathogens (Enterobacteriaceae) except Pseudomonas; high degree of resistance may develop rapidly during therapy.	1 g q6h	Oral	GI hypersensitivity, fever, eosinophilia, photosensitivity, neurologic disturbances (malaise, drowsiness, dizziness, visual disturbances); convulsions pseudomotor cerebri (?); mild leukopenia, thrombocytopenia, hemolytic anemia; can produce false elevations of 17-ketosteroids and 17-ketogenic steroids in urine.

TABLE 28-24 Nursing Process Related to Acute Infectious Diseases

ASSESSMENT	MANAGEMENT	EVALUATION
	Pneumonia	
Note quantity and quality of respirations; check for presence of expiratory grunt; auscultate lungs for abnormal breath sounds; note amount, color, and tenacity of sputum. Check temperature, blood pressure, and arterial blood gas reports. Check blood cultures, WBC, and leukocyte count. Take sputum and throat culture if ordered. Check on allergy and medication history.	Keep patient in most comfortable position for breathing; elevate head of bed and support back with pillows; turn and reposition every 2 h. Use proper aseptic technique in disposal of contaminated waste. Observe patient for abdominal distention due to paralytic ileus (distention pushes the diaphragm up so that it presses on the base of the lungs and does not allow the lung to expand). Protect against drafts and chills. Check that oxygen therapy is instituted as ordered; give antibiotics on schedule. Check vital signs q2–4h; assist patient to cough productively by helping splint patient's chest. Offer 2000–3000 mL of fluid daily. Offer oral hygiene every few hours, more often if herpetic lesions are present.	Observe for adverse reaction to antibiotic: nausea, vomiting, diarrhea, pruritus, skin rash, soft tissue reaction. Use analgesics with caution to prevent depression of cough reflex and respiratory rate. Be alert for complications such as pleural effusion, delayed resolution, superinfection and delirium, empyema, septicemia, atelectasis and shock. Watch for signs of fluid and electrolyte imbalance. Measure abdominal girth to evaluate increase or decrease in distention. Observe for sharp increase or decrease in circulatory or respiratory rate. Encourage gradual increase in activity during convalescence but remind patient of lowered resistance and susceptibility to secondary infection.
	Meningitis	
Assess for presence of nuchal rigidity, headache, photosensitivity, positive Kernig and/or Brudzinski sign. Determine level of consciousness; assess for signs of increased intercranial pressure. Ask children's parents for preceding events, such as otitis media or *H. influenzae* exposure; obtain list of possible contacts. Check that all cultures are obtained before starting antibiotic therapy. Check on medication and allergy history.	Assist physician with lumbar puncture. Monitor intake and output, body weight with children (with young children weigh each used diaper and then subtract diaper weight for I&O measurement). Observe isolation techniques as ordered; keep siderails elevated. Position for maximum comfort without pressure or flexion of neck. Support shoulders and neck when repositioning. Decrease stimuli in room (darken, keep quiet) Do neurological and pupil check every 2–4 h; give antibiotics as scheduled.	Observe for adverse reaction to antibiotics: hypokalemia, hypernatremia, nephrotoxicity, ototoxicity, and blood dyscrasias. Observe for changes in level of consciousness and for seizures or convulsions. Observe for sharp increase or decrease in vital signs; may be indicative of shock. Watch for signs and symptoms of increasing intercranial pressure, manifested by slowly falling pulse and respirations, accompanied by a rise in blood pressure. Observe for neurological complications such as damage to the cranial nerves and/or visual or auditory deterioration. Observe for terminal rise in temperature due to failure of the thermoregulatory mechanism.
	Endocarditis	
Check for "Osler's nodes" on the tips or lateral borders of the fingers and toes; petechial hemorrhage on skin or conjunctiva; clubbing of fingers; weight loss; skin color (often called "cafe au lait"); quality and quantity of pulse. Check on medication and allergy history; check that all cultures are taken before antimicrobial therapy started.	Auscultate breath sounds every 2–4 h to detect early signs of failure or secondary respiratory infections. Monitor I&O; give adequate oral and IV hydration. Give frequent small feedings when able to take oral nourishments. Reposition frequently if on bed rest. Apply antiembolitic hose; give antibiotics as scheduled. Monitor activities when allowed out of bed and promote planned rest periods. Check on serum electrolytes.	Observe for adverse effects of antibiotics: hyperkalemia, neurotoxicity, superinfection. Observe for signs of emboli in lower extremities: pain, pallor, coolness and loss of leg pulses; pulmonary emboli: dyspnea shortness of breath, cyanosis, and frothy or blood-tinged sputum; and of brain emboli: CVA, paralysis, aphasia. Observe for early signs of cardiac involvement: irregular pulse, tachycardia, chest discomfort, dypsnea on exertion. Educate patient to prevent recurring infection; may need prophylactic antibiotics during procedures likely to cause transient bacteremia (dental work

493

TABLE 28–24 Nursing Process Related to Acute Infectious Diseases (*Cont.*)

ASSESSMENT	MANAGEMENT	EVALUATION
		or any GI or GU procedure) and to seek medical treatment for persistent sore throats or bacterial infections such as boils on the skin.
	Sexually Transmitted Diseases	
Check for medication and allergy history, with emphasis on reactions to penicillin or procaine. Assess genital area for surface infections, rashes; urinary frequency; dysuria; vaginal or urethral discharge; all skin areas for lesions and drainage; chancres on lip, tongue, fingers, eyelids, nipples; condylotoma on moist skin surfaces (mucous membrane of mouth, tongue or anus). Identify all sexual contacts.	Observe caution when handling pads or objects potentially contaminated by drainage from genital tract; wash hands thoroughly after contact. Secretion precautions should be taken until 24 h after initiation of effective therapy. Use nonjudgmental attitude while interviewing and examining the patient. Monitor patient closely for 30 min after receiving any injection. Properly instruct patient if going home on oral self-medication. Treat all sexual partners, if necessary.	Observe for adverse effects of antibiotic therapy: skin rash and potential anaphylactic shock. Instruct patients in the importance of protecting their eyes from contamination and of maintaining adequate cleanliness. Educate patient to potential involvement of all body systems if disease not fully treated or patient is not compliant with complete dosage and duration of antibiotic therapy. Advise patient of importance of follow-up visits for culture and antimicrobial therapy. Caution patient not to become reinfected by sexual contact with untreated previous sexual partners.
	Urinary Tract Infections	
Assess for urinary frequency, oliguria, dysuria, urgency; back pain; fever; assess urine for color and odor, volume, specific gravity, and presence of casts or particulate matter; assess for medication and allergy history; obtain urine cultures before beginning antimicrobial therapy.	Monitor I&O; provide at least 3000 mL of fluid daily; give acid fluids for a strongly acid urine (cranberry juice). Provide warm sitz baths for relief of discomfort. Observe for electrolyte or water imbalance; keep covered bedpan or urinal easily within reach of patient. Give antiseptic drugs, if ordered, to relieve bladder pain. Use aspirin, heat lamps, and hot tub baths for relief of discomfort. Monitor BUN and creatinine.	If antibiotic is effective, urine should be clear of original organisms within 72 h. Watch for signs and symptoms of renal failure. Continue to observe color, consistency, and content of urine; check for sediment, clots, and shreds of material. Observe for hematuria. Instruct patient in importance of fluid hydration and personal hygiene, particularly to cleanliness of perineum with respect to fecal contamination. Observe for adverse effects of antibiotics: rash, sore throat, purpura, crystalline urine, renal toxicity, and vitamin K deficiency.

therapy is necessary to confirm absence or recurrent infection. Chronic suppression of bacteriuria can also be treated with a urinary antiseptic, e.g., **nitrofurantoin, methenamine mandelate** or **hippurate, nalidixic acid,** or acidifying agents (Table 28-23). Urinary pH must be adjusted to the optimum for the drug selected and usually should be held below pH 6.0. Treatment is continued for 6 months to 1 year, after which point renal function and bacteriuria are reevaluated.

NURSING PROCESS RELATED TO COMMON ACUTE INFECTIOUS DISORDERS

The nursing process in pneumonia, meningitis, endocarditis, STDs, and UTI are summarized in Table 28-24.

REFERENCES

Abramowicz, M.: "Adverse Interactions of Drugs," *Med Lett Drugs Ther,* 23:17–28, 1983.

Altman, L., and L. Tompkins: "Toxic and Allergic Manifestations of Antimicrobials," *Postgrad Med,* 54:157, 1978.

Anderson, A. C., G. R. Hodges, and W. G. Barnes: "Determination of Serum Gentamicin Sulfate Levels Ordering Patterns and Use as a Guide to Therapy," *Arch Intern Med,* 136:785–787, 1926.

Appel, G. B., and H. C. Neu: "The Nephrotoxicity of Antimicrobial Agents," *N Engl J Med,* **296**:663–670, 1977.

Arko, R. J., W. P. Duncan, W. J. Brown, W. L. Peacock, and T. Tomizawa: "Immunity in Infections with *Neisseria Gonorrhoeae,* Duration and Serologic Response in the Chimpanzee," *J Infect Dis,* **133**:441–447, 1976.

Austrian, R., R. M. Douglas, G. Schiffman, A. M. Coetzee, H. J. Koornhof, H. Smith, and D. W. Reid: "Prevention of Pneumococcal Pneumonia by Vaccination," *Assoc Am Physician,* **89**: 1977.

Barry, A: *The Antimicrobic Susceptibility Test: Principles and Practice,* Philadelphia: Lea & Febiger, 1976.

Baumens, E., and C. Clemmons: "Foods That Foil Drugs," *RN,* **41**:79–81. 1978.

Benet, L. Z.: "Effect of Route of Administration and Distribution on Drug Action," *Pharmacokinet Biopharm,* **6**:559, 1978.

Bennett, W: "Drug Therapy in Renal Failure: Dosing Guidelines for Adults," *Ann Intern Med,* **93**:262–286, 1980.

Bennett, W. M.: "Principles of Drug Therapy in Patients with Renal Disease," *West J Med,* **123**:372–375, 1975.

Bogart, D. B., C. Liu, Roth, G. R. Kerby, and C. H. Williams: "Rapid Diagnosis of Primary Influenza Pneumonia," *Chest* **68**.513–517, 1975.

Brunner, L., and D. Suddarth: *Textbook of Medical-Surgical Nursing,* 3d ed., Philadelphia: Lippincott, 1975.

Cockeril, F. R., and R. S. Edson: "Mode of Action of Sulfamethoxazole and Trimethoprim in the Inhibitions of Production of Folinic Acid," *Mayo Clin Proc,* **58**:148–156, 1983.

Coleman, D. L., R. I. Horwitz, and V. T. Andriole: "Association Between Serum Inhibitory Bactericidal Concentration and Therapeutic Outcome in Bacterial Endocarditis," *Am J Med,* **73**:260–267, 1982.

Collier, J., E. M. Calhoun, and P. L. Hill: "A Multicenter Comparison of Clindamycin and Metronidazole in the Treatment of Anaerobic Infections," *Scand J Infect Dis* [Suppl.], **26**:96–100, 1981.

Davies, J.: "General Mechanisms of Antimicrobial Resistance," *Rev Infect Dis,* **1**:23, 1979.

Dilworth, J. A., P. Stewart, J. M. Gwaltney, Jr, J. O. Handley, and M. A. Sands: "Methods to Improve Detection of Pneumococci Respiratory," *J Clin Microbiol,* **2**:453–455, 1975.

Eickhoff, T. C., P. Z. Brachman, J. U. Bessett, and J. F. Brown: "Surveillance of Nosocomial Infections in Community Hospitals: Surveillance Methods, Methods Effectiveness and Initial Results," *J Infect Dis,* **120**:305–317, 1969.

Erchenwald, H. F., and G. McCracken: "Antimicrobial Therapy in Infants and Children," *J Pediatr,* **93**:337–341, 1978.

Finland, M.: "Changing Ecology of Bacterial Infections as Related to Antimicrobial Therapy," *J Infect Dis,* **122**:419–431, 1970.

Galgiani, J. N., D. F. Busch, C. Brass, L. W. Rumans, C. W. Mangels, and D. A. Stevels: "*Bacteroides fragilis* Endocarditis, Bacteremia and Other Infections Treated with Oral or Intravenous Metronidazole." *Am J Med,* **65**:284–289, 1978.

Gilium, R. F., and A. J. Barsky: "Diagnosis and Management of Patient Noncompliance," *JAMA,* **228**:1563, 1974.

Gleckman, R., and O. DeTorres: "Antibiotic Prescribing," *Postgrad Med,* **72**:223–230, 1982.

———, G. Alvarez, and D. W. Joubeat: "Drug Therapy Reviewed: Trimethoprim-sulfamethoxazole," *Am J Hosp Pharm,* **36**:893, 1929.

Hermans, P. E.: "Symposium Antimicrobial Agents: Foreword," *Mayo Clin Proc,* **58**:3–6, 1983.

Jick, H.: "Adverse Reactions to Trimethoprim Sulfamethoxazole in Hospitalized Patients," *Rev Infect Dis,* **4**:426–428, 1982.

Kaplan, E. L., A. F. Bascom, A. Bisno, D. Durack, and H. Houser: "Prevention of Bacterial Endocarditis," *Circulation,* **56**:139A, 1977.

Kaufman, R. E., R. Johnson, H. W. Jaffe, C. Thornsberry, and G. M. Reynolds: "Cooperative Study Group: National Gonorrhea Therapy Monitoring Treatment Results," *N Engl J Med,* **294**:1–4, 1976.

Knoben, J. E., and P. O. Anderson: *Handbook of Clinical Drug Data,* 5th ed., Hamilton, Ill.: Drug Intelligence Publication Press, 1983.

Kucers, A., and M. M. C. K. Bennett: *The Use of Antibiotics: A Comprehensive Review with Clinical Emphasis.* 2d ed., Philadelphia: Lippincott, 1975, pp. 417–423.

Levin, H. S., and B. M. Kagan: "Antimicrobial Agents, Pediatric Dosages, Routes of Administration and Preparation Procedures for Parenteral Therapy," *Pediatr Clin North Am,* **15**:275–290, 1968.

Lorian, V., and C. C. DeFreitas: "Minimal Antibiotic Concentrations of Aminoglycosides and B-Lactam Antibiotics for Some Gram Negative Bacilli and Gram Positive Cocci," *J Infect Dis,* **139**:599–603, 1979.

Mandell, G. L., and M. A. Sands: "Antimicrobial Agents Penicillins and Cephalosporins," in A. G. Gilman, L. S. Goodman, and A. Gilman (eds.), *Goodman and Gilman's The Pharmacological Basis of Therapeutics,* 6th ed., New York: Macmillan, 1980, pp. 1126–1161.

Mead, P. B.: "Practical Applications of Antibodies in Preventing and Treatment of Pelvic Infection," *Reproduct Med,* **13**:135–141, 1974.

Meade, R. H.: "Drug Therapy Review: Antimicrobial Spectrum, Pharmacology and Therapeutics Use of Erythromycin and Its Derivatives," *Am J Hosp Pharm,* **36**:1185–1190, 1979.

Meyers, B. R., S. Z. Hirchman, L. Strougo, and E. Srulevitch: "Comparative Study of Piperacillin, Ticarcillin and Carbenicillin," *Pharmacokinet Antimicrob Agents Chemother* **17**:608–611, 1980.

Murillo, J: "Gentamicin and Ticaricillin Serum Levels," *JAMA,* **241**:2401–2404, 1979

Murray, H. W., H. Masul, L. B. Senterfil, and R. B. Robert: "The Protean Manifestations of *Mycoplasma pneumoniae* Infections in Adults," *Am J Med,* **58**:229–242, 1975.

Newton, D. W.: "Physiochemical Determinants of Incompatibility and Instability in Injectable Drug Solutions and Admixtures," *Am J Hosp Pharm,* **35:**1213–1222, 1978.

Newton, M., et al.: "Parenteral Antibiotics: The Hazards to Watch For," *RN,* **44:**44–51, 1981.

Nightingale, D., M. French, and R. Quintitani: "Cephalosporins," in J. J. Scherthag and W. J. Jusko (eds.), *Applied Pharmacokinetics Principles of Therapeutics and Drug Monitoring,* San Francisco: Applied Therapeutics, 1980, pp. 174–239.

Polk, R.: "Moxalactam (Moxam)," *Drug Intell Clin Pharm,* **16:**104–112, 1982.

Poporad, G. A., and E. Abrutyn: "The Third Generation Cephalosporins: Cefotaxime, Moxalactam, and Cefoperazone," *Hosp Formul,* **17**(11):1458–1465, 1982.

Reller, L. B., and C. W. Stratton: "Serum Dilution Test for Bacterial Activity: Standardization and Correlation with Antimicrobial Assays and Susceptibility Tests," *J Infect Dis,* **136:**196–204, 1977.

Sande, M. A., and W. M. Scheld: "Combination Antibiotic Therapy of Bacterial Endocarditis," *Ann Intern Med,* **92:**390–395, 1980.

——, and G. L. Mandell: "Antimicrobial Agents: General Considerations," in A. G. Gilman, L. S. Goodman, and A. Gilman (eds.), *Goodman and Gilman's The Pharmacological Basis of Therapeutics,* 6th ed., New York: Macmillan, 1980, pp. 1080–1106.

——, and ——: "Antimicrobial Agents: The Aminoglycosides," in A. G. Gilman, L. S. Goodman, and A. Gilman (eds.), *Goodman and Gilman's The Pharmacological Basis of Therapeutics,* 6th ed. New York: Macmillan, 1980, pp. 1162–1181.

—— and ——: "Antimicrobial Agents: Tetracyclines and Chloramphenicol," in A. G. Gilman, L. S. Goodman, and A. Gilman (eds.), *Goodman and Gilman's The Pharmacological Basis of Therapeutics,* 6th ed., New York: Macmillan, 1980, pp. 1181–1199.

Sarubbi, F. A., Jr., and J. H. Hull: "Amikacin Serum Concentrations Prediction of Levels and Dosage Guidelines," *Ann Intern Med,* **89:**612–618, 1978.

Schenthag, J. J.: "Aminoglycosides," in J. J. Schenthag and W. J. Jusko (eds.), *Applied Pharmacokinetics Principles of Therapeutics and Drug Monitoring,* San Francisco: Applied Therapeutics, 1980, pp. 174–239.

Schneider, P.: "Drug Therapy in Patients Receiving Total Parenteral Nutrition," *Infusion,* **7:**8–10, 1983.

Siegel, D.: "Tetracyclines: New Look at Old Antibiotic," *NY State J Med,* **78:**950–956, 1978.

Souney, P., and B. F. Polk: "Single Dose Antimicrobial Therapy for Urinary Tract Infections in Women," *Rev Infect Dis,* **4:**29–34, 1982.

Stramm, W. E., K. F. Wasner, and R. Amsel: "Causes of the Acute Urethral Syndrome in Women," *N Engl J Med,* **303:**409–415, 1980.

Tager, I., and F. E. Speizer: "Role of Infection in Chronic Bronchitis," *N Engl J Med,* **292:**563–571, 1975.

Tipper, D. J.: "Mode of Action of Beta Lactam Antibiotics," *Rev Infec Dis,* **1:**39, 1979.

Trissel, L. A.: *Handbook of Injectable Drugs,* 3d ed., Bethseda, Md.: American Society of Hospital Pharmacists, 1983.

White, S., and K. Williamson: "What to Watch for When You Give Penicillin," *RN,* **44:**21–23, 1979.

—— and ——: "What to Watch for When You Give Cephalosporins," *RN,* **44:**29–31, 1979.

—— and ——: "What to Watch for When You Give Tetracycline," *RN,* **44:**31–33, 1979.

—— and ——: "What to Watch for When You Give Aminoglycosides," *RN,* **44:**73–75, 1979.

Wilson, W. R., et al.: "Short Term Therapy for Streptococcal Infective Endocarditis Combined Intramuscular Administration of Penicillin and Streptomycin," *JAMA,* **245:**360–363, 1981.

29

INFECTIOUS DISORDERS II: MYCOBACTERIAL AND NONBACTERIAL INFECTIONS*

SHELDON LEFKOWITZ
SANDE JONES
CATHERINE JOHNSON

MYCOBACTERIAL INFECTIONS

LEARNING OBJECTIVES

Upon mastery of the contents of this section, the reader should be able to:

1. Describe two stages of tuberculosis (TB).
2. Explain three problems in the therapy of tuberculosis.
3. List which drugs can be used in the short course of tuberculosis therapy.
4. List the primary and secondary drugs used in the treatment of tuberculosis, and for each drug give an adverse effect and the dosage.
5. Describe a method to prevent peripheral neuritis, an adverse effect of using isoniazid.
6. List the drug of choice for the treatment of Hansen's disease.

TUBERCULOSIS

Tuberculosis is a communicable chronic bacterial infection caused by *Mycobacterium tuberculosis*. Tuberculosis was once the leading cause of death throughout the world. The advances in detection, treatment, and prevention have dra-

matically decreased the incidence of this infection. However, the problem of tuberculosis has not been eradicated, and there are still approximately 30,000 new cases of tuberculosis diagnosed each year in the United States. The treatment of tuberculosis presents special therapeutic problems for two reasons: the organism is slow-growing and there is a need for chronic multiple drug therapy because mycobacteria develop resistance to the various single agents.

Tuberculosis presents with many problems related to the lungs, but extrapulmonary tuberculosis is also common. *Mycobacterium avium-intracellulare* and *Mycobacterium kansasii* have also been associated with chronic pulmonary infections and are often referred to as "atypical mycobacteria." *M. kansasii* responds well to antituberculosis therapy, but *M. avium–intracellulare* does not respond to drug therapy.

Tuberculosis can present in two stages: (1) the patient is asymptomatic but has evidence of *M. tuberculosis*, and (2) the patient has clinical disease. The use of the tuberculin skin test is helpful in screening the patient population for tuberculosis.

Clinical Pharmacology and Therapeutics of Tuberculosis

Principles of Therapy
Prior to the understanding that tuberculosis was a disease caused by mycobacteria, the therapy was diet, rest, exercise, surgery, and fresh air. With the discovery that tuberculosis was an infectious disease, the effectiveness of therapy was then limited by the availability of antimicrobial agents.

---

*The editors thank Arthur G. Lipman and Susan I. Molde, who contributed the chapter on infectious disease in the first edition.

The treatment of mycobacteria should be guided by the same principles used in the treatment of any infectious disease (see Chap. 28). Principles that are specific to the therapy of tuberculosis are as follows:

1. Drugs that kill the bacillus (bactericidal agents) are preferred.

2. Combination therapy should always be used. The risk of a resistant organism in a susceptible bacillus population is about 10 in a million. When two or more drugs are used, the risk decreases to 10 in a trillion.

3. In certain parts of the world mycobacteria are resistant to isoniazid and streptomycin. Patients exposed to tuberculosis in those areas should be assumed resistant to those drugs, and different drugs should be utilized.

4. Failure of the patient to take the medication as prescribed (noncompliance) is a major factor in treatment failure.

5. Therapy is continued for a minimum of 9 months but in many cases may be continued for 18 to 24 months.

6. To improve compliance, the treatment program should be simple. When possible, the medication should be given as a single dose after breakfast.

Prior to the start of drug therapy, a culture for mycobacteria should be taken. Therapy should be initiated before the results of the culture are known, since it takes from 6 to 8 weeks to grow the organism. Drugs should be started based on the suspected susceptibility patterns. Cultures should be taken, but sensitivity testing does not have to be done during the course of treatment. Cultures are useful in monitoring the progress of the therapy.

The most common drugs used in the treatment of tuberculosis are **isoniazid, ethambutol, rifampin,** and **streptomycin.** These agents are often referred to as the primary, first-line, or major drugs. The secondary, or second-line, drugs include **para-aminosalicylic acid, ethionamide, pyrazinamide, cycloserine, kanamycin, capreomycin,** and other investigational drugs. In general, second-line drugs are more toxic and may be less effective than the first-line drugs (see Table 29-1).

Patients become noninfectious after a few weeks of drug therapy. The bacteriologic cultures usually become negative after a few months of therapy. However, therapy is continued for 18 to 24 months to prevent a relapse of the disease.

Initial Treatment

The initial drug program usually consists of the bactericidal combination of **isoniazid-rifampin** or **isoniazid-ethambutol.** If the disease is more extensive, it may require the use of a three-drug program: **isoniazid-rifampin-ethambutol** or **iso-**

TABLE 29-1 Drugs Used in the Treatment of Tuberculosis

DRUGS	DAILY ADULT DOSAGE	COMMON ADVERSE REACTIONS
First-Line Drugs		
Ethambutol (EMB)	15–25 mg/kg PO	Optic neuritis, allergic reactions
Isoniazid (INH)	5–10 mg/kg PO or IM	Hepatitis, peripheral neuropathy, hypersensitivity
Rifampin (RM)	10–20 mg/kg (max. 600 mg/day) PO	Hepatitis, fever, thrombocytopenia
Streptomycin (SM)	15–20 mg/kg (max. 1 g/day) IM	Ototoxicity, nephrotoxicity
Second-Line Drugs		
Capreomycin (CM)	15–30 mg/kg (max. 1 g/day) IM	Ototoxicity, nephrotoxicity
Cycloserine (CS)	10–20 mg/kg (max. 1 g/day) PO	Personality alterations, psychoses, seizures, rash
Ethionamide (ETA)	15–30 mg/kg (max. 1 g/day) PO	GI intolerance, hepatotoxicity, hypersensitivity
Kanamycin (KM)	15–30 mg/kg (max. 1 g/day) IM	Ototoxicity, nephrotoxicity
Para-aminosalicylic acid (PAS)	150 mg/kg (max. 12–15 g/day) PO	GI intolerance, hypersensitivity, hepatotoxicity, sodium overload
Pyrazinamide (PZA)	15–30 mg/kg (max. 2 g/day) PO	Hepatotoxicity, hyperuricemia

niazid-rifampin-streptomycin. Depending on the results of susceptibility tests, additional secondary agents may be utilized.

Short-Course Therapy

Tuberculosis can now be treated for 9 months using the combination of isoniazid-rifampin. Therapy should be continued for at least 6 months following the last negative bacteriologic culture. The short-course treatment program must be modified if the clinical status of the patient is not improved.

Treatment Failures

Treatment failure may occur when a patient with clinical tuberculosis does not demonstrate a negative culture or when, after a standard therapeutic course, a patient relapses. When therapy is restarted, the selection of drugs should be based on the in vitro sensitivity testing. Drugs that are no longer sensitive should be discontinued. In many cases new drugs are added to the initial drug program. The retreatment program should consist of at least three drugs and in some case may include six or more drugs.

Antimycobacterial Drugs

Isoniazid

Mechanism of Action   The exact mechanism of action of isoniazid (INH, Nydrazid) has not been determined. One of the proposed mechanisms is interference with the metabolism of the proteins, carbohydrates, nucleic acids, and lipids of the mycobacteria.

Isoniazid inhibits synthesis of mycolic acids. The mycolic acids are constituents of the bacterial cell wall. Their loss affects the integrity of the cell wall and, hence, cell stability. Isoniazid has no value in treating infections caused by organisms other than mycobacteria, since mycolic acid is found only in this genus of microorganisms. Depending on the concentration, isoniazid can be either bacteriostatic or bactericidal. Isoniazid in a concentration of 0.2 μg/mL or less inhibits most tubercle bacilli. When isoniazid resistance occurs, it is due to the failure of the drug to enter the bacterial cell.

Pharmacokinetics   Isoniazid is rapidly and completely absorbed following intramuscular (IM) or oral administration. The drug is widely distributed throughout the body, including in the cerebrospinal fluid (CSF), maternal milk, and placenta. It is not bound to plasma protein.

In patients with normal renal and hepatic function, the elimination half-life ranges from 1 to 4 h. Liver and renal disease increase the half-life of isoniazid. Isoniazid is metabolized in the liver by acetylation and dehydrazination. Acetylation rate is genetically determined; persons may be rapid or slow acetylators. The rate of metabolism does not appear to alter the efficacy of the drug when it is given on a daily basis. Attempts have been made to correlate the hepatotoxic effects of isoniazid with the rate of acetylation. Rapid acetylation is not a good indicator of potential hepatic problems.

Clinical Use   Isoniazid is among the safest and most active of the antimycobacterial agents. The high levels achieved in all body fluids, including CSF, make it appropriate for most types of clinical tuberculous infections. It is included in all first-line drug combinations, and it is also the drug of choice when single-agent therapy is employed as chemoprophylaxis in persons who convert from a negative to a positive purified protein derivative (PPD) skin reaction but who lack radiographic or other clinical evidence of tuberculosis.

Adverse Effects   The most common adverse effect of isoniazid is peripheral neuritis, which is usually preceded by paresthesia of the feet and hands. Peripheral neuritis is most common in patients who are malnourished, alcoholic, or diabetic. The neurotoxicity may be prevented by giving pyridoxine hydrochloride (vitamin B_6) 10 to 100 mg daily.

Isoniazid may produce elevations in aspartate aminotransferase (SGOT), alanine aminotransferase (SGPT), and serum bilirubin in approximately 10 to 20 percent of patients, usually within the first 6 months of therapy. These values usually return to normal even if therapy is continued. The incidence of isoniazid-induced hepatitis is more common in patients over the age of 35.

Additional adverse effects include convulsions, optic neuritis with atrophy, muscle twitching, fever, rash, a systemic lupus erythematosus–like syndrome, and rheumatic syndrome with arthralgia.

Isoniazid may decrease the elimination of **phenytoin** (Dilantin), and patients should have their phenytoin dosage adjusted. Aluminum-containing antacids may decrease the absorption of isoniazid and should be administered separately.

Dosage   The treatment of clinical tuberculosis includes isoniazid along with other drugs for 18 to 24 months. The usual dosage is 5 to 10 mg/kg/day of isoniazid, which is usually given as a single daily dose of 300 mg. When used in the prevention of tuberculosis, the usual dosage is 300 mg daily for 1 year.

Rifampin

Mechanism of Action   Rifampin (Rimactane; Rifadin) is a semisynthetic antimicrobial agent derived from rifamycin B, one of the rifamycins produced by *Streptomyces mediterranei*. Its mode of action involves inhibition of RNA synthesis through the formation of a stable complex with DNA-dependent RNA polymerase, thereby preventing the action of the enzyme. Inhibition of RNA polymerase prevents all reproduction.

Rifampin may be bacteriostatic or bactericidal, depending on the dosage or the organism. Rifampin is active against *tuberculosis* and other mycobacteria including *M. bovis, M. marinum, M. fortuitum, M. leprae, M. kansasii, M. avium,* and *M. intracellulare.* Rifampin also has activity against some bacteria, including *Staphylococcus aureus, Neisseria, Haemophilus influenzae,* and *Legionella pneumophila.* High concentrations are necessary when rifampin is used in the treatment of *Chlamydia trachomatis,* poxvirus, and adenoviruses.

Pharmacokinetics Rifampin is administered orally and is well absorbed from the gastrointestinal (GI) tract, with peak levels achieved 2 to 4 h after a 600-mg dose. Drug absorption is impaired if rifampin is taken either immediately after meals or concomitantly with para-aminosalicylic acid. Rifampin penetrates tissues well, and therapeutic levels are achieved in the lungs, bronchial secretions, CSF, pleural fluid, liver, bile, urine, and the tuberculosis cavity.

The plasma half-life of rifampin is approximately 3 h. Plasma concentrations are increased in patients with impaired hepatic function. Renal dysfunction has no effect on the plasma concentrations of rifampin. Rifampin is deacetylated in the liver, and most of the drug (60 percent) is excreted in the feces, with a smaller amount appearing in the urine. The urine and feces may take on a harmless orange to red-brown coloration. Unlike many other antimicrobial agents, this drug is active when deacetylated. Rifampin administration can result in the induction of liver enzymes and enhancement of drug metabolism.

Clinical Use Rifampin is a first-line antituberculosis drug used in the treatment of clinical tuberculosis. Rifampin can also be used in the treatment of asymptomatic meningococcus carriers, with dapsone in the treatment of Hansen's disease, and in the treatment of some bacterial infections. The main limitation to the use of rifampin is its cost.

Adverse Effects The most commonly observed side effects of rifampin involve GI disturbances and nervous system complaints such as headache, drowsiness, ataxia, dizziness, and fatigue. The most serious problem is liver damage, expressed as jaundice. Rifampin can induce liver enzymes that are responsible for the metabolism of **digitalis derivatives, methadone, oral hypoglycemic agents, estrogens, warfarin,** and **corticosteroids.** Patients on these drug combinations should be closely monitored.

Dosage The usual dosage for adults is 600 mg/day as a single daily dose in combination with at least one other antituberculosis drug. The usual pediatric dosage for patients over 5 years is 15 mg/kg/day as a single daily dose, to a maximum of 600 mg/day, in combination with at least one other antituberculosis drug.

The treatment for prophylaxis of meningococcal meningitis in children less than 1 year old uses rifampin in a dosage of 5 mg/kg twice daily for 2 days. For children between 1 and 12, the dosage is 10 mg/kg, to a maximum of 600 mg, twice daily for 2 days.

Ethambutol

Mechanism of Action The mechanism of action of ethambutol is not completely understood. It is believed to inhibit the cellular metabolism of the bacteria. Ethambutol is bacteriostatic in action. Ethambutol (Myambutol) is active against only the organisms of the genus *Mycobacterium* and not other bacteria.

Pharmacokinetics Ethambutol is administered orally and is readily absorbed (about 80 percent) from the GI tract. Absorption is not affected by food.

Concentrations in plasma are maximum 2 to 4 h after the drug is taken and are proportional to the dose. A single dose of 15 mg/kg produces a plasma concentration of about 5 μg/mL at 2 to 4 h. The drug has a half-life of 3 to 4 h. About 50 percent of the peak concentration is present in the blood at 8 h, and less than 10 percent at 24 h. One to two times as much ethambutol is present in the erythrocytes as in the plasma.

Ethambutol is partially metabolized in the liver. About 50 percent of the nonmetabolized drug, and 8 to 15 percent of the metabolized drug, is excreted in the urine.

Adverse Effects Ethambutol is usually well-tolerated. The major side effect associated with its use is optic neuritis of the central fibers of the optic nerve, resulting in loss of central vision and an impaired red-green discrimination. The optic neuritis occurs in approximately 3 percent of patients and is almost totally avoidable by using a maintenance dosage of 15 mg/kg/day. Mild GI upset, allergic reactions, fever, headache, malaise, and dizziness have also been reported.

Dosage Treatment of tuberculosis in adults uses 25 mg/kg/day orally for up to 12 weeks, then 15 mg/kg/day for a total of 18 to 24 months, in combination with rifampin or isoniazid.

Ethambutol has replaced para-aminosalicylic acid as a first-line drug for use in combination with isoniazid. It is better tolerated than para-aminosalicylic acid, and it carries less risk of toxicity. Before treatment is initiated, the patient should undergo an ophthalmologic examination and be questioned carefully concerning any impairment of visual acuity or inability to distinguish green from red, because of the potential for drug-induced neuritis.

Streptomycin and Kanamycin

Streptomycin and kanamycin (Kantrex) are both aminoglycoside antibiotics, and their pharmacology is discussed in

Chap. 28. These agents are usually administered IM in a dosage of 15 to 25 mg/kg/day with a maximum of 1 g daily. The drugs are usually given five times a week or less frequently to decrease the risks of adverse effects. Patients should be monitored for renal and eighth cranial nerve damage.

Capreomycin Sulfate

Capreomycin sulfate (Capastat) is a polypeptide antibiotic. Its mechanism of action is still unknown. The drug is not absorbed orally and must be given IM. Following a 1-g IM injection, the peak levels range from 20 to 47 μg/mL. In patients with normal renal function the half-life is between 4 and 6 h. The adverse effects of capreomycin are similar to those of the aminoglycosides, with nephrotoxicity and ototoxicity being the most serious effects. Capreomycin may also produce pain at the site of injection. The usual dosage of capreomycin is 15 mg/kg or 1 g daily.

Para-aminosalicylates

Aminosalicylic acid and its salts (para-aminosalicylic acid, or PAS) are closely related to para-aminobenzoic acid. The mechanism of action of para-aminosalicylic acid is similar to that of the sulfonamides in that it inhibits folic acid synthesis. It is bacteriostatic in action. It is indicated only in the treatment of *M. tuberculosis*. Prior to the introduction of ethambutol and rifampin, it was widely used.

The most common adverse effects of para-aminosalicylic acid are GI problems, including nausea, vomiting, abdominal pain, anorexia, and diarrhea. The problems may require stopping use of the medication. Prior to stopping the drug, aluminum hydroxide gel should be administered in an attempt to alleviate the GI problems. More serious side effects include hypersensitivity reactions (fever, joint pains, skin rashes, leukopenia, etc.). If a hypersensitivity reaction occurs, use of the drug should be stopped. It may be restarted in low doses and then in gradually increased doses.

The usual adult dosage of para-aminosalicylic acid is 10 to 12 g daily given in two or three divided doses. The pediatric dosage is 200 to 300 mg/kg daily in three or four doses.

Ethionamide

The exact mechanism of action of ethionamide (ETA, Trecator-SC) is still unknown. Its action in vivo may be bacteriostatic or bactericidal. Ethionamide is rapidly and completely absorbed. It is distributed throughout the body, including in the CSF and placenta. The half-life of ethionamide is about 3 h.

The most disturbing adverse effects include nausea, vomiting, abdominal pain, anorexia, weight loss, and diarrhea. In an attempt to reduce these adverse effects, the drug has been given in lower doses, given more frequently, given along with antiemetics, and administered rectally (this dos-

age form is not commercially available). Hepatitis has occurred in 5 percent of the patients receiving ethionamide. It is more common in diabetic patients, who also have more difficulty in controlling their disease when on ethionamide. The drug has caused neurotoxicity in the forms of depression, restlessness, and paresthesia. The neurotoxicities may be prevented or alleviated if pyridoxine is given. The neurotoxicity of ethionamide may be additive with the neurotoxicities of cycloserine and isoniazid.

The usual adult dosage is 500 to 1000 mg given in one to three divided doses. The maximum daily dosage should be 1 g.

Pyrazinamide

Pyrazinamide has bacteriostatic or bactericidal action. Its exact mechanism of action is unknown. Pyrazinamide is rapidly and completely absorbed and then widely distributed throughout the body, including in the CSF. The plasma half-life is 9 to 10 h in patients with renal and hepatic function. The half-life may be increased in patients with renal or hepatic disorders.

The most frequent adverse effect of pyrazinamide is hepatotoxicity, which appears to be dose-related. When a dosage of 3 g/day is given, the incidence of hepatotoxicity is 15 percent. Other adverse effects include anorexia, nausea, fever, malaise, hepatomegaly, and splenomegaly. Pyrazinamide frequently causes hyperuricemia, which is usually asymptomatic. Acute gout may develop in some patients. If the gout is severe or is accompanied by acute gouty arthritis, pyrazinamide should be discontinued.

The usual adult dosage is 20 to 35 mg/kg/day given orally in three to four divided doses. The maximum daily dosage should not exceed 3 g.

Cycloserine

Cycloserine (Seromycin) may be bacteriostatic or bactericidal in its action. It is a competitive inhibitor of D-alanyl-D-alanine synthetase and alanine racemase; both enzymes are required for bacterial cell wall synthesis. Cycloserine inhibits the growth of *Mycobacterium* and other bacteria (*Enterobacteriaceae, Escherichia coli, S. aureus*).

Cycloserine can be administered orally and is rapidly absorbed from the stomach and small intestines. It is widely distributed throughout the body. Its plasma half-life is 10 h. In patients with normal renal function 60 to 80 percent of the dose is excreted unchanged in the urine.

The frequent adverse effects are on the nervous system, including headaches, tremors, seizures, agitation, confusion, and hallucinations. Psychosis, hyperirritability, and aggression have all been associated with the use of cycloserine. Patients who present with frequent use of alcohol, depression, epilepsy, renal dysfunction, or cycloserine serum levels above 30 μg/mL are at a greater risk for the nervous system adverse effects.

The dosage of cycloserine is started at 250 mg every 12 h. Dosage adjustments are then made to keep the serum concentration below 30 µg/mL.

Investigational Drugs

The introduction of new antituberculosis medication is limited because of small potential for profit in the United States. Additional drugs have been used outside the United States and may be indicated in certain patients. The drugs include clofazimine, thiacetazone, and ansamycin. There has also been research interest in using some of the second- and third-generation cephalosporins in the treatment of certain mycobacteria.

NURSING PROCESS RELATED TO TUBERCULOSIS

The nursing process in the pharmacologic treatment of tuberculosis is outlined in Table 29-2.

CASE STUDY

G.G., a 76-year-old male American Indian from a rural area, reported to the medical center for evaluation of a chronic cough and a 20-lb weight loss. Both symptoms had gradually progressed over a 4- to 5-month period.

When questioned carefully, he also reported night sweats, anorexia, and fatigue. The remainder of the review of systems was totally negative, as was his family history. The patient had had a partial gastrectomy 30 years earlier, and he had smoked one to two packs of cigarettes per day for almost 50 years.

The patient lived in a six-room apartment with his wife, aged 72, who had hypertension and diabetes mellitus. His son, aged 38, his son's wife, aged 36, and their three daughters, aged 14, 8, and 2, also shared the same apartment. The son and his family were all reported to be healthy.

Assessment

On physical examination the patient appeared chronically ill. His temperature was 37.8°C orally, pulse 92, and respirations 22. The middle lobe of his right lung had rales and was also dull to percussion, as was the apex of the right lung. The heart sounds were normal. The liver was slightly enlarged but not tender. The stool was negative for occult blood. The skin and extremities were unremarkable.

The chest x-ray showed an infiltrate in the right middle lobe, with apical scarring in the right apex and a Ghon complex at the right hilus. The left lung had scattered fibronodular densities. The white blood count was 4300. Ziehl-Neelsen stains of sputum showed numerous acid-fast bacilli.

Management

The patient was admitted to the hospital for treatment of his active tuberculosis. He was begun on isoniazid 300 mg/day orally, ethambutol 24 mg/kg/day orally, pyridoxine 50 mg daily, and streptomycin 500 mg/day intramuscularly for 8 weeks, then 500 mg intramuscularly twice weekly for 2 months.

After 3 weeks of therapy clinical improvement was manifested by a normal temperature, a decrease in cough, and a 4-lb weight gain. He attended group classes on tuberculosis.

After 4 weeks sputum cultures were reported growing *M. tuberculosis*. The patient was then discharged to a chronic disease hospital. Three months after the initial diagnosis the patient was discharged to his home to continue the isoniazid, pyridoxine, and ethambutol until a 24-month course of therapy had been completed.

The public health nurse performed and evaluated intermediate-strength PPD testing on all family members and all were reactive. Arrangements were made to have chest x-rays done, all of which were negative. After examinations were done, no family members were found to have signs of active tuberculosis.

Two of the granddaughters, aged 2 and 8, were begun on prophylactic isoniazid 300 mg/day orally and pyridoxine 50 mg/day orally. Because of her debilitated condition the patient's wife was also placed on this regimen, which was continued for 1 year. Both the grandchildren received treatment for 3 years.

Evaluation

The public health nurse continued to follow the family for 3 years. Clinical evaluation and yearly chest x-rays revealed no active disease, and the patient had no symptoms.

TABLE 29-2 Nursing Process Related to Tuberculosis

ASSESSMENT	MANAGEMENT	EVALUATION
	General Aspects	
Assess patient for unexplained malaise, loss of appetite, productive cough, elevated afternoon temperature, night sweats, hemoptysis. Assess level of understanding of disease process. Assess socioeconomic factors that may affect therapeutic plan. Identify personal contacts for follow-up care.	Explain drug therapy, drugs usually used in combination to delay appearance of resistant organisms. Stress need for proper rest and nutrition. Explain infectious nature of disease. Administer drugs with consideration of the patient's comfort. It is imperative that patients take prescribed medications regularly and without interruption.	Effectiveness of drug therapy—signs and symptoms of improvement include decreased fever and malaise, increase in appetite and weight gain, decreased cough and production of sputum, negative sputum culture, and regression in size of lesion on x-ray. Emphasize necessity of periodic medical evaluation.
	Isoniazid	
Use with caution in patients with history of epilepsy, seizures, or convulsions.	Give on empty stomach, since food decreases absorption.	Adverse effects—Watch for anorexia; weight loss; symptoms of pyridoxine deficiency, which can be controlled by daily administration of vitamins; headache; vertigo; peripheral neuritis; convulsions in patients with previous history of seizures.
	Rifampin	
Assess for impaired liver function.	Urine, saliva, sputum, sweat, tears, and feces may become red-orange in color. Monitor liver function tests. Do not give immediately after meals or with para-aminosalicylic acid, which decreases quinidine clearance.	Adverse effects—Watch for liver dysfunction and jaundice, GI disturbances, drowsiness, fatigue, ataxia, pain in extremities, and menstrual disturbances. When drug is discontinued, quinidine dosages may need to be reduced to avoid quinidine toxicity.
	Streptomycin	
Assess for history of impaired kidney function, present levels of hearing.	Watch for signs of ototoxicity and nephrotoxicity. Give 1 h after oral medications.	Adverse effects—Watch for tinnitus, damage to eighth cranial nerve, elevated blood urea nitrogen, and kidney dysfunction.
	Para-aminosalicylic Acid	
Assess for history of sensitivity to salicylates.	Give with food or after meals. Antacids may be needed to counteract gastric discomfort. Check expiration date. Drug must be stored away from heat and humidity in tightly sealed container. Avoid concurrent use with other salicylates.	Adverse effects—Watch for anorexia, gaseous distention, nausea, vomiting, diarrhea, hepatitis, dermatitis, drug fever, goitrogenic effects due to inhibition of iodine accumulation in the thyroid gland. Allergic reactions appear to be most common between the 2d and 7th week of treatment. Drug may interfere with results of Benedict's test for glycosuria.
	Ethambutol	
Assess visual acuity and for color blindness.	Give with food to prevent nausea and vomiting. Monitor patient's eyesight and color perception.	Adverse effects—Watch for visual and muscular incoordination, optic neuritis and loss of central vision, loss of red-green color sense.
	Ethionamide	
Give with caution to patients with diabetes mellitus.	Give with food to minimize gastric irritation. Monitor blood sugar and urine glucose.	Adverse effects—Watch for severe GI symptoms, postural hypotension, depression, drowsiness, peripheral neuropathy, dermatoses, and hepatitis.

TABLE 29-2 Nursing Process Related to Tuberculosis (*Cont.*)

ASSESSMENT	MANAGEMENT	EVALUATION
	Pyrazinamide	
Assess for history of liver damage or gout.	Monitor blood uric acid levels. Give after meals.	Adverse effects—Watch for hepatotoxicity, hyperuricemia. Drug may increase uric acid enough to precipitate attack of gout.
	Cycloserine	
Use with caution in patients with history of epilepsy or renal insufficiency.	CNS effects may be minimized by giving pyridoxine anticonvulsants, tranquilizers, and sedatives.	Administration of 1 g or more daily causes drowsiness, allergic reactions, hyperreflexia, and convulsions.

Leprosy (Hansen's Disease)

Leprosy affects between 10 and 20 million individuals throughout the world. Leprosy is a chronic granulomatous infection which causes problems with the skin, nasal mucosa, and peripheral nerves. The two types of leprosy are lepromatous and tuberculoid. Hansen's disease is caused by *Mycobacterium leprae*.

The treatment of leprosy in the United States is usually under the care of a specialist. The drug choice in the therapy of leprosy is **dapsone** (Avlosulfon). Dapsone can also be used in the treatment of dermatitis herpetiformis and of malaria. The usual dosage in the treatment of leprosy is 1 to 1.5 mg/kg daily in children and 50 to 100 mg daily in adults. Additional drugs used in the treatment of leprosy include rifampin and clofazimine. For additional information the National Hansen's Disease Center in Carvill, Louisiana, can be contacted.

FUNGAL INFECTIONS

LEARNING OBJECTIVES

Upon mastery of the contents of this section, the reader should be able to:

1. List three drugs that can be used in the treatment of systemic mycoses.
2. Give a drug that can be used topically and orally in the treatment of dermatophytes.
3. List four adverse effects of amphotericin B.
4. Give two drugs that can be used in the treatment of oral candidiasis.
5. Explain the mechanism of action of amphotericin B, griseofulvin, and ketoconazole.

Fungal infections can be classified into three groups:

1. Systemic infections such as cryptococcosis, blastomycosis, histoplasmosis, coccidioidomycosis, candidiasis, aspergillosis, sporotrichosis, and others

2. Local infections caused by *Candida albicans*
3. Infections due to dermatophytes, which affect the hair, skin, and nails

The diagnosis of fungal infections is dependent on culturing the organism from an appropriate patient specimen.

SYSTEMIC MYCOSES

Systemic mycoses are infections that include blastomycosis, coccidioidomycosis, cryptococcosis, histoplasmosis, paracoccidioidomycosis, aspergillosis, and others. These infections are more common in patients who are immunocompromised congenitally (hypogammaglobulinemia), by disease (Hodgkin's, diabetes mellitus, lymphoma), or by drugs (corticosteroids, azathioprine, or antineoplastics).

There are major endemic areas for the occurrence of mycoses. Coccidioidomycosis is most common in Arizona, the southern two-thirds of California, the western half of Texas, and northern New Mexico. The occurrence of histoplasmosis and blastomycosis are most common in the central and southeastern states. The treatments of these infections are presented in Table 29-3.

CANDIDIASIS (MONILIASIS)

The yeastlike fungus *Candida albicans* prefers a humid, moist environment, usually found in intertriginous, interdigital, or mucous membrane sites. Infections are aggravated by heat, perspiration, occlusive clothing, and repeated exposure to water, which promotes tissue maceration. Predisposing factors include diabetes mellitus, hypothyroidism, percutaneous anemia, and defects in cell-mediated immunity. Obesity, pregnancy, old age, and infancy also predispose to *Candida* infections. Glucocorticosteroids and broad-spectrum antibiotics will promote *Candida* colonization. The primary lesion of *Candida* infections is a superficial pustule with erythema. This may progress to weeping, erythematous, and denuded dermatitis.

Clotrimazole 1% or **miconazole** 2% are effective against *Candida* organisms. They should be applied two or three times daily. Lotions are effective on dry lesions but may sting when applied to weeping, denuded lesions. Application should continue for 1 week after resolution of the lesions. In severely inflamed cases, wet soaks or compresses will alleviate discomfort and dry the skin. Patients with mixed *Candida* and bacterial infections should receive systemic antibiotics, e.g., **erythromycin**. The single most important aspect of therapy is to keep the skin dry. Environmental factors such as chronic exposure of hands to water, tight-

fitting clothing, and warm or humid conditions should be avoided.

In most instances, oral anticandidiasis agents are not needed. Oral **nystatin** may reduce *Candida* colonization of the GI tract and may reduce the recurrence of *Candida* vaginitis. In severe refractory cases, and in chronic mucocutaneous candidiasis, the use of **ketoconazole** (200 mg/day) is beneficial and may be preferable to systemic **amphotericin B** therapy.

TABLE 29-3   Chemotherapy of the Systemic Mycoses

INFECTION	PRIMARY THERAPY	SECONDARY THERAPY
Actinomycosis*	Penicillin	Tetracycline, rifampin
Aspergillosis		
Allergic bronchopulmonary	Corticosteroids	
Aspergilloma, pulmonary	Observation	Surgery, amphotericin B transtracheally or percutaneously
Systemic	Amphotericin B IV	Ketoconazole or flucytosine†
Blastomycosis		
Acute pulmonary (especially in localized outbreaks)	Observation	Amphotericin B IV
Invasive, progressive, or systemic	Amphotericin B IV	Hydroxystilbamidine isothionate or ketoconazole†
Candidiasis		
Chronic mucocutaneous	Ketoconazole	Amphotericin B IV
Septicemia	Amphotericin B IV	Flucytosine†
Meningitis	Flucytosine†	Amphotericin B IV
Endocarditis	Amphotericin B IV	Surgery
Bladder infection	Amphotericin B IV with or without intravesicular use	Flucytosine† or ketoconazole
Chromomycosis	Flucytosine	Amphotericin B intralesionally
Coccidioidomycosis		
Progressive	Amphotericin B IV	Ketoconazole
Meningitis	Amphotericin B intrathecally	Amphotericin B IV or miconazole or ketoconazole or transfer factor
Cryptococcosis		
Pulmonary	Observation	Flucytosine,† amphotericin B IV
Meningitis	Amphotericin B IV combined with flucytosine	Amphotericin B IV or intrathecally, or flucytosine separately, or miconazole
Other	Flucytosine†	Combined therapy
Histoplasmosis		
Progressive disseminated and chronic cavitary	Ketoconazole	Amphotericin B IV
Mycetoma	Amphotericin B† or flucytosine† or ketoconazole†	Surgery
Nocardiosis*	Sulfonamide	Co-trimoxazole or amikacin
Paracoccidioidomycosis	Ketoconazole	Amphotericin B IV or sulfonamide
Phycomycosis	Amphotericin B†	Surgery and correction of diabetic ketoacidosis

*Not a mycosis, but historically dealt with by mycologists.
†Based on in vitro sensitivity.
   Source: J. P. Utz: *The Systemic Mycosis in Current Therapy of Infectious Diseases, 1983–1984,* H.E. Koss and R. Platt (eds.), Philadelphia: B.C. Decker; St. Louis: C.V. Mosby, 1983.

FUNGAL INFECTIONS OF THE SKIN

Dermatophytosis (ringworm) is caused by the *Microsporum, Epidermophyton,* and *Trichophyton* genera of fungi, which are superficial pathogens that subsist on keratin of the skin, hair, and nails. Therefore, infections with these organisms are confined to the keratinized layers of the skin and do not invade deeper tissue except under extraordinary conditions.

Tinea pedis, dermatophytosis of the feet, can be divided into the common "athlete's foot," on the instep and toe webs, and the less common "moccasin foot," which involves the entire sole and sides of the feet. *Athlete's foot* is effectively treated with most topical antifungal therapy. Clotrimazole 1% or miconazole 2%, as a cream or lotion, applied twice daily for 4 weeks is usually sufficient. *Moccasin foot* is usually chronic and subject to relapse. Topical preparations (clotrimazole or miconazole) applied twice daily will usually provide temporary improvement. In such cases topical preparations are combined with orally administered **griseofulvin** (microsize) 250 mg two to four times daily in adults, and treatment lasts from 2 to 6 months.

Tinea cruris ("jock itch") is characterized by a pruritic erythematous scaling eruption in the inguinal crease. The scrotum may be involved. Topical application of clotrimazole 1% or miconazole 2% twice daily for 4 weeks is adequate for acute infections. This may be combined with systemic griseofulvin or ketoconazole in refractory cases.

Tinea unguium, a yellow discoloration of the distal and lateral margins of the nails with subungual keratotic debris, is characteristic of onychomycosis in the soft keratin of the nail bed. Topical preparations of clotrimazole 1% or miconazole 2% and combination therapy with griseofulvin may be indicated.

Tinea corporis, dermatophytosis of the body surfaces, is more prevalent in hot, humid climates. **Griseofulvin** (microsize) 250 mg two to four times daily for 1 to 3 months, in combination with topical miconazole twice daily for a minimum of 4 weeks, should be used.

Tinea capitis, patchy hair loss with or without inflammatory changes, may be produced by *Microsporum* and *Trichophyton* dermatophytes. Treatment for adults is **griseofulvin** (microsize) 250 mg two to four times daily for 4 weeks. Children under 50 lb may be given 125 mg twice daily; children 50 to 100 lb, three times daily. Topical preparations of **miconazole** may be applied twice daily.

Tinea versicolor is a common superficial fungal infection seen in all age groups, but it is typically encountered in young adults. The causative agent, *Pityrosporum orbiculare,* is a component of normal skin flora. It is transformed into a filamentous pathogen that is restricted to the outermost layers of the lipid-rich stratum corneum. During the winter months the lesions are asymptomatic. During sun exposure in the summer, the affected areas filter out the tanning spectrum of sunlight and leave relatively hypopigmented patches amid uninvolved normally tanned skin. This color reversal with seasons provides the description "versi-color," and the uneven tanning of the skin is the chief complaint. Treatment is usually with **selenium sulfide** lotion 2.5% (Selsun), applied to all affected areas, left on overnight, and washed off in the morning. Topical preparations may be helpful in treating this condition; miconazole 2% can be applied twice daily for 10 days. Sodium thiosulfate (Tinver Lotion), **tolnaftate,** and **haloprogin** may all be used for topical treatment of tinea versicolor. Systemic therapy is usually not effective.

CLINICAL PHARMACOLOGY AND THERAPEUTICS OF FUNGAL INFECTIONS

Antifungal Drugs

Amphotericin B

Mechanism of Action Amphotericin B (Fungizone) works by altering cell permeability by binding to the sterol moiety (ergosterol) of the fungus or yeast. This results in loss of intracellular components from the cell, producing irreversible damage. Amphotericin B may be fungicidal or fungistatic in action.

Pharmacokinetics Amphotericin B is poorly absorbed from the GI tract and must be given parenterally. Once absorbed, amphotericin B is 90 to 95 percent protein-bound. It is poorly distributed to the CSF and must be given intrathecally to achieve levels in the CSF. Amphotericin B is administered chronically, drug concentrations can be detected in the urine for 2 weeks after the drug is stopped. The slow elimination may be due to the slow release of the drug from its peripheral stores. Amphotericin B is not hemodialyzable.

Clinical Use Amphotericin B should be used only in the treatment of severe fungal infections caused by susceptible fungi. All patients on amphotericin B should be hospitalized. Prior to the use of amphotericin B many of these fungal infections were fatal.

Adverse Effects The incidence of adverse effects with amphotericin B is extremely high. Patients receiving intravenous (IV) amphotericin B will usually experience fever, chills, headaches, malaise, muscle and joint pain, weight loss, and vomiting. The adverse effects are considered dose-related and may be reduced by giving a lower dose and/or by dosing on alternate days. The reactions may be treated with meperidine, antipyretics, antihistamines, and antiemetics.

Nephrotoxicity occurs in the majority of patients receiving IV amphotericin B. This may be dose-related, and giving a smaller dose may decrease the renal problems. The renal problems in patients will usually improve after use of the drug is stopped. Patients should have their renal function monitored prior to the start of amphotericin B and during its use.

Other adverse effects include hypokalemia; cardiac enlargement; reversible normocytic, normochromic anemia; a shocklike fall in blood pressure; and others. Amphotericin B may cause pain at the injection site.

Dosage Amphotericin B is given by a slow intravenous infusion. Amphotericin B is commercially available as 50 mg of powder, which must be reconstituted prior to use. Amphotericin B should be mixed with 10 mL of sterile water that is preservative-free. This gives a concentration of 5 mg/mL, which is further diluted by adding 500 mL of D_5W to give a concentration of 0.1 mg/mL. This concentration of amphotericin B can be administered. It is usually recommended that while the drug is being infused, it should be protected from light.

The dosage of amphotericin B is based on the ability of the patient to tolerate the drug. The initial dosage is 0.25 mg/kg infused over a 6-h period. The dosage can then be increased over 7 days to 0.5 mg/kg. The maximum daily dosage is 1.5 mg/kg. Therapy with amphotericin B is usually over several months and is based on the severity and the type of infection.

Flucytosine

Mechanism of Action After entering the fungal cell, flucytosine (Ancoban) is deaminated to fluorouracil. The fluorouracil acts as an antimetabolite and interferes with RNA and protein synthesis. The principal antifungal activity of flucytosine is against *Cryptococcus* and *Candida*.

Pharmacokinetics Flucytosine is rapidly and completely absorbed when the drug is given orally. Patients with normal renal and hepatic function will achieve a peak serum concentration of 30 to 45 μg/mL following a 2-g oral dose. It has been recommended that the therapeutic range be considered to be between 25 and 100 μg/mL.

The elimination half-life of flucytosine is between 2.5 and 6 h in patients with normal renal function. In patients with renal disorders the half-life increases and is proportional to the creatinine clearance. The majority of flucytosine is excreted unchanged in the urine.

Clinical Use Flucytosine is indicated for serious infections caused by *Candida* and *Cryptococcus* organisms. In most cases amphotericin B is considered the drug of choice in these infections. In the treatment of certain infections the use of the combination of **amphotericin B** and flucytosine is indicated (cryptococcal meningitis).

Adverse Effects Flucytosine affects the rapidly growing cells of the bone marrow (causing hypoplasia) and GI tract (causing nausea, vomiting, anorexia, etc.). These adverse effects occur more frequently when the concentration of flucytosine is over 100 μg/mL. Less-frequent adverse effects include confusion, hallucinations, vertigo, rashes, etc.

Dosage The adult daily dosage is usually 50 to 150 mg/kg/day in divided doses every 6 h. In severe infections, and to prevent the emergence of resistant organisms, higher doses are recommended. The dosage for children weighing less than 50 kg is 1.5 to 4.5 g/m^2.

Griseofulvin Microsize or Ultramicrosize

Mechanism of Action Griseofulvin (Fulvicin-U/F, Grifulvin V) has fungistatic activity inhibiting cell division. It inhibits mitosis in a manner similar to that of colchicine, but its mechanism is probably different. Griseofulvin is deposited in the hair, nails, and skin and makes the environment unfavorable to the growth of the fungus. Griseofulvin inhibits the growth of dermatophytes, including *Epidermophyton*, *Microsporum*, and *Trichophyton*, in concentrations of 0.5 to 3 μg/mL. It has no effect on bacteria, the fungi producing deep mycoses in humans, or certain fungi producing superficial lesions. Resistance can emerge among susceptible dermatophytes.

Pharmacokinetics Absorption of griseofulvin depends greatly on the physical state of the drug and is aided by high-fat foods. Preparations containing microsize particles of the drug are absorbed twice as rapidly as those with larger particles. Adults given microsize griseofulvin, 1 g daily, develop blood levels of 0.5 to 1.5 μg/mL. Ultramicrosize griseofulvin is absorbed twice as fast as microsize and gives twice the blood levels. The absorbed drug has an affinity for diseased skin and is deposited there, bound to keratin.

Griseofulvin is distributed mainly to the skin, hair, nails, liver, and skeletal muscles. The elimination half-life of griseofulvin is approximately 9 to 24 h.

Clinical Use Griseofulvin is indicated in the treatment of mycoses of the hair, nails, and skin. It is used when topical therapy has proven ineffective. Griseofulvin is not effective against deep mycotic infections or bacterial infections. It can be used to treat tinea corporis, tinea pedis, tinea cruris, tinea barbae, tinea capitis, and tinea unguium.

Adverse Effects The overall incidence of adverse effects due to griseofulvin is low. Adverse effects include headaches, epigastric distress, nausea, vomiting, diarrhea, hepatotoxicity, photosensitivity, and mental confusion.

Griseofulvin may increase the metabolism of **warfarin** (Coumadin) and may require an increase in warfarin doses. **Phenobarbital** may reduce the absorption of griseofulvin. When **alcohol** and griseofulvin are taken together, the combination may cause tachycardia and flushing (disulfiram-like reaction).

Dosage The particle size of griseofulvin has been reformulated since it was first introduced. Griseofulvin ultramicrosize 250 mg is equivalent to 500 mg of the microsize, which is equivalent to 1000 mg of the original formulation.

The usual adult dosage is 250 to 500 mg of the ultramicrosize preparation, or 500 to 1000 mg of the microsize preparation, given once a day. The microsize preparation can be given in a dosage of 300 mg/m^2 to children. Treatment is usually continued for 3 to 6 weeks if only hair or skin is involved.

Imidazole Antifungal Agents

The imidazole agents are all fungistatic in action. Their mechanism of action is altering cell membranes and interfering with intracellular enzymes.

Clotrimazole Clotrimazole (Mycelex-G, Gyne-Lotrimim) can be used to treat oral candidiasis and vaginal candidiasis (discussed in Chap. 46). It is not used systemically. The dose in the treatment of oral candidiasis is one troche five times a day. Clotrimazole is usually well tolerated but may cause topical irritation.

Miconazole Miconazole (Monistat IV) is active against most fungi and gram-positive bacteria. Its main use is in the treatment of severe systemic fungal infections and not bacterial infections. Candidiasis, cryptococcosis, coccidioidomycosis, and others appear to be inhibited by a concentration of 1 to 2 µg/mL.

Miconazole is well distributed to most body tissues. The level in the CSF is unpredictable, and the drug should be given intrathecally in the treatment of meningitis. Miconazole is primarily metabolized through the liver and then excreted in the urine.

Systemic miconazole produces severe adverse effects, including thrombophlebitis, vomiting, anemia, thrombocytosis, hyponatremia, hyperlipidemia, and occasionally, leukopenia and hypersensitivity. It also interacts with warfarin and increases the anticoagulant effect of warfarin.

Miconazole can be administered intravenously (with slow infusion), intrathecally, and by bladder irrigation. The usual dosage by IV infusion in the treatment of candidiasis is 600 to 1800 mg daily for 1 to 20 weeks, cryptococcosis 1.2 to 2.4 g daily for 3 to 12 weeks, and coccidioidomycosis 1.8 to 3.6 g daily for 3 to 20 weeks. The intrathecal dosage is usually given undiluted in a dose of 20 mg given every 1 to 2 days but this may vary. When miconazole is used in bladder irrigation, 200 mg is diluted and instilled two to four times a day. Miconazole vaginal cream is also used in the treatment of vaginal candidiasis.

Ketoconazole Ketoconazole (Nizoral) is the first antifungal drug effective in systemic mycoses that can be given by mouth. A single daily dose of 200 to 400 mg is taken with food. The drug is well absorbed and widely distributed, but concentrations in the central nervous system are low. Daily dosage suppresses *Candida* infections of the mouth or vagina in 1 to 2 weeks, and dermatophytosis in 3 to 8 weeks. Mucocutaneous candidiasis in immunodeficient children responds in 4 to 10 months.

Ketoconazole is reported to suppress the clinical manifestations of systemic paracoccidioidomycosis, blastomycosis, or histoplasmosis in 2 to 6 months. Fungal meningitis usually fails to respond. With oral doses of 200 mg, peak levels of ketoconazole may be 2 to 3 µg/mL, persisting for 6 h or more. The major toxic effects thus far are referable to the GI tract, but some hepatic toxicity has been observed with high doses.

Nystatin Nystatin (Mycostatin) has no effect on bacteria or protozoa, but in vitro it inhibits many fungi, including *Candida*, dermatophytes, and organisms producing deep mycoses in humans. In vivo, its action is limited to surfaces where the nonabsorbed drug can be in direct contact with the yeast or mold.

The mode of action is similar to that of amphotericin B. It involves binding of nystatin to fungal membrane sterols, principally ergosterol. There it disturbs membrane permeability and transport features. This results in loss of cations and macromolecules from the cell. Resistance is due to a decrease in membrane sterols or a change in their structure and binding properties.

Nystatin is not significantly absorbed from skin, mucous membranes, or the GI tract. Virtually all nystatin taken orally is excreted in the feces. There are no significant blood or tissue levels after oral intake.

Nystatin can be applied topically to the skin or mucous membranes (buccal, vaginal) as a cream, ointment, suppository, suspension, or powder for the suppression of local *Candida* infections. Nystatin may be given orally for the suppression of *Candida albicans* (Monilia) in the lumen of the bowel. Topical nystatin preparations often contain antibacterial drugs [nystatin, neomycin, gramicidin, triamcinolone (Mycolog); see Chap. 38].

NURSING PROCESS RELATED TO FUNGAL INFECTIONS

Assessment

Infection usually occurs by inhalation, traumatic implantation, or the pathologic takeover of a normal inhabitant when resistance of the host is lowered. Superficial infections of the skin and its appendages (hair and nails) rarely cause temporary disability and usually respond to treatment. However, if internal organs are involved, fungal disease may be so serious as to constitute a threat to life.

Assessment of the patient's age and social environmental history may help determine which type of fungal infection is present. Histoplasmosis is often transmitted by inhalation of spore-bearing dust. The partially decayed droppings of pigeons, chickens, and birds offer an excellent medium for the growth of this fungus. Actinomycosis is a disease of young adult males and may be acquired from chewing on a pencil or straw on which the fungi or spores have settled. Tinea capitis is a common problem of young children. Tinea circinata is often secondary to an infection of the scalp, feet, or nails and may be due to an infected pet. Tinea cruris and tinea pedis are common problems of athletes.

The systemic mycoses have become more frequent in occurrence, with the increased availability and use of potent antibiotics, antimetabolite therapy, and cancer chemotherapy. Patients who are on these medications or who are debilitated or severely ill have reduced host defenses, and they become prey to invasion by fungi which healthy people could normally withstand.

The diagnosis of fungal infection is made by direct microscopic examination of the infected skin and by growth of the offending organism in culture.

Management

Nursing management will relate directly to the type and location of the fungal infection. During the acute vesicular stage of tinea pedis wet dressings and soaks are used to remove the crusts, scales, and debris and to reduce the inflammation. Fungistatic creams or lotions are applied to the involved areas. If superimposed infection is present, a systemic antibiotic may be used. Treatment of tinea cruris consists of keeping the area dry and frequently applying **amphotericin B.** Tinea versicolor is treated by application of a fungicidal cream or **selenium sulfide** shampoo to the affected area. Tinea capitis is usually treated with **griseofulvin,** frequent shampooing of the hair with 2% selenium sulfide, and a topical antifungal preparation applied to reduce dissemination of the organism. Shampoo is necessary, since griseofulvin kills the vegetative hypha but not the reproductive spores. Griseofulvin and a topical antifungal medication are also used to treat tinea corporis.

Actinomycotic lesions respond to **penicillin,** with large daily doses given over 4 to 6 weeks. Surgical drainage and excision of localized lesions may be necessary. Histoplasmosis is treated with **amphotericin B** and may need surgical intervention in chronic cavitary disease.

Superficial fungal infections usually respond quite well to treatment. Prevention of reinfection, however, is an important aspect of patient teaching.

Since tinea capitis is spread by direct contact with an infected person or articles such as caps or combs of the infected person, children must be taught not to use each other's clothes. Each member of the family should have his or her own brush and comb. The nurse, being aware of the infectious nature of tinea, may assist the patient and family in setting up a hygienic regimen for home use. All infected household members and pets must be treated, since familial infections are relatively common.

Patients with tinea pedis should be instructed to keep their feet as dry as possible, since moisture encourages the growth of fungi. Areas between the toes must be dried thoroughly; small pieces of cotton can be placed between the toes at night to absorb moisture. The patient may need to discard shoes, socks, or slippers that may be fungally infected and/or contain spores, since the risk of reinfection is high. The patient should be advised not to go barefoot if using a shared locker or shower room, such as in school or sports facilities. Powdering between the toes and wearing clean, dry socks is also helpful in keeping the feet healthy. Perforated, light shoes should be worn. At home, towels should not be shared, and a disinfectant should be used to clean the tub and shower after each use.

Nail infections are particularly hard to treat, and response is often poor. Toenails grow so slowly that the medication may have to be used for a year or more with only a 20 percent rate of cure.

Fungal infections may be difficult to correct because of the tendency of fungi to form spores.

Evaluation

Patients need support and encouragement during prolonged courses of treatment. The nurse must work with the patient and family and continue to discuss with them the importance of good personal hygiene to prevent reinfection or further spread of the infection.

PARASITIC INFECTIONS

LEARNING OBJECTIVES

Upon mastery of this section, the reader should be able to:

   1.   List two parasitic infections caused by protozoa and two caused by helminths.

   2.   Correlate pharmacologic intervention with the life cycle of *Plasmodium* in humans and in mosquitoes.

   3.   Give the drug and its dosage used for (a) suppressive therapy of malaria due to *Plasmodium malariae,* (b) radical cure of infection due to *Plasmodium ovale,* and (c) treatment of the clinical attack of *Plasmodium vivax.*

   4.   Discuss the therapy of *Plasmodium falciparum* which is resistant to chloroquine.

   5.   Give two methods that may help to control malaria worldwide.

   6.   Give the causative organism for amebiasis.

7. List two drugs that can be used in the treatment of extraintestinal amebiasis.

8. List three indications for the use of metronidazole, and give two drugs that it can interact with.

9. Give a drug that can be used in the treatment of infection with *Leishmania donovani* (kala azar).

10. List two drugs that can be used in the treatment of giardiasis.

11. Describe two methods for the prevention of giardiasis.

12. Give a drug that can be used in the treatment of each of the following helminthic infestations: roundworm, whipworm, hookworm, and threadworm.

13. Give a source for drugs and information for the treatment of parasitic diseases.

Parasitic infections still remain a leading cause of sickness and death throughout the world. Malaria, amebiasis, trypanosomiasis, leishmaniasis, and giardiasis are parasitic diseases caused by protozoa. Schistosomiasis and filariasis are examples of parasitic infections caused by helminths (worms). The Centers for Disease Control (CDC) are an important source of information on parasitic diseases and of drugs not commercially available (see Table 29-4).

MALARIA

It is estimated that malaria infects between 125 and 200 million individuals and that approximately 1 billion people live in endemic areas. The greatest advances in reducing the disease have been made in Europe and North America. Probably the most important agents that have been used in the control of malaria are the insecticides which control the mosquito vector. Recently, there have been increased problems with the control of malaria because of the development of chloroquine-resistant strains of *falciparum,* increasing resistance of the mosquito to insecticides, the reduction of worldwide malaria control programs, and the increase in international travel.

Malaria is characterized by paroxysms of severe chills, fever, and profuse sweating. In some patients the development of symptoms can be coordinated with the life cycle of the *Plasmodium.* Human malaria can be caused by one of four *Plasmodium* species: *P. vivax, P. ovale, P. falciparum,* and *P. malariae.*

Life Cycle of the Plasmodium

The therapy of malaria is based on the life cycle of the plasmodia (see Fig. 29-1). The vector for malaria is the mosquito *Anopheles,* which becomes a carrier of the disease by ingesting the blood of a host which contains both sexual forms of the parasite. In the mosquito the sporozoites form and migrate to the salivary glands of the mosquito. The sporozoites are transmitted to the bloodstream of a suitable host

TABLE 29-4   Drugs Available from CDC for Treatment of Parasitic Diseases*

DRUG	INDICATION AND ADULT DOSAGE
Bithionol (Bitin)	Alternative in fluke infections: 30–50 mg/kg qod for 10–15 days
Dehydroemetine	Amebiasis: 1–1.5 mg/kg IM up to 5 days
Diloxanide furoate (Furamide)	Amebiasis: 500 mg tid for 10 days
Melarsoprol (Arsobal)	Trypanosomiasis with CNS involvement: 2–3.6 mg/kg/day for 3 days; 7 days later, 3.6 mg/kg/day for 3 days; 21 days later, 2d dosage repeated
Nifurtimox (Lampit)	Trypanosomiasis (Chagas' disease): 5 mg/kg/day in four divided oral doses; every 14 days, dosage increased 2 mg/kg until it reaches 15–17 mg/kg/day
Niridazole (Ambilhar)	Dracunculiasis: 25 mg/kg/day for 10 days
Pentamidine isoethionate	Leishmaniasis: 2–4 mg/kg/day IM for 14 days Pneumocystosis: 4 mg/kg/day for 14 days Trypanosomiasis: 4 mg/kg/day for 10 days
Quinine dihydrochloride	Severe malaria: 600 mg q6–8h
Sodium stibogluconate (Pentostam)	Leishmaniasis (kala azar and cutaneous): 10 mg/kg/day IM or IV for 6–10 days
Suramin (Germanin)	Filariasis: 100–200 mg (test dose) IV, then 1 g IV weekly for 5 weeks, preceded by diethylcarbamazine Trypanosomiasis with CNS involvement: given with tryparsamide

*Information about drugs for parasitic diseases can be obtained by calling the Parasitic Disease Drug Service, (404) 329-3670, or by writing to the Centers for Disease Control, 1600 Clifton Road, Atlanta, GA 30333.

when the insect bites. The sporozoites go to the parenchymal cells of the host's liver. In the liver they divide to form hepatic (exoerythrocytic) schizonts, which contain numerous merozoites. During the hepatic phase of the disease the patient (host) is asymptomatic. Then affected hepatic cells release merozoites into the bloodstream. These merozoites

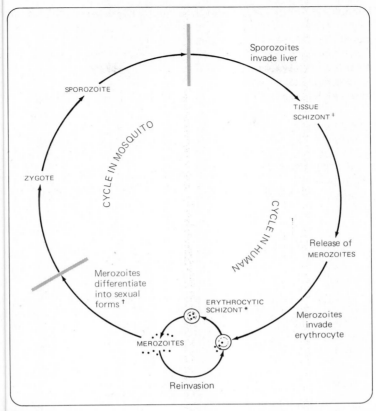

FIGURE 29-1

Life Cycle of the Malarial Parasite. Parasites of the genus *Plasmodium* have a complex life cycle, part of which occurs in humans. (*) The erythrocytic shizontocidal suppressive agents (chloroquine, quinacrine, pyrimethamine, chloroguanide, quinine) eliminate the asexual erythrocyte form of the organism. (†) The sexual forms are eliminated by pyrimethamine and primaquine, preventing transmittal of disease to the vector. (‡) Primaquine is used to eliminate exoerythrocytic tissue schizonts and prevent relapse.

may reinvade the liver, but most commonly they affect the erythrocytes. They again multiply, this time in the erythrocytes, to form mature erythrocyte schizonts which again release merozoites. When the erythrocytes burst, they release pyrogenic substances, which cause the characteristic fever of malaria. The released merozoites can then reinvade the erythrocytes producing the cyclic pattern of fever. The other fate of the merozoites is to undergo sexual division to form the male and female gametocytes. These gametocytes can be ingested by mosquitoes and the cycle is completed.

Clinical Pharmacology and Therapeutics of Malaria

The erythrocytic stage of the life cycle is the most sensitive to drug therapy. The exoerythrocytic (liver) stage is harder to treat because the sporozoites are resistant to most forms of drug therapy. The therapy of the erythrocytic stage will make the patient asymptomatic, but it does not produce a cure, since the liver is still releasing merozoites. For patients who reside in endemic areas, it may never be possible to rid the body of the plasmodia, and therapy will then be only suppressive.

Suppressive Therapy

Chloroquine phosphate (Aralen) is effective against the erythrocytic phase of the disease. It is usually administered once a week to patients who reside in endemic areas. (When the exposure to the disease is terminated, **primaquine** is given to eliminate the liver phase of the disease.) In certain areas *P. falciparum* can be resistant to chloroquine, and various other combinations have to be used. The most common drug combination is **pyrimethamine** 25 mg and **sulfadoxine** 500 mg (Fansidar), but others can be recommended.

Persons traveling to areas where malaria is endemic will

need chemoprophylaxis (see Table 29-5). It is important to check with the local public health authorities prior to travel, to determine the frequency of chloroquine-resistant strains of *Plasmodium*.

The disease affects such a large number of individuals that research efforts have been directed at developing a vaccine to control the disease and a biologic control of the mos-

quito. These research efforts are still in the experimental stages.

Treatment of Acute Attack

The clinical attack is treated with drugs that affect the erythrocytic stage. With *P. vivax* and *P. ovale* the drug of choice is **chloroquine phosphate**. In *P. falciparum* resistant to

TABLE 29-5   Drugs and Doses for Malaria Chemoprophylaxis

GENERIC NAME	BRAND NAMES	ADULT DOSAGE	PEDIATRIC DOSAGE
Amodiaquine*	Camoquin Flavoquin Basoquin	520 mg (400-mg base) once weekly and continued for 6 weeks after last exposure in a malarious area	<1 year: 65 mg (50-mg base) 1–3 years: 130 mg (100-mg base) 4–6 years: 195 mg (150-mg base) 7–10 years: 260 mg (200-mg base) 11–16 years: 390 mg (300-mg base)
Chloroquanide* (proguanil)	Paludrine	100–200 mg daily and continued for 6 weeks after last exposure in a malarious area	2 years and under: 25–50 mg 3–6 years: 50–75 mg 7–10 years: 100 mg
Chloroquine phosphate	Aralen Avloclor Resochin	500 mg (300-mg base) weekly and continued for 6 weeks after last exposure in a malarious area	<1 year: 62 mg (37.5-mg base) 1–3 years: 125 mg (75-mg base) 4–6 years: 165 mg (100-mg base) 7–10 years: 250 mg (150-mg base) 11–16 years: 375 mg (225-mg base) or 5 mg/kg as base
Chloroquine sulfate*	Nivaquine	500 mg (300-mg base) weekly and continued for 6 weeks after last exposure in a malarious area	<1 year: 62 mg (37.5-mg base) 1–3 years: 125 mg (75-mg base) 4–6 years: 165 mg (100-mg base) 7–10 years: 250 mg (150-mg base) 11–16 years: 375 mg (225-mg base) or 5 mg/kg as base
Hydroxychloroquine	Plaquenil	400 mg (310-mg base) weekly and continued for 6 weeks after last exposure in a malarious area	<1 year: 50 mg (37.5-mg base) 1–3 years: 100 mg (75-mg base) 4–6 years: 130 mg (100-mg base) 7–10 years: 200 mg (150-mg base) 11–16 years: 280 mg (225-mg base) or 5 mg/kg as base
Primaquine	(None)	26.3 mg (15-mg base) daily for 14 days or 79 mg (45-mg base) once weekly for 8 weeks; started during last 2 weeks of exposure or following a course of suppression with chloroquine or a comparable drug	0.3 mg/kg/day as base for 14 days or 0.9 mg/kg/day as base weekly for 8 weeks
Pyrimethamine*	Daraprim	25 mg weekly and continued for 8 weeks after last exposure in a malarious area	2 years and under: 6.25 mg 3–10 years: 12.5 mg Over 10 years: adult dosage
Pyrimethamine-sulfadoxine†	Fansidar Falcidar Antemal Methipox	25 mg pyrimethamine and 500 mg sulfadoxine weekly and continued for 6 weeks after last exposure in a malarious area	(In terms of sulfadoxine) 6–11 months: 125 mg 1–3 years: 250 mg 4–8 years: 500 mg 9–14 years: 750 mg

*Available from CDC.

†Countries where pyrimethamine-sulfadoxine can be obtained: Belgium, Brazil, Burma, West Germany, Hong Kong, Indonesia, Kampuchea, Laos, Malaysia, Philippines, Singapore, Switzerland, Thailand, United States, Venezuela, Vietnam.

Source: Modified from MMWR, March 10, 1978. **27**:(Supp) 1981.

chloroquine, the combination of **pyrimethamine and sulfadoxine** is recommended. In life-threatening *P. falciparum* infections, IV **quinine** may be indicated.

Radical Cure

In order to prevent relapse, it is necessary to treat the hepatic form of the disease. The drug usually used for this purpose is **primaquine phosphate**. A radical cure of *P. falciparum* can be achieved by just treating the erythrocyte phase, since the plasmodia do not reinvade the liver.

Antimalarial Drugs

The pharmacology of the antimalarial drugs used in the prophylaxis, treatment, and suppression of malaria are outlined in Table 29-6.

Chloroquine

From 1946 to 1966, chloroquine (Aralen) was the drug of choice for the treatment of malaria the world over. In 1966, chloroquine-resistant malaria began to appear in southeast Asia.

Mechanism of Action Chloroquine is one of several 4-aminoquinoline derivatives displaying antimalarial activity. Chloroquine is particularly effective against the erythrocytic form of malaria because it is concentrated within the parasitized erythrocyte. This preferential drug accumulation appears to occur as a result of specific uptake mechanisms or binding sites present in the parasite. Chloroquine phosphate may inhibit nucleic acid synthesis and other metabolic activity of the parasite.

Pharmacokinetics The absorption of chloroquine from the GI tract is rapid and complete. The drug is widely distributed and is extensively bound to body tissue, with the liver containing 500 times the blood concentration. The plasma half-life of chloroquine is 72 to 120 h. The primary pathway involved in the hepatic metabolism of chloroquine is desethylation. **Desethylchloroquine** is the major metabolite. Both the parent compound and the metabolites are slowly eliminated by renal excretion.

Clinical Use The drug is effective against all four types of malaria, but many species of *P. falciparum* may have become chloroquine-resistant. Chloroquine destroys the erythrocytic stages of the infection and therefore ameliorates the clinical symptoms seen in *P. vivax* and *P. ovale* malaria. The disease will return, however, unless the liver stages are sequentially treated, first with chloroquine and then with primaquine. Chloroquine may also be used prophylactically for individuals traveling to endemic areas.

TABLE 29-6 Properties of Antimalarial Agents

AGENTS	CLASS OF AGENT BY ACTION	SITE OF ACTION	THERAPEUTIC USE	RESISTANCE	TOXICITY
4-Aminoquinolines (chloroquine, amodiaquine)		Not definitely known; strongly bound to nucleic acids; protein synthesis and glycolysis reduced	Acute attack, chemoprophylaxis	*Plasmodium falciparum* from southeast Asia, South America	Minimal
Quinine	Blood schizonticide*		Acute attack caused by chloroquine-resistant *P. falciparum*	Recrudescence in strains of *P. falciparum*	Cinchonism, immune hemolysis
Quinacrine			None (replaced by chloroquine)	Cross-resistance with chloroquine–*P. falciparum*	Dermatitis
8-Aminoquinolines (primaquine, quinocide)	Hepatic schizonticide,† gametocide, sporonticide‡	Not definitely known; block glycolysis	Radical cure in *P. vivax, P. ovale*; chemoprophylaxis in combination with chloroquine	Strains of *P. vivax*	Hemolysis in G6PD deficiency
Chlorquanide, pyrimethamine, trimethoprim	Primary hepatic schizonticide, sporonticide‡	Block dihydrofolate reductase	Chemoprophylaxis; acute attack in chloroquine-resistant *P. falciparum*	Readily developed in all *Plasmodium* sp.	Minimal; thrombocytopenia with pyrimethamine
Sulfonamides, sulfones	Blood schizonticide	Block utilization of paraaminobenzoic acid	Acute attack in chloroquine-resistant *P. falciparum*; chemoprophylaxis	Readily developed in all *Plasmodium* sp.	Minimal; agranulocytosis (sulfones)

*Blood schizonticide eradicates asexual erythrocytic forms.
†Hepatic schizonticide eradicates exoerythrocytic (hepatic) schizonts and prevents relapses (radical cure).
‡Sporonticide inhibits development of the form infectious for the mosquito.

Chloroquine also possesses anti-inflammatory properties and is used in the treatment of rheumatoid arthritis and lupus erythematosus (see Chap. 26). Chloroquine also has been found useful in treating extraintestinal amebiasis caused by *Entamoeba histolytica*.

Adverse Effects The toxicity of chloroquine is related to dose and duration of treatment. When used for suppressive purposes, chloroquine causes few untoward effects, although dizziness, headache, itching, skin rash, vomiting, and blurring of vision may occur. In higher doses these symptoms are more common, and some effects in skin, blood, and eyes can occur. Chloroquine should not be used in the presence of retinal or visual-field changes.

Dosage The usual adult oral dosage in the treatment of clinical malaria is 600 mg followed by 300 mg 6 h later, and then 300 mg daily for 2 days. The children's dosage is 25 mg/kg, which is given in four divided doses. For the prophylaxis of malaria the phosphate salt (300 mg) is given once weekly, beginning 2 weeks prior to the expected exposure and extending through a period of 6 weeks after exposure. The children's prophylactic dosage is 5 mg/kg once a week. Chloroquine hydrochloride can be given for severe malaria by the IM route in an initial dose of 200 to 300 mg, which is repeated every 6 h, but the dosage should not exceed 800 mg in the first 24 h.

Quinine

Quinine is an alkaloid derived from the bark of the South American cinchona tree. Despite the fact that its use has been largely superseded by other, more effective antimalarial agents, quinine is still the standard of comparison in evaluating antimalarial drugs.

Mechanism of Action The exact mode of action of quinine is not known, but it appears to alter the action of DNA in the plasmodia. **Quinine**, along with **quinacrine** and chloroquine, is classed as a "blood schizonticide." It has no effect on the primary or secondary exoerythrocytic (tissue) forms of the parasites and, therefore, cannot bring about a radical cure of malaria caused by *P. vivax, P. malariae*, or *P. ovale*. It is neither effectively gametocidal nor sporonticidal to *P. falciparum*. Although quinine cannot prevent infection, it can suppress the symptoms of malaria and also bring about rapid control of an acute attack.

Pharmacokinetics Quinine is rapidly and completely absorbed following oral administration. The absorption of quinine is mainly in the upper portion of the small intestines. It is widely distributed in the body, and it crosses the placenta and is transferred into milk. It is approximately 70 percent bound to plasma proteins. The plasma half-life of quinine is 4 to 5 h.

Clinical Use Quinine is used for chemoprophylaxis and to treat the acute attack of malaria due to all four *Plasmodium* species. Although it is not considered the first-line drug, it is extremely useful when treating *P. falciparum* resistant to chloroquine and pyrimethamine-sulfadoxine. Intravenous quinine is currently the treatment of choice for severe *P. falciparum* which is resistant to chloroquine.

Quinine is also effective in the treatment of night leg muscle cramps. Quinine sulfate should be used after stretching exercises have proven ineffective.

Adverse Effects Quinine can give rise to a group of side effects collectively known as cinchonism. Cinchonism can produce tinnitus, blurred vision, dizziness, and headache. These adverse effects are troublesome to the patient but seldom require stopping use of the drug. Tinnitus will rarely occur if the serum concentration is kept below 10 μg/mL. Additional adverse effects of quinine include hypersensitivity reactions, GI effects (nausea, vomiting, and abdominal discomfort), hematologic effects [thrombocytopenic purpura, hypoprothrombinemia, and hemolysis in patients with glucose-6-phosphate dehydrogenase (G6PD) deficiency], and hepatic effects (granulomatous hepatitis).

Dosage Quinine, when used for chemoprophylaxis or suppressive therapy, is given to adults in a dosage of 325 mg twice a day for at least 6 weeks after exposure. When used in the treatment of *P. falciparum* resistant to chloroquine, quinine is given in a dosage of 650 mg orally every 8 h for 72 h. This can be given in conjunction with (1) oral **tetracycline**, (2) **pyrimethamine-sulfadoxine**, or (3) **pyrimethamine-sulfadiazine**.

The usual pediatric dosage for the treatment of an acute attack is 25 mg/kg daily given every 8 h for 3 days.

The IV dosage of quinine dihydrochloride is 600 mg every 6 to 8 h administered slowly (over 1 h) by infusion. The patient should be switched to oral therapy as soon as possible.

The usual dosage in the therapy of nocturnal leg cramps is 325 mg given once a day at bedtime.

Hydroxychloroquine (Plaquenil)

Hydroxychloroquine, like chloroquine, is a 4-aminoquinoline derivative. Its mechanism of action and clinical uses are similar to those of chloroquine. It is used for suppressive and acute treatment of malaria caused by *P. vivax, P. malariae, P. ovale*, and susceptible strains of *P. falciparum*. Hydroxychloroquine has not been proven to be more effective than chloroquine.

Adverse reactions associated with its use are similar to those described for chloroquine. This drug should not be used in patients with psoriasis or porphyria, since it may exacerbate these conditions.

Hydroxychloroquine sulfate is available in 200-mg oral

tablets, which are equal to 155 mg of the hydroxychloroquine base. For suppressive or chemoprophylactic therapy 400 mg is administered once a week beginning 1 to 2 weeks prior to the patient's entering the endemic area and continuing until 6 weeks after she or he leaves the area. The pediatric dosage is 6.5 mg/kg of hydroxychloroquine sulfate. The treatment of acute attack is 800 mg of hydroxychloroquine initially, then 400 mg 6 to 8 h later; 18 h after the second dose, another 400 mg is given; the final dose of 400 mg is given 24 h after the third dose.

Primaquine

Mechanism of Action Primaquine is the least toxic and most effective of the 8-aminoquinoline antimalarial compounds. The mechanism by which 8-aminoquinolines exert their antimalarial effects is unknown.

Pharmacokinetics Primaquine is readily absorbed from the GI tract and, in contrast to chloroquine, is not bound extensively by tissues. It is rapidly metabolized, and the metabolites are reported to be as active as the parent drug. Peak plasma levels are reached 4 to 6 h after an oral dose, with almost total drug elimination occurring in 24 h.

Clinical Use Primaquine is an important antimalarial drug because it is essentially the only one effective against the liver (exoerythrocytic) forms of the malarial parasite. The drug also kills the gametocytes, and patients recovering from *P. falciparum* malaria can be given primaquine for its gametocidal properties. Primaquine is relatively ineffective against the asexual forms of *P. falciparum*. Primaquine is useful for the treatment of *P. vivax* malaria.

Adverse Effects In individuals with a genetically determined G6PD deficiency, primaquine can cause lethal hemolysis of red cells. With higher doses or prolonged drug use, GI distress, nausea, headache, pruritis, and leukopenia can occur.

CASE STUDY

W.M., a 38-year-old white male, came to the emergency room (ER) complaining of frequent episodes of severe chills, intense headaches, and nausea and vomiting. The symptoms began a week prior to his arrival in the ER. The history taken by the ER nurse showed that W.M. had served in Vietnam 10 years previously and was now working in construction. He was on no medication except aspirin for his headaches and flulike symptoms.

Assessment

On physical examination W.M. was febrile, with a temperature of 40°C. His blood pressure was 150/70, and

Dosage Primaquine phosphate is administered orally, and 26.3 mg of the salt is equivalent to 15 mg of the primaquine base. The usual adult dosage of primaquine is 15 mg once a day for 14 days. The pediatric dosage is 0.3 mg/kg of primaquine given daily for 2 weeks.

Pyrimethamine and Pyrimethamine-Sulfadoxine

Pyrimethamine (Daraprim) is a folic acid antagonist with similar activity to trimethoprim. Pyrimethamine-sulfadoxine (Fansidar) is similar in activity to other sulfonamides. Pyrimethamine and sulfadoxine are both well absorbed following oral administration. The half-lives of both drugs are long, with that of pyrimethamine being 111 h and that of sulfadoxine being 169 h.

Pyrimethamine-sulfadoxine is indicated in the treatment of *P. falciparum* that is resistant to chloroquine. Pyrimethamine is seldom used alone, and if sulfadoxine cannot be used, other combinations with dapsone or quinine or sulfadiazine may be used. Pyrimethamine with a sulfonamide (sulfadiazine or others) is the treatment of choice for toxoplasmosis.

The adverse effects of pyrimethamine and sulfadoxine are usually mild and infrequent when they are used in the treatment of malaria. When they are used in the treatment of toxoplasmosis, adverse hematologic effects (blood marrow depression) can occur because of prolonged folic acid deficiency.

The usual dosage for chemoprophylactic and suppressive therapy is a weekly tablet (25 mg of pyrimethamine and 500 mg of sulfadoxine) during and for 6 weeks after exposure. The treatment of the acute attack is 2 to 3 tablets as a single dose.

NURSING PROCESS RELATED TO MALARIA

Table 29-7 summarizes the nursing process relevant to drug therapy of malaria.

he was tachycardic with a heart rate of 115. His lungs and abdomen were unremarkable. The liver and spleen were not enlarged or tender. His skin was intensely hot and flushed and diaphoretic. He was complaining of severe chills and nausea.

Management

W.M. was admitted to the hospital. Blood tests were done and a peripheral smear showed a *Plasmodium* malarial parasite present. W.M. stated that he had never taken any malaria-suppressive drugs while in Vietnam.

TABLE 29-7 Nursing Process Related to Malaria

ASSESSMENT	MANAGEMENT	EVALUATION
	General Aspects	
Assess for history of travel in endemic areas, sudden onset of chills with cyclic occurrence (paroxysms). Diagnosis is established by finding plasmodia in patient's blood. Most favorable time for discovery is during a chill and 12 to 18 h after a chill.	Observe strict blood precautions during hospitalization. Use disposable needles, lancets, and syringes, and properly dispose of or sterilize all contaminated items. During chills, keep patient as comfortable as possible, covered with blankets and warmed with hot-water bottles. When fever begins, remove coverings and sponge bathe. Keep patient dry, and change linen frequently during periods of perspiration. Give support during chills to alleviate apprehension, and do not leave alone. After paroxysm, patient will need period of uninterrupted rest. Monitor for darkened urine, a sign of blackwater fever.	Complications of malaria include fatigue, changes in blood viscosity, water and electrolyte imbalance, GI disturbances. Blackwater fever is a sometimes fatal complication of *P. falciparum* infection. Relapses may continue to occur over the years. Infection may be transmitted through blood transfusions of infected donors. Complications of chronic malaria include congested and enlarged liver and spleen, anemia and cachexia, depression, loss of ability to concentrate, and deterioration of memory.
	Hydroxychloroquine Sulfate	
Drug is contraindicated in presence of retinal or visual-field changes attributed to any 4-aminoquinoline compound or of known sensitivity to this compound. Do not use for long-term therapy in children. Use with caution in patients with psoriasis, porphyria, hepatic disease, alcoholism, G6PD deficiency, or concurrent use of hepatotoxic drugs.	Warn patients to keep this drug out of the reach of children; a number of fatalities have been reported following accidental ingestion, sometimes in small doses (1 g in a 3-year-old). Monitor blood cell counts. Drug may precipitate severe attack in psoriasis patients and may exacerbate condition when used in patients with porphyria. Give adults medication on same day of each week.	Adverse effects—Watch for mild and transient headache, dizziness, and GI complaints. With an overdose or hypersensitivity reaction, toxic symptoms may occur within 30 min and include headache, drowsiness, visual disturbances, cardiovascular collapse, and convulsions, followed by sudden and early respiratory and cardiac arrest.
	Quinine	
Assess for present level of visual and hearing acuity. Check for sensitivity.	Drug must be given daily and has a bitter taste. Give IV slowly. Causes dangerous lowering of blood pressure. Place patient on monitor to detect arrhythmias. IV administration may also cause irritation of intima, resulting in thrombosis. Given IM, drug may cause sterile abscess. Observe for signs of cinchonism—ringing in ears, headache, nausea, dizziness, and disturbance of vision. Drug has analgesic effect similar to that of aspirin.	Adverse effects—Watch for dizziness, tinnitus, palpitations and tremors, disturbances of sight and hearing, allergic responses. Symptoms of cinchonism are likely to occur when maximum therapeutic dosage is administered.
	Chloroquine	
Use caution in patients with history of liver damage, neurologic disorders, or hematologic disorders. Assess visual acuity.	GI disturbances can be minimized by giving drug during meals or with a glass of milk or piece of bread. Eye exams should be done at least every 3 months.	Adverse effects resemble mild cinchonism. High doses of this drug can cause severe toxic effects. Watch for dermatologic problems, toxic psychoses, and peripheral neuropathies or permanent nerve deafness. Prolonged use can cause severe, permanent eye damage with corneal or retinal changes.
	Primaquine	
Check for sensitivity to drug and for G6PD deficiency.	Stop drug stat on any sign of darkening of urine or a sudden drop in hemoglobin concentration or leukocyte count.	Adverse effects—Watch for epigastric distress, nausea, vomiting, and abdominal pain. Drug can cause bone marrow depression, hemolytic anemia, and agranulocytosis. Large doses result in hemolytic effects, particularly in persons belonging to the deeply pigmented races.

He was immediately started on chloroquine 1 g (loading dose), then 500 mg in 6 h, then 500 mg for 2 succeeding days. Therapy also included primaquine 15 mg daily for 14 days. Treatment was also supplemented with iron therapy and dietary measures as indicated.

AMEBIASIS

Amebiasis is an infection caused by the protozoan *Entamoeba histolytica*. The organism is in the asymptomatic carrier state in most individuals, but it can present as mild diarrhea to severe dysentery. The most common extraintestinal effects are caused by invasion by the organism into the liver (hepatic abscess). The diagnosis of amebiasis is made by identification of *E. histolytica* in the stool.

Clinical Pharmacology and Therapeutics of Amebiasis

Drugs available for therapy can be classified according to their site of antiamebic action (Table 29-8). Luminal amebicides such as **diiodohydroxyquin** and **diloxanide furoate** are active against luminal organisms but are ineffective against parasites in the bowel wall or tissues. The parenterally administered tissue amebicides **dehydroemetine** and **emetine** are effective against parasites in the bowel wall and tissues but not against luminal organisms. **Chloroquine** acts only against organisms in the liver. Antibiotics taken orally are direct-acting luminal amebicides that exert their effects against bacterial associates of *E. histolytica* in the bowel lumen and in the bowel wall but not in other tissues. Parenteral antibiotics have little antiamebic activity at any site. **Paromomycin**, however, has a direct effect on amoebas. **Metronidazole** is uniquely effective against organisms at three sites: the bowel lumen, bowel wall, and tissues. However, metronidazole used alone is not sufficient as a luminal amebicide.

Amebicidal Drugs

Metronidazole (Flagyl)

Mechanism of Action Metronidazole is batericidal, amebicidal, and trichomonicidal in its action. Clinically the drug is reduced (the nitro is removed), and it is this reduced preparation that kills the organisms by interaction with various cellular macromolecules. The development of resistance to metronidazole is uncommon.

Pharmacokinetics The drug is well absorbed following oral administration. Food delays the absorption but does not alter the extent of absorption. The drug is widely distributed throughout the body, including in bone, saliva, CSF, pleural fluids, seminal fluids, milk, the placenta, and other body tissues and fluids. The normal plasma half-life of metronida-

Evaluation

W.M. was discharged to home care after 10 days of hospitalization. He continued on his full course of drug therapy and all symptoms subsided. Arrangements were made for further doctor's office visits.

zole is 6 to 8 h but it may be prolonged due to hepatic disorders. Decreased renal function does not appear to alter the elimination of metronidazole.

Clinical Use Metronidazole can be used in the treatment of acute intestinal amebiasis and in the therapy of hepatic amebic liver abscess. It may be necessary to use a luminal amebicide for the treatment of symptomatic amebiasis in association with metronidazole.

Metronidazole is used orally in the treatment of trichomoniasis. When trichomonal therapy is indicated, all sexual partners should be treated. Metronidazole can also be used in the treatment of giardiasis.

Metronidazole is used in the treatment of severe anaerobic bacterial infections. It can be used orally or intravenously in the treatment of intraabdominal, gynecologic, bone, skin, joint, lower respiratory tract, central nervous system, and other infections.

TABLE 29-8 Drug Therapy of Amebiasis

DRUG	DOSAGE
Asymptomatic Intestinal Carrier	
Diiodohydroxyquin	650 mg tid for 20 days
or diloxanide furoate*	500 mg tid for 10 days
Mild to Moderate Intestinal Disease	
Metronidazole	750 mg tid for 5–10 days
plus diiodohydroxyquin	As above
or diloxanide furoate*	As above
or tetracycline	500 mg qid for 5 days
Severe Intestinal Disease	
Above regimen	1.0–1.5 mg/kg/day IM
plus dehydroemetine*	(max. 90 mg/day) for up to 5 days
or emetine	1 mg/kg/day IM (max. 60 mg/day) for up to 5 days
Extraintestinal Disease	
Metronidazole	As above
or chloroquine phosphate	1 g/day for 2 days, then 500 mg/day for 4 weeks
plus dehydroemetine*	As above for 10 days
or emetine	As above for 10 days

*Investigational drug available through the Parasitic Disease Drug Service, CDC.
Source: Petersdorf et al. (eds.), *Harrison's Principles of Internal Medicine,* 10th ed., New York: McGraw-Hill, 1983.

Adverse Effects Metronidazole can produce the following adverse effects: nausea; vomiting; headaches; dry mouth with a sharp unpleasant metallic taste; and epigastric distress. The IV dosage form has also been associated with GI problems and the metallic taste. More-serious side effects that have been reported but are usually rare include peripheral neuropathy, dizziness, ataxia, leukopenia, and thrombophlebitis (with IV administration).

Carcinogenicity and mutagenicity have been reported in laboratory animals, but similar results in humans have not been documented. More clinical evaluation of the problem is needed. It is recommended that the drug be avoided unless the benefit of use outweighs the potential risks.

Metronidazole increases the activity of warfarin. If possible the two drugs should not be used together. When metronidazole is taken along with alcohol, a mild disulfiram-like reaction can occur.

Dosage

1. For urogenital trichomoniasis, adults are given 250 mg orally three times daily for 7 days. A single dose of 2 g (eight tablets) orally is also effective. Sexual partners should be treated simultaneously.

2. For giardiasis, adults are given 250 mg orally three times daily for 7 days. Children are given 5 mg/kg orally three times daily for 5 days.

3. For amebiasis, if the patient has severe intestinal disease (amebic dysentery), the suggested dosage is 750 mg three times daily for 10 days plus a course of a luminal amebicide. For the treatment of liver abscess, a standard regimen is 750 mg three times daily for 10 days; a course of a luminal amebicide should be added to enhance eradication of luminal organisms.

4. For balantidiasis if tetracycline is ineffective, the dosage is 750 mg three times daily for 7 days.

5. For *Gardnerella (Haemophilus) vaginalis,* for refractory infections only, the dosage is 500 mg orally twice a day for 5 days.

6. For anaerobic infections, the usual adult dosage of metronidazole IV is 15 mg/kg as a loading dose, followed by a 7.5-mg/kg maintenance dose given every 6 h. The IV metronidazole is given over 1 h. Patients should be switched to oral therapy as soon as it is appropriate. The maximum daily IV dosage is usually 4 g. Therapy is usually continued for 1 to 3 weeks.

Chloroquine

In the treatment of amebiasis, chloroquine (Aralen) is used both to eradicate and to prevent amebic liver abscess. Chloroquine reaches high liver concentration, which makes it effective when used in conjunction with emetine in the treatment of amebic liver abscess. Chloroquine is not used in the treatment of the intestinal phase of amebiasis because the drug is not active against luminal organisms.

Chloroquine is given in a loading dose of 500 mg twice daily for 2 days and is followed by 250 mg twice daily for 1 to 3 weeks. When chloroquine is used for prophylaxis against liver abscess, a 1-week course is recommended during the treatment of mild to moderate intestinal infection.

Emetine

Emetine hydrochloride, used for more than 70 years for the treatment of *E. histolytica* infection, still remains a principal drug used for the treatment of severe intestinal infections (amebic dysentery), liver abscess, and other forms of extraintestinal amebiasis. Emetine should not be used in the treatment of asymptomatic or mild intestinal infections.

Emetine is administered parenterally, not orally, because it is absorbed erratically from the GI tract and may induce emesis. Emetine may be an extremely toxic drug to the liver, heart, kidneys, skeletal muscles, and GI tract if given in larger than recommended doses for greater than 10 days. The most-serious adverse effects are cardiotoxic. GI effects include nausea, vomiting, diarrhea, and epigastric distress. The local injection is associated with pain, tenderness, and muscle weakness. The **dehydroemetine dihydrochloride,** which is available from the Centers for Disease Control (CDC), may be associated with less toxicity.

The daily dosage of emetine for adults and children is 1 mg/kg intravenously or intramuscularly. The maximum daily dosage for adults is 65 mg. For children under 8 years, the maximum is 10 mg.

Diloxanide Furoate

Diloxanide furoate (Furamide) was introduced in 1957 and has since been extensively used outside the United States for the treatment of intestinal amebiasis. The drug is not effective in the treatment of extraintestinal amebiasis. In the United States diloxanide is available only from the Parasitic Disease Drug Service at the CDC.

It is given in a dosage of 500 mg orally three times daily, for 10 days. The dosage for children is 20 mg/kg orally divided into three doses and given for 10 days.

Halogenated 8-Hydroxyquinolines

Diiodohydroxyquin (Yodoxin) and **iodochlorhydroxyquin** were among the first drugs used in the treatment of amebiasis. Diiodohydroxyquin is currently the only 8-hydroxyquinoline preparation available for the treatment of amebiasis. The mechanisms of action of these compounds are not completely understood. The drugs are classified as luminal amebicides, since the drugs are not absorbed from the GI tract. In the treatment of mild cases or in the therapy of an asymptomatic carrier, diiodohydroxyquin may be used as the only form of therapy. In the treatment of more severe disease a tissue amebicide such as metronidazole should also be used.

The most serious adverse effects are neurotoxic effects, which are related to large doses given for a long period of time. These adverse effects include optic neuritis, optic atrophy, and peripheral neuropathy. Loss of vision has also occurred. Adverse GI effects may include diarrhea, vomiting, nausea, constipation, pruritus ani, and abdominal discomfort. Iodism (increase in iodine) can produce various skin eruptions. Diiodohydroxyquin can also cause discoloration of the hair and nails and may interfere with thyroid function tests.

The usual adult dosage is 650 mg orally given three times a day for 3 weeks. The pediatric dosage is 30 to 40 mg/kg given in three divided doses for 3 weeks.

Paromomycin Sulfate

Paromomycin sulfate (Humatin) is an aminoglycoside antibiotic which is useful in the treatment of intestinal amebiasis. In the treatment of severe infections paromomycin should be used in conjunction with other tissue amebicides, **metronidazole**, **chloroquine**, or **emetine**. The most common adverse effects are GI effects, including nausea, vomiting, anorexia, diarrhea, and epigastric distress. Paromomycin is also associated with adverse effects similar to those of the other aminoglycosides (see Chap. 28).

The dosage of paromomycin is 25 to 35 mg/kg given in three divided doses after meals for 5 to 10 days for both adults and children.

NURSING PROCESS RELATED TO AMEBIASIS

Assessment

Although amebiasis exists chiefly in the tropical countries, it also prevails wherever sanitation is poor. It is estimated that at least 10 percent of the population of the United States have amebiasis in the acute, chronic, or asymptomatic stage. It occurs particularly where human excreta is used as the chief fertilizer for vegetables and wherever fecal contamination of drinking water occurs.

Although the disease varies in severity, the onset is usually acute, with symptoms developing within 2 to 4 days of exposure. Weakness, prostration, nausea, vomiting, and a gripping pain in the right lower quadrant of the abdomen, and tenesmus usually occur. Each day the patient has frequent, small, semifluid, foul-smelling stools containing blood and mucus, the latter laden with amoebas. A positive diagnosis can be made if either the trophozoite or cyst can be found in the stool. It is easier to find the parasite in the stool during the acute stage of the disease than later on in its course. Immediately after defecation, a warm stool should be sent to the laboratory for examination. Several stool specimens from consecutive bowel movements may be requested. To keep the specimen warm, the container should be kept, and transported, with a hot-water bottle or in a pan of warm water.

Signs of hepatic involvement may appear several months after an attack of amebic dysentery. Amebic liver abscesses differ from those caused by bacteria in that they are more often single than multiple, are always large, have little evidence of real inflammation in their walls, and give surprisingly few symptoms. The patient may complain of nausea, vomiting, and jaundice. This is sometimes followed by chills and sweats, temperature elevation, malaise, and constant dull pain in the area of the liver, which is full of necrotic and liquified liver tissue, the walls of which contain hosts of amoebas.

In the patient interview it is important to determine a history of thyroid disorder or iodine sensitivity, since these would contraindicate use of **diiodohydroxyquin**. The antibiotic **paromomycin** should not be used if the patient has an intestinal obstruction. **Emetine** is usually not used when the patient has heart disease or liver or kidney disorder, or if the patient is aged, debilitated, or pregnant. **Metronidazole** should be administered with caution to patients with central nervous system diseases or severe hepatic disease.

Management

The patient with a mild form of amebiasis can be treated on an outpatient basis. **Metronidazole** is one of the most effective and least toxic intestinal amebicides available. It produces prompt cessation of diarrhea and discharges parasites from stools in 24 h. However, serial follow-up of the stools is necessary because the disease can recur. Patients receiving metronidazole should be instructed to stop taking the drug immediately and call a physician if any neurologic symptoms develop, since convulsive seizures have occurred during metronidazole therapy. The patient should also call the doctor on the occurrence of peripheral neuropathy, characterized by numbness or paresthesia of an extremity. Metronidazole may cause a darkening of the urine and does produce a bitter metallic taste. "Furry" tongue, glossitis, and stomatitis may occur associated with a sudden overgrowth of *Candida*. If patients drink alcoholic beverages while taking metronidazole, they may experience a modification of taste, plus suffer abdominal discomfort, nausea, vomiting, flushing, and headache, so this information must be included in patient education.

If the halogenated hydroxyquinolines such as **diiodohydroxyquin** are given, the patient should be monitored for iodism (symptoms include itching, dermatitis, headache, rhinitis, abdominal discomfort, and furunculosis).

The patient should be hospitalized if placed on emetine, since it is a general protoplasmic poison and causes a variety of toxic reactions. It is administered by deep subcutaneous and deep IM injection. Pain, local edema, and necrosis can occur at the injection site, so sites of injection need to be rotated. Care should be taken to aspirate before injecting, since IV administration is dangerous. The patient should be placed on strict bed rest, and pulse rate and blood pressure should be watched carefully. A decrease in blood pressure and an elevated pulse may indicate toxicity to cardiac muscle. Cardiac changes may vary from disturbance in rhythm to acute myocarditis and heart failure. The drug is given over a period of 5 to 10 days. However, it is so slowly eliminated from the body that it can be found in the urine 40 days after a single dose is administered. Therefore, the patient must remain on restricted activity for some time after therapy has stopped, because cardiovascular symptoms may be late in appearing.

Severe diarrhea can cause fluid and electrolyte imbalances, in which case the patient should be hospitalized and placed on IV infusions. The patient should remain on bed rest during the acute phase of diarrhea and should receive a nonirritating, low-residue, bland diet containing weak tea, rice, broth, toast, and plenty of fluids. The diet should later be increased to include high calorie value.

In caring for a patient with amebiasis, the nurse should remember to use careful hand-washing techniques and to explain to the patient the role of hand washing in preventing reinfection and spread of the disease. Since cysts can be excreted in the stool, fecal material should be flushed immediately, and the bedpan should be sterilized. The number and character of stools should be documented, with observation for the presence of cysts, mucus, and blood.

Evaluation

Therapy with the amebicides should result in a decrease of diarrhea. However, amebiasis is a disease with remissions and exacerbations, and it may persist for years. The patient must continue with medical follow-up and stool checks. During acute exacerbations the patient may become dehydrated, exhausted, or anemic and require hospitalization for IV fluid replacement and blood transfusions. The patient with a liver abscess may need surgical drainage if drug therapy fails or if the abscess is quite large.

Patients need to understand the importance of cleanliness, proper sanitation habits, and disposal of waste materials. They must wash their hands well before eating meals or touching any food, to prevent reinfecting themselves or infecting others through the ingestion of foods contaminated with cysts. It is extremely important that persons who are carriers (who have only mild GI distress and unknowingly pass cysts) be located and restricted from jobs associated with food handling.

MISCELLANEOUS PROTOZOAL INFECTIONS

Leishmaniasis

Leishmaniasis in humans is a disorder that is produced by one of four protozoa: *Leishmania donovani* causes visceral leishmaniasis, or kala azar; *Leishmania tropica* and *Leishmania mexicana* produce cutaneous leishmaniasis; and *Leishmania braziliensis* causes mucocutaneous leishmaniasis. The parasites are usually transmitted to humans from animals by the bite of the phlebotomic sand flies.

Sodium stibogluconate, or **antimony gluconate** (Pentostam), is the treatment of choice for visceral leishmaniasis and cutaneous leishmaniasis. It is given in dosages of 600 mg/day intramuscularly or intravenously for 6 to 10 days. It is rapidly excreted; toxicities usually include GI disturbances, jaundice, weakness, rash, and albuminuria. Other drugs that have been used are **stiboten** (Fuadin) and **pentamidine**.

Giardiasis

Giardiasis is caused by the protozoan *Giardia lamblia*, which parasitizes the small intestines. Patients with giardiasis may be asymptomatic, or they may be symptomatic with explosive watery diarrhea. The acute symptoms usually resolve, and then there occurs a chronic phase, where the patient has no symptoms or only mild symptoms of epigastric distress, flatulence, or soft stools. The protozoan is waterborne, and the common source of the infection is contaminated drinking water.

Patients who have giardiasis should be treated. The most common drugs used are **quinacrine** (Atabrine) and **metronidazole** (Flagyl). Quinacrine is given in a dosage of 100 mg orally three times a day for 5 to 7 days, and metronidazole is given in a dosage of 250 mg three times a day for 10 days.

Chemoprophylactic drugs cannot prevent the development of giardiasis. Giardiasis can be prevented by avoiding contaminated water or by treating the water (boiling or using halogen disinfectant tablets).

Trypanosomiasis (Sleeping Sickness)

African trypanosomiasis is a disease caused by *Trypanosoma brucei*, which is transmitted to humans by the tsetse fly. The easiest form of therapy is to prevent the bite of the insect by the use of screens and insect repellents. Pentamidine in a dosage of 3 to 4 mg/kg (of base) as a single IM dose can be used in the treatment of the infection.

HELMINTHIC INFECTIONS

Worm infections represent the most common parasitic diseases in humans. It has been estimated that in various parts of the world more than 800 million persons are infected with helminths. Helminthic infections may be limited solely to the intestinal lumen, or the immature worm may move through the body prior to localization in a particular tissue. Complicating the host-parasite relationship and the role of chemotherapy in helminth-induced infections is the complex life cycle of many of these organisms. Whereas some helminths may have a simple cycle of egg deposition and hatching of the egg to produce a mature worm, others must progress through one or more hosts and one or more morphologic stages before emerging as adults. Furthermore, the infective form may be either an adult worm or an immature worm. Not uncommonly, treatment is further complicated by infection with more than one genus of helminth. Helminths can be divided into three groups: cestodes (tapeworms), nematodes (roundworms), and trematodes (flukes).

Clinical Pharmacology and Therapeutics of Cestode Infections

Cestodes (tapeworms) that parasitize humans have complex life cycles usually requiring development in a second or intermediate host. Following their ingestion, the infected larvae develop into adults in the host's small intestine. Although a majority of patients remain symptom-free, others experience a vague abdominal discomfort, hunger pains, indigestion, and anorexia and may develop a vitamin B deficiency. In some cestode infections, eggs containing larvae are ingested; the larvae invade the intestinal wall, enter a blood vessel, and lodge in tissue such as muscle, liver, or one eye. Symptoms are associated with the particular organs affected.

Human tapeworm infections can be classified into three groups. For the first group, humans act as the hosts and have the adult tapeworms in the intestines. This group includes infections of *Taenia saginata* (beef tapeworm), *Diphyllobothrium latum* (fish tapeworm), *Hymenolepis* sp., and *Dipylidium caninum* (dog tapeworm). For the second group, humans harbor the larval forms in their tissues. This group includes eshinococcosis, sparganosis, and coenurosis. The last group is a combination of the first two groups and includes infection with *Taenia solium* (pork tapeworm).

Niclosamide

Niclosamide (Yomesan) is an insoluble chlorosalicylamide derivative that inhibits the uptake of glucose and the production of energy derived from anaerobic metabolism. The ability of niclosamide to inhibit the anaerobic incorporation of inorganic phosphate into adenosine triphosphate (ATP) is detrimental to the parasite. The drug affects the scolex and proximal (tail) segments of the cestode. This results in a detachment of the cestode's scolex from the host's intestine by the normal peristaltic action of the host's bowel.

The broad range of activity of niclosamide against cestodes, and the absence of significant side effects associated with its use, make it valuable in the treatment of *T. saginata* (beef tapeworm), *Hymenolepis nana* (dwarf tapeworm), and *T. solium* (pork tapeworm) infestations.

Adverse effects are usually uncommon but may include abdominal discomfort.

Niclosamide is available as 500-mg tablets for oral use and may be obtained from the Parasitic Disease Drug Service of the CDC (see Table 29-4). A single dose of four tablets (2 g) of niclosamide is chewed thoroughly. The dose for children 11 to 34 kg is two tablets; children over 34 kg get three tablets.

Paromomycin Sulfate

Paromomycin (Humatin), an aminoglycoside antibiotic, is an alternative drug choice for treating tapeworm infections. It is given in an oral dosage of 1 g every 15 min for four doses. The children's dosage is approximately 11 mg/kg in the same dosage schedule.

Clinical Pharmacology and Therapeutics of Nematode Infections

Nematodes, because of their shape, are commonly referred to as roundworms. Some of the nematodes (filarial worms and quinea worms) live in blood, lymphatics, and other tissues and are referred to as blood and tissue nematodes. Others are found primarily in the intestinal tract. Other intestinal nematodes are acquired by ingestion of their eggs from soil. The intestinal nematodes can cause enterobiasis (pinworm or seatworm), strongyloidiasis (threadworm), trichuriasis (whipworm), and ascariasis (roundworm). The tissue nematodes can cause strongyloidiasis, gnathostomiasis, and dracunculiasis.

Piperazine

Piperazine tartrate and citrate (Antepar) acts on the musculature of the helminth, causing a flaccid paralysis and thereby permitting expulsion of the worm by the normal peristaltic action of the host's intestine. The drug increases the resting potential of the helminth muscle in such a way that the pacemaker presumably present in the muscle membrane is suppressed.

Piperazine is administered orally and is readily absorbed from the intestinal tract. Most of the drug is excreted in the urine within 24 h of its administration.

Piperazine is used to treat infection with *Ascaris lumbricoides* (roundworm) and with *Enterobius vermicularis* (pinworm). A 7-day course of treatment results in cure rates approaching 95 percent. A repeat course after 2 weeks is sometimes recommended. Other household members should be treated simultaneously, since pinworm infestations usually involve several persons, many of whom will be asymptomatic.

Side effects occasionally include GI distress, urticaria, and dizziness. Neurologic symptoms of ataxia, hypotonia, and visual disturbances, and exacerbations of epilepsy, can occur in patients with preexisting renal insufficiency.

Piperazine is considered an alternative agent to mebendazole and **pyrantel pamoate**. The drug may be as effective clinically, but it has a less convenient dosage schedule. When used in the treatment of pinworm, a single daily dose of 65 mg/kg (maximum dose of 2.5 g) for 7 days is needed for adults and children. In treatment of roundworm the adult is given a single dose of 3.5 g, and pediatric patients are given 75 mg/kg for 2 consecutive days.

Pyrvinium Pamoate

Pyrvinium pamoate (Povan) is a basic cyanine dye which interferes with the absorption of exogenous glucose in intestinal helminths. It is an alternative agent for treating *E. vermicularis* (pinworm). The drug is administered orally. It is not absorbed from the intestinal tract and therefore is eliminated in the feces. Single-dose therapy, repeated after 2 weeks to eliminate any worms that have matured from residual ova, is usually effective. Other members of the household should also be treated.

Pyrvinium pamoate will stain the stools and vomitus bright red. Although quite harmless, this coloration may cause the patient some concern. GI intolerance occurs occasionally.

The adult and pediatric dosage for the treatment of pinworms is 5 mg/kg, to a maximum of 350 mg, in a single dose, which is repeated in 2 weeks.

Pyrantel Pamoate

Pyrantel pamoate (Antiminth) is a depolarizing neuromuscular blocker that produces specific paralysis of the parasite after oral use. Pyrantel pamoate and piperazine have opposing mechanisms of action and therefore should not be administered together. Pyrantel pamoate is active against several nematodes: *A. lumbricoides* (roundworm), *Ancylostoma duodenale, Necator americanus* (hookworm), and *E. vermicularis* (pinworm). The drug is administered orally because very little is absorbed. Less than 15 percent of the drug and its metabolites are excreted in the urine.

The adverse effects include occasional headache, dizziness, drowsiness, and GI problems.

Pyrantel pamoate is available as a suspension (250 mg/5 mL) and may be mixed with fruit juices or milk. In treatment of pinworm and roundworm it is extremely effective but has been reported to produce more adverse effects than mebendazole. The adult and pediatric dosage is 11 mg/kg (maximum 1 g) taken once daily. In the treatment of pinworm the dose must be repeated in 2 weeks.

Thiabendazole

Thiabendazole (Mintezol) is a benzimidazole derivative with an unknown mode of action. It shows a broad spectrum of activity against the following nematodes: *A. lumbricoides* (roundworm), *N. americanus* (hookworm), *A. duodenale, E. vermicularis* (pinworm), *Strongyloides* (threadworm), and *Trichuris trichiura* (whipworm). Its primary use is in the treatment of strongyloidiasis.

Thiabendazole is administered orally and is rapidly absorbed from the intestinal tract, with peak plasma levels achieved in about 1 h. The drug is metabolized in the liver and then excreted by the kidney.

Thiabendazole is the drug of choice for treatment of cutaneous larva migrans (creeping eruption), strongyloidiasis, trichostrongyliasis, and trichinosis. Severe forms of visceral larva migrans also can be treated with this drug.

Frequent side effects such as anorexia, nausea, vomiting, drowsiness, and vertigo occur in up to one-third of patients treated with thiabendazole.

For treating threadworm, cutaneous larva migrans, hookworm, and whipworm infestations, the usual dosage is 25 mg/kg twice daily for 1 to 2 days.

Mebendazole

Mebendazole (Vermox) is also a benzimidazole. It inhibits glucose uptake in helminths, resulting in a depletion of glycogen and, consequently, decreased synthesis of ATP. Utilization of glucose is not affected. The drug is used for the treatment of infections caused by *E. vermicularis* (pinworm), *T. trichiura* (whipworm), *N. americanus* (hookworm), and *A. duodenale*. A large number of nematodes and cestodes from several species of animals are susceptible to mebendazole.

Mebendazole is given orally. It is poorly soluble, with only 5 to 10 percent of the drug being absorbed from the intestinal tract. Principally, the decarboxylated derivative is recovered in the urine. Most of the orally administered drug is found in the feces within 24 h.

Mebendazole is primarily used for the treatment of *T. trichiura* and *E. vermicularis* infections, in which it produces high cure rates. Because of its broad-spectrum antihelminthic effect, mixed nematode infections, as well as roundworm, hookworm, or pinworm infestations, frequently respond to therapy.

The drug is poorly absorbed and therefore is well tolerated. Abdominal discomfort and diarrhea may occur. Its use in pregnancy is contraindicated.

Mebendazole is available as 100-mg chewable tablets. The dosage for children and adults is the same. Its broad spectrum of activity against numerous worms and its convenient dosage schedules make this the drug of choice in many infestations. In the treatment of pinworm a single 100-mg dose is given. In the treatment of whipworm, hookworm, roundworm, and mixed infestations a dosage of 100 mg twice a day for 3 consecutive days is administered. A second course of therapy may be required 3 to 4 weeks later.

Clinical Pharmacology and Therapeutics of Trematode Infections

Trematodes (flukes) are nonsegmented, flattened helminths that are often leaflike in shape. The eggs, which are passed out of their hosts in sputum, urine, or feces, undergo several stages of maturation in other hosts before the larvae enter humans. The larvae are acquired either through food (aquatic vegetation, fish) or by direct penetration of the skin. After ingestion, most trematodes mature in the intestinal tract (intestinal flukes); others will migrate and mature in the liver and bile duct (liver flukes); still others penetrate the intestinal wall and migrate through the abdominal cavity to the lung (lung flukes). Diarrhea, abdominal pain, and anorexia are common symptoms associated with trematodes.

Schistosomiasis (bilharziosis) is a group of diseases caused by five different species of trematodes which belong to the genus *Schistosoma*. These helminths are cylindrical at the anterior end and flattened at the posterior end. The larvae penetrate skin that is in contact with contaminated water and then migrate through the host's lymphatics and blood vessels to the liver or lung. Approximately 3 weeks after trematode penetrations, patients complain of malaise, fever, and vague intestinal symptoms. Diarrhea or dysentery is associated with infestations by *Schistosoma mansoni* and

Schistosoma japonicum whereas hematuria and dysuria are commonly caused by *Schistosoma haematobium*.

The treatment of schistosomiasis is usually with praziquantel given in a dose of 40 mg/kg once. The treatment of *S. mansoni* will require a dosage of 20 mg/kg given three times a day for 1 day.

Paragonimus westermani and *Paragonimus kellicotti* are two species of lung flukes. Paragonimiasis therapy is with praziquantel (Biltricide) or bithional (Acetamer).

NURSING PROCESS RELATED TO HELMINTHIC INFECTIONS

The nursing process related to the use of antihelminthic drugs is outlined in Table 29-9.

CASE STUDY

S.N. is a 6-year-old white male who was referred to the hospital outpatient clinic by his school nurse. The school nurse had noticed S.N. acting "out of character" for him; he displayed unusual irritability and nervous habits such as nail biting and constant itching, especially of the anus. After discussion with S.N.'s mother, it was found she too had noticed the persistent itching, more so at night. They were referred to the outpatient clinic.

Assessment

S.N. presented as an apparently healthy, well-nourished 6-year-old boy. The physical examination was unremarkable except for reddened areas, especially around the anus, from repeated scratching.

Management

Pinworm was suspected; however, for a confirmed diagnosis, S.N.'s mother was instructed on obtaining anal

impressions on cellophane tape before her child rose in the morning and placing the impressions on glass slides. These slides were then examined under a microscope, where a definitive diagnosis of pinworm was made.

S.N. was instructed to fast and was given a single dose of pyrvinium pamoate suspension 10 mg. His parents were alerted to the fact that his stools would acquire a bright-red color following the medication. All his bed linens and clothing were boiled, and the family used good hand washing before eating and after defecating.

Evaluation

S.N.'s entire family was treated for pinworm, and his school was notified and a check of his schoolmates was done.

VIRAL INFECTIONS

LEARNING OBJECTIVES

Upon mastery of the contents of this section, the reader should be able to:

1. Explain the fundamental differences in the therapies of bacterial and viral infections.

2. Give one indication for the use of idoxuridine.

3. Give two indications and two experimental uses for acyclovir.

4. Discuss the therapy of encephalitis due to herpes simplex virus.

5. Describe two methods of increasing human interferon.

6. Give two disorders where interferon may be useful.

The basic principles that apply to the treatment of most infectious diseases unfortunately cannot always be applied in the therapy of viral infections. The use of culture and sen-

TABLE 29-9 Nursing Process Related to Antihelminthic Therapy

ASSESSMENT	MANAGEMENT	EVALUATION
	Pyrvinium Pamoate	
Used in treatment of pinworm. Contraindicated in any condition in which GI absorption might take place (denuded intestinal epithelium) or with intestinal obstruction or acute abdominal disease.	Tablets should be taken while fasting and swallowed whole to avoid staining of teeth. Liquid preparation will stain clothing if spilled on it. Stools will be colored bright red and, if emesis occurs, vomitus will be colored bright red and will stain most materials. Examine patient's fingernails for eggs; reinfection can occur from scratching anal area. Nail-biting children should wear gloves until infection has been controlled.	Adverse effects—Watch for nausea, vomiting, diarrhea, cramping, photosensitivity. About 90% or more of patients treated with pyrvinium pamoate are cured when a single effective dose is given. Since pinworm infection is so easily passed on, treatment of all members of family or group should be considered, for complete eradication of the organism.
	Mebendazole	
Indicated for whipworm, pinworm, roundworm, common hookworm, American hookworm. Contraindicated in pregnancy. Use with caution in children under 2.	Tablets may be chewed, swallowed, or crushed and mixed with food.	Adverse effects—Watch for transient symptoms of abdominal pain and diarrhea, which have occurred in cases of massive infestation and expulsion of worms. If patient is not cured 3 weeks after therapy, a second course of treatment is advised.
	Niclosamide	
Indicated for all tapeworms. Contraindicated in patients who show hypersensitivity.	Tablets should be chewed thoroughly and swallowed with a small amount of water. They should be taken after a light meal. Excretion precautions are required only for patients with pork tapeworm. Patients with fish tapeworm may need supportive therapy with vitamin B_{12} and folic acid.	Adverse effects—Watch for nausea and vomiting (low incidence), loss of appetite, abdominal discomfort, diarrhea, drowsiness, headache. Need for follow-up dosage is rare. Patients need education on adequate inspection, refrigeration, and thorough cooking of fish, beef, and pork products.
	Piperazine	
Administer with caution in presence of renal disease. Drug is not recommended in presence of epilepsy. Use with caution in severe malnutrition or anemia. Indicated for pinworm and *Ascaris* infestations.	If hypersensitivity reactions or significant CNS or GI disturbances occur, drug should be discontinued.	Adverse effects—Watch for mild nausea, vomiting, diarrhea, abdominal pain, and headache. Excessive, large doses may produce urticaria, muscle weakness, blurred vision, and vomiting. Symptoms disappear when drug use is stopped. To prevent reinfection, patient must be educated in good personal and sanitary habits, plus environmental hygiene.
	Pyrantel Pamoate	
Drug is useful against pinworm and common roundworm. Use with caution in pregnancy, in children under age 2, and in presence of liver dysfunction.	Monitor SGOT for elevation. Drug may be taken with milk or fruit juices.	Adverse effects—Watch for mostly GI symptoms, anorexia, nausea, vomiting, gastralgia.
	Thiabendazole	
Drug is effective in treatment of threadworm, cutaneous larva migrans, pinworm, trichinosis, hookworm, whipworm, and *Ascaris* infections. Use with caution in patients who have renal or hepatic dysfunction.	Side effects are decreased if drug is given after meals. Monitor blood count for leukopenia. If hypersensitivity reaction occurs (erythema multiforme), drug use should be discontinued.	Side effects occur 3–4 h after ingestion and last for 2–8 h. They include dizziness, anorexia, nausea and vomiting, abdominal cramping, diarrhea, headache, drowsiness, lethargy, and pruritus. Because CNS side effects may occur quite frequently, activities requiring mental alertness should be avoided.

sitivity tests to select the appropriate antimicrobial drugs cannot always be used in the therapy of viral infections. The use of antimicrobial agents in the treatment of other infectious diseases is based on the differences between the host cells and the invading organisms (e.g., penicillins inhibit the cell walls of the bacteria; sulfonamides inhibit the formation of folic acid). The fundamental difference between bacterial infections and viral infections is that viruses are dependent on the metabolic processes of the host cells. Therefore, many chemicals that inhibit the growth of the virus will also inhibit the host cells.

In many infections the growth of the virus reaches its maximum near the time clinical symptoms first appear or even prior to the development of symptoms. In order for antiviral agents to be clinically effective, they must be administered before the onset of disease (chemoprophylaxis). This is the case when **amantadine** is used to treat influenza A infections. In other viral infections (herpetic keratitis, disseminating herpes simplex or zoster) the replication of the virus continues after the appearance of clinical manifestations of the disease. In the treatment of these infections the inhibition of the virus replication may promote healing.

The prevention of viral replication can theoretically be achieved by inhibiting any one of the following steps:

1. Adsorption to and penetration of host cells
2. Synthesis of early, nonstructural proteins (nucleic acids polymerase)
3. Synthesis of RNA and DNA
4. Synthesis of late, structural proteins
5. Assembly (maturation) of viral particles and their release from the cell

CLINICAL PHARMACOLOGY AND THERAPEUTICS OF VIRAL INFECTIONS

Vaccines

Edward Jenner almost 200 years ago developed the first and most successful vaccine against smallpox. Now in the twentieth century smallpox is almost completely eradicated, and the principles developed with the smallpox vaccine are being used to treat other viruses and to develop other vaccines. It is hoped that the advances in vaccine technology will help to eliminate or treat viral diseases such as herpes, hepatitis, influenza, cholera, and some infections linked to cancer.

Advances in the development of biologicals were initiated by discoveries in molecular cellular biology and, in particular, in the techniques of recombinant DNA technology known as gene splicing. By taking apart the genes of the virus, biologists can alter the virus so that it can cause a body's immunologic system to develop protection against a disease without having the disease. Newer work includes the development of a single vaccine that would contain numerous messages to protect the body against multiple diseases.

The development of a multiple-purpose vaccine would have great worldwide therapeutic implications.

As with any therapeutic modality, vaccines are not totally harmless; about 1 patient in 100,000 develops a severe infection. The newer technology also is extremely expensive, which makes the newer vaccines expensive. Some people have raised objections to the research efforts involving recombinant DNA techniques. Their objections center around gene-splicing technology, which some feel may cause changes in the normal order of the universe and lead to a new form of biologic pollution. As with any treatment modality, the benefit of the treatment of the disease must be weighed against the adverse effects of the therapy.

Antiviral Drugs

Amantadine

Amantadine (Symmetrel), a tricyclic symmetric amine, inhibits penetration of the virus into susceptible cells or the uncoating of certain myxoviruses, e.g., influenza A (but not influenza B), rubella, and some tumor viruses. It therefore inhibits the replication of these viruses in vitro and in experimental animals. In humans, a daily dose of 200 mg of amantadine hydrochloride for 2 to 3 days before and 6 to 7 days after influenza A infection reduces the incidence and severity of symptoms and the magnitude of the serologic response.

When given orally, amantadine is almost completely absorbed from the gut. The drug is largely excreted by the kidneys into the urine. In persons with renal failure, amantadine may accumulate and cause toxicity.

Chemoprophylaxis with amantadine can be effective in reducing infection rates among household contacts of those with virus infections, in limiting institutional spread of infection, and in protecting adults at high risk during influenza outbreaks. Amantadine also has beneficial effects in some cases of Parkinson's disease.

Adverse effects include insomnia, slurred speech, dizziness, ataxia, and other central nervous system signs. The drug can cause release of stored catecholamines.

Idoxuridine

Idoxuridine (Stoxil) is incorporated into viral DNA, and it inhibits the replication of herpes simplex virus (HSV) in the cornea and thus aids in the healing of herpetic keratitis in humans. Idoxuridine applied to the corneal epithelium remains local and is not rapidly removed by the bloodstream. For treatment of herpes simplex keratitis, idoxuridine is applied to the cornea every 2 h around the clock by instilling 1 drop of 0.1% aqueous solution into the conjunctival sac. This tends to accelerate spontaneous healing. Ointments containing 0.5% idoxuridine have been prepared to provide higher drug concentrations.

DNA synthesis by the host cells is also affected by idoxuridine, and some toxic effects on corneal cells are occasionally observed. Idoxuridine may induce allergic contact dermatitis. Topically applied idoxuridine has limited effect on skin lesions of herpes simplex or herpes zoster.

Cytarabine

Cytarabine (cytosine arabinoside or Ara-C; Cytosar-U) inhibits DNA synthesis and interferes with the replication of DNA viruses. The toxicity is about 10 times that of idoxuridine. Because of its higher toxicity for the cornea, cytarabine has been employed topically only for patients with herpetic keratitis who have failed to respond to idoxuridine. Cytarabine 0.3 to 2 mg/kg IV as a single daily dose for 5 days has been used in severe disseminated herpes simplex.

Vidarabine

Vidarabine (adenine arabinoside or Ara-A; Vira-A) is phosphorylated in the cell to the triphosphate derivative, which inhibits viral DNA polymerase much more effectively than it inhibits mammalian DNA polymerase. In vivo, vidarabine is rapidly metabolized to arabinosylhypoxanthine (Ara-Hx), which has only slight antiviral action.

Vidarabine can be used in the treatment of encephalitis caused by the herpes simplex virus. The drug may reduce the number of deaths associated with the infection, but the neurologic complications may not be reduced. It has been used experimentally with varying results in the therapy of other viral infections. Immunocompromised patients who have varicella zoster infections respond to vidarabine, but patients with varicella zoster encephalitis do not.

The most common adverse effects are nausea, vomiting, diarrhea, anorexia, and weight loss. Pain and thrombophlebitis at the injection site may also occur.

It is recommended that vidarabine be administered IV over 12 to 24 h using an in-line membrane filter (0.45 μm or smaller). The usual dosage for adults and children with normal renal function is 15 mg/kg daily for 10 days.

Acyclovir

Mechanism of Action   Acyclovir (acycloguanosine sodium or ACV; Zovirax) has an antiviral effect due to the inhibition of DNA synthesis and the prevention of viral replication. Acyclovir inhibits the replication of herpes simplex virus and varicella zoster virus. The pharmacologically active form is acyclovir triphosphate in the treatment of herpes simplex. Its mechanism of action against other viruses (Epstein-Barr and cytomegalovirus) is not completely understood but appears to be different from that against herpes simplex.

Pharmacokinetics   After IV administration acyclovir is widely distributed to body tissues and fluid, including the CSF. In patients with normal renal function the elimination of acyclovir is biphasic, with an initial phase of 0.35 h and a terminal phase of 2 to 3.5 h. In renal disease the half-lives of both phases increase. The drug is primarily excreted unchanged in the urine. The plasma half-life of acyclovir can be increased by the administration of **probenecid** prior to the IV infusion.

Clinical Use   Acyclovir is given IV in the treatment of mucosal and cutaneous herpes simplex infections in immunocompromised patients. It can be used topically in the treatment of nonimmunocompromised patients with genital herpes (first-episode infections). It has been used experimentally in the prevention of herpes simplex infection in bone marrow transplant patients and leukemic patients and in the therapy of localized and disseminating herpes zoster infections, of varicella zoster (chicken pox) infections in immunocompromised patients, of infections caused by Epstein-Barr virus, and of infections caused by cytomegalovirus.

Acyclovir (Zovirax 5% ointment) can be applied topically to treat first-episode genital herpes. The preparation will decrease the duration of viral shedding and the number of days required for healing. Acyclovir does not modify the recurrence rate subsequent to herpes infections. It is usually applied every 4 h to the affected area. Nurses applying acyclovir cream should use an applicator or finger cot.

Adverse Effects   The adverse effects of acyclovir are usually minor following IV therapy. Most reactions are due to local effects at the site of administration. These reactions include pain, phlebitis, and inflammation. Care should be taken to prevent the extravasation of acyclovir.

Additional adverse effects include renal damage (renal tubular necrosis), nervous system effects (presenting as nervousness, jitters, delirium, dizziness, confusion, hallucinations, etc.), hematologic effects (thrombocytosis, thrombocytopenia, leukopenia, etc.), and others. The topical dosage forms appear to cause no adverse effects beyond occasional skin irritation.

Dosage   IV acyclovir should be administered by slow infusion, usually over 1 h. The usual adult dosage for patients with normal renal function is 5 mg/kg given every 8 h. In children under 12 years of age the usual dosage is 250 mg/m² given every 8 h. In patients who are immunocompromised, therapy is continued for 7 days, while nonimmunocompromised patients' therapy is for 5 days.

Interferon

Interferons are proteins which have antiviral activities. Interferons are produced in response to many viral infections. Among human interferons (IFN) three main substances are described:

1. IFN-α represents human leukocyte interferon (type 1).
2. IFN-β represents human fibroblast interferon (type 1).
3. IFN-γ represents human immune interferon (type 2).

In view of the broad range of viruses that are susceptible to inhibition by interferon, this agent can be considered a potentially valuable antiviral drug.

Many inducers of endogenous interferon (e.g., double-stranded RNA, synthetic polymers, small molecules such as tilorone) have been tested—as topical agents applied to mucous membranes or as systemic agents given by injection—for use in the therapy of viral infections. In general, the results have been less than satisfactory. While harmless and potent inducers of endogenous interferon are still being sought, the research emphasis has been to increase production of exogenous human interferon. Human interferon is now being produced in milligram quantities in pooled blood leukocytes, in fibroblasts in culture, in lymphoblastic cells in culture, or increasingly, by recombinant DNA technology, with bacteria acting as the producing cells.

Clinical studies have been performed mainly with human leukocyte interferon. When given early, interferon has prevented dissemination of herpes zoster in cancer patients, reduced cytomegalovirus shedding after renal transplantation, and prevented reactivation of herpes after trigeminal root section. In chronic active hepatitis, interferon has suppressed viremia with hepatitis B virus. Currently, the suggestion is being explored that interferon might have an adjunctive role in the management of certain neoplasms and might provide effective therapy in rabies and hemorrhagic fevers. The ultimate role of interferons in the treatment of human disease remains to be established.

The doses used have been a million to a trillion IV units daily. Adverse effects have included fatigue, weakness, anemia, and GI disturbances.

NURSING PROCESS RELATED TO ANTIVIRAL THERAPY

The nursing process with antiviral drugs is outlined in Table 29-10.

TABLE 29-10 Nursing Process Related to Antiviral Therapy

ASSESSMENT	MANAGEMENT	EVALUATION
	Amantadine	
Administer with caution to patients with any disease affecting CNS, with history of peripheral edema or with congestive heart failure, or with renal impairment, orthostatic hypotension, or liver disease.	If CNS effects develop on a once-a-day dosage schedule, a split dosage schedule may reduce complaints. Observe patients with seizure history for increased seizure activity. Monitor closely for signs of heart failure. Monitor I&O. Monitor for hypotension when patient changes position. Patients who report CNS effects or blurring of vision should be cautioned against driving or working in situations where alertness is important.	Adverse effects—Watch for CNS disturbances, depression, CHF, orthostatic hypotensive episodes, psychoses, urinary retention, and light-headedness. High doses may cause convulsions. Drug should not be discontinued abruptly, since patients with Parkinson's disease have experienced parkinsonian crisis when drug was stopped suddenly.
	Idoxuridine	
Used primarily for treatment of herpes simplex keratitis, characterized by redness of the eye, tearing, photophobia, and pain.	Hot compresses to the eye may relieve some discomfort. Hands should be washed well before and after touching the eye. Frequency of use of eye drops will decrease as symptoms improve.	May induce allergic contact dermatitis. May cause toxic effect on corneal cells.

REFERENCES

Abramowicz, M.: "Drugs for the Treatment of Tuberculosis," *Med Lett Drugs Ther,* **19**:97, 1977.

Adams, E. G., et al.: "Invasive Amebiasis-Amebic Dysentery and its Complications," *Medicine,* **56**:315, 1977.

Addington, W. W.: "Treatment of Pulmonary Tuberculosis: Current Options," *Arch Intern Med,* **139**:1391–1395, 1979.

Allen, H. et al.: "Selenium Sulfide: Adjunctive Therapy for Tinea Capitis," *Pediatrics,* **69**:81–83, 1982.

Bennett, J. E.: "Infections Caused by Higher Bacteria and Fungi," in H. Petersdorf et al. (eds.), *Principles of Internal Medicine,* 10th ed., New York: McGraw-Hill, 1983.

Brunner, L., and D. Suddarth: *Textbook of Medical-Surgical Nursing,* 3d ed., Philadelphia: Lippincott, 1975.

Buchanan, R. A.: "Pyruvium Pamoate," *Clin Pharmacol Ther,* **16**:716–719, 1974.

Byrd, R. B.: "Toxic Effects of Isoniazid in Tuberculosis, Chemoprophylaxis," *JAMA,* **241**:1239–1244, 1979.

Halloran, T.: "Convulsions Associated with High Cumulative Doses of Metronidazole," *Drug Intell Clin Pharm,* **16**:409–412, 1982.

Harland, P. S. E. G., and R. H. Meakins: "Treatment of Cutaneous Larva Migeans with Local Thiabendazol," *Br Med J,* **2**:772, 1977.

Hirsch, M. S., and M. N. Schwartz: "Antiviral Agents," *N Engl J Med,* **302**:903–949, 1980.

Johnson, F., and K. H. Wildrick: "State of the Art Review: The Impact of Chemotherapy on the Care of Patients with Tuberculosis," *Am Rev Respir Dis,* **109**:636–664, 1974.

Knight, R.: "The Chemotherapy of Amebiasis," *J Antimicrob Chemother,* **6**:577, 1980.

——, et al.: "Intestinal Parasites," *Gut,* **14**:145–168, 1973.

Lefkowitz, M. S.: "The Antimycobacterial Drugs," *Semin Respir Med,* **2**:196–201, 1981.

Lester, T. W.: "Drug Resistant and Atypical Mycobacterial Disease Bacteriology and Treatment," *Arch Intern Med,* **139**:1399–1401, 1979.

McEvoy, G. K. (ed.): "Amebicides," in *American Hospital Formulary Service, Drug Information 84,* Bethesda, Md.: American Society of Hospital Pharmacists, 1984.

——: "Antihelminths," in *American Hospital Formulary Service, Drug Information 84,* Bethesda, MD: American Society of Hospital Pharmacists, 1984.

——: "Antimalarial Agents," in *American Hospital Formulary Service, Drug Information 84,* Bethesda, MD: American Society of Hospital Pharmacists, 1984.

——: "Antiviral Agents," in *American Hospital Formulary Service, Drug Information 84,* Bethesda, MD: American Society of Hospital Pharmacists, 1984.

Mandell, G. L. (ed.): *Principles and Practice of Infectious Diseases,* vols. 1 and 2, New York: Wiley, 1979.

Plorde, J. J.: "Amebiasis," in Petersdorf et al. (eds.), *Principles of Internal Medicine,* 10th ed., New York: McGraw-Hill, 1983.

——: "Malaria," in Petersdorf et al. (eds.), *Principles of Internal Medicine,* 10th ed., New York: McGraw-Hill, 1983.

Rollo, I. M.: "Drugs Used in Chemotherapy of Amebiasis," in A. G. Gilman, L. G. Goodman, and A. Gilman (eds.), *Goodman and Gilman's The Pharmacological Basis of Therapeutics,* 6th ed., New York: Macmillan, 1980.

——: "Drugs Used in Chemotherapy of Helminthiasis," in A. G. Gilman, L. S. Goodman, and A. Gilman (eds.), *Goodman and Gilman's The Pharmacological Basis of Therapeutics,* 6th ed., New York: Macmillan, 1980.

——: "Drugs Used in Chemotherapy of Malaria," in A. G. Gilman, L. S. Goodman, and A. Gilman (eds.), *Goodman and Gilman's The Pharmacological Basis of Therapeutics,* 6th ed., New York: Macmillan, 1980.

——: "Miscellaneous Drugs Used in the Treatment of Protozoal Infections," in A. G. Gilman, L. S. Goodman, and A. Gilman (eds.), *Goodman and Gilman's The Pharmacological Basis of Therapeutics,* 6th ed., New York: Macmillan, 1980.

Sanders, W. F. "Rifampin," *Ann Intern Med,* **85**:82–86, 1976.

Trenhome, G., and P. E. Carson: "Therapy and Prophylaxis of Malaria," *JAMA,* **240**:2293–2295, 1978.

Turim-Barima, Y., and S. Carruthers: "Quinidine-Rifampin Interaction," *N Engl J Med,* **304**:1466–1469, 1981.

Wolinsky, E.: "Nontuberculosis Mycobacteria and Associated Diseases," *Am Rev Respir Dis,* **119**:107–159, 1979.

Young, L. S.: "Nosocomial Infections in the Immunocompromised Adult," *Am J Med,* **70**:398–404, 1981.

30

DISORDERS OF THE ALIMENTARY TRACT*

ANITA G. LORENZO
ANNA M. TICHY

LEARNING OBJECTIVES

Upon mastery of the content of this chapter, the reader will be able to:

1. List three common types of drug-induced gastrointestinal problems and an example of a drug that has the potential to cause each type.

2. Compare and contrast the prognosis and clinical findings of gastric versus duodenal ulcers.

3. State the mechanism of action for and the efficacy of the following modalities in the management of peptic ulcer disease: histamine (H_2) blockers, anticholinergics, antacids, sucralfate, sedatives, dietary modification, and surgery.

4. List the most common adverse effects for each agent utilized for peptic ulcer disease, including cimetidine, ranitidine, antacids, sucralfate, and anticholinergics.

5. Compare the appropriate dosage regimen and instructions that should be explained to the patient upon administration of aluminum- versus magnesium-containing antacids.

6. Indicate the nursing interventions and monitoring parameters to be utilized in the management of peptic ulcer disease patients.

7. Compare and contrast the pathology, and clinical findings of ulcerative colitis versus Crohn's disease.

8. State the rationale for and the efficacy of the following modalities in the management of inflammatory bowel disease: sulfasalazine, corticosteroids, immunosuppressants, parenteral/enteral nutrition, antidiarrheals, and surgery.

9. List the most common adverse effects for each agent utilized for inflammatory bowel disease, including sulfasalazine, antidiarrheals, and metronidazole.

10. State the appropriate dosage regimen and instructions that should be explained to the patient upon administration of sulfasalazine and corticosteroids.

11. Indicate the nursing interventions and monitoring parameters to be utilized in the management of inflammatory bowel disease patients.

12. Define the two types of hemorrhoids and clinical findings of each type.

13. State three goals of therapy for the general medical management of hemorrhoids.

14. State three cautionary instructions that should be explained to the patient upon administration of hemorrhoidal preparations.

15. Indicate the general nursing interventions in the management of patients with hemorrhoids.

16. Describe the therapeutic goals and modes of treatment for irritable bowel syndrome and gastroesophageal reflux.

ANATOMY AND PHYSIOLOGY

The alimentary tract, an epithelial-lined hollow tube which extends from the mouth to the anus, serves the important functions of digestion and absorption of nutrients and drugs (see Fig. 30-1). Ingested materials are mechanically moved through the 9 m of tract while appropriate levels of digestive enzymes and acid are secreted to break down complex biochemical structures and facilitate absorption. The secretory and contractile activities of the gastrointestinal tract are regulated by the nervous system. Intrinsic neuronal synapses enable activity initiated in one segment of the alimentary tract to influence contractility and secretion in another. The extrinsic parasympathetic influence mediated by two branches of the vagal nerve is primarily excitatory, augmenting peristalsis, muscle tone, and secretion. The sympathetic splanchnic innervation, mediated by branches from the celiac plexus, is primarily inhibitory to secretion and motility. The activity within the alimentary tract, therefore,

*The editors thank Kenneth J. Bender, who was a cocontributor of the chapter on this subject in the first edition.

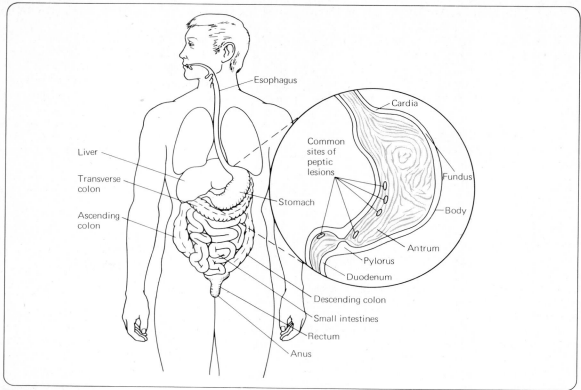

FIGURE 30-1

Structures of the Alimentary Tract. Common sites of peptic ulcer formation are illustrated in relation to the anatomy of the stomach and duodenum.

may be influenced by receptors within the tract responding to local stimuli such as mechanical distention and chemical composition of luminal contents, as well as by external factors such as emotional and behavioral stimuli.

Gastric Secretory Activity

The stomach epithelium has a unique regenerative capacity, undergoing a complete turnover every 5 days. The epithelial lining forms invaginations or gastric pits into which numerous glands empty their secretions. The cell type determines the nature of the secretory products. An alkaline, viscid fluid which protects against autodigestion is secreted by the surface epithelial cells and by mucous neck cells. The gastric glands of the fundus and body of the stomach contain parietal cells, which are responsible for hydrochloric acid secretion, and chief cells, which are the source of the proteolytic enzyme pepsin. Pepsinogen, the inactive precursor of pepsin, is continuously synthesized and stored intracellularly in zymogen granules. The accumulated granules are discharged in response to stimuli such as the cholinergic mediator acetylcholine, gastrin, histamine, and caffeine. An acidic pH of

2 is optimal for a rapid conversion of pepsinogen to the active form, pepsin. Pepsin is autocatalytic in that it initiates the activation of more pepsinogen. As an endopeptidase, pepsin cleaves bonds within a polypeptide chain. The antral region of the stomach is the site of gastrin production. Following absorption into the bloodstream, gastrin stimulates the parietal and to a lesser degree the chief cells to induce acid-pepsin secretion. Vagal impulses, mechanical distention of the antrum, an alkaline environment, and certain secretagogues such as caffeine, protein digestion products, meat extracts, and alcohol are potent stimulants of gastrin release.

The parietal cells secrete an isotonic solution which contains a hydrogen ion concentration of approximately 160 meq/L. This concentration remains constant regardless of the rate of secretion. The determinants of secretory rate are the numbers of parietal cells, the degree of gastric distention, the presence of stimulants such as vagal impulses, gastrin, and histamine, and the amount of inhibitory forces, which include secretin and cholecystokinin. The intake of food is followed by a large secretory response, in contrast to the small basal secretion which occurs during interdigestive periods. Although the gastric secretion of hydrochloric acid is not essential to digestion, it serves such important functions as the activation of pepsinogen, denaturation of proteins, and destruction of some bacteria. Intrinsic factor, necessary for vitamin B_{12} absorption in the small intestine, is also secreted by the parietal cells. A deficiency of intrinsic factor results in pernicious anemia (see Chap. 36).

DRUG-INDUCED GASTROINTESTINAL DISEASE

Drug-induced diseases and adverse drug reactions must be considered whenever a patient complains of gastrointestinal symptoms. Patients may exhibit mild but annoying side effects such as nausea and constipation. However, severe pathologic conditions, including small bowel perforation and pseudomembranous colitis, may be manifestations of drug therapy. A complete drug history is essential to rule out drug-induced gastrointestinal (GI) disease in these patients (see Table 30-1 for drug-induced effects).

Pseudomembranous colitis is a drug-induced problem manifested by fever, abdominal pain, and mild to severe diarrhea. The most plausible mechanism is proliferation of colonic clostridia during administration of broad-spectrum antimicrobials. The clostridia produce a toxin which locally injures the colonic mucosa. Management includes stopping the antibiotic. If the diagnosis is confirmed and the organism is sensitive, oral **vancomycin** (Vancocin) or **metronidazole** (Flagyl) is administered. **Cholestyramine** (Questran) may be helpful in mild cases.

PEPTIC ULCER DISEASE

It is estimated that peptic ulcer disease occurs in approximately 10 percent of the population. A peptic ulcer is a circumscribed epithelial defect which extends through the muscularis mucosa and the submucosa, and can penetrate the muscularis propria. The lesions, which can be single or multiple, can occur in any region exposed to the acid-peptic proteolytic activity of gastric juice, such as the gastric or duodenal mucosa.

It is useful clinically to classify peptic ulcers according to anatomic location (see Fig. 30-1). Although gastric and duodenal ulcers are similar pathologically, the prognostic and therapeutic implications are different.

Duodenal ulcers are usually located within 3 cm of the pylorus. They are the most common type, making up 80 percent of all peptic ulcers. Duodenal ulcer disease is a chronic condition with irregular periods of remission and exacerbation. The majority of patients have relatively benign disease that only requires medical management during the periods of exacerbation. About 10 to 20 percent of patients

with duodenal ulcer disease develop intractable symptoms or severe complications.

Gastric ulcers are usually located in the antrum or near the antral-fundic junction and may occur in patients with preexisting duodenal ulcers. Unlike duodenal ulcers, many gastric ulcers are asymptomatic, and may be first diagnosed with the onset of severe complications such as perforation. Patients with symptoms of gastric ulcer tend to have a chronic condition that responds poorly to medical management. In addition, about 7 percent of cases originally diagnosed as gastric ulcer disease are later found to be gastric carcinoma.

Zollinger-Ellison syndrome is a condition of excessive secretion of gastrin from a pancreatic tumor. The high gastrin levels result in profound gastric hypersecretion and fulminant peptic ulceration. The presentation of Zollinger-Ellison syndrome is similar to duodenal ulcer disease except that the condition is commonly resistant to medical and/or surgical therapy, resulting in death secondary to ulcerative complications.

Etiology

The causes and pathogenetic mechanisms of peptic ulcer remain unexplained despite numerous theories and investigative studies. Current concepts deal with this disease as a localized disruption of the gastric or duodenal mucosa resulting from a physiologic disturbance in the balance of aggressive and defensive factors. The aggressive factor is the acid-pepsin component of gastric juice, which is the immediate agent of mucosal damage. The defensive factor, the gastric mucosal barrier (GMB), consists of a layer of surface columnar epithelial cells and a coating of mucus. These components impede diffusion of acid (hydrogen ion) from the gastric lumen into the mucosa.

GMB integrity may be impaired by chemical or mechanical agents that loosen tight junctions between cells, disrupt the lipid layer of epithelial cells, or lyse cells. Agents such as taurocholic acid, alcohol, and acetylsalicylic acid (aspirin) have been experimentally shown to increase mucosal permeability and hydrogen ion back diffusion (see Table 30-1 for drug-induced effects).

The relation of emotions to ulcerogenesis is not clear. It has been postulated that psychologic stress induces ulcer formation neurally through thalamic vagal stimulation and hormonally via the hypothalamic or hypophyseal-pituitary-adrenal axis. Stress situations are characterized by both elevated adrenocorticotropic (ACTH) hormone levels and cortisol secretion. The mechanisms by which these hormones may induce peptic ulcer are not clear.

Preventive or treatment modalities will ultimately depend on a definitive theory for the etiology and pathogenesis of ulcer disease which can satisfactorily explain the complex interrelationships of psychosocial and physiologic factors.

TABLE 30-1 Drug-Induced Gastrointestinal Disease*

DRUG	COMMENT
Malabsorption	
Alcohol	Direct effect of chronic alcohol abuse on the GI tract causing malabsorption of protein, thiamine, folic acid, vitamin B_{12}, sodium, water, fat, and D-xylose.
Cholestyramine	Binds bile acid anions, resulting in steatorrhea and malabsorption of fat and the fat-soluble vitamins D and K.
Neomycin	Mild malabsorption of a variety of nutrients and impaired absorption of digoxin.
Aluminum hydroxide antacids	Bind phosphate in the GI lumen, resulting in decreased absorption of dietary phosphate.
Laxatives containing bisacodyl, phenolphthalein	Laxative abuse may result in mild malabsorption of a variety of nutrients.
Colchicine	Mild steatorrhea and vitamin B_{12} malabsorption.
Antineoplastics	Lactose malabsorption and milk intolerance.
Drug-Induced Ulcers	
Salicylates, phenylbutazone, ibuprofen, and other nonsteroidal anti-inflammatory agents	Gastric bleeding and dyspepsia reported. Mechanisms include back diffusion of hydrogen ions and mucosal injury, altered mucous secretion and composition, as well as inhibition of prostaglandins with increased gastric acid secretion.
Corticosteroids	Not associated with peptic ulcer disease except in high-dosage and chronic regimens or in patients with prior ulcer disease.
Potassium salts (slow-release forms, e.g., Micro-K, Slow-K)	Local tissue damage may result in erosions or ulcerations of the esophagus, stomach, or duodenum.
Antineoplastics (methotrexate, bleomycin, 5-fluorouracil)	Gingivitis, glossitis, pharyngitis, stomatitis, and ulcerations with bleeding of the mucosal membranes of the mouth or other portions of the GI tract may occur.
Drug-Induced Colitis	
Antimicrobials Penicillin, amoxicillin, ampicillin, lincomycin, nafcillin, clindamycin, cephalexin, cefazolin, cephalothin, cefoxitin, tetracycline, chloramphenicol, metronidazole, cotrimoxazole, erythromycin, and aminoglycosides (oral)	Pseudomembranous colitis most likely caused by clostridial toxins.
Antineoplastics Bleomycin, methotrexate, 5-fluorouracil, 6-mercaptopurine	Hemorrhagic enterocolitis due to destruction of rapidly dividing GI tract cells may lead to intestinal perforation.

*Drugs which induce constipation and diarrhea are discussed in Chap. 20.

Clinical Findings

History

The outstanding symptom of peptic ulcer disease is an episodic, epigastric pain that occurs most frequently 1 to several hours after meals. In contrast to the 2- to 3-h postprandial pain characteristic of duodenal ulcer, gastric ulcer pain is manifested 30 to 90 min after ingestion of a meal. Nocturnal discomfort between midnight and 3 A.M., when acid secretion is at its peak, is of diagnostic importance in duodenal ulcer disease. The discomfort varies in intensity from a hunger pang to more severe forms such as gnawing, aching, burning, and cramping. Relief may be obtained by buffering the gastric secretions with food, by removing the gastric content by vomiting or aspiration, and by the administration of certain drugs.

Complications of ulcers include pyloric obstruction (resulting from edema or scarring), perforation, and hemorrhage. The nurse must be aware of the features of these possible complications in order to assess the patient's condition and initiate appropriate interventions.

Physical Examination

Since the major physical sign of uncomplicated peptic ulcer disease is a well-localized epigastric tenderness, the patient should be asked to indicate areas of tenderness. Gentle percussion, rather than palpation, may be more useful in localizing this site, and the patient's facial expression should be monitored for the duration of the examination period. Once peptic ulcer disease is suggested by subjective symptoms and clinical manifestations, confirmation must come from diagnostic laboratory procedures, including upper-gastrointestinal x-rays and gastroscopy.

A perforated ulcer will cause severe generalized abdominal pain with the characteristic facial expressions of agony. The pain may radiate to the shoulder or back. A boardlike, abdominal rigidity is characteristic of peritonitis. The patient may guard against or resist any positional change. The rigidity may be so severe as to preclude effective palpation. "Rebound" tenderness may also be present. On auscultation, bowel sounds may not be audible, indicating cessation of peristalsis. However, with pyloric obstruction, 50 percent of the cases are characterized by visible peristaltic waves and audible, hyperactive bowel sounds. Complications such as hemorrhage may be manifested by abdominal distention, which may or may not be accompanied by tenderness.

Clinical Pharmacology and Therapeutics

Attenuating the effects of acid secretion is the current cornerstone of medical therapy for peptic ulcer disease. Histamine H_2 blockers, antacids, and sucralfate are all effective modes of therapy for duodenal ulcers, gastric ulcers, and Zollinger-Ellison syndrome. Adjunctive therapy for peptic ulcer disease includes anticholinergic drugs, antianxiety agents, and dietary adjustments. Surgery may be necessary for disease refractory to medical therapy or for life-threatening complications.

Histamine H_2 Receptor Antagonists

Histamine-induced responses are mediated by at least two known receptors. H_1 receptors are antagonized by conventional antihistamines such as **diphenydramine** (Benadryl) which are used in the treatment of allergies. H_2 receptors are blocked by a class of agents which includes **cimetidine** (Tagamet) and **ranitidine** (Zantac), used in the treatment of peptic ulcers. A new era in the treatment of peptic ulcer disease is apparent with the discovery of H_2 receptors in 1972.

Mechanism of Action Cimetidine and ranitidine inhibit basal and nocturnal gastric acid secretion stimulated not only by histamine but also by pentagastrin, food, or a physiologic vagal reflex. One theory postulates that H_2 antagonists inhibit acid secretion by blocking the effects of histamine on its receptor and eliminating the potentiating effect of histamine on gastrin and acetylcholine. A 300-mg dose of cimetidine before a meal raises the mean gastric pH to a value of 3 to 5 for 3 h and to a value of 6 in 4 h. Ranitidine, on a weight basis, is about 5 to 10 times more potent than cimetidine in blocking gastric acid secretion. Both drugs reduce pepsin secretion but have little or no effect on secretion of intrinsic factor, gastrin, or mucus.

Pharmacokinetics **Cimetidine** can be administered orally, intravenously, or intramuscularly. Bioavailability is 60 to 70 percent for an oral dose. Most of the drug is excreted unchanged by the kidney, with only 20 percent metabolized in the liver. Patients with decreased renal function require either a decreased dosing frequency or a decreased dosage. The manufacturer recommends administering 300 mg every 12 h if creatinine clearance is less than 30 mL/min. The drug is removed by hemodialysis and should be given just after completion of the procedure. Adequate inhibition of gastric acid secretion is maintained for 6 to 8 h, although the serum half-life of cimetidine is 2 to 3 h.

Ranitidine is well-absorbed orally; however, oral bioavailability is about 50 percent due to first-pass metabolism. About 50 to 70 percent of an oral dose is excreted unchanged in the urine. The serum half-life after a single oral dose is 2 to 2½ h. Ranitidine is metabolized to three metabolites which are weak H_2 antagonists and are considered to have no significant pharmacologic effect. Patients with decreased renal function require a reduced total dosage. Adequate inhibition of gastric acid secretion is maintained for 8 to 12 h.

Adverse Effects The incidence of adverse effects during short-term treatment (less than 3 months) for peptic ulcer disease is relatively small. Minor reactions occur more frequently with longer therapy. The most common side effects are gastrointestinal (2.1 percent), such as diarrhea and dyspepsia, and central nervous system reactions (1.2 percent). Central nervous system effects include somnolence, confusion, restlessness, lethargy, agitation, visual hallucinations, seizures, and slurred speech. These side effects are more frequent in high-dosage regimens, in the elderly or young, or in renal or hepatic disease. **Cimetidine** is reported to have caused granulocytopenia in rare instances. A common adverse reaction to cimetidine is a small, reversible rise in the serum creatinine. Endocrine effects include development of gynecomastia. Gynecomastia is probably due to an antiandrogen property and occurs infrequently. Other reported adverse effects are rare, including interstitial nephritis, bradycardia, hepatitis, and cholestasis.

Ranitidine, unlike cimetidine, is reported to lack antiandrogenic effects. Other reported side effects include bradycardia, increased serum creatinine, decreased white blood cell count, skin rash, diarrhea, dyspepsia, impotence, dizziness, headache, and mental confusion.

Drug Interactions   Cimetidine may potentially interact with many drugs because it inhibits the hepatic microsomal oxidative system, reduces hepatic blood flow, and increases the pH of the gastrointestinal tract. Clinically important interactions include cimetidine's inhibition of the elimination of **warfarin** (coumarin anticoagulants), benzodiazepines (**diazepam**, **chlordiazepoxide**), **theophylline**, **phenytoin**, β-adrenergic antagonists (**propranolol**, **metoprolol**), and **lidocaine**.

Ranitidine does not inhibit the cytochrome P450 mixed function oxygenase enzyme system in the liver. However, there are reports of inhibition of several drugs that are metabolized in the liver, and considerably more research is indicated on the drug interactions of this newer agent.

Clinical Indications   Cimetidine is effective in healing duodenal and gastric ulcers; however, the ulcers may reoccur. Maintenance therapy is useful to prevent the recurrence of duodenal ulcers and may be useful for gastric ulcers. The Zollinger-Ellison syndrome is also treated with cimetidine. The use of cimetidine to treat upper-gastrointestinal bleeding, reflux esophagitis, acute pancreatitis, acid aspiration syndrome, or nonulcer dyspepsia is not supported with scientific data, although it is frequently used for these conditions. Cimetidine is less effective than antacids in maintaining a gastric pH greater than 4 and preventing gastrointestinal bleeding from any cause, including peptic and stress ulcers.

Clinical trials show **ranitidine**, a newer drug, to be effective in the treatment of duodenal ulcers, gastric ulcers, and Zollinger-Ellison syndrome. The drug appears to be as effective as cimetidine in the prophylaxis of duodenal ulcers. Ranitidine is reported to heal duodenal ulcers in some patients who failed to heal on cimetidine therapy.

Dosage and Preparations   The usual dosage regimen for treatment of duodenal and gastric ulcers is 300 mg of **cimetidine** (Tagamet) four times a day (with meals and at bedtime) for 6 to 8 weeks. Prophylaxis for duodenal ulcers requires a single 400-mg dose at bedtime. For treatment of Zollinger-Ellison syndrome, 1200 to 2400 mg of the drug is given daily in divided doses. The dosage in renal failure should be reduced. Cimetidine is available in tablets, liquid for injection, and in oral liquid. Clinical experience with the use of cimetidine in children is very limited, although doses of 20 to 40 mg/kg/day have been used when benefits clearly outweighed the risks.

The usual dosage regimen of **ranitidine** (Zantac) for treatment of duodenal and gastric ulcers is 150 mg two times a day. Prophylaxis for duodenal ulcer requires a single 150-mg dose at bedtime. For treatment of Zollinger-Ellison syndrome, 600 to 900 mg of the drug is given daily in divided doses. The dosage in renal failure should be reduced. Ranitidine is available in the solid oral and injectable dosage forms. Safety and efficacy of the use of ranitidine in children have not been established.

Antacids

Antacids are prescribed in large quantities as effective therapy for peptic ulcer disease. Commercially available products vary greatly in their ingredient formulation, buffering capacity, regimen expense, and adverse effects.

Mechanism of Action   The primary mechanism by which antacids reduce ulcer pain is elevation of gastric pH. Adding alkali raises the gastric pH above the optimum for pepsin activity. Pepsin activity is completely inhibited between pH 4.0 and 5.0. Therefore, the goal of antacid therapy is to maintain a gastric pH between 4.0 and 5.0.

Other mechanisms for pain relief are proposed as patients with achlorhydria also obtain benefit from antacid therapy. These mechanisms include tightening of the mucosal barrier and increasing lower-esophageal sphincter tone. Antacids do not absorb acid or coat the ulcer.

The antacid regimens are formulated to maintain an elevation of gastric pH in order to promote healing. The effectiveness of antacids in raising gastric pH in vivo is correlated with their ability to neutralize acid in vitro (buffering or neutralizing capacity). As shown in Table 30-2, the neutralizing capacity of antacids varies as much as fivefold.

Pharmacokinetics   Insoluble antacids depend on particle size for neutralization of acid. A smaller particle size increases the surface area of the antacid; an increased surface area optimizes the effectiveness of the antacid. Tablet antacids must be thoroughly masticated to decrease particle size. Liquid antacid suspensions already have a fine particle size and a large surface area. Liquid antacids are more effective than tablet antacids in neutralizing acid on a milligram for milligram basis.

The four major types of antacids have significantly different pharmacokinetic properties. **Sodium bicarbonate** is highly soluble with a rapid onset, but a short duration of action. The drug is completely absorbed, which causes a sodium and alkali load to the system that makes it contraindicated for chronic therapy.

Calcium carbonate exerts a rapid, prolonged, and potent neutralization of gastric acid. The drug reacts with hydrochloric acid to form calcium chloride, which may be absorbed while in the stomach. Approximately 5 to 10 percent of the calcium dose may be absorbed systemically; the rest is converted back to insoluble calcium salts in the small intestine and excreted in the feces.

Aluminum may be formulated as the hydroxide, carbonate, phosphate, or aminoacetate salts. The drug is a relatively weak antacid. The aluminum can be absorbed systemically and accumulate in bone and brain, especially in patients with diminished renal function.

Magnesium is the fourth major type of antacid. The salts of magnesium include the oxide, hydroxide, and trisilicate. **Magnesium hydroxide** is the most commonly used and the most potent of the three salts. The drug has a rapid onset and somewhat prolonged duration. Magnesium salts react with hydrochloric acid to form magnesium chloride. About 15 to 30 percent of the total dose is absorbed in this form. Usually the magnesium is then rapidly eliminated by the kidneys. In renal failure, caution must be exercised to prevent accumulation and hypermagnesemia.

Adverse Effects The adverse effects of antacids depend upon the ingredients in the commercial formulation, the pharmacokinetics of the drug, and the concomitant diseases of the patient. The most serious adverse effects include electrolyte distrubances, gastric hypersecretion, and milk-alkali syndrome. Constipation and diarrhea are common side effects of aluminum and magnesium antacids, respectively.

Electrolyte disturbances are a common side effect of all the antacids. **Sodium bicarbonate** ingestion may lead to systemic alkalosis and sodium retention. Each gram of sodium bicarbonate contains 12 meq of sodium. Large daily intakes may cause sodium and water retention, especially in patients with cirrhosis, heart failure, or renal disease. The normal

TABLE 30-2 Liquid Antacid Preparations

BRAND NAME	Ingredients (mg/5 mL)			Dosage (mL) USUAL[1]/HIGH[2]	NEUTRALIZING CAPACITY (meq)[3]	SODIUM (mg/5 mL)
	AlOH	MgOH	OTHER			
AlternaGel	—	600	—	5–10/60	12	2
Amphojel	320	—	—	10/110	13	7
Basaljel	400[4]	—	—	10/50	28	2
Basaljel Extra	1000[4]	—	—	5/30	22	23
Bisodol	—	475[5]	644[6]	5/45	15	196
Delcid	600	665	—	5/15	42	15
Di-Gel	282	87	20[7]	10/80	18	9
Gelusil	200	200	25[7]	10/60	24	1
Gelusil II	400	400	30[7]	10/30	48	1
Maalox	225	200	—	10–20/50	27	1
Maalox Plus	225	200	25[7]	10–20/50	27	1
Maalox T.C.	600	300	—	5–10/25	28.3	1
Mylanta	200	100	20[7]	5–10/55	12.7	1
Mylanta II	400	400	30[7]	5–10/30	25.4	1
Riopan	—	—	480[8]	5–10/50	13.5	1
Titralac	—	—	1000[9]	5/35	20	11

[1]Recommended by the manufacturer.

[2]The number of milliliters (to the nearest teaspoonful) required to neutralize 140 meq of acid (see text).

[3]The meq of acid neutralized in a 15-min standardized test by the lowest usual dose recommended by the manufacturer, which is the basis for the statement of acid neutralizing capacity in the labeling of antacid products required by the United States Food and Drug Administration (*Federal Register,* **39:**19862, 1974).

[4]Aluminum carbonate gel.

[5]Magnesium carbonate.

[6]Sodium bicarbonate.

[7]Simethicone.

[8]Magaldrate.

[9]Calcium carbonate.

Source: Adapted from *The Medical Letter,* **24:**62, June, 1982. Used by permission.

daily sodium intake should be 50 to 70 meq/m² of body surface area. Manufacturers have reformulated most other antacids to contain minor amounts of sodium as listed in Table 30-2.

Aluminum antacids bind phosphate in the gastrointestinal tract. The decreased absorption of this electrolyte may result in significant *hypophosphatemia*. Phosphate depletion may be manifested by anorexia, malaise, muscle weakness, and osteomalacia. Serum phosphate levels should be monitored at least every 2 weeks to prevent this complication during chronic therapy.

Any antacids containing calcium, aluminum, or magnesium may accumulate in the body and cause toxicity. *Hypercalcemia* may induce neurologic, gastrointestinal, or renal symptoms. *Accumulation* of *aluminum* in the brain causes a neurologic syndrome. *Elevation* of *magnesium* levels is manifested by hypotension, gastrointestinal, and neuromuscular side effects. These problems are accentuated in renal failure. Patients who have decreased renal function should be administered aluminum and magnesium antacids only with careful monitoring.

Gastric hypersecretion is another major side effect of antacids. **Sodium bicarbonate** and **calcium bicarbonate** have both been implicated in causing an acid rebound phenomenon. Sodium bicarbonate reacts with hydrochloric acid to form carbon dioxide and gastric distention. Gastric distention results in further release of acid. Calcium seems to have a local effect on gastrin-producing cells resulting in hypergastrinemia and hypersecretion. Neither of these antacids should be used for chronic therapy of peptic ulcer disease.

Finally, the *milk-alkali syndrome* has been reported with **sodium bicarbonate** and **calcium carbonate**, although more commonly with the former. The syndrome consists of hypercalcemia, renal insufficiency, and metabolic alkalosis. The symptoms of nausea, vomiting, headache, mental confusion, and anorexia should reverse when the antacid is discontinued.

Drug Interactions Antacids have the potential for interacting with many other drugs. The alkali can raise the pH of the gastrointestinal tract and the urine, which may alter absorption and/or excretion of drugs. The antacids contain polyvalent cations (e.g., calcium, magnesium, and aluminum) which are capable of forming insoluble chelates with other drugs. An important and well-documented interaction is the impaired absorption of **tetracycline** by antacids containing polyvalent cations. Tetracycline should not be administered within an hour or two of the administration of these antacids. Other drug interactions are not well-documented or the clinical significance has not been established. Close monitoring should be undertaken when antacids are concomitantly administered with **iron, isoniazid, phenothiazines, quinidine, salicylates,** or **sodium polystyrene sulfonate resin.**

Clinical Indications Antacids are effective in healing duodenal and gastric ulcers. They are utilized prophylactically to maintain a gastric pH greater than 5.5 units in critically ill patients in order to prevent stress-induced ulcers. Antacids (given in doses of 140 meq of neutralizing capacity seven times a day) are as effective as cimetidine in healing duodenal ulcers.

Dosage and Preparations The antacid of choice for peptic ulcer disease is a high-potency antacid containing a combination of magnesium hydroxide and aluminum hydroxide. The combination of aluminum and magnesium decreases the potential for adverse effects from either drug. The intensive dosage regimen proven to be effective in peptic ulcer disease is the equivalent of 140 meq of neutralizing capacity administered seven times per day. The doses are usually given 1 and 3 h after meals and before bedtime. Using Table 30-2 as a guide, one can determine that 15 mL of Delcid, 30 mL of Gelusil II, or 110 mL of Amphojel are required for one dose. It is apparent that many of the products require large volumes to be administered and are expensive (range of $40 to $70 for 1 month of therapy). Therefore, a concentrated formula requiring less volume and expense is preferred.

Most of the manufacturers' "recommended or usual doses" are much lower than the equivalent of 140 meq of neutralizing capacity. In addition, the intensive dosage regimens for treatment of peptic ulcer disease differ significantly from the prescriptions written "antacids to be given as needed for pain," which are employed only to achieve symptomatic relief.

Antacids are available as chewing gums, tablets, lozenges, powders, and liquids. Tablets are convenient for symptomatic relief of pain. However, a very large number of tablets are required to neutralize 140 meq of acid. For example, a patient would need to take 17 Gelusil II tablets per dose for treatment of peptic ulcer disease. Liquid antacids are always preferred for intensive therapy.

Anticholingerics

Mechanism of Action Anticholinergic agents competitively inhibit the effect of acetylcholine at the parasympathetic junctions. Medium to large doses reduce gastric acid secretion, gastrointestinal motility, and bladder contractility. Lower doses dry respiratory tract secretions, dry the mouth, and dilate the pupils.

Adverse Effects At the dosages necessary to affect peptic ulcer disease, anticholinergic side effects will accompany therapy. The common adverse reactions include dry mouth, urinary retention, constipation, blurred vision, drowsiness, dizziness, and tachycardia. Elderly patients are especially sensitive to the anticholinergic side effects; these agents should be used with caution in this population. These drugs are contraindicated in cases of preexisting narrow-angle glaucoma, obstructive uropathy, intestinal obstruction, paralytic ileus, unstable cardiovascular status, severe ulcerative colitis, toxic megacolon, reflux esophagitis, toxemia of pregnancy, and myasthenia gravis.

Drug Interactions Anticholinergic agents may interact with other drugs possessing anticholinergic properties such as phenothiazines and tricyclic antidepressants to increase the incidence or severity of these side effects. By slowing gastric emptying, anticholinergics may decrease the rate of absorption of other drugs; but the total amount of drug absorbed is probably not affected. The combination of anticholinergic drugs with sedatives or alcohol may increase drowsiness.

Clinical Indications The anticholinergic agents have been used in treating peptic ulcer disease for many years. However, there are no controlled clinical trials proving the efficacy of anticholinergics as *single* agents for the treatment or prevention of duodenal and gastric ulcers. Anticholinergics are not effective therapy for peptic ulcer disease compared with antacids or cimetidine. They may be useful as *adjunctive therapy* in the Zollinger-Ellison syndrome, in patients with nonhealing ulcers, and for peptic ulcer disease. Anticholinergics should not be used alone or recommended as first-line drugs in the treatment of ulcers.

Dosage and Preparations An optimum schedule for dosing anticholinergic drugs is 30 min prior to meals and at bedtime. This spacing with meals allows peak action of the anticholinergic to occur at approximately the time that acid secretion is maximal. Bedtime administration minimizes nocturnal basal gastric acid secretion. Table 30-3 lists several anticholinergic agents presently available.

Combination anticholinergic preparations are often prescribed in peptic ulcer disease. These products contain various ingredients including antianxiety agents, barbiturates, ergot alkaloids, antihistamines, and kaolin, as well as one or more anticholinergic drugs (e.g., Cantil with phenobarbital, Donnatal, Librax, Bellergal). None of these preparations is indicated in the rational therapeutics of peptic ulcer disease, because they increase the cost of therapy and the incidence of adverse effects. If the patient needs a sedative or antianxiety drug, a single agent with the dosage titrated to that appropriate to the individual should be used rather than one of these fixed-dosage combination preparations.

The nurse should warn the patient of the potential for drowsiness and blurred vision with anticholinergic drugs. These side effects may make the operation of a car or hazardous machinery dangerous. Dry mouth and photophobia may be somewhat relieved by chewing sugarless gum and wearing sunglasses, respectively.

Sucralfate

Sucralfate (Carafate) is a unique addition to the therapeutic armamentarium of peptic ulcer disease. It is the only drug presently on the market that enhances mucosal defense.

Mechanism of Action Sucralfate is a complex salt of aluminum hydroxide with a sulfated sucrose skeleton. When the drug encounters acid in the stomach, it becomes a highly condensed adhesive substance. This property is maintained as it moves through the alkaline duodenum. As sucralfate goes into solution, it becomes a highly polar anion

TABLE 30-3 Anticholinergic Agents

GENERIC NAME	TRADE NAME	ADULT DOSAGE*	CHILD DOSAGE†
Anisotropine	Valpin 50	50 mg	
Belladonna			
Extract	—	15 mg	
Tincture	—	0.6–1.0 mL	0.03 mL/kg
Clidinium	Quarzan	2.5–5.0 mg	
Glycopyrrolate	Robinul	1.0–2.0 mg	
Hyoscyamine (L)	Levsin, Cystospaz	0.125–0.25 mg‡	
Isopropamide	Darbid	5.0–10 mg§	
Mepenzolate	Cantil	25–50 mg	
Methantheline	Banthine	50–100 mg	12.5–50 mg
Methscopolamine	Pamine	2.5–5.0 mg	
Oxyphenonium	Antrenyl	5.0–10 mg	
Propantheline	ProBanthine	7.5–30 mg	1.5–3.0 mg/kg/day

*All doses are to be given three to four times daily by mouth unless otherwise noted.
†Only a few of these drugs are approved for use in children.
‡Hyoscyamine (L) is to be given every 4 h.
§Isopropamide is to be given every 12 h.

which binds positively charged protein molecules to prevent peptic hydrolysis. The drug also directly adsorbs pepsin and inhibits peptic activity. Finally, sucralfate adsorbs bile salts from the gastric lumen. In summary, sucralfate acts in three ways to heal ulcers; (1) by forming a protective barrier at the ulcer site, (2) by preventing diffusion of hydrogen ions, and (3) by inhibiting the action of pepsin.

Pharmacokinetics Sucralfate is nonsystemic in action. Less than 5 percent of an oral dose is absorbed. More than 90 percent of the drug is recovered unchanged in the stool; the rest of the dose is excreted unchanged in the urine. Sucralfate has a prolonged duration of action. Binding to gastric ulcers is demonstrated up to 6 h after dosing.

Adverse Effects and Drug Interactions Sucralfate is minimally absorbed and has minimal side effects. The most common side effect is constipation, which occurs in less than 3 percent of patients. Other reported side effects are usually minor and occur rarely, including diarrhea, nausea, indigestion, dry mouth, rash, pruritus, back pain, dizziness, sleepiness, and vertigo. The physiologic function of the gastrointestinal tract remains virtually unchanged during therapy. There are no known contraindications to the use of sucralfate. To date, there are no clinically significant drug interactions with sucralfate; although careful surveillance is suggested.

Clinical Indications Sucralfate is effective in the treatment of duodenal ulcers. Healing rates for gastric ulcers are less impressive. The efficacy of sucralfate in peptic ulcer disease is comparable with that of H_2 blockers. The use of sucralfate in the prevention of peptic ulcer disease requires further study at this time. An additive or synergistic effect with cimetidine or intensive antacids and sucralfate has not been studied. Sucralfate is approved by the Food and Drug Administration for short-term (up to 8 weeks) treatment of duodenal ulcers.

Dosage and Preparations The recommended dose of sucralfate is 1.0 g four times a day on an empty stomach. The drug should be taken 1 h before each meal and at bedtime. The tablet is scored and may be broken in half for easier swallowing. Antacids may be prescribed as needed for relief of pain but should not be taken within ½ h before or after sucralfate. Treatment should be continued for 4 to 8 weeks unless healing has been demonstrated by x-ray or endoscopic examination.

Adjunctive Therapy
Early medical literature often states that the typical ulcer patient is high-strung, hard-driving, and anxious. In fact, peptic ulcer disease occurs in a wide variety of individuals with no signs or symptoms of anxiety or hyperactivity. Psychotherapy does not promote or prevent the recurrence of peptic ulcers. Bed rest is advised only in patients with intractable symptoms. Sedatives are adjunctive therapy and prescribed for a few, selected patients.

There is no evidence of the effectiveness of frequent soft, bland meals with high milk or cream content in the treatment of ulcers. In fact, such a diet may potentially be harmful. There is evidence that milk may be detrimental to ulcers because the calcium and protein stimulate increased gastric acid secretion. Elimination of roughage produces constipation, and withdrawal of spices sharply decreases palatability. Neither has been shown to affect the clinical course of peptic ulcer disease.

Patients should be encouraged to eat as normal a diet as possible and avoid offending agents. Patients who report that certain foods irritate their stomach should eliminate these foods. **Alcohol** and **caffeine** are known stimulants of gastric acid secretion and need to be discontinued. Caffeine is an ingredient in many soft drinks as well as in tea and coffee. The association between **nicotine** and peptic ulcer disease is controversial, but smoking should be avoided, if possible.

NURSING PROCESS RELATED TO PEPTIC ULCERS

The nursing process associated with the care of the person with ulcer disease is outlined in Table 30-4.

CASE STUDY

A 33-year-old white male, J.D., with a diagnosis of recurrent duodenal ulcer, presented to the medical clinic with a complaint of moderate but persistent "gnawing" pain focused near the midline in the epigastrium near the xiphoid process. He described the pain as becoming worse as the day progressed and complained further of constantly being tired. The admitting nurse reviewed his chart and examined him, gathering the data which follows.

Assessment
J.D. presented with slight pallor and exhibited superficial and deep epigastric tenderness. His stool guaiac test was

TABLE 30-4   Nursing Process Related of Peptic Ulcer Disease

ASSESSMENT	MANAGEMENT	EVALUATION
	General Aspects	
Ascertain what dietary and environmental factors exacerbate symptoms. Note duration, location, timing of pain; what relieves pain; associated symptoms, vomiting, stool characteristics. Determine vital signs, hematocrit, hemoglobin, stools for occult blood.	Emphasize need to stay on regimen for 4–8 weeks even if symptom-free. Adjust regimen to be compatible with lifestyle. Eliminate ulcerogenic drugs (aspirin, phenylbutazone, indomethacin—see Table 30-1). Smoking may be prohibited.	Routine evaluation should include observation of vital signs, stool guaiac, hematocrit, symptoms, abdominal examination. Observe for hemorrhage manifested by hematemesis, melena, faintness, shock. Observe for perforation manifested by sudden onset of pain, acute abdomen. Observe for obstruction manifested by constipation, nausea, vomiting.
	H$_2$ Blockers	
Screen for drug interactions with cimetidine: warfarin, theophylline, phenytoin, and lidocaine. Use with caution in the elderly or young, or in renal or hepatic disease.	Increase dosage interval in renal failure for cimetidine and ranitidine.	Observe for side effects including diarrhea, dyspepsia, headache, somnolence, confusion, agitation, or gynecomastia.
	Sucralfate (Carafate)	
See General Aspects, above.	Administer dose 1 h before meals and at bedtime. Tablets may be broken in half for easier swallowing. Instruct patient not to take antacids within a ½ h before or after sucralfate.	Observe for side effects such as constipation.
	Anticholinergics	
Use with caution in elderly patients. Screen patients for narrow-angle glaucoma, obstructive uropathy, gastrointestinal disease, myasthenia gravis, or unstable cardiovascular status. These drugs may have additive side effects with phenothiazines and tricyclic antidepressants.	Should be given ½ h before meals and if needed before bedtime. Frequent sips of water, ice chips, sugarless candy may minimize dry mouth discomfort. Good oral care needed. Shade eyes in bright light. Instruct patient that sedative or alcohol use may increase drowsiness and make driving hazardous.	Observe for urinary retention, constipation, tachycardia, dizziness, blurred vision, drowsiness, diminished bowel sounds.
	Antacids	
Assess patient's ability to self-administer proper dosage (i.e., eyesight, dexterity, cognitive function). Ascertain whether equipment is available to self-administer at home (e.g., measuring device with proper volume). Assess use of commonly used over-the-counter and home remedies in all drug histories. For patients with renal or cardiac disease, care is required in selection of antacid (see text).	Make sure patient understands how to take medication. Liquids must be shaken. Tablets must be chewed thoroughly. Follow with a small amount of water (2–4 oz). Instruct not to change antacid type without consulting prescriber. May need to alternate antacids to control diarrhea and constipation. Teach to self-medicate. Supply cups at bedside to measure doses. If patient usually awakens at night with pain, can set alarm and take antacid 1 h before usual occurrence.	See General Aspects, above. Antacids can decrease absorption of some drugs, such as tetracycline. Check for patient acceptance and compliance. Note number and consistency of stools.

1+, and the hemoglobin concentration and hematocrit were lowered. The lowered mean corpuscular hemoglobin concentration and serum iron level, and the increased total iron-binding capacity, confirmed iron-deficiency anemia. Vital signs were blood pressure, 130/76; temperature, 98.8°F; pulse, 88; and respirations, 24.

Endoscopy revealed a 2-cm ulcer in the duodenal bulb with sharp margins and base consisting of some granulation and significant fibrous tissue indicative of previous healing. Results of cytologic study of the lesion were normal.

Prior to coming to the clinic, J.D. was taking 1 tsp of an aluminum magnesium hydroxide antacid three to four times daily, a "health tonic" from a natural foods store when he felt tired, and an occasional aspirin for headache.

The patient, an advertising executive, was living in an upper middle class suburb with his wife and three children, all of whom were well. Having recently begun his own advertising agency, he expressed concern that he might be hospitalized, which would interfere with maintaining his business.

The nurse diagnosed the following problems: pain and bleeding from recurrent ulcer; iron-deficiency anemia secondary to bleeding; high environmental stress level related to business concerns; and fatigue related to the anemia.

Management

To counter gastric acid–pepsin secretion, the physician increased the antacid dosage to 1 tbsp given 1 and 3 h after meals and before bedtime. An anticholinergic, propantheline bromide (ProBanthine), 30 mg, was ordered at bedtime. The nurse instructed J.D. on the importance of adhering to medication orders to ensure healing in spite of possible cessation of epigastric pain. The patient was observed while measuring his correct dosage of antacid. He was further advised that a small amount of liquid may be taken with the antacid to ensure its transport to the gastric lumen, but that the antacid should not be followed by a full glass of water, which would increase the rate of gastric emptying and decrease the efficacy of the antacid. Possible adverse effects of the antacid (constipation or diarrhea) and the anticholinergic (dry mouth, blurred vision, drowsiness, urinary retention, or dizziness) were reviewed with the patient. He was instructed to utilize ice chips or sugarless hard candy to counteract the dry mouth and to wear sunglasses for light sensitivity. He was asked to call the clinic if there were signs of urinary retention. He was cautioned that operation of a car or hazardous machinery is dangerous if drowsiness or blurred vision occur. The nurse and dietician reviewed dietary measures with J.D. and his wife, recommending that the intake of foods which stimulate gastric secretion, e.g., alcohol, coffee, and tea, be decreased or eliminated. Acetaminophen was suggested to replace the occasional use of aspirin. Promotion of physical, gastric, and emotional rest was the goal of suggesting that attempts be made to minimize emotional episodes which might exacerbate the condition.

To correct the iron-deficient state, the patient was asked to discontinue the "tonic," and a total-iron dose was calculated and administered by an IV drip iron-dextran solution following an initial test dose for allergy to the iron preparation.

Evaluation

Upon return to the clinic for follow-up 2 weeks later, J.D. was noted to have a guaiac test–negative stool and an improvement in hematocrit. He stated that he had noted a decrease in ulcer symptoms during the first week and had noted no ulcer symptoms or adverse drug effects for the second week during the day or night. The nurse stressed the need to continue to follow the prescribed regimen until his next visit in 3 weeks, as well as the need to continue to minimize environmental stress and alcohol intake.

INFLAMMATORY BOWEL DISEASE

Two forms of chronic nonspecific inflammatory bowel disease based upon distinct histopathologic features, clinical manifestations, and patterns of morbidity and mortality have been identified. *Ulcerative colitis* is a diffuse inflammatory disease affecting the rectal mucosa and varying portions of the proximal colon. The other major chronic inflammatory bowel disease is granulomatous colitis or *Crohn's disease* of the colon. This disease may affect any area of the small or large intestine in a segmental fashion but is most frequently confined to the terminal ileum, cecum, and ascending colon. Crohn's disease can be differentiated from ulcerative colitis with regard to depth of involvement and other pathologic features.

Ulcerative colitis is characterized by alterations in the mucosa which consist of ulceration, edema, and loss of mucosal detail and haustration. The inflamed mucosa, irritated by secondary infection, bleeds readily with the passage of luminal contents. Involvement proceeds proximally in a contiguous, diffuse manner without "skip" areas. The ulcers may perforate with resultant abscess formation. In chronic cases, the length and internal diameter of the colon may be decreased secondary to muscle spasm and thickening. Though predominately a disease of the bowel, ulcerative colitis is associated with a number of systemic extracolonic manifestations affecting the integument, eye, cardiac, renal, hepatobiliary, and musculoskeletal systems.

In Crohn's disease, the relative sparing of the mucosal layer accounts for the infrequent development of hemorrhagic ulceration. Transmural involvement of the bowel wall with submucosal fibrosis and edema may result in chronic partial intestinal obstruction. Though free perforations are rare, deep fissure ulcers have a tendency to lead to fistula and abscess formation. The spectrum of systemic extracolonic manifestations associated with ulcerative colitis occur less frequently in patients with Crohn's disease.

Although ulcerative colitis is most common in young and middle adulthood, approximately 20 percent of the patients are in the pediatric age group. The incidence of Crohn's disease has a bimodal distribution, occurring most commonly in the adult between the ages of 20 to 30 years and 40 to 50 years.

Etiology

Although a specific causative agent in the pathogenesis of ulcerative colitis has not been identified, it appears that a multiplicity of factors may be implicated. A genetic predisposition is evidenced by the fact that 10 to 15 percent of ulcerative colitis patients have a relative with inflammatory bowel disease. In addition, serum colon antibodies are frequently found in healthy relatives.

Psychologic evaluation of colitis patients has revealed certain personality traits held in common. Patients are often described as having difficulty expressing ideas and anger, and are immature, meticulous, conscientious, and perfectionistic. Though psychologic factors may not be causative, emotions such as anxiety and resentment result in such physiologic colonic alterations as hyperemia, lysozyme secretion, increased tone, and secretion of thick, tenacious mucus. These functional alterations, induced by psychogenic factors, may exacerbate or prolong the course of ulcerative colitis.

It has been hypothesized that autoimmune mechanisms may be involved in ulcerative colitis, as autoimmune diseases such as rheumatoid arthritis, erythema nodosum, and iritis frequently accompany colitis. Glucocorticoids, which are therapeutic in autoimmune diseases, are utilized in the treatment program of ulcerative colitis.

Other theories suggest a defect in the connective tissue of the bowel, destructive activity of enzymes, hereditary deficiency of lactase, and bacterial infection. In addition, some drugs may produce an ulcerative colitis–like syndrome (see Table 30-1).

The etiology of Crohn's disease is also unknown; however, as in ulcerative colitis, patients with this disease frequently demonstrate the presence of anticolon antibodies and circulating lymphocytes which are cytotoxic for colon epithelial cells.

Clinical Findings

The patient with ulcerative colitis may present with one of three different patterns of the disease: remitting, chronic, and fulminant. The remitting course occurs in 65 percent of the patients and is characterized by frequent remissions and exacerbations. The disease gradually progresses in severity. In 30 percent, the disease is chronic, and the intestinal symp-

toms may be mild but continuous and may be accompanied by malnutrition and anemia. The acute fulminant type is characterized by a sudden development and progressively rapid course including elevated temperature, frequent diarrhea, rectal bleeding, abdominal pain, and abdominal distention. About 13 percent of these patients develop *toxic megacolon,* in which the transverse colon becomes markedly dilated with thinning of all coats of the bowel wall. Excessive use of narcotic antidiarrheal agents may result in this complication, and severe hemorrhage and perforation contribute to the high (20 to 30 percent) mortality rate from this adverse development. Medical therapy and decompression of the small intestine by intubation is successful in about two-thirds of the cases. If perforation occurs, surgical intervention with ileostomy and colectomy is mandatory.

The major symptoms of ulcerative colitis are rectal bleeding and diarrhea. The initial episode and subsequent exacerbations of the disease are often precipitated by incidents or experiences that have emotional implications for the patient. Infection, illness, fatigue, and the ingestion of laxatives or dietary irritants are also associated with exacerbations.

Crohn's disease has been described as a chronic condition of low mortality and high morbidity. The acute form is characterized by severe, cramping abdominal pain in the right lower quadrant, mild diarrhea, fatigue, and moderate fever. The patient with the chronic form of Crohn's disease has a long history of diarrhea. The semisolid stools, which number three to four per day, contain mucus and pus, but no blood. If ulceration occurs high in the small intestine, steatorrhea may also be present. Bowel movements relieve the colicky abdominal pain. Chronicity is accompanied by weight loss, anemia, fever, decreased food intake, malabsorption, and malaise. Anorectal abscesses, fissures, and fistula are common findings.

Clinical Pharmacology and Therapeutics

The goal of therapy is to treat the symptoms and complications, treat any deficiency states, and arrest the disease process. Like the etiology of the disease, the mechanisms of therapeutic action remain to be fully elucidated. Agents used for the inflammatory disease process include anti-inflammatory agents, antimicrobials, corticosteroids, and immunosuppressants. Symptomatic therapy may be achieved with antispasmodics and opiates, and deficiency states may be corrected by diet adjustments and nutritional supplements. Medical management must be complemented by rest and adequate psychologic and emotional support. In cases not responsive to therapy, surgical intervention may be necessary.

Sulfasalazine

Sulfasalazine (Azulfidine) is a combination of 5-aminosalicylic acid and the sulfonamide antimicrobial sulfapyridine chemically bonded together. This drug is the most commonly prescribed medication for patients with inflammatory bowel disease.

Sulfasalazine is effective in the treatment of mild to moderate inflammatory bowel disease, and is commonly administered as the initial therapeutic agent. The combination of sulfasalazine and prednisone is no better than prednisone alone in the treatment of active Crohn's disease. Sulfasalazine is not as effective as corticosteroids in rapidly inducing remission in the acute phase of ulcerative colitis. However, the drug will significantly reduce the relapse rate in ulcerative colitis.

Mechanism of Action   The mechanism of action of sulfasalazine is not completely understood. Recent evidence shows that **5-aminosalicylic acid** is the active moiety that is delivered to the site of inflammation by the parent compound. Prostaglandins are mediators of the inflammatory process. The active moiety inhibits prostaglandin synthesis in the gastrointestinal tract, suggesting one mechanism for the beneficial effects of sulfasalazine. The antimetabolic and antibacterial properties of the drug are limited and probably do not account for the efficacy of sulfasalazine.

Pharmacokinetics   When taken orally, sulfasalazine is not completely absorbed in the GI tract. After absorption, some of the drug recirculates into the intestines with bile. As the drug enters the colon, it is split by bacteria to form sulfapyridine and 5-aminosalicylic acid. Sulfapyridine is well-absorbed into the systemic circulation and is excreted with its metabolites in the urine. The second moiety, 5-aminosalicylic acid, remains in the colon and is excreted in the feces.

Adverse Effects   The clinical benefits of sulfasalazine are limited by the common adverse effects. Dose-dependent reactions correlate with the serum level of sulfapyridine. These side effects include nausea, vomiting, fever, headache, arthralgias, and reticulocytosis. Hypersensitivity reactions to sulfasalazine are not dose-related and may involve many body systems including the skin, lung, blood, kidneys, and liver. Excess sun or sunlamp exposure may cause severe sunburn. Administration of this drug may produce an orange-yellow color in alkaline urine.

Drug Interactions   Drugs reported to interact with sulfasalazine include **tetracycline, iron, folic acid,** and **digoxin**. The only interaction that seems to be clinically significant is sulfasalazine and digoxin. Since sulfasalazine may decrease the bioavailability of digoxin, it is recommended that digoxin levels be monitored when a patient is taking both of these drugs.

Dosage and Preparations   Adults should be given 0.5 to 1 g of **sulfasalazine** four times a day for treatment of active inflammatory bowel disease. By starting at a low dose and increasing in daily increments of 0.5 to 1.0 g, the incidence of GI effects should be diminished. After remission is achieved, the optimal maintenance dose for ulcerative colitis is 0.5 g four times a day. Children are given 40 to 60 mg/kg/day and then 30 mg/kg/day for treatment and maintenance, respectively.

Antibiotics

Antibiotics are utilized for the management of inflammatory bowel disease based on the evidence suggesting an infectious etiology. However, there are no conclusive data to show that a particular microbial agent is responsible. Long-term antibiotic therapy is associated with numerous side effects including changes in host defense mechanisms, bacterial resistance, and gastrointestinal tract flora. The risk versus benefit of such therapy must be taken into account. The value of adequate antibacterial therapy for infectious complications of inflammatory bowel disease such as abscess or sepsis is lifesaving and unquestioned. The use of antibiotics for active inflammatory bowel disease without infectious complications remains controversial.

Uncontrolled studies report the beneficial effects of metronidazole in Crohn's disease. **Metronidazole** (Flagyl) is bacteriocidal against several gut anaerobes including *Bacteroides fragilis*. The Cooperative Crohn's Disease Study Group conducted a controlled study involving 89 patients. The researchers concluded that metronidazole is slightly more effective than sulfasalazine in the treatment of Crohn's disease. In addition, it is beneficial to switch from sulfasalazine to metronidazole when initial treatment fails, but not vice versa. There was no difference in the frequency or type of adverse reactions between the two drugs in this study. However, adverse reactions due to metronidazole therapy for infections include paresthesias, neuropathy, seizures, and mutagenicity. The use of metronidazole for Crohn's disease is considered investigational.

Corticosteroids

Corticosteroids, including **hydrocortisone, methylprednisolone, prednisone,** and **prednisolone**, are the most effective therapy available for the management of acute inflammatory bowel disease. The mechanism of action is not clearly defined, but the agents exert anti-inflammatory effects via multiple mechanisms. Rectal corticosteroid (Cortenema, Rectoid) instillation may be beneficial for proctitis. As much as 50 percent of the steroid dose administered rectally may be absorbed systemically. Corticosteroids do not cure inflammatory bowel disease, nor do they prevent recurrence of disease. Numerous complications can result from the overuse of these drugs (see Chap. 35, "Endocrine Disorders").

For the treatment of severe, acute inflammatory bowel disease, parenteral corticosteroid therapy is recommended in doses equivalent to 60 to 80 mg/day of prednisone. The total daily dosage should be tapered and discontinued as rapidly as the disease process allows. Alternate-day therapy is advantageous whenever possible, especially in children, in whom it may reduce growth retardation. Rectal solutions and foam preparations are administered in doses of 100 mg hydrocortisone or equivalent corticosteroid by slow rectal drip or retention enema once or twice daily.

Immunosuppressants

Azathioprine (Imuran) and **mercatopurine** (Purinethol) have been investigated for the management of inflammatory bowel disease. The efficacy of these agents is controversial, and the mechanism of action is unexplained. A major problem is that nearly all patients experience side effects. The indication for use of immunosuppressants must remain empirical until the role of immunity as an etiology is resolved. Similarly, further definition is required of the dosage regimens for optimum therapeutic response with minimum adverse effects. These agents are discussed further in Chapters 31 and 37, respectively.

Antidiarrheal Agents

The use of antispasmodics and opiates in controlling the diarrhea associated with ulcerative colitis is common, but should be tempered by certain considerations. In severe colitis, diarrhea is symptomatic of an inflamed, rather than hypermotile bowel, and the effectiveness of these drugs may be marginal. Further, acute dilation of the colon, or toxic megacolon, is a life-threatening complication of severe colitis and has been reported to be precipitated by injudicious use of opiates or antispasmodics. Therefore, it is recommended that these drugs be used sparingly in mild to moderate cases of colitis, and avoided in severe, fulminant colitis. The combination of **diphenoxylate** 2.5 mg and **atropine** 0.025 mg (Lomotil) is used in a daily range between 5 and 20 mg (of diphenoxylate). Alternative approaches to diarrhea include restriction of oral intake to medications and clear fluids, and administration of such bulk-forming agents as **methylcellulose** or **psyllium**.

Parenteral and Enteral Nutrition

Due to gastrointestinal inflammation, rapid transit time, surgical bowel resections, and fistula formation, together with increased nutrient requirements, patients with inflammatory bowel disease often present to the hospital with protein-calorie malnutrition. Common dietary problems include malabsorption of vitamins A, D, E, K, and B_{12} as well as malabsorption of carbohydrates, fat, and protein. In the face of these complications, total parenteral nutritional support may be necessary and lifesaving. Parenteral nutrition also allows complete bowel rest and decreases fistula drainage. However, whenever the GI tract may be utilized, the enteral route is preferred, whether by mouth or tube feedings. A low-residue, low-fat, lactose-free diet, or an elemental formula is ideal during acute exacerbations of inflammatory bowel disease (see Chap. 25).

Surgery

Total colectomy with ileostomy may be performed if there is severe involvement of colon and rectum or complications refractory to medical management. Providing psychologic support to the patient prior to and following this procedure will be important in the acceptance of the ileostomy. Careful follow-up for the first several months will enable early detection of such complications as obstruction, dehydration, electrolyte imbalance, bleeding, and maladjusted ostomy appliances. Special therapeutic considerations after the ileostomy include avoiding enteric-coated tablets, which will not be absorbed, and timed-released capsules, which will be only partially absorbed; using oral antibiotics with caution because of the abrupt changes in gastrointestinal flora; using diuretics with caution because the patient is at increased risk of electrolyte imbalance; and omitting the use of either laxative or enema preparations for diagnostic procedures as such preparations are unnecessary after the lower bowel has been removed.

NURSING PROCESS RELATED TO INFLAMMATORY BOWEL DISEASE

The use of the nursing process in patients with inflammatory bowel disease is summarized in Table 30-5.

CASE STUDY

S.C., a 13-year-old female, was admitted to the pediatric medicine unit because of a 2-day history of frequent and severe diarrhea with bright-red blood in the feces and rectal tenesmus. Other complaints included cramping in the lower abdomen and increasing weakness and anorexia for 10 days prior to admission.

Assessment

S.C. appeared pale, debilitated, frail, and small for her age, with an absence of overt signs of reproductive maturation. She measured 56 in tall, weighed 75 lb, and was reported to have lost 5 lb in the preceding week. Dry, turgorless skin, dry mucous membranes, and chapped lips were found on physical examination. She sat clutching her abdomen with a drawn expression. Vital signs were blood pressure, 85/50; temperature, 102.8°F; pulse, 120/min; respirations, 28/min.

Stool specimens revealed blood, pus, and mucus, but were negative for pathogenic organisms. Sigmoidoscopy showed hyperemic mucosa which was edematous and

TABLE 30-5   Nursing Process Related to Inflammatory Bowel Disease*

ASSESSMENT	MANAGEMENT	EVALUATION
Number and character of stools. Signs of fluid and electrolyte imbalance, including laboratory tests, skin turgor, condition of mucous membranes, weight, vital signs, oliguria, and respiratory rate. Abdominal pain: location and character. Events precipitating episode. Extracolonic manifestations: skin lesions, ocular disorders, liver pathology, or arthritis.	To minimize GI adverse effects, give sulfasalazine with meals and / or gradually increase the dosage to therapeutic levels. The patient should be told that the urine may turn orange-yellow in color. Well-balanced low-residue, high-protein diet. May require vitamin and iron supplementation. Avoid excessive use of antispasmotics and antidiarrheals, which may precipitate megacolon. Rest after meals may decrease peristalsis and diarrhea. Patient may experience mood swings, dependency, sensitivity, and aggressive behavior. Nurses should recognize needs, and develop trust relationship, give support, encourage patients to verbalize, and let them know their complaints are understood.	Monitor abdominal girth—enlargement may indicate megacolon. Note appetite, mood, temperature, number and character of stools. Monitor vital signs, intake and output. Evaluate hematocrit and stool guaiac test results.

*Nursing processes for specific agents used to treat ulcerative colitis are discussed elsewhere in text. For corticosteroids see Chap. 35; immunosuppressants, Chap. 26; antidiarrheals, Chap. 20; vitamins, Chap. 25.

showed multiple, minute ulcerations without presence of polyps or perforation. Carcinoma was ruled out by subsequent radiologic and cytologic studies. The inflammatory process was differentiated from Crohn's disease by full-thickness biopsy and determined to be ulcerative colitis.

The nursing diagnosis included pain, diarrhea with perianal irritation, dehydration, and compromised nutritional status.

Management

In order to correct the dehydration, the physician ordered an intravenous (IV) line and blood chemistries to determine the quantity and type of fluids to be used. The nurse explained to the patient and her family that the IV fluid would provide nutrients and medication during the acute phase when the patient was not tolerating fluids orally. The nurse initiated intake and output measurements to monitor fluid status. On the second day, a low-residue, low-fat, lactose-free liquid oral diet as tolerated was added to the parenteral fluids. Liquids were offered in frequent small amounts, because large quantities of hot or cold fluids could stimulate peristalsis.

Hygiene and physical comfort measures were provided by using a small fracture bedpan and by having a washcloth available for perineal care following defecation. The rectal area was coated with petrolatum to minimize the potential for excoriation, and soft facial tissues were used instead of the coarser toilet paper. The nursing care plan included provision for sitz baths to stimulate circulation and relieve discomfort if excoriation did occur.

Hydrocortisone was prescribed to attenuate the disease process in doses of 75 mg administered intravenously every 6 h during the first 48 h. Nurses monitored for symptoms of peritonitis by careful observation of the abdomen, since corticosteroids may impart a general feeling of well-being and mask initial discomfort from this complication. Other parameters monitored due to the corticosteroid therapy included intake and output, blood glucose, blood pressure, and signs of infection such as white blood cell count and fever. Two tablets of diphenoxylate / atropine (Lomotil) were administered four times daily for 2 days, requiring careful observation of the abdomen for megacolon.

To address emotional factors which may exacerbate the disease, S.C. was referred for follow-up counseling. Attention was given to the stressful adolescent period and the feelings of modesty and embarrassment which are generated in the patient by the illness, weight loss, and frequent bloody stools. The patient and her family were made cognizant of the possibility that stressful situations may precede and exacerbate the illness.

Evaluation

After 48 h, there was a decrease in the number of stools and discomfort in the lower abdomen. Vital signs, intake and output, and laboratory evaluations revealed that fluid and electrolyte homeostasis had been reestablished and was not adversely affected by the hydrocortisone administration. No excoriation of the perineum occurred. The Lomotil was discontinued as the cramping and diarrhea were controlled.

Following a sigmoidoscopy and x-ray with results approaching normal limits and determination of a guaiac test–negative stool, the patient was prepared for discharge and given a prescription for 0.5 g four times a day of sulfasalazine. S.C. and her mother were informed of the adverse effects of the drug and how to take the drug to minimize side effects. Sulfasalazine is best taken after meals or with food to lessen stomach upset. Each dose should be taken with a full glass (8 oz) of water. Tablets should be swallowed whole and not crushed or broken, since they are enteric-coated. If a dose is missed, the patient should take it as soon as possible. S.C. was told to stop taking this medicine and check with her doctor if any of the following side effects occurred: continuous headache, joint pains, vomiting, fever, rash. The drug may cause sensitivity to sunlight, and too much sun (or sun lamps) should be avoided. Urine may turn orange-yellow in color. She was instructed to return to the clinic in 1 week and maintain bed rest at home until the clinic appointment.

HEMORRHOIDS

The anal canal, the terminal 3 cm of rectum, connects the distal end of the gastrointestinal tract with the outside of the body. The boundary between the anal canal and the rectum is marked by the anorectal (pectinate) line. At this line, the lining of the canal changes from the columnar epithelium of mucous membrane to the stratified squamous epithelium identical with skin. A number of plexuses of veins are present in this area. The internal hemorrhoidal plexus is located in the submuscosal space above the anorectal line, while the external hemorrhoidal plexus is located in the subcutaneous base below the anorectal line. Anal continence is maintained by two sphincters encircling the anal canal. The internal sphincter is an involuntary smooth muscle of the rectum which extends from the rectum to within 1 cm of the anal orifice. The external sphincter is a voluntary striated muscle which lies outside the internal sphincter and extends subcutaneously to end at the terminal portion of the anal canal.

Hemorrhoids are anorectal swellings composed of varicosities involving one or more of the hemorrhoid plexuses of veins. Hemorrhoids may be classified according to location and degree of severity. *Internal hemorrhoids* are varices occurring above the anorectal line. A distended internal hemorrhoid may on occasion prolapse below the anorectal line external to the sphincter. The prolapsed hemorrhoid is associated with pain and the possibility of hemorrhage and strangulation with subsequent thrombosis. *External hemorrhoids* are varices located below the anorectal line external to the sphincters. An acute, external thrombotic hemorrhoid is a hemorrhoidal vessel that has ruptured and formed a hematoma. This acute form is associated with considerable discomfort. A chronic external hemorrhoid or cutaneous skin tag is a sequel to a hematoma in which the clot has become organized and replaced by fibrous connective tissue which is covered by anal skin. Mixed internal-external hemorrhoids occur most commonly.

Etiology

Hemorrhoids are a common problem afflicting 35 percent of the population over the age of 25 years. Interference with venous return from the hemorrhoidal veins results in venous congestion and subsequent varicosity. A number of etiologic factors have been identified including hereditary predisposition, gravitational pressure, increased abdominal or portal pressure, and low-fiber diets. Factors such as prolonged sitting or standing, pregnancy, constipation, coughing, heart failure, portal hypertension, and physical exertion increase hemorrhoidal pressure.

Clinical Findings

The symptoms of hemorrhoids vary with location. Internal hemorrhoids most frequently present with painless bright-red bleeding upon defecation. Other manifestations include pruritis, burning, pain, inflammation, irritation, swelling, discomfort, seepage, protrusion, and thrombosis.

Clinical Pharmacology and Therapeutics

The therapy of hemorrhoids may be directed at symptomatic relief, avoidance of precipitating or aggravating factors, or surgical intervention. Patients should avoid constipation and straining when defecating, since both will precipitate or aggravate the development of the symptoms of hemorrhoids. Diets should contain adequate amounts of fiber and fluids. Other conservative measures include sitz baths, warm compresses, bed rest, and bulk stool softeners. Suppositories should be administered gently because hemorrhoids are easily traumatized. Surgical intervention is indicated when there is bleeding, thrombosis, infection, or ulceration. Newer techniques involve internal hemorrhoidectomy, in which the hemorrhoid is tied off and as the blood supply decreases, the hemorrhoid tissue sloughs. Other methods used include cryodestruction, where the hemorrhoid is destroyed by freezing.

The general medical management of hemorrhoids includes several important recommendations to maximize therapeutic benefit. First, wash the anorectal area with warm water. Anorectal products should be used after bowel movements. Pregnant and nursing women are cautioned to use only external products or internal protectants. Internal (intrarectal) products should contain recommended ingredients as outlined in Table 30-6. Any product that causes pain is to be discontinued. The patient should be under the care of a physician for severe manifestations including bleeding, seepage, prolapse, or persistent pain (greater than 1 week).

TABLE 30-6 FDA-Recommended Hemorrhoidal Ingredients

CATEGORY	INGREDIENTS	TRADE NAME OF TYPICAL PRODUCT CONTAINING THE INGREDIENT
Anesthetics	Benzocaine, pramoxine*	Tronolane, BiCozene, ProctoFoam/Nonsteroid
Astringents	Calamine,* zinc oxide,* witch hazel (hamamelis water)	Gentz, Tucks pads/ointment/cream
Counterirritants	Menthol, phenol	Tanurol, Hemocaine
Keratolytics	Alcloxa, resorcinol	BiCozene, Perifoam
Protectants	Petrolatum,* aluminum hydroxide, cocoa butter, cod liver oil, glycerin, shark liver oil, kaolin, lanolin, wood alcohols, zinc oxide,* calamine*	Vaseline jelly, Anusol, Tucks cream/ointment, Preparation H
Vasoconstrictors	Epinephrine HCl solution, ephedrine sulfate solution,* phenylephrine HCl solution*	Wyanoids, Rectagene balm, A-Caine Rectal, Emeroid, Epinephricaine Rectal
Corticosteroids	Hydrocortisone	Proctacort, Anusol-HC, Dermolate Anal-Itch, Cortef Rectal Itch

*May be used by external or intrarectal administration.

Dosage and Preparations

Most of the hemorrhoidal preparations that are commercially available contain a combination of drugs that are directed at relieving the patient's symptoms, i.e., the swelling, pain, and itching (see Table 30-6). Hemorrhoidal preparations may contain anesthetics, vasoconstrictors, protectants, counterirritants, keratolytics, anticholinergics, corticosteroids, antiseptics, and/or astringents. There is a lack of evidence that any of these ingredients or combinations is effective. The Food and Drug Administration (FDA) advisory review panel on nonprescription hemorrhoidal drugs does not recommend wound-healing agents, antiseptics, anticholinergics, or corticosteroids. Products containing vasoconstrictors should be avoided in patients with hypertension and other cardiovascular disease, diabetes, hyperthyroidism, or patients taking monoamine oxidase inhibitors. A safe, intrarectal product for pregnant or lactating women consists of 100 percent petrolatum. The use of corticosteroids is recommended in the treatment of perirectal itching.

Hemorrhoidal preparations are available in various forms, including suppositories, ointments, foams, and pads. For anal hygiene, hygienic wipes or pads are practical and convenient methods to help prevent perianal itching. Suppositories may have a beneficial psychologic effect; however, their usage is not recommended in the treatment of anorectal disease. In prone patients, the suppository may ascend into the rectum and lower colon. Foams have no proven advantage over ointments. In general, ointments are the optimal vehicle and should be applied sparingly to the perianal area and anal canal with one's finger. For intrarectal administration of ointments, pile pipes with a well-lubricated tip and side holes are recommended (see Fig. 30-2).

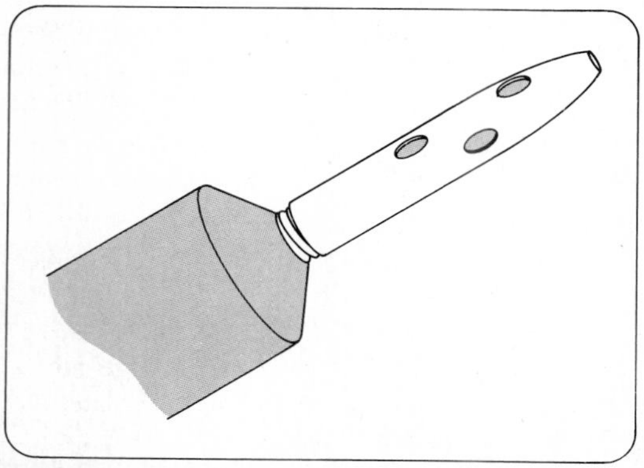

NURSING PROCESS RELATED TO HEMORRHOIDS

The nursing process in the care of the patient with hemorrhoids is outlined in Table 30-7.

MISCELLANEOUS DISORDERS

Irritable Bowel Syndrome

The most commonly diagnosed gastrointestinal disease is irritable bowel syndrome, which causes considerable distress for those afflicted with the disorder and constitutes a complex management problem for the clinician. Patients with irritable bowel syndrome usually present with one of three clinical patterns: (1) chronic abdominal pain with constipa-

FIGURE 30-2

Pile Applicator for Intrarectal Administration of Ointments.

TABLE 30-7   Nursing Process Related to Care of Persons with Hemorrhoids

ASSESSMENT	MANAGEMENT	EVALUATION
Check etiologic factors including diarrhea, constipation, congestive heart failure, portal hypertension. Check stools for blood. Observe anal area for edema and inflammation. Hematocrit may drop due to bleeding. Assess subjective statements regarding pain, bleeding, etc. Assess use of medication or other self-treatment.	Use fiber, fluid, and bulk-stool softeners as needed to maintain regular soft-formed stools. Patient may be embarrassed about condition. Patient education: Wash anal area after defecation, avoid use of dry paper after defecation, use heat or cold applications to reduce pain, elevate buttocks to assist in reduction of prolapse or swelling. Instruct in proper use of suppositories, cream, or other application.	Preparations applied to hemorrhoids should give symptomatic relief; evaluate subjective statements and observe hemorrhoids. Increased discomfort may indicate complication: Thrombosis, prolapse, strangulation. Bowel routine and character of stool should be noted. Placebo effect may be significant.

tion, (2) chronic watery diarrhea with or without abdominal pain, or (3) alternating constipation and diarrhea. Symptoms occur intermittently, lasting for weeks or months per episode.

The mechanism of irritable bowel syndrome is altered intestinal motility. It has been proposed that an increased response to the normal release of cholecystokinin after meals, an exaggerated colonic reaction to psychologic stress, and/or altered contractions of the intestinal smooth muscle contribute to the pathogenesis of the disorder.

Clinical Pharmacology and Therapeutics

The goals of the therapy in irritable bowel syndrome are to reassure patients of the usual nonprogressive nature of the disorder and to help patients to identify the relationship between emotional stress and the onset and severity of the symptoms and to adjust their lifestyles accordingly. Drug therapy is largely empirical and is directed at altering gastrointestinal tract motility. Patients with constipation may respond to increased bulk in dietary form or as bulk-forming laxatives, while severe diarrhea may be treated with diphenoxylate/atropine (Lomotil) or paragoric (see Chap. 20, "Constipation and Diarrhea.") Sedatives or antianxiety agents are useful when specifically indicated for psychoemotional target symptoms. Antispasmotics sometimes provide symptomatic relief.

Antispasmotics   Antispasmotics are anticholinergic drugs having pharmacology and precautions similar to the anticholinergics used as adjuncts in the treatment of peptic ulcer disease (see above). They are employed to decrease intestinal motility and secretion, although their efficacy in treating irritable bowel syndrome is questionable. **Dicyclomine hydrochloride** (Bentyl, Antispas, others), available as capsules, tablets, syrup, and injectable, is given in doses of 10 to 20 mg for adults and 10 mg for children. Infant colic, also thought by some to represent altered intestinal motility, is treated by doses of 5 mg of the syrup form diluted with an equal volume of water. Dicyclomine is dosed three to four times daily. Other antispasmotics include **methixene hydro-**

chloride (Trest), used in adult doses of 1 to 2 mg tid, **oxyphencyclimine hydrochloride** (Daricon), used in adult doses of 5 to 10 mg bid, and **thiphenamil hydrochloride** (Trocinate), used in doses of 400 mg every 4 h.

Gastroesophageal Reflux and Esophagitis

Reflux esophagitis consists of esophageal damage resulting from the reflux of gastric or intestinal contents into the esophagus and inadequate esophageal mucosal defenses. *Gastroesophageal reflux* is normally prevented by the lower-esophageal sphincter and the anatomic configuration of the gastroesophageal junction. This antireflux mechanism can be compromised by disease or pseudoobstruction of the intestine (scleroderma-like diseases, pregnancy, myopathy, hiatal hernia, surgical destruction) and drugs, including methylxanthines (**aminophylline, theophylline, caffeine**), tobacco smoke, and other smooth muscle–relaxing agents (**anticholinergics, β-receptor blockers, nitrates, calcium channel antagonists**). In the presence of an incompetent antireflux mechanism, gastrointestinal contents will reflux when gastric volume is increased, when bending or reclining causes gastric contents to be near the gastroesophageal junction, or when gastric pressure is increased by pregnancy, obesity, ascites, or tight clothing.

The characteristic symptom of gastroesophageal reflux or reflux esophagitis is heartburn. Dysphagia occurs if strictures develop, and severe reflux can be complicated by aspiration pneumonia.

Clinical Pharmacology and Therapeutics

The goals of therapy in reflux esophagitis are to prevent the reflux and to neutralize any refluxed material. Patients should be advised to elevate the head of their beds, eliminate foods that exacerbate the symptoms (orange juice, mint, alcohol, caffeine-containing beverages, chocolate, and fatty foods are frequent offenders), avoid anticholinergic prescription and nonprescription drugs (see Table 12-5), reduce weight if overweight, and stop smoking. Bile esophagitis may be treated with **cholestyramine** (Questran) and **alumi-**

num hydroxide antacids. In peptic reflux neutralization may be accomplished by antacids and H_2-receptor antagonists. Although not approved by the Food and Drug Administration for this use, both H_2-receptor blockers have been used to treat reflux esophagitis. Some clinicians prefer **ranitidine** (Zantac) over **cimetidine** (Tagamet) because of its longer duration of action. A high-potency antacid is considered most effective to neutralize peptic reflux. **Gaviscon**, although a low-potency antacid of high cost, is promoted for use in reflux esophagitis. Gaviscon liquid contains aluminum hydroxide, magnesium carbonate, and sorbitol. Gaviscon chewable tablets, containing aluminum hydroxide, magne-sium trisilicate, alginic acid, and sodium bicarbonate, should be chewed thoroughly and followed by a glass of water or milk.

If the patient does not respond to conservative management and neutralization, **metoclopramide** (Reglan; see Chap. 19) in doses of 10 mg qid or **bethanechol** (Urecholine; see Chap. 11) in doses of 25 mg qid may be added. These two drugs raise sphincter control, hasten gastric emptying, and improve esophageal clearance, but their effectiveness is limited and may be complicated by adverse effects. Antireflux surgery is reserved for complicated cases that do not respond to drug therapy.

REFERENCES

Abramowicz, M. (ed.): "Ranitidine (Zantac)," *Med Lett Drugs Ther,* 24:111–113, 1982.

——: "Antacids," *Med Lett Drugs Ther,* 24:61–62, 1982.

Berner, B. D., C. S. Conner, D. R. Sawyer, and J. K. Siepler: "Ranitidine: A New H_2-Receptor Antagonist," *Clin Pharm,* 1:499–509, 1982.

Bramble, M. G., and C. O. Record: "Drug-Induced Gastrointestinal Disease," *Drugs,* 15:451–463, 1978.

Brogden, R. M., A. Carmine, R. C. Heel, T. M. Speight, and G. S. Avery: "Ranitidine: A Review of its Pharmacology and Therapeutic Use in Peptic Ulcer Disease and Other Allied Diseases," *Drugs,* 24:267–303, 1982.

Danilewitz, M., L. O. Tim, and B. Hirschowitz: "Ranitidine Suppression of Gastric Hypersecretion Resistant to Cimetidine," *N Eng J Med,* 306:20–22, 1982.

Drake, D., and D. Hollander: "Neutralizing Capacity and Cost Effectiveness of Antacids," *Ann Intern Med,* 94:215–217, 1981.

"Drugs For Esophageal Reflux," *Med Lett Drugs Ther,* 22:26, 1980.

Fieshler, B., and E. Achkar: "An Aggressive Approach to the Medical Management of Peptic Ulcer Disease," *Arch Intern Med,* 141:848–851, 1981.

Freston, J. W.: "Cimetidine: Developments, Pharmacology, and Efficacy," *Ann Intern Med,* 97:573–580, 1982.

——: "Cimetidine: Adverse Reactions and Patterns of Use," *Ann Intern Med,* 97:728–734, 1982.

Gardner, R. C.: "Pharmacotherapy of Inflammatory Bowel Disease," *Am J Hosp Pharm,* 33:831–838, 1976.

Garnett, W. R.: "Antacid Products," in *Handbook of Nonprescription Drugs,* Washington: American Pharmaceutical Association, 1982.

——: "Sucralfate—Alternative Therapy for Peptic Ulcer Disease," *Clin Pharm,* 1:307–314, 1982.

Given, B. A., and S. J. Simmons: *Gastroenterology in Clinical Nursing,* 2d ed., St. Louis: Mosby, 1975.

Glickman, R. M.: "Inflammatory Bowel Disease," in R. G. Petersdorf et al. (eds.), *Harrison's Principles of Internal Medicine,* 10th ed., New York: McGraw-Hill, 1983.

Goyal, R. K.: "Diseases of the Esophagus," in R. G. Petersdorf et al. (eds.), *Harrison's Principles of Internal Medicine,* 10th ed., New York: McGraw-Hill, 1983.

Green, P. H. R., and A. R. Tall: "Drugs, Alcohol, and Malabsorption," *Am J Med,* 67:1066–1076, 1979.

Grossman, M. I.: "New Medical and Surgical Treatments for Peptic Ulcer Disease," *Am J Med,* 69:647–649, 1980.

——: "Peptic Ulcer: New Therapies, New Diseases," *Ann Intern Med,* 95:609–627, 1981.

Guyton, A. C.: "The Gastrointestinal Tract," in *Textbook of Medical Physiology,* 6th ed. Philadelphia: Saunders, 1981.

Henry, D. A., and M. J. S. Langman: "Adverse Effects of Anti-ulcer Drugs," *Drugs,* 21:444–459, 1981.

Hodes, B.: "Hemorrhoidal Products," in *Handbook of Nonprescription Drugs,* 7th ed., Washington: American Pharmaceutical Association, 1982.

Jacknowitz, A. I.: "Ulcerative Colitis and Its Treatment," *Am J Hosp Pharm,* 37:1635–1646, 1980.

Khan, A. K., J. Piris, and S. C. Truelove: "An Experiment to Determine the Active Therapeutic Moiety of Sulphasalazine," *Lancet,* 1:892–894, 1977.

Kirsner, J. B.: "Observations on the Medical Treatment of Inflammatory Bowel Disease," *JAMA,* 243:557–562, 1980.

——, and R. G. Shorter: "Recent Developments in 'Nonspecific' Inflammatory Bowel Disease," *N Eng J Med,* 306:775–785, 837–848, 1982.

Klotz, U., K. Maier, C. Fischer, and K. Heinkel: "Therapeutic Efficacy of Sulfasalazine and its Metabolites in Patients with Ulcerative Colitis and Crohn's Disease," *N Eng J Med,* 303:1499–1502, 1980.

Kodner, I. J. et al.: "Inflammatory Bowel Disease," *Clin Symp,* 34:3–32, 1982.

Korelitz, B. I.: "Therapy of Inflammatory Bowel Disease, Including Use of Immunosuppressive Agents," *Clin Gastroenterol,* 9:331–349, 1980.

LaMont, J. T., and K. J. Isselbacher: "Disorders of the Colon and Rectum," in K. J. Isselbacher et al. (eds.), *Harrison's*

Principles of Internal Medicine, 9th ed., New York: McGraw-Hill, 1980.

MacFadyen, B. V.: "The Role of IVH in Gastrointestinal Diseases," *Clin Consultations Nutr Support,* 2:1–4, 1982.

Malagelada, J. R.: "Medical Versus Surgical Therapy for Duodenal Ulcer," *Mayo Clin Proc,* 55:25–32, 1980.

Mangini, R. J.: "Clinically Important Cimetidine Drug Interactions," *Clin Pharm,* 1:433–440, 1982.

Marks, I. N.: "Current Therapy in Peptic Ulcer," *Drugs,* 20:283–299, 1980.

McGuigan, J. E.: "Peptic Ulcer," in R. G. Petersdorf et al. (eds.), *Harrison's Principles of Internal Medicine,* 10th ed. New York: McGraw-Hill, 1983.

Myers, S. A.: "The Chronic Threat of Crohn's Disease: How to Help Your Patients Cope," *RN,* 41:65–71, 1978.

——: "Crohn's Disease," *Crit Care Update,* 7:12–30, 1980.

Panter, C. G.: "Varicose Veins and Hemorrhoids," *Parents,* 56:120, 1981.

Parker, M.: "Crohn's Disease: A Vicious Circle," *Nurs Mirror,* 154:41–43, 1982.

Richardson, C. T.: "Sulcralfate," *Ann Intern Med,* 97:269–272, 1982.

Rosen, A., B. Ursing, T. Alm, F. Barany, I. BErgelin, K. Ganrot-Norlin, J. Hoevels, B. Huitfeldt, G. Jarnerot, U. Krause, A. Krook, B. Lindstrom, and O. Nordle: "A Comparative Study of Metronidazole and Sulfasalazine for Active Crohn's Disease: The Cooperative Crohn's Disease Study in Sweden—Design and Methodologic Considerations," *Gastroenterology,* 83:541–549, 1982.

Singleton, J. W.: "Medical Therapy of Inflammatory Bowel Disease," *Med Clin North Am,* 64:117–1133, 1980.

Spiro, H. M.: "Pharmacology, Clinical Efficacy, and Adverse Effects of Sucralfate, A Nonsystemic Agent for Peptic Ulcer," *Pharmacotherapy,* 2:67–71, 1982.

Ursing, B., T. Alm, F. Barany, I. Bergelin, K. Ganrot-Norlin, J. Hoevels, B. Huitfeldt, G. Jarnerot, U. Krause, A. Krook, B. Lindstrom, O. Nordle, and A. Rosen: "A Comparative Study of Metronidazole and Sulfasalazine for Active Crohn's Disease: The Cooperative Crohn's Disease Study in Sweden—Result," *Gastroenterology,* 83:550–562, 1982.

31

RENAL DISORDERS*

H. KATHERYN TATUM
AGATHA A. QUINN

LEARNING OBJECTIVES

Upon mastery of the contents of this chapter, the reader will be able to:

1. Name the kidney function test used for adjusting therapy with renally excreted drugs in patients with renal failure.

2. List drugs which may promote kidney stone formation.

3. Identify the type(s) of nephrolithiasis treated with each of the following: urinary acidification, urinary alkalinization, penicillamine, acetohydroxamic acid, allopurinol, thiazide diuretics, and sodium cellulose phosphate.

4. Describe the mechanism of action, proper administration, and adverse effects of penicillamine, acetohydroxamic acid, thiazide diuretics, sodium cellulose phosphate, and urinary pH modifiers in the treatment of nephrolithiasis.

5. List drugs which may induce acute renal failure.

6. List drugs which may induce chronic renal failure.

7. Explain the mechanisms by which drugs cause nephrotoxicity.

8. Distinguish among prerenal, intrarenal, and postrenal failure according to cause and treatment.

9. Describe the goals of therapy and related management of acute renal failure.

10. Explain the nursing processes associated with the use of the following in acute renal failure: fluids, diuretics, diet, sodium polystyrene sulfonate, and antacids.

11. Describe the causes and therapy for anemia due to chronic renal failure.

12. Describe the causes and treatment of osteodystrophy due to chronic renal failure.

13. List the drugs used to suppress the immune response in renal transplantation.

14. Describe the adverse drug effects and associated nursing care in immunosuppression following renal transplantation.

15. Describe the ways in which renal failure leads to alterations in drug handling.

16. Identify drugs which should not be used in patients with renal failure.

17. Identify drugs which need no dosage change in patients with renal failure.

18. Identify drugs requiring dosage modification with renal failure and the techniques used to adjust dosage.

Aside from their role in excreting waste products of metabolism, the kidneys are essential in maintaining the body's fluid and chemical composition within a very narrow range. This remarkable capacity of the kidneys to preserve the internal milieu of the body, however, can be disrupted by a number of disease processes which impair their functional capacity. Such a loss of renal function, which is defined as *renal failure,* can lead to profound alterations in body composition. Waste products of the body's metabolism, particularly of protein metabolism, accumulate in renal failure. Many of these are toxic to various organ systems. Further, the kidneys function as glands to synthesize the most active form of the hormone vitamin D. They store and release substances for such diverse functions as blood pressure control (angiotensin I) and red blood cell synthesis (*erythropoietin*). These synthetic functions are also impaired in renal failure, as is the ability of the kidneys to eliminate many drugs. The role of pharmacotherapeutics in renal disorders is the prevention and treatment of diseases that may result in renal impairment; this includes minimizing exposure to nephrotoxic drugs and chemicals; correction of metabolic derange-

*The editors thank William A. Handelman, who cocontributed the chapter on this subject in the first edition.

ments that result from renal failure; suppression of the immunologic response to transplantation; and modification of drug regimen when impaired renal function alters the pharmacokinetics of a drug.

DETERMINING RENAL FUNCTION

It is possible for one component of the nephron to function abnormally without affecting the remainder of the nephron, but most diseases which affect the kidney involve the loss of entire nephron units. Therefore, tests which measure total renal function are an indirect means of assessing the remaining percentage of normally functioning nephrons. The tests most commonly used to assess overall renal function are the *serum creatinine* and the *creatinine clearance* (C_{cr}). Creatinine is a metabolic product of muscle catabolism. As such, it has the advantage of being produced by the body in a remarkably constant amount from day to day. More important, for purposes of assessing renal function, it is not metabolized, secreted, or reabsorbed to any significant degree. Thus, the amount filtered at the glomerulus is equal to the amount excreted in the urine. The determination of creatinine clearance, therefore, is an indirect measurement of glomerular filtration rate (GFR) and therefore of renal function. Normal creatinine clearances are approximately 100 to 400 mL/min. Values, however, are normally lower in women than in men because of less muscle mass, and values for both sexes decrease above age 60. Adjustment in dosage of renally excreted drugs during renal function impairment is commonly based upon the creatinine clearance level. Changes in serum creatinine *over time* are an accurate reflection of change in overall renal function, so the following formula is reliable for predicting creatinine clearance for males when the serum creatinine in milligrams per deciliter (creat), weight in kilograms (wt), and age in years are known (Brater, 1983a).

$$C_{cr} \text{ (estimated)} = (140 - \text{age}) \times (\text{wt}/72) \times (\text{creat})$$

The estimated creatinine clearance for females is 85 percent of that calculated using this formula for males. In addition, nomograms are available for estimating renal function (see Fig. 31-1).

Blood urea, or blood urea nitrogen (BUN), has long been used clinically as an index of renal function, partly because elevations in BUN are closely correlated with symptoms of renal failure. When the BUN is elevated (above 25 mg/dL), a patient is said to be *azotemic,* and when symptomatic from such elevation, that patient is *uremic* (generally at BUN levels above 100 mg/dL). The usefulness of the BUN as an index of renal function is limited by the fact that in conditions characterized by low urine volumes (e.g., dehydration and congestive heart failure), the BUN will be elevated disproportionately to any true decrement in renal function.

NEPHROLITHIASIS

Nephrolithiasis (renal stones) is a heterogeneous disorder associated with considerable morbidity from pain, hematuria, infection, and obstruction which can even lead to kidney damage. Most patients with renal stones have been found to suffer from one or more metabolic disturbances (e.g., hypercalciuria, hyperparathyroidism, cystinuria, hyperoxaluria, hyperuricosuria). Proper management of nephrolithiasis requires identification of the chemical composition of the stones and of the type of underlying metabolic disorder(s).

Etiology and Clinical Findings

In North America more than two-thirds of all renal stones are calcium-containing, either as pure calcium oxalate or as hydroxyapatite (calcium phosphate). Hypercalciuria (excess calcium in urine), hyperoxaluria (excess oxalic acid in urine), and hyperuricosuria (excess uric acid in urine) have each been associated with calcium stones. Primary hyperparathyroidism, vitamin D overdose, neoplasia, intestinal hyperabsorption of calcium, and renal tubular leak of calcium are causes of hypercalciuria. Genetic inheritance, high dietary intake, and ileal disease are factors in hyperoxaluria and/or hyperuricosuria associated with calcium-containing stones.

Noncalcium stones include struvite calculi (20 percent of all stones), uric acid stones (5 percent), and cystine stones (1 percent). *Struvite calculi* (magnesium ammonium phosphate) occur in persistently alkaline urine which is produced by urea-splitting bacterial infections, such as *Proteus, Pseudomonas, Klebsiella,* and some strains of *Staphylococcus.* Struvite stones can contain calcium phosphate, so they are also called infection stones and triple phosphate stones. Cystinuria is an inherited metabolic disorder which may result in cystine stones. Uric acid stones typically occur with persistently acidic urine (pH <5.5) and/or hyperuricosuria, which may or may not be accompanied by clinical gout.

Crystallization of renal stones depends upon (1) concentration of the crystalloid in the tubular urine, (2) pH of the urine, (3) presence of nucleation sites, and (4) the concentration of inhibitors to crystal formation (e.g., citrate, magnesium, pyrophosphate). Hypersaturation of a specific crystalloid, pH conducive to crystallization (e.g., acid for uric acid stones, alkaline for struvite stones), presence of foreign bodies in urine, and low levels of inhibitors promote calculi formation.

Specific diagnostic data needed in nephrolithiasis include review of the patient's history for genetic and dietary factors, as well as other symptoms of the underlying metabolic disorder. Laboratory determination of serum calcium, phosphorus, and uric acid is performed. Urine specimens collected for 24 h, after fasting, and following high intake of calcium may be evaluated for infection, pH, calcium, sodium, uric acid, oxalate, and cystine. The chemical composition of any stones strained from the urine should be determined. Roentgenologic appearance of the stones may also aid diagnosis, as calcium, cystine, and struvite stones are

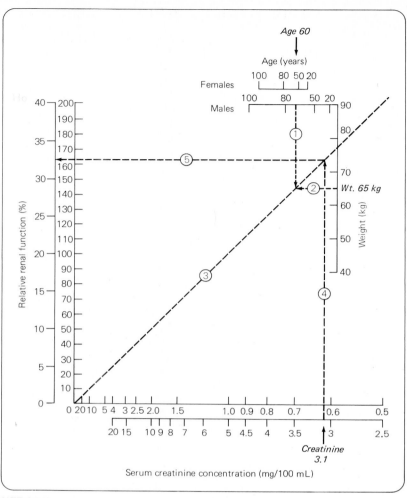

FIGURE 31-1

Nomogram for Estimating Renal Function. Determine relative renal function from serum creatinine concentration in adults by first defining the point where lines perpendicular to the patient's age (1) and weight (2) intersect. Draw a line from the origin through that point (3). Construct a line perpendicular to the point representing the patient's serum creatinine (4) to line 3. From this intercept point, run a line horizontally to the relative renal function scale (5). The outer scales are used for serum creatinines higher than 2.5 mg/dL. The example lines on the figure for a 60-year-old woman weighing 65 kg demonstrate that her renal function is about 33 percent of normal when her serum creatinine is 3.1 mg/dL. *(From T. D. Bjorsson: Clinical Pharmacokinetics, 4:216, 1979. Used by permission.)*

radiopaque (appear light like bones on x-ray) and uric acid stones are radiolucent (appear as dark areas on x-ray when contrast medium is used). However, often stones are present but not visualized on x-ray.

Drug-Induced Nephrolithiasis

A number of drugs predispose to urinary stone formation. Adrenocorticosteroids, **furosemide** (Lasix), aluminum-containing antacids which bind phosphate (e.g., Amphojel), and vitamin D can cause hypercalciuria. Vitamin D can also be

associated with increased oxalate excretion. **Acetazolamide** (Diamox) can impair renal acidification and promote formation of calcium phosphate stones. Any drug which alters urinary pH (see Table 31-1) can predispose to certain types of stone formation. **Triamterene** (Dyrenium) has been associated with calcium stone formation.

Clinical Pharmacology and Therapeutics

The treatment of nephrolithiasis depends upon the composition of the calculi and the underlying metabolic abnormality. In a few situations the cause of the stone formation can be corrected (e.g., diet modification in cases of excess intake, parathyroidectomy in primary hyperparathyroidism). However, in most cases therapy is aimed at altering the conditions which promote stone formation: reduction of the concentration of the crystalloid in the urine, alteration of urine pH, promotion or replacement of inhibitors, and removal of infection and other foci of precipitation. Table 31-2 outlines the treatment of the prevalent types of nephrolithiasis. The pharmacology and nursing process with most of these agents are discussed elsewhere in this text, as appropriate to their primary indication [e.g., **allopurinol** (Zyloprim) and **penicillamine** (Cuprimine) in Chap. 26; urinary antimicrobials in Chap. 28; thiazide diuretics in Chap. 23; drugs to treat acute pain during passage of a stone in Chap. 17].

Acetohydroxamic Acid (Lithostat)

Acetohydroxamic acid (Lithostat), or AHA, is indicated as an adjunct in the treatment of struvite renal stones which occur as a complication of renal infections with urea-splitting organisms. A persistent alkaline urine, which results when ammonia is liberated from urea by the bacterial enzyme urease promotes precipitation of struvite. Antimicrobial therapy of these infections frequently fails to eradicate bacteria within the calculi, resulting in recurrent infection and further calculus formation.

Mechanism of Action Acetohydroxamic acid inhibits the activity of bacterial urease, resulting in a normalization of urine pH. Stone formation is retarded or prevented and small preexisting stones may regress. Surgery is often required, however, to remove larger preexisting stones prior to long-term therapy. While acetohydroxamic acid lacks antimicrobial activity, many antibiotics are more effective after normalization of the urine pH.

Pharmacokinetics Acetohydroxamic acid is well-absorbed after oral administration, although it chelates and decreases the absorption of dietary iron. The drug is distributed throughout body water and reaches peak blood levels within 1 h of oral administration. Up to two-thirds of AHA is eliminated unchanged in the urine, so dosage adjustment is required in the presence of renal insufficiency. Half-life in normal renal function is 5 to 10 h.

Adverse Effects Mild headaches and gastrointestinal symptoms (nausea, vomiting, anorexia) occur in 30 percent of patients on acetohydroxamic acid. Psychiatric symptoms (malaise, anxiety, nervousness) have been reported in 20 percent of the patients. While 15 percent develop a reversible Coombs'-negative hemolytic anemia, most patients on AHA develop a mild reticulocytosis. Superficial thrombophlebitis of the legs and a rash associated with concurrent alcohol ingestion have been reported. Adverse effects are more common in patients with renal insufficiency, but do

TABLE 31-1 Drugs Used to Alter Urine pH

DRUG	USUAL DOSAGE RANGE*
Alkalinizers	
Acetazolamide (Diamox)	250–1000 mg daily
Potassium citrate and citric acid (Polycitra-K)	5–20 mL diluted in 150–250 mL water after meals and at bedtime
Potassium citrate and sodium citrate (Citrolith, Polycitra)	1–4 g (10–30 mL syrup) qid
Sodium bicarbonate	325 mg–2 g qid
Sodium citrate and citric acid solution (Shohl's solution; Bicitra)	5–30 mL diluted in 30–90 mL water after meals and at bedtime
Acidifiers	
Ammonium chloride	1–3 g bid–qid
Ammonium biphosphate, sodium biphosphate, and sodium acid pyrophosphate (pHos-pHaid)	1 g qid followed by glassful of water
Ascorbic acid (vitamin C)	>2 g daily in divided doses
Potassium acid phosphate (K-Phos Original)	1 g dissolved in 180 to 240 mL water with meals and at bedtime
Potassium acid phosphate and sodium acid phosphate (K-Phos M.F., K-Phos No. 2)	1–2 tablets qid–q2h with a glassful of water

*Shown for adults and children. Pediatric dosages should be on lower end of range.

not seem to increase with long-term therapy. AHA should not be used during pregnancy.

Dosage and Administration The daily dosage of 10 mg/kg for children and 10 to 15 mg/kg for adults should be administered on an empty stomach at intervals of 6 to 8 h. Adult dosage should not exceed 1.5 g daily. In the presence of impaired renal function lower doses and 12-h dosing intervals are recommended. Complete blood count should be performed after 2 weeks of therapy and at 3-month intervals thereafter, with dosage reduced if reticulocytes (immature red blood cells) exceed 6 percent.

Sodium Cellulose Phosphate

Sodium cellulose phosphate (Calcibind), or SCP, reverses the intestinal hyperabsorption of calcium in absorptive hypercalciuria by exchanging sodium for calcium ions in the intestine and binding the calcium so that it is eliminated in the feces. The drug is not absorbed. SCP is indicated for absorptive hypercalciuria, type I, characterized by recurrent calcium oxalate or calcium phosphate stones, but not for absorptive hypercalciuria, type II, which corrects readily with moderate dietary restriction of calcium (i.e., avoiding dairy products).

Adverse Effects Diarrhea and dyspepsia are associated with sodium cellulose phosphate. Secondary hypoparathyroidism occurs if calcium absorption is excessively depressed, so parathyroid hormone (parathormone) levels should be determined initially between the third and twelfth weeks of therapy. Elevated parathormone levels require discontinuation or dosage reduction. Hypomagnesemia and hyperoxaluria, as well as depletion of iron and trace metals (copper, zinc), can occur. Dietary restriction of oxalates, calcium, vitamin C (metabolized to oxalate), and sodium (<150 meq/day); supplementation of magnesium; and a high fluid intake should be encouraged for patients taking this drug. Children and pregnant women should not take SCP.

Dosage and Administration Dosage of SCP is regulated by urinary calcium levels. The recommended initial dose is 5 g with each meal for patients on a moderate calcium restricted diet having a daily urinary calcium in excess of 300 mg. When the daily urinary calcium declines to less than 150 mg, dosage of SCP is reduced to 2.5 g with breakfast and lunch and 5 g with supper. The drug is supplied as a powder which should be suspended in water or juice and taken within 30 min of the meal. The drug has an unpleasant taste.

TABLE 31-2 Treatment of Common Types of Nephrolithiasis

STONE CONTENT	TYPE/METABOLIC MECHANISM	TREATMENT
Calcium phosphate or calcium oxalate	Absorptive hypercalciuria, type I	Sodium cellulose phosphate (Calcibind) Calcium-restricted diet
	Absorptive hypercalciuria, type II	Moderate dietary calcium restriction Fluid intake sufficient to produce >2 L urine daily
	Renal hypercalciuria	Thiazide diuretic
	Hyperuricosuric calcium oxalate nephrolithiasis	Allopurinol 100 mg tid Eliminate excessive high-purine foods
	Primary hyperparathyroidism	Parathyroidectomy
	Enteric hyperoxaluria (e.g., following ileal bypass surgery)	Calcium 0.25–1 g qid
	No metabolic abnormality	Fluids sufficient to produce >2 L urine daily
Uric acid	Hyperuricemia with acid urine	Allopurinol 100 mg tid Urinary alkalinization
Cystine	Cystinuria	Alkalinization of urine Penicillamine 1–4 g daily divided into four doses (children 30 mg/kg/day) Adequate fluid to ensure >2 L urine daily
Struvite (magnesium ammonium phosphate)	Infection with urea-splitting bacteria	Antimicrobial drug Acetohydroxamic acid (Lithostat) Surgery (?)

Urinary pH Modifiers

Alkalinization of urine retards the precipitation of cystine uric acid stones, while struvite and calcium phosphate stones are less likely to form in acid urine. Phosphates, pyrophosphate, and citrate in these agents (Table 31-1) increase levels of inhibitors to stone formation. Liquid forms are diluted in water or juice, which may be chilled to increase palatability.

Thiazide Diuretics

Thiazide diuretics are useful in treatment of renal hypercalciuria, correcting the renal leak of calcium by promoting reabsorption of calcium at the renal tubule (see also Chap. 23). In addition, urinary inhibitor activity is increased by the thiazides, although the mechanism has not been elucidated. **Hydrochlorothiazide** (HydroDiuril), others) 50 mg twice a day, **chlorthalidone** (Hygroton) 50 mg daily, or an equivalent dose of any related thiazide diuretic will accomplish the desired effect.

Penicillamine

Penicillamine (Cuprimine) is thought to prevent cystinuria by forming a complex with cystine which is more water soluble than cystine alone. It decreases crystalluria and stone formation and may decrease the size of preexisting stones. The usual adult dosage is 2 g daily in four divided doses, while the daily dose for children is 30 mg/kg. Adverse effects can be minimized by beginning with low doses and gradually titrating to levels (up to 4 g daily in adults) which maintain urinary cystine below 100 mg/day (see also Chap. 26).

NURSING PROCESS RELATED TO NEPHROLITHIASIS

Assessment

While many stones are initially detected on x-ray or as the cause of asymptomatic hematuria, the pain of nephrolithiasis is typically located in the flank. The pain may spread downward into the loins, testicle, or vulva as the stone migrates. Frequency, urgency, and dysuria may result from a stone in the ureter or bladder. Explanation to the patient of the numerous tests and meticulous collection of urine samples is important to diagnosis of nephrolithiasis. The nurse should instruct these patients to strain all urine through four layers of gauze and to show any solid material strained from the urine to their health care provider.

Management

Increasing water intake to 4 to 6 L daily to achieve a urine output of *at least* 2 L/day (preferably 3 to 4 L) is appropriate in all forms of nephrolithiasis. It is particularly important to maintain high urine flow at night and for 3 h after meals. Dietary manipulation may serve as an adjunct to pharmacotherapy or may minimize adverse effects of drug therapy. Avoidance of dairy products will maintain a calcium intake of 400 to 500 mg/day. While this moderate restriction is beneficial in most calcium stone formers, further restriction has little value. Dietary calcium restriction may be detrimental in renal hypercalciuria and in children. Since increased urinary oxalate excretion accompanies dietary calcium restriction, oxalate restriction should be initiated concomitantly (i.e., avoidance of spinach and similar greens, vitamin C supplements, rhubarb, chocolate, cranberry juice, tea).

The adverse effects of most of these drugs can be quite serious. Patients taking **acetohydroxamic acid** (Lithostat) should be encouraged to inform their health care providers if they experience jaundice, malaise, joint pain, or decreased urine output. Those on **sodium cellulose phosphate** (Calcibind) should report blood in urine, tetany or tremors, confusion, muscle weakness, or diarrhea accompanied by significant fluid loss. Women should take precautions to avoid pregnancy when taking these drugs.

Evaluation

Urine pH determinations should be performed for patients taking urinary alkalinizers and acidifiers. Since these drugs can also modify systemic pH, changes in respiration and cognitive status should be evaluated and investigated.

The effect of drugs used to treat nephrolithiasis is often based upon measuring some constituent of a 24-h urine collection, so accurate and complete collection is crucial. Determination of urine pH, serum creatinine, and a complete blood count should be obtained regularly for patients on acetohydroxamic acid, with discontinuation or modification of dosage if there is evidence of hemolytic anemia, renal impairment, or a high urine pH indicating inadequate effect (see above). With sodium cellulose phosphate, therapy is evaluated by urine calcium and oxalate levels, serum parathormone levels, serum magnesium, and complete blood counts. Hypomagnesemia, oxaluria, elevated parathormone, and iron-deficiency anemia require investigation and corrective therapy.

RENAL FAILURE

Renal failure (or *renal insufficiency*) occurs when kidneys are no longer able to perform their functions adequately in the maintenance of normal body homeostasis and excretion of waste products of metabolism. There are two classifications of renal failure. In *acute renal failure* cessation of renal function is sudden, can often be pinpointed as to onset and etiology, and is usually complete. *Chronic renal failure* progresses gradually over months or years. The two types of renal failure have quite different etiologies, prognoses, and management.

Drug-Induced Nephrotoxocity

Many drugs can cause renal impairment, precipitating acute or chronic renal failure, as well as other renal dysfunction. In the presence of preexisting renal impairment, such drugs frequently have an increased capacity to damage renal structures. Similarly, the risk is higher for renal dysfunction if two nephrotoxins are used concurrently.

The two mechanisms of drug nephrotoxicity which can result in acute renal failure are *direct toxicity* and *immunologic response,* or hypersensitivity. The more common type of drug injury is *direct,* or *dose-related,* nephrotoxicity, in which excessive dosage and duration of therapy are implicated in causing *acute tubular necrosis.* This is particularly common for drugs which are concentrated by the kidney, resulting in greater concentrations of drug in the renal tissue than in plasma. The aminoglycoside antibiotics (see Chap. 27), particularly gentamicin (Garamycin), are the most frequent cause of renal failure in the hospitalized patient. The risk of developing renal failure is greatly reduced if gentamicin dosage is individualized for body weight and renal function, if serum levels are monitored at the peak and trough blood levels, and if the drug is stopped as soon as possible. Other substances with dose-related nephrotoxicity include **amphotericin B, tetracyclines,** some heavy metals (gold, mercury, lead, *cis-*platinum), radiographic contrast media, and organic solvents (see Table 31-3).

TABLE 31-3 Drug-Induced Nephrotoxicity

SYNDROME	ASSOCIATED DRUGS AND CHEMICALS
Acute tubular necrosis	Antibiotics: aminoglycosides (amikacin, gentamicin, kanamycin, neomycin, netilmicin, streptomycin, tobramycin), cephalosporins, polymixins (sodium colistimethate, polymixin E), tetracyclines
	Heavy metals: *cis-*platinum (antitumor drug), gold (including oral and parenteral antirheumatoid drugs), mercury, lead, arsenic, copper
	Organic solvents: ethylene glycol (in automobile antifreeze), carbon tetrachloride, trichloroethylene, toluene, gasoline, turpentine
	Radiographic contrast media, e.g., diatrizonate sodium (Hypaque-NA), diatrizonate meglumine (Renografin-M)
Proteinuria and nephrotic syndrome	Penicillamine, phenytoin, heroin
Acute interstitial nephritis	Methicillin, penicillin, cephalothin, ampicillin, ibuprofen, naproxen, fenoprofen, sulfonamides, rifampin, thiazide diuretics, phenindione, oxacillin, furosemide
Chronic tubulo-interstitial nephritis	Phenacetin, aspirin, acetaminophen, lithium, nitrosoureas (CCNU, BCNU)

Immunologic nephrotoxicity occurs irrespective of the dose or duration of therapy and may manifest as acute interstitial nephritis, arteritis, or glomerulopathy (acute glomerulonephritis, proteinuria, nephrotic syndrome). Such reactions are believed to be allergic in nature and are often heralded by fever, skin rash, and eosinophilia, which are soon followed by deteriorating renal function. The most frequently implicated drugs are the penicillins, followed by the cephalosporins, anticonvulsants, and nonsteroidal antiinflammatory drugs (see Table 31-3).

Chronic renal failure can result from *tubulointerstitial nephritis.* The best example is analgesic abuse nephropathy (renal papillary necrosis) from the heavy consumption of phenacetin-containing drugs. **Phenacetin** has been withdrawn from analgesic preparations in the United States. **Aspirin** and **acetaminophen** (Tylenol, Datril, others) have been associated with papillary necrosis much less frequently. Additionally, chronic lead poisoning can cause arteriolar nephrosclerosis, and heroin addiction is associated with chronic glomerulonephritis, both of which can result in chronic renal failure.

Aside from causing renal failure, drugs can impair specific renal functions. **Amphotericin B, penicillamine,** and outdated **tetracyclines** have caused renal tubular acidosis. **Chlorpropamide** and **clofibrate** potentiate the action of antidiuretic hormone, resulting in hyponatremia, while **lithium** and **demeclocycline** inhibit the action of antidiuretic hormone, resulting in a diabetes insipidus–like syndrome.

ACUTE RENAL FAILURE

Acute diminution or cessation of renal function can be caused either by factors originating in the kidney (*intrinsic renal failure*), by factors which interfere with the supply of blood to the kidney (*prerenal failure*), or by blockage to the exit of urine (*postrenal* or *obstructive failure*). All three types are usually characterized by a decrease in urine flow, but their treatment differs.

Etiology and Clinical Findings

Prerenal Failure

Conditions characterized by actual or effective intravascular volume depletion (shock, burns, dehydration, congestive heart failure, surgery, etc.) or by mechanical impairment of blood flow to the kidney cause prerenal failure. Since renal tubular function is preserved, the kidney avidly retains sodium and water in an attempt to maintain intravascular volume, causing low urine volumes with high specific gravity. If treatment of the dehydration (Chap. 24), shock (Chap. 48), congestive heart failure (Chap. 44), or obstruction results in an increase in urine flow and return of the BUN and creatinine toward normal, it is assumed that prerenal factors played a major role in the renal function impairment.

However, if not treated rapidly, prerenal failure may lead to renal damage, and intrinsic renal failure can result.

Postrenal Failure

Obstruction of the urine flow of both kidneys somewhere within the urinary tract causes postrenal failure. The obstruction can be intrarenal (e.g., obstruction of the renal tubules by uric acid crystals); within the renal pelvis, ureters, or bladder (obstruction by stone, tumor, clot, or infarcted renal papilla); or most commonly, within the urethra (obstruction by stones or prostatic tissue). Prolonged unrelieved obstruction will lead to intrinsic, and often irreversible, renal failure. Treatment involves removal of the obstruction.

Intrinsic Renal Failure

Severe prerenal or postrenal abnormalities along with renal failure secondary to drug administration account for the majority of cases of intrinsic renal failure. Therefore, the most important factors in its prevention include the recognition and correction of these abnormalities as well as knowledge of the nephrotoxic potential of drugs.

Although it is doubtful that therapeutic maneuvers can alter the duration or severity of intrinsic renal failure once it is established, several steps are often taken to determine whether the renal failure has progressed to the point of impaired tubular function. Any patient with a sudden decrease in urine output should be catheterized in order to accurately assess urine volume. A sample of urine should be sent to the laboratory for measurement of osmolality, urine sodium, and creatinine concentrations, and a simultaneous plasma creatinine should be measured. *Prerenal factors should be corrected and adequate hydration ensured,* preferably with monitoring of central venous or pulmonary artery pressure. If such measures do not restore urine flow, loop diuretics (furosemide, bumetanide, or ethacrynic acid; see Chap. 23) in high doses (equivalent to 40 to 100 mg furosemide) or an osmotic diuretic such as mannitol (see Chap. 39) may be ordered as a "challenge" to test renal function. Careful monitoring is necessary since the loop diuretics are nephrotoxic and ototoxic, and mannitol can result in volume overload and serum hyperosmolality, especially in patients with preexisting heart failure. If these measures fail to restore urine flow rates to normal, it is assumed that intrinsic renal failure is established and must be treated.

Clinical Pharmacology and Therapeutics

The goals of therapy in established acute renal failure are (1) regulation of fluid and electrolyte balance, (2) control of nitrogen retention, and (3) provision of adequate nutrition. The therapy required to accomplish this depends upon the stage of renal failure. The *oliguric phase,* usually beginning within hours of the inciting event and heralded by a decrease in urine volume, lasts about 7 to 14 days. (Some patients with

renal failure never develop oliguria, such as those with renal failure induced by gentamicin and radiographic contrast materials, which is called *nonoliguric renal failure*). This initial phase, whether oliguric or nonoliguric, is the most critical period since renal function is minimal and profound alterations in body chemical composition occur. The *diuretic phase,* which begins as early as 7 days or as long as 6 weeks after the onset of renal failure, is characterized by urine volumes of 4 to 6 L/day (occasionally up to 20 L/day) and excessive losses of water and electrolytes. The *recovery phase,* which may require weeks or months, is a period of gradual return of renal function to normal, although some deficit may persist.

Regulation of Fluid Balance

Since little urine is excreted during the oliguric phase, meticulous care should be taken with volume replacement, limiting fluids to urine volume plus insensible fluid loss (500 mL/day; more if patient has burns, fever, or is on a respirator) and the volume of drainage from nasogastric tubes, ileostomies, etc. A balance of fluid intake must be maintained during the diuretic phase to ensure adequate hydration without excess, since too much fluid can stimulate incremental urine volumes and excess electrolyte losses. Fluid therapy adequate to maintain urine output at 3 to 4 L/day is considered optimal in the diuretic phase.

Electrolyte abnormalities are universal in patients with acute renal failure. The most common of these is *hyponatremia,* as fluid is retained in excess of sodium because the kidneys are unable to correct the imbalance during the oliguric phase. The treatment is to decrease the patient's fluid intake below maintenance requirements. Correction with hypertonic saline is not indicated except in a neurologic emergency (e.g., seizures) because of the risk of severe volume overload. If used, it should be followed immediately with dialysis. During the diuretic phase sodium is washed out with the large urine volume, so oral or parenteral replacement may be needed.

Hyperkalemia occurs during the oliguric phase in renal failure patients for two reasons. First, renal potassium excretion diminishes markedly. In a patient without renal function, serum potassium rises 1.0 to 1.5 meq/L/day. However, this may be markedly accelerated in patients with excessive catabolism, particularly those with crush injuries in which large amounts of potassium are released from injured muscle (*rhabdomyolysis*). In such cases, potassium increments of 4 meq/L or more in several hours can occur and are often fatal. Second, acidosis results in a shift of potassium out of cells and into the extracellular volume (including the blood) without changing body potassium content. Treatment of hyperkalemia (oral or rectal cation exchange resins, glucose and insulin, calcium gluconate, sodium bicarbonate, and/or diuretics; see Chap. 24) should be instituted prior to dialysis whenever hyperkalemia results in ECG changes, since dialysis is a relatively slow and inefficient method of correcting hyperkalemia. *Hypokalemia* requiring potassium supplementation can occur during the diuretic phase.

Hyperphosphatemia results from an inability to excrete phosphate as well as excessive release of phosphate from damaged muscle in patients with rhabdomyolysis. This hyperphosphatemia results in *hypocalcemia*. Aluminum-containing antacids can be administered by mouth to bind the phosphate in the gut (see Chap. 24). Severe hyperphosphatemia (greater than 10 mg/dL) is best managed by dialysis. The hypocalcemia is rarely symptomatic, since acidosis helps protect against tetany by increasing the proportion of ionized to bound calcium. Administration of calcium in the presence of hyperphosphatemia is quite hazardous, as it can lead to extensive intravascular, intrarenal, and soft tissue deposition of calcium phosphate. *Hypermagnesemia* can occur in renal failure, particularly in patients in whom magnesium-containing antacids have been administered. If neuromuscular toxicity occurs, dialysis is indicated.

Control of Nitrogen Retention

In a patient with sudden cessation of renal function the products of protein breakdown accumulate and BUN concentration will rise approximately 20 mg/dL/24 h. Patients who are excessively catabolic, such as those with severe burns or rhabdomyolysis, may have much more rapid increments. Therefore, after 1 to 5 days of renal failure, BUN concentrations are greater than 100 mg/dL and the clinical syndrome of *uremia* occurs. Uremia is a constellation of symptoms associated with severe renal failure, the most prominent of which are neurologic and gastrointestinal. Other prominent symptoms include generalized skin itching and inflammation of the pericardium, peritoneum, and lung. The accumulation of a number of uremic toxins (by-products of protein metabolism) has been implicated in causing these symptoms. Management of acute renal failure, therefore, includes removal of these toxins by dialysis, symptomatic treatment of the uremic manifestations, and limitation of protein intake and catabolism.

Dialysis

Dialysis is based upon the physical principle that substances in solution will pass along a semipermeable membrane from the side containing the higher concentration of the substance to the side containing the lower concentration until a new equilibrium is reached. It is a technique used to rid the blood of substances that have accumulated in excessive concentrations, resulting in some toxic effect on the body. These substances include electrolytes, toxic metabolites (urea and other products of protein catabolism), drugs (e.g., barbiturates and other depressants), and poisons (e.g., ethylene glycol).

Two methods of dialysis are generally available in the treatment of acute renal failure. *Peritoneal dialysis* uses as its semipermeable membrane the large surface area of the body's own peritoneal cavity. The dialysis solution is infused into the peritoneal cavity through a catheter and drained off after a variable period, with this cycling continued for 36 to 72 h. *Hemodialysis* involves circulating the blood outside the body into a machine where the semipermeable membrane is a cellophane-like material. This treatment lasts 4 to 6 h and requires access to the patient's circulation either through catheters placed into a subclavian or femoral vein or by surgical connection of an artery and vein (arteriovenous fistula). The blood must be heparinized to prevent clotting in the dialysis tubing. The composition of the dialysis solution is adjusted according to the patient's blood chemistry, and dialyzable drugs (such as some antibiotics) may be added to the solution to prevent loss of therapeutic effect during the procedure.

Management of Uremic Symptoms

Uremic pruritis may be controlled by cleansing of the skin and application of an emollient cream or calamine lotion. **Diphenhydramine** (Benadryl) 25 to 50 mg has also been used to relieve itching. If *nausea and vomiting* is not adequately controlled by limitation of oral intake, **prochlorperazine** (Compazine) in a dose of 10 mg every 8 to 10 h may be ordered. Overdosage of prochlorperazine is associated with hypotension and extrapyramidal signs. *Gastrointestinal bleeding* is serious in uremic patients since it constitutes a hypercatabolic state, so some physicians use **cimetidine** (Tagamet) in doses of 300 mg IV every 12 h to control stress ulcers. As cimetidine is excreted unchanged in the urine, careful dosage selection and monitoring of the leukocyte count for neutropenia is required in renal failure patients. *Delirium* and *acute psychosis* may require sedation with paraldehyde or short-acting barbiturates, such as **secobarbital**, **pentobarbital**, and **amobarbital**, which are preferred over **phenobarbital** since they are primarily inactivated in the liver and can be used in normal doses. **Phenytoin** (Dilantin) in usual dosage ranges can be used to control *seizures* until dialysis can correct the underlying cause.

Provision of Adequate Nutrition

For those patients who can tolerate an oral diet, protein should be restricted to 20 to 30 g of high-quality protein per day. Caloric intake in the form of carbohydrates should be kept high (2000 to 3000 kcal/day). However, most patients cannot be fed, usually because of the severity of their underlying disease and uremic gastrointestinal symptoms. Because poor nutrition is associated with impaired immunity, poor wound healing, and catabolism of the body's own protein, the prognosis of these patients is improved if they receive intravenous hyperalimentation (see Chap. 25). Special solutions (e.g., Nephramine) have been designed for the renal failure patient. These generally provide essential amino acids, which can be converted directly into protein; low concentrations of sodium, potassium, and magnesium; and high calorie content. In addition, water-soluble vitamins are dialyzable and should be supplemented (folate, B vitamins, vitamin C).

Prognosis

The prognosis of acute renal failure depends upon the initiating cause. Obstetric and medical cases have the lowest mortality, while burns and surgically related cases have the highest mortality. It is thought that adequate nutrition is crucial to reducing deaths from acute renal failure. Some patients with an initial course compatible with acute renal failure fail to recover renal function and after several months are considered to have chronic renal failure.

CHRONIC RENAL FAILURE

Chronic renal failure exists in any patient whose baseline renal function is less than normal. It may be stable for many years, or may progress over a period of weeks, months, or years to *end-stage renal failure,* resulting in death unless dialysis or transplantation is provided. Unlike acute renal failure, patients with chronic renal failure do not have spontaneous reversal of their disease.

Etiology and Clinical Findings

Chronic renal failure is the result of damage to both kidneys as a consequence of chronic glomerulonephritis, immune diseases, hereditary disorders, infection, or obstruction. Chronic renal failure is divided into mild (creatinine clearance greater than 50 mL/min), moderate (creatinine clearance 15 to 50 mL/min), and severe or end-stage failure (creatinine clearance less than 15 mL/min). Only the patient with severe renal failure is likely to be symptomatic from the renal failure.

Clinical Pharmacology and Therapeutics

Although the pathophysiologic alterations in chronic renal failure are similar to those seen in acute renal failure, the duration of the illness results in differing manifestations. In addition to disturbances of fluid balance and uremia, chronic renal failure patients develop bone disease and anemia.

Fluid Balance

Sodium and *water imbalances* occur, although urine volumes are well-maintained even in advanced renal failure. However, water balance can be modulated only over a very narrow range, usually a fluid intake of 2 to 4 L/day. Most patients with chronic renal failure require moderate salt restriction (1 to 2 g of sodium per day) to control edema. Fluid and salt allowances must be tailored individually for each patient by closely following the patient's weight, electrolytes, and physical signs (blood pressure, edema) for evidence of fluid overload. When urine output declines in patients with end-stage renal failure, salt and water intake must be reduced proportionately.

About 80 percent of patients with severe chronic renal failure will have *hypertension,* usually secondary to a chronic state of volume overload. Therefore, the first line of therapy is salt and fluid restriction, diuretic therapy, and dialysis. Most patients will require additional antihypertensive therapy (see Chap. 40). Adequate therapy for blood pressure is important, since uncontrolled hypertension invariably leads to more rapid acceleration of renal deterioration and additional complications such as stroke and coronary disease. For patients on hemodialysis, the predialysis dose of the antihypertensive medication is usually omitted, since it may precipitate hypotension during dialysis.

Hyperkalemia is rarely a problem in chronic renal failure patients except in the very final stages. However, patients with severe renal failure should be warned against eating foods with high potassium content (citrus fruits, bananas, potatoes, chocolate), since a sudden load may precipitate severe hyperkalemia. Patients with potassium concentrations greater than 5.5 meq/L should be placed on long-term sodium polystyrene sulfonate (Kayexalate) therapy by mouth, with doses individualized to control the serum level of potassium (see Chap. 24).

Uremic Symptoms

Due to the duration of uremia in chronic renal failure, deposition of calcium, urea crystals, and other toxic substances in the tissues compounds the symptoms of uremia seen in acute renal failure. Adequate dialysis is the best way to control the symptoms, although symptomatic treatment (see above) may also be employed.

Renal Osteodystrophy

Reduction of nephron mass results in phosphate retention in chronic renal failure. The resultant hyperphosphatemia causes a fall in serum levels of calcium, which stimulates the parathyroid gland to release parathyroid hormone. This hormone acts on the kidney to increase excretion of the excess phosphorus and retain calcium, and it mobilizes calcium from bone stores to restore serum levels. However, this normalization of serum levels of phosphate and calcium is performed at the expense of an elevated (and constantly increasing) level of parathyroid hormone. When this occurs chronically, severe bone resorption results. The problem is compounded by the fact that the kidneys fail to convert vitamin D to its most active form (1,25-dihydroxyvitamin D_3) in severe renal failure. Since vitamin D is necessary for both calcium absorption from the gut and incorporation of mineral into bone, this combination of *secondary hyperparathyroidism* and vitamin D deficiency results in a severe form of bone disease called *uremic osteodystrophy.* In its most severe form it can be totally disabling, with spontaneous fractures of bones (the "brittle bone" syndrome), bone deformities, severe pain, and neurologic complications from vertebral compression.

Since it is difficult to lower phosphate by dietary means, phosphate-binding antacids [**aluminum hydroxide** gel (Amphojel) or **aluminum carbonate** (Basaljel)] are used instead. Magnesium-containing antacids must not be used because of the risk of causing hypermagnesemia. Therapy is aimed at keeping the serum phosphate below 4.5 meq/L, but hypophosphatemia (less than 2.0 meq/L) should be avoided. Once the serum phosphate is controlled in patients with symptomatic osteodystrophy, vitamin D can be added. 1,25-Dihydroxyvitamin D_3 (calcitriol; Rocaltrol) should be reserved for those patients who do not improve with other forms of vitamin D, since it can cause sudden and severe hypercalcemia. Calcium carbonate can be supplemented at doses of 2 to 10 g/day. For patients on dialysis, a dialysate with a high calcium concentration can be used. However, patients with hyperphosphatemia should not be given vitamin D or calcium supplements, since metastatic calcification can result. In patients with medically uncontrollable hyperphosphatemia and symptomatic osteodystrophy, particularly if they are hypercalcemic, parathyroidectomy may be indicated.

Anemia

Almost all patients with chronic renal failure are anemic, with the hematocrit in dialysis units averaging about 25 percent. The cause of this anemia is multifactorial. *Erythropoietin*, a potent stimulus of bone marrow erythropoiesis, has decreased production in severe chronic renal failure. *Iron-deficiency anemia* is quite common in advanced renal faliure due to a combination of gastrointestinal blood loss, abnormal absorption of iron from the gut, and chronic blood loss during dialysis. Oral iron therapy often is not effective, and intravenous iron dextran complex (Imferon) is given in such cases. *Hemolysis* is often a problem in chronic renal failure patients. Red blood cell turnover is increased in uremia owing to red blood cell metabolic abnormalities due to uremic toxins and to red blood cell antibodies which may form in reaction to impurities in the dialysis machine.

In many centers, patients are routinely treated with anabolic steroids (see Chap. 35), e.g., **nandrolone** (Deca-Durabolin), 100 mg given intramuscularly weekly. These agents directly stimulate erythropoiesis and, unlike testosterone, produce only mild virilization. Hematocrit levels often increase by several percentage points in such patients.

Transfusion therapy is discouraged in dialysis patients, and is reserved only for patients who are symptomatic from their anemia owing to the decreased oxygen-carrying capacity of their blood. The patients requiring most frequent transfusion are those with angina pectoris and children with renal failure (in whom hematocrits tend to run quite low).

Prognosis

Availability of dialysis and transplantation have considerably improved the prognosis of end-stage chronic renal failure, which was once virtually universally fatal. Both hemodialysis and peritoneal dialysis are adaptable to long-term therapy and can be performed in the home or dialysis center. Lack of donors, the phenomenon of kidney graft rejection, and concomitant disease present in many recipients and transplant candidates have limited the impact of transplantation on the prognosis of chronic renal failure.

Suppression of Graft Rejection

Great advances in tissue typing have been made in the past 15 years to improve the tissue "match" between donor and recipient. However, unless the transplant is from an identical twin, the recipient's body will invariably reject the donor kidney, no matter how good the match. Thus, renal transplant recipients must remain on lifelong therapy directed at suppressing graft rejection. If the graft fails, the patient must either be retransplanted or return to dialysis. Drugs used to suppress graft rejection include corticosteroids, immunosuppressants, and antilymphocyte globulins.

Corticosteroids

Corticosteroid therapy (see Chap. 35) is given to fight rejection, usually 1 g of methylprednisolone hemisuccinate (Solu-Medrol) intravenously daily for several days after transplant, then tapered rapidly to 80 to 100 mg of prednisone daily for several weeks. If no rejection episodes intervene, this dosage is then tapered more slowly over several months. If a rejection episode occurs (which is common), additional large-pulse doses of steroids are given in an attempt to reverse the rejection. Corticosteroids must be maintained indefinitely after transplantation; rejections have occurred many years after transplantation when therapy was stopped.

Immunosuppressants

Three drugs, **azathioprine** (Imuran), **cyclosporine** (Sandimmune), and **cyclophosphamide** (Cytoxan) are used to suppress cell-mediated immunity after transplantation. The precise mechanisms by which these drugs suppress homograft rejection is unknown, but each decreases T-lymphocyte activity. **Cyclophosphamide** is an antineoplastic agent whose pharmacology is presented in Chap. 37. **Azathioprine** and **cyclophosphamide** are also used to treat rheumatoid arthritis and other immune diseases (see Chap. 26).

Pharmacokinetics   **Azathioprine** is well-absorbed following oral administration. It is metabolized to mercaptopurine, which is rapidly degraded in erythrocytes and liver. Blood levels have little value in predicting therapeutic outcome.

Cyclosporine has incomplete and variable gastrointestinal absorption. It is 90 percent protein-bound in plasma, primarily to lipoproteins. The drug is extensively metabolized and eliminated in the bile. Blood levels correlate with clinical effect, and levels of 50 to 300 ng/mL appear to minimize both adverse effects and rejection.

Adverse Effects   **Azathioprine** may cause nausea and vomiting during the first few months of therapy. Its principal and most serious adverse effects are leukopenia and thrombocytopenia. On the other hand, **cyclosporine** rarely causes bone marrow or gastrointestinal toxicity, but is nephrotoxic and has been associated with hepatotoxicity and hypertension. All immunosuppressants appear to increase the risk of neoplasia, especially lymphomas. Immunosuppressed patients are at high risk for infection. These drugs may be teratogens.

Dosage and Administration   Initial dosage of **azathioprine** to suppress transplant rejection is 3 to 5 mg/kg daily at the time of transplant with maintenance dose in the range of 1 to 3 mg/kg as a single daily dose.

Oral therapy with **cyclosporine** is initiated 4 to 12 h prior to transplantation in doses of 8 to 15 mg/kg/day and continued for 1 to 2 weeks, after which it is tapered by 5 percent per week to maintenance doses of 5 to 10 mg/kg/day. The oral solution should be mixed in a glass container with room temperature milk, chocolate milk, or orange juice and drunk immediately; the glass is then rinsed with more milk or juice which is drunk to ensure that the entire dose is taken. An IV solution (50 mg/mL) is available for those unable to take the oral solution. IV doses, which are one-third the oral dose, are given over a 2- to 6-h period diluted in 20 to 100 mL of normal saline or 5% dextrose.

Other Agents

Antilymphocyte and antithymocyte globulin (Atgam), or ALG, is an adjunctive agent in the prevention and treatment of graft rejection which delays the onset and reduces the incidence of graft rejection and improves patient survival. The usual dose is 10 to 30 mg/kg daily (5 to 25 mg/kg for children) given intravenously for 2 to 4 weeks following transplantation. The globulin, which impairs T-lymphocyte function, is obtained from equine sources, so skin testing for hypersensitivity should precede therapy. Anaphylactic reactions, increased viral infections, fever, and joint pain are adverse effects associated with therapy.

Irradiation of the graft or recipient's blood, heparinization, and antiplatelet therapy have been shown to be without benefit in suppressing rejection. Thymectomy and maternal γ globulin are currently experimental treatments.

NURSING PROCESS RELATED TO RENAL FAILURE

Assessment

It is probably impossible for the nurse to recognize every drug that is nephrotoxic. However, the nurse should recognize the most common nephrotoxins and the need to evaluate any unexplained decrease in urine output, as well as the accumulation of fluid (increasing weight, sacral or peripheral edema, dyspnea, signs of congestive heart failure, and elevation in blood pressure) in any hospitalized patient. In addition, a gradual change in neurologic status, particularly sonnolence, mental confusion, or asterixis, should prompt evaluation of renal function. A detailed drug history is essential to assess possible nephrotoxic drug reactions.

Because patients with chronic renal failure often live at home, it is the community health nurse or the dialysis nurse who routinely assesses the physical status of such a patient. Vital signs, blood pressure readings, fluid intake and output, signs of electrolyte imbalance, and body weight are all parameters of renal function assessed at each visit. Auscultation of the heart and lungs by the nurse enables detection of congestive heart failure, pulmonary edema, or pericarditis. Clotting times are checked before, during, and after each hemodialysis.

It is important for the nurse to assess the safety of the environment at home and in the dialysis unit. Is the patient able to take his or her own medications? Is the patient drinking the required amount of fluid? Are there factors which increase the exposure to infection? Only by establishing a close one-to-one relationship with the patient and the family can the nurse guide the patient toward independence.

Management

Discriminate use of ice chips, which contain less fluid volume than water, may be satisfying to fluid-restricted patients who are thirsty. Oral hygiene should be thorough and gentle since decreased oral intake and uremia cause dryness, a bad taste, and uriniferous smell to the breath. The patient may need support in adjusting to the dietary restrictions and must be counseled against eating food brought in by visitors (chocolate, for instance, is extremely high in potassium). Hard candy may be a well-tolerated source of calories.

Careful observation should be made for symptoms of uremia. Chest pain that increases in severity when the patient lies down or a friction rub on auscultation may be the first signs of pericarditis, which should be *reported immediately* in dialysis patients who are heparinized. Increasing lethargy may be a sign of uremia or may represent an adverse drug reaction. Uremic patients may not exhibit fever as a sign of infection, the complication which carries the highest mortality for patients in renal failure. Tachypnea, mental confusion, hypotension, and even hypothermia may be the first signs of sepsis in these patients.

Patients with acute renal failure undergoing peritoneal dialysis therapy present their own special nursing problems. The nurse must be familiar with the procedure. The bottles must be warmed to body temperature both for patient comfort and to increase the efficiency of dialysis. Sterile technique must be maintained. An accurate record must be kept of the amount of fluid entering and leaving the peritoneal cavity. Changes in rates of inflow or outflow, or abdominal discomfort on inflow, may indicate poor catheter position. Abdominal tenderness and clouding of the dialysis outflow fluid are early indicators of peritonitis.

Nurse specialists are commonly directly involved with the dialysis procedure for patients on hemodialysis, but all nurses caring for the patient must pay careful attention to the catheter site. Pain, bleeding, serous or purulent drainage, and hematomas are all signs of problems and should be immediately brought to the attention of the physician. Antibiotic therapy and removal of the catheter is the usual treatment. A new catheter can be inserted in the opposite femoral or subclavian vein. Once a surgical fistula has been produced, it should be assessed by auscultation at the incision site for a bruit, and blood pressure readings should not be performed in that limb until healing is complete.

Those in chronic renal failure must be thoroughly educated as to their disease, particularly in the importance of dietary control of fluid, salt, potassium, and protein, and must be given strict and concrete guidelines to follow. Patients who have little understanding of the reasons behind dietary management are most likely to develop serious problems. In this regard, the aid of a trained renal dietitian is essential in helping the patient plan a diet. The patient must also be warned that salt substitutes contain potassium and are therefore dangerous. Any dietary changes should be discussed with the dietitian.

These patients are chronically ill and, as a result, often have serious psychologic and social problems. Many of the patients on long-term in-center dialysis are unemployed. Children are often particularly resentful of their disease. Patients should constantly be encouraged to seek employment, and children must attend school and other peer-group activities. Positive reinforcement should be emphasized; e.g., a patient who normally has excessive weight gain between dialysis treatments should receive praise on any occasion in which weight gains are acceptable. The dialysis nurse must be cognizant of what is happening in the patient's private life, since this is often crucial in understanding the way in which the patient reacts to the disease and therapy.

Before deciding to undergo a kidney transplant, these patients must be aware of the risks of transplantation, including the possibility of rejection, the risks of surgery, and the need to reliably take medications for the rest of their lives. In addition, patients should be aware of the hazards of immunosuppression, including life-threatening infection, steroid side effects, and a greatly increased cancer risk in transplant recipients. Despite these problems, a functioning transplanted kidney is by far the most acceptable outcome in patients with end-stage renal failure.

A nursing guideline to some of the more common drugs used in treatment of renal failure is presented in Table 31-4. The next section, Use of Drugs in Renal Failure, discusses modification of drug therapy for patients in renal failure, a crucial consideration in nursing management.

Evaluation

The nurse must monitor vital signs, weight, blood chemistries, and fluid intake and output to evaluate the effectiveness of the medical and nursing regimen and drug therapy. Whether certain drugs are aiding the patient may be difficult to ascertain, as their side effects may be similar to symptoms of renal failure. Complications such as congestive heart failure, hypertension, and infection are a constant threat, and it is the nurse who frequently interprets their symptoms first.

Following transplant the nurse must recognize the signs of graft rejection: fever, warmth over the graft, malaise, abdominal pain in the area of the graft, edema, and decreased urine output. Immunosuppressed patients must be observed for atypical signs of infection. Those on azathioprine or cyclophosphamide should also have regular complete blood counts and be observed for easy bruising. For those on cyclosporine it is important to evaluate creatinine clearance, liver function tests, and blood pressure.

CASE STUDY

R.L., a 27-year-old divorced accountant, was admitted to the hospital with complaints of fatigue, anorexia, swelling in his legs, headaches, and generalized itching. He had been hospitalized at 11 years of age with acute glomerulonephritis. Since that time, he has had persistently abnormal urinalyses, and was rejected for military service. However, he had felt well until 2 years ago, when he sought medical attention for severe headaches and epistaxis. At that time, a blood pressure of 220/140 was noted, and his serum creatinine level was 4.5 mg/dL. He responded well to antihypertensive medication. He lives alone, but near his mother and three teenage siblings.

Physical Examination

The patient's blood pressure was 180/100; pulse, 100; respirations, 28. He had pale, dry, yellowish skin. His breath had a uriniferous odor, and the tongue was heavily coated. Fine rales were heard on auscultation in both lung fields. An S_4 gallop was heard, along with a cardiac murmur. Pitting edema was present in both lower extremities to midthigh. On neurologic evaluation, he was oriented to time and place but had difficulty in subtracting serial sevens and could not recall five numbers in sequence. Deep tendon reflexes were 3+, and mild, unsustained asterixis was present.

Laboratory Data

On admission, blood analysis showed the following: sodium, 150 meq/L; potassium, 5.8 meq/L; phosphate, 8.2 meq/L; pH, 7.25; BUN, 140 meq/L; creatinine, 14 mg/dL; hematocrit, 18 percent. Urinalysis showed a specific gravity of 1.010, 3+ proteinuria, 3 to 5 RBC, 5 to 10

TABLE 31-4 Drugs Used in Renal Failure

DRUG	ASSESSMENT	MANAGEMENT	EVALUATION
Diuretics Furosemide (Lasix), ethacrynic acid, bumetanide (Bumex)	Check degree of edema, daily weight, fluid intake and output, serum potassium and sodium levels, history of diabetes or gout.	Teach patient possible fluid restrictions, avoid giving fluids at bedtime; if diagnostic or "challenge dose" results in large diuresis, the need for fluid replacement should be considered (in prerenal failure).	Observe degree of edema; check weight, serum glucose, frequency of stools; evaluate hearing changes or ringing in ears.
Antiemetics Prochlorperazine	Take blood pressure, record fluid intake and output, note any abnormal muscle movement.	Administer before patient becomes very nauseated; give rectally or intramuscularly.	Check blood pressure for signs of orthostatic hypotension; check sclera for jaundice; may have skin reactions or motor symptoms; may aggravate restless limb syndrome of uremia; measure and describe emesis.
Anabolic steroids Nandrolone decanoate (Deca-Durabolin), testosterone propionate	Check red blood cell count, weight, fluid intake and output.	Female patients should be told that excessive hair growth, deepening of the voice, or baldness may occur.	Unusual bleeding may occur if patient is on anticoagulants; check urine and stool for blood; check hematocrit, hemoglobin counts.
Antacids Amphojel, Basaljel	Check phosphate levels; check for constipation.	Teach patients to take medication without fail (patient may stop taking medication because of taste); do not substitute magnesium antacids.	Check phosphate level; give mild cathartic or stool softener for constipation.
Miscellaneous Kayexalate	Check serum potassium and sodium levels; check for constipation or diarrhea; check for signs of hyperkalemia; weakness, fatigue, ileus, peaked T waves, and wide QRS, bradycardia.	In enema, warm Kayexalate and sorbital (mix at patient's bedside, because it becomes thick paste quickly); give slowly; patient to retain enema 1 h; may cause diarrhea; patient may need cleansing enema prior to Kayexalate.	Check serum potassium and sodium levels; check number of stools.
Potassium preparations (K-Ciel, K-Lor, etc.)	Check serum potassium levels. Check for signs of hypokalemia; muscle weakness, arrhythmias, flat or inverted T waves, and heart block. Hypokalemia may predispose patient to digitalis toxicity.	Teach patient to take medication with meals.	Check potassium levels; signs of hyperkalemia.
Vitamin D (1,25-dihydroxyvitamin D_3 or Rocaltrol)	Check serum calcium and blood urea nitrogen.	Do not use over-the-counter preparations containing vitamin D.	Check for symptoms of hypercalcemia—lassitude, anorexia, nausea, and diarrhea; if increase in blood urea nitrogen or serum calcium, stop drug.
Miscellaneous supplements (iron, vitamins, folic acid)	Check laboratory tests (complete blood count, folate levels, serum, iron, etc.).	Teach patient to take medications at same times each day.	Check patient compliance and understanding.
Phenytoin (Dilantin), diazepam (Valium): as anticonvulsant	Check rate and depth of respirations, pulse rate, blood pressure; assess previous convulsions.	Provide for safety of patient (padded side rails), since excitement and discoordination can occur when drug is given intravenously.	Chart accurate degree and number of convulsions; check blood pressure, pulse rate, and respirations.

WBC, and 3 to 5 broad waxy and granular casts. Chest x-ray revealed cardiomegaly and interstitial edema. ECG demonstrated a sinus rhythm, with mildly peaked T waves.

Based upon this data and previous hospital records, the physician's diagnosis was chronic renal failure (severe) secondary to chronic glomerulonephritis. Orders included the following: methyldopa (Aldomet), 500 mg PO qid; furosemide (Lasix), 40 mg IV bid; aluminum hydroxide gel (Amphojel), 30 mL PO qid and PRN at bedside; Kayexalate, 30 g PO in 50 ML sorbitol, to be repeated if serum potassium remained greater than 5.0 meq/L 4 h after the first dose; type and cross-match for 2 units of packed red blood cells; oxygen per nasal cannula at 2 L/min PRN; daily measurement of serum electrolytes; 24-h urine collection for creatinine and protein excretion; diet containing 20 g of protein, 1000 mg of sodium, and 1500 mg of potassium. Fluid restricted to 1000 mL/24 h; strict charting of fluid intake and output; daily weight measurement and bed rest with bathroom privileges. In addition, a surgery consultant was asked to see the patient to place an arteriovenous fistula for dialysis.

Assessment

Upon his admission to the unit, the nurse took R.L.'s vital signs. After being weighed, R.L. appeared distressed and stated, "I've gained 10 pounds in the last 3 weeks." His temperature was normal at 36.8°C. Rales were heard in both lower lobes, and slight distention of the neck veins was noted. The patient had difficulty in removing his shoes, and both calves, ankles, and feet were edematous. Both eyes appeared puffy.

R.L. appeared alert and knowledgeable when questioned about his past medical history. He admitted that he sometimes forgot to take his medication and found it difficult to stay on a low-protein diet. He stated that he felt lethargic and useless. The nursing diagnosis included fluid retention and electrolyte imbalance due to severe renal failure, mild respiratory distress due to congestive heart failure, and depression.

Management: Initial 24 h

A primary goal of the nurse was to monitor fluid and electrolyte imbalances and reestablish homeostasis. R.L.'s limited fluid intake was equally distributed throughout the day to reduce thirst. R.L. actively participated in calculating his intake. Because of his dry mouth, gentle mouth care was given, and the patient was allowed to suck on ice chips, which were included in his intake allowance.

He was placed in Fowler's position, and the foot of the bed was elevated to increase venous drainage of the extremities. Because of the edema and dry scaly condition of his skin, special care was given and included bathing with Alpha-Keri oil. Calamine lotion was used to provide comfort and reduce itching. A foot cradle and special linen were placed on the bed to protect edematous lower extremities.

Because the patient was right-handed, it was likely that the surgeon would place the arteriovenous fistula for dialysis in his left forearm. The nurse therefore placed a sign over the bed noting that blood pressure readings and blood samples were not to be taken from the left arm and explained the reason for this to the patient.

The nurse observed the patient taking his medications and questioned him to see if he complied with therapy and understood its importance. R.L.'s blood pressure was taken while he was sitting and lying down prior to administration of his antihypertensive drugs.

As R.L.'s serum potassium level was elevated, the nurse monitored his pulse. He was placed on a cardiac monitor. After the first intravenous dose of furosemide was given, the nurse maintained an hourly determination of intake and output.

Oxygen therapy was begun. After 2 h the respiratory rate had decreased to 18/min and the patient removed the oxygen himself.

The patient began to verbalize his feelings of inadequacy as well as his fears about starting hemodialysis. The nurse allowed the patient to express his feelings and acted as a sounding board. In addition, the nurse arranged for him to visit the dialysis unit and to talk to a long-term dialysis patient who worked as a social worker at the hospital. Long-term goals were identified to help the patient accept his disease process, promote independence, and prevent complications.

Evaluation: Initial 24 h

R.L.'s weight increased by ½ lb, and his urine output was only 800 mL/24 h despite the intravenous furosemide therapy. His hematocrit and electrolyte status remained the same. However, his respirations were decreased to 14/min and were not as labored. His blood pressure decreased slightly to 160/100. He was sent to the operating room, where an arteriovenous fistula was placed under local anesthesia. Upon return to the floor, the nurse heard a loud bruit by auscultating at the incision site. This area was marked and auscultated every 2 h. Acetaminophen (Tylenol) was prescribed for pain. The next morning R.L. was taken to the dialysis unit for insertion of a left subclavian catheter for his first dialysis. Upon his return, he seemed somewhat depressed and complained of a headache. but he did note that his breathing was much better. He told the nurse that he "was just going to have to get used to it" and that the procedure wasn't nearly as bad as he expected. The nurse recognized the patient's beginning acceptance of his need for dialysis therapy, and expanded the care plan to include the probability of long-term home hemodialysis. The patient was told that after his fistula was developed, the subclavian catheter would be removed and dialysis would then be initiated via the fistula.

USE OF DRUGS IN RENAL FAILURE

Nearly all drugs or their metabolites are excreted by the kidney. Therefore, the onset of renal failure results in major alterations in drug clearance. This is compounded by the fact that because of the serious nature of their disease, patients with renal failure are usually on a large number of drugs. It is estimated that more than 25 percent of hospitalized patients with severe renal failure will have an adverse drug reaction.

Pharmacokinetics in Renal Failure

Absorption from the gastrointestinal tract in chronic renal failure may be impaired for drugs that require an acidic gastric pH, since the conversion of excess urea to ammonia raises gastric pH. Impaired oral iron absorption is the best example of such poor drug absorption in uremia. Presystemic metabolism may also be decreased in renal failure, resulting in increased bioavailability, as has been noted with **propranolol** (Inderal).

Distribution of drugs can be altered by uremic acidosis. **Digoxin** shows a decreased volume of distribution in end-stage renal disease, requiring smaller loading doses. Protein binding may be profoundly altered in uremia, due to hypoalbuminemia or displacement of the drug from binding sites by uremic toxins. As a result, toxic effects may be observed despite normal serum drug concentrations. Table 31-5 lists some drugs with decreased protein binding in uremia.

The kidneys have a small role in drug *metabolism,* although **insulin** requirements may decline in renal failure because a considerable amount (25 percent) of insulin is metabolized by the kidneys. Renal failure may impair hepatic elimination of some drugs, by a mechanism which is currently unknown. In addition, some drugs are biotransformed by the liver to active metabolites which require renal excretion. For example, **procainamide** (Pronestyl) is metabolized to **N-acetylprocainamide** (NAPA), which has antiarrhythmic activity and may reach toxic levels in patients with renal failure.

Impaired *elimination* is the most important alteration

that occurs in renal failure for drugs that are primarily excreted in unchanged form by the kidney. Drug half-life is therefore markedly increased for such drugs in renal failure. Knowledge of this alteration in drug half-life allows specific guidelines to be established for drug dosage and the interval between doses in patients with renal failure.

Renal failure can effect the drug-receptor interaction or *pharmacodynamics* of drugs. Electrolyte alterations alter response to cardiovascular drugs (e.g., **digoxin**, **quinidine**, **pindolol**). Urinary tract anti-infective drugs, such as **nitrofurantoin** (Furadantin), **nalidixic acid** (NegGram), and **methenamine** (Mandelamine) should not be used in renal failure, since they fail to reach adequate urinary concentrations even in moderate renal failure.

Guidelines in Drug Dosages

Recognizing that renal function is impaired in a patient is the first step in realizing that drug therapy must be altered. With this in mind, the following principles may greatly reduce the incidence of adverse drug reactions in patients with renal failure:

1. No drug should be given unless specifically indicated. "Routine" orders for sleeping pills, laxatives, and antacids may have disastrous consequences.

2. Awareness of the pharmacology and potential side effects of any drug used is critical.

3. Drug dosages should be altered according to specific published guidelines and should be based on timed creatinine clearances, with revision of doses as needed for patients with changing renal function.

4. Drugs for which guidelines for use in renal failure are not available should not be used.

5. If possible, drug blood levels should be monitored. This is particularly important for any drug with a *narrow therapeutic index,* in which toxic effects occur at levels only slightly higher than therapeutic effects (e.g., **digoxin**, **gentamicin**, **phenobarbital**, and **phenytoin**). However, since renal failure may alter the relationship between serum concentration and drug effect, *clinical monitoring* of efficacy and toxicity must accompany blood level determinations.

6. Metabolic loads administered along with the drugs, for example, carbenicillin used in a dose of 16 g/day results in the administration of 75 meq of sodium. Other drugs contain magnesium, potassium, or phosphate or can cause fluid retention.

7. For drugs that are significantly removed during dialysis, additional doses must be given at the end of dialysis or added to the dialysate (dialysis solution).

TABLE 31-5   Drugs with Decreased Protein Binding in Renal Failure

Barbiturates
Penicillin G
Clofibrate (Atromid-S)
Diazoxide (Hyperstat)
Dicloxacillin
Furosemide (Lasix)
Phenylbutazone (Butazolidin)
Phenytoin (Dilantin)
Salicylates
Warfarin
Diazepam (Valium)
Morphine
Triamterene (Dyrenium)

Methods of Dosage Adjustment

Selection of a dose and dosing interval to produce the desired clinical effect in a patient in renal failure requires knowledge of the patient's level of renal function (measured or estimated creatinine clearance) and data from the literature on the usual half-life of the drug in those with that level of renal function. *Increasing the interval* between standard doses is one technique to prevent drug accumulation, but in severe renal impairment this method increases the duration of time during which the serum drug concentration is below the minimally effective level. *Decreasing the amount of drug* administered at standard intervals prevents accumulation and decreases fluctuation in blood levels, but can result in elevated trough levels. Therefore, the *combined approach* of decreasing the dose and at the same time increasing the interval between doses for those in severe renal failure more closely approximates the normal peak, average, and trough blood levels. For some drugs, it is sufficient to alter only the dosage interval or the dosage amount, but the combined approach is suggested for those with narrow therapeutic ranges. Nomograms have been developed for drugs like **digoxin** and the **aminoglycosides** to show recommended dosage adjustments at various levels of renal impairment (see Fig. 28-1).

Table 31-6 is summary of some commonly used drugs, indicating the major route of elimination, changes in half-life in severe renal failure (glomerular filtration rate <15 mL/min), and recommended dosage changes with various degrees of renal failure. In addition, the dializability of each drug is indicated.

CASE STUDY

A.P., a 72-year-old widow, was admitted to the hospital with lower abdominal pain, loss of appetite, and fever and chills of 24-h duration. Initial evaluation revealed a blood pressure of 120/70, temperature of 38.6°C, pulse of 120, marked tenderness in the left lower quadrant of the abdomen, and a guaic-positive stool. The white blood cell count was 16,000, with 60 percent polymorphonuclear cells and 32 percent band cells. Initial serum creatinine was 1.8 mg/dL. The physician diagnosed diverticulitis and ordered cephalothin (Keflin), 500 mg IV q6h, and gentamicin (Garamycin), 80 mg IV q8h. The patient rapidly improved, and was afebrile 48 h after admission. Antibiotics were continued. On the fourth hospital day, the nurse noted that the patient had not voided in the previous shift despite adequate fluid intake, and urine output in the previous 24 h had been only 400 mL.

Assessment

The nurse, aware that the patient was taking two antibiotics with the potential for additive or synergistic nephrotixic effects, noted that the patient's weight had increased from an admission weight of 48 kg to 50 kg. Her blood pressure was 170/98, and the patient denied any previous history of hypertension. The patient noted some shortness of breath and on auscultation of her lungs had scattered bibasilar rales. Upon notification, the physician asked the nurse to obtain a urine specimen. The patient was unable to void spontaneously, and the nurse informed the patient that it would be necessary to catheterize her. The nurse reassured the patient and explained the procedure to her as it was being performed. The catheterization resulted in 50 mL of dark urine, which was sent to the laboratory along with a blood specimen. The urinalysis showed a specific gravity of 1.010, 2+proteinuria, 0 to 5 white blood cells per high-power field, many epithelial cells, and 3 to 5 coarse granular casts per high-power field. The urinary sodium concentration was 60 meq/L. The serum creatinine was 4.8 mg/dL; BUN 62 mg/dL; serum sodium, 132 meq/L; serum potassium, 5.0 meq/L; serum chloride, 92 meq/L; CO_2 content, 20. The physician diagnosed acute renal failure secondary to gentamicin therapy. A blood level of gentamicin drawn 4 h after the last dose was elevated to 10 μg/mL.

Initial Management

The patient was informed that her kidneys were not functining properly and that certain procedures were necessary in order to prevent any serious complications. A Foley catheter was inserted to accurately monitor urine output. The physician inserted a subclavian catheter to accurately measure the central venous pressure (CVP). Since the initial reading was elevated at 10 cmH2O, furosemide was given intravenously at a dose of 80 mg. Vital signs and urine output were monitored continuously. Since the output was only 30 mL over the ensuing 2 h, a second furosemide dose of 200 mg was given. The nurse inquired if the patient had any hearing difficulties after this dose. Two-hour output was again only 30 mL. A third furosemide dose of 600 mg IV was given, again with no results. At this point, the physician concluded that acute renal failure was established. The gentamicin was discontinued, and cephalothin continued at a reduced dose of 500 mg q12h IV. Fluids were reduced to the amount needed only for cephalothin infusion, plus an oral allowance of 500 mL. The nurse kept exact records of fluid intake and output. Oxygen was ordered and improved the patient's dyspnea. When the patient complained of thirst, ice chips were administered and their volume estimated. The subclavian dressing was changed daily to minimize the risk of infection. Breath sounds were checked hourly for 4 h after the subclavian placement because of the risk of a pneumothorax. A chest x-ray was ordered to assess the position of the catheter.

Evaluation

The patient's weight increased by 0.5 kg the next day, and sacral edema was noted. However, breathing was unchanged. A diet restricted to 1 g of sodium, 1.5 g of

TABLE 31-6 Drug Dose Modification in Renal Failure

DRUG	MAJOR ELIMINATION ROUTE	t½ (h) NORMAL	t½ (h) RENAL FAILURE†	Dosage Change In Renal Failure* MILD	Dosage Change In Renal Failure* MODERATE	Dosage Change In Renal Failure* SEVERE	DIALIZABILITY‡
Acetaminophen	Hepatic	2	2	None	None	None	Yes
Amikacin	Renal	2	30–50	50% normal dose	35% normal dose	25% normal dose	Yes
Amoxicillin	Up to 90% renal	1	6–18	None	q6–12h	q12–48h	Yes
Ampicillin	Up to 90% renal	1	6–20	None	q6–12h	q12–24h	Yes
Aspirin	Hepatic	2–19	2–19	q4h	q4–6h	Avoid	Yes
Azathioprine	Hepatic; 20% renal	N/A§	N/A	None	None	Slight decrease	Yes
Cefoxitin	90% renal	0.7	7–30	q8h	q8–12h	q12–24h	Yes
Cephalexin	90% renal	1	20–30	None	q6–12h	q12–36h	Yes
Cephalothin	66% renal	0.5	3–15	None	None	q 8–12h	Yes
Chlorpropamide	Hepatic; 25% renal	25–42	44–85	Decrease	Avoid	Avoid	No
Cimetidine	Up to 80% renal	1.5–2.5	3–10	300 mg/6 h	300 mg/8 h	300 mg/12 h	Slight
Cyclophosphamide	Hepatic; up to 20% renal	5	Prolonged	None	None	Slight dose decrease	Yes
Cyclosporine	Hepatic	19	Prolonged	None	None	None	No
Diazepam	Hepatic	20–90	20–90	None	None	None	No
Digitoxin	Hepatic	180	180	None	None	None	No
Digoxin	70% renal	6	100	None	50% dose decrease	50–70% dose decrease	No
Diphenhydramine	Hepatic	3–8	Unknown	None	None	Increase interval	No
Doxycycline	50% hepatic; 50% renal	15–24	25	None	None	None	No
Furosemide	Up to 70% renal	½–1	Prolonged	None	None	None	None
Gentamicin	Renal	2	30–60	75–100% normal dose	35–75% normal dose	25–35% normal dose	Yes
Heparin	Hepatic	0.5	½–1	None	Ineffective	Ineffective	No
Hydrochlorothiazide	Renal	2.5	24	None	None	None	No
Ibuprofen	Hepatic	15–3	Unknown	None	None	None	No
Lidocaine	Hepatic	1.5	1.5	None	None	None	No
Methyldopa	Renal; up to 40% hepatic	1	3–6	None	q9–18h	q12–24h	Yes
Nalidixic acid	Hepatic; 15% renal	1.5	21	None	Ineffective	Ineffective	Yes
Nitrofurantoin	Up to 50% renal	0.3	1	None	Ineffective	Ineffective	Slight
Oxazepam	Hepatic	20	20	None	None	None	Unknown
Penicillin G	Up to 90% renal	0.5	6–20	None	q8–12h	q12–18h	Yes
Phenytoin	Hepatic	15	8	None	None	None	No
Prednisone	Hepatic	1	1	None	None	None	No
Prochlorperazine	Hepatic	20	20	None	None	None	No
Propoxyphene	Hepatic	9–15	Unknown	None	None	Slight dose decrease	No
Propranolol	Hepatic	4	2–3	None	None	None	No
Quinidine	Hepatic; up to 25% renal	3–16	3–16	None	None	None	No
Tetracycline	60% renal	6–15	7–75	Avoid¶	Avoid¶	Avoid¶	Slight
Tolbutamide	Hepatic	4–8	4–8	None	None	None	No
Triamterene	Hepatic	2	2	None	Avoid	Avoid	No

*Mild renal failure (GFR > 50 mL/min); moderate renal failure (GFR = 15–50 mL/min); severe renal failure (GFR < 15 mL/min).   †Severe renal failure (GFR < 15 mL/min).   ‡Hemodialysis.   §N/A = Not applicable, since azathioprine is a prodrug.   ¶Use doxycycline.

Sources: R.J. Anderson and R.W. Schrier (eds.): *Clinical Use of Drugs in Patients with Kidney and Liver Disease*, Philadelphia: Saunders, 1981; W.M. Bennett et al.: *Drugs and Renal Disease*, New York: Churchill Livingston, 1978; B.G. Kastrup (ed.): *Facts and Comparisons*, Philadelphia: Lippincott, 1984; G.B. Appel and H.C. Neu: "Infections and Antibiotic Usage in Patients with Renal Disease," in M. Martinez-Maldonado, *Handbook of Renal Therapeutics*, New York: Plenum, 1983.

potassium, and 40 g of protein was ordered; however, the patient refused all food. Hard candies were offered by the nurse to provide some carbohydrate intake. After consultation with the physician and dietitian, Nephramine was ordered to be given intravenously at 25 mL/h, plus urine output. On the third day after the discovery of renal failure, the creatinine peaked at 8.2 mg/dL, with BUN of 92 mg/dL. However, that day the urine increased to 50 mL/h, and the following day the 24-h urine output increased to 3.5 L. Over the next 24 h, weight decreased to 26.5 kg and the patient complained of dizziness when sitting up. The nurse noted a 40 mmHg fall in blood pressure on standing. The intravenous rate was increased to match the urine output with 0.45% normal saline in D_5W. The Nephramine was discontinued and the patient's diet was changed to 2 g of sodium and 80 g of protein. The urine output gradually decreased over the next 2 days to 2 L/day, and the creatinine fell to 2.2 mg/dL. The Foley catheter, CVP line, and all medications were discontinued.

The nurse's role throughout the illness was to accurately assess the renal status of the patient by monitoring both the patient's volume and electrolyte status and fluid intake and output. In addition, many procedures with potential for serious complications were performed to aid in the patient's management. It was the nurse's role to check for the presence of these complications as well as to ensure that all catheters were placed aseptically and frequently checked for the presence of infection in this high-risk patient. The nurse also correctly assessed that the patient's caloric intake was inadequate at the height of the renal failure, and an intravenous alimentation solution specially designed for renal failure patients was supplemented. Expert nursing care helped this patient recover from a very serious complication of therapy.

REFERENCES

"Acetohydroxamic Acid (Lithostat by Mission)—New Therapy for Struvite Renal Stones," *Facts and Comparisons Drug Newsletter,* **2**:49, July 1983.

Anderson, R. J., and R. W. Schrier (eds.), *Clinical Use of Drugs in Patients with Kidney and Liver Disease,* Philadelphia: Saunders, 1981.

Bagby, S. P.: "Drug Therapy in Renal Stone Disease," *Drugs and Renal Disease,* in W. M. Bennett, G. A. Porter, S. P. Bagby, and W. J. McDonald (eds.), New York: Churchill Livingstone, 1978.

Bennett, W. M.: "Drug Therapy in Reduced Renal Function," in W. M. Bennett, G. A. Porter, S. P. Bagby, and W. J. McDonald (eds.), *Drugs and Renal Disease,* New York: Churchill Livingstone, 1978.

Bjornsson, T. D.: "Use of Serum Creatinine Concentration to Determine Renal Function," *Clin Pharmacokinet,* **4**:200–222, 1979.

Brater, D. C.: "Drugs and the Kidney: Adjusting Drug Regimens in Patients with Renal Disease," in M. Martinez-Maldonado (ed.), *Handbook of Renal Therapeutics,* New York: Plenum, 1983a.

————: "Drugs and the Kidney: Renal Contribution to Handling of Drugs," in M. Martinez-Maldonado (ed.), *Handbook of Renal Therapeutics,* New York: Plenum, 1983b.

Brundage, D. J.: *Nursing Management of Renal Problems,* 2d ed., St. Louis: Mosby, 1980.

Castro, J. E.: *The Treatment of Renal Failure,* New York: Appleton-Century Crofts, 1982.

Gutch, C. F., and M. H. Stoner: *Review of Hemodialysis for Nurses and Dialysis Personnel,* 4th ed., St. Louis: Mosby, 1983.

Hekeleman, F. P., and C. A. Ostendarp: *Nephrology Nursing: Perspectives of Care,* New York: McGraw-Hill, 1979.

Jackle, M., and C. Rasmussen: *Renal Problems: A Critical Care Nursing Focus,* Bowie, MD: Brady, 1980.

Kastrup, B. G. (ed.); *Facts and Comparisons,* Philadelphia: Lippincott, 1984.

Lewis, S. M.: "Pathophysiology of Chronic Renal Failure," *Nurs Clin North Am,* **16**:501–513, 1981.

Oestreich, S. J.: "Rational Nursing Care in Chronic Renal Disease," *Am J Nurs,* **79**:1096–1099, June 1979.

Orr, M. S.: "Drugs and Renal Disease," *Am J Nurs,* **81**:969–971, May 1981.

Pak, C. Y. C.: "Diagnosis and Therapy of Nephrolithiasis," in M. Martinez-Maldonado (ed.), *Handbook of Renal Therapeutics,* New York: Plenum, 1983.

Rao, K. V., C. E. Pru, and C. M. Kjellstrand: "Care of the Transplant Recipient," in M. Martinez-Maldonado (ed.), *Handbook of Renal Therapeutics,* New York: Plenum, 1983.

Roberts, S. L.: "Renal Assessment: A Nursing Point of view," *Heart Lung,* **8**:105–113, January–February 1979.

Stark, J. L.: "BUN/Creatinine: Your Keys to Kidney Function," *Nursing 80,* **10**:33–38, May 1980.

Tichy, A. M.: "Renal Failure," *Crit Care Update,* **9**:7–21, August 1982.

32

HEPATOBILIARY DISORDERS

IRA A. COHEN
ROSEMARY R. BERARDI
PATRICIA A. SARAN

LEARNING OBJECTIVES

Upon mastery of the contents of this chapter, the reader will be able to

1.   Explain why routine liver enzyme determinations and liver function tests are of limited use in predicting alterations in drug metabolism resulting from liver disease.

2.   State the three types of acute hepatic injury caused by drugs.

3.   Describe two mechanisms by which drugs produce hepatic damage.

4.   Identify those drugs most commonly associated with liver injury.

5.   Describe the indications, adverse effects, administration techniques, mechanisms of action, and monitoring parameters for the following drugs used in the treatment of hepatobiliary disease: vitamin K, cholestyramine, vasopressin, spironolactone, lactulose, neomycin, immune globulin, hepatitis B immune globulin, hepatitis B vaccine, prednisone, azathioprine, iopanoic acid, and chenodeoxycholic acid.

6.   Identify drugs which should be used with caution or are contraindicated in patients with specific major manifestations or complications of hepatobiliary disease.

7.   Identify those forms of hepatitis for which drug therapy has been proved effective in preventing or altering the course of the disease.

8.   Describe the nature of pain associated with cholelithiasis and the use of narcotic analgesics in treating biliary colic.

9.   List the major aspects of a medication history which should be elicited from patients with (1) cirrhosis, (2) acute hepatitis, and (3) chronic hepatitis.

Diseases of the liver and biliary tract are common causes of morbidity and may be associated with serious and poten-

tially fatal outcomes. Therapeutic implications related to hepatobiliary disease are myriad, since these diseases (1) are often induced by drugs and other chemicals, (2) frequently require preventive and/or active drug therapy, (3) are often associated with or cause concurrent related problems requiring drug therapy, and (4) alter the metabolism, pharmacologic effects, and adverse reactions of many drugs. Therefore, this chapter will focus on the role of the liver in drug metabolism, hepatic factors which influence drug effects, drug-induced liver disease, and the treatment of cirrhosis, hepatitis, and cholelithiasis.

ROLE OF THE LIVER IN DRUG METABOLISM

Although many drugs and by-products of body chemistry are eliminated partially or predominantly in an unchanged form, others must undergo one or more biotransformation steps to a more water-soluble compound in order to be excreted in the urine and/or bile. A variety of enzyme systems mediate biotransformation. The liver is the predominant site of production of drug-metabolizing enzymes and is the major site of drug metabolism and drug detoxification (see Chap. 5).

Factors Influencing Drug Metabolism

A variety of factors influence the ability of the liver to metabolize drugs. These include (1) the rate at which the drug reaches the liver via the blood (hepatic blood flow), (2) the ability of the hepatocytes to extract the drug from the blood, and (3) the ability of the various hepatic enzyme systems to metabolize the drug. Drug interactions, surgical procedures, and diseases (including various types of liver disease) are capable of altering the relative concentrations of unchanged drug and its hepatic metabolites (Table 32-1). The direction, magnitude, and duration of these changes in drug metabolism depend upon whether hepatic function and metabolic pathways are enhanced or inhibited, whether the

TABLE 32-1   Drugs Whose Effects Are Altered by Liver Disease

DRUG	LIVER DISEASE(S)[1]	MECHANISM(S)	CLINICAL IMPLICATIONS
Acetaminophen[2]	Severe CAH, cirrhosis, acute alcoholic hepatitis, hepatic necrosis following acute overdose of acetaminophen	Decreased metabolism	Avoid or decrease dose.
Barbiturates Phenobarbital	Cirrhosis, CSLD	Decreased metabolism	Avoid[3] or decrease dose; monitor serum concentrations.
Amobarbital	Cirrhosis, CSLD,[4] AVH	Decreased metabolism	Avoid[3] or decrease dose.
Benzodiazepines Diazepam and chlordiazepoxide	Cirrhosis, AVH, CAH[4]	Decreased metabolism of parent compound and active metabolite	Avoid[3] or use oxazepam[3] or lorazepam[3] instead.
Chlorpromazine	Cirrhosis	Increased CNS sensitivity	Avoid.[3]
Digitoxin	CAH[4]	Diminished protein binding, increased free (active) drug concentration	Avoid or use digoxin instead.
Lidocaine	Cirrhosis, CAH, passive liver congestion[5]	Decreased metabolism	Decrease initial maintenance dose and monitor serum concentrations.
Meperidine	Cirrhosis, AVH	Decreased metabolism, increased CNS sensitivity (?)	Avoid[3] or decrease dose.
Meprobamate	Cirrhosis, AVH, cholestatic hepatitis	Decreased metabolism (?)	Avoid[3] or use oxazepam[3] instead.
Morphine	Cirrhosis	Increased CNS sensitivity	Avoid.[3]
Pentazocine	Cirrhosis	Decreased metabolism	Avoid.[3]
Phenytoin	Cirrhosis[4]	Decreased metabolism, saturated enzyme pathway	Decrease dose, monitor serum concentrations.
Propranolol	Cirrhosis, CSLD[4]	Decreased metabolism	Decrease dose or change to renally eliminated beta blocker.
Prednisone	CSLD	Decreased metabolism of prednisone to active metabolite, prednisolone	None or use prednisolone.[6]
Theophylline and aminophylline	Cirrhosis, passive liver congestion,[5] AVH	Decreased metabolism	Decrease dose; monitor serum concentrations.

[1]CAH = chronic active hepatitis; CSLD = chronic severe liver disease (multiple type or unspecified); AVH = acute viral hepatitis.

[2]Massive overdoses can also *cause* acute hepatic necrosis by saturation of a major biotransformation pathway.

[3]Many of these agents are CNS depressants and should be avoided whenever possible in patients with prehepatic encephalopathy.

[4]Especially pronounced in presence of concurrent hypoalbuminemia.

[5]Due to right-sided heart failure or cor pulmonale.

[6]Although prednisone conversion to active prednisolone may be diminished in some types of CSLD, the metabolism of whatever prednisolone is present is inhibited, too, and in the presence of frequently concurrent hypoalbuminemia, concentrations of free prednisolone are usually adequate to promote the desired therapeutic effect.

intervention is acute or chronic, the magnitude and duration of the intervention, and the pharmacologic properties of the specific drug requiring metabolism [e.g., which enzyme system(s) are necessary for metabolism of that agent, whether the drug is "activated" or detoxified by the altered biotransformation step].

HEPATIC FACTORS INFLUENCING DRUG EFFECTS

Predictors of Hepatic Metabolizing Capabilities

Compared with our knowledge of the influence of renal dysfunction on drug effects, very little is known about the ability of various forms of liver disease to alter the metabolism, efficacy, and adverse reactions associated with drugs. Unlike the case of renal disease (in which the magnitude of alteration in drug elimination capacity often correlates with the degree of elevation of several easily measured laboratory parameters, such as serum creatinine and blood urea nitrogen), there are no reliable predictive laboratory tests to assess hepatic drug-metabolizing capabilities. For example, tests for intracellular enzymes, such as glutamic oxaloacetic and pyruvic transaminases (SGOT and SGPT), can indicate the presence of hepatocellular destruction. However, in the presence of even severe acute or chronic liver cell damage, these tests do not accurately reflect the ability of the liver to metabolize drugs. A prolonged prothrombin time and a decreased serum albumin are often noted in patients with many types of liver disease and, in the absence of nutritional deficiencies or other reasons for the abnormalities, are indicative of a diminished ability of the liver to synthesize proteins. Although these abnormalities often occur in patients with altered hepatic drug elimination, defects in protein synthesis can occur in the presence of good drug-metabolizing capabilities, and occasionally the opposite is also true.

Influence of Hepatic Blood Flow

Metabolism of drugs which undergo significant "first pass" changes by the liver (e.g., **propranolol, lidocaine, pentazocine, meperidine**) is generally highly sensitive to alterations in hepatic blood flow. Factors which can diminish hepatic perfusion, such as severe cirrhosis, surgical or pathologic shunts of liver blood flow, passive liver congestion due to right-sided heart failure or cor pulmonale, and some drugs (e.g., **cimetidine**) have been shown to decrease the metabolism of some of these agents, leading to increased concentrations of the drugs and a potential increase in pharmacologic action and side effects. Acute viral hepatitis, however, does not usually decrease hepatic perfusion and, as expected, has not been associated with a decreased elimination of those agents.

Influence of Microsomal Enzyme Concentrations

The metabolism of other drugs is relatively independent of changes in liver blood flow and influenced more by alterations in hepatic microsomal enzyme concentrations. A number of drugs can influence the concentrations of those metabolizing enzymes by increasing (inducing) their production (e.g., **barbiturates, alcohol, phenylbutazone, phenytoin**) or inhibiting their production (e.g., **cimetidine, influenza vaccine**). Enzyme inducers may enhance both their own metabolism and the metabolism of other agents which undergo biotransformation by affected enzyme systems (see Chap. 6). Liver disease, such as severe cirrhosis, chronic active hepatitis, and acute hepatitis, has also been shown to decrease the metabolism of some drugs (e.g., **theophylline, diazepam, chlordiazepoxide**), presumably by decreasing the concentrations of the hepatic microsomal enzymes responsible for detoxifying these agents.

Other Factors Affecting Metabolism

Although some properties of a drug may occasionally allow prediction of whether a particular type of liver disease might influence its metabolism, many other factors besides the pathway of metabolism of the drug and the type of liver disease affect the likelihood and magnitude of altered metabolism. These include the duration and severity of the liver disease (often hard to ascertain), the presence or absence of hypoalbuminemia (for those drugs highly bound to albumin), the presence of other concurrently administered drugs which might augment or inhibit metabolism, and a variety of either unproven or unknown sources of variability. Although the recommendations indicated on Table 32-1 may prove helpful in planning or adjusting the drug regimen for a specific patient, it must be realized that the information known about the limited number of hepatically metabolized drugs studied is subject to great interpatient variability. Even the parameters determining the handling of a particular drug for a given patient change over time, and the duration and magnitude of altered drug metabolism caused by liver disease is highly unpredictable.

Pharmacodynamic Changes with Liver Disease

It should be noted that even in the absence of altered drug metabolism, patients with some types of liver disease have been reported to manifest enhanced central nervous system (CNS) effects to certain agents, such as the phenothiazines (e.g., **chlorpromazine**) and some of the narcotic analgesics (e.g., **meperidine, morphine**). Enhanced CNS sensitivity to benzodiazepines has also been reported in patients with liver disease–related pharmacodynamic alterations and appear independent of changes in the pharmacokinetics (e.g., metabolism) of those drugs.

DRUG-INDUCED LIVER DISEASE

Drug-induced liver disease may follow the inhalation, ingestion, or parenteral administration of a number of drugs. Although adverse drug effects on the liver represent only a minor segment of liver disease, special populations such as the elderly and patients receiving antituberculosis or psychoactive drugs appear to be at greater risk.

Classifications and Mechanisms

Drugs may lead to acute or chronic hepatic injury. Acute hepatic injury can be cytotoxic, cholestatic, or mixed forms with both features. *Cytotoxic* injury refers to direct damage of the liver cell. *Cholestatic* injury refers to arrested bile flow accompanied by jaundice. Chronic hepatic disease can also occur during a course of drug therapy leading to *chronic active hepatitis, steatosis,* or *hepatic tumors.*

Drugs can produce hepatic damage by two general mechanisms:

1. By acting as an intrinsic hepatotoxin.
2. By inducing an idiosyncratic or unpredictable reaction.

The hepatotoxins produce a predictable, dose-dependent, and reproducible reaction in exposed individuals. Alcohol is frequently included in this category. Idiosyncratic drug reactions are unpredictable, not dose-dependent, and may occur at any time during, or shortly after, drug exposure. Hepatic injury due to idiosyncrasy can be caused by hypersensitivity reactions and may include extrahepatic manifestations such as arthralgias, fever, rash, leukocytosis, and eosinophilia. The exact mechanism by which a drug induces hepatic injury is often difficult to assess in the clinical setting.

Clinical Pharmacology and Therapeutics

The diagnosis of drug-induced hepatic disease is often presumptive, since detection of the causative agent is difficult. Patients should be carefully questioned for a history of exposure to any drug, particularly drugs known to produce hepatic injury. Information should be obtained regarding the duration of exposure to a specific drug and its relationship to the onset of symptoms. Predisposing factors (e.g., alcoholism, preexistent liver or kidney disease, previous history of drug exposure) and nutritional status should also be noted. The presence of liver injury accompanied by jaundice, fever, rash, and eosinophilia suggests the likelihood of drug-induced liver disease, although lack of these features does not exclude the possibility. Mild elevations of SGOT and SGPT occur with many drugs, the majority of which do not produce signs and symptoms of hepatotoxicity. Recurrence of hepatic dysfunction after giving a rechallenge dose often offers support for the diagnosis. Since rechallenge may be potentially dangerous, the risk must be weighed against the benefit.

The treatment of drug-induced hepatic injury consists of removal of the responsible agent and provision of supportive care. Maintenance of caloric intake and or fluid and electrolyte balance is essential. Corticosteroid (e.g., prednisone) therapy is largely empirical, with some evidence of success.

Drugs Reported to Cause Clinically Significant Liver Injury

Although numerous drugs have been reported to cause liver injury, the drugs listed in Table 32-2 have an increased incidence of producing clinically significant hepatotoxicity.

NURSING PROCESS RELATED TO DRUG-INDUCED LIVER DISEASE

Assessment

The nurse can play an important role in promoting the early diagnosis and treatment of drug-induced liver disease. The diagnosis, however, is often difficult due to a number of variables. First of all, there is no "classical" presentation for most drug-induced hepatotoxicity. The clinical spectrum ranges from asymptomatic individuals with serum transaminase elevations to patients who present with fulminant hepatic failure. Hepatotoxicity often mimics viral hepatitis or biliary tract obstruction. Once there is a suspicion of drug-induced hepatic diseae, it is imperative to immediately discontinue all implicated causative agents and prohibit further exposure. Modification of drug therapy in liver disease is a related area for which the nurse must be able to identify

---

TABLE 32-2   Drugs Causing a Relatively High Incidence of Significant Hepatotoxicity

Acetaminophen	Contraceptive steroids	Phenylbutazone
Alcohol	Dantrolene	Phenytoin
Androgens	Erythromycin estolate	Rifampin
Aspirin	Isoniazid	Sulfonamides
Bacillus Calmette-Guérin vaccine (BCG)	Mercaptopurine	Tetracycline
Carmustine	Methotrexate	Tricyclic antidepressants
Chlorpromazine	Methyldopa	Valproic acid
Chlorpropamide	Mithramycin	Vitamin A

(1) drugs whose effects may be altered by disease, (2) drugs which should be avoided in patients with liver disease, and (3) methods to monitor drug therapy (i.e., identify drug response and side effects) in the patient with liver disease.

A thorough history is mandatory to ascertain information about exposure to environmental toxins (chemicals in work or hobbies) and drug ingestion (including alcohol, prescription drugs, over-the-counter drugs, and home remedies). It is important to inform the patient about the reason for such questions.

It is often impossible to detect hepatotoxicity in susceptible patients merely by observational methods, since numerous causative agents as well as idiosyncratic reactions can induce the disease. There are, however, two clinical presentations that indicate a high probability of drug-induced hepatic injury:

1.   Transaminase elevations greater than 5000 IU/L (although liver injury secondary to shock may also cause this high an elevation).

2.   Hypersensitivity phenomena (e.g., fever, rash, and eosinophilia).

The nurse should detect early signs of jaundice in the conjunctiva and buccal cavity. These areas are particularly helpful when assessing the black population. Evidence of jaundice in the skin and sclera is apparent at a later stage. Other objective signs include an enlarged and potentially painful liver on deep palpation, darkened urine, light-colored stools, fever, and elevated serum liver enzyme tests. Nausea, vomiting, anorexia, arthralgias, and abdominal pain are symptoms that often precede jaundice.

In specialty settings, where the number of medications used may be more limited, the nurse should be aware of the drugs that are hepatotoxic. Patients receiving such drugs should be specifically observed for signs and symptoms of drug-induced liver disease. In patients with current liver disease or a history of liver disease, the nurse should assess the safety and efficacy of each drug added to the patient's regimen. The nurse should consult with the physician if an alteration in the drug treatment plan seems justifiable. The following guidelines should be applied in assessing the potential safety and efficacy of a drug order for the patient with liver disease:

1.   All unnecessary drugs, both prescription and nonprescription, should be avoided, especially if the drug is partially or predominantly hepatically metabolized.

2.   When given a choice between two therapeutic agents of comparable efficacy and similar spectrums and incidence of side effects, it is advisable to choose the drug whose activity and elimination is less reliant upon hepatic metabolism, especially if the alternative agent is primarily eliminated unchanged in the urine.

3.   When no such choice exists, with the exception of life-threatening situations, a conservative initial dosing reg-imen (i.e., empirically lowered dose and/or increased dosing interval) is advisable.

4.   Even when conservative dosing is practiced, vigorous monitoring of the patient for signs and symptoms of drug toxicity is essential. Since the drug may still circulate for relatively long periods of time, and since drug accumulation can occur and may be delayed even with a conservative regimen, monitoring of the patient should be continued past the point at which one would expect the drug's effects to be diminished in the normal patient.

5.   Even for those drugs known to be influenced by a particular type of liver disease, there is no reliable index to use as a guide for prospectively calculating the dose of a drug in a patient with hepatic dysfunction. Therefore, even when empiric dosage alterations have been made, it is important to monitor the effectiveness of the drug by establishing a therapeutic goal and assessing whether the patient has achieved that goal within a reasonable duration of treatment. Failure to reach that therapeutic goal could indicate that an empiric dosage decrease was too drastic for the degree of liver dysfunction. When available for a specific drug, measurement of serum drug concentrations can aid in dosage adjustment.

6.   Pharmacists or drug information centers should be consulted whenever possible concerning drug dosage in hepatic disease and the measurement and interpretation of serum drug concentrations.

Management

When symptoms indicative of hepatotoxicity are present, the nurse should contact the physician immediately and seek prompt resolution of questionable medication orders. Drugs which are known hepatotoxins should be withheld until the physician has reviewed the patient's drug regimen. If there are signs of an allergic reaction, such as rash, fever, or eosinophilia, the nurse should anticipate the withholding of all medications while the benefits and risks for each drug are weighed. Subsequent changes in drug or dosage should be discussed with the patient. Despite the fact that there is no specific treatment, the nurse should take an active role in the education of the patient and reinforcement of the supportive recommendations.

The patient will need to be informed about the reaction and instructed to make future health care workers aware of this problem. If the agent is not positively identified, the patient should still inform others of the incident. The education process should also include the avoidance of other known hepatotoxins (including alcohol) while liver function tests remain abnormal. The patient should be instructed further to keep scheduled appointments for follow-up clinic visits and laboratory tests. Management of the complicated case of hepatic injury may require that the patient be hospitalized. Documentation of the patient's signs, symptoms, laboratory tests, suspected diagnosis, follow-up plans, and education received should be a permanent part of the medical record. Documentation should be made by all health professionals who have had contact with the patient.

Jaundice is a highly visible sign of illness to the patient. It can become a stigma and consequently have a considerable emotional impact on the patient. These feelings need to be acknowledged. Ongoing explanations reduce unfounded fears that may seem very real to the patient. Further supportive care for uncomplicated cases includes avoidance of fatigue. One to two weeks of rest without strenuous exercise should be encouraged, although strict bed rest is not mandatory. In addition to a diminished level of activity, an adequate caloric intake is essential. The frequent incidence of nausea, vomiting, and anorexia associated with many types of liver disease promotes the need for creative feeding approaches for these patients. Antiemetics offer little relief, and phenothiazines should be avoided in these patients, if possible, since there may be increased CNS sensitivity.

Evaluation

Providing supportive care and discontinuing use of the suspected responsible agent(s) are the primary treatment modalities for drug-induced liver disease. Once the diagnosis has been made and recommendations given to the patient, the plan of care does not end. Diligent follow-up must be undertaken to evaluate the patient for signs and symptoms indicative of the progression, stabilization, or regression of liver damage, and to determine if further intervention is necessary. Subsequent clinic visits should include liver function tests, a physical examination, a thorough reassessment of current drug therapy, and recording the patient's responses to any changes made. Liver function tests should be monitored until they return to normal or until such time (approximately 6 months) that persistently abnormal liver function tests warrant a liver biopsy to document possible chronic hepatitis or cirrhosis.

CIRRHOSIS AND LIVER FAILURE

Cirrhosis may be defined as a chronic disease of the liver characterized by diffuse and progressive destruction of liver parenchymal cells and their replacement with fibrotic connective tissue. The advancing fibrosis is usually accompanied by nodular regeneration with resultant distortion of normal lobular structure and eventual liver cell necrosis. In the later stages of cirrhosis, these processes may lead to distortion of liver shape, hepatic insufficiency, and interference with the circulation of blood and bile to and from the liver.

Complications

Advanced cirrhosis with progressive liver necrosis, scarring, and nodularity eventually lead to obstruction of portal circulation and increased portal pressure. Portal hypertension

may contribute to life-threatening complications, including variceal hemorrhage, ascites, and hepatic encephalopathy coma.

Massive hemorrhage from the esophageal and gastric varices can occur abruptly and usually presents as painless hematemesis or melena. Bleeding can be complicated by an impaired clotting system and alcohol-induced gastritis.

Increased portal pressure, increased flow of hepatic lymph, hypoalbuminemia, secondary hyperaldosteronism, and impaired water excretion due to excessive serum levels of antidiuretic hormone lead to avid sodium and water reabsorption and loss of fluid into the extravascular space. The development of ascites is usually accompanied by increased abdominal girth, edema, and decreased urinary output.

In hepatic encephalopathy, ammonia formed by the action of bacteria and enzymes on protein is absorbed from the intestine and accumulates within the brain. This is thought to be due to the shunting of portal blood directly into the systemic circulation and to impaired liver metabolism. Other factors which may contribute to hepatic coma include changes in plasma levels of amino acids and the accumulation of mercaptans, short-chain fatty acids, and false neurotransmitters. Hepatic encephalopathy may be precipitated by gastrointestinal bleeding, increased dietary protein, constipation (including that caused by oral iron supplements), fluid and electrolyte disturbances, acute infections, surgery, deterioration of liver function, and drugs (e.g., sedatives, tranquilizers, and narcotic analgesics) which cause CNS depression.

Clinical Pharmacology and Therapeutics

Cirrhosis is a serious illness that requires continued medical attention. Because there is no specific drug therapy, successful recovery depends upon two important factors: (1) abstinence from alcohol (or removal of other offending agents) and (2) prevention or treatment of complications. Vitamin and mineral supplementation is essential in cirrhotic patients when there is a history of dietary insufficiency, blood loss anemia, and alcoholism. The cirrhotic patient is likely to require the following vitamins and minerals: folic acid, thiamine, iron, and vitamin K (see Chap. 25, "Nutritional Disorders" and Chap. 36, "Hematologic Disorders"). If intensive pruritis accompanies jaundice, topical lotions, antihistamines, or cholestyramine may provide relief.

Treatment of Pruritis

Chronic biliary obstruction leads to the deposition of bile salts in the skin. The clinical manifestation of this development in the jaundiced patient is intense itching. Various therapeutic maneuvers, including the application of topical preparations and the administration of antihistamines and corticosteroids, have been tried in an attempt to provide relief. The use of such agents is not likely to benefit the patient since they do not correct the underlying pathologic mechanism. Cholestyramine and cholestipol are anion exchange resins which are occasionally given to relieve these symptoms.

Cholestyramine Cholestyramine (Questran) is a quaternary ammonium anion exchange resin that exchanges chloride for cholates. The exchange process binds bile salts in the intestine, forming an insoluble, nonabsorbable complex which is then excreted in the feces. This action disrupts the enterohepatic circulation of bile salts and thereby reduces their serum concentration. Bile salts are then mobilized from the skin into the serum, resulting in decreased itching. The efficacy of cholestyramine depends upon the ability of the bile salts to reach the duodenum, where the exchange takes place. Patients with total biliary obstruction will, therefore, not respond to cholestyramine therapy.

Adverse effects The main side effects of cholestyramine include constipation, nausea, and abdominal cramping. The gastrointestinal symptoms usually occur early in therapy and subside with continued administration. Constipation may be alleviated by concurrent administration of stool softeners. The unpleasant odor and taste of the drug make it difficult for patients to take; however, these can be masked by mixing the drug with a thick juice, such as orange or apricot juice. Carbonated beverages should be avoided since they can cause excessive foaming. Absorption of the fat-soluble vitamins A, D, E, or K may also be impaired by the drug.

Drug interactions Cholestyramine may bind weakly acidic drugs such as **warfarin, digitoxin, tetracycline, phenobarbital**, and **thiazides**, possibly resulting in their decreased absorption. As a general rule, drugs should be given at least 1 h before or 4 h after the resin is administered.

Dosage and administration The usual oral dose of cholestyramine is 1 teaspoonful (5 g of dried resin) given three to four times daily before meals for at least 3 to 4 weeks. Daily doses of more than 24 g are associated with increased gastrointestinal side effects and malabsorption of fat-soluble vitamins. The resin should be mixed with 60 to 180 mL of water or juice immediately prior to administration.

Response to therapy Relief from pruritis usually requires 1 to 3 weeks of cholestyramine therapy. Response to treatment has occurred after several days; however, in these cases it is difficult to separate the drug effect from the natural abatement of the disease process.

Colestipol Colestipol (Colestid) is an anion exchange resin similar to cholestyramine. It binds approximately the same amount of bile salts per gram of resin. Since colestipol is odorless and tasteless, it may be better tolerated than cholestyramine; however, it is slightly more expensive. Both drugs are primarily indicated for the treatment of hypercholesterolemia. Dosage is usually 15 to 30 g daily in two to four divided doses. Colestipol should be mixed with at least 90 mL of water or juice just prior to administration.

The pharmacology of **cholestyramine** and **colestipol** is discussed further in Chap. 41.

Treatment of Variceal Hemorrhage

Acute variceal hemorrhage is a medical emergency and requires prompt and effective care. Initial treatment consists of the evacuation of gastric contents and cold saline irrigation of the stomach through a nasogastric tube to induce local vasoconstriction. Bleeding from gastritis or peptic ulcer is usually treated with **cimetidine** or **antacids**. Replacement of lost blood is essential if there are signs of hypovolemia or if blood loss is severe. Emergency endoscopy is critical to locating the actual bleeding site and exclusion of other causes of gastrointestinal hemorrhage. Once the diagnosis of bleeding varices is made, several treatment methods may be chosen to temporarily control bleeding.

The Sengstaken-Blakemore tube permits balloon tamponade and provides local compression of the esophageal and gastric varices. Although usually effective in producing temporary control of massive hemorrhage, this procedure is uncomfortable for the patient and is often complicated by rebleeding, esophageal erosions, airway obstruction, or aspiration. Intravenous or intraarterial **vasopressin** may also be administered to control bleeding.

Surgical management of acute bleeding varices includes the direct injection of sclerosing agents such as **ethanolamine oleate** into each varix to induce hemostasis. Various types of portacaval shunting procedures can also be performed to arrest bleeding.

Vasopressin Vasopressin (Pitressin) is postulated to produce a significant decrease in portal blood flow and pressure through vasoconstriction of the mesenteric arterioles. This results in decreased collateral flow to the varices, which in turn slows or stops bleeding long enough to allow a clot to form at the bleeding site. Temporary control of variceal hemorrhage may be achieved by vasopressin infusions. However, therapeutic doses are often associated with potentially serious side effects.

Adverse effects Frequent side effects from vasopressin therapy include skin blanching, phlebitis, abdominal cramps, mild hypertension, and fecal incontinence. Cardiac complications related to its intense vasoconstriction action include angina, acute myocardial failure, and arrhythmias. Bowel necrosis, water intoxication, and tachyphylaxis can also occur with vasopressin therapy.

Dosage and administration Continuous intravenous infusion of 0.2 to 0.4 U of vasopressin per minute through a peripheral vein is usually recommended as the starting dose. Vasopressin dosage may be increased to 0.9 U/min if necessary. The lowest effective dose should be used since many of the side effects are dose-related. When bleeding is controlled, the rate of vasopressin infusion is usually tapered over the next 24 to 48 h prior to discontinuation. Intraarterial infusions into the superior mesenteric artery, at a rate of 0.1 to 0.5 U/min have been given in an attempt to reduce the systemic adverse effects of vasopressin. Because of catheter-associated complications, intraarterial infusion appears to offer no clear advantage over peripheral vein infusion.

Response to therapy The results of studies with vasopressin have been varied, with some investigators claiming that vasopressin infusions neither control bleeding nor alter outcome. Unfortunately, even if the bleeding is temporarily controlled, the long-term mortality rate associated with bleeding varices does not significantly improve.

Methods to Minimize Recurrence Propranolol has been given investigationally in oral daily doses of 40 to 360 mg to prevent the recurrence of variceal hemorrhage. This action is thought to be related to the drug's ability to decrease portal venous pressure. Prophylactic use of antacids to prevent mucosal irritation and stool softeners to minimize straining and intraabdominal pressure can also be employed. Patients should be instructed to avoid alcohol, salicylates, and other drugs capable of irritating the gastric and esophageal mucosa.

Treatment of Ascites

Bed rest and sodium restriction are usually the first therapeutic measures to be tried in the cirrhotic patient with ascites. Bed rest increseas the glomerular filtration rate and enhances the diuretic action of the kidneys. Sodium restriction helps prevent the formation of ascites and edema. Fluid intake should be limited to 1500 mL/day in the presence of marked hyponatremia. Diuretic therapy should be initiated if these measures fail to produce adequate weight loss.

The goals of diuretic therapy are to mobilize ascitic and edema fluid to achieve a weight loss of 0.5 to 1 kg/day and to prevent the major complications caused by overly aggressive diuresis. This gradual controlled diuresis allows equilibration of ascitic fluid with plasma volume. Overly aggressive diuresis may be complicated by intravenous volume depletion, hypokalemia, hyponatremia, metabolic alkalosis, and azotemia and may lead to compromised renal function, hepatic encephalopathy, hepatorenal syndrome, and death. It is, therefore, imperative to monitor diuretic therapy by carefully assessing weight loss, fluid and electrolyte balance, blood pressure, and changes in mental status.

A minority of patients with advanced cirrhosis fail to respond to intensive medical therapy. Paracentesis or surgical implantation of a peritoneovenous shunt (LeVeen) has been useful in obtaining short-term control of ascites in these patients. However, both of those procedures can lead to significant complications and have not been shown to prolong the survival of the patient with end-stage cirrhosis.

Spironolactone The initial diuretic of choice in cirrhotic patients with normal renal function is spironolactone (Aldactone), an aldosterone antagonist. Spironolactone is a weak, slow-acting diuretic which is less likely to induce hypovolemia than the more potent diuretics. The drug specifically antagonizes the effects of hyperaldosteronism that exists in most cirrhotics, and it does not cause potassium depletion.

Dosage and administration Spironolactone is often begun at 100 mg/day when treating patients with ascites. If diuresis is inadequate, the dosage should be increased slowly (every 2 to 4 days) in a stepwise increment, until a maximum dose of 100 mg four times a day is reached. Although daily doses of up to 1 g have been used, other diuretics are usually added before increasing the spironolactone dose above 400 mg/day.

Response to therapy A 2- to 4-day period is usually required in order to achieve the maximum diuretic response with any given dose of spironolactone. Frequent dosage adjustments should be avoided for this reason.

Additional Diuretics Occasionally diuresis with **spironolactone** remains insufficient and the addition of more potent diuretics such as **hydrochlorothiazide, furosemide,** or **metolazone** may be warranted on an intermittent or a continuous basis. The dose should be started low and then cautiously increased to promote an appropriate diuresis. Patients should be monitored closely to prevent the diuretic-induced complications associated with depletion of plasma volume.

Other potassium-sparing diuretics such as **triamterene** and **amiloride** do not competitively inhibit aldosterone and are of questionable efficacy in the treatment of cirrhotic ascites.

The mechanism of action, adverse effects, drug interactions, dose, and other complications of diuretic therapy are discussed in the chapter on edema (see Chap. 23).

Albumin Parenteral albumin may be required to increase the plasma colloid oncotic pressure. The administration of albumin provides only temporary improvement at a high cost and has the added disadvantage of possibly increasing portal pressure.

Treatment of Hepatic Encephalopathy

Therapeutic management of hepatic encephalopathy is aimed at the identification and correction of precipitating events and the reduction of ammonia produced in the colon. Dietary protein should be restricted for several days and gradually reinstituted in a stepwise manner depending on the patient's clinical response. Fluid and electrolyte abnormalities should be corrected. Sedatives, tranquilizers, and narcotic analgesics should be discontinued. Gastrointestinal bleeding, if present, should be controlled and antibiotics administered if evidence of infection exists. Prevention of constipation and bowel "sterilization" with **laxatives, lactulose,** or **neomycin** help decrease ammonia production and absorption.

Laxatives Mild laxatives and stool softeners are used routinely to ensure daily bowel movements and to prevent the accumulation and absorption of nitrogenous waste. Because chronic diarrhea can produce hypokalemia, doses should be titrated to give several soft stools per day. Vigorous catharsis or enemas may only be necessary in the acute phase of encephalopathy.

Lactulose Lactulose (Cephulac, Chronulac) is a synthetic disaccharide used to treat hepatic encephalopathy by virtue of its effect on colonic pH and its ability to induce osmotic diarrhea. The disaccharide passes unchanged into the colon, where intestinal bacteria convert it to lactic and acetic acids which acidify the colon to a pH of 5. Acidification of colonic contents reduces the absorption of nonionized ammonia and favors the diffusion of ammonia from the blood into the colon, thereby decreasing the blood ammonia concentration. Unless acidification of the stool can be accomplished, therapeutic efficacy cannot be fully achieved.

Adverse effects The most common adverse effect of lactulose is the induction of excessive diarrhea, which could lead to dehydration and hypokalemia, both of which have been identified as precipitants of hepatic encephalopathy. Additional adverse effects include abdominal cramping and flatulence. The excessive sweetness of the syrup can occasionally cause nausea or vomiting.

Precautions Lactulose is a sugar and should be used with caution in diabetics. Concomitant administration of other laxatives should be avoided when titrating the dose, since they may mask the endpoint of therapy.

Dosage and administration Lactulose syrup (10 g/15 mL) may be mixed with fruit juice or other foods to improve its palatability. The drug is given orally in doses of 30 to 45 mL three or four times daily and titrated to the production of two to three soft stools per day or a colonic pH of 5. Rapid laxative effect can be obtained by administering an initial loading dose of 30 to 45 mL hourly until catharsis occurs. Rectal administration may be indicated in the treatment of comatose patients. A retention enema of 300 mL of lactulose in 700 mL of tap water or equal parts of lactulose and normal saline can be given for 1 h.

Response to therapy Improvement in mental status usually occurs within 24 to 48 h for oral lactulose. The beneficial effect of the enema may be seen within 12 h. The drug is usually effective for both acute and chronic encephalopathy.

Neomycin Neomycin is a relatively nonabsorbable antibiotic which inhibits colonic ammonia production by decreasing the normally occurring ammonia-producing bacteria in the colon. As a consequence of its antimicrobial activity, neomycin also causes loose stools which enhance the removal of nitrogenous waste from the colon.

Adverse effects Approximately 1 to 3 percent of orally administered neomycin is absorbed and rarely may lead to ototoxicity and nephrotoxicity, especially in patients with renal insufficiency. Long-term neomycin therapy may cause staphylococcal enterocolitis and suppress the absorption of

fat, glucose, iron, vitamin B$_{12}$, and various drugs such as **vitamin K**, **digoxin**, and **penicillin**.

Dosage and administration Neomycin may be administered either orally or rectally. In patients with normal renal function, 4 to 8 g/day should be administered in divided doses four times a day at the onset of therapy. Chronic encephalopathy may respond to a maintenance dose of 2 to 4 g/day. A 1% neomycin solution may be administered as a retention enema four times a day.

Response to therapy Lactulose and neomycin appear to be equally effective in the treatment of hepatic encephalopathy. Neomycin may produce a more rapid response in patients with acute episodes. Although controversial, there is some evidence to suggest that the combination of lactulose and neomycin may be more effective than either drug alone. Initial therapy should be instituted with lactulose, since it is less toxic and more desirable for long-term use. If a patient does not respond to lactulose, the drug should be discontinued and neomycin should be given.

Additional agents **Levodopa** and **bromocriptine** have been investigated for the treatment of hepatic encephalopathy. Their action is based on the theory that false neurotransmitters accumulate in cirrhotic patients and interfere with synaptic transmission. These drugs are thought to displace the false neurotransmitters and improve synaptic transmission. Their exact role in therapy awaits further evaluation.

Intravenous or oral administration of keto-analogs of corresponding essential amino acids or branched-chain amino acids appears to effectively reverse the course of hepatic encephalopathy.

Prognosis

The prognosis for patients with cirrhosis depends upon the stage of advancement and the appearance of complications. Abstinence from alcohol and a nutritious diet will usually improve the prognosis in patients without major complications. Continued alcohol ingestion in the presence of variceal hemorrhage, ascites, and hepatic encephalopathy usually results in irreversible liver disease and death.

NURSING PROCESS RELATED TO CIRRHOSIS AND LIVER FAILURE

Assessment

Nurses in community settings (e.g., mental health clinics, outpatient clincs, public health agencies) are in a particularly favorable and responsible position to identify cases of cirrhosis in its early stages. Evidence of clinical signs of cirrhosis, particularly when combined with a history of excessive alcohol intake, contact with another hepatotoxin, or a history of past liver disease, requires careful evaluation and referral to a physician.

The phrase "critically ill" is never more appropriate than when applied to the patient with liver failure, a condition that adversely affects nearly every vital function. Skilled nursing interventions which help liver failure patients include (1) promptly recognizing developing encephalopathy and combating its progression, (2) knowing how to control upper gastrointestinal (GI) bleeding, which is so common in these patients, (3) knowing ways to inhibit the breakdown of protein and other sources of excessive nitrogenous waste accumulation, and (4) knowing how to treat and monitor ascites and edema.

Nursing assessment of these patients focuses particularly on gathering complete data on nutritional requirements, bowel habits, fluid balance, circulatory function, skin, and comfort status. In conditions associated with alcohol or drug abuse, sensitive psychosocial and environmental assessment is vital (see Chap. 49). Nursing assessment of fluid retention, ascites, and nutritional status should include measurement of the following parameters used to determine patient status and drug effects:

1. Weight—should be ascertained daily, on the same scale, at the same time of day, and with similar clothing whenever possible.

2. Abdominal girth—the patient's position should be the same with each measurement (usually every 8 h); an indelible marker should be used on the initial assessment to indicate the placement of the tape measure.

3. Circumference of the extremities—degree of pitting at the ankles. Once again, consistency is of the utmost importance, whether it is in reference to the level of measurement or the kind of scaling system utilized to assess the degree of pitting present.

4. Fluid intake and output—records of this are mandatory and essential to patient management. Consideration should be given to blood products given [not just intravenous (IV) solutions], blood loss (via hematemesis or melena), diarrhea, estimated ascitic fluid leakage through skin from paracentesis sites or injection sites, and medications given in liquid form (e.g., antacids). Frequent monitoring of vital signs and scrutiny of the laboratory data will help establish specific nursing plans for further assessment of the patient's fluid and electrolyte balance.

5. Mental status—observation of mental status changes is most important, because subtle changes may indicate hepatic encephalopathy and serious deterioration of the patient. Manifestations of encephalopathy progress from early prehepatic coma with mild mental confusion to deep hepatic coma (see Table 32-3).

Management

Ongoing serial assessment of the above parameters is required due to rapidly changing patient condition. Some patients may require placement in an intensive care unit.

When inserting a nasograstric (NG) tube or when using cleansing or **neomycin** enemas, it should be assumed that patients with cirrhosis have esophageal varices and hemorrhoids, even if this has not yet been confirmed. Mechanical trauma from an NG tube or an increase in intraabdominal pressure from enemas can cause the rupture of varices. Irritating drugs given orally should be avoided when possible or buffered with food or antacids. **Aspirin**, in particular, should be avoided not only because of the gastric irritation, but also because of its platelet-inhibiting effects that could increase the risk of bleeding. Since numerous over-the-counter products contain aspirin, the patient should be cautioned not to use them unless the product's content has been assessed and approved by a physician, nurse, or pharmacist. Another precaution when the prothrombin time is prolonged is to avoid all unnecessary injections. When injections are unavoidable, the subcutaneous route is preferred for some drugs (e.g., vitamin K). Small-gauge needles should be selected and gentle pressure applied to the site after injection in order to decrease bleeding. Guaiac tests to detect blood in NG aspirate and stool should be done routinely. New or recurrent bleeding should be promptly and thoroughly investigated. **Ferrous sulfate**, **folic acid**, and **thiamine** are often given as supplements to cirrhotics, who frequently have a poor nutritional status. Iron will often cause the stool to become black and may lead the nurse to believe falsely that the patient has had an upper GI bleed.

The control of sodium and water retention through dietary restriction and diuretics is a major goal for reducing the amount of ascitic fluid. While the exact restrictions for sodium and water and protein vary from patient to patient, they have been shown to be effective, although ongoing consultation with a dietitian is essential to maintain palatability

TABLE 32-3 Staging of Mental Status

Stage 1—Prodromal

Mild confusion, euphoria or depression, vacant stare, inappropriate laughter, forgetfulness, inability to concentrate, slow mentation, slurred speech, untidiness, lethargy, belligerence, minimal asterixis. These signs are not necessarily present concurrently.

Stage 2—Impending

Obvious obtundation, aberrant behavior, definite asterixis, constructional apraxia (impairment of the ability to use objects correctly). Keep a record of the patient's handwriting and stick figure configuration.

Stage 3—Stuporous

Marked confusion, stupor (but patient arousable), incoherent speech, asterixis, noisiness, abusiveness, violence. Restraints may be necessary at this stage. Do not sedate; a sedative could be fatal.

Stage 4—Comatose

Unarousable, patient responds only to painful stimuli, no asterixis, positive Babinski sign, hepatic fetor (correlates with the degree of somnolence and confusion).

of food and patient understanding and motivation. Reduction of mechanical pressure imposed by the ascites, which may force the diaphragm upward and restrict lung expansion, is aided by placing the patient in a high Fowler's position. Frequent turning and positioning are vital to prevent prolonged external pressure and skin breakdown from compromised cellular perfusion due to interstitial edema.

The nurse should plan care to avoid factors that precipitate hepatic coma. Constipation is prevented by the routine use of stool softeners and mild laxatives. The stage of encephalopathy often dictates the nursing interventions which are aimed at ammonia detoxification, the primary one being the use of **lactulose**. The number and character of all stools should be carefully recorded. Excessive stooling or frank diarrhea is an indication for reducing the dosage of lactulose. Any other laxatives or agents that alter the nature of bowel movements, such as antacids, should be avoided or used concurrently only with caution and vigorous monitoring of the patient. Since the main goal of lactulose therapy is the reduction of nitrogenous waste accumulation, its effectiveness may allow for the liberalization of the dietary protein intake. As an alternative to lactulose, **sorbitol** may be given orally or administered via a high-colonic enema. Due to its high osmolality, large quantities of water should be given. Fluid intake and output, electrolytes, and blood urea nitrogen levels must be monitored during therapy.

The cirrhotic patient is always in danger of potential bleeding. The nurse as well as the patient and family should be aware of the behaviors that will decrease this risk, including the avoidance of **aspirin**, **alcohol**, constipation, heavy lifting, severe coughing, and large meals. Food should be chewed well to decrease trauma to the mucosa.

Evaluation

Dependent on the stage of advancement and the presence of complications, the nurse must be capable of evaluating effectiveness of therapy and other management procedures, either from hour to hour in an intensive care unit setting or by evaluation in the home or clinic. An appreciation for the chronicity of this disease, major complications, and factors that will usually improve the prognosis is of vital importance. Provision for the continuity of care is also imperative. Regardless of the stage of the disease or clinical setting the following factors should be regularly addressed:

1. Laboratory tests (SGOT, SGPT, hematocrit, hemoglobin, sodium, potassium, creatinine, blood urea nitrogen)
2. Physical examination
3. Mental status
4. Stool changes: number, volume, consistency, color, etc.
5. Nutritional status
6. Alcohol and other drug intake
7. Evidence of bleeding

CASE STUDY

J.H., a 52-year-old white male, was admitted with the complaint of "vomiting blood." He had a 22-year history of alcohol abuse. The patient appeared sluggish and confused.

Assessment

Three weeks prior to admission, J.H. started feeling fatigued and had nausea, upset stomach, and headaches which he treated with aspirin. Three days prior to admission, J.H. began vomiting blood. He admitted his daily alcohol intake had increased over the past month to approximately "a quart of whiskey a day." He was hospitalized 3 months prior to this admission with worsening abdominal swelling and shortness of breath and was placed on a salt-restricted diet and treated with spironolactone. His discharge weight was 180 lb.

Examination on his current admission included these findings: height 5'8"; weight 200 lb; blood pressure 90/60 with orthostatic changes; pulse 130; temperature 99.4°F; respirations 28 and shallow; jaundiced skin; icteric sclera; distended abdomen with small sucussion splash; dilated superficial abdominal veins and vascular spiders; palpable liver beyond the right costal margin; evidence of gynecomastia; pitting edema of both lower extremities; hemorrhoids and guaiac-positive stools. Gastric aspirate contained bright red blood. Laboratory tests included the following: total bilirubin 6.1 mg/dL; SGOT 50 IU; serum albumin 2.7 g/dL; prothrombin time 17 s (control of 12 s); hemoglobin 10.5 g/dL; hematocrit 30 percent.

J.H. was admitted to the intensive care unit with a preliminary diagnosis of active upper GI bleeding possibly secondary to esophageal varices. His physician diagnosed cirrhosis with complicating portal hypertension, hypoalbuminemia, ascites, edema, hypoprothrombinemia, peripheral neuropathy, and acute hepatic encephalopathy.

Management

Admitting orders included IV infusion of D_5W with 30 meq KCl and multivitamins; typing and cross matching for two units of whole blood, one of which was to be given stat; vitamin K 10 mg subcutaneously (SC) daily; thiamine 100 mg intramuscularly (IM) stat; furosemide 40 mg IV daily; high colonic enema stat; bed rest; an indwelling urinary catheter; insertion of a subclavian catheter; iced saline lavage of the stomach via an NG tube; insertion of an arterial line.

Nursing priority goals and approaches for J.H. were established. The first priority goal was to detect the site of GI bleeding and to control blood loss. The NG tube was passed with extreme care to avoid trauma to possible varices. All stools and NG aspirate were observed for gross blood and were chemically tested for occult blood. Initial NG drainage was positive for blood necessitating iced saline lavage to temporarily control the bleeding. The patient was at additional risk of bleeding due to hypoprothrombinemia and therefore received whole blood (which contains necessary clotting factors) and vitamin K. To decrease the chance of bleeding, small-bore (25-gauge) needles were used for the vitamin K and thiamine injections. Efforts were made to prevent physical trauma that could lead to further bleeding. For example, oral care was given with a soft swab instead of a toothbrush.

The second priority was to decrease the respiratory effort associated with J.H.'s distended abdomen and accumulated ascitic fluid, since hypoxia could contribute to hepatic encephalopathy. He was placed in a high Fowler's position and observed for signs of increased respiratory effort that would indicate the need for oxygen therapy. After giving the initial dose of furosemide, the nurse maintained hourly evaluations of vital signs, central venous pressure, and fluid intake and output. Abdominal girth, daily weight, serum electrolytes, and mental status changes were also monitored. The patient's position was rotated every 2 h to redistribute the area of dependence and fluid pressure.

A third priority was to monitor those factors that could contribute to worsening of the patient's mental status. The high-colonic enema removed nitrogenous waste responsible for the production of ammonia and other toxins associated with hepatic encephalopathy. Lactulose therapy was deferred since the patient was to remain with nothing by mouth (NPO) until his condition stabilized. Careful records of fluid intake and output of urine, stool, and nasogastric drainage were maintained in order to estimate fluid and electrolyte losses and assess renal func-

tion. Since infection could also precipitate hepatic coma, careful handwashing and aseptic technique were maintained.

Additional goals included the improvement of the patient's nutritional status, continued loss of accumulated edema and ascitic fluid, prevention of recurrent encephalopathy and avoidance of drugs which could cause gastritis and/or liver disease. Another important goal was to counsel the patient to abstain from alcohol upon discharge.

Evaluation

Gastroscopy revealed marked gastritis with points of hemorrhage but no evidence of ulcers or varices. Intensive antacid therapy was initiated. The administration of whole blood and vitamin K improved the prothrombin time to 14 s.

During the initial 24 h, the patient became less restless; his respirations stabilized at 20 per minute and were no longer labored. The abdominal girth had decreased by 2 in, and his weight was down by 7 lb. Vital signs remained stable and the serum electrolytes were normal, with a potassium of 4.0 meq/L.

Six hours after the second dose of furosemide, J.H.'s mental status began to decline. The furosemide was discontinued, and spironolactone therapy was reinstituted at 100 mg/day. He became less oriented and developed asterixis. The patient's status later returned to admission level with decreased confusion and lethargy.

Approaches to other goals included the provision of adequate calories and the advancement of dietary protein. Enemas were discontinued and lactulose therapy was titrated to three soft stools per day to prevent recurrent encephalopathy. The pharmacist recommended acetaminophen for headaches because of the GI irritation and bleeding associated with the use of aspirin. At discharge an appointment was made for J.H. with the alcoholic rehabilitation clinic.

VIRAL HEPATITIS

Hepatitis literally means "inflammation of the liver" and may be caused by a variety of factors including viral infections, alcohol, drugs, and other chemicals (see "Drug-Induced Liver Disease" in this chapter). Viral hepatitis may be acute or chronic. Acute viral hepatitis (AVH) may be caused by any of three viral subtypes: (1) hepatitis A virus (HAV), (2) hepatitis B virus (HBV), or (3) non-A, non-B viruses. The management of acute viral hepatitis, regardless of type, is primarily a question of prevention. Specific preventive measures, signs and symptoms, clinical manifestations, histopathologic findings, sequelae (including the development of chronic hepatitis), vectors of spread, populations at risk, incubation periods, and prognoses, however, vary greatly according to the causative virus.

Hepatitis A

Formerly known as "infectious hepatitis," hepatitis A is primarily transmitted by the fecal-oral route, usually in the presence of poor hygiene and sanitation. There is no chronic carrier state associated with the hepatitis A virus, and it is usually transmitted during the last 2 weeks of the typical 4-week incubation period, prior to the onset of clinical manifestations of the disease. Recovery from acute hepatitis A is usually rapid and complete, and patients typically require only supportive care measures. Life-long immunity from further infection with HAV is subsequently conferred.

Treatment of Acute Hepatitis A

There is no specific drug therapy for the treatment of any type of AVH. Supportive therapy and, when necessary, hospitalization is important to better ensure that the recovery is uneventful. Drugs and other substances with the potential to cause liver damage, and therefore exacerbate or confuse the clinical picture, should be avoided during the active and recovery phases of AVH (see Table 32-2).

Prevention of Acute Hepatitis A

Immune Globulin (IG, Immune Serum Globulin, ISG)   Adherence to strict standard guidelines governing personal hygiene (including hand washing) and the handling of potentially contaminated equipment and body fluids is the foundation for preventing the spread of HAV infections. In addition, prophylaxis with immune globulin (IG) should be utilized to prevent or diminish the severity of infection in those individuals likely to be exposed to HAV (including handlers of nonhuman primates and persons traveling for extended periods to parts of the world where HAV is endemic) and those who have been definitely or presumably exposed to the virus. Routine prophylaxis of hospital personnel is not necessary or recommended as a substitute for or adjunct to the proper handling of the HAV-infected patient.

Postexposure prophylaxis with IG is recommended as soon as possible after intimate or prolonged exposure to a person with an active HAV infection. This would include close family members, household and sexual contacts of infected persons, as well as exposed staff and inmates of institutions having an HAV outbreak, (e.g., day-care centers where diapered infants are cared for, prisons, centers for the mentally retarded).

Immune globulin is a sterile solution of antibodies from human plasma which is free of live virus. It is derived from the blood of professional donors and imparts passive, relatively short-lasting, immunity. Given within 2 weeks of probably exposure or infection with HAV, it has been reported to be 80 to 90 percent effective in preventing hepatitis. Except for the rare potential to promote acute hypersensitivity reactions in those persons with a history of allergic reactions to human source vaccines and immunoglobulins, IG-related side effects are uncommon and are usually limited to soreness at the site of the IM injection. The usual IG dose for preexposure and postexposure HAV prophylaxis is 0.02 mL/kg given as a deep IM injection. Travelers intending to stay in HAV-endemic areas for more than 3 months may receive 0.06 mL/kg of IG every 5 months. Since IG may interfere with the ability of live vaccines to promote active immunity, it is recommended that at least several months elapse between the administration of IG and the administration of a live vaccine.

Hepatitis B

Formerly known as "serum hepatitis," hepatitis B usually occurs secondary to parenteral transferance of the hepatitis B virus (HBV) or by exposure of a mucous membrane or bro-ken skin to infected blood derivatives or other contaminated body fluids. HBV infection is, therefore, relatively common in patients who have been transfused, among the patients and staff of hemodialysis units, in parenteral drug abusers, in sexually active male homosexuals, and among health personnel whose professional activities promote exposure to HBV-infected blood or blood products and equipment. This, of course, includes health personnel having accidental finger-sticks with blood-tainted needles. Immunosuppressed patients, such as renal transplant recipients and cancer patients, are also at higher risk of developing HBV infections. HBV is also transmitted by the perinatal route since the hepatitis B surface antigen (HBsAg) positive mother is likely to infect her newborn. The mean incubation period for HBV is long, 75 days, and peak infectivity occurs from 3 to 11 weeks post exposure. The vast majority of acute hepatitis B infections resolve without complications and confer immunity to future HBV infection. However, 1 percent of exposed patients will die of fulminant hepatitis, 5 to 10 percent progress to a chronic hepatitis, and an estimated 5 percent become chronic asymptomatic infectious carriers of the virus.

Treatment of Acute Hepatitis B

As in the case of infections with HAV, management of AHB, with or without acute complications, is supportive. Although corticosteroid therapy has been attempted in the past, there is no evidence that prednisone treatment decreases the severity, morbidity, or mortality of the disease. Once more, the focus of management is placed on the prevention of the infection.

Prevention of Acute Hepatitis B

Infection with HBV entails the adherence to strict guidelines in the handling of potentially infected patients, equipment, and blood products. Careful screening of blood donors and the avoidance of paid donors are also essential. The transfusion of most blood products should be carefully monitored, performed only when essential, and should be substituted by transfusion of lower-risk alternatives whenever appropriate.

Postexposure prophylaxis for HBV was in the past accomplished with IG injections and has been reported to prevent up to 75 percent of HBV infections if administered soon after exposure. The content of antibodies to hepatitis B surface antigen (HBsAg) (anti-HBsAg) contained in IG, varies greatly, depending on the population whose pooled plasma was used to prepare a given lot of the product. Minimum titers of anti-HBsAg in recent years, however, have been high enough to justify its use in certain populations, especially since IG is very inexpensive compared to the alternative drug for passive immunization against HBV, hepatitis B immune globulin (HBIG). IG is still indicated (1) when exposure to HBV is likely, but the diagnosis has not yet been serologically confirmed, (2) when a decision to provide prophylaxis is made despite a low suspicion that exposure was from an HBsAg-positive source, (3) when the source of blood exposure is unknown, or (4) as a potential alternative when HBIG is unavailable. The IM dose of IG used in these situations is 0.06 mL/kg.

Hepatitis B Immune Globulin (HBIG)   HBIG is prepared from the pooled plasma of persons who have been infected with HBV and have high titers of anti-HBsAg. It usually confers passive immunity to HBV infections if treatment is initiated soon after exposure. Due to the relative scarcity of acceptable donor plasma, the cost of each adult dose is very high ($150 to $200). Adverse reactions and cautions are rare and are comparable with those described for IG. HBIG is indicated following percutaneous (i.e., needle-stick, transfusion, or direct mucous membrane) exposure to HBsAg-containing material. Within 24 h of exposure, adults should receive 0.06 mL/kg by IM injection into the deltoid or gluteal muscle. The dose should be repeated one month later. As an alternative, hepatitis B vaccine may be used in combination with HBIG to enhance post-percutaneous exposure efficacy. In this case, the second costly dose of HBIG is not required. The combination is now uniformly recommended for perinatal prophylaxis, where 0.5 mL of the HBIG should be administered to the neonate by the IM route within 12 h of birth. The CDC also recommends that adults who have been previously uninfected with HBV and who have not been adequately vaccinated be given a single dose of HBIG within 14 days of sexual contact with an HBsAg-positive person.

Hepatitis B Vaccine (Heptavax)   Preexposure prophylaxis is recommended for those health personnel, patients, and others at high risk of exposure to HBV (e.g., hemodialysis staff, blood bank technicians, phlebotomists, operating room nurses and surgeons, dentists, family and close contacts of HBV carriers, sexually active homosexual males). Prophylaxis is not recommended for general health care personnel, since these relatively lower risk individuals are more reasonably protected by good technique in the handling of laboratory specimens, equipment, and patients, and since most acute hepatitis patients are usually no longer infectious by the time they are seen by these individuals. Preexposure prophylaxis used to be accomplished using passive immunization (i.e., IG 0.05 to 0.07 mL/kg every 4 months). This therapy has recently been replaced by active immunization using hepatitis B vaccine, which contains chemically inactivated HBsAg from the plasma of chronic carriers. The usual dose of the vaccine is 20 μg (1 mL) IM with repeated injections administered 1 month and 6 months later. It is recommended that children less than 10 years old receive 10 μg per injection. Revaccination (booster shots) should probably be administered once every 5 years. Patients who are relatively immunosuppressed (e.g., renal transplant, hemo-

dialysis, and oncology patients) respond relatively poorly and may require twice the dose and/or IG prophylaxis. As discussed earlier, hepatitis B vaccine may also be utilized in combination with HBIG for postexposure prophylaxis. Although the preparation is not a live vaccine and does not interfere with response to HBIG, it is recommended that the sites of IM injections of the two agents be different. When administered for this indication, the first dose of vaccine should be given within 7 days of exposure. The doses and schedule for the series of three vaccinations are identical to those previously described for preexposure prophylaxis of adults and children. No significant side effects have been reported; however, the theoretical risk of contracting AIDS from HBIG vaccination is a source of controversy. The current cost for the initial series of vaccinations in the United States is approximately $100.

Non-A, Non-B Hepatitis

Non-A, non-B hepatitis is caused by at least several different viruses and is an entity which has only recently been defined. It is currently thought to account for at least 90 percent of the cases of posttransfusion hepatitis and is thought to be spread by vectors similar to those of HBV. The exact incidence of non-A, non-B hepatitis in the population is poorly defined, since there are currently no serologic tests to identify the presence of the virus in infected patients. The diagnosis is therefore one of exclusion (i.e., ruling out a HAV, HBV, or drug-induced etiology). Patients with non-A, non-B infections are more likely to develop chronic hepatitis than their HBV counterparts.

Management of Non-A, Non-B Viral Hepatitis

There is no effective drug therapy to treat acute hepatitis, and the management must focus on preventive methods, including exercising great care in interpatient hand washing and the handling of blood, blood products, and specimens. Preexposure immunoprophylaxis recommendations are controversial, poorly defined, and unproven. Prompt postexposure prophylaxis with 0.02 to 0.06 mL/kg of IG has been proposed following a needle-stick infected by a suspected non-A, non-B acute hepatitis patient or during institutional outbreaks of apparent non-A, non-B disease.

Chronic Hepatitis

Sustained laboratory and clinical evidence of inflammatory liver disease can occur in the case of drug-induced hepatitis (see "Drug-Induced Liver Disease" in this chapter); HBV or non-A, non-B viral hepatitis, and "lupoid"-type chronic hepatitis (i.e., liver disease presumably linked to autoimmune phenomena). There are two subcategories of chronic hepatitis: chronic persistent hepatitis (CPH) and chronic active hepatitis (CAH). The chronic persistent type generally follows a benign (nonaggressive) course, doesn't usually lead to cirrhosis, and requires no definitive treatment. On the other hand, CAH can progress to cirrhosis, liver failure, and death.

Treatment of Chronic Active Hepatitis

Drug-induced CAH should be managed by prompt withdrawal of the offending agent and supportive care. CAH due to viral infection and the lupoid type of CAH may be managed with corticosteroids and other immunosuppressive agents. Prednisone or prednisolone, often in combination with azathioprine (see Chap. 26), has been shown to suppress the clinical manifestations and prolong life of patients afflicted with these types of CAH (especially the lupoid type). They are especially indicated if the liver biopsy is consistent with progressive severe hepatocellular damage.

Corticosteroids It is assumed that the hepatocellular damage from CAH is caused by an immune-mediated inflammatory response within the liver and that corticosteroids (prednisone or prednisolone) inhibit that response by decreasing (1) deposition of fibrin, (2) the phagocytic activity of white cells, and (3) the migration of white cells into the affected area. The exact mechanism of immunosuppressive drugs in CAH or the reason why they appear to be effective in CAH and not in other inflammatory diseases of the liver is, however, unknown.

Pharmacokinetics The pharmacokinetics of prednisone and prednisolone and the controversy regarding the selection of one of these compounds in a patient with liver dysfunction is addressed in Table 32-1. Prednisone is considered by many to be the drug of choice for CAH due to its lower cost.

Prednisone is often initiated at a dose of 30 mg/day for the first week and then tapered to a maintenance dose of 10 to 15 mg/day for an initial 6-month course. If benefits are obtained from treatment (based upon an improvement or halt in the progression of symptoms and liver biopsy findings with concurrent normalization of serum laboratory tests), treatment is usually continued for 2 to 3 years. This is the time most associated with disease progression and death in untreated or nonresponding patients. Relapse is common after discontinuation of therapy. The dosage should be carefully tapered prior to discontinuation, and monitoring should be close to assess worsening of the patient of Addisonian-type complications. Therapy should be discontinued after 6 months in the HBV-positive nonresponder, but should continue in the HBV-negative nonresponder in hopes of eliciting improvement with a higher dose. If dose-related complications occur in a responder, the corticosteroid dose can usually be halved by adding 50 to 100 mg/day of azathioprine to the regimen. Of responders 20 percent will relapse after the first few months of therapy, and 75 percent of these individuals will die if treatment is not

enhanced by an increase in the prednisone dose (to 60 mg/day) or by using 30 mg/day of prednisone plus 150 mg/day of azathioprine.

NURSING PROCESS RELATED TO HEPATITIS

Assessment

The assessment of the hepatitis patient does not differ significantly from that of the patient with drug-induced liver disease, since the findings are often similar. The primary focus of the assessment should be on a thorough drug, social, and family history to ascertain information on exposure to drugs, alcohol, chemicals, contaminated needles, transfusions, and potential hepatitis carriers and infected persons. Further questions should assess whether the patient's profession or social habits predispose the person to a high risk of viral hepatitis.

Management

Despite the fact that there is no specific drug therapy for treating active disease, emphasis should be placed on pre- and postexposure prevention (i.e., prophylaxis). Infectious patients should be advised to avoid blood donations and contact of their blood with other persons. In general, treatment is directed at relieving symptoms and helping the patient maintain good nutrition despite anorexia. Food can be eaten as tolerated, but alcohol should be avoided for at least 6 months.

Health professionals in high-risk areas previously described require preexposure immunization with hepatitis B vaccine and postexposure immunization with either IG or HBIG or a combination of HBIG and hepatitis B vaccine. As recommended for most immunizations, deep intramuscular injections in adults and children should be made in the anterolateral aspect of the thigh or in the deltoid muscle of the upper arm. The former site is recommended for infants. When necessary, adults may receive the injection in the upper outer quadrant of the gluteal muscle.

For each case of documented or suspected hepatitis, the nurse should consult the institution's or agency's policy and/or procedure manuals for specific management recommendations. The serologic assessment of hig-risk individuals to detect exposure is often recommended. This mandates scrupulous record keeping. All prophylactic immunizations should also be documented. The nurse should be aware of all patients with the potential for hepatitis or exposure, particularly in the clinic setting. All new patients with renal transplants, on dialysis, or with cancer or other cause to be immunosuppressed should be assessed for immunization requirements.

Staff education programs that include the proper handling of equipment, secretions, isolation techniques (when appropriate), and the obligation for reporting of cases should be mandatory.

Evaluation

Periodic evaluation of the patient's clinical status and serologic documentation are absolutely necessary. Further preventive measures, clinical manifestations, sequelae, and prognosis vary according to the causative virus. Continued evaluation and care can be accomplished by a multidisciplin-

ary and interdepartmental and/or agency approach; public health agencies are specifically designed for follow-up. Patients deemed appropriate for HBIG and hepatitis B vaccine injections should be given specific appointment dates and times for future injections. Reports of liver biopsies must be made known to the primary physician so that the appropriate patient information can be communicated. Continuity of care, which necessitates reevaluation until deemed unnecessary, includes laboratory studies and an updated drug history.

CASE STUDY

S.B., a 45-year-old registered nurse, joined the staff of her hospital's hemodialysis unit 4 months ago. The last few days, she had called in sick with progressively worsening "flu-like" symptoms.

Assessment

The head nurse of the dialysis unit contacted S.B. She questioned her regarding her past medical history and about her "flu-like" symptoms and other potential signs and symptoms associated with hepatitis, exposure to hepatitis virus, and the use of potentially hepatotoxic drugs. Except for diet-controlled diabetes mellitus, S.B. reported that she had been in very good health until several weeks earlier. She said her social habits included having several drinks a day after work and smoking about one pack per day. She said that the odors of both burning tobacco and food have recently made her feel nauseated. She denied taking regularly scheduled medications, except for aspirin, which she was taking frequently for her recent "flu symptoms." When asked about exposure to specific hepatotoxins, S.B. mentioned that she had taken isoniazid (INH) for tuberculosis and had finished her therapy 3 years earlier. She had not recently had her ears pierced and was not a user of injectable drugs. None of her friends or family members had a history of hepatitis. She was married and had two children away at college. Upon close questioning, S.B. acknowledged that in her first week in the unit she had gotten a patient's blood into a slight open cut on her ungloved hand. She immediately washed her hands and since it was a "small amount" of blood, felt it was unnecessary to report the incident or take any other preventive measures. She said she had never received immunization against viral hepatitis, and didn't recall being tested for the presence of antihepatitis antibodies.

Because of the responsibility to S.B. and other employees and patients in the unit, the head nurse required that S.B. be examined and tested. S.B. was reluctant because she didn't seem "ill enough," but was seen the next morning at the employee health service.

A history confirmed the information the head nurse had elicited, and revealed additional findings, including dark urine color, intermittent low-grade fevers, and a recent 5-lb weight loss. Physical examination revealed a tired-looking, weak, jaundiced woman with right upper quadrant abdominal tenderness, hepatomegaly, and conjunctival and sublingual icterus. Laboratory data at this time included a total serum bilirubin of 5.6 mg/dL, a direct serum bilirubin of 4.8 mg/dL, an SGOT of 850 IU/mL, an SGPT of 940 IU/mL, an alkaline phosphatase of 150 mU/mL, and a 4+ urine bilirubin. She was found to be hepatitis B surface antigen (HBsAg)–positive and had an elevated anti-HBsAg titer (i.e., hepatitis B antibody–positive). It was, therefore, almost certain that S.B. had contracted hepatitis B and that after an approximate 14-week incubation period she had manifested prodromal signs and symptoms of infection and had subsequently become jaundiced.

Management

At this time, S.B. required no specific treatment for her apparently uncomplicated case of hepatitis B. She was placed on several weeks of bed rest until she felt capable of resuming nonstrenuous activities. S.B. was also placed on a high-protein, high-calorie diet and advised to eat most of her meals in the morning when she was less likely to feel nauseated. She was told to avoid her typical daily ingestion of alcohol for the next few months (until clinical evidence of her hepatitis completely resolved), advised to avoid all unnecessary prescription and over-the-counter medications (especially those associated with hepatotoxicity), and cautioned to avoid contact of her blood with other persons (especially until it was verified that the infection was resolved and that she had not become a carrier).

Evaluation

It was too late to use HBIG (or IG followed by HBIG) when it was confirmed that the source was HBsAg-positive. These measures should have been administered immediately after her exposure to the contaminated blood.

Once S.B. was jaundiced, it was unlikely that she was still infectious. She was informed of the necessity to keep her follow-up appointments for reexamination and laboratory reassessment.

As is the case with the majority of patients who develop acute infections with HBV, S.B.'s liver enzymes (drawn biweekly) declined rapidly and were normal at the end of 3 months. As required, her case was reported to the appropriate public health authorities. Once recovered, S.B. will be immune from further infection from HBV and will not require future immunization against hepatitis B.

Should S.B. have become a chronic carrier of HBV, she would be restricted from future work with high-risk patients. In the event that she developed chronic active hepatitis as a sequela from the HBV infection, she would be at high risk of developing severe glucose intolerance if placed on prednisone therapy since she is a diabetic.

It must be noted, however, that upon her employment in the hemodialysis unit she should have been screened for past infection with HBV, and once she was found to be anti-HBsAg–negative, S.B. should have received hepatitis B vaccinations. Hence, her case of hepatitis B could have been prevented by either appropriate preexposure prophylaxis with the vaccine or postexposure prophylaxis with HBIG.

S.B.'s case had far-reaching effects on the dialysis unit. Strict policies and procedures to avoid and detect the spread of hepatitis had been in effect for years. Procedures for routine hepatitis screening of employees, however, had been relaxed due to a low incidence rate of hepatitis in the recent past and the subsequent impression that screening would not be cost-effective. Consultation and coordination with the infectious disease, environmental control, and employee health departments was instituted. Policies and procedures were scrutinized, reviewed with employees, and enforced.

GALLSTONES (CHOLELITHIASIS)

Gallstone Formation

The primary bile acids in humans are cholic acid and chenodeoxycholic acid. Cholesterol serves as a precursor of bile salts and is made more soluble by the proper ratio of bile acids, lipids, and lecithin. An abnormal ratio of these constituents allows for saturation of the bile with cholesterol and favors the formation of cholesterol crystals or, less commonly, other types of crystals in the bile. These crystalline masses grow and become gallstones. Several drugs (e.g., **clofibrate, estrogens**) may potentially contribute to the formation of gallstones.

Clinical Findings

Only 10 to 15 percent of gallstones contain enough calcium to be visualized by regular abdominal x-rays. Therefore, diagnosis is often aided by the use of radiopaque contrast media (e.g., **iopanoic acid**) that are administered orally to detect abnormal filling of the gallbladder (oral cholecystogram, or OCG) or bile ducts (oral cholangiogram). Alternatives to the OCG include the use of ultrasound, percutaneous transhepatic cholangiography, or endoscopic retrograde cholangiopancreatography (ERCP).

Iopanoic Acid   Iopanic acid (Telepaque) is an iodinated compound that is variably absorbed from the GI tract after oral administration and is metabolized by the liver, and a significant percentage concentrates in the gallbladder and is excreted in the bile. Its maximum concentration in the bile is obtained 10 to 20 h after dosing. If the bilirubin is greater than 2 mg/dL or if the cystic duct is obstructed, the drug may never reach the gallbladder in high enough concentrations to be useful and the drug should not be utilized. When used for an OCG, visualization of the gallbladder is achieved with serial x-rays of the abdomen taken during the time when peak concentrations of the radiopaque metabolite should be in the bile (approximately 14 h post dose). This procedure is sufficient to diagnose cholelithiasis in the vast majority of patients receiving one dose of the agent. In the absence of significant liver disease, failure to visualize the gallbladder is usually due to cystic duct obstruction, failure of the patient to take the dose of the contrast medium, or inadequate absorption of the drug. Therefore, following a nonvisualizing first test, the procedure is repeated 24 h later (after the administration of a second 3-g dose or a double dose). Failure to visualize after a second dose is usually indicative of cholelithiasis with chronic inflammation of the gallbladder and/or cystic duct obstruction.

Adverse effects   Approximately one-fourth of patients will experience transient GI side effects including nausea and vomiting (which can promote inadequate iopanoic acid absorption and nonvisualization of the gallbladder). Patients who are sensitive to iodine may experience an allergic reaction to the drug, and, if they require an OCG, should be premedicated with antihistamines and corticosteroids and monitored closely with appropriate emergency drugs available. Since iopanoic acid has an uricosuric effect, it may precipitate urate nephropathy in previously untreated hyperuricemic patients, and if used in that population, vigorous hydration and adequate urinary output must be promoted. Other forms of renal toxicity have been reported to occur rarely. The drug is, therefore, relatively contraindicated in patients with significant renal or hepatic disease. It should also be avoided in patients with severe hyperthyroidism, cholangitis, or coronary artery disease. Iopanoic acid may also interfere with thyroid function tests.

Dosage and administration For the performance of an OCG, six 500-mg tablets are usually administered 14 h prior to the procedure following several days of a fat-containing diet. The patient should receive vigorous hydration but no food between the time of the dose and the x-rays. If the examination requires repeating, another 3 g may be administered a day after the first dose, or 6 g may be administered a few days later. No more than 6 g of the drug should be given within a 24-h period.

Clinical Pharmacology and Therapeutics

Once diagnosed, the decision of when and how to treat gallstones in a particular patient is dependent upon multiple factors, including:

1. Whether the patient is symptomatic or asymptomatic.
2. The frequency and severity of biliary colic attacks and the degree to which the disease interferes with the patient's daily activities.
3. The age of the patient.
4. The presence or absence of complications associated with cholelithiasis.
5. The size of the stone(s).

The treatment of choice in the symptomatic patient is removal of the gallbladder, which yields a high cure rate and is performed on an estimated 350,000 Americans each year. Although usually well-tolerated, as with any surgical procedure, perioperative complications can arise, and several thousand cholecystectomy-related deaths occur annually. Drugs which dissolve gallstones have been developed in an effort to provide a medical alternative to an operation for patients (1) at high risk of surgical complications, (2) who have postoperative retained stones in the remaining biliary tree, or (3) who have asymptomatic disease which may become active in the future.

Chenodeoxycholic Acid Chenodeoxycholic acid (Chenix), which is also called chenodiol and CDCA, is a naturally occurring bile acid which is used to treat susceptible gallstones in symptomatic patients with functioning gallbladders. In those cases it may serve as an alternative to surgery. Although its mechanism of action is not yet totally defined, it has been tested in humans with asymptomatic cholelithiasis and has promoted enhanced solubility (desaturation) of bile cholesterol and a subsequent partial or total dissolution of many stones. CDCA is most effective in the dissolution of relatively small, lower-density radiolucent stones ("floaters") composed primarily of cholesterol. It is relatively ineffective in dissolving stones that are (1) primarily composed of bile pigments, (2) high in calcium (radiopaque), (3) larger than 1.5 cm in diameter, and (4) in obese

patients. In addition to these limitations of therapy, beneficial effects of CDCA may dissipate upon discontinuation of treatment, leading to "regrowth" of stones and necessitating indefinite treatment or repeated courses of the drug.

Adverse effects The drug seems to be generally well tolerated, although it may cause dose-related diarrhea and serum transaminase elevations. Potential long-term side effects have not yet been adequately studied.

Dosage and administration The recommended daily maintenance dosage for *chenodiol* is 13 to 16 mg/kg. The dosage must be rounded off so that the drug can be given twice a day as the appropriate number of 250-mg tablets. Dosing may be initiated with 250 mg given twice a day and gradually increased as tolerated over a few weeks until the recommended maintenance dose is achieved. Diarrhea or significant liver enzyme elevations may necessitate temporary dosage alterations or discontinuation of treatment, respectively. At least several years of treatment with these relatively expensive agents are usually required to attain the desired response.

Ursodeoxycholic acid Ursodeoxycholic acid (UDCA) is an investigational semisynthetic congener of CDCA. Although there is less clinical experience with UDCA when compared to CDCA, it appears to be more potent (dose of 8 to 10 mg/kg/day), of comparable efficacy and limitations, and less likely to cause diarrhea and liver enzyme abnormalities.

The long-term usefulness, future role, and indications of CDCA, UDCA, and similar agents in the treatment of gallstones currently remains controversial pending the outcome of further clinical studies.

Symptomatic Management of Cholelithiasis

The majority of patients with an intermittent attack of biliary colic will improve in less than a week with only supportive therapy. Prolonged symptoms and, especially, the presence of fever and chills may indicate a serious complication of gallbladder disease (e.g., cholecystitis, cholangitis, pancreatitis) and deserve immediate medical attention. Severe pain due to biliary colic is common and is secondary to increased pressure, inflammation, and dilation of the bile duct proximal to an obstruction from a stone. It often presents as a steady aching or may be referred to the epigastrum, right upper quadrant, or right shoulder. It usually requires parenteral treatment with potent narcotic analgesics. Morphine and many other narcotics have been reported to increase intrabiliary pressure and cause spasm of the spincter of Oddi, thereby exacerbating the symptoms. The incidence and magnitude of these adverse effects of narcotics are highly variable. Although documentation is lacking, pentazocine and meperidine have been reported to be less likely to influence biliary pressure or sphincter constriction and have, therefore, been promoted as the drugs of choice for managing biliary colic. Regardless of which analgesic is used, the patient should be monitored for evidence of pain exacerbation, which often occurs within the first half-hour post injection, and should be assessed for adequacy of pain relief.

Bilirubin elevations are rarely great enough in uncomplicated cholelithiasis to cause pruritis and necessitate treat-ment. In those cases and in the rare situations in which related gallbladder disease causes sustained symptomatic hyperbilirubinemia due to partial obstruction of bile flow, antipruritic therapy may be instituted. These measures are discussed under "Cirrhosis" in this chapter.

REFERENCES

Beck, M. L.: "Gastrointestinal Basics," in K. W. Carey (ed.), *Ensuring Intensive Care*, Springhouse, PA: Springhouse Intermed, 1981.

Bond, W. L.: "Clinical Relevance of the Effect of Hepatic Disease on Drug Disposition," *Am J Hosp Pharm,* **35**:406–414, 1978.

Bongiovanni, G. L.: *Manual of Clinical Gastroenterology,* New York: McGraw-Hill, 1983.

Centers for Disease Control: "Immune Globulins for Protection Against Viral Hepatitis," *Ann Intern Med,* **96**:193–197, 1982.

——: "Inactivated Hepatitus B Virus Vaccine," *Ann Intern Med,* **97**:379–383, 1982.

——: "General Recommendations on Immunization," *Ann Intern Med,* **98**:615–622, pt. 1, 1983.

——: "Update: Postexposure Prophylaxis of Hepatitis B," *Ann Intern Med,* **101**:351–354, 1984.

"Chenodial for Dissolving Gallstones," *Med Lett Drug Ther,* **25**:101–102, 1983.

Czaja, A. J.: "Current Problems in the Diagnosis and Management of Chronic Active Hepatitis," *Mayo Clin Proc,* **56**:311–323, 1981.

Dienstag, J. L.: "Diagnosis and Prevention of Viral Hepatitis," in K. J. Isselbacher, et al., (eds.), *Principles of Inter-nal Medicine, Update IV,* New York: McGraw-Hill, 1983.

Fogel, M. R., et al.: "Continuous Intravenous Vasopressin in Active Upper Gastrointestinal Bleeding," *Ann Intern Med,* **96**:565–569, 1982.

Gannon, R. B., and K. Pickett: "Jaundice," *Am J Nurs,* **83**:404–407, 1983.

Lebrec, D., et al.: "Propranolol for Prevention of Recurrent Gastrointestinal Bleeding in Patients with Cirrhosis," *N Engl J Med,* **305**:1371–1374, 1981.

Ludwig, J.: "Drug Effects on the Liver: A Tabular Compilation of Drugs and Drug-Related Hepatic Disease," *Dig Dis Sci,* **24**:785–795, 1979.

Maynard, J. E.: "Prevention of Hepatitis B Through the Use of Vaccine," *Ann Intern Med,* **97**:442–444, 1982.

Petersdorf, R. G., et al: *Principles of Internal Medicine, 10th ed.,* New York: McGraw-Hill, 1983.

Schiff, L., and E. R. Schiff: *Diseases of the Liver, 5th ed.,* Philadelphia: Lippincott, 1982.

Thompson, M. A.: "Managing the Patient with Liver Dysfunction," *Nursing 81,* **11**:101–107, 1981.

Zimmerman, H. J.: *Hepatotoxicity: The Advance Effects of Drugs on the Liver,* New York: Appleton-Century-Crofts, 1980.

33

NEUROLOGIC DISORDERS*

ROBERT W. PIEPHO
LAURA K. NEILLEY

LEARNING OBJECTIVES

Upon mastery of the contents of this chapter the reader will be able to:

1. Explain the composition and significance of the blood-brain barrier.
2. Relate the neurochemical basis of parkinsonism to the action of antiparkinsonian drugs and the mechanisms of drug-induced parkinsonism.
3. Compare the indications for levodopa, amantadine, bromocriptine, and anticholinergic drugs in parkinsonism.
4. Name two anticholinergic drugs used to treat parkinsonism.
5. Describe the adverse effects of and dietary modifications for levodopa therapy.
6. Explain the importance of monitoring postural blood pressure, cognitive and affective status, bowel function, and ability to operate machinery safely when patients are taking antiparkinsonian drugs.
7. Explain the rationale for the combination of a decarboxylase inhibitor and levodopa.
8. Relate the pathophysiology of myasthenia gravis to the mechanisms of drugs used in its treatment.
9. Name three types of drugs which are contraindicated in myasthenia gravis.
10. Differentiate the cause and nursing management of cholinergic crisis and myasthenic crisis.
11. Relate the pathogenesis of seizures to the action of antiepileptic drugs.
12. List four groups of drugs used in seizure disorders and give one example of each.
13. State five common adverse effects of antiepileptic drugs and the measures to minimize or monitor for these effects.

14. Describe the benefits and cautions in the use of blood levels in monitoring anticonvulsant therapy.
15. List skeletal muscle relaxants effective at three sites of action.
16. Describe adverse effects common to skeletal muscle relaxants.
17. Explain the appropriate indications for and titration of dosage for skeletal muscle relaxants.
18. List adverse effects unique to cyclobenzaprine (Flexeril) and orphenadrine (Norflex) compared to other skeletal muscle relaxants.
19. Describe the nursing responsibilities in monitoring mannitol, dexamethasone, and pentobarbital therapy for cerebral edema.
20. Explain why intravenous 5% dextrose in water (D_5W) is contraindicated in increased intracranial pressure.
21. Indicate the role of the nurse in preventing and monitoring the adverse effects of ergotamine and methysergide.
22. List at least two drugs used for each: acute treatment of migraine and prophylaxis of migraine.
23. Explain what is meant by the paradoxical effect of amphetamines in attention deficit disorder.
24. Describe how the nurse can work with parents and teachers to ensure maximum benefit of drugs used in attention deficit disorder.
25. Indicate the symptoms of senile dementia which might be improved by vasodilators, ergot alkaloids (Hydergine), and antipsychotic drugs.
26. Explain the nursing techniques to minimize adverse effects and monitor the efficacy of vasodilators and ergot alkaloids used to treat dementia.

The nervous system consists of several subdivisions: the central nervous system (CNS) composed of the brain and spinal cord, the peripheral nervous system, and the autonomic nervous system. Neurologic disorders can result from altered

*The editors thank Melvin H. Van Woert, M.D., who cocontributed the chapter on this subject in the first edition.

structure or function of the nervous system, and the clinical manifestations are largely dependent upon the location of the lesion. Etiology of neurologic disorders can be nutritional, toxic, degenerative, vascular, neoplastic, traumatic, congenital, metabolic, infectious, electrophysiologic, genetic, behavioral, or iatrogenic (see Table 33-1 for drug-induced neurologic defects or diseases).

This chapter will deal with a select group of neurologic conditions that are seen by the health care provider. Drugs presented in this chapter will be discussed as they relate to these specific conditions. Pharmacotherapy of several important neurologic disorders is discussed in other chapters. Neurologic deficits with a nutritional basis are overviewed in Chap. 25. Use of corticotropin (ACTH) and corticosteroids in multiple sclerosis and other neurologic conditions is referenced in Chap. 35. Anticoagulants and platelet function inhibitors in the prevention and treatment of stroke and transient ischemic attack are discussed in Chap. 42.

DRUG PENETRATION INTO THE CENTRAL NERVOUS SYSTEM

In order to gain access to brain tissue, drugs that alter CNS function must cross from the bloodstream into the cerebrospinal fluid (CSF) or into the interstitial fluids of the brain.

TABLE 33-1 Drug-Induced Neurologic Disorders

PROBLEM	POTENTIAL AGENT	PROBLEM	POTENTIAL AGENT
Seizures	Insulin, penicillin (IV), oxacillin, carbenicillin, phenothiazines, tricyclic antidepressants, maprotiline, halothane, vincristine, cycloserine, isoniazid, lithium carbonate.	Dyskinesias	Antipsychotic drugs, reserpine, methyldopa, antidepressants (amoxapine), levodopa, phenytoin.
Syncope	Parasympathomimetics, anticholinesterases, nitrate preparations, antihypertensive agents, antipsychotic drugs, antidepressants, monoamine oxidase (MAO) inhibitors.	Peripheral neuropathies	Streptomycin, colistin, isoniazid, demethylchlortetracycline, sulfamethoxypyridazine, nalidixic acid, nitrofurantoin, phenelzine, isocarboxazid, tricyclic antidepressants, phenytoin, propranolol, chlorpropamide, tolbutamide, ergotamine, methysergide, digitalis preparations, chloroquine, procarbazine, vincristine, vinblastine, disulfiram, glutethimide.
Stroke	Oral contraceptive agents.		
Headache	Nitrate preparations, hydralazine, indomethacin, nalidixic acid, tetracycline, corticosteroids, oral contraceptives. Withdrawal of amphetamines or methysergide, or the interaction of MAO inhibitors with tyramine from foodstuffs will also cause headache.		
		Myopathies	Corticosteroids, amphotericin B, carbenoxolone (or licorice), clofibrate, chloroquine.
Optic neuropathy	Ethambutol, isoniazid, chloramphenicol, penicillamine, quinine, quinidine, chloroquine, chlorpromazine, thioridazine, chlorpropamide, tolbutamide, phenylbutazone, ergotamine.	Malignant hyperthermia	Any potent inhalation anesthetic (e.g., halothane, ether) or any skeletal muscle relaxant (e.g., tubocurare, succinylcholine).
		Impotence	Thiazide diuretics, spironolactone, furosemide, hydralazine, reserpine, clonidine, guanethidine, methyldopa, MAO inhibitors, tricyclic antidepressants, antipsychotic agents (e.g., thioridazine), estrogenic compounds (in males), benzodiazepines, barbiturates, anticholinergic agents, digitalis, clofibrate, alcohol, marijuana, heroin.
Amblyopia	Parasympatholytics (e.g., propantheline), antipsychotic drugs, antidepressants, antiparkinsonian agents, antihistamines.		
Ototoxicity	Capreomycin, colistin, gentamicin, kanamycin, polymyxin B, viomycin, amikacin, co-trimoxazole, acetazolamide, ethacrynic acid, furosemide, quinidine, quinine.		
		Psychotic behavior	Anticholinergics (particularly in the elderly), tricyclic antidepressants, antiparkinsonian drugs, antipsychotic agents, antihistamines (more commonly in children), CNS stimulants (e.g., amphetamine), pentazocine, digitalis, corticosteroids.
Vestibular toxicity (ataxia)	Streptomycin, phenytoin, clonazepam, phenobarbital, carbamazepine.		
Cochlear toxicity (tinnitus)	Dihydrostreptomycin, neomycin, paromomycin, vancomycin, chloroquine, chloramphenicol, aspirin, phenylbutazone.	Depressive behavior	Reserpine, prazosin, methyldopa, beta blockers, guanethidine, oral contraceptives (10 to 40 percent incidence), chronic amphetamine usage, indomethacin.

This is not feasible for all pharmacologic agents. The capillary walls of the cerebral vessels are structurally different from capillaries in other organs, having endothelial cells which are closely adhered to each other and not porous as in the case of most other body capillaries. Some of these capillaries are further surrounded by projections from adjacent glial cells. The CSF, which is a special fluid system that supports the brain in the cranial vault, is formed by the group of cerebral blood vessels called the choroid plexus.

Many large molecular substances hardly pass at all from blood into the CSF or into interstitial fluids even though these same substances pass readily into the usual interstitial fluids of the body. Hence, the terms *blood-CSF barrier* and *blood-brain barrier* are used. These barriers are found in the choroid plexus and all brain parenchyma except the hypothalamus. Drugs which do pass readily through these barriers and reach brain tissue do so because these barriers are highly permeable to water, oxygen, carbon dioxide, and most lipid-soluble substances (e.g., anesthetics and alcohol) and are slightly permeable to electrolytes (sodium, potassium, and chloride).

The blood-CSF and blood-brain barriers are almost totally impermeable to substances like gold, sulfur, and arsenic. Powerful synaptic transmitter substances like acetylcholine, norepinephrine, dopamine, and glycine are prevented from entering brain tissue even though their concentrations in the blood may become quite high. Other factors which influence the type of drug crossing these barriers are the degree of protein binding of the drug and the presence of specialized transport systems in the capillary walls.

If the blood-brain barrier did not exist, many drugs currently used would have additional toxic effects. For example, the anticholinergic drugs used to treat peptic ulcer and diarrhea can be used in high dosage since they do not penetrate into the brain. Other anticholinergic drugs which are used to treat parkinsonism penetrate the blood-brain barrier; the major side effects of high doses are mental confusion and hallucinations. On the other hand, the blood-brain barrier may create problems by barring certain antibiotics and anticancer agents from gaining access to infections or tumors in the CNS, making it impossible with systemic administration to achieve effective concentrations of these drugs in the CSF or brain parenchyma.

PARKINSONISM

Parkinson's disease, or parkinsonism, is one of the more common degenerative diseases of the nervous system in persons over 40 years of age. The major symptoms are poverty of movement (akinesia or bradykinesia), increased muscle tone (rigidity), resting tremor, and disturbances of posture.

Clinical Findings

The patient with parkinsonism characteristically performs very little spontaneous movement and is slow in initiating voluntary movements. The general muscle immobility, particularly in the face ("masked" facies), is a diagnostic sign of the disease. The muscles are rigid and resistant to passive movement of a joint. The increased muscle tone in parkinsonism is typically present throughout the passive movement with occasional catching known as *cogwheeling*. The tremor is a rhythmical alternating contraction of a muscle group and its antagonists, typically three to five times per second, which is usually present while the patient is resting and is aggravated by emotional stress. The parkinsonian patient typically has a stooped posture, walks with a slow, shuffling gait, and has great difficulty turning around.

Etiology and Pathogenesis

Although the causes of parkinsonism can be identified in a limited number of patients, most patients are diagnosed as having idiopathic parkinsonism (unknown etiology). Some of the causative factors that have been identified include encephalitis, carbon monoxide poisoning, aggressive neuroleptic drug therapy (e.g., phenothiazines, butyrophenones), and chronic manganese poisoning.

The neurochemical basis of parkinsonism is a deficiency of the neurotransmitter dopamine, which stimulates the

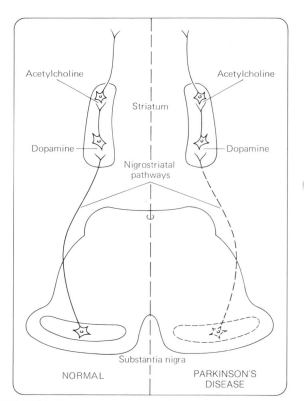

FIGURE 33-1

Pathologic and Biochemical Changes in Parkinson's Disease. The nigrostriatal pathway is partially degenerated resulting in a decreased dopamine release in the striatum (see text for full explanation).

dopamine receptor in a region of the extrapyramidal system of the brain called the striatum. Although the etiology of parkinsonism often remains a mystery, aging is known to be associated with decreased activity of the enzyme tyrosine hydroxylase, which is the rate-limiting enzyme for the biosynthesis of dopamine. The striatum regulates the coordination of muscle movement which is essential to the performance of intricate tasks. In both idiopathic *Parkinson's disease* and *postencephalitic parkinsonism,* there is a degeneration of an important nerve pathway which projects from the substantia nigra to the striatum (the nigrostriatal pathway) (Fig. 33-1). The nerves in this pathway produce dopamine. The nigrostriatal dopaminergic neurons synapse with cholinergic nerves (nerves synthesizing acetylcholine) in the striatal region of the brain. Dopamine released from the nigrostriatal nerve endings *inhibits* impulse flow in the striatal cholinergic neurons. The loss of dopamine due to death of the nigrostriatal neurons results in a loss of inhibition

(stimulation) of the striatal cholinergic neurons. In *drug-induced parkinsonism,* the nigrostriatal dopaminergic neurons remain intact, but the amount of dopamine reaching the dopamine receptors on the cholinergic neurons is reduced just as in idiopathic and postencephalitic parkinsonism. **Reserpine** causes the release of dopamine, which results in a depletion of dopamine in the nigrostriatal pathway. Antipsychotic drugs such as **phenothiazines** and **butyrophenones** block the dopamine receptors in the striatum, thus preventing dopamine action.

Clinical Pharmacology and Therapeutics

Antiparkinsonian drugs either restore dopamine action to the striatum or block the effects of the overactive cholinergic neurons in the striatum. Levodopa, amantadine, bromocriptine, anticholinergics, and MAO inhibitors are the five types of drugs employed (Table 33-2).

TABLE 33-2   Antiparkinsonian Drugs: Indications, Dosage, Adverse Effects

DRUG	TRADE NAME	AVERAGE DAILY DOSAGE RANGE (mg)	INDICATIONS (TYPES OF PARKINSONISM)	ADVERSE EFFECTS
		Anticholinergics		
Benztropine mesylate	Cogentin	1–6	Postencephalitic, arteriosclerotic, idiopathic, drug-induced	Drowsiness, dry mouth, acute glaucoma attack, increased intraocular pressure, constipation, toxic psychosis (central cholinergic deficit), constipation, urinary retention, dizziness, postural hypotension.
Biperiden	Akineton	2–8		
Chlorphenoxamine	Phenoxene	150–180		
Cycrimine	Pagitane	3.75–20		
Diphenhydramine	Benadryl	10–400		
Ethopropazine	Parsidol	100–600		
Orphenadrine hydrochloride*	Disipal	150–250		
Procyclidine	Kemadrin	10–20		
Trihexphenidyl	Artane, Tremin	6–10		
		Dopaminergic		
Levodopa (L-dopa)	Dopar, Larodopa, Bendopa	2000–8000	Postencephalitic, arteriosclerotic, idiopathic	Dyskinesias, on-off phenomenon, nausea, vomiting, blurred vision, postural hypotension, arrhythmias, gout, confusion, agitation.
Levodopa / carbidopa	Sinemet	See individual drugs; decreases levodopa to 75% single-agent dose.	Postencephalitic, idiopathic	See levodopa.
Amantadine	Symmetrel	200–600	Postencephalitic, idiopathic, arteriosclerotic, drug-induced	Depression, congestive heart failure, edema, urinary retention.
Bromocriptine mesylate	Parlodel	10–100	Postencephalitic, idiopathic	Nausea, vomiting, postural hypotension, aggression, hallucinations.
		Other		
Carbidopa	Lodosyn	10–150	Used only with levodopa	Dyskinesias occur sooner and at lower levodopa dose.

*Not effective in drug-induced parkinsonism.

Levodopa

Mechanism of Action Dopamine does not pass the blood-brain barrier, and, therefore, has no therapeutic effect in parkinsonism. The precursor of dopamine is levodopa (L-dopa; Dopar, Larodopa) which is an amino acid that crosses the blood-brain barrier and is converted to dopamine (Fig. 33-2). Presumably, most of the levodopa is converted to dopamine in the remaining nigrostriatal dopaminergic neurons of the parkinsonian patient.

Levodopa is the most effective treatment presently available for idiopathic Parkinson's disease and postencephalitic parkinsonism, as it alleviates all of the symptoms of parkinsonism. However, the bradykinesia and rigidity respond somewhat better than the tremor. About two-thirds of parkinsonian patients derive a significant improvement from levodopa therapy.

Pharmacokinetics Levodopa is absorbed by the small intestine, and the peak blood levels are usually reached within 30 to 90 min after an oral dose, although food may decrease its absorption. Less than 1 percent of administered levodopa actually reaches the brain because the decarboxylase enzyme converts levodopa to dopamine in other organs such as the gut, liver, and kidney. It is excreted in the urine as dopamine and homovanillic acid.

Adverse Effects There are many side effects associated with levodopa therapy and constant regulation of dosage is necessary to maintain the optimal risk-benefit ratio. Anorexia, nausea, and vomiting frequently occur during initiation of therapy and their severity is dependent, to a great extent, upon the rate of increase of the daily dose of levodopa. It is believed that these side effects are due to increased dopamine formation in the vomiting center of the brain. Levodopa is often tolerated better if given immediately after meals.

Another common side effect of levodopa therapy is involuntary body movements which are called *dyskinesias*. Levodopa-induced dyskinesias may consist of facial grimacing, head nodding, tongue protrusion, exaggerated gestures, and rocking movements of muscles of the head, tongue, arms, legs, and trunk. The dyskinesias can be minimized by reducing the total daily dose of levodopa or by increasing the frequency of administration to six to eight times per day.

Other, less frequent side effects are lightheadedness due to a fall in blood pressure, cardiac arrhythmias, and mental changes such as aggressive behavior, hallucinations, delusions, and hypomania.

After 1 to 2 years of therapy with levodopa some patients develop transient episodes of severe exacerbation of parkinsonian symptoms ("on-off" effect). The patient's performance may oscillate from bradykinesia with other severe parkinsonian symptoms to dyskinesia with only transient periods of good control in between. This may occur several times during the day. In some patients, the dyskinesia phase may be associated with high plasma concentrations of levodopa and the bradykinesia with lower levels of levodopa.

Pyridoxine (vitamin B$_6$) should be avoided during levodopa therapy. Pyridoxine is a cofactor for dopa decarboxylation and can enhance the extracerebral decarboxylation of levodopa. Thus, administration of pyridoxine in conjunction with levodopa increases dopamine formation from levodopa in tissues such as the liver and kidney, leaving less levodopa available to cross the blood-brain barrier. Clinically, pyridoxine markedly antagonizes or totally abolishes the therapeutic effect of the drug. The patient should be advised to avoid multivitamin preparations that contain pyr-

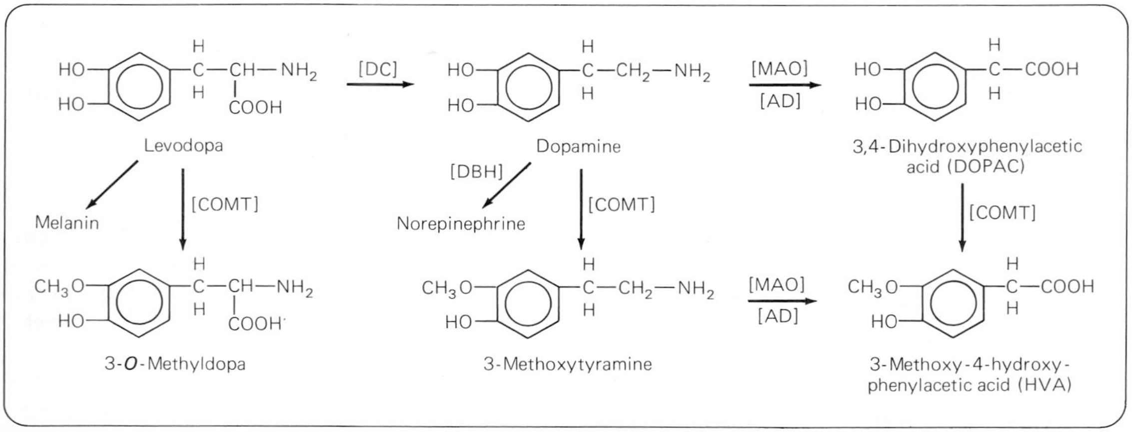

FIGURE 33-2

Catabolic Pathways of Levodopa. The pathway of levodopa metabolism is shown. The abbreviations represent the following enzymes: AD = aldehydrodehydrogenase; COMT = catechol-*O*-methyltransferase; DBH = dopamine β-hydroxylase; DC = aromatic L-amino acid decarboxylase or dopa decarboxylase; MAO = monoamine oxidase.

idoxine. A preparation like Larobec can be recommended, since it is a multivitamin preparation without vitamin B_6.

Levodopa is a precursor of the catecholamines, dopamine, norepinephrine, and epinephrine, which can elevate blood pressure. Some **MAO inhibitors** (type A, or nonselective) enhance the effects of catecholamines by inhibiting the enzymes which inactivate them. Levodopa should not be given with MAO inhibitors, because this combination can produce dangerous elevations of blood pressure.

Dosage and Administration The most important principle of levodopa therapy is to begin with small doses to avoid adverse effects. Daily doses are gradually increased until satisfactory clinical results are achieved or until the occurrence of side effects prevents further increases. The drug should be taken with food to decrease gastric irritation.

Parkinsonian patients are usually started on 125 to 250 mg of levodopa (Dopar, Larodopa) orally two or three times daily. The dose is usually increased by 250 g every 4 to 7 days until an average total dose of 3 to 4 g in divided doses is reached. The short half-life of the drug (approximately 2 h) results in a need for multiple daily doses.

Carbidopa

Mechanism of Action Because dopamine is unable to cross the blood-brain barrier, dopa decarboxylase, which catalyzes the decarboxylation of dopa to dopamine in various body tissues, effectively limits the amount of levodopa available to enter the brain. Drugs such as carbidopa that inhibit dopa decarboxylase in the extracerebral organs but do not cross the blood-brain barrier can be used in conjunction with levodopa to allow a greater percentage of levodopa to get into the brain (Fig. 33-3).

Adverse Effects The major advantage of the combination of **levodopa** with **carbidopa** is a reduction in certain side effects, such as anorexia, nausea, and vomiting. The decrease in side effects permits a more rapid increase in dosage of levodopa during the initial phase of therapy. Dyskinesias, mental side effects, and orthostatic hypotension are not modified by using this drug combination.

Dosage and Administration At the present time, **carbidopa** (Lodosyn) is the only dopa decarboxylase inhibitor available in the United States. Carbidopa is combined with **levodopa** in a single tablet (Sinemet), which is the preferred dosage form, although a few patients require titration of the individual agents. There are three sizes: **carbidopa/levodopa** 10/100, 25/100, and 25/250. Generally, therapy is initiated with the smaller dose of Sinemet four times a day, and the dosage gradually increased to a maximum of about 1500 mg levodopa with 150 mg of carbidopa daily. Conversion of a patient on levodopa alone to carbidopa/levodopa therapy is done by decreasing the total daily levodopa intake by 75 to

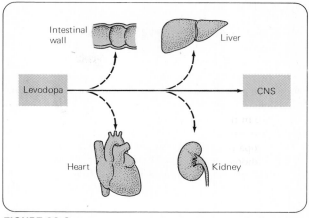

FIGURE 33-3

Effect of Carbidopa on Levodopa Distribution. Carbidopa prevents metabolism of levodopa by peripheral organs, as indicated by the dashed lines, thereby allowing the total dose of levodopa to reach the CNS.

80 percent and initiating this dose of levodopa as Sinemet therapy the next morning; dosage is adjusted according to response.

Amantadine

Mechanism of Action Amantadine (Symmetrel) is an antiviral drug which exhibits antiparkinsonian effects. Amantadine increases the release of dopamine from dopaminergic neurons. Therefore, its antiparkinsonian action may be due to an enhancement of the amount of dopamine released from the remaining nigrostriatal neurons in patients with Parkinson's disease. This drug is less effective than levodopa and is generally only effective in the early stages of the disease.

Pharmacokinetics Amantadine is rapidly absorbed from the GI tract and has a long duration of action. It is excreted unchanged in the urine and requires dosage reduction in the presence of renal disease.

Adverse Effects Adverse effects include dizziness, mental confusion, nausea, headache, drowsiness, congestive heart failure, and livedo reticularis, a purplish meshwork pattern of cutaneous discoloration. Mild anticholinergic effects also occur.

Dosage The usual dosage is 100 mg orally twice a day. Improvement may be seen within a few days, but after 1 to 2 months the therapeutic efficacy may diminish. In an effort to maintain the therapeutic effect, a "washout" period of 1 month every 6 months should be utilized in the patient's regimen.

Bromocriptine

Mechanism of Action   Bromocriptine (Parlodel) is an ergot derivative that directly stimulates dopamine receptors, including those present in the striatum. Although some parkinsonian patients have responded better to bromocriptine than to levodopa, levodopa or levodopa/carbidopa remain the most efficacious drugs for most patients. However, the encouraging experience with bromocriptine suggests that with further research an even more potent dopamine-receptor stimulant may eventually be found to replace levodopa as the treatment of choice. Dopaminergic agonists, such as **lisuride, pergolide,** and **lergotrile** are currently being investigated for this purpose.

Pharmacokinetics   Bromocriptine is less than 30 percent absorbed after oral administration. It is highly bound to plasma albumin and completely metabolized prior to excretion, primarily in the bile.

Adverse Effects   The main side effects are anorexia, nausea, vomiting, hypotension, lightheadedness, hallucinations, ataxia, depression, psychosis, and dyskinesias. Clinically insignificant and transient elevations in blood urine nitrogen (BUN), serum glutamic oxaloacetic transaminase (SGOT), creatinine phosphokinase (CPK), and alkaline phosphatase can occur.

Dosage   The usual dosage of bromocriptine ranges from 10 to 100 mg daily in divided doses. Average daily dosages are 40 to 80 mg.

Anticholinergic Drugs

Mechanism of Action   Striatal nerve cells which synthesize acetylcholine are thought to be hyperactive in parkinsonism due to the loss of dopamine. Drugs which block the acetylcholine (muscarinic) receptor in the brain also ameliorate the rigidity and tremor in Parkinson's disease. These anticholinergic (also called antimuscarinic) drugs have minimal effect on the bradykinesia, and their use is limited by anticholinergic adverse effects (see Chap. 12).

Dosage and Administration   Many anticholinergic drugs are available, but there is no evidence that one is more effective than another. **Trihexphenidyl** (Artane) is usually started at 2 mg/day and increased by 2 mg daily each week until maximum benefit is obtained with tolerable side effects. Other common anticholinergic drugs which are used to treat parkinsonism are **benztropine** (Cogentin); which has the advantage of being available for parenteral administration as well as orally; **ethopropazine** (Parsidol), which is a phenothiazine derivative; and antihistamines such as **diphenhydramine** (Benadryl), which also have strong anticholinergic action in the CNS (see Table 33-2 for a complete listing of drugs of this type).

Although the anticholinergic drugs are much less effective than levodopa for treating idiopathic and postencephalitic parkinsonism, they are the treatment of choice for drug-induced parkinsonism. Levodopa, amantadine, and anticholinergic drugs can be administered in combination for maximum therapeutic benefit in idiopathic or postencephalitic parkinsonism.

MAO Inhibitors

Monoamine oxidase (MAO) inhibitors were used in the treatment of parkinsonism in the early 1960s but fell into disuse due to the serious adverse effects and drug interactions associated with their use. An investigational selective MAO type B inhibitor **deprenyl** does not appear to have the potential for toxicity of the nonselective MAO inhibitors. Hence, it has been used successfully as an adjunct to levodopa therapy and will extend the duration of action of levodopa. In addition, it also appears to provide a mood-elevating effect that is desirable in many parkinsonian patients. The usual daily dose is 10 mg.

THE NURSING PROCESS RELATED TO PARKINSONISM

As the anticholinergic agents are discussed in Chap. 12, this discussion mainly relates to the use of levodopa, carbidopa, amantadine, and bromocriptine.

Assessment

Baseline assessment of the degree of bradykinesia, tremor, and rigidity, as well as the ability to perform the activities of daily living, is made before therapy is initiated. Marked improvement in the patient's condition and ability to function may alter interactional patterns within the family and the patient's social community, so the interpersonal environment should also be considered.

The care provider should elicit the names of other drugs the patient may be taking, since Parkinson's disease is aggravated by certain agents and toxicity can result. If the patient has other medical problems necessitating the use of neuroleptic and antihypertensive agents, a multidisciplinary approach may be warranted for optimal patient care.

As cardiac disease, liver disease, renal impairment, psychosis, and orthostatic hypotension may contraindicate the use of the antiparkinsonian drugs or require dosage adjustment and special monitoring, the patient's history, physical condition, and emotional status should be evaluated. **Bromocriptine** should not be prescribed to those with sensitivity to ergot preparations. Pregnancy and lactation contraindicate the antiparkinsonian drugs, and exposure to bromocriptine can be hazardous to both mother and fetus.

Those patients who are depressed require careful observation during therapy with antiparkinsonian drugs. Since these drugs cause visual disturbances and drowsiness, the patient's ability to operate machinery safely should be assessed.

Management

All antiparkinsonian drugs should be taken with food or after meals to minimize gastric irritation and anorexia, as well as to avoid dry mouth from parasympatholytic drugs during meals. Absorption of levodopa is inhibited by protein in the diet. The best approach is to instruct the patient to decrease the number of high-protein foods (milk, meat, fish, eggs, poultry, nuts, beans) in the diet and to spread protein intake over four or more smaller meals. This may reduce the "on-off" phenomenon. The patient who is stabilized on levodopa before the change in diet may need to decrease the dosage level to prevent dyskinesias. When the patient takes a combination product (Sinemet), there is no need to limit **pyridoxine**. However, with the plain levodopa, use of multivitamin preparations containing pyridoxine are to be avoided. Levodopa may darken urine or sweat, but this does not represent a serious problem.

The patient and family members should have a thorough education about the drug and the disease. In spite of the patient's slow movement and speech impairment, nursing personnel and family members should understand that intelligence is not necessarily impaired. Prior education and functioning should help the nurse determine an appropriate level for the teaching program. Since the maximal effectiveness of **levodopa** may not be realized for 2 to 6 months, the patient and family should understand that the benefits of the drug may not be immediate.

Other components in patient education should include methods to avoid orthostatic hypotension by rising slowly from a lying or sitting position, sitting down if one feels dizzy, avoiding standing still for long periods, and wearing support stockings. Exercise, conscious posture control, and management of constipation (when anticholinergic drugs are taken) are vital components of a thorough education plan. Dyskinesias should be explained, as well as methods to alleviate them by modification in drug therapy.

Adverse effects that may occur with **amantadine** administration can be managed by dosage reduction or, in the case of congestive heart failure, by traditional measures (diuretics, digoxin, rest). Livedo reticularis, although benign, can contribute to a patient's feeling stigmatized and efforts should be directed toward improving self-image and elevating the legs, which diminishes its appearance. In those with renal impairment, drug blood levels should be monitored frequently, and elderly patients should be observed very closely for amantadine toxicity. Amantadine should not be discontinued abruptly, as symptoms can exacerbate (parkinsonian crisis).

Adverse effects of **bromocriptine** can be minimized by starting with small doses and increasing gradually to effective levels, giving the drug with food in the evening. The nurse needs to be alert for central nervous system aberrances (confusion, delusions, nightmares, depression, and suicidal ideation). Hypotension and angina may become emergent problems. Bromocriptine may be additive with levodopa in Parkinson's disease, requiring a reduction of levodopa dosage. For patients receiving antihypertensives along with bromocriptine, additive hypotension may result, requiring antihypertensive dosage adjustment.

Evaluation

Improvement of rigidity, bradykinesia, tremor, and ability to function are the basis of evaluation for therapeutic effect. Activities of daily living should be used to measure improvement. Presence of anticholinergic symptoms, severe gastric distress, dyskinesia may require dosage adjustment. An increase in problems such as falls or trauma may require either an increase in medication or a dosage reduction. Blood pressure should be evaluated lying and standing for hypotension and the heart auscultated for arrhythmias. Any symptoms of difficult urination should be noted, and regular laboratory evaluation of hepatic and renal function is indicated. Evaluation of emotional status and interpersonal relations should not be overlooked. Every attempt should be made to maintain the patient as a functioning member of society.

CASE STUDY

A.J., aged 72, was brought to the long-term care facility by his wife, who stated he had become too difficult for her to manage. She indicated that he had parkinsonism which was diagnosed 8 years prior to his admission. Problems which were difficult for the wife to handle and caused her to seek assistance were severe constipation, falls, mood disturbances, and inability to feed, dress, or toilet himself without assistance. Mrs. J. requested that the house physician–geriatric nurse practitioner (GNP) team assume the care of her husband, since the family physician had

recently retired. A.J. was receiving biperiden (Akineton) 2 mg qid and a stool softener prior to admission.

Assessment

The geriatric nurse practitioner interviewed both A.J. and his wife. Other than the parkinsonism, A.J.'s history was remarkably negative for severe or chronic disorders. A.J. and his wife were depressed by the separation caused by his institutionalization, but both felt that the requirements of his complete care were too demanding for Mrs. J. The couple had lived comfortably on his pension since his retirement from the vice presidency of a large corporation 7 years earlier. Their two children resided several thousand miles away. A.J. had never been on levodopa therapy.

On physical examination, the nurse noted cogwheel rigidity, immobility of facial expression, slowness of movement, stooped posture, extreme instability on standing, and a tendency to break into a trot when walking. The tremor, at 3 per second, was a pill-rolling type and increased at rest. His voice was weak, low, and lacked expression. Vital signs were blood pressure 128/82, pulse 80 and regular, respiration 22. Auscultation of the heart revealed regular sinus rhythm with no murmurs or other adventitious sounds. While difficult to evaluate due to the rigidity, range of motion appeared decreased no more than 10 percent in any joint. The rest of the examination was noncontributory.

Management

After the physician had examined the patient, she and the geriatric nurse practitioner discussed the possibility of levodopa therapy. Except for his depression, which would require close observation, there seemed to be no contraindication for the therapy. The physician and nurse presented this option to Mr. and Mrs. J., who agreed to try the drug. Mrs. J. asked the GNP if it were true that the drug was an aphrodisiac. The nurse explained that much of the increased sexual drive noted in some patients had been attributed to the decrease in parkinsonism symptoms and resulting euphoria, although theories exist that dopamine levels in the brain do affect sexual drive directly.

The GNP and physician worked with the clinical pharmacist to develop a dosing protocol for gradually increasing the doses of levodopa/carbidopa (Sinemet), under the supervision of the GNP, to a level of optimum balance between adverse and therapeutic effects, and for tapering the Akineton to a lower dose. The physical therapist and dietitian were also consulted; an exercise program and a diet with the minimum daily protein requirement spread over four small meals were established.

A.J. and his wife were very interested in the drug, and the nurse supplied reading material and spent time discussing the drug and other aspects of the management plan with the patient.

After a month, the drug regimen of the patient was adjusted to Akineton 1 mg tid and Sinemet 250/25 qid. Both drugs were taken after meals.

The patient was supplied with a warming plate so that his food would not become cold during the extended time it took him to eat. To treat the persistent constipation from the anticholinergic drugs, high fluid and bulk intake were given to complement the actions of the stool softener and exercise program.

Evaluation

While the patient showed decreased rigidity and bradykinesia after a week of therapy, maximal effect was not achieved until the fourth month of therapy, when rigidity and bradykinesia were nearly absent. The tremor persisted, but was severe only when the patient was fatigued. The patient was able to resume independent functioning in activities of daily living (ADL). He experienced some orthostatic hypotension in the morning, but this was alleviated by rising slowly. His blood pressure dropped to 108/72, but his pulse and heart sounds remained normal. Constipation remained an occasional problem.

A.J. was discharged from the long-term care facility and the next year he and his wife were able to take the ocean cruise they had always put off until retirement. During the cruise, A.J. began to experience exacerbation of symptoms until he secured an appropriate low-protein diet.

MYASTHENIA GRAVIS

Myasthenia gravis (MG) is a peripheral neurologic disorder that is characterized by skeletal muscle weakness secondary to a defect in neuromuscular transmission. The muscle weakness is sporadic and characteristically intensifes upon prolonged or repetitive exercise. This results in easy fatigability, ocular ptosis, hoarseness, difficulty in swallowing, nasal speech, double vision, and shortness of breath. All these features may vary from minute to minute during the examination, or from hour to hour throughout the patient's day. Respiratory muscle involvement can be dramatic and life-threatening. Myasthenia gravis is twice as common in women as in men. Although it may develop at any age, the most common age of onset is between the ages of 20 and 30 years in women and 60 and 70 years in men.

Etiology and Pathophysiology

The integrity of the neuromuscular junction depends on the neuronal manufacture and release of the neurotransmitter acetylcholine (ACh) from the axonal terminals into the synapse adjacent to the muscle end plate. ACh then binds to specific end plate receptor molecules, depolarizes the membrane, and initiates cell contraction. This process is terminated by the enzyme acetylcholinesterase (AChE), which quickly frees the end plate for another signal (see Chap. 10 for more details).

The defect in neuromuscular transmission in myasthenia gravis is not known. Several hypotheses have been proposed. One hypothetical set suggests that the production and/or the amount of ACh is reduced, that some factor impairs ACh's ability to induce muscle contraction, that there is a shortage of ACh receptors on the end plate, that breakdown of ACh is faulty, or that some combination of these factors is the cause of the problem. The net result is a decrease in neural impulses to the terminals of the finest branches of the motor nerves in the muscle fibers.

Another hypothesis is that myasthenia gravis is an autoimmune disease in which there is generation of serum antibodies and activation of complement at the receptor protein of the neuromuscular junction. A high percentage of myasthenic patients have associated thymic hyperplasia and/or thymus tumor (thymoma). The thymus is the site for maturation of lymphocytes, which play a role in cell-mediated immunity. A substantial number of myasthenic patients have circulating antimuscle antibodies and anti–acetylcholine receptor antibodies. The histocompatibility antigen HL-AB is found in younger female myasthenic sera. Myasthenic syndromes occur in disseminated immunologic disorders (e.g., thyroiditis), and as complications of certain drugs (e.g., D-penicillamine).

Clinical Findings

Whether the defect is presynaptic, postsynaptic, immunologic or genetic, pathologic findings are few. Diagnosis is confirmed by giving a subcutaneous injection of the short-acting AChE inhibitor **edrophonium chloride** (Tensilon) intravenously. An unequivocal improvement in muscle strength in 5 to 20 min is diagnostic for the disease.

Most patients with active myasthenia gravis will have detectable levels of acetylcholine receptor antibodies in their sera. Concurrent thyroid disease should be excluded once the diagnosis is established. Mediastinal x-rays may exclude thymoma.

Clinical Pharmacology and Therapeutics

Spontaneous remission occurs in about 25 percent of patients. Treatment is with acetylcholinesterase inhibitors, thymectomy, corticosteroids, and immunosuppressives (Table 33-3). **Potassium supplements, ephedrine sulfate,** and **calcium** have been used as adjuncts to the anticholinesterases to improve therapeutic response. More recently, plasmapheresis has been used in those refractory to standard therapies.

Acetylcholinesterase Inhibitors

Neostigmine bromide (Prostigmin) is a short-acting anticholinesterase inhibitor. Oral forms are used for long-term therapy when no difficulty in swallowing exists. The initial dose is 15 mg one to three times daily. This dose is gradually

increased to an average daily dose of 150 mg, according to therapeutic response and adverse effects. **Neostigmine methylsulfate** can be given by subcutaneous, intramuscular, or intravenous routes in myasthenic crisis.

The advantages of **pyridostigmine** (Mestinon) and **ambenonium** (Mytelase) over neostigmine are the longer durations of action and reduced severity of side effects. Patients taking one of these drugs at bedtime need not be awakened during the night to take more medication.

Edrophonium chloride (Tensilon) can be used to determine whether the myasthenic patient is receiving adequate anticholinesterase medication. If during treatment with other anticholinesterase agents, a 2-mg intravenous test dose of edrophonium increases muscle strength, the patient is being undertreated. Excessive anticholinesterase medication can produce muscle weakness by binding to the ACh receptors; in this situation (cholinergic crisis) an injection of edrophonium chloride will increase muscle weakness and indicate the need for reducing the oral anticholinesterase dose. If the patient shows no change in strength, the current dose is optimal. (See Chap. 11 for description of individual drugs.)

Adverse Effects   The major adverse effects from cholinergic overstimulation include increased salivation, miosis, wheezing due to bronchial secretion and bronchospasm, nausea, abdominal pain, and diarrhea. Atropine sulfate 0.6 mg two to four times daily can be used to control excessive muscarinic effects and to treat cholinergic crisis.

TABLE 33-3   Dosages of Drugs Used for Myasthenia Gravis

DRUG	AVERAGE DAILY DOSE RANGE
ACTH gel	80–120 units gel IM
Ambenonium (Mytelase)	2–10 mg/injection
Azathioprine (Immuran)	Initial: 60 mg/kg or 50–100 mg
	Maximum: 25 mg/kg or 125–250 mg
Cyclophosphamide (Cytoxan)	1–5 mg/kg
Edrophonium chloride (Tensilon)	Used only for testing (see text)
Ephedrine sulfate	100 mg
Guanidine	1.5–2.5 g
Neostigmine bromide (Prostigmin)	15–200 mg
Neostigmine methylsulfate (Prostigmin)	initial: 0.5 mg. Repeat doses titrated to response
Prednisone	100 mg on alternate days
Pyridostigmine bromide (Mestinon)	600 mg

Suppression of the Immune Reaction

ACTH ACTH treatment has been used mainly in severely ill patients, especially those who have not had satisfactory results from thymectomy. A typical course of treatment consists of single daily injections of 100 to 160 units of ACTH gel (see Chap. 35) intramuscularly for 10 days. Ventilatory support and nasogastric tube feeding may be necessary because skeletal muscle weakness can occur after the second or third day of therapy. After the course of ACTH therapy, some improvement will occur in about 92 percent of patients, usually lasting about 60 to 90 days. Additional courses of ACTH or single injections of ACTH at 1- to 3-week intervals may be administered to prolong the therapeutic benefit.

Adrenocorticosteroids A typical program for myasthenia is **prednisone** 100 mg as a single dose every other day. Muscle weakness (myopathy) may also occur initially with the use of the corticosteroids. This may be avoided by gradually increasing corticosteroid therapy, starting with low doses, or administering drugs every other day instead of daily. The prednisone dose can be gradually reduced as improvement occurs, and remissions are frequently maintained with doses of 20 to 40 mg of prednisone on alternate days.

Thymectomy Surgical removal of the thymus is indicated in all cases of thymoma and in those patients who have a poor response to anticholinesterase drugs. The myasthenic symptoms are improved in about two-thirds of the patients who have undergone thymectomy.

Immunosuppressants **Azathioprine** (Immuran) and **cyclophosphamide** (Cytoxan) are the most commonly used immunosuppressives in the treatment of MG. These drugs (see Chaps. 31 and 37, respectively) are considered after steroid therapy and thymectomy have been unsuccessful, and, preferably, for patients beyond the reproductive years, since both agents are considered teratogenic in women and men. When used for long periods, both agents are considered to be oncogenic as well. All immunosuppressant drugs render the patient more susceptible to infection.

Azathioprine is generally preferred over **cyclophosphamide** even though it is slower-acting, because it is milder and lacks the side effects of alopecia, hemorrhagic cystitis, and secondary malignancies associated with the latter.

Drugs Contraindicated in Myasthenia Gravis

Patients with myasthenia gravis are particularly sensitive to neuromuscular blocking agents like curare, succinylcholine, and gallamine. Drugs which depress membrane excitability, such as anticonvulsants, antiarrhythmics, and quinine (including tonic water) should be avoided or used with great caution. Local anesthetics warrant cautious use, whereas ether as a general anesthetic is contraindicated in myasthenics.

Centrally acting narcotic analgesics should be avoided because of respiratory depression. Certain antibiotics can block neuromuscular transmission, probably by blocking ACh release from the nerve terminals (see Table 33-4).

NURSING PROCESS RELATED TO MYASTHENIA GRAVIS

Assessment

As the degree of pathologic involvement will vary at different points in the illness due to the characteristic pattern of remission and exacerbation, the nurse will need to assess the patient's functional abilities for safety and ability to perform activities of daily living. To prevent the dangerous complication of aspiration pneumonia it is particularly important to note choking and aspiration of food. It is also necessary to note the patient and family adjustment to the illness and the potential ability of the family to manage the illness in later stages.

A complete nursing assessment should also look at a myasthenic's other health factors and the medications being used for such. Diabetes, hypothyroidism, alcoholism, corti-

TABLE 33-4 Drugs Contraindicated in Myasthenis Gravis

Neuromuscular blocking agents
 Curare
 Succinylcholine
 Gallamine
Membrane excitability depressants
 Quinidine
 Quinine
 Phenytoin
 Propranolol
 Procainamide
Analgesics
 Morphine
 Meperidine
Anesthetics
 Local: Procaine, lidocaine
 General: Ether
Antibiotics
 Streptomycin
 Kanamycin
 Gentamicin
 Tetracycline
 Neomycin
 Tobramycin
 Polymixin group
 Bacitracin
 Paromomycin
 Colistin

costeroid therapy can themselves cause myopathy or exacerbate myasthenia gravis and can make a nursing assessment even more confusing.

Management

Myasthenia gravis is a chronic disorder that will require lifelong treatment and evaluation. This involves considerable patient and family teaching. The drug dosage may be difficult to regulate, and the family members and patient will need to know how to adjust the medication dosage and schedule based upon the pattern of symptoms, as well as what developments require that the nurse or physician be contacted.

The nurse needs to look at the patient's dosage schedule of medications. Neostigmine needs to be given regularly day and night over a 24-h period to prevent cholinergic crisis. The larger portion may be distributed at a time when the patient is more fatigued, like afternoons or after meals. The nurse can educate the patient to keep a daily record of status in relation to medications and dosage times.

Nursing plans for the myasthenic patient should always include instruction of the patient and family as to avoidance of illness (avoiding large crowds, exposure in bad weather, and contact with sick people). Febrile illness can aggravate myasthenia gravis, especially if the infection involves the respiratory system. Patients on steroids and immunosuppressants need to have a complete blood and platelet count done periodically in order to monitor early hematologic side effects. Nurses working in outpatient settings or as visiting nurses may have a different perspective from which to assess the patient's living environment and family involvement in the educational plan.

A total team approach is necessary to adequately manage this rare but complex disorder that has major psychosocial as well as physiologic impact upon the patient and the family unit. The Myasthenia Gravis Foundation is a valuable source of educational material for the patient and family, the general public, and for health professionals.

Evaluation

Very astute observational skills are needed to evaluate the adequacy of the treatment of myasthenia gravis, as the symptoms of overdosage (*cholinergic crisis*) and undertreatment (*myasthenic crisis*) are similar, that is, muscular weakness. Since the requirements for cholinesterase-inhibiting drugs will vary depending upon whether the disease is in remission or progression, either situation can occur at any time. When muscle weakness occurs, the physician should be contacted. The nurse who assists during the administration of the **edrophonium** challenge to differentiate between the two problems should monitor the patient's circulatory and respiratory status throughout the procedure and should be prepared to institute emergency treatment for circulatory collapse or respiratory arrest.

EPILEPTIC SEIZURE DISORDERS

Seizures result from excessive synchronous discharge of neurons in the brain. There is a sudden, transient disturbance of consciousness and/or motor function which tends to recur. Seizures occur as a symptom in many types of diseases of the brain (e.g., biochemical, traumatic, neoplastic, infectious, and vascular). In many patients, however, the etiology of the seizures is unknown (idiopathic). The neurologic signs and symptoms may vary in different types of epileptic seizures depending on location of the initial discharging neurons and how the discharge spreads over the brain. The electroencephalogram (EEG) may be helpful in localizing the lesion and sometimes gives an indication of etiology.

Clinical Findings

The choice of antiseizure drug depends primarily upon the type of seizure the patient has (Table 33-5). There are several types of seizures which are classified according to their clinical picture.

The generalized tonic/clonic (*grand mal*) seizure consists of tonic and clonic muscle spasms associated with loss of consciousness, tongue biting, and urinary and fecal incontinence.

Partial seizures with elementary symptomatology (*focal seizures*) are usually due to a localized lesion in the brain which produces sudden, involuntary movements in one part of the body, such as an arm or leg, or a localized change in sensation. The patient usually remains conscious. However, if the convulsion progressively spreads to involve other bilateral parts of the body (Jacksonian seizures), consciousness is lost and a grand mal seizure ensues.

Simple absence (*petit mal*) attacks consist of a sudden loss of consciousness, without falling, which lasts only 5 to 30 s. Occasionally there may be some minor muscle movements of the eyes, head, or extremities. Petit mal epilepsy is a childhood disease which rarely persists beyond the age of 20.

Partial seizures with complex symptomatology (*psychomotor seizures* or *temporal lobe seizures*) are characterized

TABLE 33-5 Treatment of Seizure Disorders

Tonic-Clonic (Grand Mal; Focal)
Drug of choice: Phenytoin
Alternatives: Phenobarbital, primidone, carbamazepine
Absences (Petit Mal)
Drug of choice: Ethosuximide
Alternatives: Valproic acid, clonazepam, trimethadione
Complex Partial Seizures (Temporal Lobe; Psychomotor)
Drug of choice: Carbamazepine, primidone
Alternatives: Phenytoin, phenobarbital, methsuximide
Status Epilepticus
Drug of choice: Diazepam, IV
Alternatives: Phenytoin, IV; phenobarbital, IV

by sudden episodes of behavioral changes or mood alterations. There may be moaning, inappropriate laughing, or grimacing. Usually the patient is amnesic about the attack.

The therapeutic objective in treating seizure disorders is to prevent seizures without adverse effects, most notably CNS impairment. Drug therapy remains the principal means of treatment. Surgery, psychotherapy, and diet and fluid balance are adjuvant methods. It was once thought that anticonvulsant therapy was always lifelong, but individuals who are seizure-free for a period of years and who have been slowly tapered off anticonvulsant therapy may still remain seizure-free.

Clinical Pharmacology and Therapeutics

Mechanism of Anticonvulsant Action

Although this is not completely understood, it is felt that the mechanism of action of most anticonvulsant drugs is to modify the ability of the brain tissue to respond to seizure-provoking stimuli. Specific neurophysiologic changes include elevation of excitatory synaptic threshold, potentiation of pre- and postsynaptic inhibition, and prolongation of the refractory period.

Blood Levels of Anticonvulsants

The monitoring of blood levels of antiepileptic drugs has enabled clinicians to determine the optimum dose for each individual patient, determine compliance, and identify the agent producing toxicity in patients receiving multiple drugs. Blood levels will also identify patients with unusual rates of metabolism of antiepileptic drugs due to genetic or disease-induced abnormalities.

The most effective blood levels and pharmacokinetics of some anticonvulsants are listed in Table 33-6. The final adjustment of the dose of these drugs should be determined by measurement of plasma concentration. Initially, therapy with a single antiepileptic agent is started and the dose adjusted until effective blood levels are obtained. If no improvement is seen, another drug should be substituted. If only partial improvement is obtained, a second drug should be added and monitored by blood levels if possible.

When the patient's seizures are poorly controlled and the blood level of the antiepileptic drug is low, the dosage should be increased. When seizures are completely controlled and the blood level is less than that found effective in the majority of patients, there is no need to increase the level just to agree with the pharmacologic standards.

Phenytoin and Other Hydantoins

Mechanism of Action Hydantoins, such as **phenytoin** (Dilantin), **mephenytoin** (Mesantoin), and **ethotoin** (Peganone), cause membrane stabilization by altering ion movement across cell membranes, an effect which may be due to their action on Na^+-K^+-ATPase. Hydantoins are used to treat grand mal, focal, and psychomotor seizures. Mephenytoin and ethotoin are seldom used, so phenytoin will be considered as a prototype.

Pharmacokinetics Phenytoin appears to be slowly though completely absorbed from the gastrointestinal tract, although malabsorption has been reported in a few patients. Peak plasma levels usually do not occur for several hours after an oral dose with an "extended" dosage form, but occur sooner with "prompt" dosage forms. The intramuscular route has been shown to be a slow and unreliable route of absorption.

Phenytoin is primarily metabolized through a dose-dependent metabolism (also called zero-order kinetics; see Chap. 5). Dose-dependent metabolism means that a change in the daily dose will result in a disproportionate change in the plasma level, making dose adjustment difficult. In addition, the dose-dependent process causes the half-life to be longer with higher plasma levels and shorter with lower plasma levels. The average half-life is approximately 24 h for a plasma concentration in the range of 10 μg/mL. Therefore, several days are required to achieve steady-state concentrations.

Phenytoin is 70 to 95 percent bound to plasma protein and is widely distributed throughout the body, including to the CNS. Serum concentrations between 10 and 20 μg/mL are considered therapeutic.

Adverse Effects Nystagmus has occurred with plasma concentrations of 8 to 20 μg/mL and is almost always present with higher levels. Nystagmus on far lateral gaze has been used by some clinicians to estimate when a plasma level of approximately 20 μg/mL has been achieved. Ataxia occurs at levels about 30 μg/mL while lethargy, with slurred speech, occurs at levels greater than 40 μg/mL. Other adverse effects include nausea, vomiting (rare), rash, pseudolymphoma, gingival hyperplasia, megaloblastic anemia secondary to folate depletion, hirsutism, peripheral neuropathies, osteomalacia, hyperglycemia, and even paradoxical seizures at extremely high plasma levels. A lupus erythematous–like syndrome and a morbilliform rash, which will rarely progress to Stevens-Johnson syndrome, can occur. If a rash appears, the drug should be discontinued.

Other drugs administered in conjunction with phenytoin may modify its metabolism and thereby alter its therapeutic or toxic effects (see Table 33-7). **Phenobarbital** can significantly lower circulating blood levels of phenytoin by enhancing its metabolism in the liver. On the other hand, such drugs as **isoniazid, aspirin, cycloserine, disulfiram, dicoumarol,** and **methylphenidate** depress the metabolism of phenytoin, raise serum levels of phenytoin, and may induce serious side effects.

Dosage Since **phenytoin** has such a long half-life, control of seizures can usually be achieved by once-per-day dosing, if an "extended" dosage form is used (Dilantin Kapseals are the only FDA-approved dosage form of this type). Other generic phenytoin preparations are termed "prompt" and are not intended for once-a-day dosage, as they may provide such a rapid release of phenytoin that toxic serum levels would be attained. The daily dosage range for phenytoin is 200 to 600 mg (adult) or 50 to 300 mg (4 to 8 mg/kg) in children.

Barbiturates

The bartiburates used to treat seizure disorders include **phenobarbital, mephobarbital** (Mebaral), and **metharbital** (Gemonil). Phenobarbital represents one of the most effective, least expensive, and least toxic of all agents used. Barbiturates and deoxybarbiturates are used to treat grand mal, focal, and psychomotor seizures. Phenobarbital and other barbiturates limit the spread of seizure activity and also elevate the seizure threshold.

Adverse Effects Common side effects include drowsiness, but nystagmus, ataxia, megaloblastic anemia, rashes, and osteomalacia may also develop. The shorter-acting mephobarbital and metharbital are sometimes recommended for those who cannot tolerate phenobarbital, but this is rare. The pharmacology of barbiturates is considered in detail in Chap. 22, and dosages are shown in Table 33-6.

Primidone

Primidone (Mysoline) is similar to phenobarbital. Although it can be used as a first-line agent, it is usually reserved for patients who do not respond to phenobarbital or phenytoin. The mechanism of action of primidone is similar to that of phenobarbital and phenytoin.

Pharmacokinetics Primidone is converted in the liver to two active metabolites, phenobarbital and phenylethylmalonamide, both of which have long plasma half-lives. When plasma levels are monitored, both the parent drug and phenobarbital levels should be checked.

Adverse Effects The most common complaints are sedation, dizziness, vertigo, nausea and vomiting, diplopia, and nystagmus. Serious adverse effects of leukopenia, morbilliform rash, and systemic lupus erythematosus have been reported.

Dosage This medication is usually started in small doses, 50 to 125 mg daily at bedtime, which is then gradually increased to two or three doses of 250 mg or even 500 mg daily. Children under 8 years old should be treated with one-half of the adult dosage.

Carbamazepine

Mechanism of Action Carbamazepine (Tegretol) has similar effects to those of phenytoin. It has been demonstrated to inhibit electrically induced seizures and to suppress localized brain discharge. However, the molecular basis for these actions has not been elucidated. This drug is also used in the treatment of trigeminal neuralgia.

Pharmacokinetics Carbamazepine is rapidly absorbed following oral administration, but peak plasma concentrations are reached between 2 to 6 h due to individual patient variation. The drug is approximately 80 percent bound to plasma proteins. It is metabolized in the liver to an active metabolite which also has anticonvulsant activity. The half-life of the parent compound is 13 to 17 h and that of the metabolite is 5 to 8 h. Following further metabolism, inactive products are excreted in urine and bile.

Adverse Effects The most common adverse effects of carbamazepine are diplopia, blurred vision, dizziness, drowsiness, ataxia, nausea, and vomiting. These may decrease in severity with continued dosing and may be limited by gradually increasing dosage to attain the desired therapeutic action. Several more serious adverse effects have been reported, including aplastic anemia and other hematologic insults, jaundice, acute oliguria with hypertension, cardiovascular collapse, and skin rashes including Stevens-Johnson syndrome. Therefore, the complete blood count (CBC) and liver function should be monitored four times yearly, with closer (weekly) monitoring of the CBC during the first 2 months.

Dosage The drug is usually started at a dose of 200 mg bid to minimize side effects. Daily dose is gradually increased to 600 to 1200 mg/day (adults) or 20 to 30 mg/kg/day (children) and should be divided in two to four doses to minimize plasma level variations.

Oxazolidinediones

Trimethadione (Tridione), although no longer the agent of choice, has been used to treat petit mal seizures. The other agent in this class, **paramethadione** (Paradione), is less frequently prescribed. Due to the lack of methods to determine plasma concentration and because of toxicity potential, these agents are infrequently used. The pharmacokinetics and dosage of these agents is outlined in Table 33-6.

Adverse Effects The side effects of the oxazolidinediones include sedation and hemeralopia (blurring of vision in bright light or a glaring effect). Diplopia, vertigo, irritability, aplastic anemia, and pancytopenia also have been reported.

TABLE 33-6 Dosage, Therapeutic Concentration, and Pharmacokinetics of Some Anticonvulsants

DRUG	TRADE NAME	Usual Daily Dosage, mg ADULT	Usual Daily Dosage, mg PEDIATRIC	THERAPEUTIC PLASMA CONCENTRATION,[1] µg/mL	BIO-AVAILABILITY, %	PROTEIN BINDING, %	PLASMA HALF-LIFE, h	ELIMINATION	ACTIVE METABOLITES
Hydantoins									
Phenytoin (diphenylhydantoin)	Dilantin Diphenylan, Ditan	200–600[2]	6–8/kg[2]	10–20	80–95[1]	87–93	20–30[2]	Hepatic metabolism; 1–5% unchanged in urine	No
Mephenytoin	Mesantoin	200–600	100–400	10–20	*	*	*	Hepatic metabolism	No
Ethotoin	Peganone	1000–2000	500–1000	15–50	*	*	3–9[2]	Hepatic metabolism	No
Barbiturates and Related Drugs									
Phenobarbital	Luminal, Barbita, others	60–400	2–5/kg	10–30	80	50–60	4–120[3]	Hepatic metabolism (50–80%)[1] and renal excretion of unchanged drug (20–50%)	No
Mephobarbital	Mebaral	400–600	50–250	*	*	*	*	Hepatic metabolism	No
Metharbital	Gemonil	100–300	5–15/kg	*	*	*	*	Hepatic metabolism	No
Primidone	Mysoline	500–1500	5–20/kg	5–12[5]	*	Negligible	6–12	Hepatic metabolism	Yes
Succinimides									
Ethosuximide	Zarontin	15–30/kg	20–60/kg	40–100	100	None	≤60[3]	Hepatic metabolism; 10–20% unchanged in urine	No
Methsuximide	Celontin Kapseals	600–2400	20–60/kg	10–40	*	Negligible	≤36–45[4]	Hepatic metabolism; 1% unchanged in urine	Yes
Phensuximide	Milontin	1000–4000	Not used	*	*	Negligible	*	Hepatic metabolism	Yes

Benzodiazepines

Diazepam	Valium	5–30	0.1–1/kg	100–200 (ng/mL)	≤75	97–99	≤24–48	Hepatic metabolism; about 2% unchanged in urine	Yes
Clonazepam	Clonopin	10–15	0.1–0.2/kg	20–80 (ng/mL)	*	≤80	20–60[3]	Hepatic metabolism; 1–2% unchanged in urine	No
Chlorazepate	Tranxene	22.5–90	15–60	*	*	*	30–100	Hepatic metabolism	Yes

Oxazolidinediones

Trimethadione	Tridione	600–1800	20–60/kg	>700	*	Negligible	≤16	Hepatic metabolism; 1% unchanged in urine	Yes
Paramethadione	Paradione	900–2400	300–900	*	*	Negligible	*	Hepatic metabolism	Yes

Miscellaneous

Carbamazepine	Tegretol	400–1600	100–600	4–12	70+	70–80	10–20	Hepatic metabolism; 1–2% unchanged in urine	Yes
Valproic acid derivatives	Depakene Depakote	1000–2000	15–40/kg	40–120	*	≤90	13–21	Hepatic metabolism	No

*Not well-studied or documented.

[1]High variability.

[2]Half-life may vary manyfold between individuals (e.g., 8 to 60 h) and is dose-dependent. At higher plasma concentrations dose increases must be small.

[3]Half-life is shorter in children.

[4]Half-life of the active metabolite.

[5]Metabolized to phenobarbital, so phenobarbital levels should be monitored as well.

Source: Modified from H. Kutt and F.H. McDowell: "Neurological Diseases," in G.S. Avery (ed.): *Drug Treatment,* 2d ed., Sydney, Australia: ADIS Press (Australasia Pty Ltd., 404 Sydney Road, Balgowlah, New South Wales, 2093), 1980. Used by permission.

TABLE 33-7   Drugs Which Cause Changes in Phenytoin Plasma Concentration

INCREASE PLASMA CONCENTRATION	DECREASE PLASMA CONCENTRATION
Alcohol	Alcohol
Chloramphenicol*	Carbamazepine
Chlordiazepoxide*	?Clonazepam
Chlorpromazine	Diazepam
Cimetidine	Diazoxide*
Diazepam*	Phenobarbital
Dicoumarol*	Primidone
Disulfiram*	Tolbutamide
Halothane	Valproate sodium
Isoniazid (slow acetylators)*	
Methylphenidate*	
Phenobarbital	
Phenylbutazone*	
Primidone	
Prochlorperazine	
Sulfamethizole	
Valproate sodium	

*May cause marked changes.

Succinimides

The succinimide anticonvulsants were developed in the search for agents effective against petit mal seizures. **Ethosuximide** (Zarontin) is the agent of choice for this type of seizure. The exact mechanism of action of ethosuximide is still unknown.

Pharmacokinetics   Ethosuximide is completely absorbed from the intestines. It is not extensively bound to plasma proteins and is distributed to most body compartments. Only 10 to 20 percent of the drug is excreted unchanged in the urine; the remainder is metabolized in the liver to an inactive metabolite. The plasma half-life of ethosuximide is 30 h in children and 60 h in adults.

Adverse Effects   Gastrointestinal upset, fatigue, lethargy, headaches, and dizziness are common adverse effects. Eosinophilia, isolated blood dyscrasias, and lupus erythematosus syndrome have also been reported but are rare. Because of the gravity of these effects, a complete blood count should be done every 3 months with liver function monitored every 6 months.

Dosage and Preparations   Dosage is usually begun with 250 mg daily for children and 500 mg for adults and then increased at weekly intervals to 250 to 500 mg two or three times daily for adults. Other succinimides are **methsuximide** (Celontin) and **phensuximide** (Milontin). These agents are similar to **ethosuximide** but are usually less effective and are reserved for those patients who do not respond to ethosuximide. **Phensuximide** and **methosuximide** are also used for refractory seizure disorders.

Benzodiazepines

Clonazepam (Clonopin) is an agent which has been shown to be useful in petit mal and myoclonic seizures, while **diazepam** (Valium) has been shown to be effective when given intravenously for the treatment of status epilepticus. **Clorazepate** (Tranxene) is used in Jacksonian seizures. The benzodiazepines may lose their anticonvulsant activity with continuous dosage (tolerance). See Chap. 34 for a detailed discussion of this drug group.

Valproic Acid and Derivatives

Mechanism of Action   **Valproic acid** (sodium valproate, sodium di-*n*-propylacetate; Depakene) is useful in many types of epilepsy, but its approved indication in the United States is for simple absence seizures. Although its mechanism of action has not been fully elucidated, valproate increases CNS concentrations of the inhibitory neurotransmitter, γ-aminobutyric acid (GABA), which may account for its therapeutic effect.

Pharmacokinetics   The drug is rapidly absorbed, but peak concentrations are delayed several hours if the drug is taken with meals. Valproic acid is highly protein bound (80 to 94 percent) and is extensively metabolized with a half-life of approximately 15 h.

Adverse Effects   Although the drug has a low incidence of side effects (mostly gastrointestinal, e.g., nausea, vomiting, and anorexia), fatal hepatotoxicity has been reported. **Divalproex sodium** (Depakote), which has similar antiepileptic activity to valproic acid, causes less gastrointestinal irritation. Liver function tests should be done before starting therapy and every 2 months thereafter to monitor for hepatotoxicity, which represents a potentially fatal reaction. Caution should also be exercised when phenobarbital is used concurrently with valproate, or blood levels of phenobarbital may increase by as much as 40 percent.

Dosage   The recommended initial dose is 25 mg/kg/day, with increases of 5 to 10 mg/kg/day at 1-week intervals until seizures are controlled or side effects preclude further increases. The maximum daily dose is 60 mg/kg/day in children or 3 g in adults.

Miscellaneous Agents

Acetazolamide   The carbonic anhydrase inhibitor acetazolamide (Diamox) has been used in conjunction with other anticonvulsants in treating all types of seizures. See Chap. 39 for a detailed discussion of its pharmacology.

Ketogenic Diet

A ketogenic diet, which will result in systemic ketone buildup and metabolic acidosis, has also been used in the treatment of simple absence seizures. Results of this approach are equivocal at best, but this dietary protocol can mimic the systemic effects of acetazolamide.

NURSING PROCESS RELATED TO SEIZURE DISORDERS

Assessment

A primary nursing responsibility when a patient has an epileptic seizure is to observe the course of the seizure, as this may assist with the diagnosis. Whether the seizure is local or generalized, its duration, associated pupil changes, and occurrence of incontinence should be observed during the seizure. State of consciousness and presence of Babinski reflex following the seizure should be noted, as should the presence and type of aura before the seizure. If the patient does not regain consciousness between seizures, the physician should be notified immediately, since the patient may be in status epilepticus.

Nurses may also assist in case finding. For example, school nurses can identify students whose behavior could be indicative of epilepsy and refer them to the family physician. Since many conditions, including anoxia, drugs, diabetes, and head trauma, can cause *symptomatic epilepsy,* the nurse must also observe factors from the historical, physical, and psychologic findings that could relate to the seizure disorder. Symptomatic epilepsy is treated differently from idiopathic epilepsy; since management of the underlying disorder as well as possible use of drugs to control the seizures may be indicated.

Management

As there is a social stigma attached to epilepsy, nursing's educative role is twofold: to support public education about epilepsy and to teach patients and families about the disease. There are many misconceptions about epilepsy, such as that it causes mental retardation, that people with epilepsy must severely restrict their activities, and that it is caused by insanity.

Patients need to understand that they must continue to take medication even if seizure-free for a long period. Medication should be changed or decreased only by a prescriber and not by patients who believe they are cured. It should be emphasized that there is no medical cure for idiopathic epilepsy, and spontaneous cures are rare over 5 years of age.

The adult or adolescent patient should know the names and important effects of the drugs being taken. The nurse can assist the patient to comply with the drug regimen by making it as easy as possible to follow. For example, some of these agents, such as some forms of **phenytoin** and **phenobarbital**, have long half-lives and can be given once daily. Only Dilantin Kapseals should be used for once-daily dosing; other forms may cause toxicity. Even children can learn to take the medication by associating it with some routine activities. Although overexertion or excessive fatigue should be avoided, the patient should maintain a normal exercise and activity pattern. Patients should be instructed to wear and carry identification which indicates they have epilepsy and states the drug and dosage they are taking. During the early therapy, gastric irritation can be minimized by taking drugs with meals.

Seizure activity can be stimulated by excess fluid intake. Patients should avoid medications which can cause fluid retention (e.g., **oral contraceptives**, certain anti-inflammatory drugs such as **prednisone**). The fluid retention associated with premenstrual edema may be treated by a diuretic or adjustment in the anticonvulsant dosage. Emotional stress, fever, fatigue, and electric shock have also elicited seizures in patients on anticonvulsant therapy. A flickering light, such as that associated with a poorly functioning television, may trigger a seizure. Alcohol lowers the threshold for seizure activity, but most patients can tolerate occasional cocktails. Sudden cessation of excessive alcohol intake can also precipitate seizures.

Patients should be educated as to signs and symptoms of drug toxicity and to notify their care provider as soon as possible for follow-up. The care provider should be aware of other drugs given concomitantly with phenytoin; **cimetidine** (Tagamet), **disulfiram** (Antabuse), and **methylphenidate** (Ritalin), and other drugs listed in Table 33-7, can raise serum phenytoin levels to toxic points.

Good oral care and gum massage are important in those patients, especially children, taking phenytoin, in order to minimize the effects of hyperplasia of the gums. An oral water jet (e.g., Water Pik) may aid in gum care.

Family members should be taught what to do if a seizure occurs and what to observe as the seizure progresses. While the patient's safety should be ensured to prevent self-inflicted injuries, the patient should never be restrained. A padded tongue blade or rolled piece of cloth can be inserted between the teeth to prevent tongue biting only if this can be done without force. After the seizure, a side lying position can prevent aspiration of secretions.

In status epilepticus, the nurse should establish and maintain the airway, including suctioning of secretions to prevent aspiration. Drugs given intravenously during status epilepticus should be injected slowly (over 3 to 5 min).

Evaluation

A recently developed technique for determining the blood concentration of antiepileptic drugs requires only a finger-stick blood sample, and results are available in minutes. This test is useful not only in adjusting dosages but also can be used when there is a question of patient noncompliance to drug therapy. Failure to take the drug as prescribed is a major cause of therapeutic failure in epilepsy.

The use of blood level tests complements clinical evaluation of seizure control. Records should be maintained of the type and frequency of seizure activity.

Nystagmus and ataxia are signs of toxicity of phenytoin which the nurse should be able to identify. The drowsiness that may accompany most types of therapy will usually diminish after the first few days of drug therapy. Children who experience paradoxical excitement with phenobarbital may be very difficult for parents to handle, and a change of therapy is indicated. Since blood dyscrasias and hepatotoxicity may occur, a complete blood count and liver function tests are performed every 6 months by some clinicians.

Since phenobarbital is known to induce hepatic enzymes and some antiepileptic drugs are protein-bound in the plasma, patients require meticulous evaluation of therapeutic and toxic effects of drug therapy during periods of drug change or dosage adjustment.

CASE STUDY

The first grade teacher noted that Debbie P., age 7, had severe problems following directions and had begun to suspect that the child was mentally retarded. However, after a faculty workshop in which the school nurse practitioner had discussed organic problems which can interfere with learning, the teacher wondered if Debbie might have a problem which could be treated and referred her to the nurse.

Assessment

The school nurse practitioner examined Debbie and performed screening tests for vision, hearing, and developmental level. No physical or sensory deficit was noted, and the child seemed within normal ranges in growth and development. However, when the nurse had D.P. hyperventilate, she developed a dazed appearance, staring eyes, and immobility lasting 4 s. The nurse suspected simple absence seizures.

Management

The school nurse practitioner called Debbie's parents and recommended she be taken to her pediatrician for an examination and contacted the physician to explain the results of the assessment. After examining Debbie and securing an electroencephalogram (EEG), which showed 3-per-second wave and spike dysrhythmias synchronous over both frontal lobes upon hyperventilation, the physician diagnosed petit mal epilepsy and prescribed ethosuximide (Zarontin) 0.5 g daily.

In a second telephone contact of the parents by the nurse, arrangements for a home visit were made. Finding the parents distressed by the diagnosis, the nurse explained what epilepsy is and discussed some commonly believed myths about the disorder. The EEG was explained to the parents, who were unsure what kind of data the doctor had obtained from this test. The child's and parents' other questions were explored and answered.

The nurse stressed that while Debbie should be allowed to grow up as normally as possible, medication and regular medical supervision were required. Since the drug was in the syrup form, the nurse explained the importance of shaking the medication and secured pediatric dosing spoons to ensure accurate dosing. The parents demonstrated the administration technique correctly. They were given a list of adverse signs and symptoms that warranted contacting the physician. These included sore throat, fever, rash, uncoordination, lethargy, and increased seizure activity.

Evaluation

The teacher and parents were able to report to the nurse practitioner that no signs of seizure activity had been noted and that her school performance had improved. The physician indicated that he was satisfied with the therapeutic serum level of ethosuximide at 50 μg/mL and a normal blood count. However, 3 months later, Debbie had a grand mal seizure requiring addition of phenobarbital elixir, 30 mg daily, and additional parent education.

SPASTICITY AND MUSCLE SPASM

Spasticity is a type of increased muscle tone resulting in enhanced resistance to passive movement of a joint or extremity. Increasing force applied by the examiner is matched by increasing resistance to movement. Sometimes there may be sudden muscle relaxation after the initial resistance, which is known as the clasp-knife phenomenon. Drugs which decrease muscle tone may be used to treat spasticity or muscle spasm which may follow trauma or inflammation.

Clinical Findings

Spasticity is usually associated with muscle weakness, increased tendon reflexes, absent abdominal reflexes, clonus, extensor plantar responses, and flexor or adductor spasms. Spasticity is a prominent neurologic sign in many diseases of the central nervous system, including cerebral palsy, cerebral vascular disease, brain injuries, brain tumors, multiple sclerosis, spinal injuries, spinal cord tumors, and amyotrophic lateral sclerosis.

Spasm may also accompany many acute or chronic recurrent musculoskeletal conditions in which the pain–muscle tension–pain cycle appears. Chief among such conditions is low back pain, a very common presenting complaint affecting 80 to 90 percent of all individuals at some time in their lives. Accounting for industrial absenteeism second only to the common cold, impairment of the back and spine is the most frequent chronic cause of disability.

The nurse needs a comprehensive approach to patients with spasticity or spasm. These patients require a thorough history and physical as well as time-consuming patient education, which is critical to the success of the therapy.

Clinical Pharmacology and Therapeutics

Marked spasticity may interfere with such rehabilitative measures as therapeutic exercise programs, utilization of braces, transfer maneuvers, posture and equilibrium, ambulation, and activities of daily living. Furthermore, spasticity may lead directly or indirectly to muscle and soft tissue contracture, pain, and psychologic problems. Drug therapy, by reducing muscle tone, may alleviate some of these problems.

Although spasticity presents many problems for the patient, it may also serve a useful purpose. This is seen in the increased tone found in the antigravity muscles in weak but spastic lower extremities. For example, it is to the advantage of a hemiplegic or paraplegic to ambulate with the lower limbs in spastic extension rather than flexed or flaccid. If spasticity is reduced too much, these patients may be unable to walk at all. However, it might be useful to reduce the spasticity sufficiently to enable the patient to sit in a wheelchair in comfort.

Drug treatment can help prevent contractures and grotesque posturing by reducing muscle tone and permitting more effective physical therapy. Without therapy the spastic paraplegic often becomes emaciated, develops pressure sores and contractures of the hip and knee joints, and may have painful muscle spasms day and night.

The proper approach to drug therapy is to set functional goals which the patient might be able to accomplish if spasticity were reduced and to continue medications only if these goals are attained. The goal should never be to reduce muscle tone just for the sake of decreasing spasticity. For patients with spasticity, the major criterion of drug effectiveness should be, "What can the patient do now that was impossible before?"

For the treatment of the acute phase of low back pain and similar mechanical musculoskeletal disorders, the major management emphasis is to provide rest and relaxation of the area involved. Bed rest is the chief treatment modality and should be encouraged for 2 to 7 days after an acute episode. Adjunctive therapies include heat applications, hot tubs, linaments, and a firm mattress. Analgesia may be necessary, usually consisting of intensive **aspirin** or **acetaminophen** therapy or use of a **nonsteroidal anti-inflammatory agent**. No analgesic or anti-inflammatory medication is clearly superior to aspirin for the relief of low back pain except narcotics, which have little role in low back pain and should be confined to the first 24 to 48 h in patients with severe pain. Muscle relaxants remain a controversial remedy, since **diazepam** (Valium), the most commonly prescribed muscle relaxant, has not been proved superior to aspirin for low back pain. Although low back pain is common in pregnancy, muscle relaxants are contraindicated in this condition.

Mechanisms of Action of Skeletal Muscle Relaxants

Skeletal muscle tone can be reduced by the administration of drugs that interfere at some point in the transmission of nerve impulses from the cerebral cortex to the muscle (Fig. 33-4). Interference with neuromuscular transmission can be accomplished by (1) affecting impulse traffic within the CNS; (2) blocking transmission at the neuromuscular junction; or (3) interfering with the contractile process within the muscle itself. Drugs that block transmission at the neuromuscular junction, such as **succinylcholine** or **d-tubocurare** are too potent for chronic use in treatment of spasticity (see Chaps. 16 and 47 regarding use of these drugs in surgery). However, drugs that interfere with CNS pathways, such as **diazepam** or **methocarbamol**, and drugs that affect the muscle directly, such as **dantrolene**, are useful (Table 33-8).

Centrally Acting Muscle Relaxants

Agents which affect impulse transmission in the CNS can be divided into two groups based on their primary site of action. The group which has a greater effect on the neurons in the brain than on those in the spinal cord includes **diazepam** (Valium), **meprobamate** (Miltown, Equanil), **carisoprodol** (Soma), and **metaxalone** (Skelaxin). A second group of centrally acting muscle relaxants block spinal interneurons as well as neurons in the brain. These are the mephenesin derivatives, including **methocarbamol** (Robaxin), **chlorzoxazone** (Paraflex), and **chlorphenesin** (Maolate). **Cyclobenzaprine** (Flexeril), **orphenadrine citrate** (Norflex, others), and **baclofen** (Lioresal) are thought to be centrally acting, but the precise site is unknown. Several of these agents are combined with analgesics as fixed dose preparations (Table 33-9).

Diazepam and Meprobamate
The main use of **diazepam** (Valium) and **meprobamate** (Miltown, Equanil) are as anx-

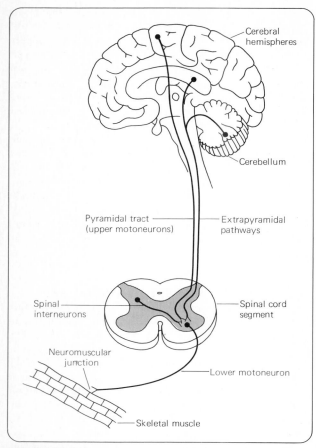

FIGURE 33-4

Pathways Involved in Skeletal Muscle Control. Skeletal muscle relaxants work in the brain, in the spinal cord segment, or at skeletal muscle. Neuromuscular blockers such as tubocurarane and succinylcholine produce blockade at the neuromuscular junction (see Chaps. 16 and 47).

iolytics, so the pharmacology of these agents is discussed in detail in Chap. 34. Diazepam is also the most frequently prescribed drug for the treatment of spasticity and muscle spasms associated with sprains, arthritis, and other musculoskeletal disorders. A usual starting dose of diazepam for a healthy young adult is 5 mg twice daily, increasing the dose by 5 mg every 3 to 4 days until the symptoms are alleviated or sedation occurs. The maximum tolerated intake of diazepam varies considerably, but the elderly are quite sensitive to this drug. Dosage for elderly adults is started at 2 mg tid, and dosage increments should be initiated no more frequently than every 2 weeks. The dosage and time course of action (onset, peak, half-life) of diazepam and other skeletal muscle relaxants are shown in Table 33-8.

Both meprobamate and diazepam produce drowsiness as the major factor limiting dosage. Meprobamate has other adverse effects, may be less effective, has greater dependence potential, and may affect the metabolism of other drugs by inducing hepatic microsomal enzymes. For these reasons many prescribers avoid meprobamate.

Carisoprodol and Metaxalone The precise mechanism of action of these two chemically unrelated drugs is unknown; skeletal muscle relaxation may be the result of generalized CNS depression. **Carisoprodol** (Soma, Rela, Soprodol) is chemically related to meprobamate and appears in high concentrations in breast milk. Both drugs are metabolized in the liver to inactive metabolites which are excreted in the urine and are used with extreme caution in those with hepatic impairment. **Metaxalone** (Skeaxin) causes a false positive in reducing tests for glucosuria (e.g., Clinitest). Adverse effects of both agents include dizziness, drowsiness, nausea, vomiting, and headaches. Neither drug should be taken concurrently with other CNS depressants or alcohol. Dosage and pharmacokinetics of both drugs are outlined in Table 33-8.

Mephenesin Derivatives The mephenesin derivatives include **methocarbamol** (Robaxin, Mebaxin, others), **chlorzoxazone** (Paraflex), and **chlorphenesin** (Maolate). These drugs are primarliy used as adjuncts to rest, heat, and physical therapy for the relief of muscle spasm and pain in skeletal muscle secondary to sprain, trauma, fibrositis, myositis, and bursitis. These drugs selectively block internuncial neurons in the spinal cord. Their muscle relaxation may also be due to general central nervous system depression.

Pharmacokinetics All of these drugs are rapidly absorbed and are converted in the liver to inactive metabolites. These drugs have similar time courses of activity, although the onset and peak activity of chlorzoxazone may be slightly slower (see Table 33-8).

Adverse effects Drowsiness, dizziness, gastrointestinal upset, skin rash, and anaphylactic reactions can occur with these drugs in oral doses. These drugs should not be taken concurrent with alcohol or other CNS depressants. **Methocarbamol** (Robaxin) may also cause fainting, hypotension, bradycardia, blurred vision, pain, or thrombophlebitis at the injection site, and fever when given parenterally. **Clorzoxazone** has been associated with liver damage in a few cases.

Dosage and administration As with other muscle relaxants, dosage is generally begun at the low end of the dosage range and gradually increased until symptoms are controlled. However, some prescribers used large initial doses in acute conditions. As improvement occurs, the dosage is sometimes decreased to a maintenance level which is about one-half to two-thirds peak dosage. These drugs should be taken with meals if they cause gastrointestinal irritation. **Chlorzoxazone,** the only oral agent for use in children, is given in doses of 125 to 500 mg three to four times daily, depending upon the age and weight of the child. **Methocarbamol** is approved for parenteral use in tetanus in

TABLE 33-8 Skeletal Muscle Relaxants

DRUG	TRADE NAME	AVERAGE DAILY ADULT DOSAGE RANGE, mg	ONSET/PEAK, h	HALF-LIFE, h
Centrally Acting at Brain or Brain Stem				
Diazepam	Valium, Val Release	6–40	0.5–1/2–3	20–50*
Meprobamate	Equanil, Miltown	1200–2400	1/1–3	6–17†
Carisoprodol	Soma, Rela, Soprodol	1050–1400	0.5/4‡	8
Metaxalone	Skelaxin	2400–3200	1/2‡	2–3
Centrally Acting at Spinal Cord				
Chlorphenesin	Maolate	1600–3200	0.5/1–3	3.5
Chlorzoxazone	Paraflex	1000–3000 (Children: 375–2000)	1/3–4	1
Methocarbamol	Robaxin	4000–8000	0.5/2	2
Centrally Acting—Site Unknown				
Cyclobenzaprine	Flexeril	20–60	1/12–24§	24–72
Orphenadrine citrate	Norflex, Marflex, Flexoject, others	200 (PO) 120 (IV or IM)	1/2‡	14*
Baclofen	Lioresal	40–80	1/2	2–4
Direct-Acting at Muscle				
Dantrolene sodium	Dantrium	50–400¶	2–3/4–6	9¶
Quinine sulfate	Quinine, others	200–300(hs)	0.5/2–6§	1–3

*For parent drug. Active metabolites are produced.
†Increases two to four times with multiple doses.
‡Duration of action is 4–6 h.
§Approximate duration of action.
¶IV doses may be higher, especially for prevention or treatment of malignant hyperthermia. IV half-life 5 h.

doses of 15 mg/kg q7h for children and 1 to 2 g every 6 h for adults. **Methocarbamol** may be given intravenously or intramuscularly, but subcutaneous injection should be avoided.

Cyclobenzaprine and Orphenadrine The common characteristics of these two skeletal muscle relaxants are that both are centrally acting and both produce anticholinergic adverse effects. **Cyclobenzaprine** (Flexeril) is structurally related to the tricyclic antidepressants (see Chap. 34) and has a similar adverse effect profile, such as sedation, potent anticholinergic effects, and norepinephrine potentiation. The mechanism of skeletal muscle relaxation is unknown for these agents.

Pharmacokinetics The half-life of these agents is shown in Table 33-8. **Cyclobenzaprine** is metabolized to inactive conjugates which are eliminated in the urine. The two active metabolites of **orphenadrine** (Norflex), with half-lives of 2 to 25 h, are eliminated in the urine and feces.

Adverse effects Dry mouth, tachycardia, palpitations, urinary hesitancy, blurred vision, dizziness, constipation, and mental confusion (especially in the elderly) are anticholinergic effects of these drugs. They should be used with caution in cardiac decompensation, narrow-angle glaucoma, arrhythmias, and coronary insufficiency. **Cyclobenzaprine** probably has the same drug interactions as discussed in Chap. 34 for the tricyclic antidepressants. Dosage of these agents is shown in Table 33-8.

Baclofen γ-Aminobutyric acid (GABA) is a neurotransmitter in the brain and spinal cord which may be important in the regulation of muscle tone. Baclofen (Lioresal) is a derivative of GABA used in the treatment of spasticity, although it is not known whether it acts like GABA or has another unrelated mechanism of action. However, its muscle relaxant effect is apparently superior to the other drugs presently available for use in spinal cord injury and multiple sclerosis. Stroke patients tolerate the drug poorly.

Pharmacokinetics Baclofen is rapidly absorbed, although absorption is reduced with increasing doses. It is primarily excreted by the kidneys in unchanged form, and dosage reduction may be necessary in those with renal impairment.

Adverse effects   Baclofen is contraindicated in persons with seizure disorders since it produces a deterioration of the electroencephalographic tracing in epileptic subjects and has produced seizures in others. Some other side effects have been sedation, nausea, vomiting, muscle hypotonia (in overdose), diarrhea, vertigo, fecal or urinary urgency, and mental confusion.

Dosage   Therapy with baclofen is usually started by giving 5 mg tid during the first 2 days and then increased over 1 to 2 weeks to about 60 mg daily in divided doses. Abrupt withdrawal can result in hallucinations or psychosis.

Direct-Acting Skeletal Muscle Relaxants

Two skeletal muscle relaxants, quinine and **dantrolene** (Dantrium), act directly on the muscle. **Quinine** (Quide, others) and **quinine combined with aminophylline** (Quinite) are used in the treatment of nocturnal recumbency leg cramps and "restless leg syndrome," including those associated with arteriosclerosis, diabetes, arthritis, varicose veins, and thrombophlebitis. Quinine is further discussed as an antimalarial drug in Chap. 29; dosages are shown in Tables 33-8 and 33-9.

Dantrolene   Dantrolene (Dantrium) is recommended for the treatment of spasticity resulting from stroke, spinal injuries, multiple sclerosis, or cerebral palsy. It is used in the prevention and treatment of malignant hyperthermia. The action of dantrolene is confined to the contractile mechanism of skeletal muscle and it does not affect the brain or spinal cord. It appears to cause muscle relaxation by dissociating the excitation-contraction coupling, probably by interfering with the release of calcium from the sarcoplasmic reticulum.

Pharmacokinetics   Peak blood levels are obtained 4 to 6 h after a single dose. Dantrolene is highly bound to plasma albumin and is metabolized by hepatic microsomal enzymes to two inactive metabolites, which are eliminated in the urine with a small amount of the parent drug. Beneficial effects of dantrolene may not become apparent for a week or more after institution of therapy.

Adverse effects   The most common side effects of dantrolene is muscle weakness, which rarely may result in slurring of speech, drooling, and enuresis. Other common side effects are drowsiness, dizziness, lightheadedness, diarrhea, nausea, malaise, and fatigue. These side effects are usually transient, lasting up to 4 days after the initiation of therapy, and are generally related to the rate of increase in dosage and total daily dose. Severe weakness or diarrhea may necessitate decreasing the dosage or discontinuing the drug. If diarrhea recurs after reinstitution of dantrolene at a lower dose, the drug probably should be discontinued.

Abnormal liver function tests have occurred in patients on dantrolene, and these should be monitored during therapy. Recently there have been reports of hepatitis from dantrolene, resulting in fatality in some cases.

Dantrolene should be used with caution in patients with severely impaired pulmonary function (particularly those with obstructive pulmonary disease) or preexisting liver disease. Dantrolene may cause photosensitivity reactions, so patients should be warned against excessive exposure to sunlight.

Dosage and administration   The starting dose is 25 mg twice a day, which is increased weekly by increments of 50 to 100 mg/day to a maximal dose of 400 mg daily, given in four divided doses. For children, the recommended starting dose of 1 mg/kg twice a day is gradually increased to a maximum of 3 mg/kg four times a day but not to exceed 400 mg daily.

The drug tends to induce a generalized muscle weakness at high doses that can be detrimental to functional improvement. The desirability of long-term dantrolene therapy in ambulatory patients depends on a balance between the weakness and other side effects caused by the drug and the functional improvement obtained from its use. Long-term

TABLE 33-9   Combination Skeletal Muscle Relaxants

TRADE NAME(S)	SKELETAL MUSCLE RELAXANT	ANALGESIC, OTHER	USUAL DOSAGE
Parafon Forte, Blanex, Flexaphen, others	Chlorzoxazone, 250 mg	Acetaminophen, 300 mg	2 qid
Norgesic	Orphenadrine, 25 mg	Aspirin, 385 mg Caffeine, 30 mg	1–2 tid to qid
Soma Compound, Soprodol Compound	Carisoprodol, 400 mg	Aspirin, 325 mg	2 qid
Robaxisal	Methocarbamol, 400 mg	Aspirin, 325 mg	2 qid
Quinite	Quinine, 260 mg	Aminophylline, 195 mg	1 hs and/or with evening meal

administration of dantrolene is considered justifiable if the drug produces a significant reduction in pain and/or disabling spasticity or a reduction in the intensity of nursing care needed, or if annoying manifestations of spasticity are eliminated as judged by the patient.

NURSING PROCESS RELATED TO SPASTICITY

Assessment

The nurse is often in a key position to assess factors that will determine rehabilitation goals and selection of appropriate drug therapy. Since skeletal muscle relaxants are sedating, these agents may be inadvisable for patients with depressed consciousness or who are taking other CNS depressants. Patients with concurrent anxiety and spasm may benefit from **diazepam** (Valium). Glaucoma, chronic lung disease, prostatism, and cardiac disease require extra caution with the use of **cyclobenzaprine** (Flexeril) or **orphenadrine** (Norflex) due to their anticholinergic effects. Hepatic disease is an important consideration with all skeletal muscle relaxant drugs except **baclofen** (Lioresal); with this drug adequate renal function is a crucial consideration. Pregnancy and lactation contraindicate all skeletal muscle relaxants.

Management

The information in Table 33-8 can be used by the nurse to plan drug administration schedules so that peak drug effects will coincide with physical therapy sessions or other times when maximal drug effects are needed. Because these drugs are often initiated at low doses and titrated up to maximal benefit, the nurse must monitor for both therapeutic and adverse effects. After the drug plasma levels approximate steady state (i.e., after four or five half-lives), the nurse may request an order for an increase in dosage if (1) the patient is still experiencing pain and/or dysfunction from spasticity, (2) the maximal daily dosage has not been attained, and (3) the patient has not developed dangerous or unacceptable adverse effects. If gastric irritation occurs, these drugs should be taken with food. Because of the sedative quality of skeletal muscle relaxants, the patient should be cautioned about the operation of motor vehicles and dangerous machinery. Alcohol and other CNS depressants should be avoided due to additive effects with skeletal muscle relaxants.

In lifelong pain or spastic conditions the chief role of the care provider is to educate the patient regarding the condition and to assist in the management of chronicity as a lifestyle. Patients should be counseled that medications are adjuvants to other treatments, particularly exercise, posture control, good body mechanics, and physical therapy. Nerve stimulators, ultrasound, massage and manipulation, surgery, and acupuncture are effective in some cases.

To prevent lower back pain, exercises which will strengthen abdominal, gluteal, and back muscles are advised. Exercises like pelvic tilt, knee-to-chest, and sit-ups may be helpful. It should be stressed to the patient that these exercises are for the *prevention* of lower back pain, not for treatment of acute episodes. Mild warm-up exercises prior to vigorous physical exercise are advisable.

Drug-seeking behavior often presents itself to the practitioner, especially if the patient has perceived that satisfactory medical care means obtaining a prescription. In dealing with the complex needs of a patient with spasticity and/or pain with spasm, clinicians need to clarify such expectations and clearly relate their own. Because many patients are financially unable to stay at home in bed and fear job loss if their employers learn of their medical problem, requests for analgesia are frequent and may, indeed, be warranted to provide quick relief while maintaining activity.

Evaluation

If a particular drug agent does not help the patient (as judged by whether the patient's physical functioning or quality of life improves), or if side effects warrant discontinuance, withdrawal of the drug should be done slowly since many of these agents can cause hallucinations, seizures, tremor, abdominal and muscle cramps, nausea, vomiting, sweating, and other withdrawal symptoms if stopped abruptly. If, however, drug therapy helps the patient achieve maximal function with minimal or no adverse effects, continuance may be indicated. Ongoing surveillance of liver function, cognitive status, mood changes, paresthesias, visual complaints, hypotension (including determination of postural changes in blood pressure) and gastrointestinal complaints should continue as well.

CEREBRAL EDEMA

Cerebral edema (increased fluid content within the brain parenchyma) can result from a variety of assaults to the brain, including anoxia, hypercapnia, fluid-electrolyte imbalance, hypertension, hemorrhage, necrosis, and trauma. After the cranial sutures close in childhood, cerebral edema will cause increased intracranial pressure ($\uparrow$ICP) because the skull is nonexpansible. The increased ICP can result in pressure on vital structures and herniation of the brain over the tentorium or through the foramen magnum, ultimately resulting in death. Because even moderately increased ICP causes impairment of the brain's mechanisms for autoregulating blood flow, anoxia, and hypercapnia (which results in further cerebral edema), it is crucial that cerebral edema be treated at its onset.

Clinical Findings

Increases in intracranial pressure from cerebral edema cause decreases in level of consciousness, beginning with flattened affect and progressing to somnolence, stupor, and coma. Pupil changes in size, equality, and reactivity occur, with fixed and dilated pupils being an ominous sign. Papilledema (swelling of the head of the optic nerve seen on fundoscopic examination), headache, vomiting, elevated temperature, and seizures are early signs, while muscle rigidity, decorticate and decerebrate posturing, low blood pressure, and bradycardia are late signs of increased ICP.

Clinical Pharmacology and Therapeutics

The cause of the increased ICP must be identified and treated. Meticulous attention is given to adequate respiratory function, limitation of fluid intake (usually output plus 500 mL daily), and sound nutritional support, since acidosis, hypoxia, hypervolemia and malnutrition can further elevate intracranial pressure. If seizures are present, the anticonvulsant **phenytoin** (Dilantin) usually is administered. Cerebral edema and increased ICP are treated with osmotic diuretics, **dexamethasone** (Decadron), and **pentobarbital** (Nembutal). Surgical decompression and cerebral spinal fluid evacuation may also be used.

Osmotic Diuretics

Mannitol (Osmitrol) decreases cerebral edema by elevating the osmolarity of the plasma, which draws water from the extracellular spaces of the brain. A total dose of 1.5 to 2 g/kg is infused intravenously over 30 to 60 min as a 15 to 25% solution. Intracranial pressure should begin to decline within 15 min of the initiation of the infusion. Mannitol can cause fluid and electrolyte imbalance, fluid overload with congestive heart failure, and osmotic nephrosis. A *rebound* of intracranial pressure above pretreatment levels may occur when the mannitol is discontinued.

Other osmotic diuretics which are occasionally used in cerebral edema are intravenous **urea** (Ureaphil) and oral 50 to 75% **glycerin** solutions (Glyrol, Osmoglyn) in doses of 1.5 g/kg/24 h in three doses. Glycerin is metabolized by the brain and may have beneficial metabolic, as well as osmotic, effects. With urea it is necessary to document adequate renal and hepatic function prior to administration and to avoid extravasation. Glycerin (also called **glycerol**) can cause hyperosmolar nonketotic coma and is used with extreme caution in diabetics. See Chap. 39 for more complete discussion of osmotic diuretics, since they are also used to reduce ocular pressure in acute glaucoma.

The loop diuretic **ethacrynic acid** (Edecrin; see Chap. 23) is under investigation for use in cerebral edema. Research shows that it decreases astroglial swelling.

Dexamethasone

Dexamethasone (Decadron) is commonly used to reduce cerebral edema. An initial intravenous dose of 10 mg is fol-lowed by 2 to 4 mg q4–6h until maximum response is noted or as long as edema persists. Children's dosages should approximate 0.2 mg/kg in divided doses over 24 h. The pharmacology and clinical use of dexamethasone and other corticosteroids is presented in Chap. 35.

Pentobarbital-Induced Coma

Recent clinical studies show that pentobarbital (Nembutal) will reduce increased ICP even in cases refractory to other drugs and evacuation of cerebral spinal fluid. It may even exert a protective effect on the brain against the complications of increased ICP. An intravenous loading dose of 3 to 5 mg/kg is given, followed by a continuous infusion of 1 to 3 mg/kg hourly. During therapy the patient will remain in a drug-induced coma, so direct measurement of intracranial pressure is generally used to monitor therapy; the goal is to keep pressure below 15 or 20 mmHg (normal pressure in the reclining position is 0 to 15 mmHg). Serum levels of 2.5 to 3.5 mg/dL are considered effective. The pharmacology of parenteral pentobarbital is covered in Chap. 47, since it is also used as a general anesthetic for surgery.

NURSING PROCESS RELATED TO CEREBRAL EDEMA

Assessment

Small changes in neurologic signs can herald the onset of increased ICP, so clinical assessment of neurologic status is an important nursing function. Even minor deterioration in neurologic signs should be reported to the physician for patients with cerebral hemorrhage, head trauma, stroke, brain tumor, or any other condition at risk for the development of cerebral edema.

Prior to administering mannitol the nurse should analyze the patient's serum chemistry reports for electrolyte balance (especially normal serum sodium), determine the patient's weight, and assess intake and output to establish that cardiopulmonary and renal function are adequate. Diabetes, peptic ulcer, infection, renal disease, and hypertension require cautious use of **dexamethasone**. The nurse should question family members about whether the patient has had any hypersensitivity reaction to barbiturates, if **pentobarbital**-induced coma is considered.

Management

Positioning and movement can affect intracranial pressure. Unless it is otherwise ordered, the patient should be positioned in the supine or lateral position with the head of the bed elevated 30°. The prone position, neck flexion, severe hip flexion, abrupt movements, and high Fowler's position (90° sitting upright) should be avoided. Adequate respiratory function must be maintained; patients on ventilators are often hyperventilated to decrease Pa_{CO_2}, since high levels promote cerebral vasodilation and increase cerebral edema.

When drugs such as antibiotics are given by IV piggyback to the patient with cerebral edema, **dextrose solutions**, such as D_5W, should not be used, since free water is liberated when the glucose is metabolized. Balanced salt or normal saline solutions are indicated instead. Parenteral nutrition is required for the comatose patient; adequate protein intake is particularly important for the patient receiving corticosteroids like **dexamethasone** due to their catabolic effects.

Evaluation

CNS depressant drugs are to be avoided in those with increased ICP as they obscure neurologic signs. If severe pain exists, small doses of **codeine** are sometimes prescribed. If direct monitoring of intracranial pressure is instituted, the nurse should immediately report to the physician if intracranial pressure does not decline within 15 min of the initiation of a mannitol infusion. Weight gain or poor urine output after **mannitol** indicates cardiac decompensation or renal impairment. When mannitol therapy is discontinued, the nurse should observe for rebound increased ICP to above pretreatment levels or deterioration of neurologic status. Hyponatremia or dehydration can result from mannitol infusions, so serum sodium and skin turgor should be evaluated regularly. It is advised that the patient have an indwelling urinary catheter during mannitol therapy.

Since dexamethasone (Decadron) suppresses immune function and causes glucose intolerance, patients should be monitored for signs of infection, hyperglycemia, and glucosuria. The nurse should also observe for increased blood pressure, gastric distress, blood in vomitus or nasogastric aspirant, occult blood in the stool, and adequate urine output. Dexamethasone should be switched to oral dosage as soon as possible and the dosage tapered gradually to minimize adrenal suppression and to avoid adrenal insufficiency.

Pentobarbital-induced coma is virtually a form of long-term general anesthesia. Monitoring of cardiac, respiratory, and renal status, as well as neurologic signs and intracranial pressure, is constant and intensive. The nurse must be able to accurately interpret the wave forms on the intracranial pressure monitor. Only the most well equipped units with well-trained and sufficiently numerous nursing staff should attempt this type of therapy.

MIGRAINE HEADACHE

Migraine is a type of vascular headache in which the pain is usually unilateral and throbbing in nature and is generally associated with anorexia, nausea, and, sometimes, vomiting. Migraine is twice as common in women as in men. In some patients the headaches are preceded by sensory, motor, and mood abnormalities. These *prodromal symptoms* have been

attributed to intracranial vasoconstriction which produces ischemia in certain regions of the brain. The migraine headache is thought to be due to dilation of the extracranial arteries. It has also been noted that *serotonin* levels are elevated during the preheadache phase of a migraine and decline during the actual attack.

Clinical Pharmacology and Therapeutics

Some patients do not require pharmacologic treatment for migraines after they are reassured as to the nature of the disorder. Avoidance of certain foods or activities, use of a contraceptive method other than oral estrogens, biofeedback, psychotherapy, or new contact lenses or glasses are effective for others. The pharmacotherapy of migraine headache can be divided into agents effective for the acute attack and those intended for prophylaxis (Table 33-10).

Acute Migraine Treatment

Ergotamine Tartrate   If given at the onset of the migraine, ergotamine tartrate (Gynergen, Ergomar, Ergostat) is the drug of choice for acute migraine headache. It is also used to abort cluster headaches.

Mechanism of action   Ergotamine is an α-adrenergic blocking agent which directly stimulates the muscles of extracranial and intracranial blood vessels, producing vasoconstriction. It also has serotonin antagonist properties.

Pharmacokinetics   Ergotamine is poorly absorbed orally, although caffeine increases the rate and extent of absorption. Sublingual absorption is dependent on the pH of the mouth. Ergotamine is metabolized in the liver and excreted in the bile.

Adverse effects   The side effects of ergotamine include anorexia, nausea, vomiting, diarrhea, paresthesia, muscle aches, angina pectoris, and occasionally, ischemia of the extremities. Ergotamine therapy is contraindicated in patients with occlusive arterial disease, severe pruritis, and severe liver disease, and in pregnancy. It should be used with extreme caution in hypertensive patients.

Dosage   Ergotamine may be administered orally, sublingually, rectally, and by aerosol inhalation. Ergotamine is commonly administered by the sublingual route with an initial dose of 2 mg followed by 2 mg every 30 to 60 min until headache is relieved or a total of 6 mg/24 h has been administered. Oral and rectal preparations of **ergotamine with caffeine** (Cafergot, others) are used in doses of 1 to 2 mg (one or two tablets or suppositories) every 15 min to 1 h. The aerosol form (Medihaler ergotamine) dosage begins with one inhalation which may be repeated every 5 min, but no more than six doses should be used in 24 h.

Other Agents for Acute Treatment   **Dihydroergotamine mesylate** (D.H.E. 45) is similar to ergotamine, but must be given parenterally. Its onset is in 15 to 30 min, and it persists for 3 to 4 h. Dosage of 1 mg IM may be repeated hourly

TABLE 33-10 Drugs Used to Treat Migraine

DRUG	TRADE NAME	DOSAGE FORM / ROUTE	USUAL DOSAGE	MAXIMUM DOSAGE*
		Acute Treatment		
Ergotamine tartrate	Gynergan	Tablet	2–6 tablets / attack	10 tablets / week
	Ergomar, Ergostat	Sublingual tablet	1 tablet / 30 min	3 tablets / 24 h, 5 tablets / week
	Medihaler Ergotamine	Aerosol inhalant	1 inhalation / 5 min	6 inhalations / 24 h
Dihydroergotamine mesylate	D.H.E. 45	IM IV	1 mg; repeat q1h 2 mg	3 mg / attack 6 mg / week
Ergotamine tartrate / caffeine	Cafergot, Ercaf, others	Tablet, suppository	2 at onset, repeat in 1 h	6–10 / week
Promethazine	Phenergan	Tablet	50 mg / attack	
Codeine		Tablet	30 mg / attack	
Meperidine	Demerol	IM	50 mg / attack	
		Prophylaxis		
Methysergide maleate	Sansert	Tablet	2 mg tid to qid	5 months maximum†
Propranolol	Inderal	Tablet	40 mg tid	
Amitriptyline	Elavil	Tablet	30 mg / day	
Hydrochlorothiazide	Hydrodiuril, others	Tablet	50 mg / day	
Ergot / atropine / phenobarbital	Bellergal	Tablet	One bid or tid	3–6 weeks
Diazepam	Valium	Tablets	20–40 mg / day	

*Relates to ergot preparations only.

†If therapy continues longer than 4 to 5 months, patients should have a drug-free month or two every 6 months.

until the attack subsides up to a total of 3 mg. Intravenous dosage of up to 2 mg (maximum 6 mg/week) is used for speedier onset of action. Severe, protacted migraine unresponsive to other drugs may respond to corticosteroids (e.g., **hydrocortisone, prednisone**) which reduce periarterial inflammation. **Promethazine** (Phenergan) 50 mg PO is useful in controlling nausea and inducing sleep, which terminates attacks in some people. Once the headache is established (after 30 min), **codeine sulfate** or **meperidine** (Demerol) may be needed to terminate the pain.

Prophylaxis of Migraine

Methysergide Maleate Methysergide maleate (Sansert) is used on a prophylactic basis to reduce the frequency and severity of migraine headaches. Protective effects require 1 to 2 days to develop.

Mechanism of action Methysergide blocks serotonin receptor sites. Serotonin is a vasoactive chemical and has

been postulated by some investigators to be involved in the vascular changes during migraine headache.

Adverse effects Side effects include edema, numbness and paresthesia of the extremities, cramps, abdominal pain, and depression. Rarely, fibrosis of the retroperitoneal, pulmonary, and cardiac tissues may develop during long-term therapy with methysergide, resulting in severe morbidity, including kidney failure. For this reason methysergide is recommended only in severe cases of migraine when the patient can be kept under close supervision to detect any evidence of fibrosis. Intravenous pyelograms should be obtained yearly to detect any sign of retroperitoneal fibrosis such as ureteral obstruction and hydronephrosis. Methysergide is given for 6 months followed by 2 months off the drug before resuming therapy in an effort to avoid the fibrotic complications.

Dosage The usual daily dose of methysergide is 2 to 6 mg orally. Dose should be tapered by 2 mg/week when discontinuing or approaching the "drug holiday" for this agent, so that precipitation of migraine status can be avoided.

Other Agents for Prophylaxis   Many other drugs have been tried as antimigraine agents in an effort to reduce both frequency and severity of these episodes. **Amitriptyline** (Elavil) is almost as effective as methysergide maleate, but does not have the specter of retroperitoneal fibrosis associated with its use. It is dosed initially at 50 mg daily in divided doses and may be increased to 25 mg tid if the patient doesn't respond to the lower dosage. Patients seem to either respond very well to this drug or not at all, so continued dosing in a nonresponder is fruitless (for further details on amitriptyline, see Chap. 34).

Propranolol (Inderal) may also be of benefit in migraine prophylaxis, but primarily reduces the severity and frequency of the headache rather than rendering patients headache-free. Dosage is quite variable, but therapy is usually initiated with 40 to 80 mg daily in two or three divided doses, and is rapidly titrated to the maximum range of 120 to 320 mg/day (further information on propranolol can be found in Chap. 14).

Many other drugs are currently being tested in migraine prophylaxis. These include calcium channel blockers (e.g., **verapamil**; see Chap. 43), **flunarizine**, **pizotyline**, **lisuride**, and oral **dihydroergotamine**.

In women whose migraine attacks are related to menstruation, diuretics [e.g., **hydrochlorothiazide** (Hydrodiuril) 50 mg daily] given for a few days prior to the menstrual period may decrease the frequency of headaches. Since anxiety and emotional stress may also precipitate migraine, administration of the antianxiety agents, e.g., diazepam (Valium), may be helpful. A combination of **ergotamine**, 0.3 mg, **belladonna**, 0.1 mg, and **phenobarbital**, 20 mg (Bellergal) two or three times daily for a few weeks has proved effective for some patients.

NURSING PROCESS RELATED TO MIGRAINE

Assessment

Due to the many functional and organic causes for headaches, a thorough assessment including history and physical examination should be done. Family history and personality factors are also assessed, as there is a genetic factor in the etiology of migraine. Adults with migraine headaches frequently show characteristic personality patterns (rigid, perfectionistic, and ambitious). A description of the nature of the migraine headache, precipitating factors, and prodrome should be elicited. The nurse may suggest that the patient keep a daily events chart looking for a possible stress-relief

pattern that may be associated with onset and amelioration of symptoms.

Management

Sometimes effective in aborting the acute migraine attack is the administration of **ergotamine** during the prodromal phase. Relaxation in a warm bath followed by bed rest in a quiet, darkened room may also help avert the attack.

Due to poor absorption and the difficulty estimating the amount of the drug remaining when the patient vomits, the oral route is less desirable for **ergotamine** administration during the acute attack. Patients should be taught to keep a record of the medication taken during an attack so that the recommended maximum cumulative dosages are not exceeded. The dangers associated with therapy should be thoroughly explained to ensure informed consent and careful compliance.

If the attack has persisted for 2 h before the **ergotamine** is taken, the medication will usually be ineffective, so patients should be told to take the medication as soon as they feel an attack beginning. Until the drug relieves the migraine, the patient should rest in a chair. Once the headache is relieved, at least 2 h of bed rest in a quiet, darkened room without food or drink will promote the relaxation needed to prevent another attack from occurring immediately.

Patients on long-term prophylactic therapy require continued medical follow-up. All those on any ergot derivatives should be told to report nontransient claudication or coldness of the extremities as well as Raynaud's symptoms, while those on **methysergide** are instructed to report promptly dysuria or back or chest pain. Since migraine symptoms may be stress-related, the nurse can educate the patient as to relaxation techniques, biofeedback therapy, and modifications in lifestyle.

Evaluation

The frequency, duration, and severity of migraine will establish the therapeutic effectiveness of the drug. Detection of side effects before permanent damage occurs requires ongoing follow-up, specifically directed at the known adverse effects.

ATTENTION DEFICIT DISORDER (HYPERKINETIC SYNDROME)

Attention deficit disorder (ADD), also termed minimal brain dysfunction (MBD), is a poorly defined disorder in children which may be characterized by involuntary persistent overactivity, learning difficulties, short attention span, and impaired powers of concentration. Attention deficit disorder is an overly diagnosed and treated disease, and psychologic therapy may be more effective than drug therapy. The etiology of this so-called hyperkinetic syndrome is not known.

Clinical Pharmacology and Therapeutics

Paradoxically, the most effective drugs for this condition (see Table 33-11) have been the CNS stimulants **dextroamphetamine** (Dexedrine), **methylphenidate** (Ritalin), and **pemoline** (Cylert). All these drugs increase the level of catecholaminergic (adrenergic) transmission within the CNS, but their actual mechanism of action in the treatment of ADD has not been elucidated. The starting dose of dextroamphetamine is 2.5 to 5.0 mg daily with increments of 2.5 to 5.0 mg daily at weekly intervals up to a maximum of 40 mg daily. The starting dose of methylphenidate is 5 mg twice a day with increments of 5 to 10 mg at weekly intervals up to a maximum of 60 mg daily. Usually dextroamphetamine and methylphenidate are discontinued after the onset of puberty in the child with ADD. A more complete discussion of amphetamines is presented in Chaps. 13 and 25.

Pemoline

Mechanism of Action Pemoline (Cylert) acts as a central nervous system stimulant but it has little sympathomimetic action. Its effectiveness in the treatment of ADD is slightly less than that of the other CNS stimulants mentioned above.

Pharmacokinetics Pemoline produces a peak serum level in about 2 to 4 h and has a serum half-life of approximately 12 h. Pemoline and its active metabolites are primarily excreted in the urine. Its onset of action in children is delayed, and optimal effects may not be evidenced until the third or fourth week of therapy.

Adverse Effects The most common adverse effects include insomnia and anorexia, which are usually transient and will respond to a dosage reduction. Other adverse effects include skin rash, depression, hallucinations, irritability, and nausea. A delayed hypersensitivity reaction involving the liver, with elevated SGOT and SGPT without clinical effects, rarely occurs.

Dosage The recommended starting dose is 37.5 mg daily in the morning. It then may be increased by 18.75 mg/week at weekly intervals until desired response is observed. The usual dosage range for clinical effectiveness is 56.25 to 75 mg/day. The maximum recommended dosage is 112.5 mg daily.

NURSING PROCESS RELATED TO ATTENTION DEFICIT DISORDER

Assessment

The data base should include more than the complaints of the parent or teacher. A thorough examination of the child and environment are warranted to rule out other physical and psychosocial factors.

Management

The parents should be assisted in coping with the side effects of the psychostimulant drugs. To avoid insomnia, the drug may be taken in the early morning and late afternoon. Anorexia may be a problem and can be helped by having the child eat breakfast before the onset of drug action. Small, frequent meals with emphasis on high caloric foods can improve nutrition.

The use of these drugs should not preclude or replace other therapy, such as special education and psychiatric approaches. Parents and teachers should understand that the drug therapy is symptomatic treatment and not a cure. The nurse may be able to assist the parents and teachers to define the goals to be achieved through a combination of approaches.

Evaluation

Children treated with psychostimulants often show reduced weight gain and stature because of appetite suppression and the reduction in the growth hormone level caused by these drugs. Height and weight graphs on these children, secured as part of a health maintenance program, acquire special significance in evaluation of the overall effects of drug therapy.

Problems of drug abuse may appear at about the junior high school age, so the medication usage of young person taking the drugs at this age should be evaluated carefully to ensure they are taken properly and not "shared" with schoolmates. If possible, it is best to discontinue drugs before this age.

The subjective statements of parents, teachers, and the child are a major source of data for evaluation of the therapeutic efficacy, although the nurse's observation of the child's behavior is also important.

TABLE 33-11 Drugs Used in Treatment of Attention Deficit Disorder

GENERIC NAME	TRADE NAME	HALF-LIFE, h	AVERAGE DAILY DOSE RANGE
Dextroamphetamine sulfate	Dexedrine	5	10–40 mg
Methylphenidate	Ritalin	2–7	15–60 mg
Pemoline	Cylert	12	56.25–75 mg

SENILE DEMENTIA

Dementia is characterized by deterioration in cognition, intellect, behavior, and emotion. It is noted in 5 percent of the population at 65 years of age, and has a 20 percent incidence in the 75-year-old population.

Etiology

Approximately 50 percent of the dementia that occurs in the elderly patient population is of the *alzheimer type* (primary degenerative dementia). The precise etiology of Alzheimer's disease is not defined, but many causes (decreased cholinergic function due to decreased activity of choline acetyltransferase, exposure to heavy metals or aluminum, slow viruses, genetic factors, or chromosomal abnormalities) have been suggested. Other types of dementia are associated with:

1. Arteriosclerotic or multi-infarct dementia, which is caused by small vessel occlusion in the CNS
2. Metabolic disorders such as hepatic failure
3. Alcoholism or other drug abuse
4. CNS infection, such as syphilis
5. Selected intracranial lesions, such as subdural hematoma or brain tumors

Very commonly dementia is iatrogenic (induced by prescribed medication). Drugs listed in Table 33-1 can cause sensory alteration, syncope, depression, or psychosis and have been implicated as causal factors in dementia.

Clinical Pharmacology and Therapeutics

Obviously, the treatment of dementia should be handled by treating the primary cause if this can be identified. However, most cases of dementia do not have a clear-cut etiology, so treatment is symptomatic and somewhat conjectural.

Vasodilators

Vasodilators have been used based on the potential of these agents to dilate cerebral vessels and reduce local cerebral ischemia (Table 33-12). The most commonly used agents of this type are **papaverine** (Pavabid) and **cyclandelate** (Cyclos-

pasmol); the Food and Drug Administration conducted a review of the clinical studies with these agents and concluded that there is no evidence supporting the efficacy of these agents. However, some subsequent studies have shown papaverine to be effective in improving psychologic test scores in patients with dementia. These agents are also used in peripheral vascular disease and other occlusive disorders.

Mechanism of Action **Papaverine, ethaverine** (Cebral), and **cyclandelate** relax all smooth muscle, including vascular smooth muscle, by acting directly on the muscle. Cerebral blood flow increases as a result. **Isoxsuprine** (Vasodilan) primarily relaxes skeletal smooth muscle. Some of these drugs have adrenergic effects, but the precise mechanism of vasodilation is not known.

Pharmacokinetics The pharmacokinetics of **cyclandelate** and **isoxsuprine** are not well-studied. **Papaverine** and its derivative, **ethaverine**, are highly bound to plasma protein and localize in fat deposits and in the liver. They are metabolized by the liver. Half-life varies widely, but effective blood levels can be maintained by q6h dosing or use of sustained release forms.

Adverse Effects and Dosage The usual dosage and major adverse effects of these drugs are shown in Table 33-12.

Dihydrogenated Ergot Alkaloids

The dihydrogenated ergot alkaloids (Hydergine; **DHEA**) or **ergoloid mesylates** have also been shown to be useful in improving both mood and self-care in patients with dementia. The ergot preparations are claimed to have positive effects on both cerebral metabolic disruptions and alterations in capillary blood flow. Use of DHEA should be restricted to patients with minimal to moderate symptomatology, since it has little therapeutic effect in florid cases.

Mechanism of Action Initially it was thought that this agent worked by α-adrenergic blockade resulting in vasodilation. More recent studies show that the drug increases metabolism and that vasodilation is secondary to this effect.

TABLE 33-12 Cerebral Vasodilators

DRUG	TRADE NAME(S)	USUAL DOSAGE	ADVERSE EFFECTS
Cyclandelate	Cyclospasmol, Cydel, Cyvaso	Initial: 400 mg tid to qid Maintenance: 200 mg bid to qid	GI distress, flushing, dizziness, headache, tachycardia.
Isoxsuprine hydrochloride	Vasodilan, Vasoprine	PO: 10–20 mg tid to qid IM: 5–10 mg bid to tid	Hypotension, tachycardia, nausea, dizziness, rash.
Papaverine hydrochloride	Pavabid, Cerespan, others	PO: 60–300 mg 1–5 times/day Timed release: 150–300 mg q12h IM, IV: 30–120 mg q3h	Nausea, abdominal distress, anorexia, sedation, malaise, flushing, vertigo, jaundice.
Ethaverine	Ethaquin, Cebral, others	PO: 100 mg tid Timed release: 150 mg q12h	See papaverine.

Other theories postulate that the drug's benefits are directly related to restoration of metabolism in brain cells which results in improved cerebral function.

Pharmacokinetics   The drug undergoes considerable first-pass metabolism when taken orally. Peak levels occur at 1 h, and the half-life is approximately 3.6 h. Results may not be apparent for 3 to 4 weeks after therapy begins.

Adverse Effects   Serious adverse effects are rare. Transient gastric upset or sublingual irritation occurs occasionally. Unlike the natural ergots discussed in the section on migraine headache, this agent apparently does not cause vasoconstriction or any serious sequelae with long-term use.

Dosage and Administration   DHEA is available in several dosage forms and under numerous brand names, including Hydergine, H.E.A., Circanol, Deapril-ST, Gerimal, and Trigot. Oral tablets and oral liquid, sublingual tablets, and capsules containing liquid are available. Usual initial dosage is 1 mg tid.

Miscellaneous Agents

Lecithin (phosphatidyl choline) and **choline** have also been used in treatment of dementia, but their efficacy is equivocal. These compounds, which are acetylcholine precursors, have been used in an attempt to replace the acetylcholine deficit that is believed to occur in Alzheimer's disease. In spite of the attractiveness of this approach, most studies indicate that no significant improvement is obtained, even at doses of choline up to 200 mg/kg/day. Other agents currently being investigated for treatment of Alzheimer's disease include **centrophenoxime, piracetam, physostigmine,** and **vasopressin** analogs, but definitive studies are needed to evaluate the usefulness of these agents. Antipsychotic drugs, such as **haloperidol** (Haldol) and **thioridazine** (Mellaril), may be used symptomatically for their antiparanoia and sedative effects. Results are variable and often do not warrant the potential adverse effects (see Chap. 34).

NURSING PROCESS RELATED TO SENILE DEMENTIA

Assessment

Nursing assessment of the patient with organic brain syndrome includes a careful history of medical illness, substance abuse, diet, trauma, familial disease, and drugs, including over-the-counter medications. Since some dementia may be reversible, such a history proves invaluable. Specifically, intellectual status should include evaluation of calculation ability, judgment, memory, and orientation. Particular attention should be paid to association of symptoms with life events, especially loss of job, loved ones, and/or health. Depression can make the diagnosis and treatment of dementia difficult.

Management

Drug therapy with cerebral activators, oxygen, antidepressants, and antipsychotics involves very close monitoring for improvement in mood and mental status as well as adverse effects. The prescriber does well to follow the adage of "start low and go slow," especially with an elderly population. The nurse who is familiar with goals of therapy can assist with observation of progress during dosage titration.

Signs and symptoms such as dizziness, confusion, unsociability, and lack of self-care often associated with the elderly may be helped by vasodilators like **cyclandelate** (Cyclospasmol) or ergot derivatives such as **DHEA** (Hydergine). Side effects of vasodilation can be very annoying; those related to gastrointestinal origin can be relieved by giving the oral agent with food or antacid.

Extreme caution should be taken in patients with severe obliterative coronary artery disease or cerebrovascular disease since blood flow is compromised by vasodilator effects of the drug elsewhere. Patients with bleeding diasthesis should be monitored carefully if on **cyclandelate** as there is a possibility of large doses causing bleeding. Glaucoma patients should also have cyclandelate administered with caution.

Nondrug therapy within the nurse's realm includes close attention to intercurrent illness, minimizing sensory deprivation (e.g., cataract surgery, hearing aids, radio/TV/reading material), orientation exercises (calendars, naming objects and people, repetition), home services, short-term nursing home placement to relieve stress on relatives, and behavior modification techniques. Rehabilitation of the elderly should include efforts to improve nutrition and diminish feelings of loneliness and the effects of idleness.

Evaluation

The nurse can gauge improvement in self-care by observing eating, bathing, dressing, and toileting. Cognitive and affective capacity is evaluated by mental alertness, motivation, sociability, emotional stability, and cooperation.

MISCELLANEOUS NEUROLOGIC DISORDERS

Other neurologic disorders are listed in Table 33-13.

TABLE 33-13   Miscellaneous Neurologic Disorders

DESCRIPTION	TREATMENT

Benign Essential (Familial) Tremor

Characterized by a regular, rhythmic shaking of the extremities and head. Inherited as a Mendelian dominant trait. In patients over 60 years of age, it is called senile tremor.	Therapy may be with diazepam or chlordiazepoxide. Alcohol also produces some relief. Some patients also receive benefit from propranolol and metoprolol. Dosage is started with propranolol at 10 mg four times a day then gradually increases until tremors are controlled or adverse effects are noticed.

Eaton-Lambert Syndrome

Skeletal muscle weakness similar to myasthenia gravis which is usually associated with malignant neoplasm (most often bronchial carcinoma). It does not respond to acetylcholinesterase inhibitors and is only slightly improved after removal of carcinoma.	Treatment is usually with guanidine, which increases release of acetylcholine. The dosage is 250 mg three times a day (maximum 2.5 g/day). Adverse effects include paresthesias, anorexia, vomiting, abdominal pain, diarrhea, excessive sialorrhea, anxiety, tremors.

Gilles de la Tourette Syndrome

Chronic neurologic disorder consisting of involuntary muscle movement and various types of vocalizations. Frequently misdiagnosed as a psychiatric disorder.	Haloperidol (Haldol) dose based on adverse effect range from 2–180 mg/day. The drug is started at low doses then gradually increased. After stabilization, the drug dosage is decreased over 1–2 years. Pimozide (Orap) is an orphan neuroleptic agent approved in 1984 for patients who fail to respond to other therapy.

Huntington's Chorea

A progressive genetic disease inherited in an autosomal dominant pattern; about one-half of the offspring of an affected parent will develop the disease. Involuntary choreiform movements and mental deterioration are observed signs. The involuntary movements are similar to those of tardive dyskinesia, both are aggravated by levodopa and anticholinergic drugs.	Therapy is with agents that block dopamine receptors. Fluphenazine (Prolixin), haloperidol, and prochlorperazine (average daily dosages are 15 mg, 2–15 mg, and 2–20 mg, respectively).

Intention (Action) Myoclonus

A form of irregular, stimulus-sensitive, uncontrollable skeletal muscle jerking movements which occur at onset of sleep and at times during the sleep period. Stimuli are frequently loud noises, bright lights, attempts to sit up and other voluntary actions. It is a symptom of a variety of brain lesions.	Therapy consists of the anticonvulsants phenytoin, phenobarbital, diazepam, and clonazepam. Clonazepam is commonly given in daily doses of 2–20 mg. Also carbidopa 50 mg qid and L-5HTP (1–2 g) in divided doses have been used, since these increase serotonin levels.

Narcolepsy

Rare chronic syndrome characterized by sleep attacks. Sudden loss of muscle tone and sleep paralysis. Phenomenon of unknown etiology.	Stimulant drugs like dextroamphetamine or methylphenidate may help. Imipramine and MAO inhibitors are useful but must not be combined with an amphetamine.

Wilson's Disease

Rare inborn error of copper metabolism which is inherited. Neurologic symptoms include athetosis, dysarthria, tremor, and rigidity. An associated liver cirrhosis is usually present. There is an excess of copper which can be deposited in the liver, brain, and kidney.	Therapy is directed at removal of copper usually by penicillamine. The daily dose of penicillamine is 1–2 g in divided doses; also need to supplement with pyridoxine, 50–100 mg daily. Can also prevent the absorption of copper by giving potassium sulfide 20 mg with each meal.

REFERENCES

Ambielli, M., "Migraine Headache: Current Therapy," *J Neurosurg Nurs*, 14:203–206, August 1982.

American College of Neuropsychopharmacology Food and Drug Administration Task Force: "Neurologic Syndromes Associated with Antipsychotic Drug Use," *N Engl J Med*, 289:20–23, 1973.

Amery, W. K., et al.: "The Anti-migrainous Pharmacology of Flunarizine (R 14950), A Calcium Antagonist," *Drugs Exptl Clin Res*, 71:10, 1981.

Biederman, J.: "New Directions in Pediatric Psychopharmacology," *Drug Ther*, 12:147–170, 1982.

Browne, T. R.: "Drug Therapy Reviews: Clinical Pharmacology of Antiepileptic Drugs," *Am J Hosp Pharm*, 35:1048–1056, 1978.

Bruya, M., and R. H. Bolin: "Epilepsy: A Controllable Disease: II. Drug Therapy and Nursing Care," *Am J Nurs*, 76:392–397, March 1976.

Cailliet, R.: *Low Back Pain Syndrome*, Philadelphia: Davis, 1981.

Chadwick, D., R. Harris, P. Jenner, E. H. Reynolds, and C. D. Marsden: "Manipulation of Brain Serotonin in the Treatment of Myoclonus," *Lancet*, 1:434–435, 1975.

Cooper, C.: "Anticonvulsant Drugs and the Epileptic's Dilemma," *Nursing*, 6:44–51, January 1976.

Corbett, M., H. L. Frankel, and L. Michaelis: "A Double Blind Cross-Over Trial of Valium in the Treatment of Spasticity," *Paraplegia*, 10:19–22, 1972.

Duvoisin, R., "Parkinson's Disease: A Review," *US Pharm*, 4:63–84, 1979.

Eisler, T., et al.: "Deprenyl in Parkinsons Disease," *Neurology*, 31:19–23, 1981.

Engel, W. K., et al.: "Myasthenia Gravis," *Ann Intern Med*, 81:225–246, 1974.

Finnerty, F. A.: "Hypertensive Emergencies," *Crit Care Update*, 9:7–17, July 1982.

Fishman, R. A.: *Cerebrospinal Fluid in Diseases of the Nervous System*, Philadelphia: Saunders, 1980, pp. 43–54.

Flacke, W.: "Treatment of Myasthenia Gravis," *N Engl J Med*, 288:27–31, 1973.

Gallagher, B. B.: "Clinical Pharmacology and Rational Prescribing," *Epilepsia*, 23(Suppl. 1):S19–S28, 1982.

Gary, R.: "Cerebral Vasospasm: Process, Trends and Interventions," *J Neurosurg Nurs*, 13:256–264, October 1981.

Goldberg, H. A., and J. D. Dorman: "Intention Myoclonus: Successful Treatment with Clonazepam," *Neurology*, 26:24, 1976.

Hier, D. B., and L. R. Caplan: "Drugs for Senile Dementia," *Drugs*, 20:74–80, 1980.

Hrovath, M.: "Myasthenia Gravis: A Nursing Approach," *J Neurosurg Nurs*, 14:7–12, February 1982.

Johnston, M. V., and J. M. Freeman: "Pharmacologic Advances in Seizure Control," *Pedatr Clin North Am*, 28:179–194, 1981.

Kerner, K. F.: "Management of Headache in the Emergency Department," *Top Emerg Med*, 4:19–32, July 1982.

Lance, J. W.: *The Mechanism and Management of Headache*, London: Butterworth, 1969.

Langun, R. J., and G. C. Cotzias: "Dos and Don'ts for the Patient on Levodopa Therapy," *Am J Nurs*, 76:917–918, June 1976.

Lieberman, A. M., Zolfaghari, D. Boal, et al.: "The Antiparkinsonian Efficacy of Bromocriptine," *Neurology*, 26:405–409, 1976.

Lisak, R.: "Myasthenia Gravis—Mechanisms and Management," *Hosp Pract*, 18:101–1090, March, 1983.

MacDougall, V.: "Epilepsy: Teaching Children and Families About Seizures," *Can Nurse*, 78:30–36, April 1982.

Nowakowski, J. F., et al.: "Myasthenia Gravis," *Ann Emerg Med*, 11:272–275, May 1982.

Parkes, J. D.: "Adverse Effects of Antiparkinsonian Drugs," *Drugs*, 21:341–352, 1981.

Peipho, R. W., and A. S. Lorenzo: "Therapeutic Management of the Epilepsies," *US Pharm*, 4:36–50, 1979.

Raskin, N. H.: "Pharmacology of Migraine," *Annu Rev Pharmacol Toxicol*, 21:463–478, 1981.

Reese, T. S., and M. J. Karnovsky: "Fine Structural Localization of a Blood-Brain Barrier to Exogenous Peroxidase," *J Cell Biol*, 34:207–217, 1967.

Reynolds, E. H., and S. D. Shorvon: "Single Drug or Combination Therapy for Epilepsy?" *Drugs*, 21:374–82, 1981.

Saccar, C.: "Pharmacological Approaches to Minimal Brain Dysfunction," *Drug Ther*, 9:107–120, 1979.

Scheife, R. T., and J. R. Hills: "Migraine Headache: Signs and Symptoms, Biochemistry, and Current Therapy," *Am J Hosp Pharm*, 37:365–74, 1980.

Sethy, V. H: "Therapy of Intention Myoclonus with L-5-Hydroxytryptophan and a Peripheral Decarboxylase Inhibitor, MK 486," *Neurology*, 25:135–140, 1975.

Seybold, M. E., and D. B. Drachman: "Gradually Increasing Doses of Prednisone in Myasthenia Gravis: Reducing the Hazards of Treatment," *N Engl J Med*, 290:81–94, 1974.

Shapiro, A. K., E. Shapiro, and H. Wayne: "Treatment of Tourette's Syndrome with Haloperidol, Review of 34 Cases," *Arch Gen Psychiatry*, 28:92–97, 1973.

So, E. L., and J. K. Penry: "Epilepsy in Adults," *Ann Neurol*, 9:3–16, 1981.

Sweet, R. D., J. Blumberg, J. E. Lee, and F. H. McDowell: "Propranolol Treatment of Essential Tremor," *Neurology*, 24:64–67, 1974.

"The Older Adult and Drug Therapy," *Geriatric Nursing*, 2:411–416, pt. 1, November–December 1981; 3:31–33, pt. 2, January–February 1982.

"Valproic Acid Hyperammonemic Stupor," *Nurses Drug Alert*, 6:17–18, March 1982.

Van Woert, M. H.: "Myasthenia Gravis, Eaton Lambert Syndrome and Familial Dysautonomia," in A. M. Goldberg and I. Hanin (eds.), *Biology of Cholinergic Function,* New York: Raven, 1976, pp. 567–581.

——, R. Jutkowitz, D. Rosenbaum, and M. B. Bowers, Jr.: "Gilles de la Tourette's Syndrome: Biochemical Approaches," in M. D. Yahr (ed.), *The Basal Ganglia,* New York: Raven, 1976, pp. 459–465.

——, ——, ——, and ——: "Serotonin and Myoclonus," in M. M. Cohen (ed.), *Monographs in Neural Sciences,* vol. 3, Basel: Karger, 1976, pp. 71–80.

Wiley, L.: "Epilepsy Nursing," *Nursing,* 4:30–45, January 1974.

Yarh, M. D.: "Overview of Present Day Treatment of Parkinsons Disease," *J Neurol Transm,* 43:227–38, 1978.

Yesavage, J. A., J. R. Tinklenberg, L. E. Hollister, and P. A. Berger: "Vasodilators in Senile Dementias: A Review of the Literature," *Arch Gen Psychiatry,* 36:220–224, 1979.

Zarcone, V.: "Narcolepsy," *N Engl J Med,* 288:1156–1166, 1973.

34

PSYCHIATRIC DISORDERS

ROSWELL LEE EVANS
NANCY A. RICHART

LEARNING OBJECTIVES

Upon mastery of the contents of this chapter, the reader will be able to:

1. Relate theories of the biochemical etiology of schizophrenia to the proposed mechanism of action of the antipsychotic drugs.

2. State at least four clinical indications for antipsychotic drugs.

3. Describe the use of the nursing process in the detection, management, and prevention of adverse drug effects of the antipsychotics, including neurologic, autonomic, cardiovascular, allergic, and endocrine reactions.

4. Explain the guidelines for selection of anxious patients to be treated by drug therapy.

5. Name at least four groups of drugs used to treat anxiety.

6. Give examples of criteria based on target symptoms for evaluating the effectiveness of antianxiety drug therapy.

7. Explain the efficacy of the following groups of drugs as antianxiety agents: antihistamines, antidepressants, antipsychotics, barbiturates, and β-adrenergic blockers.

8. Give at least four examples of benzodiazepines.

9. Based on pharmacokinetics, give guidelines for selecting among benzodiazepines.

10. Compare the benzodiazepines to other antianxiety drugs with respect to mechanism of action and adverse effects.

11. Describe the nursing process relative to the treatment of anxiety disorders.

12. Differentiate between endogenous and exogenous depressions according to presentation and treatment.

13. List the symptoms of bipolar affective disorder which could be used as guides for assessment and for evaluation of the effectiveness of drug therapy.

14. List three types of drug therapy useful in affective psychoses.

15. Relate the biogenic amine hypothesis to the etiology and treatment of depression.

16. Discuss the efficacy of antidepressants in depression, anxiety, phobic anxiety, and enuresis.

17. List at least five groups of adverse effects of antidepressants and the use of the nursing process in detecting, preventing, and treating these effects.

18. Compare the phenothiazines according to indications, adverse effects, half-life, and dosage schedules.

19. Compare the tricyclic and related antidepressants according to efficacy, adverse effects, and indications.

20. Describe the adverse effects of monoamine oxidase (MAO) inhibitors.

21. Indicate the clinical uses for lithium carbonate.

22. Define the stabilization and maintenance phases of therapy with lithium carbonate and explain use of serum lithium levels in each.

23. Outline a teaching plan for the patient given lithium carbonate; a MAO inhibitor; a phenothiazine; an antidepressant; a benzodiazepine.

Drugs to treat emotional disturbances are among the most frequently used agents on the market today. While it could be logically inferred from this that a large portion of the population is emotionally disturbed, it is more likely that the rational use of these drugs is simply not understood by those who prescribe and those who use them. Furthermore, emotional disturbances themselves are relatively ill defined and misunderstood. Too readily, perhaps, the prescriber chooses to use a psychotropic drug (i.e., a pharmacologic agent which will affect mood and behavior) for a patient who exhibits unexplained behavior or vague symptoms. It is imperative that nurses and other health professionals understand the basic concepts of emotional disturbances, the principles of rational drug therapy to apply in treating these problems, and the relationship between psychotherapy and pharmacotherapy in emotional problems. Further, they must use this knowledge to educate the public and to solve the individual patient's medication problems.

In this chapter an overview of three major groups of emotional disturbances, schizophrenic disorders, anxiety disorders, and affective disorders, is presented. The pharmacology and therapeutics of psychotropic drugs commonly used in these three disorders are discussed.

SCHIZOPHRENIA

In this country, the probability is that 1 out of every 100 people will be diagnosed at some point during their lifetime, but generally between the ages of 20 and 40, as having a schizophrenic illness. Approximately 23 percent of these individuals will require hospitalization.

Schizophrenia (from the Greek for "split mind" or "split personality") is a broad category of illnesses made up of a large number of subgropus, e.g., simple, paranoid, catatonic, and disorganized. Throughout the ages, schizophrenia has been a feared and misunderstood illness. Treatment modalities have been diverse and variously successful. Hydrotherapy, electroconvulsive therapy, insulin coma, hypnosis, psychoanalysis, behavioral therapy, group therapy, and family therapy are but a few of the treatment methods attempted. Not until the introduction of chlorpromazine in the 1950s was there an efficacious pharmacologic approach to treatment. Pharmacotherapy is now the most efficacious and rapid approach in resolving symptoms of schizophrenia.

Etiology

Speculation about the etiology of schizophrenia and other mental illnesses has included analytic and family theories, psychosocial theories, genetic theories, and organic theories, including the biochemical theories which have contributed to the understanding of the effects of psychopharmaceutics in these disorders.

Biochemical Theories

A biochemical etiology helps to explain the mechanisms of action of the psychotropic agents used in the treatment of schizophrenic disorders. The dopamine hypothesis for the etiology of schizophrenia is perhaps the most widely accepted theory for explaining the disorder and the actions of the antipsychotic agents. This theory was developed as a result of the introduction of drugs that control psychoses and drugs that mimic the symptoms of schizophrenia (amphetamines, LSD). It is postulated that since the antipsychotics antagonize the actions of dopamine as a neurotransmitter in the forebrain, there may be a functional overactivity of dopamine in the limbic system or cortex of the schizophrenic. Psychomimetic effects of amphetamines and LSD, induced by the drugs' effects on endogenous dopamine, can be blocked by the dopamine-blocking effects of the anti-

psychotics. In vitro models using an enzyme, adenylate cyclase, from stimulated basal ganglia demonstrate blocking of the increased ganglionic activity when an antipsychotic compound is added. Many other approaches seem to support this hypothesis for the biochemical basis of schizophrenia and the postsynaptic dopamine blockade mechanism of action of the antipsychotics; however, there continues to be uncertainty regarding these theories.

Clinical Findings

The diagnosis of schizophrenia may be difficult because of the variety of symptoms and variations in their severity. The clinician must also rule out a number of disease states that can manifest like schizophrenia (see Table 34-1).

Symptoms

The schizophrenic has defects in four main areas, often referred to as "Bleuler's four As": affect, association, autism, and ambivalence. The emotion (*affect*) of the schizophrenic typically shows some degree of inappropriateness. Either the kind of feeling displayed by the schizophrenic is not in tune with the ideas being expressed or the amount of emotion shown is discrepant. The second general characteristic is a peculiarity in thought processes and in the handling of words, called *associative looseness*. *Autistic thinking* is characterized by personalized, esoteric thought processes that are hard for the observer to follow. The schizophrenic often has very intense opposing feelings about the same object (*ambivalence*). These intense ambivalent feelings contribute greatly to the inactivity and seeming apathy of the schizophrenic patient.

Hallucinations and delusions, which are secondary symptoms of the disorder, generally occur later in the nat-

TABLE 34-1 Causes of Schizophrenic Symptoms

Drugs	
Alcohol	Indomethacin
Antidepressants	Isoniazid
Cimetidine	Levodopa
Sympathomimetics (amphetamines)	Barbiturates
Corticosteroids	Antipsychotics
Anticholinergics	Digitalis glycosides
Hallucinogens (LSD, PCP)	Disulfiram
Antimalarials (quinacrine)	Bromides
Diseases	
Ventricular arrhythmias	Pituitary adenoma
Hemodialysis	Addison's disease
Thyroid disorder	Cushing's syndrome
Parkinsonism	Hypoglycemia
Hyponatremia	Lupus arteritis (CNS)
Acute porphyria	Seizure disorders
Dementia	Neoplasms

ural progression of the disease and are often the only ones that can be identified. Schizophrenics are also known to exhibit social withdrawal, difficulties developing interpersonal relationships and managing anxiety, and failure to learn from past experiences.

Schizophrenic patients may exhibit a number of other symptons which are not pathognomonic of the diagnosis. These include abnormal motor movements such as bizarre posturing, grimacing, smiling, mute stares, catatonic posture, and repetitious motor rituals such as rocking of the upper trunk while sitting. Symptomatic physical symptoms, panic, anxiety, chaotic sexuality, depersonalization, and impulsivity are also seen.

As understanding of the illness has increased, many definitions and diagnostic criteria have evolved including those in *The Diagnostic and Statistical Manual of Mental Disorders* (see References). The basic deficits observable in the schizophrenic involve alterations in mood, thought, and behavior. The course of a patient's illness fluctuates; remissions from acute symptoms for periods of time are common. There is interpatient variation of illness presentations. All patients do not demonstrate all of the signs and symptoms of schizophrenia.

Clinical Pharmacology and Therapeutics of Schizophrenia

A mentally ill patient's chances of being discharged from the mental institution have doubled since the introduction of psychotropic medications. Utilization of psychotropics has enabled clinicians to implement additional psychotherapeutic approaches (such as psychoanalysis, behavioral therapy, psychodrama, group therapy, and milieu therapy) at an early stage of hospitalization. Drugs seem to speed recovery from the acute episodes of mental illness and allow patients to return to the community to continue their normal routines. It is important to remember, however, that these drugs are not curative and give only symptomatic relief from mental illness.

Antipsychotic Agents

The term *tranquilizer* is often used, by both the lay public and the medical profession, as a synonym for all psychotropic agents, with "major tranquilizer" representing primarily the phenothiazine-like agents used in psychotic illnesses, and "minor tranquilizer" representing agents for treating anxiety. In this chapter, drugs used to treat schizophrenia are called *antipsychotic agents,* but they have also been called neuroleptics, major tranquilizers, and ataractic agents. In keeping with this system of classification, other agents used to treat psychiatric disorders would be antidepressants, antimanic agents, and antianxiety (anxiolytic) agents.

Since the introduction of the first antipsychotic, chlorpromazine (Thorazine), a large number of other agents have been introduced (see Table 34-2). Chemical classes of anti-

psychotics include the phenothiazines, thioxanthenes, butyrophenones, dihydroindolones, and dibenzoxazepines. All of these agents possess common pharmacologic properties.

Mechanism of Action Antipsychotics are nonselective in their actions. They affect not only the brain and central nervous system (CNS), but most organ systems of the body. All of the drugs share two common pharmacologic properties: first, they all have the ability to ameliorate the course of schizophrenia, and second, they all evoke *extrapyramidal symptoms* (EPS), such as muscle spasms and abnormal movements. It used to be felt by most clinicians that EPS must be exhibited before the drug exerted its antipsychotic effect. This is no longer considered a valid therapeutic endpoint, since it is now known that the antipsychotic action and EPS are separate effects.

The exact mechanism of action for the antipsychotic drugs is not known. Strong evidence indicates that these drugs act by affecting the neurotransmitters dopamine, norepinephrine, and serotonin, and their respective activities in neural transmission. In relieving symptoms of schizophrenia they are suspected of blocking postsynaptic dopamine receptors. Observation of schizophrenic behavior correlates with known functions of certain areas of the brain, providing clues to the mechanism of action of the antipsychotic agents. The action of antipsychotic agents implicates four anatomic sites in the midbrain:

1. The reticular activating system of the midbrain, where sensory input is monitored
2. The structures of the amygdala, hippocampus, and limbic system, which provide emotional coloring for incoming messages
3. The hypothalamus, which governs peripheral responses to sensory information
4. The globus pallidus and corpus striatum, where extrapyramidal symptoms are elicited

Other significant pharmacologic properties of the antipsychotic agents include marked α-adrenergic blockade, anticholinergic activity, CNS sedation, decrease of seizure threshold, and alteration of temperature regulation. These pharmacologic effects explain most of the common unwanted side effects and other therapeutic uses of these agents. α-Adrenergic blockade of the vasculature may lead to postural hypotension. Blockade of dopamine receptors in the hypothalamic-pituitary-adrenal axis is responsible for rises in prolactin and subsequent endocrine abnormalities. Dopamine blockade in the nigrostriatal structures of the brain causes extrapyramidal side effects. Dopamine blockade in the hypothalamus can cause hyper- and/or hypothermia in some patients.

Researchers feel that the effects mediated by psychotropic agents in these areas influence the major integrating systems of the brain by reducing extraneous or distracting sensory information, both internal and external, thereby reducing the somatic responses to them.

TABLE 34-2 Selected Antipsychotic Drugs: Potencies, Doses, and Side Effects

CLASS AND NONPROPRIETARY NAME	TRADE NAME†	RELATIVE POTENCY‡	Dose			Adverse Effects*		
			Antipsychotic Dose Range—Daily Dosage (mg)		SINGLE INTRAMUSCULAR DOSE¶	SEDATIVE EFFECTS	EXTRAPYRAMIDAL EFFECTS	HYPOTENSIVE EFFECTS
			USUAL	EXTREME§				
Phenothiazines								
Aliphatic								
Chlorpromazine	Thorazine	100	200–800	25–2000	25–50	+++	++	IM +++
Triflupromazine	Vesprin	25–50	50–200	50–400	20–50	++	+++	++
Piperidine								
Thioridazine	Mellaril	100	100–600	50–800		+++	+	++
Piperazine								
Perphenazine	Trilafon	8	8–32	4–64	5–10	++	+++	+
Prochlorperazine edisylate	Compazine (edisylate and maleate)	25	75–100	15–150	5–10	++	+++	+
Prochlorperazine maleate								
Fluphenazine hydrochloride	Permitil, Prolixin (hydrochloride, enanthate, and decanoate)	4	2–10	1–60	1.25–4 (decanoate or enanthate 25–50 every 2 weeks)	+	+++	+
Fluphenazine enanthate								
Fluphenazine decanoate								
Acetophenazine	Tindal	20	40–80	20–150	—	++	++	++
Trifluoperazine	Stelazine	5	4–15	2–64	1–2	+	+++	++
Nonphenothiazines								
Thioxanthenes								
Chlorprothixene	Taractan	100	50–400	30–600	25–50	+++	++	++
Thiothixene	Navane	5	6–60	6–60	2–6	+ to ++	++	++
Butyrophenones								
Haloperidol	Haldol	5	2–6	1–100	3–5	+	+++	+
Dihydroindolones								
Molindone	Moban	10	15–40	60–400		+ to ++	+++	+
Dibenzoxazepines								
Loxapine	Loxitane	10	20–50	60–400		+ to ++	++	++

*Less intense +, ++, +++, more intense.

†Only representatives from the various groups are presented; the trade name list is noninclusive.

‡Dosage (in mg) which gives efficacy comparable to 100 mg chlorpromazine.

§Extreme dosage ranges should not be exceeded except when all other appropriate measures have failed.

¶Except for the enanthate and decanoate forms of fluphenazine, dosage is given IM every 4 to 6 h for agitated patients.

625

Indications   Two specific indications for the antipsychotics are the treatment of schizophrenia and the treatment of the manic phase of bipolar affective illness. These drugs have very little, if any, use in treating depression and nonpsychotic anxiety. Specific target symptoms of schizophrenia that would be most likely to improve with the use of antipsychotics include hyperactivity, tension, hostility, combativeness, hallucinations, negativism, and poor sleep. Lack of insight, poor judgment, impaired memory, and disorientation are less likely to improve with drug therapy, but are indications for treatment.

Besides antipsychotic effects, these agents possess other clinically useful pharmacologic properties (see Table 34-3). Although the phenothiazines that are used as antipsychotics have some antihistaminic activity, they are less active than those that are used strictly as antihistamines, such as **promethazine** (Phenergan). Many of the phenothiazines, except **thioridazine** (Mellaril), show antiemetic properties. Apart from the phenothiazines, **haloperidol** (Haldol), a butyrophenone, is also an antiemetic and has been used clinically for refractory vomiting.

Chlorpromazine and **haloperidol** have been used in the treatment of hiccoughs. Antipruritic activity is exhibited by the phenothiazines, and they have been used clinically for pruritis. Nonphenothiazine agents show little antipruritic activity and are not clinically useful for this purpose. Some of the phenothiazines (**promethazine**) are used to potentiate the effects of narcotic analgesics in order to decrease the dose of the narcotic.

These drugs are also used as sedatives, especially in crisis situations such as grief reactions and acute anxiety episode. While it is common to see the phenothiazines used for this purpose, the use of these agents instead of antianxiety drugs is questionable.

Choice of Drug   The similarities between the various antipsychotic groups of drugs might lead one to ask how one drug is chosen over the others for a particular patient. Even with the advent of nonphenothiazine antipsychotics, there is no evidence that any of these drugs has superiority over the others (in equivalent doses) in the resolution of psychotic symptoms. Rational selection of a psychotropic agent should

TABLE 34-3   Clinical Uses of Antipsychotic Agents

Schizophrenia
Bipolar affective disorder
Antihistamines
Antiemetic
Hiccoughs
Antipruritic
Analgesia (to potentiate narcotics; preprocedural medication)
Sedative
Shivering
Organic brain syndrome
Gilles de la Tourette's syndrome

be based on the consideration of the pharmacologic properties and adverse effects, as well as the patient's past experience with the drug. If a particular drug has produced significant adverse effects, consideration should be given to cross-sensitivities that exist within the same chemical group of drugs, and a member of another group should be chosen. For example, if the patient becomes very sedated on one antipsychotic, changing to an agent rated as less sedating may be appropriate, e.g., from chlorpromazine to haloperidol (see Table 34-2). Problems secondary to extrapyramidal or hypotensive effects may be handled in a similar manner. If a drug has worked for the patient in the past, it is a good choice with which to begin treatment. Clinicians should alsp keep in mind that there is apparently great variation in drug effects among patients: some react much differently than others to the same drug. A patient who fears a certain agent is likely not to take it, and another drug would be a better choice.

Pharmacokinetics   All of the psychotropic agents share similar pharmacokinetic characteristics. Oral administration of these drugs provides incomplete absorption from the gastrointestinal tract. Interpatient variation in bioavailability results in a broad range of response to equal doses. Taking the drug with food or other drugs may slow absorption. Administration of antiparkinsonian drugs, which is quite common in this patient population, slows the motility of the gastrointestinal tract and decreases absorption. Most of these drugs are extensively (90 percent) bound to body protein. Total body stores build slowly over the first 2 to 4 weeks of therapy.

These drugs are highly concentrated in the brain and to a lesser extent in other vital organs such as the lungs and muscle tissue. There is a great intersubject variability in blood levels after the same dose. Correlating blood levels with specific drug doses and clinical response has not been satisfactory and is still considered experimental. **Haloperidol** has shown the most consistent correlation between blood level and response. Research in this area is promising, and as assay technology improves, it is anticipated that dosing antipsychotics based on blood levels may be possible.

Antipsychotic drugs are metabolized almost completely by the liver. Metabolism begins very quickly after the administration of the drug. Over 150 metabolites of **chlorpromazine** have been identified to date. All of the phenothiazines have some metabolites with antipsychotic activity, complicating the utilization of blood levels for the adjustment of dosage regimens. **Haloperidol** is the only agent for which no active metabolites have been reported. Excretion of the conjugated metabolites and free drug is through the feces and urine. Use of these agents, especially phenothiazines, in liver disease should be approached with caution; conceivably, these drugs would require dosage reductions since their metabolism may be altered. **Haloperidol** may be the drug of choice in liver disease. Drug levels can be detected in the urine for up to 6 months after a dose of a phenothiazine. The slow release of protein-bound drug is responsible for this phenomenon and may account for some patients remaining stable for several months after discontinuing medications and then abruptly becoming psychotic again.

Adverse Effects The most common adverse effects of the psychotropic drugs involve the CNS, autonomic nervous system (ANS), and cardiovascular system.

Central nervous system Sedation is the most common CNS side effect of all the antipsychotics. Table 34-2 indicates the relative sedative effects of these drugs. This *sedation* is nonspecific and refers to the control of agitation, hyperactivity, and disordered sleep patterns commonly seen in schizophrenic patients. Use of these agents as hypnotics in normal patients is not recommended. However, the antipsychotics with sedative properties (e.g., **thioridazine**) are extremely useful for emotionally disturbed patients who have problems with insomnia, eliminating the need for hypnotics.

Researchers have postulated that nonspecific sedation is due in part to the amelioration of underlying thought disorders prevalent in the schizophrenic patient. Some patients respond to certain of the antipsychotics by exhibiting insomnia, an individual variation which should be taken into consideration when selection of a drug is made. In clinical practice, **haloperidol** exhibits a *bimodal action*. If given to an agitated, combative patient, it produces sedation, but it elicits nonsedative effects when given to a nonpsychotic patient. Tolerance to the sedative effect develops in most patients over several weeks.

Psychomotor retardation Psychomotor functions, including reaction time, dexterity or coordination, speed of activity, and steadiness, are adversely affected by the administration of antipsychotic agents, antianxiety drugs, and antidepressants. No specific agent seems more offensive than the others. Some attention should be given to advising patients about these particular side effects if they drive or work with machinery. Concomitant use of alcohol and other CNS-depressant drugs can intensify psychomotor problems.

Seizure threshold Caution should be exercised when administering phenothiazines to patients with preexisting convulsive disorders, since all phenothiazines can lower the seizure threshold, disposing patients to seizures. The older agents, especially the "high-dose" or less potent phenothiazines such as **chlorpromazine** (Thorazine) and **chlorprothixene** (Taractan), have been implicated in causing these problems. Butyrophenones and the more potent "low-dose" phenothiazine drugs are less likely to lower the seizure threshold than are high-dose phenothiazine drugs. If treatment with antipsychotic drugs is considered necessary for patients who are predisposed to seizures, prophylactic anticonvulsive therapy should be initiated.

Iatrogenic depression Antipsychotic drugs have been implicated in exogenous depression in patients treated for both psychotic and nonpsychotic disorders. Clinical depression in the psychotic patient can be a manifestation of psychotropic drug therapy or of the illness itself, and often prompts the clinician to institute antidepressant therapy. Drug-induced depression is transitory and reversible on discontinuance of the offending drug, and antidepressant therapy is not often required. Addition of an antidepressant to the existing antipsychotic therapy often creates more intense drug-related problems and has been associated with precipitating further psychotic symptoms.

Autonomic nervous system Autonomic nervous system effects are caused by either the anticholinergic (atropine-like) activity of the antipsychotic drugs or by α-adrenergic blockade. Table 34-4 lists the most common of these side effects. Generally the incidence of autonomic side effects of the various agents parallels their sedative effects: those with a high incidence of sedation (see Table 34-2) have a correspondingly high incidence of autonomic nervous system side effects.

One of the more serious adverse effects is *orthostatic hypotension*. **Chlorpromazine** and **chlorprothixene** tend to be the most significant offenders, especially in elderly patients. Tachycardia has been attributed to the reflex mechanisms activated by hypotension. The patient should report episodes of tachycardia to the clinician, and baseline electrocardiograms should be performed. Some of the phenothiazines, especially **thioridazine**, have been reported to be cardiotoxic, causing myocardial infarctions and a "sudden death" phenomenon.

The α-blocking activities of the antipsychotic drugs are responsible for the *inhibition of ejaculation* in the male. **Thioridazine** is commonly implicated. This side effect is an alarming prospect for both the male and his sexual partner; both should be reassured that the problem is drug-induced and that it is reversible upon discontinuance of the drug or on switching to a drug in a different group.

Initially, all patients will exhibit *dry mouth* when any of the psychotropics is given. This is a transitory effect and should disappear over several weeks. Patients often complain that their mouths feel like cotton and their speech is slurred because of the dryness. Patients can use sugarless hard candies, chew gum, or use **artificial saliva** to make the adverse effect more tolerable.

Constipation and urinary retention are very common adverse effects of therapy, especially in older patients. *Constipation* should *not* be ignored. Increasing diet fiber, ensur-

TABLE 34-4 Autonomic Nervous System Adverse Effects of Antipsychotic Drugs

Blurred vision	Mydriasis, miosis
Dental caries	Nausea, vomiting
Diarrhea	Pallor
Dry mouth	Paralytic ileus
Edema	Rhinitis
Ejaculation inhibition	Tachycardia
Hypotension	Urinary hesitancy

ing proper hydration, and encouraging exercise are the best methods of preventing constipation secondary to these agents. Stool softeners such as **docusate calcium** (Surfak) or **docusate sodium** (Colace) should be utilized, rather than stimulant laxatives. Bowel training for patients who feel that a daily bowel movement is the only normal pattern is extremely helpful in controlling indiscriminate laxative use in this population.

Elderly men with prostatic hypertrophy commonly have symptoms of urinary hesitancy when taking a phenothiazine. In these patients the dosage should be reduced or the drugs discontinued, since *urinary retention* leading to renal damage, a potentially lethal complication can ensue. Difficulty with micturition has also been reported in the young and is quickly reversible with a reduction in dose or discontinuance of medication.

Patients should also be advised to avoid over-the-counter preparations that contain anticholinergic agents (e.g., atropine or scopolamine) since they tend to aggravate the autonomic effects of the antipsychotic agents.

Neurologic syndromes Neurologic syndromes are the most dramatic side effects of the antipsychotics. Extrapyramidal symptoms (EPS), characterized by uncontrollable, bizarre, involuntary movements, are side effects that are more frightening to patients than they are dangerous. It is believed that the blockade of dopamine receptors in the basal ganglia is the primary etiology of these symptoms. The normal catecholamine balance between acetylcholine and dopamine is disrupted, allowing a relative increase in the acetylcholine effects which cause the extrapyramidal symptoms.

Dystonic reactions are the most alarming EPS, usually occurring within the first 5 days, and sometimes within an hour after administration of the drug. They are more common in the young and generally do not occur after the first 3 months of antipsychotic therapy. Acute dystonic reactions are often induced when children are administered antiemetic phenothiazines or after accidental ingestion of these agents. **Prochlorperazine** (Compazine) suppositories are notorious for this side effect. Dystonias include muscle spasms of the eye (ocylogyric crisis), jaw (trismus), neck (torticollis), and back (opisthotonos).

Whereas dystonias are prolonged abnormal tonic contractions of muscle groups, the other group of hyperkinetic reactions, *dyskinesias,* is characterized by tics, spasms, and other clonic types of muscular contractions. Rhythmic, involuntary movements such as flailing of the arms, grimacing, and extruding the tongue are common characteristics of this type of dystonic reaction.

If these reactions should occur, serum electrolytes should be measured to rule out hypocalcemia, which can predispose the patient to dystonic reactions. In addition, hypocalcemic tetany can be almost indistinguishable from dystonic reactions. Dystonic reactions also mimic symptoms of tertiary meningitis, encephalitis, diphtheria, and acute psychosis.

Acute dystonic symptoms should be treated as a medical emergency to alleviate the patient's fear and discomfort. **Diphenhydramine** (Benadryl) is the drug of choice. Antiparkinsonian drugs administered intramuscularly or intravenously also relieve the condition. See Chap. 33 on neurology for a discussion of the use of antiparkinsonian agents in the treatment of drug-induced EPS.

Tardive dyskinesia is a persistent dyskinesia characterized by hyperkinetic activity in the oral region, and by choreiform and possibly athetoid jerking movements. It is usually irreversible and most frequently occurs in elderly patients who have been treated with psychotropic agents for long periods of time. Tardive dyskinesia may also occur in young patients and in patients on antipsychotics for short periods of time. Organic brain syndrome and other neurologic lesions have been reported to predispose patients to tardive dyskinesia; however, there has been little evidence to support these claims. Treatment for this disorder has not been uniformly reliable. Withdrawal of the drug is occasionally successful; in most patients it only worsens the problem. Increasing the dosage of the drug has occasionally relieved some patients but generally only for a short while. Other drug treatments have been attempted, including **reserpine, deanol, lithium carbonate, lecithin, choline, physostigmine, clonidine,** etc.; however, these approaches have not proved useful. The best treatment is prevention through the use of the minimum effective doses of phenothiazines.

Akathisia is an extrapyramidal symptom that is characterized by the patient's inability to sit still. Akathisia constitutes 50 percent of the EPSs that patients experience with antipsychotic drugs. All of the antipsychotic drugs produce these symptoms. Patients express the feeling that they are driven and cannot concentrate. Insomnia, pacing, and constant leg and finger movements are common manifestations of akathisia. These symptoms closely mimic those of many of the psychiatric disorders, especially schizophrenic symptoms, and therefore are detected only by careful observation. If the symptoms are reduced by administration of an antiparkinsonian drug in combination with the phenothiazine for several days, the diagnosis of akathisia is almost certain. Reduction of the dose of phenothiazine will also alleviate this side effect, and it will be corrected on discontinuance of drug therapy. Increasing the dosage of the antipsychotics may improve the symptoms temporarily but they soon will return.

Pseudoparkinsonism accounts for about 40 percent of the EPSs exhibited by patients. Clinically it presents similarly to true parkinsonism. Patients have a triad of symptoms: dyskinesia, rigidity, and resting tremor (pill-rolling). Accompanying these symptoms are drooling, a masklike face, shuffling gait, and loss of associative movements such as the arm swing during walking. Symptoms are rapidly amenable to treatment with anticholinergic antiparkinsonian drugs.

Much controversy has arisen concerning the prophylactic use of antiparkinsonian drugs before EPSs occur. Unless the patient has a history of exhibiting EPS on initiation of therapy, there is no rationale for the addition of antiparkinsonian drugs to the patient's antipsychotic regimen. These drugs are not without their own side effects, including increased anticholinergic effects, possible toxic psychosis, and interference with absorption of the phenothiazine. If a clinician feels that an antiparkinsonian drug is necessary, the drug should be discontinued in 2 to 4 weeks, since occurrence of parkinsonism after that period of time is unusual.

Many patients who are told that they will be taking medication for extended periods of time worry about dependence. Mild withdrawal symptoms occur after a long period of high doses, but there is no evidence that physical dependence results. Patients should be reassured that these drugs are *not* physically addicting.

Cardiovascular manifestations Although the incidence is low, cardiac toxicity does occur with antipsychotic drugs. Sudden deaths have been reported to be caused by phenothiazines, and abnormal ECGs are seen in some patients receiving high-dose medications. **Thioridazine, chlorpromazine**, and **trifluoperazine** are the most commonly implicated drugs. ECG abnormalities resemble those of hypokalemia and are often reversed by the administration of potassium. Fatalities from ventricular tachycardias have been reported. In light of the existing evidence, periodic electrocardiographic examination is certainly warranted for patients taking long-term high-dose psychotropics.

Hematologic changes Hematologic changes occur with the use of psychotropic agents; *leukopenia* and *agranulocytosis* are the most common. Agranulocytosis occurs most often within 3 to 8 weeks of the initiation of therapy and can have a very sudden onset. Older women are at greatest risk for this toxicity. Close attention should be paid to minor symptoms while patients are taking these drugs, especially shortly after their initiation; fever, increased weakness, fatigue, and sore mouth and throat are symptoms of both agranulocytosis and severe leukopenia. If these conditions are confirmed by laboratory tests (including a white blood count below 3500/mm³) vigorous therapy with antibiotics, reverse isolation, and discontinuance of the antipsychotic drug should be instituted, as these blood dyscrasias can be fatal.

Dermatologic reactions Dermatologic reactions involving the skin are not uncommon and generally occur within 2 to 8 weeks after the initiation of therapy. Dermatoses are nonfatal and present as *maculopapular eruptions* involving most of the body. *Photosensitivity* reactions, characterized by general erythema, occasionally involving the nonexposed parts of the body, are common and can be precipitated by a brief exposure to direct sunlight. **Chlorpromazine** is a principal offender, but all of the phenothiazine derivatives are suspect. Another skin-related toxicity is *oculocutaneous pigmentation,* in which the skin takes on a slight gray or purplish hue. This reaction is often associated with the formation of minute deposits of pigment on the lens and cornea, causing complaints of blurring or brownish discoloration of vision. Patients taking high doses of **chlorpromazine** or

thioridazine are susceptible to this toxicity. Occurrence is generally within 20 to 50 days after the start of high-dose therapy. Immediate discontinuation of the drug is warranted. Unless the condition is far advanced, it is reversible within several weeks.

In *pigmentary retinopathy,* a process separate from the more common oculocutaneous pigmentation, there is deposition of pigment in the retina. Impaired vision occurs and smaller doses are involved.

Allergic or hepatotoxic reactions Fever and other symptoms resembling virus infections, upper-quadrant pain, and malaise followed by pruritus and jaundice are the progression of symptoms which indicate hepatotoxicity in patients receiving psychotropic agents. This is a sensitivity reaction producing obstructive jaundice, usually occurring within 3 to 4 weeks after the initiation of treatment. A drug-free trial period of several weeks should be completed before treatment is reinstituted. Cross-sensitivity to hepatotoxicity from related drugs is rare; however, it would be advisable to continue therapy with a drug from a different chemical group.

Endocrine changes Patients show much concern over metabolic and endocrine changes caused by phenothiazines. *Weight gain* can be expected in patients under **phenothiazine** therapy. (**Molindone**, however, is reported to cause no increase in weight and, in fact, may facilitate weight loss.) The mechanism for this change is unknown and little can be done about the problem. Patients should be advised to diet and to exercise regularly.

Galactorrhea and *breast engorgement* are usually accompanied by amenorrhea. *Gynecomastia* occurs occasionally in male patients. These side effects are thought to be caused by increased prolactin secretion by the anterior pituitary, a result of suppression of the prolactin-inhibiting factor produced by the hypothalamus. If amenorrhea occurs, it is appropriate to perform a pregnancy test, using serum since urine tests are invalidated by the presence of phenothiazine. If the patient is not pregnant, she should be reassured that the amenorrhea is harmless, but that birth control precautions and periodic gynecologic checkups are advisable. *Decreased libido,* in both male and female patients, may be a result of phenothiazine therapy, particularly with **thioridazine**. Butyrophenones and antidepressants will also produce these endocrine problems. A reduction in dosage or a change to another drug group corrects the problem in several weeks.

Dosage The use of antipsychotic agents is rather empirical. Doses should begin at a low level, 200 to 800 mg of **chlorpromazine**, or the equivalent of the selected drug, and be titrated upward until the target symptoms are resolved. See comparative doses in Table 34-2. In patients who are acutely psychotic it is often reasonable to begin doses at a higher level, 600 to 1200 mg of **chlorpromazine** or equivalent. Evidence is not conclusive, but in medication-resistant patients with chronic psychoses, so-called megadose therapy may have some validity. "Low-dose" nonphenothiazine drugs (e.g., **haloperidol**) have been given in very large doses to resistant patients, typically those described as "back ward" chronic patients, but "high-dose" drugs like **chlorpromazine** should not be used in megadose therapy because of their toxicity.

Acute stabilization   In the acute stages of schizophrenia, it is difficult to obtain the patient's cooperation, and intramuscular or oral liquid dosage forms of the psychotropics may be used to initiate therapy. Cooperation should be acquired within 1 to 5 days, when motor excitement and hyperactivity will generally have ceased. Rapid tranquilization has been attempted in many institutions in an attempt to control the acute psychotic patient; antipsychotics are given either intramuscularly or orally at regular intervals (e.g., 5 to 10 mg **haloperidol** IM qh) until improvement is observed.

Within 2 months the patient should begin to interact in daily activities in either the inpatient or the outpatient environment. Complete resolution of symptoms may not have occurred yet, but the patient should have regained enough control that socialization is possible. If this has not occurred, some consideration should be given to increasing the dose of the prescribed drug or switching to a different drug. Although all of the psychotropic drugs are purported to have equivalent antipsychotic effects, it has been observed empirically that some patients respond to one better than to another. Many clinicians believe that it is appropriate to increase a dose to the maximum and maintain that level for several months before switching to another agent.

Maintenance   After initiation of therapy and stabilization of thought disorders, maintenance therapy should begin. Dosage should be slowly decreased in order to find the minimum dose that will control symptoms. A drug-free trial should not be attempted in most cases of newly diagnosed schizophrenia until the illness has been in remission for at least 6 to 8 months. Chronic schizophrenics present a different problem, since the relapse rate is high (greater than 40 percent). Treating this group as maintenance patients indefinitely, without stopping the medication, may be indicated. This preventive measure does not guarantee that the psychotic symptoms will not recur, but the probability is much smaller.

In unreliable patients, long-acting dosage forms like **fluphenazine enanthate** (Prolixin enenthate) or **fluphenazine decanoate** (Prolixin decanoate) are given intramuscularly to facilitate maintenance therapy. Effects from a single injection last 2 to 4 weeks and eliminate the need for patients to take oral medication. Fluphenazine enanthate and fluphenazine decanoate are supplied in solutions with 25 mg/mL. Conversion from oral to intramuscular enanthate or decanoate can be accomplished by rounding the daily oral dose, expressed in equivalent milliliters of injection, up to the next 0.5 mL and administering the IM dose weekly or every 2 weeks. For example, if a patient taking the equivalent of 40 mg of fluphenazine hydrochloride orally each day is to receive the long-acting form, the dosage of the enanthate or

decanoate preparation would be 50 mg IM every 2 weeks (because 40 mg PO = 1.6 mL IM; rounded up to the next 0.5 mL, this is 2.0 mL, and there are 50 mg in 2.0 mL).

If the dosage of a drug is to be reduced, it should be done slowly. This practice prevents the possible rebound symptoms of the psychotic episode, although the rebound phenomenon is not well-explained. Intervals for reduction of dosage should be between 2 weeks and several months, with close observation to identify returning symptoms. Patients should be warned against abruptly discontinuing their medication.

Polydrug therapy   Polydrug therapy is another area which can precipitate problems. A drug should be given at its maximum dosage rather than add additional antipsychotic agents. If the prescribed antipsythotic does not produce resolution of symptoms, a new drug entity should be instituted and the original drug discontinued. Combination use of antipsychotics, antidepressants, or lithium accomplishes nothing more than increasing the side effects, thus complicating therapy and decreasing the patient's compliance.

A precaution in switching from one drug to another is worthy of note. One method that is utilized is to slowly reduce the dose of the undesirable drug while increasing the dosage of the new drug. When the dose of the new drug is at the appropriate level, the first drug can be discontinued.

Drug Administration   Establishing rational dosage schedules of the psychotropic drugs offers the nurse an opportunity to help patients. Traditionally, antipsychotics have been given on a multiple-dose schedule (e.g., qid or q4h). This practice is appropriate for psychotic patients who require the secondary effect of sedation to control agitation and symptomatic motor abnormalities. However, it wastes nursing time, inconveniences patients, decreases compliance, increases the patient's discomfort, and increases the cost of drug therapy. In most cases, multiple doses are unnecessary after the initial 48 to 72 h, and giving one daily dose of the antipsychotic may be possible.

Once-daily dosage is possible because all the psychotropic agents have long half-lives (10 to 20 h). In fact, for most of the psychotropic agents the duration of action is greater than 24 h. Large doses are well-tolerated when given at one time. Bedtime is often the best time of day to administer the total dose of the drug. This allows the patient to take advantage of the sedative effects of the drug and may obviate the need for a hypnotic. Having the side effects occur during the night while the patient is asleep is also an advantage. Patients should be educated concerning once-a-day dosing; many feel that taking the full dose at one time is dangerous.

Since the half-life and the duration of action of the antipsychotic agents are so long, the only purpose that slow-release forms serve is to prolong the sedation, which is usually unwarranted. If some sedation is called for during the day, a fraction of the total dose can be given in the morning.

The routine use of intramuscular preparations for agitated patients is not rational. Many of the injectable pheno-thiazines are painful on injection and may cause sterile abscesses. Oral liquid dosage forms are absorbed almost as fast as the injection and are better accepted by the patient.

NURSING PROCESS RELATED TO SCHIZOPHRENIA

Assessment

The assessment by the psychiatric nurse follows the process of diagnosis generally used by all types of therapists. While nurses in other specialty areas may encounter the psychotic patient in a nonpsychiatric setting, they usually should not attempt to diagnose the problem. However, it is important for them to recognize characteristic symptoms of thinking disturbances during the interview and the mental status examination in order to make appropriate referrals to psychiatric specialists.

Management

While few nurses actually assume responsibility for the adjustment of drug therapy, nearly every nurse may be called upon to monitor the effects of these agents. These effects, both therapeutic and adverse, must be considered in order to arrive at appropriate management goals and specific target symptoms for patients on antipsychotic drugs.

Double-blind studies have shown that patients who take their medications as prescribed or who continue other forms of therapy show a much lower relapse rate. It usually requires considerable effort on the part of the therapist to ensure compliance in patients taking antipsychotics. Education of the patient, rational drug therapy, the patient's trust, and the patient's involvement in his or her outcome are valuable factors in ensuring compliance.

Table 34-5 summarizes the nursing process relative to adverse effects of the antipsychotic drugs.

Evaluation

The evaluation of therapy is facilitated by setting specific goals with respect to target symptoms and the patient's ability to function. Otherwise, "success" may be difficult to define in this complex area.

Detection, prevention, and appropriate approaches to management of the adverse effects of the antipsychotics are an important part of nursing care for all patients receiving these agents.

CASE STUDY

J.D. is a 23-year-old white married female and mother of two. J.D. initially made contact with the mental health center "because," she said, "I am one of God's chosen; I have to bear persecution from the whole world." Her husband stated that her condition had rapidly deteriorated in the last 3 weeks. She lacked both insight and the capacity to make responsible decisions, and relied on religion to take care of all her needs. When things did not work out well for her, she rationalized that it was "God's will" and that she was being punished for her sins and the sins of the world. J.D. cried frequently for no apparent reason. The physician made the diagnosis of acute psychotic episode with secondary depression, admitted the patient to the adult psychiatric unit, and ordered chlorpromazine 100 mg PO initially and q4h for agitation.

Assessment

During the first day the nurse on the psychiatric ward collected the following basic data from the patient and her husband. J.D. is the older of two children of a dominating, critical mother and an irresponsible father. She described her father as a drunkard who didn't support his family, was unpredictable and violent, and engaged in homosexual activities to which she was exposed. Her mother was seen as hard-tempered, restrictive, and threatening. J.D.'s mother imposed strict religious practices upon her children and used threats of the supernatural to control their behavior.

Her parents were divorced when she was 14 years old. Her first sexual experience occurred when she was 11 years old. She was seduced by a 51-year-old man who later paid her for this act. She told her father, but no action was taken. Her development between 11 and 17 was unremarkable. She became extremely dependent on her mother and on her religious activities. She had little or no contact with her father until she was 17, when she quit school and moved in with her father "to find out what he was really like."

At 17 she began to lead a very promiscuous life, suffering from severe guilt feelings about her actions. When J.D. was 19 years old, she married her husband, who is 30 years her senior, after a courtship of 3 weeks. Mr. D. works as a waiter. Their children are a boy and a girl, aged 4 and 2 respectively. Both J.D. and her husband have engaged in numerous extramarital affairs. Her marriage is characterized by fears, unhappiness, infidelity, and remorse. The couple share no common goals, friends, or ideas. J.D.'s friendships are mainly with older women and are superficial in nature.

J.D.'s living conditions are totally inadequate—the entire family lives in a one-room kitchenette apartment. Any attempts on her part to be "a good housewife and

TABLE 34-5 The Nursing Process Related to Adverse Effects of Antipsychotic Drugs

ADVERSE REACTION	ASSESSMENT/EVALUATION	MANAGEMENT
Central Nervous System		
Sedation Impaired motor function Depression	Subjective statement. Activity level, participation in environment. No. of hours asleep/24 h. Reaction time, dexterity in performing tasks (threading needle, craft project, etc.). Review concurrent medication for other sedating drugs. Liver function; history of liver disease. Prior seizure history.	Encourage active participation in environment. Do not allow isolation. Suicide precautions for depression. Patient education: avoid concurrent alcohol, other CNS depressants. Caution against driving or working around machinery until drug effects are evaluated.
Lowered seizure threshold	History of seizures.	Avoid antipsychotics or use prophylactic anticonvulsants.
Autonomic Nervous System		
Dry mouth	Subjective statement.	Frequent sips of water. Good oral hygiene. Suck on sugar-free candy, chew sugar-free gum, or use artificial saliva.
Dental caries	Examine mouth for caries, condition of mucous membranes.	Dental examination every 6 months.
Hypotension Tachycardia	Age; history of cardiovascular disease. Subjective statement of palpitations, dizziness, syncope. Pulse, blood pressure lying and standing. Review concurrent medications for other hypotensives.	Patient education: take medication at bedtime. Arise slowly from lying, sitting, squatting. Use support stockings. Report palpitations, syncope. Safety precautions to prevent falls. Levarterenol for hypotensive crisis. Lie flat ½–1 h with parenteral dose; give deep IM and massage site well. Do not mix other drugs in same syringe.
Constipation Paralytic ileus	Auscultate bowel sounds; inspect and palpate abdomen for masses, distention, etc. Record of bowel movements; prior history.	Prevent by high-bulk diet, fluids, activity, use of stool softener. Patient education: how to prevent. Principles of bowel hygiene. Report constipation. May slow absorption of drugs.
Urinary hesitancy or retention	Subjective statement. Age. History of benign prostatic hypertrophy. Palpate prostate; percuss bladder for distention. Fluid intake and output; frequency of voiding.	Reduce dose or stop antipsychotic. Elderly men stand to void; adequate fluids. Catheter for severe distention. Phenothiazines may color urine reddish or brown.
Blurred vision	Subjective statement. History of glaucoma. Differentiate from toxic effects (oculocutaneous pigmentation, retinopathy).	Orient to environment; adequate light. Teach to avoid driving if vision blurred. Take precautions for patient's safety. Use antipsychotic with caution in patient at risk for acute angle closure glaucoma.
Rhinitis	Subjective statement of nasal stuffiness. Examine nasal mucosa.	If severe, may require nasal decongestant (phenylephrine). Explain cause of rhinitis.
Neurologic		
Dystonias	Age (usually children). Spasms of eyes, neck, jaw, shoulder, back muscles.	Prevent accidental poisoning by proper storage. Conservative treatment, withdraw drug. Administer diphenhydramine.
Tardive dyskinesia	Hyperkinesia of mouth, choreiform and athetoid movements. History of organic brain lesions. Early recognition.	Prevent by using lowest effective dose. May be irreversible. Stopping antipsychotic may help.
Akathisia	Insomnia, pacing, constant movement.	Trial of antiparkinsonian drug. Stop antipsychotic drug or reduce dose.
Pseudoparkinsonism	Rigidity, dyskinesia, tremor, masklike facies, shuffle, loss of associative movements.	Tolerance often develops after weeks. Antiparkinsonian drug for several weeks. Take measures for patient's safety. Explain cause and transient nature.

TABLE 34-5 The Nursing Process Related to Adverse Effects of Antipsychotic Drugs (*Cont.*)

ADVERSE REACTION	ASSESSMENT/EVALUATION	MANAGEMENT
Cardiovascular		
ECG changes Cardiac irregularities	Baseline and periodic ECG; flattening of T wave. Heart sounds, pulse—note arrhythmias. History of heart disease, arrhythmia.	Sudden onset of tachyarrhythmia may require cardiopulmonary resuscitation.
Hematologic		
Leukopenia Agranulocytosis	Periodic complete blood count. Note bruising, bleeding; lethargy; mouth sores.	Stop drug if white blood count below 3500/mm^3. Teach to report bruising, bleeding, increased weakness and fatigue, sore mouth or throat. Vigorous therapy required if infection occurs.
Dermatologic		
Maculopapular rashes	Involves most of body. Nonfatal.	Discontinue drug immediately.
Ophthalmic		
Oculocutaneous pigmentation Photosensitivity	Gray or purplish skin. Blurred vision; normal acuity. Slit-lamp ophthalmoscopy. Sunburn on exposed areas.	Avoid sunbaths, exposure to sun. Wear long sleeves, hat, gloves. Change drugs for ocular involvement.
Pigmentary retinopathy	Impaired acuity. Pigment deposits on retina on ophthalmoscopy.	Stop or change drug. May cause blindness if not detected.
Hepatobiliary		
Cholestatic jaundice	Laboratory tests show liver obstruction. Jaundice. Subjective statement of pruritus, malaise, nausea.	Stop or change drug. Symptomatic treatment.
Metabolic and Endocrine		
Weight gain	Baseline and periodic weights.	Proper diet and exercise. Support and reassurance.
Lactation Menstrual abnormalities	Serum (not urine) test for pregnancy if indicated by age, history, symptoms. Examine breasts for masses.	Explain and reassure. Birth control continued. Gynecologic checkups annually or semiannually.
Gynecomastia (male)	Subjective statement. Examine breasts.	Stop or change drug.
Decreased libido Failure to achieve orgasm	Subjective statement of patient or partner.	Explain transient nature. Support and reassurance. Stop or change drug.

mother'' are frustrated by the conditions in which she lives.

The medical history and the physical examination revealed no physical abnormalities. J.D. is thin, weighing 15 lb under her normal weight. The mental status examination revealed the following: vacillates in attitudes toward others; relates in a timid manner; shows some rigidity in manners and in current thought; is well-oriented; has attention lapses, preferential ideas, hallucinations, and a poor level of abstraction. The patient's clothing was dirty and unkempt. Her husband indicated she had not been eating, drinking, sleeping, or bathing herself or the children.

The nurse made the following nursing diagnosis: depressive affect, irrational fears (of storms, of being alone), and poor personal hygiene.

Management

The initial oral dose of chlorpromazine was administered and J.D. was instructed that the medication might make her sleep. She was encouraged to sleep as much as possible on the day of admission, since rest and fluids were priority needs. Plans were established to reevaluate J.D.'s needs in 24 h, in order to discourage isolation and withdrawal. The PRN chlorpromazine was administered three or four times daily.

The nurse temporarily assumed the responsibility of assisting the patient with personal hygiene and also instituted measures that also could prevent the adverse effects of the chlorpromazine. J.D. was offered at least 8 oz of juice or water with each dose of the medication and every hour when awake. Because of potential dizziness, the patient was assisted to the bathroom, and staff recorded intake and output, as well as frequency of urination and bowel movements. Food was offered, but she was not forced to eat. The nursing staff observed the patient every half hour, recording her symptoms on a flow sheet.

Blood pressure was measured twice daily in lying and standing positions. The patient was observed for abdominal distention, tremor, or abnormal movements at these times. Daily weights were taken.

J.D. was encouraged to participate in ward activities and group discussions. However, she would discuss her problems only with the staff. The nurse referred the husband to the social worker for assistance in locating child care agencies during J.D.'s hospitalization. The medication was explained to J.D. and she was taught how to prevent or minimize side effects, and what to report to her therapist on discharge.

Evaluation

J.D.'s psychotic symptoms cleared rapidly and there was a marked and noticeable change at the end of 72 h. Her personal hygiene rapidly improved and she soon assumed responsibility for her hygiene and nutrition. Although her depressive symptoms improved as the psychosis cleared,

J.D. still evidenced some depression. Perhaps thioridazine or haloperidol might have been a better drug for J.D., since these exert less depressive effects than chlorpromazine.

The ward milieu was an effective treatment agent for this patient. She interacted easily with other patients and seemed to gain some insight into her own behavior through her association with them. She was willing and cooperative in participating in ward activities and discussions.

Four days after the initiation of pharmacotherapy, J.D. began to exhibit restlessness and inability to concentrate. She also complained of an inability to sleep, even with a sedating medication. When asked to sit, J.D. moved her legs and feet constantly. It was suspected that she was experiencing extrapyramidal symptoms, and trihexyphenidyl (Artane) therapy was initiated, 2 mg twice a day. The symptoms cleared in 24 h.

Blood pressure remained stable. No problems with elimination or orthostatic hypotension were noted. Dry mouth was present, but was controlled by frequent sips of water.

Eight days after admission, J.D. was discharged to the day care center of the mental health center, with a prescription for chlorpromazine 300 mg at bedtime and trihexyphenidyl 2 mg daily. Group therapy, to assist J.D. in dealing more effectively with her low self-concept, and couples therapy with her husband, to allow them to begin dealing with their marital difficulties, were part of the discharge plan.

ANXIETY

Anxiety may be a symptom of many illnesses or disorders, including the psychoses and affective disorders, as well as many organic illnesses. Manifestations of anxiety are familiar to everyone and in most circumstances cannot be considered pathologic. Common symptoms include shakiness, tension, muscle aches, restlessness, sweating, clammy hands, dry mouth, dizziness, upset stomach, flushing, worry, rumination, anticipation of misfortune, difficulty in concentrating, insomnia, and irritability. These symptoms become pathologic when social or occupational functioning is impaired.

Two major diagnostic categories hallmarked by anxiety include adjustment disorders and anxiety disorders. If an individual with a relatively healthy personality develops symptoms of anxiety as a result of extreme environmental stress, the diagnosis is likely to be an "adjustment disorder." Such stress could be associated, for example, with war, natural disasters (flood, earthquake, fire), and rape. "Anxiety disorders" refer to the development of anxiety symptoms in

a basically unhealthy personality. Anxiety disorders are subdivided into several categories (see Table 34-6).

Clinical Pharmacology and Therapeutics of Anxiety

Drug therapy for the symptoms of anxiety is palliative and does not cure the underlying psychopathology. The antianxiety agents as a class are the most commonly prescribed drugs in this country. Surveys conducted several years ago indicated that 15 percent of the adult population in the United States takes one of this group of drugs to treat anxiety. The overwhelming majority of the drugs are prescribed by medical practitioners not involved in psychiatry or neurology.

Nonpharmacologic forms of therapy should constitute the primary treatment plan for patients suffering from anxiety. Efforts are made to uncover the characteristic mechanisms that the patient has utilized to handle unpleasant experiences, and his or her present emotional state (e.g., anxiety and/or depression). As therapy continues, patients gain insight into their behavior patterns and can use this information to form new methods of coping with life's experiences.

Some patients experience such trauma and pain from the symptoms of anxiety that the benefits of nonpharmacologic treatment are difficult to obtain. The form of nonpharmacologic treatment itself may create additional anxiety, preventing patients from coping with their problems. Under such circumstances, drug therapy is indicated.

TABLE 34-6 Categories of Anxiety Disorders

CATEGORY	DESCRIPTION
Phobic disorders	Persistent and irrational fear of object or situation despite recognition that it is of no real danger. Characterized by anxiety, apprehension, feeling of impending disaster, and even panic.
Panic disorder	Recurrent episodes of anxiety that occur unpredictably; however, they may be associated with certain situations. Sudden onset of intense apprehension, fear, or terror, often associated with feelings of impending doom, characterize this disorder.
Generalized anxiety disorder	Essential feature of persistent unremitting anxiety of long duration. Symptoms include signs of motor tension, autonomic hyperactivity, apprehension and vigilance, and scanning.
Obsessive-compulsive disorder	Recurrent thoughts or compulsion to perform ritualized acts to decrease anxiety, in spite of the fact that they are purposeless or unreasonable.
Posttraumatic stress disorder	Resultant from experiencing psychologically traumatic event outside the range of usual human experience. Hallmark of the disorder include numbing of responsiveness to or reduced involvement with the external world, a variety of autonomic, dysphoric, or cognitive symptoms.

Indications for Drug Treatment

Anxiety symptoms resulting from generalized anxiety, panic, and posttraumatic stress disorders (see Table 34-6) can be relieved by antianxiety agents, but they generally remit promptly without drug treatment. If distress continues and is severe, drug treatment is certainly indicated and will often facilitate attempts at psychotherapy; pharmacologic therapy should be terminated as soon as the acute symptoms are controlled. The use of antianxiety agents in the treatment of anxiety resulting from phobic or obsessive-compulsive disorders is of little or no benefit. Tricyclic antidepressants may be more helpful for these individuals.

Whenever antianxiety drugs are used in the treatment of anxiety, assessment of their efficacy should be based on the alleviation of *target symptoms* of anxiety. Examples of target symptoms include muscular tension, restlessness, tremor, excessive perspiration, fatigue, insomnia, and sexual dysfunction. If the patient's condition worsens, it may be that the medication is exacerbating the problem.

Pharmacologic Agents

A number of agents are used to treat anxiety: benzodiazepines, barbiturates, propanediol carbamates, antipsychotics, tricyclic antidepressants, antihistamines, and β-adrenergic blocking agents (see Table 34-7). Because of the chemical dissimilarities of these drugs, we will discuss each group individually after a discussion of their common mechanisms of action.

All these drugs exert their action by lessening learned avoidance responses or by diminishing anticipatory responses to external or imagined danger or to unpleasant situations. Each of these clinical classes, except the β-adrenergic blockers, possesses general *central nervous system depressant effects* which partially account for their antianxiety effects. With the advent of the benzodiazepines, however, it has become evident that the antianxiety effects are independent of sedative effects, although the locus of the pharmacologic action, beyond the immediate sedation, is not yet definable. Ideally, an antianxiety agent should reduce or eliminate a patient's symptoms without causing drowsiness or impairment of psychomotor function.

Benzodiazepines

Benzodiazepine derivatives (listed in Table 34-7) are among the most widely used drugs in clinical medicine today. One study reported that 30 percent of all hospitalized patients receive one member of this group, **diazepam** (Valium). There are many reasons for its popularity, including efficacy, wide margin of safety, and acceptance by patients. Benzodiazepines are the most efficacious group of drugs in the treatment of anxiety.

The benzodiazepines have many other clinical uses besides the treatment of anxiety. They are used as muscle relaxants, anticonvulsants, hypnotics, and in the treatment of alcohol withdrawal.

Mechanism of Action The precise mechanism of action of the benzodiazepine derivatives is not known. It is proposed that these agents enhance γ-aminobutyric acid (GABA) activity. GABA potentiation at presynaptic nerve endings and via postsynaptic influence causes muscle relaxation; anticonvulsant effects by a general inhibiting effect; and arousal-lowering by effects on the catecholamine-activating system in the brain. The influence on the catecholamines in the higher centers of the brain (cerebral cortex) may account for the specific antianxiety effects of the benzodiazepines. Evidence indicates that their anxiolytic effects seem to be more specific than the effects of barbiturates and other central nervous system depressants. Furthermore, the effects are not completely dependent on sedation, as they are with antihistamines, propanediol carbamates, and barbiturates, since the benzodiazepines suppress anxiety for extended periods beyond their initial sedative effects. In comparison to other agents, the benzodiazepines do not sig-

nificantly alter normal sleep patterns (during a short course of therapy). Benzodiazepines raise the seizure threshold (anticonvulsant properties).

Pharmacokinetics The primary differences between the benzodiazepines are reflected in the way they are absorbed, distributed, and metabolized. Table 34-8 lists the differences in these benzodiazepine properties. Figure 34-1 reflects the biotransformation pathways of the benzodiazepines; many available benzodiazepines are either precursors or metabolites of desmethyldiazepam. Benzodiazepines metabolized to desmethyldiazepam or other active metabolites generally have long durations of action. Those metabolized by conjugation and those lacking active metabolites generally have short durations of action and do not tend to accumulate.

Chlordiazepoxide (Librium) This drug is well-absorbed from the gastrointestinal (GI) tract, with total absorption in an hour. Blood levels peak 2 to 4 h after oral administration. Intramuscular administration is not recommended because of unpredictable, incomplete absorption and pain at the

TABLE 34-7 Antianxiety Agents

NONPROPRIETARY NAME	TRADE NAME	INITIAL SINGLE ADULT DOSE, mg	USUAL RANGE DAILY DOSAGE, mg
Benzodiazepines			
Alprazolam	Xanax	0.5	0.5–1.5
Chlordiazepoxide HCl	Librium	10	20–60
Chlordiazepoxide	Libritabs		
Clorazepate dipotassium	Tranxene	7.5	15–60
Diazepam	Valium	5	5–40
Flurazepam	Dalmane	15	15–30
Halazepam	Paxipam	60	80–160
Lorazepam	Ativan	1	20–60
Oxazepam	Serax	10	30–90
Prazepam	Centrax, Verstran	20	20–60
Temazepam	Restoril	15	15–30
Triazolam	Halcion	0.25	0.125–0.5
Barbiturates			
Phenobarbital, sodium	Luminal	15	45–200
Butabarbital, sodium	Butisol	15	45–200
Amobarbital, sodium	Amytal	65	45–200
β-Adrenergic Blockers			
Propranolol HCl	Inderal	10	30–120
Propanediol Carbamates			
Meprobamate	Equanil, Miltown, and others	600	400–1200
Tybamate	Solacen, Tybatran	500	500–1500
Antihistamines			
Hydroxyzine HCl	Atarax	25	25–150
Hydroxyzine pamoate	Vistaril	25	25–150

TABLE 34-8 Pharmacokinetic Profile of Benzodiazepines*

DRUG	ELIMINATION HALF-LIFE, h	PEAK BLOOD LEVEL, h	PERCENT BOUND†
Alprazolam	12–15	1	80
Chlordiazepoxide	5–30	2–4	98
Clorazepate	24–200	1	NA
Diazepam	20–50	1	75
Flurazepam	50–100	1	NA
Halazepam	14	2	NA
Lorazepam	10–20	3	NA
Oxazepam	5–20	4	NA
Prazepam	24–200	1	NA
Temazepam	10–15	2–3	NA
Triazolam	2.7–4.5	1–1.5	89

*See Fig. 34-1 for metabolites.
†NA = Not available.

injection site. A long-acting benzodiazepine, chlordiazepoxide is stored in adipose tissue, bound to plasma protein, and slowly released. This accounts for the traces of drug that can be found in the urine long after discontinuation of the drug. The half-life of chlordiazepoxide is 5 to 30 h. It exerts clinical effects for 12 to 24 h after administration of a single dose. After prolonged use, the half-life and clinical effect are extended. Chlordiazepoxide is metabolized in the liver and excreted via the urine as a glucuronide conjugate. The metabolites are as active as the parent compound (see Fig. 34-1); therefore, cumulative effects can be produced by repeated administration. Elderly patients and those with

hepatic dysfunction require close monitoring and possibly reduced dosages.

Because of the long half-life, frequent administration is not necessary; one or two doses daily often prove sufficient. With chlordiazepoxide and other long-acting benzodiazepines it may be advantageous to prescribe a small dose in the early part of the day and the remainder of the total daily dose at bedtime, taking advantage of the drug's sedative-hypnotic effects.

Diazepam (Valium) This drug is more rapidly absorbed than chlordiazepoxide and clinical effects can usually be demonstrated within 30 min. Peak serum levels are reached faster and the half-life is longer than with chlordiazepoxide. The duration of clinical effect, dosage administration, and problems from active metabolite accumulation are similar to those of chlordiazepoxide. Intramuscular administration is not recommended as it results in peak serum levels that are significantly lower than from oral administration; IV use gives excellent results.

Oxazepam (Serax) and Temazepam (Restoril) Oxazepam is a metabolite of diazepam. It is absorbed well from the GI tract, yielding a peak plasma level in about 4 h. The half-life of oxazepam is 3 to 20 h, with the clinical effects correspondingly shorter-lived than those of diazepam. Due to this shorter half-life, more frequent administration is necessary. There are no active metabolites or cumulative effects. Oxazepam and other drugs with no active metabolites are preferable when patients with impaired liver function require treatment for anxiety. Temazepam is a precur-

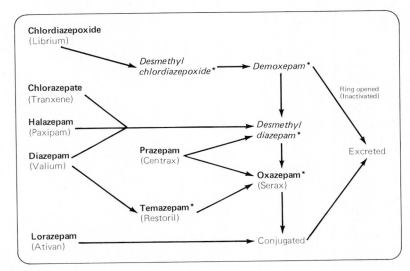

FIGURE 34-1

Metabolic Pathways of Some Benzodiazepines. Note that diazepam (Valium), chlordizepoxide (Librium), and others are metabolized to various active metabolites (*), whereas oxazepam (Serax) and lorezepam (Ativan) have no active metabolites.

sor of oxazepam (see Fig. 34-1), and has been marketed as a hypnotic. Since it has a relatively short half-life and no active metabolites, it is expected to cause few problems with hangover. Temazepam reaches peak blood levels in 2 to 3 h and may not assist patients experiencing difficulty with sleep latency.

Lorazepam (Ativan)   Lorazepam is similar to oxazepam in its pharmacokinetic properties. Lorazepam's longer half-life is the primary difference.

Clorazepate (Tranxene) and Prazepam (Centrax)   These drugs are precursors of desmethyldiazepam. As noted in Table 34-8, both of these agents have long half-lives and active metabolites similar to diazepam. Clorazepate must be hydrolyzed in the stomach to desmethyldiazepam before reaching the systemic circulation. Prazepam is slowly absorbed and must be dealkylated by the liver to desmethyl-diazepam to be active. Clinical efficacy of these agents is identical to diazepam; however, prazepam, due to its slow absorption, is not a good choice for a hypnotic.

Triazolobenzodiazepine Derivatives   **Alprazolam** (Xanax) and **triazolam** (Halcion) are relatively new antianxiety/hypnotic agents. Alprazolam's pharmacokinetic properties are not significantly different from those of previously mentioned benzodiazepines; however, alprazolam may possess antidepressant properties in addition to antianxiety effects. The antidepressant effects of alprazolam require more investigation. Triazolam is a unique benzodiazepine due to its extremely short half-life and absence of active metabolites. Triazolam has either no active metabolites or insignificant metabolites, making it a good choice as a hypnotic. The lack of active metabolites and the shorter half-lives of alprazolam and triazolam prevent the hangover and psychomotor retardation that result from longer-acting agents.

Adverse Effects   Remarkably, the benzodiazepines exhibit few adverse effects. Drowsiness or ataxia is commonly reported, particularly with **diazepam**. Psychomotor retardation and hangover are common side effects. Tolerance to drowsiness, ataxia, psychomotor retardation, and hangover can be expected but may require reducing the dose or switching to an agent with a different pharmacokinetic profile. Paradoxic insomnia, hyperexcitability, hyperactivity, increased agitation, rage, and hostility may develop after the initial administration. These resemble alcohol-induced paradoxic reactions. Some authorities believe the drugs "disinhibit" the defense mechanism and allow patients to release their feelings. **Chlordiazepoxide** has been associated with these reactions most frequently. Psychotic episodes and the number of suicidal attempts have been exacerbated after administration of these drugs, but generally with higher than usual doses.

Headache, vertigo, and dizziness are reactions that seem to be dose-related and are most common in the geriatric population. Mental confusion and slurred speech may be an indication to decrease the dose. Autonomic side effects are not common, but can occur especially in the debilitated patient; these include mild hypotension, dry mouth, constipation, retarded ejaculation, and sexual impotence. Hematologic problems (agranulocytosis) are rare, but have occurred, and are similar to those of the barbiturates. Weight gain has been attributed to these drugs, but whether the drugs cause an endocrine disturbance or whether the weight gain results from increased appetite due to the improvement of the patient's outlook is not known. Amenorrhea is common with the use of the benzodiazepines; however, this can generally be alleviated by dose reduction. The safety of benzodiazepines during pregnancy has not been established; therefore, benzodiazepines should be avoided during pregnancy. Secretion into breast milk has been established and often causes the nursing infant to be sluggish and slow to feed.

One of the factors that has encouraged the use of benzodiazepines has been their low suicide potential. However, an increasing number of fatalities from overdoses of benzodiazepines as single agents have occurred. Fatalities from the combination of benzodiazepines and alcohol or other CNS depressants are common. Clinicians should monitor the patient's compliance in taking these drugs as prescribed. Prescription refills without reevaluation should be avoided. Few people benefit from long-term benzodiazepine therapy.

Patients tend to develop tolerance quickly to the sedative and euphoric effects of the benzodiazepines. Tolerance to the clinical effect on anxiety does not occur, but physical dependence does develop and is quite common. Since some of the benzodiazepines have long half-lives, a withdrawal syndrome may not appear for 1 week after cessation of therapy. Evidence of a withdrawal syndrome can be seen after a relatively short course of therapy employing dosages within the normal range. Symptoms seen in this case are usually short-lived and benign.

Barbiturates

Use of this group of drugs for anxiety should be historical in contemporary medical practice. Unfortunately, they are still used. Overall, the pharmacologic effect is that of generalized central nervous system depression with a large sedative component. Studies comparing the barbiturates with placebos have shown them to have little or no effect upon anxiety. Efficacy tends to be highly variable and often unsatisfactory.

Some of the problems associated with their use are an unacceptable daytime drowsiness and somnolence that interferes with the patient's daily routine; a rapid addiction potential; depressive symptoms that complicate the treatment of anxiety; and a potential for suicide from overdose that is greater than with other agents. Further, barbiturates induce hepatic microsomal enzymes, which can accelerate the metabolism of other drugs metabolized in the liver; they are tightly bound to plasma proteins and displace other drugs; and they significantly alter rapid eye movement (REM) sleep, leaving the patient fatigued and "hung over" after their use, especially with long-term therapy.

All of these problems make barbiturates unacceptable for treating anxiety. Their only advantage is their low cost, which is greatly outweighed by the potential problems, some of which are life-threatening (see also Chaps. 22 and 37, since barbiturates are also used in sleep disturbances and as anesthetics).

Propanediol Carbamates

Characteristic of the group of propanediol carbamates are **meprobamate** (Equanil, Miltown) and **Tybamate** (Solacen). The drugs of this group were the first nonbarbiturates used to treat anxiety. The effectiveness of the benzodiazepines has rendered these compounds obsolete, and research has demonstrated questionable efficacy as antianxiety agents. Normal therapeutic doses of the drugs tend to impair learning, motor coordination, and reaction time. REM sleep is suppressed by the propanediol carbamates, as by the barbiturates, leaving the patient with a barbiturate type of hangover on arising, which may result in further anxiety and depression. Meprobamate is commonly used as a muscle relaxant, but controlled clinical trials do not substantiate beneficial results.

Pharmacokinetics Propanediol carbamates are well-absorbed from the gastrointestinal tract. **Meprobamate** exhibits peak blood levels in 1 to 3 h, while **tybamate** reaches its peak somewhat faster. Onset of action is therefore intermediate, usually in less than 1 h. The plasma half-life of meprobamate is about 10 h; tybamate has a short half-life of 3 h. These drugs are distributed throughout the body. Propanediol carbamates cross the placental barrier and are present in the umbilical cord at levels close to maternal levels. Birth defects have been associated with their use during the first and third trimester of pregnancy. Respiratory depression at birth has also been a problem in infants. The drugs are present in the milk of nursing mothers at concentrations two to four times maternal blood levels.

Elimination of these drugs from the body is via metabolism by the liver. Metabolites are excreted in the urine in an inactive form. Theoretically at least, the drugs speed up their own metabolism by inducing hepatic microsomal enzymes. It is known that metabolism of other drugs (e.g., **warfarin**) is altered.

Adverse Effects Major problems with propanediol carbamates include sleepiness and ataxia. Hypotension appears frequently in the geriatric population, and is especially prominent upon initiation of therapy. Allergic reactions occur in about 3 percent of patients, who appear to be predisposed to dermatologic problems. Urticaria and erythematous rashes have occurred with the use of meprobamate.

Hematologic side effects include acute nonthrombocytopenic purpura and agranulocytosis; patients taking one of the propanediol carbamates who present with unexplained bruises and fever should be evaluated carefully for these hematologic problems.

Tolerance and physical dependence occur with these drugs, as with the barbiturates. The margin of safety and the therapeutic dosage range are extremely narrow when compared with the benzodiazepines. Tolerance to the antianxiety effect develops rapidly; patients will often increase the dose to obtain the desired effect. Physical dependence has been demonstrated at the upper end of the dosage range.

Patients taking doses of 1600 to 2000 mg of **meprobamate** have experienced delirium and convulsions upon withdrawal. Symptoms generally begin to occur 36 to 48 h after termination. When patients learn of the drug's addiction potential, they often stop taking it themselves, producing the abstinence phenomenon (agitation, insomnia, and tachycardia). (**Tybamate** has *not* been associated with this phenomenon.) Clinicians should encourage patients to taper the dose of meprobamate.

Suicide potential is great with the propanediol carbamates. Suicide has been successful with a 12-g dose of meprobamate. Deep coma is associated with plasma levels of 100 to 200 μg/mL and respiratory collapse generally ensues with plasma levels over 200 μg/mL.

Antipsychotics

The use of the antipsychotic agents for the treatment of anxiety is a source of much controversy. In certain situations these agents may be more useful than others: in anxious and agitated geriatric patients; anxious persons who have a high degree of distractibility, racing thoughts, or periods of thought blocking; obsessional patients with strong imaginations, marginal thinking, and poor reality testing; and in patients for whom other antianxiety regimens have failed. In essence, the patients who fit these criteria often seem prepsychotic or borderline psychotic. In these cases, anxiolytic drugs only complicate the problems or will not control symptoms.

All of the antipsychotics listed in Table 34-2 have been utilized for treating anxiety. The most popular drugs are the oral forms of **chlorpromazine** and **thioridazine**, in doses starting at 10 to 25 mg tid, increased slowly until symptoms are controlled. If the dose must be increased beyond 75 to 100 mg of chlorpromazine (or its equivalent), the patient's diagnosis should be reevaluated.

Antipsychotic drugs should be avoided, if possible, in the treatment of anxiety. Generally this group of drugs should be second-choice and should not precede a trial of a benzodiazepine. Even at low doses, side effects are common, especially in the elderly. Antipsychotics can also create further agitation and confusion. Tolerance and physical dependence do not develop, perhaps supplying a rationale for their use in patients prone to dependency. Reliable clinical trials have not substantiated efficacy superior to the benzodiazepines. The pharmacokinetics, adverse effects, and nursing process of antipsychotics were discussed earlier in this chapter.

Antihistamines

The antihistamines should also be reserved as second-choice agents in anxiety. Since the introduction of the benzodiazepine derivatives, the use of antihistamine drugs has decreased in use. The most commonly used of this group are **hydroxyzine hydrochloride** (Atarax) and **hydroxyzine pamoate** (Vistaril). Both of these drugs have less severe anticholinergic effects that the other antihistamines and a greater sedative effect. These agents have been useful as sedative-hypnotic agents owing to this sedative property, but more effective agents are now available. Many nonprescription antianxiety products contain an antihistamine in a low dose. Generally, these are more hypnotic than antianxiety agents and are worthless in the treatment of anxiety. The antianxiety effects of antihistamines are due to the secondary pharmacologic effects of nonspecific CNS depression. No specific effect beyond this mechanism has been demonstrated, and their use as antianxiety agents has little rationale. The only definite indications for their use as an antianxiety agent is in treating anxiety associated with pruritic dermatoses. Certain patients who are predisposed to physical dependence may be offered some benefit from the use of these drugs, since tolerance and physical dependence do not develop with the antihistamine drugs.

Side effects are prominent with these agents. Anticholinergic effects much like those described for the antipsychotic agents are the most frequent and troublesome.

Antidepressants

Imipramine and **amitriptyline**, in low doses, are the antidepressants most widely used for their antianxiety effects. No proven efficacy of one tricyclic antidepressant (TCAD) over another has been demonstrated for this purpose, and benzodiazepines are more efficacious in the treatment of anxiety. The use of the tricyclic antidepressants should be almost exclusively reserved for the treatment of affective disorders.

It is not known whether the antianxiety effects of antidepressants are due only to the general depressant effects on the CNS or whether a specific antianxiety effect exists. Some clinical trials indicate that the antidepressants are useful for treating patients with panic attacks due to phobic anxiety. This condition is not very common and the reliability of the small clinical trials is questionable. Phobic anxiety, whether from school phobia, acrophobia, or any other phobias, responds poorly to any pharmacotherapy. Behavioral modification techniques give results much faster and are a much more acceptable treatment, especially in children. Monoamine oxidase inhibitors have been used with some success in the phobias. Side effects, toxicity, and pharmacokinetics of antidepressants will be discussed below in the section on affective disorders.

β-Adrenergic Blocking Agents

These agents, of which **propranolol** (Inderal) was the first available in the United States, represent an alternative pharmacologic approach for treating anxiety disorders. Many of the somatic manifestations of anxiety may result from excess β-adrenergic activity. Peripheral somatic manifestations of anxiety such as tachycardia, palpitation, tremor, and hyperventilation improve with the use of propranolol. The drug's effects are attributable to its peripheral β-adrenergic antagonism and not to its CNS effects.

Presumably there are no criteria for the utilization of propranolol in the treatment of anxiety, and its use must be considered investigational. Patients with diabetes, congestive heart failure, asthma, or obstructive lung disease should never be given propranolol in the treatment of anxiety.

NURSING PROCESS RELATED TO ANXIETY

The nursing process in neurotic anxiety is summarized in Table 34-9.

CASE STUDY

M.E., a 24-year-old woman, was brought to the emergency room by the police after she was sexually assaulted by two men.

Assessment

The ER nurse obtained the following information from the patient: M.E. was employed as an assistant buyer for a large department store located in a suburban shopping center. About 9:30 P.M., as she was leaving work and going to her car parked in the underground lot, she was suddenly confronted by two men, one of whom was armed with a knife. At knifepoint, M.E. was forced into the back seat of their car, blindfolded, and forced to lie on the floor of the car while she was driven to another location. She had no idea where she was taken; she believes the men drove around in an effort to confuse her. She was taken into an apartment where she was sexually assaulted by both men for approximately the next 3 h. During the course of the sexual assault M.E. was struck several times in the face by one of the men. She suffered numerous lacerations on the face, including one on the eyelid and one below the left eye, both requiring sutures.

TABLE 34-9 Overview of Nursing Process Related to Treatment of Anxiety

ASSESSMENT	MANAGEMENT	EVALUATION
	General Aspects	
Assess predisposing and precipitating factors. Symptoms and amount of interference with normal activities (e.g., phobias, compulsions, physical symptoms, amnesia, sleep disturbances, etc.). Distinguish category and type of anxiety.	Many anxiety reactions resolve spontaneously. Nondrug therapy: supportive relationships, group therapy, psychoanalysis, etc. Drug therapy useful for generalized anxiety, panic, and posttraumatic disorders.	Alleviation of target symptoms (e.g., muscular tension, restlessness, tremor, excess perspiration, fatigue, insomnia, sexual dysfunction).
	Related to Antianxiety Drugs	
Elderly or debilitated may have increased drug reactions. Elderly, those with psychotic history, or patients subjected to extreme pain or stimulation may have paradoxical reaction. Check for impaired hepatic and renal function. Note any concurrent administration of CNS depressants or drugs whose metabolism is altered if liver enzymes are induced propanediols and barbiturates only. Allergy to other sedative-type drugs, pregnancy, lactation require caution. Previous dermatologic problems (propanediols only). Caution should be exercised when using β blockers in the following: pregnancy and lactation, depressed patients, chronic obstructive pulmonary disease, asthma, and congestive heart failure.	Wean from antianxiety drug; avoid abrupt withdrawal. Instruct to avoid driving or operating machinery if drugs cause dizziness, drowsiness, impaired performance. Teach to avoid concurrent use of other CNS depressants, alcohol. Parenteral benzodiazepines: IV may cause phlebitis. Do not mix with other drugs or save previously prepared drug. Have patient remain recumbent after injection; assist with ambulation if unstable or dizzy. Diazepam, chlordiazepoxide, clorazepate, lorazepam, prazepam, paxipam, and alprazolam have long half-lives, may be given twice daily.	See above. Drowsiness may be cumulative; watch for increasing ataxia, somnolence, or "hangover." Carefully evaluate for drug abuse, suicide potential. Withdrawal state: Convulsions, agitation may occur up to 1 week after abruptly stopping long-acting benzodiazepines; sooner after other drugs. Check for hypotension. All effects increased if taking another CNS depressant concurrently. Other adverse reactions include headache, dizziness, orthostatic hypotension, allergic rashes and weight gain. Blood dyscrasias: periodic complete blood count, bruising, sore throat, mouth sores.

She also sustained several superficial lacerations on her hands and forearms.

In the ER, M.E. was assigned a registered nurse who would stay with her, provide emotional support, explain procedures, and answer any questions. The nurse also contacted the local sexual assault center at M.E.'s request and asked that a victim advocate be sent to the hospital. M.E.'s emotional response at this point was dull and flat, indicating that she was in a state of emotional shock. M.E. was examined and her injuries were treated. When all the medical procedures were completed, she went home, accompanied by three friends, who had been called at the patient's request. The discharge planning for M.E. included a return appointment with the plastic surgeon and instructions for contacting the sexual assault center.

Assessment

The following day M.E. contacted the sexual assault center and received information about a weekly support group for rape victims. The next group would meet on the following night. The next night, M.E. attended the support group and became very agitated and upset as she related the details of her assault. She stated that she had not eaten or slept since the assault and was so frightened she would not have attended the group if two friends had not accompanied her. The registered nurse group facilitator assessed M.E.'s reaction and determined that she could go home after the group and contact the nurse at the mental health center the next day.

The next day M.E. came to the mental health center after contacting the nurse by phone. The data base included sleep pattern disturbances, eating pattern disturbances, symptoms specific to the focus of the attack, plus an emotional response of feeling ashamed, guilty, and extreme fear, fear of physical injury, mutilation, and death. M.E. exhibited an acute stress reaction (acute posttraumatic stress disorder) secondary to the assault. She had not been to work since the assault. At this point she was feeling exhausted from the lack of sleep and poor nutrition and hydration of the last several days. The nurse, in consultation with the psychiatrist, suggested that diazepam 10 mg qid be ordered for M.E. for specific target symptoms of insomnia and extreme fear. Also the nurse explained the side effects of the drug and cautioned the patient about driving a car, ingesting alcohol, and taking any other medications without checking with the nurse. The follow-up plans included (1) short-term issue-oriented crisis intervention with the mental health nurse, (2) continued attendance at the victim support group, (3) medication as ordered. Another appointment was scheduled with the nurse for the following Monday (3 days away), and M.E. was instructed to contact the sexual assault center victim advocate or the mental health center if she needed to.

Evaluation

The following Monday (1 week after the attack) M.E. returned for her appointment with the mental health nurse. She related that she had been able to get some sleep,

was able to eat, and in general was feeling much less anxious. She stated that she had one very bad period on Saturday night, when she awakened suddenly and found her roommate gone. She called the crisis line and talked with a victim advocate, who reassured her until her roommate returned home about 20 min later.

Generally M.E. was feeling more in control of herself and requested the medicine dosage be lowered because she was returning to work the next day. Dosage was changed to diazepam 10 mg at 6:00 P.M., and at bedtime. She had confided in her supervisor, who was understanding and empathetic. M.E. would not work in the evening again until she felt she could handle it.

Within 2 weeks M.E. no longer required any medication. She would continue outpatient crisis intervention with the mental health nurse on a weekly basis plus weekly meetings with the victim support group.

AFFECTIVE DISORDERS

Depression

Like schizophrenia, the various affective disorders, particularly the depressive disorders, are poorly defined, and the diagnostic methodology lacks standardization. Many classifications or subtypes of depression have been proposed, but for the purposes of discussing drug therapy, depressions are classified as endogenous and exogenous. Common characteristics associated with each of these classifications are summarized in Table 34-10. The distinction between endogenous and exogenous depressions is essential. Treatments for the two types of depression are different, and empirical treatment is inappropriate, since it can prolong the patient's therapy and discomfort. Often a key in the differentiation of endogenous from exogenous depression is the fact that patients with an endogenous depression have generally per-

TABLE 34-10 Characteristics of Depression

Endogenous Depression

Allegedly biochemical in origin
Equated with psychosis by some clinicians, but can be psychotic or nonpsychotic
Autonomous: independent of environmental stimuli
Symptoms seem alien to the individual
Symptoms are continuous
Early awakening; symptoms worse in the morning
Responds to electroshock and pharmacotherapy

Exogenous Depression

Caused by external stress
Fluctuates according to psychologic factors
Hysterical postures
Initial insomnia; symptoms worse in evening
Does not respond to electroshock or pharmacotherapy

formed well in previous life experiences and lead a well-adjusted life, while exogenous depression is generally associated with a lifelong character disorder. Extensive research into the patient's background and activities is helpful in determining whether the episodes are exogenous or endogenous.

Clinical depression is also associated with a number of disease states, including both hypo- and hyperfunction of the adrenal, thyroid, and parathyroid glands. Uremia, anemia, and cancer may also produce a clinical depression. Patients exhibiting depressive disorders should receive a thorough physical and psychological evaluation. Depression may also be drug-induced, by such agents as **reserpine, propranolol, methyldopa, diazepam, levodopa,** and antineoplastic agents (see Table 34-11). These syndromes are readily reversible upon withdrawal of the offending agents. Patients may self-medicate in order to counteract effects of depression: amphetamines to overcome the chronic fatigue, narcotic and nonnarcotic agents to relieve the physical pain, antipsychotic and antianxiety agents for the chronic tension, hypnotics and CNS depressants for the insomnia, recreational drugs, and others. This form of therapy only temporarily stops the symptoms, which return as soon as the drugs are withdrawn.

Bipolar Affective Disorders

Bipolar affective disorders are characterized by recurrent psychotic episodes of an affective nature. Any given episode of this condition can present as either of two sets of symptoms: depression or mania (elation). Both sets of symptoms involve disturbances in mood and self-esteem, with signs of aggression lying just beneath the surface. Although a patient may experience only one episode of either manic or depressive symptoms, the typical course in manic-depressive psychosis is for repeated episodes of the illness to occur. Often, recurring episodes of psychotic depression alternate with periods of mania (bipolar illness). There may or may not be intervals of comparatively normal behavior and mood.

In a patient suffering from a depressive episode, normal symptoms of sadness become greatly intensified. There are three classic types of symptoms: depressed mood, retarded motor activity, and disturbances in the thinking process. The patient's appearance is one of extreme sadness and

TABLE 34-11 Drugs That May Cause Depression

Analgesics and Nonsteroidal Anti-inflammatory Drugs

Ibuprofen (Motrin, Advil, others)	Opiates (morphine, meperidine, others)
Indomethacin (Indocin)	Pentazocine (Talwin)
Phenylbutazone (Butazolidin)	Phenacetin

Antihypertensives

Clonidine (Catapres)	Propranolol (Inderal)
Guanethidine (Ismelin)	Reserpine
Hydralazine (Apresoline)	
Methyldopa (Aldomet)	

Antimicrobials

Ampicillin	Streptomycin
Clotrimazole (Lotrimin)	Sulfonamides
Griseofulvin (Fulvicin P/G)	Tetracycline
Nalidixic acid (NegGram)	Isoniazid (INH)
Nitrofurantoin (Furadantin)	

Antineoplastics

Azathioprine (Imuran)	Vincristine (Oncovin)
L-Asparaginase (Elspar)	Bleomycin (Blenoxane)

Antiparkinsonian Agents

Amantadine (Symmetrel)	Levodopa (Dopar, Larodopa)
Carbidopa (Lodosyn)	Levodopa/Carbidopa (Sinemet)

Antipsychotics

Phenothiazines	Haloperidol (Haldol)

Cardiac Drugs

Digitalis glycosides	Procainamide (Pronestyl)
Lidocaine (Xylocaine)	

Sedative Hypnotics

Benzodiazepines	Ethanol
Barbiturates	Chloral hydrate

Steroids and Hormones

ACTH	Oral contraceptives
Corticosteroids	

Stimulants and Appetite Suppressants

Amphetamines	Phenmetrazine
Fenfluramine	Diethylpropion

Miscellaneous

Cyproheptadine (Periactin)	Lysergide (LSD)
Diphenoxylate/atropine (Lomotil)	Cannabis
	Cimetidine (Tagamet)
Disulfiram (Antabuse)	

dejection. The energy level is low and appetite is poor. Sleep is restless and disturbed. Somatic complaints may make normal functioning difficult, if not impossible. The patient looks and feels utterly depressed, hopeless, and helpless. Suicide must be considered an ever-present danger.

In a manic episode symptoms are reversed. Instead of depression, the patient experiences an elated but unstable mood, pressure of speech, and increased motor activity. In the hypomanic phase, the patient is light, talkative, humorous, and witty. It is only after association over a period of time that one notices that the patient is overly friendly, easily distracted, impatient, impulsive, and disregarding of reality. In acute mania, patients are constantly moving, never completing anything they start. They are demanding and can become viciously angry if thwarted in their desires. Disregard of others is striking. Patients may fluctuate between tears and smiles in just a moment. As the symptoms progress, patients lose control and contact with reality. They seem consumed with purposeless activity that can lead to collapse from exhaustion, and even to death, if the mania is not controlled.

Clinical Pharmacology and Therapeutics of Affective Disorders

Drug therapy in the treatment of affective disorders has received a great deal of attention in the last decade, stimulated by new theories concerning the etiology of depression (catecholamine and serotonin theories) and the positive correlations that have been demonstrated with various forms of drug therapy. Reclassification of depressions, based on the normal metabolic byproducts of catecholamines, has provided evidence that clinicians can predict drug response. Although replication of studies is required, a depressed patient with decreased levels of 3-methoxyhydroxyphenylglycol (MHPG) may respond best to antidepressants that block reuptake of norepinephrine (NE) whereas a low level of 5-hydroxyindoleacetic acid (5-HIAA) may indicate the need for a serotonin (5-hydroxytryptamine, 5-HT) uptake blocker. Other biologic markers, results of dexamethasone suppression tests (DST) and thyroid-stimulating hormone tests, have been utilized to establish optimum antidepressant response. Patients whose plasma cortisol levels are not depressed after being administered dexamethasone tend to respond better to antidepressant treatment. After drug treatment, DST results showing suppression of cortisol levels indicate return to normal function. Therefore, the test may be used to confirm clinical observation. Even with all the interest and new information concerning affective disorders, however, therapy still remains extremely empirical.

Endogenous depressions are best treated with a combination of drug therapy and psychotherapy. When the decision is made that the patient is suffering from an endogenous depression, selection of an appropriate pharmacologic agent is the next step.

Patients with *exogenous depression* benefit minimally

from drug therapy. It is generally felt that any effects from drug therapy in these patients come from a placebo effect, and long-term therapy is felt to be detrimental to the overall recovery of the individual.

Clinicians should approach the treatment of the depressed patient with a great deal of caution regardless of the mode of therapy utilized. All types of depression are catastrophic experiences that make it difficult for the patient to reestablish normal activity for fear of failing again. As a defense, in order not to exacerbate the illness again, patients lead restricted lives. Patients' feelings of demoralization and incompetence are a part of the normal process of the illness. Demoralization can be confused with the depressive illness itself, but it is a result of the illness and is not responsive to medication.

Appropriate nonpharmacologic treatment is to give supportive, directive, and remobilizing psychotherapy. Clinicians should avoid telling patients that they can control their feelings, or that they should just try to forget their symptoms and proceed with their activities. Although meant to encourage the patient in returning to some purposeful activity, such approaches can only reinforce the patient's sense of inadequacy and potentiate the demoralization. On the other hand, telling patients to take a rest or a vacation may only be giving them more time to brood about their feelings.

The primary drugs used in the treatment of affective disorders are tricyclic and tetracyclic antidepressants, monoamine oxidase inhibitors, and lithium carbonate.

Tricyclic and Related Antidepressants

Tricyclic, tetracyclic, and triazolopyridine-structured drugs make up the most commonly employed antidepressants. The *tricyclic antidepressants* (TCADs) are structurally similar to the phenothiazines with the exception of their stereochemistry, which changes the receptor affinity. Tetracyclics and triazolopyridines are structurally dissimilar to TCADs; however, they are pharmacologically and therapeutically similar. The derivatives available for clinical use in the United States are listed in Table 34-12.

Mechanism of Action One theory of the etiology of affective disorders, the biogenic amine hypothesis, is helpful in explaining the action of antidepressants. These amines include norepinephrine, dopamine, and 5-hydroxytryptamine (5-HT, serotonin), which are chemical transmitters of electrical impulses that maintain affective homeostasis. Simply stated, in their absence, clinical depression may occur; if their metabolism is suppressed or their release enhanced, or

TABLE 34-12 Antidepressant Drugs: Preparations, Dosage Forms, Doses, Therapeutic Plasma Levels

NONPROPRIETARY NAME	TRADE NAME	DAILY DOSE FIRST 2 WEEKS, mg	USUAL RANGE OF DAILY DOSE AFTER FIRST 2 WEEKS, mg	RESPONSE RANGE (SERUM LEVELS), ng/mL
		Tricyclics		
Amitriptyline	Elavil, Endep	50–100	75–300	125–250*
Doxepin	Sinequan, Adapin	50–100	75–300	75–200*
Imipramine	Presamine, Tofranil	50–100	75–300	150–300*
Imipramine pamoate	Tofranil-PM	50–100	75–300	150–300
Trimipramine	Surmontil	50–100	75–300	180*
Amoxapine	Asendin	50–150	150–600	30–120*
Desipramine†	Norpramin Pertofrane	50–150	75–300	150–300
Nortriptyline	Aventyl	25–50	50–100	50–100
Protriptyline†	Vivactyl	10–30	15–60	50–150
		Tetracyclic		
Maprotiline	Ludiomil	75–150	75–300	180–450*
		Triazolopyridine		
Trazodone	Desyrel	50–150	150–600	800–1600
		Monoamine Oxidase Inhibitors		
Isocarboxazid	Marplan	10–30	10–50	
Phenelzine	Nardil	30–45	45–90	
Tranylcypromine	Parnate	20–30	20–60	

*Parent compound plus active metabolite.
†Desmethylated derivatives.

if there is an alteration of their receptors, mania or psychotic behavior may result.

Mechanisms of action of the antidepressants remain unclear; however, the biogenic amine hypothesis offers two distinct possibilities.

1. These agents may enhance the activity of norepinephrine by blocking its reuptake into the storage granules of nerve endings.

2. The antidepressants may potentiate 5-HT by blocking its reuptake or its metabolism.

However, research has shown that neither action alone will resolve depression.

All of these drugs have effects on the CNS similar to those seen with the phenothiazines. Sedation is common with all of these agents. REM sleep is affected by the antidepressant agents. EEG results show desynchronization, increased theta activity, and sometimes epileptic discharges.

Perhaps the most notable pharmacologic feature of the TCADs and tetracyclic compounds is their anticholinergic effects, which are about 100 times as potent as those of the antipsychotics. Mydriasis, tachycardia, decreased salivation, sweating, and disturbances of accommodation are the commonest anticholinergic effects. The triazolopyridines, on the other hand, have virtually no anticholinergic effects.

Indications Antidepressants have several indications: depression, anxiety, phobic anxiety, enuresis, chronic pain states, and panic disorders. In endogenous depression, beneficial results are achieved within 2 to 4 weeks after the initiation of therapy in about 70 percent of the cases treated. This percentage increases with the addition of psychotherapy. In exogenous depression, the response to antidepressants is similar to the response to a placebo. Depressions associated with schizophrenia, paranoia, or other psychoses may not show any benefit from antidepressants; in fact, the symptoms of these illnesses could be exacerbated. This is especially true for manic or hypomanic patients.

Until the etiology of depressive disorders can be identified by laboratory methods, and the correlation of drug therapy with diagnosis becomes more sophisticated, there will be no clinically significant difference between any of the antidepressants. Choice should be based on the patient's tolerance of the adverse effects, the results of prior exposure to a particular drug, and the outcome of a clinical trial of a chosen drug. Highly agitated or hyposomnic patients may respond better to a more sedating agent. Patients who are overly sensitive to the sedative properties of these drugs may respond better to a drug such as **desipramine** or **amoxapine** (Asendin) which causes less sedation.

The use of antidepressants for the treatment of anxiety is discussed in the section on anxiety disorders. Drug treatment of enuresis is largely empiric and lacks support from statistical trials. Enuresis in children is rarely a result of clinical depression. Behavioral conditioning is a much faster and

generally more acceptable form of treatment. The antidepressants, especially imipramine, do work, but with the risk of a number of side effects. Withdrawal of the drug usually results in relapse within 1 to 2 months.

Pharmacokinetics All of these drugs are rapidly and completely absorbed from the GI tract. There is a great variability among patients in absorption and in the blood levels achieved with a dose. Plasma levels are low, which has complicated research in correlating blood levels with clinical effects. These drugs are highly protein bound and are rapidly distributed to the body tissues. The antidepressants are long-acting drugs, the half-lives approaching those of the phenothiazines. When steady-state blood levels are achieved, the clinical effect can be maintained with one daily dose. The exception to this generalization is **trazodone** (Desyrel), which has a shorter half-life and must be dosed more frequently.

Onset of action is of particular concern to both clinician and patient. Usually 7 to 21 days of therapy are required to obtain the maximum clinical effect from antidepressants. Clinicians have attempted to shorten this lag period by the concomitant use of thyroid preparations and diuretics. Results have been extremely erratic and this practice should be avoided.

Metabolism occurs in the liver and produces a number of metabolites. Urinary excretion is the primary route of elimination of the drug. Small amounts of unchanged drug and metabolites may be excreted in the feces via the bile. The rate of elimination is relatively rapid; after a single dose one-third to one-half of the drug can be found in the urine within 24 h. However, once steady-state levels of the drug are achieved, the drug may be found in the urine months after administration is terminated.

Adverse Effects Most side effects of the antidepressants can be corrected by a dosage adjustment. Anticholinergic side effects are the most commonly occurring problems. Dry mucous membranes are the most frequent. Dry mouth, blurred vision due to decreased accommodation, tachycardia, palpitations, adynamic ileus, constipation, urinary retention, delayed micturition, and exacerbation of hiatal hernia are all anticholinergic side effects. These effects occur early in therapy and generally clear after 2 to 4 weeks of therapy. If they become chronic problems, the patient is less likely to continue therapy; therefore, some alleviation of these symptoms should be attempted. Adynamic ileus, tachycardia, and urinary retention can be special problems for the elderly patient and can be life-threatening. Trazodone is without significant anticholinergic problems.

CNS and neuromuscular effects are also common. Drowsiness is the adverse effect reported most frequently, especially early in treatment. This can be used to the patient's advantage if the total dose is given at night to assist with sleep. However, REM sleep is affected by the use of all of the antidepressant agents. This effect decreases with time. A rebound increase in REM sleep may occur when these drugs are discontinued.

Weakness and fatigue are also early therapy problems that improve with continued therapy. Occasionally, CNS stimulation occurs, and psychotic episodes have been initiated. Psychomotor excitement such as agitation, tremor, and insomnia, may occur. Hallucinations and exacerbations of other emotional disturbances have been reported and indicate reduction or withdrawal of the drugs. Occasionally, the temporary addition of an anxiolytic drug may be helpful. Extrapyramidal symptoms, although not as common as with the phenothiazines, do occur, especially in the very young and in the elderly. Antidepressants can cause an abnormal EEG and may lower the seizure threshold.

Cardiovascular side effects have recently received increased attention. T-wave flattening and inversion, as well as bundle branch block, atrioventricular block, tachycardia, bradycardia, ventricular extrasystoles, congestive heart failure, and myocardial infarction have occurred with the use of TCADs. The clinician should approach the use of these agents in patients with cardiovascular problems with *extreme caution;* many clinicians feel that the risks involved do not warrant their use. **Trazodone** appears to cause fewer cardiovascular problems.

Gastrointestinal effects can be attributed to the use of those antidepressants with significant anticholinergic effects. Anorexia, nausea and vomiting, diarrhea, cramps, increased appetite, stomatitis, peculiar taste (often described as a metallic taste), and black tongue have all been reported. These side effects normally remit with continued therapy, but may require decreasing the dose or discontinuing the drug. Some of the GI problems may be treated with additional drugs, but caution should be exercised. As an example, the use of kaolin antidiarrheals may retard the absorption of the TCAD and the clinical effect may be lost. Concomitant use of an anticholinergic or antispasmodic agent may potentiate side effects of blurred vision, dry mouth, or adynamic ileus.

Hematologic problems from antidepressants are similar to those from the phenothiazines. Eosinophilia, leukopenia, purpura, thrombocytopenia, and agranulocytosis have been reported. Leukocyte and differential counts should be performed on patients who develop sore throats and fever. The offending agent should be immediately discontinued if abnormal laboratory results are found.

On rare occasions, patients may develop allergic manifestations much like those seen with the phenothiazines. Photosensitization, rashes, urticaria, edema, and drug fevers may occur. Endocrine alterations from antidepressants, such as decreased libido, impotence, galactorrhea, breast engorgement, and weight gain, occur with less frequency than with phenothiazines.

Antidepressants have been implicated in causing birth defects. However, definite cause-effect relationships have not been established, and effects, if they occur, do not seem to be dose-related. Although the risks from using an anti-

depressant during pregnancy are not clearly defined, the clinician should carefully weigh the risk to the fetus versus the potential benefit to the patient.

Nursing mothers excrete these drugs in breast milk. Infants are especially susceptible to the adverse effects of the TCADs.

Drug Interactions Since the antidepressants are extensively metabolized, both liver enzyme induction and protein-binding competition may occur, making drug interactions possible (see Table 34-13). **Barbiturates** may enhance liver enzyme activity, thereby reducing plasma concentrations of antidepressants. **Phenothiazines** may compete with antidepressants and elevate both drugs' plasma concentrations. Combinations of these agents may potentiate the anticholinergic effects and lead to an anticholinergic toxic psychosis.

TABLE 34-13 Drugs that Interact with TCAD

DRUG	EFFECT

Central nervous system depressants
  Benzodiazepines
  Meprobamate
  Barbiturates
  Alcohol
	Increase CNS depression and psychomotor retardation.

CNS stimulants
  Amphetamine
  Methylphenidate
	Increase therapeutic and toxic effects. TCAD may inhibit metabolism of amphetamine.

MAO inhibitors	May result in increased excitation, hyperpyrexia, convulsions; may be fatal.
Anticonvulsants	TCAD may increase metabolism.
Phenothiazines	Combination may result in increased serum levels of both drugs.
Barbiturates	May increase metabolism.
Diuretics	Increase risk of orthostatic hypotension.

Centrally acting antihypertensives
  Methyldopa
  Clonidine
  Guanethidine
  Reserpine
	TCAD may block the uptake of these drugs, resulting in reduced hypotensive effect.

Oral anticoagulants	TCADs may decrease metabolism of dicoumarol.

Vasopressors
  Epinephrine
  Norepinephrine
  Phenylephrine
	TCADs may enhance pressor effect.

Estrogens	Combination has resulted in lethargy, nausea, headache, tremor, and hypotension. TCAD effects may be blocked by estrogens.

Antidepressants may block the activity of other drugs, such as **guanethidine**.

Drug Choice and Dosage Theoretically the choice of an antidepressant could be made on the basis of catecholamine metabolite studies. However, the invasiveness of the studies and the absence of supportive replication have not encouraged routine use. Furthermore, clinical studies do not support differences in efficacy between agents. Therefore, as for the phenothiazines, the choice is based on tolerance of side effects, historical response, and the patient's willingness to take a specific drug. For example, if a depressed patient demonstrates significant psychomotor retardation, the clinician may opt to use **desipramine**, which is less sedating than **amitriptyline**; or if a patient cannot tolerate anticholinergic effects, **trazodone** may be a good choice.

Dosage determination for the antidepressants, based on the available pharmacokinetic information, is very similar to that which was discussed for the phenothiazines. Doses should start at the level indicated in Table 34-12 and be increased or decreased according to the patient's tolerance until at least 150 mg/day of **imipramine** (or equivalent) is reached. Several weeks at this dose should elapse with no results before further increases are prescribed.

Steady-state antidepressant levels to determine whether patients have therapeutic serum concentrations are often helpful (see Table 34-12). After the maximum dose or therapeutic plasma concentrations have been maintained for 4 to 6 weeks, a decision concerning the continuation of this therapy or a change to an alternate therapy should be made on the basis of clinical effects of the drug. Some patients will benefit from the initial sedative effects provided during the day by multiple doses, but once-a-day doses can be implemented initially, except with **trazodone**, which must be dosed multiply.

Doses required for the mood-elevating effect in the endogenously depressed patient generally exceed 150 mg/day of **imipramine** or its equivalent. Doses exceeding 300 mg/day of imipramine or its equivalent generally require hospitalization of the patient for proper monitoring. The efficacy of exceeding 300 mg/day has not been established and should only be attempted in hospitalized patients resistant to therapy.

Imipramine is the TCAD which is commonly used to treat enuresis. There is, however, no evidence that other agents are not equally effective. Children receiving TCADs for enuresis usually require 75 to 100 mg of imipramine nightly. Doses should not exceed 2.5 mg/kg/day. The clinician should remember that tolerance to the clinical effect does develop, and discontinuing the drug and restarting again may be required.

Use of antidepressants in chronic pain states seems justified, since dopamine is decreased during pain and antidepressants increase this neurotransmitter. Clinical trials are limited, but results support their use in doses similar to those used in the treatment of depression.

Investigational Agents A group of so-called second generation antidepressants including **bupropion** (Wellbutrin) and **zimelidine** (Zelmid) are currently under investigation for the treatment of depression. These agents are structurally unrelated to the tricyclics, appear to have a different mechanism of action, and may have an improved side effect profile. These agents have stimulatory rather than sedating effects, a lesser incidence of anticholinergic effects, and minimal cardiovascular effects. Bupropion has been used in doses of 150 to 750 mg/day with an onset of therapeutic effect within 5 to 21 days. Zimelidine is used in dosages of 100 to 300 mg daily but has been associated with potentially severe adverse effects.

Monoamine Oxidase Inhibitors

Monoamine oxidase inhibitors (MAOIs) are effective in the treatment of endogenous depression, but since the tricyclics, tetracyclics, and triazolopyridine derivatives are more effective and the MAOIs carry more risk with their use, they are not considered agents of choice. The MAOIs used in clinical practice are listed in Table 34-12.

Mechanism of Action Like the other antidepressants, these drugs also affect norepinephrine and other biogenic amines. MAOIs block the action of a number of enzymes. One such enzyme is monoamine oxidase (MAO), which is responsible for the degradation of biogenic amines. Blocking the action of MAO increases the activity of the biogenic amines at receptor sites, providing a lift in mood.

Indications MAOIs provide a rapid effect; some effect should be seen within 24 h. MAOIs should be reserved for the patient who is resistant to the effects of tricyclic, tetracyclic, or triazolopyridine therapy, especially if the patient responded well to previous MAOI therapy; who can be trusted with an extremely toxic drug; and for whom electroconvulsive therapy is contraindicated. **Tranylcypromine** (Parnate) is thought to be the most effective MAOI.

Adverse Effects Hypertensive crisis is the most serious adverse effect of the MAOIs and may be produced when they are taken in combination with any of the agents listed in Table 34-14. These agents are rich in tyramine, a precursor of biogenic amines. Agitation, hallucinations, hyperreflexia, hyperpyrexia, convulsions, tremors, and insomnia are CNS effects that are possible with MAOIs; the rapid availability of more catecholamines at the receptor sites can occasionally precipitate toxic agitation and manic attacks. Orthostatic hypotension appears frequently and generally requires dose reduction. Headache, inhibition of ejaculation, hyperhidrosis, difficulty in urination, and dry mouth are common results of the use of MAOIs. Chronic use may also produce hepatic damage.

In spite of their potential for toxicity, MAOIs are still used frequently in medical practice. Many of the serious

TABLE 34-14 Foods and Drugs That Can Produce Hypertensive Crisis in Patients Taking Monoamine Oxidase Inhibitors

Cheddar cheese
Alcohol (beer, Chianti wine)
Chicken liver
Yeast products
Cream
Broad beans
Pickled herring
Coffee
Chocolate
Amphetamines
Narcotic analgesics
Phenylpropanolamine (often in over-the-counter cold remedies)
Tricyclic antidepressants

drug reactions previously reported with MAOIs have not been supported in recent studies, and their significance has been challenged.

Lithium Carbonate

Lithium is a unique psychotropic agent in that it is a naturally occurring element which can be used to control behavioral problems. Lithium has neither the sedative properties of the antipsychotic drugs nor the same kind of antidepressant action as the antidepressants. It is the only drug that is specifically indicated for the treatment of bipolar affective disorders.

Mechanism of Action Lithium's precise mechanism of action has not been elucidated; however, it is known that at the cellular level the lithium ion crosses the cell membrane like the sodium ion. The current hypothesis is that lithium replaces intracellular sodium, thereby stabilizing the axonal membrane. Supposedly, this activity decreases the amplitude of the action potential, thus reducing CNS activity by regulating catecholamines. Lithium also inhibits the release of norepinephrine and 5-HT, increases the reuptake of norepinephrine, and possibly increases the turnover rate of 5-HT. These activities explain the effect of the drug in controlling manic behavior and the stabilization effects that prevent the severe depression episodes of manic-depressive disorders.

Indications Clinical use of lithium carbonate is restricted to the treatment of the manic-depressive disorders. Attempts to use the drug for other disorders such as premenstrual tension, anxiety disorders, and hyperthyroidism have given inconsistent results. Patients who experience episodes of both mania and depression (bipolar illness) and those who experience recurrent major depressive episodes benefit from the use of lithium carbonate.

Pharmacokinetics The short-acting dosage forms are rapidly and completely absorbed, with a peak plasma level reached in 1 to 3 h, as compared to 4 to 5 h for the slow-release preparations. Slowing absorption decreases the peak blood levels, thereby possibly reducing the side effects. Lithium is not bound to plasma protein. Excretion of the drug is totally through renal mechanisms; therefore, the renal function of a patient is of primary concern to the clinician. Elimination is biphasic: there is a rapid drop in plasma level 5 or 6 h after administration, and then a very slow excretion over the next 24 h due to the slow shift of lithium from intracellular to extracellular sites (half-life is about 24 h and may be as long as 36 h for elderly). Measuring the plasma level of the drug during the second phase of excretion more closely estimates the steady-state concentration; therefore, blood levels should be tested 10 to 12 h after the last dose of the drug. Serum levels should be 0.6 to 1.5 meq/L.

Adverse Effects All patients experience some discomfort upon initiation of lithium therapy. Table 34-15 is a list of side effects and toxicities that have been reported with lithium use. Initially, patients may experience diarrhea, vomiting, drowsiness, muscular weakness, and lack of coordination. These problems are usually short-lived and require no treatment. Some side effects that may or may not subside shortly after the start of treatment include tremors, polyuria, thirst, and mild nausea. These problems are not harmful, but may require reduction or discontinuation of the dose if they prove disabling to the patient. Lithium carbonate irritates the mucosa of the GI tract, causing the various intensities of nausea. Taking the medication after meals often resolves this problem. While patients are taking lithium, a normal diet, especially sodium intake, should be maintained. Lithium readily replaces sodium, and the absence of sodium can cause toxicity.

When serum lithium levels exceed 1.5 to 1.8 meq/L, the adverse effects begin to appear, indicating that the patient may be developing toxic levels of lithium. The first toxic signs are blurred vision, ataxia, tinnitus, increased urination, and diarrhea. Patients should be instructed to inform the clinician if these sypmtoms occur. If the serum level continues to increase, CNS and cardiovascular toxicity ensue. Blackouts, seizures, hyperactive movements, stupor, coma, arrhythmias, hypotension, and peripheral circulatory failure make up the most common symptoms of acute toxicity. The drug should be withdrawn immediately and measures taken to quickly reduce the concentration of lithium in the body. Osmotic diuresis, urinary alkalinization, and dialysis are effective in reducing lithium blood levels.

Some chronic effects are seen after the long-term use of lithium. Thyroid disturbances, syndromes resembling diabetes insipidus, elevation of blood glucose, and elevated white blood cell counts have been described. Goiter is the most common problem. Patients experiencing this effect remain euthyroid, and the condition is reversible with the discontinuance of the drug or the addition of a thyroid hormone. A decrease in glucose tolerance is also documented in many patients. It, too, is completely reversible upon discontinuance of the drug. The change does not indicate a pathologic disturbance in carbohydrate metabolism, but a physiologic effect exerted by the lithium ion. Use of lithium during pregnancy is not recommended.

Dosage **Lithium carbonate** is available in single-release dosage forms (Eskalith, Lithonate, Lithotabs, others) and a slow-release dosage form (Lithobid, Eskalith CR). **Lithium citrate** is available as a syrup. The slow-release preparations may offer some advantages over the single-release products since patients may experience fewer side effects, and a reduced frequency of administration may ease compliance problems. Dosing of lithium carbonate is based entirely on measurement of lithium plasma concentration. Initiating the dose with 30 mg/kg/day based on lean body weight will achieve steady-state plasma concentrations of 0.8 to 1.2 meq/L. The usual dosage requirements are between 600 and 3600 mg/day. In order to maintain a constant steady-state plasma concentration, doses should be taken throughout the day, most appropriately on a schedule of three or four times a day. Slow-release products may be administered twice a day as long as the dose does not exceed 1800 mg/day.

In the therapy of the manic-depressive patient, there are two phases of treatment with lithium carbonate. The first is the stabilization phase and the second is the maintenance phase. During stabilization of the acutely manic patient, concomitant therapy is advised, since lithium takes 7 to 14 days to begin to control manic symptoms. The addition of an antipsychotic drug will control the patient's behavior in this stage, particularly the physically exhausting symptoms. If the hyperactive stage is allowed to continue, the patient may suffer harm from extreme weight loss, physical injuries, and loss of sleep. As soon as the acute symptoms subside, the antipsychotic should be discontinued gradually.

In this stage of treatment dosage should begin with serum lithium of 1 to 1.5 meq/L and should continue until the manic symptoms have resolved. It normally takes 5 or 6 days for enough lithium to accumulate to produce these blood levels. During this phase, serum lithium levels should be determined every 1 to 2 days. If the level exceeds 1.5 meq/L or if toxic signs appear, the dose should be reduced.

TABLE 34-15 Side Effects and Toxicity of Lithium

Cardiovascular System	*Mental Symptoms*
Pulse irregularities	Mental retardation
Fall in blood pressure	Somnolence
ECG changes	Confusion
Peripheral circulatory failure	Restlessness and disturbed behavior
Circulatory collapse	Stupor
	Coma
Central Nervous System	*Neuromuscular Symptoms and Signs*
Anesthesia of skin	General muscle weakness
Incontinence of urine and feces	Ataxia
Slurred speech	Tremor
Blurring of vision	Muscle hyperirritability
Dizziness	Fasciculation (increased by tapping muscle)
Vertigo	Twitching (especially of facial muscles)
Epileptiform seizures	Clonic movements of whole limbs
	Choreoathetoid movements
	Hyperactive deep tendon reflexes
Gastrointestinal Symptoms	*Miscellaneous*
Anorexia	Polyuria
Nausea	Glycosuria
Vomiting	General fatigue
Diarrhea	Lethargy and tendency to sleep
Thirst	Dehydration
Dryness of mouth	
Weight loss	

Source: R. I. Shader, *Manual of Psychiatric Therapeutics: Practical Psychopharmacology and Psychiatry*, Boston: Little, Brown and Company, 1975.

TABLE 34-16   Overview of Nursing Process Related to Affective Disorders

ASSESSMENT	MANAGEMENT	EVALUATION
General Aspects		
History of previous episodes. Retarded motor level or manic activity. Sleep patterns, bowel patterns, diurnal cycles, anorexia. Manic: Talkative, witty, pacing, impulsive, distractible, constant purposeless activity. Depressive: Low energy level, somatic complaints, demoralization. Depressed mood. Disturbed thinking process. Suicide potential. Distinguish endogenous from exogenous. Analyze family / support systems.	Nondrug therapy: Supportive, optimistic; suicide precautions (continued during early improvement), therapeutic milieu; reactivation; avoid approaches that reinforce inadequacy and demoralization. Drug therapy, electroshock therapy (endogenous).	Improved appetite, sleeping, personal appearance. Decreased constipation. Normalization of activity, thinking process (reality focus), mood. Able to complete normal daily activities, increased interest in environment.
Tricyclic Antidepressants (TCADs), tetracyclics, triazolopyridines		
Prior exposures to TCADs and outcomes. History of cardiovascular disease, seizure disorder, benign prostatic hypertrophy, hiatal hernia, current pregnancy or lactation, glaucoma, constipation, organic CNS lesions. Concurrent drugs, especially with anticholinergic effects. Age, especially child or elderly. Baseline ECG, weight, vital signs.	Tell patient about side effects factually without overemphasis. Teach how to detect and prevent. Explain may require up to 3 weeks for maximal effects; alcohol may potentiate adverse effects. Taper dosage; do not stop abruptly. Administration once daily is appropriate in many patients. Encourage appropriate diet and exercise to prevent weight gain.	See above description of general aspects. Note conversion to manic state or appearance of delusions, hallucinations. Evaluate for adverse effects, including weight gain, vital signs (for arrhythmia, tachycardia, hypotension), especially in early therapy.

During maintenance therapy, the patient should continue to take lithium prophylactically for an indefinite period of time. After acute symptoms clear, dosage reduction is appropriate. The daily dosage, usually about 1200 mg/day in four divided doses, should be correlated with clinical assessment of adverse effects and with serum lithium levels. Serum levels in the maintenance stage should remain between 0.9 and 1.2 meq/L. After a maintenance dose has been established, serum lithium levels should be monitored monthly or bimonthly. Future episodes of mania or depression may occur while the patient is taking maintenance therapy, but generally they will be less severe; an increase in lithium dosage and the addition of an antipsychotic or antidepressant drug, depending on the phase of the illness, is appropriate.

Planned follow-up is extremely important in manic-depressive illness. Monitoring of lithium levels can be of assistance in determining compliance, and the therapeutic effects and toxicity of the drug should be closely observed. If possible, the patient's family should be involved in the follow-up process. If mood swings start to occur, the patient frequently stops the medication, paving the way for a full-blown episode; patients and family should be told to contact the clinician if they notice mood swings.

NURSING PROCESS RELATED TO AFFECTIVE DISORDERS

Table 34-16 outlines the nursing process in affective disorders.

TABLE 34-16 Overview of Nursing Process Related to Affective Disorders (*Cont.*)

ASSESSMENT	MANAGEMENT	EVALUATION
Monoamine oxidase Inhibitors (MAOIs)		
Age, especially child or elderly. Note history of hypertension, cardiovascular disease, epilepsy, diabetes, impaired liver function. Concurrent drug therapy for interactions (narcotics, sedatives, sympathomimetics).	Abstain from tyramine-containing foods, sympathomimetics. Teach to rise slowly from lying position to avoid orthostatic hypotension. Teach to report headaches (may be first sign of hypertensive crisis), pruritus, CNS adverse effects. Stop drug approx. 2 weeks before surgery.	See above description of general aspects. Watch vital signs, especially blood pressure, frequently during early therapy. Side effects: Hypotension, psychomotor stimulation, atropine-like effects, insomnia, euphoria. Toxic effects: Hypertensive crisis; overdose (toxic psychosis, stupor, coma); hepatotoxicity (jaundice, pruritus); swing between depression and manic states.
Lithium Carbonate		
Note history of impaired renal function, cardiovascular disease, current pregnancy, lactation, restricted diet, fluid loss, concurrent drug therapy: diuretics, theophylline	Normal diet and salt intake, adequate fluids (2000–3000 mL/day); educate patient. Control takes 7–14 days, so may require an antipsychotic initially; taper with improvement. Inform patient that mild adverse effects usually diminish. Teach how to identify and report severe effects.	Serum lithium levels taken 10–12 h after last dose: Stabilization, <1.5 meq/L (monitor every 3–4 days). Maintenance, 0.9–1.5 meq/L (monitor monthly or bimonthly). Recurrence of depression during maintenance may require increased or added drugs. Monitor fluid intake and output when ill or losing fluid from any site. Mild toxicity: Nausea, anorexia, vomiting, thirst, polyuria, tremor, muscle weakness. Severe toxicity (withhold drug): Chorea, athetosis, confusion, convulsions, coma. Goiter, ECG changes may occur.

CASE STUDY

The fourth admission to the mental health center of C.D., a 27-year-old, 140-lb, married male and father of two children, was precipitated by his swing into the manic phase of his illness. C.D.'s symptoms on admission consisted of hyperactivity, talkativeness, and suspicion of people.

Assessment

The psychiatric nurse-clinician gathered the following data from C.D., his wife, and the previous charts.

Prior to his first hospitalization 1 year ago, Mr. D. was a fourth-year law student with the highest scholastic average in his class. He was editor of the university newspaper and very active in school affairs on campus. Feeling inadequate to maintain his high scholastic level, he found it increasingly difficult to keep up with his studies and campus involvement, so he dropped out of school. Since that time he worked sporadically at several menial jobs, but his ability to function was severely impaired by alternating moods of elation and depression.

His psychiatric illness includes three previous admissions to the mental health center and two admissions to a private hospital. During the second hospitalization he demonstrated hypomanic symptoms, while on the third admission his symptoms were depressive. During his first three admissions, the patient was treated with chlorpromazine 1000 to 1200 mg daily. This met with success; however, relief was short-lived after discharge.

C.D.'s childhood development seems to have been

unremarkable, except that he was always a high achiever. C.D. saw this as the only way to please his father, which had always been important to C.D.

One of C.D.'s recurrent concerns was about being a "good provider" for his family. This was especially difficult for him because he and his family had always been financially dependent on his parents, who were now in their middle 60s. The patient's father was paying for the fourth mental health center hospitalization, as he had for all the previous admissions to psychiatric hospitals.

On this fourth admission, C.D. reported that the mania began, like other episodes, with a conflict at home. As his manic behavior rose, C.D.'s wife became afraid of him. He spoke to her in a loud and angry tone of voice, cursing her and calling her names.

In the initial interview, C.D. paced the room, spoke rapidly, and tended to dominate the conversation if allowed to do so. The examiner noticed hostility and suspicion during the interview. C.D. frequently made mention of the fact that the examiner was "only a nurse." He reported that he really did not need sleep any more and only went to bed for 2 or 3 h each night to get his wife to quit nagging him.

Health history, physical examination, medication history, and routine laboratory studies were otherwise noncontributory.

The nurse-clinician's impression was manic-depressive psychosis in the manic phase, resulting in hyperactivity, accelerated speech activity, disturbed sleep habits, suspicion, and irritability.

After reviewing the nurse's data base and interviewing the patient, the physician ordered lithium carbonate, 600 mg tid; daily blood lithium levels; thyroid-stimulating hormone (TSH), ECG, and serum creatinine; and chlorpromazine 200 mg tid.

Management

The nurse's initial plans included orienting C.D. to the ward as tolerated, observation every half hour for symptoms, which were recorded on a flow sheet, and reduction of external stimuli as much as possible. The approach taken by the staff was one of firm, matter-of-fact, passive friendliness, with necessary limits to control combative behavior. Contact with other patients was minimized during the initial hospitalization period.

C.D.'s hyperactive behavior increased. The day after admission he awakened all of the patients on the ward at 5 A.M. While the staff was settling down the rest of the patients, C.D. dressed himself like an Indian and began running up and down the hall. It was necessary to medicate C.D. with chlorpromazine 100 mg IM. In the afternoon, after being expelled from the community meeting, he went to the day room and proceeded to dismantle the piano. Several other times he became hostile and belligerent and required chlorpromazine.

The lithium was administered with the regular diet at breakfast, supper, and a bedtime snack, and blood samples for the daily serum lithium level were drawn at 7 A.M. each morning. The patient was encouraged to drink lots of fluids by providing him several times daily with juices he liked. During the next 2 weeks C.D.'s lithium dosage was raised four times until C.D. was taking 2400 mg daily. Nurses observed C.D. for minor and severe toxic effects. Within 1 month of his admission, C.D. was stabilized on his medication. After education regarding the lithium, he was discharged from the inpatient service to return every week to the medication clinic for a check on his medication. At the time of his discharge, C.D. refused any other form of therapy.

Evaluation

Although the chlorpromazine, given on a PRN basis, was somewhat effective in calming C.D., he was extremely hyperactive and hyposomnic during the initial days of his hospitalization. The regular dosage schedule of chlorpromazine should have been increased to control the hyperactive behavior. Nurses should have consulted with the physician regarding this, since they found it difficult to get the patient to avoid physical exhaustion and to take adequate food and fluid, because of his hyperactivity and suspicion. Additionally, the need for intramuscular admission could have been eliminated with the greater cooperation from the patient.

C.D.'s lithium dosage was advanced slowly and he experienced few side effects. Polyuria, vomiting, and tremor were transient; although the patient continued to experience nausea even after his discharge. The serum lithium level throughout the stabilization and early maintenance phases never exceeded 1.5 meq/L.

Six Months Post Discharge

Approximately 6 months after discharge from the inpatient service, C.D.'s attendance at the lithium clinic became sporadic and finally ceased altogether. After missing his second clinic appointment, a referral was made to the community mental health nurse, who made a home visit.

Assessment

The nurse obtained the following information from C.D. and his wife, who had stayed home from work because of her concern for him. About 4 weeks ago, C.D. began to experience a recurrence of depression which progressively interfered with his normal functioning. He was staying in bed about 18 out of every 24 h, was not eating or consuming adequate fluid, and had no concern for his personal hygiene (he had not bathed in 4 days). At the nurse's urging and with Mrs. D's assistance, C.D. bathed and drank 6 oz of orange juice. Mr. and Mrs. D. accompanied the nurse to the mental health center.

Management

The mental health nurse, in consultation with the psychiatrist, recommended inpatient hospitalization for C.D. Upon admission to the unit the data base included severely depressed affect, delusional thinking, impaired somatic and motor activity, and severely retarded communication and social participation. The nursing care plan initially focused on C.D.'s inability to eat and to maintain self-care. Medication included continuation of the maintenance level of lithium carbonate 2400 mg daily. Imipramine hydrochloride 150 mg at bedtime was added to treat his depression. Prior to ordering the imipramine hydrochloride, a DST (dexamethasone suppression test) was ordered. Dexamethasone 1 mg was given orally at bedtime. The following day serum cortisol levels were drawn at 4:00 P.M. and 11:00 P.M. Test results were nonsuppressive, and the imipramine hydrochloride as ordered was begun. Upon admission, and following the routine ward orientation, the nurse, Ms. R., explained his medication regime to C.D. Ms. R. indicated that she would be offering him fluids every hour to lessen the constipating effects of imipramine hydrochloride and also because he was poorly hydrated on admission. She explained to C.D. that he might experience some drowsiness or dizziness and that these signs usually subside after a few weeks. She also offered C.D. a supply of sugarless candy to help relieve any dryness of his mouth. C.D. adjusted marginally to ward routine, and there was no significant improvement in his depressive symptoms over the next 2 weeks. The doctor ordered an increase of imipramine hydrochloride to 300 mg at bedtime. His lithium level remained the same. The nursing staff noticed an improvement within another week (3 weeks after admission and beginning medication). C.D. was taking more responsibility for his activities of daily living and indicating more interest in the unit routine. He continued to meet three times per week with the clinical nurse specialist and participate in group therapy. As C.D.'s depression lessened, he began to assume the role of leader in the daily unit government meetings.

After 1 month of treatment his depression was resolved. The nursing staff and C.D. began planning his discharge. Discharge plans included an appointment in the lithium clinic in 1 week. C.D. was discharged on the following medications: lithium carbonate 2400 mg daily, and imipramine hydrochloride 300 mg at bedtime.

Evaluation

One week later, when C.D. returned to the lithium clinic, another DST was done. Because he was an outpatient, only one serum cortisol level was drawn, at 4:00 P.M. the next day. The results of the DST were normal, and the decision was made to discontinue the tricyclic antidepressant. Lithium carbonate was continued as ordered with a return appointment in the lithium clinic in 1 week, and individual psychotherapy weekly with the clinical nurse specialist.

REFERENCES

Amdisen, A.: "Sustained Release Preparations of Lithium," in F. N. Johnson (ed.), *Lithium Research and Therapy,* New York: Academic Press, 1975.

Bryant, S. C., and L. Ereshefsky: "Antidepressant Properties of Trazodone," *Clinical Pharm,* 1:406–417, 1982.

Carroll, B. J., M. Feinberg, J. F. Greden, et al.: "A Specific Laboratory Test for the Diagnosis of Melancholia," *Arch Gen Psychiatry,* 38:15–22, 1981.

Cluff, L. E., G. J. Caranasos, and R. B. Stewart: *Clinical Problems with Drugs,* vol. V, Philadelphia: Saunders, 1975.

Cole, J., and L. Hollister: *Schizophrenics,* New York: Medcom, 1972.

Cooper, T. B.: "Plasma Level Monitoring of Antipsychotic Drugs," *Clinical Pharmacokinet,* 3:14–38, 1978.

Davis, J. M.: "Theories of Biological Etiology of Affective Disorders," *Int Rev Neurobiol,* 12:145–175, 1970.

———: "Overview: Maintenance Therapy in Psychiatry: 2. Affective Disorders," *Am J Psychiatry,* 133:1–13, 1976.

Diagnostic and Statistical Manual of Mental Disorders, 3d ed., American Psychiatric Association, 1980.

Fann, W. E., W. M. Pitts, and J. C. Wheless: "Pharmacology, Efficacy, and Adverse Effects of Halazepam, a New Benzodiazepine," *Pharmacotherapy,* 2:72–79, 1982.

Freedman, A., H. Kaplan, and B. J. Saddock: *Modern Comprehensive Textbook of Psychiatry II,* Baltimore: Williams and Wilkins, 1976.

Gaultieri, G. T., and S. F. Powell: "Psychoactive Drug Interactions," *J Clin Psychiatry,* 39:720–729, 1978.

Gilman, A. G., L. S. Goodman, and A. Gilman: *Goodman and Gilman's The Pharmacological Basis of Therapeutics,* 6th ed., New York: Macmillan, 1980.

Gram, L. F., et al.: "Drug Level Monitoring in Psychopharmacology: Usefulness and Clinical Problems, with Special Reference to Tricyclic Antidepressants," *Therapeutic Drug Monitoring,* 4:17–25, 1982.

Hansten, P. P.: *Drug Interactions,* 4th ed., Philadelphia: Lea & Febiger, 1979.

Hollister, L. E.: "Clinical Use of Psychotherapeutics: Current Status," *Clin Pharmacol Ther,* 10:170–198, 1969.

———: *Clinical Use of Psychotherapeutics,* Springfield, Ill.: Thomas, 1973.

Kyes, J., and C. K. Hofling: *Basic Psychiatric Concepts in Nursing,* Philadelphia: Lippincott, 1974.

Lande, N.: "Extrapyramidal Parkinson-Like Reactions to Phenothiazines," *Drug Intell Clin Pharm,* **8:**166–170, 1974.

Meyler, L., and A. Herxheimer: *Side Effects of Drugs,* vol. 9, Amsterdam: Excerpta Medica, 1980.

Schildkraut, J. J.: "Current Status of Biological Criteria for Classifying the Depressive Disorders and Predicting Responses to Treatment," *Psychopharmacol Bull,* **10:**5–25, 1974.

——: "Neuropharmacology of Affective Disorders," *Am Rev Pharmacol,* **13:**427–454, 1977.

Shader, R., and A. DiMascio: *Psychotropic Drug Side Effects: Clinical and Theoretical Perspective,* Baltimore: Williams and Wilkins, 1970.

Van Praag, H. M.: "Neurotransmitters and CNS Disease: Depression," *Lancet,* **2:**1259–1264, 1982.

35

ENDOCRINE DISORDERS

JOANN GANJE CONGDON
CELESTE MARTIN MARX

OVERVIEW OF THE ENDOCRINE SYSTEM

LEARNING OBJECTIVES

Upon mastery of the content of this section, the reader will be able to:

1. Describe the mechanisms of action of two types of hormones.
2. Explain how hormone secretion is regulated.
3. Differentiate pharmacologic and physiologic uses of hormones.
4. Characterize the pharmacokinetics of hormones.

Many adaptive processes work continuously to maintain physical and psychologic integration and stability. This adaptation to a constantly changing environment is mediated by both the nervous system and the endocrine system. The nervous system detects changes in the environment and transmits this information through sensory pathways to the hypothalamus where endocrine and autonomic activity are generated and relayed to the pituitary gland, adrenal medulla, and other organs. The neuroendocrine system regulates and coordinates the various organ systems to meet the body's need for: (1) energy production; (2) chemical homeostasis (fluid and electrolyte balance, adaptation to stress); (3) growth and development; and (4) reproduction. Disruption in components of these control systems will result in a divergence from the normal adaptive processes.

ENDOCRINE GLANDS

The endocrine system is composed of glands which secrete biologically active chemical substances called *hormones* into the bloodstream. These glands include the pituitary, thyroid, parathyroids, adrenals, pancreas, ovaries, testes, and thymus. Once released into the bloodstream, hormones are transported to specific target tissues where they exert their regulatory effect. The physiologic action of a hormone is ultimately the result of its interaction with a specific receptor.

Common Characteristics

Although each endocrine gland possesses individual characteristics (Table 35-1), endocrine glands share some of the following:

1. Since hormones circulate in the blood, they affect many organs and systems. For example, hypothyroidism changes can be found in the central nervous system, the skin, the muscles, the gastrointestinal system, the heart, and the blood vessels.

2. Many common signs and symptoms may be manifestations of endocrine disease. For example, serious psychologic disturbances can be an important manifestation of pituitary insufficiency, hypo- or hyperthyroidism, hyperparathyroidism, hypoglycemia, Addison's disease, or Cushing's syndrome.

3. Hormones are secreted cyclically in response to certain body and environmental rhythms. For example, adrenocorticotropic hormone (ACTH) production reaches a peak in the early morning, diminishes during the day, and is lowest by evening. Also, estrogen secretion levels vary during the menstrual cycle.

4. Hormones are secreted in small amounts and do not accumulate because they are rapidly inactivated and excreted. For example, the plasma half-life of endogenous cortisol is only 30 min. Only 15 μg of triiodothyronine (T_3), the most active thyroid hormone, is produced daily.

5. Endocrine hormones act in a catalytic manner by stimulating a physiologic response; they do not themselves initiate new biochemical reactions. For example, the anabolic androgens *promote normal mechanisms* for body tissue building and for reversing the catabolic, or tissue-depleting, process.

TABLE 35-1 Summary of the Major Hormones

GLAND	HORMONE	MAJOR FUNCTION/CONTROL OF:
Hypothalamus	Releasing hormones	Secretions of the anterior pituitary
	Oxytocin	(See posterior pituitary)
	Antidiuretic hormone	(See posterior pituitary)
Anterior pituitary	Growth hormone (GH, somatotropin, STH)*	Growth; organic metabolism
	Thyroid-stimulating hormone (TSH)	Thyroid gland
	Adrenocorticotropic hormone (ACTH, corticotropin)	Adrenal cortex
	Prolactin (PRL)	Breasts (milk formation)
	Gonadotropic hormones: Follicle-stimulating hormone (FSH), Luteinizing hormone (LH)	Gonads
	Melanocyte-stimulating hormone (MSH)	Pigmentation
Posterior pituitary†	Oxytocin	Milk secretion; uterine motility
	Antidiuretic hormone (ADH, Vasopressin)	Water excretion
Adrenal cortex	Cortisol (hydrocortisone)	Organic metabolism; response to stress
	Androgens	Growth and, in women, sexual activity
	Aldosterone	Sodium and potassium excretion
Adrenal medulla	Epinephrine, norepinephrine	Organic metabolism; cardiovascular function; response to stress
Thyroid	Thyroxine (T_4), triiodothyronine (T_3)	Energy metabolism; growth and development
	Calcitonin	Plasma calcium
Parathyroids	Parathyroid hormone (parathormone, PTH, PH)	Plasma calcium and phosphate
Gonads		
Female: ovaries	Estrogen	Reproductive system; growth and development
	Progesterone	Reproductive system; growth and development; breasts
Male: testes	Testosterone	Reproductive system; growth and development
Pancreas	Insulin, glucagon	Organic metabolism; plasma glucose
Thymus	Thymus hormone (thymosin)	Lymphocyte development
Pineal	Melatonin	?Sexual maturity

*The names and abbreviations in parentheses are synonyms.

†The posterior pituitary stores and secretes these hormones; they are synthesized in the hypothalamus.

Source: Adapted from D. S. Luciano et al.: *Human Function and Structure,* New York: McGraw-Hill, 1978. Reprinted from J. G. Congdon: "Endocrine System," in S. Lewis and I. Collier (eds.), *Medical Surgical Nursing: Assessment and Management of Clinical Problems,* New York: McGraw-Hill, 1983.

HORMONES

General Mechanisms of Action

The chemical nature of hormones is variable, but most are either steroids or proteins.

Steroid Hormones

Steroid hormones, which are derived from cholesterol in the body, differ from each other in the number and nature of chemical groups appended to the ring-shaped nucleus (Fig. 35-1). The steroid hormones are lipid-soluble and are able to penetrate the cell membranes of their target tissues. Once inside the cell, they move to the nucleus and there influence the rate of protein and enzyme synthesis, which alters the activity level of the cell (Fig. 35-2a). The response to steroid hormones is relatively slow (45 min to several hours). Examples of steroid hormones are those produced by the adrenal cortex and gonads—cortisol, aldosterone, progesterone, and testosterone.

Protein Hormones

While steroid hormones have important functions, most hormones are protein, composed of amino acids connected together in chains. Protein hormones do not appear to interact with the nucleus of the cell body. Because of their size and insolubility, protein hormones do not penetrate cell membranes, but interact with specific membrane receptors that are linked with cellular enzymes (Fig. 35-2b). Hormone-receptor complexes produce the common responses within the cell such as the stimulation of protein synthesis, enzyme

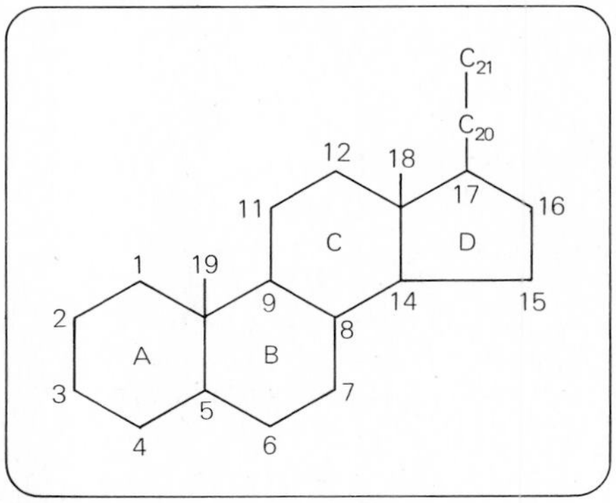

FIGURE 35-1

A Steroid Nucleus. The four rings are identified by letters, while the numbers designate the locations where chemical groups are appended and result in the characteristic activity of the particular steroid hormone. For example, the only difference between the female hormone progesterone and the mineralocorticoid, deoxycorticosterone, is that the latter has a hydroxyl (OH) group at position 21. Such similarity of structure in steroid hormones accounts for their frequent overlap of function (e.g., progesterone and estrogens in oral contraceptives have some aldosterone-like activity and cause fluid retention).

activation, secretion of hormones, or alteration of cell membrane permeability. These responses occur quite rapidly compared with those of the steroid hormones. Examples of protein hormones are those produced by the pancreas, thyroid, parathyroid, pituitary, and the adrenal medulla—insulin, thyroxine, parathormone, growth hormone, and epinephrine, respectively.

Control of Hormone Secretion

Control of hormone interaction, secretion, and release is usually best understood in terms of feedback, particularly *negative feedback*. In negative feedback, the rising concentration of a specific hormone inhibits the mechanism of release of that hormone. An example is excretion of ACTH (from the pituitary), which regulates the secretion of cortisol by the adrenal glands. In turn, cortisol controls the secretion of ACTH by the pituitary gland. Whenever cortisol levels fall, ACTH levels rise, and whenever cortisol levels rise, ACTH levels fall. (See Fig. 35-3.) Hormone secretion can also be controlled by changes in the *blood level of a substance*. For example, insulin is secreted in response to increased glucose in the blood, while a decreased level of blood glucose inhibits insulin secretion. The posterior pituitary and the adrenal medulla are endocrine glands which are directly *stimulated by the nervous system*.

Indications for Hormonal Drugs

Hormone preparations are given for physiologic and pharmacologic use. *Physiologic use* involves replacement therapy or the use of drugs which interfere with hormone production either by blocking or destroying the tissue that makes the hormone. Replacement therapy is indicated when a gland is unable to secrete an adequate amount of hormone, such as the administration of insulin in diabetes mellitus. The use of radioactive iodine (^{131}I) is an example of a (non-hormone) drug that permanently reduces thyroid hormone production by destroying thyroid glandular tissue. The physiologic need for hormones fluctuates with such variables as age, sex, state of health, activity level, stress level, reproductive status, endogenous hormone production, and hormone antibody level. Therefore, dosages may vary from person to person and ongoing assessment of a person's status and response to therapy is crucial.

Pharmacologic use involves the administration of supraphysiologic doses to alter normal responses, as in the use of corticosteroids for their anti-inflammatory effects and for their control of allergic reactions. The potential for adverse effects is much greater in pharmacologic, as opposed to physiologic, uses of hormones, due to the unnaturally high blood levels and abnormal rhythmicity of therapy.

Pharmacokinetics

While many natural and synthetic hormones are well-absorbed after oral administration, parenteral administra-

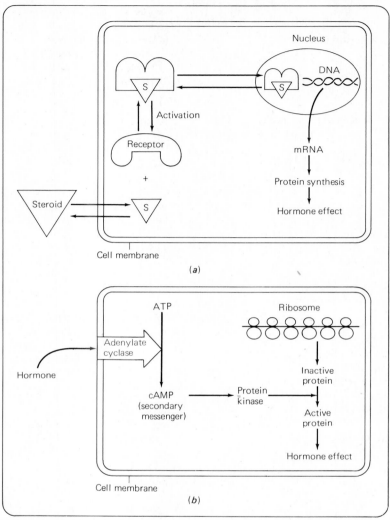

FIGURE 35-2

Mechanisms of Hormone Action. (*a*) Steroids penetrate the cell membrane and bind to a receptor protein in the cytoplasm. This hormone-receptor complex is transported to the nucleus where it modifies the formation of messenger RNA and, hence, protein synthesis. (*b*) Protein hormones activate the enzyme adenylate cyclase, which catalyzes the synthesis of cAMP. This "secondary messenger," in turn, stimulates a protein kinase that activates certain proteins and alters the rate at which the reactions involving these proteins occur.

tion is used for some hormonal drugs due to desired rapid onset of action (or prolonged effect as with depot intramuscular injections), first pass metabolism, or breakdown of protein chains by gastrointestinal enzymes (e.g., insulin). Many hormones circulate in the blood primarily bound to albumin and/or plasma proteins, and the administration of exogenous drugs which bind to the same sites on plasma proteins can alter hormonal balance or the interpretation of plasma hormone measurement because the fraction of free (active) hormone is increased. Similarly, diseases (e.g., renal and hepatic) or physiological states (e.g., pregnancy) which alter plasma protein concentration or binding affinity can alter the proportion of free hormone. Steroid hormones are primarily excreted into the bile and urine after metabolism in the liver by conjugation, and several undergo enterohepatic recycling. Protein hormones are metabolized in the liver and other tissues, and the mostly inactive metabolites and small amounts of active hormone are excreted in the urine.

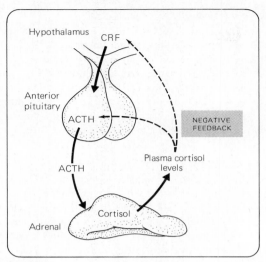

FIGURE 35-3

Feedback Inhibition. Negative feedback functions to control the hypothalamic–pituitary–adrenal (HPA) axis and regulate plasma cortisol levels. Negative feedback (dashed lines) is important in the regulation of many hormones.

THE HYPOTHALAMUS AND THE PITUITARY

LEARNING OBJECTIVES

Upon mastery of the content of this section the reader will be able to:

1. Give two synonyms for vasopressin and for growth hormone.

2. List the clinical uses for the available pituitary hormones.

3. Describe the physiologic effects of growth hormone and vasopressin.

4. Outline the nursing process related to the administration of growth hormone and vasopressin.

The pituitary gland, a bilobed organ located at the base of the brain and connected to the median eminence of the hypothalamus by the pituitary stalk, is composed of two embryologically distinct tissues, the adenohypophysis and the neurohypophysis. The *anterior pituitary,* derived from the adenohypophysis, produces and secretes seven peptide (short-chain protein) hormones (Table 35-1) under the control of hypothalamic releasing and inhibiting factors. The *posterior pituitary,* a part of the neurohypophysis, stores and releases under neural control two hormones, *vasopressin (antidiuretic hormone, ADH)* and *oxytocin.*

Recently it has been possible to isolate, characterize, purify, and even synthesize hypothalamic releasing and inhibiting factors. These hormones, such as somatotropin-releasing hormone (SRH), thyrotropin-releasing hormone (TRH), and gonadotropin-releasing hormone (GnRH), are currently under investigation for the treatment of a wide variety of endocrine disorders. While short elimination half-lives limit their present application to diagnostics, it is anticipated that other uses will be developed and that these agents will become commercially available during the next decade.

All of the pituitary hormones except melanocyte-stimulating hormone and prolactin are currently available and have approved clinical applications (Table 35-2). Since several of these applications are related to reproductive functions, the use of gonadotropins, oxytocin, and the stimula-

TABLE 35-2 Uses of Available Pituitary Hormones

HORMONE	USES
Corticotropin (ACTH)	Diagnostic testing of adrenal function Multiple sclerosis exacerbations Nonsuppurative thyroiditis Hypercalcemia associated with cancer Inflammatory and immune diseases
Thyrotropin (TSH)	Diagnosis of hypothyroidism Adjunct in thyroid carcinoma Enhancement of ^{131}I uptake
Gonadotropins (FSH, LH)	Female infertility Male hypogonadism, cryptorchidism
Somatotropin (growth hormone, GH)	Growth failure due to GH deficiency
Oxytocin	Stimulate labor Control postpartum bleeding Abortifacient Stimulate lactation (letdown) Antepartum fetal heart rate testing* Breast engorgement*
Vasopressin (antidiuretic hormone, ADH)	Diabetes insipidus Paralytic ileus and abdominal distention Nocturnal enuresis* Prevent alcoholism in beer drinkers (produces nausea due to water intoxication)* Reduction of hepatic portal pressure/control of bleeding esophageal varices* Delay absorption of local anesthetics* Reduction of hemorrhage in bleeding disorders*

*Investigational; not FDA approved.

tion and suppression of prolactin secretion are discussed in Chap. 46, "Women's Health Care." ACTH and TSH are presented here with the discussions of the adrenal cortex and thyroid, respectively.

ANTERIOR PITUITARY DISORDERS

The diagnosis and treatment of disorders associated with anterior pituitary dysfunction is complicated by the fact that the pituitary usually occupies an intermediate position on the axis between hypothalamic control and the observed effect. This means not only that pituitary dysfunction must be inferred indirectly from dysfunction of the target system(s), but also that the cause of such dysfunction may be any place along the hypothalamic–pituitary–target gland axis. To further complicate differential diagnosis, most endocrine functions are under the control of several hormones. For example, anovulatory infertility may be due to primary ovarian failure, deficiency of gonadotropin release from the pituitary, failure of hypothalamic releasing factors, or even excess prolactin secretion due to pituitary or hypothalamic factors. Many drugs without obvious endocrine activity and psychobiologic factors can alter hypothalamic functions. Therefore, thorough medication and psychosocial histories and the use of pharmacologic agents as part of *stimulation tests* and *suppression tests* are an important part of endocrinology.

Hyperpituitarism

Gigantism and Acromegaly

Although any or all of the pituitary hormones may be secreted in excess, the effects of hyperfunction of the anterior pituitary are most closely associated with overproduction of growth hormone, which is manifested as *gigantism* in children and *acromegaly* in adults. Hypersecretion of growth hormone generally occurs due to the presence of pituitary adenoma. When surgical resection of the tumor is not feasible, drugs may be used to decrease growth hormone release. Two ergot derivatives, **bromocriptine** and **lergotrile mesylate**, are under investigation for this effect. Bromocriptine (Parlodel; see the discussion of lactation suppression in Chap. 46) in doses of 1.25 to 5.0 mg one to four times daily can result in sustained decline in growth hormone levels in acromegaly.

Hyperprolactinemia

Galactorrhea, amenorrhea, and female infertility can result from high levels of prolactin, which may be associated with a pituitary tumor (craniopharyngioma). In the absence of a demonstrable pituitary tumor, **bromocriptine** (Parlodel; see Chap. 46) in doses of 2.5 mg, two or three times daily with meals, may reverse the hyperprolactinemia and associated symptoms within 6 to 12 weeks; therapy should not be continued longer than six months.

Other Syndromes

Ectopic tumors, such as lung tumors, are common sources of hypersecretion of pituitary hormones. GH, ACTH, and TSH have been produced by nonpituitary tumors.

Chronic primary hypothyroidism may lead to sustained excessive thyrotropin production and hyperplasia of the pituitary. Resultant excessive release of the other pituitary hormones causes sexual precocity, galactorrhea, and growth, for which the treatment is thyroid replacement.

Hypopituitarism

Panhypopituitarism, a complete loss of pituitary function associated with decrements in growth hormone, ACTH, gonadotropins, and TSH, may be induced by tumors, surgical ablation, irradiation, or postpartum pituitary necrosis. Adults with hypopituitarism can be adequately maintained with replacement of thyroid, glucocorticoids, and appropriate sex hormones. Hypopituitarism in the young is associated with the development of *dwarfism* and sexual infantilism due to lack of growth hormone and the other adenohypophyseal hormones, and so the treatment of panhypopituitarism in children requires human growth hormone (HGH) therapy.

Growth Failure

While failure to attain normal growth patterns can be caused by drugs or by chromosomal, cardiac, pulmonary, gastrointestinal, orthopedic, thyroid, and central nervous system disorders, growth failure due to growth hormone deficiency is the most frequent manifestation of inadequate pituitary function. In addition to decreased growth, hypoglycemia and delayed tooth eruption accompany this condition. Growth hormone deficiency is diagnosed by ruling out other causes of growth failure and by the lack of elevation in plasma growth hormone levels in response to stimulation testing (Table 35-3). Once low growth hormone levels are documented, treatment of growth failure involves supplementation with human growth hormone.

Growth Hormone

Human growth hormone, also called somatropin, somatotropin, and HGH, is a simple polypeptide hormone with complex physiologic activity. The availability of HGH as a therapeutic agent (Asellacrin, Crescormon) is a major endocrinologic advance, since animal-derived growth hormones are not active in humans.

Control of GH Output Release of growth hormone does not occur with diurnal variation, but rather in short bursts stimulated by sleep. Growth hormone is also increased by exercise, hypoglycemia, acute stress, and high protein dietary intake. A number of drugs influence growth hormone release, including **levodopa, clonidine, dopamine, glucagon**, and β-endorphins, which constitutes the rationale for the stimulation testing discussed above. Hyperglycemia, thyroid deficiency, chronic emotional stress, and other drugs (e.g.. **fenfluramine, ethanol, cyproheptadine**) inhibit growth hormone release. Some drugs which stimulate the release of growth hormone in the normal individual decrease its output in patients with acromegaly (e.g., **bromocriptine**).

Physiologic Activity   The actions of growth hormone include induction of longitudinal bone growth, increasing skeletal and muscle mass, and retarding fat deposition. These effects of HGH are accompanied by positive nitrogen and phosphorus balance with reduced urinary loss of these elements; positive calcium balance also is produced despite continuing urinary losses. Anabolic effects on cartilage, bone, muscle, and kidney are seen. Increased protein synthesis and tissue DNA content are indicative of cellular multiplication. Growth hormone elevates blood sugar, which is called *diabetogenic action*. Hyperlipidemia, perhaps

TABLE 35-3   Growth Hormone Stimulation Procedures

STIMULANT	PROCEDURE / RESPONSE
Exercise	Vigorous and continuous exercise for 20 min should elevate HGH levels.*
Sleep	Blood sampled through an indwelling catheter q20min for 2 h during sleep should demonstrate normal HGH levels for age.
Arginine†	Arginine HCl, 300 mL (or 5 mL/kg) is infused over 30 min. Plasma HGH should rise 10–20 ng/mL over preinfusion baseline by 2 h. Allergic reactions (headache, nausea, vomiting, flushing, nervousness) should be treated with parenteral antihistamines, such as diphenhydramine (Benadryl).
Insulin†	Insulin (0.075–0.1 U/kg) is infused IV. Should cause hypoglycemia (blood glucose < 45 mg/100 mL) and increase of HGH within 90 min.* Test contraindicated in elderly and cardiac patients.
Levodopa†	Oral levodopa dose of 125 mg (500 mg if weight > 12 kg) should increase HGH levels within 90 min.* Propranolol enhances test response, but may increase nausea, vomiting, and hypoglycemia.
Glucagon†	IV infusion of 15 µg/kg should raise HGH levels within 90 min.*
Clonidine†	Oral clonidine (0.005 mg/kg, 0.15 mg/m², or 25 µg) should raise HGH levels within 90 min.* Drowsiness may occur.

*Normal response is an increase in plasma HGH levels of 6–8 ng/mL.

†Preparation for test includes normal night's sleep and overnight fast. Patient is to rest 30 min to reduce apprehension prior to baseline blood sample.

due to increased fat breakdown to free fatty acids and decreased amino acids in the serum, are also observed.

Adverse Effects   Adverse effects associated with the administration of somatotropin include hyperglycemia, so that regular urine glucose testing is required. Hypothyroidism may also develop during HGH therapy, and preexistent hypothyroidism impairs response to HGH. Baseline and periodic thyroid function tests are done. Lipodystrophy, lipoatrophy, and an increased frequency of antibody production to the hormone have been seen when subcutaneous administration is used, and so injections must be given intramuscularly.

Dosage and Administration   HGH is supplemented by thrice weekly IM injections of 2 IU. In older children or after prolonged therapy dosage increase may be necessary. If growth during therapy is less than 2.5 cm (1 in) in height in a six-month period, the dose is doubled for the next six months. When the epiphyses close, indicated by sexual maturity, the injections are stopped. If the patient has panhypopituitarism, estrogen or androgen therapy is started and somatotropin therapy is stopped after adequate height has been achieved. These hormones, as well as corticosteroids, may impair the response to HGH if given earlier. Corticosteroid therapy should be limited to less than 10 to 15 mg/m² of hydrocortisone equivalent daily during HGH therapy.

POSTERIOR PITUITARY DISORDERS

While *antidiuretic hormone* (vasopressin, ADH) is not necessary to survival, it does have dramatic physiologic actions. ADH controls reabsorption of sodium-free water in the collecting duct of the nephron and is a potent vasoconstrictor. Clinical syndromes are associated with deficient activity (diabetes insipidus) and excess activity (SIADH) of this hormone.

Diabetes Insipidus

In neurogenic diabetes insipidus the deficiency of ADH activity results in the loss of large volumes of fluid in the urine and secondary polydipsia. Hypophysectomy, head trauma, congenital deficiency, and surgical transection of the pituitary stalk are the most common causes of diabetes insipidus. Hormonal replacement of vasopressin and use of nonhormonal drugs which increase ADH release are the two approaches to treating diabetes insipidus.

Vasopressin

Vasopressin is available in several forms: **vasopressin injectable** (Pitressin Synthetic), **vasopressin tannate** injection in oil, **lypressin** capsules for inhalation (Diapid), and **desmopressin acetate** nasal solution (DDAVP). The **extract of posterior pituitary** (Pitressin), which contains both oxytocin and vasopressin, is available for injection and as capsules for inhalation. Vasopressin is indicated in the treatment of diabetes insipidus and postoperative paralytic ileus; other uses are listed in Table 35-1.

Control of ADH Output   The primary control of the production and release of vasopressin is plasma osmolarity, which is sensed by hypothalamic osmoreceptors. Increased plasma osmolarity increases ADH output, while decreased osmolarity has the opposite effect. Volume depletion also increases ADH production and release. Pain, emotion, stress, and certain drugs also increase vasopressin output (Table 35-4).

Physiologic Activity   Vasopressin is active in the epithelium of the renal collecting tubule, promoting resorption of water. It also causes vasoconstriction through its effect on smooth muscle of the vascular bed. Gastrointestinal motility and tone are enhanced by vasopressin.

Pharmacokinetics   Aqueous vasopressin has a short half-life of about 2 to 3 h. This may be advantageous in labile diabetes insipidus and for postoperative ileus. Vasopressin tannate in oil is the injectable form with a long (24 to 72 h) duration of action. **Lypressin** must be administered every 3 to 6 h, while **desmopressin** has an average duration of action of 12 h (range, 8 to 20 h).

Adverse Effects   Overdosage may cause water intoxication manifested as apathy, headache, stupor, muscle twitching,

TABLE 35-4   Drugs Which Alter Endogenous Vasopressin Activity

Increase ADH Release

Anesthetics
Carbamazepine (Tegretol)
Chlorpropamide (Diabinese)
Cholinergic drugs
Clofibrate (Atromid-S)
Cyclophosphamide (Cytoxan)
Morphine
Nicotine
Tricyclic antidepressants

Decrease ADH Release

Chloral hydrate (Noctec, others)
Chlorpromazine (Thorazine)
Ethanol
Furosemide (Lasix)
Phenytoin (Dilantin)

Alter Response at Nephron

Colchicine
Glyburide (Dibeta)
Magnesium (high dose)
Propoxyphene (Darvon)
Tetracyclines [especially demeclocycline (Declomycin)]

weight gain, hyponatremia, and seizures. Adverse effects include local irritation from injection or nasal administration, vulvar pain, circumoral pallor, nausea, vomiting, hypertension, cramping, flatus, frequent defecation, vertigo, and angina. Vasopressin should be used with caution in conditions where vasoconstriction and/or fluid retention are contraindicated, e.g., coronary heart disease, congestive heart failure, and pulmonary edema. Allergic reactions, such as anaphylaxis, urticaria, and bronchospasm, have occurred.

Dosage and Administration   Dosage is titrated to normalization of urine output, thirst, and sensorium. **Aqueous vasopressin** is given IM or SC every 6 to 8 h in doses of 0.25 to 0.5 mL. **Pitressin tannate** must be warmed and thoroughly mixed before the dose of 0.5 to 1.0 mL every one to three days is administered. For chronic use, nasal insufflation forms are preferred. **Lypressin**, which contains 2 U per squirt may require 2 to 3 squirts three times daily and at bedtime while **desmopressin** is inhaled through the plastic catheter two to three times daily. Loss of control can result if the internasally administered drug washes away during swimming.

Nonhormonal Therapy

Chlorpropamide, an oral antidiabetic agent (see below), appears to augment ADH action in the kidney and to promote the release of ADH. It is usually effective for neurogenic diabetes insipidus in daily doses of 125 to 250 mg, although 500 mg/day is sometimes required. Concomitant thiazide diuretic therapy may potentiate the antidiuretic effect of chlorpropamide and counteract its hypoglycemic action. Prompt reversal of the signs of diabetes insipidus generally results with therapy of 400 to 800 mg of the anticonvulsant **carbamazepine** (Tegretol) daily (see Chap. 33). **Clofibrate** (Atromid-S) is a lipid-lowering drug which, at 1.5 to 2.25 g/day, markedly decreases the urine volume in diabetes insipidus (see Chap. 41).

Nephrogenic Diabetes Insipidus

Kidney resistance to normal levels of ADH, called nephrogenic diabetes insipidus, can be inherited, due to metabolic derangements, or drug-induced. **Lithium** therapy, employed in manic depressive illness, has been associated with one-eighth of the reported cases of diabetes insipidus. Lithium purportedly inhibits the subcellular mechanism by which ADH exerts its effect in the kidney. Other drugs (Table 35-4) may have similar effects. The differentiation of nephrogenic diabetes insipidus from true ADH deficiency is established by administering **pitressin** (ADH), because nephrogenic diabetes insipidus does not respond to **pitressin**. The **thiazide diuretics** *reduce* urine output in nephrogenic diabetes insipidus; the mechanism of this paradoxical effect is not clear (see Chap. 23).

Syndrome of Inappropriate Secretion of ADH

In times of great stress, ADH may be released in amounts which are far in excess of those indicated by the plasma osmotic pressure. This syndrome of inappropriate secretion of ADH (SIADH) has been observed following head trauma, with pulmonary and cerebral disorders, and in patients with malignant tumors. It is also associated with those agents which increase ADH release (Table 35-4). Laboratory criteria for diagnosis of SIADH in a patient not taking diuretics include hyponatremia with low serum osmolality, urine which is less than maximally dilute relative to the low plasma osmolality, inappropriately large urinary sodium loss, normal renal function, normal thyroid function, normal adrenal function, no evidence of fluid overload or dehydration, and recovery with fluid restriction. When a patient cannot tolerate fluid restriction, **demeclocycline** (Declomycin) 300 to 600 mg daily may be used. If the patient has liver dysfunction, demeclocycline toxicity is increased. Alternative agents include **lithium, phenytoin, furosemide,** and oral **urea.**

NURSING PROCESS RELATED TO THE PITUITARY HORMONES

The nursing process related to growth hormone and to the vasopressin analogs is shown in Table 35-5.

THE ADRENAL CORTEX

LEARNING OBJECTIVES

Upon mastery of this section the reader will be able to:

1. Explain the regulation of ACTH and corticosteroid hormone secretion, including diurnal rhythm and stress responses.
2. List the clinical uses of corticotropin and the corticosteroids.
3. Name the three types of hormones secreted from the adrenal cortex.
4. State the physiologic functions of mineralocorticoids and glucocorticoids.
5. List two mineralocorticoids and at least four glucocorticoids available for therapeutic use.
6. Describe the assessment and management associated with the adverse effects of corticosteroids.
7. Explain why cortisone and prednisone are not to be used for topical or intraarticular administration or for those with severe hepatic dysfunction.
8. Explain the rationale for the following during corticosteroid therapy: tapered withdrawal, alternate day dosing, supplemental doses in times of stress.
9. Indicate the symptoms and treatment of Addison's disease.
10. Indicate the symptoms and treatment of Cushing's syndrome.
11. List conditions that contraindicate or require caution in the use of corticosteroid drugs.
12. Outline a teaching plan for the patient taking corticosteroids.

TABLE 35-5   Nursing Process Related to Use of Pituitary Hormones

THERAPY	ASSESSMENT	MANAGEMENT	EVALUATION
Growth hormone	Height and weight baseline; compare to age norms. Diet, drug, and psychosocial history for contributing factors. Use with caution if family history of diabetes. Explain stimulation testing; help to minimize patient's anxiety.	Assure that injection is intramuscular Teach patient/family how to monitor for glucosuria; signs of hyperglycemia	Monitor every 6 to 12 months for growth, onset of puberty, hypoglycemia, hypothyroidism.
Vasopressin	Baseline weight, vital signs, input/output volumes, sensorium, serum and urine electrolytes. Baseline bowel sounds and record of stools, if given for ileus.	Teach proper method of nasal insufflation. Use short-acting aqueous vasopressin intramuscular for postoperative ileus; hemorrhage. Insure adequate fluid intake, availability.	Evaluate desired outcome: bowel activity, decreased urine output, or decreased hemorrhage, etc. Check weight, vital signs, input/output volumes, sensorium, serum and urine electrolytes, vulvar pain, gastrointestinal distress, flatus, injection site or nasal mucosa for irritation, angina.

PHYSIOLOGY OF THE ADRENAL GLANDS

The end organs of the *hypothalamic-pituitary-adrenal axis (HPA axis)*, the adrenal glands, normally contain two types of endocrine tissues. The chromaffin cells in the center of the gland (adrenal medulla) are derived from the neural tissue and release catecholamines (epinephrine, norepinephrine). Surrounding that tissue is the cortex of the adrenal gland (adrenal cortex) in which steroid hormones are formed; hence the common name *corticosteroids*. These two different tissues are physiologically as well as anatomically related; the enzyme responsible for catalyzing the synthesis of epinephrine is induced by high corticosteroid concentrations. The pharmacology of the catecholamines is discussed in Unit III. Three distinct hormone types are produced in the adrenal cortex: *mineralocorticoids* (aldosterone and deoxycorticosterone), *glucocorticoids* (cortisol and corticosterone), and *androgens*.

Control of Adrenocortical Function

The production and release of adrenocorticosteroids is under the control of corticotropin (adrenocorticotropic hormone, ACTH) from the pituitary, which is, in turn, regulated by corticotropin-releasing hormone (CRH) from the hypothalamus and negative feedback from circulating levels of corticosteroids (Fig. 35-3). Because their activities are not required in constant amounts throughout the day, the adrenocorticosteroids are secreted in *response to stressful events* (injury, pain, exercise, fear, infection, flight, or strong emotions) and on a *regular circadian rhythm* (24-h cycle). In humans over 3 years old this secretion is usually on a *diurnal* basis, with the gradual rise of serum and urinary corticosteroid concentrations beginning at 3 to 4 A.M., peaking at approximately 8 A.M., and gradually declining to a minimum around midnight. Adults who work at night and sleep by day show a reversal to a *nocturnal* pattern. However, with an abrupt change in sleeping or working hours, several weeks may be needed to reestablish adrenocortical cycling.

Corticotropin has only minor influence on the production and release of aldosterone. Activation of the *renin-angiotensin system* (see Chap. 40) by conditions which cause decreased renal blood flow (hemorrhage, hypotension, standing, hyponatremia, vasodilator drugs, exercise, etc.) stimulate aldosterone output. In addition, factors such as hyperkalemia, salt loss, and standing posture directly stimulate the output of aldosterone.

Production of Adrenocorticosteroids

The adrenal steroids are produced from cholesterol in a series of common metabolic pathways (Fig. 35-4). Congenital absence of one of the enzymes in this synthetic network results in a deficit of some hormones and an overproduction of others. For example, congenital absence of 11β-hydroxylase results in adrenogenital syndrome manifested by viril-ization (from the overproduction of androgens) and hypertension (due to accumulation of 11-deoxycorticosterone which has aldosterone-like activity). Because of the common chemical structure of these hormones, there is some overlap in function. Thus, androgens and glucocorticoids have weak salt- and water-retaining effects (aldosterone-like activity) and, as a result, side effects of the therapeutic use of these agents can be increased blood pressure, weight gain, and edema.

Actions of the Adrenocorticosteroids

Glucocorticoids Cortisol (hydrocortisone), the primary natural glucocorticoid, has diverse effects in the metabolism of carbohydrates, fats, and proteins. In general, the effects of cortisol are to prepare the body for fasting during stress, as it increases the production of glucose (gluconeogenesis), decreases glucose use in muscle, and promotes glycogen storage. Muscle and adipose tissue are broken down to provide amino acids, fatty acids, and triglycerides as energy substrates. Fat deposition is redistributed from the extremities to the face, neck, and trunk.

Cortisol markedly inhibits the normal inflammatory response and breaks down lymphoid tissues of the thymus, spleen, lymph nodes, and circulating lymphocytes (*lympholytic effects*). It decreases vascular permeability, response to lymphokines, and complement synthesis. Polymorphonuclear neutrophils (PMNs) in the blood are increased by glucocorticoids due to demargination of bone marrow stores, but fewer eosinophils, PMNs, and monocytes are found at inflammation sites.

Other systems influenced by cortisol include the cardiovascular system, kidney, and central nervous system. Blood volume, cardiac output, glomerular filtration rate, and blood flow to muscles are increased by glucocorticoids. Cortisol increases brain excitability and affects mood. Glucocorticoids are necessary for the action of a number of hormones; thus they are said to have a "permissive effect" for glucagon and catecholamines. The action of other hormones, such as insulin and growth hormone, are antagonized by glucocorticoids.

Mineralocorticoids Mineralocorticoids regulate the ability of the body to retain sodium and excrete potassium. The kidney is the organ most profoundly affected, but aldosterone, the primary natural mineralocorticoid, also acts on the intestines, salivary glands, and sweat glands. This salt-retaining function of mineralocorticoids helps to maintain blood volume and blood pressure; hypertension and edema can result from excess mineralocorticoid activity.

Sex Hormones The adrenal androgenic sex hormones are normally prominent only in the fetus and infant, and at puberty. During puberty, androgens stimulate the growth of pubic and axillary hair (thelarche). Female psychosexual behavior may also be influenced by the adrenal androgenic steroids. Androgens are discussed in detail in a subsequent section of this chapter.

CLINICAL PHARMACOLOGY OF CORTICOSTEROIDS

Because of their diverse physiologic activity, numerous adverse effects, which are extensions of the drugs' pharmacologic actions, can accompany the therapeutic use of adrenocorticosteroids. In order to maximize therapeutic potency and minimize these undesired effects, pharmaceutical chemists have studied the structure-activity relationships (see Chap. 5) of the steroids and synthesized a number of agents with more specific pharmacologic activity. The glucocorticoid and mineralocorticoid activity can be separated. (Table 35-6 shows the relative anti-inflammatory and salt retention activity of the natural and synthetic corticosteroids.) As yet the anti-inflammatory and the carbohydrate-protein (glucocorticoid) effects have not been separated. Two mineralocorticoids are available: **deoxycorticosterone**, which must be parenterally administered, and **fludrocortisone**. Numerous glucocorticoids of varying potency and durations of action are available (see Table 35-7).

Indications

Both glucocorticoids and mineralocorticoids are used physiologically for *replacement therapy* in the adrenalectomized or adrenal-insufficient patient. Glucocorticoids administered in pharmacologic doses have *therapeutic application* in suppressing the immune and inflammatory responses (Table 35-8). The use of glucocorticoids in most cases is palliative or symptomatic rather than curative, except in replacement therapy.

Pharmacokinetics

With the exception of **deoxycorticosterone** (Doca. Percorten), the corticosteroid preparations are well absorbed and effective orally. They are extensively bound to plasma proteins; cortisol is 90 percent bound to the alpha-2-globulin (cortisol-binding globulin, CBG, or transcortin). If all the hormonal binding sites on CBG are occupied, cortisol will bind to albumin. In conditions where there is an increase in CBG (e.g., pregnancy, oral contraceptive therapy), measurement of plasma cortisol gives the false impression of hypercorticism, but the free cortisol level (which is the pharmacologically active component) remains unchanged. Synthetic glucocorticoids are protein-bound to a lesser degree than cortisol.

TABLE 35-6   Relative Mineralocorticoid and Glucocorticoid Activity of Corticosteroid Preparations

CORTICOSTEROID	RELATIVE GLUCOCORTICOID ACTIVITY	RELATIVE MINERALOCORTICOID ACTIVITY	EQUIVALENT ANTI-INFLAMMATORY DOSE
Short-Acting Glucocorticoids (Biologic Half-Life of 8–12 h)			
Hydrocortisone* (cortisol)	1	1	20
Cortisone*	0.8	0.8	25
Intermediate-Acting Glucocorticoids (Biologic Half-Life of 18–36 h)			
Prednisone	4	0.8	5
Prednisolone	4	0.8	5
Methylprednisolone	5	0.0–0.5	4
Triamcinolone	5	0	4
Paramethasone	10	0	2
Long-Acting Glucocorticoids (Biologic Half-Life of 36–54 h)			
Dexamethasone	25	0	0.75
Betamethasone	25	0	0.6
Agents with Primarily Mineralocorticoid Activity			
Fludrocortisone	10	125–400	—†
Deoxycorticosterone*	0	10–20	—
Aldosterone*	0.35–0.0	300	—

*Natural corticosteroid endogenous to humans. Aldosterone is not available for clinical use due to its short duration of action.

†Although fludrocortisone has significant glucocorticoid activity, its potent mineralocorticoid effects preclude its use as an anti-inflammatory drug. At doses of fludrocortisone necessary for salt-retaining activity, little glucocorticoid effect is manifest.

TABLE 35-7 Glucocorticoids and Mineralocorticoids

GENERIC NAME	TRADE NAME	DOSAGE FORMS*
	Glucocorticoids	
Cortisone acetate	Cortone acetate	Tablets; injection
Hydrocortisone (cortisol)	Cortef, Hydrocortone, Cortaid, others	Tablets; injection; topical ointment, cream, gel, spray, lotion; retention enema
Hydrocortisone acetate	Biosone, Fernisone, Cortef Acetate, others	Injection; topical ointment, cream, foam; ophthalmic ointment
Hydrocortisone cypionate	Cortef Fluid	Oral suspension
Hydrocortisone sodium phosphate	Hydrocortone Phosphate	Injection
Hydrocortisone sodium succinate	Solu-Cortef	Injection
Prednisolone	Delta-Cortef, Cortalone, others	Tablets, topical cream
Prednisolone acetate	Meticortelone Acetate, Niscort, others	Injection; ophthalmic drops
Prednisolone acetate with prednisolone sodium phosphate	Due-Pred, Panacort RP, others	Injection
Prednisolone sodium phosphate	Hydeltrasol, others	Injection; ophthalmic drops
Prednisolone tebutate	Hydeltra-TBA, others	Intraarticular injection
Prednisone	Meticorten, Deltasone, others	Tablets, syrup
Triamcinolone	Aristocort, Kenacort	Tablets; syrup
Triamcinolone acetonide	Kenalog-10, Trilog, others	Injection; topical ointment, cream
Triamcinolone diacetate	Aristocort Forte, Triamolone, others	Injectable
Triamcinolone hexacetonide	Aristospan Intralesional, Aristospan Intra-articular	Intralesional; intraarticular
Methylprednisolone	Medrol	Tablets
Methylprednisolone acetate	Depo-Medrol, others	Injectable; topical ointment; retention enema; intrarectal foam
Methylprednisolone sodium succinate	Solu-Medrol, A-methaPred, others	Injectable
Fluprednisolone	Alphadrol	Tablets
Dexamethasone	Decadron, Hexadrol, others	Tablets, elixir
Dexamethasone acetate	Decadron-LA, others	Injectable for soft tissue or intraarticular
Dexamethasone sodium phosphate	Decadron Phosphate, Decadron Phosphate Respihaler, Turbinaire Decadron Phosphate, others	Injectable; aerosol for inhalation; ophthalmic drops, ointment; metered nasal spray
Beclomethasone dipropionate	Beclovent, Vanceril	Aerosol for inhalation
Betamethasone	Celestone	Tablets, topical cream
Betamethasone acetate and betamethasone sodium phosphate	Celestone Soluspan	Injectable
Betamethasone sodium phosphate	Celestone Phosphate, others	Injectable
Paramethasone	Haldrone	Tablets

TABLE 35-7 Glucocorticoids and Mineralocorticoids (*Cont.*)

GENERIC NAME	TRADE NAME	DOSAGE FORMS*
	Mineralocorticoids	
Deoxycorticosterone acetate	Doca Acetate and Percorten Acetate	Injection, pellets for implant
Deoxycorticosterone pivalate	Percorten Pivalate	Repository injection
Fluorocortisone acetate	Florinef	Tablets

*A number of glucocorticoids are available only for topical use: betamethasone dipropionate (Diprosone, Vancenase, or Beconase nasal inhalers), betamethasone valerate (Valisone, others), betamethasone benzoate (Uticort, others), desonide (Tridesilon), flumethasone pivalate (Lorcorten), flurandrenolide (Cordran, others), fluorometholone (Halog, others), amcinonide (Cyclocort), clocortolone pivalate (Cloderm), medrysone (HMS Liquifilm Ophthalmic), flunisolide (Nasalide).

Corticosteroids are metabolized by the microsomal enzymes in the liver with the inactive metabolites excreted in the urine. The duration of action of the glucocorticoids is much longer than their plasma half-life, and so the term *biologic half-life* is used to reflect the duration of glucocorticoid activity (Table 35-6). Similarly, plasma concentrations do not directly correlate with therapeutic activity, and so clinical status. rather than blood levels, is used in monitoring therapy.

Several of the steroids must be metabolized to be active; **prednisone** is converted in the body to **prednisolone**, the active form. **Cortisone** is converted to cortisol (**hydrocortisone**), also the active form. Inactive forms of the drug are not used for topical or intraarticular administration, because activating enzymes are not present at the administration site. Similarly, active forms are generally used in patients with severe hepatic dysfunction, since conversion from the inactive forms may be impaired.

Altering the drug solubility changes the duration of drug action, so corticosteroids are available as a variety of salts, suspensions, and esters in nearly every conceivable dosage form (Table 36-7) and as one ingredient in a number of combination products for topical use.

Adverse Effects

Corticosteroids can adversely affect almost every organ system. These adverse effects can be related to the physiologic activity of the corticosteroids and to extensions of desired pharmacologic effects. Some of these effects can be prevented or ameliorated through proper dosing and administration (see below) and through nursing interventions. Table 35-9 relates the major adverse effects of the corticosteroids to the underlying physiologic mechanisms and lists the techniques for detection and management of each.

Drug Interactions Drugs which are taken concurrently can affect response to glucocorticoid therapy. **Phenytoin** (Dilantin), the **barbiturates**, and **rifampin** induce microsomal enzymes and may enhance the elimination of corticosteroids, increasing their dose requirement or altering the interpretability of steroid suppression tests. Conversely, **erythromycins**, **oral contraceptives**, and **troleandomycin** (TAO) inhibit microsomal enzymes; patients taking these drugs at the same time as corticosteroids may need a decreased dosage of corticosteroids to avoid adverse effects. The interaction between troleandomycin and corticosteroids is used therapeutically to reduce the dosage of corticosteroid required in certain respiratory disorders (see Chap. 27).

Thiazide diuretics, **furosemide** (Lasix), **bumetanide** (Bumex), or **amphotericin B** use may potentiate the potassium wasting which occurs with corticosteroids, and hypokalemia can result. **Indomethacin** (Indocin) can increase the risk of gastrointestinal ulceration in patients taking corticosteroids. Corticosteroids may antagonize the response to the oral anticoagulant **warfarin**. The physiologic action of glucocorticoids in elevating blood glucose antagonizes the action of **oral antidiabetic agents** and **insulin** therapy; increased doses of these drugs may be required to stabilize diabetes control. Immunosuppression from steroids may compromise response to antibiotics, particularly **tetracycline**, causing superinfection.

Corttiicosteroids may induce the microsomal enzymes which metabolize **cyclophosphamide**, salicylates, and **isoniazid** (INH). As a result the serum salicylate levels achieved by a specific dose of aspirin may be reduced, and abrupt decreases in the corticosteroid dose could result in salicylism. The antitubercular action of isoniazid could be compromised in those taking corticosteroids.

Dosing and Administration

Dosage requirements for corticosteroids vary widely among patients, so individualization of dosage is crucial. The *initial dosage* in chronic therapy depends upon the disease state being treated. Once the desired therapeutic endpoint (relief of symptoms) is achieved, this initial dosage is titrated downward to the *least amount of drug* required for the desired level of clinical control, which is the *maintenance dose*. Changes in patient situation, such as exacerbation or

TABLE 35-8   Indications for the Use of Glucocorticoids

Replacement Therapy

Primary insufficiency (acute or chronic)
Congenital adrenal hyperplasia
Adrenal insufficiency secondary to anterior
pituitary insufficiency

Ophthalmic Indications

Diffuse posterior uveitis and choroiditis
Allergic conjunctivitis*
Keratitis*
Allergic corneal marginal ulcers*
Chorioretinitis
Herpes zoster ophthalmitis*
Iritis/Iridocyclitis*
Optic neuritis
Sympathetic ophthalmia
Anterior segment inflammation*

Endocrine Indications

Diagnosis of adrenal disorders
Nonsuppurative thyroiditis
Hypercalcemia due to malignancies

Respiratory Diseases

Symptomatic sarcoidosis
Berylliosis
Fulminating or disseminated tuberculosis
Bronchial asthma/status asthmaticus
Allergic rhinitis (hay fever)*
Loeffler's syndrome
Prevention of hyaline membrane disease

Gastrointestinal Indications

Hepatic cirrhosis
Ulcerative colitis*
Regional enteritis (Crohn's disease)
Idiopathic steatorrhea
Intractable sprue

Hematologic Indications

Idiopathic thrombocytopenic purpura
Secondary thrombocytopenia (IV form only)
Acquired hemolysis and anemia
Erythroblastopenia; congenital hypoplastic anemia

Collagen Diseases

Ankylosing spondylitis
Bursitis†
Systemic lupus erythematosis
Acute rheumatic carditis
Polymyositis
Acute nonspecific tenosynovitis†
Acute gouty arthritis
Rheumatoid arthritis
Osteoarthritis
Epicondylitis†
Psoriatic arthritis

Skin Disorders

Erythema multiforme*
Exfoliative dermatitis*
Angioedema
Atopic dermatitis*
Contact dermatitis*
Bullous dermatitis herpetiformis
Severe cystic acne†
Mycosis fungoides*
Pemphigus*
Psoriasis*
Seborrheic dermatitis*

Indications for Use of Intraarticular Injection

Osteoarthritis-associated synovitis
Rheumatoid arthritis
Acute gouty arthritis
Epicondylitis
Acute nonspecific tenosynovitis
Posttraumatic osteoarthritis

Malignancies

Acute and chronic myelocyte and lymphocytic leukemias
Chronic Hodgkin's disease
Breast cancer
Prostate cancer

Nervous System Indications

Antiemetic therapy
Cerebral edema
Diagnosis of depression
Multiple sclerosis
Tuberculous meningitis with subarachnoid or impending block
Trichinosis

Miscellaneous Indications

Allergic disorders
Transfusion reactions
Serum sickness
Drug hypersensitivity
Prevention of transplant rejection
In septic shock to prevent "shock lung" (adult respiratory distress syndrome)
Nephrotic syndrome
Post–myocardial infarction syndrome

---

*Topical therapy may be employed in these conditions.
†Local injection often employed in these conditions.

TABLE 35-9   Adverse Effects of Glucocorticoids in Pharmacologic Dosages

ADVERSE EFFECTS	PHYSIOLOGIC MECHANISM	DETECTION	PREVENTION/MANAGEMENT
Edema, hypertension, congestive heart failure in susceptible persons	Mineralocorticoid activity to increase retention of sodium and water	1. Weight 2. Blood pressure 3. Palpate for edema 4. Auscultate heart and lungs	1. Low sodium diet 2. Use of drug with weak mineralocorticoid activity
Hyperglycemia, exacerbation of diabetes mellitus, insulin resistance	Promotion of gluconeogenesis, decreased glucose utilization, antagonism of growth hormone	1. Blood glucose or urine for glycosuria 2. Symptoms of hyperglycemia: hunger, polyuria, thirst	1. Teach patient to evaluate urine or blood sugar, symptoms of hyperglycemia 2. Insulin dosage of diabetics may need to be increased
Hypokalemia, metabolic alkalosis, hypocalcemia	Enhanced excretion of potassium, hydrogen, and calcium	1. Serum chemistries 2. Muscle cramps, diarrhea, nausea, vomiting, tetany, arrhythmias, paresthesias	1. Avoid concurrent potassium-depleting diuretics 2. High potassium and calcium foods in diet, supplementation PRN
Muscle wasting, myopathy, weakness	Inhibition of protein synthesis, proteolysis	1. Hand grip strength 2. Measure muscle mass	1. Encourage exercise 2. High protein and calcium diet
Peptic ulceration, pancreatitis, gastrointestinal upset	Proteolysis, impaired immune reaction	1. X-rays or gastroscopy in susceptible or symptomatic 2. Epigastric pain, tarry stools, vomiting blood 3. Check stools for occult blood	1. Avoid concurrent use of known gastric irritants (aspirin, indomethacin, caffeine) 2. Give antacids when high dose therapy 3. Take drug with meals
Euphoria, insomnia, "steroid psychosis"	Excitation of brain cells	History of depression or psychosis, question significant others	1. Inform patient about cause of symptoms 2. Sedatives may be needed; reduce or discontinue corticosteroid if severe
Adrenal insufficiency on abrupt drug withdrawal or high stress situation	Suppression of HPA axis by endogenous corticosteroids	Nausea, anorexia, fatigue, malaise, myalgia, depression, hypoglycemia, and hypotention on drug withdrawal	1. Use lowest effective dose 2. Alternate day dosing, give before 9 A.M. 3. Tapered withdrawal if doses equivalent to or more than 10 mg prednisone for 13 days or 25 mg prednisone for 5 to 10 days. 4. Supplementary doses in stress situation
Cushingoid body habitus: moon face, buffalo hump, trunchal obesity	Mobilization of fatty acids and glycerol via lipolysis	Physical examination	1. Lowest effective dose 2. Alternate day doses
Growth failure in children	Inhibited protein synthesis, antagonism to growth hormone	Low height and weight compared to age norms	1. High protein diet 2. Alternate day dosing
Hirsutism, irregular menses in females	Androgenic effects, pituitary inhibition	History and physical examination	1. Use of depilatories 2. Inform woman that menses may be affected
Striae, thin fragile skin, impaired wound healing, easy bruising, thrombophlebitis, thromboembolism	Proteolysis, impaired protein synthesis	History and physical examination	1. Safety precautions to prevent injuries 2. Have patient report bruising, calf pain, etc.
Activation of latent infections, increased susceptibility to infection	Lympholytic activity, impaired inflammatory response	1. Chest x-rays if activation of tuberculosis suspected 2. Careful history and physical	1. Tell patient to report cold, sore throat, fever 2. Decrease exposure to infection
Cataracts, increased intraocular pressure, exacerbation of glaucoma	Mobilization of fats, amino acids, glucose; (?) mineralocorticoid effect in glaucoma	Periodic eye examination including tonometry and fundoscopic	1. Have patient report any visual problems

remission of the disease process, increased exposure to stress, or a change in patient responsiveness to the drug, often require adjustment of this maintenance dose or supplemental doses. After long-term therapy, which results in suppression of the HPA axis, the drug must be *withdrawn slowly* (tapered doses) to avoid potentially life-threatening adrenal insufficiency. Following withdrawal, patients are observed carefully for disease recurrence and may require supplemental corticosteroids if subjected to stressful situations, such as surgery, during the time that the HPA axis is recovering function.

When corticosteroids are used in a life-threatening situation, large parenteral doses, as a single large dose or at frequent intervals, are administered depending upon the clinical condition of the patient. For example, in septic shock **hydrocortisone** 50 to 150 mg/kg, **dexamethasone** 6 mg/kg, or **methylprednisone** 30 mg/kg is administered. A single large dose is relatively devoid of the chronic adverse effects discussed above. Short-term therapy, particularly with low doses, results in only transient suppression of the HPA axis, and tapered withdrawal may not be required. HPA suppression occurs when **prednisone** in a dose of 7.5 to 10 mg (or the equivalent) is given on a daily basis for 14 days or longer. If suppression is suspected, a tapering dosage schedule should be employed.

Because the HPA axis is least susceptible to suppression at its peak activity, once daily doses should be given before 9 A.M. This dose also mimics the diurnal secretion of endogenous corticosteroids. Multiple daily doses are given at evenly spaced intervals. Giving oral corticosteroids with meals or a snack minimizes gastrointestinal upset. Regular antacid doses between meals may be initiated as a prophylaxis to peptic ulcers.

Alternate Day Therapy Alternate day therapy is a dosing regimen in which twice the daily dosage of a *shorter acting* corticosteroid (short- and intermediate-acting agents; see Table 35-6) is given every other morning to minimize HPA suppression, growth suppression, and altered habitus. It is recommended in *most* cases that will require long-term glucocorticoid therapy, even for those patients who have previously received daily therapy for a long period. Alternate day dosing is only indicated for pharmacologic uses of glucocorticoids and *not when corticosteroids are given for physiologic replacement.*

For a few patients therapy can be initiated on an alternate day schedule, but most will need to begin with once daily doses, or even multiple daily doses, until clinical symptoms are controlled. Transition to alternate day dosing may be slow, with gradual tapering down of the "off" day dose, usually accompanied by concurrent increases in the "on" day dose. However, since corticosteroid doses equivalent to 10 mg of prednisone daily are considered suppressive to the HPA axis, some prescribers make the switch to alternate day dosing all at once. Patients undergoing tapering of corticosteroid doses may experience fatigue, joint pain, "flulike"

symptoms, or depression. If the patient experiences these symptoms or symptoms of the disease process under treatment during the switch to alternate day dosing or tapered withdrawal, additional doses may be given or the tapering process deferred or performed at a slower rate.

NURSING PROCESS RELATED TO CORTICOSTEROIDS

Assessment

The nurse must be aware of the condition for which the patient is receiving corticosteroids and the desired level of clinical control. Complete obliteration of disease symptoms is not always the desired therapeutic endpoint as this may require unacceptably high doses of corticosteroids. Baseline observations of the signs and symptoms of the disease process should be recorded.

A number of conditions contraindicate corticosteroids or require extra caution in their use. Patients with latent infections, such as ocular or systemic fungal infections, tuberculosis, or amebiasis, are at risk for exacerbation of their disease during corticosteroid therapy. Corneal perforation has occurred in patients with ocular herpes simplex who were given corticosteroids. A history of peptic ulcer disease or concurrent use of other gastric irritants requires that the nurse be aware of the potential for peptic ulcer formation. Patients should not be vaccinated with live viruses, including smallpox, while on immunosuppressive doses of a corticosteroid. Since corticosteroids suppress growth, mothers on pharmacologic doses of corticosteroids are advised not to nurse their infants. The adverse effects of corticosteroids may be particularly dangerous for patients with the following: active or latent diabetes, osteoporosis, congestive heart failure, hypertension, renal insufficiency, thromboembolitic tendencies, convulsive disorders, or a family history of psychiatric illness.

Management

Prevention and management of adverse effects of the corticosteroids (Table 35-9) is a crucial nursing activity. Patients on long-term corticosteroids must receive thorough educational preparation in managing their illness and its therapy. This educational program should include an explanation of the role of corticosteroids as palliative treatment of their disease. Patients on long-term therapy should understand the need for adequate protein, potassium, and calcium in the diet, as well as the value of avoiding excessive sodium intake. Females should be informed that menstrual irregularities may occur, and if so, they should be reported to the physician or nurse. The importance of wearing or carrying identification that they are on long-term corticosteroid therapy and the need to inform any health care providers of this fact should be emphasized. Patients should be taught to call their care provider immediately if they experience signs of infection (prolonged sore throat or cold, fever), gastrointestinal ulceration (epigastric burning; black, tarry stool; vomiting of blood), fluid retention (high blood pressure, edema of face or extremities, weight gain), or unusual physical or psychosocial stress. The dangers of stopping the drug abruptly must be presented. The signs of adrenal insufficiency (fatigue, nausea, vomiting, diarrhea, weight loss, and dizziness) and the need to inform the physician of their occurrence should be known to anyone for whom the drug dosage is tapered or discontinued.

In administering these drugs, the nurse must double-check the label to ensure that the proper agent and route of administration are selected. Preparations meant for intraarticular injection may be harmful if given systemically, while the injection of shorter-acting aqueous preparations into the joint may mean that efficacy is lost sooner than anticipated. Oral agents should be taken with food, and, if given once daily or in alternate day doses, prior to 9 A.M.

Since these patients are immunosuppressed, exposure to infection must be minimized. Good aseptic technique and avoiding contact with personnel and other patients with infections are required.

Evaluation

Periodic evaluation should include the status of the disease process, blood pressure, body weight, and a check for edema. The nurse should consider laboratory data on blood glucose and serum potassium, as well as evaluation of stools for occult blood.

DISORDERS OF ADRENOCORTICAL FUNCTION

Adrenal Insufficiency

When steroid production does not meet physiologic needs, the symptoms of this deficiency may include weakness, hypoglycemia, hypotension, weight loss, nausea, vomiting, anorexia, abdominal pain, fluid and electrolyte disturbances (hypovolemia, hyponatremia, and hyperkalemia due to inadequate mineralocorticoid action), and eosinophilia. These symptoms are most often seen in times of stress, including infection, when corticosteroid needs are highest.

Etiology and Clinical Findings

Failure to produce adequate adrenal steroids may occur for three reasons. The adrenal gland may not respond to normal or even increased amounts of ACTH, which is called *primary adrenal insufficiency* or Addison's disease. Patients with this disease have increased pigmentation due to the

lack of feedback inhibition by cortisol of pituitary melanocyte-stimulating hormone. *Secondary adrenal insufficiency* results when the pituitary gland does not stimulate the normal adrenal to produce corticosteroids. The most common cause of adrenal insufficiency is the suppression of the HPA axis by *pharmacologic doses of corticosteroids.*

The simplest laboratory test of adrenal function is a fasting morning plasma cortisol, but a variety of factors can complicate interpretation of this test. These include circadian rhythms varying from the normal diurnal patterns, the use of drugs which increase physiologic release of cortisol (see Table 35-10), or the use of **heparin** which invalidates the assay for cortisol.

ACTH Stimulation Tests

Stimulation testing is used in the differential diagnosis of primary and secondary adrenal insufficiency as an indicator of the stress response. Natural or synthetic corticotropin (ACTH) is administered parenterally and plasma cortisol levels drawn 60 min later. If the plasma cortisol does not increase above 20 mg/dL, primary adrenal insufficiency is diagnosed. Continuous infusions of ACTH (for 8 h, repeated daily for 3 to 5 days) may be used as a stimulation test, followed by daily plasma cortisol and 24-h urinary 17-hydroxycorticosteroids, when it is suspected that the adrenal cortex is refractory to stimulation due to prolonged suppression. ACTH is also used in diagnosis of adrenal hyperfunction,

TABLE 35-10 Drugs Which Interfere with Plasma and Urine Tests for Corticosteroids

FALSELY HIGH RESULT	FALSELY LOW RESULT
Plasma Cortisol	
Amphetamines	
Calcium supplements	
Estrogens	
Ethanol	
Lypressin (Diapid)	
Methoxamine (Vasoxyl)	
Nicotine	
Urinary 17-Hydroxycorticosteroids	
Chloral hydrate (Noctec)	Estrogens
Chlordiazepoxide (Librium)	Phenytoin (Dilantin)
Chloramphenicol	Reserpine
Chlorpromazine (Thorazine)	
Meprobamate (Equanil)	
Quinidine	
Spironolactone (Aldactone)	
Urinary 17-Ketosteroids	
Chlorpromazine (Thorazine)	Chlordiazepoxide (Librium)
Erythromycins	Estrogens
Meprobamate (Equanil)	Phenytoin (Dilantin)
Penicillins	Quinidine
Spironolactone (Aldactone)	Reserpine

since the response to ACTH is exaggerated in Cushing's disease (see below).

Pharmacokinetics of ACTH ACTH is destroyed by the enzymes of the gastrointestinal tract and therefore cannot be given orally. ACTH is rapidly inactivated, having a plasma half-life of about 10 to 15 min; thus, prolonged infusions are used when a long duration of action is desired. Zinc and gelatin-diluted repository injections are also used to lengthen activity.

Indications Although the main use of ACTH is as a diagnostic tool in the determination of adrenal function (see above), ACTH has been used therapeutically in secondary adrenal insufficiency and in many conditions where glucocorticoids are used. Experimental uses of ACTH include therapy of infantile spasms and multiple sclerosis. ACTH has disadvantages in that it must be given parenterally, causes an increased level of all adrenal steroids (glucocorticoids, mineralocorticoids, and androgens), and is therapeutically *ineffective* in the treatment of primary adrenal insufficiency.

Adverse Effects ACTH from porcine sources may cause hypersensitivity reactions; this is less common with **cosyntropin** (Cortrosyn), the synthetic subunit of ACTH. Cosyntropin is preferred for adrenal function testing, since it is the most accurately dosed ACTH preparation. Therapeutic use of ACTH can result in the same adverse effects as corticosteroid therapy (see Table 35-9).

Preparations and Dosing The usual diagnostic dosage of **corticotropin injection** (ACTH, Acthar) is 10 to 25 U. Replacement or pharmacologic use generally requires 20 U, four times daily. Diagnostic doses of the synthetic agent, **cosyntropin** (Cortrosyn), is 250 μg.

Repository injections of **corticotropin zinc hydroxide** (Corticotropin-Zinc) and **corticotropin gel** (H.P. Acthar Gel, Cortigel-40, others) are employed only for replacement and pharmacologic uses. Usual daily doses are 40 to 80 U IM or SC q24–72h.

Clinical Pharmacology and Therapeutics

The treatment of adrenocortical insufficiency relies on replacement of the most physiologic glucocorticoids available. **Hydrocortisone** is given in doses of 25 mg/m²/day or 10 to 15 mg/kg/day, titrated to normoglycemia, remittance of azotemia, and normal plasma cortisol levels. Additional mineralocorticoid activity is provided by **fludrocortisone** at doses of 0.5 to 2.0 mg daily, titrated to the normalization of sodium and potassium balance. To mimic the natural circadian variation in plasma hormone levels, the dose may be divided to provide two-thirds in the morning and one-third in the afternoon. The patient must be provided with extra exogenous steroids for use in severe, acute stress; **dexameth-**

asone, 4-mg injection is usually provided for this purpose, with the patient instructed to keep the syringe with him or her at all times. For less acute stress, such as acute illness, minor infections, and hospitalization, the dosage of **hydrocortisone** and **fludrocortisone** may be titrated upward, then gradually tapered downward after the acute stress has resolved.

Cushing's Syndrome

The physical signs of adrenal excess, *Cushing's syndrome,* are those of overexposure to glucocorticoids: rounded "moon" face (from fat deposition), red skin (steroid rosacea), glassy eyes, puffy eyelids (from fluid retention), pouting mouth, and deposition of fat on the jawline and back of the neck ("buffalo hump"). The arms and legs are thin and the skin is prone to bleeding, acne, poor wound healing, and hirsutism. The abdomen is obese, often with striae. Psychological abnormalities, weakness, hypertension, renal calcification, and amenorrhea in females may occur. On laboratory examination, hyperglycemia, hypernatremia, hypokalemia, polycythemia, eosinopenia, and lymphopenia are found.

Etiology and Clinical Findings

The principal causes of Cushing's syndrome are Cushing's disease (overstimulation of the adrenal by ACTH of pituitary origin), iatrogenic Cushing's (due to high doses of exogenous steroids), adrenal tumor, or ectopic ACTH production (as in bronchogenic carcinoma). The differentiation of the cause of the overfunction is accomplished by the measurement of plasma cortisol and urinary metabolites of corticosteroids (17-hydroxycorticosteroids and 17-ketosteroids) before and after stimulation and suppression tests. A number of drugs can compromise the accuracy of these measurements (Table 35-10).

Dexamethasone Suppression Tests Administration of the glucocorticoid, **dexamethasone** (Decadron), tests the responsiveness of the HPA axis to feedback inhibition, since there is impaired suppression in patients with Cushing's syndrome. Dexamethasone suppression tests are also used in the diagnosis of depressive psychosis (see Chap. 34). For screening purposes in hypercorticism the *overnight dexamethasone suppression test* is used with 1 mg dexamethasone given at 11 P.M.; the plasma cortisol drawn at 8 A.M. the next day will suppress to less than 5 mg/100 mL in the normal person without hypercorticism. For greater accuracy a *low-dose dexamethasone suppression test* (0.5 mg dexamethasone every 6 h for a 48-h period) will distinguish Cushing's syndrome due to pituitary ACTH excess from Cushing's syndrome due to other causes, as suppression will result with high dexamethasone doses only in the former.

Metyrapone Test **Metyrapone** (Metopirone) is a drug which reduces cortisol production by inhibiting the enzyme

11β-hydroxylase in the adrenal (see Fig. 35-4) resulting in increased ACTH secretion (lack of feedback inhibition) and acceleration of the output of 11-deoxycorticosterone and deoxycortisol, which increases urinary 17-hydroxycorticosteroids and 17-ketosteroids. The urinary steroids will rise if pituitary hyperfunction is the cause of the Cushing's syndrome, but tumor-induced corticosteroid or ACTH synthesis is not responsive. Metyrapone is also used to diagnose adrenal hypofunction, but care must be taken since adrenal crisis can be induced. Use of metyrapone in treating Cushing's syndrome is not successful, since compensatory ACTH release causes adrenal hyperplasia and overrides the inhibition of cortisol synthesis. The usual metyrapone dosage for HPA testing is 750 mg (15 mg/kg) orally every 4 h for six doses. Adverse effects include nausea, abdominal discomfort, headache, allergic rash, and sedation. **Cyproheptadine** (Periactin), **phenytoin** (Dilantin), and **estrogens** can interfere with interpretation of the metyrapone test.

Clinical Pharmacology and Therapeutics

The treatment of choice for Cushing's syndrome is the removal of any tumor source of ACTH or of the adrenal glands if they are the source of overproduction. After adre-

nalectomy, the patient will require full replacement of corticosteroids and mineralocorticoids (see "Adrenal Insufficiency" above).

When surgery is not recommended, the production of adrenal steroids can be reduced by therapy with either of two agents. **Mitotane** (o′, p′-DDD; Lysodren) or **aminoglutethimide** (Cytadren). Although onset of action of aminoglutethimide is more rapid, its high incidence of dermatologic reactions make **mitotane** the drug of choice for inoperative Cushing's syndrome. Patients on either of these therapies must be monitored for signs of adrenocortical insufficiency, which is the major adverse effect. If patients do not respond after 4 to 5 weeks of mitotane therapy, the prognosis for control is poor. These agents are discussed further in Chap. 37.

Hyperaldosteronism

Hyperaldosteronism is often seen as a compensatory mechanism in low-output congestive heart failure (*secondary hyperaldosteronism*). When it occurs due to adrenal adenoma, it is called *primary hyperaldosteronism* or Conn's disease, which accounts for about 1 percent of the cases of hypertension. Childhood-onset hyperaldosteronism is most

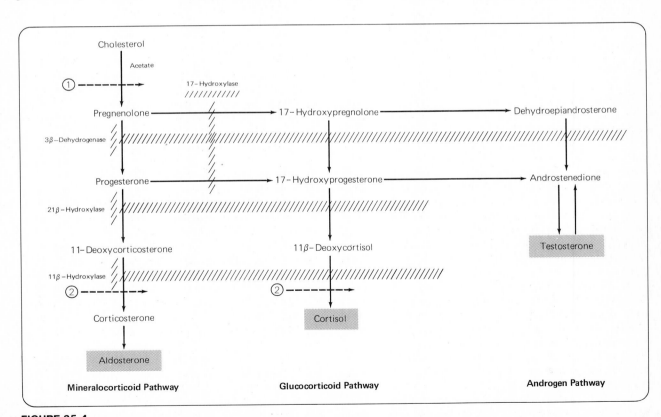

FIGURE 35-4

Synthesis of the Adrenocorticosteroids. Slashes indicate that several reactions in the pathway are catalyzed by the same enzyme. Numbers indicate the sites of action of two inhibitors of corticosteroid synthesis: (1) aminoglutethimide, and (2) metyrapone.

often due to bilateral adrenal hyperplasia, usually caused by the congenital absence of an enzyme involved in corticosteroid synthesis.

Hypertension accompanied by unexplained hypokalemia, muscle weakness, tetany, and electrocardiographic abnormalities are seen in Conn's syndrome. Some types of congenital adrenal hyperplasia produce virilization of the child.

The management of the increased blood pressure caused by hyperaldosterone states with potassium-depleting diuretics (**thiazides, furosemide,** etc.; see Chap. 23) requires scrupulous monitoring of potassium levels. The acute electrolyte imbalance seen in Conn's disease can be corrected by the administration of **spironolactone** (Aldactone), a competitive inhibitor of aldosterone activity (see Chap. 23). The onset of action of spironolactone is several days, the time required to attain sufficient levels of the active metabolite, **canrenone.** After electrolyte balance is restored, surgery is performed in cases with tumors. Congenital adrenal hyperplasia is managed by replacement of the deficient corticosteroids.

CASE STUDY

W.C., a 28-year-old telephone operator, came to the clinic for evaluation of easy fatiguability, back and stomach aches, poor appetite, and vomiting, which worsened during her change from night (11 P.M. to 7 A.M.) to day shift. four weeks previously. During her physical examination, she suddenly asked if her symptoms could be related to the dextroamphetamine sulfate (Dexedrine) she had used for two days prior to coming to the clinic to ease her transition to day work. Upon further questioning, she also described self-medication with No-Doz (caffeine 100 mg/tablet) and Dietac (phenylpropanolamine 50 mg and caffeine 200 mg/capsule). Her only prescribed medication was Demulen oral contraceptives (ethinyl estradiol and ethinodiol diacetate) for the past five years. Her social use of drugs included: three to six cups of coffee daily, one-half pack of cigarettes daily, and an average of three beers weekly.

Assessment

W.C.'s medical and surgical histories were noncontributory. Her examination was entirely normal, except for a temperature of 96°F, darkly pigmented axillae, areolae, and labia, decreased general muscle tone; and sparse pubic hair. Height was 63 in, weight was 45 kg (99 lb), down 3 kg over the previous week. Blood pressure in the right arm (sitting) was 90/50, which fell to 72/50 upon standing. Her laboratory tests demonstrated nonfasting blood sugar of 50 mg/100 mL, serum sodium 125 meq/L, potassium 6 meq/L. Liver enzymes and renal function studies were normal. Blood count showed mild anemia, hemoglobin 8.5 mg/100 mL, and eosinophilia to 12 percent. Urinalysis showed dark yellow color, specific gravity of 1.027, 10 to 12 white blood cells per high power field, and gram-negative rods on gram stain. Endocrine studies included a 4 P.M. plasma cortisol determination, which was "borderline normal" at 3.0 mg/100 mL (expected 3 to 12 mg/100 mL).

From these data the physician recognized signs and symptoms consistent with adrenal insufficiency. The nurse noted that the worsening of her status (adrenal crisis) could have been precipitated by the recent stressful change in her working hours and her bacteriuria/cystitis. Interpretation of her near-normal cortisol level was aided by recognition of the many pharmacologic stimuli to increase cortisol levels (caffeine, amphetamine, alcohol, estrogen, nicotine) and the fact that the 4 P.M. level should be expected to be a near-peak level in this night-waking telephone operator and was thus falsely normal. The oral contraceptives have the additional effect of increasing plasma cortisol-binding globulin, providing a higher total cortisol concentration in plasma without a similar increase in free (active) cortisol. Thus, the use of oral contraceptives could mask some of the laboratory evidence of adrenocortical insufficiency.

Management

The therapeutic plan for this patient included admission for emergent management of the near adrenal crisis (postural hypotension, electrolyte and fluid imbalance, and steroid deficiency), as well as treatment of the infection which may have overwhelmed her borderline compensatory mechanisms.

Injectable hydrocortisone sodium succinate (Solu-Cortef) 100 mg was administered intravenously immediately, followed by 100 mg more in the first liter of intravenous fluids. After this, 100 mg were given every 8 h. No specific mineralocorticoid replacement was needed with this high-dose therapy. Intravenous fluids with dextrose in normal saline were given to replete the intravascular volume, sodium, and glucose deficits. The nurse observed blood pressure meticulously, since a vasopressor (e.g., dopamine) might have been required if volume replacement did not satisfactorily restore blood pressure. A warming blanket was used to maintain body temperature. Ampicillin was given intravenously to treat the cystitis, as oral tolerance of medications was still limited.

Following stabilization and improvement in urinalysis, the patient was to be discharged on hydrocortisone 20 mg daily, with oral ampicillin 250 mg q6h for a total of 10 days. The nurse counseled the patient on the importance of avoiding excessive stimulant intake (caffeine, nicotine, phenlypropanolamine, amphetamines). W.C. was concerned about the need to discontinue the oral contraceptives, but the nurse explained that these are not contraindicated in patients with adrenocortical insufficiency. A note was made in her medical record regarding potential false elevation in cortisol concentrations due to the estrogens in the oral contraceptives. W.C. was given a syringe containing 4 mg of dexamethasone, taught how to self-administer it, and instructed to carry it at all times. The drug's use in the event of acute stress or adrenal crisis was explained, as were the signs of adrenal insufficiency (hypotension, fatigue, nausea, vomiting, abdominal pain) and the need to wear identification indicating her condition. W.C. found the hyperpigmentation disfiguring, but the nurse explained that this would remit with adequate treatment of the disease.

Evaluation

W.C. was instructed to return to the clinic for 8 A.M. plasma cortisol levels once a stable work pattern had been maintained for at least two weeks. When the patient returned the nurse questioned her about clinical symptoms of adrenal insufficiency or corticosteroid excess and reviewed serum electrolytes. As a result, the nurse judged that replacement therapy was currently adequate. It was suggested that W.C., who was working the day shift, take 15 mg hydrocortisone in the morning with breakfast and 5 mg at 2 P.M. with a snack, to stimulate normal diurnal variation.

THE PANCREAS

LEARNING OBJECTIVES

Upon mastery of the content of this section, the reader will be able to:

1. Describe the homeostatic mechanisms that control blood glucose levels and the variations that occur in Type I and Type II diabetes mellitus.

2. Describe the consequences of insulin deficiency in diabetes mellitus.

3. Discuss the advantages and disadvantages of two methods of urine glucose testing.

4. Identify the commonly used insulins and indicate their onset, peak, and duration.

5. Explain the recent developments in insulin therapy.

6. Explain the mechanism and action of the sulfonylureas.

7. State a minimum of four adverse effects of insulin and the sulfonylureas.

8. Describe the role of the glycosylated hemoglobin test in the management of diabetes mellitus.

9. State the nursing responsibilities associated with the use of pharmacologic interventions in the treatment of diabetes mellitus.

The endocrine functions of the pancreas are located in the islets of Langerhans. These islets are highly vascularized masses of cells scattered throughout the pancreatic tissues. The islets of Langerhans contain alpha, beta, and delta cells that secrete glucagon, insulin, and somatostatin, respectively, directly into the bloodstream.

Glucagon raises the blood sugar by converting glycogen to glucose (within the liver), thus acting as a hyperglycemic agent. *Insulin* promotes the process that lowers blood sugar (hypoglycemia). Although the exact role of *somatostatin* has not been clearly defined, it is thought to have an inhibitory effect on both insulin and glucagon. Somatostatin directly influences the secretion of glucagon and insulin by the alpha and beta cells.

The beta cells are the most numerous, making up about 75 percent of the islet cell population. It is the dysfunction of these cells that leads to insufficient secretion of insulin or abnormal insulin metabolism that results in diabetes mellitus.

PHYSIOLOGY OF INSULIN

Insulin is a small protein molecule (molecular weight of about 6000) composed to two chains (A and B) of amino acids loosely held together by disulfide bonds. It is derived from a large polypeptide precursor, *proinsulin,* which is synthesized in the beta cells of the pancreas. Proinsulin is transformed into insulin within the beta cells and the insulin is then stored in membrane-bound granules and eventually secreted.

Control of Insulin Release

Glucose is the most profound stimulus for insulin release. The elevation of blood glucose increases both the production and the release of insulin. Other stimuli include fructose, certain amino acids, hormones (ACTH, growth hormone, glucocorticoids, thyroxin, estrogens), vagal stimulation, potassium, and oral hypoglycemic agents (e.g., **tolbutamide, chlorpropamide**). Inhibitors of insulin secretion are hyperglycemia, somatostatin, epinephrine, norepinephrine, **thiazide diuretics, phenytoin,** and **diazoxide.**

Glucose is a more potent stimulus if ingested orally than if intravenously administered because the presence of glucose in the duodenum stimulates several gastrointestinal hormones that also promote insulin release. These include gastrin, pancreazymin, secretin, and glucagon.

Physiologic Activity of Insulin

Postprandial (Fed State)   Normally, when food is ingested and absorbed, blood glucose levels rise, stimulating the release of insulin from the beta cells of the pancreas. Insulin then promotes the uptake of glucose, amino acids, and fatty acids, and their conversion to storage forms in tissue cells. As glucose is transported into tissues (facilitated by insulin), blood glucose levels decrease. In muscle cells, insulin facilitates the uptake of glucose and its conversion to glycogen (the storage form of glucose) and also promotes the uptake of amino acids and their conversion to proteins. In adipose tissue, glucose is converted to free fatty acids and stored as triglycerides. In the presence of insulin the rate of breakdown of triglycerides to free fatty acids is decreased.

Fasting State   In a fasting individual blood glucose is low and insulin release is not stimulated. As a result the available glucose is utilized mainly by the brain (which does not require insulin for glucose transport). The relative hypoglycemia in the fasting state leads to the release of hormones, such as glucagon, glucocorticoids, epinephrine, and growth hormone, that act to increase blood glucose levels. In addition, this relative lack of insulin leads to a breakdown of glycogen to glucose in the liver, a conversion of amino acids to glucose via gluconeogenesis, and a breakdown of triglycerides to free fatty acids, which are used as an energy source primarily by muscle.

Alterations in Diabetes Mellitus   When food is ingested by a diabetic, there is insufficient insulin to facilitate glucose transport. As glucose entry into the cell diminishes, the body signals for fuel, and glycogen is released from the liver. As a result, blood glucose continues to rise and as it exceeds the renal threshold (around 180 mg/dL of blood) glucose is excreted into the urine (glucosuria). High urinary glucose leads to an increased osmotic pressure of the urine, resulting in an osmotic diuresis that is manifested as excessive urination (polyuria). The resulting water and electrolyte loss causes increased thirst (polydypsia); the caloric loss causes increased hunger (polyphagia) and fatigue. Thus the classic symptoms of diabetes mellitus are experienced: glucosuria, polyuria, polydypsia, and fatigue. In addition, because of the absence of insulin, the body attempts to supply energy by mobilizing free fatty acids and protein drawn from adipose tissue and muscle stores. The resultant oxidation of fat leads to ketoacid accumulation and a drop in blood pH. The metabolism of protein results in the liberation of amino acids which are converted into urea in the liver and excreted, resulting in a negative nitrogen balance and muscle wasting. If left untreated, this diabetic ketoacidosis state can lead to coma and death (see Fig. 35-5).

DIABETES MELLITUS

It is estimated that there are 10 million diabetics in the United States. Epidemiological studies report that increasing numbers of the United States population are developing diabetes mellitus. The following reasons for this are suggested: the increase in life expectancy, the numbers of diabetic children who have survived to have children, the increasing incidence of obesity, and the increased use of diabetic screening drives.

Etiology and Classification

Evidence is growing that diabetes mellitus is not a single disease, but a series of disorders or a group of diseases with diverse etiologies. Current theories link the causes solely or in combination to a genetic defect in the immune system, viruses, diet and obesity, drugs (see Table 35-11), and/or autoimmune processes. The classification of diabetes mellitus which has been approved by both the American Diabetes Association and the World Health Organization is shown in Table 35-12.

Complications

The complications of diabetes mellitus are many in number, potentially disabling or life-threatening in severity, and common in occurrence. There is no agreement regarding the pathogenesis of some of these complications. For example, the vascular disease, which causes most of the morbidity and mortality from diabetes mellitus, may be a genetic concomitant of the disease and unrelated to blood sugar, or it may be a complication of diabetes that is related to insulin

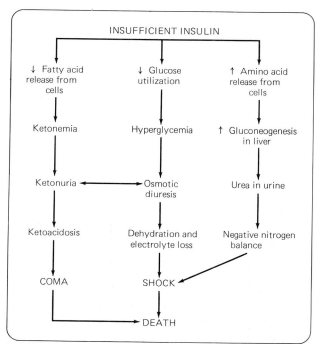

FIGURE 35-5

Pathophysiology of Insulin Deficiency. The three major mechanisms are fatty acid release leading to ketoacidosis, hyperglycemia leading to fluid loss, and protein breakdown leading to negative nitrogen balance. The results of these processes are coma, shock, and death.

TABLE 35-11 Causes of Drug-Induced Diabetes Mellitus*

Phenytoin (Dilantin) and other hydantoins
Thiazide diuretics
Furosemide (Lasix)
Ethacrynic acid (Edecrin)
Estrogens (including oral contraceptives)
Progestagens
Corticosteroids
Diazoxide (Hyperstat)
Lithium

*Usually by unmasking latent disease in those with impaired glucose tolerance. Can also aggravate existing diabetes mellitus.

TABLE 35-12 Classification of Diabetes Mellitus

CLASS	DESCRIPTION
Type I or insulin-dependent diabetes mellitus (IDDM)	Previously called "juvenile diabetes." Insulin-dependent and ketosis-prone. Can occur at any age.
Type II or non-insulin-dependent diabetes mellitus (NIDDM)	Most common form. Formerly called "adult" or "maturity onset." Can occur at any age, but is predominantly in those over 40 years of age. Subdivided into (a) obese non-insulin-dependent, and (b) nonobese non-insulin-dependent (65 percent of all diabetics).
Secondary diabetes	Named according to the condition (medication, surgery, illness) that brought on the disease.
Gestational diabetes	Discovered during pregnancy.
Impaired glucose tolerance	Previously called borderline, chemical, latent, or subclinical. Blood sugar levels between those considered normal and those considered diabetic.

deficiency and/or hyperglycemia and thus, preventable by blood sugar control.

The complications are usually divided into (1) acute complications: hypoglycemia, ketoacidosis, and hyperglycemic hyperosmolar nonketotic coma (see Table 35-13), and (2) chronic complications: large vessel disease and small vessel disease.

Acute Complications

Acute hypoglycemic states occur when blood glucose falls abnormally low. Possible causes include glucose deficiency, insulin excess, insulin reaction, or excess exercise. The sign and symptoms reflect depression of the central nervous system and activation of the autonomic nervous system. This condition can progress rapidly to a life-threatening state.

Ketoacidosis This is an acute complication that occurs with severe insulin deficiency and that worsens as the compensatory mechanisms fail. The clinical signs and symptoms vary but become progressively more severe. (See Fig. 35-5.)

Hyperglycemic Hyperosmolar Nonketotic Coma (HHNK) This condition occurs in the diabetic who is able to provide enough insulin to prevent the acidotic cycle but not enough to correct hyperglycemia, osmotic diuresis, and extracellular fluid depletion. The diabetic is usually elderly, noninsulin dependent, and is under severe stress. As the condition worsens, there are increasing CNS abnormalities. Once coma has occurred, death is common. This condition should be considered a medical emergency.

Chronic Complications

Diabetes is sometimes defined not only as a lack of insulin, but also as a premature aging of the blood vessels. This accounts for the majority of the chronic complications with diabetes. The development of complications seems to be promoted by the altered lipid metabolism common to diabetes. The initial lesion is a thickened basement membrane

in the capillaries and arterioles, which results in vascular changes. The belief that tight control of blood sugar may help to delay this process is becoming more widely accepted.

The chief vessels affected by large vessel disease (macroangiopathy) are those of the heart, brain, and the periphery, principally the lower extremities. Small vessel disease (microangiopathy) can be found throughout the body, but the problems most commonly seen are retinopathy, nephropathy, and the neuropathies.

Clinical Findings

The most sensitive method for detecting diabetes mellitus, if done correctly, is the oral glucose tolerance test (OGTT) in combination with the serum insulin value. Other laboratory tests that can aid in the diagnosis are the two-hour postprandial blood (2hPP) glucose test and the fasting blood sugar (FBS). These should be considered along with the signs and symptoms attributable to osmotic diuresis.

Urine Tests

Urine tests for glucose are the quickest and least expensive, but also the least effective methods of screening for diabetes. The urine tests will be positive for glucose only after the blood glucose levels have become sufficiently elevated to allow glucose to spill into the urine, usually at 180 mg/dL. The urine tests cannot measure for hypoglycemia and may give a negative reading for urine glucose in persons with an elevated renal threshold. Renal threshold for glucose can vary according to age, current health status, and

TABLE 35-13 Signs, Symptoms, and Treatment of Acute Complications of Diabetes Mellitus

HYPOGLYCEMIA	KETOACIDOSIS	HHNK
	Onset	
Rapid (minutes–hours)	Gradual (days)	Gradual (days)
	Causes	
Insulin excess	Food excess	Severe stress (infection, surgery, trauma, psychological factors)
Insulin reaction	Insufficient insulin	
Omission or delay of meals	Neglect of therapy (diet, exercise, insulin)	Food excess
Excess exercise	Stress (infection)	
	Symptoms	
"Inward nervousness," hunger, weakness	Thirst	Thirst
Cold, clammy, sweat	Headache	Polyuria—leading to concentration of urine
Nausea, dizziness	Polyuria	
Double or blurred vision	Nausea, vomiting	Vomiting
Psychopathic behavior†	Abdominal pain	Dim vision
Lethargy*	Blurred vision	As condition progresses: confusion, lethargy, weakness, paralysis, seizures
Stupor	Numbness of fingers and toes	
Convulsions		
	Signs	
Pallor	Florid face	Severe dehydration: dry skin and mucosa; dry tongue; shrunken, soft eyeballs
Sweating	Dehydration	
Normal respirations	Kussmaul's respirations	Respirations ↓
Normal pulse	Rapid pulse	Pulse ↑
Normal or ↑BP	BP↓	BP ↓
Temperature normal or ↓	Temperature ↑	Temperature ↑
Tremors	Soft eyeballs	
	Acetone breath	
	Normal or absent reflexes	

activity level. For accuracy, urine tests rely on normal renal thresholds, complete bladder emptying, and precise testing procedure according to the test product used.

Two methods of testing urine glucose concentrations are the copper reduction method (Clinitest) and the glucose oxidation method (Clinistix, Diastix, Test-Tape). All of these products must be protected from moisture, heat, and direct light. In order to assure uniformity among the results on all products, *all urine test results should be recorded in percentages of glucose in the urine*, rather than the "plus" system used prior to 1980 (e.g., +, ++, +++, etc.).

Copper Reduction The Clinitest method has replaced the older Benedict's test. The Clinitest tablet contains anhydrous copper sulfate which generates heat when combined with water and urine. Careful adherence to specific directions in the Clinitest kit must be followed to assure accurate readings. Clinitest procedures can be done as either a five-

or a two-drop method. The two-drop method is quantitative for larger amounts of sugar. The nurse should be sure that the proper color chart is used for the method selected. The major advantage of the Clinitest is that it is more quantitative for larger amounts of glucose urine concentrations (> 1%). This is important for the diabetic with glucosuria who adjusts his insulin dosage according to the degree of glucosuria. **Salicylates, ascorbic acid, nalidixic acid** (NegGram), **probenecid,** and the **cephalosporins** may cause false positive results with Clinitest testing.

Glucose Oxidase The glucose oxidase methods are simple to use and more sensitive to low urine glucose concentrations. The enzyme glucose oxidase converts urine glucose to gluconic acid. It is the method of choice for non-insulin-dependent diabetics who are rarely glucosuric. Diastix has a color chart which is more quantitative at the higher glucose concentrations than Test-Tape or Clinistix. The glucose

TABLE 35-13 Signs, Symptoms, and Treatment of Acute Complications of Diabetes Mellitus (*Cont.*)

HYPOGLYCEMIA	KETOACIDOSIS	HHNK
Chemical Features		
Urine glucose negative	Urinary glucose positive—5%	Urinary glucose positive—5%
Urinary ketones positive		Urinary ketones negative
Blood glucose usually 60 mg/dL or ↓	Urinary ketones negative	Blood glucose ↑ 1000 mg/dL
Blood ketones negative	Blood glucose ↑ 250 mg/dL	Blood ketones usually negative
	Blood ketones positive	
Blood Miscellaneous		
Normal	↓ pH	↑ Na, ↑ BUN
	↓ Bicarbonate,	↑ Hct, ↑ Hgb (because of volume depletion)
	↓ K⁺	
	↓ Hct, Hgb	K⁺ normal or ↑
	↑ BUN	Bicarbonate normal
Treatment		
Oral glucose (orange juice 120 mL; 2 tsp sugar, honey, corn syrup; candy)	↑ Regular insulin (SQ or IV)	↑ Fluids rapidly—IV
		Electrolytes
IV glucose (10–50%)	Fluids	Small doses regular insulin (5–10 U)
IV glucagon	Electrolytes	
Response to Treatment		
Rapid	Slow	Slow

*More common in elderly.
†More common in young.

oxidase methods are subject to interference from high doses of **ascorbic acid** (vitamin C), **salicylates**, and **levodopa**.

Other Diagnostic Tests
In vitro diagnostic tests are available for testing ketones in the urine. Acetest Reagent Tablets can be used to evaluate the urine or blood, while Chemstrip-K and Ketostix are reagent strips for urine testing only. Reagent strips are also available to check blood glucose (Chemstrip bG Strips, Dextrostix, and Visidex II). Many clinicians consider blood testing the preferred method for home monitoring of diabetes.

Clinical Pharmacology and Therapeutics
Management of diabetes mellitus varies depending on the classification of the disease. In Type I, or insulin-dependent diabetes, the only effective treatment measures are insulin, diet, and exercise. In Type II, the treatment of choice is diet therapy, weight control, stress reduction, and exercise. However, insulin or the oral hypoglycemic agents may be used. There is accumulating evidence that some of the complications of diabetes may be prevented or delayed by normalization or near normalization of plasma glucose concentrations.

Insulin
The physiology and activity of insulin is discussed above. The precise mechanism of action of insulin is not known, but it may be mediated through cyclic AMP or some other secondary messenger such as cyclic GMP, K⁺, or Mg⁺.

Types of Insulin Available
Exogenous insulin preparations are purified extracts from beef or pork pancreas. This insulin possesses biologic effects qualitatively identical to those of human insulin. *Pork insulin* differs from human insulin by only one of the amino acids in the B chain. *Beef insulin* differs in four amino acids from human insulin.

Due to improved purification procedures, insulin has changed dramatically within the past few years. The insulin available up to about a decade ago contained 10,000 to 50,000 parts per million (ppm) of proinsulin and other contaminants. The development of a single peak insulin reduced that figure to about 3000 ppm. These have since been improved and that figure has dropped to 50 ppm.

Today, a new class of further purified single-peak insulins are available. These products, indicated by the term *purified insulin* on the label, contain less than 10 ppm of proinsulin, with some preparations containing less than 1 ppm. The purified preparations produce less fat atrophy and hypertrophy, less incidence of local skin allergy, less anti-insulin antibody formation, and less insulin resistance. In addition, they also seem to increase the incidence of the "honeymoon" phase (temporary period of remission during which time the islet cells are producing some insulin, which occurs most frequently in children) in the newly diagnosed Type I diabetic. Because the daily requirement of insulin may fall as much as 10 to 20 percent when a diabetic is changed from conventional to a highly purified insulin, home blood glucose monitoring is advised. The increase in purity has not been without expense. At present the cost of the purified insulins is double that of the other insulins. However, with increased use that price difference is expected to narrow.

With the exception of one concentrated dosage form, *insulins contain* 100 U/mL. The concentrated form contains 500 U/mL.

Biosynthetic *human insulin* (Humalin), the first drug product developed through recombinant DNA techniques, became available in 1983. The diabetic research centers presently using this product see very little difference between it and the newer purified insulins. However, it is cautioned that diabetics who are changed from animal insulins to human insulins be followed carefully during the first few weeks to determine whether the dosage needs adjustment.

Pharmacokinetics

Because insulin is inactivated by the gastrointestinal enzymes, it cannot be administered orally. Insulin is generally administered by the subcutaneous route, although for rapid effect regular insulin may be administered intravenously or intramuscularly, as may be done in emergency situations. Insulin is metabolized in the liver (50 percent), kidneys (25 percent), muscles, and other tissues. These inactive metabolites are excreted in the urine.

Insulin preparations may be modified to affect the time course of action and are divided into three groups based upon their onset peak and duration of action: rapid-acting, intermediate-acting, and long-acting. This classification is outlined in Table 35-14. Current available insulin options are presented in Table 35-15.

Rapid-Acting Insulin

Regular or crystalline insulin is the only form that can be given intravenously, although when given as an intravenous infusion it is somewhat unreliable because the drug adheres to the bottle and tubing. For this reason some physicians may increase the desired dose by 10 U per infusion bottle.

Because of its rapid action and prompt dissipation, regular insulin provides the most accurate control in unstable clinical situations. It is the insulin of choice during diabetic ketoacidosis, illness, and surgery. Its dose is often adjusted according to the results of blood glucose levels or urine sugar results ("sliding scale"). When used in chronic management it is commonly given 20 to 30 min before a meal.

Intermediate-Acting Insulin

These insulins have a fairly rapid onset and moderately prolonged duration of action. They are the insulin of choice for most diabetics. For some, a combination of rapid-acting and intermediate-acting insulins provides more consistent control of blood glucose levels. NPH insulin or isophane is a primary intermediate-acting insulin. NPH means *neutral protamine Hagedorn*. (The letters signify properties of the preparation and its origin: neutral solution; protamine, which is added to extend the length of time for absorption and action; and Hagedorn, the laboratory of origin.)

The Lente insulins are similar to NPH except that they do not contain protamine; therefore, the potential for inducing insulin allergy is reduced. Semilente is the rapid-acting form, and ultralente is the long-acting form. Lente insulin is a mixture of semilente and ultralente types.

Intermediate-acting insulins are usually given 30 to 60 min before breakfast and, if given twice a day, 30 to 60 min before the last meal of the day. It is important to give supplemental snacks at the peak activity time if hypoglycemic reactions are a problem.

Long-Acting Insulin

PZI, or protamine zinc, is a major long-acting insulin. It is prepared by reacting insulin and zinc with protamine. It absorbs at a slower but steady rate. Long-acting insulins are rarely used at the present time.

Adverse Effects

Hypoglycemia

Mild to marked hypoglycemic reactions are most likely to occur during the peak activity time of the

TABLE 35-14 Classification and Action Time of Insulin

TYPE	EXAMPLE	ONSET (h)	PEAK (h)	DURATION (h)
Rapid acting	Regular	¼–1	2–4	5–7
Intermediate acting	NPH, Lente	1–3	6–12	12–24
Long acting	Ultralente, Protamine zinc	4–6	14–24	36+

TABLE 35-15   Insulin Preparations and Pharmacokinetics

PRODUCT	SOURCE	ONSET (h APPROX.)	PEAK (h APPROX.)	DURATION (h APPROX.)
Regular	Beef, pork, or beef-pork	¼–1	2–4	5–7
Humulin-R	DNA recombinant	¼–1	2–4	5–7
Regular	Pork*	¼–1	2–4	5–7
Velosulin	Pork*	¼–1	2–4	5–7
Actrapid	Pork*	½–1	2½–5	8
Semilente	Beef-pork or beef	1–3	2–8	12–16
Semitard	Pork*	1½	5–10	16
Protaphane	Pork*	1–1½	4–12	24
NPH	Pork, beef, or beef-pork	1–3	6–12	24–28
Humulin-N	DNA recombinant	1–3	6–12	24–28
Monotard	Pork*	2½	7–15	22
Insulatard	Pork*	2–4	4–12	24–28
Lente	Pork, beef, or beef-pork	1–3	6–12	24–28
Lente	Beef*	1–3	6–12	24–28
Lentard	Beef-pork*	2½	7–15	24
PZI	Pork, beef, or beef-pork	4–6	14–24	36+
Ultralente	Beef-pork or beef	4–6	18–24	36+
Ultratard	Beef*	4	10–30	36
Mixtard (premixed, Regular 30%, NPH 70%)	Pork*	Like Regular and NPH when mixed		
Regular (concentrated 500 U/mL) Ilentin II	Pork*	Single dose frequently acts over a long period, sometimes as long as 24 h		

*Purified.

insulin given. (See Table 35-13 for signs and symptoms and Table 35-15 for peak times.) Meals, snacks, and exercise should be coordinated with the insulin activity. Diabetics should carry identification that indicates their disease and any hypoglycemic medication in use. A fast-acting carbohydrate should also be carried. Hard candy or sugar (not chocolate because its fat content makes it absorb slower) is most effective. Glutose, Monojel, and glucose tablets are commercially prepared simple sugars that are available for use. When in doubt about whether a diabetic is having an insulin reaction or a hypoglycemic reaction, the *initial treatment should be for hypoglycemia.*

In the event of an emergency hypoglycemic reaction, or a hypoglycemic reaction with loss of consciousness, intravenous dextrose or glucagon can be administered. **Glucagon** 0.5 to 1 mg can be given SC, IM, or IV. It may be repeated after 20 min if the patient's response is unsatisfactory. In order to prevent secondary hypoglycemic reactions, additional carbohydrates should be given as soon as the patient regains consciousness.

Allergy   The most common evidence of allergy is a transient, local itching, swelling, or erythema at the site of injection. The incidence of this reaction has decreased with the use of purified insulin.

Insulin Resistance   Insulin resistance is manifested by the requirement of massive doses of insulin. It is most likely caused by the development of antibodies. Corticosteroids are sometimes given to reduce antibody formation, but must be monitored closely as severe hypoglycemia could occur. If the insulin resistance has occurred as a response to acute stress, treatment should be directed at the precipitating cause.

Lipodystrophy   Lipodystrophy is manifested by changes in subcutaneous fat (atrophy or hypertrophy) at the site of injection. Rotation of sites and use of the purified insulins can aid in more reliable absorption.

Somogyi Effect   This syndrome is a hyperglycemic response to the administration of too much insulin. Despite large doses of insulin, hyperglycemia persists. The body's normal defense mechanisms overreact to hypoglycemia caused by overinsulinization and secrete large amounts of epinephrine, glucagon, and glucocorticoids into the bloodstream, which significantly raises the blood sugar. Improvement is seen with a decrease in insulin.

Dosage and Administration

The timing of the insulin dosage should depend upon the onset and duration of the insulin used, but this may vary from diabetic to diabetic, and can also be affected by the route of administration and the dose.

Most normal adults secrete 30 to 40 U of insulin daily and many diabetics require this amount of replacement on a daily basis. The average maintenance dose is 0.5 to 1 U/kg of body weight daily, but this will vary among diabetics. The amount of insulin is usually started out low and then increased by 20 percent each day until the plasma glucose is normal and the urines are negative for glucose. After stabilization, it is not uncommon for a drop in insulin requirement to occur. Depending on the degree of islet cell damage, the pancreas may make a temporary recovery. The dosage in insulin is reduced to prevent the occurrence of hypoglycemia, but insulin is not eliminated. Interruption of insulin therapy during this temporary remission could increase the risk of antibody formation and thus the development of hypersensitivity. Small amounts of insulin may also extend this remission period.

Type II diabetics have some endogenous secretion of insulin, and so their exogenous dose may be small. However, some individuals are insulin resistant and may require fantastically large doses—sometimes as much as 1000 U daily—to achieve control.

Storage and Mixing   Although insulin is a heat-labile protein, current preparations are stable so that the vial in use can be stored out of the refrigerator, provided it is not exposed to extreme temperatures or light. Extra bottles may be stored in the refrigerator but not in the freezer. The injection of cold insulin may be irritating to the tissues and may contribute to lipodystrophy.

Agitation, violent shaking, or dropping a vial of insulin can cause the loosely bound polypeptide chains to break apart. This will inactivate the insulin. Diabetics should never shake a vial to dissolve a precipitate, but should be taught to gently rotate the vial between their hands to resuspend any particles that have precipitated. Regular insulin will remain clear, but modified insulin should look cloudy or milky after mixing. Frothing indicates the beginning of protein breakdown.

When it is necessary to prefill syringes for a diabetic, the syringe should be stored tip up. This will avoid plugging of the needle and will also make easier the gentle rolling needed to restore the solution within the syringe to a homogenous state.

When mixing two insulins, such as regular and NPH or Lente, it is less important in which order the insulins are drawn into the syringe than it is that the *same pattern* be used each time. The dead space in the syringe will then be occupied by the same type of insulin each time, avoiding fluctuations in dosage. Further, since some regular insulin will combine with the excess protamine when mixed with NPH or protamine zinc insulin, and will then absorb more slowly and peak later, insulin should be injected within 1½ min of mixing. When this is not possible, exactly the same amount of time should pass between mixing and injection of each dose, especially if this interval is less than 20 min. Since the reaction between the protamine and the regular insulin is usually complete in less than 20 min, syringes filled hours or days in advance (as is often done for the visually impaired diabetic) can be assumed to be equivalent. Because it is possible to inadvertently inject some of the insulin first drawn into the syringe into the bottle of the insulin drawn second into the syringe, many clinicians will teach the diabetic to draw up the regular insulin first. That way, if a small amount of regular insulin gets into the NPH or other modified insulin, it will react with the excess protamine or other additive and assume the pharmacokinetic characteristics of that insulin. If the regular insulin is drawn up second, there may (after a number of doses) be considerable contamination and change in onset and duration of action of the insulin from the bottle assumed to be regular insulin.

Site and Injection Technique   The desired site for insulin injection is an area with substantial fatty layers. Intramuscular injections will cause the insulin to be absorbed too rapidly, and is avoided unless it is specifically ordered in an emergency. Only U-100 insulin syringes should be used, because these are calibrated to measure the specific insulin concentration of U-100 insulin. Most disposable syringes are one-half or five-eighths of an inch, 25 or 27 gauge, silicone coated needles. The needle should be aspirated before injection in order to avoid inadvertent intravascular injection. Suitable injection sites include the surfaces of the upper arms, abdomen, thighs, and upper back. When diabetics are hospitalized, nurses can focus on using sites that are difficult for self-administration. Injection sites should be rotated systematically to avoid tissue hypertrophy, atrophy, and erratic absorption. Repeated injections into the same site makes the site less sensitive to pain but also decreases insulin absorption and delays action. Diabetics should be made aware that this practice may provoke unexpected hypoglycemia when sites are subsequently changed. Rotation guides or drawings can help keep track of injection sites. Areas that are about to be exercised should be avoided, as injection into these areas can result in rapid absorption and cause hypoglycemia. For diabetics who are insulin resistant and using the concentrated form of regular insulin, care must be taken to avoid errors in measurement of the dosage as small errors may result in significant overdosage.

Oral Hypoglycemic Agents: The Sulfonylureas

In addition to insulin, only two classes of drugs have been used therapeutically to control hyperglycemia: the sulfonylureas and the biguanides. The biguanides were removed from the market in 1978 because of reported serious side effects associated with their use.

Mechanisms of Action

The sulfonylureas act primarily by stimulating the beta cells of the pancreas to secrete insulin. Research indicates that they may also increase the number of insulin cell membrane receptors, secondarily decrease glucose output by the liver, increase insulin sensitivity in peripheral tissue, and have other extrapancreatic effects. They will not lower blood sugar in persons who have no functioning beta cells. They are *not* oral insulin products and should not be labeled as such.

Pharmacokinetics

The sulfonylureas are well absorbed when taken orally. The onset of action, peak, and duration vary among the drugs (see Table 35-16), but their therapeutic responses are similar. Dosages should be adjusted according to blood glucose levels.

Tolbutamide Tolbutamide (Orinase) was the first of the sulfonylureas to be used clinically. It is rapidly absorbed and has the shortest duration of action. It is highly protein-bound to plasma albumin, is metabolized in the liver, and is excreted in the form of inactive metabolites in the urine. About 75 percent of the metabolites are excreted within 24 h.

Tolazamide Tolazamide (Tolinase) is more slowly absorbed and has an intermediate duration of action. It is metabolized in the liver to six major metabolites, half of which are active (possessing hypoglycemic activity). About 85 percent of the dose is excreted in the urine.

Acetohexamide Acetohexamide (Dymelor) is an intermediate-acting drug. It is metabolized in the liver to hydroxyhexamide, a metabolite whose hypoglycemic activity persists longer than that of the parent drug. It is excreted primarily

TABLE 35-16 Oral Hypoglycemic Agents

NAME	ONSET (h)	PEAK (h)	DURATION (h)	HALF-LIFE (h)	USUAL DOSAGE
Tolbutamide (Orinase)	½–1	3–5	24	6	0.5–2 g, single or divided doses
Tolazamide (Tolinase)	4–6	4–8	15	7	0.1–1 g, single or divided doses
Acetohexamide (Dymelor)	1	3	12–24	5–6	0.25–1.5 g, single or divided doses
Chlorpropamide (Diabinese)	1	2–4	72	36	0.1–0.5 g, single dose
Glipizide (Dibeta) *	1–1½	2	10–24	2–4	2.5–40 mg, single or divided doses (average dose = 17 mg daily)
Glyburide (Microanse) *	2–4	3–5	24	10	2.5–20 mg, single or divided doses (average dose = 15 mg daily)

*Second generation sulfonylureas.

through the urine. It should be used with caution in renal insufficiency because accumulation of the metabolite may cause hypoglycemia. It also has uricosuric activity.

Chlorpropamide Chlorpropamide (Diabenese) is the longest acting sulfonylurea. It is extensively metabolized, but 20 percent is excreted unchanged by the kidney. Due to its long half-life, a maximum blood level (steady state) may not be achieved for 3 to 4 days after the initiation of therapy. Thus, dose advancements should not be made any earlier than at 3- to 4-day intervals. Within 96 h about 80 to 90 percent of the drug is excreted in the urine. Because of its prolonged activity hypoglycemic reactions, if they occur, may last for 3 to 5 days. Care should be taken when this drug is given to the elderly. It is highly bound to plasma albumin.

Glyburide and Glipizide Glyburide (Dibeta, Micronase) and glipizide (Glucotrol) are two second-generation sulfonylureas marketed in 1984. Based upon clinical trials, these agents are effective in small doses and appear to have high therapeutic effects and low toxicity. Both agents are metabolized by the liver to inactive metabolites and, like the other sulfonylureas, are highly bound to plasma albumin. **Glipizide** should be given 30 min before a meal to achieve greatest postprandial reduction in blood sugar. The initial dosage is 5 mg daily, but geriatric patients and those with liver disease should have therapy initiated at 2.5 mg daily. Dosage is adjusted in increments of 2.5 to 5 mg with several days between titration steps. Daily doses of glipizide above 15 mg should be given in divided doses. **Glyburide** is initiated at 2.5 to 5 mg daily in single or divided doses with increments no more frequently than 2.5 mg at weekly intervals based on blood glucose response.

Indications

The sulfonylureas should be used in the treatment of Type II diabetics who cannot be treated with diet alone or who are unable or unwilling to take insulin if weight reduction and diet approaches fail. They should not be used in ketosis-prone diabetes, in the presence of serious endocrine, renal, or liver dysfunction, in pregnancy, or during stress periods (surgery, infection, fever, trauma) complicated by ketoacidosis.

Elderly persons should be started on about half the usual daily dose as some are very sensitive and may develop severe hypoglycemic reactions. During the beginning treatment phase all persons should monitor urines four times daily for glucosuria.

There continues to be controversy about the safe and judicious use of these drugs, led by the reports of the University Group Diabetes Program (UGDP), which was designed to evaluate the long-term effects of drug therapy. However, the study was terminated prior to completion because the subjects in the tolbutamide- and phenformin-treated groups had a higher incidence of cardiovascular deaths. Although the study design has been criticized, it has led many physicians and diabetics to avoid these agents. Many feel the risk of complications is too high unless all other measures to control the disease have been exhausted.

Adverse Effects

Diabetics who do not respond to these drugs can have either primary or secondary failures. With primary failures the blood glucose levels remain high (unchanged) when therapy is initiated; there is no response. Secondary failure usually occurs after a few months of responsive therapy; it is most often precipitated by stress and the failure is permanent. This type is more common in the nonobese diabetic and is an indication to discontinue the oral drugs and begin insulin therapy.

The overall incidence of undesirable effects in the sulfonylureas is low. Gastrointestinal reactions are secondary to an increase in gastric acid secretion and are manifested as heartburn, nausea, vomiting, abdominal pain, or diarrhea. These effects can usually be alleviated by decreasing the dose. Central nervous system effects include confusion, vertigo, atoxia, tinnitus, headache, and weakness. These are more often seen with large doses of **chlorpropamide**.

A more commonly seen adverse effect occurs when the sulfonylureas are combined with ethyl alcohol. A result that is similar to a disulfiran (Antabuse)-alcohol reaction takes place. Flushing, headache, nausea, vomiting, tachycardia, shortness of breath, and photosensitivity can occur. These symptoms usually disappear within an hour and more frequently occur with **chlorpropamide**.

Hypoglycemia can occur with overdosage, missed meals and snacks, weight loss, increased activity, or impaired renal and liver function. These reactions tend to occur more often in the elderly, and with those who consume alcohol. Some drugs trigger a synergistic effect when given in combination with the sulfonylureas (see Table 35-17).

NURSING PROCESS RELATED TO DIABETES MELLITUS

Assessment

Important factors in the assessment of the diabetic include a health history, physical exam, and an appraisal of attitude and knowledge of the disease process. If diagnosed, assess the patient's concept of diabetes:

What does the patient know and practice about diabetes?

What are the complications (especially hyperglycemia and hypoglycemia) previously experienced?

Can the patient explain his or her treatment and management modalities, including how to manage complications?

Table 35-17   Drug Interactions with Hypoglycemic Agents

DRUGS THAT INCREASE EFFECTS OF INSULIN	DRUGS THAT DECREASE EFFECTS OF INSULIN	DRUGS THAT INCREASE EFFECTS OF ORAL HYPOGLYCEMIC AGENTS	DRUGS THAT DECREASE EFFECTS OF ORAL HYPOGLYCEMIC AGENTS
Alcohol	Corticosteroids	Alcohol*	Alcohol*
Anabolic steroids	Diazoxide	Allopurinol	Corticosteroids
Anticoagulants	Epinephrine	Anabolic steroids	Diuretics
Antineoplastics	Estrogens	Anticoagulants (oral)	Glucagon
Isoniazid (INH)	Glucagon	Ascorbic acid	Epinephrine
Methamphetamine	Lithium	Chloramphenicol	Estrogens
Monoamine oxidase	Oral contraceptives	Clofibrate	Nicotinic acid
(MAO) inhibitors	Phenothiazines	Cyclophosphamide	Oral contraceptives
Oral hypoglycemics	Phenytoin	Guanethidine	Phenytoin
Phenylbutazone	Propranolol*	MAO inhibitors	Rifampin
Propranolol*	Thiazide diuretics	Phenylbutazone	Thyroid preparations
Salicylates	Thyroid preparations	Probenecid	
		Salicylates	
		Sulfinpyrazone	
		Tetracyclines	

*Interaction varies.

Questions concerning social and cultural factors should be included. Most health care facilities have some form of diabetes assessment guide to follow in this initial interview.

Management

Diabetic education is the key to diabetic management. Based on the previous assessment, an organized teaching plan can be constructed. The overall goal of management is to maintain blood glucose levels within normal limits and to allow the diabetic to live as normal a life as possible. The diabetic needs to know that control is dependent on diet, medication (for some), weight control, and exercise (see Table 35-18).

Evaluation

After a reassessment of the diabetic's understanding of the management plan, a standard approach for monitoring the diabetic condition can be developed. Each time the diabetic is seen for diabetes evaluation, a review of this plan is needed. Further teaching or reinforcement of previous teaching will strengthen the skills of self-management. To facilitate this process, a copy of the assessment sheet or guide should be available for use by the physician, clinic nurse, or visiting nurse.

Other laboratory tests, such as the *HbA*$_{1c}$ (*glycosylated hemoglobin*), can further evaluate blood glucose control. The glycosylated hemoglobin test indicates the plasma glucose concentration over a 4- to 12-week period, and is not affected by short-term fluctuations in the plasma glucose levels. Glycosylated hemoglobins are products of the hemoglobin chain and make up about 4 to 8 percent of the total hemoglobin. After hemoglobin is produced it remains in the red blood cell for the approximate life of the cell. As the hemoglobin circulates in the blood, glucose molecules grad-

TABLE 35-18   A Diabetic Teaching Guide

1. Physiology
   Anatomy
   Causes
   Symptoms
2. Medications
   A. Insulin
      Injection technique
      Type
      Dose
      Time
      Onset, peak, duration
      Site rotation
      Dystrophy
      Care of supplies
   B. Oral hypoglycemic
      Type
      Dose
      Action
      Time
3. Acute complications
   A. Hypoglycemia
      Symptoms
      Causes
      Treatment
   B. Hyperglycemia
      Symptoms
      Causes
      Treatment
4. Blood sugar monitoring
   A. Urine testing
      Reason
      Time
      Method
      Equipment
      Record keeping
      Management of results
   B. Home glucose monitoring
      Reason
      Time
      Method
      Equipment
         Visual
         Meter
      Record keeping
      Management of results
5. Diet
6. Exercise
   Type
   Amount
7. Hygiene
   Oral
   Foot
   Skin
8. Sick day rules
9. Stress management
10. Health maintenance
11. Drug interactions
   Alcohol
   Other

ually attach to it; thus, the glycosylated hemoglobin reflects the mean plasma glucose levels over the previous 1 to 3 months. Studies show that the glycosylated hemoglobin levels are reliable indicators of the degree of diabetic control. If the levels are 7.5 percent or lower, diabetic control is considered good.

Home blood glucose monitoring is believed to be a more accurate indicator of metabolic control than urine testing. This home management technique should be considered, especially if

1. Consistent control is a problem.
2. Renal thresholds are high or low.
3. Hypoglycemia is difficult to interpret.
4. The diabetic is pregnant.
5. The patient has difficulty voiding.

However, in order to be effective, the home blood glucose monitoring equipment must be accurate. The diabetic must be motivated and able to understand the correct use of the materials and what his or her role is in achieving glycemic control.

There are several types of blood glucose monitoring machines and reagent strips available today (see section "Clinical Findings" above). Choosing one can be a complex task. Selection will depend on product availability, expense, specific individual limitations, and clinician and patient preferences.

Evaluation of compliance and the identification of any new problems need to be accomplished with each outpatiet visit. The inpatient should be evaluated for indications of hyperglycemia and hypoglycemia. Subjective data and review of signs should be supplemented by blood glucose and/or urine glucose determinations. Education can be evaluated by patient demonstration, paper and pencil test, or interview.

CASE STUDY

R.C., a 48-year-old white man with a positive family history of diabetes mellitus (father and paternal grandfather), was an insulin-dependent diabetic for 18 years. He came to the clinic for routine evaluation and was seen by the physician who referred him to the Diabetic Nurse Clinician whose assessment follows.

Assessment

R.C. had been instructed to eat an 1800-calorie diet containing no free sugar; however, he admitted to frequent dietary indiscretion and irregular eating habits. He had not had any recent weight change.

He was currently using NPH-U-100 insulin, 55 U every morning along with 15 U regular U-100 insulin every morning. He had never been treated with oral hypoglycemics.

R.C.'s history was positive for the following diabetic complications: three hospital admissions in the prior two years for ketoacidosis; amputation of all toes of the right foot two years earlier; chronic renal failure (serum creatinine 3.1 mg% and 4+ proteinuria); and numbness and burning pain in both feet for several years. R.C. had no history of heart attack, angina pectoris, hypertension, diarrhea, cataracts, glaucoma, vision changes, or kidney infections.

R.C. worked as a long-haul truck driver and was frequently out of town and on the road. He had a wife and two children. He denied chronic alcohol use or use of street drugs. He was on no other medications. He smoked one and one-half packages of cigarettes per day.

On physical exam, R.C. weighed 170 lb and was 65 in tall. His blood pressure (right arm, seated) was 140/85. Fundoscopic exam showed exudates and microaneurysms on both fundi. Pedal pulses were absent bilaterally, and there was decreased vibratory sense and pinprick bilaterally. No skin lesions were noted, but both feet were dry and dirty with fungal infections in the left toenails.

Laboratory studies revealed a fasting blood sugar of 345 mg%, consistent with determinations over the prior year which ranged from 250 to 350 mg%. Chest x-ray and ECG were within normal limits. Urinalysis revealed 5% glucose, negative acetone, 4+ protein; the microscopic analysis was within normal limits. Patient's home urine tests had averaged before breakfast, 5%; before lunch, negative to trace; before dinner, 0.5 to 1%; and before bedtime, 0.5 to 1%.

The patient's wife stated that her husband frequently got agitated, sweaty, nervous, and confused in the middle of the day. During this clinic visit the patient experienced a hypoglycemic reaction at 11:30 A.M.

From these data the nurse clinician drew the following conclusions: R.C. was not well-controlled and tended to have large swings between hyperglycemia and hypoglycemia. His hypoglycemic reactions tended to occur when his regular insulin dose was having peak effect, and he was inconsistent in his eating habits (both in type of food and time of meals). Although he had already had an amputation, he still had poor foot hygiene, and was overweight (at 5 ft 5 in tall, his ideal weight was about 136 lb).

R.C. demonstrated diabetic retinopathy, as well as chronic renal failure, which would affect his urinary threshold for sugar and the duration of action of his insulin. His occupation was potentially very hazardous to himself and others in view of his tendency toward hypoglycemic reactions.

Management

The physician and nurse clinician conferred and defined the therapeutic plan for this patient. A major goal was to ascertain what factors contributed to the patient's poor management of his illness. The nurse interviewed R.C. and administered the standard pretest used in the course which the nurse taught to newly diagnosed inpatients. The test revealed that R.C. had a very low-level understanding of his illness and its therapy. He indicated that he had received some instruction when he was first diagnosed, but that he was so overwhelmed by the diagnosis that he remembered very little and was embarrassed to admit it by asking questions. R.C. also expressed extreme fear of "being a cripple" and "losing his manhood."

The nurse initiated a complete diabetic education program, emphasizing foot care and dietary instruction for weight loss and disease control. The importance of a regular eating pattern (morning, noon, and evening, with a small bedtime snack) was stressed.

The physician decreased the regular insulin dose to 10 U in the morning in an attempt to smooth out the patient's blood sugar response and prevent midday hypoglycemia. The physician indicated he would later attempt to adjust the NPH dosage to control the hyperglycemia. A referral to an ophthalmologist for evaluation of the diabetic retinopathy was made to determine if any of the lesions could be treated with photocoagulation. He was also referred to a podiatrist.

The nurse observed R.C. draw up and self-administer the insulin to verify proper dosing; it was necessary to emphasize the necessity for accuracy, since the patient was somewhat inexact in his measurements.

Evaluation

The patient was seen at two-week intervals for two months. No further hypoglycemic reactions occurred. With regular meals, improved eating patterns, and an increased NPH dosage, R.C. not only lost 6 lb but also brought his hyperglycemia under control. Fasting blood sugars ranged from 160 to 210 mg% and urine sugars were trace to 0.5%.

The condition of the patient's feet also improved, and so he was scheduled to be seen at less frequent intervals of every three months with specific instructions to contact the clinic if foot lesions, symptoms of hypoglycemia or hyperglycemia, infections, or a positive urinary acetone occurred.

THE THYROID

LEARNING OBJECTIVES

Upon mastery of the content of this section the reader will be able to:

1. Describe the physiologic mechanisms which regulate the level of thyroid hormone.
2. List the physiologic effects of the thyroid hormones.
3. Compare the common pharmacologic therapies used for the treatment of hypothyroidism.
4. Indicate three approaches to the treatment of hyperthyroidism.
5. Identify two types of antithyroid drugs, their actions, indications, and related nursing care.
6. Name some drugs that have a synergistic effect when combined with the thyroid hormones.

PHYSIOLOGY OF THE THYROID GLAND

The thyroid gland is a two-lobed organ located in the front of the trachea in the anterior portion of the neck. The major function of the gland is to synthesize, store, and secrete the hormones *triiodothyronine* (T_3) and *thyroxine* (T_4). The synthesis of these hormones is dependent on the anterior pituitary hormone, thyrotropin (thyroid-stimulating hormone, TSH). TSH is in turn regulated by the thyrotropin-releasing hormone (TRH) that is formed in the hypothalamus. Thyroid-stimulating hormone is regulated by negative feedback, since high levels of thyroid hormone suppress the release of TSH and make the anterior pituitary less responsive to TRH. Calcitonin is also produced by the thyroid gland. Calcitonin is released in response to increased levels of calcium; thus, it inhibits the release of calcium from bone and renal tubular reabsorption of calcium (see next section on the parathyroids).

Synthesis of T_3 and T_4

The production of T_3 and T_4 depends on the presence of iodine and tyrosine in the thyroid gland. Iodine and tyrosine (an amino acid) are derived from dietary sources. Iodine is absorbed from the GI tract as iodide and then is dispersed throughout the body (Fig. 35-6). The thyroid gland traps the iodide and then converts it to iodine by oxidation. At the same time tyrosine is iodinated to monoiodotyrosine (MIT) and diiodotyrosine (DIT). The last step in the synthesis of thyroid hormone requires the coupling of MIT and DIT to form triiodothyronine (T_3) and the coupling of two DIT molecules to form thyroxine (T_4). The T_3 and T_4 are then stored in the cells of the gland until their release by proteolytic enzymes.

Once the hormones are released they are bound extensively to plasma proteins. Thyroxine is bound mostly to thyroid-binding globulin (TBG) and thyroid-binding prealbu-

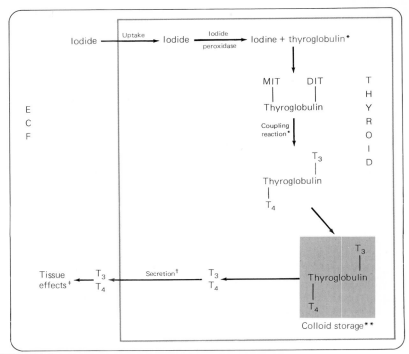

FIGURE 35-6

Production of Thyroid Hormone and Sites of Drug Action. Synthesis of thyroid hormones begins with iodide uptake into the follicular cells of the thyroid from the extracellular fluid (ECF) by an active transport mechanism. The iodide is converted to iodine, a reaction catalyzed by iodide peroxidase. Precursors to thyroid hormone are formed by the inclusion onto the amino acid tyrosine of one iodine (monoiodotyrosine; MIT) or two iodines (diiodotyrosine; DIT). The iodinated tyrosine residues, located in a large protein (thyroglobulin), are coupled: two diiodotyrosines to form thyroxine (T_4), or one monoiodotyrosine plus one diiodotyrosine to form triiodothyronine (T_3). Thyroglobulin is stored in the colloid area of the thyroid until proteolytic attack liberates T_3 and T_4 into the ECF, where they elicit their tissue effects. (*)Antithyroid drugs—propylthiouracil, methimazole—work by preventing iodination of tyrosine and the coupling reaction. (†)Iodide and lithium prevent secretion of T_3 and T_4 into the ECF. (‡)β-Adrenergic blockers—propranolol, metoprolol—reverse tissue effects at the cardiovascular system. (**)Radioactive iodine (^{131}I) concentrates in colloid storage and selectively damages the follicular cells of the thyroid.

min (TBPA), and to some extent to albumin. However, triiodothyronine binds less to TBG and albumin and does not bind at all to TBPA. The serum half-life of T_4 is approximately 6 days and that of T_3 is 1 day.

Effects of Thyroid Hormones

Thyroid hormones increase the basal metabolic rate of all body cells. They aid in the regulation of lipid and carbohydrate metabolism, are essential for normal growth and development (increase rate of bone growth and epiphyseal closure), effect respiratory rate and oxygen consumption, maintain cardiac output, regulate heat production, and stimulate the development of the central nervous system. Thyroid hormones increase the synthesis of cholesterol but also increase its metabolism. The net result is a decrease in cholesterol.

HYPERTHYROIDISM

Hyperthyroidism (thyrotoxicosis) is a condition resulting from increased activity of the thyroid gland. It is second only to diabetes mellitus among the naturally occurring endocrine disorders. Excess secretion of thyroid hormones results in generalized symptoms that may affect every organ system, but especially the cardiovascular, neuromuscular, and gastrointestinal systems. Frequently encountered symptoms of thyrotoxicosis include palpitations, nervousness, irritability, fatigue, tachycardia, and weight loss. Since these general symptoms can represent many other disease states, proper diagnosis requires demonstration of an overactive thyroid gland.

Etiology and Clinical Findings

Graves' disease, or acute toxic goiter, is a syndrome of thyroid enlargement, exophthalmos, and thyrotoxicosis. *Toxic nodular goiter* is less severe and usually occurs in older persons with preexisting goiter. *Iatrogenic thyrotoxicosis* occurs due to excess intake of thyroid medication. Less commonly, hyperthyroidism is caused by a thyroid tumor or a TSH-secreting pituitary adenoma. Demonstration of increased serum T_3 and/or T_4 and decreased thyroid-binding capacity (T_3 uptake) are common in hyperthyroidism.

Clinical Pharmacology and Therapeutics

Hyperthyroidism can be treated with antithyroid drugs, radioactive iodine, or surgery. The method used will depend on patient variables such as the cause of hyperthyroidism, the age of the patient, the severity of the disease, the presence or absence of other complications. In clinical practice a combination of the three methods may be used.

Antithyroid Drugs

The antithyroid drugs control hyperthyroidism by depressing the synthesis of the thyroid hormones T_3 and T_4 in the thyroid gland. They do not inactivate previously formed thyroid hormones; therefore, their effects are usually delayed until the bodily stores of existing T_4 and T_3 are depleted. It may take up to three months to achieve a euthyroid state. They also do not interfere with the action of exogenously administered thyroid hormones. Drug therapy is usually the treatment of choice in hyperthyroidism. Antithyroid drugs are listed in Table 35-19. The thioamides are the most commonly used clinically.

Thioamides

These agents interfere with the organification of iodine. Adverse effects of these agents occur in about 3 to 5 percent of patients treated with them. Any symptom of illness, such as sore throat, enlargement of cervical lymph nodes, GI disturbance, fever, skin rash, headache, unusual bleeding or bruising, or jaundice, may necessitate either a reduction in dosage or withdrawal of the drug. They should be used with caution in pregnancy. Agranulocytosis is the most serious effect of overdosage. Prolonged therapy may result in hypothyroidism.

Iodide

Although iodides are necessary for thyroid hormone production, in large doses they suppress the function of the gland. Iodide specifically reduces the size, vascularity, and friability of the thyroid gland before thyroidectomy. In addition, it can shorten the onset of action of other antithyroid drugs.

Iodine is contraindicated in pulmonary tuberculosis, because it may interfere with the healing of lesions, and in hypokalemic states. Serious adverse reactions are uncommon. Skin rash, mucous membrane ulceration, salivary gland swelling, metallic taste, and gastric distress, if they occur, will subside when iodine is discontinued. Iodine poisoning can result from overdosage. Symptoms mainly result from irritation to the GI tract: vomiting, diarrhea, abdominal pain. Clients should also be cautioned against indiscriminate use of over-the-counter drugs containing iodide (e.g., cough medicines), as these may negate the iodine therapy.

The maximal effect of these preparations is usually seen within two weeks, and after that time an escape from therapeutic effect may be evident. For that reason iodide therapy is not a primary method of therapy and is usually used in association with surgery.

Radioactive Iodine

Radioactive iodine (RAI) remains an effective method of treatment for hyperthyroidism, especially in adults with serious cardiac complications, adult Graves' disease, and thyroid carcinoma. The most frequently used preparation is ^{131}I. Tracer doses are used in diagnostic tests for thyroid function. Treatment need not involve hospitalization and often eliminates the need for hospitalization.

Mechanism of Action   Radioactive iodine limits the secretion of thyroid hormones by damaging and destroying thyroid tissue.

Adverse Effects   When used in tracer doses there is little radiation hazard. In therapeutic doses there is a risk of increased mutation to normal exposed cells. Because of this, it is contraindicated in children, pregnant women, and nursing mothers. Tenderness, soreness, swelling of the gland, and skin rashes have been reported. The incidence of iatrogenic hypothyroidism is high when large doses have been used. Iodide preparations should be avoided before treatment with radioactive iodine since the nonradioactive iodide preparations will compete with the radioactive iodine for entrapment in the thyroid gland. After administration of the radioactive iodine exacerbation of hyperthyroidism sometimes occurs because of leakage of the stored thyroid hormones. These problems can be managed clinically with **propranolol** (Inderal).

Dosage   Radioactive iodine is measured by the curie (Ci). The dose varies depending on the thyroid weight, radioactive iodine uptake, and the rate of release of radioactive

Table 35-19 Antithyroid Drugs

DRUG	ROUTE AND DOSE	COMMENTS
	Thioamides	
Methimazole (Tapazole)	*Adults:* 15 mg for mild symptoms; 30–40 mg for moderate symptoms; 60 mg for severe symptoms. Give in three divided doses at 8-h intervals. Maintenance dose is 5–15 mg/day. *Children:* 0.4 mg/kg initially in three divided doses at 8-h intervals. Maintenance dose is one-half the initial dose.	More potent than propylthiouracil and longer duration of action. Store in dark container. *Minor reactions:* skin rash, urticaria, GI disturbance, arthralgia, hair loss, decreased taste. *Major reactions:* hepatic damage, inhibition of myelopoiesis, drug fever, a lupus-like syndrome, and hypoprothrombinemia.
Propylthiouracil (Propacil, PTU)	*Adults:* 300 mg/day in three divided doses at 8-h intervals. Maintenance 100–150 mg/day. *Children* 10 yr and up: 150–300 mg/day 6–10 yr: 50–150 mg/day in three divided doses at 8-h intervals.	Administer with meals to decrease GI distress. May increase effect of anticoagulants. Adverse effects the same as above, but less severe.
	Iodine Products	
Strong iodine solution (Lugol's solution)	5% iodide and 10% potassium iodide in solution. Dose 0.3 mL tid. (Usually 10–14 days before thyroidectomy)	Administer diluted with milk, orange juice, or water to decrease bitter taste. Decreases vascularity and increases firmness of thyroid to ease in surgical removal. Used with antithyroid drugs for treating thyrotoxic crisis.
Sodium iodide	1–3 g IV infusion for treatment of thyroid crisis.	Used for acute treatment of thyroid crisis. Disrupts release of hormones.
Iodo-Niacin	Tablets of 135 mg potassium and 25 mg niacinamide HCl. *Adults:* 2 tab tid *Children* (above 8 yr): 1 tab tid.	For the prophylaxis of goiter and management of hyperthyroidism. Take after meals with water.
Potassium iodide	*Adults:* 300–650 mg q4–6h. *Children:* 250–1000 mg daily in divided doses.	Induction of thyroid involution before surgery. Facilitates bronchial drainage and cough in chronic pulmonary conditions.
Saturated solution potassium iodide (SSKI)	0.3–0.6 mL, 4–12 times/day.	Induction of thyroid involution prior to surgery. Expectorant. Keep bottle cap closed tightly.
	Others	
Propranolol (Inderal)	*Adults:* 20–80 mg, q4–6h PO. May give IV 1–3 mg at rates of 1 mg/min.	Beta-adrenergic blocker. Use in thyroid storm and severe hyperthyroidism. Blocks peripheral effects of thyroid hormone. Monitor respiratory status. Causes bronchoconstriction.
Lithium carbonate	*Adults:* 300–600 mg up to qid. Titrated according to serum lithium levels.	Blocks thyroid hormone release. Does not increase glandular hormonal storage. Potential for toxicity—narrow margin of safety.
Perchlorate, sodium or potassium	Maximum of 250 mg PO qid.	Interferes with iodide trapping. Nausea, vomiting, skin rash, leukopenia, aplastic anemia, agranulocytosis, and lymphadenopathy are possible adverse effects.

iodine from the gland. It is administered orally in a glass of water or by intravenous route. Average doses are:

Diagnostic	2 to 10 μCi
Hyperthyroidism	4 to 10 mCi
Thyroid cancer	50 to 150 mCi

Radioactive iodine is rapidly absorbed and radioactivity can be detected in the thyroid within minutes. Thyroid function begins to decrease in two weeks, with maximum effect occurring at about 10 weeks. RAI is excreted in the urine.

Surgery

Surgery is indicated in pregnancy (antithyroid drugs should be avoided since they cross into fetal circulation), multinodular goiter, and in children. Surgery involves a subtotal thyroidectomy. The procedure is associated with low mortality and morbidity. The patient should be euthyroid at the time of the procedure and should be treated with antithyroid drugs prior to surgery.

HYPOTHYROIDISM

Etiology and Clinical Findings

Hypothyroidism is a clinical state that results from a variety of causes and that leads to a decrease in the amount of thyroid hormone produced, as evidenced by decreased serum T_3 and T_4 and increased RT_3U (T_3 uptake). It may be due to the thyroid gland's inability to secrete an adequate amount of thyroid hormone (primary hypothyroidism) or to failure of the pituitary to produce a sufficient amount of TSH (secondary hypothyroidism). Hypothyroidism that develops at birth and results in developmental abnormalities is termed *cretinism*. A severe form of hypothyroidism is called *myxedema* and is associated with thickening of the facial features and doughy induration of the skin. The hypothyroidism may also be drug-induced (sulfonamides, lithium carbonate, perchlorates, and thioamides).

The signs and symptoms of cretinism may be present at birth, but more commonly they develop in the first months of life. The first sign may be failure of the child to feed properly. Additional signs are persistence of jaundice, a hoarse cry, sleepiness, and constipation. Later the more classical signs of cretinism may appear including short stature, coarse features with protruding tongue, sparse hair, dry skin, "pot belly," umbilical hernia, and cold skin. Mental development is delayed, and the severity of this and other signs and symptoms will depend on how soon replacement therapy is started.

In the adult the signs of hypothyroidism are less specific but may include lethargy, constipation, cold intolerance, decrease in appetite, and dryness and loss of hair. Later the clinical picture of myxedema becomes evident with dull, expressionless face, sparse hair, large tongue, and pale and cool skin which feels rough and doughy. If left untreated the patient may proceed into a myxedema coma characterized by hypothermia, coma, and respiratory depression.

Thyroid Stimulation Test

Differential diagnosis of primary and secondary hypothyroidism can be accomplished by administering 10 IU of **thyrotropin** (thyroid-stimulating hormone, TSH; Thytropar) for one to three days followed by measurement of serum T_3 and T_4. Thyrotropin is also used to enhance the uptake of ^{131}I in thyroid carcinoma and in the diagnosis of thyroid cancer remanant after surgery. It can cause menstrual irregularities, thyroid swelling, nausea and vomiting, cardiac arrhythmias, and hypersensitivity reactions manifested as hypotension, urticaria, and fever.

Thyroid Hormone Replacement

Replacement with thyroid hormone is commonly indicated in states where there is diminished or absent thyroid function: hypothyroidism, cretinism, and myxedema. The objective of treatment is to return the patient to a normal metabolic (euthyroid) state. This is usually accomplished with a full replacement dose of any of the preparations listed in Table 35-20.

The patient's response to therapy in conjunction with the laboratory results usually determine the therapeutic maintenance dose. However, in all cases, the overall impression of the client's well-being will take priority over the laboratory tests in establishing individual therapy.

The age and general physical condition of the client, the severity of the disease, manifested signs and symptoms, and evidence of complications influence the starting hormonal dosage and the rate of incremental advancement until a maintenance dose is reached.

A relatively healthy adult can be initiated at higher dosages and raised to maintenance in about two to three weeks. In infants and children there is a sense of urgency to achieve full replacement because of the critical role thyroid hormone has in growth and development. In the elderly, or those with cardiac complications, a small initial dose is used. A larger dose may stimulate metabolic activity, stressing the circulatory system to the point of heart failure. Generally thyroid therapy is increased in low increments at spaced intervals until the desired response is obtained. It is most often given as a single dose before breakfast.

Adverse Effects

Unless clearly indicated, thyroid replacement therapy should not be used in clients with known cardiovascular disease and/or hypertension. Any signs of chest pain or aggravated cardiovascular signs necessitate immediate reduction in dosage.

The adverse reactions are usually as a result of overdosage or of a too rapid increase in dosage. If these occur, it is recommended that the hormone be stopped for several days and that therapy begin again at a lower dose. Significant adverse reactions include: headache, palpitations, cardiac arrhythmias, angina, tremors, sweating, insomnia, weight loss, heat intolerance, menstrual irregularities, and diarrhea (symptoms similar to hyperthyroidism), as well as allergic skin reactions. Severe overdosage may result in symptoms resembling thyroid storm.

Drug Interactions Thyroid hormones can enhance the effects of catecholamines and potentiate the effects of **digitalis glycosides**, **anticoagulants**, and **indomethacin** (Indocin).

TABLE 35-20 Thyroid Replacement Drugs

DRUG	ROUTE AND DOSE	COMMENTS
Natural Thyroid Hormones		
Thyroid desiccated (Lannett, Amour, Thyrar, Thyrocrine)	*Adult myxedema:* 16 mg/day for 2 weeks, increase to 32 mg/day for 2 weeks, then 65 mg/day. Increase according to lab tests and clinical response. Usual maintenance dose: 65–195 mg/day PO. *Adult hypothyroidism without myxedema:* 65 mg/day. Increase monthly by 65 mg/day until desired response. *Children:* Dose similar to adults. Final maintenance dose may be higher in growing child than in adult.	Low cost. Standardized according to iodine content. Contains varying amounts of T_3 and T_4 and benefits may be unpredictable. Store in dark, dry container to delay degradation.
Thyroglobulin (Proloid)	Start with small amounts and increase gradually at 1–2 week intervals. Maintenance dose is 32–200 mg/day.	Action is similar to desiccated thyroid, but purer and biologically standardized. Degrades on prolonged storage. High cost.
Levothyroxine (T_4, L-thyroxine; Synthroid, Levothroid, Noroxine)	*Adults:* 0.05–0.1 mg daily. Increase every 1–3 weeks until desired response. Usual maintenance dose 0.1–0.2 mg daily. In *elderly* with long-standing disease, starting dose may be as little as 0.025 mg/day. Increase 0.025 mg/day at 3–4 week intervals, depending on response. *Myxedema coma:* 0.2–0.5 mg IV first day, 0.1–0.3 mg second day if needed. Daily IV administration may be necessary until oral dose can be given. *Children:* Initial dose 0.025–0.05 mg/day with increments of 0.05–0.1 mg every 2 weeks until desired response. Range up to 0.3–0.4 mg/day.	In order to sustain growth, dosage is higher in infants and children than in adults.
Synthetic Thyroid Hormones		
Liothyronine sodium (T_3; Cytomel)	*Mild hyperthyroidism:* 25 µg/day. Increase by 12.5–25 µg every 1–2 weeks. Usual maintenance dose is 25–75 µg/day. *Myxedema and simple goiter:* 5 µg/day. Increase by 5–10 µg/day every 1–2 weeks. Usual maintenance dose 50–100 µg/day. *Cretinism:* 5 µg/day. Increase 5 µg every 3–4 days until desired response. Doses as high as 20–80 µg/day may be required. Above 3 yr give full adult dose.	Synthetic preparations of T_3 contain uniform amounts of thyroid hormone. More rapid onset and shorter duration of action than other thyroid preparations, so will require more frequent administration. Monitor for cardiac side effects.
Liotrix (Euthroid, Thyrolar)	*Adults:* 15–30 mg/day, increase gradually every 1–2 weeks until response is achieved. *Children:* Same as adult, increase dosage every 2 weeks. *Older adult:* One-fourth to one-half of the normal adult dose. Double dose every 8 weeks if necessary.	A mixture of synthetic T_4 and T_3 in a 4:1 ratio by weight. 60 mg = 1 g thyroid. Usually given as a single dose before breakfast. Predictable content. More expensive. No advantage over other thyroid hormones.

In diabetes, the dosage of **insulin** or the **oral hypoglycemics** may need to be increased because the addition of thyroid hormones can increase blood sugar levels. The reverse is also true; decreasing the dose of thyroid hormone may cause hypoglycemic reactions.

DISORDERS OF CALCITONIN ACTIVITY

Patients with medullary carcinoma of the thyroid will secrete excessive amounts of calcitonin. Calcium balance is not disrupted and bone metabolism appears normal, perhaps because of compensatory overactivity of the parathyroid glands. The tumor releases other substances as well: ACTH, 5-hydroxytryptamine, and histaminase. These substances are commonly associated with diarrhea and cushingoid signs. The diarrhea appears to be prostaglandin-mediated, as it can be inhibited by the administration of **indomethacin** (Indocin). Diagnosis is made by stimulating calcitonin release by an infusion of calcium, pentagastrin, or ethanol. Treatment is surgical thyroidectomy. A true calcitonin deficiency state has not been recognized.

NURSING PROCESS RELATED TO THYROID DISORDERS

The nursing process in hyperthyroidism and hypothyroidism is outlined in Table 35-21.

TABLE 35-21   Nursing Process in Thyroid Disorders

ASSESSMENT	MANAGEMENT	EVALUATION
	Hyperthyroidism	
Skin: warm, moist. Dependent edema. Nervous system: agitated mood swings, tremor, irritability, increased tendon reflexes; insomnia. Cardiac: increased BP, P; arrhythmias, palpitations. Exophthalmos: Check for pregnancy. Loose bowel movements, diaphoresis, ravenous appetite, weight loss. Musculoskeletal: weakness, fatigue. Increased sensitivity to warm room.	Teach to take drug as ordered. For exophthalmos, methycellulose drops qid, wear protective glasses, tape eyes shut at night or use sleep mask, exercise ocular muscles, restrict sodium intake. Cool, restful environment. Avoid stress. Well-balanced diet—at least six meals daily. Avoid bulk foods, caffeine. Explain reason for abnormal behavior to family/friends. ^{131}I: Usually no need for isolation; (for large doses isolate 8 days). Tell patient he is not dangerous. Methimazole and thiouracil—teach to report sore throat, fever, rash.	Therapeutic effects: decrease in nervous system symptoms, decreased pulse, appetite, etc. Remission: 4–8 wk with drugs. Adverse effects: All drugs may produce hypothyroidism (headache, fatigue, weight gain, etc.). Iodine-headache, salivation (iodism); "escape" (recurrence of hyperthyroidism). Methimazole and thiouracil—hold drug and report decreased CBC, fever, rash, sore throat. Weigh daily—report daily loss greater than 1.5 kg. In stress, infection, watch for thyroid storm (tachycardia, delirium, irritability).
	Hypothyroidism	
Skin: thick, dry, flaky; appears puffy and edematous. Dry hair, brittle nails. Nervous system: lethargic, forgetful. Personality changes, slowed mental process. Gastrointestinal: constipation, decreased appetite, often weight gain. Check for pregnancy. Cardiac: increased capillary fragility, decreased pulse, BP changes. Distant heart sounds. Musculoskeletal: fatigue, weakness. Others: increased sensitivity to infection, narcotics, barbiturates, and anesthesia.	Warm environment. Measures to prevent skin breakdown. May require controlled caloric intake. Prevent constipation; fluids, bulk, exercise, drugs if necessary. Avoid enemas due to vagal stimulation. Avoid or reduce dose of sedative drugs (narcotic, barbiturate, anesthetics). Patient education: Stress need for life-long drug. Give list of symptoms of hyperthyroidism and hypothyroidism.	Therapeutic effects: improved vital signs, increased physical and mental activity, decrease in edematous appearance. Improvement should appear in 2–14 days. Daily weight. May develop cardiac complications from too rapid replacement—hold drug and report angina, orthopnea, dyspnea, etc.

CASE STUDY

J.G., a 28-year-old married mother of two girls (ages 7 and 4) reported for her annual gynecologic checkup to the nurse practitioner at the family practice clinic with a complaint of infertility. Mrs. G. indicated that she and her husband had been attempting to conceive for over two years.

Assessment

J.G. was para 2 gravida 2; both pregnancies and deliveries had been completely normal, and she had had no difficulty in conceiving either time. She had ceased to use contraception (a diaphragm) two years earlier and had never used oral contraceptives. The patient indicated that her menstrual cycle had lengthened from the previous 28 days to 33 to 40 days. J.G. also complained of extreme fatigue, decreased libido, constipation, muscle weakness, and aches and pains. She was further distressed by forgetfulness.

Vital signs were: blood pressure 98/60; temperature 96°F, pulse 62, and respirations 16. J.G. sat slumped in the chair and spoke slowly in a hoarse tone. Her skin, hair, and nails were dry and flaky, but her face, hands, and feet appeared swollen and puffy. The hematocrit was 35 percent. The remainder of the physical examination, including pelvic examination, was normal.

The nurse practitioner suspected that the patient's complaints were caused by hypothyroidism.

Management

J.G. was referred by the nurse to the physician, who reviewed the nurse's examination findings and ordered a T_3 uptake, serum T_3 and T_4 concentrations, and serum cholesterol. Results of all tests were normal except for an elevated cholesterol and low serum T_3 concentration. The physician verified the diagnosis of hypothyroidism. In order to differentiate primary from secondary hypothyroidism a serum TSH was drawn and results indicated primary hypothyroidism. The physician ordered 10 μg of sodium liothyronine (Cytomel) daily and asked the nurse to follow J.G. until signs of myxedema were alleviated.

The nurse explained the functions of the thyroid to J.G. and the expected course of therapy. It was stressed that she might need to take the drug for the rest of her life. Methods of preventing constipation were outlined, and the patient was advised to limit caloric intake until her next clinic visit and to keep warm.

J.G. was warned to avoid sedative drugs and to report any chest pain or difficulty in breathing. Due to her forgetfulness all instructions were supplied in writing, including a list of the symptoms of hyperthyroidism and hypothyroidism, and the nurse contacted the patient's husband to explain the situation to him as well.

Evaluation

J.G. began to experience improvement within 3 days, and all symptoms were alleviated without adverse effect by the third week. At that time the physician increased the dosage to 25 μg of Cytomel daily. When the patient returned to the clinic two months later for evaluation, she complained of having begun to feel nervous and jittery and she had lost 5 lb in 10 days without dieting. Since her symptoms were indicative of iatrogenic hyperthyroidism, the physician decreased the dosage of the Cytomel. From then on J.G. showed no further signs of thyroid disorder.

THE PARATHYROIDS

LEARNING OBJECTIVES

Upon mastery of the content of this section, the reader will be able to:

1. Explain the actions of parathyroid hormone and calcitonin.

2. List the drugs used to normalize serum calcium in hypoparathyroidism and hyperparathyroidism.

3. State the mechanisms of action of corticosteroids, nonsteroidal anti-inflammatory drugs, and salmon calcitonin in hypercalemia.

PHYSIOLOGY OF CALCIUM REGULATION

The function of the parathyroid glands is to maintain serum calcium concentrations. There are usually four small parathyroid glands in the neck region, located close to the thyroid gland. When the fraction of ionized (unbound) calcium in the blood falls, *parathyroid hormone* (PTH) is secreted. Parathyroid hormone decreases urinary calcium loss, increases absorption of calcium from the diet, enhances metabolic activation of vitamin D, mobilizes the bone stores of calcium, and promotes urinary phosphate excretion.

The effect of PTH is balanced by the activity of *calcitonin* from the thyroid. High ionized calcium levels in the blood stimulate the secretion of calcitonin, which inhibits the reabsorption of calcium from bone, inhibits renal phosphate reabsorption, and promotes urinary calcium loss.

DISORDERS OF PARATHYROID FUNCTION

Hypoparathyroidism

Hypoparathyroidism usually occurs when the parathyroid glands are removed during thyroid surgery, which manifests (within days to years) as the inability to maintain adequate levels of free calcium. The disorder may present as acute hypocalcemia (tetany, muscle overactivity, seizures) or as chronic hypoparathyroidism (mental symptoms of psychosis and depression, loss of hair, dry skin, weak teeth and nails, cataracts, and calcium deposits in soft tissues). Pseudohypoparathyroidism is said to be present when serum PTH levels are normal, but end-organ responsiveness is reduced.

Clinical Pharmacology and Therapeutics

Vitamin D is used to manage the decreased intestinal absorption of calcium. The active forms have a more rapid onset of action; synthesized active vitamin D (**calcitriol**) is preferred, although other forms are used (see Chap. 25). **Calcium** is given to supplement losses. Increased serum phosphate (which tends to depress serum calcium) is controlled by the administration of **aluminum antacids** to bind phosphates in the gastrointestinal tract and increase fecal loss. These drugs are discussed in the section on hypocalcemia in Chap. 24.

Hyperparathyroidism

Hyperparathyroidism may be caused by the oversecretion of PTH independent of serum calcium concentrations (*primary hyperparathyroidism*), which is usually caused by a tumor of one or more of the parathyroid glands. Because the skeleton is demineralized to provide much of the calcium, osteomalacia may occur. In addition, urinary phosphate wasting may cause kidney stones or renal calcification. A medical emergency may be precipitated by acute worsening of the hypercalcemia (parathyroid crisis), with symptoms of severe hypercalcemia.

Secondary hyperparathyroidism occurs when chronically low serum calcium levels lead to a physiologic increase in PTH secretion, accompanied by hyperphosphatemia. This disorder may be seen in vitamin D deficiency states such as dietary insufficiency, failure to absorb adequate dietary vitamin D, failure to metabolize dietary forms to active vitamin D (as in renal failure), enhanced metabolic deactivation [as with adverse reaction to **phenytoin** (Dilantin)], or in patients who are resistant to normal doses of vitamin D.

Clinical Pharmacology and Therapeutics

Treatment of primary hyperparathyroidism usually involves surgery with subsequent supplementation of calcium, phosphorus, and vitamin D to restore mineralization of the bones and guard against postoperative hypocalcemia due to iatrogenic hypoparathyroidism. Nonsteroidal anti-inflammatory drugs may be used in primary hyperparathyroidism not amenable to surgery, since they inhibit prostaglandins which have parathormone-like activity to mobilize calcium from the bone. With doses of **indomethacin** (Indocin) at 25 to 50 mg tid or **aspirin** at 600 to 1200 mg tid, the onset of activity is approximately three days with maximal hypocalcemic

effect by approximately 11 days. An initial 3-day trial is advised to ascertain if the serum calcium will respond to the nonsteroidal anti-inflammatory drugs, since the doses are high enough to cause significant adverse effects (listed in Chap. 26); this therapy should be discontinued if ineffective during the trial.

Secondary hyperparathyroidism is managed by supplementing vitamin D, preferably in active forms such as **calcitriol** (Rocaltrol). Calcium is given to suppress further parathormone release (see Chaps. 25 and 31).

Hypercalcemic emergencies are treated with fluids (to elicit forced caluresis); loop diuretics (see Chap. 23) such as **furosemide** (Lasix; 20 to 100 mg q1–2h) or **bumetanide** (Bumex; 50 mg q2h); oral phosphates (see Chap. 24); corticosteroids; and/or **calcitonin**. Corticosteroid doses in acute treatment are 200 to 500 mg **hydrocortisone sodium succinate** tid by infusion. Maintenance doses of 10 to 80 mg of **prednisone** daily are gradually decreased as tolerated. Onset of corticosteroid activity is slow due to its mechanism of action in hypercalcemia, which is to slow calcium turnover by inhibiting osteoclast activity, decreasing intestinal calcium absorption, and decreasing renal tubular calcium reabsorption. Corticosteroids are often used concurrently with calcitonin.

Salmon Calcitonin

Commercially available **calcitonin** is derived from salmon sources, but human and porcine calcitonin are used investigationally. Salmon calcitonin (Calcimar) appears to act on bone, renal tubules, and the GI tract to reduce serum calcium levels by a mechanism identical to mammalian calcitonin (see above), but its potency is greater and it has a longer duration of action. It is probably inactivated by metabolism in the kidney and other tissues to smaller, inactive segments.

Indications   Salmon calcitonin is a good drug for treatment of hypercalcemic emergency in patients with uremia or heart failure, since it has no fluid-retention effect. However, its effect is not as profound or persistent as other modalities. It is also used in treatment of Paget's bone disease (osteitis deformans).

Adverse Effects   Hypersensitivity reaction, including anaphylactic response, can occur as with any animal-derived protein. Nausea, vomiting, flushing, skin rashes, and local inflammatory reactions at the site of injection also occur. "Calcium escape" may take place after a few days of therapy, resulting in hypercalcemia unresponsive to calcitonin. Combination therapy with corticosteroids or phosphate may prevent this. For long-term therapy, periodic microscopic examination of the urine for casts is recommended.

Use of salmon calcitonin with the antineoplastic drug **mithramycin** (Mithracin; see Chap. 37), which is used in hypercalcemia related to neoplasms, may produce recurrent hypocalcemia.

Dosage and Administration Prior to use of salmon calcitonin, a test for hypersensitivity is performed by injecting 1 MRC U (0.1 mL of a 1:10 dilution) intradermally or subcutaneously on the inner aspect of the forearm. A positive reaction consists of more than mild erythema within 15 min of the injection.

For hypercalcemia the dose of salmon-derived **calcitonin** given by intramuscular injection is 2 to 8 MRC U/kg q12h. Subcutaneous administration may also be used for volumes of less than 2 mL. Paget's disease requires 50 to 100 MRC U daily.

NURSING PROCESS RELATED TO PARATHYROID DISORDERS

Abnormal calcium balance is the cardinal feature of parathyroid disorders. The nursing process related to pharmacologic agents used to treat hypocalcemia and hypercalcemia is outlined in Chap. 24.

THE GONADS (ANDROGENS)

LEARNING OBJECTIVES

Upon mastery of the content of this section, the reader will be able to:

1. Explain the physiologic functions of the androgens and the mechanisms which control androgen secretion.

2. Compare the indications for androgens and anabolic steroids.

3. Describe the nursing process related to the adverse effects of androgens and anabolic steroids.

PHYSIOLOGY OF GONADAL HORMONES

A balance of hypothalamic and pituitary stimulation and end-organ responsiveness is necessary to control the processes of sexual development and function. The production of *gonadotropin-releasing hormone (GnRH)* by the hypothalamus governs the release of hormones which stimulate the gonads (testes in the male, ovaries in the female) and other sexual organs. In both sexes two *gonadotropins* ("gonad growers") are released from the pituitary after stimulation by GnRH (see Fig. 35-7). *Follicle-stimulating hormone (FSH)* induces ripening of the female ovarian follicle and causes spermatozoa formation in the seminiferous tubule of the male. *Luteinizing hormone (LH)* effects ovulation and supportive hormone synthesis from the remnants of the follicle in the female and stimulates androgen synthe-

sis by the interstitial tissue of the testicle (Leydig cells) in the male.

The gonads contain enzymes which give them specificity in metabolizing adrenal steroid precursor pregnenolone to progesterone, estrogen, and testosterone. While the former two hormones predominate in the female and the latter in the male, both sexes produce some of each. In addition, the adrenal gland produces some androgen, in a pathway related to cortisol synthesis. The physiologic activity and clinical use of the gonadotropins, estrogens, and progestins are discussed in Chap. 46, "Women's Health Care."

Actions and Control of Androgens

Androgens produce dramatic growth in the skeletal and cardiac muscle, bone, kidney, and brain. Their presence at a critical time in fetal development causes male genital differentiation. At puberty androgens are responsible for growth and maturation of the genitalia. The skin on the body thickens, and greater pigmentation and oil production are seen; male hair patterns (chest, pubic, and beard hair growth, and recession of temporal hairline) develop.

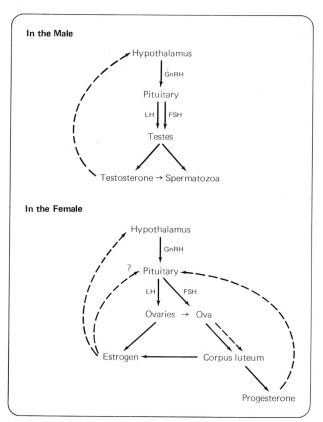

FIGURE 35-7

The Hypothalamic-Pituitary-Gonadal Axis in the Male and Female. Solid arrows indicate positive influence while broken arrows indicate negative influence or feedback inhibition.

Androgens promote growth of muscle and long bones. Continued production causes fusion of the epiphyses and halts growth. The size of the kidneys and cartilage formation are enhanced. Androgens have an erythropoietic effect to stimulate red blood cell formation. The brain is affected to allow tonic (noncyclical) male sexual drive. Androgens do promote spermatogenesis in low doses; however, large amounts may cause feedback inhibition of FSH and LH, interrupting sperm generation. The nonspecificity of feedback inhibition explains some of the difficulty in developing a male contraceptive; the same axis which maintains fertility (spermatogenesis) also controls virility (sexual drive and potency: see Fig. 35-7).

Androgenic Versus Anabolic Effects As shown in Table 35-22, the activities of the male sexual hormones may be divided into two types: *androgenic* (including male sexual characteristics or function) and *anabolic* (promoting growth of muscle, bone, or skin changes). Knowledge of the structural characteristics of the part of the hormone which provide receptor specificity for each of these actions has allowed the development of synthetic hormones which provide relatively specific therapy for particular indications and adverse effects: the *androgens* and the *anabolic steroids*.

ANDROGENS

Mechanism of Action

In the body, testosterone is converted to 5α-dehydrotestosterone (DHT), the most active form of the hormone, which combines with cytoplasmic receptors. The interaction of androgens with cytosolic receptors appears to affect the formation of messenger RNA, inducing protein synthesis and the generation of phospholipids.

Indications

Replacement therapy with androgens is used in hypogonadal states (cryptorchidism, bilateral torsion, orchitis, orchidectomy, GnRH deficiency, pituitary dysfunction, delayed puberty, male climacteric, oligospermia, impotence due to androgen deficiency, etc.) where androgens are not being synthesized or are present in inadequate amounts. Unfortunately, although the replacement hormones maintain many physiologic activities, the testicles may atrophy due to feedback inhibition of FSH and LH, preventing the stimulus to the maintenance of their interstitial tissue and impairing spermatogenesis. Androgens are used *pharmacologically* in females in metastatic breast cancer, postpartum breast engorgement, and endometriosis.

Pharmacokinetics

Testosterone is eliminated rapidly after oral administration by first pass metabolism, and so it is generally administered parenterally. Synthetic androgens (e.g., **fluoxymesterone**, **methyltestosterone**, and the anabolic steroids) are less avidly metabolized, have longer half-lives, and can be given orally. Aqueous suspensions of testosterone may be irritating and are variably absorbed after IM injection. Testosterone and esters of testosterone (**testosterone cypionate** and **testosterone enanthate**) in oil are effective if injected IM every two to four weeks. Testosterones are 98 percent bound to sex hormone–binding globulin in the plasma. They are eliminated primarily by conjugation in the liver. The elimination half-life of testosterone has variously been reported at between 10 and 100 min.

Adverse Effects

In the female the major adverse effect of androgens is masculinization (hirsutism, acne, clitoral enlargement, menstrual irregularity, deepening of voice). Oral dosage forms may cause gastrointestinal upset, while inflammation at the site of injection or implantation of the pellet occurs with parenteral forms. Retention of sodium and water, as well as hypercalcemia, can occur. Males may experience gynecomastia, excessive frequency and duration of penile erections, testicular atrophy, and, at high doses, oligospermia. Methyltestosterone has been associated with liver dysfunction.

Drug Interactions Androgens and anabolic steroids may potentiate the effects of oral anticoagulants and diabetes therapies. The use of **methandrostenolone** may increase the sensitivity to therapeutic and toxic effects of glucocorticoids. These agents may alter laboratory tests of thyroid function (decreased protein-bound iodine, thyroxine-binding capacity, uptake of radioactive iodine and resin triiodothyronine uptake; free thyroxine levels are unaffected), liver function

TABLE 35-22 Biological Actions of Androgens

ANDROGENIC ACTIVITY	ANABOLIC ACTIVITY
Differentiation of fetus to male	Stimulation of growth of muscle and long bone
Growth and maturation of the genitalia and secondary sexual characteristics: thickened, oily skin, recession of temporal hair, pubic and axillary hair patterns, development of beard, enhanced pigmentation, growth of the larynx; deepening of the voice	Induction of positive nitrogen, sodium, calcium, potassium, chloride, and sulfate balances.
	Increased size of kidneys
Maintenance of libido and aggressiveness	Increased red blood cell and hemoglobin levels
Spermatogenesis	
Inhibit release of pituitary gonadotropins	

(demonstration of liver toxicity of these agents), electrolytes (due to sodium and water retention and calcium and potassium loss), clotting times, serum cholesterol (elevated), and creatinine (increased).

Preparations and Dosage

Available androgen preparations and replacement dosages are listed in Table 35-23. Dosages in breast cancer are discussed in Chap. 37, while the dosages and androgen/estrogen combination products employed in endometriosis and postpartum breast engorgement are covered in Chap. 46.

ANABOLIC STEROIDS

These drugs are synthetic derivatives of testosterone, and so they have variable androgenic effects in addition to their anabolic effects. Anabolic steroids promote protein synthesis, positive nitrogen balance, erythropoiesis, and stimulate growth of muscle, kidney, and long bones.

Indications

Anabolic hormones have an erythropoeitic effect which is valuable in treating aplastic anemia, Fanconi's anemia, and anemia due to chronic renal failure. They have doubtful efficacy in postmenopausal osteoporosis (see Chap. 46). While anabolic hormones induce growth, development, and hypertrophy of skeletal muscle, muscle strength is not increased proportionally to muscle bulk. Therefore, their use by athletes for muscle-building is highly questionable. Malnourished and anorectic patients, who may benefit from the sense of well-being and enhanced appetite once the diet is corrected, are treated with anabolic steroids. These agents may hasten acquisition of normal height without disturbance of sexual maturation. This effect is useful in children who have growth retardation due to pituitary insufficiency. Because androgens hasten epiphyseal closure and limit ultimate height achieved, they are either employed for only short periods (6 weeks to 6 months at a time) or, preferably, not used until the therapy with growth hormone produces the desired height and until sexual development is accomplished.

TABLE 35–23 Androgen Preparations

GENERIC NAME	TRADE NAME(S)	DOSAGE FORM*	USUAL DOSAGE
Short-Acting Agents			
Testosterone	Testaqua, Histerone, others	Aqueous suspension	10–25 mg IM, 2 to 3 times weekly
Testosterone propionate	Testex	Injection in oil	10–25 mg IM, 2 to 3 times weekly
		Buccal tablet	5–50 mg held against buccal mucosa daily
Fluoxymesterone	Halotestin, Android-F, Ora-Testryl	Tablets	2–10 mg orally daily†
Methyltestosterone	Android, Virilon, Testred, others	Tablets, capsules	10–40 mg orally daily†
		Buccal tablets	5–20 mg held against buccal mucosa daily
Long-Acting Agents			
Testosterone cypionate (in oil)	Depo-Testosterone, Andro-Cyp, others	Repository injection	50–400 mg deep IM every 2–4 weeks
Testosterone enanthate (in oil)	Delatestryl, Android-T, others	Repository injection	50–400 mg deep IM every 2–4 weeks
Testosterone pellets	Oreton	Pellet	150–450 mg implanted subcutaneously every 3–6 months

*Testosterone is *never* given intravenously; should be injected intramuscularly.
†Divided dosage improves oral tolerance; q6h dosing is generally used.

Pharmacokinetics and Drug Interactions

The pharmacokinetics and drug interactions are comparable to those listed for the androgens (above). The half-life of these synthetic steroids exceeds that for **testosterone**, and they are bound to plasma proteins and primarily eliminated by hepatic conjugation.

Adverse Effects

The most serious adverse effect is hepatotoxicity which appears to be dose-related and occurs early in therapy. While the hepatic effects are usually reversible, continuation of therapy can result in hepatic necrosis, hepatic coma, and even death. Virilization is the most common adverse effect. In women this presents as menstrual abnormalities, hirsutism, hoarseness, and reversible clitoral enlargement. Prepubertal males may experience hirsutism, penile enlargement, skin pigmentation, and increased frequency of erection, while inhibition of testicular function (oligospermia, gynecomastia, testicular atrophy), chronic priapism, male pattern baldness, and impotence occur in the postpubertal male. Both sexes may notice acne and altered libido. As with androgens, fluid and sodium retention, edema, hypercalcemia, premature closure of the epiphyses in children, virilization of the fetus (if taken during pregnancy), and GI irritation may occur.

Preparations and Dosages

Table 35-24 lists the available preparations and usual dosages of the anabolic steroids.

NURSING PROCESS RELATED TO ANDROGENS AND ANABOLIC STEROIDS

The nursing process related to the physiologic and pharmacologic use of anabolic steroids is shown in Table 35-25.

Nursing process for specific uses such as osteoporosis (Chap. 46), breast engorgement (Chap. 46), cancer (Chap. 37), and endometriosis (Chap. 46) is covered in other parts of this text.

DISORDERS OF MALE REPRODUCTIVE REGULATION

Male Hypogonadism

Deficiency of the end product sexual hormones in the postpubertal male is called male hypogonadism. Symptoms of hypogonadism in the pubertal-aged male are seen as failure of sexual development: impaired growth of body hair, lack of genital maturation, and continued long-bone growth due to absence of epiphyseal closure. In the adult, symptoms include lack of sexual desire, frequent impotence, and infertility due to inadequate sperm production. There may also be reversal of the physical signs of male hormone activity: muscular atrophy, alteration of fat deposition and hair growth patterns, change in voice (higher pitch). Psychosocial changes may also occur, diminishing aggressive tendencies and promoting submissiveness.

Etiology and Clinical Findings

Primary hypogonadism is an inability of the end organ (testes) to produce hormone and reproductive cells in the presence of adequate amounts of stimulating hormones from the pituitary and hypothalamus. It is seen when the testicles have been removed (surgical castration for cancer management, accidents), fail to develop in utero (congenital anorchia), or degenerate in later life. Testicular function may be assessed by evaluating plasma testosterone levels, semen quality, and FSH plasma levels, which correlate inversely with spermatogenesis. If plasma testosterone levels are low, stimulation testing is performed by administering

TABLE 35-24 Anabolic Steroids

GENERIC NAME	TRADE NAME	DOSAGE FORMS	USUAL ADULT DOSAGE
Ethylestrenol	Maxibolin	Tablets, elixir	Up to 0.1 mg/kg/day
Oxandrolone	Anavar	Tablets	2.5–5 mg, 2 to 4 times daily for 2–4 weeks
Oxymetholone	Anadrol-50	Tablets	Osteoporosis: 5–30 mg daily (21-day maximum duration)
			Anemia: 1–5 mg/kg/day for 3–6 months
Stanozolol	Winstrol	Tablets	2 mg, 2 to 3 times daily
Nandrolone phenpropionate	Androlone, Durabolin	Injection	25–50 mg deep IM weekly
Nandrolone decanoate	Deca-Durabolin, others	Injection in oil	50–100 mg deep IM every 3–4 weeks
Methandriol	Anabol, others	Aqueous injection	10–40 mg deep IM daily
		Injection in oil	50–100 mg deep IM 1 to 2 times weekly

human chorionic gonadotropin (HCG; Glucor, Pregnyl, others; see Chap. 46) in doses of 2000 IU IM daily for four days. Plasma testosterone should rise to about 300 mg/dL 24 h after the last dose in normal prepubertal boys. Plasma LH concentration may also be determined following HCG stimulation.

Inadequate synthesis of testosterone and spermatozoa caused by insufficient stimulation of the testes by gonadotropins is called *hypogonadotropic hypogonadism*. This may occur after surgical hypophysectomy or with panhypopituitarism. If inadequate release of GnRH is responsible for the hypogonadal state, it is termed *hypothalamic hypogonadism*. In addition to inadequate stimulation by GnRH or gonadotropins, *secondary hypogonadism* may also occur from the administration of estrogens or androgens (which may be converted to estrogens), because their feedback effect inhibits gonadotropin release. By blocking dopamine receptors and increasing prolactin levels, phenothiazine tranquilizers such as **chlorpromazine** (Thorazine) and **thioridazine** (Mellaril) may block gonadotropin release. **Alcohol, marijuana**, and **heroin** may also decrease gonadotropin release. When alcoholic cirrhosis develops, portal shunting leads to an increased exposure of testosterone to the systemic circulation and increased conversion to estrogen. Thus, the action of synthesized testosterone is decreased and feedback inhibition of gonadotropins occurs due to the estrogen generation.

GnRH has been used investigationally to test the respon-

TABLE 35-25   Nursing Process Related to Androgens and Anabolic Steroids

ASSESSMENT	MANAGEMENT	EVALUATION
Observe for conditions which contraindicate or require cautious use of these agents: benign prostatic hypertrophy, breast cancer, diabetes, heart disease, concurrent anticoagulant use, history of myocardial infarction (hypercholesterolemic effects), hepatic dysfunction, pregnancy.	Take oral forms with food to decrease GI upset.	Periodic evaluation for jaundice and liver function test. Discontinue if signs of hepatotoxicity.
	Low salt diet may decrease fluid retention. If persistent, a diuretic order may be requested.	Observe for hypercalcemia (anorexia, nausea, abdominal pain, dry mouth, polyuria). Periodic serum calcium levels.
	Tell women to report virilization: hoarseness, voice change, change in menstruation, hirsutism. May improve with decreased dose, but does not always reverse even with discontinuation.	Monitor urine sugar and report abnormalities to physician.
Baseline body measurements in children (height, weight, sexual development).	Informed consent should include knowledge that ultimate height may be limited by use of these drugs in children (premature skeletal maturation).	Observe for virilization in women and prepubertal males.
		Periodic weights and check for edema.
If used for anemia, baseline hematocrit and hemoglobin levels. Other pharmacologic uses: record baseline status and target symptoms.	Males should discontinue drug if fertility desired, but antispermatogenic effects may be slow to reverse.	Check implants for sloughing, injection sites for irritation. Ask about GI upset with oral forms.
	Males should be instructed to report priapism, gynecomastia, testicular atrophy.	Replacement therapy: check effectiveness by evaluating development of secondary sex characteristics
	Both male and female patients should be told to report edema, acne, changed libido, GI distress, jaundice.	Pharmacologic therapy: Evaluate target symptoms.
	Exercise (active or passive) will increase anabolic effects.	
	Diet should have adequate calories to assure positive nitrogen balance. Sufficient quantities of iron and protein are important.	
	Note use of these agents on requests for thyroid function tests.	
	Consumer education: These drugs have not been proven to enhance athletic ability, but have significant adverse effects.	
	Concurrent use of furosemide (Lasix) or corticosteroids allow continued therapy if hypercalcemia is a risk.	

siveness of the pituitary, when the testicles are known to be responsive to adequate gonadotropin stimulation. A 1000-U bolus of GnRH should lead to a doubling to tripling of FSH and a four- to eightfold increase in LH by 45 min after injection. However, this test does not reliably differentiate hypothalamic from pituitary failure.

Clinical Pharmacology and Therapeutics

Hypogonadism is generally treated by replacement with a long-acting testosterone, an ester of testosterone, or an oral synthetic androgen (Table 35-7). Because testicular atrophy andd oligospermia can result from long-term androgen therapy, it is anticipated that in the future commercial availability of GnRH and pure forms of FSH and LH at a reasonable cost may provide a more physiologic replacement for patients with secondary hypogonadism.

Occasionally, inadequate GnRH stimulation of the pituitary and testes may occur due to disordered feedback stimulation by inadequate testosterone levels. This insensitivity of the hypothalamus may be corrected by the administration of **clomiphene citrate** (Clomid; see Chap. 46), restoring fertility and virility.

Male Hypergonadism

True hypergonadism is rarely diagnosed clinically. One condition which occurs in 70 percent of elderly men and may be caused by locally excessive testosterone metabolism, is benign prostatic hypertrophy (BPH). This overgrowth of the prostate gland impedes micturition, an effect which is magnified by the use of common drugs with anticholinergic effects (see Table 12-5). At present, surgical prostatectomy is the principal treatment of this condition, although estrogens (**stilbestrol**) and the investigational antiandrogenic agent **cyproterone acetate** have been employed.

Antiandrogenic therapy has also been used in the management of males with persistent severe deviations of sexual behavior (rape, sexual abuse of children, etc.), as a reversible "pharmacologic castration." **Cyproterone acetate, estrogens,** and the investigational phenothiazine-like drug **benperidol** have been used for this purpose. Cyproterone acetate has also been considered for treatment of precocious puberty.

Excessive androgen activity has been associated with severe cases of cystic acne. The administration of **corticosteroids** and **oral contraceptives** have been purported to ameliorate this condition, perhaps by feedback inhibition of androgen synthesis.

REFERENCES

Arcangelo, V.: "Simple Goiter," *Nursing 83,* **13**:47, 1983.

Bentley, P. J.: *Endocrine Pharmacology, Physiological Basis and Therapeutic Applications,* Cambridge: Cambridge University Press, 1980.

Blevins, D.: *The Diabetic and Nursing Care,* New York: McGraw-Hill, 1979.

Boyd, A.: "Diabetic Retinopathy," *Postgrad Med,* 73:279–291, 1983.

Burke, M. D.: "Adrenal Dysfunction: Test Strategies for Diagnosis," *Postgrad Med,* 69:155–170, 1981.

Cavalier, J.: "Crucial Decisions in Diabetic Emergencies," *RN,* 43:32–37, 1980.

Depew, C. C., and R. J. Auricchio: "Intensive Care Therapeutics," in B. S. Katcher, L. Y. Young, and M. A. Koda-Kimble (eds.), *Applied Therapeutics, The Clinical Use of Drugs,* San Francisco: Applied Therapeutics, 1983.

Dillon, R. S. (ed.): *Handbook of Endocrinology, Diagnosis and Management of Endocrine and Metabolic Disorders,* 2d ed., Philadelphia: Lea Febiger, 1980.

Elliot, G. T., and M. W. McKenzie: "Treatment of Hypercalcemia," *Drug Intell Clin Pharm,* 17:12–22, 1983.

Essig, M.: "Oral Antidiabetic Agents," *Nursing 83,* **13**:59–63, 1983.

Evangelisti, J., and C. Thorpe: "Thyroid Storm—A Nursing Crisis," *Heart Lung,* 12:184–194, 1983.

Friedman, A. L., and W. E. Segar: "Antidiuretic Hormone Excess," *J Pediatr,* 94:521–526, 1979.

Garofano, C.: "Helping Diabetics Live with Their Neuropathies," *Nursing 80,* **10**:43–44, 1980.

Guthrie, D., and R. Guthrie: *Nursing Management of Diabetes Mellitus,* 2d ed., St. Louis: Mosby, 1982.

Itami, R. M., M. E. Geffner, S. M. Kaplan, and B. M. Lippe: "The Levodopa-Propranolol Test for Growth Hormone Screening," *J Pediatr,* 100:838–839, 1982.

Joyce, M., C. Kuzick, and D. Murphy: "Those New Blood Glucose Tests," *RN,* 46:46–52, 1983.

Kastrup, E. K., J. R. Body, and B. R. Olin (eds.): "Hormones," in *Facts and Comparisons,* Philadelphia: Lippincott, 1984.

Kiser, D.: "The Somogyi Effect," *Am J Nurs,* 80:236–238, 1980.

Koda-Kimble, M. A., and M. D. Rotblatt: "Diabetes Mellitus," in B. S. Katcher, L. S. Y. Young, and M. A. Koda-Kimble (eds.), *Applied Therapeutics: The Clinical Use of Drugs,* 3d ed., San Francisco: Applied Therapeutics, 1983.

Lanes, R., and E. Hurtado: "Oral Clonidine, An Effective Growth Hormone Releasing Agent in Prepubertal Subjects," *J Pediatr,* 100:710–714, 1982.

Lewis, M. J., G. V. Groom, R. Barber, and A. H. Henderson: "The Effects of Propranolol and Acebutolol on Overnight Plasma Levels of Anterior Pituitary and Related Hormones," *Bri J Clin Pharmacol,* **13**:737–742, 1981.

Lewis, S., and I. Collier: *Medical-Surgical Nursing,* New York: McGraw-Hill, 1983.

Lundin, D.: "Reporting Urine Test Results: Switch from + to %," *Am J Nurs,* **78:**878–879, 1978.

McConnell, E.: "Diabetes and Surgery," *Nursing 81,* **11:**118–123, 1981.

Malseed, R.: *Pharmacology: Drug Therapy and Nursing Considerations,* Philadelphia: Lippincott, 1982.

Murray, P.: "When Hyperglycemia Goes Critical," *RN,* **46:**55–60, 1983.

Muthe, N.: *Endocrinology: A Nursing Approach,* Boston: Little, Brown, 1981.

Nemchik, R.: "The News About Insulin," *RN,* **45:**49–54, 1982.

Nyberry, K.: "When Diabetes Complicates Your Pre- and Post-op Care," *RN,* **46:**42–47, 1983.

Ohlsen, P.: "Discrepancies between Glycosuria and Home Estimate of Blood Glucose in Insulin-Treated Diabetes Mellitus," *Diabetes Care,* **3:**178, 1980.

Rodman, J.: "Switch to Human Insulin Will Be Slow," *RN,* **46:**139, 1983.

Slater, N.: "Insulin Reaction vs. Ketoacidosis: Guidelines for Diagnosis and Intervention," *Am J Nurs,* **78:**875–877, 1978.

Surr, C.: "New Blood-Glucose Monitoring Products," *Nurs 83,* **13:**42–45, 1983.

White, J., E. Martin, and C. Fetner: "Treatment of the Syndrome of Inappropriate Secretion of Antidiuretic Hormone with Lithium Carbonate," *N Engl J Med,* **292:**390–392, 1975.

White, N., and B. Miller: "Glycohemoglobin," *Nursing 83,* **13:**55–57, 1983. op. no. 99

36

HEMATOLOGIC DISORDERS

CARY E. JOHNSON
MARY J. WASKERWITZ

This chapter deals with the hematologic system which consists of many individual components, including bone marrow, liver, spleen, lymph nodes, and blood and can be divided into three functionally specialized systems: the erythropoietic, the leukopoietic, and the hemostatic.

The erythropoietic system is concerned with the production and function of erythrocytes, or red blood cells (RBC). The major site for erythrocyte production is the bone marrow of the long bones, ribs, vertebrae, and skull. The leukopoietic system is specifically involved with the production of leukocytes (white blood cells), whose function involves the body's immune system. The hemostatic system is responsible for coagulation; the major components of this system are the circulating blood platelets and the coagulation factors in the plasma. The functions and abnormalities of the immune system and the coagulation system are presented in more detail in Chaps. 26 and 42.

ANEMIAS

LEARNING OBJECTIVES

Upon mastery of the contents of this section, the reader will be able to:
1. Describe the general symptoms of anemia.
2. State five important parameters of nursing assessment in anemia.

Anemia is a condition in which the number of red blood cells per cubic milliliter, the quantity of hemoglobin, and the volume of packed red cells per 100 mL of blood are below normal, lowering the oxygen-carrying capacity of the blood. Anemia is not a primary disease but rather a symptom complex.

Classification

Anemias can be classified in several ways, one of which is by cause, or etiology. Three major causes of anemia are blood loss, decreased red blood cell production, and increased red blood cell destruction. A second method of classifying anemia is by the form and structure of the red blood cell, or morphology. The various types of anemia cause characteristic changes in the size and hemoglobin content of the red blood cell. These morphologic changes can be useful in differentiating the anemias and in monitoring therapy, as the red blood cells should return to normal if the treatment has been successful.

Clinical Findings

The general symptoms of anemia depend mainly on the rate and amount of change in the total blood volume and the reduction in the oxygen-carrying capacity of the blood. If the anemia becomes severe and compensatory systems fail, certain characteristic signs and symptoms will develop, including increased pulse and respiratory rate, shortness of breath, and chronic fatigue. The anemic patient may appear pale, with a loss of the normal pinkish color of the skin, mucous membranes, and nail beds. Further symptoms of anemia result from decreased oxygen supply to the neuromuscular system and include faintness, headache, drowsiness, and muscular weakness.

IRON-DEFICIENCY ANEMIA

LEARNING OBJECTIVES

Upon mastery of the contents of this section, the reader will be able to:
1. Explain the mechanisms involved in each of the following aspects of iron metabolism: (1) absorption, (2) transport, (3) storage, and (4) excretion.
2. State the normal daily iron requirements for the adult male and female.
3. List three causes of iron-deficiency anemia.
4. Explain the therapeutic goals for the patient with iron-deficiency anemia.
5. Describe the major side effects of oral iron ther-

703

apy and discuss ways to lessen or avoid these problems through patient education.

6. Explain the methods used to monitor patient response to iron therapy.

7. Differentiate between the elemental iron content of 300 mg of each: ferrous sulfate and ferrous gluconate.

8. Discuss the length of therapy required with oral preparations used in the treatment of iron-deficiency anemia.

9. List and discuss each step in the education of the patient to receive long-term therapy for iron-deficiency anemia with an oral preparation.

10. List four indications for parenteral iron therapy.

11. Describe the side effects and precautions for intramuscular and intravenous iron injections.

12. Describe the symptoms and treatment of iron poisoning.

Pathogenesis

Iron-deficiency anemia is the most common disorder of the erythropoietic system. A review of the features of normal iron metabolism (see Fig. 36-1) is helpful in understanding the various aspects of this anemia. The total body content of iron in an average adult male is approximately 4 g. The greater part of this, about 70 percent, is in the form of hemoglobin; about 25 percent is in the form of storage and transport iron. The remaining iron is intracellular, in the form of myoglobin and enzyme iron.

Iron absorption is variable and seems to be influenced by many factors involving the degree of erythropoietic activity, the status of the body iron stores, and the intake of food sources of iron. Absorption is increased when iron stores are depleted or when red blood cell production is active. The average diet of an adult in the United States contains about 10 to 20 mg of elemental iron in the form of various salts and complexes in food sources. About 5 to 10 percent of the iron in this form is absorbed by healthy persons, with an increase to 20 to 40 percent absorption in the presence of iron deficiency.

The actual process of iron absorption is complex and involves several steps. Food sources of iron are digested to release the available inorganic iron, which is primarily absorbed in the small intestine. Depending upon need, iron can be absorbed from the gastrointestinal tract into the intestinal mucosal cells and stored as *ferritin,* an iron storage complex, or be delivered to the plasma. Iron entering the plasma is bound to a protein molecule, called *transferrin,* which transports the iron to the erythrocyte precursors in the bone marrow for hemoglobin synthesis. Transferrin is also involved in transporting iron to and from iron storage sites in the liver, spleen, bone marrow, and other tissues. In addition to ferritin, iron may also be stored in the form of *hemosiderin.*

Iron is carefully conserved, especially from red cells which have been broken down at the end of their life cycles,

and is reutilized or stored. Normal daily iron losses in the adult male are estimated to be 0.5 to 1.0 mg. Most iron is lost in sweat and in feces. Normal menstruation increases the average daily losses of iron in women by 0.5 to 1.0 mg, representing a monthly blood loss of 30 to 60 mL. The average dietary intake of iron is, therefore, sufficient to maintain iron homeostasis only in males and nonmenstruating females. Increased iron demands during pregnancy and lactation, and in rapidly growing newborns and adolescents can result in iron deficiency if iron supplements are not added to the diet. After the age of 60, the iron requirement for both sexes becomes nearly equal (see Table 25-2).

Etiology

The causes of iron deficiency may be grouped into several categories, including those associated with insufficient dietary intake, those associated with abnormal blood losses, and those associated with an increased physiologic need for iron.

Achlorhydria, lack of gastric acid, can reduce iron absorption. Gastric acid has a major effect in facilitating the absorption of food sources of iron as well as in converting ferric iron to ferrous iron, a more absorbable form of iron. Decreased iron absorption is associated with gastric surgery involving total or partial removal of the stomach, resulting in the loss of essential gastric acid and other secretions and decreased intestinal transit time.

Blood loss is the most common cause of iron-deficiency anemia in adults. Hemoglobin contains 3.4 mg iron/g, and so a person with a normal hemoglobin concentration of 15 g/dL will have 0.5 mg iron in each milliliter of whole blood. A chronic daily blood loss of as little as 3 to 4 mL may result in iron deficiency. One of the major sites for chronic, and sometimes asymptomatic, blood loss is the gastrointestinal tract. Chronic aspirin and corticosteroid therapy may significantly increase gastrointestinal blood loss. Excessive menstrual blood loss may also lead to iron deficiency.

The rapid growth of infants causes a high demand for iron. The general diet of the infant is iron-poor and should be supplemented to prevent deficiency. Pregnancy also results in a major drain on body iron stores, the greatest iron requirement occurring during the third trimester.

Clinical Findings

Most patients are asymptomatic and laboratory tests are normal until the iron stores have been depleted, making early diagnosis difficult. An examination of a peripheral blood smear shows characteristic pale (hypochromic) small (microcytic) erythrocytes varying widely in size and shape. The hemoglobin is generally less than 8 g/dL and the hematocrit reading is less than 25 percent. The *serum iron* concentration is decreased, the *total iron-binding capacity* (TIBC), which measures the amount of transferrin in the plasma, is increased, and the serum ferritin concentration is decreased.

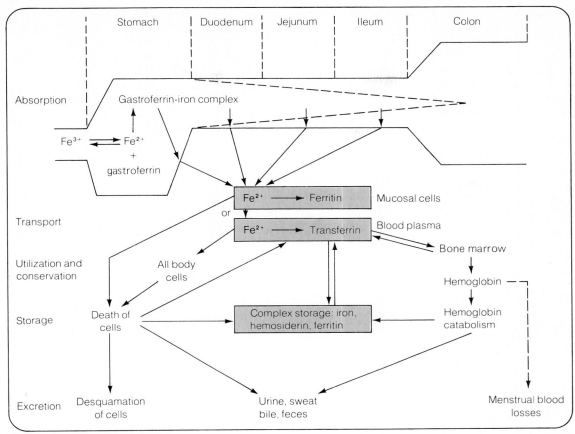

FIGURE 36-1

Schematic Outline of Iron Metabolism.

Clinical Pharmacology and Therapeutics

Therapeutic Goals

The goals of therapy for iron-deficiency anemia are to identify and correct the cause of the anemia and to restore the total body iron content to normal and return hemoglobin synthesis to normal. If the cause of the iron deficiency remains unidentifiable or uncorrectable, as in malabsorption or certain carcinomas, the patient must receive continuing iron replacement.

Iron can be administered orally, intramuscularly, or intravenously, but the oral route is preferred, as it is less expensive, produces fewer adverse reactions, and is generally most acceptable to the patient. An agent that tends to stimulate blood cell formation or to increase hemoglobin in the blood is said to be a *hematinic*.

Oral Iron Therapy

Preparations and Dosage Forms

Ideally, an iron preparation should be well tolerated, inexpensive, safe, effective, and readily absorbable. Dosage is determined by the elemental iron content of the preparation (Table 36-1). Many products differ only in the type of iron salt that is used, and so it is important to recognize that 325 mg of **ferrous gluconate**, containing 37 mg of elemental iron, and 325 mg of **ferrous sulfate**, containing 65 mg of elemental iron, are not equivalent. These two forms of iron are equal in the amount of iron salt present but different in the amount of elemental iron that each provides.

The standard preparation used in the oral management of iron-deficiency anemia is **ferrous sulfate**. Other salts, such as **ferrous gluconate** and **ferrous fumarate**, are as effective as ferrous sulfate when administered in equivalent amounts but offer no therapeutic advantage and may be more costly.

In an attempt to decrease the gastrointestinal irritation often associated with iron administration, and to improve compliance, various sustained-release dosage forms have been designed. These preparations release the iron slowly as they pass through the gastrointestinal tract. However, maximal iron absorption occurs in the duodenum and proximal small bowel, and iron salts released distal to these areas are only minimally absorbed. Consequently, sustained-release preparations are generally about one-fourth to one-sixth as effective as ferrous sulfate solutions in providing absorbable iron and also are much more costly.

Chemical agents such as ascorbic acid and polysorbate have been added to ferrous sulfate preparations to enhance iron absorption. However, in order for absorption to be increased significantly, a large amount of ascorbic acid must be used, and the increased cost to the patient is not warranted. Other combination products which contain multivitamins and minerals in addition to the iron contribute nothing but cost to the treatment of iron-deficiency anemia.

Oral Dosages

The dosage of oral iron preparations is based on the need to provide the body with sufficient elemental iron to sustain maximal hemoglobin regeneration. Hemoglobin contains an iron concentration of 0.34 percent and is synthesized at a maximal rate of 0.3 g/100 mL of blood/day. One can calculate that an adult with a 5000-mL blood volume has a maximal daily hemoglobin regeneration of 15 g and would

require 50 mg of elemental iron. The absorption of iron salts in iron deficiency is increased and generally exceeds 20 percent of the oral intake. Therefore, to provide 50 mg of iron for maximal hemoglobin regeneration, approximately 250 mg of elemental iron would have to be administered daily. Considering the variations in blood volume, hemoglobin synthesis, and iron absorption from patient to patient, 195 to 260 mg of elemental iron is usually sufficient to meet the maximal requirements. Because a 325-mg **ferrous sulfate** tablet contains 65 mg of elemental iron, a dosage regimen of one tablet three or four times daily will supply an adequate amount of iron.

Adverse Effects

The major patient complaints associated with oral iron therapy are a result of the irritating effects of iron salts on the gastric and intestinal mucosa. Abdominal cramps, nausea, vomiting, diarrhea, or constipation can occur. A gradual increase in the daily dosage of the iron preparation over a 3- to 4-day period may prevent many of these unpleasant side effects. Patients receiving oral iron treatment should be advised that iron preparations may cause the stool to become black in color and that this color change is normal. Although iron absorption is increased when the stomach is empty, gastric irritation is also increased. This problem can be lessened if iron medications are taken with meals, and the increased patient compliance is more important than a slight reduction in iron absorption. If the patient cannot tolerate the prescribed amount of iron each day, the dosage can be decreased to an amount that will cause fewer problems.

About 1 percent of patients treated with oral iron medications develop side effects severe enough to warrant the discontinuation of treatment. These patients, as well as those who refuse oral iron therapy, require treatment with parenteral iron preparations.

Liquid preparations are available for use in pediatric therapy. The liquid preparations may cause teeth staining, which can be avoided by giving the preparation through a straw, or placing the drops on the back of the tongue, and brushing the teeth after administration. If taste is a problem, the liquid iron preparations can be mixed with milk or fruit juices to increase palatability. Concomitant therapy with antacids or tetracycline should be avoided to prevent binding and decreased iron absorption.

Iron Toxicity

Oral iron preparations are a serious cause of poisoning in children. As little as 10 tablets (3 g) ingested at one time can be lethal.

Symptoms The symptoms of acute iron intoxication proceed in stages, beginning 30 to 60 min following ingestion. Initial symptoms include vomiting, diarrhea, and dark black stools (melena). These symptoms may be followed in 12 to 24 h by shock, coma, and metabolic acidosis. Death may

TABLE 36-1 Iron Content of Commonly Used Iron Medications

PRODUCT	IRON SALT AND ADDITIVES	ELEMENTAL IRON PER TABLET (mg)
Ferrous sulfate (generic)	Ferrous sulfate	65
Feosol	Ferrous sulfate	65
Ferrous gluconate (generic)	Ferrous gluconate	37
Fergon	Ferrous gluconate	37
Ferrous fumarate (generic)	Ferrous fumarate	107
Ircon	Ferrous fumarate	66
Feosol spansule (sustained release)	Ferrous sulfate	50
Simron	Ferrous gluconate and polysorbate 20	10
Theragran Hematinic	Ferrous fumarate and multivitamins	67
Fero-Grad 500 (sustained release)	Ferrous sulfate and sodium ascorbate	105
Ferro Sequels (sustained release)	Ferrous fumarate and docusate sodium	50
Imferon, parenteral	Iron dextran	50 mg/mL

occur 12 to 48 h after ingestion. These toxic effects are a result of hemorrhage from the ulcerogenic action of iron on the mucosa of the gastrointestinal tract. High concentrations of unbound ionic iron in the plasma cause metabolic disturbances, shock, and liver damage.

Treatment The two major goals in the management of acute iron poisoning are to remove the ingested iron and to combat shock. In order to remove iron tablets and any unabsorbed iron, the stomach is aspirated and lavaged with a 1% **sodium bicarbonate** solution. **Deferoxamine**, an antidote which complexes iron, is administered orally by nasogastric tube, and intravenously. In order to avoid hypotension, an adverse effect of intravenous deferoxamine, the infusion rate should not exceed 15 mg/kg body weight/h. In addition, general supportive measures for shock and acidosis should be maintained.

Patient education in the prevention of iron poisoning is essential for all patients receiving oral iron medications. They must be cautioned about the importance of protecting small children from discovering and ingesting the candylike iron tablets.

Parenteral Iron Therapy

The major indications for the use of parenteral iron products are (1) a noncompliant patient; (2) a patient unable to absorb iron from the gastrointestinal tract; (3) a patient having iron losses that are too great to be replaced by oral therapy; (4) a patient with a gastrointestinal disorder, such as inflammatory bowel disease, in which symptoms may be aggravated by iron preparations; (5) a patient who cannot tolerate oral iron preparations. Parenterally administered iron does not give a faster response than that obtained from oral iron; therefore, the rate of recovery from anemia should be the same. Because ferrous irons are toxic in their free forms, parenteral iron products must contain iron which is bound or complexed with another substance, such as dextran (see Table 36-1).

Parenteral Dosage and Administration

The exact calculation of the dosage of parenteral iron needed for replacement is important because of the limited ability of the body to excrete iron. If excess iron is administered, it is retained and deposited in certain tissues, causing the complications of iron overload known as *hemochromatosis*. The following equation is used for an adult to calculate the approximate total amount of elemental iron required to restore an initially low hemoglobin value to the average normal value of 14.8 g/100 mL and to replenish iron stores:

$$\text{Total iron (mg)} = 0.3 \times \text{weight (lb)} \times \left(100 - \frac{100 \text{Hgb}}{14.8}\right)$$

The patient's hemoglobin value in g/dL is substituted into the equation for Hgb. This yields the required dose of parenteral iron in milligrams of elemental iron.

Since iron dextran complex will be used as the replacement form of iron, the volume to be injected, in milliliters, can be calculated by dividing the total milligrams of iron derived from the formula by 50, as the preparation has a concentration of 50 mg elemental iron/mL.

Z-Track Intramuscular Because parenteral iron solutions may stain the skin, separate needles should be used for withdrawing the solution from the vial or ampul and for injecting it intramuscularly deep into the buttock. To prevent leakage of the solution from the intramuscular injection site, which could stain the subcutaneous tissue, the Z-track intramuscular method should be used for injection. The Z-track method involves displacing the tissues laterally prior to insertion of the needle. Because superficial tissue layers are more elastic and are less anchored than deeper tissues, they will displace further than the deeper layers. Hence, there will be no contiguous track through which the iron can backtrack to the subcutaneous layers once the needle is removed and the tissues are released to return to their normal positions. Because the iron must be deposited *deep* within the muscle, a 2½- to 4-in needle will be required. Generally, no more than 2 mL (100 mg) is given in a single injection.

Intravenous Methods Iron dextran can also be given intravenously, and this route of administration has several advantages over intramuscular injections. Because larger doses of iron may be given in a single injection via the intravenous route, the discomfort and inconvenience of multiple intramuscular injections can be avoided. This method should only be used when specifically indicated. At present, one technique for the intravenous administration of iron has been approved by the U.S. Food and Drug Administration. If no adverse reaction occurs within 30 to 60 min following a 0.5-mL (25-mg) IM or IV test dose, a 2-mL (10-mg) intravenous dose may be administered daily until the total calculated amount of iron has been given.

Another technique is the *total dose infusion method*. In this procedure, the total calculated dose of iron dextran is diluted in a ratio of 250 mg iron dextran to 100 mL normal saline solution and infused initially at a rate to deliver a test dose of 25 mg over 5 min. If no adverse reaction occurs, the infusion rate can be increased to 10 to 15 mg/min. It is most important that the iron dextran used for intravenous administration be obtained from *single-dose ampuls* rather than multidose vials, as the vials contain 0.5 phenol as a preservative substance, which should not be injected intravenously because of the high incidence of adverse reactions. Due to a high incidence of adverse reactions associated with the total dose infusion method, the manufacturer of iron dextran recommends that this method of administration be avoided.

Adverse Effects

Adverse reactions to parenterally administered iron may be immediate or delayed in onset and include flushing, joint pain, nausea, fever, bronchoconstriction, headache, and urticaria. Anaphylactoid reactions have also occurred and may be fatal. For this reason, epinephrine should be immediately available when iron is being administered parenterally. Intramuscular iron preparations may stain the skin if not injected properly, and intravenous iron administration may cause phlebitis at the infusion site. The overall incidence of adverse reactions to either intravenous or intramuscular iron dextran is about 1 to 2 percent.

Monitoring Therapy

Uncomplicated iron-deficiency anemia in which the cause has been identified and corrected has an excellent prognosis with adequate iron replacement. Certain laboratory parameters can be used to monitor the response to iron therapy. One of the first changes is an increase in the percentage of immature red blood cells (reticulocytes), beginning in 4 to 6 days and reaching a maximum value of 4 to 6 percent in 9 to 12 days after the initiation of iron therapy. The hemoglobin value may also be monitored and should increase in concentration by 2 g/100 mL at the end of 3 weeks. Both the reticulocyte response and the rate of hemoglobin increase are proportional to the severity of anemia: the patient with a mild anemia may have little or no reticulocyte response and will have a slow increase in hemoglobin concentration while the patient with severe anemia will have a rapid response to iron therapy. The serum iron will gradually rise, and the initially elevated iron-binding capacity will return to normal in about a month. Iron therapy should be continued until all blood values have returned to normal and iron stores have been replenished, often requiring a treatment period of 4 to 6 months. Recurrence of anemia is common with shorter treatment programs that do not allow sufficient time for the replacement of iron stores. If the underlying cause of anemia is not found or is uncorrectable, the therapy will be only minimally successful and continuing therapy may be required.

VITAMIN B_{12}-DEFICIENCY ANEMIA

LEARNING OBJECTIVES

Upon mastery of the contents of this section, the reader will be able to:

1. List three causes of vitamin B_{12}-deficiency anemia.
2. Define pernicious anemia as it relates to vitamin B_{12} deficiency.
3. Explain the therapeutic goals for the patient with vitamin B_{12}-deficiency anemia.
4. Describe the side effects and precautions for the parenteral administration of vitamin B_{12}.
5. List the indications for oral vitamin B_{12} therapy.
6. Explain the methods used to monitor patient response to vitamin B_{12} therapy.
7. Explain the importance of patient education for the patient requiring lifelong vitamin B_{12} replacement therapy.

Vitamin B_{12} deficiency is a clinical condition in which the total body supply of vitamin B_{12} has been exhausted or is inadequate to maintain the necessary bodily functions. Erythropoiesis is greatly affected, and a megaloblastic (large cell) anemia will develop in the absence of this essential vitamin. The most common cause of vitamin B_{12} deficiency is impaired absorption due to a lack of gastric intrinsic factor, a condition known as *pernicious anemia.*

Pathogenesis

Vitamin B_{12} is generally absent in plants but is found in most foods of animal origin, such as eggs, meat, fish, milk, and cheese. The recommended daily adult intake of vitamin B_{12} is approximately 2 to 3 μg. This amount is present in most diets containing animal products and will maintain normal red blood cell production and body stores of the vitamin.

If a deficiency of vitamin B_{12} occurs, normal deoxyribonucleic acid (DNA) synthesis cannot proceed. Red blood cell production in the bone marrow is affected, resulting in the formation of abnormally large erythrocytes known as *macrocytes.* Vitamin B_{12} is also an essential factor in nerve cell myelin synthesis, and an uncorrected deficiency can result in irreversible neurologic damage.

The absorption of vitamin B_{12} is dependent on the gastric secretion of *intrinsic factor,* which is a complex glycoprotein produced by the parietal cells of the stomach. Intrinsic factor binds with vitamin B_{12} to form a complex of which approximately 70 percent is absorbed by special receptors on the brush border of mucosal cells in the ileum. This process requires a pH greater than 5.7 and the presence of calcium ions. Only 2 percent of uncomplexed vitamin B_{12} is absorbed, and this quantity is not sufficient to maintain body stores in the absence of intrinsic factor. The absorbed vitamin B_{12} is bound in the plasma to transcobalamin, a carrier protein which transports the vitamin to the tissues for use or storage.

Etiology

The three major causes of vitamin B_{12} deficiency are dietary deficiency, small-bowel malabsorption, and lack of gastric intrinsic factor. A dietary deficiency of vitamin B_{12} is rare in the United States, as the many food sources of this vitamin are common in the diet; only strict vegetarians who avoid meat and all animal products are likely to develop a dietary deficiency.

Clinical Findings

Examination of a peripheral blood smear will show the characteristic macrocytic erythrocytes and hypersegmented granulocytes associated with a megaloblastic anemia. If the symptoms of anemia are present, the hemoglobin concentration is usually less than 8 g/100 mL. The anemia is classified as macrocytic and normochromic and must be differentiated from folate deficiency, which causes the same morphologic changes in the red blood cells. This differentiation can be accomplished by measuring the serum concentration of vitamin B_{12} and folate. The serum vitamin B_{12} level is usually less than 100 pg/mL in the deficiency state, in comparison with a normal level in the range of 200 to 900 pg/mL. The serum folate concentration is normal.

Schilling Urinary Excretion Test   In order to differentiate small-bowel malabsorption of vitamin B_{12} from pernicious anemia due to a lack of intrinsic factor, the *Schilling urinary excretion test* is useful. In this test the patient is first given an intramuscular "flushing dose" of 1000 μg of vitamin B_{12}. About 2 h later, an 0.5-μg oral dose of radiocobalt-labeled vitamin B_{12} is administered to the patient, and the urine is then collected for 24 h. The initial intramuscular dose of vitamin B_{12} will prevent normal retention of the labeled vitamin, and therefore the greater part of labeled vitamin B_{12} absorbed will be excreted in the urine. If the patient has normal vitamin B_{12} absorption, approximately 10 to 35 percent of the labeled oral dose will be excreted in the urine. If less than 5 percent is excreted in the urine, malabsorption must be considered. The test is then repeated, but the patient is given intrinsic factor with the labeled oral dose of vitamin B_{12}. If the urinary recovery of the labeled vitamin B_{12} is increased to the normal range, a diagnosis of pernicious anemia is made.

Clinical Pharmacology and Therapeutics

Therapeutic Goals

The therapeutic goals in the treatment of vitamin B_{12}–deficiency anemia include correcting, if possible, the underlying cause of the anemia, returning the hematologic status to normal, and replacing the body stores of the vitamin. Bacterial overgrowth associated with blind-loop syndrome should be corrected surgically or with appropriate antibiotics. Strict vegetarians can be educated as to the dietary cause of their anemia, but generally they do not change their eating habits and must receive a supplement of oral vitamin B_{12}. Persons with uncorrectable malabsorption syndromes or pernicious anemia require lifelong parenteral therapy with vitamin B_{12}.

Cyanocobalamin (Vitamin B₁₂)

Parenteral Therapy   Two forms of vitamin B_{12} available for therapeutic use are *cyanocobalamin* and *hydroxocobalamin*. Hydroxocobalamin produces higher blood levels of longer duration, as it is retained in the body more efficiently than cyanocobalamin. Both these preparations only rarely cause allergic reactions. A depot, long-acting preparation of cyano-cobalamin in a sesame oil–aluminum monostearate gel is available but offers no advantages over hydroxocobalamin.

Dosage recommendations for the treatment of vitamin B_{12} deficiency vary slightly. Initially, 100 μg of cyanocobalamin is given intramuscularly daily for 6 or 7 days. After initial therapy, intramuscular injections of 100 μg of cyanocobalamin should be continued three times a week until the hematologic status of the patient has returned completely to normal. This process generally takes 2 months and requires a total dose of approximately 2000 μg of cyanocobalamin. It is important to use a frequent, intermittent dosage schedule, as the body retains only a portion of an injected dose, that amount being inversely related to the size of the dose. For example, 95 percent of a 100-μg dose is retained in 48 h but only 15 percent of a 1000-μg dose, so large doses of cyanocobalamin are wasted. The cyanocobalamin maintenance program consists of a 100-μg intramuscular injection on a once-a-month schedule for life. Hydroxocobalamin may be given in a dose of 1000 μg intramuscularly q2–4 months, because of the better retention of this form of vitamin B_{12}. Patients with vitamin B_{12}–deficiency anemia must be evaluated at least every 4 months to be sure that remission is being maintained.

Oral Therapy   Oral therapy is generally not satisfactory for the treatment of pernicious anemia, since only 1 to 2 percent of the orally administered dose is absorbed in the absence of intrinsic factor. In certain circumstances, however, oral therapy may be warranted, as in patients who refuse parenteral therapy, in patients with underlying bleeding disorders in whom repeated intramuscular injections would be hazardous, or in patients who have had a hypersensitivity reaction to a parenteral form of vitamin B_{12}. Oral therapy can also be used as a dietary supplement for the strict vegetarian. Because the absorption of oral vitamin B_{12} in pernicious anemia is low, large doses, in the range of 500 to 1000 μg/day, are needed. Several oral products are available which contain porcine (pig) intrinsic factor in addition to vitamin B_{12}. Absorption will be adequate for a short time, but because the intrinsic factor is from an animal source, antibodies will develop and the patient will become refractory to treatment and will relapse. Parenteral therapy will then be required.

Monitoring Therapy

With adequate therapy, symptomatic improvement may be observed within several days. The reticulocyte response, the most useful parameter to monitor the hematologic response of the patient, should rise significantly within 2 to 3 days. The hemoglobin and the hematocrit values usually return to normal after 6 to 8 weeks of therapy.

Untreated vitamin B_{12} deficiency is fatal because of the progressive degeneration of the central nervous system. With treatment, neurologic symptoms of short duration are reversible. However, if such symptoms have been present for more than 6 months, some residual dysfunction must be expected. To avoid the expense of multiple return visits to the physician for vitamin B_{12} injections, a family member can be trained to give the patient intramuscular injections. However, the importance of routine follow-up examinations must be stressed to ensure that the anemia is being controlled and that other complications are not developing.

FOLIC ACID DEFICIENCY ANEMIA

LEARNING OBJECTIVES

Upon mastery of this section, the reader will be able to:

1. Explain the metabolic function of folic acid in normal cell growth and division.

2. List three causes of folate-deficiency anemia.

3. List two types of drugs which may lead to folic acid deficiency.

4. Explain the use of laboratory tests to distinguish folate-deficiency anemia and vitamin B_{12}–deficiency anemia.

5. Explain the therapeutic goals for the patient with folate-deficiency anemia.

6. Explain the danger of folic acid therapy in a patient with vitamin B_{12}–deficiency anemia.

Folic acid deficiency is second only to iron deficiency in incidence and importance and causes a megaloblastic anemia which is indistinguishable from the anemia of vitamin B_{12} deficiency. *Folic acid* is a specific synthetic chemical compound, pteroylglutamic acid, whereas the term *folate* is used for naturally occurring compounds from dietary sources with similar nutritional activity.

Pathogenesis

Unlike vitamin B_{12}, folates are produced by plants and are found in high concentration in green leafy vegetables, yeast, and liver. Folate is heat-labile and water-soluble, and so the method of cooking foods greatly affects the dietary content of folate. Boiling green vegetables in large amounts of water can remove most of the folate not destroyed by heat, and the loss is even greater if the water is discarded.

The recommended daily folate intake for normal adults is 200 μg. Folate requirements are doubled to 400 μg/day during pregnancy, and clinical deficiency can develop in women receiving an inadequate diet without supplementation. The active growth of infants and young children also increases the need for folate to an amount four to ten times greater than the adult requirement on a microgram per kilogram (μg/kg) basis.

Folates found in food products are converted to an absorbable form by enzymes in the small intestine and approximately 80 percent of the dietary intake is absorbed. The total body content of folate is estimated to be 5 to 10 mg, with the largest quantity being stored in the liver. This amount is sufficient to maintain normal metabolic functions for only 2 to 4 months, if a decrease in intake or absorption should occur.

Absorbed folate is converted to tetrahydrofolate, which is the active form found in coenzymes. The conversion process is a two-part reduction reaction that requires the enzyme *dihydrofolate reductase*. The coenzymes of tetrahydrofolate are involved in purine and pyrimidine synthesis, necessary for DNA production and amino acid interconversions. With failure to produce adequate DNA, erythropoiesis is affected, and the red blood cells become macrocytic; granulocytes (white blood cells) are also affected and become hypersegmented. These changes are characteristic of megaloblastic anemia and are similar to the changes induced by vitamin B_{12} deficiency.

Etiology

The disorders which can cause folate deficiency include dietary deficiency, increased requirements, malabsorption, and inhibition of folate metabolism. Nutritional folate deficiency can be a problem, as body stores are sufficient to last for only a few months. The major causes for dietary deficiency of folate are diets lacking in fresh green vegetables or generally poor diets associated with chronic illness, alcoholism, or food faddism. Cooking methods can also greatly reduce the dietary intake of folate.

Increased requirements of folate occur during pregnancy because of the rapid growth of the fetus, with the sharpest drop in the serum folate level occurring in the third trimester. Lactation also increases the folate requirement, and the milk of folate-deficient women, being low in folate, may cause a deficiency to develop in breast-fed infants. The incidence of folate deficiency in pregnancy is second only to that of iron deficiency, so prophylaxis with iron and folate supplements is an important part of a prenatal care program. Active growth during infancy and childhood increases the need for folate, although dietary intake is generally sufficient.

Inflammatory bowel disease affecting the major absorptive sites of folate in the small intestine or surgical removal of these absorptive areas can lead to malabsorption of folate. Anticonvulsants such as **phenytoin** or **phenobarbital**, and the **oral contraceptives**, can increase the daily requirements for dietary folate.

Inhibition of folate metabolism by folate analogs or other inhibitors can also cause the megaloblastic anemia of folate deficiency. Drugs such as **methotrexate** competitively inhibit dihydrofolate reductase and prevent dietary folate from being converted to its active form. **Triamterene** and **trimethoprim** may also cause a folate deficiency by the same mechanism but are much less potent antagonists than **methotrexate**. Alcohol has also been shown to inhibit folate metabolism.

Patients with renal disease who are being dialyzed on a chronic basis have a significant increase in folate losses. Water-soluble folate is removed from the blood by the dialysis procedure and should be replaced by a daily oral supplement to prevent the development of deficiency.

Clinical Findings

The examination of the peripheral blood smear shows macrocytic erythrocytes and hypersegmented white blood cells. The values for the mean corpuscular indices are consistent with megaloblastic anemia and cannot be differentiated from the values associated with vitamin B_{12} deficiency. The principal means of distinguishing folate deficiency from vitamin B_{12} deficiency is the measurement of the serum level of folates and vitamin B_{12}. The normal serum folate level is more than 7 μg/mL; it is generally less than 3 μg/mL in folate deficiency. One method of diagnosing folate deficiency anemia is the oral administration of small, physiologic daily doses of folate to the patient. If the reticulocyte count subsequently increases, the diagnosis is confirmed; if not, a course of **parenteral vitamin B_{12}** should be administered to the patient.

Clinical Pharmacology and Therapeutics

Therapeutic Goals

The therapeutic goals for folate deficiency involve correcting the cause of the deficiency, returning the body stores to normal, and correcting the anemia. Patients with a folate-deficient diet from alcoholism or other causes may require special counseling in an attempt to correct these factors.

Folic Acid

Dose   The initial treatment for folate deficiency consists of a dose of 1 mg of folic acid daily for 2 to 3 weeks. This dose is sufficient to replace stores and correct the anemia. Higher amounts are unnecessary, as most of the dose is excreted in the urine. While only 6 percent of a 1-mg dose is excreted, 80 percent of a 15-mg dose is excreted and not utilized. The parenteral use of folic acid is generally not required; even patients with malabsorption will respond to high oral doses. However, if the patient is unable to take oral medications, parenteral folic acid is indicated.

Once folate stores have returned to normal, maintenance therapy should be considered. In most patients, normal dietary sources of folate are sufficient and continued maintenance is not required. If the underlying cause cannot be corrected, appropriate daily maintenance supplements of **folic acid**, in the range of 0.1 to 0.5 mg, must be given. The prophylactic dose of folic acid during pregnancy is usually 0.3 mg/day.

Adverse Effects   Oral and parenteral folic acid preparations only infrequently cause hypersensitivity reactions. The major *contraindication* that must be stressed is the use of folic acid alone in the treatment of vitamin B_{12} deficiency. If folic acid is used to treat the anemia symptoms of a patient with vitamin B_{12} deficiency, the clinical signs and symptoms of the anemia will be corrected; however, the neurologic degeneration will progress. Vitamin B_{12} deficiency can also develop after folate deficiency has been diagnosed and treated. For this reason, it is important to evaluate vitamin B_{12} absorption periodically in patients for whom long-term maintenance therapy with folic acid is necessary.

Monitoring Therapy

A response to **folic acid** treatment is indicated by a rise in the reticulocyte count in 2 to 3 days, and subjective improvement may occur even sooner. The hemoglobin and hematocrit values will return to normal after 6 to 8 weeks of therapy. Patient education and counseling are important, especially when an inadequate diet is the cause for the deficiency. Pregnant women must be aware of the importance of taking oral folate and iron preparations daily throughout pregnancy even though they may "feel fine." All patients should have periodic follow-up examinations to prevent an unrecognized recurrence of the anemia and to confirm that the cause of the deficiency has been correctly diagnosed and adequately treated.

APLASTIC ANEMIA

LEARNING OBJECTIVES

Upon mastery of the contents of this section, the reader will be able to:

1. Define *aplastic anemia.*
2. List four examples of drugs which may cause aplastic anemia.
3. Describe the characteristic signs, symptoms, and laboratory findings of aplastic anemia.
4. List and explain the therapeutic goals for the patient with aplastic anemia.
5. Name two classes of drugs used in the treatment of aplastic anemia.
6. Describe the process of bone marrow transplantation.

Aplastic anemia is a disease characterized by severe and generalized reduction or depletion of erythroid, myeloid, lymphoid, and megakaryocytic elements in the bone marrow with resultant pancytopenia. The bone marrow fails to produce red blood cells, white blood cells, and platelets.

Etiology

Aplastic anemia can be acquired or constitutional (congenital). Most cases of acquired aplastic anemia are idiopathic but the cause can be related to exposure to radiation or a variety of chemicals or drugs such as the antibiotic **chloramphenicol**, the anticonvulsant **trimethadione**, and the arthritic analgesic **phenylbutazone** (see Table 36-2). Chemotherapeutic agents are drugs which, if given in high enough doses, will regularly cause bone marrow failure or a decrease in bone marrow activity. This effect may be profound but is usually transitory. Most pharmacologic agents that have been implicated in the etiology of acquired aplastic anemia do not suppress bone marrow function when given in therapeutic doses. Aplastic anemia is a rare complication of the normal use of drugs that is not related to the route of administration or to cumulative dosage. This complication may be attributed to an idiosyncratic drug reaction, especially considering that the anemia often develops after treatment with the drug has ceased.

Aplastic anemia may also occur as a complication of infections such as infectious hepatitis, infectious mononucleosis, or other viral infections.

Most patients with congenital aplastic anemia suffer from a disease that is more specifically known as Fanconi's anemia. Fanconi's anemia is distinguishable from acquired aplastic anemia by the presence of distinct physical anoma-

lies that include café au lait spots, skeletal deformities, short stature, microcephaly, renal abnormalities, and mental deficiency. This disease has an autosomal recessive mode of inheritance, and persons with it have a predisposition to certain malignancies. Treatment with androgens may be beneficial to patients with Fanconi's anemia. This disease is very rare and hence will not be discussed in this chapter.

Clinical Findings

Signs and Symptoms

The signs and symptoms of aplastic anemia are directly related to the degree of pancytopenia. The anemia may cause fatigue, pallor, dyspnea, and tachycardia. The thrombocytopenia may cause bleeding, petechiae, ecchymoses, purpura, and epistaxis. The neutropenia may result in the development of systemic or local infection accompanied by fever or mouth sores.

Laboratory Findings

Laboratory test results are consistent with pancytopenia. Patients with the severe form of aplastic anemia present

TABLE 36-2 Drugs and Chemicals Frequently Associated with Aplastic Anemia and Hemolytic Anemia*

AGENT	PANCYTOPENIA	Hemolytic Anemia G6PD	Hemolytic Anemia IMMUNE
Aspirin		+++	
Benzene (organic solvents)	++		
Cephalosporins			++
Chloramphenicol	++++	+++	
Gold compounds	+++		
Hair sprays	++		
Insecticides (chlorinated)	+		++
Isoniazid		++	+
Levodopa			+++
Mefenamic acid			++
Mephenytoin	+++		
Methyldopa			+++
Nalidixic acid		++	
Naphthalene (moth balls)		+++	
Nitrofurantoin		+++	
Penicillin	+		+++
Phenacetin		++	+++
Phenylbutazone	+++		
Phenytoin	++		
Primaquine		++++	
Quinacrine	+++	++	
Quinidine		++	++
Quinine		++	++
Sulfonamides	+	+++	++
Sulfonylureas	++	++	+
Trimethadione	+++		

*The plus signs indicate the relative frequency of reported cases. Other drugs have been reported in a limited number of case reports.

with hemoglobin less than 7 g/dL, reticulocyte count less than 1 percent, platelet count less than 20,000/mm³, and absolute neutrophil count (total number of neutrophils that are found in the white blood cell count differential) less than 500/mm³. Bone marrow aspiration and biopsy are consistent with hypoplasia and marked reduction in all hematopoietic precursors. Examination of the bone marrow is important to rule out the presence of a myeloproliferative disorder that may have caused the pancytopenia and to evaluate the degree of bone marrow failure.

Clinical Pharmacology and Therapeutics

There is great variability in the clinical courses for patients with aplastic anemia. Rare spontaneous recoveries or improvements in bone marrow status do occur in these patients. Some patients have a mild to moderate form of aplasia and will require only occasional therapeutic support. Patients with severe aplastic anemia (generally defined as previously described) have historically had a very grim prognosis. Some reports describe 4-month survival at only 70 percent for patients with severe aplastic anemia. Patients who develop aplastic anemia after having infectious hepatitis often have a serious form of aplastic anemia.

Therapeutic Goals

The therapeutic goals for the patient with aplastic anemia include (1) prevention and management of infection and bleeding; (2) maintenance of the hematologic status with blood and platelet transfusion as needed; and (3) stimulation of hemopoiesis and bone marrow function. Therapeutic approaches currently include (1) supportive care, (2) androgen and glucocorticoid therapy, (3) immunosuppressive therapy, and (4) bone marrow transplantation.

Supportive Care

Infusions of blood products must be utilized when clinically indicated but must be planned carefully so that immediate benefits may be achieved with minimal detriment to future therapy. Most physicians try to maintain hemoglobin 7 to 9 g/dL in these patients. Platelet concentrates can be given for active bleeding.

Although these patients tolerate common viral infections quite well, they are highly susceptible to disseminated bacterial and fungal infections. Parenteral broad-spectrum antibiotics are indicated for all cases of suspected sepsis. The prophylactic use of antibiotics should be avoided in order to not select for resistant bacterial strains or opportunistic organisms.

Androgen and Glucocortocoid Therapy

The observation that androgenic hormones increased erythropoiesis in patients being treated for advanced breast cancer led to their use in aplastic anemia. Agents that have been used include **methyltestosterone, testosterone enanthate, testosterone proprionate, oxymetholone, nandrolone deca-**

noate, and **etiocholane.** Some patients respond to one of these agents and not to another. The dose is 1 to 2 mg/kg/week intramuscularly or 2 to 5 mg/kg/day orally.

Side effects of androgen therapy include masculinization, baldness, deepening of voice, edema, hirsutism, acne, liver dysfunction, and nausea. Other late complications of long-term use of androgens include premature skeletal maturation and an increased incidence of hepatocellular carcinoma.

The effectiveness of androgen therapy remains controversial. The time that it takes for the bone marrow to respond to androgens varies. Usually red cell function returns first, followed by white cells, and perhaps months or years later, platelets.

The use of high doses of corticosteroids in patients with acquired aplastic anemia is generally ineffective as a stimulus for hematopoiesis. Such doses are immunosuppressive and increase the risk of infection. **Methylprednisolone** 40 mg/kg for 2 days followed by tapered doses for several subsequent days has been used in an attempt to stimulate bone marrow function. Some clinicians use steroids such as **prednisone** in low doses of 5 mg/day to reduce annoying episodes of soft tissue bleeding or in combination with androgens to counteract the bone maturing effects of the androgens.

Immunosuppressive Therapy

The use of immunosuppressive agents in the treatment of aplastic anemia began after bone marrow recovery was noted in aplastic patients being prepared for bone marrow transplantation who received high-dose **cyclophosphamide** or **ATG (antithymocyte globulin).** Currently many clinical trials using agents such as ATG are being conducted on patients with aplastic anemia who are not eligible for bone marrow transplantation. Since the treatment protocol is not yet standardized, the dosage and schedule of ATG that patients receive vary from 1 mg/kg/day for 40 days to 40 mg/kg/day for 4 days.

Patients who receive intravenous ATG must be monitored closely for signs and symptoms of any allergic or anaphylactic reactions during or after the infusion. Because marked swelling of the extremity with local enduration and erythema can occur, ATG is generally administered through central intravenous lines. Patients are often given steroids such as **prednisone** on infusion days in order to alleviate any symptoms of serum sickness.

The effectiveness of this treatment has yet to be determined.

Bone Marrow Transplantation

Bone marrow transplantation as treatment of aplastic anemia is reserved for patients with severe aplastic anemia, but should not be delayed for patients with histocompatible donors. Transplantation is possible only if an HLA-matched sibling or relative is available to act as marrow donor. This is a lymphocyte-typing system, genetically determined, which specifies the degree of histocompatibility (the degree of immunologic likeness between donor and recipient).

The process of bone marrow transplantation begins with suppression of the host's lymphoid system to permit engraftment of the donor's marrow. High-dose **cyclophosphamide** given over several days is the most commonly used immunosuppressive agent.

The donor's bone marrow is obtained via multiple bone marrow aspirates of the iliac crest, usually performed while the donor is under general anesthesia. The marrow is processed and then given to the recipient intravenously, in a fashion similar to that of a routine blood transfusion.

The period of engraftment (time that it takes for the patient's bone marrow to become cellular and subsequently for his or her blood counts to achieve normal levels) can be many weeks. There is much morbidity and mortality associated with bone marrow transplantation, largely caused by graft rejection, infectious complications caused by the pretreatment with immunosuppressive therapy, or a phenomenon known as graft versus host disease. Graft versus host disease (GVH) is a reaction of donor engrafted tissue against the recipient's tissue.

After marrow transplantation, **methotrexate** is often given in low dosages at defined intervals as prophylaxis against GVH. This disease occurs in varying degrees of severity in over half of the patients undergoing bone marrow transplantation. It may be lethal or produce long-term disabilities.

Monitoring Therapy

Currently bone marrow transplantation is the treatment of choice for patients with severe aplastic anemia and offers a chance of cure for as many as 50 percent of these patients. This percentage is much higher for patients receiving a transplant of marrow from an identical twin and in patients who have not received multiple transfusions prior to the transplant.

HEMOLYTIC ANEMIA

LEARNING OBJECTIVES

Upon mastery of the contents of this section, the reader will be able to:

1. Define *hemolytic anemia.*

2. List two types of inherited hemolytic anemia and explain the mechanism of each.

3. List at least six drugs which can cause hemolytic anemia.

4. Describe the characteristic signs, symptoms, and laboratory findings of hemolytic anemia.

5. Describe the therapeutic program for the patient with acute hemolytic anemia.

Hemolytic anemia is a clinical condition in which the destruction of red blood cells is increased while the bone marrow function is normal.

Etiology

Hemolytic anemia may be either inherited or acquired.

G6PD Deficiency

One inherited variety of hemolytic anemia is associated with a deficiency of *glucose-6-phosphate dehydrogenase* (G6PD), an enzyme required for the metabolic production of energy and for the maintenance of glutathione in the reduced form. Patients with a significant deficiency of G6PD are unable to generate and maintain sufficient amounts of glutathione in the reduced form; if they are exposed to an oxidizing substance, the integrity of the erythrocytes cannot be protected and hemolysis results. For this reason, it is important for patients with G6PD deficiency to avoid exposure to drugs and chemical compounds that are known to induce hemolysis in this disorder (see Table 36-2). In order to prevent drug-induced hemolytic reactions, thorough patient education is necessary, as well as awareness on the part of the health professionals involved in prescribing, dispensing, and administering medications to the patients.

The incidence of G6PD deficiency is highest in the black population and in individuals of Mediterranean descent; approximately 13 percent of black males in the United States may be affected. Screening tests are available to identify patients with G6PD deficiency and are especially important for use in high-risk populations. These tests should also be performed on all family members of a patient who is found to have a deficiency, because the condition is a sex-linked, inherited disorder. The expression of the defect in individual female heterozygotes (carriers) varies greatly. The deficiency of G6PD is not an "all or none" defect, and special assays are used to quantitate the percentage of G6PD enzyme activity present in order to classify the deficiency as mild, moderate, or severe.

Sickle-Cell Anemia

Sickle-cell anemia, another inherited variety of hemolytic anemia, is caused by an abnormal sickle-cell hemoglobin (HbS) molecule synthesized by the erythropoietic system and found in the red blood cells in varying amounts depending on the severity of the abnormality. The altered structure of the sickle-cell hemoglobin molecule allows it to bind to other sickle-cell hemoglobin molecules to form long, helical monofilaments, which distort the normal shape of the erythrocyte to form the sickled cell. Because of its abnormal shape, the sickled erythrocyte can become lodged in small capillaries, causing hemostasis, vascular occlusion, and tissue hypoxia with severe pain.

Persons with *sickle-cell trait* have erythrocytes containing 20 to 45 percent sickle-cell hemoglobin, are not anemic, have no physical abnormalities, are usually asymptomatic, and have a normal life span. Persons with sickle-cell disease, however, have erythrocytes containing 80 to 100 percent sickle-cell hemoglobin, with associated chronic hemolytic anemia, recurrent attacks of pain, frequent bacterial infections due to the loss of normal spleen function, gradual deterioration of tissue and organ functions, and hence a shortened life expectancy.

In sickle-cell anemia, the therapeutic goals are to prevent further sickling of erythrocytes and to reverse the process in red cells already affected. Of primary importance is the management of precipitating factors, such as infection and dehydration, with appropriate antibiotics and intravenous fluids. Prophylactic oral **penicillin** in a dose of 125 to 250 mg once or twice daily and vaccination with **pneumococcal vaccine** (Pneumovax) are used to reduce the incidence of infection. Oral supplements of **folic acid** are also administered due to the increased need for folic acid in patients with chronic hemolytic anemia. At present, the most effective therapeutic measure available is the transfusion of normal red blood cells.

Drug-Induced Hemolytic Anemia

Of special interest among the acquired hemolytic anemias are the drug-induced forms caused by immune and nonimmune mechanisms. The primary nonimmune mechanism of hemolysis involves the injury of erythrocytes with defective enzyme systems, such as G6PD deficiency, by certain drugs with oxidative properties. The direct Coombs' test is used to differentiate immune and nonimmune hemolytic anemias.

Drugs which may cause hemolytic anemia by an immune mechanism include: large intravenous doses of **penicillin, phenacetin, quinine, quinidine, methyldopa, levodopa,** and the **cephalosporin** group of antibiotics (see Table 36-2).

Clinical Findings

Symptoms
The clinical features of hemolytic anemia may include lethargy, fatigue, and skin pallor. Gallstones and jaundice may result from the chronic increased production of bilirubin, the primary waste product of metabolized hemoglobin from the destroyed red blood cells. Enlargement of the spleen is commonly associated with congenital hemolytic anemias.

Laboratory Findings
The general laboratory findings in hemolytic anemia are related to the increased destruction of erythrocytes and the compensatory increase in erythropoiesis. The peripheral blood smear will often contain fragments of hemolyzed erythrocytes. The serum concentration of *haptoglobin,* a carrier protein that binds free hemoglobin released from hemolyzed red blood cells and transports it to the liver for removal, is greatly reduced or may be absent in hemolytic

conditions. *Reticulocytosis,* a compensatory increase in the number of immature red blood cells in the circulation, is another laboratory finding associated with hemolytic anemia. Specific laboratory tests used in the differential diagnosis of hemolytic anemia include erythrocyte enzyme determinations to identify hereditary deficiencies, hemoglobin electrophoresis to identify abnormal hemoglobin molecules, and the direct Coombs' test to identify immune reactions.

Clinical Pharmacology and Therapeutics
The treatment of hemolytic anemia must be directed at the underlying cause. Implicated drugs must be discontinued. In addition, general supportive measures must be employed in the prevention or management of shock. If hemolysis is severe and acute in onset, transfusions of whole blood or packed red cells may be necessary. Renal function must also be maintained by the use of intravenous fluids and potent diuretics, because of the potential damage and obstruction caused by the entry into the renal tubules of massive amounts of hemoglobin from the circulation. The removal of the spleen can decrease the severity of many chronic hemolytic disorders, since it is a major site of red blood cell destruction. Corticosteroids such as **prednisone** have also been used successfully in the management of hemolytic anemias caused by immune reactions. The initial dose of prednisone in the treatment of acute hemolytic anemia should be in the range of 1.0 to 1.5 mg/kg/day. This dose is continued until the serum and urine are clear of hemolytic products and the serum hemoglobin is normal. The prednisone dose is then tapered and usually discontinued in a short period of time, depending on patient response.

NURSING PROCESS RELATED TO THE ANEMIAS

There are many aspects of nursing process common to all of the anemias regardless of cause. However, the nurse must not overlook those aspects of assessment, management, and evaluation unique to the various etiological processes in anemia.

Assessment
Patients who are anemic often state that they feel more tired than usual and may be irritable and/or have episodes of weakness. Shortness of breath with exercise and headaches are also associated with anemia. Significant findings on physical examination can include pallor (especially of the face, lips, and mucous membranes), splenomegaly, rapid heart rate that is markedly elevated by exercise, heart murmur, and a rapid respiratory rate.

Laboratory findings will include a decreased hemoglobin and hematocrit and findings specific to the type of anemia. For example, in iron-deficiency anemia there will be a decreased serum ferritin, decreased red blood cell indices (MCV, MCH, MCHC), and hypochromic microcytic cells on blood smear. In aplastic anemia there is a decrease in neutrophils and platelets as well as in red blood cells. Vitamin B_{12}–deficiency anemia is a macrocytic anemia accompanied by low serum vitamin B_{12} levels.

The nurse should also consider factors which contributed to the development of the anemia. Analysis of the nutritional history should focus on the adequacy of meat, dark green vegetables, and other sources of iron, folic acid, and vitamin B_{12}. Medication over the prior 12 months is reviewed for possible causes of hemolytic or aplastic anemia (Table 36-2). Daily intake of more than a quart of milk may predispose an infant to iron-deficiency anemia, since a large portion of the child's calories are derived from this food, which is low in iron. Pica (the eating of clay or dirt or other nonfood substances) is also indicative of iron-deficiency anemia. Other factors to consider are familial history of G6PD deficiency; gynecologic history of excessive menstrual flow, multiple pregnancies at short intervals, or lactation; gastrointestinal disorders that contribute to malabsorption; history of GI surgery; hypocoagulation as evidenced by nosebleeds or bruising; dark stools or blood in stools; and recent or current rapid growth.

Nurses must explain the laboratory procedures to patients, such as the Schilling test used to diagnose pernicious anemia and the frequent complete blood counts used to monitor the course of aplastic anemia.

Management

Patients with anemia must understand how and when to take their medications, the importance of dietary support of therapy, and how to adjust their activities appropriately for the severity of their disease. Patients on oral iron therapy must be instructed to take the full course of therapy to correct the anemia and replenish iron stores. Oral iron can be taken with meals if necessary, to decrease gastric discomfort. The dosage should be gradually increased to a full dose over a period of a few days if severe gastric discomfort occurs. The patient should know that oral iron may turn the stools dark. If parenteral **iron dextran** is required, it should be given deep into a muscle using the Z-track technique described previously in this chapter. Epinephrine and other emergency drugs should be available to treat anaphylaxis when parenteral iron is given.

Pernicious anemia is a chronic disease requiring medical supervision, repeated vitamin B_{12} injections, monitoring of laboratory values, and a proper diet. Nursing support and intervention can allow these patients to adjust to their disease without changing their lives. They must be alerted to the multiple systemic changes that can be associated with

the disease so that they can note and report all significant changes.

Patients with folic acid anemia also must understand the need to complete the entire course of therapy. Nurses must work with the patient and the person who assumes primary responsibility for cooking in the home (if it is other than the patient) to assure that they understand proper nutritional support. Directions and lists of foods high in iron, folic acid, and vitamin B_{12} must be given both verbally and in writing.

When their hemoglobin level is low, patients with aplastic anemia must learn to plan daily activities accordingly, allowing for adequate rest periods. They must also be aware of the signs and symptoms of a very low hemoglobin that may warrant red cell transfusion. Such signs and symptoms include tachycardia, shortness of breath, tachypnea, weakness, and headache. When their platelet counts are low, especially when they are less than 20,000/mm^3, patients must take measures to decrease any risk of trauma or hemorrhage. For example, contact sports must be limited, seat belts must be worn during rides in cars, and constipation must be avoided through use of stool softeners, laxatives, or high-fiber diets. Oral hygiene should include the use of soft-bristle toothbrushes or sponges that will not cause gum bleeding. Hormonal suppression of menstrual flow may be necessary. Patients should be instructed in emergency treatment of acute bleeding episodes such as the application of direct pressure for epistaxis or frank bleeding. Since severe headache could be the presenting sign of an intracranial bleed, medical attention should be sought immediately at the first sign of headache. Patients whose absolute neutrophil counts are low, especially when they are less than 500/mm^3, are highly susceptible to disseminated bacterial and fungal infections. Whenever they do not feel well, their temperature should be checked accurately. The physician must always be notified for fever greater than 101°F or any other sign of infection. Acetaminophen can be given for fever or other ailments, but aspirin-containing products should be avoided as they will interfere with platelet function. Careful hand washing is imperative for all persons who come in contact with these patients. Strict isolation to limit exposure to infection is financially and emotionally impractical.

Evaluation

With most types of anemia, patients experience subjective improvement and improved laboratory findings within a few days (see sections on monitoring therapy for each anemia). They must be encouraged to continue to take the full course of medication, however. The nurse must specifically evaluate for adverse effects, such as gastric irritation or constipation in those taking *oral iron,* that also can contribute to noncompliance.

CASE STUDY

J.S., a 26-year-old female in the fifth month of her third pregnancy, presented for her first prenatal clinic visit. Her two previous pregnancies were entirely normal. Her children were 13 months old and 2 years old. They were healthy and active. She had not been able to find a baby-sitter for them, to allow her time to come to the prenatal clinic on a regular basis. Her husband worked during the day and attended evening classes at a local college, so did not have much free time to help in caring for the children.

Assessment

The patient's chief complaint was feeling excessively tired and "run down." During an interview with the nurse, she related a history of "heavy" menstrual flow, lasting from 5 to 6 days every month. She had had a sore mouth and a poor appetite for several weeks and had had to stop her activities at times to "catch my breath." In reviewing her dietary history, the nurse noted a less than adequate intake of meat products and fresh green vegetables in comparison with accepted dietary standards for pregnant women. The nurse realized that in planning dietary interventions consideration must be given to the financial resources and nutritional status of the patient, in addition to her lack of appetite.

After interviewing and examining the patient and reviewing her laboratory data (see Table 36-3), the diagnosis of iron-deficiency anemia was confirmed. The contributing factors of multiple pregnancies within a few years, the heavy menstrual blood flow, diet deficient in adequate amounts of iron and folic acid, and inconsistency of prenatal care, which has prevented early detection and treatment of the anemia, were also noted. Further, the nurse was aware of the increased need for iron and folic acid which would occur during the third trimester of pregnancy.

TABLE 36-3   Laboratory Report, Patient J.S.

LABORATORY TEST	TEST RESULT	NORMAL VALUE
Iron	40 μg/dL	33–150 μg/dL
TIBC	500 μg/dL	250–450 μg/dL
MCV	77 μm^3	82–92 μm^3
MCH	23 pg	27–31 pg
MCHC	26%	30–34%
Hematocrit	24%	36–48%
Hemoglobin	8 g/dL	12–16 g/dL
TIBC saturation	8%	25–35%

On examination, the peripheral blood smear shows hypochromic, microcytic erythrocytes with marked anisocytosis and poikilocytosis.

Management

Following the clinic protocol, the nurse-midwife ordered ferrous sulfate 300 mg tid with meals and folic acid 1 mg daily. She recommended frequent rest periods throughout the day and asked the patient to return in 1 month.

The nurse also realized that patient education is an important part of a patient management and compliance program and therefore stressed the following considerations in her discussion with the patient:

1.   The importance of continuing to take the iron medication for the full, prescribed period, even though she would begin to feel better, in order to replace depleted iron stores in her body. She was also made aware of the importance of frequent rest periods.

2.   The dietary status of the family. After evaluation and discussion with the patient and a dietitian, a series of satisfactory menus were prepared to ensure adequate family intake of foods supplying sufficient amounts of proteins, vitamins, and iron.

3.   The possible side effects of oral iron preparations and the way to reduce some of these problems by taking the medication with meals.

4.   The danger of accidental iron poisoning in children. Since there were small children in her home, the patient was instructed to store all medications in an out-of-reach place and to ask the pharmacist for "childproof" containers.

5.   The need for continued prenatal clinic visits to monitor her progress and the status of her unborn child. Arrangements were made through the clinic social worker for the patient to utilize the facilities of a local day-care center as needed.

Only if the patient returned to the clinic for her next scheduled appointment would the nurse be able to evaluate the effectiveness of the previous patient education process. The patient's return would indicate that she realized the seriousness of her condition and was prepared to take adequate measures to improve her health. In all the the nurse's future interactions with the patient, a supportive, caring attitude must be conveyed. If at any time the nurse becomes judgmental or negative, the patient could discontinue her clinic visits and be lost from the health-care system.

Evaluation

Upon the scheduled return visit to the clinic, the patient reported that she had begun to feel less tired and short of breath. Her hemoglobin had increased to 11 g/100 mL, reticulocytes were elevated to 10 percent, and the hematocrit reading was 28 percent. She stated that she had had no gastrointestinal irritation except for the one time that she forgot to take her medication with the evening meal and took it at bedtime without food. The family had done "fairly well" in adhering to the suggested diet plan,

except that during the first weeks, the patient stated, she "was just too tired to do all that shopping and food preparation." In the last 2 weeks, as she had felt better, she had begun to enjoy preparing the meals which were suggested.

HEMOPHILIA

LEARNING OBJECTIVES

Upon mastery of the contents of this section, the reader will be able to:

1. Differentiate hemophilia A and hemophilia B.
2. Explain the varying degrees of severity of hemophilia.
3. Describe the signs, symptoms, and laboratory findings of hemophilia.
4. List two therapeutic goals in the treatment of hemophilia.
5. List and describe three therapeutic preparations used in the treatment of hemophilia A.
6. List and describe two therapeutic preparations used in the treatment of hemophilia B.
7. Discuss two parameters for monitoring patients receiving factor replacement.
8. Discuss the major risk associated with chronic administration of factor concentrates.
9. Explain two methods used in the treatment of patients with high levels of factor VIII inhibitors.

Hemophilia is a hereditary disorder of the hemostatic system characterized by delayed coagulation and excessive bleeding. The fundamental abnormality is associated with a deficiency or qualitative defect in one of the plasma proteins involved in the intrinsic system of the coagulation mechanism (see Fig. 42-1). The most common clinical condition is *hemophilia A*, or classic hemophilia, which involves a deficiency or defect in factor VIII. *Hemophilia B*, or Christmas disease, is a less common disorder and results from a deficiency or defect in factor IX.

Hemophilia is a recessive, sex-linked, hereditary disease, with the defective gene located on the X chromosome of the reproductive cells, which is clinically manifested in males; females are rarely symptomatic.

The deficiency or defect in the coagulation factors associated with hemophilia A or B is not an "all or none" condition, and varying degrees of clinical severity exist. Some persons have less than 1 percent of the normal amount of antihemophilic factor (AHF, factor VIII) or factor IX activity in their blood. These are severe hemophiliacs who may bleed spontaneously and frequently. Other persons may have

25 to 50 percent of normal factor activity and experience bleeding problems only following major trauma or surgery. The incidence of hemophilia A is estimated to be one or two in 20,000 males, while the incidence of hemophilia B is less than one in 20,000 males.

Clinical Findings

Signs and Symptoms

Patients with hemophilia are generally diagnosed early in childhood, especially if the factor deficiency is moderate to severe. They often present a history of repeated, prolonged bleeding episodes following minor injuries. A positive family history for the disease is significant in making an early diagnosis. Patients with a mild degree of hemophilia, however, can be asymptomatic and undiagnosed until a tooth is extracted or other minor surgical procedure is performed that results in an unexpected and prolonged bleeding episode.

Hemarthrosis, or bleeding into the joint spaces, is one of the most common clinical manifestations of hemophilia. This condition is extremely painful because of swelling and inflammation of the joint. Subcutaneous and intramuscular bleeding and *hematomas* are also common and can be dangerous if they compress vital structures, such as an artery or airway. Bleeding in the gastrointestinal and genitourinary tract occurs frequently and must be monitored closely and managed by factor replacement.

Laboratory Findings

The basic laboratory tests used to evaluate the coagulation mechanism (see Chap. 42) can also be used as *screening tests* in the diagnosis of hemophilia. Specific *factor assays,* which measure the actual concentration of factors VIII and IX in the plasma, are relatively simple to perform and provide important diagnostic information in differentiating hemophilia A and B.

Clinical Pharmacology and Therapeutics

Therapeutic Goals

The therapeutic goals in hemophilia include the prevention and control of bleeding episodes and the correction of the coagulation mechanism. These goals can be accomplished by replacement therapy with the specifically deficient factor.

Dosage

The concentration of coagulation factors in the normal plasma or in replacement preparations is expressed in *units* (U); 1 U represents the factor activity in 1 mL of fresh plasma from normal male donors. Therefore the concentration of all coagulation factors in normal plasma is 1 U/mL and represents 100 percent of normal factor activity. In order to maintain normal hemostasis, the concentration of factor VIII in hemophilia A must be approximately 25 to 30 percent of normal, equivalent to a plasma concentration of 0.25 to 0.3 U/mL. The hemostatic concentration of factor IX in hemophilia B is estimated to be 15 to 25 percent of normal.

Depending on the clinical condition of the patient, an initial loading dose of the specific factor may be necessary to bring the plasma concentration into the therapeutic range. The maintenance dosage and length of therapy depend upon the plasma half-life of the administered factor, the clinical condition being treated, and the response of the patient to treatment (see Table 36-4).

Preparations

Plasma Fresh or fresh-frozen plasma contains approximately 1 U/mL of the coagulation factors and can be used in the treatment of hemophilia. In order to sufficiently increase the plasma activity in patients with severe hemophilia, however, a large volume of plasma may be necessary because of the low concentration of factors and the dilutional effect of plasma administration. For this reason, more concentrated and purified preparations have been developed.

Cryoprecipitate One method of preparing a more concentrated preparation of factor VIII is *cryoprecipitation.* Plasma is rapidly frozen and slowly thawed, and the resulting precipitate is removed by centrifugation. This procedure produces a preparation which has a factor-VIII concentration that is nearly 20 times greater than plasma.

Purified factor VIII Other procedures have been developed to produce factor-VIII preparations containing up to 400 times more factor VIII than plasma. These AHF concentrates (Factorate, Hemofil) are standardized by assay, and each bottle is labeled with its factor-VIII content. The preparation is convenient for use in home care programs and in the treatment of patients requiring large doses of factor VIII.

Purified Prothrombin-Complex Factors Factors II, VIII, IX, and X are the vitamin K–dependent plasma coagulation factors and are also known as the prothrombin-complex factors. These factors have been purified to produce therapeutic preparations (Konyne, Proplex) containing a concentration of the individual factors up to 60 times greater than plasma. These preparations are used in the management of specific factor deficiencies, such as hemophilia B, and in the treatment of severe bleeding complications that may be associated with drug therapy with coumadin-type anticoagulants.

Patients receiving factor replacement therapy should be closely monitored both clinically and by specific laboratory tests. The signs and symptoms of bleeding, such as swelling, pain, or actual blood flow, should decrease and stabilize. The factor activity should not fall below 25 percent of normal, and therapy should be continued for a period of 2 to 14 days, depending upon the condition being treated.

ε-Aminocaproic Acid ε-Aminocaproic acid (Amicar) is an effective agent used in hemophiliac patients with severe

TABLE 36-4 Preparations Available for Replacement Therapy in Hemophilia

COAGULATION DISORDER	PREPARATION	Minor Hemorrhages		Major Hemorrhages and Surgery	
		INITIAL DOSE	MAINTENANCE DOSE	INITIAL DOSE	MAINTENANCE DOSE
Hemophilia A	Fresh CPD plasma (approximately 1 U factor VIII/mL)		10–15 mL/kg q12h	35 mL/kg	20 mL/kg q8h, reduced to q12h after 1–2 days
	Cryoprecipitate (averages 85 U factor VIII per bag)		1.25–1.75 bags/ 10 kg q12h	4 bags/10 kg	2.5 bags/10 kg q8h, reduced to q12h after 1–2 days
	Purified factor VIII		10–15 U/kg q12h	35 U/kg	20 U/kg q8h, reduced to q12h after 1–2 days
Hemophilia B	CPD plasma	30 mL/kg	7 mL/kg q12h	60 mL/kg	7 mL/kg q12h
	Purified prothrombin complex factors	30 U/kg	10 U/kg q12h	60 U/kg	10 U/kg q12h

mucosal bleeding episodes due to trauma or dental procedures. Amicar helps to maintain clots which have formed by inhibiting fibrinolysis. An intravenous or oral prophylactic dose of 100 mg/kg is administered every 6 h for 24 h prior to dental extraction and continued for 8 to 10 days. Side effects include nausea, cramping, diarrhea, dizziness, tinnitus, nasal stuffiness, headache, and skin rash. These side effects are generally mild and disappear on withdrawal of the drug.

Adverse Effects

The intravenous administration of factor concentrates can cause transient fever, chills, headache, nausea, flushing, and tingling. These effects are infrequent and generally mild, but the patient should be monitored closely during the infusion. The major risk associated with the administration of factor concentrates, as with all blood products, is that of viral hepatitis. These preparations are obtained from the pooled plasma of multiple donors, and every precaution is taken to screen the donors.

Complications

Factor VIII Inhibitors An acquired complication in patients with hemophilia A is the production of inhibitors to factor VIII, presumably related to factor-VIII replacement therapy. The immunologic mechanism is unclear, but the administered factor VIII acts as an antigen and the resultant antibodies inactivate it. As the plasma concentration of factor-VIII antibodies increases, bleeding episodes become more frequent and severe and less responsive to replacement therapy. The factor-VIII-inhibitor level can be measured by specific laboratory tests; the result is reported as the number of units of factor VIII neutralized by 1 mL of the plasma being treated. For example, 1 mL of plasma having an inhibitor level of 10 U/mL will neutralize 10 U of factor VIII. This means that a patient with an inhibitor level of 10 U/mL will require a replacement dose of factor VIII equivalent to 10 U/mL of plasma in addition to the normal therapeutic dose. If exposure to the antigen (factor VIII) continues, many patients will produce a high level of inhibitor, resulting in a dangerous therapeutic problem. Corticosteroids and other immunosuppressive drugs, such as **cyclophosphamide**, have been used in an attempt to decrease antibody production and thereby lower the inhibitor level in the plasma.

Another mode of therapy being used in the management of patients with excessively high levels of factor VIII antibodies is the administration of anti-inhibitor coagulant complex (Autoplex) which contains, in concentrated form, variable amounts of activated and precursor clotting factors. The activated factors allow normal coagulation to progress through the common pathway, bypassing factor VIII in the intrinsic system (Fig. 42-1). The patient must be monitored

for signs of intravascular coagulation which include changes in blood pressure and pulse rate, respiratory distress, chest pain, and cough. If any of these symptoms occur, the infusion of Autoplex should be stopped and the patient monitored for diffuse intravascular coagulation by the appropriate laboratory tests such as fibrinogen concentration and platelet count.

The recommended dosage range is 25 to 200 factor VIII correctional U/kg of body weight, depending upon the severity of hemorrhage. This dosage may be repeated as needed based on the patient's response.

In less severe cases of patients having factor VIII antibodies, very large doses of **prothrombin** complex factors have been successfully used to control bleeding episodes. Commercially available concentrates (Konyne and Proplex) contain a small concentration of activated factor X (Xa). When these preparations are administered in large enough doses, a sufficient amount of factor Xa can be supplied to the patient to activate the common pathway and correct hemostasis by bypassing factor VIII in the intrinsic system. These patients must also be carefully monitored for the signs and symptoms of intravascular coagulation.

The Hemophilic Child

Health professionals can be of great help in the education and support of children with hemophilia and their families. The hemophilic child and the family must realize that although blood loss associated with spontaneous bleeding episodes and minor trauma tends to be slow and oozing in nature and therefore can be controlled quickly enough not to become life-threatening, the degenerative arthritis associated with these episodes is a real and chronic problem. Head injuries with intracranial hemorrhage are the most common cause of death in hemophiliacs.

Information related to normal growth and development and the importance of childhood independence should be provided to the parents. These children, even if not overprotected in early childhood, may begin to limit their activities themselves. The association of pain and possible hospitalization with certain activities will act as a deterrent to them, limiting their participation, whether potentially dangerous or not. Parents should be trained to prepare and administer factor VIII concentrates at the first sign of bleeding and to recognize conditions that may warrant further treatment by a physician.

The prognosis in hemophilia has greatly improved with major therapeutic advances in recent years. With appropriate treatment and management programs, patients can expect a nearly normal life span. The complications associated with hemophilia can also be minimized. Other coagulation problems are reviewed in Chap. 42.

CASE STUDY

P.V., a 16-year-old, well-developed, well-nourished male weighing 60 kg had a medical history of hemophilia A. The diagnosis had been made by the family physician when P. V. had had repeated episodes of joint bleeding when learning to walk as a baby. His family history was positive, with a maternal grandfather and cousin having hemophilia. At that time the pediatrician evaluated his hemostatic system. Laboratory test results included a prolonged partial thromboplastin time, a normal platelet count, and a normal prothrombin time. Platelet function tests were normal. The factor-VIII assay confirmed the suspected diagnosis of hemophilia A, demonstrating the factor-VIII activity to be moderate at 3 percent of normal.

Prior to the age of 14 years, P.V. had been admitted to the hospital frequently for control of multiple bleeding episodes, and his absence from school had caused him to fall one year behind in his education. He then entered a hemophilia home-care program at a local medical center and was trained to self-administer factor VIII at home as needed. After he entered this program, the frequency of hospitalization was greatly reduced.

Several months after completing the home-care program, P.V. was hospitalized with a bleeding episode of the right hip resulting from a fall. He had self-administered 450 U of factor VIII immediately after the fall and again about 10 h later, but his hip continued to swell and became extremely painful. He was then brought to the emergency room, in accordance with previous instruction in the home-care program, and was admitted to the hospital and placed on complete bed rest. After examining the patient's hip and reviewing his history, the admitting physician ordered 900 U of factor-VIII concentrate IV q12h and Empirin #3, one tablet q4h PRN for pain.

Assessment

On reviewing the medication orders, the nurse recognized Empirin #3 as an aspirin-containing analgesic and judged it unsafe for this patient. Further, the nurse analyzed his physical needs, which primarily involved the administration of the factor VIII and the restrictions of bed rest; observed how well he was able to meet his emotional need to maintain independence; evaluated his factor-VIII self-administration technique in accordance with the procedure recommended by the home-care program; assessed his need for pain medication; and examined his right hip for signs and symptoms of continued bleeding, such as increased pain and swelling.

Management

The nurse contacted the physician about the order for Empirin #3, explaining the rationale for judging it unsafe. In its place the physician ordered Tylenol #3, which the nurse administered to P.V.

In formulating the plan relative to the emotional needs of this teenager, the nurse recalled that the major developmental task of his age group centers on a search for self and a striving for independence. The nursing staff was aware that hospitalization tends to make patients dependent and realized the possible detrimental effects this could have on this teenager. He was encouraged to self-administer his factor VIII, as prescribed, during his hospitalization. The staff also encouraged his mother and friends to visit him often and to bring him news of familiar events in his environment. The patient was frequently evaluated and consulted by the nurse as to the condition of his hip and was reminded that he might have pain medication whenever he felt it was necessary.

Evaluation

After talking to the patient and his mother and observing the patient give his own factor VIII and state why he used it and the side effects he watched for, it was apparent to the nurse that he was managing his chronic disease well and had benefited from his participation in the home-care program. He seemed to be performing well in school and to be socially well-adjusted, as he referred often to his friends, both male and female, and their many group activities. He reported to the nurse that he was active on his high school swimming team, having made his own decision to avoid contact sports.

After the patient had received 5 days of factor-VIII treatment, the bleeding stopped and the patient was discharged.

BLOOD TRANSFUSION

LEARNING OBJECTIVES

Upon mastery of the contents of this section, the reader will be able to:

1. Identify the four common blood group classifications and list the acceptable blood types that may be transfused in persons with each classification.

2. Explain the mechanism for the development of a hemolytic transfusion reaction.

3. Explain the importance of the expiration date for blood products.

4. List three indications for the transfusion of whole blood.

5. List four indications for the transfusion of packed red blood cells.

6. Review the indications for the use of platelet transfusions.

7. List two intravenous solutions that cannot be used with blood transfusions and explain why each is unacceptable.

8. Review the procedure for checking a unit of blood before administration.

9. Describe patient-monitoring procedures during a blood transfusion and explain the importance of each parameter.

10. Explain the need for a blood-warming coil when multiple units of blood are being transfused within a short period of time.

11. List and define six complications associated with blood transfusion, indicating the symptoms of each.

12. Explain why hemolytic transfusion reactions may not occur until several days after a blood transfusion.

13. Outline the drug treatment program for a patient with a severe hemolytic transfusion reaction and explain the rationale for each drug used.

14. Explain the drug therapy used in the management of febrile transfusion reactions.

15. Explain the drug therapy used in the management of an allergic transfusion reaction with possible respiratory complications.

16. Describe two methods of preventing circulatory overload with blood transfusions.

17. Explain the drug therapy used in the management of hypocalcemia associated with massive blood transfusion.

18. State three indications for the use of blood plasma.

19. List three concentrated blood products that can be derived from plasma and discuss one indication for the use of each.

BLOOD CLASSIFICATION SYSTEMS

Red blood cells can be differentiated or classified by the presence or absence of specific antigens on their surface, called *agglutinogens*. The *ABO system* of classification, which is based on the identification of these antigens, consists of four major blood groups (Table 36-5). Two major agglutinogens, identified as A and B, are used to name these blood groups. Group A blood contains red cells with agglutinogen A on their surface, and group B contains red cells with agglutinogen B. If the red blood cell contains both A and B agglutinogens, the blood group is AB; and if neither agglutinogen is present, the blood group is O. The ABO system also identifies the presence of the *agglutinins,* or antibodies, in the blood plasma. These antibodies are produced during fetal development and are directed against the agglutinogen or agglutinogens *not* present in the fetal red blood cells.

The ABO system is the universal identification system of blood groups and is used as a means to correctly match donor blood with that of the recipient for a blood transfusion. Incorrect matching, such as group A blood transfused into a group B recipient, would result in incompatibility and would cause a severe transfusion reaction. The naturally occurring anti-A antibodies of the recipient would attach to the donor group A erythrocytes, resulting in the immediate hemolysis of those red blood cells.

Another important classification system used to determine blood compatibility is the *Rh system.* Anti-Rh antibodies do not occur naturally in the plasma as do the antibodies of the ABO system. An *immunizing event* must generally take place, caused by Rh-positive red cells entering the circulation of an Rh-negative person. This immunization can result from the transfusion of mismatched red blood cells or from blood exchange during the delivery of an Rh-positive baby by an Rh-negative woman. Once the anti-Rh antibodies have been produced, a second exposure to Rh-positive red blood cells will result in the hemolysis and destruction of those red cells by the reticuloendothelial system. For this reason, Rh typing is an important part of blood-compatibility testing.

BLOOD COLLECTION AND PRESERVATION

The methods of collecting and preserving blood for transfusion have been greatly improved and have reduced the incidence of bacterial contamination and other potential hazards. Plasma collection bags have a nonwettable surface to minimize the potential for clot formation during storage. Specific *anticoagulant preservatives* are also mixed with the blood at the time of collection, to allow it to be stored for future use. Two of these substances, acid citrate dextrose

TABLE 36-5 ABO Blood Groups

PATIENT'S BLOOD GROUP	RED BLOOD CELL ANTIGENS	PLASMA ANTIBODIES	COMPATIBLE RED BLOOD CELLS	COMPATIBLE WHOLE BLOOD	COMPATIBLE PLASMA
A	A	Anti-B	A, O	A	A, AB
B	B	Anti-A	B, O	B	B, AB
AB	A, B	None	A, B, AB, O	AB	AB
O	None	Anti-A, anti-B	O	O	A, B, AB, O

(ACD) and the more common citrate phosphate dextrose (CPD), contain citric acid, which complexes with the ionic calcium present in the blood and thus prevents coagulation. CPD has proved to be somewhat better than ACD in preserving red blood cells and is used more frequently. The dextrose present in these preservatives provides an energy source to maintain the viability of the red blood cells.

It is important always to check the expiration date on the label of all blood products before administration. CPD-preserved blood can be stored under proper conditions for 21 days. After this period of time, a significant number of the red cells will no longer be viable and only the plasma can be salvaged for the production of certain plasma fractions, such as γ globulin and albumin.

Blood Donation

Four major tests are performed on blood that is collected for donation. The tests include blood grouping, antibody screening, serologic test for syphilis, and hepatitis-B surface antigen screening.

Blood donors are interviewed and screened before their blood is accepted for transfusion purposes. Donors must weigh at least 110 lb, be at least 16 years of age (a physician's permission is required after age 65 years), have blood pressure between 180–90/110–50 mmHg, have pulse rate between 100–50 beats/min, and have hemoglobin greater than 12.5 g/dL if female or 13.5 g/dL if male. Donors cannot have underlying heart disease, insulin-dependent diabetes, epilepsy, chronic renal disease, ulcers, bleeding disorders, pregnancy, hepatitis, cancer, or malaria. If a donor has an upper respiratory infection on the day of donation, he/she will be rejected.

Many medications can also affect donor status and so a careful medication history is necessary prior to donation. Persons who take anticoagulants, anticonvulsants (for seizure disorders), drugs of abuse, long-term steroids, tranquilizers, or vasodilators cannot donate blood. Under many circumstances persons who take antibiotics, antihypertensives, antimigraine agents, or fertility drugs can donate blood.

Antecubital veins are used for the phlebotomy (blood drawing). It normally takes only 15 min to complete the entire process. Fatigue and hunger contribute to donor reactions, which usually consist of shocklike symptoms. Donors are given refreshments high in glucose immediately after donation. Blood can be donated every two months.

BLOOD PRODUCTS

Whole Blood

The primary use of whole blood is for the replacement of acute blood-volume losses caused by hemorrhage or trauma. The average blood volume of an adult is 5 L. A sudden loss of 30 percent of this volume requires immediate correction.

A sudden loss of 50 percent can be fatal. Blood volume losses in the range of 500 to 1000 mL, as during surgical procedures, can be managed without blood transfusion by the use of plasma-expanding colloid solutions (dextran) or buffered saline solutions. Whole blood is also essential for exchange and partial-exchange transfusions which remove total or partial blood volume and the substances in that blood which are harmful to the patient. The volume of blood removed is replaced with new blood in increments of 10 to 50 mL depending on the size of the patient. These exchange transfusions are used in the treatment of hemolytic disease of the newborn, such as erythroblastosis fetalis, and in the management of sickle-cell crisis.

Packed Red Cells

In most clinical conditions other than those associated with acute blood-volume loss, the purpose of blood transfusion is to improve the oxygen-carrying capacity of the blood. Because the only component of whole blood having this function is the red cell, transfusion of other blood components is usually unnecessary and can be dangerous because of the presence of antigens and antibodies in the blood. For this reason, red blood cells are separated from the plasma and prepared in a concentrated form. Red blood cells are used for the transfusion treatment of most patients with anemia. Most blood transfusions administered to patients are red cell transfusions.

A hemoglobin less than 6 g/dL usually requires transfusion, although in the absence of physical stress or pulmonary or cardiac disease, most patients tolerate hemoglobin values of 3 to 6 g/dL without developing heart failure. Hence the decision to transfuse should be based on patient status and not solely on level of hemoglobin. A unit of red blood cells has a volume of approximately 300 to 450 mL. Many formulas are used to calculate the total amount of red cells to give to a patient. One simple formula is to estimate that 2 mL of red cells per kilogram of body weight will raise the hemoglobin concentration by 1 g/dL.

Red blood cells can be prepared in special ways to reduce the number of leukocytes contained in the unit in order to avoid reactions. These methods cut down the number of leukocytes contained in each unit of red cells by 50 to 90 percent.

Platelets

Platelet transfusions are usually indicated for patients with thrombocytopenia who are bleeding from their mucous membranes or into the gastrointestinal or genitourinary tract. Central nervous system bleeding requires emergency platelet transfusion. Skin bleeding, such as petechiae or ecchymoses, is so common in these patients that their presence alone is usually not an indication for transfusion. Most patients will not bleed significantly if their platelet count is greater than 50,000/mm³. The risk of serious bleeding increases dramatically as the platelet count drops below 20,000/mm³.

Platelets are usually prepared from a single unit of whole blood by differential centrifugation. The high gravitational force necessary to sediment the platelets results in the release of ADP into the plasma, causing the platelets to aggregate, and so an anticoagulant such as ACD or CPD must be added to prevent platelet clumping. After centrifuge the platelet yield from one unit of whole blood is suspended in 10 to 50 mL of plasma. Each unit of platelets will raise the platelet count of an adult approximately 5000 to 10,000/mm³ under optimal conditions.

Platelets may also be obtained directly from donors by plateletpheresis, a technique in which platelets are separated from whole blood so that the red cells and most of the plasma are returned to the donor. These single-donor platelet transfusions decrease the alloimmunization to platelet antigens that regularly develop in recipients of multiple transfusions and lead to a refractory state in which transfused platelets are rapidly destroyed. A unit of single-donor platelet concentrate contains the equivalent number of platelets contained in 6 to 8 U of random-donor platelet concentrates plus 250 to 350 mL plasma.

Because platelets clump when chilled, concentrates are usually prepared from donor blood before it is refrigerated and are most often stored at 22°C. Platelet transfusions should be administered soon after they are made available since platelet activity diminishes rapidly during storage. Likewise they should be administered at a rapid rate for maximum effectiveness. Normally, transfused platelets have a life span of about 9 to 10 days. Host factors such as sepsis, fever, splenomegaly, or alloimmunization can shorten the survival of transfused platelets. Platelet function is markedly altered following exposure to certain drugs such as **aspirin**, **antihistamines**, **sulfinpyrazone**, **phenylbutazone**, and **dipyridamole**. A sustained rise in the recipient's platelet count is the best indication that transfusion has been successful.

Although matching for ABO groups could readily be accomplished in most blood banks, "incompatible" platelets are often administered. The number of red cells that are infused in platelet packs is so low that hemolytic reactions do not occur. Likewise Rh antigens, on contaminating red cells in the platelet packs, could theoretically sensitize Rh-negative recipients. Adverse reactions to platelet transfusions include the risk of transmission of hepatitis and the risk of bacterial contamination in platelets stored at room temperature. Incompatible platelets are rapidly removed from circulation and there is little systemic reaction associated with their destruction. Symptoms of reaction include only a brief chill or slight elevation in temperature.

Platelets are usually administered through a conventional nylon blood transfusion filter. Special filters designed for platelet transfusion have no particular advantage.

White Blood Cell Transfusions

Patients who are severely neutropenic (generally following administration of chemotherapy), are febrile with documented infection, and have not responded to appropriate antibiotics may benefit from the use of white blood cell transfusions.

Granulocyte transfusion therapy began in the 1960s when large numbers of granulocytes were obtained from patients with chronic granulocytic leukemia who had very high white blood cell counts. These granulocytes were then given to infected neutropenic patients. While only a small percentage of the transfused cells subsequently appeared in the recipients' circulation, many patients responded to the transfusion with reduction in fever and/or clearing of bacteria from the bloodstream.

Because the granulocytes from 30 to 40 U of whole blood from normal donors are needed to provide enough cells for a single granulocyte transfusion, methods have been developed to selectively harvest only granulocytes from normal donors. Commonly used methods for harvesting granulocytes include differential centrifugation and use of nylon fiber filter machines. Both methods enable the same donor to be used repeatedly, even for several days in a row. Machines that employ differential centrifugation pass donor blood into centrifuge bowls that separate platelets, white cells, and red cells on the basis of cell density. The white cells are removed for patient transfusion while the platelets, red cells, and plasma are returned to the donor. Donation involves a 3- to 4-h process as 8 to 14 L of blood are processed. Sometimes donors are treated before the harvesting with corticosteroids to increase the number of circulating granulocytes in their peripheral blood. Machines with nylon fiber filters collect white blood cells as heparinized whole blood passed through the filter with selective adherence of granulocytes and monocytes to the filter fibers. Lymphocytes, red cells, plasma, and platelets are returned to the donor. Use of fiber filters results in a greater white cell yield than is achieved with differential centrifugation but sometimes this method causes cell damage resulting in diminished phagocytic and bactericidal capabilities. White cell donors do not themselves become severely neutropenic and hence are not at increased risk for infection subsequent to donation.

Granulocyte donors should be ABO compatible with the recipient since each unit of granulocytes will contain some 25 to 50 mL of red cells. Likewise, because the recipient is exposed to the donor's granulocyte antigens, the use of family members for donation is theoretically desirable.

One unit of granulocytes (generally 250 to 350 mL volume) is administered slowly over 3 to 6 h. Granulocyte transfusions normally produce chills and fever, and so the occurrence of the symptoms is not necessarily an indication for discontinuing the transfusion. Premedication with an **antihistamine**, **acetaminophen**, and **corticosteroids** may control recipient reactions. Slowing or temporarily stopping the transfusion may also control symptoms. Severe reactions such as fever as high as 105°F, disorientation, dyspnea, bronchoconstriction, or changes in blood pressure warrant cessation of transfusion.

Not all blood banks are capable of processing granulocytes for transfusion. Blood banks have set criteria for patient eligibility for granulocyte transfusion that generally includes low absolute neutrophil count with significant fever and documented infection that has not responded to an appropriate course of antibiotics.

Evaluation of the usefulness of white blood cell transfusions has been difficult because of variation in patient eligibility criteria, cell collection and transfusion procedures, and patients' hematological status. Some researchers are also evaluating the role of prophylactic white blood cell transfusions to prevent infections in neutropenic patients.

Plasma and Plasma Derivatives

Plasma, obtained by centrifugation and separation of the cellular elements from a unit of fresh whole blood, has a volume of approximately 200 mL/U. It may be frozen and stored for one year but must be used within several hours of thawing.

Fresh frozen plasma can be used as a volume expander to replace blood losses when whole blood is unavailable or cannot be properly cross-matched. Fresh plasma contains coagulation factors and can serve as an immediate source of these factors to correct a deficiency and control bleeding episodes in patients with hemophilia A or B. Plasma also contains γ globulins naturally produced by the immune system, to prevent certain infections to which the donor has been previously exposed. It can therefore be used prophylactically in the management of patients with hypogammaglobulinemia to reduce the incidence of life-threatening infections.

Albumin, the major protein in the plasma, is important in maintaining the osmotic pressure of the blood at a level necessary to keep the intravascular volume stable. It is prepared by several methods and is available in concentrations of 5 g/100 mL and 25 g/100 mL. These preparations are used in the treatment of patients in shock and those with hypoalbuminemia caused by lack of albumin production associated with liver disease or to excessive albumin losses in renal disease.

Immunoglobulins and certain **clotting factors** may also be separated from the plasma to prepare concentrated preparations for therapeutic use in deficiency states. **Hepatitis B immune globulin** (human) (HBIG) is used in the prevention of viral hepatitis in persons—e.g., health professionals—who have been exposed to contaminated blood from an infected patient most often through a cut or accidental needle puncture. The usual dose is 0.06 mL/kg of body weight as soon as possible following exposure. A second dose should be administered 28 to 30 days after exposure.

Adverse Reactions of Blood Transfusions

Hemolytic Transfusion Reactions

A hemolytic transfusion reaction is the occurrence of clinical and laboratory signs of red cell destruction following transfusion. The most common cause of a *hemolytic transfusion reaction* is the administration of ABO-incompatible blood. Naturally occurring anti-A and anti-B antibodies will rapidly destroy transfused red cells of the wrong group. The signs and symptoms associated with the administration of incompatible blood generally occur rapidly after the start of the transfusion and include chills and fever, flushing of the face, pain in the back and thighs, tachycardia, rapid respiration, and a feeling of heat along the vein being used for the infusion. If these signs and symptoms are immediately recognized and the blood transfusion stopped, adverse effects may be avoided. Nausea and vomiting with cyanosis may follow along with shock, coma, and failing pulse in severe cases. When the transfusion is discontinued the nurse should check the patient's vital signs, evaluate his or her mental status, and report this information to the physician. Intake and output measurement should be initiated. The blood bank must be informed of the type and severity of the reaction and any remaining blood or blood containers should be returned for evaluation.

Uncontrolled bleeding due to *disseminated intravascular coagulation* (DIC) may result from the release of coagulation-initiating substances from the hemolyzed red blood cells. The extensive production of microclots depletes the circulation of coagulation factors and fibrinogen and thus prevents normal hemostasis and causes profuse spontaneous bleeding. Large amounts of hemoglobin are released from the hemolyzed cells into the plasma (hemoglobinemia), and also enter the urine (hemoglobinuria). Hemoglobinemia can be detected by examining the patient's plasma for the presence of the red hemoglobin after centrifugation. *Renal failure* can result from the precipitation of hemoglobin and heme pigments in the renal tubules and from the decreased renal blood flow caused by peripheral vascular failure.

Rh-type incompatibility reactions can also occur. Rapid hemolysis generally does not occur because the anti-Rh antibodies are small. They attach to the Rh-positive red cells, which are then hemolyzed and removed by the reticuloendothelial system. These reactions are usually mild; they can however, be lethal, as in erythroblastosis fetalis.

Delayed transfusion reactions may occur between 1 and 14 days after the administration of incompatible blood, with a falling hematocrit, jaundice, and hemoglobinuria as the first signs of significant red blood cell hemolysis. The delay in the hemolytic reaction may be due to initially low antibody concentrations in the serum of the recipient which cause little or no red cell destruction. The transfused red cells will, however, stimulate antibody production, and as the antibody concentration increases over the next several days, hemolysis will increase and the signs and symptoms of transfusion reaction will develop. Most delayed hemolytic reactions are benign because of the relatively slow extravascular destruction of red cells.

The treatment of hemolytic transfusion reactions is directed at preventing the development of renal complications. This can be accomplished by maintaining renal blood flow and preventing or decreasing the precipitation of hemoglobin and heme pigments in the renal tubules. An osmotic diuretic such as **mannitol** can be used to maintain urine flow, glomerular filtration, and renal blood flow if urine output is decreasing. The dose of mannitol is approximately 25 g of a 20% solution infused over a 5-min period. This dose may be repeated if no urine flow occurs, but no more than four 25-g doses should be given in a 24-h period. The pediatric dose of mannitol is 1.5 g/kg infused over a 20-min period. Mannitol is contraindicated if the patient is in heart failure or if acute renal tubular necrosis has occurred. A potent diuretic, such as **furosemide** (Lasix), may also be used in a dose of 40 to 80 mg IV. This dose may be doubled and repeated if a satisfactory response does not occur after the initial dose. The pediatric dose for furosemide is 1 to 2 mg/kg, with a repeat dose, if necessary, of 2 to 4 mg/kg.

Adequate fluid replacement is also necessary to induce and maintain urine output. One liter of 5 **dextrose in 0.45** (½) **NS** should be infused over 1 h, with an additional 500 mL given if there is no response. Additional intravenous fluids should not be given if urine output is inadequate. If diuresis begins, the urine output can be maintained by administering intravenous fluids at a rate of 100 mL/h. The pediatric fluid dose is 3000 mL/m² of body surface area/24 h.

The precipitation of hemoglobin and heme pigments is promoted by an acid urine, and for this reason the urine should be alkalinized by the oral or intravenous administration of **sodium bicarbonate** in a dose of 4 to 5 g initially. The urine pH can then be checked and maintained greater than a pH of 7 by doses of 1 to 2 g sodium bicarbonate every 4 to 6 h.

Nonhemolytic Transfusion Reactions

A *nonhemolytic transfusion reaction* is most often due to the recipient's sensitivity to transfused donor platelets, white blood cells, or other plasma constituents.

Febrile Transfusion Reactions These reactions constitute the bulk of those reported to the blood bank and are caused by donor or recipient antibodies directed against antigens present on leukocytes or platelets. The reactions can occur during or shortly after transfusion and usually consist of shaking chills and a 2 to 3°F rise in temperature that returns to normal within a few hours. **Acetaminophen** is useful in controlling the symptoms of febrile transfusion reactions. Patients who experience these reactions should be considered as candidates for spin filter blood products in the future.

Allergic Transfusion Reactions These reactions occur most often in patients who have a history of allergy or hypersensitivity. They are most often characterized by urticaria and itching which can be managed with antihistamines such as **diphenhydramine** (Benadryl), in a dose of 50 to 100 mg orally or parenterally, depending on the severity of the reaction. The pediatric dose is 1 to 2 mg/kg.

Respiratory complications, including bronchoconstriction and anaphylaxis, due to an allergic reaction can be life-threatening but generally respond well to epinephrine 1:1000 solution in a dose of 0.1 to 0.3 mL administered subcutaneously at 15- to 30-min intervals up to a total of three doses. If bronchoconstriction continues to be a problem, a continuous intravenous infusion of **aminophylline** can be started. Parenteral corticosteroids, such as **methylprednisolone** (Solu-Medrol), may also be required in severe cases.

Miscellaneous Transfusion Complications

Circulatory Overload This situation can result when a large volume of blood is transfused in a short time period, and can be especially dangerous in the patient with compromised cardiac function and may cause pulmonary edema and death. This complication can generally be avoided by using packed red blood cells instead of whole blood and by decreasing the rate of transfusion.

Metabolic Complications These are associated with massive transfusions of CPD-anticoagulated blood, because of the effect of sodium citrate on the serum calcium concentration and the acid-base balance of the patient. The signs and symptoms of *hypocalcemia* can be minimized by the intravenous administration of 10 mL of 10% **calcium gluconate** for every two units of transfused blood. This solution, however, must not be added directly to the transfused blood and should not be administered faster than 1 to 2 mL/min. A significant increase in the serum potassium level, *hyperkalemia*, may also result from the massive transfusion of blood that is near its expiration date. A unit of blood that is 10 to 14 days old may contain up to 10 meq of potassium that has been released from hemolyzed red cells. A transfusion of multiple units of such blood may therefore cause severe hyperkalemia.

Bacterial Reactions Such reactions are caused by the transfusion of contaminated blood products. These reactions can be prevented by use of careful aseptic techniques during transfusion, proper refrigeration of blood products, and double checking the expiration date on all blood products. Signs and symptoms of a bacterial reaction include fever, shaking chills, severe hypotension, skin flushing, abdominal pain, pain in the extremities, and nausea and vomiting. If these reactions occur, the transfusion should be stopped immediately and appropriate intravenous broad-spectrum antibiotic therapy should be initiated.

The *transmission of infectious disease* is a potential complication of blood transfusions. The most common infectious disease is viral hepatitis. The amount of blood on the tip of a contaminated needle can be sufficient to cause clinical hepatitis. The serum of all blood donors is screened for the presence of viral hepatitis antibodies, but the test does not detect the presence of the actual virus. If the antibodies are not present at the time of blood donation, an infected donor can supply blood contaminated with hepatitis virus and still have a negative antibody screen. Because no completely accurate method of detecting the hepatitis virus is available, the risk associated with blood transfusions continues.

Blood products prepared from the pooled plasma of multiple donors, such as coagulation-factor concentrates, carry a much greater risk of transmitting viral hepatitis to the recipient because of the increased number of potentially infected donors.

Transmission of other infectious diseases by blood or blood products, although rare, is possible. Malaria and cytomegalic inclusion disease are examples of such diseases. Acquired immune deficiency syndrome, AIDS, can also be transmitted by blood and blood products with cases being reported in hemophilic children. Posttransfusion syphilis has been nearly eliminated by the serologic testing of donors and of all units of blood prior to their release from the blood bank.

NURSING PROCESS RELATED TO BLOOD PRODUCT TRANSFUSIONS

Nurses employ nursing process both with the donors of blood products and for patients receiving transfusions. While it is critical to the donor and the recipient that the nurse collecting blood meticulously perform the assessment described in the section on blood donation, above, this discussion will focus on the blood transfusion procedure.

Assessment

Before the transfusion is begun, the unit of blood, packed cells, or other blood product must be identified as the correct unit ordered for the patient. All forms provided by the blood bank and information on the label of the blood product must be checked by two specified persons, according to hospital policy, with the wristband of the recipient. This double check is imperative to prevent avoidable errors. The transfusion record is then signed by both persons. The baseline vital signs of the patient, including blood pressure, pulse, and temperature, are recorded before the transfusion is started.

Management

An intravenous infusion, using a blood administration set with a standard in-line filter to remove microclots and any particulate matter, is begun with an appropriate solution. Not all intravenous solutions are suitable for use with blood products. **Isotonic saline solution** is completely compatible, but **dextrose 5% in water** will hemolyze red blood cells and must never be used. Intravenous solutions containing calcium, such as **lactated Ringer's**, should also be avoided, because the calcium present can cause the blood to clot if mixing takes place. Most drugs in concentrated form may injure red blood cells and should never be added directly to blood for transfusion. Prior to administration, the unit of blood should be mixed thoroughly, by gently inverting it several times. Blood must be transfused as soon as it arrives at the patient's unit unless approved 4°C refrigeration is available.

The first 25 to 50 mL of blood should be infused slowly over approximately 30 min (a lesser amount would be given to children) as a test for an acute untoward reaction. The remainder of the blood can be infused at a faster rate since the longer the transfusion time the greater the potential for bacterial growth within the unit of blood. Children and patients with a limited cardiac reserve must receive transfusions at a slower rate, but the transfusion must be completed within no more than 4 h.

A unit of **packed red blood cells** may be mixed with 50 to 100 mL of normal saline solution at the time of administration to decrease the viscosity of the red cells and permit a more rapid infusion rate.

If multiple units of blood are to be administered in a short time, the blood can be warmed to room temperature by a blood-warming coil or other special device to prevent possible adverse cardiovascular effects that may result from a rapid decrease in the blood temperature.

The amount of whole blood or packed cells necessary to increase the hemoglobin to a desired level can be calculated from the fact that 3 mL of packed cells or 6 mL of whole blood per kilogram of body weight will raise the hemoglobin concentration by approximately 1 g/100 mL. Therefore, to raise the hemoglobin concentration of a 70-kg man by 1 g/dL, 420 mL of whole blood would be required.

Evaluation

The patient's vital signs should be recorded at 30-min intervals and the urine output and other signs monitored for signs of a transfusion reaction (nausea, vomiting, chills, fever, tachycardia, pain in the back, tachypnea, flushed face, shock, decreased urine output, etc.). The infusion rate should be checked frequently. When the transfusion has ended, the appropriate forms must be completed and returned with the empty container to the blood bank. The patient should also be monitored for several more hours for a delayed transfusion reaction.

REFERENCES

Beal, R. W.: "Hematinics: Patho-physiological and Clinical Aspects," *Drugs,* 2:190, 1971.

Buchanan, G. R.: "Hemophilia," *Pediatr Clin North Am,* 27:309–325, 1980.

Buchholz, D. H.: "Blood Groups and Blood Component Transfusion," in D. R. Miller, H. A. Pearson, R. L. Baehner, and C. W. McMillan (eds.), *Smith's Blood Diseases of Infancy and Childhood,* 4th ed., St. Louis: Mosby, 1978.

Buickus, B. A.: "Administering Blood Components," *Am J Nurs,* 79:937–941, 1979.

Charache, S.: "The Treatment of Sickle Cell Anemia," *Arch Intern Med,* 133:698, 1974.

Charlton, R. W., and T. H. Bothwell: "Iron Deficiency Anemia," *Semin Hematol,* 7:67, 1970.

Child, J., D. Collins, and J. Collins: "Blood Transfusions," *Am J Nurs,* 72:1602, 1972.

Cullins, L. C.: "Preventing and Treating Transfusion Reactions," *Am J Nurs,* 79:935–936, 1979.

Garratty, G., and L. D. Petz: "Drug-Induced Immune Hemolytic Anemia," *Am J Med,* 58:398, 1975.

Girdwood, R. H.: "Drug-Induced Anaemias," *Drugs,* 11:394, 1976.

Handin, R. I.: "Platelet Transfusions," in D. G. Nathan and F. O. Oski (eds.), *Hematology of Infancy and Childhood,* Philadelphia: Saunders, 1974.

Kazak, A.: "Processing Blood for Transfusion," *Am J Nurs,* 79:931–934, 1979.

Lipton, J. M., and D. G. Nathan: "Aplastic and Hypoplastic Anemia," *Pediatr Clin North Am* 27:217–235, 1980.

O'Reilly, R. J., and M. Sorell: "Aplastic Anemia and Bone Marrow Transplantation," in D. R. Miller, H. A. Pearson, R. L. Baehner, and C. W. McMillan (eds.), *Smith's Diseases of Infancy and Childhood,* 4th ed., St. Louis: Mosby, 1978.

Oski, F.: "Red Cell Transfusion and Phlebotomy," in D. G. Nathan and F. O. Oski (eds.), *Hematology of Infancy and Childhood,* Philadelphia: Saunders, 1974.

Parker, A. L.: "Massive Transfusion," *Am J Nurs,* 79:944–948, 1979.

Patterson, L. E., and P. G. Rigby: "Aplastic Anemia," *J Am Pharm Assoc,* NS14:417, 1974.

Rossman, M., R. Seavin, and E. G. Taft: "Pheresis Therapy: Patient Care," *Am J Nurs,* 77:1135–1141, 1977.

Rutman, R., C. Hyatt, W. V. Miller, and E. White: "Screening Donors and the Phlebotomy Procedure," *Am J Nurs,* 79:926–930, 1979.

Schreiber, A. D.: "Autoimmune Hemolytic Anemia," *Pediatr Clin North Am,* 27:253–265, 1980.

Streiff, R. R.: "Folic Acid Deficiency Anemia," *Semin Hematol,* 7:23, 1970.

Sullivan, L. W.: "Vitamin B_{12} Metabolism and Megaloblastic Anemia," *Semin Hematol,* 7:6, 1970.

Swanson, M.: "Drugs, Chemicals and Hemolysis," *Drug Intell Clin Pharm,* 7:6, 1973.

Vaz, D.: "The Common Anemias: Nursing Approaches," *Nurs Clin North Am,* 7:711, 1972.

Wintrobe, M. M., et al.: *Clinical Hematology,* 7th ed., Philadelphia: Lea & Febiger, 1974.

37

NEOPLASTIC DISORDERS

ROBERT J. STAGG
CAROL S. VIELE
ROBERT J. IGNOFFO

LEARNING OBJECTIVES

Upon completion of this chapter the reader will be able to:

1. List and describe the phases of the cell cycle and their importance to the treatment of neoplastic disorders.

2. Define the cell-kill hypothesis and how it applies to the use of chemotherapy.

3. Explain the rationale for combination chemotherapy.

4. Explain the rationale for adjuvant chemotherapy.

5. Describe the rationale of regional drug administration.

6. List the major pharmacologic classes of chemotherapeutic agents and their mechanism of action.

7. Describe the major toxicities associated with the commonly used chemotherapeutic agents.

8. Delineate the nursing role in the assessment, management, and evaluation of the major toxicities associated with chemotherapeutic agents.

9. Calculate the appropriate drug dosage for a patient by both the body surface area (mg/m^2) and body weight (mg/kg) methods.

10. List the commonly used antineoplastics which are vesicants and techniques to prevent and treat extravasation of these drugs.

Cancer is the second leading cause of mortality in the United States, accounting for approximately 400,000 deaths annually. Many therapeutic modalities have been employed in the treatment of cancer including surgical resection, radiation therapy, immunotherapy, and chemotherapy. In the past decades, chemotherapy has greatly improved the cure rate and survival of several neoplastic disorders including adult and childhood leukemias, Hodgkin's disease, non-Hodgkin's lymphoma, and testicular carcinoma. This chapter focuses on the role of the nurse in the use of chemotherapy in the management of cancer.

TYPES OF NEOPLASTIC DISORDERS

The literal translation of the Greek word neoplasia is "new form." A neoplasm may be defined as an abnormal group of cells which behave much like a parasite, enlarging in an uncontrolled manner, competing for host nutrients, developing a degree of autonomy, and ultimately threatening host survival. Neoplasms are classified as either benign or malignant based on the pathologic characteristics of the tumor (Table 37-1). The term *cancer* is reserved for those neoplasms classified as malignant. The following is a discussion of the most common cancers, including those of the skin, lung, colon and rectum, lymph nodes, and bone marrow. For a more complete review of these neoplasms and a discussion of those not mentioned, the reader is referred to other texts and references.

Skin Cancer

There are approximately 300,000 new cases of skin cancer (nonmelanoma) each year in the United States, making it the most prevalent neoplasm. There are several causes of this disorder, including chemical carcinogenesis, ultraviolet light, ionizing radiation, and immunodeficiency. Nonmelanomatous skin cancer is divided into two types, basal cell and squamous cell carcinomas. Both of these subtypes are considered curable unless diagnosed at a very advanced stage. In most instances, the cancerous lesions can be surgically excised. Curettage, cryosurgery, and radiation are useful for those lesions which are unresectable. Chemotherapy can be used in the treatment of basal cell carcinoma.

Lung Cancer

Lung cancer is the most common noncutaneous malignancy in the United States. There are approximately 130,000 new cases and 111,000 deaths annually as a result of this malignancy. The World Health Organization (WHO) has classified lung cancer into 12 subtypes. The four most common

729

TABLE 37-1 Characteristics of Benign and Malignant Neoplasms

BENIGN	MALIGNANT
Encapsulated	Nonencapsulated
Noninvasive	Invasive
Well-differentiated	Poorly differentiated
Slowly growing	Rapidly growing
Nonmetastasizing	Metastasizing

Source: Modifed from H. L. Pitot: *Fundamentals of Oncology,* New York: Marcel Dekker, 1978.

carcinomas are squamous cell, small cell ("oat cell"), adenomatous, and large cell. The development of a pulmonary neoplasm is usually the result of a repetitive injury, such as that caused by cigarette smoking or asbestos exposure. Surgical resection of the tumor is the cornerstone of therapy. Chemotherapy and radiation are used to treat those patients having unresectable tumors or disseminated disease. The therapy for lung cancer is not usually successful, since at the time of diagnosis the disease is usually too advanced.

Colorectal Cancer

Colorectal cancer is the third most common cancer in the United States, with approximately 120,000 new cases per year. Dietary and genetic factors are believed to play major roles in the etiology of this malignancy. Surgical resection of the primary tumor site is the treatment of choice. Unfortunately, metastatic disease is often found at the time of presentation or develops following surgical resection. The most common sites of metastases are the liver, lymph nodes, peritoneum, lung, and adrenals. Metastatic colorectal cancer is often refractory to all types of therapy. Recently, there has been some success in managing liver metastases with hepatic intraarterial chemotherapy.

Breast Cancer

About one in eleven women will develop breast cancer making it the most common cancer among women. There are approximately 113,000 new cases of breast cancer each year. Women at high risk include those over the age of 50, those with a family history of breast cancer, those who never had children, and those that had their first child after age 30. Breast changes which may be consistent with cancer include lumps, swelling, dimpling, pain or tenderness, retraction or scaling of the nipple, or nipple discharge. Breast self-examination remains the best method for early detection. Surgical resection of the primary tumor using mastectomy with lymph node dissection is the therapeutic modality of choice, although recently less extensive surgery has been used. Radiation, chemotherapy, and hormonal manipulation are used for those patients with a high risk of recurrence, locally unresectable disease, or distant metastases. Breast reconstruction is gaining wider application among patients who remain disease-free after therapy.

Leukemias

The leukemias are a group of hematologic malignancies of the bone marrow characterized by morphologic and quantitative alterations in the blood cells and their precursors, in particular the white blood cells. About 25,000 cases of leukemia were diagnosed in 1982. They are classified into acute and chronic types according to the predominant cell type involved and the disease characteristics. Acute leukemia is further subclassified into acute lymphocytic leukemia (ALL), which frequently occurs in children and may be curable, and acute nonlymphocytic leukemia (ANLL), which is more common in adults and has a less promising prognosis. The chronic leukemias include chronic lymphocytic (CLL), which primarily affects the elderly and has a long, slow, progressive course, and chronic myelocytic (CML). Chemotherapy (sometimes in combination with total body irradiation and bone marrow transplantation) is the cornerstone of therapy for all leukemia with the exact treatment being dictated by the type and stage of the disease. Serial bone marrow aspiration and biopsy is used to evaluate treatment response. Surgery has no utility in the management of these neoplasms, while radiation is commonly used to prevent and treat meningeal leukemia, the occurrence of leukemia cells in the cerebral spinal fluid.

Lymphomas

Primary malignancies involving the lymph nodes of a patient are called lymphomas. There are approximately 30,000 new cases of lymphomas annually in the United States. These neoplasms are subdivided into Hodgkin's disease (HL) and non-Hodgkin's lymphomas (NHL). Etiologic factors for lymphomas may include radiation exposure, certain viral infections, and hereditary predisposition. Following diagnosis, both HL and NHL are surgically staged according to the extent of organ and lymphatic involvement. Early stage lymphomas confined to a regional chain of lymph nodes are commonly treated with radiation therapy. Combination chemotherapy is used for more advanced disease.

PRINCIPLES OF CELL BIOLOGY

In order to understand the rationale for anticancer drug therapy, it is necessary to have a knowledge of some principles of cellular biology. This section includes a discussion of cell growth (kinetics), of normal and cancer cells, and drug action in relation to the cell cycle.

Normal Cell Growth

The cell cycle is depicted in Fig. 37-1. Nonproliferating cells are in the G_0 phase, or resting phase. Cells which are

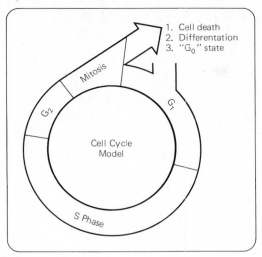

FIGURE 37-1

Phases of the Cell Cycle: G_0, resting phase; G_1, presynthetic phase, S, DNA synthesis phase; G_2, Premitotic phase, and mitosis cell division. [Source: R. J. Ignoffo: "Oncology" in B. S. Katcher, L. Y. Young, and M. A. Koda-Kimble (eds.) *Applied Therapeutics: The Clinical Use of Drugs,* 3d ed, San Francisco: Applied Therapeutics, Inc., 1983. Used by permission.]

undergoing replication proceed systematically through the four phases of the cycle. The first is the G_1 phase, or presynthetic phase, which is highly variable in length and involves the development of the many enzymes that are necessary for DNA synthesis. Next is the S phase, or synthesis phase, which lasts from 10 to 20 h. In this phase, the DNA content of the cell is doubled. The cell then enters into the G_2 phase, or premitotic phase, which is relatively short (2 to 10 h) and involves RNA synthesis and the formation of the spindle apparatus. At this point, the cell enters into the M phase, or mitotic phase, which lasts for about 1 h. In this phase, the parent cell divides into two daughter cells. The two daughter cells may then either proceed through the cell cycle or enter the G_0 phase.

Cancer Cell Growth

Two major concepts concerning the growth of malignant cells include growth fraction and doubling time. The term *growth fraction* is used to describe the percentage of tumor cells that are actively dividing. The *doubling time,* which is inversely related to the growth fraction, is the time required for a specific number of tumor cells to double their mass. In general, hematologic tumors, such as leukemias, have a high growth fraction compared to solid tumors, such as breast and colon carcinomas, or melanoma, which have low growth fractions (see Table 37-2). Response to chemotherapy generally occurs more readily in high growth-fraction tumors since chemotherapeutic agents kill tumor cells more effectively when the cells are actively dividing.

TABLE 37-2 Growth Characteristics of Various Tumors

TUMOR	GROWTH FRACTION, %	DOUBLING TIME, DAYS
Breast cancer	1	55
Colon cancer	4	13.5
Melanoma	3.3	18.5
Lymphocytic leukemia	50	4
Lymphoma	32	1.9

Source: G. Steel: "Cytokinetics and Neoplasia," in J. F. Holland and E. J. Frei (eds.), *Cancer Medicine,* Philadelphia: Lea and Febiger, 1973. (Data from G. Steel: "Cell Loss as a Factor in Growth Rate of Human Tumors," *Europ J Cancer,* **3**:381, 1967 and J. J. Fabreikant and J. Cherry: "The Kinetics of Cellular Proliferation in Normal and Malignant Tissues," *V J Surg Oncol,* **1**:23, 1969.)

As a tumor enlarges, its growth fraction decreases and its doubling time increases. This phenomenon has been demonstrated in several animal and human tumors and is called Gompertzian growth (Fig. 37-2). This is the principle behind debulking surgery, which is used to decrease the total number of malignant cells, stimulating the remaining cells in the G_0 phase to enter the cell cycle, rendering them more vulnerable to subsequent chemotherapy.

Drugs and the Cell Cycle

Antineoplastics that kill cells only during a specific phase of the cell cycle are termed *cell-cycle specific* (CCS). CCS agents are most effective when administered by continuous infusion

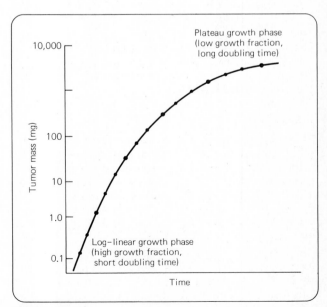

FIGURE 37-2

Gompertzian Cell Growth. The graph illustrates decreasing growth fraction and increasing doubling time.

which provides a prolonged drug exposure to the tumor. Agents that kill tumor cells in any phase of the cycle are called *cell-cycle-nonspecific* (CCNS) agents. In contrast, CCNS agents produce a more effective cell kill when administered as a large intermittent bolus. The degree of cell kill is proportional to the dose given. Table 37-3 provides a list of CCS and CCNS agents.

PRINCIPLES OF CANCER CHEMOTHERAPY

The Cell-Kill Hypothesis
The cell-kill hypothesis states that a constant fraction of tumor cells will be killed each time an antineoplastic drug is administered, provided that the dose remains the same. The essential element of this hypothesis is that some cells survive a course of treatment purely by chance, even though all cells may be sensitive. For example, if a treatment regimen decreases the tumor cell population by 50 percent on the first course of therapy, the surviving fraction of cells may be reduced again by 50 percent from each subsequent course of treatment. Continued objective remission will occur only if response is obtained with subsequent courses of treatment. Cure can be achieved when the tumor burden has become low enough for the host's own immune system to eradicate the remaining tumor cells.

TABLE 37-3 Classification of Antineoplastic Drugs by Cell-Cycle Action

CELL-CYCLE-SPECIFIC AGENTS (CCS)	CELL-CYCLE-NONSPECIFIC AGENTS (CCNS)
Asparaginase	Actinomycin D
Azathioprine	Bleomycin*
Bleomycin*	Busulfan
Cytarabine	Carmustine (BCNU)
Etoposide	Chlorambucil
Fluorouracil (5-FU)	Cisplatin
Floxuridine	Cyclophosphamide
Hydroxyurea	Dacarbazine (DTIC)
Mercaptopurine	Daunorubicin
Methotrexate	Doxorubicin
Thioguanine	Hexamethylmelamine
Vinblastine	Lomustine (CCNU)
Vincristine	Melphalan (L-PAM)
Vindesine	Nitrogen mustard
	Procarbazine
	Triethylene thiophosphoramide (TEPA)

*Bleomycin has properties of both CCS and CCNS.

Source: R. J. Ignoffo: "Oncology," in B. S. Katcher, L. Y. Young, and M. A. Koda-Kimble (eds.), *Applied Therapeutics: The Clinical Use of Drugs,* 3d ed., San Francisco: Applied Therapeutics, Inc., 1983. Used by permission.

Clinical Response to Chemotherapy
A standard set of criteria are used by the oncologist to assess patient response to chemotherapy. *Complete remission* is defined as the disappearance of all measurable disease assessed by physical examination, chest x-rays, scans, and laboratory tests. In most cases, complete remission is associated with an increased disease-free interval and survival. *Disease-free interval* is the term which describes the period of no measurable disease. *Partial remission* is defined as an objective decrease of greater than 50 percent of measurable tumor, lasting for at least one month. For some tumors, partial remission translates into a prolonged survival. Patients with stable disease have no objective change in their measurable tumor burden, which occasionally results in prolonged survival. *Progressive disease* is defined as a greater than a 25 percent increase in measurable disease.

THE CLINICAL USE OF CHEMOTHERAPEUTIC AGENTS

There are four major modalities used in the treatment of cancer: surgery, radiation, immunotherapy, and chemotherapy. Surgery and radiation are curative only for localized malignancies. Currently, in most neoplastic disorders, immunotherapy offers little benefit. Chemotherapy affords a modality of cancer treatment which can be used alone or in combination with surgery and/or radiation to achieve cure, control, or palliation of a malignancy (Table 37-4).

Single-Agent Chemotherapy
For most malignancies a combination of drugs offers the best chance for response. There are, however, some neoplastic disorders such as colorectal cancer for which single-agent therapy is as effective and is associated with fewer toxicities than combination therapy. In addition, single-agent therapy is often used to treat those patients unable to tolerate combination therapy. This includes patients who have received extensive prior radiation or chemotherapy or have a poor Karnofsky performance status. The Karnofsky performance status is a rating scale of the patient's functional level (Table 37-5).

Combination Chemotherapy
Combination chemotherapy was designed because of the poor results obtained with single-agent therapy for many neoplastic disorders. The following principles should be considered when selecting drugs for combination therapy:

1. Each drug must have demonstrated activity in the particular malignant disorder.
2. The combination should have additive or synergistic action.

3. The drugs should not have overlapping toxicities.

4. Each drug should be administered in a dose which is close to the maximum tolerated dose when administered as a single agent.

5. The drugs should be administered in the most effective schedule.

The use of these principles may be illustrated by analyzing the MOPP regimen used for Hodgkin's disease. **Nitrogen mustard** (M) is bone marrow suppressive; **vincristine** (O) is primarily neurotoxic; **procarbazine** (P) is mildly marrow suppressive; and **prednisone** (P) is mildly immunosuppressive in short-course therapy. Because each agent has different major dose-limiting toxicities, they can be used in their full "single-agent" dosage. All of these agents have limited activity when administered alone; however, when combined, a complete response rate of 60 to 80 percent is obtained.

TABLE 37-4   Neoplastic Diseases Which Respond to Chemotherapy

TYPE OF CANCER	USEFUL DRUGS
Prolonged Survival or Cure	
Gestational trophoblastic tumors	Methotrexate, dactinomycin, vinblastine, cisplatin
Testicular tumors	Dactinomycin,* methotrexate,* chlorambucil,* cisplatin, Etoposide
Wilms' tumor	Dactinomycin (with surgery and radiotherapy)
Neuroblastoma	Cyclophosphamide (with surgery and/or radiotherapy)
Acute lymphoblastic leukemia	Daunorubicin,* prednisone,* vincristine,* mercaptopurine,* methotrexate,* L-asparaginase
Hodgkin's disease Stage IIIB & IV	Mechlorethamine,* vincristine,* doxorubicin, prednisone,* procarbazine,* bleomycin, dacarbazine
Palliation and Prolongation of Life	
Prostate carcinoma	Estrogens, with orchiectomy
Breast carcinoma	Androgens, estrogens, alkylating agents,* fluorouracil,* vincristine,* prednisone,* methotrexate* (with surgery and/or radiotherapy), adriamycin
Chronic lymphocytic leukemia	Prednisone, alkylating agents
Acute nonlymphocytic leukemia	Cytarabine and 6-thioguanine, daunorubicin

*May be used as one agent in combination chemotherapy.

TABLE 37-5   Karnofsky Performance Scale

LEVEL OF ACTIVITY	RATING, %
Normal	100
Able to carry on normal activity, minor signs or symptoms	90
Normal activities with effort	80
Cares for self, but cannot do active work	70
Requires occasional assistance, but able to do most self care	60
Requires frequent assistance	50
Disabled; requires visiting nurse	40
Severely disabled, death not imminent	30
Hospitalization required	20
Moribund	10
Dead	0

Combination therapy has increased the response rate of a number of malignant disorders including leukemia, lymphoma, Hodgkin's disease, and carcinomas of the breast, testes, and lung.

Adjuvant Chemotherapy

There is a high incidence of relapse for some cancers following the irradiation of all clinically apparent disease. This is most likely due to the presence of residual microscopic malignant cells in the systemic or lymphatic circulation. Adjuvant chemotherapy is administered to patients in complete remission in an attempt to destroy these remaining undetectable cells. The two types of cancer which have shown improved survival following adjuvant chemotherapy are breast carcinoma and osteogenic sarcoma. The role of adjuvant therapy in colon cancer and various sarcomas is currently being investigated.

Regional Chemotherapy

The rationale for choosing regional administration over standard intravenous administration is that it delivers a higher drug concentration directly into the tumor tissue, while sparing normal tissue. Regional therapy includes intraarterial, intraperitoneal, intrathecal, intrapleural, and intrapericardial chemotherapy.

Intraarterial Chemotherapy

Cancers which are not adequately controlled by systemic chemotherapy may respond to chemotherapy administered directly into the artery supplying the tumor. This method of administration presents the tumor with a drug concentration severalfold higher than intravenous administration. Intraarterial treatment is most successful for tumors supplied by a single artery. In general, the smaller the artery feeding the tumor, the greater the drug concentration and thus the greater the potential therapeutic advantage. Second, by administering the drug regionally into an artery, systemic exposure, and therefore systemic toxicity, may be minimized, especially if the tumor extracts the drug. Diseases which are treated with this approach include primary or metastatic liver cancer, malignant melanoma, soft-tissue limb sarcoma, and local pelvic tumors.

Intraperitoneal Chemotherapy

Some cancers, such as ovarian carcinoma, may remain localized within the peritoneal cavity and result in morbidity and mortality through local invasion or obstruction. Intraperitoneal therapy may be used to deliver a high concentration of drug to the tumors lining the peritoneal wall. Studies using **cisplatin, bleomycin,** and **phenylalanine mustard** (L-PAM) are ongoing to determine if the response rate with intraperitoneal therapy is superior to traditional intravenous chemotherapy.

Intrathecal/Intraventricular Chemotherapy

Several malignancies, including acute lymphocytic leukemia, lymphoblastic lymphoma, and small cell lung cancer, can metastasize to the intrathecal space resulting in meningeal disease. Because most antineoplastic drugs do not cross the blood-brain barrier, direct intrathecal or intraventricular injection is used to obtain appropriate drug levels in the cerebrospinal fluid. The introduction of drugs into the intrathecal space may be accomplished by a direct lumbar injection at the third lumbar space. Some patients with meningeal disease may receive intraventricular chemotherapy through the use of an Ommaya reservoir, a 3-mL chamber connected to a short catheter that is implanted into the third ventricle. The drugs most frequently administered by this route are **methotrexate, cytarabine,** and **triethylenethiophosphoramide** (TEPA).

Intrapleural Chemotherapy

Malignancies, including lymphomas and carcinomas of the breast, lung, and ovary, commonly metastasize to the pleural cavity causing a malignant effusion. Treatment of the effusion may require systemic chemotherapy, intrapleural chemotherapy, or occasionally, surgery. For nonsymptomatic pleural effusion, systemic chemotherapy is used, especially for rapidly responsive tumors such as in Hodgkin's disease. Refractory effusions require intrapleural instillation of a sclerosing agent, resulting in an adhesive pleuritis which decreases the reaccumulation of pleural fluid and leads to pleural fibrosis. The most commonly used sclerosing agent,

tetracycline, is more efficient and less toxic than the other sclerosing agents—**mechlorethamine, TEPA,** and **bleomycin.** The dose of **tetracycline,** 500 to 2000 mg, is dissolved in 50 mL of 50% dextrose. Following drainage of the effusion, this mixture is instilled into the pleural cavity via a chest tube and the patient rotated to different positions every 15 min for 1 h in order to distribute the drug to all pleural surfaces. The dosages of **mechlorethamine, TEPA,** and **bleomycin** range from 10 to 20 mg. The major side effect of this type of local chemotherapy is pleuritic pain. It is recommended that narcotic analgesics be given prior to treatment. It must be emphasized that significant systemic absorption of both **mechlorethamine** and **TEPA** may occur resulting in hematopoetic or gastrointestinal toxicity.

Intrapericardial Chemotherapy

A variety of tumors can metastasize to the pericardium, including breast cancer, lung cancer, Hodgkin's disease, non-Hodgkin's lymphoma, melanoma, sarcoma, and leukemia. Metastatic disease to the pericardium may occur by either direct extension of an adjacent primary or by lymphatic or hematogenous spread. Pericardial metastasis commonly results in a pericardial effusion. Like intrapleural therapy, several sclerosing agents have been instilled into pericardium to control recurrent effusions. **Tetracycline, mechlorethamine, TEPA,** and **fluorouracil** (5-FU) are effective in about 50 percent of patients. External beam radiation may be effective for patients with effusions caused by lymphomatous or leukemic infiltration.

Adverse Effects

The adverse effects of cytotoxic drugs can manifest as acute, delayed, or chronic toxicities. *Acute toxicities* include emesis, hypersensitivity reactions (fever, rash, and anaphylaxis), or cardiovascular complications (arrhythmias). The most common of the acute toxicities is emesis. *Delayed toxicities* from chemotherapy may include mucositis, alopecia (hair loss), or bone marrow suppression (suppressed blood cell production). For many antineoplastic drugs, either mucositis or bone marrow suppression is the dose-limiting toxicity. Mucositis presents as mouth sores, gastric pain, or diarrhea. Bone marrow suppression is manifested by a decrease in peripheral leukocytes, platelets, or erythrocytes. The *nadir* is defined as the lowest level of the peripheral cell counts. The *chronic toxicities* caused by cytotoxic drugs involve damage to organ systems such as the heart, lung, liver, or kidney. They may limit the total lifetime dose.

CHEMOTHERAPEUTIC AGENTS

The mechanism of action, adverse effects, phase specificity, and composition of various groups of chemotherapeutic agents are summarized in Table 37-6.

TABLE 37-6 Drugs Used to Treat Neoplasms

DRUGS	PHASE ACTION	MECHANISM	ADVERSE EFFECTS
Alkylating Agents			
Nitrogen Mustards Mechlorethamine (Mustargen) Cyclophosphamide (Cytoxan) Busulfan (Myleran) Chlorambucil (Leukeran) Melphalan (Alkeran) Uracil mustard	CCNS	Add a chemical group (alkyl) to DNA causing breakage	Leukopenia, thrombocytopenia; anorexia, nausea, vomiting; vesicants; alopecia; hemorrhagic cystitis (cyclophosphamide); pulmonary fibrosis (busulfan); congestive heart failure (cyclophosphamide).
Nitrosoureas Carmustine (BCNU, BiCNU) Lomustine (CCNU) Streptozocin (Zanosar)	CCNS	Alkylators, inhibit DNA synthesis	Leukopenia, thrombocytopenia; nausea, vomiting, anorexia; confusion, lethargy; nephrotoxicity (streptozocin).
Other Alkylators Triethylenethiophosphoramide (ThioTEPA, TEPA) Dacarbazine (DTIC) Cisplatin (Platinol) Hexamethylmelamine (HMM) Pibobroman (Vercyte)	CCNS	Alkylators with some antimetabolite activity; some inhibit DNA and RNA synthesis	Leukopenia, thrombocytopenia; nausea, vomiting; vesicants; rashes; nephrotoxicity (cisplatin); neurotoxic (HMM); hepatotoxicity (dacarbazine).
Antimetabolites			
Folate Antagonist Methotrexate (Folex, Mexate; amethopterin, MTX)	CCS	Irreversibly binds to enzyme required in synthesis of folic acid	Leukopenia, thrombocytopenia; anemia; diarrhea; stomatitis; alopecia; headache, blurred vision. High doses require leukovorin rescue.
Pyrimidine Analogs Cytarabine (Cytosar; Ara-C, cytosine arabinoside) Azacitidine Fluorouracil (Adrucil, Efudex, Fluoroplex; 5-FU) Floxuridine (FUDR)	CCS	Inhibit DNA polymerase and precursors required to form the pyrimidine bases needed to synthesize DNA	Leukopenia, thrombocytopenia; nausea, vomiting; hepatotoxicity; seizures, confusion, neuromuscular weakness, ataxia; local skin irritation and photosensitivity (5-FU, Floxuridine); cholangitis (Floxuridine).
Purine Analogs 6-Mercaptopurine (6-Purinethiol, 6MP) Thioguanine (6-TG, TG)	CCS	Incorporated into DNA causing cell death	Leukopenia, thrombocytopenia; nausea, vomiting; hepatotoxicity.
Antitumor Antibiotics			
Doxorubicin (Adriamycin) Daunorubicin (Cerubidine) Bleomycin (Blenoxane) Plicamycin (Mithracin; mithramycin) Mitomycin C (Mutamycin) Dactinomycin (Cosmegen)	CCNS	Bind between DNA base pairs causing fragmentation; alkylators	Potent vesicants; leukopenia, thrombocytopenia; alopecia, skin rash; nausea, vomiting, weight loss, stomatitis, oral ulcers; cardiac toxicity (doxorubicin, daunorubicin); pulmonary fibrosis (bleomycin).
Vinca Alkaloids			
Vincristine (Oncovin) Vinblastine (Velban)	CCS	Binds to microtubules to arrest cell division	Constipation; parasthesias, cranial nerve palsies; nausea, vomiting; leukopenia and anemia (vinblastine).

TABLE 37-6   Drugs Used to Treat Neoplasms (*Continued*)

DRUGS	PHASE ACTION	MECHANISM	ADVERSE EFFECTS
Hormones			
See Table 37-7.	CCNS	Suppress immune tissue or alter hormonal environment of hormone-dependent tumors	Fluid retention, hypertension, immune deficiency (corticosteroids), adrenal insufficiency (corticosteroids, aminoglutethimide), masculinization or feminization, gynecomastia or breast pain, menopausal symptoms (Tamoxifen), many others depending on hormone type.
Miscellaneous			
Procarbazine (Matulane)	CCNS	Most are not known; most inhibit DNA or RNA synthesis. Mitotane causes adrenal inhibition without adrenal destruction	Leukopenia, anemia, thrombocytopenia (procarbazine, hydroxyurea); nausea, vomiting, diarrhea, anorexia (mitotane, procarbazine, hydroxyurea); anaphylaxis (asparginase); adrenal insufficiency (mitotane); anaphylaxis (etoposide).
Hydroxyurea (Hydrea)	CCS		
Mitotane (Lysodren; *o,p'*-DDD)	CCNS		
L-Asparaginase (Elspar)	CCS		
Etoposide (Vepesid)			
Cisplatin (*see* alkylators)			
Radiopharmaceuticals			
Sodium iodide ^{131}I (Iodotope)	CCNS	Destroy rapidly proliferating tissue in thyroid carcinoma (sodium iodide ^{131}I), leukemias (sodium phosphate ^{32}P), peritoneal or pleural effusions (chromic phosphate ^{32}P).	Leukopenia, thrombocytopenia, radiation sickness. Drugs require careful handling by health care workers (see Chap. 35).
Sodium phosphate ^{32}P			
Chromic phosphate ^{32}P (Phosphocol ^{32}P)			

Alkylating Agents

The alkylating agents are one of the oldest and most useful classes of chemotherapeutic agents. They are a diverse group of chemicals which all share the similar characteristic of being able under physiologic conditions to add an alkyl group to biologic macromolecules like DNA, which results in disruption and fragmentation (Fig. 37-3).

Mechlorethamine   Mechlorethamine (Mustargen; nitrogen mustard), the first alkylating agent, was initially developed during World War I as a chemical warfare agent. The cytotoxic action of mechlorethamine is due to its ability to alkylate DNA, leading to breakage and disruption of the DNA helix. This occurs at any stage of cell growth; thus, mechlorethamine is a CCNS agent.

Clinical use and dosage   Mechlorethamine is a constituent of the MOPP regimen which has been used for the treatment of Hodgkin's disease. The standard dose of this agent is 0.1 to 0.4 mg/kg given intravenously. Additionally, it is administered intraarterially into solid tumors in an attempt to decrease tumor size and pain. Severe tissue necrosis occurs if drug extravasates. In the event of extrav-

asation, **sodium thiosulfate** may be locally instilled as an antidote.

Adverse effects   The major toxicities associated with mechlorethamine involve the hematopoietic, gastrointestinal, and dermatologic systems. Hematologic toxicities include leukopenia and thromobocytopenia. The leukopenia has an onset at 4 to 7 days, a nadir at 10 to 14 days, and a recovery by day 21. The thrombocytopenia is less dramatic and is usually transient. Severe nausea and vomiting occur in approximately 90 percent of patients. Antiemetic therapy should be instituted at least 2 h prior to infusion of this agent and continued for at least 12 h after administration. Skin reactions may include thinning of hair or total alopecia.

Cyclophosphamide   Cyclophosphamide (Cytoxan) is a chemical analog of mechlorethamine. It is converted by the liver into two active alkylating metabolites which bind to the DNA helix, preventing further cell growth. Cyclophosphamide is a CCNS agent.

Clinical use and dosage   Cyclophosphamide is used to treat a large number of malignancies including breast can-

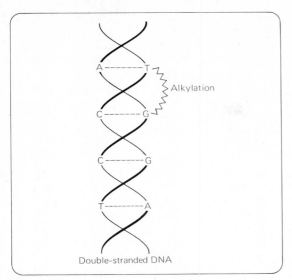

FIGURE 37-3

Intrastrand Cross-Linking of DNA by Alkylating Agents. Cross-linking either leads to mispairing in nucleic acid replication and transcription or prevents the double-stranded DNA from separating, thereby inhibiting replication.

cer, lymphomas, multiple myeloma, and small cell carcinoma of the lung. Two different dosage regimens are commonly employed. The first uses a single intravenous dose of 500 to 1500 mg/m² administered every 1 to 4 weeks. The second dosage regimen employs a lower dose, 60 to 120 mg/m² administered daily. The dose of cyclophosphamide can be increased when the drug is used as an immunosuppressive agent, for example in bone marrow transplantation.

Adverse effects Cyclophosphamide's adverse effects involve the hematopoietic, gastrointestinal, dermatologic, genitourinary, and cardiac systems. Leukopenia is observed in all patients receiving doses of 1 to 1.5 g/m². The leukopenia has an onset at day 7, nadir at day 14, and recovery by day 21. Mild thrombocytopenia occurs in about 20 percent of patients within 14 days of drug administration. Nausea and vomiting are dose-related, occurring in 90 percent of the patients receiving doses of 1 to 1.5 g/m² and in 20 percent of patients receiving 0.5 g/m² or less. Additionally, anorexia is a common complaint with this agent. Following 1 to 3 months of therapy with cyclophosphamide, total baldness occurs in about 70 to 80 percent of the patients. Genitourinary effects with this agent can be severe. Hemorrhagic cystitis occurs in about 5 percent of patients, while the incidence of nonhemorrhagic cystitis is about 4 to 35 percent. If fluids are forced (40 to 50 mL/kg/day) cystitis may be prevented. Gonadal dysfunction occurs in male patients at 1 to 3 months, and in females at 3 to 6 months. Irreversible congestive heart failure developing within 2 weeks of ther-

apy may be observed in patients receiving doses of 50 mg/kg or more.

Triethylenethiophosphoramide Triethylenethiophosphoramide (TEPA; ThioTEPA) is a polyfunctional alkylating agent, similar in action to mechlorethamine. It is a CCNS agent.

Clinical use and dosage TEPA has activity against a variety of tumors including Hodgkin's disease and carcinomas of the ovary, breast, and bladder. It has become a second-line drug for treating these disease states because of the availability of more effective agents. Currently, its most important use is as a topical irrigant for papillary tumors of the bladder. For bladder irrigation, 60 mg of the drug is diluted in 30 to 60 mL of sterile water and instilled through an indwelling catheter; the solution is retained in the bladder for 2 h. This procedure is repeated every 1 to 4 weeks. Additionally, TEPA has been used as a sclerosing agent in the local treatment of malignant effusions of the pleura and pericardium. When treating malignant effusions, 10 to 60 mg of the drug is diluted in 10 to 20 mL of normal saline and instilled into the pleural or pericardium cavity. This procedure is repeated every 1 to 4 weeks if needed.

Adverse effects TEPA's adverse effects involve the hematopoietic and gastrointestinal systems. The hematopoietic effects include moderate anemia, thrombocytopenia, and leukopenia. The onset occurs from day 14 to 21 with a prolonged recovery period to day 42. Mild nausea and vomiting may occur on the day of administration. If this is noted, prophylactic antiemetic therapy should be instituted prior to the next dose of this agent.

Busulfan, Chlorambucil, and Melphalan These three orally available agents all produce their cytotoxicity by alkylation. However, each has its own unique spectrum of antitumor activity.

Clinical use and dosage The major use of **busulfan** (Myleran) is in the treatment of chronic myelogenous leukemia. A dose of 4 to 12 mg is given orally for 2 to 3 weeks; thereafter, a dose of 1 to 3 mg/day is administered.

Chlorambucil (Leukeran) is used primarily to treat chronic lymphocytic leukemia. Additionally, this agent is used to treat the elderly or debilitated patient since it is less toxic than other alkylating agents. An induction regimen of 6 to 12 mg is administered daily until a resonse is achieved. The patient is then begun on a maintenance regimen of 2 mg daily.

Melphalan (Alkeran) is the alkylator of choice for the treatment of multiple myeloma in combination with other agents. It is administered in a dose of 0.25 mg/kg for 4 days every 4 to 6 weeks. Melphalan has also been used as adjuvant therapy for breast cancer and in the treatment of refractory ovarian carcinoma.

Adverse effects The toxicities of the oral alkylating agents are mild compared to **nitrogen mustard** and **cyclo-**

phosphamide. Bone marrow suppression resulting in leukopenia may occur, reaching a nadir by 10 to 14 days, but may continue for up to 8 weeks. These agents may produce mild nausea and vomiting. Alopecia is an uncommon side effect with these agents. A rare side effect associated with the prolonged administration of **busulfan** is pulmonary fibrosis.

Nitrosoureas   The nitrosoureas are a group of drugs which are also alkylating agents. This group includes **carmustine** (BiCNU; BCNU), **lomustine** (CeeNu; CCNU), and **streptozocin** (Zanosar). In addition to their alkylating properties, the nitrosoureas appear to inhibit several key enzymatic steps necessary for the synthesis of DNA. These agents are considered CCNS. The nitrosoureas have a high lipid solubility and are capable of crossing the blood-brain barrier which makes them useful in the treatment of meningeal leukemias and brain tumors.

Clinical use and dosage   **Carmustine** possesses activity against several tumors including acute lymphocytic leukemia, Hodgkin's disease, multiple myeloma, brain tumors, and gastrointestinal carcinomas. It is typically administered in a dose of 30 to 200 mg/m² as a 60-min intravenous infusion every 6 to 8 weeks.

Lomustine is used primarily to treat brain tumors. Additionally, it has activity against small-cell lung carcinoma and Hodgkin's disease. Lomustine is administered orally in a dosage of 100 to 130 mg/m² as a single dose which is repeated every 6 weeks.

Streptozocin is used to treat islet cell tumors of the pancreas and gastric carcinoma. As a single agent, streptozocin is administered intravenously at a dose of 1 to 1.5 g/m² every 3 to 4 weeks. Additionally, it has been used in combination regimens at dosages of 500 to 1000 mg/m² for 3 to 5 days every 4 to 6 weeks. This drug is not available commercially and must be obtained from the National Cancer Institute in Bethesda, Maryland.

Adverse effects   The nitrosoureas may produce toxicities involving the hematopoietic, gastrointestinal, dermatologic, neurologic, and renal systems. Hematopoietic reactions include leukopenia and thrombocytopenia. Leukopenia has an onset at days 21 to 28 of therapy, reaching a nadir by day 42, and recovery by day 56. Thrombocytopenia occurs by day 28 of therapy with a median nadir of 90,000 platelets/mm³. Gastrointestinal side effects commonly include nausea, vomiting, and anorexia. Prophylactic antiemetics should be administered. Stomatitis and alopecia can occur but are uncommon. Neurologic reactions are rare and include confusion and lethargy. Infrequent hepatic or renal damage may occur with long-term administration of these agents. Streptozocin appears to be the most nephrotoxic nitrosourea causing kidney damage in about one-third of patients. This is usually reversible with discontinuation of the drug. Patients should be well-hydrated prior to receiving streptozocin.

Dacarbazine   Dacarbazine (DTIC; DTIC-Dome) is activated by liver microsomal enzymes and then functions as an alkylating agent. It appears to inhibit the synthesis of RNA and protein more than DNA. It kills cells slowly and is considered a CCNS agent.

Clinical use and dosage   DTIC is used in the therapy of malignant melanoma, Hodgkin's disease, and sarcoma. When used in the treatment of Hodgkin's disease it is frequently used with **doxorubicin**, **bleomycin**, and **vinblastine**. It is recommended to be given intravenously in a dose of 3.5 mg/kg/day. This is given for 10 days, a cycle which is repeated every 28 days. An alternative dosage administration schedule is to give 250 mg/m² for 5 days and then repeat the dosing in 3 weeks.

Adverse effects   Toxicities include gastrointestinal symptoms of nausea and vomiting which develop in almost 90 percent of patients. The nausea and vomiting usually occur within 1 to 3 h after the treatment. Myelosuppression can also occur with leukopenia and thrombocytopenia. Additional less common adverse effects include hepatotoxicity, fever, malaise, alopecia, neurotoxicity, facial flushing, and dermatologic problems. Extravasation of dacarbazine during intravenous administration can cause severe pain and necrosis.

Antimetabolites

The antimetabolites are agents which inhibit important biochemical reactions required for DNA synthesis and cell growth by interfering with or substituting for normal metabolites. These agents include folate antagonists, pyrimidine analogs, and purine antagonists.

Folate Antagonists

Methotrexate   Methotrexate (MTX, amethopterin; Folex, Mexate) is a cell-cycle-specific agent and was the first antimetabolite used in the treatment of neoplastic disorders. Methotrexate inhibits cell growth by substituting for folic acid, binding tightly but reversibly to dihydrofolate reductase (DHFR). DHFR is necessary for the synthesis of DNA and vital proteins. Methotrexate is highly CCS, acting primarily during the S phase.

Clinical use and dosage   Methotrexate has been used in the treatment of acute lymphocytic leukemia, lymphomas, breast carcinoma, lung carcinoma, sarcomas, and head and neck tumors. Nonneoplastic proliferative disorders, such as psoriasis, have also been effectively controlled by methotrexate therapy. Methotrexate is used in three dosage regimens: low-dose, moderate-dose, and high-dose therapy. Low-dose therapy consists of 2.5 to 5 mg/day orally. Some tumors, such as osteogenic sarcoma and lung carcinoma are relatively resistant to low-dose methotrexate because of reduced cell-membrane transport of the drug. The use of moderate- to high-dose regimens with **leucovorin rescue** overcomes this drug resistance. Moderate doses (1 to 2 g/m²) and very high doses (3 to 20 g/m^2) are usually administered intravenously every 3 to 4 weeks. Certain drugs (**aspirin, phenylbutazone, probenecid,** and **sulfonamides** should not be administered concurrently with methotrexate, because they enhance toxicity by inhibiting excretion of drug into the urine or displace MTX from plasma-binding sites. In addition, methotrexate can displace **insulin** from its binding site, leading to hypoglycemia.

Leucovorin (citrovorum) "rescue" The cytotoxicity of **methotrexate** can be reversed by the oral or intravenous administration of **folinic acid** (leucovorin, citrovorum factor LV; Wellcovorin), which bypasses the methotrexate block of DHFR. Plasma concentrations of methotrexate are usually measured at 0, 6, 24, 48, and 72 h after infusion and can be used to predict impending toxicity. If the concentrations of MTX are above 10^{-5} M at 24 h, 10^{-6} M at 48 h, or 10^{-7} M at 72 h, bone marrow suppression or gastrointestinal side effects are likely to occur. The primary consideration in rescue is to maintain adequate leucovorin concentrations as long as the methotrexate level exceeds 10^{-8} M. Toxicity can be prevented with 6 to 15 mg/m^2 of leucovorin given every 6 h for 2 to 3 days, starting within 24 h of treatment. Delaying the administration of leucovorin longer than 42 h usually results in irreversible toxicity, especially to the bone marrow and gastrointestinal tract.

Adverse effects Methotrexate's adverse effects involve the hemotopoietic, gastrointestinal, dermatologic, neurologic, and renal systems. Leukopenia, thrombocytopenia, and anemia have a rapid onset occurring between days 4 to 7, a nadir at day 14, and recovery by day 21. Nausea and vomiting are dose-related, occurring in about 20 percent of patients receiving low to moderate doses, and in about 50 percent of patients receiving high doses. Diarrhea and stomatitis are frequent side effects. Prophylactic antiemetics, antidiarrheals, and mouth care should be instituted in this patient population. Low-dose regimens may cause mild alopecia beginning by week 4. Total baldness may be noted with high doses, but reverses after therapy is discontinued. Neurologic effects following intrathecal administration may be manifested by headache, blurred vision, and meningismus (symptoms of meningeal irritation in the absence of infection). Nephrotoxicity, caused by crystallization of methotrexate in the renal tubules, occurs in approximately 5 percent of patients receiving high-dose therapy. With high-dose therapy, the urine must be alkalinized with **acetazolamide** (Diamox) or **sodium bicarbonate** to maintain a pH above 6.5 during the entire course of administration. Patients should be encouraged to drink 3 L/day and void every 3 h. Lastly, hepatic failure can occur in patients receiving high-dose therapy.

Pyrimidine Analogs

Cytarabine Cytarabine (cytosine arabinoside, ARA/C; Cytosar) has been shown to be exceedingly active in the treatment of acute nonlymphocytic leukemia (ANLL). Cytarabine, a CCS agent, exerts its cytotoxic effects through the inhibition of DNA polymerase, an enzyme that catalyzes the formation of DNA. It must first be converted in the cell to its active metabolite, arabinosylcytosine triphosphate (ara-CTP). Antitumor activity correlates with the intracellular concentration of ara-CTP.

Clinical use and dosage Currently, there are several combination regimens which include cytarabine that have consistently produced complete remissions in over 50 percent of adult patients with ANLL. Cytarabine is usually given in doses of 100 mg/m^2/day in 5- to 10-day courses by either the subcutaneous or intravenous route. High-dose therapy, 3000 mg/m^2, is being investigated for the management of refractory disease.

Adverse effects The major adverse effects associated with cytarabine involve the hematopoietic, gastrointestinal, and dermatologic systems. Cytarabine-induced bone marrow suppression depends on the dose of drug and the frequency of administration. Since one of the objectives of therapy is to produce moderate to severe myelosuppression, white blood cell and platelet counts will often be depressed to below 1000 and 20,000, respectively. The onset of pancytopenia is seen at days 4 to 7, the nadir at days 10 to 14, and the recovery by day 21. Supportive therapy with packed red blood cells, platelets, and antibiotics is essential. Severe gastrointestinal toxicity occurs in 25 to 75 percent of patients and presents as stomatitis and/or diarrhea. Nausea and vomiting are common with cytarabine, especially in combination therapy regimens, and may be minimized by the use of antiemetics. Alopecia occurs rarely in standard dose therapy and frequently with high-dose regimens.

Other toxicities noted with this agent involve the liver, central nervous system, and eyes. Hepatic toxicity may include hyperbilirubinemia, and slight elevations of the transaminases and alkaline phosphatase. Central nervous system reactions are noted with high-dose therapy and may manifest as tonic/clonic seizures, confusion, somnolence, impaired mental function, and grand mal seizures. Coma leading to death occurs in up to 60 percent of patients who receive a lifetime dose exceeding 48 g/m^2. Conjunctivitis due to cytarabine being secreted into the lacrimal fluid occurs in patients receiving high-dose regimens. Prophylactic corticosteroid eye drops (see Chap. 39) should be instituted prior to high-dose cytarabine and continued for at least 3 days after cytarabine therapy is discontinued.

5-Azacitidine 5-Azacitidine (5-azacytidine, 5-AZC; Ladakamycin) is a cell-cycle-specific agent which inhibits nucleic acid metabolism. It is an investigational agent available from the National Cancer Institute.

Clinical use and dosage 5-Azacitidine may be used to treat refractory ANLL. This investigational agent is available from the National Cancer Institute in 100-mg vials. Azacitidine must be given within 8 h of reconstitution because of rapid decomposition. The method of administration is by continuous intravenous infusion of 50 to 200 mg/m² in three divided daily doses for 5 days.

Adverse effects The major toxicities with this agent involve the hematopoietic, gastrointestinal, neurologic, and hepatic systems. Leukopenia is the most significant toxicity with onset at days 14 to 17, nadir at days 25 to 40, and recovery in 1 to 3 weeks after treatment is completed. Nausea and vomiting occur in 70 percent of the patients. Neuromuscular toxicities include muscle tenderness, weakness, and lethargy occurring on days 2 to 3 of therapy. Hepatic toxicity with elevation of liver enzymes, confusion, somnolence, rash, fever, phlebitis, and transient hypotension have also been reported.

Fluorouracil Fluorouracil (5-fluorouracil, 5-FU; Adrucil, Efudex) is one of the most commonly used agents in chemotherapy. A CCS agent, it inhibits DNA synthesis by blocking thymidylate synthesis.

Clinical use and dosage There are two commonly used dosage regimens: (1) weekly intravenous bolus injections of 12 to 15 mg/kg, and (2) 12 mg/kg IV infusion for 3 to 5 days every 2 to 4 weeks. Fluorouracil has also been given in similar doses by direct hepatic artery infusion in patients with hepatic metastases secondary to carcinomas of the breast or colon. The topical preparations (Efudex, Fluoroplex) are used to treat active keratosis and superficial basal carcinoma. For basal carcinoma the 5% cream is applied twice daily with therapy continuing as long as 10 to 12 weeks.

Adverse effects The toxicities associated with fluorouracil administration involve the following organ systems: hematopoetic, gastrointestinal, neurologic, and dermatologic. Moderate to severe leukopenia occurs in 100 percent of patients. The onset is usually noted at days 7 to 10, nadir occurring at day 14, and recovery by day 24. Thrombocytopenia occurs rarely and reverses more slowly. Mild nausea, vomiting, stomatitis, and diarrhea occur frequently with this agent. Central ataxia has been noted in 5 percent of patients. Mild alopecia occurs in 5 to 50 percent of patients and dry scaling dermatitis in 10 to 20 percent. Hyperpigmentation of nails and nail beds is common. Pruritic maculopapular rash has also been noted. Patients should be instructed not to sunbathe while receiving this therapy. The most frequent adverse effects of topical agents are pain, pruritis, and severe inflammation at the site of application.

Floxuridine Floxuridine (FUDR) is a fluoropyrimidine similar to fluorouracil which was first introduced in 1960. Floxuridine, which itself is cytotoxic, is converted by the liver into two active metabolites, 5-fluorouracil and floxuridine monophosphate, which are CCS and act by inhibiting DNA synthesis.

Clinical use and dosage Floxuridine is most commonly infused directly into the hepatic artery for the treatment of primary and metastatic tumors of the liver. The intraarterial dose ranges from 0.1 to 0.3 mg/kg/day for 14 days and is usually repeated every 4 weeks. More recently, the drug has been administered intravenously in doses of 0.05 to 0.1 mg/kg/day.

Adverse effects The most serious toxicity associated with the use of FUDR is cholangitis (inflammation of the bile ducts). This is manifested by elevations in liver function tests, bilirubin and alkaline phosphatase. Rare hematologic reactions include anemia, thrombocytopenia, and altered prothrombin time. Mild nausea, vomiting, diarrhea, or stomatitis (inflammation of the mouth) may occur. Rare dermatologic effects include alopecia, dermatitis, rash, and photosensitivity. Patients should be warned to avoid prolonged exposure to direct sunlight. Fever, malaise, lethargy, and weakness have also been reported with the use of this agent.

Purine Analogs

6-Mercaptopurine and 6-Thioguanine 6-Mercaptopurine (Purinethol; 6 MP) and thioguanine (6-TG) are analogs of the physiologic purine compounds hypoxanthine and adenine, respectively. **Mercaptopurine** and **thioguanine** are inactive and must be converted intracellularly to their respective 5′-phosphate ribonucleotides, which then inhibit a number of vital metabolic reactions necessary for DNA synthesis. The 5′-phosphate ribonucleoside of thioguanine is incorporated directly into DNA, thereby causing cell death. Both of these agents are CCS.

Clinical use and dosage **Mercaptopurine** is primarily used to maintain patients with acute lymphocytic leukemia in remission. It is administered orally in a dose of 2.5 mg/kg/day. Because the metabolism of mercaptopurine is inhibited by **allopurinol**, the dosage of mercaptopurine must be reduced when both drugs are administered concomitantly. **Thioguanine** has been used orally in a dose of 2 mg/kg/day in combination with **cytarabine** in the treatment of acute myelogenous leukemia.

Adverse effects The adverse effects of mercaptopurine and thioguanine can be grouped into hematologic, gastrointestinal, and hepatic toxicities. Bone marrow suppression, manifested by leukopenia, thrombocytopenia, and anemia has an onset at 7 to 10 days, nadir at day 14, and recovery by day 21. Additionally, mild nausea, vomiting, and anorexia are occasionally observed with the use of these agents. Abnormal liver function may occur 1 to 2 months after the initiation of therapy. **Thioguanine** produces hepatotoxicity less frequently than **mercaptopurine**.

Antitumor Antibiotics

Doxorubicin and Daunorubicin Doxorubicin (Adriamycin; ADR) and **daunorubicin** (Cerubidine; DNR, daunomycin) are anthracycline antibiotics that differ chemically by only one hydroxyl group. However, this results in a significant difference in their pharmacology and clinical activity. Both doxorubicin and daunorubicin are cytotoxic by virtue of binding between DNA base pairs.

Clinical use and dosage   **Doxorubicin** has a wide spectrum of antitumor activity which includes breast carcinoma, medullary thyroid carcinoma, testicular carcinoma, lymphomas, multiple myeloma, soft-tissue sarcomas, gastric carcinoma, and acute leukemias. In contrast, **daunorubicin** has activity only in the acute leukemias. The kinetic differences between the two drugs have led to different dosage schedules. Doxorubicin is administered at a dose of 30 to 90 mg/m^2 IV every 3 to 4 weeks. Daunorubicin is most commonly administered IV at a dose of 45 mg/m^2 for 3 consecutive days. Both drugs are potent vesicants, and if extravasated may cause severe pain, induration, and local tissue necrosis. Local measures, such as applying ice packs and local injection of **hydrocortisone**, may minimize the extent of tissue damage. **Sodium bicarbonate** 5 mL injected locally may prevent severe tissue damage.

Adverse effects   The major toxicities associated with **doxorubicin** and **daunorubicin** involve the hematopoietic, gastrointestinal, dermatologic, and cardiac systems. Severe bone marrow aplasia is noted with an onset at days 7 to 10, a nadir at days 10 to 20, and recovery by day 28. Nausea, vomiting, and abdominal pain often occur on the day of administration. Dermatologic effects include alopecia, inflammation, and skin rashes. Reversible alopecia usually occurs after the initial dose and results in total hair loss for the period of treatment. Cardiac toxicity is the major dose-limiting factor with these agents. There are two types of cardiac toxicities, an acute form and a delayed dose-related form. The acute form of cardiac toxicity usually presents as an arrhythmia and does not preclude further drug administration. The delayed form presents as congestive heart failure and occurs when the total dose exceeds 550 and 750 mg/m^2 for doxorubicin and daunorubicin, respectively. There are several methods for monitoring the myocardial effects of these agents. One method utilizes the echocardiogram to measure systolic time intervals and ejection fraction. The electrocardiogram may also be helpful in that a decrease in voltage suggests decreased myocardial contractility. Patients with preexisting cardiac disease, prior chest irradiation, or prior exposure to an alkylating agent are at greater risk and should be monitored closely while receiving these agents. It is important to instruct the patients receiving these that their urine will be reddish orange for approximately three days after drug administration, so as to prevent unnecessary concern about changes in urine color.

Bleomycin   Bleomycin (BLM; Blenoxane) is an antitumor antibiotic which is a mixture of polypeptides. Bleomycin A$_2$ is the principal polypeptide in the mixture and comprises at least 50 percent of the marketed preparation. Bleomycin binds to DNA causing scission and fragmentation of the DNA molecule. In addition, the DNA repair mechanisms are disrupted by the drug. Although bleomycin is considered CCNS, its primary action is on cells in the G$_2$ phase.

Clinical use and dosage   **Bleomycin** has activity against several tumors including head and neck carcinoma, squamous cell carcinoma of the lung, Hodgkin's disease, lymphomas, and testicular cancer. Since bleomycin is not irritating to tissues, it may be administered by the intramuscular, subcutaneous, or intravenous routes. Bleomycin is most commonly administered in a dose of 2 to 15 mg/m^2 twice weekly as an intravenous bolus. In addition, it may be given as a 24-h continuous infusion in a dose of 15 to 30 mg/m^2.

Adverse effects   The toxicities associated with this agent involve the gastrointestinal, dermatologic, and pulmonary systems. **Bleomycin** does not have significant hematopoietic toxicity. Nausea, vomiting, anorexia, weight loss, and mucosal ulceration are common gastrointestinal complications. Oral ulceration occurs in 50 percent of patients within 4 to 5 weeks but usually resolves in 2 months. Inspection of mucosa is mandatory in patients receiving bleomycin. Severe buccal pain may occur and is indicative of complete gastrointestinal mucositis, precluding further therapy. Dermatologic side effects include palmar erythema, pruritis, vesicles, hyperpigmentation, and alopecia. Pulmonary toxicity, presenting as pneumonitis or fibrosis, can be a life-threatening complication. Clinical signs include basilar rales, shortness of breath, cough, and weakness. Pulmonary function tests should be monitored on a regular basis. Because bleomycin is a polypeptide mixture, hypersensitivity reactions, including urticaria, facial edema, and frank anaphylaxis can occur. Hypersensitivity reactions occur most frequently with lymphoma patients. Small test doses of 1 mg may be given prior to the administration of full dosage in order to detect potential acute hypersensitivity reactions. Lack of hypersensitivity to the test dose, however, does not preclude subsequent reactions. Other toxicities include hypertension, hypotension, dysuria, and mental confusion. Fever and chills are common and usually begin 2 to 6 h after drug administration and last for 4 to 6 h. Pretreatment with **diphenhydramine** (Benadryl) and acetaminophen may minimize these disturbing effects.

Plicamycin   Plicamycin (Mithracin) is an antitumor antibiotic derived from a *steptomyces tanashiensis*. This drug was formerly called mithramycin. The mechanism of this CCNS agent is not fully understood; however, it may be inserted into DNA and inhibit DNA-directed RNA synthesis.

Clinical use and dosage   **Plicamycin** has activity against metastatic embryonal testicular carcinoma. Dosage regimens vary greatly but generally alternate daily doses of 25 to 50 μg/kg for eight to ten doses are administered IV. In addition, plicamycin has the ability to reduce elevated serum calcium caused by metastatic bone disease. For hypercalcemia a dose of 15 to 25 μg/kg is given every third day until a response is obtained. Extravasation of mithramycin is associated with severe local pain and phlebitis. The surrounding tissue may slough and require grafting. If extravasation occurs, 1 mL of **EDTA** (150 mg/mL) should be injected into the surrounding tissue followed by an ice pack.

Adverse effects The major adverse effects associated with plicamycin involve the hematopoetic, gastrointestinal, hepatic, and renal systems. Thrombocytopenia is common with this agent, while leukopenia is uncommon. Thrombocytopenia may be severe with an onset at day 7, nadir at day 14, and recovery by day 28. In addition, plicamycin inhibits coagulation. The combined effect of drug-induced thrombocytopenia and coagulopathy leads to hemorrhage in 33 percent of patients. Nausea, vomiting, anorexia, malaise, diarrhea, and stomatitis are common. Reversible hepatic toxicity presents as elevated SGOT and lactic dehydrogenase. The degree of lactic dehydrogenase elevation can be significant—up to 4000 IU/L. Nephrotoxicity presents as proteinuria along with elevated blood urea nitrogen (BUN) and creatinine. In addition, plicamycin may cause electrolyte abnormalities including hypocalcemia, hypokalemia, and hypophosphatemia. These may result in depression and confusion. Hypersensitivity reactions including fever and severe facial flushing have been noted.

Dactinomycin Dactinomycin (Cosmegen; actinomycin D) is an antitumor antibiotic derived from *Streptomyces parvullus*. Dactinomycin, a CCNS agent, binds to DNA resulting in the inhibition of DNA and RNA synthesis.

Clinical use and dosage Dactinomycin has established activity in several neoplastic disorders: methotrexate-resistant choriocarcinoma, soft-tissue sarcomas, metastatic testicular carcinomas, and Wilms' tumor. Regimens vary considerably but the usual daily dose is 15 μg/kg administered IV for 5 days every 4 to 6 weeks. Dactinomycin is extremely irritating to subcutaneous tissues. If extravasation occurs, 4 mL of 10% **sodium thiosulfate** may be injected into the surrounding area to prevent further damage. Ice or warm packs may be applied to increase patient comfort.

Adverse effects The major toxicities with this agent involve the hematopoietic, gastrointestinal, and dermatologic systems. Bone marrow suppression consists of anemia, leukopenia, and thrombocytopenia with an onset at day 7, nadir at day 14, and recovery by day 28. Commonly, nausea and vomiting occur 1 to 3 h after administration. Stomatitis often occurs requiring frequent mouth care. Dermatologic side effects include alopecia or skin eruptions in the form of pustules or papules. In areas where skin has been exposed to radiation, erythema may be noted.

Mitomycin C Mitomycin C (Mutamycin) is an antitumor antibiotic derived from *Streptomyces caespitosus*. This CCNS agent is activated in vivo to an alkylating agent which inhibits DNA synthesis.

Clinical use and dosage Mitomycin C has activity in gastrointestinal, breast, and pancreatic carcinomas. This drug is administered in a dose of 10 to 20 mg/m² IV every 4 to 8 weeks. Mitomycin C is a potent vesicant and may cause severe tissue necrosis if infiltrated. If extravasation occurs, 4 mL of 10% **sodium thiosulfate** or **pyridoxine hydrochloride** (50 mg/mL) 1 mL should be injected locally. Warm or cold compresses may be used for patient comfort.

Adverse effects Mitomycin C's toxicities involve the hematopoietic, gastrointestinal, renal, and pulmonary systems. Bone marrow suppression is observed in all patients, with onset at days 10 to 14, nadir at days 14 to 28, and recovery by days 35 to 56. Additionally, nausea, vomiting, diarrhea, and stomatitis are common with this agent. Occasionally, renal failure and interstitial pneumonia may be observed.

Vinca Alkaloids

Vincristine Vincristine (Oncovin), an alkaloid derived from the periwinkle plant (*Vinca rosea*), has been used clinically since 1960. Vincristine is a CCS agent which binds to the microtubules and spindle proteins in the S phase causing arrest of cellular division.

Clinical use and dosage Vincristine is used to treat a wide variety of malignancies including leukemias, lymphomas, neuroblastomas, Wilms' tumor, testicular carcinoma, breast carcinoma, and Hodgkin's disease. The therapeutic dose of vincristine is 1 to 2 mg/m² administered intravenously once a week. If signs of neurotoxicity are evident, the dose should be decreased by 50 percent. Extravasation of this agent may cause severe tissue sloughing and necrosis. In the event of infiltration **hyaluronidase** (Wydase) 150 U/mL, 1 mL should be injected locally. Heat is applied to enhance systemic absorption of the drug.

Adverse effects The major toxicities associated with vincristine involve the gastrointestinal and neurologic systems. The most troublesome GI side effect is constipation, which occurs most often in patients over the age of 50. All patients receiving this agent must be placed on stool softeners and a stimulant laxative of choice. Fluids should be encouraged in order to enhance stool softening. Neurologic toxicity presents primarily as peripheral neuropathy with paresthesia of the hands and feet, absence of deep tendon reflexes, decreased muscle strength, and lower extremity weakness. Muscle weakness precludes further therapy. Central nervous system neuropathy is uncommon, but if present manifests as cranial nerve palsies. The cranial nerves most frequently affected are III, V, VI, and VII, leading to facial and jaw pain. Rarely, an increase in antidiuretic hormone may occur 1 to 10 days following therapy with this drug.

Vinblastine Vinblastine (Velban), a derivative of the periwinkle plant, differs chemically only slightly from **vincristine**. Vinblastine is a CCS agent having a mechanism of action which is essentially the same as vincristine's.

Clinical use and dosage Vinblastine is used to treat breast carcinoma, Kaposi's sarcoma, lymphomas, choriocarcinoma, testicular carcinoma, and Hodgkin's disease. Its potency is one-tenth that of vincristine, being administered IV at a dose of 0.1 to 0.2 mg/kg every 2 to 3 weeks. Vinblastine may cause cellulitis or tissue sloughing if extravasation occurs. The antidote for this agent is 1 mL **hyaluronidase** (Wydase) 150 U/mL injected into the area. Heat may be applied to enhance the systemic absorption of the drug.

Adverse effects Vinblastine's toxicities consist of hematopoietic, gastrointestinal, dermatologic, and neurologic system alterations. Leukopenia and anemia are common with this agent, with an onset at days 4 to 7, a nadir at day 10, and recovery by day 17. Severe nausea and vomiting can occur with this agent, specifically when doses exceed 0.2 mg/kg/day. Rare dermatologic toxicities include alopecia, rashes, and photosensitivity. Peripheral neurologic side effects include paresthesia, neuritis, decrease in muscle strength, and absence of deep tendon reflexes. Mild neurologic symptoms occur in 90 percent of the patients receiving this agent and disappear after discontinuing therapy. Uncommonly, neuropathy involving the central nervous system occurs and presents as jaw pain, headache, depression, orthostatic hypotension, or convulsions.

Hormonal Therapy

Hormonal therapy may be used in the management of a variety of neoplasms. Several classes of steroids are used, including the estrogens, antiestrogens, glucocorticosteroids, progestins, androgens, and antiadrenal agents. Table 37-7 provides a list of the commonly used agents. A complete discussion of these agents is presented in Chap. 35. The tumors of some organs, mainly the prostate and mammary glands, are dependent on hormones for their growth. By altering the

TABLE 37-7 Hormonal Agents Used in Cancer Therapy

TYPE OF AGENT	PREPARATIONS
Estrogens	Diethylstilbestrol (DES) Ethinyl estradiol
Antiestrogens	Tamoxifen (Nolvadex)
Glucocorticosteroids	Hydrocortisone Prednisone Dexamethasone
Progestins	Medroxyprogesterone Acetate (Depo-Provera) Hydroxyprogesterone Caproate (Delautin)
Androgens	Testosterone esters Fluoxymesterone (Halotestin) Calusterone (Methosarb) Nadrolene decanoate (Deca-Durabolin) Testolactone (Teslac)
Antiadrenal	Aminoglutethimide

hormonal environment it may be possible to alter the growth of the neoplasm.

Estrogens

Estrogens are useful in the management of cancer of the breast and prostate. Two agents which are frequently used are **diethylstilbestrol** (DES) and **ethinyl estradiol**. Estrogens inhibit protein synthesis by binding to estrogen receptors (ER) within the tumor. Patients with ER-positive tumors respond more frequently to estrogens (60 percent) than those with ER-negative tumors.

Clinical Use and Dosage **Diethylstilbestrol** and **ethinyl estradiol** are effective in treating breast carcinoma in postmenopausal patients and carcinoma of the prostate. Dosage of diethylstilbestrol in breast cancer is 15 mg/day in three divided doses. The current recommended dosage of diethylstilbestrol in prostatic carcinoma is 1 to 3 mg/day. Ethinyl estradiol is most frequently administered in a dose of 3 mg daily for both breast and prostatic cancer.

Adverse Effects The estrogens commonly cause gynecomastia in men which can be prevented by giving a small dose of radiation to each breast prior to treatment with the hormone. Side effects in both sexes include nausea, vomiting (dose-related), fluid retention, changes in libido (in women), and thromboembolic disease. The nausea and vomiting can be controlled through the use of antiemetics prior to administration. Patients need to monitor weight gain and notify physicians if edema occurs. Thromboembolic disease may present as thrombophlebitis, pulmonary embolism, stroke, or myocardial infarction.

Antiestrogens

The most commonly used hormonal agent for breast cancer is **tamoxifen** (Nolvadex). Because breast cancer is closely linked with estrogen balance, it seems obvious that an antiestrogen such as tamoxifen may be effective in inhibiting its growth. Tamoxifen binds to estrogen receptors (ER) in tumor tissue, blocking the effect of estrogen and leading to altered DNA synthesis. However, this mechanism alone cannot account for the dramatic response seen in postmenopausal (estrogen-deficient) patients with metastatic breast cancer.

Clinical Use and Dosage **Tamoxifen** has traditionally been used to treat postmenopausal patients with ER-positive breast cancer. More recently, premenopausal patients with ER-positive tumors have responded to tamoxifen. The partial remission rate ranges from 40 to 60 percent, which is similar to that observed with estrogen therapy. The usual dose of 10 mg administered orally twice daily may be escalated to 20 mg twice daily if response is not initially observed. Occasionally, patients may experience a "flare" of their disease during the first few weeks of tamoxifen therapy. This presents as increased bone pain or local swelling and erythema. A transient flare may be an indication of a therapeutic response, but flares lasting longer than 30 days usually represent disease progression. Tamoxifen is preferred over estrogens for initial therapy because it produces a similar response with fewer side effects.

Adverse Effects Toxicities associated with **tamoxifen** administration involve the hematopoietic, gastrointestinal, gynecologic, dermatologic, and neurologic systems. Transient thrombocytopenia, leukopenia, and anemia may be noted. The blood counts usually revert to normal even while the patient continues therapy. Blood counts should be monitored on a regular basis during therapy. The gastrointestinal side effects include nausea and vomiting occurring in approximately 25 percent of patients. Gynecologic problems such as vaginal bleeding and menstrual irregularities occur infrequently, with the noted exception of hot flashes occurring in 25 percent of patients receiving therapy. Dermatologic side effects include skin rashes and pruritus vulvae. Neurologic side effects are rare and include dizziness, headache, and depression.

Glucocorticosteroids

Glucocorticosteroids are synthetic derivatives of the natural adrenal hormone, cortisol (hydrocortisone). The commonly used agents include **hydrocortisone, prednisone,** and **dexamethasone.** Glucocorticosteroids appear to inhibit DNA synthesis by decreasing intracellular energy stores. Additionally, these agents retard mitotic division and cellular protein synthesis.

Clinical Use and Dosage Corticosteroids produce lymphocytopenia and thus are used in the treatment of acute lymphoblastic leukemia, chronic lymphocytic leukemia, lymphomas, and multiple myeloma. The most commonly used corticosteroid is **prednisone,** which is given orally in doses of 60 to 100 mg for 5 to 7 days. **Hydrocortisone** is reserved for replacement therapy or parenteral administration. **Dexamethasone** is used to treat cerebral edema secondary to brain metastases.

Adverse Effects Toxicity from corticosteroids can be divided into short- and long-term side effects. Short-term effects include salt and water retention, occasional potassium loss, gastric irritation, insomnia, and psychotic disturbances. **Dexamethasone** is less salt- and water-retaining than **hydrocortisone** or **prednisone** and may be substituted in equivalent doses. Several long-term side effects have been reported after 6 months of daily therapy and include osteoporosis, pigmented striae, poor wound healing, truncal obesity, moon facies, cataracts, or open-angle glaucoma. Corticosteroid regimens that utilize 5- to 14-day courses usually do not suppress the adrenals, and thus no taper is required. If, on withdrawal, the patient exhibits muscle weakness, dizziness, hypotension, or lethargy, corticosteroids should be reinstituted and tapered more slowly (see Chap. 35).

Progestins

Progestins are compounds related to the endogenous steroid, **progesterone.** Although its antitumor activity is unclear, progestins appear to bind to cellular receptors, similar to the estrogens, inhibiting DNA synthesis. Approximately 40 percent of patients with estrogen receptor (ER) positive tumors will also have progesterone receptors. Patients with both estrogen and progesterone receptor-positive tumors have a 77 percent response to hormonal therapy.

Clinical Use and Dosage The major use of progestins is in the treatment of carcinomas involving the endometrium, kidneys, and breasts. The three most commonly used agents are: (1) **medroxyprogesterone** acetate (Depo-Provera), 600 to 1000 mg given IM once or twice a week; (2) **hydroxyprogesterone caproate** (Delalutin), 500 to 1000 mg given IM once a week; and (3) **megestrol acetate** (Megace), 40 mg given orally once a day.

Adverse Effects The most severe toxicity of the progestins is the increased incidence of thromboembolism. This may present as thrombophlebitis, cerebrovascular accident, or pulmonary emboli. These complications preclude treatment in patients with a history of thromboembolic episodes. Hypersensitivity reactions occur occasionally, manifesting as pruritis, urticaria, generalized rash and, rarely, anaphylaxis. Rare psychic disturbances include nervousness, insomnia, somnolence, fatigue, or dizziness. Other toxicities include nausea, vomiting, and headache.

Androgens

Androgens are steroidal derivatives of the endogenous hormone, testosterone. The antitumor effects of androgens are not understood but may be due to their ability to suppress pituitary function. Additionally, they inhibit DNA synthesis by binding to specific intracellular hormone receptors.

Clinical Use and Dosage Androgens are primarily used in the treatment of postmenopausal metastatic breast carcinoma. They produce regression in approximately 25 to 30 percent of patients with metastatic lesions of soft tissue or bone. Metastatic visceral lesions are generally less responsive. The most commonly used androgen is **fluoxymesterone** (Halotestin), which is given orally in doses of up to 30 mg/ day for at least 2 months or until response or progression is evident. Other androgens include **testosterone** and its esters, **nandrolone decanoate** (Deca-Durabolin), **dromostanolone propionate** (Drolban), and **testolactone** (Teslac).

Adverse Effects Toxicities involve the gastrointestinal, hepatic, gonadal, and renal systems. Nausea and vomiting are usually dose-related, which can be minimized by starting with low doses and titrating to full dosage. Cholestatic hepatotoxicity and jaundice are uncommon side effects associated with androgens (e.g., **fluoxymesterone**). If patients have preexisting hepatic metastases or parenchymal disease, dosage must be adjusted. Gonadal dysfunction in the form of enhanced libido and virilization is more common with **testosterone** and its esters than with oral agents. Salt and water retention are common with these agents. Hypercalcemia may be seen with the first two weeks of therapy if bone lesions are activated.

Aminoglutethimide

Aminoglutethimide (Cytadren) is an antiadrenal drug. It was originally introduced as an anticonvulsant. The finding that patients receiving aminoglutethimide developed adrenal insufficiency led to the removal of this agent from the market. It has recently been rereleased as an antineoplastic agent. Aminoglutethimide blocks adrenal steroidogenesis resulting in the decreased production of glucocorticoids, mineralocorticoids, androgens, progestins, and estrogens. This produces a chemical adrenalectomy which is reversible upon withdrawal of the drug.

Clinical Use and Dosage **Aminoglutethimide** is used in the management of prostatic cancer and advanced hormonally responsive breast cancer. The starting dose of aminoglutethimide is 250 mg twice daily for 2 weeks. The dose is then escalated to 1000 mg administered in divided doses.The response rate associated with this agent in ER-positive patients is approximately 50 percent. Replacement corticosteroid therapy is given by administering 30 to 40 mg of **hydrocortisone** daily. Mineralocorticoid replacement therapy is usually unnecessary.

Adverse Effects Toxicities associated with **aminoglutethimide** administration involve the hematopoietic, dermatologic, neurologic, and cardiovascular systems. Hematologic reactions are uncommon and include leukopenia and agranulocytosis, which are usually reversible within 10 days of stopping therapy. Dermatologic effects are uncommon and include rash, pruritus, and urticaria. Neurologic side effects include vertigo, lethargy, drowsiness, nystagmus, and ataxia which tend to be more severe during the initial 14 days of therapy. Patients should be warned not to attempt to drive a car or operate machinery which requires concentration during this period. Cardiovascular side effects include hypotension and tachycardia occurring in approximately 10 percent of the patients.

Miscellaneous Agents

Procarbazine Procarbazine (Matulane), in addition to its antineoplastic activity, is a mild monoamine oxidase inhibitor. This CCNS agent is rapidly metabolized in the liver to hydroxyl radicals which inhibit the synthesis of DNA, RNA, and essential proteins.

Clinical use and dosage Procarbazine is an oral agent primarily used in Hodgkin's disease. It also possesses activity against non-small-cell carcinoma of the lung and brain tumors. As a single agent, it is administered in doses of up to 200 mg/m^2/day. In the MOPP regimen for Hodgkin's disease, it is administered in doses of 100 mg/m^2 for 14 days. Due to procarbazine's inhibition of monoamine oxidase, patients should be advised against ingesting beverages and foods with a high tyramine content, such as cheese, bananas, beer, red wine, and yogurt. Procarbazine also potentiates tranquilizers, hypnotics, and narcotics. Tricyclic antidepressants are contraindicated during procarbazine administration.

Adverse effects The toxicities associated with this agent involve the hematopoietic, gastrointestinal, neurologic, and dermatologic systems. Hematologic effects include leukopenia and thrombocytopenia, occurring in approximately 60 to 70 percent of patients with an onset at day 14, a nadir at day 21, and recovery by day 28. Gastrointestinal toxicities may present as nausea, vomiting, anorexia, stomatitis, dysphagia, or diarrhea. These are dose-related, occurring in approximately 75 to 80 percent of patients. Fortunately, these side effects usually subside with continued therapy. Neurologic reactions are uncommon and present as mild paresthesias, ataxia, dizziness, headaches, insomnia, and hallucinations. These may be related to the depletion of pyridoxine; therefore, replacement therapy with **pyridoxine hydrochloride** 50 mg/day is indicated. Dermatologic effects noted with this agent include macropapular rash, urticaria, flushing syndrome, and erythematous facies.

Hydroxyurea Hydroxyurea (Hydrea) is a CCS agent. It inhibits ribonucleoside diphosphate reductase (RDR), an enzyme necessary for DNA synthesis.

Clinical use and dosage Hydroxyurea is an effective agent in chronic myelogenous leukemia. The drug is given orally in a daily dose of 20 to 30 mg/kg in two divided doses.

Adverse effects Toxicities with this agent involve hematopoietic, gastrointestinal, dermatologic, and renal organ systems. Hematopoietic effects include leukopenia and, less commonly, anemia and thrombocytopenia with an onset at days 5 to 7, a nadir at days 7 to 10, and recovery by days 21 to 30. Mild nausea and vomiting occur in most patients and, therefore, prophylactic antiemetics should be administered. Stomatitis and ulceration are uncommon and may respond to dosage reduction. Dermatologic complications can occur including rash, facial erythema, recall of radiation, and, rarely, partial alopecia. Hydroxyurea should be used cautiously in patients with renal or hepatic dysfunction.

Mitotane Mitotane (Lysodren, o',p'-DDD) exerts its cytotoxic effect on the mitochondria of adrenocortical cells. It reduces the production of corticosteroids and alters the peripheral metabolism of cortisol.

Clinical use and dosage Since mitotane kills adrenocortical cells, it is useful in the treatment of inoperable adrenocortical carcinoma. Usual therapeutic doses range from 8 to 10 g/day, given orally in three or four divided doses. The drug is better tolerated if therapy starts with an initial dose of 2 g/day and gradually is increased over several days to 8 to 10 g/day.

Adverse effects The major adverse reactions of this agent involve the gastrointestinal, neurologic, and dermatologic systems. Gastrointestinal reactions include anorexia, nausea, vomiting, and diarrhea which occurs in 80 percent of patients receiving this agent. Neurologic side effects include depression, dizziness, and vertigo in approximately 40 percent of patients. Skin rashes occur in about 15 percent of patients. Adrenal insufficiency may develop in patients treated with this agent; thus, corticosteroid replacement may be necessary.

L-*Asparaginase* L-**Asparaginase** (Elspar) is an enzyme which hydrolyzes the essential amino acid, asparagine, to nonfunctional aspartic acid and ammonia. Normal cells possess the ability to synthesize their own asparagine, while tumor cells are dependent on the serum pool for their supply. The administration of asparaginase deprives tumor cells of asparagine, resulting in cell death.

Clinical use and dosage The only application for L-asparaginase is in the treatment of acute lymphocytic leukemia. It produces complete responses in 30 to 60 percent of patients resistant to **vincristine** and **prednisone**. The usual dosage schedule is 200 IU/kg administered IM or IV for 14 to 21 days.

Adverse effects In contrast to most chemotherapeutic agents, L-asparaginase does not cause significant myelosuppression. However, severe hepatic, renal, pancreatic, gastrointestinal, neurologic, and coagulation disorders are common. Changes in liver function tests frequently occur, but return to normal once therapy has been discontinued. Rare oliguric renal failure has been observed. Decreased insulin synthesis with subsequent hyperglycemia may occur in a significant number of patients. Approximately 5 percent of patients may develop pancreatitis. Thus, frequent blood sugar and serum amylase monitoring is recommended. Nausea occurs in 50 percent of patients. Central nervous system toxicities occur in 30 to 60 percent of patients, presenting as depression, malaise, or personality changes. These effects rapidly disappear after completion of therapy. In addition, encephalopathy is occasionally reported and is most often seen in patients over 50 years of age. Coagulation defects such as hypofibrinogenemia are common and may require replacement therapy. Hypersensitivity demonstrated by itching, urticaria, bronchial spasm, hacking cough, and swelling of neck and lips occurs in 15 percent of patients. Anaphylaxis has been reported in approximately 10 percent of patients and is most common with intravenous adminis-

tration. When this agent is given **epinephrine** should be available and the patient closely monitored.

Cisplatin Cisplatin (Platinol) is the only heavy metal (platinum) compound which has been marketed as an antineoplastic. It is unclear how this CCNS agent produces its cytotoxicity, but it appears that the drug binds to base pairs on DNA and RNA inhibiting cellular reproduction. Many additional mechanisms have been postulated such as the inhibition of DNA precursors and RNA synthesis.

Clinical use and dosage Cisplatin is active against a variety of malignancies including non-small-cell cancer of the lung and carcinomas involving the ovaries, testes, prostate, and the head and neck. This agent is most often administered intravenously in doses of 100 mg/m² once every 3 to 4 weeks or 10 to 20 mg/m² daily for 5 days. Cisplatin is eliminated by the kidneys and therefore dosages must be reduced in patients with renal failure.

Adverse effects The major toxicities associated with cisplatin involve the gastrointestinal, hematologic, and renal systems. Gastrointestinal toxicities include nausea, vomiting, and anorexia which occur in almost all patients within 6 h of therapy. Less frequently, diarrhea is observed with the use of this agent. All patients must be premedicated with antiemetics prior to cisplatin administration. The hematologic toxicities, including leukopenia, thrombocytopenia, and anemia, are first noted at days 10 to 14, with nadir at days 14 to 21, and recovery by day 28. Nephrotoxicity is often the major dose-limiting toxicity with this drug. Creatinine clearance must be monitored prior to each cisplatin dose. In an attempt to minimize nephrotoxicity, all patients should be well hydrated prior to administration to ensure a urine output of at least 125 mL/h. Patients with a creatinine clearance of less than 50 mL/min should not receive cisplatin. In addition, tinnitus and hearing loss may occur. A baseline audiogram should be obtained prior to initiating therapy. In addition, peripheral neuritis has been reported in approximately 10 percent of patients receiving cisplatin.

Hexamethylmelamine The mechanism of action of hexamethylmelamine (HMM) is largely unknown. Alkylation, inhibition of DNA and RNA precursors, and inhibition of DNA and RNA synthesis have all been proposed as possible mechanisms. It is an investigational agent available from the National Cancer Institute.

Clinical use and dosage Hexamethylmelamine has activity in carcinomas of the lung, breast, uterus, ovaries, testes, and liver. The ultimate role for this wide-spectrum antitumor agent has not yet been determined, but its lack of myelosuppression makes it an ideal agent for combination chemotherapy. Hexamethylmelamine is most commonly administered in a dose of 6 to 12 mg/kg/day in four divided doses for 21 days.

Adverse effects The major side effects with this agent involve the hematopoietic, gastrointestinal, and neurologic systems. The GI side effects include anorexia, nausea, vomiting, abdominal cramps, and diarrhea. These occur a few days after beginning treatment in 50 to 70 percent of patients. Hematologic toxicities include mild myelosuppression manifesting as leukopenia and thrombocytopenia in 10 to 30 percent of patients. Neurotoxicity may present as peripheral neuropathy, sleep disturbances, depression, Parkinson's disease–like syndrome, hallucinations, or seizures. This toxicity is reversible when therapy is discontinued. In the event of neurotoxicity, pyridoxine 100 mg tid may relieve symptoms and allow for the continued use of this agent.

Etoposide   Etoposide (VP-16; Vepesid) is a semisynthetic podophyllotoxin derived from the May apple plant. The exact mechanism by which **etoposide** produces its cytotoxic effect is somewhat unclear at this time. It was initially believed to be a mitotic inhibitor but was subsequently found to act in the cell cycle prior to mitosis. Additionally, etoposide has been shown to produce breakage of DNA strands. This occurs primarily in the G_2 and S phases of the cell cycle.

Clinical use and dosage   Etoposide has activity against a number of tumors including testicular cancer, non-Hodgkin's lymphoma, small-cell lung cancer, and the leukemias. The recommended IV dose is 50 to 100 mg/m²/day for 5 days, or 100 mg/m²/day on days 1, 3, and 5 in combination therapy. The drug should be diluted in normal saline to a concentration of 0.2 to 0.4 mg/mL and administered over 30 to 60 min. Severe hypotension occurs following rapid intravenous administration.

Adverse effects   Toxicities from etoposide involve the gastrointestinal, hematopoietic, and dermatologic systems. The gastrointestinal side effects include nausea, vomiting, and infrequent diarrhea. Myelosuppression manifesting as leukopenia and thrombocytopenia is the principal dose-limiting toxicity of etoposide. The onset of leukopenia is at days 5 to 7, nadir at days 7 to 14, and recovery by day 20. Reversible alopecia occurs in 20 to 90 percent of patients, sometimes progressing to total baldness. Hypersensitivity reactions characterized by chills, fever, and tachycardia have also been reported. These reactions generally respond to stopping the infusion and administering steroids and antihistamines.

NURSING PROCESS RELATED TO CANCER CHEMOTHERAPY

Assessment

Case finding and referral are important assessment responsibilities of the nurse. The nurse must be aware of cancer risk factors, including drugs which are carcinogenic (Table 37-8). Since nearly every organ or tissue type can develop a

cancerous growth, the symptoms of the cancer will be dependent on the location of the neoplasm. The "Guidelines for the Cancer Related Checkup: Recommendations and Rationale" (American Cancer Society, 1980) affords the health professional a reasonable protocol for the assessment of the signs and symptoms of cancer.

The nurse also needs to assess how the cancer affects normal physiologic functioning, the patient's ability to perform usual activities of daily living, and the psychological response of the patient and his or her significant others. Nursing has a unique role in patient education related to the prevention, detection, and management of cancer, but all health professionals have a responsibility in this area. The American Cancer Society and other organizations provide numerous resources for the education of both the public and of health care professionals.

Management

Understanding Drug Selection and Dosage   The nurse who cares for the cancer patient must understand the process involved in drug and dosage selection. The selection of a drug regimen for an individual patient should be based on the factors summarized in Table 37-9. Once the regimen has been selected, the dosage of each drug must be determined. The dosage of an antineoplastic may be calculated by two different methods. The first method derives the dosage by multiplying the patient's weight in kilograms (kg) by the number of milligrams per kilograms per day (mg/kg/day) to be administered. For example, **floxuridine** 0.3 mg/kg/day is to be administered for 14 days to an 80-kg male. The daily dose of floxuridine is calculated by multiplying the patient's weight, 80 kg, by 0.3 mg/kg/day to obtain a dose of 24 mg/day. The second method of dosage calculation may be difficult for those unfamiliar with the concept of body surface area (BSA). This method of calculation is widely used in oncology because it has been shown that drug serum levels correlate better when the dosage is based on BSA rather than on milligrams per kilogram. Figure 7-3 is a nomogram for determining a patient's BSA. The patient's height and weight are all that is needed to utilize this nomogram. For example, Adriamycin 30 mg/m² is to be administered to a 155-cm female weighing 60 kg. The dose of Adriamycin is calculated by multiplying the 30 mg/m² by the BSA obtained from the nomogram, 1.58 m², to obtain a dose of 47.4 mg, which should be rounded to the nearest whole number. Fractional doses are used for more potent drugs, such as **vincristine**.

Toxicity Management

The nurse who is caring for the cancer patient should be familiar with the toxicities associated with each antineoplastic agent. The management of these toxicities is of primary concern to the oncology nurse. This section discusses the management of the common hematologic, gastrointes-

TABLE 37-8 Drugs Established as Human Carcinogens

DRUG	MALIGNANCY
Radioactive drugs [phosphorus (^{32}P), radium, mesothorium, thorotrast]	Organs where concentrated (acute leukemia, osteosarcoma, nasal sinus carcinoma, angiosarcoma of the liver)
Chlornaphazine	Bladder cancer
Arsenic	Skin cancer
Methoxypsoralen	Skin cancer
Phenacetin-containing drugs	Renal pelvis carcinoma Bladder cancer (?)
Alkylating agents (melphalan, cyclophosphamide, chlorambucil, dihydroxybusulfan, and others)	Acute nonlymphocytic leukemia Bladder (cyclophosphamide) Other sites (?)
Immunosuppressive agents (Azathioprine)	Lymphoma Skin cancer Soft-tissue sarcoma Melanoma (?) Liver and gall bladder (?) Lung adenocarcinoma (?)
Androgen-anabolic steroids	Hepatocellular carcinoma
Estrogen-containing drugs Prenatal (DES) Postnatal (DES, conjugated estrogens, oral contraceptives)	Vaginal adenocarcinoma Endometrial carcinoma Breast cancer (?) Cervical cancer (?) Ovarian cancer (?) Choriocarcinoma (?) Melanoma (?) Liver tumors (benign)

Source: R. Hoover and J. F. Fraumeni: *Cancer,* **47**:1074, 1981. Used by permission.

TABLE 37-9 Factors Influencing Drug Selection and Response to Chemotherapy

FACTOR	SIGNIFICANCE
Type of cancer	Natural history—rapid-growing vs. slow-growing
Extent of disease stage	More advanced—less responsive
Responsiveness to chemotherapy	Inherent tumor sensitivity
Prior chemotherapy	Resistance mechanisms
Prior radiotherapy	Lower drug dosage usually required because of myelosuppression
Karnofsky status	Higher rating means better drug tolerance
Renal or hepatic function	Dysfunction alters drug clearance from the body
Pharmacokinetics	Drug distribution and site of action

Source: R. J. Ignoffo: "Oncology," in B. S. Katcher, L. Y. Young, and M. A. Koda-Kimble (eds.), *Applied Therapeutics: The Clinical Use of Drugs,* 3d ed., San Francisco: Applied Therapeutics, Inc., 1983. Used by permission.

tinal, dermatologic, and neurologic toxicities associated with the administration of neoplastic agents.

Leukopenia The hematologic toxicity of leukopenia is the most serious consequence of the generalized bone marrow suppression associated with the use of most antineoplastic agents (Table 37-10). The onset, nadir, and duration of the leukopenia depend upon the drug, the dose, and the schedule of administration. White blood counts of 1000 to 2000/mm^3 are commonly seen, and a count of less than 1000 is not unusual. Additionally, the neutrophil counts in these patients are frequently very low, predisposing these patients to severe infections. Temperatures should be taken at 4-h intervals in all leukopenic patients. A slight temperature elevation should be rechecked after an hour and any elevation over 38°C orally should be brought to the physician's attention immediately unless otherwise specified.

The most serious threat to a leukopenic patient is from the bacteria which normally inhabit the body surface. Nasal, rectal, and cutaneous abscesses are common in these patients and can be the cause of dramatic temperature elevations. Abscess formation in these patients does not show the characteristic accumulation of pus because of the absence of granulocytes. In addition, an infection which would remain localized in the normal patient can be the cause of a septicemia in the neutropenic patient. The importance of routine examination of all orifices as well as the skin cannot be overemphasized. Checking of these areas each shift by the nurse, with repeated explanations of the rationale for careful examination, will alert the patient to the necessity for continued observation. Routine mouth care with **sodium bicarbonate** 1 tbsp and **sodium chloride** (table salt) 1 tbsp in 1 qt of water for oral lavage should be instituted. Mouth lavage should be completed after each meal and at bedtime. Soft toothbrushing, or toothettes, should be used to clean teeth, tongue, and hard palate prior to lavage. Scrupulous cleansing of the rectal area should be completed after each bowel movement, and Tucks may sooth rectal discomfort. Because rectal trauma increases the likelihood of sepsis, patients with neutrophil counts of less than 1000 should not receive rectal suppositories or have rectal temperatures taken.

A second source of infection for the leukopenic patient is from the environment. Whether the patient is at home or in the hospital, contact with anyone having an infection should be avoided. The technique of total reverse isolation has been abandoned because the incidence of infection is not significantly decreased when the gown, mask, and glove precautions are maintained. At the same time, the unnecessary isolation of a patient may have a negative psychologic effect. Using good hand-washing technique upon entering and leaving the patient's room is the most important factor with these patients. Visitors should be screened by the nurse and instructed in the precautionary measures and the reason for their use.

Thrombocytopenia   Thrombocytopenia is another common side effect associated with cancer chemotherapy. Platelet counts may decrease to 50,000/mm³ and lower. When bleeding occurs or platelet counts are below 20,000/mm³, platelet transfusions may be required. Routine hematests of the urine and guaiac testing of stools are recommended. The skin should be checked frequently for petechiae or bruising. Intramuscular injections should be avoided. Pressure should be applied for 3 to 5 min to any puncture site, and rechecked for hematoma or continued bleeding. These patients need to take precautions to avoid unnecessary trauma. Injuries to the skin such as cuts and bruising should be noted when they occur and watched carefully. Bleeding from the nose and gums may be observed in these patients. A soft toothbrush or toothettes will be sufficient to clean the teeth when mouth lavages are used. Flossing of the teeth should be avoided. When patients have nosebleeds, they should pinch the nostrils for a full 10 min, applying sufficient pressure to stop the bleeding. They should avoid blowing the nose, since this will loosen a clot and restart the bleeding.

Nausea and vomiting   Nausea and vomiting are the most commonly observed gastrointestinal toxicities. Vomiting may occur within 1 h of drug administration and persist for up to 24 h. The severity of emesis depends on the particular agent administered (Table 37-11). There are several antie-

TABLE 37-10   Leukopenia with Chemotherapeutic Agents

DRUG	ONSET, DAYS	NADIR, DAYS	RECOVERY, DAYS
Bleomycin	4–7	10	18
Busulfan		10–14	28–42
Carmustine	21–28	42	56
Chlorambucil	7	10–14	28–42
Cisplatin	10–14	14–21	28
Cyclophosphamide	7	14	21
Cytarabine	4–7	10–14	21
Dacarbazine	7	14	28
Dactinomycin	7	14	21–28
Daunorubicin	7–10	10–20	28
Doxorubicin	7–10	10–20	28
Etoposide	5–7	7–14	20
Fluorouracil	7–10	14	24
Hydroxyurea	5–7	7–10	21–30
Lomustine	21–28	42	56
Mechlorethamine	4–7	10–14	21
Melphalan	7	10–18	42–50
Mercaptopurine	7–10	14	21
Methotrexate	4–7	14	21
Mitomycin-C	10–14	14–28	35–56
Plicamycin	7	14	28
Procarbazine	14	21	28
Streptozocin	7	14	21
Thiotepa	14–21	28	42
Vinblastine	4–7	10	17

metics available. (See Chap. 19, "Nausea and Vomiting.") The appropriate antiemetic should be administered 1 h prior to drug administration and continued for at least 24 h. If the antineoplastic has strong emetogenic properties, the use of combination antiemetic therapy may be necessary, such as the use of concurrent **metoclopramide** (Reglan), **dexamethasone** (Decadron), and **diphenhydramine** (Benadryl) for patients receiving cisplatin.

Diarrhea Diarrhea is another gastrointestinal side effect frequently encountered. Skin breakdown about the anus must be prevented, especially in the neutropenic patient, since infection can readily occur at this site. Antidiarrheal medication may be employed, i.e., **atropine** with **diphenoxylate** (Lomotil) or **loperamide** (Imodium). Patients should be taught rectal care if the antineoplastic prescribed is known to cause diarrhea. Symptomatic relief may be obtained through the use of astringent pads (e.g., Tucks) or an emolient cream applied to the anus.

Mucositis Mucositis is another common side effect of chemotherapy, and may be severe. Mouth sores (stomatitis) are most frequently seen, but any mucous membrane can be affected. Stomatitis cannot be prevented but some measures to promote comfort may be helpful and good oral hygiene is imperative. Frequent mouth lavage may be the best tolerated method for keeping the mouth clean and free of food particles. Bland food served at a medium temperature will minimize irritation as much as possible. A topical anesthetic such as Cetacaine or viscous **lidocaine** (Xylocaine) used before meals will numb the mouth so that the patient can better tolerate eating. Candidiasis is the most common infection seen in patients with stomatitis. Therefore, routine use of **nystatin** suspension (Mycostatin, Nilstat), or oral **ketoconazole** (Nizoral) is a good preventive measure. The patient should be told to swish 5 to 10 mL of the nystatin around the mouth and then swallow. This should be done at least

four times per day. Ketoconazole is administered in a dose of 200 to 400 mg orally daily. The antifungal **clotrimazole** (Mycelex-T) is available as a troche given five times daily to treat oral candidiasis.

Dermatologic Toxicity Alopecia is seen with almost all chemotherapeutic agents. **Cyclophosphamide, doxorubicin, dactinomycin,** and **daunorubicin** have the most dramatic effect on the hair follicles. While alopecia is the least significant of the systemic effects of chemotherapy, it can be one of the most emotionally disturbing. The patient's body image is threatened by the loss of hair, which is sometimes radical. A scalp tourniquet, applied prior to administration and for up to 30 min after, can sometimes limit the alopecia. The use of wigs, scarves, or hats should be discussed and encouraged with these patients. At the same time, they need the opportunity to ventilate their feelings about the change in their self-image. It is important to reiterate to patients that the hair loss is usually reversible following discontinuation of therapy.

Neurotoxicity Neurotoxicity is a special consideration when administering the vinca alkaloids **vincristine** and **vinblastine,** as well as some other agents. Minor neuropathies, such as tingling in the hands and feet and a decrease or loss of the deep tendon reflexes, are generally seen in all patients. The more serious toxic reactions include weakness of hand strength, ataxia and loss of coordination, foot drop or wrist drop, and paralytic ileus. Because the neurotoxicity of the vinca alkaloids can be irreversible in more severe reactions, education of the patient concerning the early and transient signs of neurotoxicity is necessary. Constipation from a high impaction of the bowel can be a severe problem in these patients. Dietary control of bowel movements can help, as can appropriate stool softeners and laxatives to pro-

TABLE 37-11 Emetic Potential of Antineoplastic Drugs

SEVERE*	MODERATE*	MILD-TO-NONE*
Azacitidine (rapid injection)	Azacitidine (slow infusion)	Bleomycin
Carmustine	Cytarabine	Busulfan
Cisplatin	Etoposide	Chlorambucil
Cyclophosphamide (high-dose parenteral)	Hexamethylmelamine	Fluorouracil
Dacarbazine	Mitotane	Hydroxyurea
Dactinomycin	Procarbazine	L-Asparaginase
Daunorubicin	Thiotepa	Melphalan
Doxorubicin	Vinblastine	6-Mercaptopurine
Lomustine		Methotrexate
Mechlorethamine		Mitomycin C
Plicamycin		Thioguanine
Streptozocin		Vincristine

*The listing of agents is based on the frequency and severity of nausea and vomiting. That is, severe includes a frequency of greater than 75 percent incidence of vomiting, usually with retching; moderate is between 25 and 75 percent vomiting; and mild is less than 25 percent vomiting.

Source: K. See-Lasley and R. J. Ignoffo: *Manual of Oncology Therapeutics,* St. Louis: Mosby, 1981.

TABLE 37-12 Vesicant Anticancer Drugs

Carmustine
Dacarbazine (DTIC)
Dactinomycin
Daunorubicin
Doxorubicin
Etoposide
Mechlorethamine
Mitomycin C
Plicamycin
Vinblastine
Vincristine

mote daily evacuations. Even minor paresthesias may be anxiety-producing if they are unexpected and patients need to know that they may occur. Patients should also be instructed to report any increase in symptoms of neurotoxicity to the physician or nurse.

Extravasation Management

One of the major concerns of the nurse when administering an antineoplastic drug intravenously is whether it will irritate the vessel wall, or worse, cause local tissue necrosis upon accidental extravasation. Many of the antineoplastic agents are vesicants (Table 37-12). A *vesicant* is an agent which, when accidentally infiltrated into the skin, causes severe local tissue breakdown and necrosis. The degree of irritation to the tissues is dependent on the particular antineoplastic being administered and the amount extravasated. The best way to prevent extravasation is to adhere to a strict guideline for antineoplastic drug administration (Table 37-13). If extravasation does occur, the nurse must take the appropriate measures to minimize tissue damage. Table 37-14 provides sample guidelines for treating extravasations. Many institutions now require that an extravasation treatment kit be available. Such a kit contains the appropriate recommended antidotes needed to treat an extravasation (Table 37-15).

Evaluation

Ascertaining the effectiveness of the nursing care and drug therapy of the cancer patient is dependent upon the therapeutic goals. Criteria of evaluation will depend upon whether the goal is cure, remission, or palliation. It is important to weigh the risk-benefit ratio of administering an antineoplastic drug to ensure that the net effect is favorable. The nurse should evaluate the effectiveness of nursing measures undertaken to relieve the discomfort of the side effects. It may be necessary to reevaluate and modify the plan many times before the optimum management regimen for a given patient is found.

TABLE 37-13 Guidelines for Administering Chemotherapy

1. Dilute the drug in the appropriate amount of diluent to avoid high concentrations.
2. Select an infusion site in the following order of preference: forearm > dorsum of hand > wrist > antecubital fossa.
3. Insert a 21- or 23-gauge "butterfly" needle (one venipuncture only) into the vein.
4. Lightly tape the tubing of the "butterfly" distal to the needle. Do not obscure the injection site by covering it with tape.
5. Administer 5 mL of normal saline solution (NS) and withdraw a small amount of blood to test vein integrity and flow. Observe for extravasation.
6. If extravasation of NS is obvious, select another site (the other arm, or lateral or proximal to the initial site in that arm). Avoid a distal point on the same vein because of the potential for extravasation "upstream."
7. If multiple drugs are prescribed, some clinicians prefer to inject the vesicant agents first. If all drugs are vesicants, inject the one with the least amount of diluent first. Separate each administered drug with 3 to 5 mL of saline.
8. Administer the drug over at least 3 min or approximately 5 mL/min. Withdraw blood once for each 1 to 2 mL of solution administered to assure proper needle placement. Repeatedly ask the patient if he/she feels any pain, burning, or tingling.
9. Follow the drug injection with 5 to 10 mL or more of normal saline to flush tubing and needle of all drug.

Source: K. See-Lasley and R. J. Ignoffo: *Manual of Oncology Therapeutics,* St. Louis: Mosby, 1981. Used by permission.

TABLE 37-14 Management of Chemotherapy Extravasations

1. Stop injection immediately, leaving needle in place.
2. Withdraw 3 to 5 mL of blood and solution (if possible).
3. Administer 25 mg hydrocortisone into the needle (optional) and remove needle.
4. With a 27-gauge TB syringe, aspirate any extravasated solution not removed by procedure (2).
5. Purposely administer the antidote subcutaneously in a "pincushion" manner in the extravasated area (use four to five injections).
6. Apply cold compresses for 1 h to allow time for the antidote to interact with the vesicant.
7. Apply warm compresses at the extravasated site for 1 h.*
8. Follow-up should be obtained weekly (or earlier if mechlorethamine), observing for signs of inflammation and necrosis.
9. Surgical excision should be considered at the first sign of tissue breakdown or ulceration.

*It is well known that drug absorption from subcutaneous or intramuscular injections is enhanced in the presence of heat and decreased by cold. Some clinicians prefer cold over heat in the setting of extravasation. In our opinion, a combination of initial cold compresses followed by heat may be more rational than either method alone.

Source: K. See-Lasley and R. J. Ignoffo: *Manual of Oncology Therapeutics,* St. Louis: Mosby, 1981. Used by permission.

TABLE 37-15   Table of Antidotes for Extravasated Antineoplastic Drugs

EXTRAVASATED DRUG	ANTIDOTE	DOSE OF ANTIDOTE, mL
Actinomycin D	Sodium thiosulfate 10%	4
Carmustine	$NaHCO_3$ (8.4%)	5
Daunomycin	$NaHCO_3$ (8.4%);	5
	Dexamethasone (4 mg/mL)	1
Doxorubicin	$NaHCO_3$ (8.4%)	5
	Dexamethasone (4 mg/mL)	1
Mitomycin C	Sodium thiosulfate 10% or	4
	Pyridoxine (50 mg/mL)	1
Mechlorethamine	Sodium thiosulfate 10%	4
Plicamycin	EDTA (150 mg/mL)	1
Vinblastine	Hyaluronidase 150 U/mL + heat	1
Vincristine	Hyaluronidase 150 U/mL + heat	1

CASE STUDY

H.R., a 52-year-old married female, noticed a lump in the upper outer quadrant of her left breast and went to her physician to have it evaluated. She was admitted to the hospital for a biopsy. Frozen section revealed stage II adenocarcinoma: The tumor was 4 cm in diameter, with involvement of two lymph nodes. A modified radical mastectomy was performed. H.R. was perimenopausal, having ceased to menstruate two years prior. However, hormonal treatment was not initiated because studies indicated that the breast tissue was estrogen receptor-negative. Plans were made for the patient to begin combination chemotherapy following surgery.

The physicians recommended to H.R. that she receive six cycles of adjuvant chemotherapy with cyclophosphamide, fluorouracil, and methotrexate. She received her first doses consisting of 5-FU 600 mg/m² IV, methotrexate 40 mg/m² IV, and cyclophosphamide 100 mg/m² orally prior to her discharge from the hospital. The intravenous drugs were given by the physician and the patient started her oral cyclophosphamide; she would continue the course (days 2 to 14) at home.

Assessment

Four weeks after the initial course, H.R. reported to the oncology clinic for the next cycle of chemotherapy. The nurse recorded her height (165 cm) and weight (58 kg) and calculated her body surface area at 1.63 m². Since all three drugs can cause bone marrow suppression, a CBC with differential and platelet count were obtained. The white cell count was 5800/mm³, and the differential count and platelet count were within normal limits. The patient reported that she had no adverse effects from the initial course of therapy except for nausea lasting for 24 h. H.R. was then asked about any history of renal or ulcer disease, and reported none.

The nurse inspected the incision and found it to be clean and well healed. Minimal lymphedema was noted in the left arm and the shoulder showed good range of motion. H.R. indicated she had been doing "wall-climbing" and "sweeping" exercises regularly. She had been fitted for a breast prosthesis at a special shop. The nurse indicated that it might take time for the size to stabilize and that several fittings over the next few months might be required.

A discussion of the adaptation of H.R. and her family to the diagnosis and the surgery revealed that H.R. felt that her husband and two children, who were college students, had been very supportive and helpful. She felt that many of her friends had been oversolicitous; she found this very depressing and still found herself occasionally bursting into tears at times for no specific reason. However, she stated that she looked forward to returning to her job as a high school counselor, so that friends would begin to treat her normally and she could avoid the long days at home alone. She had a good understanding of the disease and the goals of chemotherapy.

The nurse's impression was that H.R. did not demonstrate any signs or symptoms which would contraindicate continuation of the drug regimen and that she was progressing satisfactorily both physically and psychologically after the surgery.

The physician examined the patient, reviewed the laboratory data, and ordered cyclophosphamide 150 mg orally days 1 to 14, methotrexate 65 mg IV day 1, 5-FU 980 mg IV day 1, and prochlorperazine (Compazine) 25 mg administered every 4 h rectally as needed.

Management

The nurse administered prochlorperazine 10 mg intramuscularly in an attempt to prevent the nausea and vomiting which the chemotherapeutic agents could cause; the intramuscular route was chosen to ensure rapid effect.

H.R. was instructed to lie quietly after the injection and her blood pressure was assessed for hypotension from the prochlorperazine. H.R. was also given a prescription for prochlorperazine suppositories to take at home.

After 30 min, the nurse inserted a 23-gauge "butterfly" in the right hand and injected the methotrexate. After flushing the line with normal saline and checking for the blood return, the fluorouracil was given. The line was flushed after the fluorouracil and the butterfly removed. The time for each of the injections was 3 min.

Following the injections the nurse explained to H.R. the important measures she should take to minimize adverse effects and what signs and symptoms she should report to the clinic. The nurse reinforced this teaching with the following written information:

1. To prevent irritation of the bladder from the cyclophosphamide you should drink at least 10 to 12 glasses (40 to 50 mL/kg) of fluid per day. You should void at least every 2 h during the day. Report any painful or bloody urine if it occurs.

2. You may experience some hair loss from the therapy, but this is only temporary and your hair will return upon completion of the therapy. If your hair is long, you might wish to change it to a short haircut so that any loss will be less noticeable.

3. Call the clinic if you experience a fever over 37.5°C (99°F) for more than 24 h, nausea unrelieved by the antiemetic, diarrhea, mouth sores, or difficulty swallowing.

4. Try to avoid exposure to infections. Report any sore throat, cold or flu symptoms, bruising, or bleeding.

In future teaching sessions, the nurse planned to instruct H.R. on the signs and symptoms of recurrent breast cancer and to advise regular follow-up for H.R.'s daughter, who is at increased risk of breast cancer.

Evaluation

On subsequent visits, H.R. complained of nausea and thinning of her hair. In addition, she had slight leukopenia and thrombocytopenia. She had no mucositis, stomatitis, diarrhea, or painful urination. The nurse explained at this time about the hair loss and reminded the patient that her hair would return after the therapy was completed. Her antiemetic therapy was also changed from prochlorperazine to thiethylperazine (Torecan) 10 mg administered orally or rectally every 4 h as needed. After three months, H.R. was back at work and functioning well. She had no signs or symptoms of recurrence, but regular follow-up and chemotherapy were to continue.

REFERENCES

Aherne, G., E. Piall, V. Marks, G. Mould, and W. F. White: "Prolongation and Enhancement of Serum Methotrexate Concentrations by Probenecid," *Br Med J*, 1:1097–1099, 1978.

American Cancer Society: "Guidelines for the Cancer-Related Checkup: Recommendations and Rationale," *Cancer J Clinicians*, 30(4):193–210, 1980.

Cadman, E.: "Toxicity of Chemotherapeutic Agents," in F. F. Becker, *Cancer: A Comprehensive Treatise*, vol. 5, New York: Plenum, 1977.

Chatner, B.: *Pharmacologic Principles of Cancer Treatment*, Philadelphia: Saunders, 1982.

Dedrick, R. L., C. E. Myers, and A. M. Guarinot: "Pharmacokinetic Rationale for Peritoneal Drug Administration in Treatment of Ovarian Cancer," *Cancer Treat Rep*, 62:1–11, 1978.

DeVita, V. T.: "The Consequences of the Chemotherapy of Hodgkin's Disease: The 10th Annual David A. Karnofsky Lecture," *Cancer*, 47:1–13, 1981.

——, S. Hellman, and S. A. Rosenberg: *Cancer Principles and Practice of Oncology*, Philadelphia: Lippincott, 1982, chaps. 4, 8, and 9.

——, R. C. Young, and G. P. Canellas: "Combination Versus Single Agent Chemotherapy: A Review of the Basis for Selection of Drug Treatment of Cancer," *Cancer*, 35:98–110, 1975.

Dorr, R. T., and W. L. Fritz: *Cancer Chemotherapy Handbook*, New York: Elsevier, 1980.

Evans, W. E., C. B. Pratt, R. H. Taylor, L. F. Barker, and W. R. Crom: "Pharmacokinetic Monitoring of High-Dose Methotrexate: Early Recognition of High-Risk Patients," *Cancer Chemother Pharmacol*, 3:161–166, 1979.

Friedman, M. A., and E. Slater: "Malignant Pleural Effusions," *Cancer Treat Rev*, 5:49–66, 1978.

Ignoffo, R. J., and M. A. Friedman: "Therapy of Local Toxicities Caused by Extravasation of Cancer Chemotherapeutic Drugs," *Cancer Treat Rev*, 7:17–27, 1980.

Jaffe, N., E. Frei, III, D. Traggis, and Y. Bishop: "Adjuvant Methotrexate and Citrovoroum-Factor Treatment of Osteogenic Sarcoma," *N Engl J Med*, 291:994, 1974.

Liegler, D. G., E. S. Henderson, M. A. Hahn, and V. T. Oliverio: "The Effect of Organic Acids on Renal Clearance of Methotrexate in Man," *Clin Pharmacol Ther*, 10:849–857, 1969.

Mauch, P. M.: "Treatment of Malignant Periocardial Effusions," in N. T. DeVita, S. Hellman, and S. A. Rosenberg (eds.), *Cancer Principles and Practice of Oncology,* Philadelphia: Lippincott, 1982, pp. 1571–1573.

Mellett, L. B.: "Physicochemical Considerations and Pharmacokinetic Behavior in Delivery of Drugs to the Central Nervous Ssytem," *Cancer Treat Rep,* 61:527–531, 1977.

Norton, L., and R. Simon: "Tumor Size, Sensitivity to Therapy, and Design of Treatment Schedules," *Cancer Treat Rep,* 61:1307–1317, 1977.

Pitot, H. L.: *Fundamentals of Oncology,* New York: Dekker, 1978.

Schabel, F. M.: "Rationale for Adjuvant Chemotherapy," *Cancer,* 39:2875–2882, 1977.

See-Lasley, K., and R. J. Ignoffo: *Manual of Oncology Therapeutics,* St. Louis: Mosby, 1981.

Skipper, H. E.: "Combination Therapy: Some Concepts and Results," *Cancer Chemother Rep,* 4:137, 1974.

Steel, G. G.: *Growth Kinetics of Tumours,* Oxford: Clarendon, 1977, pp. 286–287.

Theologides, A.: "Neoplastic Cardiac Tamponade," *Semin Oncol,* 5:181, 1978.

Tubiana, M., and E. P. Malaise: "Growth Rate and Cell Kinetics in Human Tumors: Some Prognostic and Therapeutic Implications," *Scientific Foundation of Oncology,* Chicago: Year Book, 1976, pp. 126–136.

Tyson, L. B., R. J. Gralla, R. A. Clark, and M. G. Kris: "Combination Antiemetic Trials with Metaclopramide (MCP)," *Proc Am Soc Clin Oncol,* 2:91, 1983.

38

DERMATOLOGIC DISORDERS*

RICHARD A. F. CLARK
MARCIA G. TONNESEN

LEARNING OBJECTIVES

Upon mastery of this chapter, the reader will be able to:

1. Describe the structure and functions of the skin.
2. List the most frequent types of dermatologic reactions to drugs and give an example of each.
3. List at least three factors which influence percutaneous absorption of drugs.
4. Describe why permeability and solubility are important in the use of topical preparations.
5. List the goals for the use of topical preparations.
6. Give examples of agents that are used to relieve itching and describe their mechanism of action.
7. Discuss the conditions where use of antipruritics should be avoided and why.
8. List causative factors leading to dehydration of the skin.
9. Discuss measures to prevent dry skin and ways to correct dryness.
10. List agents used to reduce moisture and friction.
11. Discuss commonly used agents to cleanse and debride the skin.
12. List the categories of agents used to kill or reduce cutaneous microorganisms.
13. State the desired characteristics of an antiseptic.
14. List adverse effects of topical corticosteroid therapy to reduce inflammation.
15. Discuss why fair skin should be protected from the sun and explain what is meant by sun protection factor.
16. Describe patient education associated with (a) the use of isotretinoin and tetracycline in acne, (b) the management of dry skin, (c) PUVA therapy in psoriasis, and (d) skin infections.

ANATOMY AND PHYSIOLOGY OF THE SKIN

Although the skin is the largest organ of the body, it is normally only 3 to 5 mm thick. Skin over the palms and soles is thickest while that portion covering eyelids and genitalia is thinnest. The three main layers of skin are epidermis, dermis, and subcutis (Fig. 38-1), each of which will be described in more detail below.

The epidermis is composed of keratinocytes which provide a protective covering for the body, melanocytes which form pigment called melanin that protects the body from ultraviolet irradiation, and Langerhans cells which are macrophagelike cells that protect the body from foreign particles. Keratinocytes proliferate in the basal layer of the epidermis and move upward as they produce large quantities of keratin, a specific cytoskeletal protein which provides the epidermis with its tensile strength, and secrete a cement substance which forms the permeability barrier of the skin (Table 38-1). Subsequently, keratinocytes finally slough or desquamate. Melanocytes reside in the basal layer of skin but have long dendritic processes which extend to keratinocytes in upper layers of the skin. Melanocytes produce and package melanin into melanosomes and transfer these melanosomes into keratinocytes to form a protective barrier to the ultraviolet rays of the sun. Langerhans cells are found in the upper layers of the skin where they act as sentry cells for foreign particles that penetrate the epidermis.

The dermis contains major structural elements such as collagen, elastin, hyaluronic acid, and proteoglycans; singly disposed cells such as fibroblasts, fixed tissue histiocytes, and mast cells; as well as nerves, blood vessels, lymphatics, and appendages. There are four major appendages within the dermis and subcutis: hair follicles, sebaceous glands, eccrine

*The authors are grateful to Evelyn J. Whelan, Susan K. Warner, and Jacki Kinoshito for review of the nursing process implications and for text contributions to this chapter. The editors thank Joseph A. Romano, Catherine Clayton, and Joseph Bertino, who contributed the chapter on this subject in the first edition.

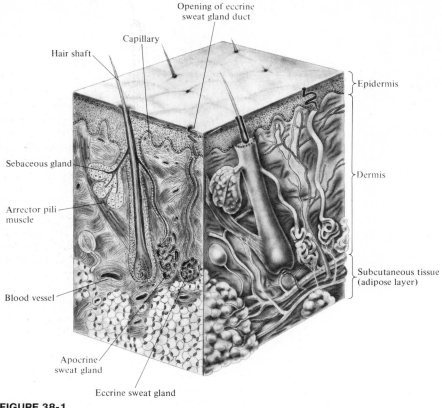

FIGURE 38-1

Diagrammatic Cross Section of Normal Skin. (*Source: J. Parrish, Dermatology and Skin Care, New York: McGraw-Hill Book Company, 1975.*)

glands, and apocrine glands. Hair provides a warm covering for mammals but has become rather rudimentary in man. Most sebaceous (sebum producing) glands connect into the upper portion of hair follicles. Sebum which is secreted by sebaceous glands onto the surface of the skin has antibacterial and antifungal properties and lubricates the skin to help prevent moisture loss and to ensure cutaneous suppleness. Eccrine sweat glands are independent of hair follicles with secretory epithelium located in the subcutis and ducts ascending as coiled loops through the dermis and epidermis.

TABLE 38-1 Functions of the Skin

Permeability barrier
Fluid balance (hydroregulation)
Waste elimination
Temperature regulation
Sensation (temperature, touch, itch, pain)
Surface lubrication
Protection against pathogenic organisms
Protection against physical and chemical injury
Protection against solar radiation

Excess body heat can be dissipated through sweat formation and evaporation. In addition, the acidic pH of sweat contributes to the antibacterial and antifungal properties of secretory components covering the skin surface. Apocrine sweat glands like sebaceous glands are connected to hair follicles but are found only around the nipples, in the axillae, and in the anogenital region. They do not participate in body temperature regulation but may have some residual function in the mating responses of humans similar to their role in lower mammals.

The subcutis, composed of relatively loose connective tissue and fat cells, provides necessary pliability and cushioning of the skin. It also facilitates thermal control and acts as a food reserve.

DRUG-INDUCED DISORDERS OF THE SKIN (DERMATITIS MEDICAMENTOSA)

Adverse drug reactions are frequently manifested as skin eruptions. Although there is lack of data on the exact incidence of these reactions, it is estimated that 1 to 5 percent of hospitalized patients experience rashes secondary to medications. Dermatitis medicamentosa is a term used to describe skin rashes induced by the internal administration of certain drugs. Almost any reaction pattern that can occur in the skin (see Table 38-2) may be drug-related and most drugs can provoke several types of eruptions.

The most common drug-related reaction pattern is a *maculopapular* or *morbilliform rash.* Clinical and histologic features alone do not allow differentiation of a drug-induced maculopapular rash from that due to other causes, most commonly viral infections. A maculopapular drug rash itself has relatively little associated morbidity; however, on rare occasions it can progress to exfoliative dermatitis.

Urticaria (hives) and *angioedema* are frequent skin manifestations of drug hypersensitivity and may be associated with systemic symptoms: arthritis, arthralgias, fever, and leukocytosis (especially eosinophilia). In an extremely allergic patient, a fulminant anaphylactic syndrome may develop within minutes after drug administration, manifested by urticaria, hypotension, severe asthma, and possibly laryngeal edema. This is a medical emergency. Any patient who has developed urticaria to a medication is at risk for having an anaphylactic attack if the same or related drug is administered again. It is essential for the nurse to *independently* obtain a careful history of drug hypersensitivity before administering *any* drug to a patient for the first time even though this history may have already been given to a physician.

Photosensitivity may occur when a patient on certain drugs is exposed to artificial ultraviolet light or sunlight. Photosensitive reactions can be subdivided into two types: *phototoxic,* which have a nonimmunologic basis, and *photoallergic,* which have an immunologic basis.

Purpura and *petechiae* are signs of bleeding into the skin. They can be caused by drug-induced thrombocytopenia or drug-induced vasculitis. When the latter is associated with IgA immune complexes and glomerulonephritis it is called Henoch-Schönlein purpura; otherwise drug-induced vasculitis is often referred to as allergic angiitis. When medium-size arteries are involved, the term polyarteritis nodosa is used to denote the disorder. Drug-induced thrombocytopenia may be due to bone marrow suppression, immunologic platelet destruction, or direct destruction of platelets by the drug.

Erythema multiforme consists of a symmetrical eruption of erythematous papules which develop central blisters and may expand with concentric rings of color to form classic "target" lesions. The severe febrile form of erythema multiforme, called *Stevens-Johnson syndrome,* involves multiple mucous membranes as well as other organs and may be life-threatening.

Skin rashes due to drug reactions are usually generalized in nature; however, *fixed drug eruptions* may occur in the same local site each time the patient is exposed to the drug. Initially the eruption consists of an erythematous plaque. After repeated exposures, blistering and hyperpigmentation occur.

PRINCIPLES OF TOPICAL THERAPY

The skin is ideally suited for the topical administration of medication in the treatment of dermatologic conditions. However, in some cases this is not always satisfactory and systemic administration may be needed.

When topical therapy is used several principles should be

TABLE 38-2   Drugs Potentially Causing Dermatologic Eruptions

Maculopapular, Morbilliform Eruption	*Erythema Multiforme*	*Photosensitive Eruptions*
Ampicillin	Barbiturates	Griseofulvin
Antihistamines	Hydantoins	Nalidixic acid
Antimalarials	Penicillins	Phenothiazines
Barbiturates	Phenolphthalein	Psoralens
Gold salts	Phenylbutazone	Sulfonamides
Griseofulvin	Sulfonamides	Sulfonylureas
Insulin		Tetracyclines
Penicillins	*Urticaria, Angioedema*	Thiazides
Phenothiazines	Barbiturates	
Phenylbutazone	Griseofulvin	*Fixed Drug Eruption*
Sulfonamides	Insulin	Barbiturates
Thiazides	Opiates	Phenacetin
	Penicillins	Phenolphthalein
Purpura	Phenothiazines	Salicylates
Gold salts	Salicylates	Sulfonamides
Hydantoins	Sulfonamides	Tetracyclines
Phenothiazines		
Quinidine		
Sulfonamides		
Thiazides		

followed. Foremost is that therapy should do no harm. Therapy should consist of appropriate medications and should avoid chemicals or drugs that cause skin eruptions themselves. Since the type of lesion, in most cases, is more important than the cause of the lesion, once therapy has begun the lesion may change and the therapy will need to be modified. Therefore, the nurse will need to report such changes to the prescriber, or instruct the patient to follow the eruption closely and report changes. The nurse should also be able to instruct the patient in the use of topical medication according to the principles stated here, i.e., how much to apply, how often, how long, and whether to hydrate the skin.

Release from Vehicle

A drug must be released from the vehicle in which it has been compounded (manufactured) if it is to have the desired effect. The rate and amount of drug released from the vehicle is determined by the physical–chemical relationship between the drug and the vehicle (the solubility of the drug in the vehicle). A drug with a stronger affinity for the vehicle than the skin will be released more slowly. Although drug penetration into the skin can be greatly facilitated with the use of vehicles like **acetone, alcohol, ether, chloroform,** or **dimethylsulfoxide** (DMSO), these vehicles are avoided due to their adverse effects. The rule that the vehicle should be free of "sting, stench, or stain" should be adhered to. Several important additional factors must be considered for the vehicle of a topical medication. The compound must be stable and soluble in the vehicle and the vehicle should be soluble in the base as well as in the stratum corneum (see below).

Percutaneous Absorption

After a drug has been released from its vehicle, the major route for its absorption is through the epidermis, not the hair follicles or eccrine glands. The rate-limiting step to percutaneous absorption of a drug is the *stratum corneum,* the uppermost layer of the epidermis. Sebum only provides a minor resistance to drug absorption. There are regional differences in the thickness of the stratum corneum; thus the palms and soles are more resistant to percutaneous absorption than the face or genitalia. In general the skin of the very young and old is more permeable to drug absorption.

When the stratum corneum is well hydrated, penetration of a drug occurs more rapidly. Wrapping the treated area with an occlusive dressing or using a base such as hydrocarbon ointment (petrolatum) will increase the hydration of the skin and thus the percutaneous absorption of the drug. When the integrity of the skin is altered (wounds, burns, chafed areas, or lesions of some dermatoses) drugs are rapidly and uncontrollably absorbed. The use of topical medications in this situation should be extremely cautious.

Nature of the Base

The terms for the various dermatologic bases are often used interchangeably, i.e., cream and ointment, but the various dermatologic dosage forms have different advantages, disadvantages, and indications (see Table 38-3). Factors that influence the selection of the various topical bases include: the type of lesion, the effect desired, the condition of the patient, and the area to be treated.

Additional factors which affect topical therapy include drug concentration in the base and the amount of drug applied to the skin surface.

AGENTS USED IN TOPICAL THERAPY

Topical therapy can be used to meet one or more of the following objectives:

1. To alleviate symptoms such as itching
2. To restore hydration
3. To cleanse and debride
4. To eradicate causative organisms with specific agents such as antibiotics
5. To reduce inflammation
6. To protect the skin
7. To reduce scale and callus

The successful treatment of a particular skin lesion may require achievement of some or all of these objectives and any one form of therapy may achieve one or several of these goals. If an eruption does not respond in the expected time, the nurse must consider the possibility of another diagnosis or the existence of a complication such as secondary fungal or bacterial infection, or contact sensitivity to one of the ingredients of the topical preparation.

Agents to Relieve Itching, Burning, and Pain

Pruritus, or itching, is one of the most common symptoms of dermatologic disorders and is one of the least tolerated by most patients.

The agents used in the treatment of pruritus include **camphor, menthol,** and **phenol.** Camphor, in concentrations of 0.5 to 1.0%, produces a cooling effect by causing evaporation from the skin. Menthol is used in concentrations of 0.1 to 0.25%, also for its cooling effect. Phenol, which is used in a concentration of 1%, produces its effects by local anesthetic action. These agents should be avoided when lesions are raw, weeping, or ulcerated, since there is a greater amount of percutaneous absorption in these circumstances. Several of these compounds are often incorporated into the same preparation with good clinical results. For example: 0.5% menthol 0.25% camphor in Aquaphor.

Dry skin is one of the most common causes of skin itching in the absence of disease. Patients with dry skin should

TABLE 38-3   Topical Bases

	Indications		
	ADVANTAGES	DISADVANTAGES	EXAMPLES
Ointments and Creams			
Semisolid preparations used for skin hydration and increased penetration of topical medicine			
Hydrocarbon bases (ointments)	Alleviate dryness (emollient). Good base for drugs that undergo hydrolysis (e.g., antibiotics, bacitracin). Good percutaneous absorption.	Greasy, nonwashable. Not good to apply to hairy areas. Skin must be hydrated first with wet compresses or immersion in water for 5 to 10 min.	White petrolatum Yellow petrolatum
Absorption bases (ointments)	Emollient, lubricating. Absorb water and allow incorporation of aqueous solution to form emulsions.	Greasy, nonwashable.	Aquaphor Polysorb
Water-removable bases (creams)	Easily removed from skin and clothing; can be used in hairy areas	Lower percutaneous absorption which can be increased with occlusive dressing (e.g., plastic wrap).	Eucerin cream Nivea cream Cold cream
Water-soluble bases (gels)	Low skin toxicity, water soluble, and easy to remove. Nongreasy; stable.	May be removed by perspiration. Can be drying.	Polyethylene glycol (PEG)
Lotions			
Various combinations of water, oil, alcohol, humectants such as glycerin and propylene glycol, and keratin softeners such as urea and lactic acid	Easily applied and removed, can be used in hairy areas. Alleviate dryness and remove scales depending on preparation.	May be removed by perspiration. May be drying depending on preparation.	Keri Lotion Lubriderm Neutraderm
Powders			
Solid dosage form	Absorbent, cooling, reduce friction.	Wear off easily; may be difficult to apply.	Talcum powder
Shake Lotions and Liniments			
Insoluble powder dispersed in water, oil, or alcohol	Used for protection and for drying.	May overdry skin. Not used on abraded skin.	Calamine lotion Camphor liniment
Pastes			
Semisolid preparations containing large portions of powder	Used with crusted or scaly dermatoses. Absorbs serous secretions. Less macerating, occlusive, and penetrating than ointments.	Difficult to remove. Cannot be used in hairy areas.	Zinc oxide paste
Plasters			
Solid or semisolid adhesive masses on suitable backing.	Protectant, mechanical support, and supply prolonged skin contact of medication.	Irritating; prevent evaporation of skin moisture. Can cause sensitization of skin.	Mustard plaster Unna boot

receive an emollient lotion or ointment designed to retain skin moisture and rehydrate the skin. Cool, moist compresses or wet dressings can also be used to treat itching.

Systemic antihistamines and antianxiety agents are used to treat pruritus but these agents may cause excessive sedation and are often ineffective. The topical use of antihistamines and local anesthetics should be avoided because of their adverse effects. These agents can cause hypersensitivity reactions which may also sensitize patients to future systemic use of these agents and to similar compounds (e.g., sulfonamides, thiazides, and oral hypoglycemic agents).

The local application of a corticosteroid preparation should only be used when other forms of antipruritic therapy have been ineffective.

Agents to Hydrate the Skin (Emollients)

Dry skin is a common problem, especially in older patients during the winter months. Skin is not dry because it lacks grease or oil, but because it lacks water. To maintain normal skin hydration, the water content of the stratum corneum must remain at approximately 10%. Therefore, the goal of therapy is to replace water in dry skin.

Measures to prevent xerosis (skin dryness) include elimination of soaps, solvents, and other drying compounds and frequent use of emollients such as humectants, occlusive agents, and keratin-softening agents. Soaps should have minimum defatting activity and have a neutral pH. Examples include Dove, Alpha Keri, Basis, and Neutrogena. *Humectants* are substances that promote retention of water in the skin by their ability to absorb water. Humectants commonly included in dermatologic topical preparations are glycerin and propylene glycol. Lotions and creams such as Aquacare, Extra Strength Vaseline Intensive Care, Keri Lotion, Lubriderm, and Sofenol contain humectants as well as lubricating oils that lessen skin friction without necessarily increasing skin moisture.

The primary means for correcting dryness, however, is to add water to the skin and then apply a hydrophobic occlusive substance to retain the absorbed water. In vitro the stratum corneum can absorb as much as five to six times its own weight and increase its volume threefold when soaked in water. In vivo this can be accomplished by either soaking the affected area or bathing for 5 to 10 min and then immediately applying a water-in-oil or fatty hydrophobic base (Aquaphor, Eucerin, lanolin, white petrolatum). Use of petrolatum alone is only moderately effective since it does not hydrate the skin but only prevents further transepidermal water loss. Maximum hydration can be accomplished by the use of 40 to 60% **propylene glycol** in water applied under a plastic occlusion dressing and allowed to remain on overnight.

Keratin-softening agents that are used to hydrate and to promote removal of scales and crusts include: **urea-containing creams** (Aquacare, 2% urea; Aquacare/HP, 10% urea; Calmurid, 10% urea; Carmol, 20% urea) and **lactic acid** preparations (Lacticare, Purpose Dry Skin Cream). If 6% **salicylic acid** is added to 60% propylene glycol and applied under plastic occlusion overnight, an extremely effective keratolytic and hydrating gel is formed.

Agents to Reduce Perspiration and Maceration

Intertriginous areas and palms and soles often become macerated secondary to friction and excess hydration of the skin. Gentle cleansing and ventilation of the skin are first priorities followed by application of a dusting powder containing one or more of the following agents: **talc, calcium carbonate, kaolin, zinc stearate, microporous cellulose,** or **magnesium stearate.** Talc is a natural hydrous magnesium silicate that prevents chafing and irritation by reducing friction. Magnesium stearate promotes adherence of the powder preparation to the skin and serves as a mechanical barrier to irritants. Calcium carbonate, kaolin, zinc stearate, and microporous cellulose provide moisture-absorbing properties. Powders should be used with care since inhalation of the dust can lead to chemical pneumonia. Powders should never be applied to acute oozing dermatitis since they can promote crusting and infection.

Recurrent maceration of intertriginous areas or palms and soles may be secondary to hyperhidrosis (excess sweating). In these instances once the maceration has resolved, a variety of antiperspirants may be tried to reduce the excessive sweating. **Aluminum chloride** 20% in 80% absolute ethyl alcohol (Drysol) or **scopolamine hydrobromide** (0.025%) are effective for axillary hyperhidrosis. **Glutaraldehyde** 2% (Cidex) is effective for hyperhidrosis of the palms and soles and probably works by producing a blockage of sweat ducts within the stratum corneum. A 10% solution of Cidex may be necessary for the feet but this will cause a temporary brown discoloration of the soles. **Methenamine** hydrolyzes to ammonia and formaldehyde when applied to the skin and reduces hyperhidrosis by a mechanism similar to glutaraldehyde.

Agents to Cleanse and Debride

Wet compresses are useful for weeping, pustular, and ulcerated lesions, producing a cooling, cleansing, and soothing effect. What is mixed with the water (Table 38-4) to form the wet compress seems to be less important than the method of application. The most frequently used preparation is **normal saline** (0.9% sodium chloride) which possesses mild antipruritic, cleansing, and debridement properties. **Boric acid** is not recommended as a topical agent because of potential systemic toxicity due to percutaneous absorption especially in children and on abraded skin. Tepid water is recommended for most wet compresses while warm soaks are better for furuncles and cellulitis. A clean soft white cloth is soaked in the solution, the excess solution is removed, and the cloth is then applied to the lesion. The process is repeated every 2 to 3 min for 5 to 15 min as frequently as every 2 to 6 h depending on the response desired. The solutions have a marked drying effect and should be stopped before causing excess xerosis. If lesions are too generalized to be effectively treated by using wet compresses, a colloidal bath may be employed. The patient should remain in the bath for 20 to 30 min and then pat the body dry, repeating the process two to six times daily. Commonly used bath preparations are **colloidal oatmeal** (Aveeno) and **oilated colloidal oatmeal** (Oilated Aveeno). To use these preparations mix one cupful of the preparation in two cups of water and then add the mixture to the bath water. The patient should be warned to exercise caution in getting into and out of the tub, since it may become slippery.

At times enzyme preparations are used for debridement such as **streptokinase-streptodornase** (Varidase), **subtilisin** (Travase), **collagenase** (Santyl, Collagenase ABC), **fibrinolysin**, and **deoxyribonuclease** (Elase); however, their efficacy is questionable and marked irritation and sensitization may occur. If enzyme preparations are used it is essential for the nurse to apply the medication to the affected lesion so as not to irritate the surrounding healthy tissue.

Agents to Treat Infection

A variety of agents are available that can kill or reduce cutaneous microorganisms. They include: antiseptics, disinfectants, sanitizers, fungicides, sporicides, topical antimicrobial agents, and others. *Antiseptics are agents that kill or inhibit the growth of microorganisms on living objects, while disinfectants kill or inhibit the growth of microorganisms on nonliving objects. Sanitizers* are agents that reduce the bacterial count to acceptable levels as determined by public health standards. *Fungicides* and *sporicides* kill fungi and spores, respectively. *Topical antimicrobials* are used to treat infections of the skin and mucous membranes.

Antiseptics and Disinfectants

The mechanisms of action of some antiseptics and disinfectants are listed in Table 38-5. In general, the desired characteristics of an antiseptic are that it: (a) should be immediately effective, (b) have a long-lasting effect on a wide range of microorganisms, (c) be inexpensive, and (d) have few adverse effects. The most effective antiseptics now available are the **iodophors** and **chlorhexidine** (Hibiclens).

A 4% solution of **chlorhexidine** has been proven effective for hand washing, as a skin and wound cleanser, and as a surgical scrub. It is effective against gram-positive and gram-negative organisms, and its action is cumulative.

Iodophors (Betadine, Iodine, Povidine) are complexes of **iodine** which slowly release the iodine. The iodophors are less irritating to the skin than tincture of iodine. They are effective against gram-positive and gram-negative organisms, but they do *not* have a cumulative effect. Prolonged use may have a drying effect upon the skin.

Hexachlorophene (pHisohex) is more effective against gram-positive organisms (e.g., staphylococcus) than against gram-negative organisms. It has the disadvantage that its onset of action is delayed, and that it has to be used for three to five days before it becomes effective. Once effective, however, its action persists. Hexachlorophene used in high concentration, especially in the newborn and infants, may be absorbed and has caused toxicity. Therefore, the 3% solution requires a prescription.

Isopropyl alcohol and **ethanol** (70 to 95%) are very effective against gram-positive and gram-negative organisms, but

TABLE 38-4   Solutions for Wet Compresses

AGENT	RANGE OF CONCENTRATION USED, %	HOW PREPARED
Acetic acid	1	1 tsp of concentrated acetic acid to 1 L of water
Aluminum acetate (Burow's solution)	5–10	1 part solution in 10 parts tepid water or 1 or 2 Domeboro tablets to 1 pint of water
Magnesium sulfate (Epsom salt)	2–4	8 tsp to 1 L of water
Potassium permanganate	0.03	1 crushed 65-mg tablet to 250 mL of water
Silver nitrate	0.1–0.5	1 tsp of 50% stock to 1 L of water
Sodium bicarbonate	2–5	8 tsp to 1 L of water
Sodium chloride	0.6–1.5 (usually normal saline: 0.9)	2 tsp to 1 L of water

TABLE 38-5 Commonly Used Antiseptics and Disinfectants

PROTEIN DENATURANTS	PROTEIN PRECIPITANTS	INTERFERE WITH BACTERIAL METABOLISM	OTHER MECHANISMS
Phenol	Resorcinol	Silver nitrate	Chlorhexidine (Hibiclens)
Creosol solution (Lysol)	Isopropanol (isopropyl alcohol)	Silver sulfadiazine (Sulfamylon)	Acetic acid
Parabens	Ethanol (ethyl alcohol)	Nitrofurantoin (Furacin)	Gentian violet (Methylrosaniline chloride)
	Formalin or formaldehyde	Merbromin (Mercurochrome)	
	Zinc sulfate	Thimerosal (Merthiolate)	Potassium permanganate
	Zinc oxide	Iodine	Benzoic acid
			Hydrogen peroxide
	Benzalkonium chloride (Zephiran)	Povidine iodine (Betadine, Prepodyn, Septodyne)	Sodium hypochlorite solution (Dakin's)

will dry the skin when used in routine hand washing or for surgical skin preparation.

Benzalkonium chloride (Zephiran) is not as effective as other agents, since it has little action against gram-negative organisms.

Benzoyl peroxide has proved efficacious in acne vulgaris, probably through a mechanism of action related to its bacteriostatic activity against *Propionibacterium acnes*.

Topical Antimicrobial Agents

The use of antibacterial, antifungal, and antiviral agents in the treatment of topical infections (Table 38-6) follows similar principles as when these agents are employed systemically (see Chap. 28). For severe topical infections it may be necessary to use systemic antimicrobial therapy in lieu of, or in addition to, topical therapy. When used topically all antimicrobial preparations have the potential to cause superinfection. **Chloramphenicol, sulfonamides** (except Sulfamylon), and **penicillin** should be avoided as topical dermatologics because of their potential adverse effects, as well as the danger of causing sensitization to future systemic use of the drug, which may result in severe allergic reactions.

An increased incidence of adverse reactions to **neomycin** (when used topically) has been reported, especially in patients with decreased renal function. Ototoxicity and nephrotoxicity have been reported, as has contact dermatitis. Therefore, many clinicians now avoid neomycin-containing ointments, such as Neosporin G, in favor of combinations like **polymixin B** and **bacitracin** (Polysporin).

Agents to Reduce Inflammation

There are a wide variety of preparations that are used topically to reduce inflammation. They include corticosteroids, tar and tar extracts, and halogenated quinolones. The most widely used are topical corticosteroids.

Topical Corticosteroids

Corticosteroids possess anti-inflammatory, antipruritic, and vasoconstrictive activity when used topically. Fluorinated and/or esterified corticosteroids (Table 38-7) are more potent on a milligram to milligram basis than are nonfluorinated and nonesterified compounds. Although the presence of infection requires cautious use of corticosteroids, bacterial, viral, and fungal infections are *not* absolute contraindications for the use of topical steroid preparations. Adverse effects of topical steroids include skin atrophy, depigmentation, acneiform eruptions, and, rarely, systemic effects (see Chap. 35 for more details on systemic effects). These preparations should be applied sparingly two or three times a day. The patient may be instructed to cover these preparations with an occlusive dressing to increase absorption for recalcitrant lesions. Increased absorption may occur without occlusion when corticosteroids are applied to abraded areas, to the skin of infants and small children, and to the face and intertriginous areas of adults. Therefore, corticosteroids in the lowest potency category in Table 38-7 are used in these circumstances. In contrast, corticosteroids in the lowest and low potency categories are ineffective for the treatment of many dermatoses on the glabrous skin of adults. As a general rule the lowest potency corticosteroid that is effective should be used. Topical corticosteroids are available in various dosage forms. The ones that are the most to the least lubricating are hydrocarbon ointment bases, water in oil ointment bases, creams and gels, aerosols, and lotions. The nurse should be able to assess whether the dermatologic condition is responding to therapy and whether cutaneous side effects have occurred.

Tars and Tar Extracts

Tars and extracts of crude coal tar have been used for many years for their anti-inflammatory properties. Preparations commonly used are **crude coal tar** (1 to 5%), **coal tar distillate** (1 to 3%), LCD (**liquor carbonis detergens,** 3 to 15%), and **ichthammol** (3%). Crude coal tar consists of a hetero-

TABLE 38-6   Topical Antimicrobial Preparations

AGENT	TRADE NAME	CONCENTRATIONS
Antifungal Agents		
Calcium undecylenate	Cruex	10% in talc base
Zinc undecylenate and undecylenic acid	Desenex	Ointment and powder: 5% undecylenate and 20% zinc undecylenate Aerosol powder: 20% concentration of each component
Triacetin	Enzactin	Aerosol: 1% Cream: 1% Powder: 1% Gel: 1%
Iodochlorhydroxyquin	Vioform and others	Cream and ointment: 3%
Miconazole	Micatin	Cream: 2%
	Monistat	Vaginal preparation
Acrisorcin	Akrinol	Cream: 2 mg/g
Haloprogin	Halotex	Cream and solution: 1%
Tolnaftate	Tinactin	Cream, powder, and solution: 1%
	Aftate	Powder aerosol: 72 mg/120 g
Clotrimazole	Mycelex, Lotrimin	Cream and solution: 1%
Nystatin	Mycostatin, Nilstat	Ointment, cream, powder: 100,000 U/g
Amphotericin B	Fungizone	Cream and ointment: 3%
Antibacterial Agents		
Neomycin	Myciguent	Ointment: 5 mg/g
Bacitracin	Baciguent	Ointment: 500 U/g
Polymyxin B		Ointment: 5000–10,000 U/g
Gentamicin	Garamycin	Ointment and cream 0.1%
Tetracycline	Achromycin and others	Ointment: 1% and 3%
Chlortetracycline	Aureomycin	Ointment: 3%
Chloramphenicol	Chloromycetin	Ointment: 1%
Erythromycin	Ilotycin	Ointment: 1%
Combination Agents (**Cont.**)		
Oxytetracycline and polymyxin B	Terramycin	Ointment: 30 mg oxytetracycline and 10,000 U polymyxin B per gram
Bacitracin and neomycin	Bacimycin	Ointment: 500 U bacitracin and 5 mg neomycin per gram
Neomycin and gramicidin	Spectrocin	Ointment: 25 mg neomycin and 0.25 mg gramicidin per gram
Polymyxin B, neomycin, and gramicidin	Neosporin G	Cream: 10,000 U polymyxin B, 5 mg neomycin, and 0.25 mg gramicidin per gram
Polymyxin B and bacitracin	Polysporin	Ointment: 10,000 U polymyxin B and 500 U bacitracin per gram
Polymyxin B, neomycin, and bacitracin	Mycitracin	Ointment: 5000 U polymyxin B, 5 mg neomycin, and 5000 U bacitracin per gram
Polymyxin B, neomycin, and bacitracin	Neosporin, Neo-Polycin	Ointment: 5000 U polymyxin B, 5 mg neomycin, and 4000 U bacitracin per gram
Dexamethasone and neomycin	Neo-Decadron	Cream: dexamethasone 0.1% and neomycin 0.5%

TABLE 38-6 Topical Antimicrobial Preparations (*Continued*)

AGENT	TRADE NAME	CONCENTRATIONS
		Combination Agents (Cont.)
Fluocinolone and neomycin*	Neo-Synalar	Cream: fluocinolone 0.025% and neomycin 0.5%.
Flurandrenolide and neomycin*	Cordran-N	Cream and ointment: flurandrenolide 0.05% and neomycin 0.5%.
Hydrocortisone and neomycin*	Neo-Cortef	Cream: hydrocortisone 1 or 2.5% and neomycin 0.5%.
Hydrocortisone and oxytetracycline*	Terra-Cortril	Ointment: hydrocortisone 1% and oxytetracycline 3%.
Hydrocortisone, neomycin, polymyxin B, and bacitracin*	Cortisporin	Cream: hydrocortisone 0.5%, neomycin 0.5%, polymyxin B 5000 U, and bacitracin 400 U per gram.
Hydrocortisone, neomycin, polymyxin B, and bacitracin	Cortisporin	Ointment: hydrocortisone 1%, neomycin 0.5%, polymyxin B 5000 U, and bacitracin 400 U per gram.
Triamcinolone, neomycin, gramicidin, and nystatin*	Mycolog Mytrex	Cream and ointment: triamcinolone acetonide 0.1%, neomycin 0.25%, gramicidin 0.25%, and nystatin, 1000 U per gram.

*Although combinations of steroids and antibiotics are commonly used, they are not recommended. If an anti-inflammatory agent is needed for a few days in conjunction with an antibacterial agent, it should be prescribed separately.

geneous mixture of compounds, and its mechanism of action, although not known, has been attributed to antiseptic, antipruritic, anti-inflammatory, and photosensitivity effects. Crude coal tar (1 to 5%) and ultraviolet light (UVB) therapy have been used for the treatment of psoriasis since 1925 in a method known as the *Goeckerman regimen.* Attempts have been made to develop coal tar products that are cosmetically acceptable through masking the unpleasant odor, color, and staining properties of crude coal tar. LCD is a 20% tincture of coal tar that has acceptable cosmetic properties. Tar gel products (Estar and psoriGel) represent a formulation of crude coal tar that is both convenient and cosmetically acceptable. Tar gels are best applied under an emollient because of their drying properties. Side effects associated with tars include folliculitis, photosensitization, and contact dermatitis. Crude coal tar is thought to have carcinogenic potential but no reports have occurred of increased frequency of skin cancer in psoriatic patients treated many years with coal tar and ultraviolet light.

Halogenated Quinolones

Iodochlorhydroxyquin (Vioform), containing 40% **iodine,** was originally developed as a substitute for the antiseptic iodoform. This preparation, however, has anti-inflammatory as well as antibacterial effects. Iodochlorhydroxyquin is commonly used alone or in combination with corticosteroids for nummular or hand eczema. This agent should be used with discretion, however, since a recent report documented systemic absorption which could result in adverse effects such as neurotoxicity. Another similar preparation, **diiodohydroxyquin,** is combined with 0.5 or 1% **hydrocortisone** (Vytone) and has similar properties to Vioform except it does not stain the skin and clothing as Vioform does.

Agents to Protect the Skin

Various topical preparations are available that protect the skin from noxious stimuli including insect bites, trauma, excess moisture, and sunlight. The most effective method for protecting the skin from noxious agents is to prevent their contact with the skin either by protective clothing, avoidance, repellents (in the case of insects), or sunscreens.

Insect Repellents

These agents do not kill insects but instead repel them from treated areas. Most repellents are volatile and when applied to skin or clothing, their vapors tend to prevent insects from alighting, and thus, protect the skin against bites. Although many compounds have been tested, only a few are effective as well as safe for use on the skin. The ideal repellent should have an inoffensive odor, protect for several hours, be effective against a wide spectrum of insects, withstand weather conditions, and be cosmetically appealing. The best all-purpose repellent is *N,N*-diethyl-*m*-toluamide. **Ethohexadiol, dimethyl phthalate, dimethyl carbate,** and **butopyronoxyl** are effective but against a small range of insects; thus, a mixture of two or more is desirable. Repellents are toxic if taken internally, may cause itching, burning, and swelling when applied on the skin of patients who are sensitive to these chemicals, and cause a burning sensation and an irritant response when applied to broken skin, mucous membranes, or the eyes.

Sunscreens

Patients with fair skin should be protected against the ultraviolet irradiation of the sun, not only for prevention of sunburn but also for reduction of the incidence of long-term

TABLE 38-7 Topical Corticosteroid Preparations

PERCENT	CORTICOSTEROID	VEHICLE
	Lowest Potency	
0.25	Hydrocortisone	Cream, lotion
0.5	Hydrocortisone	Cream, ointment, lotion
1.0	Hydrocortisone (Hytone)	Cream, ointment, lotion
2.5	Hydrocortisone (Hytone, Cortef)	Cream, ointment
0.5	Prednisolone (Meti-Derm)	Cream
0.25	Methylprednisolone acetate (Medrol)	Ointment
1.0	Methylprednisolone acetate (Medrol)	Ointment
0.04	Dexamethasone (Hexadrol)	Cream
0.1	Dexamethasone (Decadron, Decaderm)	Cream, gel
0.1	Betamethasone	Cream
0.2	Betamethasone	Cream
	Low Potency	
0.01	Fluocinolone acetonide (Fluonid, Synalar)	Cream, lotion
0.2	Hydrocortisone valerate (Westcort)	Cream
0.01	Betamethasone valerate (Valisone)	Cream
0.025	Flurandrenolide (Cordran)	Cream, ointment
0.025	Fluorometholone (Oxylone)	Cream
0.025	Triamcinolone acetonide (Kenalog, Aristocort)	Cream, ointment
0.03	Flumethasone pivalate (Locorten)	Cream
	Intermediate Potency	
0.025	Halcinonide (Halog)	Cream, ointment
0.025	Betamethasone benzoate	Cream, gel, lotion
0.1	Betamethasone valerate (Valisone)	Cream, ointment, lotion
0.05	Desonide (Tridesilon)	Cream, ointment
0.025	Fluocinolone acetonide (Synalar)	Cream, ointment
0.1	Amcinonide (Cyclocort)	Cream
0.05	Flurandrenolide (Cordran)	Cream, ointment, lotion
0.1	Triamcinolone acetonide (Kenalog, Aristocort)	Cream, ointment, gel, lotion
	High Potency	
0.05	Betamethasone dipropionate (Diprosone)	Cream, ointment, lotion
0.5	Triamcinolone acetonide (Kenalog, Aristocort)	Cream, ointment
0.2	Fluocinolone (Synalar HP)	Cream
0.25	Desoximetasone (Topicort)	Cream
0.05	Diflorasone diacetate (Florone)	Cream, ointment
0.1	Halcinonide (Halog)	Cream, ointment, lotion
0.05	Fluocinonide (Lidex, Topsyn)	Cream, ointment, gel

Source: Adapted from *The Medical Letter on Drugs and Therapeutics,* **22**:52, 1980.

hazards such as skin cancer (basal cell epithelioma, squamous cell carcinoma, and melanoma) and premature aging of the skin. It is important to apply sunscreens even on cloudy days since ultraviolet rays can penetrate the clouds and still cause skin damage. Sunscreen agents exert their effect by either physical or chemical means. Physical sunscreens, such as **titanium dioxide** or **zinc oxide,** scatter and reflect ultraviolet radiation while chemical agents, such as **aminobenzoic acid** (*p*-aminobenzoic acid, PABA), **cinnamates,** and **padimate,** absorb ultraviolet radiation. Sunscreen products are rated on the basis of their sun protection factor (SPF). This factor is derived by dividing the exposure dose of UV-B (sunburn radiation) that will elicit a minimal erythema response (MED) in sunscreen-protected skin by the MED of unprotected skin. SPF can be interpreted as representing the ratio of the amount of time one can spend in the sun with a sunscreen to time without a sunscreen to obtain a mild sunburn reaction. The higher the SPF the more effective the agent is in preventing sunburn. The relationship of skin type to recommended sunscreen SPF is presented in Table 38-8. The ability of a sunscreen to remain effective under the stress of prolonged exercise, sweating, and swimming is a function of both the ultraviolet absorbing agent and the vehicle/solvent system of the preparation. Two

TABLE 38-8 Skin Types and Recommended Sunscreen Products

SKIN TYPE	SUNBURN AND TANNING HISTORY	SUN PROTECTION FACTOR (SPF)	PRODUCT CATEGORY DESIGNATION (PCD)
I	Always burns easily Never tans (sensitive)	15	Maximal, ultra
II	Always burns easily Tans minimally (sensitive)	15	Maximal, ultra
III	Burns moderately Tans gradually (light brown—normal)	8 or more	Extra
IV	Burns minimally Always tans well (moderate brown—normal)	4–7	Moderate
V	Rarely burns Tans profusely (dark brown—insensitive)	2–3	Minimal
VI	Never burns Deeply pigmented (insensitive)		

Source: Modified from *American Pharmaceutical Association Handbook of Nonprescription Drugs,* 7th ed., 1982. Reprinted with permission of the American Pharmaceutical Association.

chemical absorbing agents may be more effective than any one compound. Some commonly used sunscreen products and their active ingredients are listed in Table 38-9. A variety of lipsticks containing these agents are also available.

Protectants Against Trauma

To protect small areas of eczematous skin, **zinc oxide** (Lassar's) paste, **zinc oxide ointment,** or paste-impregnated bandages may be used. Some of these topical products are astringents as well as protectants. Preparations such as bandages impregnated with zinc oxide paste (Unna's boot), commercially available as Dome-Paste and Gelcast, are useful as protectants and for providing mechanical support in the treatment of stasis ulcers. Caution must be taken in using any of these occlusive coverings since they may increase tissue maceration and prevent heat loss and thus contribute to discomfort of the affected area or promote infection.

Agents to Reduce Scale and Callus

In some cases scaling and callus formation are due to rapid proliferation of epidermal cells, thus these processes can be

TABLE 38-9 Sunscreen and Suntan Agents

PRODUCT TRADE NAME	SUNSCREEN AGENT	SPF
Maximal (Ultra) Protection		
Block Out (cream lotion)	Octyldimethylaminobenzoic acid (Padimate O) 8%; oxybenzone, 6%	15
Coppertone Supershade	Padimate O, 7%; oxybenzone, 3%	15
Eclipse	Padimate O, 7%; oxybenzone, 3%	15
PreSun 15 Lotion	Aminobenzoic acid, 5%, padimate O, 5%; oxybenzone 3%	15
Extra Protection		
Block Out (clear lotion)	Padimate O, 8%; oxybenzone, 6%	10
Coppertone Nose Kote	Homosalate, 8%; oxybenzone, 3%	8
Maxafil Cream	Menthylanthranilate, 5%; cinoxate, 4%	8
Pabafilm	Padimate O, 5.5%; oxybenzone, 3%	10
Pabanol	Aminobenzoic acid, 5%	14
PreSun 8 Creamy, Gel, or Lotion	Aminobenzoic acid, 5%	8
Solbar	Oxybenzone, 3%, dioxybenzone, 3%	8
RVPaque	Cinoxate; red petrolatum	10
Moderate Protection		
Pabagel	Aminobenzoic acid, 5%	6
PreSun 4 Lotion	Padimate O, 4%	4
RVP	Red petrolatum	4
Shade Extra Protection	Homosalate, 8%; oxybenzone, 3%	6
SunDare, clear and creamy lotions	Cinoxate, 1.75–2%	4–6
Minimal Protection		
Coppertone Lite Oil	Homosalate, 4%	2
Q.T. Quick Tanning, foam and lotion	Padimate O, 1.5%	2
Tropical Blend Dark Tanning Lotion and Oil	Homosalate, 4%	2

Source: Reprinted from the *American Pharmaceutical Association Handbook of Nonprescription Drugs,* 7th ed., 1982. Reprinted with permission of the American Pharmaceutical Association.

reduced with various combinations of keratolytics (agents that remove the horny layer of skin) and of agents that suppress the rate of epidermal proliferation. Keratolytics are agents that loosen keratinocyte cohesion, thereby facilitating desquamation. There are many types of keratolytics with distinctly different mechanisms of action. **Resorcinol** and **urea** are presumed to act as keratolytics by their irritant effect, **sulfur** is believed to function by eliciting an inflammatory reaction that causes an increase in cell sloughing, **tretinoin** increases epidermal mitosis and cell turnover, and **salicylic acid** lowers skin pH causing increased hydration and thus facilitates loosening and removal of scale or callus. Salicylic acid has emerged as the most effective and least toxic of the keratolytics. Vehicle composition, contact time, and concentration of keratolytic agent are important considerations to the success of a keratolytic preparation as they are to all dermatologic topical preparations.

Commonly used keratolytic preparations contain 2 to 20% **salicylic acid**, 16% **urea**, 2 to 4% **resorcinol**, 4 to 10% **sulfur**, or 0.025 to 0.5% **tretinoin.** Tretinoin (Retin A), a derivative of vitamin A, is sometimes effective in keratiniz-ing disorders but is most commonly used topically in the treatment of acne. **Isotretinoin** (Accutane), another vitamin A derivative, is used orally in the treatment of severe nodu-locystic acne. The drug has caused major fetal abnormalities when used by pregnant women. Additional adverse effects of isotretinoin include abnormal liver function tests, musculoskeletal symptoms, dry skin, cheilitis, and elevated blood lipids. The drug is highly effective in the treatment of nodulocystic acne and other severe forms of acne but its toxicities require close monitoring prior to and during therapy.

The other keratolytics are included in preparations used for treatment of verrucae (warts), seborrheic dermatitis (dandruff), psoriasis, and acne. Keratolytic agents can cause a primary irritant response especially on mucous membranes or in eyes. Resorcinol and salicylic acid can cause systemic toxicity if used in large amounts on abraded or broken skin.

Agents that suppress the rate of proliferation include 3 to 5% **sulfur,** 3 to 5% ammoniated mercury, 0.1 to 1% **anthralin** and tars, and are most often used in the treatment of psoriasis.

CASE STUDY

T.A., a 16-year-old female, came to the dermatology clinic with the complaint of severe acne of an eight-month duration.

Assessment

T.A. told the nurse that she had attempted to control the acne with dietary management and a variety of over-the-counter agents. She reported washing her face at least six times daily and avoided consuming any cola beverages, chocolate, or fried foods with no improvement. T.A. denied the use of any other drugs including oral contraceptives.

The nurse noted upon examination that T.A. exhibited moderately severe papules, pustules, and open come-dones distributed over the face, chest, and back. After the dermatologist saw the patient and prescribed tetracycline 500 mg PO bid, benzoyl peroxide 5% gel in A.M., and Retin A 0.05% cream at hs, T.A. was referred to the nurse for management and follow-up.

Management

The nurse explained that the topical medicine was used to open clogged pores and fight bacteria and indicated that T.A. should contact the clinic if any excessive skin irritation occurred. T.A. was advised to avoid excessive exposure to sunlight while using the Retin A treatment. The nurse explained to T.A. that low-dose tetracycline therapy suppresses the growth of *Propioni bacterium* *acnes,* a bacteria found in hair follicles that contributes to acne pustule formation. The nurse instructed her to take the tetracycline with a full glass of water about 1 h before meals and told her that taking the medication with milk or antacids could inhibit absorption of the drug. The nurse also explained that vaginal monilia and gastric distress were common side effects of tetracycline. If pregnancy was planned or occurred, the tetracycline must be stopped immediately.

The patient was encouraged to eat a well-balanced diet and told that no foods were prohibited. However, during the process of cooking, aerosolized oils and greases could exacerbate acne.

The nurse then cleaned the patient's face with acetone and used a comedo extractor to remove the blackheads and open the pustules. A corticosteroid, triamcinolone acetonide (Kenalog), was injected into the area of a cystic lesion. This procedure was repeated monthly.

The nurse also allowed T.A. time to discuss her reactions to the disfigurement and reassured her that acne is a transient condition that could be controlled until she grew out of it.

Evaluation

After six weeks there was a noticeable decrease in new eruptions and the tetracycline was reduced to 250 mg bid. The skin of the patient's face showed dryness, but no excessive erythema was noted. Wibi, a noncomedogenic moisturizer, was recommended.

CLINICAL ENTITIES

As a guide to appropriate therapy for dermatologic disorders it is helpful to classify skin eruptions into reaction patterns since the response of skin to therapy is often more related to the reaction pattern than to the underlying etiology or pathogenesis of the skin disease. Notable exceptions to this approach are many bacterial and parasitic infections that should be treated with specific systemic and topical antibiotics, cutaneous manifestations of systemic disease in which the underlying problem must be identified and treated, and skin tumors which are ablated by a variety of surgical or radiological techniques. A discussion of diagnosis and treatment of these more specialized dermatologic problems is beyond the scope of this chapter; however, the large majority of cutaneous disorders which the nurse not specialized in dermatology must assess and help treat are classified below by reaction patterns.

Reaction Patterns

Maculopapular

Morbilliform (measleslike) reactions consist of generalized, erythematous, flat or minimally raised, blanchable eruptions which may be extremely pruritic and may resolve with scaling. A *viral infection* or *drug reaction* is most likely to be the underlying cause. Therapy should include agents to relieve itching when present and, in severe cases, to reduce inflammation.

Urticaria

The characteristic skin lesion of urticarial reactions is the wheal, a pale red, rounded or flat-topped, well-demarcated elevation which is the result of edema in the upper dermis. Wheals are evanescent, lasting less than 24 h, vary in size from several millimeters to several centimeters, occur anywhere on the skin surface, and are usually pruritic. Wheals are the hallmark of classic urticaria, an allergic response to any of a vast number of initiating agents such as drugs, infections, foods and food additives, inhalants, or insect bites. Therapy should include systemic antihistamines and topical antipruritic agents as well as efforts directed toward identification and avoidance of the precipitating factor.

Papulosquamous

Papulosquamous reactions are characterized by the presence of erythematous papules and plaques with a superficial scale which is often typical of the underlying etiology. Numerous diverse dermatologic disorders may manifest as papulosquamous eruptions. One of the most common and important is *atopic dermatitis* which often appears in infants as a generalized, ill-defined, inflamed eruption with fine scale, in children as a dry, pruritic, excoriated, and lichenified rash with a predilection for flexor folds, and in adults as a persistent hand dermatitis with excoriations and fissures. Therapy should include topical hydrating and anti-inflammatory agents, and systemic antipruritic and antibacterial agents if superinfection intervenes.

Seborrheic dermatitis appears as erythema and greasy scaling in a typical distribution which includes the scalp, eyebrows, eyelids, nasolabial and postauricular folds, moustache, beard, presternal and occasionally genital areas. Keratolytic and mild anti-inflammatory agents are the mainstay of therapy.

Psoriasis is characterized by sharply circumscribed, erythematous plaques covered by loosely adherent silvery scales, which may be generalized but frequently occur in areas of repetitive mild trauma such as the elbows, knees, scalp, genitalia, and gluteal fold. Since psoriasis is a hereditary, chronic, proliferative disease of the epidermis, treatment should consist of topical anti-inflammatory (corticosteroids, tar), keratolytic, and hydrating agents as well as antiproliferative therapy such as ultraviolet light and, in severe otherwise refractory cases, drugs such as **methotrexate** or PUVA therapy. PUVA is an acronym for photosensitizing *psoralens* (**methoxsalen**) plus ultraviolet light (UV-A).

Pityriasis rosea, presumed to be viral in origin, is a transient (six- to eight-week) eruption consisting of an initial erythematous scaling plaque, the "herald patch," followed by crops of small oval papular lesions with a peripheral rim of fine scale distributed in a characteristic "firtree" pattern on the trunk, parallel to the ribs. Antipruritic and hydrating agents are useful, when indicated, but the rash will resolve without specific treatment. *Fungal infections* manifest as scaling erythematous lesions which often have a raised red advancing border. Therapy consists of appropriate topical antifungal agents as well as prophylactic measures to decrease excess moisture, maceration, and reinfection.

Vesiculobullous

Vesicles (small blisters, 0.5 cm) and bullae (large blisters) are predominant lesions in a wide variety of skin diseases. Filled with clear fluid, they ooze and weep when broken and result in denuded, often painful, crusted, eroded lesions which heal slowly and are prone to superinfection. *Acute contact dermatitis,* such as poison ivy, manifests as vesicles and bullae associated with erythematous pruritic papules and plaques in localized areas where contact with the allergen occurred. Topical therapy should consist of cleansing compresses, antipruritic agents, and anti-inflammatory agents once the lesions no longer ooze. Oral antihistamines and occasionally systemic corticosteroids (**prednisone**) are necessary. *Herpes virus infections* are characterized by clusters of vesicles on an erythematous base (herpetiform arrangement) which are localized in herpes simplex but which follow a dermatome in herpes zoster (zosteriform distribution). Therapy should include cleansing and gentle debridement of crusts, antibacterial agents to prevent superinfection, and avoidance of topical steroids which may worsen the infection.

Pustular Ulcerative

Pustules (small blisters containing a purulent exudate) and ulcers (deep craters resulting from epidermal and dermal tissue necrosis) signify the presence of an inflammatory and usually infectious process. The coexistence of papules, pustules, and cysts on the face, chest, or back is the hallmark of *acne vulgaris.* Treatment should consist of systemic and topical antibacterial agents as well as topical keratolytics. Follicular pustules are usually the result of folliculitis, best treated with topical antibacterial agents as well as measures to decrease maceration and friction. Satellite pustules are seen in *cutaneous candidiasis,* usually responsive to broad-spectrum topical antifungal agents and to drying agents. Chronic pressure and inadequate peripheral venous circulation contribute to the generation of *chronic ulcers,* many of which become superinfected. Therapy should consist of measures to cleanse and debride the ulcer followed by topical antiseptic or antibacterial agents.

Photosensitive

Photosensitivity induced by exposure to ultraviolet and/or visible light may be caused by varied etiologic factors and manifested by varied morphologic forms. An "allergic" response of the skin to light might result in solar urticaria, with the presence of wheals, or polymorphous light eruption, usually appearing as papulovesicles or plaques. A photosensitive eruption might be the consequence of a drug reaction. The cutaneous manifestations of porphyria, which include skin fragility and blister formation, are the result of light-induced excitation of porphyrin molecules in the skin which cause distinctive cutaneous changes. Lupus erythematosus is a systemic autoimmune disease frequently associated with skin lesions which may be exacerbated by exposure to light. Treatment of photosensitive disorders should be directed primarily toward correcting the underlying disease mechanism but should also include sunscreens and not infrequently topical anti-inflammatory agents.

NURSING PROCESS RELATED TO DERMATOLOGIC DISORDERS

The role of the nurse is extremely important when dealing with the disorders of the integumentary system. It is the nurse practitioner, school nurse, community health nurse, clinic nurse, or acute hospital staff nurse who frequently detects the dermatologic disorder, and so each nurse must be knowledgeable and skillful in the observation and description of dermatologic conditions.

The nursing process in a variety of common dermatologic disorders is outlined in Table 38-10.

Assessment

Observation and history taking are the main tools of dermatologic assessment. Observation of the skin should begin with a general survey of the skin color, texture, turgor, and temperature, as well as condition of the hair, scalp, and nails. If rashes, lesions, or injuries are present, their color, type (e.g., papule, macule, vesicle, etc.), grouping or configuration, distribution over the body, and associated symptoms should be noted. The identification and diagnosis of skin disorders is basically accomplished by careful observation of the individual lesion and the distribution of the lesions.

The history should include the types of symptoms and their duration, what has been done to treat the disorder, and how effective treatment has been. The nurse should also note the patient's emotional status and whether there is a patient or familial history of serious systemic diseases, since dermatologic symptoms may be a manifestation of an underlying disease.

Management

Following assessment and diagnosis it is the nurse's function to obtain the participation of the patient in the plan of care. Since many skin diseases are chronic, patients can learn to monitor their own symptoms and treatment. Education of the patient is of prime importance; patients must know the rationale for treatments and how they can maximize the effects of the treatment. The fact that patients frequently undertreat or overtreat skin disorders might be a reflection of their lack of understanding of the skin disorder. Further, the treatment process may be bothersome or unesthetic, and compliance may be a problem. If the nursing staff show revulsion, the patient's well-being may be jeopardized.

The nurse must be particularly aware of the psychological needs of the patient who experiences disorders of the skin. We live in a society in which smooth, unblemished skin is touted by the advertising media as a mark of beauty. Therefore, patients with disfiguring skin disorders may feel ugly, depressed, and shunned by society. Such psychological factors may aggravate many skin diseases and contribute to noncompliance with the therapeutic regimen. Thus proper management may require elimination or control of these factors.

Lack of patience with the slow progress seen with chronic skin conditions is often a difficult patient problem. An accepting attitude on the part of the nurse is essential in assisting the patient to deal with his or her condition, especially when it is chronic. Cosmetics (Erase and Covermark) may be recommended to patients since these agents successfully camouflage many types of dermatologic lesions.

A therapeutic modality important in the care of the patient with a dermatologic disorder is touch, which portrays to the patient that he or she is not repulsive. With the exception of those few conditions where the disorder is

TABLE 38-10   Nursing Process Related to Selected Dermatologic Disorders

DISORDER	ASSESSMENT	Management		EVALUATION
		MEDICAL/ PHARMACOLOGIC	NONPHARMACOLOGIC	
		Papulosquamous		
Contact dermatitis (irritant, i.e., dishpan hands, or allergic, i.e., poison ivy)	Lesions are erythematous and weeping (acute), dry scaling papules or macules (chronic). Acute or chronic in nature depending on contact. Distribution is important clue to diagnosis and etiology. Ascertain causal factor by history/patch testing.	Treat acute with wet dressings or lotions like calamine; chronic with creams or ointments. Secondary infections treated with antibiotics; severe disease may require topical or even systemic steroids.	Avoid contact with the specific local agent. Sometimes requires change in lifestyle, employment, or recreation.	Note change in lesion from exudative (or wet) to dry, lichenified (leathery). Note impact of required lifestyle changes. Recurs with each contact with irritant or allergen.
Seborrheic dermatitis (severe dandruff)	Dry scales with or without erythema in areas where sebaceous glands are present (scalp, back, face, body folds). Assess environmental stress level.	Scalp: shampoos containing selenium sulfide (1–2.5%); other agents in seborrheic preparations are keratolytics, astringents, drying agents, and emollients. Severe cases may require shampoos containing tars and topical steroids.	Avoid excess stress. Explain chronicity of disorder.	Observe for rashes caused by medications and excess drying with some agents. Frequently recurs.
Atopic dermatitis (eczema) and hand dermatitis (dyshidrosis)	Lesions are dry and leathery. Acute lesions are erythematous and weeping. Check for familial history of dermatitis, asthma, hayfever. Assess for symptoms of asthma, hayfever, allergic rhinitis, and urticaria, which are often associated. Ascertain environmental irritants that induce rash formation, degree of itching/scratching, and secondary infection.	Topical steroids or tar. Oral antihistamines. Antibiotics for secondary bacterial infection.	Minimize exposure to irritants. Avoid soap. Minimize scratching by cutting nails and using cotton gloves at night. Encourage use of emollients frequently. Psychologic support for patient and family.	Frequency of recurrence. Ability to control rash and discomfort. Precipitating factors.
Stasis dermatitis	Lesions begin around ankles but may involve entire lower leg. They are dry and leathery with abnormal pigmentation. Acute lesions are erythematous and weeping. Ascertain status of venous return and patient's lifestyle.	Topical steroids. Antibiotics for secondary bacterial infection. Unna boot for protection of macerated or ulcerated lesions.	Support stockings to promote better venous return. Educate patient in ways to promote venous return, i.e., to elevate legs, avoid standing, and possibly change lifestyle. Encourage frequent use of emollients.	Chronic disease. Monitor patient compliance. Observe area for bacterial infection or ulceration. Monitor legs for venous thrombosis.

TABLE 38-10 Nursing Process Related to Selected Dermatologic Disorders (*Continued*)

DISORDER	ASSESSMENT	Management MEDICAL/ PHARMACOLOGIC	NONPHARMACOLOGIC	EVALUATION
		Papulosquamous (Cont.)		
Psoriasis (mild to moderate)	Epidermal hyperplasia with high rate of epidermal turnover. Lesions are discrete erythematous papules and plaques covered with silver-white scales; often on elbows, knees, scalp. Familial history. Concurrent arthritis common. Environmental stress level.	Suppress rapid proliferation with anti-inflammatory agents (tar, steroids), or with ultraviolet light treatments. If disease is severe and persistent psoralens (methoxsalen) plus ultraviolet light or antineoplastics (methotrexate) may be used. Keratolytics.	Much emotional support due to chronicity and disfigurement. With PUVA therapy (psoralens plus ultraviolet) burns can result because methoxsalen is a photosensitizer. Take oral methoxsalen with food to decrease nausea.	Observe for adverse drug effects of potent agents used to treat the disorder. Often recurs. With PUVA therapy, observe for nausea, pruritus, and severe erythema. Erythema peaks at 48 h after therapy.
Pityriasis rosea	Papulosquamous erythematous lesions on trunk of adults.	Control symptoms of itching. Tepid colloidal baths (Aveeno oatmeal bath) for 10–15 min daily.	Explain it is noninfectious and will resolve spontaneously. Caution about slippery tub with colloidal baths.	Resolves in 6 weeks with or without treatment.
		Acne		
Acne vulgaris	Lesions are inflamed pilosebaceous follicles with formation of cysts, papules, nodules, on face, neck, and back. Present in 90% of teenagers. May have significant psychosocial implications. Emotional stress level.	Prevent blockage of pilosebaceous opening with keratolytics (benzoyl peroxide, retinoic acid). Counteract inflammation secondary to *P. acnes* with oral or topical antibiotics (tetracycline, clindamycin, erythromycin). Estrogens. Isotretinoin (Accutane; 13-*cis*-Retinoic acid) for severe cystic acne.	Emotional support. Sunlight. Dietary control (the role of diet in acne is dubious). Draining of pustules and removal of blackheads by nurse or physician: warn patient that picking can cause scarring and abscesses. Warn females that isotretinoin and tetracycline are teratogens; contraception crucial. Take isotretinoin with food.	Observe for side effects of the systemic agents. Check for excessive irritation or dryness of skin secondary to topical agents or oral isotretinoin. Evaluate for pregnancy (isotretinoin and tetracycline must be *stopped* at first suspicion of pregnancy). Monitor constipation, myalgia, arthalgia, hypertriglyceridemia, eye irritation, and skeletal hypertrophy with isotretinoin.

TABLE 38-10 Nursing Process Related to Selected Dermatologic Disorders (*Continued*)

DISORDER	ASSESSMENT	Management MEDICAL/ PHARMACOLOGIC	NONPHARMACOLOGIC	EVALUATION
Bacterial Infections				
Impetigo	Honey-colored, crusted erythematous macules with pustules or blisters. Culture for possible infection with nephrogenic streptococcus. Predisposing factors are trauma, poor hygiene, contagion, poor host defense, or other skin disease.	Topical and systemic antibiotics.	Compresses prior to application of topical antibacterial agents. Prevent spread of infection on patient and to others.	Monitor resolution of lesions.
Furunculosis (boils)	Warm, tender, red nodules. Culture for organism. Predisposing factors include trauma, poor hygiene, contagion, poor host defense, or other skin disease.	Incision and drainage. Systemic antibiotics.	Hot compresses to keep lesion draining.	Monitor lesion for resolution or exacerbation.
Folliculitis	Small pustules in hair follicle usually on face, arms, back, buttocks, or legs. Culture for organism. Predisposing factors include trauma such as shaving, poor hygiene, hot tubs, poor host defense, or other skin disease.	Systemic and topical antibiotics.	Frequent scrubs with antiseptic solution such as Hibiclens.	Monitor for resolution of lesions.
Viral Infections				
Herpes simplex (cold or fever sore)	Lesions are recurrent small groups of vesicles on erythematous base on lip or genital area. Predisposing factors are sun, trauma, infection, emotional stress, sexual contact with carrier.	Nonspecific drying agents. Idoxuridine (Stoxil) for eye involvement. Acyclovir for primary genital herpes. Systemic Ara-A or Acycloviv for herpes in neonate and immunocompromised host.	Remove or minimize precipitating factor. Counsel regarding abstinence from sexual contact when infection is active. Educate the carrier of genital herpes of danger to fetus during pregnancy and delivery.	Often recurring. Observe for eye involvement. Observe for systemic involvement in immunocompromised host.
Herpes zoster (shingles)	Vesicles on red base that follow distribution of a nerve root; painful. Assess for other infection or malignancy since herpes zoster can be associated with these.	Symptomatic treatment for fever and pain. Passive immunity for high-risk persons attained with zoster immune globulin. Idoxuridine (Stoxil) or Acyclovir for eye involvement.	Care to avoid secondary infection. Isolate from nonimmune persons during stage of vesicle formation.	Resolution in 7–14 days. Observe for development of secondary infection. Observe for eye involvement.

TABLE 38-10 Nursing Process Related to Selected Dermatologic Disorders (*Continued*)

DISORDER	ASSESSMENT	MEDICAL/ PHARMACOLOGIC	NONPHARMACOLOGIC	EVALUATION
		Management		
		Viral Infections (Cont.)		
Warts (verrucae, condylomata accuminata, molluscum)	Papillary growths raised above the skin. Note if single or multiple, size, location.	Should be removed surgically, mechanically, or chemically (salicylic acid 10–40%) by trained health personnel.	Contagious; avoid direct contact with others, picking, excessive use of nonprescription drugs.	Observe for resolution and recurrence.
		Parasitic Infections		
Scabies (mites)	Pruritus of interdigital folds, wrists, elbows, axilla, nipples, navel, other skin folds. Manifestations vary with individual sensitivity, duration of infestation, hygiene.	Soak in soap and water followed immediately by application of benzyl benzoate (10%) or Kwell lotion which is left on 24 h. Oral antihistamines and emollients for pruritus. Topical steroids for severe eczematous reactions.	Educate in good hygiene. Wash clothes and bed sheets at same time as Kwell application. Treat family members and sexual contacts.	Resolution of pruritus and rash.
Pediculosis (lice or crabs)	Minute red noninflammatory points with flush of skin and pruritus. May become inflamed with scratching. Usually associated with poor hygiene.	Benzyl benzoate (10%)	Education in hygiene and prevention. Clothes and bedding should be treated with insecticide.	Resolution of rash and pruritus.
		Fungal Infections		
Candidiasis (moniliasis)	Acute or chronic infection of skin or mucous membrane, especially mouth, GI tract, vagina. Predisposed are infants, elderly, women, those on broad-spectrum antibiotics.	Antifungal creams, ointments, lotions: nystatin (Mycostatin), clotrimazole. Ketoconazole for severe infections.	Educative measures on prevention of spread with sexual contact, infection may spread to partner.	Resolution of pruritus, exudate, rash.
Tinea infections: tinea capitis (scalp ringworm), onychomycosis (nail ringworm), tinea corporis (body ringworm), tinea cruris (jock itch), tinea pedis (athlete's foot)	Scaly red macules, crusting, alopecia on scalp, white or brown area at nail border. Sometimes itches. Ascertain source of infection (e.g., tinea capitis often from other persons or animals; tinea pedis from shower or locker room floor).	Oral griseofulvin for 4–8 weeks or longer depending on site and organism. Give after high fat meal to avoid GI upset. Ketoconazole for recalcitrant infections. Topicals: clotrimazole (Lotrimin), tolnaftate (Tinactin), keratolytics (sulfur, salicylic acid, undecylenic acid, etc.).	Keep area clean and dry. Educate in prevention of exposure and infection of others.	Good prognosis for cure.

infectious or when the therapeutic agent causes staining or irritation, many prescribers recommend that the nurse apply topical medications with clean bare hands. This may be particularly therapeutic when the disorder is disfiguring, as may occur in psoriasis.

Since there are many over-the-counter preparations available for treating minor skin lesions, people tend to treat themselves rather than seeking medical advice. There is a definite risk of compounding the original problem by adding an allergic reaction from the self-prescribed medication. Additionally, family and friends frequently advise favorite home remedies which may further damage and irritate sensitive skin. Nurses may assist patients in choosing soaps and preparations which will cleanse, hydrate, and protect sensitive skin as well as counseling avoidance of irritants and allergens. Persons should be encouraged to seek medical advice when skin problems develop.

When the dermatologic disease is infectious in nature the nurse must often educate the patient and family regarding the transmission of the fungus, parasite, virus, or bacteria.

Rashes occurring in the hospitalized patient or outpatient may be due to a drug the patient is taking. If the patient who develops skin lesions is taking a medication known to cause serious dermatologic disorders, the medication should be discontinued and the physician notified. All rashes must be carefully assessed and reported, even if a probable cause is not identified.

Evaluation

As a dermatologic disorder resolves, the nature of the manifestation may change, and so the nurse should carefully observe the lesions and report any changes. Lack of improvement within a reasonable length of time for the particular disorder indicates a need for review of the diagnosis and the treatment plan.

Many of the preparations used to treat dermatologic disorders cause rashes as their major adverse effect, and so new eruptions may be indicative of the need to reconsider the treatment mode.

CASE STUDY

J.S., a 34-year-old female, presented to the Dermatology Clinic with the chief complaint of cracks in the skin of both hands which had persisted for six months.

Assessment

J.S. was a housewife and mother of two preschool children with jogging as her only hobby. Her normal day consisted of jogging 4 miles, cooking three meals, washing one load of laundry, general upkeep of the house, and bathing the children. She stated that she washed her hands with soap frequently and did not wear protective gloves when exposing her hands to household cleansers or solvents. She usually applied a lubricating lotion at bedtime. She recalled that when the problem began she developed very small 'scattered vesicles on the sides of her fingers, which appeared "tapioca-like." She complained of moderate pruritus and fairly marked tenderness in the fissured areas.

She denied a personal or family history of psoriasis, hay fever, asthma, or other skin dermatoses. She also denied the use of any drugs.

On examination of her hands, the skin was found to be moderately erythematous, slightly edematous, and uniformly very dry with scaling and accentuated skin lines. In addition there were fissures in the fingertips and web spaces between the thumb and index finger. No vesicles, papules, exudate, or crusting were noted.

Management

J.S. was informed that the cause of her symptoms was excessive dry skin, which probably was secondary to repeated exposure to chemical irritants such as soaps, detergents, and solvents, and is a common problem among housewives, food handlers, bartenders, nurses, dentists, and surgeons.

The main objectives of therapy are hydration of the skin and avoidance of irritants. The patient was told that skin becomes dry due to a lack of water, not oil. Thus, she was instructed to stop the use of soaps as this disrupts the protective barrier of the stratum corneum and allows for increased water loss. It was recommended, instead, that she use a soap substitute, i.e., Cetaphil lotion, and that she wash only when necessary. If a soap was needed, a very mild one like Dove should be used with thorough rinsing. For hydration of the skin, a bland emollient was to be applied several times a day and always after exposure to water or if itching occurred.

A medium potency topical corticosteroid ointment, fluocinolone acetonide, 0.025%, was prescribed to reduce inflammation. J.S. was instructed to soak her hands in tepid water for 10 min, to pat dry only, and then immediately to apply a thin layer of the steroid ointment. By hydrating the skin, penetration of the medication would be enhanced. The immediate application of ointment would trap water in the skin.

Finally, great emphasis was placed on preventive measures. J.S. was told to protect her hands always from any chemical irritant with vinyl gloves. If sweating and maceration become a problem, she was advised to wear a pair of disposable cotton gloves inside the vinyl gloves.

It was stressed that resolution might be slow but that with good skin care on her part positive changes would be seen.

Evaluation

J.S. was seen four weeks later with a moderate amount of improvement. The erythema and edema had resolved along with a slight decrease in the depth and amount of tenderness of the fissures. She stated she had been able to adhere to the instructions fairly consistently. The topical corticosteroid was discontinued but the application of emollients was continued.

REFERENCES

Arndt, K. A.: *Manual of Dermatologic Therapeutics with Essentials of Diagnosis,* 3d ed., Boston: Little, Brown, 1983.

——, and H. Jick: "Rates of Cutaneous Reactions to Drugs," *JAMA,* **235**:918–923, 1976.

Billow, J. A., and R. E. Hopponen: "Acne Products," in *Handbook of Nonprescription Drugs,* 7th ed., Washington: American Pharmaceutical Association, 1982, pp. 547–559.

Bond, C.: "Burn and Sunburn Products," in *Handbook of Nonprescription Drugs,* 7th ed., Washington: American Pharmaceutical Association, 1982, pp. 485–498.

DeSimone II, E. M.: "Sunscreen and Suntan Products," in *Handbook of Nonprescription Drugs,* 7th ed., Washington: American Pharmaceutical Association, 1982, pp. 449–511.

Fitzpatrick, T. B., A. Z. Eizen, K. Wolff, I. M. Freedberg, and K. F. Austen: *Dermatology in General Medicine,* New York: McGraw-Hill, 1979.

Lawlor, Jr., G. J., and T. J. Fischer (eds.): *Manual of Allergy and Immunology, Diagnosis and Therapy,* Boston: Little, Brown, 1981.

Marko, J.: "Skin Disorders," in G. S. Avery (ed.), *Drug Treatment Principles and Practice of Clinical Pharmacology and Therapeutics,* 2d ed., New York: ADIS, 1980.

Osol, A., and J. E. Hoover: *Remington's Pharmaceutical Sciences,* 15th ed., Boston: Mack, 1975.

Parrish, J. A.: *Dermatology and Skin Care,* New York: McGraw-Hill, 1975.

"Proceedings of Workshop in Dermatopharmacology," *Clin Pharmacol Ther,* **16**:861–988, 1974.

Robinson, J. R., and L. J. Gauger: "Dermatitis, Dry Skin, Dandruff, Seborrhea, and Psoriasis Products," in *Handbook of Nonprescription Drugs,* 7th ed., Washington: American Pharmaceutical Association, 1982, pp. 561–592.

Sadik, F., and J. C. Delafuente: "Insect Sting and Bite Products," in *Handbook of Nonprescription Drugs,* 7th ed., Washington: American Pharmaceutical Association, 1982, pp. 473–483.

Skierkowski, P., and N. Lublanezki: "External Analgesic Products," in *Handbook of Nonprescription Drugs,* 7th ed., Washington: American Pharmaceutical Association, 1982, pp. 513–523.

Smith, G. H.: "Diaper Rash and Prickly Heat Products," in *Handbook of Nonprescription Drugs,* 7th ed., Washington: American Pharmaceutical Association, 1982, pp. 605–614.

Wormser, H.: "Poison Ivy and Poison Oak Products," in *Handbook of Nonprescription Drugs,* 7th ed., Washington: American Pharmaceutical Association, 1982, pp. 593–603.

Zanowiak, P., and M. R. Jacobs: "Topical Anti-infective Products," in *Handbook of Nonprescription Drugs,* 7th ed., Washington: American Pharmaceutical Association, 1982, pp. 525–546.

39

OPHTHALMOLOGIC DISORDERS

MARY JO SAGATIES
JOHN B. CONSTANTINE

LEARNING OBJECTIVES

Upon mastery of the content of this chapter, the reader will be able to:

1. Describe a proper method for administration of eye drops and eye ointment, including measures to minimize systemic absorption.

2. List the drug groups used in ophthalmic diagnostics and in the treatment of glaucoma and external ocular inflammation.

3. Explain the nursing process related to agents used in ophthalmic diagnostics, glaucoma, and external ocular inflammation.

4. Compare the usual treatment for the two types of primary glaucoma.

5. Explain why mydriatic drugs are not contraindicated for all persons with glaucoma.

6. Indicate the classification (drug group), mechanism of action, indications, and adverse effects for the following drugs used to treat glaucoma: (1) pilocarpine, (2) physostigmine, (3) mannitol, (4) epinephrine, (5) timolol, and (6) acetazolamide.

7. Describe the role of the nurse in instructing the patient regarding self-care in ophthalmic disorders, including self-administration of topical ophthalmics and over-the-counter preparations.

8. List ophthalmic diseases and symptoms which can be induced by the administration of systemic drugs.

9. Describe the local adverse effects of topical corticosteroids and antimicrobials.

Although the science of ophthalmology is considered to be a medical and nursing specialty, the ocular structures should not be viewed as isolated organs. Various types of systemic disease often present initially or simultaneously with involvement of the ocular structures. In addition, many preparations used to treat ophthalmic disorders may have systemic effects, just as many drugs used to treat systemic diseases may have ocular side effects. Further, it should be realized by the care giver that vision is a precious sense. Emotional support of the patient experiencing a temporary or permanent visual loss, or even the threat of visual impairment, is an essential component of the therapeutic regimen which should not be neglected. The most common ocular conditions requiring drug therapy are increased intraocular pressure, inflammation, and dry eyes.

NURSING TECHNIQUES IN EYE CARE

In order to adequately care for patients with symptoms and diseases of the ocular structures, the nurse should be able to properly administer topical ophthalmic preparations, participate in educating the patient for self-care, and knowledgeably advise patients about the proper use of over-the-counter ophthalmic preparations.

Administration of Ophthalmic Drugs

Topical application of the appropriate solution or ointment is the most common method of providing pharmacologic therapy to the ocular structures. Drugs also gain entrance to the eye through systemic administration, intraocular injection, or periocular injection.

The efficacy of any ophthalmic preparation depends on its ability to reach the appropriate structures or receptors in adequate concentrations, which is determined by the principles of drug biotransport across membranes discussed in Chap. 5. Characteristics of the preparation affecting its absorption include lipid and water solubility, pH, ionization, tonicity, concentration, and duration of contact with the cul-de-sac and/or cornea. Contact of the drug can be prolonged by administering the medication as an ointment or continuous irrigation. Surfactants like **benzalkonium chloride** reduce surface tension and improve absorption. The integrity of the corneal epithelium and the lacrimal drainage system may have implications for the effectiveness of treatment and systemic adverse effects. In choosing the appropriate drug regimen to treat any inflammation or infection of the deep ocular structures, it should be considered that most topical agents (e.g., most direct-acting anticholinergics and antibiotics) and many systemic drugs (e.g., most oral antimicrobials and some parenteral antimicrobials) do not reach therapeutic levels in the internal eye and may require direct intraocular injection.

The general principles of administration of ophthalmic drops and ointments are similar. The eyelids and lashes should be cleansed with sterile water or irrigating solution on a cotton ball by wiping across the closed eye from the inner to the outer canthus. The patient should be sitting with the head tilted slightly backward or lying down on his/her back. The nurse should instruct the patient to look up while the lower lid is pulled away from the eye to form a pouch.

Ophthalmic Drops

When administering ophthalmic drops, the appropriate amount of solution is dispensed into the pouch without touching the lid with the dropper (Fig. 39-1). The patient should gently close the eyes for a few seconds without squeezing the lids. To avoid systemic absorption of the drug through the vascular nasal mucosa, gentle pressure for 1 to 2 min may be applied to the lacrimal sac which is the upper dilated portion of the nasolacrimal duct located in the groove of the lacrimal bone.

Ophthalmic Ointment

In the administration of an eye ointment the medication is applied as a thin ribbon along the inner aspect of the lower lid with care taken not to touch the globe or lid with the end of the tube. While the ointment form of the medication protects the eye, softens discharge, is undiluted by tears, and keeps the drug in contact with the eye for longer periods of time than do liquid drops, it has a tendency to form a film over the eye which interferes with vision. The ointment form of some ophthalmic preparations has also been associated with a higher incidence of contact dermatitis and delayed healing through inhibition of mitosis of corneal epithelial cells and so are avoided prior to and following surgical procedures.

Patient Education

In the discussion of any ophthalmic condition, it should be kept in mind that ocular disease ususally brings on fears of blindness. Anxiety levels may be high and instructions can be easily misinterpreted or forgotten unless the directions are clearly and concisely reinforced and supplied in written form.

Patients should be taught the signs and symptoms which indicate an exacerbation or worsening of their specific disorder. Instructions should be given about the action to be taken in an emergency. Patients with glaucoma or postoperative patients should be made aware of activities which

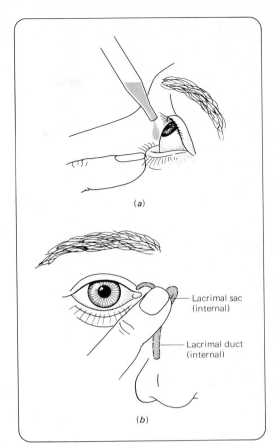

FIGURE 39-1

Proper Administration of Eye Drops. (*a*) The patient looks upward and the drop is aimed toward the conjunctival pouch. (*b*) Pressure is applied to the area overlying the lacrimal sac after administration to decrease systemic absorption through the lacrimal duct.

increase intraocular pressure (e.g., lifting, straining to defecate) and how to avoid them if possible. There may also be a need to decrease the intensity of the patient's activities of daily living for a time after a diagnosis is made or after surgery. Those patients with infections must be taught proper hand-washing techniques and the importance of not touching the unaffected eye. Medication instructions for the patient must be explicit as to the dosage, frequency, and adverse effects of the medication to be used. Since allergic reaction to eye drops is fairly common, the patient should be instructed to examine the eye daily for increased redness, lid swelling, or itching.

Patients who will need eye drops on a continuing basis should be taught the proper technique of self-administration with follow-up demonstrations to ensure proper use. It is helpful if family members are also taught the technique of instillation in order to help the patient if difficulty is encountered, since self-administration of ocular medication can be a frustrating task for the patient. Patients should be warned not to put any medication in their eyes that is not sterile, particle-free, and labeled specifically for ophthalmic use.

Patient compliance to any therapeutic regimen is difficult to control, especially once the condition begins to improve. The importance of following the plan of treatment should be emphasized. The patient should also be aware of the importance of not using "old" medications in the eye; medications should be discarded when they have been discontinued by the physician. The patient should be instructed also to check solutions for cloudiness or discoloration before use and to discard any solutions so affected.

Since written communication is generally more effective than verbal, it is helpful for patients to receive written instructions upon discharge from the hospital or when seen in an outpatient department. Instructions regarding medications and procedures should be included, as well as the name of the physician or institution to contact if any problems should arise.

Finally, the nurse should be aware of organizations and community resources available to persons with ocular disorders. (List is available from the American Foundation for the Blind, Inc., 15 West 16th St., New York, NY 10011.) Individual needs must be identified and referral to the appropriate organization should be made when necessary. Nurses should also support community education programs that inform the public of the importance of seeking diagnosis and treatment of ophthalmic disorders.

Over-the-Counter (OTC) Ophthalmic Preparations

People may self-medicate for various "minor" ophthalmic disorders. For self-limiting conditions, such as stinging, tearing, itching, "tired eyes" or "eye strain," the use of OTC preparations may be appropriate. In conditions where the patient is experiencing pain or blurred vision, self-medication is not advisable. OTC ophthalmic preparations should not be used consecutively for longer than 48 h.

All ophthalmic preparations are initially sterile and contain ingredients to maintain sterility, as well as ingredients to adjust tonicity and pH to approximate that of tears. Ophthalmic preparations have expiration dates and the patient should discard any medication not used within three months of opening the package. Crystals of drug may form around the lid of the bottle and care must be taken not to introduce these into the eye during administration.

Contact Lens Products

Contact lenses are broadly classified as hard or soft depending on their chemical and physical properties. Contact lenses are used for cosmetic as well as therapeutic purposes (e.g., keratoconus, aphakia, etc.). The care and storage of hard contact lenses requires use of cleansing products, wetting solutions, and soaking solutions. These can be pur-

chased as separate agents or as a single multifunctional product. Soft contact lenses contain a larger portion of water and are more susceptible to bacterial contamination, thus require disinfection. Disinfection can be achieved by heat (thermal) or by chemicals. For both hard and soft contact lenses a rewetting solution can be used as a lubricant during insertion. Products for use with hard contact lenses can not be used with soft contact lenses and many solutions are incompatible with other solutions. The manufacturer's instructions or a pharmacist should be consulted before any preparation is used. Nurses assisting patients in the care of their contact lenses during illness, disability, or confinement to bed should be very certain that appropriate techniques and solutions are employed.

Most contact lens products contain preservatives which may cause allergic responses in some people. Preparations which are preservative-free and considered hypoallergenic are available (e.g., Unisol, saline solution, others).

Irrigation Solutions

Isotonic salt solutions (e.g., Eye-Stream, Dacriose) and boric acid solutions (e.g., Collyrium, Blinx, Trisol, Lauro) are available over-the-counter as "eye washes" for use in soothing the eyes and removal of foreign bodies from the eyes. Several come with eye cups or an eye irrigator to facilitate washing of the eye. The patient should be instructed to avoid cross-contamination of the eyes and to seek medical assessment if the eye irritation or sensation of a foreign object does not rapidly abate. Routine irrigation of the eyes is not indicated and may be harmful by introducing infection or foreign bodies into the eyes.

Artificial Tears

Artificial tear preparations are commonly indicated in the treatment of keratoconjunctivitis sicca, or dry eye, a condition which results from deficient precorneal tear film. Symptoms include a gritty, sandy, or foreign body sensation in the eye or general eye irritation which may be aggravated by a smoky environment or a dry, hot atmosphere. These agents are indicated when neurologic disease impairs tear production and/or the corneal relfex.

Artificial tear preparations sooth and lubricate dry eyes by blending with the precorneal tear film to promote corneal wetting and tear film stability. The ingredients generally include salts in concentrations balanced to match the tonicity of the eye, buffers to adjust pH, viscosity agents to prolong contact time with the eye (e.g., **methylcellulose, polyvinyl alcohol**), and preservatives to maintain sterility (e.g., **benzalkonium chloride, povidone**). The usual dosage is 1 to 3 drops three or four times daily, as necessary. Tears Plus, Liquifilm Tears, Lyteers, Methulose, Tears Naturale, and Hypotears are examples of these agents.

A slow-release insert of **hydroxypropyl cellulose** (Lacrisert) is available by prescription, requiring daily or twice-daily insertion into the inferior cul-de-sac of each involved eye. Mild transient adverse effects consisting of local irritation, photophobia, matting of the eyelashes, and hyperemia have been reported. This preparation is for use by patients with moderate or severe keratoconjunctivitis sicca or recurrent corneal erosions.

Lubricants

Several petrolatum based emollients (e.g., Duratears, Duolube, Nu-Tears, Lacri-Lube S.O.P.) are available for protection and lubrication of the eye, particularly at night, in recurrent corneal erosions, keratoconjunctivitis sicca, and exposure keratitis.

Vasoconstrictors

In addition to their moisturizing quality, these preparations have a vasoconstrictor effect which diminishes conjunctival redness due to fatigue, overwear of contact lenses, colds, and extensive reading or close work. The vasoconstrictors are sympathomimetics which stimulate α-adrenergic receptors. Systemic absorption can result in interactions with other drugs or disease states (see Chap. 13 and the sections in this chapter on ophthalmic diagnostics and glaucoma). The consumer should be aware that ocular redness may be a sign of serious eye disorders, such as corneal abrasions, corneal erosions, acute iritis, or acute glaucoma, which require medical attention. The use of vasoconstrictors is contraindicated in these condition. Three sympathomimetics, **naphazoline hydrochloride** (Clear Eyes, Vaso Clear, Allerest Eye Drops), **phenylephrine hydrochloride** (Phenylzin, A.K.-Nefrin, Optised) and **tetrahydrozoline hydrochloride** (Visine, Murine Plus, Soothe Eye Drops) are commonly used in these preparations, along with buffers, viscosity agents, and preservatives.

Antiseptics

A mercury-containing ophthalmic antiseptic agent, **yellow mercuric oxide** ointment, is available without prescription in 1 and 2% concentrations. This agent is active against many common bacterial and fungal pathogens, but may cause serious rash or irritation, particularly in those sensitive to mercury. The preferred therapy for conjunctivitis and corneal ulcer is with specific antimicrobial therapy based upon culture and susceptibility studies. Because the risks of adverse reaction outweigh the potential benefit, the nurse should explain the hazards associated with the use of these agents, especially for prolonged periods, as mercury poisoning can result.

DRUG-INDUCED OPHTHALMIC DISORDERS

Information about ocular toxicology is accumulating rapidly. The nurse should be aware that many systemic drugs have ocular side effects. These ocular reactions may be reversible or irreversible depending on the type of pharmaceutical agent involved, dosage, and duration of therapy. Table 39-1 includes examples of ocular adverse effects of several common systemic preparations. The reader is referred to the National Registry of Drug-Induced Ocular Side Effects for further information on this subject (see References).

OPHTHALMOLOGIC DIAGNOSTICS

Mydriatics and Cycloplegics

Diagnostic agents which dilate the pupil are called *mydriatics* while those that interfere with the accommodative process are called *cycloplegics*. Mydriatics are sympathomimetics most commonly used to produce pupillary dilation for ophthalmoscopic examination and include phenylephrine hydrochloride and hydroxyamphetamine. **Phenylephrine hydrochloride** (Neo-Synephrine, others) acts directly on the

TABLE 39-1 Drug-Induced Ocular Adverse Effects

OCULAR COMPLICATION	AGENT/DRUG
Lacrimation	Fluorouracil, hydralazine, reserpine
Decreased tear production	Propranolol
Cataracts	Allopurinol, corticosteroids, radiation
Myopia	Hydralazine, oral contraceptives, tetracycline
Accommodative changes	Narcotic analgesics, phenothiazines, tricyclic antidepressants
Retinal edema	Chloramphenicol
Corneal deposits*	Plaquenil
Retinal pigmentation*	Methanol, plaquenil, quinine
Papilledema	Tetracycline, sulfonamides, vitamin A
Optic neuritis*	Chloramphenicol, ethambutol, isoniazid, methanol
Central scotoma	Ethyl alcohol
Nystagmus	Phenytoin, diazepam, oral contraceptives
Photophobia	Ethambutol, fluorouracil, gold, tetracycline
Toxic amblyopia	Ethanol, ethambutol, ketamine, quinine
Elevated intraocular pressure	Corticosteroids
Oculogyric crisis	Chlorpromazine, diazepam, haloperidol

*Usually irreversible.

α-adrenergic receptors to produce pupillary dilation. **Hydroxyamphetamine** (Paredrine) is an indirect-acting sympathomimetic which causes the release of norepinephrine from adrenergic nerve endings.

Cycloplegic mydriatics dilate the pupil and interfere with accommodation by paralyzing the ciliary muscles. These anticholinergic agents act as competitive inhibitors of endogenous acetylcholine on the muscarinic receptors of the iris sphincter muscle, thus producing pupillary dilation. Paralysis of the ciliary muscle interferes with the ability to accommodate vision to focus on near objects. **Atropine sulfate, cyclopentolate hydrochloride** (Cyclogel), **homatropine hydrobromide, scopolamine hydrobromide** (Isopto Hyoscine), and **tropicamide** (Mydriacyl) are representatives of this class which are commonly used clinically. These agents are often indicated in a thorough examination of the fundus of the eye, in evaluation of refractive and accommodative disorders, after certain operative procedures, in treatment of some corneal diseases, and to prevent or release adhesions in inflammatory diseases of the iris and ciliary body. Dosages may vary depending upon the condition for which the drug has been prescribed (see Table 39-2). For eye examination, the drugs with the shortest durations of action are preferred.

Dyes

The diagnosis of several external ocular disorders of the conjunctiva, cornea, and lacrimal apparatus is facilitated by the use of **fluorescein sodium** and **rose bengal** (see Table 39-3). Fluorescein sodium is also used in examination of the iris, retina, and choroid.

Fluorescein Sodium (Topical)

Fluorescein sodium in solution and ophthalmic strips provide uniform fluorescence to the corneal epithelium and the bulbar and palpebral conjunctiva. It is used in the diagnosis of corneal or conjunctival injury. Fluorescein sodium stains abraded or ulcerated areas of the corneal epithelium a bright green when viewed with a cobalt blue filter and stains lesions of the conjunctiva a yellow-orange due to the acidity of this tissue. Hard contact lenses that are improperly fitted may also be recognized by evaluation of the fluorescein pattern. The solution form of fluorescein sodium contains **benoxinate hydrochloride** which is a topical anesthetic of rapid onset (15 s or less after administration) and short duration (15 min after administration). This solution can therefore be used in ophthalmic procedures in which a topical

TABLE 39-2 Common Mydriatics and Cycloplegics*

	DOSAGE†	COMMENTS‡
Mydriatic		
Phenylephrine hydrochloride (Neo-Synephrine, Efricel, others)	2.5–10.0%; 1–2 drops for pupillary dilation	Lower concentrations minimize cardiovascular side effects, especially drug-induced hypertension.
Hydroxyamphetamine (Paredrine)	1.0%; 1–2 drops for pupillary dilation	
Cycloplegic		
Atropine sulfate	1.0–3.0%; 1 drop tid for 3 days	Prolonged duration (2–4 weeks). Systemic effects include hyperactivity, facial flushing, elevated body temperature.
Cyclopentolate hydrochloride (Cyclogel)	0.5–2.0%; 2 drops 5 min apart	Rapid onset (25–60 min); moderate duration (24 h)
Homatropine hydrobromide (Homatropine, Homatrocel)	2.0–5.0%; 6–8 drops 15 min apart	Onset 60 min; moderate duration (24–48 h)
Scopolamine hydrobromide (Isopto Hyoscine)	0.25%; 2 drops 30 min apart	Fewer side effects and shorter duration than atropine (8 days)
Tropicamide (Mydriacyl)	0.5–1.0%; 2 drops 5 min apart	Onset 20–30 min; short duration (2–6 h)

*Combination agents are available which contain two or more different mydriatics, local anesthetics, antihistamines, and/or corticosteroids.

†Dosage of cycloplegic mydriatics applies to refraction only. Dosages for other conditions depend on the concentration of the solution, frequency of administration, and nature of condition.

‡Onset of action refers to onset of cycloplegia.

anesthetic and fluorescent agent is indicated, such as applanation tonometry and removal of foreign bodies.

Adverse effects include burning, stinging, and conjunctival injection which have occasionally been reported upon administration. Severe allergic corneal reaction with a diffuse epithelial keratitis, sloughing of necrotic epithelium, and iritis have rarely been reported. These agents should not be administered to patients who have a known hypersensitivity to fluorescein sodium or who are wearing hydrogel (soft) contact lenses.

Fluorexon   Fluorexon (Fluoresoft) is a large molecule of fluorescein used in the fitting of hydrogel (soft) contact lenses which are discolored with the use of topical fluorescein sodium. It is not recommended for use with highly hydrated "extended wear" lenses. Fluorexon is applied topically with or without the lens in place. Adverse effects are comparable to those with topical fluorescein sodium.

Fluorescein Sodium (Injectable)

Fluorescein sodium injectable is used as an intravenous diagnostic aid which demarcates the vascular area under investigation. It is used in ophthalmic angiography, including evaluation of the integrity of the retinal and choroidal circulation, since defects in the retinal vessels or pigmented epithelium permit leakage of fluorescein from the intravascular system. Fluorescein sodium may also be used in examination of iris vasculature, delineation of the pattern of aqueous flow, determination of tissue viability, identification of malignant tumors, and determination of the arm-to-retina circulation time (the appearance of fluorescence at the optic disc approximately 9 to 14 s after injection of a fluorescein bolus in the antecubital vein). This agent is helpful in determining the patency of the nasolacrimal system or as an antidote to aniline dyes.

Gastrointestinal distress, nausea, and vomiting are common adverse effects after intraveneous administration. Headache, syncope, hypertension, urticaria, pruritus, and

TABLE 39-3   Common Diagnostic Dyes

DRUG	DOSAGE	COMMENTS
Fluorescein sodium ophthalmic strips (Flo-Glo Strip; Fluor-I-Strip)	0.6-mg impregnated strip	The strip should be moistened with sterile irrigating solution and then applied to the fornix or conjunctiva. The patient should blink frequently after the moistened strip has touched the cornea or conjunctiva to circulate the fluorescent material
Fluorescein sodium solution (Fluress)	1–2 drops of a solution containing 0.25% fluorescein sodium and 0.4% benoxinate hydrochloride	Aseptic technique must always be used in administration since the solution is easily contaminated by *Pseudomonas aeruginosa*. Opacities of the cornea and visual loss may result from prolonged use.
Fluorexon (Fluoresoft)	0.35%; 1–2 drops	Used in fitting soft contact lenses to avoid discoloration of the lens. Repeated rinsing of lens with normal saline will remove any dye.
Fluorescein sodium injectable (Fluorescite injection; Funduscein injection)	Children: 35 mg per 10 lb body weight Adults: 10 mL of 5% solution, 5 mL of 10% solution, or 2 mL of 25% solution	The antecubital vein is the preferred site of administration. If an allergic reaction is suspected, a test dose of 0.05 mL may be injected ID and evaluated 30–60 min following the injection.
Rose bengal	1–2 drops of 1% solution 1.3-mg-impregnated strip	The patient should blink frequently to circulate the material. Staining of clothing should be avoided. A topical ophthalmic anesthetic may be administered prior to the instillation of rose bengal to prevent irritation to the ocular tissues. The impregnated strip should be moistened with sterile normal saline and applied to the fornix or conjunctiva.

angioneurotic edema occasionally occur. Cardiac arrest, basilar artery ischemia, transient dyspnea, convulsions, and severe shock rarely occur. The drug should not be administered to patients who are pregnant or who have a known hypersensitivity to fluorescein sodium.

Prior to the administration of the drug, this diagnostic procedure and its possible adverse effects should be explained to the patient. Proper technique should be used in administering the drug so as to prevent extravasation and thrombophlebitis at the injection site. After administration the skin usually takes on a yellowish discoloration for 6 to 12 h and the urine will be bright yellow for 12 to 36 h. Fluorescein sodium should be administered with caution (emergency tray available) in patients with a history of allergy or bronchial asthma.

Rose Bengal

Rose bengal is used mainly in the diagnosis of suspected keratitis and keratoconjunctivitis sicca (dry eye), but it is also indicated in the detection of foreign bodies or in the delineation of the margins of ulcers and corneal or conjunctival erosions. This diagnostic agent stains dead and degenerated corneal and conjunctival epithlial cells, including the nuclei and cell walls and the mucus of the precorneal tear film, a bright pink to red. Adverse effects include irritation, burning, stinging, and discoloration which are more frequently reported than with fluorescein.

Topical Anesthetics

Use of ophthalmic topical anesthetics is indicated in foreign body removal, applanation tonometry, suture removal, and ocular surgery. Common agents include tetracaine (**Pontocaine** 0.5%), **proparacaine** (Ophthaine 0.5%) and **cocaine** (2.0 to 4.0%), which must be made sterile for ophthalmic use. These agents should not be prescribed for prolonged anesthesia since they retard epithelization of the cornea (see Chap. 47).

NURSING PROCESS RELATED TO OPHTHALMIC DIAGNOSTICS

Assessment

Prior to any ophthalmic diagnostic procedure the nurse should assess for allergies or other contraindictions to the use of the drug. Since some of the topically applied agents will be systemically absorbed, it is important to identify diseases such as hyperthyroidism and cardiac disorders which may be adversely affected by mydriatics or local anesthetics. Drug interactions may also occur, so sympathomimetic mydriatics should not be used prior to surgical procedures with agents (e.g., **halothane**) that sensitize the myocardium

to adrenergic effects. Concomitant use of these mydriatics and **monoamine oxidase inhibitors, tricyclic antidepressants, reserpine, guanethidine,** or **methyldopa** could result in exaggerated systemic adrenergic symptoms. Elderly patients may be more susceptible to the systemic adverse effects of the drugs, as well as more prone to acute angle closure glaucoma. Since pupil dilation may precipitate angle block in eyes capable of angle closure (as determined by gonioscopy), drugs with mydriatic activity should not be used in susceptible patients unless a peripheral iridectomy has been performed. The nurse should also assess for history of cardiac disease, asthma, or allergies prior to intravenous administration of fluorescein.

Management

Explanation of diagnostic procedures and sensory experience to be anticipated will usually facilitate patient cooperation. Following local anesthetic administration, care should be exercised to avoid damage to the cornea by advising the patient not to rub the eye and covering it with an eye patch until the corneal ("blink") reflex returns. Those patients who have received topical mydriatics should be informed that some pupillary dilation and photosensitivity may persist for a short time. Sunglasses will help minimize discomfort and the patient may want to arrange alternate transportation to avoid the need to drive.

The most common reaction to intravenous fluorescein is nausea and vomiting approximately 15 s after injection. The patient should also be informed that the skin will take on a yellowish discoloration for 6 to 12 h and the urine will be bright yellow for 12 to 36 h.

Evaluation

Many diagnostic agents cause irritation of the ocular structures. The patient should be informed that any irritation, discomfort, or discoloration of the eye is usually transient, but that the physician should be notified if these symptoms persist for more than 24 h.

GLAUCOMA

Glaucoma is an ophthalmic disorder characterized by an increase in intraocular pressure above normal levels which may result in progressive irreversible loss of vision if untreated. Since this condition is often asymptomatic, elevation of intraocular pressure is usually the first manifestation of the disease.

Etiology and Classification

The intraocular pressure is a reflection of the rate of production and the rate of outflow of aqueous humor. Aqueous humor is produced by the ciliary body and bathes the ante-

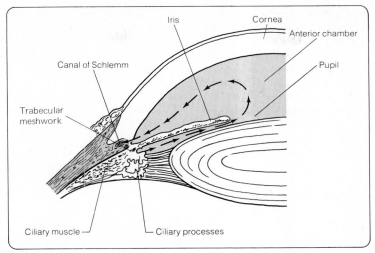

FIGURE 39-2

Normal Flow of Aqueous Humor.

rior chamber of the eye and its associated structures. After its synthesis, the aqueous humor is secreted by the ciliary processes and floats forward between the lens and the iris into the anterior chamber. It drains into the venous system of the eye via the trabecular meshwork and the canal of Schlemm which are located near the junction of the cornea and sclera (Fig. 39-2). Since overproduction by the epithelium of the ciliary processes is a rare occurrence, glaucoma is usually attributed to an interference in the outflow of aqueous humor from the anterior chamber of the eye.

Glaucoma is classified as primary, secondary, or congenital. *Primary glaucoma* includes acute or angle-closure glaucoma and chronic or open-angle glaucoma (Fig. 39-3). Chronic glaucoma is more common than acute glaucoma. There is an established genetic component in the manifestation of glaucoma.

In *primary angle-closure glaucoma* (narrow-angle glaucoma) the root of the iris is displaced anteriorly, which results in a narrowed filtration angle and shallow anterior chamber. It is an acute or subacute process characterized by

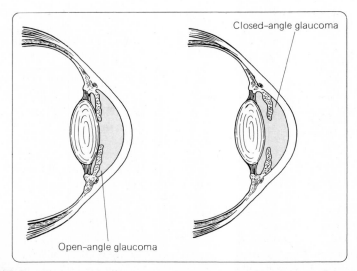

FIGURE 39-3

Comparison of Open-Angle and Angle-Closure Glaucoma.

severe ocular and facial pain, ocular inflammation, nausea, and vomiting. The patient may notice a decrease in visual acuity and the presence of halos or rainbows. Such an attack may be precipitated by pupil dilation associated with pharmacologic mydriasis, a darkened room, or emotional stress. Treatment of the acute attack includes administration of topical miotics (cholinergic agents) and systemic medications such as carbonic anhydrase inhibitors and osmotic diuretics. Surgery is usually performed after the attack has subsided to prevent the occurrence of subsequent episodes. A peripheral iridectomy, in which a portion of the iris is removed, results in an increase in aqueous humor outflow and reduction of intraocular pressure.

Primary open-angle glaucoma (wide-angle glaucoma) is a chronic progressive process characterized by cupping of the optic disc which may be associated with atrophy and visual field loss. Drug therapy may include administration of cholinergic drugs, β-adrenergic blocking agents, an oral carbonic anhydrase inhibitor, or topical sympathomimetics. Surgical intervention may be necessary if medical management does not result in adequate pressure control. The majority of these surgical procedures attempt to promote the drainage of aqueous humor from the anterior chamber by creating an opening between this chamber and the subconjunctival space. Once the fluid is drained into the subconjunctival space, it is transported by episcleral or conjunctival veins or escapes through the conjunctiva. Although these procedures usually result in adequate control of the intraocular pressure, drug therapy may still be necessary.

Secondary glaucoma may occur with an increase in size of the lens or ciliary body, with adhesions between the lens and iris after the administration of topical or systemic corticosteroids, after cataract extraction, or following trauma. The nature of the causative factor determines the type of drug therapy and/or surgical treatment employed.

Congenital glaucoma usually results from a structural anomaly of the anterior chamber in which the trabecular meshwork is covered by a membrane or attached to the iris. This type of glaucoma is characterized by photophobia, tearing, and blepharospasm (spasmotic contraction of the orbicularis oculi muscle). It is a rare disease. The treatment usually involves surgical incision of the tissue lying in front of the trabecular meshwork, possibly followed by drug therapy.

Clinical Findings

Since glaucoma usually presents as an asymptomatic disease, it is commonly diagnosed during routine examination. Tonometry (measurement of intraocular pressure), ophthalmoscopic evaluation of the optic nerve, visual field examination, and gonioscopy (examination of the filtration angle) are the techniques used in determining the presence of this disease. If primary open-angle glaucoma is allowed to progress without treatment, the patient may notice a reduction in periph-

eral vision. Tonometry usually reveals an intraocular pressure which is elevated above 21 mmHg in persons with glaucoma.

Clinical Pharmacology and Therapeutics

Direct-Acting Cholinergics

Cholinergic or miotic agents are used in the treatment of glaucoma and can be classified as direct- or indirect-acting agents. In the treatment of glaucoma the shortest acting agent in the lowest concentration that is effective should be used to lower the intraocular pressure. In general, the direct-acting agents have shorter durations of action than the indirect-acting agents. If intraocular pressure cannot be reduced with the shorter acting preparations, then the concentration can be increased or a longer acting agent substituted. If once per day dosing can be employed, administration of the drug at bedtime will reduce the discomforts of miosis. With all of the cholinergic agents systemic absorption of the drugs should be avoided or minimized by proper administration techniques. If toxicity develops, **atropine sulfate** may be used to reverse the adverse effects of the cholinergic agents.

The *direct-acting cholinergic* agents function like acetylcholine at the junction of parasympathetic nerve endings of muscle cells to cause contraction of the ciliary and sphincter muscles of the iris. The resulting miosis due to the contraction of the pupil and ciliary body facilitates the drainage of aqueous humor by opening the angle in the anterior chamber in angle-closure glaucoma and decreasing the resistance to outflow through the trabecular meshwork, subsequently reducing the intraocular pressure. The most common direct-acting cholinergics presently in use include **pilocarpine** and **carbachol** (Table 39-4).

Pilocarpine **Pilocarpine hydrochloride** (Adsorbocarpine, Almocarpine, Akarpine, Isopto Carpine, Pilocar, Pilocel, others) and **pilocarpine nitrate** (P.V. Carpine Liquifilm) may be used to reverse the mydriasis caused by cycloplegic mydriatic agents or during an acute attack of narrow-angle glaucoma, but their primary use is in the maintenance control of intraocular pressure in glaucoma. Pilocarpine should not be used in cases with acute iritis or active inflammatory disease of the anterior segment. The appropriate concentrations should be individually titrated for each patient, but the drops are usually instilled two or four times daily. **Epinephrine, β-adrenergic blocking agents**, or a **carbonic anhydrase inhibitor** may be administered concurrently with pilocarpine.

Browache, eyeache, and dull headaches are common adverse effects of pilocarpine. Blurring of vision due to miosis and accommodative spasm, poor dark adaptation due to failure of pupillary dilation in decreased illumination, and conjunctival injection and irritation are occasionally noted. Abdominal cramps, bronchiolar spasms, pulmonary edema, and lens opacities with prolonged use have been reported. Other systemic symptoms are rare but include salivation, lacrimation, sweating, nausea, vomiting, and diarrhea in pilocarpine toxicity.

The **pilocarpine ocular therapeutic system** (Ocusert Pilo-20, Ocusert Pilo-40) is a drug-delivery system consisting of a clear waferlike disc which permits continuous release of pilocarpine for one week. The Ocusert Pilo-20 releases pilocarpine at a rate of 20 μg/h for one week; the Ocusert Pilo-40 at a rate of 40 μg/h for one week. Patients should be instructed on the insertion, removal, and manipulation of the Ocusert system and be cautioned that the insertion of the system into the cul-de-sac of the eye is often accompanied by ciliary spasm, severe miosis, and/or systemic signs of toxicity due to the fact that the initial burst of the drug is approximately three times the normal per-hour rate. To minimize the dimness and blurring of vision which accompanies the initial insertion of the system, the Ocusert should be placed in the eye at bedtime. If well tolerated by the patient, the advantages of the system include greater convenience and better patient compliance. Constant therapeutic levels of the drug are attained even though a lower quantity of the preparation is administered overall, thereby decreasing undesirable side effects. The patient should be instructed to check for the presence of the system upon arising in the morning and retiring at night.

It is suggested that therapy be initiated with the Ocusert Pilo-20 system regardless of the concentration of pilocarpine previously used to maintain satisfactory control of the intraocular pressure. Conjunctivitis or keratitis may be aggravated by the presence of the system in the eye. Blurred vision, foreign body sensation, tearing, stinging, itching, bulbar and palpebral conjunctival injection, headache, and increased mucous discharge have been reported.

Carbachol Carbachol (Isopto Carbachol, Carbacel; Miostat Intraocular) has a double action in that it is known to stimulate the motor end plate of the muscle cell and inhibit the action of cholinesterase. Carbachol is used in treatment of chronic open-angle glaucoma and to produce pupillary miosis during ocular surgery. It is also indicated as a replacement drug in eyes which have become allergic or resistant to pilocarpine. Since the duration of action is longer than pilocarpine, carbachol is usually administered every 8 h.

Carbachol should be administered with caution to patients with acute heart failure, peptic ulcer, hyperthyroidism, bronchial asthma, gastrointestinal spasm, Parkinson's disease, and urinary tract obstruction. Conjunctival injection

TABLE 39-4 Cholinergic (Miotic) Agents Used in Glaucoma

AGENT	USUAL CONCENTRATIONS	USUAL DOSAGE	Activity	
			ONSET	DURATION*
Direct-Acting				
Pilocarpine (Isopto Carpine, Pilocar, others)	0.5, 1.0, 2.0, 3.0, 4.0%	1 drop q4–6h	30 min	4–6 h
Ocusert-Pilo	20 μg/h, 40 μg/h	1 Ocusert/week	10–15 min	
Carbachol (Carbacel, Isopto Carbachol)	0.75, 1.50, 2.25, 3.0%	1 drop q8–12h	10–20 min	4–8 h
Indirect-Acting				
Physostigmine (eserine sulfate, Isopto Eserine)	0.25, 0.50% solution 0.25% ointment	1 drop q4–8 h (solution); ¼ in of ointment applied at night	10–20 min	24–48 h
Demecarium bromide (Humorsol)	0.125, 0.25%	1 drop twice weekly to twice daily	20–30 min	12 h to 4 days
Isoflurophate (Floropryl)	0.025, 0.05, 0.1%	1 drop q8–12 h	15–30 min	1–2 weeks
Echothiophate iodide (Phospholine iodide)	0.03, 0.06, 0.125, 0.25%	1 drop twice daily	15–30 min	1–2 weeks

*Duration of miosis.

and eye and brow pain are common adverse effects. Accommodative spasm, headache, and blurred vision are frequently noted with initial therapy, although blurred vision usually subsides with prolonged use. Abdominal cramps, diarrhea, sweating, and flushing are rarely reported.

Indirect-Acting Cholinergics (Acetylcholinesterase Inhibitors)

The indirect-acting cholinergic (parasympathomimetic) drugs, or anticholinesterase agents, increase the amount of acetylcholine available at the synapse by inactivating cholinesterase, the enzyme that destroys acetylcholine. This leaves acetylcholine free to act on the effector cells of the sphincter and ciliary muscles, causing pupillary constriction and accommodative spasm. This indirect action yields the same therapeutic effect as that achieved by other cholinergic agents. Because of their side effects, these drugs are usually reserved for patients with primary open-angle glaucoma in which other preparations are not effective.

Administration of anticholinesterase agents is accompanied by a reduction in blood cholinesterases which are required for inactiviation of **succinylcholine.** If surgery under general anesthesia with succinylcholine is planned, the anesthesiologist should be informed of the patient's use of anticholinesterases and the drug may be discontinued 4 to 6 weeks prior to surgery to prevent severe respiratory distress due to prolonged depolarization at the motor end plate. If emergency surgery is needed, a muscle relaxant other than succinylcholine should be used.

Common anticholinesterase agents used in the treatment of glaucoma include **physostigmine, demecarium bromide, insoflurophate,** and **echothiophate iodide** (see Table 39-4).

Physostigmine   Physostigmine, or **eserine sulfate,** is a short-acting cholinesterase inhibitor which inactivates cholinesterase by forming a temporary chemical combination. Physostigmine solution and ointment cause intense miosis within 10 to 30 min. The duration of miosis ranges from 24 h to 2 days, although the reduction in intraocular pressure only lasts 4 h. Because of this long activity, physostigmine ointment applied at bedtime will allow for continuous aqueous outflow throughout the night. The normal dose ranges from 2 to 3 drops tid for the solution; a small quantity of the ointment is applied at bedtime.

The most common side effects reported with physostigmine are twitching of the eyelids (due to the percutaneous absorption of the drug), chronic conjunctival irritation, contact allergic dermatitis, and changes in the pigmented epithelium of the iris. It should be noted that physostigmine solution will oxidize on exposure to light and air. If the solution turns pink or brown it should be discarded.

Demecarium   Demecarium bromide (Humorsol) is a long-acting cholinesterase inhibitor. Its application in the eye results in intense miosis, ciliary muscle contraction, and decrease in intraocular pressure. Following the instillation of 1 to 2 drops of demecarium bromide, a decrease in intraocular pressure will occur within 1 h. The duration of action is from 12 h to several days. The preferred dosage for most cases of open-angle glaucoma is 1 drop of a 0.125% solution bid. This will maintain smooth diurnal control of the intraocular pressure.

Echothiophate iodide   Echothiophate iodide (Phospholine iodide) is a longer-acting cholinesterase inhibitor with prolonged effects (up to 96 h for reduction of intraocular pressure) similar to **demecarium bromide.** A dosage schedule of two doses a day should never be exceeded because of the prolonged activity of this drug.

Echothiophate is marketed as a dry powder which is indefinitely stable when dry. After reconstitution with the accompanying diluent, however, the unused portion should be discarded after 2 months. Under no circumstances should the powder be applied directly to the patient's eye; transconjunctival absorption is rapid, and serious systemic poisoning will result.

Isoflurophate   Isoflurophate (Floropryl) is a long-acting cholinesterase inhibitor. It has a duration of action ranging from days to weeks. Whenever possible, isoflurophate ointment, like echothiophate solution, should be applied at night for greater convenience to the patient and to minimize side effects. For initial therapy in glaucoma, a ¼-in strip of ointment is placed in the eye every 8 to 72 h. Systemic toxicity associated with excessive absorption of isoflurophate may result in nausea, vomiting, abdominal cramps, diarrhea, urinary incontinence, salivation, profuse sweating, respiratory difficulties, or cardiac irregularities.

Adrenergic (Sympathomimetic) Agents

Although the complete mechanism of action is not quite understood, it is believed that sympathomimetic agents stimulate adrenergic receptors in the ciliary body of the eye to increase the facility of outflow of aqueous fluid. In addition, production of aqueous humor is reduced with the overall therapeutic effect of lowering the intraocular pressure. Adrenergic agents also cause dilation of the pupil and a reduction in blood flow by constricting conjunctival blood vessels. **Epinephrine, phenylephrine,** and **dipivefrin** (a prodrug) are the most common adrenergic agents (see Table 39-5). The precautions, drug interactions, and systemic effects of these drugs are discussed in Chap. 13.

Adrenergic agents should not be used in the treatment of narrow-angle glaucoma, since the pupil dilation may precipitate acute angle closure. These agents can discolor soft contact lenses, and so the patient should not let the solution come in contact with the lens. If the solution becomes discolored or shows a precipitate, it should be discarded.

Epinephrine **Epinephrine bitartrate** (Epitrate), **epinephrine hydrochloride** (Epifrin, Glaucon), and **epinephrine borate** (Epinal, Eppy) stimulate α- and β-adrenergic receptors to decrease the aqueous inflow in open-angle glaucoma and promote aqueous outflow.

Eye pain or ache, browache, headache, allergic lid reactions, and conjunctival injection and swelling have been reported. With prolonged therapy, adrenochrome deposits may appear in the cornea and conjunctiva. Reversible macular edema has been noted in aphakic patients (those in whom the lens is absent). Systemic effects such as palpitations, tachycardia, hypertension, pallor, diaphoresis, trembling, and cardiac arrhythmia may occur.

Phenylephrine Phenylephrine hydrochloride (Efricel, Neo-Synephrine, AK-Dilate, others) is a sympathomimetic agent which is an α-receptor stimulator producing pupil dilation and vasoconstriction. The pupil dilating effect as used in diagnostic procedures was previously discussed. It is also used in the management of open-angle glaucoma and uveitis.

Dipivefrin Dipivefrin hydrochloride (Propine) is a prodrug which is administered as an inactive form of **epinephrine** and subsequently converted to epinephrine inside the eye by enzyme hydrolysis. This modified form of epinephrine promotes absorption, stability, and comfort of the drug, results in a decrease in the number and severity of side effects, and reduces the concentration of the drug necessary to produce the desired therapeutic effect. Once it is converted to epinephrine, the drug exerts its adrenergic effect by decreasing aqueous fluid production and promoting aqueous outflow.

Erythema, burning, and stinging have been noted upon administration. Photophobia and glare are less frequently noted. Adrenochrome deposits in the conjunctiva and cor-nea have been noted with prolonged use. Systemic effects include hypertension, tachycardia, and arrhythmias. Mascular edema has been reported in aphakic patients.

β-Adrenergic Blocking Agents

The precise mechanism of action of the β-blocking agents in glaucoma has not been clearly established, but a reduction in aqueous formation and a slight increase in aqueous outflow has been attributed to blockage of β_1- and β_2-adrenergic receptors. One of the major advantages is that, unlike miotics, control of the intraocular pressure is obtained with little effect on pupil size or accommodation. Dimming or blurring of vision, night blindness, changes in visual acuity due to increased accommodation and inability to see around lenticular opacities with a constricted pupil are not reported as side effects. The patient wearing hard contact lenses constructed of polymethyl methacrylate is able to tolerate this therapy without difficulty. **Timolol maleate** is the β-adrenergic-blocking agent used in glaucoma therapy, but clinical trials with the investigational selective β_1 blocker **betha-kanol** indicate that this agent may have advantages for those who cannot tolerate the β_2 effects that accompany nonselective agents like **timolol** (see Chap. 14).

Timolol Timolol maleate (Timoptic) is used in cases of chronic open-angle glaucoma, aphakic glaucoma, and selected cases of secondary glaucoma. The normal dosage is 1 or 2 drops of a 0.25 or 0.50% solution once or twice a day. Visual disturbances and refractive changes have infrequently been reported. Blepharitis, dermatitis, conjunctivitis, and blepharoptosis have occasionally been noted. Important systemic adverse effects include hypotension, syncope, bronchospasm, bradyarrhythmia, congestive heart failure, respiratory failure, and masked symptoms of hypoglycemia in insulin-dependent diabetics. Timolol maleate is not for

TABLE 39-5 Sympathomimetic Agents Used in Glaucoma

DRUG	AVAILABLE CONCENTRATION, %	DOSAGE	COMMENTS
Epinephrine bitartrate (Epitrate)	0.50, 1.0, 2.0	1 drop qd or bid	Solution should be discarded if a precipitate develops or if it turns brown.
Epinephrine hydrochloride (Epifrin, Glaucon)	0.25, 0.50, 1.0, 2.0	1 drop qd or bid	
Epinephrine borate (Epinal, Eppyln)	0.25, 0.50, 1.0, 2.0	1 drop qd or bid	
Phenylephrine hydrochloride (AK-Dilate, Efricel, others)	2.5, 10.0	1 or 2 drops qd or bid	Decreased intraocular pressure when applied topically; although there are less side effects associated with the 2.5% solution, it is often necessary to administer the 10.0% solution to obtain the desired effect.
Dipivefrin hydrochloride (Propine)	0.1	1 drop q12h	Prodrug form of epinephrine with decreased side effects upon topical administration.

use in patients with uncontrolled cardiac failure or severe chronic obstructive pulmonary disease.

Carbonic Anhydrase Inhibitors

Carbonic anhydrase inhibitors are used in the treatment of chronic open-angle glaucoma, preoperative acute angle-closure glaucoma, and secondary glaucoma. Long-term use in chronic noncongestive angle-closure glaucoma is not recommended. The agents used in glaucoma are **acetazolamide** (Diamox), **dichlorphenamide** (Daranide), and **methazolamide** (Neptazane) (see Table 39-6). They may be used in conjunction with miotics, osmotic diuretics, and **epinephrine**. These agents have the ability to reduce aqueous production by approximately 60 percent and are useful when patients do not respond to miotics.

Mechanism of Action   Carbonic anhydrase inhibitors lower intraocular pressure by noncompetitively inhibiting carbonic anhydrase, an enzyme that plays a role in the formation of aqueous humor. This enzyme is also found in the kidney tubule, and so the inhibitor also causes mild diuresis.

Pharmacokinetics   Acetazolamide is well absorbed after oral administration and is excreted unchanged by the kidney by a process involving both tubular secretion and passive reabsorption. **Dichlorphenamide** and **methazolamide** are inactive as administered and must be biotransformed to active metabolites which are excreted by the kidney. These drugs are given several times daily depending on their rate of onset and duration of action (see Table 39-6).

Adverse Effects   Adverse reactions include loss of appetite, tingling of extremities, drowsiness, hypokalemia, and confusion with short-term therapy. Acidosis may develop with long-term use. Transient myopia, urticaria, melena, glycosuria, hematuria, convulsions, flaccid paralysis, and hepatic insufficiency have occasionally been reported. Adverse effects common to sulfonamides have been reported such as rash, fever, renal calculi, bone marrow depression, leukopenia, hemolytic anemia, crystalluria, pancytopenia, agranulocytosis, and thrombocytopenia purpura and are an indication to stop therapy. Because they alkalinize the urine, carbonic anhydrase inhibitors can prolong the half-life of **quinidine**. They will also enhance the potassium-depleting effects of **ACTH** or **corticosteroids**.

Hyperosmotic Agents

Intraocular pressure can be reduced by altering the serum osmolarity. Osmotic diuretics shift fluid from the anterior chamber of the eye to the plasma. Thus the effect on the eye is to render the ciliary processes unable to secrete aqueous humor against the increased ocular gradient. Among the hyperosmotic agents most often used in glaucoma are **mannitol**, **glycerin**, and **urea**. They are used when a temporary but rapid drop in intraocular pressure is required, such as in acute glaucoma and prior to certain ocular surgical procedures (e.g., cataract and glaucoma surgery, see Table 39-7). Intravenous osmotic agents undergo little metabolism and are excreted rapidly in the urine to produce an osmotic diuresis, which also increases the excretion of sodium and potassium.

Mannitol   Mannitol (Osmitrol) is an inert sugar alcohol found in many fruits and vegetables. It is used IV as a 20% solution in a dosage from 1 to 3 g/kg over 30 to 60 min. Since the drug may crystallize, an in-line filter should always be used during its administration. The cardiovascular status of the patient should be carefully evaluated before administer-

TABLE 39-6 Carbonic Anhydrase Inhibitors Used in Glaucoma

| GENERIC NAME | TRADE NAME | DOSAGE | Activity | | COMMENTS |
			ONSET	DURATION, h	
Acetazolamide	Diamox, Cetazol				
Tablets		250 mg qid	2 h	6–8	
Capsules		500 mg bid	2 h	22–30	
Injectable		500 mg IV	5–10 min	2	Reconsitute the 500-mg vial with 5 mL of sterile water for injection prior to use.
Dichlorphenamide	Daranide, Oratrol	25–50 mg qd to tid	30 min	6–12	Potassium excretion is increased with use of this drug, therefore serum potassium levels should be monitored. A priming dose of 100 to 200 mg is usually administered.
Methazolamide	Neptazane	50–100 mg bid to tid	2 h	10–20	Usually administered with a miotic agent.

TABLE 39-7   Hyperosmotic Agents Used in Glaucoma

AGENT	DOSAGE	COMMENTS
Mannitol (Osmitrol)	1.5–2.0 g/kg of a 20% solution given IV over 30–60 min.	Drug of choice for intravenous use; solution should be inspected for crystals and administered with the appropriate in-line filter.
Urea (Ureaphil, Ureavert)	1.0 g/kg. over 2½ h. Pediatric: 0.1–1.5 g/kg IV in 24 h.	Rarely used due to severe local necrosis which may occur if solution extravasates.
Glycerin (Glyrol, Osmoglyn)	1.0 to 1.5 g/kg of 50% solution over ice orally.	Used in patients with renal insufficiency; major disadvantages are hyperglycemic effects in patients with diabetes mellitus and the gastrointestinal side effects.

ing mannitol. Rapid infusion may lead to congestive heart failure.

Adverse effects related to mannitol use include nausea, vomiting, headaches, electrolyte imbalance, circulatory overload, pulmonary edema, intraocular hemorrhage, and water intoxication. Pain and irritation occur with extravasation at the injection site. Urinary catheterization may be necessary if the patient is elderly, comatose, has difficulty voiding, or is preoperative.

Glycerin   Glycerin (Glyrol, Osmoglyn) is another sugar alcohol which produces a marked reduction in intraocular pressure. It is given orally in a dose of 1 to 2 g/kg (preferably in juice) and may not be tolerated by the nauseated patient having an acute closed-angle attack. Because of its rapid metabolism, it has less diuretic effect than mannitol. Glycerin should be administered cautiously to diabetic patients.

Urea   Urea (Ureaphil, Urevert), a protein catabolism end product, is given intravenously in a dosage of 1 g/kg, using a 30% solution, at a rate not exceeding 4 mL/min. As with mannitol, electrolyte depletion can result in hyponatremia and hypokalemia. Urea should not be administered to patients who have impaired renal, hepatic, or cardiac function, active intracranial bleeding, severe dehydration, or congestive heart failure. Nausea, vomiting, headache, electrolyte imbalance, water intoxication, pulmonary edema, circulatory overload, intraocular hemorrhage, hypotension, dehydration, syncope, confusion, acute psychosis, nervousness, and hyperthermia have been reported. Thrombophlebitis may occur at the injection site. Extravasation should be avoided as it can result in tissue necrosis. Urea should not be administered intravenously in the lower extremities of

the elderly due to the fibrinolytic effect of this agent. Urinary catheterization may be necessary in patients who have difficulty voiding or who are elderly, comatose, or preoperative.

NURSING PROCESS RELATED TO GLAUCOMA

Assessment

Primary open-angle glaucoma is usually an asymptomatic process. Gradual reduction in peripheral vision occurs late in the disease. The nurse should stress the importance of routine measurement of the intraocular pressure in all persons, especially those over the age of 35 years.

The nurse should be aware that attacks of acute glaucoma are characterized by severe ocular pain, redness of the eye, blurred vision, and perception of colored haloes around lights. The pain is often not localized to the eye but involves the entire head and may be accompanied by nausea and vomiting. Those with these symptoms should be advised to seek immediate medical attention.

It is frequently stated that drugs which dilate the pupil are contraindicated in glaucoma. This would include the sympathomimetics (Chap. 13), the parasympathetic blockers (Chap. 12), and drugs with anticholinergic adverse effects (Table 12-5). However, these agents are contraindicated only in *primary* angle-closure glaucoma, in which they may precipitate an acute attack. They are used with caution in the elderly, a population at risk for angle-closure glaucoma. However, in open-angle glaucoma or following peripheral iridectomy for angle-closure glaucoma, drugs with mydriatic effects can be used safely.

Management

Patients should be advised to wear a Med-Alert bracelet or carry some identification indicating that they have glaucoma. Encouraging good elimination patterns is important, since straining during a bowel movement can increase intraocular pressure. Keeping the home well lighted may complement the therapeutic effects of miotics. During the first 2 h after patients use miotics, they may experience blurring of vision and driving may be dangerous. Other important aspects of patient education and drug administration will be found under "Patient Education" and "Administration of Ophthalmic Drugs" in this chapter.

In acute angle-closure attacks, the objectives are not only to rapidly reduce the eye pressure, but also to treat the nausea, vomiting, and pain that may accompany the increased intraocular pressure. The patient is usually placed in a well-lighted room to encourage miosis. Simple analgesics may be administered, and the patient should receive emotional support and explanations of procedures, since anxiety may further elevate ocular pressure.

Evaluation

Once treatment of glaucoma has been initiated, patients should be monitored by tonometry for changes in intraocular pressure. Compliance with the plan of treatment should be emphasized as the only way to avoid progressive visual impairment. Prognosis is good if the eye pressure remains controlled, but progressive visual field constriction and eventual blindness can be anticipated if the pressure is not maintained near normal levels.

The nurse should note whether the miosis induced by the drugs is sustained or abates before the next dose; the latter may be an indication for dosage change. Redness of the conjunctiva and decreased or increased lacrimation are also noted to evaluate the adverse effects of the drugs. Long-term therapy with miotics can cause cataracts, and so observation of the lens for opacities is indicated.

Monitoring blood pressure, pulse rate, urine output, and signs of electrolyte imbalance are important during the use of mannitol because of the rapid, copious diuresis.

During therapy with carbonic anhydrase inhibitors, it is important to note signs of acidosis, electrolyte imbalance, or drowsiness. Caution in operating machinery or a vehicle is required if drowsiness occurs. The drug may be taken with meals if GI distress occurs. Patients on chronic therapy should be evaluated for signs of blood dyscrasias (sore throat, easy bruising) and periodic complete blood counts should be performed.

The nursing process related to the β-adrenergic blocking drugs is presented in Chap. 14. The nursing process related to sympathomimetics is summarized in the diagnostics section of this chapter and is detailed in Chap. 13.

CASE STUDY

Mrs. H.F., a 62-year-old white widow accompanied by her daughter, was admitted to the ophthalmology unit via the emergency room with a diagnosis of acute angle-closure glaucoma of the left eye. Tonometry showed intraocular pressures of 55 mmHg (left) and 20 mmHg (right). H.F. also had a history of heart disease and was taking digoxin 0.25 mg daily and furosemide 40 mg daily. She was under the care of a cardiologist, and her condition was considered stable.

The medical orders included the following: IV (keep open) with 5% dextrose/0.25% normal saline; bed rest; low-sodium diet; routine admission blood chemistry and urinalysis; ECG: pilocarpine 4%, 1 drop os q5min for three doses, 1 drop qh for three doses, and then 1 drop q6h; mannitol 20%, 500/mL IV to run over 30 min; digoxin 0.25 mg PO daily; furosemide 20 mg IV now and 40 mg PO daily; potassium chloride 20 meq PO daily in orange juice.

Assessment

Mrs. H.F. was holding the left side of her face and described the pain in her left eye as "stabbing." The left eye was reddened, with a dilated pupil and excessive lacrimation. Vital signs were: blood pressure 180/100, pulse 100, temperature 98.8°F, respiration 22. Mrs. H.F. complained of nausea and vomited twice. She seemed tense and fidgety. The nurse checked the results of the electrolyte studies which were normal before administering the mannitol, furosemide, and digoxin. Oral drugs were withheld until she was no longer nauseous.

The nurse arrived at the following diagnoses: (1) pain, nausea, and vomiting, secondary to increased intraocular pressure; (2) elevated blood pressure due to pain and anxiety or to cardiac problem; (3) anxiety.

Management

The nurse defined the following goals: (1) to decrease intraocular pressure; (2) to provide maximal comfort by decreasing pain, nausea, and vomiting; (3) to ascertain the cause of the abnormal blood pressure and prevent further complications from drug therapy.

To accomplish the first two goals the patient was placed in a quiet, well-lighted room. The pilocarpine and mannitol were administered. Ongoing observation of the eye tension, pupil size, lacrimation, and redness was maintained.

Careful monitoring of cardiac status was a priority. During the mannitol administration the nurse took the blood pressure and pulse every 5 to 10 min to observe for circulatory overload and maintained accurate intake and output records. The lungs were auscultated for the appearance of rales and the heart for the abnormal S_3 that is associated with heart failure. The nurse also asked the patient to inform the nursing staff if she felt short of breath or had chest pain.

The staff informed the patient of the purpose of each procedure, maintaining a calm and confident atmosphere. The patient was encouraged to verbalize her fears, and the daughter was allowed to stay with her mother. Both were interested in the prognosis of glaucoma and were told that the disease need not and should not result in blindness if correctly treated.

During the discussions with the daughter and the patient, the nurse was also able to gather information about the patient's occupation, living arrangements, and lifestyle for discharge planning.

Evaluation

The pain, lacrimation, and redness of the left eye decreased within 1 h of the initiation of mannitol. Immediate miosis was noted at the first instillation of pilocarpine. The nurses continued to observe for return of the symptoms.

During the administration of mannitol and the following hour, the blood pressure decreased to 138/86 and no signs of circulatory overload were noted. The lungs remained clear and there was no S_3, shortness of breath, or chest pain. The patient urinated 750 mL in 3 h. Tonometry revealed a pressure of 21 mmHg in both eyes.

EXTERNAL OCULAR INFLAMMATION

Inflammation of the ocular structures can be the result of invasion by an infectious organism, secondary to an allergic response, or numerous other conditions. It can be manifested by redness, swelling, and exudate associated with one or more eye structures.

Blepharitis is an inflammation of the eyelid margins which may be acute or chronic. It is usually a result of seborrheic dermatitis and staphylococcal infection. *Conjunctivitis* is an inflammation of the palpebral and/or bulbar conjunctiva of the eye most commonly the result of a bacterial, viral, fungal, allergic, chemical, mechanical, or parasitic agent. *Keratitis* is an inflammation of the cornea most commonly due to invasion by a bacterial, fungal, viral, mechanical, chemical, or radiational agent. Keratitis may also be the result of corneal exposure due to inadequate lid closure or to inadequacy of the tear film. *Hordeolum* is a facial acute infection within the meibomian glands and other glands at the margin of the eyelid, commonly caused by staphylococcus. *Chalazion* is a focal chronic inflammation of a meibomian gland and may occur as the chronic result of a resolved hordeolum.

Etiology

External ocular inflammation may be caused by bacterial, fungal, or viral organisms, chemical or mechanical irritants, allergic responses, or systemic disease. Acute conjunctivitis is most commonly caused by bacterial or fungal organisms and usually involves both eyes. Among the causes of chronic conjunctivitis are viruses, chemical and physical irritants such as cosmetics and eyedrops, and excessive lacrimation. Systemic disease accounts for a small percentage of cases. An example of this is gonococcal urethritis, which may be complicated by bacteremia.

Ocular inflammation is usually a self-limited condition, resolving in 3 to 5 days with treatment and in 7 to 10 days if left untreated. Chronic conjunctivitis may be minimized by removal of the irritants, if possible.

Clinical Findings

Patients usually present with a fullness of the eyelids and a diffuse, gritty, foreign-body sensation. Vision is usually normal except for slight blurring. The patient may give a history of involvement with family or community members who have similar symptoms.

Involvement of both eyes usually indicates infectious disease, whereas unilateral involvement is more suggestive of chemical, mechanical, or lacrimal origin. The exudate may be purulent, mucopurulent, membranous, or catarrhal. An exudate which is sparse is indicative of an allergy or a viral infection. A copious exudate is usually the response to a bacterial infection. The intraocular pressure is normal and the cornea is clear.

Prior to treating an ocular infection other than a superficial conjunctivitis, cultures should be taken from the conjunctiva, cornea, or anterior chamber and sensitivity testing done. The more common infectious organisms are *Escherichia coli, Pseudomonas aeruginosa, Proteus, Chlamydia;* pneumococcus, streptococcus, staphylococcus, *Haemophilus aegyptius* (Koch-Weeks bacillus), *Haemophilus influenzae* (in children), *Neisseria gonorrheae* (in the newborn), *Herpes simplex* and other viruses, and fungi. Once the organism is isolated and sensitivity tests completed, the appropriate antimicrobial agent can be prescribed.

Clinical Pharmacology and Therapeutics

To obtain therapeutic results, effective concentration of the drug must be achieved and maintained in the intraocular fluid, which may require the administration of medication by one or more routes, including intramuscular, intravenous, or subconjunctival injection. Table 39-8 lists common drugs used topically to treat external ocular inflammation and infections. Since some of the drug will be absorbed, the adverse effects and pharmacokinetic considerations are the same as when the agent is administered systemically, although local reactions also occur. (See Chaps. 26 and 27 for the pharmacology and antimicrobial spectrum of the antibiotics, sulfonamides, and the antifungal and antiviral agents. Chapter 35 presents the systemic effects of corticosteroids.)

Local Adverse Reactions

Blurring of vision and stinging may occur transiently after the administration of topical ophthalmics used to treat

TABLE 39-8 Topical Drugs Used to Treat External Ocular Inflammation*

DRUG	TRADE NAMES	REMARKS
Antibiotics		
Chloramphenicol	Chlormycetin Ophthalmic, Chloroptic, Ophthochlor Ophthalmic	Topical antibiotics and sulfonamides are indicated only for superficial infection by susceptible strains of organisms. In serious infections, systemic therapy is indicated.
Tetracycline	Achromycin Ophthalmic	Prolonged or frequent use of topical antibiotics can stimulate hypersensitivity reactions, including hypoplasia of bone marrow with chloramphenicol.
Polymixin B	Aerosporin Sterile	
Gentamicin	Garamycin Ophthalmic, Genoptic	Dosage of solutions is 1–2 drops 2–4 times qd, or more often depending upon the severity of the infection. Dosage of ointment is a small ribbon q3h or more often, depending upon the severity of the infection. Dosages are adjusted based on patient response.
Tobramycin	Tobrex	
Erythromycin	Ilotycin Ophthalmic	
Bacitracin	Baciguent Ophthalmic	
Sulfonamides		
Sodium sulfacetamide	Bleph-10 Liquifilm, Ophthacet, Sulf 10, Isopto Cetamide, Cetamide	Dosage of solutions is 1–2 drops q1–2h initially. Ointment is applied 1–3 times qd and hs.
Sulfisoxazole	Gantrisin	
Antifungals		
Natamycin; 5% suspension	Natacyn	Used for susceptible organisms in fungal blepharitis, conjunctivitis, and keratitis. Dosage for keratitis is 1 drop q1–2h for 3–4 days, then 1 drop 6–8 times qd. Drug should be continued for 14–21 days. Conjunctivitis may require less frequent dosing. There is negligible systemic absorption.
Antivirals		
Idoxuridine (IDU); 1% solution; 0.5% ointment	Dendrid, Herplex Liquifilm, Stoxil	Mechanism of antiviral action is interference with DNA synthesis. Indicated for treatment of keratitis caused by *Herpes simplex* virus types 1 and 2. If there is no improvement in 7 days, another treatment should be tried. *Idoxuridine:* (Solution) 1 drop qh during day and q2h at night until improved, then 1 drop q2h during day and q4h at night. (Ointment) five doses qd. Continue 3–5 days after healing.
Vidarabine (Adenine arabinoside, ARA-A); 3% ointment	Vira-A	*Vidarabine:* ½-in ribbon q3h for five doses qd. After reepithelialization, continue treatment 7 days at reduced frequency.
Trifluridine; 1% solution	Viroptic	*Trifluridine:* 1 drop q2h while awake (up to 9 drops qd until reepithelialization), then 7 days at 1 drop q4h with a minimum of 5 drops daily.
Antibiotic Combinations		
Polymixin B/neomycin/bacitracin	Neosporin Ophthalmic, Neotal Ophthalmic, Mycitracin Ophthalmic	See discussion of combination antibiotic therapy, Chap. 27. Dosage: Same as single agent antibiotics
Polymixin B/oxytetracycline	Terramycin Ophthalmic	
Polymixin B/neomycin	Statrol	
Polymixin B/bacitracin	Polysporin	
Antibiotic–Corticosteroid Combinations		
Hydrocortisone/neomycin	Neo-Cortef Suspension, Cor-Oticin Suspension	Dosage: 1–2 drops 3–4 times qd or more often depending on severity of infection.

TABLE 39-8   Topical Drugs Used to Treat External Ocular Inflammation* (*Cont.*)

DRUG	TRADE NAMES	REMARKS
Antibiotic-Corticosteroid Combinations (Cont.)		
Hydrocortisone/ neomycin/ polymixin B	Cortisporin Suspension	
Hydrocortisone/chlor- amphenicol	Chloromycetin Hydrocortisone	
Prednisolone/neomycin	Neo-Delta-Cortef Oint- ment, Neo-Hydeltrasol	
Sulfonamide-Corticosteroid Combinations		
Prednisolone/sulfacet- amide	Metimyd Suspension, Metimyd Ointment, Sulphrin Suspension, Blephamide S.O.P. Ointment, Isopto Cetrapred Suspension	Dosage: 1–2 drops qh during day and q2h during night, increasing interval as improvement occurs.

*Selected list of available agents.

external ocular inflammation. In addition, these agents can cause local inflammation and irritation. Allergic reactions consisting of itching, injection, and swelling of the lid and conjunctiva may occur, especially with sulfonamide-containing preparations. If the reaction does not resolve with discontinuation of the drug, ophthalmic corticosteroids or systemic antihistamines may be required.

Healing of the cornea may be delayed by topical ointments. Both antimicrobials and corticosteroids can result in bacterial or fungal overgrowth leading to a secondary infection. With antimicrobials this is a result of superinfection with nonsusceptible organisms, while corticosteroids suppress protective anti-inflammatory response.

Topical corticosteroids can cause a number of other severe ocular adverse effects, including glaucoma, cataract formation, secondary infection with *Herpes simplex* virus, and perforation of the globe.

Other local adverse effects including photophobia, clouding of the cornea, and punctate defects have been reported with **vidarabine** and **idoxuridine.** Sunglasses may ease the discomfort of photophobia.

Use of Corticosteroids and Antimicrobial–Corticosteroid Combinations

Indications for these agents include treatment of inflammation of the exterior ocular structures in allergic conjunctivitis, vernal conjunctivitis, superficial punctate keratitis, iritis, cyclitis, herpes zoster keratitis, and corneal injury. Topical corticosteroids are prescribed, usually in conjunction with an antibiotic or sulfonamide, in superficial ocular infections to decrease edema and inflammation. Such combination

therapy should be used only if benefits from improved comfort outweigh the serious dangers of secondary infection and ocular damage. Some combination corticosteroid-antibiotic agents are shown in Table 39-8.

Ophthalmia Neonatorum

Ophthalmia neonatorum is acute conjunctivitis in the newborn which can be caused by a number of organisms, such as *Chlamydia trachomatis, Staphylococcus aureus, Haemophilus influenza, Herpes simplex virus,* and *Neisseria gonorrhea.* The Crede method of prophylaxis at birth has nearly eliminated gonorrheal ophthalmia. It consists of the instillation of a 1% **silver nitrate** solution into the eyes of the newborn by the procedure outlined in Table 39-9. *A mild chemical conjunctivitis will result from the proper administration of the solution.* The parents should be told that this will resolve in a week or less and requires no care beyond the usual external cleansing procedures that accompany the infant's bath.

Due to changing patterns of infection in neonatal conjunctivitis, the emergence of β-lactamase-producing gonococcal strains, and the chemical conjunctivitis obligate with **silver nitrate** therapy, other methods of prophylactic eye care of the newborn are under investigation. Topical **erythromycin** is effective against *Neisseria gonorrheae* and *Chlamydia trachomatis,* currently the most common cause of neonatal conjunctivitis, and causes a low incidence of chemical conjunctivitis. Topical **tetracycline** and intramuscular **penicillin** have also been employed in the prophylaxis of neonatal conjunctivitis.

NURSING PROCESS RELATED TO EXTERNAL OCULAR INFLAMMATION

Assessment

Conjunctivitis is the most common cause of erythema of the eye structures but not the only cause. While the conjunctivitis will usually resolve even if untreated, conditions involving other structures, such as iritis and glaucoma, require rapid treatment. It is therefore necessary to encourage patients with "pink eye" to seek medical care. The nurse should note the distribution of the redness and swelling and the type and amount of exudate. The state of dilation or constriction of the pupil is also important.

Management

Bacterial conjunctivitis is highly contagious, and good hand-washing technique is necessary to prevent transmission of the organisms. Patients should have their own towels and should be instructed not to use those used by other family members.

Gonorrheal conjunctivitis, which is not self limiting, requires treatment, and the unaffected eye is often covered to prevent contamination. The patient with any type of conjunctivitis may be more comfortable in a darkened room.

Patient education and drug administration techniques, which are important aspects of the management of conjunctivitis, were discussed above.

Evaluation

The evaluation is based on a decrease in redness, swelling, and exudate. If only one eye is initially involved, the unaffected eye is also observed for contamination.

TABLE 39-9   Procedure for Newborn Prophylactic Eye Care

1. Using a separate absorbent cotton or gauze pledget for wiping each eye, clean the newborn's eyelids of all mucus, blood, and meconium. Cleanse the unopened lids from the inner to the outer canthus.

2. Separate the lids and instill 2 drops of a 1% silver nitrate solution into the eye. Then hold the eyelid elevated away from the eyeball so that a pool of the drug lies in contact with all parts of the conjunctival sac for at least 30 s. This should be done immediately after birth. Handle the silver nitrate carefully as it will stain skin and equipment.

3. It is not necessary that the eyes be irrigated with normal saline after instillation of the silver nitrate as this tends to dilute the drug and compromise its effectiveness.

CASE STUDY

Mrs. S.A., a 35-year-old white female, presented to the ophthalmology clinic with a two-day history of marked "redness of the eyeball" of both eyes accompanied by severe itching, copious mucopurulent discharge, and upper lid swelling. No pain, photophobia, or decrease in visual acuity was reported. She stated that one of the children she took care of had "pink eye" the previous week. She denied any history of drug allergy.

Assessment

Upon the initial examination redness of the bulbar and palpebral conjunctiva, a moderate amount of mucopurulent discharge, and upper lid swelling of both eyes were noted. There were no palpable preauricular lymph nodes. Conjunctival scrapings were obtained and sent to the laboratory for organism identification and susceptibility.

An empiric diagnosis of bacterial conjunctivitis was made and the patient was instructed to administer sulfacetamide 10% ophthalmic solution, 1 drop in each eye q2h during the day. While the recommended dosage at night is q2h, Mrs. S.A. felt she would be unable to fulfill her responsibilities as a day care mother if she did not sleep well for at least six uninterrupted hours.

Management

The nurse demonstrated the proper method of self-administration of eye drops and emphasized the need for careful hand washing to avoid spread of the infection to her family or among the day care children. It was explained that she might experience transient stinging and blurred vision immediately after instilling the solution and that she should call the clinic if these sensations persisted, irritation developed, or the symptoms did not improve within three days. Once the condition improved, the patient was told to increase the dosage interval.

Evaluation

The culture results confirmed the empiric diagnosis. On the second day after her clinic visit, Mrs. S.A. contacted the nurse by telephone. She indicated that the condition had improved and that only a little redness and itching remained. Since the frequent dosing was time-consuming, she asked for an ointment form of the drug. The nurse explained that ointments often interfere with vision, but the patient felt that this was preferable to frequent dosing, so sulfacetamide 10% ointment was ordered. Mrs. S.A.

was instructed in the proper administration of ointments and told to apply the ointment twice daily and at bedtime. The nurse also stressed the importance of disposing of left over drugs after the course of treatment was completed.

REFERENCES

Alward P. D., and J. T. Wilensky: "Determination of Acetazolamide Compliance in Patients with Glaucoma," *Arch Ophthalmol,* 99:1973–1976, 1981.

Avery G. S. (ed.): *Drug Treatment: Principles and Practice of Clinical Pharmacology and Therapeutics,* 2d ed., New York: ADIS, 1980.

Bernstein, G. A., J. P. Davis, and M. L. Katcher: "Prophylaxis of Neonatal Conjunctivitis: An Analytic Review," *Clin Pediatr,* 21:545–554, 1982.

Berson F. G., et al.: "Acetazolamide Dosage Forms in the Treatment of Glaucoma," *Arch Ophthalmol,* 98:1051–1054, 1980.

Carmine A. A., et al.: "Trifluridine: A Review of Its Antiviral Activity and Therapeutic Use in the Topical Treatment of Viral Eye Infections," *Drugs,* 23:329–353, 1982.

Crom, D. B.: "Dexamethasone Sodium Phosphate Ophthalmic Solution (Decadron): A Review of Its Use, and Guidelines for Administration," *Ophthalmol Technol,* 1:48–49, 1982.

———: "Topical Ophthalmic Anesthetics," *Ophthalmol Nurs Technol,* 1:57–59, 1982.

———, and W. R. Crom: "Atropine Sulfate and Homatropine Bromide: Common Mydriatic/Cycloplegic Agents," *Ophthalmol Nurs Technol,* 1:38–40, 1982.

Friedlaender, M. H.: "Corticosteroid Therapy of Ocular Inflammation," *Int Ophthalmol Clin,* 23:175–182, 1983.

Goodman, A., L. S. Goodman, and A. Gilman (eds.): *Goodman and Gilman's The Pharmacological Basis of Therapeutics,* 6th ed., New York: Macmillan, 1980.

Grabie, M. T., et al.: "Contraindications for Mannitol in Aphakic Glaucoma," *Am J Ophthalmol,* 91:265–267, 1982.

Hass, I., and S. M. Drance: "Comparison between Pilocarpine and Timolol on Diurnal Pressures in Open-Angle Glaucoma," *Arch Ophthalmol,* 98:480–481, 1980.

Henkind, P., J. B. Walsh, and A. W. Berger: *Physicians' Desk Reference for Ophthalmology,* 11th ed., Oradell, N.J.: Medical Economics, 1982.

Jeffers, F. B.: "When to Use Topical Steroids in the Treatment of Eye Disease," *Ocup Health Nurs,* 29:31, 45, 1982.

Jeglum, E. L.: "Ocular Therapeutics," *Nurs Clin North Am,* 16:453–477, 1981.

Kass, M. A., et al.: "Patient Administration of Eyedrops: 1. Interview," *Ann Ophthalmol,* 14:775–779, 1982.

Kastrup, E. K. (ed.): *Facts and Comparisons,* Philadelphia: Lippincott, 1982.

Kersten, R. C.: "Ophthalmic Drugs," *Primary Care,* 9:743–756, 1982.

Korey, M. S., et al.: "Timolol and Epinephrine: Long-Term Evaluation of Concurrent Administration," *Arch Ophthalmol,* 100:742–745, 1982.

Leeds, N. H., and M. Gravdal: "Ocular Pharmacotherapy," in G. A. Peyman, et al. (eds.), *Principles and Practice of Ophthalmology,* Philadelphia: Saunders, 1980.

Mausolf, F.: *The Eye and Systemic Disease,* 2d ed., St. Louis: Mosby, 1980.

National Registry of Drug-Induced Ocular Effects, F. T. Fraunfelder, M. D., Director, Department of Ophthalmology, University of Oregon Health Sciences Center, 3181 S. W. Sam Jackson Park Road, Portland, OR 97201.

Norell, S. E.: "Monitoring Compliance with Pilocarpine Therapy," *Am J Ophthalmol,* 92:727–731, 1981.

Phillips, M.: "Ophthalmic Preparations," *Nurs Mirror,* 155:69–71, 1982.

Soll, D. B.: "Evaluation of Timolol in Chronic Open-Angle Glaucoma: Once a Day vs. Twice a Day," *Arch Ophthalmol,* 98:2178–2181, 1980.

Zimmerman, T. J., B. Leader, and H. E. Kaufman: "Advances in Ocular Pharmacology," *Annu Rev Pharmacol Toxicol,* 20:415–428, 1980.

40

HIGH BLOOD PRESSURE

DAVID S. ROFFMAN
SUE ANN THOMAS

LEARNING OBJECTIVES

Upon mastery of the content of this chapter, the reader will be able to:

1. Identify populations at risk for developing hypertension.
2. List at least five physiologic mechanisms responsible for the control of blood pressure.
3. Describe the relationship between cardiac output, total peripheral resistance, and arterial pressure.
4. State the relationship between the degree of blood pressure elevation and the development of hypertensive cardiovascular complications.
5. Define hypertension based on the criteria established by the American Heart Association.
6. Differentiate "essential" and "secondary" forms of hypertension.
7. List at least three factors which contribute to the pathogenesis of essential hypertension and three drugs which can cause hypertension.
8. State four complications of uncontrolled hypertension.
9. Describe the relationship between mild or moderate hypertension and symptoms of dizziness, headaches, and nosebleeds.
10. State at least three behavioral approaches to lowering blood pressure.
11. Describe the role of sodium, alcohol, and weight control on the regulation of blood pressure in hypertensive patients.
12. Describe the step care approach to drug therapy in the treatment of hypertension.
13. State two mechanisms of antihypertensive action for thiazide diuretics.
14. Differentiate among the antihypertensive mechanisms of various central and peripheral sympathoplegic agents.
15. List three potential mechanisms of antihypertensive action for β-adrenergic blocking agents.

16. Describe the syndrome associated with acute withdrawal of β-blocking agents.
17. State the mechanisms of action of hydralazine, minoxidil, and prazosin.
18. Describe the factors which determine the severity of hypertensive emergencies.
19. State the immediate endpoint of therapy in the treatment of hypertensive emergency.
20. List the side effects associated with nitroprusside and diazoxide therapy.
21. Give an indication for using a potent diuretic such as furosemide over a thiazide diuretic in the treatment of high blood pressure.
22. List three adverse effects for each of the following drugs: methyldopa and clonidine (central sympathoplegics) and reserpine and prazocin (peripheral sympathoplegics).
23. Describe the acute withdrawal syndrome associated with clonidine and relate this to patient education.
24. List which antihypertensives should be used with caution in elderly patients.
25. Describe how prazocin-related syncope can be controlled or avoided.
26. Explain why the dose of β-blocking agents will vary between patients in the treatment of high blood pressure.
27. Describe the adverse effects of the vasodilating antihypertensive hydralazine.
28. Describe the administration of the antihypertensives nitroprusside and diazoxide in the treatment of hypertensive emergencies.
29. Describe the adverse effects of minoxidil which limit the drug's clinical usefulness.
30. Describe the nursing process associated with the management of the adverse effects of guanethidine.
31. Differentiate the mechanism of labetalol from the mechanism of other drugs with β-adrenergic blocking activity.

Hypertension is a disease which affects approximately 60 million Americans. It is labeled the "silent killer" because the majority of patients have no symptoms until the process has been present long enough or is severe enough to cause potentially catastrophic consequences. Because of the asymptomatic nature of the disease, adequate detection, treatment, and follow-up programs are essential to decrease the cardiovascular complications of this common problem.

High blood pressure becomes more common as people get older. Below age 50 more males have hypertension, above age 50 males and females are equally affected. Males and blacks also tend to develop cardiovascular complications of high blood pressure more frequently and with greater severity than do females and whites. Additional risk factors for the development of hypertension include obesity, high sodium intake, labile blood pressure, and diabetes mellitus. Despite the fact that hypertension cannot be cured in the majority of patients, adequate control of blood pressure has been demonstrated to significantly decrease the occurrence of the cardiovascular complications, especially stroke.

Since hypertension is such a major public health issue, it is the responsibility of all health care providers to assure adequate access to appropriate medical care, patient education, and follow-up so that the complications can be prevented. *Patient education and follow-up* are especially important because many patients view the undesirable effects associated with drug or dietary therapy to be more disruptive to their lives than the disease process itself. Through education and counseling, the nurse plays a vital role in assuring patient safety, capacity for self-care, and compliance.

Patients need constant reassurance that good blood pressure control is one of the major contributors to the decrease in premature cardiovascular morbidity observed over the past decade.

REGULATION OF BLOOD PRESSURE

A multitude of physiologic mechanisms are responsible for blood pressure regulation (Table 40-1). Some of these mechanisms control blood pressure during routine daily activities while others are involved only in situations of stress or major trauma. The major contributor to systolic blood pressure is cardiac output (CO), while the major determinant of diastolic pressure (DP) is total peripheral resistance (TPR). Mean arterial pressure (MAP) is therefore determined by both output and resistance components, and can be expressed by the formula:

$$MAP = CO \times TPR$$

Mean arterial pressure can also be expressed as:

$$MAP = DP + \tfrac{1}{3} PP$$

where PP = pulse pressure (systolic pressure − diastolic pressure). Substituting a numerical example (140/80) into this relationship one observes that the mean arterial pressure (100 mmHg) is mathematically closer to the diastolic pressure (80 mmHg) than it is to the systolic pressure (140 mmHg). This observation leads to the longstanding but erroneous belief that the diastolic pressure is more important as a predictor of cardiovascular complications. Actuar-

---

TABLE 40-1 Mechanism of Blood Pressure Control

Baroreceptor Reflex

Increased arterial pressure stretches baroreceptors located in carotid and aortic arches. Impulse relayed to brainstem causes dilation of peripheral vessels and decreased cardiac output.

Chemoreceptor Reflex

Decreased arterial pressure causes decrease in oxygen and increase in carbon dioxide content in chemoreceptors in carotid and aortic bodies. Impulse relayed to brainstem to increase pressure.

Central Nervous System Ischemia

Arterial pressure less than 60 mmHg causes brainstem ischemia. Stimulates sympathetic nervous system resulting in vasoconstriction and increased heart contractility and rate.

Renin-Angiotensin Vasoconstrictor

Decreased pressure causes renal renin release. Renin causes conversion of angiotensinogen to angiotensin I which is converted to angiotensin II, a potent vasoconstrictor.

Aldosterone Pressure Regulating Mechanism

Decreased intravascular volume and pressure causes release of aldosterone from adrenal resulting in renal salt and water retention. Results in increased volume and pressure.

Capillary Fluid Shift

Flow of fluid into and out of capillaries due to acute changes in volume.

Renal Body Fluid Pressure Regulating Mechanism

Decreased arterial pressure directly affects renal salt and water retention resulting in a decreased GFR and increased tubular sodium reabsorption.

ial data has demonstrated that patients with systolic hypertension (greater than 160 mmHg) suffer the same deleterious effects as do patients with diastolic pressure elevations.

PATHOPHYSIOLOGY OF HIGH BLOOD PRESSURE

Pathogenesis

Although a variety of physiologic controls regulate blood pressure levels from time to time, there is no single abnormality which can be identified as the cause of hypertension. There is, however, a well-known sequence of physiologic changes which develop in untreated hypertensives. Early in the course of hypertension, cardiac output may be normal or mildly elevated. As the disease progresses, cardiac output returns to normal and peripheral resistance becomes consistently elevated. In the late stages of the disease, peripheral resistance remains elevated and cardiac output declines—sometimes to the point of symptomatic congestive heart failure.

Recent investigative work has centered on the vascular response to salt and the sensitivity of the arterioles to ingested salt. Additional research has been directed toward the role of the renin–angiotensin–aldosterone system. Patients with essential hypertension can be separated in high, normal, and low renin groups. Despite the fact that patients with more severe forms of hypertension tend to be in the high renin group, and that patients with low renin tend to have an elevated intravascular volume, there is currently no proven cause and effect relationship between renin and hypertension in the majority of patients.

Defining High Blood Pressure

Debate has existed for many years as to whether the *hypertensive population* can be separated from the *normotensive population* on the basis of a specific level of blood pressure. Some believe that these are in fact two separate populations, while others view blood pressure as a variable normally distributed throughout the population. Irrespective of whether or not delineation can be established between normotensive and hypertensive populations based on a specific blood pressure level, it is well established that there is a strongly positive correlation between the level of blood pressure elevation and the presence of hypertensive cardiovascular complications. The normal response of transiently elevated blood pressure in the presence of stress, trauma, anxiety, infection, and other exogenous factors have relatively little effect on morbidity and should not become the basis for either labeling patients "hypertensive" or for treating patients with drugs which they do not chronically need.

The criteria for defining hypertension established by the American Heart Association are based on the demonstration of consistently elevated blood pressure readings. Hypertension can be diagnosed in a patient whose average resting diastolic blood pressure readings exceed 90 mmHg on three

consecutive visits. A systolic blood pressure consistently greater than 160 mmHg has also been associated with significant morbidity and is more often seen in the elderly or in patients with advanced atherosclerotic cardiovascular disease.

Etiology

Between 90 and 95 percent of patients with hypertension have *essential hypertension*. In this group of patients the pathophysiologic cause of the blood pressure elevation has not been identified. Several factors which seem to have some role in the pathogenesis of essential hypertension include genetic predisposition, dietary sodium intake, body weight, and environmental stresses. In approximately 5 percent of hypertensive patients there is an identifiable cause which can explain the hypertensive condition. These *secondary* causes of hypertension can be categorized into cardiovascular, renal, endocrine, and neurogenic etiologies (Table 40-2). The

TABLE 40-2 Etiologic Classification of Hypertension

I. Arterial Hypertension (elevation of systolic and diastolic blood pressures)
  A. Essential hypertension
    1. Labile (intermittent)
    2. Established (fixed)
  B. Secondary hypertension
    1. Renal hypertension
      a. Kidney disease (pyelonephritis, glomerulonephritis, diabetic glomerulosclerosis, etc.)
      b. Renal artery disease
      c. Compression of the kidney
    2. Endocrine hypertension
      a. Pheochromocytoma
      b. Aldosteronism
      c. Cushing's syndrome
      d. Oral contraceptive use
      e. Thyroid disorders
    3. Neurogenic hypertension
      a. Anxiety states
      b. Intracranial diseases
      c. Vasomotor center disturbances
      d. Spinal cord and peripheral nerve diseases
    4. Coarctation of the aorta
    5. Toxemia of pregancy
II. Systolic Hypertension
  A. Increased stroke volume
    1. Complete heart block
    2. Aortic regurgitation
    3. Patent ductus arteriosus
    4. Thyrotoxicosis
    5. Paget's disease
  B. Decreased distensibility of aorta
    1. Arteriosclerosis of aorta
    2. Coarctation of aorta

Source: Adapted from W. A. Sodeman and T. M. Sodeman: *Pathologic Physiology: Mechanisms of Disease,* Philadelphia: Saunders, 1979.

majority of these patients can be identified through the signs and symptoms associated with their disease states (e.g., edema, fat redistribution, and electrolyte abnormalities in Cushing's syndrome). Unlike patients with essential hypertension, some patients with secondary hypertension can be cured if underlying pathology is reversed.

Drugs which can cause hypertension include **oral contraceptives, sympathomimetics** (see Chap. 13), **corticosteroids** and **ACTH** (see Chap. 35), and **phenylbutazone.** Hypertension can also result from the combination of sympathomi-

metics and antidepressants (monoamine oxidase inhibitors and tricyclic antidepressants).

Complications

Untreated hypertension leads to cardiovascular complications which affect the heart, kidneys, and central nervous system. Hypertension is the leading cause of both hemorrhagic and thrombotic stroke in the United States. Both ischemic heart disease (angina and myocardial infarction)

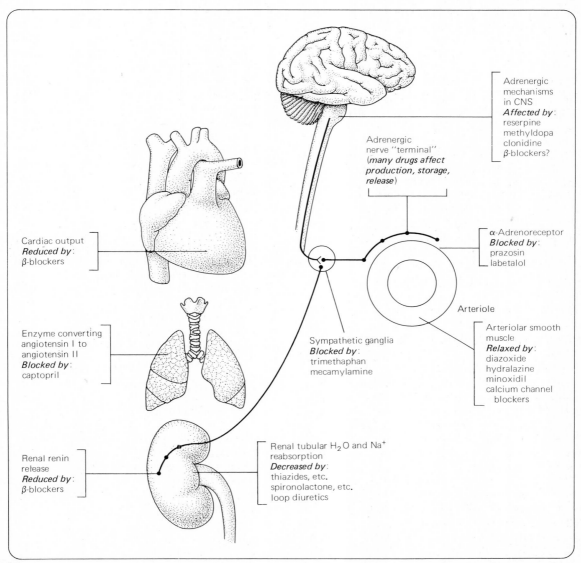

FIGURE 40-1

Schematic Representation of Various Pharmacologic Mechanisms by Which Antihypertensive Drugs May Work. [*Adapted from F. O. Simpson, "Hypertension Disease" in G. S. Avery (ed.), Drug Treatment (2nd ed.), ADIS Press, Australasia Pty Ltd., 404 Sydney Rd, Balgowlah, New South Wales, 2093, Australia.) 1980.*]

and congestive heart failure can result from uncontrolled hypertension. Finally, chronic renal failure requiring either chronic dialysis or renal transplantation can result from longstanding uncontrolled hypertension. The majority of these complications are the result of the accelerated atherosclerosis which is associated with chronic hypertension. Both cigarette smoking and hypercholesterolemia increase the morbidity associated with untreated hypertension.

Hypertensive patients have a morbidity risk twice that of normotensive patients, while hypertensive patients who smoke cigarettes or have hypercholesterolemia have a risk three times that of normotensive patients. Hypertensive patients who smoke and have an elevated serum cholesterol are at five times the risk of cardiovascular morbidity as normotensive patients.

CLINICAL FINDINGS

Accurate diagnosis of hypertension involves the documentation of three resting blood pressure readings on three separate visits. The last two readings from each visit are averaged, the first reading is ignored. Hypertension can be defined when the three averaged diastolic readings are consistently above 90 mmHg. Alternatively, any patient with a resting diastolic pressure on a single reading exceeding 105 mmHg in the presence of cardiac, renal, or neurologic disease is at greater risk and should be diagnosed as hypertensive. *Accurate* determination of blood pressure is a crucial component of detection and proper management of hypertension.

There are no symptoms associated with mild or moderate hypertension. Patients usually develop symptoms of the complications after longstanding elevations of blood pressure. Headache, dizziness, and nosebleeds do not correlate with the presence of mild or moderate pressure elevations. These symptoms are more often associated with hypertensive emergencies.

Baseline history should focus on existing identifiable risk factors such as salt intake, cigarette smoking, family history of early cardiac mortality, previous antihypertensive therapy, and symptoms of cardiovascular complications such as chest pain, dyspnea, edema, and altered neurologic or renal function. Physical examination should focus on the cardiovascular system as well: vital signs, examination of the fundi, heart, lungs, and neurologic system. Laboratory data should evaluate the status of those organs most likely to be affected by the disease or its treatment. Baseline and follow-up data should include serum electrolytes, tests of renal function, ECG, and check x-ray.

CLINICAL PHARMACOLOGY AND THERAPEUTICS

Multicenter cooperative trials have demonstrated that drug therapy which decreases blood pressure can decrease the risk of cardiovascular morbidity and mortality associated with chronic hypertension. In addition, decreasing the presence of known risk factors has been shown to lower blood pressure and to be adjunctive to drug therapy, often decreasing the number of pharmacologic agents required to adequately control blood pressure. The therapeutic objective in hypertension is to decrease the blood pressure to below 90 mmHg diastolic in the absence of undesirable side effects of therapy.

Nondrug Modalities

Behavioral Approaches

In the last two decades there have been an increasing number of studies evaluating nonpharmacologic approaches to lowering blood pressure. These treatment regimens have used a wide variety of relaxation, meditation, and biofeedback techniques. The success of these approaches has varied, but the most successful approach has been a form of biofeedback-assisted relaxation. This treatment combines the use of computerized physiologic feedback with an individualized understanding of a person's response to stress.

Hypertensive patients are frequently unaware of the stresses in their lives which are related to elevations in blood pressure. In counselor-facilitated treatment sessions, patients and their families (if appropriate) are able to observe their own pressures digitally displayed while they discuss their life situations. These sessions give the individual and his/her family the opportunity to observe and understand the relationship of life events to their own blood pressure.

During these sessions the patient is also taught to breath deeply, relax, and speak slowly. The hypertensive (and family) gradually learn what triggers the rise in blood pressure and gain the ability to lower blood pressure through behavior modification. Medications can be slowly tapered or even discontinued when blood pressures have become consistently decreased.

Exercise

Regular, aerobic exercise has been shown to lower blood pressure. Exercise may also help protect hypertensive patients from coronary artery disease by elevating blood high density lipoprotein (HDL) levels. Patients on β-blocking drugs (e.g., **propranolol** and others) should be especially cautioned to start slowly with gradual increases in exercise because of decreased endurance in these individuals. Regular exercise can also contribute to maintenance of a normal weight.

Salt Restriction

There is much controversy over the role of salt in hypertension. Studies conducted in animals have shown that excessive salt intake can cause hypertension. While it has been demonstrated that lowering salt intake significantly lowers blood pressure, recent studies in patients have shown that lowering salt intake may not be an effective treatment for all hypertensives.

Nurses should assess the salt intake of the entire family. Since Americans have such a high salt intake, it seems reasonable to advise a lowering of salt intake. A moderate salt intake using no salt in cooking and no additional salt at the table is a wise health precaution, despite the unanswered role of salt intake in the etiology of hypertension.

Alcohol Intake

Heavy drinking (intake of five or more alcohol drinks per day) has been associated with higher blood pressures. Since moderate alcohol intake (1 to 2 ounces per day) also raises the cardioprotective HDL cholesterol levels, hypertensives can drink in moderation if they desire.

Obesity Control

Obesity is closely associated with elevations of blood pressure, although not every overweight person is or becomes hypertensive. The correlation between obesity and hypertension has been long established and demonstrated in many studies of adults.

There have been extensive clinical observations correlating weight reduction with the lowering of blood pressure levels. All hypertensive patients should be encouraged to maintain an ideal weight, and those who are overweight should reduce.

Stepped Care Approach to Drug Therapy

The approach to drug therapy in hypertension should be systematic, based on the use of least toxic agents first, and should take advantage of multiple pharmacologic mechanisms (Fig. 40-1) to lower blood pressure. The stepped care approach advocated by the American Heart Association is one such approach (Fig. 40-2). Drugs are used in order of those drugs or combinations of drugs least likely to cause adverse effects as first step agents; those in subsequent steps are added to or substituted for the initial agents until the desired blood pressure is attained, the maximum effective dose has been reached, or the patient experiences an intolerable adverse effect. The choice of an agent depends mostly on the risk of predictable adverse effects in specific patients. For example, β-adrenergic receptor blocking agents such as propranolol should be avoided in patients with asthma. On the other hand, β-blockers are indicated for patients at risk of thiazide-induced toxicity and for their cardioprotective effects in patients who have had a myocardial infarction. Step three and step four agents are reserved for those patients who cannot be controlled on step one and step two agents, since these agents are associated with a higher incidence of severe adverse effects. In nonemergency cases, decreasing the blood pressure to an acceptable level can be gradually accomplished in the majority of patients within

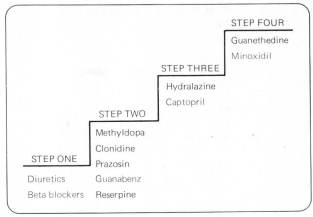

FIGURE 40-2

Stepped Care Approach to the Treatment of High Blood Pressure. If drugs in one step are ineffective, agents from the subsequent step are added or substituted.

six months of initiating therapy, barring significant adverse effects.

Diuretics

The traditional first agents in the management of hypertension are the oral diuretics (Table 40-3). Of the available agents, the thiazide diuretics are employed most frequently in hypertension. There is little difference in antihypertensive efficacy between the numerous available thiazides, despite their differences in pharmacokinetic characteristics. The high potency diuretic agents **furosemide** and **ethacrynic acid** are useful in patients with renal failure in whom intravascular volume overload is a prominent feature. The less potent diuretics **spironolactone, triamterene,** and **amiloride** are used most frequently in patients who require agents which prevent renal potassium loss (see Chap. 23). They are slightly less effective than the thiazides when used alone in the treatment of hypertension.

Thiazide Diuretics

Mechanism of Action   There are two mechanisms which contribute to the blood pressure lowering effect of thiazide diuretics. They are volume depletion and a direct action on arterioles causing dilation. Thiazides block reabsorption of sodium in the proximal portion of the distal tubule in the kidney. This action produces an increase in sodium concentration in the urine and is accompanied by an increased water loss resulting in a lowered blood pressure. In addition, there is a shift in intracellular sodium concentration in the walls of the arterioles which has been postulated to cause vascular relaxation, thereby decreasing peripheral resistance. The direct arteriolar dilating effects persist with chronic thiazide use despite the return to normal of extra-

TABLE 40-3   Diuretic Agents in Hypertension

GENERIC NAME	TRADE NAME	DAILY ANTIHYPERTENSIVE DOSE RANGE, mg
Chlorothiazide	Diuril	500–1000
Hydrochlorothiazide	Hydro-Diuril	50–100
Chlorthalidone	Hygroton	50–100
Methychlothiazide	Enduron	5–10
Metolazone	Zaroxolyn	5–10
Triamterene	Dyrenium	100–200
Amiloride	Midamor	5–10
Furosemide	Lasix	40–80
Ethacrynic acid	Edecrin	50–100

Combination Products

TRADE NAME	DIURETIC COMPOSITION	DAILY DOSE RANGE (TABLETS)
Moduretic	Amiloride 5 mg, hydrochlorothiazide 50 mg	1–2
Aldactazide	Spironolactone 25 mg, hydrochlorothiazide 25 mg	2–4
Dyazide	Triamterene 50 mg, hydrochlorothiazide 25 mg	1–2
Maxide	Triamterene 75 mg, hydrochlorothiazide 50 mg	1

vascular and plasma volume within a few weeks of the initiation of therapy.

One of the major advantages of the use of thiazide diuretics as step one agents is the fact that most other antihypertensive agents which cause arteriolar dilation result in renal fluid retention with chronic use. The use of diuretics with these other agents prevents fluid accumulation which can lead to tolerance to the antihypertensive effects of agents in other classes.

Pharmacokinetics   The major difference among the thiazides and related diuretics is their serum half-lives, reflected mostly in the duration of *diuretic* effect produced by the various agents. Antihypertensive effect, however, persists for up to 24 h even for those agents with a short half-life (e.g., **hydrochlorothiazide**). As a result, thiazide diuretics need only be administered on a once a day basis for hypertension. The thiazides are renally excreted and may therefore be less effective as diuretic agents in some patients with chronic renal failure.

Adverse effects   The most common side effects of diuretics are volume depletion and electrolyte disturbances. These effects are discussed in Chap. 23.

Dosage   **Hydrochlorothiazide** is administered 50 mg once a day for hypertension. Recent data indicates that the antihypertensive effect of 50 mg bid is no greater than 50 mg daily. Since electrolyte disturbances and volume depletion are dose dependent, especially in the elderly, the 50-mg daily dose is currently the maximum accepted dose. Other diuretics used in the treatment of hypertension, either for their potassium-sparing effects or for patients with renal insufficiency, are listed in Table 40-3.

Central Sympathoplegics

Methyldopa

Mechanism of Action   The primary mechanism of action of methyldopa (Aldomet) is to decrease sympathetic nervous system activity through a central nervous system effect. Methyldopa administration results in the formation of α-methylnorepinephrine in the peripheral circulation as well as in the central nervous system. This neurotransmitter has much less sympathetic activity than the endogenous neurotransmitter norepinephrine. The antihypertensive efficacy of methyldopa results from the action of this *false neurotransmitter* to decrease sympathetic outflow from the brain resulting in a decreased sympathetic tone in the periphery and therefore less arteriolar vasoconstriction. Although the false neurotransmitter is present in the peripheral circulation, it probably plays a minor role in the antihypertensive activity of methyldopa. The current theory for methyldopa action is that the α-methylnorepinephrine in the CNS causes stimulation of the α-adrenergic receptors which inhibits the sympathetic outflow.

Pharmacokinetics   The absorption of methyldopa is rapid but it probably undergoes first-pass metabolism. The serum half-life is biphasic with the elimination phase being about 2 h, although its antihypertensive effect persists up to 24 h. The renal clearance of methyldopa accounts for 66 percent of the unchanged drug's removal from plasma, and so those in renal failure may require lower doses. Its duration of action allows for twice daily dosing.

Adverse Effects   The most common side effects associated with **methyldopa** are sedation and nasal stuffiness. They are usually observed with initial therapy or with dosage increases. Patients should be advised of the potential for these side effects and that they will usually become tolerant to those symptoms with continued therapy. Less frequent side effects include postural hypotension, development of positive direct Coombs' test, gastrointestinal cramping, blurred vision, and failure of ejaculation which may lead to erectile impotence. Although these side effects can sometimes be managed by decreasing the dose, alternative drug therapy is most often chosen.

The positive direct Coombs' test itself usually does not cause any clinical problems; the only difficulty is when trying to cross match blood. Rarely, patients may develop febrile reactions or hepatitis as a result of methyldopa therapy. Hemolytic anemia can develop in less than 5 percent of patients who develop positive direct Coombs' test. If hemolysis is detected in a patient the drug should be stopped. The hemolytic anemia and the positive Coombs' test usually reverses after the methyldopa is stopped but this may require several weeks. Methyldopa can induce lactation in either sex, which is related to the high serum concentration of prolactin. Sudden stopping of methyldopa can cause rebound hypertension but the incidence of this is less than it is with **clonidine.**

Dosage   **Methyldopa** is added to a step one agent beginning with 250 mg bid. Dosage is then gradually increased at biweekly intervals to a maximum effective dose of 2 g/day. Some practitioners use a 3-g maximum daily dose but there is little added benefit above 2 g/day despite the increased side effects noted at higher doses.

Clonidine

Mechanism of Action   Clonidine (Catapres) exerts its antihypertensive effect through a slightly different central mechanism than does **methyldopa.** Instead of the false neurotransmitter inhibiting sympathetic outflow, clonidine itself stimulates presynaptic (inhibitory) α-adrenergic (α_2) receptors in the brain. Stimulation of these receptors causes a decrease in sympathetic tone in the peripheral arterioles and thereby a decrease in resistance, lowering the blood pressure and decreasing heart rate and cardiac output.

Pharmacokinetics   Approximately 75 percent of a single dose of clonidine is absorbed from the gastrointestinal tract. The majority of the drug is excreted unchanged in the urine with an elimination half-life of 8 to 9 h. The duration of antihypertensive effect is between 4 and 24 h, allowing the drug to be dosed on a twice a day basis in the majority of patients.

Adverse Effects   Dry mouth and sedation are frequently encountered side effects of clonidine and occur most often at the onset of therapy or when the dose is increased. Like methyldopa, these side effects often improve with continued therapy.

A severe withdrawal reaction has been observed in patients receiving more than 1.2 mg daily who abruptly discontinue clonidine. Within 8 to 12 h blood pressure may begin to rise, eventually reaching levels in excess of pretreatment values. Symptoms of headache, nervousness, abdominal pain, tachycardia, and sweating accompany the elevated pressure. Without intervention these symptoms may lead to life-threatening hypertensive crisis. Reinstitution of clonidine or use of α- and β-adrenergic blocking agents can reverse the withdrawal phenomenon. The syndrome can be avoided by educating patients about the importance of not abruptly discontinuing clonidine. Despite early claims to the contrary, clonidine can produce sexual dysfunction with a frequency similar to methyldopa.

Dosage   Clonidine therapy is initiated with a bedtime dose of 0.1 mg, increasing to 0.1 mg bid the following day. The dosage can be gradually increased in 0.1- to 0.2-mg increments in weekly or biweekly intervals to a maximum dose of 2.4 mg daily in divided doses. The investigational **transdermal clonidine** (Catapress-TTS) requires that the patch be replaced weekly.

Guanabenz

Guanabenz (Wytensin) has not been included in the traditional stepped care agents proposed by the American Heart Association because of its recent introduction. It appears most likely to be classified as a step two agent, similar to **clonidine.**

Mechanism of Action   Guanabenz is an antihypertensive agent whose mechanism closely resembles that of clonidine. The drug stimulates central nervous system α receptors leading to a decreased sympathetic outflow to the peripheral circulation. Although clinical experience is limited, guanabenz appears to be as effective an antihypertensive as methyldopa.

Pharmacokinetics   Guanabenz is well absorbed orally and is extensively metabolized by the liver. Only 1 percent of the drug is eliminated unchanged by the kidney. The average half-life of the drug is 5 h with an effective duration of action of 10 to 12 h with chronic dosing.

Adverse Effects   Clinical experience is insufficient for a complete profile of the side effects of guanabenz to be presented. However, based on data from about 850 patients, the most frequent side effects appear to be sedation in 20 to 40 percent of patients, dry mouth, dizziness, and generalized weakness. Less frequent side effects include headache, palpitations, gastrointestinal disturbances, and sexual dysfunction.

Dosage A starting dose of 4 mg bid is recommended with dosage increments of 4 to 8 mg day as required to control blood pressure. A maximum dose of 32 mg is suggested.

Adrenergic Neuron Blockers

Reserpine

Mechanism of Action The rauwolfia alkaloids, of which reserpine is the most commonly used, act primarily by interfering with peripheral sympathetic nervous system activity. Some central sympathetic depletion also plays a role in lowering blood pressure. Reserpine depletes norepinephrine from its storage granules in the presynaptic nerve ending. The decrease in norepinephrine-mediated α stimulation results in decreased peripheral resistance and lowering of blood pressure.

Pharmacokinetics Because of the indirect effect of reserpine to decrease blood pressure, its onset of maximal antihypertensive action after oral administration is delayed for up to three weeks. Antihypertensive effects may persist for a week or two after the drug has been discontinued. Reserpine is metabolized extensively with only 1 percent excreted unchanged in the urine.

Adverse Effects Because of the frequency of troublesome side effects at doses which effectively lower blood pressure and the availability of newer less toxic effects, reserpine use has decreased in recent years. The adverse effect most frequently associated with reserpine use is mental depression. This effect is reported most often in the elderly and in patients with a history of depression. Reports of suicide and increased suicidal tendency have been associated with reserpine use. The mental depression may be dose-dependent and so when used in low doses in addition to a diuretic the incidence is relatively small.

Other common side effects include sedation, nightmares, increased gastrointestinal motility which produces cramps and diarrhea, and increased gastric acid secretion. The gastrointestinal effects preclude the use of reserpine in patients with a history of peptic ulcer disease. Cardiovascular effects include bradycardia and nasal stuffiness (vasodilation of vessels of nasal mucosa). Controversy exists over the reported increased incidence of breast cancer associated with reserpine use.

Because of the effect of reserpine in depleting norepinephrine, vascular target organs including sympathetic receptors on arterioles are hyperreactive to sympathetic stimulation. As a result, administration of agents which contain sympathomimetic compounds such as nasal decongestants in over-the-counter cough and cold preparations (e.g., Dristan and others) and monamine oxidase inhibitors (e.g., Parnate) have the potential to produce extreme elevations of blood pressure. Patients should be told to avoid these drugs when taking reserpine.

Dosage Reserpine is usually administered in doses of between 0.1 and 0.3 mg daily. Dosage should be increased only after maximal effectiveness from a given dose can be assessed, usually after several weeks. The long duration of action allows for once daily dosing, an advantage for compliance. In addition, the drug is inexpensive when compared to newer antihypertensive agents. A number of preparations of reserpine or other rauwolfia alkaloids are available (Table 40-4).

Guanethidine

Mechanism of Action Guanethidine (Ismelin) is a potent sympatholytic agent which acts to decrease the response of the sympathetic nerve terminal to stimulation and to deplete the norepinephrine stores in the sympathetic nerve terminals. Guanethidine effectively replaces the norepinephrine stored in the nerve terminals which leads to inactivation (metabolism) of the displaced norepinephrine. Blood pressure is decreased by a general loss of sympathetic tone resulting in decreased peripheral resistance and a decrease in cardiac output. Because of the potency of guanethidine as a sympathetic nervous system depressant, the drug has been reserved for patients who do not respond to agents in the first three steps. Guanethidine can be added to the regimen of patients on diuretics, central sympatholytics, and vasodilators. Use of guanethidine in patients on other peripheral sympatholytics (e.g., **reserpine**) is not pharmacologically appropriate.

Pharmacokinetics Oral absorption of guanethidine varies greatly from 3 to 30 percent among patients. The drug is cleared by the kidney (35 to 50 percent excreted unchanged in the urine) but the effect of norepinephrine depletion can persist for several days after the drug has been discontinued.

Adverse Effects The major dose-limiting side effect is postural hypotension. This effect can be minimized by cautioning patients to sit up slowly on arising, dangle the legs over the edge of the bed for several minutes, and then slowly arise. The hypotension may also be accentuated by exercise, hot weather or hot showers, alcohol, and in the elderly.

Many patients describe a "generalized weakness" especially early in therapy which may not be associated with postural hypotension. As a potent sympatholytic guanethidine can precipitate heart failure in patients with poor ventricular function and can cause diarrhea in a number of patients. The diarrhea responds to small doses of anticholin-

TABLE 40-4   Rauwolfia Derivatives

GENERIC NAME	TRADE NAME	DAILY DOSE RANGE, mg
Rauwolfia	Raudixin and others	50–300
Reserpine	Serpasil and others	0.1–0.25
Deserpidine	Harmonyl	0.25

ergic agents or to **kaolin-pectin** (Kaopectate) mixtures. Male patients report impotence and retrograde ejaculation more frequently than with other antihypertensive agents. Retrograde ejaculation may be reported as a decrease in the volume of semen produced, or "dry orgasm."

Administration of decongestants or cold remedies can precipitate hypertensive crisis in patients receiving guanethidine and should therefore be avoided. Concurrent administration of tricyclic antidepressant drugs (e.g., **amitriptyline**) or the phenothiazines (e.g., **chlorpromazine**) can antagonize the effect of guanethidine.

Dosage   Guanethidine is administered initially in a 10-mg daily dose. The dosage can be increased gradually at biweekly intervals until the blood pressure is controlled or intolerable side effects intervene. Because of the extended effect of guanethidine the drug need only be administered once a day, a positive factor for patient compliance.

Guanadrel Sulfate

Guanadrel sulfate (Hylorel) is another drug which has not yet been classified according to the stepped approach to treating blood pressure. It is anticipated that it will be a step two agent, although its adverse effect profile parallels that of the step four agent, guanethidine, another peripherally acting antiadrenergic drug.

Mechanism of Action   Guanadrel blocks the adrenergic neuron by inhibiting norepinephrine release and by depleting norepinephrine stores in the nerve ending. Its antihypertensive effect is greater in the standing than in the supine position. Guanadrel does not decrease cardiac output or renal blood flow, but it does decrease heart rate and lead to fluid retention if not given with diuretic therapy.

Pharmacokinetics   Guanadrel is well absorbed after oral administration and has a half-life of about 10 h. It is 40 percent eliminated unchanged in the urine.

Adverse Effects   Like **guanethidine**, guanadrel frequently causes orthostatic hypotension, diarrhea, abdominal cramps, and gas pain. Fatigue, headache, drowsiness, and dizziness are also common, but less frequent than with methyldopa. Other significant adverse effects include dyspnea on exertion, visual disturbances, paresthesias, nocturia, urinary frequency, peripheral edema, leg cramps, and weight gain.

Tricyclic antidepressants and indirect-acting sympathomimetics (e.g., **phenylpropanolamine** and **ephedrine** in over-the-counter decongestants; **amphetamines**), and possibly **phenothiazines** may impair the effectiveness of guanadrel. Other drugs that affect sympathetic function (direct-acting sympathomimetics, α- or β-adrenergic blocking agents) may have increased effect when given concurrently with guanadrel.

Dosage   Guanadrel is usually given in doses of 10 to 25 mg three or four times daily. Because response to this drug is quite variable, doses usually begin at 10 mg/day and are increased at intervals of a week or more until the effective dose is reached.

α-Adrenergic Receptor Blocker

Prazosin

Mechanism of Action   Prazosin (Minipress) is an α-adrenergic blocking agent which is selective for the postsynaptic α receptor, α_1 (Fig. 14-2). When prazosin is used, the presynaptic α_2 receptor remains unblocked and when stimulated prevents the further release of the neurotransmitter. The effect of α_1 blockade and α_2 activation leads to vasodilation. Prazosin reduces peripheral vascular resistance without secondary reflex tachycardia. The effect of prazosin in dilating the venous beds leads to maximal antihypertensive efficacy when the patient is in the upright position. The choice of prazosin as an antihypertensive is especially appropriate in patients with concurrent congestive heart failure because of prazosin's ability to reduce both preload and afterload (see Chap. 44).

Pharmacokinetics   Prazosin is rapidly and completely absorbed when given orally. Peak plasma concentrations are achieved in 2 to 3 h. The drug is extensively metabolized in the liver and has a serum half-life of approximately 3 to 4 h. Its pharmacologic effect, however, persists for much longer, allowing prazosin to be effectively administered on a twice daily basis. Food does not appear to influence the plasma level or the time required to reach peak concentration.

Adverse Effects   Prazosin has fewer adverse effects than the other sympathoplegic agents. Because it dilates both arterial and venous beds, reflex tachycardia is not as much of a problem as it can be with **hydralazine**. Likewise, orthostatic hypotension is not a common problem as it is with drugs that deplete norepinephrine. Reported side effects include headache, fluid retention when used without a diuretic, dry mouth, mental depression, and skin rash.

When prazosin was initially introduced in the United States concern was expressed over reported cases of first-dose syncope. This phenomenon, characterized by dizziness, transient faintness, palpitations, and rarely overt syncope, is associated with large initial doses of prazosin more likely to produce acute postural hypotension. This condition is also likely to be more common in patients who are previously volume-depleted as a result of diuretic therapy. The first-dose phenomenon can be circumvented by initiating therapy with small doses and by administering the first dose at bedtime. Likewise, any succeeding increase in dosage should be initiated with the bedtime dose.

Dosage   The drug is started with 1 mg twice a day beginning with the bedtime dose and gradually increasing in biweekly intervals until the blood pressure is controlled or side effects intervene. Most patients require less than 20 mg daily but doses of up to 40 mg have been used.

β-Adrenergic-Receptor Blockers

Of all the recent developments in antihypertensive drug therapy the class of agents that has expanded most dramatically has been the β-adrenergic blocking agents. Since the introduction of **propranolol** as the first β blocker, numerous other agents with slightly different potency, selectivity, and pharmacokinetic properties have been introduced. Not only have these agents become widely used in the treatment of hypertension but also they have numerous other FDA approved and nonapproved indications.

As antihypertensive agents, β blockers were originally classified as step two agents in the American Heart Association stepped care approach. However with the recent data implicating diuretic agents as potentially more toxic than previously assumed, and with additional information on the potential benefit of β blockers in improving myocardial salvage in patients with ischemic heart disease, these drugs have become first step agents in the treatment of hypertension.

Mechanism of Action   The precise mechanism of antihypertensive action of β-blocking agents is unknown. Several pharmacologic effects would contribute to the blood pressure lowering action of these agents, but no one mechanism has proven to be the primary cause of the antihypertensive effect. Three major mechanisms include a decrease in cardiac output, a decreasing effect of the renin–angiotensin–aldosterone system, and a central nervous system effect.

β-blocking agents decrease myocardial contractility, thereby lowering stroke volume (negative inotropic effect). Since cardiac output is dependent upon the product of stroke volume and heart rate, and since β-blocking agents result in a decreased heart rate, cardiac output drops. This decreased output should primarily lead to a decreased systolic pressure, but β-blocking agents also effectively decrease diastolic pressure. Thus the depressant effect on cardiac output can not be implicated as the primary antihypertensive mechanism. Some β-blocking agents (**propranolol, timolol, metoprolol**) cause a marked decrease in plasma renin activity. This effect would result in a decreased production of angiotensin II, the potent vasoconstrictor, and a decrease in aldosterone release causing a decrease in renal sodium and fluid accumulation. The dual action to decrease angiotensin and aldosterone production and secretion causes a decrease in peripheral vascular resistance and lower intravascular volume, both of which lead to a decrease in blood pressure. Other β-blocking agents (**pindolol, atenolol**) which are as effective in lowering blood pressure do not decrease plasma renin activity as much as agents in the previously mentioned group. It therefore seems likely that other mechanisms are as important as decreasing plasma renin in causing the antihypertensive effect.

The central antihypertensive effect of β-blocking agents is related to their lipid solubility and thus to their ability to cross the blood-brain barrier. The precise central mechanism is not fully understood but it probably contributes somewhat to the overall antihypertensive efficacy of this class of agents.

Although in any individual patient, one of the three mechanisms proposed may predominate, most likely a combination of the three contributes to the overall antihypertensive effect of the β-blocking agents. One of the pharmacologic differences between the various β-blocking agents is their degree of receptor selectivity. There are two types of β-adrenergic receptors—β_1 and β_2. β_1 receptors are located primarily in the myocardium while the β_2 receptors are located in the bronchioles, arterioles, and several glands. β-blocker selectivity refers to the ability of a drug to induce sympathetic blockade at one type of receptor to a greater extent than at the other type. **Metoprolol** and **atenolol** selectively block β_1 receptors resulting in less bronchospasm on exertion in asthmatics than does a comparable dose of any of the other available β blockers such as **propranolol**, since they are all nonselective β blockers. Selectivity is a dose-dependent phenomenon, however, and *at higher doses the cardioselectivity is lost.*

Pharmacokinetics   The major differences in pharmacokinetic characteristics among the β blockers relates to their bioavailability, route of elimination, and duration of action (Table 40-5). Bioavailability problems are significant with some agents like propranolol in which the *first-pass phenomenon* plays a significant role. Once absorbed from the gastrointestinal tract, a large percentage of the drug is metabolized by the liver to less active or inactive metabolites. Also, the capacity of the liver to metabolize propranolol varies greatly between patients and results in a 10- to 40-fold difference in propranolol serum concentration in patients receiving a similar oral dose. This large effect can also be demonstrated by observing the difference between the oral dosage range (10 to 160 mg per dose) and the intravenous dosing range (1 to 5 mg per dose).

Most of the β-blocking agents are metabolized in the liver while others, such as **nadolol** (Corgard), are renally eliminated and have a more prolonged duration of action. In hypertension, even β blockers with a short serum half-life have been demonstrated to have a longer pharmacologic effect and can therefore be dosed on a twice-a-day basis. Nadolol and metoprolol can be administered once a day.

Adverse effects   The side effects of β blockers are most significant in patients with preexisting disease states in whom β-adrenergic stimulation plays an important physiologic role. These include congestive heart failure, obstructive lung disease, diabetes mellitus, and peripheral vascular disease. Because of the negative inotropic effect, β blockade can precipitate heart failure in patients with poor ventricular function. This effect is most likely to be observed early in therapy but can occur at any time as dosage is increase. Digitalis glycosides overcome some of this negative inotropic effect.

Asthma is an absolute contraindication to the use of β blockers because of the dependence of the bronchioles on β_2 sympathetic stimulation. Because there are so many other pharmacologic classes of antihypertensives to choose from in step two, there is no reason to use even a cardioselective β blocker in the treatment of patients who are asthmatic. Patients with irreversible airway disease (chronic bronchitis) alternatively can tolerate low doses of cardioselective β blockers if carefully monitored for symptoms of dyspnea.

Patients with claudication or peripheral vascular disease may have more symptoms of arterial insufficiency with β blockade, although cardioselective agents may be better tolerated. Diabetic patients, especially those who are insulin-dependent, can experience either hypoglycemia or hyperglycemia from β blockers. More importantly, however, β blockers have the potential to mask the early warning symptoms and signs of hypoglycemia. Such patients can be treated with β blocker therapy but they should perform blood glucose testing several times daily to assure that hypoglycemia does not exist.

Less common side effects of β blocker therapy include symptomatic bradycardia, hypotension, nausea, vomiting, diarrhea, and central nervous system symptoms. The central nervous system side effects, including nightmares, depression, insomnia, and hallucinations, may be more common with lipid-soluble compounds such as propranolol and metoprolol.

There are numerous reports of an acute withdrawal reaction associated with sudden discontinuation of β blockers, especially when high doses have been administered. The reaction is characterized by severe hypertension, tachycardia, worsening angina, myocardial infarction, and several cases of sudden death. If therapy is to be stopped on an outpatient basis, it should be done by gradually tapering the dosage over several weeks.

Dosage Commonly used antihypertensive doses of β-blocking agents are listed in Table 40-5. The minimum effective dose of propranolol is 40 mg daily (20 mg bid). Most patients demonstrate pharmacologic β blockade at approximately 160 mg daily. Some patients require up to 640 mg daily but doses over 320 mg daily may not lower blood pressure more effectively than will the addition of another antihypertensive agent.

α-β Adrenergic Receptor Blocker

Labetalol

Labetalol (Normodyne, Trandate) is a unique adrenergic blocking agent in that it blocks both α and β receptors. It is a nonselective β blocker and blocks both β_1 and β_2 receptors. Labetalol is as effective as the β blockers but does not appear to cause bradycardia. It has been effective for hypertensive crisis and in patients resistant to other forms of antihypertensive therapy. Labetalol has not yet been classified on the stepped care approach. The ratios of α to β blockade are 1:3 and 1:7 following oral and IV administration, respectively.

Pharmacokinetics Labetalol has 25 percent oral bioavailability, as it undergoes significant first-pass metabolism. Absorption is increased by **cimetidine**, food, and chronic liver disease. It is metabolized by the liver, and the metabolites are excreted in the bile and urine. It is 50 percent plasma protein bound and crosses the placenta and appears in breast milk. The half-life averages 5.5 h after oral administration and 6 to 8 h after IV administration.

Adverse Effects Labetalol is associated with nausea, indigestion, impotence, scalp tingling, dizziness, tiredness, depression, postural hypotension, claudication, and bronchospasm. Other effects include drug-induced lupus syndrome, eye irritation, and myalgia.

Dosage Labetalol is used for hypertension in oral doses of 200 to 800 mg daily. It is administered in two doses daily.

TABLE 40-5 Pharmacokinetic Characteristics of β-Blocking Agents

GENERIC NAME	TRADE NAME	EXTENT OF BIO-AVAILABILITY, % OF DOSE	VARIATION IN PLASMA LEVEL	β-BLOCKING CONCENTRATIONS	USUAL DOSAGE RANGE, mg	ELIMINATION HALF-LIFE, h	ACTIVE METABOLITES	CARDIO-SELECTIVE
Atenolol	Tenormin	40	Low	0.2–0.5 mg/mL	50–100	6–9	No	Yes
Metoprolol	Lopressor	50	7-fold	50–100 ng/mL	100–450	3–4	No	Yes
Nadolol	Corgard	75	5–8-fold	~200 ng/mL	80–320	14–24	No	No
Oxyprenolol	Trasicor	30	—*	—*	—*	1.5	No	No
Pindolol	Visken	100	4-fold	50–150 ng/mL	20–60	3–4	No	No
Propranolol	Inderal	30	20-fold	50–100 ng/mL	160–480	3.5–6	Yes	No
Timolol	Blocadren	50	7-fold	5–10 ng/mL	20–40	4–5	No	No

*New pharmacologic agent; approved in 1984 but not marketed. Some pharmacokinetic and dosing data not available.

Intravenous bolus doses are 20 to 80 mg at 10-min intervals or 2 mg/min by continuous infusion, up to a maximum of 300 mg.

Direct Vasodilators

Hydralazine

Mechanism of Action Hydralazine (Apresoline), a step three agent, is a direct-acting vasodilator which reduces arterial tone and thereby decreases peripheral resistance. It does not interfere with sympathetic nervous system function. Hydralazine preferentially dilates arterioles as compared to veins which minimizes postural hypotension and promotes an increase in cardiac output. Combinations of β blockers or other sympatholytic agents and hydralazine not only overcome the reflex tachycardia but also provide for additive antihypertensive efficacy.

Pharmacokinetics Hydralazine undergoes significant first pass hepatic metabolism and therefore has relatively low bioavailability. The drug is acetylated by the liver at a rate that is genetically predetermined. Patients who are slow acetylators tend to accumulate the parent compound more than do rapid acetylators. The rate of acetylation may have an effect on both the bioavailability and the adverse effects of the drug. The elimination half-life of hydralazine ranges from 2 to 8 h.

Adverse Effects Side effects of hydralazine include tachycardia, headache, gastrointestinal disturbances, and arthralgias. A syndrome resembling systemic lupus erythematosis consisting of skin rash, arthralgias or arthritis, alopecia, and a decrease in leukocyte count has been rarely associated with daily doses in excess of 200 mg. The incidence increases sharply when the daily dose exceeds 400 mg. Because of the availability of other effective antihypertensive agents, the maximum daily dose in hypertension should not exceed 200 mg.

Patients with ischemic heart disease who are not receiving β blockers or sympatholytic agents such as methyldopa may develop angina as a result of the reflex tachycardia induced by hydralazine. Such patients should receive alternative drugs to treat their blood pressure.

Dosage Hydralazine dosage should begin with 25 mg bid. Dosage can be titrated in 50-mg daily increments at biweekly intervals until a maximum dose of 200 mg daily is reached or side effects intervene. Higher doses can be used in congestive heart failure.

Minoxidil

Mechanism of Action Minoxidil (Loniten) is a potent, direct-acting vasodilator which decreases peripheral vascular resistance, thereby lowering blood pressure. The drug causes marked sodium retention and edema formation and must therefore be administered with a potent diuretic such as **furosemide.** Minoxidil has found its greatest use in patients with hypertension associated with chronic renal failure or in patients with malignant hypertension associated with renal failure.

Pharmacokinetics Minoxidil is completely absorbed from the gastrointestinal tract. Its maximal antihypertensive effect is seen in 4 h. The drug is predominantly metabolized by the liver to compounds with much less antihypertensive effect than occurs with the parent compound. The metabolites are renally eliminated. The elimination half-life of minoxidil is 4 h but the blood pressure lowering effect may persist for 10 to 72 h after a dose.

Adverse Effects Minoxidil produces frequent troublesome side effects including edema formation, reflex tachycardia, and increased hair growth in the majority of female patients. The edema can be controlled in some patients with vigorous diuretic therapy and is more common if there was pretreatment cardiac enlargement and preexisting renal insufficiency. Tachycardia can be controlled by coadministration of β-blocking agents or centrally acting sympatholytics such as **clonidine.** Rarely the drug can cause tachyarrhythmias, pericardial effusions, or reversible T-wave changes on ECG. The unsightly hair growth can be managed in some women with depilatories or by shaving, although a number of women will discontinue the drug because of this effect. Finally, although renal function may improve in some patients as a result of minoxidil therapy, in others, renal function deterioration has continued despite an improvement in blood pressure control. Patients on α-adrenergic blocking agents such as **prazosin** or **guanethidine** and those on **captopril** have a higher incidence of hypotension when placed on minoxidil than patients on other types of antihypertensive drugs.

Dosage The initial single daily dose of minoxidil is 5 to 10 mg depending on the rapidity of blood pressure control required and the degree of pressure elevation. The dosage can be increased in 5- to 10-mg increments weekly. Since the magnitude of within-day fluctuation of blood pressure is greater when there has been greater pressure reduction, the drug should be administered in two daily doses if the supine diastolic blood pressure is reduced by 30 mmHg or more. The majority of patients are controlled with doses of 40 mg or less. Doses up to 100 mg daily have been used.

Angiotensin-Converting Enzyme Inhibitor

Captopril

Mechanism of Action Captopril (Capoten) interferes with the renin–angiotensin–aldosterone system by inhibition of the enzyme which converts angiotensin I to angiotensin II

(Fig. 40-3). Captopril inhibits the powerful vasoconstrictive property of this substance. In addition, inhibition of angiotensin decreases the release of aldosterone from the adrenal cortex preventing sodium and water retention. The drug should be reserved for patients with severe or resistant hypertension or for patients with renovascular hypertension.

Pharmacokinetics   Approximately 75 percent of a dose of captopril is absorbed on an empty stomach after oral administration. Absorption is decreased to 30 to 40 percent by food. The drug is rapidly metabolized and approximately 40 percent is excreted unchanged in the urine after 24 h. The dose should be decreased in patients with renal insufficiency.

Adverse Effects   Side effects commonly associated with other antihypertensive agents such as orthostatic hypoten-

sion, sexual dysfunction, and tachycardia are rare with captopril. It does not depress cardiac function and has been used successfully as an afterload reducing agent in patients with congestive heart failure. However, uncommon but serious side effects have limited the usefulness of captopril in the treatment of hypertension.

Neutropenia (decreased white blood cell count) has been reported in 0.3 percent of patients within the first several months of therapy. Most of these cases have been in patients with multiple medical problems including immune complex and neoplastic disease. Blood counts should be obtained during the first several months of therapy and periodically thereafter.

Patients with preexisting renal failure may develop a rise in serum creatinine and cases of acute renal failure have been reported. More commonly patients develop a renal glomerular lesion manifest as proteinuria (about 1

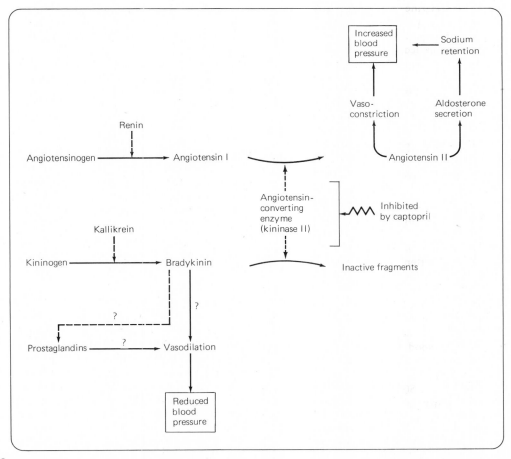

FIGURE 40-3

Mode of Action of Catopril. The renin-angiotensin-aldosterone and the kallikrein-kinin-prostaglandin systems have interrelated effects on blood pressure hemostasis. Angiotensin-converting enzyme (kininase II) converts angiotensin I to angiotensin II which can increase blood pressure. Captopril inhibits the effects of the angiotensin-converting enzyme. *(Modified from R. C. Heel et al., R. N. Brogden, et al., "Captopril: A Preliminary Review of Its Pharmacological Properties and Therapeutic Efficacy," Drugs **20**: 409, 1980.)*

to 2 percent of patients). Some of these develop nephrotic syndrome.

Rashes, fever, and allergic manifestations can occur in up to 10 percent of patients receiving captopril. Some of these reactions appear dose-dependent and may appear during the first several weeks of therapy. About 5 percent of patients report a change or loss of taste.

As an inhibitor of aldosterone release, captopril can increase serum potassium levels. It should not therefore be administered with **potassium** supplements or potassium-sparing diuretics. **Indomethacin** has been shown to decrease the effectiveness of captopril.

Dosage   In the treatment of hypertension, a starting dose of 25 mg three times a day is recommended. The dose can be increased in weekly intervals to a maximum dose of 150 mg three times daily. Other antihypertensive medications should be discontinued for several days to a week prior to the initiation of captopril to avoid acute hypotensive reactions. If captopril therapy alone is ineffective, a diuretic or β-blocking agent should be added to the regimen. The drug should be taken 1 h before meals.

Hypertensive Emergencies

Patients with malignant or accelerated hypertension or those with hypertensive crisis need aggressive intravenous antihypertensive therapy. The severity of the situation depends on the degree of blood pressure elevation and the evidence of acutely deteriorating end organ function. Patients with diastolic pressures in excess of 130 mmHg with either papilledema, acute left ventricular failure, neurologic impairment, acute renal failure, or acute myocardial ischemia are at risk for a life-threatening event. These patients need immediate lowering of the blood pressure. Patients with diastolic pressures above 120 or 130 mmHg without evidence of acutely changing end organ function can be treated more conservatively but should have their pressures lowered within a period of hours. In general, reducing the diastolic pressure to 100 mmHg acutely in these situations is acceptable. Obviously oral therapy to further reduce and maintain the blood pressure should be instituted as soon as possible.

Several antihypertensive drugs are available for parenteral administration. Of these, the two agents which are most frequently used to treat hypertensive emergencies are **nitroprusside** and **diazoxide**. **Trimethophan** (Arfonad), a rapidly acting agent which must be carefully titrated, is less frequently used (see Chap. 14). **Labetalol** is a new agent whose value in hypertensive crisis remains to be determined in clinical practice (see above). Parenteral **hydralazine** administration, by the intramuscular or intravenous route, is used when there is less urgency in lowering the pressure and is effective within 20 min. Parenteral **methyldopa** has a delayed onset of action, but can be used in hypertensive emergencies without impending end organ catastrophy.

Nitroprusside

Mechanism of Action   Nitroprusside (Nipride) produces rapid and profound dilation of both arterioles and venous capacitance vessels which results in an immediate drop in blood pressure. Because of its action to decrease both preload (venous blood return to the heart) and afterload (peripheral vascular resistance), there is little activation of the sympathetic nervous system to produce reflex tachycardia like that seen with other direct vasodilators such as **hydralazine** or **minoxidil**. Nitroprusside also improves cardiac output in patients with hypertension complicated by congestive heart failure. Myocardial ischemia and anginal pain associated with hypertensive emergencies are also improved with nitroprusside, although there is evidence to suggest that nitroprusside may steal blood away from ischemic tissue and shunt it to nonischemic tissue.

Pharmacokinetics   The drug has an immediate onset of action, and its effect is dissipated within minutes of discontinuation of the infusion. Nitroprusside combines with sulfhydryl groups in red blood cells and tissues to form cyanide which is then converted in the liver to thiocyanate. The thiocyanate is renally eliminated and has a serum half-life of approximately 5 days. Patients with renal insufficiency may accumulate thiocyanate to levels which may produce toxicity.

Adverse Effects   Hypotension is the most common adverse effect of nitroprusside and careful dosage titration can prevent or reverse this effect. Cyanide toxicity can be lethal but is fortunately a rare complication of nitroprusside therapy. Thiocyanate serum concentrations in excess of 10 μg/mL are associated with weakness, nausea, hypoxia, disorientation, psychotic behavior, and muscle spasm. These effects are most frequently reported in patients receiving the drug continuously for several days or in patients with renal failure.

Dosage   Nitroprusside is administered by intravenous infusion at an initial rate of 1 μg/kg/min. The average dose is about 3 μg/kg/min and the maximal dose is dependent upon the blood pressure response and probably should not exceed 800 μg/min. Preparations of nitroprusside are stable for 24 h. When the drug is being administered the infusion bottle should be wrapped in a light-protective covering. A light-protective wrapping is supplied with the drug by the manufacturer, but any other opaque material can be used.

Diazoxide

Mechanism of Action   Diazoxide (Hyperstat) is chemically related to the thiazide diuretics but possesses no diuretic effect. Its antihypertensive properties are due to direct arteriolar dilation. Due to its lack of effect on the venous bed an increase in cardiac output and heart rate are commonly seen.

Pharmacokinetics   Diazoxide is ineffective orally and must be administered intravenously. The drug should be given in a rapid bolus (less than 30 s) with the patient in a recumbent position for maximal efficacy. It is highly bound to serum proteins and approximately one-third of the drug is excreted renally. Uremic patients have a greater than usual response to diazoxide and a lower dose is indicated in these patients.

Adverse Effects   Excessive hypotension sometimes resulting in myocardial ischemia and infarction has been reported with rapid administration of 300-mg doses of diazoxide. Patients with a history of ischemic heart disease are at greatest risk. Administration of 100-mg bolus doses may decrease the risk of hypotension and ischemia.

Multiple doses of diazoxide commonly produce marked sodium and water retention, causing edema. This effect should be anticipated and treated with **thiazide diuretics** or **furosemide**.

Diabetics may exhibit hyperglycemia when given multiple doses of diazoxide; an increased dose of insulin may be temporarily necessary. Other side effects include gastrointestinal disturbances, headaches, and localized pain if the drug extravasates on administration.

Dosage   **Diazoxide** may be administered as rapid bolus injections in 100- to 300-mg doses. The recommended dose of diazoxide by rapid IV injection is 1 to 3 mg/kg up to a maximum of 150 mg. This dose can be repeated in 15 to 30 min until a satisfactory reduction in blood pressure has been achieved. This minibolus dosing may produce less adverse effects than will rapid administration of 300 mg in a single dose.

NURSING PROCESS RELATED TO HYPERTENSION

Assessment

The nurse has a unique opportunity to work with the hypertensive patient and family to contribute to the control of elevated blood pressure. Identification of specific factors which produce blood pressure elevation can lead to appropriate intervention which will in turn eliminate or reduce the impact of these factors. Smoking, obesity, lack of exercise, excessive sodium intake, stressful interpersonal relationships, and complex drug regimens can all impact negatively on the patient's blood pressure. The degree to which any of these factors triggers a loss of blood pressure control must be carefully evaluated on an individual basis. The nurse should assist the patient in discovering which of these "triggers" is most important and how several of these can interact. For example in a period of increased personal stress, it is likely that hypertensive patients may forget to take their medications and/or increase their food intake. The patient then comes to the practitioner and finds an elevated blood pressure. The nurse can help the patient understand how each of these factors can contribute to the loss of blood pressure control. All of this should be accomplished through a thoughtful, calm discussion between nurse and patient.

Involvement of a spouse or significant other is very valuable in the assessment of contributing factors in elevated blood pressure. Adherence to the planned regimen is also increased if the spouse or significant other is involved. Home monitoring of blood pressure helps hypertensives observe their own responsiveness. Patients can learn what factors are contributing to their change in blood pressure by home measurement.

Management

The nurse should inform the patient about environmental factors which contribute to changes in blood pressure. Talking rapidly, lack of sleep, and strenuous exercise all contribute to elevations in blood pressure. Deep breathing, adequate sleeping, relaxation, and meditation can help lower blood pressure. The measurement of blood pressure itself can effect the blood pressure level. In a stressed environment blood pressures are higher than in a relaxed, calm atmosphere.

Tangible social support, patient education, a simple medical regimen, and few side effects increase compliance in blood pressure management. The nurse has a vital role in each of these processes. Negotiating a plan of care that is acceptable and understood by the patient and family helps to insure the patient's adherence to the plan. Patient education and good interpersonal relationships between the nurse and the patient allow a reasonable, safe plan to be negotiated. Open communication allows the patient to discuss any difficulties with the drug regimen with the nurse. Specific measures can be employed to decrease unpleasant side effects or increase the chance of patient compliance. For example, most antihypertensive drugs can be administered once or twice a day. Diuretic drugs which initially cause increased urinary frequency should be administered in the morning to prevent nocturia. Multiple drug regimens, when required, can be established by combining drugs with differing mechanisms of action (e.g., **hydrochlorothiazide** and **propranolol**) and side effects so that two drugs with sedative properties (**methyldopa** and **clonidine**) are not used in the same regimen.

When blood pressure control requires more than one

TABLE 40-6 Antihypertensive Combination Preparations*

PREPARATION	DIURETIC, mg	RAUWOLFIA DERIVATIVE, mg	OTHER, mg
Serpasil-Esidrix #2 tabs	Hydroclorothiazide (50)	Reserpine (0.1)	
Serpasil-Esidrix #1 tabs	Hydrochlorothiazide (25)	Reserpine (0.1)	
Hydropres-50 tablets	Hydrochlorothiazide (50)	Reserpine (0.125)	
Diutensen-R tabs	Methyclothiazide (2.5)	Reserpine (0.1)	
Demi-Regroton tablets	Chlorthalidone (25)	Reserpine (0.125)	
Renese-R tablets	Polythiazide (2)	Reserpine (0.25)	
Enduronyl tablets	Methyclothiazide (5)	Deserpidine (0.25)	
Ser-Ap-Es tablets	Hydrochlorothiazide (15)	Reserpine (0.1)	Hydralazine (25)
Inderide tablets 80/25	Hydrochlorothiazide (25)		Propranolol (80)
Inderide tablets 40/25	Hydrochlorothiazide (25)		Propranolol (40)
Aldoclor-250 tabs	Chlorothiazide (250)		Methyldopa (250)
Aldoclor-150 tabs	Chlorothiazide (150)		Methyldopa (250)
Timolide	Hydrochlorothiazide (25)		Timolol (10)
Esimil tablets	Hydrochlorothiazide (25)		Guanethidine (10)
Combipres 0.2 tablets	Chlorthalidone (15)		Clonidine HCl (0.2)
Corzide	Bendroflumethiazide (5)		Nadolol (40)
Minizide 2 capsules	Polythiazine (0.5)		Prazosin (2)

*Selected preparations; numerous other combinations are marketed.

agent, it may be possible to utilize fixed combination drug products. However, such products should only be used when blood pressure control has been previously achieved by individual titration of one drug at a time resulting in the desired therapeutic effect. Use of fixed drug combination products before achieving adequate blood pressure prevents the adjustment of the dosage of one drug at a time, a decided therapeutic disadvantage. Some combination products are listed in Table 40-6.

CASE STUDY

Mr. D.M., a 40-year-old salesman, was diagnosed as having high blood pressure two years earlier.

Assessment

In reviewing the patient's past history, the nurse noted that Mr. M. had changed jobs just prior to his last appointment one month earlier. His blood pressure had been stable at 130/86 for one year prior to his last appointment. At his last appointment his blood pressure was 156/110. His medications were hydrochlorothiazide 50 mg daily and clonidine 0.4 mg bid. At that time, propranolol 20 mg bid was added to his regimen. He was instructed to continue on his moderate salt diet.

His medical workup revealed no hypercholesterolemia,

Evaluation

Accurate blood pressure measurement at home and by the nurse provides an objective assessment of the treatment plan. Evaluation of a patient's difficulties with the planned regimen allows for renegotiation of the treatment. Changes in the plan of care are quickly and effectively negotiated when the patient is allowed to freely discuss problems with the nurse.

obesity, myocardial infarction, diabetes mellitus, or symptoms consistent with a secondary form of high blood pressure. The patient gave a positive family history of cardiovascular disease, with both his mother and his father having died of a heart attack. D.M. did not smoke or drink. Chest x-ray, ECG, and fundoscopic examination were normal.

The patient's blood pressure at this visit was 160/110 with a pulse rate of 85. The nurse asked the patient if he had been taking his medicines as prescribed. D.M. replied that he "couldn't take the medicines and do my job." He then described the changes that had occurred in his life over the previous two months. In his new job he was working at least a 10-h day. He felt fatigued and was sleeping poorly prior to the last visit. Since his medication was increased, he felt even more exhausted. He stated that he was irritable and had not been able to function sexually with his wife. He then stopped taking his clonidine and propranolol. After he discontinued these medicines he felt better and had more energy. He stated that he had been carefully watching his diet.

Management

The nurse recognized that a complex interaction of factors had resulted in uncontrolled hypertension. After her explanation D.M. stated, "I can't live my life with the medicines, but I'll die without them." The nurse and patient then discussed the factors involved in his increase in blood pressure. The nurse consulted with the pharmacist and physician and a change in drug regimen was planned. His medicines were altered to hydrochlorothiazide 50 mg daily and prazosin 2 mg bid. He was told to begin the prazosin with the first dose at bedtime to avoid the first dose syncope phenomenon and that he should take his diuretic early in the day to avoid drug-induced nocturia during the first few weeks of therapy. In addition, he was reeducated about the need for uninterrupted therapy in the treatment of hypertension and about the necessity of seeking professional guidance from the nurse, physician, or pharmacist when new symptoms which he could attribute to drug therapy occurred.

Mr. M. then discussed with the nurse his usual day. They agreed that his extended hours were contributing to his exhaustion. He agreed to cut back to an 8-h work day. He reviewed his diet with the nurse and showed an excellent understanding of a low sodium diet. He also agreed to monitor his blood pressures at home.

Evaluation

At the next clinic visit, two weeks later, D.M.'s blood pressure was 136/84 and pulse was 85. His home pressures ranged from 128 to 134/78 to 82 after shortening his hours, and he actually was accomplishing more work. His sleep pattern and sexual function had returned to normal. He was enthusiastic over the new drug regimen and delighted at his blood pressure control. He planned to continue to monitor his blood pressure at home and return to the clinic in one month.

REFERENCES

Brunner, H. R., H. Gavras, and B. Waeber: "Oral Angiotensin-Converting Enzyme Inhibitor in Long Term Treatment of Hypertensive Patients," *Ann Intern Med,* **90:**19–23, 1979.

Caplan, R., R. Van Harrison, R. V. Wellons, and B. French: "Social Support and Patient Adherence," Ann Arbor, Mich.: The University of Michigan, Institute for Social Research, 1980.

Cohn, J. N., and L. P. Burke: "Nitroprusside," *Ann Intern Med,* **91:**752–757, 1979.

Colluci, W. S.: "Alpha-Adrenergic Receptor Blockade with Prazosin," *Ann Intern Med,* **97:**67–77, 1982.

Dasta, J. F.: "Metoprolol," *Drug Intell Clin Pharm,* **13:**320–322, 1979.

Dyer, A. R., J. Stamler, O. Paul, D. M. Berkson, M. K. Lepper, H. McKean, R. B. Shekelle, H. A. Lindberg, and D. Garside: "Alcohol Consumption, Cardiovascular Risk Factors, and Mortality in Two Chicago Epidemiologic Studies," *Circulation,* **56:**1067–1074, 1977.

Ferguson, R. K., and P. H. Vlasses: "Clinical Pharmacology and Therapeutic Applications of the New Oral Angiotensin Converting Enzyme Inhibitor, Captopril," *Am Heart J,* **101:**650–656, 1981.

Frishman, W. H.: "Nadolol: A New Beta-Adrenoreceptor Antagonist," *N Engl J of Med,* **305:**678–681, 1981.

———: "Atenolol and Timolol, Two New Systemic Beta-Adrenoreceptor Antagonists," *N Engl J Med,* **306:**1456–1462, 1982.

Graham, R. M., and W. Pettinger: "Prazosin," *N Engl J Med,* **300:**232–235, 1979.

Hill, M, and J. W. Fink: "In Hypertensive Emergencies Act Quickly But Also Act Cautiously," *Nursing 83,* **13:**34–42, 1983.

Johnson, G. P., and B. C. Johanson: "β Blockers," *Am J Nurs,* **83:**1034–1043, 1983.

Kamada, S. A., D. J. Kanada, R. A. Hutchinson, and D. Wu: "Angina-Like Syndrome with Diazoxide Therapy for Hypertensive Crisis," *Ann Intern Med,* **84:**696–699, 1976.

Kaplan, N. M.: *Clinical Hypertension,* 2d ed., Baltimore: Williams and Wilkins, 1978.

———: "New Approaches to the Therapy of Mild Hypertension," *Am J Cardiol,* **51:**621–627, 1983.

Koch-Weser, J.: "Hydralazine," *N Engl J Med,* **295:**320–322, 1976.

Long, J. M., J. J. Lynch, N. M. Machiran, S. A. Thomas, and K. L. Malinow: "The Effect of Status on Blood Pressure During Verbal Communication," *J Behav Med,* **5:**165–172, 1982.

Longsworth, D. L., J. I. Drayer, M. A. Wever, and J. H. Laragh: "Divergent Blood Pressure Responses During Short Term Sodium Restriction in Hypertension," *Clin Pharmacol Ther,* **27:**544–546, 1980.

MacCarthy, E. P., and S. S. Bloomfield: "Labetalol: A Review of Its Pharmacology, Pharmacokinetics, Clinical Uses, and Adverse Effects," *Pharmacotherapy,* 3:193–219, 1983.

Mroczek, W. J., B. A. Liebel, and F. A. Finnerty: "Comparison of Clonidine and Methyldopa in Hypertensive Patients Receiving a Diuretic," *Am J Cardiol,* 29:712–717, 1972.

Multiple Risk Factor Intervention Trial Research Group: "Multiple Risk Factor Intervention Trial," *JAMA,* 248:1465–1477, 1982.

Palmer, R. F., and K. C. Lasseter: "Sodium Nitroprusside," *N Engl J Med,* 292:294–297, 1975.

Reisin, E., R. Abel, M. Modal, D. S. Silverberg, H. E. Eliahou, and B. Modan: "Effect of Weight Loss without Salt Reduction or Reduction of Blood Pressure in Overweight Hypertensive Patients," *N Engl J Med,* 298:1–6, 1978.

Shoback, D. M., and G. H. Williams: "Potassium Sparing Diuretics: Clinical Pharmacology and Therapeutic Uses," *Drug Ther,* 13–23, 1982.

Tobian, L.: "Obesity and Hypertension," *N Engl J Med,* 248:46, 1978.

Venkata, S. R., and N. M. Kaplan: "Individual Titration of Diazoxide Dosage in the Treatment of Severe Hypertension," *Am J Cardiol,* 43:627–000, 1979.

Vidt, D. G., E. L. Bravo, and F. M. Fouad: "Captopril," *N Engl J Med,* 306:214–219, 1982.

Wade, D. W.: "Teaching Patients to Live with Chronic Orthostatic Hypotension," *Nursing 82,* 12:64–65, 1982.

Walker, B. A., B. E. Schneider, and J. A. Gold: "A Two Year Evaluation of Guanabenz in the Treatment of Hypertension," *Curr Ther Res,* 27:784–796, 1980.

——, R. S. Rajnikant, and K. B. Ramanathan: "Guanabenz and Methyldopa on Hypertension and Cardiac Performance," *Clin Pharmacol Ther,* 22:868–874, 1977.

Woolsey, R. L., and A. S. Nies: "Guanethedine," *N Engl J Med,* 295:1053–1057, 1976.

41

DISORDERS OF LIPOPROTEINS

ARTHUR F. HARRALSON
DOROTHY L. DIEHL

LEARNING OBJECTIVES

Upon mastery of the content of this chapter, the reader will be able to:

1. Identify the categories of patients that should be screened for hyperlipidemia.
2. Describe the significant items of the medical history which should be obtained from patients screened for hyperlipidemia.
3. Recognize the common manifestations of hyperlipidemia.
4. Assess the patient's understanding of the etiology, effects, and management of hyperlipoproteinemia and its relationship to other cardiac risk factors.
5. List the medication of choice in treatment of each type of hyperlipidemia.
6. Describe the mechanism of action, dosage, and adverse effects for the following antilipid drugs: clofibrate, nicotinic acid, bile acid sequestrant agents, probucol, and gemfibrozil.
7. Describe the nursing management and patient education related to the administration of the antilipemic drugs.

Hyperlipidemia is a disorder characterized by elevation of the plasma cholesterol and triglycerides. *Primary familial hyperlipoproteinemia* refers to the elevation of plasma cholesterol and triglycerides as a result of a hereditary abnormality of lipid metabolism. *Secondary hyperlipidemia* may result from a number of causes including alcoholism, hypothyroidism, nephrotic syndrome, diabetes mellitus, pregnancy, biliary obstruction, dysglobulinemia, and certain drugs (**thiazide diuretics, estrogens, corticosteroids,** chronic **alcohol** intake). The clinical manifestation of hyperlipidemia may include episodic abdominal pain, hepatosplenomegaly, pancreatitis, ischemic heart disease, claudication, and various forms of xanthoma (yellow nodules on skin).

The relationship between coronary artery disease and hyperlipidemia has led to the development of numerous drug and diet regimens that are effective in correcting hyperlipidemias. Many of the clinical abnormalities associated with hyperlipidemias, such as xanthomas and episodic abdominal pain, can be effectively treated with agents that lower plasma lipids. The efficacy of any given drug depends on its effect on the production or removal of the particular lipoproteins present in excess for each type of hyperlipoproteinemia. Although evidence is accumulating, it remains to be conclusively proved whether correcting elevated plasma lipids will prevent the development or further progression of coronary artery disease and whether all methods of reducing plasma lipids (diet, various drugs) will have equal beneficial effects.

LIPOPROTEIN COMPONENTS OF PLASMA

Plasma lipoproteins are complex macromolecules composed of varying amounts of cholesterol, triglyceride, and phospholipid noncovalently bound to protein. The lipoprotein macromolecule acts as a carrier to transport water-insoluble lipids through the bloodstream. The varying proportions of cholesterol, triglycerides, phospholipids, and protein found in lipoproteins impart different chemical and physical properties to the macromolecule. These differences permit identification of various classifications of lipoproteins by ultracentrifugation and electrophoresis (Table 41-1). Once the specific type of hyperlipidemia is identified, a numerical classification is used to indicate which lipoproteins are elevated (Table 41-2).

Premature atherosclerosis is thought to be associated with those hyperlipoproteinemias involving very-low-density lipoproteins (VLDL), intermediate-density lipoproteins (IDL), and low-density lipoproteins (LDL). In contrast, increased levels of high-density lipoproteins (HDL) may retard atherogenesis and do not represent a risk factor for the development of coronary artery disease.

TABLE 41-1 Lipid Composition of the Various Lipoprotein Classifications

CLASSIFICATION	CHOLESTEROL, %	TRIGLYCERIDES, %
Chylomicrons	5	90
Very-low-density lipoproteins	12	60
Intermediate-density lipoproteins	30	40
Low-density lipoproteins	50	10
High-density lipoproteins	20	5

CLINICAL FINDINGS

Patients with hyperlipidemia are often asymptomatic and the abnormality is identified after a random screening procedure or as part of the workup of some other symptom complex. In most clinical situations, the initial screening involves the measurement of cholesterol and triglycerides. This test is performed after a week of normal dietary intake and a 12-h fast, if possible. The use of oral contraceptives, estrogens, and lipid-lowering drugs should be discontinued a week or more before the test to avoid misinterpretation of the results. The test results should always be interpreted in terms of the patient's age and gender. The levels of cholesterol and triglycerides are generally higher in men than in premenopausal women. Postmenopausal women, however, have cholesterol levels similar to men of the same age. Although the values generally rise with age, elevated values should not be considered "normal" in the older population. The risk of myocardial infarction appears higher in patients with cholesterol levels above 220 mg/mL. Likewise, fasting triglyceride levels above 150 mg/mL may represent a risk factor in the development of coronary artery disease.

The second stage of the laboratory diagnostic procedure, typing by lipoprotein electrophoresis, is generally carried out only if there is a good chance that one of the familial

TABLE 41-2 Classification of Hyperlipidemia by Hyperlipoprotein Type

HYPERLIPOPROTEIN TYPE	CLASS OF LIPOPROTEIN FOUND ELEVATED
I	Chylomicrons
IIa	Low-density lipoproteins
IIb	Low-density and very-low-density lipoproteins
III	Intermediate-density lipoproteins
IV	Very-low-density lipoproteins
V	Very-low-density lipoproteins and chylomicrons

disorders will be discovered. In these instances, typing can serve as a guide to specific dietary and drug management. In the average patient population, where most cases of hyperlipidemia are found on random screening surveys in asymptomatic adults, typing is probably not indicated.

A thorough review of the possible secondary causes of the lipoprotein abnormality, such as diabetes, hypothyroidism, and liver disease, must be undertaken since drug treatment with antilipemic agents may not be indicated in these situations. The patient should also be questioned to determine whether they are taking any medications which may produce or exacerbate lipoprotein abnormalities.

CLINICAL PHARMACOLOGY AND THERAPEUTICS

The treatment of hyperlipidemia should always begin with appropriate modification of the patient's diet. Specific diets for each hyperlipoprotein type are used in the primary familial disorders and in severe cases of the secondary forms (Table 41-3). For most patients with slight to moderate elevation of lipid levels, a general diet with control of excessive carbohydrate intake, decreased cholesterol intake, and substitution of polyunsaturated for saturated fats suffices. If the diet does not produce an acceptable decrease in the plasma lipid levels or if the initial lipid level is very high, as in certain familial hyperlipoproteinemias, the addition of a lipid-lowering drug may be necessary. Selection of the appropriate drug is based on identification of the type of lipoprotein that is elevated. Continued therapy with a particular drug depends upon an acceptable reduction in lipids as well as the absence of significant adverse effects. A reduction of less than 15 percent in lipid levels is probably not sufficient to justify long-term therapy.

The drugs currently available for the treatment of hyperlipidemia vary markedly in their mechanisms of action, clinical effects, and adverse effects. Despite this variation, they can generally be placed into three different categories based on their clinical effect or mechanism of action. These three basic categories include (1) drugs that alter lipoprotein production (**clofibrate, probucol, gemfibrozil**); (2) drugs that alter lipoprotein metabolism (**nicotinic acid, dextrothyroxine**); (3) drugs that alter the removal of lipoprotein from the circulation (**bile acid sequestrants, β-sitosterol**).

Clofibrate

Clofibrate (Atromid-S) is effective in several types of hyperlipidemia. It is well tolerated by most patients even with prolonged use.

Indications Clofibrate is the drug of choice in the treatment of types III and IV hyperlipoproteinemia. It is somewhat less effective in the treatment of type V and is not indicated in type I. Its effect on type II hyperlipoproteinemia is variable and in some patients may even produce an increase in the cholesterol component of LDL.

TABLE 41-3 Nondrug and Drug Management of Hyperlipoproteinemia

TYPE	GOAL	CALORIES	FAT	CARBOHYDRATE	CHOLESTEROL	SATURATED FATS*	DRUGS†
I	Maintain free of abdominal pain	Unrestricted	Restrict to 25–35 g/day	Higher because of fat restriction	Unrestricted	P/S ratio not important	None
II	Decrease serum cholesterol	Unrestricted	Unrestricted	Unrestricted	300 mg/day	High P/S ratio	Primary: bile acid sequestrants Secondary: probucol or β-sitosterol
III	Decrease serum cholesterol and triglycerides	Restricted	40% of daily calories	35% of daily calories (eliminate concentrated sugars)	<300 mg/day	High P/S ratio	Primary: clofibrate Secondary: nicotinic acid
IV	Decrease serum triglycerides	Restricted	40% of daily calories	45% of daily calories (restrict concentrated sugars)	300 mg/day	High P/S ratio	Primary: clofibrate Secondary: nicotinic acid or gemfibrozil
V	Decrease serum triglycerides and eliminate abdominal pain	Restricted	30% of daily calories	50% of daily calories	Moderately restricted	High P/S ratio	Primary: nicotinic acid Secondary: clofibrate

*Ratio of polyunsaturated to saturated fat.
†Primary drug is the drug of choice. Secondary drug is used if the primary drug is contraindicated or ineffective.

Mechanism of Action   Clofibrate acts to decrease the concentrations of endogenously synthesized triglycerides of VLDL primarily through the inhibition of synthesis or secretion by the liver. Several peripheral mechanisms, however, have also been postulated. Clofibrate generally reduces plasma triglycerides by approximately 25 percent. Its effect on plasma cholesterol is somewhat less pronounced, generally producing no more than a 5 to 10 percent reduction.

Pharmacokinetics   Clofibrate is completely absorbed following oral administration and is rapidly metabolized to an active metabolite, *p*-chloroisobutyric acid (CPIB). CPIB reaches peak concentrations in the plasma within 3 to 6 h following administration of clofibrate and approximately 95 percent is bound to plasma albumin. The majority of CPIB is excreted in the urine as the glucuronide conjugate and marked accumulation of CPIB can occur in patients with renal impairment. Following the peak concentration, the plasma concentrations of CPIB exhibit a biphasic decline with half-lives of 15 and 54 h, respectively.

Adverse Effects   Clofibrate is well tolerated by most patients, and the incidence of serious side effects appears to be relatively low. The most common side effects reported are abdominal discomfort, nausea, and diarrhea. Breast tenderness and a decrease in libido are also among the more frequent complaints reported by males taking clofibrate. Urticaria, alopecia, brittle hair, skin eruptions and dryness, and weight gain have all been reported as side effects associated with clofibrate. Transient changes in liver function tests and a myositis-like syndrome have been reported, but are rare and usually reversible on discontinuation of the drug. The myositis-like syndrome consists of muscular stiffness, pain, malaise, and an increased serum creatinine phosphokinase. Other serious side effects that have been reported with clofibrate use include an increase in the incidence of cholelithiasis, nonfatal pulmonary emboli, angina pectoris, intermittent claudication, and cardiac arrhythmias.

Clofibrate interacts with numerous other medications. The action of the oral anticoagulant **warfarin** may be potentiated by the concomitant use of clofibrate. The presumed mechanism for this interaction involves displacement of warfarin from plasma protein binding sites. The overall effect of clofibrate on anticoagulation may also involve an increase in fibrinolytic activity, as well as an alteration in platelet adhesiveness. With concomitant use of clofibrate and oral anticoagulants, the anticoagulant dosage should be decreased by one-half and prothrombin time should be monitored. Because of its high degree of plasma protein binding, clofibrate has the potential for interacting with other drugs which are also highly bound to albumin (listed in Table 6-6).

Dosage   Clofibrate is given orally in doses of 500 mg, two to four times a day, usually with meals.

Nicotinic Acid

Nicotinic acid, or niacin, is one of the B vitamins which had its first clinical use in the treatment of pellagra. When used in doses much higher than necessary for its effect as a vitamin, it has been shown to have a significant hypolipemic effect. However the side effects and adverse reactions of nicotinic acid occur relatively frequently and limit its use.

Indications   Because nicotinic acid lowers cholesterol, triglycerides, and LDL and VLDL levels, it will reduce plasma lipid levels in all types of hyperlipoproteinemia except type I. Nicotinic acid is very effective in types III, IV, and V hyperlipoproteinemia. Its use in type II probably is of most benefit when it is combined with **cholestyramine**.

Mechanism of Action   The mechanism of action of nicotinic acid in reducing lipid levels is not completely understood, although a number of hypotheses have been proposed. Nicotinic acid depresses the level of circulating free fatty acids by inhibiting their mobilization from adipose tissue. The reduction in the quantity of free fatty acids available for triglyceride synthesis in the liver would be expected to decrease the plasma triglyceride levels.

There is also evidence that there may be a direct hepatic depression of VLDL synthesis. The reduction in plasma cholesterol levels produced by nicotinic acid occurs at a slower rate than that of triglycerides and may be a result of the slower turnover rate of LDL. It is also suggested that nicotinic acid acts to inhibit certain coenzymes involved in cholesterol synthesis. A catabolic effect of nicotinic acid with an increase in the oxidation of cholesterol has also been observed.

Pharmacokinetics   Nicotinic acid is rapidly absorbed from the gastrointestinal tract and peak plasma concentrations are reached within 45 min. Approximately 70 percent of the drug is metabolized and the remainder is excreted unchanged in the urine. Despite a short half-life of 45 min, decreases in plasma triglycerides occur in 1 to 4 days and decreases in plasma cholesterol occur in 5 to 7 days of continuous therapy.

Adverse Effects   Nicotinic acid produces a number of side effects, the most frequent being an intense cutaneous flushing and pruritus that appear a few hours after administration of the drug. The flush generally occurs in the upper part of the body and usually disappears after several days of taking the drug. Some patients, however, report recurrent episodes of cutaneous flushing with prolonged use of nicotinic acid. Increased pigmentation of the skin and skin dryness are seen less frequently and are reversible on discontinuation of the drug.

Gastrointestinal symptoms such as nausea, diarrhea, and abdominal pain are frequently reported with the use of nicotinic acid. These side effects are generally self-limited, but nicotinic acid may aggravate preexisting peptic ulceration.

Taking the drug with meals may be of some benefit. Among the more serious side effects of nicotinic acid is an impairment of liver function. In patients who develop abnormalities in liver function tests, liver biopsies have shown ultrastructure alterations in the mitochondria and endoplasmic reticulum. A few cases of jaundice have also been reported. Most liver function abnormalities appear to regress a few weeks after the drug is discontinued. Nicotinic acid has been noted to induce other metabolic abnormalities, including glucose intolerance and hyperuricemia. In patients with preexisting hyperuricemia, nicotinic acid can precipitate acute gout. Patients with overt diabetes may become more difficult to control. In patients without overt diabetes, nicotinic acid may produce an abnormal glucose tolerance test and, occasionally, glycosuria. Preexisting liver disease, hyperuricemia, diabetes mellitus, and peptic ulcer disease may be considered relative contraindications to the use of nicotinic acid. Although drug interactions are not common with nicotinic acid, it may enhance the hypotensive effects of ganglionic blocking agents.

Dosage   The usual adult maintenance dose of nicotinic acid is 3 g/day orally, divided in three doses. Administration at meal times reduces gastric irritation and may enhance absorption. Better patient acceptance may be achieved by starting with low doses (100 to 250 mg tid) and progressing to full maintenance doses over a period of 1 to 3 weeks.

Bile Acid–Sequestering Resins (Cholestyramine, Colestipol)

Bile acid sequestrants (BAS), such as **cholestyramine resin** (Questran) and **colestipol** (Colestid), are high-molecular-weight anion exchange resins. They are insoluble in water and are not absorbed from the gastrointestinal tract. These resins exchange chloride ions for bile acids, eliminating the bile acid from the enterohepatic circulation.

Indications   BAS are used almost exclusively in the treatment of type II hyperlipoproteinemia and should be considered the drug of choice in that abnormality. The effect of BAS augments that of diet, producing an additional 20 to 25 percent reduction in plasma cholesterol. Patients may exhibit an elevation in plasma triglycerides after beginning to use BAS, but this effect is generally transient.

Mechanism of Action   The major route of elimination of cholesterol from the body is biliary excretion with subsequent loss in the feces. BAS binds bile acids in exchange for chloride ions and prevents reabsorption of the bile through the enterohepatic cycle. The increased loss of acidic sterol in the feces results in a compensatory increase in the production of bile acids and a secondary increase in the conversion of cholesterol to bile acids. Although cholesterol and bile acid production increase, there also appears to be a compensatory increase in cholesterol catabolism. Whether the reduction in serum cholesterol is due to a net negative balance between cholesterol synthesis and catabolism or to a reported increase in LDL catabolism with BAS remains unclear.

Pharmacokinetics   Since BAS are not absorbed from the gastrointestinal tract, they are not metabolized or excreted in the urine. Essentially all of the administered BAS is excreted from the body in the feces.

Adverse Effects   The most frequently reported side effects with use of BAS involve the gastrointestinal tract. The complaints include constipation, nausea, vomiting, abdominal distention, and cramps. These problems usually occur early in therapy and subside with continued administration, but may be severe enough to require withdrawal of the drug or a reduction in the dosage. Constipation, probably the most common complaint, can be treated easily with stool softeners such as **docusate sodium** (DOSS). BAS-induced steatorrhea is generally not seen even at doses of 32 g/day. Another rare but serious side effect that is usually seen only in small children is hyperchloremic acidosis from the chloride ion exchange for bile acids. Other reported side effects of long-term BAS therapy may include biliary calcification and slight elevation of alkaline phosphatase levels.

Patients with malabsorption syndrome and those who have had an ileal-bypass operation should not be given BAS. In the usual dosage range, there is probably not much interference with the absorption of dietary fat, calcium, or the fat-soluble vitamins. There have, however, been some reports of impaired absorption of fat-soluble vitamins (A, D, E, and K) when BAS are taken in doses greater than 24 g/day. BAS may interfere with the absorption of a number of drugs, including **digoxin, warfarin, thiazide diuretics, phenylbutazone, phenobarbital**, and some antibiotics. To avoid possible problems with drug absorption, oral medications should be taken at least 1 h before or 4 h after BAS are administered.

Dosage   The usual adult dosage of BAS is 16 to 32 g/day orally in two to four divided doses. In most regimens, BAS are initially added to the dietary regimen in a dosage of 16 g/day and then increased until the maximu   response or 32 g/day is reached. To increase its palatability, BAS are usually mixed with fruit juice or applesauce.

Probucol

Probucol (Lorelco) is an effective agent for use in the reduction of elevated serum cholesterol. Its chemical structure is unique and it does not appear to act by a mechanism similar to that of any other cholesterol-lowering agent.

Indications   Probucol is effective in reducing elevated cholesterol in patients with primary hypercholesterolemia. Probucol may have some value in the treatment of combined hypercholesterolemia and hypertriglyceridemia. It is not indicated, however, when the principal abnormality is elevated serum triglycerides.

Mechanism of Action   Probucol appears to act by inhibiting the early stages of cholesterol biosynthesis, increasing excretion of fecal bile acids and minimally inhibiting absorption of dietary cholesterol. Since there is no increase in the cyclic precursors of cholesterol, the latter stages of cholesterol biosynthesis do not appear to be affected by probucol. Probucol lowers cholesterol in both low-density and some high-density lipoprotein fractions. The potential risk associated with the concomitant reduction in some high-density lipoproteins is not known at this time. Probucol is intended for long-term therapy and the maximal effects occur after about three months of therapy.

Pharmacokinetics   Probucol is poorly absorbed following oral administration with only 10 percent reaching the systemic circulation. Despite its limited absorption, the drug accumulates in adipose tissue and may persist in the blood for over six months after being discontinued. Probucol is primarily metabolized and very little is excreted unchanged in the urine.

Adverse Effects   The most common adverse effects reported with the use of **probucol** are diarrhea, abdominal pain, and nausea. These gastrointestinal reactions are generally transient and may not require discontinuation of the drug. Changes in laboratory tests that have been observed include elevations in serum transaminases, bilirubin, alkaline phosphatase, uric acid, blood urea nitrogen, creatine phosphokinase, and blood glucose. The relationship between these abnormal laboratory values and the use of probucol, however, has not been well defined. Some patients experience an idiosyncratic reaction to probucol that is characterized by dizziness, palpitations, syncope, nausea, and chest pain.

Dosage   The maximum adult dose of probucol is 1000 mg orally given in two divided doses. Probucol is usually given with the morning and evening meals.

Gemfibrozil

Gemfibrozil (Lopid) is used for the treatment of type IV hyperlipidemia which is characterized by very high serum triglyceride levels. Its use is limited to those patients who are at risk for developing abdominal pain and pancreatitis who have not responded adequately to dietary restrictions. Gemfibrozil does not appear to be useful for the treatment of type I hyperlipidemia and has little effect on elevated cholesterol in most patients.

Mechanism of Action   The mechanism of action of gemfibrozil in humans has not been clearly defined. From animal studies, however, gemfibrozil appears to have a number of actions including inhibition of basal lipolysis, reduction of incorporation of long-chain fatty acids into triglycerides, stimulation of liver sterol production, reduction in accumulation of dietary cholesterol, and enhanced fecal excretion of cholesterol. The net effect in humans has been shown to be a reduction in the levels of VLDL and LDL lipoproteins and an increase in HDL lipoproteins.

Pharmacokinetics   Gemfibrozil is well absorbed following oral administration. It is primarily metabolized undergoing hepatic glucuronidation and enterohepatic circulation. The glucuronide metabolite is renally excreted. The half-life of gemfibrozil is approximately 90 min.

Adverse Effects   The most frequently reported adverse reaction associated with the use of gemfibrozil involve the gastrointestinal system. Abdominal pain, epigastric pain, diarrhea, nausea, and vomiting have all been associated with gemfibrozil administration. Other side effects that have been reported include dermatitis, headaches, dizziness, liver function abnormalities, and various hematopoietic alterations.

Since gemfibrozil is pharmacologically similar to **clofibrate**, many of the problems associated with clofibrate may also apply to gemfibrozil. These problems may include a higher risk of gall bladder disease and a statistically higher mortality rate from noncardiovascular causes.

Dosage   The usual adult dose of gemfibrozil is 1200 mg/day orally given in two divided doses. Gemfibrozil is usually given 30 min before both the morning and evening meal.

Dextrothyroxin

Sodium dextrothyroxin is an isomer of the naturally occuring thyroid hormone that reportedly lowers plasma cholesterol without excessive stimulation of metabolism. All thyroid active agents act to increase both synthesis and catabolism of hepatic cholesterol. Dextrothyroxine preferentially reduces LDL, and therefore its primary use should be in patients with type II hyperlipidemia.

The clinical use of dextrothyroxines has been limited by what appears to be an increase in mortality with its use compared to placebo. Dextrothyroxine was eliminated from trial in the Coronary Drug Project (1975) when it was discovered that, with its use, there was an excess mortality and higher rate of nonfatal myocardial infarctions in patients with pretreatment evidence of old myocardial infarction, angina pectoris, hypertension, or abnormal ECG. In addition to cardiotoxicity, dextrothyroxine has also been associated with glucose intolerance, abnormal liver function tests, and neutropenia. Dextrothyroxine can also affect **warfarin** dosage and tends to potentiate the action of **digitalis** glycosides.

Although the cardiotoxicity of dextrothyroxine limits its use in patients with preexisting cardiovascular disease, it may be some use in patients who have hyperlipidemia but appear to be free from cardiovascular problems. The usual adult dosage is 4 to 8 mg/day orally given as a single dose.

TABLE 41-4   Nursing Process Related to Antilipemic Drugs

ASSESSMENT	MANAGEMENT	EVALUATION
Risk factors for heart disease (lifestyle, smoking, lack of exercise, obesity, positive family history, alcoholism, etc.).	Teach appropriate dietary regimen.	Laboratory: Lipoproteins should decrease at least 15% to justify long-term therapy.
Drug history (especially prior or present oral contraceptives, other estrogens, antilipemics, oral anticoagulants).	Explain the relationship of the laboratory finding of hyperlipoproteinemia to cardiac risk factors and incidence of vascular disorders.	All agents: Note change in bowel habits and gastrointestinal symptoms.
Screen for secondary causes of hyperlipidemia (diabetes, hypothyroidism, nephrosis, liver disease, alcoholism).	Bile acid sequestrants: Take other drugs at least 1 h prior. May be mixed with juice or applesauce to increase palatability. Give stool softener to prevent constipation.	Bile acid sequestrants: Observe pharmacologic effects of concurrent drugs for evidence of decreased effect as the result of altered absorption.
Diet history (one week recall).	Nicotinic acid: Take with meals.	Nicotinic acid: Note flushing, rash, jaundice, gout attack, symptoms of hyperglycemia. Flushing may subside with continued therapy.
Laboratory: Cholesterol and triglycerides for screening; lipoprotein typing when indicated.	Clofibrate: May require adjustment of dosage of other highly protein bound drugs (especially oral anticoagulants) taken concurrently.	Clofibrate: Note breast tenderness, changes in libido, changes in skin or hair, angina, gallbladder symptoms, edema, and others.
Presence of xanthoma, abdominal pain, hepatosplenomegaly, pancreatitis, claudication, ischemic heart disease.	Probucol: Take with meals. Discontinue drug if syncope, dizziness, or palpitations occur.	Probucol: Note symptoms associated with idiosyncratic reaction (dizziness, syncope, palpitations, nausea, and chest pain).
Assessment of patient's knowledge of disease.	Gemfibrozil: Take 30 min before morning and evening meals.	Gemfibrozil: Note changes in skin, headache, dizziness.
	β-sitosterol: Take with meals.	

Therapy is usually begun with a dose of 1 to 2 mg/day and increased in increments of 1 to 2 mg/day until the desired effect is achieved or a maximum dose of 8 mg/day is reached.

β-Sitosterol

β-Sitosterol (Dytelin) is a plant sterol which has a structure similar to cholesterol but is not absorbed by the gastrointestinal tract. Its main benefit is its ability to produce a decrease in plasma cholesterol in hypercholesterolemic patients. It has been suggested that β-sitosterol interferes with cholesterol absorption by competitive inhibition, although the exact mechanism is not known. The primary use of β-sitosterol appears to be type II hyperlipidemia. The major side effects associated with its use are diarrhea, nausea, and bloat-ing. The usual dose is 3 to 6 g before each meal. Because of the limited amount of information available about the use of β-sitosterol in a homogenous population of patients, it probably should be considered a secondary drug in the treatment of hyperlipidemia at this time.

NURSING PROCESS RELATED TO HYPERLIPIDEMIA

The nursing process in hyperlipidemia is outlined in Table 41-4.

CASE STUDY

Mrs. K, a 55-year-old white, widowed female, was seen by her private physician for gastrointestinal complaint of an upset stomach and diarrhea.

Assessment

The initial interview with Mrs. K revealed a prior history of chronic obstructive pulmonary disease, episodic gastric distress, and depression since the death of her husband two years earlier. Her present medications included theophylline and amitriptyline. Mrs. K smoked one and one-half packs of cigarettes a day and consumed as many as six cans of beer each night. Due to shortness of breath on exertion, her physical activity was limited to light housework. She had been unemployed for several years and was classified as permanently disabled. Her family history was vague, although she remembered that her father died from a stroke and her mother from cancer. She had a 50-year-old brother who had hypertension.

Upon physical examination, Mrs. K was noted to be both anxious and depressed. Her blood pressure was 120/80 mmHg and she was found to be approximately 25 lb above her ideal body weight. The only other finding was of small xanthomas on her buttocks. A review of her laboratory data revealed a slightly elevated fasting blood sugar of 160 mg/dL (normal 70 to 110 mg/dL), a serum cholesterol of 367 mg/dL (normal 135 to 315 mg/dL), and a serum triglyceride level of 640 mg/dL (normal 30 to 135 mg/dL). All other laboratory values were within normal limits. One week later, repeat triglyceride and cholesterol levels were found to be nearly identical and a subsequent lipoprotein electrophoresis showed a type III pattern.

Management

Mrs. K was instructed to keep a dietary record for one week including alcohol intake. On her follow-up exam her diet history showed a high intake of saturated fats, red meats, and carbohydrates, including alcohol. Since Mrs. K's history suggested both primary and secondary causes for hyperlipidemia, she was encouraged to attend dietary counseling and risk factor modification classes offered by a local hospital and started on clofibrate 500 mg PO tid with meals.

During the counseling sessions, Mrs. K was taught to recognize those habits which increased her risk of heart disease. Emphasis was placed on the relationship between the factors of smoking, alcohol, stress, poor diet, and state of health. She was advised to attempt to reduce her weight through caloric restriction, increasing intake of fruits and vegetables, and switching to foods high in polyunsaturated fats. The purpose and mechanism of clofibrate was explained to her and she was counseled to report breast tenderness, changes in her skin or hair, chest pain, gallbladder symptoms, or edema. Since amitriptyline is also highly bound to plasma albumin, it could be displaced from binding sites by clofibrate, and so Mrs. K was told to report any increased drowsiness, palpitations, or anticholinergic symptoms (dry mouth, constipation, blurred vision, etc.) which occurred during the initiation of clofibrate therapy.

Evaluation

After three months of participating in her treatment plan, Mrs. K's triglyceride level decreased to 401 mg/dL and her cholesterol level decreased to 246 mg/dL, justifying continued drug therapy. Her lipid levels were evaluated on a monthly basis and were noted to be gradually decreasing for five consecutive months. At the sixth month checkup, however, her triglyceride and cholesterol levels were found to have risen again. Mrs. K reported an increase in anxiety and depression at that time due to family problems. Although she had continued to comply with her dietary regimen, she had failed to renew her prescription for clofibrate. A return to her counseling programs was encouraged and she was restarted on clofibrate.

At her one year follow-up appointment, Mrs. K had stopped smoking, reduced her alcohol consumption, lost 15 lb, and had taken the clofibrate as prescribed. Her cholesterol level had decreased to 285 mg/dL and her triglyceride level to 340 mg/dL.

REFERENCES

Ahrens, E. H.: "The Management of Hyperlipidemia: Whether, Rather Than How," *Ann Intern Med,* 85:87–93, 1976.

Azarnoff, D. L.: "Individualization of Treatment of Hyperlipoproteinemic Disorders," *Med Clin North Am,* 58:1129–1131, 1974.

Civin, H., et al.: "Diet vs. Drugs in Hyperlipidemia," *Patient Care,* 10:20–59, 1976.

Connor, W. E., et al.: "Dietary Treatment of Hyperlipidemia," *Med Clin North Am,* 66:285–513, 1982.

Coronary Drug Project Research Group: "Clofibrate and Niacin in Coronary Heart Disease," *JAMA,* 231:361–381, 1975.

——: "The Coronary Drug Project Findings Leading to Further Modifications of Its Protocol with Respect to Dextrothyroxine," *JAMA,* 220:996–1008, 1972.

Fitzpatrick, T.B.: *Dermatology in Internal Medicine,* New York: McGraw-Hill, 1971, pp. 1173–1175.

Fredrickson, D. S., and R. Levy: "Familial Hyperlipoproteinemias," in J. D. Stanbury, J. B. Wyngaarden, and D. S. Fredrickson (eds.), *The Metabolic Basis of Inherited Disease,* New York: McGraw-Hill, 1972.

——, et al.: "Classification of Hyperlipidemias and Hyperlipoproteinemias," *WHO Bull,* 43:891, 1970.

Havel, R. J.: "Approach to the Patient with Hyperlipidemia," *Med Clin North Am,* 66:323–332, 1982.

Kannel, W. B., et al.: "Serum Cholesterol, Lipoproteins, and the Risk of Coronary Heart Disease," *Ann Intern Med,* 74:1–12, 1971.

Krauss, R.: "Regulation of HDL Levels," *Med Clin North Am,* 66:417–437, 1982.

Mann, G. V.: "Diet-Heart: End of an Era," *N Engl J Med,* 279:644–650, 1977.

Matter, S., et al.: "Body Fat Content and Serum Lipid Levels," *J Am Diet Assoc,* 77:149–152, 1982.

42

THROMBOEMBOLIC DISORDERS*

THOMAS P. REINDERS
VIRGINIA E. PARKER

LEARNING OBJECTIVES

Upon mastery of the content of this chapter, the reader will be able to:

1. Describe the function of platelets and clotting factors in the coagulation cascade.

2. Distinguish between the intrinsic and extrinsic clotting systems.

3. Identify the effects of anticoagulants, antiplatelet agents, and thrombolytic agents on hemostasis.

4. Identify the pharmacokinetic characteristics of anticoagulants and antiplatelet agents.

5. State the common adverse effects associated with anticoagulants, antiplatelet agents, and thrombolytic agents.

6. List the common indications and contraindications for anticoagulant therapy, thrombolytic therapy, and antiplatelet therapy.

7. Compare and contrast the advantages of intermittent and continuous intravenous heparin therapy.

8. List the laboratory tests for monitoring heparin and warfarin therapy.

9. Identify six mechanisms of drug interactions involving warfarin.

10. State the antidote for reversing excessive anticoagulation associated with heparin and warfarin therapy.

11. Describe the relationship of the dosage regimens of heparin and warfarin in relation to their respective half-lives.

12. Describe why a loading dose of warfarin should be avoided.

13. State the usually accepted anticoagulant dosage regimens for heparin, warfarin, streptokinase, urokinase, aspirin, and dipyridamole.

14. Describe a management protocol for ambulant patients maintained on warfarin therapy.

15. Prepare a teaching plan for a patient receiving warfarin therapy.

16. Identify the role of antiplatelet and anticoagulant drugs in the prevention and treatment of cerebrovascular disease.

HEMOSTASIS

The injury of a blood vessel results in the formation of a fibrin-platelet meshwork that develops as a structural barrier to prevent the loss of blood and to serve as a site for vessel repair. Hemostatic reactions are usually triggered by a disruption of blood vessel endothelium that allows flowing blood to come in contact with subendothelial tissue. Platelets are attracted to the subendothelial collagen and aggregation occurs as an initial stage of blood coagulation.

Platelets are small disc-shaped cells which circulate in the blood, after being produced in the megakaryocytes of the bone marrow. Their usual life span is about 10 days in normal blood; the platelet count ranges from 250,000 to 400,000/mm³. When platelets adhere to the site of vessel injury they release various biologically active chemicals including serotonin, adenosine diphosphate (ADP), and phospholipids. Serotonin acts as a vasoconstrictor while ADP leads to the aggregation of additional platelets. The release of phospholipids may trigger the formation of fibrin. This occurs through the sequential activation of clotting factors circulating in the blood.

The exposure of Factor XII to platelet phospholipids or exposed collagen fibers of an abnormal vessel wall will initiate the *intrinsic pathway of the clotting cascade*. The activated enzyme form of Factor XII will then activate Factor XI and other factors in a cascade sequence until a thrombus is ultimately formed (Fig. 42-1). Thrombus formation can also result from the activation of the *extrinsic pathway* when plasma is exposed to tissue thromboplastin. This sub-

*The editors thank Steve R. Kayser and Delores M. Giles, who contributed the chapter on this subject in the first edition.

823

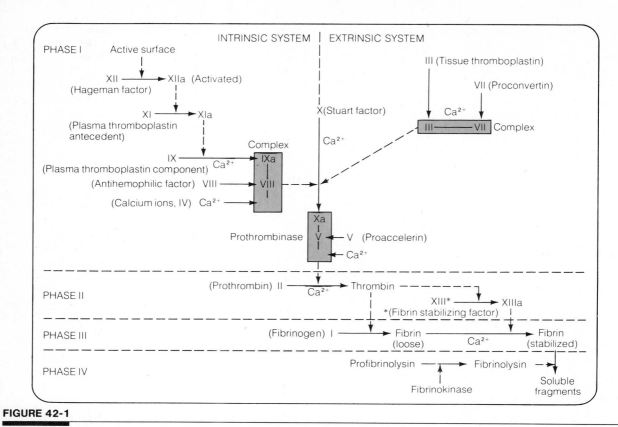

FIGURE 42-1

Simplified Diagram of the Mechanisms of Hemostasis. Phase I can be initiated by intrinsic or extrinsic mechanisms. Clot formation and maturation occurs in Phase II and Phase III. The fibrinolytic system is represented by Phase IV. *(Figure courtesy of Cary E. Johnson, Pharm.D.)*

stance is released from the injured tissue of the blood vessel wall. Again, a series of reactions will occur until fibrinogen is converted to fibrin.

Upon the initiation of the coagulation cascade, *fibrinolytic pathways* are simultaneously activated through a feedback mechanism. *Plasmin,* a proteolytic enzyme, is primarily responsible for fibrin dissolution. Plasmin is converted from *plasminogen* by the action of one or more chemical activators in the plasma or tissues.

TYPES OF THROMBOEMBOLIC DISORDERS

Deep Vein Thrombosis

Venous thrombophlebitis is a common problem in both inpatient and outpatient settings. Recognition and appropriate treatment of this condition is essential to prevent chronic venous disease or more serious sequela such as pulmonary embolism. Thrombophlebitis may occur in both superficial or deep veins. Several causes of thrombophlebitis exist, although in some patients the etiology remains undetermined. Any process that injures the vein wall may precip-

itate thrombophlebitis. These processes should alert the practitioner for early detection of thrombophlebitis and are identified in Table 42-1.

Superficial thrombophlebitis most commonly occurs in the great saphenous vein. It presents a clinical picture of pain, tenderness, erythema, warmth, and localized edema at the site of inflammation. Early recognition and prompt treatment with bed rest, elevation of the involved extremity, and warm soaks usually alleviates the pain and inflammation in seven to ten days. Anticoagulation therapy generally is not indicated.

Deep vein thrombophlebitis presents a varied clinical picture depending on the location and amount of occlusion. Sometimes there are no signs of involvement until a pulmonary embolus occurs. Recognition of deep vein thrombophlebitis depends on obtaining an accurate patient history including occurrence of any risk factors and any complaints of localized pain, tenderness, and edema. These complaints are often reported in the calf area. Physical examination may reveal signs such as warmth, erythema, edema, and measurable swelling.

Treatment of deep vein thrombophlebitis involves the

TABLE 42-1 Clinical Manifestations of Thrombophlebitis

POSSIBLE ETIOLOGY	COMMON LOCATIONS	CLINICAL SIGNS/ SYMPTOMS
Superficial		
Trauma	Saphenous veins	Erythema, pain,
Varicose veins	Forearm	tenderness, inflammation
IV therapy		of vein
Malignancies		
Deep Vein		
Trauma	Posterior tibial	Swelling, pain, tenderness,
Postoperative	Popliteal	edema, possible
state	Femoral	embolization, possible
Prolonged bed	Iliac	chronic venous
rest	Inferior vena	insufficiency
Pre/post-	cava	
partum	Superior vena	
CHF	cava	
Sepsis		
Malignancies		
Oral		
contraceptives		

use of **heparin** initially, followed by **warfarin** therapy. Use of elastic stockings and early ambulation is helpful in preventing thrombophlebitis in postoperative patients. Additionally, the use of low-dose heparin therapy in patients undergoing certain surgeries has been shown to significantly decrease the incidence of deep vein thrombosis.

Pulmonary Embolus

Pulmonary embolism may occur from thrombophlebitis when a dislodged thrombus enters the pulmonary circulation. Complete or partial obstruction of pulmonary arterial blood flow produces a sudden onset of dyspnea without obvious cause. There may also be a pleuritic type chest pain, apprehension, cough, tachycardia, and hemoptysis. Diagnosis of pulmonary embolus is supported by a variety of tests such as arterial blood gases, lung scans, and, at times, fluoroscopy.

Any patient that is at risk for development of thrombophlebitis may have the occurrence of pulmonary embolus. Most often these patients are already hospitalized at the time the nurse first sees them. However, it is important to keep in mind that young, active, healthy persons can present with pulmonary embolus without an obvious precipitating cause.

Anticoagulant therapy is indicated in the management of patients with pulmonary embolism. This therapy greatly reduces morbidity and mortality by reducing the incidence of recurrent pulmonary emboli. Ligation or clipping of the inferior vena cava or the placement of an umbrella filter in the inferior vena cava may be employed for patients with repeated embolic events despite adequate anticoagulant control or in patients with contraindications to anticoagulant therapy. Usual contraindications include: (1) preexisting bleeding tendencies such as coagulation defects, thrombocytopenia, active gastrointestinal or genitourinary bleeding; (2) hepatic insufficiency; (3) severe hypertension; (4) recent injury or surgery of the central nervous system or eye; and (5) extensive trauma. Other patients with massive pulmonary embolism may be candidates for surgical embolectomy or the use of thrombolytic therapy.

Disseminated Intravascular Coagulation (DIC)

Also known as defibrination syndrome and consumption coagulopathy, DIC is one of the most serious acquired coagulopathies. This exceedingly complex disorder is associated with widespread clotting in the microcirculation where the patient is consuming clotting factors faster than they can be released. At the same time, the fibrinolytic system is activated, with fibrinolysis accompanied by clotting. DIC is characterized by the sudden onset of hemorrhage, possibly of significant enough proportions to cause circulatory collapse. Often the predominant manifestation of hemorrhage is related to an underlying disorder. The conditions most commonly associated with DIC include:

1. Bacterial, viral, and fungal infections of the bloodstream
2. Neoplastic diseases
3. Complications of pregnancy, such as toxemia
4. Shock

Therapy consists of immediate treatment of the underlying disorder and any complications. Under some circumstances, ironically, **heparin** has been used to treat DIC, particularly with subacute or chronic problems. **Warfarin** is not useful in the treatment of this disorder.

Valvular Heart Disease

Valvular heart disease, with associated valve deterioration and cardiac failure, inevitably results in valve replacement. Mechanical valves are associated with embolization and require chronic anticoagulant therapy as a prophylactic measure. **Warfarin** therapy is extensively used for patients with mechanical devices such as cloth-covered ball and disc valves. More recently, biologic valves such as the porcine prosthesis have been developed. These valves have not been associated with embolization, thus eliminating the need for chronic anticoagulation.

Atrial fibrillation may also be associated with valvular heart disease. Cardioversion to normal sinus rhythm is sought through the use of antiarrhythmic drugs or electrical means. Generally, oral anticoagulant therapy is initiated one to two weeks prior to electrical cardioversion as prophylaxis against embolization. Patients with chronic atrial fibrillation, refractory to conventional therapy, may also be considered candidates for chronic anticoagulant therapy.

Vascular Disease

Cerebral Vascular Events

Cerebrovascular disease is the term used for a group of disorders resulting in impaired blood flow to the brain. Etiological factors in cerebrovascular disease include atherosclerosis with thrombus formation, emboli from the heart and other extracerebral sites, congenital weakness of the cerebral vasculature, hypertensive hemorrhage, or immunologic arteritis. Chronically, cerebrovascular disease has relatively nonspecific manifestations, such as cognitive impairment (see Chap. 33, "Dementia"), headache, dizziness, or stiff neck. Acute cerebrovascular events include stroke (cerebrovascular accident; CVA) and transient ischemic attack (TIA). A *transient ischemic attack* produces a brief neurologic deficit such as monocular visual impairment, slurring of speech, focal paresthesias, or weakness of the extremities. These symptoms usually last for 5 to 7 min, but may continue up to 24 h. If the deficit persists beyond 24 h it is assumed that brain infarction has occurred and the clinical condition is described as a *stroke*. The resulting neurologic deficit may resolve completely or in part over a period of weeks or may stabilize and remain unchanged.

Detailed information about the onset and course of symptoms is essential to establishing a diagnosis. Additionally, diagnostic tests including computerized tomography or lumbar puncture, electrocardiograph (ECG), brain scan, electroencephalograph (EEG), and angiography may be employed to distinguish infarct (thrombotic or embolytic) from hemorrhage, since anticoagulant therapy is contraindicated in the latter.

Prevention of stroke through blood pressure normalization and minimization of risk factors (diabetes, alcohol, smoking, obesity) is the most successful therapy. Since most people who have a TIA go on to have a completed stroke, frequently soon after the first episode, immediate treatment of TIAs is crucial. Antiplatelet therapy, consisting of **aspirin** or **dipyridamole** (Persantine) plus aspirin, effectively stops TIAs and prevents stroke in some people. If TIAs persist, some physicians will substitute oral anticoagulants for the antiplatelet therapy.

Except in the case of a *stroke in progress* (ongoing increments in neurologic deficit), where intravenous **heparin** may be useful, drug therapy is not effective in treating actual strokes. However, anticoagulant therapy is not indicated in the treatment of completed stroke because hemorrhage can occur at the site of a fresh infarct. Cerebral edema, muscle spasticity, and other complications can sometimes be managed pharmacologically (see Chap. 33).

Cardiac Events

The relationship of myocardial infarction to coronary thrombosis remains controversial. Investigators have not been able to resolve the issue of whether coronary thrombosis initiates a myocardial infarction or results from the infarction. Some evidence exists for the benefit of anticoagulant therapy in the treatment of myocardial infarction, especially for patients at risk of thromboembolic complications. Many clinicians are now exploring the benefits of antiplatelet therapy for patients with potential thromboembolic events resulting from coronary atherosclerotic heart disease.

Any myocardial or valvular condition with thrombus on the left side of the heart may result in embolization. Major causes of such thrombus formation are valvular disease, bacterial endocarditis, and atherosclerosis. Patients under 50 years of age are most likely to have valvular disease, while atherosclerosis is often implicated as the etiology of left ventricular thrombus formation in patients over 50 years of age. Warfarin therapy is generally employed in the treatment of these patients, rather than the use of antiplatelet therapy.

CLINICAL PHARMACOLOGY AND THERAPEUTICS

Anticoagulant Drugs

Heparin

Mechanism of Action Heparin is a naturally occurring mucopolysaccharide found in a variety of organs including the liver, lung, and intestine. Heparin is a large molecule with an approximate molecular weight of 12,000. The molecule has a strong electronegative charge which is thought to contribute to its anticoagulant action. Investigators have demonstrated that heparin serves as a cofactor for antithrombin III, resulting in the inhibition of thrombin. The drug also inhibits the activation of Factors IX, X, XI, and XII.

Pharmacokinetics Heparin is not absorbed by the gastrointestinal mucosa, and therefore is administered parenterally. Anticoagulant response is rapid after intravenous administration. Subcutaneous and intramuscular routes give unpredictable absorption and local hemorrhage is an added complication. The drug is largely distributed to the intravascular space and its half-life is approximately 90 min. Heparin is thought to be degraded in the liver and about 20 percent of a dose can be recovered unchanged in the urine.

Therapeutic response monitoring is limited to clotting function tests since chemical assays of heparin have not been adequately correlated with clinical response. The usual laboratory test employed for **heparin** monitoring is the activated partial thromboplastin time (APTT). Other monitoring tests include the whole blood partial thromboplastin time (PTT) and the Lee-White whole blood clotting time (LWCT). The usually accepted therapeutic endpoint for these tests is a patient response that is 1½ to 2½ times the control response.

Adverse Effects   The most frequently occurring adverse reaction with heparin therapy is bleeding. An estimated 10 percent of patients experience a bleeding episode during a course of heparin therapy. Melena, hematoma, hematuria, and ecchymosis are often reported. The dose of heparin is an important determinant of bleeding risk. Also, women have more than twice the risk of men in experiencing heparin-induced bleeding. Heavy alcohol drinkers and patients with underlying morbidity are also at greater risk. In addition to bleeding, thrombocytopenia has also been associated with heparin therapy. Prolonged use may produce osteoporosis and hair loss.

If major bleeding occurs due to excessive heparin, the effects can be reversed with **protamine sulfate**. Protamine neutralizes heparin on a milligram per milligram basis; therefore, 1 mg will neutralize 120 U of heparin sodium, U.S.P. A potential source of error is the determination of the amount of circulating heparin. Estimates based on the usual half-life of the drug and the approximate time of administration are necessary for determining an appropriate protamine dose.

Drug interactions   The concomitant administration of oral anticoagulants or antiplatelet drugs with heparin can result in a potentiated anticoagulant response. Monitoring for signs and symptoms of bleeding is routine for any of the single agents but is considered crucial when the drugs are used in combination. The incompatibilities of heparin in intravenous solutions must also be considered. When possible, heparin should be administered in dextrose 5% in water or normal saline and generally should not be mixed with other drugs in the intravenous solution.

Dosage and Administration   Due to heparin's short half-life of 90 min, a loading dose is considered desirable to achieve a therapeutic anticoagulant response. Doses ranging from 5000 to 15,000 U are employed as initial intravenous doses. Some clinicians advocate larger doses for patients with pulmonary embolism and smaller doses for patients with deep vein thrombosis. Intermittent intravenous therapy or a continuous infusion of heparin is then initiated. With intermittent therapy, the patient can be maintained at a dose of 5000 U of heparin every 4 h with dosage adjustments based on laboratory test values. Continuous administration is generally achieved through the use of an infusion pump which allows for rapid dosage adjustment. A heparin infu-sion rate of 1000 U/h is frequently suggested, with dosage adjustments based on laboratory results. Intermittent intravenous heparin is usually given through a heparin lock in a vein.

Continuous infusion provides the greatest advantage in terms of maintaining the patient in a therapeutic anticoagulant range. Fluctuations of circulating heparin are minimized and ultimately the patient receives less total heparin on a daily basis. Also, plasma samples can be taken at any time for measurement of the activated partial thromboplastin time or Lee-White clotting time. Intermittent therapy does not afford these patient benefits. However, the use of an infusion device is eliminated with intermittent therapy and the patient can easily ambulate. Additionally, electrolyte disorders are minimal due to the small solution volume administered with intermittent therapy.

Heparin may also be administered subcutaneously. This route of administration is usually reserved for prophylaxis against deep vein thrombosis. Surgery patients predisposed to thrombi formation may be given 5000 U of heparin every 8 to 12 h, starting 2 h preoperatively and continuing for 7 to 10 days postoperatively. The recommended site for subcutaneous heparin injection is the abdominal area above the anterior iliac spines. Since heparin is irritating to tissue and may cause skin necrosis, deep subcutaneous (*intrafat* and not subdermal) injection is advisable. A small gauge needle (25 or 26 gauge) is used and the subcutaneous tissue is gently pinched up before the needle is inserted at a 90° angle. Needle length should vary with the build of the patient; very thin people require a ½-in needle, while a very obese person may safely be injected with a 1-in needle. Aspiration (checking for back flow) prior to injection of the heparin or rubbing the site after injection is contraindicated, as this may promote hematoma formation. Muscle absorption is erratic and painful and hematoma formation is frequent, so the intramuscular route should be avoided unless specific indications are cited for this route. Application of ice to the site before and/or after the injection may reduce hematoma formation and irritation.

Heparin therapy is generally initiated with the onset of thromboembolic symptoms and continued for 7 to 10 days. It is usually not feasible to employ parenteral anticoagulants for maintenance therapy due to patient inconvenience and expense. Instead, the patient is converted to oral anticoagulant therapy.

CASE STUDY

G.M., a 29-year-old black female, was admitted for hospitalization after presenting in the emergency room with a seven-day duration of warmth, swelling, and pain in the lower left leg. The patient stated that on the morning of admission she experienced shortness of breath at rest and coughed up several teaspoonfuls of blood. This patient had a history of recurrent deep vein thrombosis and pulmonary embolism.

Assessment

The patient was a well-developed, slightly obese black female in no acute distress. She is alert, oriented, and cooperative. Temperature was 99°F, pulse 88/min and regular, respirations 28/min, and blood pressure 130/72 (RAL). Chest was symmetrical with good breath sounds, clear to percussion and auscultation. Extremities revealed a swollen left leg: 12 cm above knee (right equaled 58 cm, left equaled 59 cm); 12 cm below knee (right equaled 38 cm, left equaled 39.5 cm); positive Homan's sign in left leg, no cyanosis or clubbing. Neurologic examination was within normal limits. An admission roetgenogram of chest revealed clear lung fields and normal sized heart. Lung scans (^{99m}Tc-MAA) revealed multiple filling defects. ECG revealed normal sinus rhythm. Arterial blood gases (ambient air): p_{O_2} = 62 mmHg, p_{CO_2} = 36 mmHg, pH = 7.36. The patient's prothrombin time was 13 s with a control of 12 s. A medication history revealed a prescription of warfarin 10 mg daily and acetaminophen 325 mg q4h if needed for pain. Both medications were prescribed five weeks prior to this admission, for documented pulmonary embolism. The patient admitted noncompliance with the warfarin therapy for the previous two weeks. A provisional diagnosis of deep vein thrombosis and pulmonary embolism was established.

Management

Following transfer to a medical ward, anticoagulant therapy was initiated by administering heparin as a 7000-U IV bolus. A continuous infusion of heparin was ordered in a dose of 1000 U qh with daily partial thromboplastin time determinations. An automatic, self-regulating infusion pump was employed to maintain continuous heparin dosing. The heparin dosage remained constant throughout therapy and warfarin was initiated on the fourth day of hospitalization at a daily dose of 10 mg. Daily prothrombin time determinations were ordered. Heparin therapy was discontinued on the seventh day of hospitalization, when the prothrombin time remained in the therapeutic range [PT = 26 s (control-12 s)] for two consecutive days. A patient education plan was initiated during hospitalization with the objective of encouraging compliance.

Evaluation

Symptomatic improvement of the warmth, swelling, and pain in the lower left leg resolved during the hospital stay. The patient was monitored for signs and symptoms of bleeding and recurrent thromboembolism on a daily basis. The patient was discharged with a daily dose of warfarin 10 mg and a scheduled appointment with the Anticoagulant Clinic in one week for evaluation of anticoagulant control and any evidence of recurrent thrombophlebitis and pulmonary emboli.

Oral Anticoagulants

Two pharmacologic classes of oral anticoagulants are available, the **coumarin** and **indandione** derivatives. **Warfarin**, a coumarin derivative, has been the most widely used agent in the United States since the early 1950s. The indandiones were developed during the same era, but have not been widely used due to their association with hematologic, hepatic, renal, and allergic reactions. Consequently, the following discussion will be limited to the use of **warfarin sodium**.

Mechanism of Action   Warfarin inhibits the vitamin K–dependent synthesis of clotting factors II, VII, IX, and X. The anticoagulant effect is not immediate, since already formed factors must be degraded by the liver. For this reason, **heparin** is administered concomitantly for the first several days of therapy to prevent the activation of existing clotting factors. When their degradation is complete and synthesis adequately inhibited, the patient's prothrombin time determination should be within the range of 1½ to 2½ times the control value. This range of prothrombin time to control time is the generally accepted therapeutic goal. When this goal has been achieved, heparin therapy can be discontinued.

Pharmacokinetics   Warfarin is readily absorbed from the upper part of the small intestine, following oral administration. The drug is highly protein-bound, probably in excess of 97 percent. This degree of binding serves as one explanation for many of the potential warfarin interactions. Warfarin is metabolized in the liver and metabolites are excreted in the urine. The half-life of warfarin varies but usually is considered to be 44 h.

Adverse Effects   The major adverse effect associated with warfarin is bleeding. Even when initial therapy proceeds slowly and cautiously, bleeding may still occur. Macroscopic hematuria and melena are frequent signs of bleeding in patients receiving oral anticoagulants. More than half of the bleeding episodes are caused by trauma or will be localized at the sites of organic internal lesions. Minor episodes of bleeding are usually treated by withholding or reducing the warfarin dose and evaluating the potential underlying problem. Serious bleeding is generally treated with the administration of **phytonadione** (vitamin K₁). Doses of 0.5 to 5 mg will effectively reduce warfarin's anticoagulant action (see Chap. 25). Another alternative is to restore clotting factors through the infusion of plasma or whole blood.

Drug interactions   Since the interaction of warfarin with barbiturates was reported, approximately 150 other drugs have been reported to interact. Even though specific mechanisms are not identified for all warfarin interactions, general categories have been proposed to classify reported interactions (Table 42-2). Warfarin potentiation may result

TABLE 42-2   Potential Warfarin Interactions

MECHANISM	SELECTED DRUGS
Enhances Warfarin Activity	
Displacement of warfarin from protein-binding sites	Phenylbutazone, sulfonamides, chloral hydrate, sulfonylureas, clofibrate
Inhibition of warfarin metabolism	Phenylbutazone, cimetidine, clotrimazole, metronidazole, acute alcohol ingestion, allopurinol
Decreased vitamin K	Chloramphenicol, erythromycin, mineral oil
Catabolism of clotting factors	Thyroid, thyroxine
Decreases Warfarin Activity	
Microsomal enzyme induction	Barbiturates, phenytoin, carbamazepine, rifampin, griseofulvin, glutethimide
Decreased absorption	Cholestyramine, colestipol
Increased procoagulant factors	Vitamin K, estrogens
Enhances Bleeding Potential	
Inhibition of platelet function	Aspirin, phenylbutazone, dipyridamole, sulfinpyrazone, nonsteroidal anti-inflammatory drugs, dextran
Inhibition of procoagulant factors	Quinidine, alkylating agents
Production of gastrointestinal lesions	Phenylbutazone, aspirin, prednisone, potassium chloride, indomethacin

when the drug is displaced from plasma protein binding sites by drugs such as **phenylbutazone**. The concomitant administration of **barbiturates** and **warfarin** will result in microsomal enzyme induction in the liver, requiring an increased dose of warfarin for most patients. Potentiation of warfarin's anticoagulant response is also noted with the concurrent use of **antiplatelet agents**. Excessive intake of **vitamin K** can result in the need for an increased warfarin dose to achieve its therapeutic response.

Dosage and Administration   Initiation of warfarin therapy in daily oral doses of 10 mg is appropriate. Large loading doses such as 40 or 50 mg should be avoided since patients are subjected to the additional risk of bleeding without achieving an adequate therapeutic response. It takes at least five days for the levels of the vitamin K–dependent clotting factors to be suppressed to a therapeutic anticoagulant range, regardless of the dose administered. The average dose of warfarin is between 5 to 7.5 mg, yet patients will range

from 1 to 40 mg in their daily requirements. Dosage adjustments should be made on the basis of a daily prothrombin time determination while the patient is hospitalized.

Upon hospital discharge, the patient receiving warfarin should receive a prothrombin time determination within one week. One approach to the management of ambulant patients has been the creation of special clinics for patients receiving warfarin therapy. A protocol approach (Fig. 42-2) can be employed for monitoring and adjusting warfarin dosages. For example, when the patient's prothrombin time determination is within 1½ to 2½ times the control, the warfarin dose can be titrated to achieve a prothrombin time ratio of approximately twice the control. This can be achieved by altering the total weekly warfarin dose by 5 mg. Initially it is desirable to obtain prothrombin time determinations at weekly intervals and then gradually extend intervals to one month as the patient demonstrates adequate anticoagulant control.

Anticoagulant Information for the Patient
Patient education is considered essential for patients receiving anticoagulant therapy. Patient education should be provided in an attempt to motivate patients to change attitudes or behavior which might result in noncompliance with the prescribed treatment plan. Written information about anticoagulant therapy should be reinforced with verbal communication by the health care provider.

Drug Information   Patients should know the trade and generic names of their anticoagulant. Phonetic spelling may aid pronunciation of the names. Patients should know why the drug is prescribed. This will not entail a lengthy pharmacology lecture but rather a brief explanation that the drug prevents harmful clots in the blood vessels. Often the drug is described as a "blood thinner." Patients should realize this terminology refers to a decrease of blood clotting factors and not a decrease in the viscosity of the blood. **Warfarin** should be taken once each day. The time of the day is insignificant, but the dose time should be consistent to assure compliance. Warfarin is available in tablets which should be taken by mouth, with water. While commercial warfarin tablets are available in 2-, 2.5-, 5-, 7.5-, and 10-mg strengths, some clinicians will only prescribe 5-mg tablets. Patients are then instructed to use multiples or fractions of 5 mg. The tablets are easily broken by most patients by holding the tablet between the index fingers of each hand and exerting pressure against the tablet with the thumb nails of each hand. The score or indentation of the tablet should be placed on the side opposite the thumb nails. Patients should be informed that the warfarin dose is determined on the basis of their prothrombin time test and dosage changes should only be initiated by a physician. To avoid missing doses, it may be helpful to record daily dosages on a calendar, crossing through the date after a dose has been taken. Preloaded dispensing devices may also benefit selected

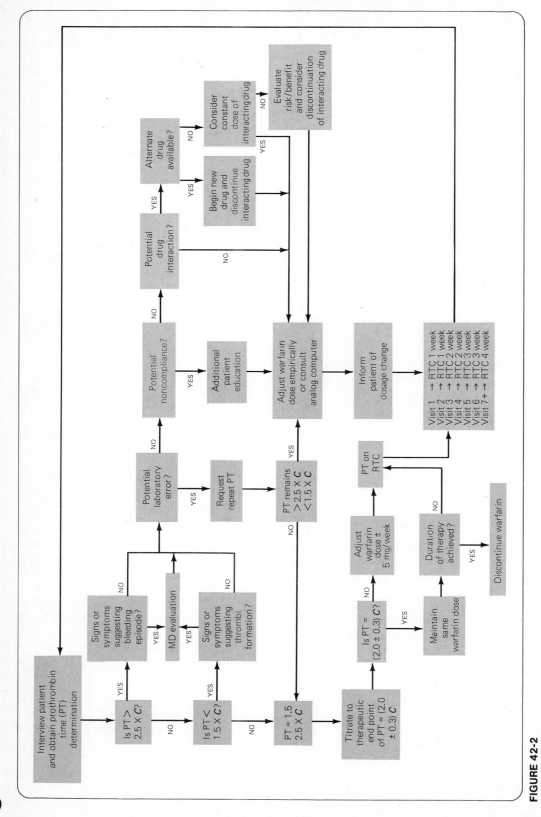

FIGURE 42-2

Warfarin Therapy Protocol for Ambulant Patients. (*From T. P. Reinders and W. E. Steinke, American Journal of Hospital Pharmacy,* **36:** *645–648, 1979. Used by permission.*)

patients. Recommendations for storage conditions pertain to keeping the drug in its original container, preferably a child-resistant one. As with all medications, the drug should be kept out of the reach of children.

Monitoring Information Patients should understand that periodic laboratory tests such as the prothrombin time will be repeated more frequently when warfarin therapy is initiated, but that the frequency will decrease as the proper dosage is established. It is also important that patients report any changes in their medications to their primary physician. Additionally, it is helpful for patients to inform all prescribers that they are receiving warfarin therapy prior to the initiation of drug treatment or dosage changes of current medications. Patients should also be advised to use caution when taking nonprescription medications, especially concerning the avoidance of **aspirin**-containing products. Diet considerations should also be discussed with patients. Large quantities of green, leafy vegetables should be avoided, yet a small daily salad is unlikely to interfere with warfarin's response. Instructions should also be given to avoid excessive amounts of alcohol. Other special instructions include avoidance of high injury risk such as contact sports. Patients may choose to carry an anticoagulant identification card on their person, or patients receiving chronic therapy may wish to purchase a medication identification necklace or bracelet. Also, female patients should inform their physician immediately if they suspect pregnancy.

Patients should be advised to record the date of any missed doses. It is not usually recommended to double doses. Instead, the physician should be notified and changes in the prothrombin time should be anticipated. Likewise, side effects should be reported to the physician or other health professionals monitoring warfarin therapy. The following signs of bleeding may be observed: (1) epistaxis, (2) ecchymoses, (3) petechiae, (4) hematuria, (5) melena, (6) hemoptysis, or (7) excessive menstrual bleeding. Persistent or excessive bleeding in spite of general first aid measures should be reported promptly. In minor bleeding episodes, dose alterations will be sufficient. In major bleeding episodes, phytonadione or replacement of clotting factors will be required. Also, patients should monitor for signs or symptoms of thromboembolism, usually consistent with their indication for anticoagulant therapy.

Thrombolytic Drugs

Mechanism of Action While **heparin** and oral anticoagulants prevent clot formation, clot dissolution occurs through the activation of the patient's fibrinolytic system. Recently, investigators have employed the exogenous use of **streptokinase** and **urokinase** to dissolve intravascular clots. Streptokinase is obtained from filtrates of Group C β-hemolytic streptococci, while urokinase is isolated from human urine or human fetal kidney tissue culture. These enzymes convert plasminogen to plasmin, which results in the degradation of fibrin clots.

Laboratory Monitoring Laboratory monitoring is employed to detect the presence of systemic fibrinolysis and not as a determinant for dosage adjustment. If lysis is detectable, then the dissolution of clots is anticipated. The tests commonly used include the *whole blood euglobulin lysis* test and the *thrombin time.*

Adverse Effects Bleeding is the most common adverse effect associated with these agents. Bleeding within 24 h occurs almost as frequently as bleeding up to two weeks after termination of therapy. Bleeding is often reported at venipuncture sites or other sites of invasive procedures. Unlike anticoagulant therapy, the frequency of bleeding is not related to excessive dose. Instead, the patients with adverse effects are those individuals with prior hemostatic defects. Severe bleeding necessitates the discontinuation of the thrombolytic agent. Due to their short half-life of approximately 10 to 15 min, lysis is rapidly halted. Whole blood can be used to restore hemostasis.

Fever and allergic reactions have also been reported. Since antibodies to streptococci are common, allergic reactions are more frequent with **streptokinase**. Patient symptoms are most appropriately treated with adrenergic agents, antihistamines, and/or intravenous corticosteroids. Fever is managed with nonprescription antipyretics such as **acetaminophen**. Streptokinase and **urokinase** should not be used concomitantly with **heparin**, oral anticoagulants, or drugs which decrease platelet function such as **aspirin** and nonsteroidal anti-inflammatory drugs.

Dosage and Administration Although thrombolytic therapy has been used in a variety of thromboembolic disorders, only small numbers of patients have been evaluated. As a result, optimal dosage recommendations are lacking. There is general agreement that both agents should be administered with a loading dose, followed by a maintenance dose. The suggested dose for **streptokinase** is 250,000 U over 20 to 30 min, with a maintenance dose of 100,000 U/h. **Urokinase** is started with 4400 IU/kg over 10 min, followed by 4400 IU/kg/h. Streptokinase is generally not readministered for six to twelve months after a course of therapy due to antigenicity.

Antiplatelet Drugs

During the past decade, agents with the ability to interfere with platelet function have been evaluated in the management of transient ischemic attacks and symptoms of progressing stroke. **Aspirin** and **dipyridamole** (Persantine) have been identified as two agents for potential use.

Aspirin irreversibly inactivates platelet cyclooxygenase for the life span of the platelet. A single dose of 325 mg daily is sufficient to produce the inhibition of thromboxane production and prevent platelet aggregation. Doses should be administered daily, since newly formed platelets are always appearing in the blood. A detailed discussion of aspirin's pharmacokinetics and adverse effects appears in Chap. 17. It is important to emphasize the potentiation of bleeding symptoms when aspirin is used concomitantly with anticoagulants or thrombolytics, necessitating careful monitoring practices.

Dipyridamole

Dipyridamole (Persantine, Pyridamole) was developed as an antianginal drug and increases coronary blood flow. It is an old drug and its pharmacokinetics have not been extensively studied.

Mechanism of Action   Dipyridamole acts on coagulation by inhibiting platelet aggregation through increasing the effects of prostacycline or by inhibiting phosphodiesterase activity. This increases the levels of cyclic AMP in platelets.

Adverse Effects   Few adverse effects occur with antiplatelet doses of pyridamole. It can cause headache, dizziness, gastrointestinal distress, skin rash, flushing, and syncope (especially in persons taking hypotensive drugs).

Dosage   The usual dose of dipyridamole is 25 mg four times daily if given with aspirin. If given alone, a dose of 100 mg four times daily is recommended. Taking the drug with a full glass of water and with meals will minimize gastrointestinal distress.

NURSING PROCESS RELATED TO THROMBOEMBOLISM

Although hospital or clinic policies may vary in the nursing management of patients on anticoagulant therapy, there are basic components which apply to most patient care settings. The following discussion is meant to serve as a general guide in patient care.

Assessment

Assessment of the patient on anticoagulant, thrombolytic, or antiplatelet therapy covers several parameters, including information on how medication is taken, new symptoms, and any changes in medications or diet. Of importance is detailed information about medication dosing, compliance, and any changes that have occurred. Eliciting symptoms will, to some extent, depend on the specific patient situation. Certainly the patient should be queried about any side effects of anticoagulants, especially those of bleeding symptoms. For example, the nurse should specifically inquire about hemoptosis, hematuria, hematemesis, heavy menses, easy bruising. In addition, symptoms that are pertinent to the particular disorder might include any leg pain, swelling, or erythema in a patient with a prior history of thrombophlebitis. Manifestation of neurologic deficits would be of utmost importance in a patient with an artificial valve, for example. Changes in medications include both prescription and nonprescription drugs. Dietary changes alone, such as increasing consumption of dark green vegetables, may be enough to change the anticoagulant therapy.

Objective information from the physical exam and laboratory findings should be compared with previous or baseline findings. Again, evidence of any bruising or bleeding should be noted immediately. Careful examination of gums, skin, and extremities must be done. Neurologic examination would be of importance in patients with previous or potential neurologic events. Standard laboratory work includes prothrombin time in warfarin patients and partial thromboplastin time for heparin patients. These should be maintained in the range of 1½ to 2½ times the control value to be considered therapeutic. Additional diagnostic tests may include hemoccult stool testing, urinalysis, complete blood count, and others, depending on the specific situation.

Management

Careful, ongoing attention is required in the management of both inpatient and outpatient situations. Monitoring laboratory values, which may include a flow chart, is the cornerstone of anticoagulant therapy. These values will predict the course of treatment continuously. Administration of anticoagulants is more mechanized with the inpatient setting and may include such devices as a heparin lock for intermittent therapy or a heparin infusion pump for continuous administration. Subcutaneous injections should be as atraumatic as possible with no aspiration or rubbing of the injection site. Patients should be well informed of the need for cooperation and compliance. Patient education (as discussed earlier) plays a major role in management and is particularly crucial with outpatients as they assume the primary responsibility for their care.

Evaluation

The process of evaluation provides feedback with regard to the success of previous interventions and the need to alter the therapeutic regimen. Evaluation continuously involves three parameters. The first is the laboratory data which is used to reflect the degree of anticoagulation that has occurred. This provides an immediate monitoring device. The second is that of recurrent symptoms or problems for which anticoagulant therapy was initiated and would necessitate further assessment. The third parameter covers any untoward effect, especially related to bleeding, for which further assessment and alteration of the therapeutic regimen would be needed.

CASE STUDY

J.T., a 53-year-old white male with an aortic valve replacement with a Starr-Edwards prosthesis, was maintained on chronic warfarin therapy for the previous seven years. During a routinely scheduled appointment at the Anticoagulation Clinic, the patient reported blood in his urine and extensive bruising of the upper right thigh.

Assessment

The patient was followed in the Anticoagulation Clinic on a monthly basis. His warfarin dose was 10 mg daily except 12.5 mg on Monday, Wednesday, and Friday. Other medications included digoxin 0.25 mg daily, hydrochlorothiazide 50 mg twice daily, and potassium chloride 40 meq daily. A careful history revealed that the patient incurred trauma to his right leg after falling on ice at a ski resort five days earlier. Due to swelling and pain in the leg, the patient was evaluated by a physician in a local hospital emergency room. He was informed that the discomfort was due to a "strained muscle" and a prescription for phenylbutazone 100 mg four times daily was initiated. The patient's prothrombin time/control time was 41 s/ 12 s. Macroscopic hematuria, petechiae on the lower extremities, and ecchymoses in the area of the right thigh were noted. The patient denied hemoptysis, gingival bleeding, epistaxis, or melena. Signs and symptoms of bleeding were attributed to the potentiation of warfarin's anticoagulant response by phenylbutazone. Phenylbutazone displaces warfarin from plasma protein binding sites, as well as inhibiting platelet aggregation and inducing potential gastrointestinal lesions.

Management

Phenylbutazone was abruptly discontinued. Additionally, the patient's warfarin therapy was temporarily discontinued for three days. A complete blood count, stool guaiac, and orthopedics evaluation were requested. The patient was instructed to return to the Anticoagulation Clinic in three days for a repeat prothrombin time determination or to come to the emergency room sooner if bleeding persisted or new evidence of bleeding signs or symptoms appeared. Specific instructions were given to the patient concerning the numerous drug interactions with warfarin. Reinforcement of previous patient information concerning the need to inform all prescribers about warfarin use was provided.

Evaluation

The patient's additional laboratory findings were negative and signs of bleeding began to disappear after three days. On the return visit the patient's prothrombin time/control time was 27 s/12 s. Warfarin therapy was restarted and the patient was instructed to return in one week for a prothrombin time determination.

REFERENCES

Breckenridge, A. M.: "Interindividual Differences in the Response to Oral Anticoagulants," *Drugs,* **14**:367–375, 1977.

Byer, J. A., and J. D. Easton: "Therapy of Ischemic Cardiovascular Disease," *Ann Intern Med,* **93**:742–756, 1980.

Chamberlain, S. L.: "Low-Dose Heparin Therapy," *Am J Nurs,* **80**:1115–1117, 1980.

Deykin, D.: "Warfarin Therapy," *N Engl J Med,* **283**:691–694, 801–803, 1970.

Evaluation of Drug Interactions, Washington: American Pharmaceutical Association, 1973.

Gallus, A. S., J. Hirsh, S. E. O'Brien, et al.: "Prevention of Venous Thrombosis with Small, Subcutaneous Doses of Heparin," *JAMA,* **235**:1980–1982, 1976.

Hand, J.: "Keeping Anticoagulants under Control," *RN,* **42**:25–29, 1979.

Hansten, P. D.: *Drug Interactions,* Philadelphia: Lea Febiger, 1979.

Harker, L. A., *Hemostasis Manual,* Philadelphia: Davis, 1974.

Hurst, J. W. (ed.): *The Heart, Arteries and Veins,* New York: McGraw-Hill, 1978.

Kelly, J. G., and K. O'Malley: "Clinical Pharmacokinetics of Oral Anticoagulants," *Clin Pharmacokinet,* **4**:1–15, 1979.

Koch-Weser, J.: "Thrombolytic Therapy," *N Engl J Med,* **306**:1268–1276, 1982.

MacLeod, S. M., and E. M. Sellers: "Pharmacodynamic and Pharmacokinetic Drug Interactions with Coumarin Anticoagulants," *Drugs,* **11**:461–470, 1976.

Mant, M. J., and E. G. King: "Severe, Acute Disseminated Intravascular Coagulation," *Am J Med,* **67**:557–563, 1979.

Medication Teaching Manual, Bethesda, MD: American Society of Hospital Pharmacists, 1980.

O'Reilly, R. A., and P. M. Aggeler: "Studies on Coumarin Anticoagulant Drugs—Initiation of Warfarin Therapy Without a Loading Dose," *Circulation,* **38**:169–177, 1968.

Raasch, R. H.: "Clinical Pharmacokinetics of Heparin," *Drug Intell Clin Pharm,* **14**:483–488, 1980.

Reinders, T. P., and W. E. Steinke: "Pharmacist Management of Anticoagulant Therapy in Ambulant Patients," *Am J Hosp,* **36**:645–648, 1979.

Salzman, E. W., D. Deykin, R. M. Shapiro, et al.: "Management of Heparin Therapy," *N Engl J Med,* **292**:1046–1050, 1975.

Thomas, D. P.: "Heparin," *Clin Haematol,* **10**:443–458, 1981.

Thompson, D. A.: "Teaching the Client About Anticoagulants," *Am J Nurs,* **82**:278–281, 1982.

Walker, A. M., and H. Jick: "Predictors of Bleeding During Heparin Therapy," *JAMA,* **244**:1209–1212, 1980.

Weiss, H. J.: "Platelet Physiology and Abnormalities of Platelet Function," *N Engl J Med,* **293**:531–541, 580–588, 1975.

43

ANGINA PECTORIS AND MYOCARDIAL INFARCTION*

THOMAS J. NESTER
JANE C. REGNIER
MOSES CHOW

LEARNING OBJECTIVES

Upon mastery of the content of this chapter the reader will be able to

1. State the predominant etiology of angina and acute myocardial infarction (AMI).

2. Relate the underlying pathophysiologic mechanism of angina to its therapy.

3. Describe how patients with angina normally characterize the symptoms.

4. Differentiate variant angina pectoris from classic angina pectoris.

5. Explain the role of calcium in the cardiovascular system.

6. State the three classes of drugs used to treat angina pectoris and how each alters the pathophysiology of angina.

7. Relative to the use of nitroglycerin, β blockers, and calcium channel blockers in angina, describe (a) mechanism of action, (b) route of administration, (c) metabolism, (d) adverse effects, (e) teaching considerations, (f) efficacy in preventing and treating acute anginal attacks, and (g) one implication for each step of the nursing process.

8. Identify the most common complications occurring post AMI.

9. Describe the general therapeutic modalities in the care of acute myocardial infarction patients.

10. List the drugs used to treat cardiogenic shock, and give one implication for nursing care relative to each agent.

11. Describe the nursing process as it pertains to analgesia, heart rhythm, sedation, and bowel function of the patient following AMI.

12. Explain the rationale and methods used for limiting myocardial infarct size.

13. Identify the agents used to limit infarct size and their proposed benefit.

14. Describe the nursing process as it pertains to the limitation of infarct size.

15. Describe the role of intracoronary thrombolysis in AMI and its therapy.

Atherosclerosis is the leading cause of death in the industrialized Western world. In the United States, the incidence of clinically detected coronary atherosclerotic heart disease has reached epidemic proportions. This disease, which narrows the lumen of the coronary arteries and reduces the supply of blood and oxygen to the myocardium, is the principal cause of angina pectoris. Progression of the atherosclerotic process can result in myocardial infarction, cardiac arrest, and sudden death. With the recognition that angina pectoris and myocardial infarction share a common etiology (i.e., ischemic heart disease) this chapter focuses on both disease entities.

ANGINA PECTORIS

Etiology and Pathophysiology

Coronary atherosclerosis is the most common etiology of angina. The less frequent causes of angina include pulmonary hypertension, valvular heart disease, cardiac hypertrophy, and disease of the cardiac microcirculation. Although usually associated with coronary artery disease, angina can occur in patients with normal coronary arteries.

*The editors thank Kim L. Kelly, Pharm. D., Joyce E. Schickler, B.S.N., and Barbara A. Voshall, M.S.N., who contributed material on these topics in the first edition.

Coronary artery vasospasm has been found to be a contributing factor in a spectrum of ischemic syndromes, including a select group of patients that were first described by Prinzmetal. Often referred to as *Prinzmetal's variant angina,* the clinical presentation differs from that seen in classic angina pectoris. The characteristic finding of *nonexertional* chest pain differentiates variant angina from *classic* or *stable* angina pectoris.

The clinical manifestation of angina is related to the imbalance between myocardial oxygen consumption and supply (see Fig. 43-1). In the presence of narrowed coronary arteries or other underlying disease, activities which increase the myocardial oxygen consumption can lead to ischemia and precipitate angina. In patients with myocardial ischemia but normal or near normal coronary arteries, the probable mechanism for ischemia is coronary artery spasm. Recent studies indicate that both coronary atherosclerosis and coronary artery spasm contribute to myocardial ischemia in some patients.

Clinical Findings

Angina pectoris is usually described as a discomfort or pain in the chest. This discomfort is often characterized by a squeezing, tightening, choking, or heavy sensation which may radiate to the neck, lower jaw, shoulder, or arm. The chest discomfort is usually precipitated by effort and relieved by rest or nitroglycerin. Symptoms which are unrelated to exercise or emotion, are unrelieved by rest, last for seconds or extended periods, are sharp or knifelike in quality, or are increased by deep inspiration or bending and twisting are not usual in the anginal syndrome. If the undiagnosed symptom is indeed angina, it is usually relieved in *less than 3 min* after the use of **nitroglycerin**, and this relief may be concurrent with a feeling of head "fullness" or headaches. Other disorders which may cause angina-like symptoms include anxiety neurosis, hiatal hernia, cervical spine disease, gallbladder disease, costochondritis, and postherpetic neuralgia.

Many people experience a particular pattern of anginal symptoms. They tend to have anginal pain more easily in the morning soon after they arise; later in the day the threshold for angina is higher, and the same level of activity may not precipitate an attack. For example, a man might experience angina in the morning while shaving or walking to his car, but later in the day the same activity or a more vigorous one will not produce an attack. Still other patients may have a normal exercise tolerance but experience chest pain at rest.

Physical examination of the person with coronary artery disease manifested by angina pectoris usually reveals no specific findings between attacks. An ECG taken during an anginal attack usually shows transient ST and T-wave changes. Stress testing is designed to uncover discrepancies between myocardial oxygen need and available supply. The stress should be sufficient to increase the heart rate to 85 to 90 percent of a predicted maximum for the patient. Coronary arteriography is usually reserved for those who are being considered for surgery but may also be indicated for the patient with rest angina to further explore coronary artery anatomy.

Clinical Pharmacology and Therapeutics

Nondrug Therapy

Angina can be precipitated by many ordinary activities, and avoidance of these activities is an important aspect in the management of angina. Examples of common precipitating factors include eating a heavy meal, getting excited or emotionally upset, or being exposed to a very cold or extremely hot, humid environment. All these events can increase myocardial oxygen consumption. Certain medications may precipitate angina and are listed in Table 43-1. Though some precipitating factors should definitely be decreased or avoided, it is important to identify those others which contribute to the person's quality of life and should be continued if at all possible. The patient should be counseled regarding measures which can be taken to prevent or diminish attacks precipitated by such activities as work and sex. The patient needs to know that an active and useful life is possible, and the nurse can help to provide this reassurance.

Cigarette smoking is another precipitating factor of angina, as well as a risk factor in the development of coronary heart disease. It increases heart rate and blood pressure, in addition to impairing myocardial oxygen delivery in some persons. Cigarette smoking should definitely be stopped if possible.

Control of risk factors and associated disease is another important measure in the management of angina. Hypertension, obesity, hyperlipidemia, anemia, hyperthyroidism, and arrhythmia should all be appropriately controlled in a patient with angina. Other specific means of managing symptoms include pacing of activities so that myocardial oxygen need is met by the supply of oxygen available and avoiding precipitating activities soon after arising, when attacks are more easily precipitated. The patient should be instructed in the use of rest to help control attacks.

TABLE 43-1 Drugs that Can Induce Angina Pectoris

Caffeine	Diazoxide
Sympathomimetics (OTC cold preparations)	Ethanol
Thyroid preparations	Methysergide
Amphetamines	Prazosin
Ergot alkaloids	Hydralazine

Drug Therapy

The three groups of drugs commonly used to treat angina are organic nitrates, β-adrenergic blockers, and calcium channel blockers.

Nitroglycerin and Other Organic Nitrates A wide variety of nitrate preparations is available (see Table 43-2), and all nitrates have similar pharmacologic action. Nitroglycerin, taken sublingually, is by far the most effective drug in relieving an acute attack of angina and may be considered the prototype of the organic nitrates.

Mechanism of action The primary pharmacologic action of nitroglycerin is the relaxation of vascular smooth muscles. This results in a reduction of peripheral resistance and a decrease in venous return. Decreased venous return, preload reduction, can influence various hemodynamic factors affecting myocardial oxygen consumption. Ventricular

TABLE 43-2 Organic Nitrates Used for Angina

GENERIC NAME	TRADE NAME	USUAL DOSAGE AND ROUTE OF ADMINISTRATION
Nitroglycerin (glyceryl trinitrate)	Nitrostat, others	1 tablet PRN sublingual but not more than 3 in 15 min
	Nitro-bid, Nitrong	2.5–9.0 mg q8–12h oral
	Nitro-bid, Nitrol	1–5 in applied to skin q3–4h PRN
	Susadrin	1 mg tid transmucosally
	Tridil, Nitro-bid IV	10–20 μg/min continuous infusion. Increased by 5–10 μg/min until clinical response occurs
Isosorbide dinitrate	Isordil, Sorbitrate	2.5–10 mg q2–3h PRN sublingual
		10–40 mg qid oral
	Isordil Tembids	40 mg q6–12 h oral
	Sorbitrate Chewable	5 mg PRN chewed
Erythrityl tetranitrate	Cardilate	5–10 mg sublingual, oral, or chewed tid and hs
Pentaerythritol tetranitrate	Peritrate	10–40 mg qid oral
	Peritrate SA, Duotrate	30–80 mg q12h oral

wall tension, a major determinant of myocardial oxygen consumption, has been shown to be decreased after sublingual nitroglycerin, whereas the heart rate and contractile state are increased. Although the latter two factors increase myocardial oxygen consumption, the net effect of nitroglycerin in most patients is a decrease in myocardial oxygen consumption, thus relieving the angina.

Although nitroglycerin causes generalized dilatation of coronary arteries in normal subjects who do not have coronary artery disease, the effects of nitroglycerin in patients with atherosclerotic coronary arteries is still questionable. In animals, nitroglycerin induces a redistribution of coronary blood flow to ischemic subendocardium. Studies in patients with coronary atherosclerosis suggested that nitroglycerin can dilate coronary arteries, and further, that nitroglycerin can improve collateral circulation even in the presence of severe coronary artery stenosis.

It has not been established whether the antianginal efficacy of nitroglycerin is primarily due to its action on the peripheral vasculature or to its effect on coronary artery blood flow. The relative contribution of each of these actions probably depends upon the degree of coronary stenosis, the presence of collateral blood vessels, and the ability of the coronary vessels to dilate in each individual patient.

Pharmacokinetics Sublingual nitrates are generally well absorbed to produce a clinical effect. The absorption is most rapid for nitroglycerin, which can relieve chest pain within 3 min in most patients, and its duration of action is short (10 to 30 min). Buccal administration of nitrates, as with chewable tablets or transbuccal tablets (Susadrin), also provides rapid absorption adequate to produce a clinical effect.

The fate of orally administered nitrates in humans is not well known. Animal studies indicate that nitrates are rapidly inactivated in the liver by the enzyme glutathione organic nitrate reductase. Pharmacokinetic data for all forms of nitroglycerin in humans are limited and difficult to interpret, as factors such as the assay procedure, interindividual variation, and blood sampling site may all affect interpretation of pharmacokinetic findings.

There appears to be no close correlation between plasma nitroglycerin concentrations, hemodynamic responses, and antianginal effects. For these reasons nitroglycerin concentrations are not utilized in clinical practice.

Stability The potency of nitroglycerin is affected by various factors; it is inactivated by heat, light, air, and moisture. Significant amounts of the drug are lost when the sublingual nitroglycerin tablet is stored in a container which is not tightly closed, when it is stored in a warm place (even close to the patient's body), when the bottle contains a large amount of cotton filler, when the drug is stored with other drugs in the same bottle, or when it is stored in a pillbox. Stability studies indicate that if the drug is stored properly in a light-resistant container with a tightly fitted metal or other suitable screw cap then it remains stable for at least

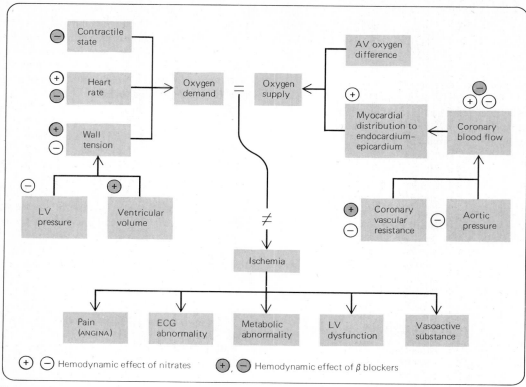

FIGURE 43-1

Pathophysiology and Therapy of Angina Pectoris. Myocardial oxygen demand is directly related to contractility, heart rate, and left ventricular (LV) wall tension. Wall tension is increased by higher left ventricular pressure (afterload) and higher ventricular volume (preload). Myocardial oxygen supply is a function of the extraction of oxygen from the blood [arteriovenous (AV) oxygen difference], coronary blood flow, and epicardial-endocardial blood distribution. Coronary blood flow is promoted by low coronary vascular resistance and high aortic pressure. A demand for oxygen by the myocardium in excess of the available supply will result in angina and its associated physiologic alterations. Nitrates and β blockers each affect several parameters in the oxygen demand and supply balance. A ⊕ denotes an increase in the parameter, while a ⊖ indicates a decrease. Notice that the deleterious effects of one type of drug (e.g., the reflex tachycardia of the nitrates or the increased coronary resistance of the β blockers) is often opposed by the effects of the other type of agent, so the β blockers and the nitrates are often coadministered for their complementary effects in angina. (*Used by permission of Alan S. Nies, M.D., from an unpublished course syllabus, University of Colorado School of Medicine, 1981.*)

five months. *A simple test of potency is that the fresh tablet taken sublingually should produce a burning sensation under the tongue or a headache.*

Intravenous nitroglycerin readily migrates into many plastics. Traditional intravenous infusion sets utilizing polyvinyl chloride (PVC) tubing absorb a greater percentage of nitroglycerin than do newer systems containing polyethylene. Many manufacturers of commercial intravenous nitroglycerin preparations now provide non-PVC-type administration sets.

Adverse effects Headache is the most common side effect of nitrates. It is usually of short duration (5 min) and seldom lasts for more than 20 min with a sublingual dose of nitroglycerin. With long-acting nitrates, headache, if it occurs, may last longer. Dizziness and syncope can also occur, especially if the patient is sensitive to nitrates, as well as tachycardia and flushing of the skin. Nausea, vomiting, and vertigo are rare.

Tolerance Tolerance is usually not a problem with nitroglycerin when it is used to treat or abort angina attacks. Cross-tolerance to the effects of sublingual nitroglycerin on blood pressure and heart rate have been reported following chronic administration on oral long-acting nitrates. However tolerance to the antianginal effects does not appear to develop.

Chronic nitroglycerin exposure of industrial workers can result in physiologic drug dependence. Five percent of workers so exposed have been shown to develop nonatheromatous ischemic heart disease after sudden withdrawal (such as when vacationing or changing jobs).

Dosage and Administration Sublingual nitroglycerin acts rapidly and effectively to treat, prevent, or abort acute attacks of angina. Other sublingual nitrate preparations offer no advantage for this purpose. The disadvantage of sublingual nitroglycerin is its short duration of action, which makes it impractical for achieving a sustained effect prophylactically. Sublingual nitroglycerin is available in several strengths (0.15-, 0.3-, 0.4-, and 0.6-mg tablets).

Intravenous nitroglycerin (Nitrol IV, Nitrostat IV, Nitro-bid IV, Tridil) has a role in treating hospitalized patients with unstable angina refractory to standard medical therapy. It has an immediate onset of action and can be titrated to treat, prevent, and terminate acute attacks of angina.

Nitroglycerin ointment (Nitro-bid, Nitrol), has been shown to be beneficial for as long as 3 h in patients with angina. It can be especially useful for prevention of nocturnal attacks. The onset of action is about 30 min. The usual dose is 1 to 2 in, spread in a thin layer over any nonhairy 6 × 6-in skin area every 3 to 4 h.

Three **transdermal nitroglycerin** delivery systems (Transderm-Nitro, Nitro-Dur, Nitrodisc) are designed to release the drug over 24 h (see Table 43-3) for prevention and treatment of angina pectoris, but they are not recommended for treatment of acute attacks. Based on the nitroglycerin concentrations they achieve in the blood they should be as effective as nitroglycerin ointment. However, the various products work by different controlled release mechanisms, and so are not interchangeable.

For many years, the efficacy of the "long-acting" oral nitrates, such as **isosorbide dinitrate, pentaerythritol tetranitrate, erythrityl tetranitrate,** or **sustained-release nitroglycerin** preparations (e.g., Klavikordal, Nitrong, Nitrostat SR, others) has been questioned. Recently, studies using direct hemodynamic measures in patients with coronary artery disease, as well as patients with congestive heart failure, showed that for many of these long-acting nitrates the effect lasted several hours. Long-acting nitrates (see Table 43-2) are likely to be effective, especially if large doses are administered.

TABLE 43-3 Transdermal Nitroglycerin (NTG) Systems

TRADE NAME	PRODUCT SURFACE AREA (cm²)	NTG CONTENT (mg)	NTG DELIVERED OVER 24 h (mg)
Transderm-Nitro 5	10	25	5.0
Transderm-Nitro 10	20	50	10.0
Nitro-Dur 5	5	26	2.5
Nitro-Dur 10	10	51	5.0
Nitro-Dur 15	15	77	7.5
Nitro-Dur 20	20	104	10.0
Nitro-Dur 30	30	154	15.0
Nitrodisc 16	8	16	11.2
Nitrodisc 32	16	32	22.4

β-Adrenergic Blocking Agents β-Adrenergic blocking agents such as **propranolol, practolol, alprenolol, sotalol, oxyprenolol, metoprolol, nadolol, pindolol,** and **timolol** have been reported to be effective in the treatment of angina pectoris. These individual β blockers differ in pharmacologic action, side effects, and metabolic disposition (see Chaps. 14 and 40). At present only propranolol (Inderal) and nadolol (Corgard) are approved by the Food and Drug Administration for use in the treatment of angina.

Mechanism of action β blockers decrease heart rate, myocardial contractility, and development of left ventricular tension. These tend to reduce myocardial oxygen consumption. β Blockers increase the ventricular ejection period and the ventricular end-diastolic pressure, and these effects tend to increase myocardial oxygen consumption. The net effect of β blockers, however, is a reduction in myocardial oxygen consumption, as demonstrated by direct measurement of oxygen consumption before and after β blockade.

Propranolol and **nadolol** are similar in the respect that they block both β_1- (cardiac) and β_2- (bronchial) adrenergic receptors equally. However, significant differences in their pharmacokinetics and adverse effects exist. The pharmacokinetics and adverse effects of these agents are presented in Chap. 40.

Dosage and administration The usual initial dose of **propranolol** is 10 to 20 mg orally tid or qid. Propranolol has been shown to be effective in stable angina pectoris when given every 12 h. Sustained release forms (Inderal LA) can be given once daily. The drug is gradually increased in increments of 40 mg/day every 3 to 5 days until the desired clinical response is achieved, the patients pulse rate falls to 55 to 60 beats per minute, or an undesirable effect occurs. There is a wide variation in effective dosages of propranolol between patients. Therapeutic response may be achieved with doses varying from 40 to 2000 mg/day.

Nadolol (Corgard) is started with an initial dosage of 40 mg of nadolol once a day for the treatment of angina. Dosage increments of 40 to 80 mg daily at 3- to 7-day intervals are recommended until an optimal clinical response or pronounced bradycardia occurs. The recommended maintenance dosage range for angina is 80 to 240 mg daily, with most patients requiring less than 160 mg/day.

If a patient has been chronically maintained on β blockers, sudden withdrawal should be avoided; rebound ischemic symptoms can occur after abrupt cessation of β blocker therapy.

Calcium Channel Blocking Agents The calcium channel blocking agents constitute the newest therapeutic modality for angina. The three calcium channel blockers approved for use in the treatment of stable, unstable, and variant forms of angina pectoris are **nifedipine** (Procardia), **verapamil** (Calan, Isoptin), and **diltiazem** (Cardizem).

Physiologic role of calcium Calcium ions play a key role in the formation of the cardiac action potential, linking excitation to contraction, and have a significant influence on the tone of the coronary and systemic arteries of the vascular tree.

In most cardiac cells, calcium ions play a role complementary to that of sodium ions. Depolarization of atrial and ventricular cells and of most of the specialized conducting cells is initiated by a rapid influx of sodium, which triggers the subsequent entrance of calcium through specific calcium channels. Calcium enters the cell at a much slower rate than that of sodium and is responsible for the plateau phase of the action potential. The influx of both calcium and sodium ions and the associated current that is produced generate the action potential and subsequent depolarization (Fig. 43-2).

Contraction of cardiac tissue and vascular smooth muscle is a result of the interaction of actin and myosin. For this process to occur in cardiac tissue, a certain amount of intracellular calcium must be present. When calcium becomes available, it binds to troponin, a regulatory protein. In the presence of adenosine triphosphate (ATP), troponin allows actin and myosin to interact, which causes the myocardial cells to contract.

In vascular smooth muscle, the actin and myosin interaction is regulated by a calcium-binding protein called calmodulin. Contraction in the vascular smooth muscle of the coronary and systemic arterioles alters tone in these vessels. Essential to both of these contractile occurrences is the availability of calcium at the site of the actin–myosin complex.

Calcium is thought to enter cells through highly selective ionic channels. One type, the voltage-dependent channel, is controlled by electric potentials and is responsible for the generation of the action potential. Passage of calcium through this channel is believed to be regulated by "gates" both outside and inside the channel, where, it is supposed, the calcium channel blockers inhibit calcium entry (Fig. 43-3).

Mechanism of action Mechanisms of action of the calcium channel blocking agents include (1) systemic vasodilation with reduction in systemic vascular resistance, (2) decreasing myocardial contractility, and (3) coronary vasodilation. Each agent manifests these effects to a different degree. The net hemodynamic effect results from direct action on the systemic vasculature and the myocardium and from evoked reflexes.

Of the currently available calcium channel blockers, **verapamil** possesses the greatest negative inotropic effect and should be used with caution in patients with preexisting heart failure or those receiving other myocardial depressants, i.e., β blockers. **Nifedipine** is the most potent systemic vasodilator of the marketed calcium channel blockers. It is generally considered to possess less negative inotropic effect than verapamil and is probably similar to **diltiazem**.

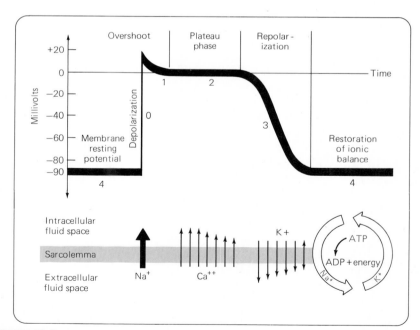

FIGURE 43-2

Generation of Cardiac Action Potential. The movement of sodium through the fast channel produces rapid depolarization. A slow inward current of calcium occurs during the plateau phase. Potassium influx causes repolarization. (*From M. B. Wiener, U S Pharmacist,* **6** *(10):45–68, 1981.*)

Although not FDA approved as antihypertensive agents, nifedipine and diltiazem are used clinically to treat high blood pressure and are under investigation for this indication.

Verapamil also decreases the rate of discharge of the sinoatrial node and slows conduction through the atrioventricular (AV) node. Like verapamil, **diltiazem** slows conduction through the AV node; an effect that is not seen with **nifedipine**. Verapamil is approved for use as an antiarrhythmic in supraventricular tachyarrhythmias.

Pharmacokinetics After oral administration of **nifedipine**, 90 percent of the administered drug is absorbed. More than 90 percent of the circulating drug is protein-bound. It is completely metabolized to inert products. Approximately 75 percent of the metabolized drug is eliminated via the kidney and up to 15 percent through the gastrointestinal tract. The plasma half-life is 4 to 5 h.

Verapamil is well absorbed after oral administration. Despite almost complete gastrointestinal absorption, the overall bioavailability of verapamil after oral administration ranges from 10 to 20 percent, indicating substantial first-pass metabolism in the liver. Ninety percent of verapamil in serum is bound to protein. The drug is primarily metabolized by the liver and up to 70 percent is eliminated via the gastrointestinal tract. The elimination half-life of verapamil varies from 3 to 7 h.

Diltiazem is absorbed rapidly and almost completely after oral administration, but only 40 percent of the dose is bioavailable after first-pass metabolism in the liver. Approximately 80 percent of the drug is bound to plasma proteins. The drug is largely metabolized by the liver and the metabolites are excreted in the urine and feces.

A summary of pharmacokinetic data is presented in Table 43-4.

Adverse effects **Nifedipine** frequently produces mild side effects which generally result from its vasodilatory effects. Headache, hypotension, flushing, dizziness, and leg edema are the more frequently reported side effects.

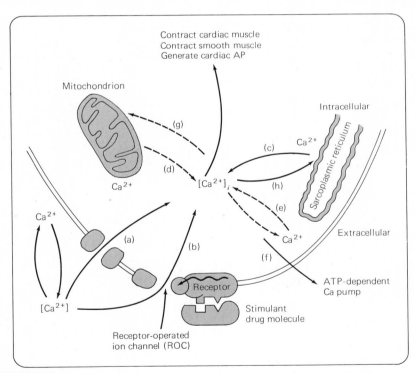

FIGURE 43-3

Movement of Calcium. Prior to the initiation of a physiologic effect (contraction of cardiac muscle, contraction of smooth muscle, or generation of cardiac action potential) the intracellular concentration of calcium must be increased. In the resting state the concentration of intracellular calcium is low. Movement of calcium into the cell can occur through two calcium-dependent channels, the receptor-oriented channel (ROC) or the action potential–dependent channel (a and b). Increased intracellular calcium can also come from internal cell storage sites like the sarcoplasmic reticulum, mitochondrion, or the internal surface of the cell membrane (c, d, and e). The removal of calcium from the cell can occur by an active extrusion pump (f) or by returning calcium to its storage sites (g, h). (*From M. B. Wiener, U S Pharmacist, 6 (10):45–68, 1981.*)

TABLE 43-4 Pharmacokinetic Characteristics of Calcium Channel Blocking Agents

CHARACTERISTIC	VERAPAMIL	NIFEDIPINE	DILTIAZEM
Absolute oral bioavailability (%)	10–35	45–65	45–67
Metabolites	Norverapamil*	Acid or lactone†	Desacetyldiltiazem‡
Excreted unchanged (%)	<5	1–2	<4
Clearance (L/min)			
Oral dosing	1.0–2.75	0.6	—
Intravenous dosing	0.5–0.9	0.8	0.9
Volume of distribution (L)	112–401	83–98	159
Elimination half-life (h)			
Single dose	1.8–5.3	1.5–5	2–6
Multiple dose	5–18	—	—
Approximate therapeutic plasma concentration (ng/mL)	50–150	25–100	40–200
Protein bound (%)	83–92	92–98	77–85

*Norverapamil has 20% of the pharmacologic activity of verapamil.
†Inactive metabolites.
‡Desacetyldiltiazem has 40–50% of the pharmacologic activity of diltiazem.
Source: From R. L. Talbert and H. I. Bussey: "Update on Calcium Channel Blockers," *Clin Pharm*, **21**:403–416, Sept.–Oct., 1983.

Oral **verapamil** is fairly well tolerated with a low prevalence of gastric intolerance and constipation, vertigo, headache, and nervousness. Verapamil prolongs conduction in the AV node and may worsen preexisting conduction disturbance. Verapamil has a negative inotropic effect and must be used with caution in patients with congestive heart failure and in patients receiving concomitant β-adrenergic blocking drugs.

Adverse effects with **diltiazem** appear fairly infrequently. Drug rash, dizziness, headaches, flushing, conduction blockade, and gastrointestinal discomfort have been reported in some patients.

Dosage and administration The usual starting dose of **nifedipine** (Procardia) is 10 mg three times a day. The dose should be increased until symptoms are relieved or undesirable side effects occur. The maximal dose generally recommended is 120 mg daily. **Verapamil** (Calan, Isoptin) is usually started in doses of 80 mg every 8 h. The dose may be increased to 360 mg daily. The usual oral dose of **diltiazem** (Cardizem) is 30 to 60 mg every 8 h.

Combination Therapy

In a patient who first presents with angina, a sublingual nitrate, preferably **nitroglycerin**, is usually the first choice. This may be adequate in some patients with mild, infrequent angina attacks. If the angina becomes worse and interrupts the daily activity, β blockers can be added, provided there is no contraindication. When nitrates and β blockers are used together, the cardiac effects are complementary (see Fig. 43-1). The increase in the heart rate induced by nitroglycerin in some patients is offset by the bradycardic effect of the β-adrenergic blocker, and the increase in ejection time and ventricular volume produced by the β-adrenergic blocker is opposed by nitroglycerin. The addition of β blockers to the nitrate therapy can reduce the need for sublingual nitrates.

In a patient who is to be treated medically but in whom the use of β blockers is contraindicated or whose angina is not well controlled with the combination of nitrates and β blockers, calcium channel blockers may be tried.

Coronary Artery Surgery

Coronary artery surgery offers an alternative approach in the management of angina. The purpose of the surgery is to increase the coronary circulation. The surgery usually involves inserting a graft (often a superficial vein such as the saphenous) between the aorta and the coronary artery beyond the occlusion, so that the lesion is bypassed. Such surgery has provided good symptomatic relief in many patients with unstable angina which has been poorly controlled by drugs. Coronary artery surgery can relieve pain in 80 to 90 percent of patients with angina, but it is not known whether it will prolong the life of patients with relatively mild disease, i.e., those with single or double coronary vessel occlusion. In those patients with occlusion of the left main coronary artery, and those with triple vessel disease, i.e., occlusion of three coronary arteries, the surgical treatment has been shown to be superior to the medical treatment.

NURSING PROCESS RELATED TO ANGINA PECTORIS

Assessment

In addition to a complete description of the angina (precipitating events; the quality, location, radiation, severity, and duration of the pain; and actions which relieve the discomfort), the history should include a careful review of systems with special attention to risk factors and the family history. The initial assessment should provide a foundation for patient teaching. Information on the meaning of the illness to the patient, family, and lifestyle will all be necessary to formulate an individualized management plan.

When patients are admitted to the hospital and state that they are taking an antianginal drug at home, the nursing history should include some information about the frequency of anginal pain and the use of the medication at home for comparison with the pattern in the hospital. The well-recognized stress associated with hospitalization may alter this pattern; the nurse should plan to initiate measures to decrease the stress. Many of these patients bring their sublingual **nitroglycerin** to the hospital with them, desiring to keep it at the bedside where it is readily accessible. The nurse should feel comfortable about allowing patients to do this with the physician's approval, unless assessment reveals that they are confused or otherwise unable to administer the drug safely.

The nurse should ascertain what patients know about the use of their antianginal medication, why they take it, how they administer it, and if they recognize the signs of adverse drug reactions. The nurse cannot assume that a patient who has taken **nitroglycerin** or any other antianginal drugs for some time understands its use or takes it properly. If assessment of the patient's knowledge or practice reveals major misconceptions or dangerous practices, self-administration cannot be judged safe until appropriate teaching has been done. It is important to ascertain if the patient taking a blocker such as **propranolol** (Inderal) or **nadolol** (Corgard) can take his pulse or knows the signs and symptoms of increased fluid retention. Patients should weigh themselves every day. Patients receiving **calcium channel blockers** should be aware of the side effects of these drugs (hypotension, irregular heartbeat, etc.) because a dose change or use of another calcium blocker may relieve the adverse effect.

It is necessary that the nurse be well aware of the characteristics of anginal pain, since it is often important to differentiate between angina and other problems which cause chest discomfort, such as coronary occlusion, heartburn, ulcer, hepatitis, hiatal hernia, and so on. If there is question about the cause of the pain, if there are unusual changes in vital signs, or if normal measures do not bring relief in the expected time, the physician must be notified.

Management

Since **nitroglycerin** and the **long-acting nitrates** are primarily self-administered and the drug therapy and modifications of lifestyle are complementary, teaching is the most important aspect of management in patients taking these agents. The fewest possible changes should be initiated in a lifestyle which has been satisfying to the patient. However, difficult choices may be required, as when there is a need to change the job or place of residence. Those caring for patients should consider ways to reduce their emotional stress.

The patient needs an understanding of the disease process, the cause of the angina, the relationship of risk and precipitating factors to symptoms and prognosis, how to use the drug, and how to store it. Patients often have misconceptions and fears about their cardiac problems. Such fears sometimes can be alleviated by an explanation of the basic underlying problem and careful instruction on how to avoid common precipitating factors. Another fear sometimes expressed by patients on **nitroglycerin** is that the drug might explode like dynamite; patients need to be assured that there is no chance of nitroglycerin exploding.

Patient education can also improve compliance with drug therapy and its efficacy. The patient should be informed as to the proper way to store the drug and how to test a **nitroglycerin** tablet for freshness. A fresh supply of nitroglycerin should be purchased every five months to ensure potency. The sublingual route of administration is quite new to most patients, and the fact that the saliva should not be swallowed until the burning sensation is gone warrants reiteration. Patients may experience syncope unless they lie or recline during use of sublingual nitroglycerin.

Patients can learn to use **nitroglycerin** prophylactically by taking it 3 to 5 min before activities that usually precipitate an attack, and so they will need guidance in identifying these factors. The method which a patient ultimately finds most successful in controlling the angina may be highly individualized.

The nurse must supply information regarding medications which may precipitate anginal attacks. This should include brand names for over-the-counter agents (see Table 43-1).

Topical nitroglycerin patches are now widely used in the treatment of angina. A discussion of special problems which may be encountered by the patient in applying, wearing, or removing the adhesive patch may be beneficial to patient understanding. Points which need to be emphasized include wearing transdermal patches continuously, 24 h a day, reapplying a fresh patch each morning to a nonhairy or shaved area, and applying the patch securely to the skin surface of the trunk or proximal limb. If nitroglycerin ointment is used, the drug will need more frequent application as ordered and the area should be cleansed before fresh ointment is applied even when rotating sites (which minimizes skin irritation). The ointment is then covered with plastic wrap to protect clothing from staining and ensure proper absorption. The fact that these forms of nitroglycerin are primarily used to prevent anginal attacks rather than alleviate an acute attack should be reinforced with the patient. The need to taper the dosage and duration of use of the transdermal preparations to avoid rebound angina when the drug is discontinued should be explained in detail to the patient.

Because **propranolol** and **nadolol** slow the heart, decrease its force of contraction, and may cause bronchial constriction, these drugs are contraindicated in bradycardia, congestive heart failure, and chronic obstructive lung disease, including asthma. Before giving each dose of the drug, the nurse should determine an apical pulse. *If the heart rate decreases to less than 55, the dosage should be reduced or withheld and the physician notified.* The nurse will therefore need to teach these patients to take their own pulse accurately. Also, the nurse must observe for respiratory distress or wheezing. If the patient is at high risk of congestive heart failure, it is also prudent to watch the intake and output, daily weight, and signs of peripheral edema and to auscultate the lungs for rales or wheezes. These observations are also important with **verapamil**, the calcium channel blocker which significantly decreases cardiac contractility.

β Blockers and calcium channel blockers may alter glucose tolerance. β **Blockers** potentiate hypoglycemia and also can mask its symptoms. A diabetic patient who is taking both a β blocker and a hypoglycemic agent (oral drugs or insulin) should be aware that signs of hypoglycemia related to the sympathetic response (tremulousness, tachycardia, sweating) cannot be relied on and should know how to identify other symptoms (generalized muscular weakness, faintness, hunger pangs, headache, numbness or tingling of tongue or lips, double vision).

Calcium channel blockers can interfere with the stimulus to endocrine and exocrine secretion. Signs and symptoms of hyperglycemia and awareness of a possible need to alter the dose of a hypoglycemic agent are nursing responsibilities. Careful watch of fasting blood sugar levels and urine sugar and acetone testing are essential.

Other nursing implications for patients receiving **calcium channel blockers** center around side effects. Hypotension can occur initially, and so it is very important that the nurse caring for these patients *check the blood pressure every half-hour for 2 h after giving the first dose of a calcium channel blocker.* Also, when the dosage is increased, especially if a patient is also on a β blocker, the same safety measure applies.

Another adverse reaction some patients experience is an increase in frequency of anginal attacks when **calcium channel blockers** are first started or when dosage is increased. The nurse should be aware of this and document each episode of pain carefully. Many adverse effects such as dizziness, lightheadedness, nausea, weakness, headache, flushing, muscle cramps, tremor, nervousness, and palpitation can occur. Many of these symptoms will disappear with continued use or reduction in dosage, but some patients require an alternative calcium channel blocker for continued therapy.

Evaluation

The patient should be instructed to keep a diary of anginal pain and its duration and relieving factors (rest, nitroglycerin, or both), so that there will be some way to judge whether the anginal attacks are becoming more frequent. In the hospital, it is the nurses' responsibility to record the amount of nitroglycerin taken and the number of anginal episodes, even if the drug is kept at the bedside for self-administration by the patient. The physician should be informed if the angina is not controlled by the prescribed therapy, and a new plan of care should be formulated.

CASE STUDY

Mr. L., a 58-year-old married male who manages a small dairy store, came to the medical clinic due to an uncomfortable intermittent chest sensation that had begun a month before the appointment. The sensation was a squeezing feeling in the substernal area, which at times radiated to his left elbow, but he stated that it was not a sensation of pain. This "squeezing" sensation always occurred in association with physical activity or emotional stress and was relieved by lying down for a few minutes.

Mr. L. had not had a complete physical examination for five years, although he had had his blood pressure taken at community screening clinics, where he had been told he had elevated blood pressure and advised to seek follow-up care but had not done so.

The initial visit was a complete diagnostic examination. His past medical history included only the untreated high blood pressure. The review of systems was negative. Significant risk factors included the following: the patient was a heavy smoker (two packs a day for 40 years), hypertensive, and obese (> 25 lb overweight for 20 years). The family history was contributory, with both heart disease and high blood pressure in several close relatives: father, brother, and grandparents. His father had died of myocardial infarction, and a 56-year-old brother was presently under treatment for postinfarction angina.

On physical examination the patient was found to be anxious appearing, and mildly obese. Blood pressure was 170/115, pulse 90, respiration 18. A few scattered wheezes, which moved or disappeared with coughing, were noted on auscultation of the chest. Otherwise, the physical examination was negative.

An electrocardiogram done during the visit was normal. The chest x-ray showed the heart size to be within the upper limits of normal, and the lungs were clear. The battery of laboratory tests, including thyroid function, were all normal except for a slightly elevated serum cholesterol. A stress electrocardiogram was discontinued before discomfort occurred when T-wave changes were noted on the monitor, but the ECG pattern returned to normal at rest.

The diagnosis of angina pectoris was made. Sublingual nitroglycerin 0.4 mg PRN, hydrochlorothiazide 50 mg qd, and propranolol 10 mg qid were prescribed for Mr. L. An appointment was made for follow-up care 4 weeks later.

Assessment

Upon interview, Mr. L. told the nurse that activities with which he had begun to associate the discomfort were walking the dog after breakfast, moving heavy objects at work, sexual intercourse, and garden work. The sensation was felt most frequently if physical exertion occurred in the morning, during exposure to cold weather, or after a meal. He had been having three to five attacks a day before coming to the clinic. The idea that there was something wrong with his heart distressed him considerably, and he expressed fear that he might have to give up the store which he had built by "hard work and the sweat of my brow" and that his wife might not consider him a "complete man" any longer. He had little understanding of the disease process. The nurse diagnosed the need for complete instruction about his medication and his condition.

Management

The goal relative to the angina was that the patient should acquire the knowledge and skill to control the anginal symptoms. He was taught about his problems of angina and hypertension. The underlying cause of the angina pectoris was described, especially as it related to the events precipitating discomfort. Modifiable risk factors were reviewed. Instructions were given about storage, transportation, and use of nitroglycerin, as well as the use of rest in conjunction with nitroglycerin to relieve the symptoms. The action and route of nitroglycerin were explained. He was advised that the onset of the action would occur in 1 to 3 min and that its duration was less than an hour. He learned that he could take up to three tablets per episode at 5-min intervals and was relieved that he could not develop a tolerance or addiction to the drug. If three tablets did not relieve the attack, he knew he was to contact the clinic promptly.

Mr. L. was also taught about taking propranolol. The action and purpose of the medication were discussed. It was stressed that propranolol should not be discontinued abruptly because of the potential rebound effect. Mr. L. was taught how to take his pulse and told to call the clinic if it should become less than 55 beats/min. He stated that he had a scale at home with which to weigh himself and was knowledgeable of the signs of increased peripheral edema.

An initial dose of nitroglycerin was given at the clinic (although the patient was feeling no discomfort then), so that he might experience the burning sensation under the tongue and the headache produced by fresh nitroglycerin. An American Heart Association booklet, entitled *Angina*, was given to Mr. L. to read at home.

Mr. L. and the nurse discussed the elimination or decrease of precipitating activities, e.g., permitting the dog to run free in the fenced yard in the morning and giving it a more leisurely walk later in the day and hiring a high school student to help in the store several hours a day to do the heavy lifting. Further, they discussed the use of nitroglycerin to prevent anginal attacks. Mr. L. was relieved to hear that this had been helpful to others in preventing anginal attacks during coitus. He also expressed interest in weight reduction, and the nurse supplied him with information about his diet.

Evaluation

When Mr. L. returned to the clinic in 4 weeks, he reported that with the nitroglycerin he had been able to prevent some probable attacks and quickly relieve others. His blood pressure was 130/90, his heart rate was 64/min, and he had lost 8 lb. He had been unable to completely eliminate coffee and cigarettes but said that he had limited himself to a cup of coffee at breakfast and a cigarette with each meal.

ACUTE MYOCARDIAL INFARCTION

Etiology and Pathophysiology

Myocardial infarction is one of the commonest diagnoses in the industrialized world. Each year about 1.5 million Americans sustain a myocardial infarction, resulting in 550,000 deaths. Mortality rates during hospitalization and during the year following infarction are 15 and 10 percent, respectively.

Almost all myocardial infarctions result from atherosclerosis of the coronary arteries. Atherosclerotic narrowing of coronary arteries reduces the blood supply to the myocardium. Acute obstruction of an atherosclerotic coronary artery results in ischemic injury to myocardial cells. When severe ischemia is prolonged, irreversible damage, i.e., cell death, occurs.

While the primary etiology of myocardial infarction is atherosclerotic disease of the coronary arteries, the contribution of arterial thrombosis, platelet aggregation, and coronary vasospasm is also of importance. Regardless of the etiology, optimal care of the patient with suspected or proven myocardial infarction requires hospitalization in an intensive care unit that has facilities for monitoring and managing potentially life-threatening complications of infarction.

Clinical Findings

The pain of acute myocardial infarction is commonly described as tight, squeezing, constricting, choking, burning, heavy, and accompanied by "a sense of impending doom." It typically lasts longer than that of angina pectoris and may become increasingly severe with time. It rarely subsides spontaneously and is not relieved by rest and nitroglycerin. The pain is frequently accompanied by sweating, nausea, vomiting, dyspnea, apprehension, weakness, or lightheadedness.

Irreversibly injured myocardial cells release a number of enzymes (LDH, CPK, SGOT) into the circulation where they can be measured. The degree of serum enzyme elevation is not prognostic, although more extensive infarctions seem to be associated with greater enzyme elevations. Other nonspecific laboratory manifestations may be recognized in patients with infarction. These include hyperglycemia, leukocytosis, and an elevated erythrocyte sedimentation rate.

In the majority of patients with acute myocardial infarction, some changes can be documented with serial 12-lead electrocardiographic (ECG) tracings. The diagnosis of myocardial infarction is confirmed by the presence of at least two of the following three features: a typical history of chest pain, ECG evidence of Q waves and/or serial repolarization (ST-T) abnormalities, and an appropriate temporal rise in cardiac serum enzyme levels.

Clinical Pharmacology and Therapeutics

Therapeutic interventions in acute myocardial infarction are primarily aimed at (1) prevention of complications and limitation of infarct size, and (2) treating the complications when they occur. Careful monitoring of cardiac rhythm and prompt treatment of arrhythmia have reduced the number of deaths resulting from intractable arrhythmias. Most deaths among post myocardial infarction patients who reach the hospital are now attributable to left ventricular failure and shock.

The extent and severity of myocardial ischemic injury, and ultimately of myocardial infarction after coronary occlusion, depend on the balance between oxygen supply and demand. The quantity of myocardium that becomes necrotic following coronary artery occlusion may be limited by interventions that favorably influence oxygen supply and demand. Protection of ischemic myocardium has been demonstrated in many animal species and is now being widely investigated in patients. Specific pharmacologic interventions will be discussed later.

General Measures

Rest and Activity   To reduce myocardial workload, activities initially should be limited to bed rest with use of bedside commode and should be coordinated in an effective rehabilitation program which continues throughout hospitalization. If arrhythmias, heart failure, or other significant complications occur, activities must be further modified.

Analgesics   The pain of myocardial ischemia contributes to excessive activity of the autonomic nervous system and the alleviation or reduction of pain is a critical factor in the routine care of patients with acute myocardial infarction. **Morphine sulfate** remains the drug of choice and is ideally administered IV in dilute solution (10 mg in 10 mL) in 2-

to 4-mg increments every 10 to 15 min until pain is relieved or toxicity (depressed respirations, hypotension, vomiting, or bradycardia) is evident. Because of its vagomimetic effects, **morphine** is not used in patients with atrioventricular (AV) block greater than first degree or in patients with sinus bradycardia. In these instances, **meperidine** (Demerol) may be used in doses of 50 to 100 mg IV. Undesirable increases in heart rate, however, may result from its vagolytic effects. **Pentazocine** (Talwin), while an effective analgesic, should not be used because its vasoconstrictive capabilities adversely affect cardiac work. All parenteral medications, including analgesics, should be administered intravenously. Intramuscular injections are avoided because they interfere with serum enzyme determinations and are erratically and unpredictably absorbed by patients with reduced cardiac output and/or blood pressure.

Sedation   Sedation is useful in reducing anxiety caused by illness and unfamiliar hospital surroundings. Nonpharmacologic methods to prevent and reduce anxiety include explanations as to what has happened and what is to happen. **Diazepam** (Valium) in divided doses through the day plus a hypnotic at bedtime may be the optimal pharmacologic therapy. Oral dosage is preferred although severe acute anxiety attacks can be managed by intravenous diazepam.

Other Therapeutic Modalities

Other general measures include:

1.   A liquid diet for 24 h because of the risk of nausea and vomiting or cardiac arrest early after infarction and the need to reduce the risk of aspiration

2.   **Docusate sodium** (Colace), 100 mg daily, to prevent constipation, Valsalva maneuver, and straining

3.   Low-flow oxygen (2 to 4 L/min) delivery by nasal prongs for two to three days to correct the hypoxemia commonly observed in acute myocardial infarction patients

4.   Full dose anticoagulation, which may be beneficial in patients with prior myocardial infarction or thromboembolism, concurrent thrombophlebitis, or complications such as congestive heart failure, hypotension, or marked obesity, and which will prevent early mobilization

In patients without a high risk of embolization, minidose heparin (5000 U subcutaneously) every 8 to 12 h diminishes the incidence of deep vein thrombosis in immobilized patients (see Chap. 42). The drug should be continued until the patient begins ambulation.

Treatment of Complications

Complications of myocardial infarction may be present at admission or develop in the early days post infarction. Common complications that may be observed include persistent or recurrent chest pain, arrhythmias, left ventricular failure, acute pulmonary edema, and cardiogenic shock. Less common complications include pericarditis, pulmonary embolism, and cardiac rupture.

Arrhythmias Rhythm abnormalities are the most frequent complications of myocardial infarction and their management depends both on the nature of the arrhythmia and on the hemodynamic consequences. Some arrhythmias require only a search for precipitating factors that can be reversed, whereas others require prompt treatment because of their ominous prognosis. Some abnormality of cardiac rhythm has been noted in 72 to 96 percent of patients with acute myocardial infarction treated in coronary care units. Moreover, many arrhythmias occur prior to hospitalization before the patient is monitored. Every known arrhythmia may be observed after acute myocardial infarction.

Bradyarrhythmias Sinus bradycardia is the commonest arrhythmia occurring during the early phases of acute myocardial infarction, and it is particularly frequent in patients with inferior infarction. When this arrhythmia is associated with hypotension, intravenous **atropine sulfate** in doses of 0.4 to 1.0 mg should be administered every 3 to 5 min (with a total dose not exceeding 2 mg) to bring the heart rate up to 60 beats/min.

First-degree atrioventricular (AV) block generally does not require specific treatment nor does second-degree AV block of the Mobitz type I (Wenckebach) variety when the average ventricular rate is adequate. However, if slowing of the ventricular rate occurs or higher degrees of AV block ensue, i.e., Mobitz type II and complete heart block, immediate treatment with a temporary transvenous pacemaker is indicated.

Tachyarrhythmias Tachyarrhythmias of any origin may be deleterious since they increase myocardial oxygen requirements, limit the time available for ventricular filling during diastole, and compromise cardiac output.

Sinus tachycardia occurs in approximately one-third of patients with acute myocardial infarction and may be associated with transient hypertension or hypotension and augmented sympathetic activity. Persistent tachycardia may increase the size of infarction and may require treatment with β-adrenergic blocking agents although in many cases pain relief, sedation, and enhanced oxygenation will correct the tachycardia.

Premature ventricular contractions The suppression of premature ventricular contractions (PVCs) is based on the concept that in the face of myocardial ischemia the threshold for ventricular fibrillation is lowered and PVCs may trigger ventricular fibrillation. Frequent PVCs ($>$6/min), multiform premature contractions, extrasystoles occurring in pairs or salvos, and early premature contractions (R on T) all constitute indications for treatment. Administration of parenteral **lidocaine** to all patients with definite or likely acute myocardial infarction is a common practice in many institutions to reduce the incidence of primary ventricular fibrillation.

Treatment of Arrhythmias Drugs utilized in the treatment of rhythm disorders are discussed in detail in Chap. 45, and are, therefore, summarized only briefly here.

Lidocaine In absence of specific, correctable factors lidocaine should be administered to patients with acute myocardial infarction and ventricular premature contractions. An initial loading dose of 200 mg may be administered as two 100-mg doses 10 min apart or four 50-mg doses, 5 min apart. All bolus injections should be given at a rate less than 50 mg/min to avoid toxicity. Subsequent infusion rates vary from 2 to 4 mg/min. In patients with shock or heart failure both loading and infusion doses should be reduced by 50 percent. Intramuscular injections of lidocaine have been utilized during the patient's transportation to the hospital but do not achieve therapeutic concentrations as promptly as those following intravenous therapy.

Procainamide When premature ventricular beats compromise hemodynamics and persist despite administration of **lidocaine**, administration of procainamide (Pronestyl) intravenously may be effective in suppressing arrhythmias caused by increased automaticity. In addition, procainamide may also suppress arrhythmias dependent upon reentry. Procainamide is also useful in the treatment of atrial arrhythmias and can be given orally to the patient who requires maintenance antiarrhythmic therapy.

Hemodynamic Disturbances

Left ventricular performance is impaired to some degree in all patients with acute myocardial infarction. The extent and degree of functional loss depend on such factors as the status of the myocardium, if there has been previous ischemia or infarction, the extent of the new infarction, and the presence of preexisting left ventricular disease as a result of hypertension or other cardiac disorders. The hemodynamic disturbances that are seen can range from transient left ventricular dysfunction with no subjective complaints to cardiogenic hypotension or shock. (For a discussion of the management of congestive heart failure see Chap. 44.)

Cardiogenic Shock Massive myocardial infarction may produce global impairment of left ventricular function which is so profound that cardiogenic shock occurs. The patient in cardiogenic shock is identified by the presence of hypotension (systolic blood pressure below 90 mmHg) in combination with a cold, clammy, vasoconstricted skin and inadequate urinary output. Cardiogenic shock may be encountered in as many as 5 to 15 percent of patients. Initial measures include assessment for and correction of hypovolemia and also control of arrhythmias. However, even aggressive therapy does little to alter the 85 to 95 percent current mortality associated with cardiogenic shock.

Inotropic agents, vasopressors (**norepinephrine**), and vasodilators are commonly employed in the treatment of cardiogenic shock. The most frequently employed inotropic agents in this setting are **dopamine** and **dobutamine**. Dopamine in an infusion rate of 1 to 5 $\mu g/kg/min$ increases cardiac contractility, cardiac output, and renal blood flow increase, with little change in heart rate and either a reduction or no change in total peripheral resistance. With higher infusion rates (10 to 15 $\mu g/kg/min$), arterial pressure, peripheral resistance, and heart rate increase and renal blood flow may decline. Dobutamine (Dobutrex) is given in doses of 2.5 to 10 $\mu g/kg/min$. Dobutamine causes peripheral vascular resistance. It does not dilate renal arteries but renal function may improve as a result of increased cardiac output (see Chap. 48, section on shock).

In addition to vasopressors and inotropic agents some patients will benefit from vasodilator therapy with IV **nitroprusside** (Nipride; see Chap. 40) or **nitroglycerin** to reduce left ventricular filling pressures as well as systemic and pulmonary vascular resistance. These agents, however, should not be given when systolic blood pressure is less than 90 mmHg or with left ventricular filling pressures of <18 mmHg.

Limitation of Infarct Size

Despite aggressive pharmacologic therapy the mortality rate associated with cardiogenic shock remains quite high. The patients who succumb from cardiogenic shock exhibit massive infarcts. Recently, therapeutic interventions designed to limit the size of infarction and decrease mortality have been assessed in both animal models and patients. In experimental myocardial infarction, myocardial necrosis begins about 20 min after the onset of ischemia and is completed over an interval of about 6 h. During the interval before necrosis is completed, therapies targeted at reducing myocardial oxygen demand, increasing oxygen and nutrient supply, favorably modifying cellular factors, or improving metabolism have been shown to reduce the amount of ischemic injury and ultimate infarct size. Although definitive answers on the efficacy of attempts to reduce infarct size in humans are not yet available, an increasing number of pilot studies have provided encouraging results. Several interventions (calcium channel blockade, β-adrenergic blockade, intravenous nitroglycerin, and intracoronary thrombolysis) appear particularly promising.

Calcium Channel Blockers Numerous regimens are being evaluated to further define the role of these agents in preserving ischemic myocardium. The effect of calcium blockade on myocardial oxygen balance is quite profound and results in both a decrease in oxygen demands and an increase in oxygen supply. The beneficial effects of calcium blockade probably underlie the high degree of effectiveness these agents have in the treatment of angina pectoris and the promise they have in salvaging ischemic myocardium.

β-Adrenergic Blocking Agents Several actions of β-adrenergic blocking agents may have favorable effects on ischemic myocardium. The principal effects of intravenous β blockers given acutely to patients are reductions in cardiac output, arterial pressure, and heart rate, with generally slight effects on left ventricular filling pressure. Reports indicate that early intervention with β blockers might limit infarct size by decreased myocardial oxygen consumption. **Metoprolol** (Lopressor) is approved for early treatment of myocardial infarction, beginning as soon after hospital admission as the patient's condition allows. Therapy is initiated with three IV bolus doses of 5 mg at approximately 2-min intervals with constant monitoring of ECG rhythm, blood pressure, and heart rate. Patients who tolerate the full 15-mg IV loading dose are placed on maintenance of 50 mg orally q6h beginning 15 min after the last IV dose and continuing for 48 h. Thereafter a maintenance dose of 100 mg twice daily is given. Those unable to tolerate the full IV loading dose are given 25 to 50 mg of metoprolol orally every 6 h beginning 15 min after the last IV dose. For severe intolerance (systolic blood pressure less than 100 mmHg, greater than first-degree heart block, heart rate less than 45, or moderate to severe heart failure), the drug must be discontinued.

In addition, β blockers are of benefit in the prevention of reinfarction and sudden death following acute myocardial infarction. **Timolol** (Blocadren) and **propranolol** (Inderal) have been approved for this indication with therapy beginning 1 to 3 weeks after the myocardial infarction and continuing up to 3 years. Timolol is given in doses of 100 mg bid, while 180 to 240 mg of propranolol are administered divided into 3 to 4 daily doses. The β blockers are discussed in Chaps. 14 and 40.

Intravenous Nitroglycerin The mechanism of the beneficial effect of **nitroglycerin** is believed to be an increase in collateral blood flow to the ischemic zone and a reduction of myocardial oxygen demand because of decreased left ventricular wall tension. Intravenous nitroglycerin has been reported to affect measurements of the infarct size in patients. However, at present, the use of intravenous nitroglycerin to reduce infarct size is still considered experimental.

Coronary Thrombolysis

Recent angiographic and intraoperative studies have shown that intraluminal coronary thrombi are present within hours of the onset of symptoms of acute transmural infarction. Several investigators have reported successful dissolution of coronary thrombi early in the course of acute myocardial infarction in humans. Angiographic evidence shows that a thrombolytic agent, usually **streptokinase** (Streptase), infused through a catheter adjacent to the thrombus, has a role in reopening the affected coronary artery. Reductions of acute ST segment elevations and relief of chest pain have been reported, and improvement in left ventricular function may result. Considerable research comparing intravenous versus intracoronary administration of this agent is being carried out at the present. See Chap. 43 for additional description of this therapy.

The above treatment modalities remain experimental at the present time. Several controlled clinical trials are underway in an effort to determine whether acute interventions with a thrombolytic agent can reduce infarct size and improve myocardial function and/or patient prognosis.

NURSING PROCESS RELATED TO MYOCARDIAL INFARCTION

The development of the coronary care unit has significantly decreased the rate of mortality from myocardial infarction. Nurses in these units use advanced skills for assessing, diagnosing, treating, and evaluating patients.

Assessment

Assessment of the patient with an acute myocardial infarction is very extensive and involves mechanical devices such as the electrocardiogram, the continuous one-lead monitor, central venous pressure, direct arterial monitoring of blood pressure, Swan-Ganz catheterization, and hourly intake and output volume measurements. The nurse must remember that these technical devices are assistive only and that the assessment of the patient as a whole is just as important.

To plan care specific to the patient's needs, the nurse should be aware of the size and location of the myocardial infarction and the complications which can be associated with it. The 12-lead ECG and the continuous 1-lead monitor can show conduction and rhythm disturbances and evolution of the myocardial infarction. Observation of the characteristics of congestive heart failure and signs of decreased tissue perfusion—confusion, low urine output, decreased blood pressure, cold, clammy skin—should be part of every patient's ongoing assessment.

Identifying the psychosocial effect of the disease on each patient and expressing an understanding of his/her needs will aid the patient in adhering to restricted activities, prescribed medications, and constant monitoring. It is often very difficult for independent patients to allow their lives to be controlled during a hospitalization.

Management

Physical and psychological rest is the primary goal immediately following an acute myocardial infarction. The nurse must appear calm and competent to reassure the patient.

All patients must have an IV site following an acute myocardial infarction because of the potential for complications. The IV site should be checked daily for patency and signs of phlebitis. In an emergency, all medications are given by the IV route for ease of access and speed of effect. **Morphine sulfate** IV is given for pain relief in doses of 2 to 4 mg every 5 to 10 min. Blood pressure, heart rate, respiratory rate, and an accurate assessment of the pain are checked before each dose is given. Morphine is given slowly over 1 to 2 min and withheld if the patient becomes hypotensive, has shallow respirations, or a respiratory rate less than 12. If this occurs the physician should be notified.

Anxiety about their illness, home responsibilities, and a new and strange environment often prevent total alleviation of pain by morphine sulfate alone. Staying with the patient and allowing him or her to express fears or administering a sedative such as **diazepam** (Valium) can help relieve pain or allow much smaller doses of the narcotic to be effective. Diazepam is very effective when given three or four times a day for the first 2 to 3 days of hospitalization. It helps patients relax and sleep and therefore lessens the workload of the heart. Before each dose is given though, it is important to assess the patient's level of consciousness because diazepam has a depressant effect on the central nervous system. Special caution should be taken with elderly patients. A smaller dose of 2.5 mg of diazepam given two or three times a day may be enough to provide a therapeutic effect without causing side effects. Orientation to time, place, and person can assist in determining a patient's level of consciousness, although many elderly patients are hard of hearing and disorientation may be mistakenly diagnosed. Patients with a prior history of affective disorders are more prone to developing depression from diazepam therapy.

Bedside commodes provide less stress to patients than do bedpans, and the use of stool softners prevents straining and constipation. Adequate fluids are also helpful if not contraindicated.

Upon arrival to an emergency room, patients who have a documeted myocardial infarction by ECG are usually started on prophylactic IV **lidocaine**. If premature ventricular beats occur with increasing frequency, additional IV lidocaine is used or the patient is changed to another IV antiarrhythmic. When giving an IV bolus of lidocaine the nurse should be monitoring the heart rate and rhythm of that patient. A 50- to 100-mg bolus should be given over a 1-to 2-min period. The patient should be informed to tell the nurse of any side effects, e.g., ringing in the ears, numbness of the tongue, and lightheadedness. If these effects occur, the bolus should be reduced or given very slowly. Hypotension can also occur if the bolus is given too fast and so blood pressure should be monitored carefully. While being maintained on a continuous infusion of lidocaine the patient may also exhibit these symptoms along with mental confusion, nausea, and vomiting. If another IV antiarrhythmic is required because of therapeutic failure or intolerable adverse effects, IV **procainamide** is often used. A patient may be bolused with 100 mg every 5 min until 1 g is given or until side effects occur. Hypotension can occur almost immediately and so the blood pressure must be checked at baseline and after each bolus. The nurse must monitor the rhythm and measure the conduction intervals. An increase in the arrhythmia or an increase in the PR, QRS, or QTc intervals must be reported to the physician immediately. The nurse must also be observant to signs and symptoms of congestive heart failure and low cardiac output. An accurately documented initial assessment is very valuable when identifying changes in the patient's condition as a result of complications or new medical treatment.

If a patient develops cardiogenic shock, medications such as **dopamine**, **dobutamine**, and **nitroprusside** are often administered. Strict blood pressure and pulmonary artery pressure parameters are ordered by the physician and constant monitoring of these pressures along with measurement of hourly urine outputs and observations of mental status, skin temperature, and peripheral perfusion are essential.

When patients are out of the acute phase of a myocardial infarction, long-term goals can be discussed. Patient education and reduction of risk factors are the primary goals. Reinforcement from private physicians, nurses, students, dietitians, and any other health professionals assist patients in modifying their lifestyles. A reminder that all patients are individuals who will require their own goals and achieve them at their own pace is important to keep in mind.

Medications such as the β-**adrenergic blocking agents** and IV **nitroglycerin**, given with the aim of limiting infarct size, require the nurse to exercise caution in observation for bradycardia, hypotension, and other adverse effects. Coronary thrombolysis, with the use of a thrombolytic agent such as **streptokinase**, is a new and experimental way to help limit infarct size. In centers where this is being done, there are protocols for the nursing staff to follow regarding postthrombolytic care. Some of these guidelines include admission to a CCU for observation and continuous anticoagulant therapy for several days.

Evaluation

The effectiveness of narcotics and sedatives in the relief of pain and anxiety must be evaluated by the nurse. Any necessary changes in the drug or dosage should be requested of the physician accordingly. Careful monitoring of patient response should be well documented.

The normal pattern of bowel function is difficult to maintain during a hospitalization that requires bed rest, limited fluids, and a less than private environment. Stool softeners are useful, but should be withheld if a patient develops frequent or loose bowel movements. A bedside commode is much less stressful than a bedpan, but constant monitoring of heart rate and rhythm is necessary because of the potential of a vasovagal response.

The fewer the premature ventricular contractions, the less irritable the myocardium will be. If a patient has no or rare PVCs 48 to 72 h after the acute myocardial infarction, the IV antiarrhythmic agent is usually discontinued and no further treatment is necessary.

Evaluating the effectiveness of dopamine, dobutamine, and nitroprusside depends largely on the reversal of cardiogenic shock symptoms. Many symptoms may have partial or transient reversal which makes evaluation difficult. Careful observation and documentation of all symptoms is the most helpful assistive device in evaluating total patient response to care.

CASE STUDY

Six months after developing angina (see previous case study), Mr. L. had an episode of severe crushing chest pain radiating down his left arm after attending the funeral of a close friend. This pain was associated with nausea and diaphoresis. He took five sublingual nitroglycerin, one every 5 min, without relief and called an ambulance. Shortly after the ambulance arrived to bring him to the hospital, Mr. L. developed ventricular fibrillation and was defibrillated. He required defibrillation again in the emergency room prior to his admission to the coronary care unit. He was given 100-mg bolus of IV lidocaine and was started on a 2-mg/min continuous infusion of lidocaine.

The ECG done in the emergency room showed significant ST elevation in leads V_2 to V_5 consistent with acute anteroseptal myocardial infarction. His blood pressure was 200/120 and his heart rate was 100/min. The CPK was slightly elevated in the initial blood sample drawn in the emergency room, although all other enzymes were normal. Other laboratory work was also normal except for a slight elevation of the white blood cell count. Mr. L. was able to state that he had faithfully been taking his hydrochlorothiazide and propranolol.

The patient was transferred to the coronary care unit with the following orders: morphine sulfate 2 to 4 mg IV q5–10 min PRN for pain, maintain lidocaine infusion at 2 mg/min, diazepam 5 mg PO q4–6h, docusate 100 mg qd, O_2 at 2L/min via nasal cannula, bed rest, low-salt soft diet, and routine standing orders (which on this unit included lidocaine bolus 75 mg for frequent PVCs and atropine sulfate 0.5 mg for significant bradycardia).

Assessment

Upon arrival in the coronary care unit, the patient appeared pale and diaphoretic. Vital signs: 170/110, pulse 104, irregular; respirations 24, temperature 99°F. The admitting nurse noted no neck vein distention; the chest was clear to auscultation although breath sounds were diminished. Heart sounds revealed normal S_1/S_2 with some PVCs but no murmurs or gallops. Abdomen was soft without organomegaly. Extremities were warm and the patient remained slightly diaphoretic. The ECG monitor showed sinus tachycardia with 4 PVCs/min.

Mr. L. was very upset when he spoke of his friend and expressed fear that he might die. The nursing diagnosis included the following areas of immediate concern: pain from an acute myocardial infarction complicated by ventricular arrhythmias, and anxiety.

Management

Mr. L. still complained of chest pain and since it had been 1 h since he had received morphine, the nurse administered the medication after she had taken the vital signs, started the oxygen, made certain the patient was positioned comfortably in bed, and attached him to the monitor. Morphine sulfate 4 mg was given over a 5-min period. The nurse was aware that Mr. L. had required defibrillation in the emergency room, and so she prepared a 100-mg bolus of lidocaine and placed it where it would be rapidly accessible. When managing a patient with an acute myocardial infarction, the nurse must anticiptate her patient's potential, as well as present, needs.

The patient's talk about his friend and his own fear of dying indicated that both emotional support and sedation were needed. The nurse listened to Mr. L.'s concerns and told him she understood his fears. She explained the equipment and each measurement performed. She also explained the need for him to rest and why sedation is important. Diazepam 5 mg was given to the patient.

The nurse also noted on the Kardex that the patient had a history of angina, hypertension, smoking, being overweight, and a positive family history of cardiovascular disease. The problems of smoking and diet control would be discussed with the patient after the acute period was over.

An accurate assessment of Mr. L.'s angina history would also be essential at this time. Often when a patient is first admitted to an emergency room or intensive care unit, an accurate assessment of the patient's angina history is difficult to obtain. When the patient is transferred to the intermediate care unit, the individual teaching plan can be completed.

Upon investigation the nurse determined that Mr. L.'s chest discomfort was brought on by activities such as walking the dog after breakfast, sexual intercourse, moving heavy objects at work, and yard work. He had had an increasing frequency of these attacks and just before his admission was taking six to seven NTG tablets to obtain partial relief. The chest discomfort was described as an anterior tightness which often extended to his left shoulder. If he was engaged in strenuous activity, he would also become short of breath.

The nurse also determined that Mr. L. had some knowledge about his condition and the proper use of nitroglycerin but needed reinforcement. When asked how old the bottle of the medication was that he was using and whether he felt the burning sensation when using it, he replied that it was some of the original batch he had purchased. He did recall that he had been taught about the potency of the drug and realized he should have remembered this when he needed more than three NTG tablets to obtain even partial relief.

Evaluation

During the acute phase, after administering the morphine IV, the nurse stayed with the patient until the pain was relieved. The diazepam helped Mr. L. and eased the stress he had experienced earlier that day. The monitor showed 1 to 2 PVCs/min with a heart rate of 80 beats/min. The IV lidocaine was maintained at 2 mg/min.

Prior to discharge evaluation of the teaching Mr. L. received occurred. Mr. L. was able to return discussion regarding his angina and its treatment. He also could relate his untreated angina to the occurrence of his heart attack. Follow-up appointments with his physician would also assist in evaluating Mr. L.'s total care during his hospitalization.

REFERENCES

Alexander, S: "Options for an Unfolding MI, Drugs to Limit Infarction," *Emerg Med,* **3**:127–132, Nov. 30, 1982.

Antman, E., J. Muller, S. Goldberg, et al.: "Nifedipine Therapy for Coronary Artery Spasm: Experience in 127 Patients," *N Engl J Med,* **302**:1269–1273, 1980.

Braun, L.T.: "Calcium Channel Blockers for the Treatment of Coronary Artery Spasm: Rationale, Effects, and Nursing Responsibilities," *Heart Lung,* **12**:226–232, May 1983.

Bussmann, W. D., D. Pasek, W. Seidel, et al.: "Reduction of CK and CK-MB Indexes of Infarct Size by Intravenous Nitroglycerin," *Circulation,* **63**:615–622, 1981.

Butler, J. D., and B. L. Harrison: "Keeping Pace with Calcium Channel Blockers," *Nursing 83,* **13**:38–43, July 1983.

Curfman, G. D., et al.: "Intravenous Nitroglycerin in the Treatment of Spontaneous Angina Pectoris: A Prospective, Randomized Trial," *Circulation,* **67**:276–282, 1983.

Fung, H.-L., E. F. McNiff, D. Ruggirello, et al.: "Kinetics of Isosorbide Dinitrate and Relationships to Pharmacological Effects," *Br J Clin Pharmacol,* **11**:579–590, 1981.

Ganz, W., N. Buchbinder, H. Marcus, et al.: "Intracoronary Thrombolysis in Acute Myocardial Infarction and Unstable Angina Pectoris," *Am Heart J,* **101**:4–13, 1981.

Gold, H. K., R. C. Leinbach, and P. R. Maroko: "Propranolol-Induced Reduction of Signs of Ischemic Injury During Acute Myocardial Infarction," *Am J Cardiol,* 38:689–695, 1976.

Greenberg, B. L., and M. S. Chow: "Angina," in B. S. Katcher, L. Y. Young, and M. A. Koda-Kimble (eds.), *Applied Therapeutics,* San Francisco: Applied Therapeutics, 1983, pp. 245–264.

Hossack, K. F., et al.: "Efficacy of Diltiazem in Angina of Effort: A Multicenter Trial," *Am J Cardiol,* 49:573–577, 1982.

Johnson, G. P., and B. C. Johanson: "Beta-Blockers, An Expert's Guide to What's on the Market," *Am J Nurs,* 83:1034–1043, July 1983.

Kissane, B. E., and L. Lemberg,: "Calcium Antagonists in Coronary Artery Disease," *Heart Lung,* 11:280–283, May–June, 1982.

Kloner, R. A., and E. Braunwald: "Review—Observations on Experimental Myocardial Ischemia," *Cardiovasc Res,* 14:371–395, 1980.

Lee, G., A. N. DeMaria, and E. N. Amsterdam: "Comparative Effects of Morphine, Meperidine and Pentazocine on Circulatory Dynamics in Patients with Acute Myocardial Infarction," *Am J Med,* 60:949–955, 1976.

Lie, K. I., H. J. Wellens, F. J. Van Capelle, et al.: "Lidocaine in the Prevention of Primary Ventricular Fibrillation," *N Engl J Med,* 291:1324–1326, 1974.

Maroko, P. R., J. K. Kjekshus, B. E. Sobel, et al.: "Factors Influencing Infarct Size Following Experimental Coronary Artery Occlusion," *Circulation,* 43:67–82, 1971.

Maseri, A., et al.: "Rational Approach to the Medical Therapy of Angina Pectoris: The Role of Calcium Antagonists," *Prog Cardiovasc Dis,* 25:269–278, 1983.

Mueller, H. S., and R. A. Chahine: "Interim Report of Multicenter Double-Blind Placebo-Controlled Studies of Nifedipine in Chronic Stable Angina," *Am J Med,* 71:645–657, 1981.

Noneman, J. W., and J. F. Rogers: "Lidocaine Prophylaxis in Acute Myocardial Infarction," *Medicine,* 57:501–515, 1978.

Rentrop, P., H. Blanke, K. R. Karsch, et al.: "Selective Intracoronary Thrombolysis in Acute Myocardial Infarction and Unstable Angina Pectoris," *Circulation,* 63:307–317, 1981.

Rossi, L. P., and E. M. Antman: "Calcium Channel Blockers, New Treatment for Cardiovascular Disease," *Am J Nurs,* 83:382–387, March 1983.

Rude, R. E., J. E. Muller, and E. Braunwald: "Efforts to Limit the Size of Myocardial Infarcts," *Ann Intern Med,* 95:736–761, 1981.

Segal, B. L., et al.: "Managing Angina with Nitrates," *Geriatrics,* 37:115–117, 1982.

Sobel, B. E., and W. E. Shell: "Serum Enzyme Determinations in the Diagnosis and Assessment of Myocardial Infarction," *Circulation,* 45:471–482, 1972.

44

CONGESTIVE HEART FAILURE

ROGER LANDER
BETH LYMAN
JOEL COVINSKY

LEARNING OBJECTIVES

Upon mastery of the content of this chapter, the reader will be able to:

1. Describe the signs and symptoms of congestive heart failure.

2. Identify factors that can aggravate congestive heart failure.

3. List the goals in the management of congestive heart failure.

4. Describe at least two methods of decreasing cardiac work load.

5. Explain the mechanism of action and clinical effect of the cardiac glycosides on cardiac inotropic state and kidney function.

6. Compare the elimination pathways, onset of action, half-life, and maintenance dose of the two major cardiac glycosides.

7. List three precautions in the administration of digitalis glycosides.

8. Describe two methods of digitalizing patients.

9. Describe the signs, symptoms, and appropriate nursing activities related to each of the common adverse reactions to the cardiac glycosides.

10. List at least six factors that predispose to digitalis toxicity.

11. State the goal of diuretic therapy in congestive heart failure.

12. Describe the beneficial hemodynamic effects of the afterload-reducing agents in heart failure, including those given intravenously and orally.

13. Explain the meaning of the acronym MOST DAMP as it relates to current practices in the treatment of acute pulmonary edema.

14. Write a teaching plan for the patient on cardiac glycosides.

15. Indicate important observational parameters relative to the assessment and evaluation of the patient in heart failure.

16. Indicate one action for each step of the nursing process for the patient receiving afterload-reducing agents.

Cardiac failure is that condition in which the heart is no longer able to pump an adequate supply of blood (provided there is adequate venous return to the heart) for the metabolic needs of the body. Cardiac failure is one of the most serious consequences of cardiovascular disease. Since the metabolic demands of the body vary widely, the myocardium must work in concert with the peripheral vascular system in order to meet these demands. When the heart can no longer pump sufficient blood to meet these demands, the *clinical syndrome* of congestive heart failure (CHF) develops.

Although most forms of heart disease can lead to CHF, in approximately 75 percent of patients the major etiologic factor is high blood pressure; careful control of blood pressure therefore is essential in preventing the development of CHF (see Chap. 40, "High Blood Pressure"). Other precipitating and aggravating factors are myocardial infarction, cardiac arrhythmias, pulmonary emboli, pulmonary infection, sudden emotional turmoil, and administration of excessive amounts of intravenous fluids. Cardiac failure may also develop gradually from extracardiac factors such as anemia, liver disease, renal disease, hormonal imbalance, and the effect of certain drugs (see Table 44-1). Adequate treatment of CHF requires detection and management of these precipitating factors.

The prognosis for patients with CHF is still poor. The Framingham study (Kannel et al., 1972) showed the 5-year survival to be approximately 40 percent for male patients and 60 percent for female patients. These figures may have

TABLE 44-1 Drugs Which May Contribute to Congestive Heart Failure

DRUG	COMMENT
Drugs Expanding Volume	
See Table 23-1.	
Drugs Directly Affecting Cardiac Performance	
Daunomycin	Has direct cardiotoxic effect, presenting as CHF, arrhythmias, or myocardial infarction.
β-Adrenergic and calcium channel blockers	Can cause negative inotropic and chronotropic effects.

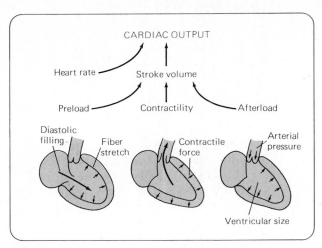

FIGURE 44-1

Determinants of Cardiac Output. The product of stroke volume and heart rate is cardiac output. Stroke volume is a function of preload (diastolic filling from venous return and resulting fiber stretch), contractility, and afterload (ventricular size and arterial pressure against which the heart must pump). [*From S. A. Price and L. M. Wilson (eds.): Pathophysiology: Clinical Concepts of Disease Processes, 2d ed., McGraw-Hill, New York, 1982.*]

improved in recent years because of the therapeutic advances (potent diuretics, vasodilating agents, and inotropic agents) made since this long-term study was performed. However, the results of large, prospective studies assessing the long-term effects of these newer treatment modalities are not yet available.

DETERMINANTS OF CARDIAC OUTPUT

Cardiac output is a function of stroke volume and heart rate. Heart rate is primarily under extrinsic neural control. Stroke volume is generally dependent on three intrinsic factors: *preload* (the amount of blood returning from the venous system), *contractility* (the ability of the heart to pump), and *afterload* (the resistance against which the heart must pump). Alteration in one or more of these variables can significantly alter cardiac output (see Fig. 44-1).

PATHOGENESIS

Many variables contribute to the clinical syndrome of congestive heart failure (CHF). There is always a defect in myocardial contractility, although the disorder may be either the result of an abnormality within the myocardium or secondary to a chronic, excessive work load (preload or afterload).

The primary cellular mechanisms responsible for depressed myocardial contractility are still unknown. Many speculate that abnormalities in calcium transport are important causes of decreased contractility, but this has yet to be demonstrated. Theoretically, reduced availability of calcium within the area of the contractile proteins would result in impaired ability to generate a contractile effort.

Compensatory Mechanisms

When the heart begins to fail, the body activates several compensatory mechanisms in order to maintain cardiac output and adequate organ function. These compensatory mechanisms include cardiac dilation, cardiac hypertrophy, increase in sympathetic tone, sodium and water retention, and increased oxygen extraction from the blood (Fig. 44-2).

If the compensatory mechanisms reach their maximum effectiveness and the heart is still failing, blood begins to back up behind the failing ventricle. Congestion of the pulmonary circulation occurs when the left ventricle fails, but most patients with left ventricular failure also develop systemic congestion. Failure of the right ventricle results in congestion of the systemic venous system which may manifest as hepatomegaly, jugular venous distention (JVD), peripheral edema, and weight gain.

CLINICAL FINDINGS

The assessment of a patient with congestive heart failure (CHF) depends on recognition of the characteristic symptoms and signs, outlined in Table 44-2.

CLINICAL PHARMACOLOGY AND THERAPEUTICS

The goals in the treatment of CHF are directed at reducing cardiac work load and improving cardiac performance. A reduction in work load, which can be accomplished by decreasing systemic demand for oxygen or by decreasing preload and/or afterload, will maximize the rate and completeness of healing. Improvements in cardiac performance achieved by increasing contractility will reverse the associated disorders of organ function and fluid balance. Often treatment involves consideration of both these goals simul-

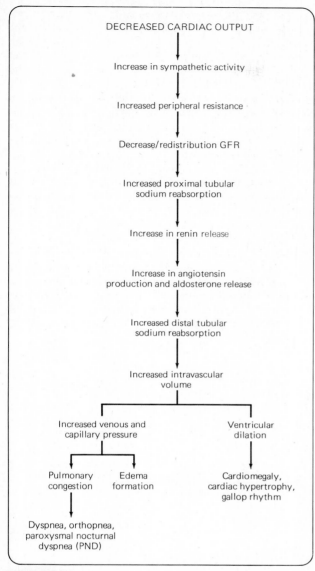

FIGURE 44-2

Pathogenesis of Symptoms in Congestive Heart Failure. Reduced cardiac output is the major pathology, leading to many of the subjective and objective findings of the syndrome.

taneously. The vigor with which modification of these variables is approached depends on the severity of the heart failure. If an acute injury such as myocardial infarction is responsible for the heart failure, approaches to improving cardiac performance must include a consideration of the rate and completeness of healing, since some interventions may temporarily improve cardiac output but in the end extend the injury and decrease patient survival time.

Reduction of Cardiac Work Load

The first step in reducing the cardiac work load is to modify the patient's physical and emotional stress. With severe forms of congestive failure, bed rest is required, and this alone may bring about diuresis. Patients with pulmonary congestion may benefit further if the head of the bed is elevated. With mild congestive failure, a reduction in daily physical activity coupled with adequate rest will often allow the patient to continue gainful employment. If the patient is obese, weight reduction will significantly reduce the cardiac work load. As the cardiac decompensation is brought under

TABLE 44-2 Signs and Symptoms of Congestive Heart Failure

RIGHT VENTRICULAR FAILURE	LEFT VENTRICULAR FAILURE
Subjective Symptoms	
Anorexia	Exertional dyspnea
Nausea	Paroxysmal nocturnal dyspnea
Bloating	Cough
Exertional right upper abdominal pain	Hoarseness
	Fatigue
Headache	Palpitations
Weakness	Cardiac dyspnea
Objective Signs	
Cyanosis	Tachypnea
Oliguria (daytime)	Orthopnea
Polyuria (nighttime)	Pulmonary edema
Mental aberration	Cough
Increased right ventricular diastolic pressure causing elevated central venous pressure	Hemoptysis
	Hoarseness
Hepatic enlargement	Cyanosis
Splenomegaly	Gallop rhythms: protodiastolic gallop (exaggerated third heart sound), atrial gallop (exaggerated fourth heart sound), summation gallop (third and fourth heart sounds superimposed because of rapid rate)
Gallop rhythms: protodiastolic gallop (exaggerated third heart sound)	
Pulmonary hypertension	
Venous engorgement: distended cervical veins, positive hepatojugular reflex	Basilar rales, fine and crepitant in early failure, coarse in later failure
Peripheral edema: dependent pretibial edema, ascites	Pleural effusion of excess fluid retained
	Cheyne-Stokes breathing
	Peripheral edema

control, the patient may gradually increase activity. However, those activities and emotional problems which precipitate symptoms should be eliminated, if possible.

Improvement of Cardiac Performance

Cardiac Glycosides

The cardiac glycosides (i.e., the digitalis drugs) have for years been considered the cornerstone of the management of CHF. They improve the contractile (positive inotropic effect) and mechanical efficiency of the failing heart, affect conduction speed within the myocardium (negative dromotropic effect), and slow the heart rate (negative chronotropic effect) (see Fig. 44-3).

Mechanism of Action   The effects of digitalis drugs seem to be due to changes in intracellular potentials and ion flux. Cardiac glycosides inhibit the action of the Na$^+$-K$^+$ ATPase (commonly referred to as the "sodium pump"). This action results in increased amounts of sodium inside the myocardial cell. Transmembrane exchange of sodium for calcium results in an increase in the amount of intracellular calcium.

This increase in calcium availability to the contractile proteins of the myocardial cell (actin and myosin) results in the increased force of contraction seen with the administration of digitalis preparations (see Fig. 44-4).

The electrophysiologic effects of digitalis drugs are also thought to be mediated through inhibition of Na$^+$-K$^+$ ATPase; however, this class of drugs also has profound effects on the autonomic nervous system. The clinical effects observed are dependent on the complex interaction of these direct effects, as well as the interaction of various indirect reflex mechanisms brought into action through the cardiovascular hemodynamic monitoring of the autonomic nervous system. The effects on refractory periods, conduction velocities, and automaticity vary in different areas of the myocardium. (For a more detailed discussion of these, see Chap. 45, "Disorders of Cardiac Rhythm.")

Diuretic action   Diuresis is often one of the first manifestations of digitalis action in patients with edema secondary to CHF. This action is mostly due to the beneficial effects of this group of drugs in improving cardiac function. Enhanced cardiac output leads to improved renal blood flow and hence increased urine output. In addition, increased renal perfusion also interrupts the compensatory cycle of

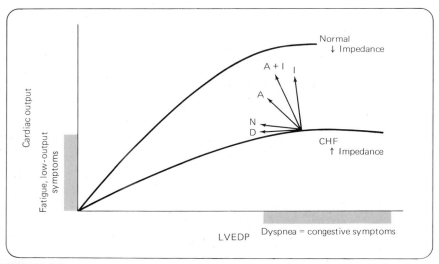

FIGURE 44-3

Ventricular Function Curves. Cardiac output is related to extent of preload, as reflected in the left ventricular end-diastolic pressure (LVEDP). The *upper curve* represents the normal heart. Cardiac output increases as the amount of venous blood returned to the heart (preload) increases, according to Starling's law of the heart. This is because as the ventricle stretches to accommodate preload, more efficient interaction of the contractile proteins occurs and stroke volume increases. The flat portion of the curve represents overstretching of the ventricle so that further increases in preload do not further increase cardiac output. The *lower curve* represents the conditions in congestive heart failure. When preload (LVEDP) and cardiac output are both low, the patient experiences confusion, oliguria, fatigue, and other low-output symptoms. Increases in preload cause little improvement in cardiac output but eventually result in edema, dyspnea, and other congestive symptoms. The effects of various therapeutic modalities on the ventricular function curve is shown. I = inotropic agents (digitalis glycosides, dopamine, and dobutamine); A = afterload reducers (hydralazine, minoxidil, and captopril); A + I = afterload reducers combined with inotropic agents; N = nitrates; and D = diuretics.

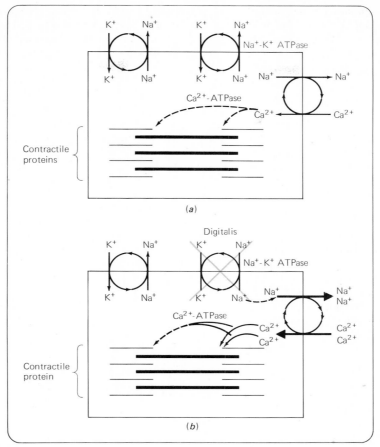

FIGURE 44-4

Mechanism of Inotropic Action of Cardiac Glycosides within Cardiac Cells. (*a*) The sodium-potassium pump catalyzed by Na^+-K^+ ATPase promotes the removal of sodium from the cardiac cell. This results in limited amounts of intracellular sodium available for exchange with calcium, which is important to the activity of contractile proteins, and normal action of sodium-potassium and sodium-calcium exchange systems. (*b*) In the presence of digitalis, the sodium-potassium exchange system is partially inhibited, and the resultant increase in intracellular sodium speeds the rate of sodium-calcium exchange and thus increases the availability of intracellular calcium to the contractile proteins, which results in a changed contraction.

renin-angiotensin-aldosterone activity. This results in a quantitative reduction of sodium reabsorption from the distal renal tubule caused by aldosterone. Animal studies have shown that a number of digitalis glycosides also inhibit tubular reabsorption of sodium directly, possibly as an effect on the NA^+-K^+ ATPase of the renal tubular cells. This direct renal tubular effect is seen after relatively large doses, and most likely contributes very little to the diuresis seen after digitalis administration in patients with CHF.

Mechanisms of toxicity In contrast to the therapeutic effects of the cardiac glycosides, toxic doses seem to cause arrhythmias by increasing automaticity (see Chap. 45), perhaps through an extension of the direct effects on membrane ATPase or through enhancement of central sympathetic outflow. Predisposing factors to toxicity include hypokalemia, hypomagnesemia, hypercalcemia, hypoxia, or acidosis. Increasing automaticity in many segments of the myocardium, along with decreased automaticity in the sinoatrial (SA) node and reduced atrioventricular (AV) nodal conduction, leads to arrhythmias of every conceivable type.

Clinical Indications The cardiac glycosides are most effective for left ventricular and biventricular failure associated with hypertension, valvular disease, and ischemic heart disease. They are less effective in diseases primarily affecting myocardial cells, such as toxic or infectious myocarditis, various forms of cardiomyopathy and endocardial fibroelastosis, and in those forms of CHF which are precipitated by acute rheumatic fever, anemia, beriberi, complete AV block, cor pulmonale, fever, infection, mitral stenosis, and thyrotoxicosis. Digitalis is contraindicated in patients with second-degree or unstable AV block and in patients with idiopathic hypertrophic subaortic stenosis (IHSS).

The use of cardiac glycosides in the presence of ischemic heart disease and following an acute myocardial infarction is controversial since they increase myocardial oxygen consumption. Digitalis drugs are also employed in some atrial arrhythmias, as discussed in Chap. 45.

Pharmacokinetics The many cardiac glycosides available include **digitalis leaf, deslanoside, oubain, digitoxin,** and **digoxin** (Table 44-3). The primary differences between the various cardiac glycosides is their pharmacokinetic characteristics: route of elimination, extent of protein binding, and elimination half-life. Since more information has been collected on digoxin and digitoxin than on the other glycosides and since in most instances the others have no real therapeutic advantages, this discussion will be limited to digoxin and digitoxin. In general, more information is available regarding the use of digoxin and the effects of various disease states on its pharmacokinetics. If toxicity occurs, it will usually be of shorter duration with digoxin as opposed to digitoxin. For these reasons, digoxin should be the cardiac glycoside of choice.

Preparations **Digoxin** is available in both intravenous and oral preparations (capsule, tablet, and elixir). Its oral absorption is variable; reports range from 50 to 100 percent. The capsules and elixir are more reliably absorbed (80 to 100 percent) than are the tablets. Bioavailability problems result from differing dissolution rates for various tablet products. Despite federal Food and Drug Administration guidelines which have reduced variability among different products, it is still wise to ensure that patients receive a preparation with proven bioavailability. Certain disease states have also been shown to alter the absorption of the tablet formulations. These include malabsorption states, such as sprue, and short bowel syndrome and situations in which gastrointestinal transit is rapid. In these conditions and in patients beginning therapy with digoxin the capsule formulation of digoxin would be recommended.

The injectable form of digoxin is available in a propylene glycol and ethanol diluent mixture. While the drug may be administered either intravenously or intramuscularly, the intravenous route is preferred, since intramuscular injection is very slowly and erratically absorbed and is extremely painful. Intravenous digoxin must be administered slowly (over several minutes), since the diluent (propylene glycol) has significant cardiac conduction toxicity if administered too rapidly. The half-life of digoxin in patients with normal renal function is approximately 1.6 days. Approximately 85 percent of the digoxin is excreted unchanged in the urine with the remaining being excreted in the stool (biliary excretion). With deterioration in renal function, a larger percentage of the drug is retained within the body, and so maintenance doses must be reduced.

With radioimmunoassay techniques, monitoring of serum digoxin levels can be a routine clinical procedure. To obtain the most accurate information, blood samples should be taken just prior to the next dose, thus avoiding the variation of levels during the distribution phase of the drug. The therapeutic range is usually considered from 0.5 to 2.0 ng/mL; concentrations in excess of 2.0 ng/mL are commonly associated with digitalis intoxication. However, in patients with decreased potassium or magnesium or in the elderly, it is not unusual to find digitalis intoxication even with serum concentrations below 2.0 ng/mL. The measurement of serum digoxin levels is useful for confirming clinical impressions with definitive data or when an unexpected drug response occurs.

Digitoxin is available in both intravenous and oral preparations. Its absorption is more complete than with digoxin; reports vary from 90 to 100 percent. Digitoxin is much more highly protein-bound (90 percent) than is digoxin (25 percent), and the elimination half-life is also much longer (7 days vs. 1.6 days). Elimination of digitoxin depends primarily on hepatic metabolism to inactive products. A small portion of digitoxin is metabolized to digoxin, which is subsequently eliminated by the kidney. The elimination of digitoxin is not changed by hepatic disease, indicating the large reserve capacity of the liver in degradation of the drug. In the anuric patient, the half-life may be as long as 9 days.

Digitoxin serum levels can be measured by radioimmunoassay. Plasma concentrations of 10 to 30 ng/mL are considered therapeutic, with levels greater than 35 ng/mL considered toxic.

Dosage The term *digitalization* is a carryover from prior times, when digitalis was administered until the signs of toxicity appeared. This approach is no longer utilized, but the term now refers to the loading dose of digitalis that is utilized to achieve a desired total body store of the drug. The speed with which digitalization is conducted depends on the clinical presentation of the patient. Normally, problems associated with congestive heart failure develop over a long period of time; thus in most cases there is no need to digitalize rapidly (in less than 24 h). A patient can be digitalized slowly over a period of 1 week or more, using the maintenance dose.

The loading dose required varies between 0.0075 and 0.02 mg/kg of body weight. The loading dose should be reduced in elderly patients, since they have been shown to have smaller distribution volumes for the cardiac glycosides, and are thought to be more sensitive to these agents because of lower total body potassium stores. Conversely, infants are often given larger loading regimens of these agents (0.02 to 0.03 mg/kg), because many experts feel that they require higher serum levels to create the same therapeutic effects. At the lower end of the dose range the primary effect seen is the increased force of contraction, while in larger doses the electrophysiologic effects become more apparent.

Since the cardiac effects of **digoxin** and **digitoxin** are

TABLE 44-3 Cardiac Glycoside Preparations

AGENT	GASTROINTESTINAL ABSORPTION	ONSET OF ACTION, min	PEAK EFFECT, h	AVERAGE HALF-LIFE	PRINCIPAL METABOLIC ROUTE (EXCRETORY PATHWAY)	Average Digitalizing Dose, mg		USUAL DAILY ORAL MAINTENANCE DOSE*
						ORAL	INTRAVENOUS	
Digoxin	50–100%	15–30	1.5–5	36 h	Renal; some GI	1.0–1.5	0.75–1.0	0.125–0.5 mg
Digitoxin	90–100%	25–120	8–12	4–7 days	Hepatic; renal excretion of metabolites	0.7–1.2	1.0	0.1 mg
Oubain	Unreliable	5–10	0.5–2	21 h	Renal; some GI	—	0.3–0.5	
Deslanoside	Unreliable	10–30	2–3	33 h	Renal	—	0.8	
Digitalis leaf	About 40%	—	—	4–6 days	Similar to digitoxin	—	—	0.1 g

*Maintenance dosage for adults; see text for dosage recommendations in the pediatric and elderly populations.

essentially equivalent on a milligram-per-milligram basis, the same guidelines apply to loading doses with both drugs. The important difference between the two drugs which must be kept in mind is their $t_{1/2}$, which affects the maintenance doses (see Table 44-3). A maintenance dose of digoxin without loading doses will achieve its full therapeutic effect within 1 week, while the full therapeutic effect of digitoxin may not be apparent for up to 1 month or more. Maintenance dosages must also be reduced in the elderly, again because of their smaller distribution space and also because of the natural decline in renal function with advancing age. This latter point is more pertinent to digoxin than digitoxin, although both must be adjusted carefully in the elderly population. The maintenance dose is usually greater (on a weight basis) for infants than for adults (0.005 vs. 0.003 mg/kg). However, the necessity for this larger dose has been questioned, and is presently somewhat of a controversial issue.

Adverse Effects Approximately 7 to 20 percent of patients receiving cardiac glycosides have clinical or electrocardiographic signs of digitalis intoxication (see Table 44-4). Cardiac glycoside intoxication is one of the most common and serious iatrogenic diseases. Most of the serious and unavoidable problems related to toxicity result from the inability to measure optimal therapeutic doses of the drug precisely. Unfortunately, the cardiac glycosides have an extremely narrow therapeutic index, which accounts for their tendency to induce intoxication. Moreover, the signs and symptoms of digitalis intoxication do not occur on a predictable basis; they may differ in different patients (at different plasma levels) and even in the same patient at different times. Patients in the elderly age groups are especially prone to intoxication, since their distribution of the drugs is reduced (due to a wasting of skeletal muscle), as is their renal elimination of these agents. Up to 18 percent of patients who develop digitalis intoxication may die from the serious digitalis-induced arrhythmias.

One of the earliest signs of digitalis intoxication is anorexia. If the patient continues to take the cardiac glycoside, the anorexia may be followed by nausea and vomiting. While the gastrointestinal signs may precede the electrocardiographic signs of digitalis intoxication, this is not always the case, and there may be no preceding GI distress.

The arrhythmogenic side effects of cardiac glycosides are related to their complex effects on the electrophysiologic properties of the heart. Almost every known type of arrhythmia may be produced through changes in impulse formation or conduction. The most common electrocardiographic indications of digitalis intoxication are premature ventricular beats and first-degree atrioventricular (AV) block (prolonged PR interval). Other arrhythmias, in order of decreasing incidence, include advanced degrees of AV block (Wenckebach phenomenon), incomplete heart block, paroxysmal ventricular, nodal, and atrial tachyarrhythmias, AV dissociation, sinus arrhythmias, SA block, and wandering

pacemaker. It is estimated that arrhythmias occur in 80 to 90 percent of glycoside intoxications.

The noncardiac symptoms of digitalis intoxication are primarily neurologic, gastrointestinal, and visual disturbances. Rare manifestations include endocrine disturbances, platelet disturbances, and allergic reactions.

Drug-drug interactions Many drugs have been shown to interact with cardiac glycosides. **Quinidine**, an antiarrhythmic agent commonly administered concurrently with digitalis preparations, has in recent years been shown to increase the serum levels and pharmacologic effect of the digitalis glycosides. The mechanism of this interaction is not completely clear, but it is of considerable clinical significance. The dosage of the digitalis preparation should be carefully monitored and will often require reduction when quinidine is added to the patient's regimen.

Several drugs may reduce the effectiveness of digitalis preparations by interfering with their intestinal absorption

TABLE 44-4 Noncardiac Manifestations of Cardiac Glycoside Intoxication

SYMPTOMS	FREQUENCY	MANIFESTATIONS
Gastrointestinal	Common	Anorexia, nausea, vomiting
	Uncommon	Diarrhea, abdominal pain, constipation
Neurologic	Common	Fatigue, headache, insomnia, malaise, lassitude, confusion, depression, vertigo
	Uncommon	Neuralgias (especially trigeminal), convulsions, paresthesias, delirium (digitalis delirium), psychosis
Visual	Common	Loss of visual acuity, color vision (usually green or yellow) with colored halos
	Uncommon	Scotomata, micropsia, macropsia, amblyopias (temporary or permanent), shimmering vision
Other	Rare	Allergic manifestations (urticaria, eosinophilia), idiosyncrasy, thrombocytopenia, gastrointestinal hemorrhage and necrosis, gynecomastia (both unilateral and bilateral), vaginal cornification in postmenopausal females

Source: E. K. Chung: "Non-cardiac Manifestations of Cardiac Glycoside Intoxication," in *Digitalis Intoxication*, Amsterdam: Excerpta Medica, 1969. Used by permission.

or hepatic recycling. These include **neomycin, cholestyramine,** and **colestipol.**

Several pharmacologic agents increase the cardiac effects of digitalis. Many of these will predispose the patient to digitalis intoxication if not properly monitored. Such agents include **amphotericin B, corticosteroids,** and **diuretics** (by producing hypokalemia), **calcium, succinylcholine,** and **sympathomimetics.** In addition to drugs, many other factors can predispose patients to digitalis intoxication, including hypomagnesemia, hypokalemia, hypercalcemia, renal disease, hypoxia, myocarditis, cor pulmonale, hypothyroidism, acute CHF, and myocardial infarction.

Management of digitalis intoxication   The treatment of digitalis intoxication varies somewhat according to the clinical presentation. If there are no life-threatening arrhythmias, discontinuance of cardiac glycoside and correction of any predisposing factors are indicated. Hypokalemia (which may be diuretic-induced) is probably one of the more common factors responsible for digitalis intoxication and in many instances can be corrected by administering an oral potassium chloride supplement. In the event that the patient is anorectic, a slow (not to exceed 20 meq/h) intravenous infusion of potassium chloride (generally not more than 80 meq/L) may be employed.

Cholestyramine and **colestipol** may be utilized in digitalis intoxication to facilitate fecal elimination of the drug. This has recently been shown to be effective not only with **digitoxin,** but also with **digoxin,** since both undergo biliary recycling. Antibodies used to bind and deactivate digoxin in toxicity cases are also being investigated.

Additional Contractility Enhancers

Today researchers are exploring the use of various agents which may increase the mechanical efficiency of the failing heart. It has been known for years that β-adrenergic catecholamines may increase contractility. Unfortunately, most catecholamines have a very short duration of action, and they cannot be administered orally. Structural relatives of the common catecholamines like **dopamine** and **dobutamine** have been used primarily as intravenous agents for emergency management of cardiac decompensation. Recently, synthetic modifications of the catecholamine family have been utilized in experimental treatment of heart failure. **Prenalterol** and **pirbuterol** are examples of experimental β-adrenergic agents which may be administered orally in patients with heart failure. The dosage of these two agents is not settled at this point. Some studies have used 10 to 20 mg/day of pirbuterol and shown clinical benefit. Investigators are also exploring the potential value of **terbutaline** and **salbutamol** (in bronchodilating doses) in the management of heart failure.

Amrinone   Amrinone (Inocor) is an inotropic (improves contractile force) and vasodilator agent approved in 1984 and indicated for the short-term treatment of congestive heart failure in patients who have not responded adequately to diuretics, digitalis, or vasodilators. It reduces both preload and afterload and is effective in patients with depressed myocardial function. Use of amrinone requires close monitoring, preferably in a critical care unit.

Mechanism of action   The mechanism of action of amrinone has not been fully elucidated but differs from that of digitalis and sympathomimetics. It appears to increase availability of calcium to contractile proteins. This agent may assist the failing heart to increase its strength of contraction at any fiber length.

Pharmacokinetics   Amrinone is metabolized by conjugation in the liver and has a half-life of 5.8 h in patients with congestive heart failure. It is 10 to 49% protein bound.

Adverse effects   Thrombocytopenia occurs in 2.4 percent of patients, requiring baseline and regular monitoring of platelet count. Less frequent are GI distress, hypotension, and arrhythmias, and a rare hypersensitivity manifested by pleuritis, pericarditis, and ascites. Amrinone is not recommended for those with valvular heart disease or recent myocardial infarction, for children, or for pregnant or lactating women. It is diluted in normal saline or 0.25% saline, because it reacts with solutions containing dextrose.

Dosage   The loading dose of amrinone is 0.75 mg/kg by IV bolus over 2 to 3 min. Maintenance dosing is accomplished by continuous infusion (usually a 1-mg/mL or 3-mg/mL solution) at 5 to 10 μg/kg/min.

Reduction of Excess Fluid

Diet

In patients with mild congestive heart failure, improvement can occur with sodium restriction and bed rest. Most patients with congestive heart failure should be managed on a 2-g salt diet. The average diet in the United States contains 6 to 15 g of salt. Not adding salt at the table reduces this to 4 to 7 g daily, and omitting salt in cooking brings further reduction to 3 to 4 g daily. The patient should be advised to avoid foods and drugs (Table 44-5) that have a high sodium content. Salt substitutes which are usually combinations of various potassium and sodium salts may be recommended. Examples of salt substitutes include Co-Salt, Morton-Lite, or Diasal.

Diuretics

Sodium retention occurs in patients with congestive heart failure as an adaptive mechanism to increase the intravascular volume. The two major mechanisms for increasing intravascular volume involve the increased sodium retention in the proximal tubules secondary to the decreased renal blood flow and the secondary hyperaldosteronism induced following the fall in cardiac output. The accompanying increase in peripheral vascular resistance presumably occurs as a consequence of the enhanced sympathetic tone.

The aim of diuretic therapy is to reduce the pulmonary venous pressure and return the blood volume to the point at which optimal filling pressure (preload) is achieved (see Fig. 44-3). A variety of diuretic agents are available, and most are effective in the milder forms of congestive failure. Their basic pharmacologic properties are discussed in Chap. 23, "Edema." Their utility in congestive failure will be addressed here. The purpose of these agents is to reduce the volume and the work load imposed on the failing myocardium. Excessive volume depletion can diminish the venous return to such an extent that the preload is reduced below the optimal level and cardiac output decreases. This probably occurs more frequently than is generally appreciated, but the decrease in pulmonary interstitial pressure results in symptomatic improvement despite the decrease in cardiac output.

Thiazide Diuretics

These are the most widely used agents because they are effective when administered orally and are relatively inexpensive. Hydrochlorothiazide (or an equivalent) may be employed in doses of 50 to 100 mg daily as a single agent, or it may be combined with a cardiac glycoside. In many instances where the patient has reduced myocardial contractility and fluid overload, these two classes of drugs complement each other very well.

An increase in potassium loss (kaluresis) occurs with the use of these agents and may further directly stimulate the increase in aldosterone secretion commonly seen in patients with CHF. The clinician should watch for signs and symptoms of potassium depletion. Periodic blood samples should be drawn to determine the serum potassium concentrations, particularly in patients who are on combination therapy with diuretics and cardiac glycosides. Intermittent administration of the thiazides on an every-other-day basis may help to avoid the problems associated with severe volume depletion and electrolyte abnormalities. Once the extracellular fluid volume is reduced, the aim of therapy is to maintain the sodium balance and to avoid electrolyte abnormalities.

Spironolactone

The aldosterone antagonist **spironolactone** (Aldactone) is a diuretic alternative which may be employed alone or in combination with the thiazide diuretics in managing CHF. On the basis of the finding of secondary hyperaldosteronism in some patients with congestive heart failure, spironolactone would seem to be an ideal diuretic in that disorder. Despite its effectiveness even when the serum aldosterone is normal, however, it is more often used as a second-line agent because of its cost and its delayed onset of action.

Spironolactone is particularly useful in patients who have difficulty maintaining adequate serum potassium. Its major adverse effects are hyperkalemia (excessive elevation of the serum potassium) and gastrointestinal upset. The therapeutic dosage range is normally between 100 and 300 mg daily. The

TABLE 44-5 Sodium Content of Selected Adult Medications

DRUG	UNIT	mg Na/UNIT	DRUG	UNIT	mg Na/UNIT
Parenteral Products			*Oral Solids*		
Amcill S	1 g per injection	71	Alka Seltzer	1 tablet	296
Dynapen	63 mg/5 mL	67	Bisodol Powder	10 g	314
Geopen	5 g	680	Bromo-Seltzer	1 capful	717
Keflin	1-g vial	62	Erythrocin Filmtabs	250 mg	70
Methicillin	1-g vial	55	Fizrin	1 packet	673
Omnipen N	2-g vial	124	Kayexelate Powder	15 g	550
Penbritin-S	1-g vial	66	Nervine Effervescent	1 tablet	544
PenG Na (Squibb)	5 mU per vial	233	Panteric Granules	1 tsp	161
Polycillin	1-g vial	68	Pasna Tri-Pak Granules	5.5-g packet	490
Principen N	1 g per injection	70	Rolaids	1 tablet	53
Prostaphlin	4-g vial	144	Sal Hepatica	1 rounded tsp	1000
Staphcillin Buff.	1-g vial	61	Sodium salicylate	10-gr tablet	97
Unipen injection	1-g vial	73	*Food Supplements*		
Ticar	3-g vial	360			
Mezlin	3-g vial	128	Carnation Slender	10-oz can	440
Azlin	3-g vial	149	Lytren	1 oz	189
Pipracil	3-g vial	137	Meritene Powder	1 oz	113
Oral Liquids			Vivonex	1000 mL	860
			Ensure	1000 mL	740
Dristan Cough Formula	5 mL	59	Osmolite	1000 mL	540
Phenergan Expectorant (plain or VC)	5 mL	51	*Miscellaneous*		
Phospho-Soda	5 mL	554	Fleet Enema	4.5 oz	5000*
Vicks Cough Syrup	5 mL	54			
Vicks Formula 44 Syrup	5 mL	68			

*Average absorption = 250–300 mg per enema

larger the dose, the more often Gl upset occurs. Since this drug has a long duration of action, a once-a-day dose schedule is satisfactory as long as Gl upset is not a problem.

Loop Diuretics In the presence of impaired renal function or when pulmonary congestion must be reduced rapidly (as in acute pulmonary edema), the loop diuretics **furosemide** (Lasix) and **bumetanide** (Bumex) should be considered. These agents appear to have the advantage of decreasing renal vascular resistance and inducing a sodium and water loss in the presence of a reduced glomerular filtration rate. With overvigorous therapy, however, volume depletion can occur, and the resulting decreased glomerular filtration rate can induce azotemia (retention of blood urea nitrogen). In acute pulmonary edema, particularly with an acute myocardial infarction, these agents have the advantage of reducing vascular resistance within minutes, thus facilitating systolic unloading (increasing cardiac output by decreasing the afterload). These potent diuretics are capable of bringing about tremendous reductions in intravascular volume which can result in a decrease in cardiac output. Patient's symptoms may be misleading, since the reduction in pulmonary congestion may produce dramatic symptomatic relief masking the decreased cardiac output. Overvigorous diuretic therapy should be avoided not only because of the risk of decreasing cardiac output but also because of the danger of electrolyte abnormalities that may predispose to dangerous digitalis-induced arrhythmias. It is important to realize that rapid depletion of intravascular volume can occur in the presence of peripheral edema if the rate of diuresis exceeds the rate of mobilization of fluid from the interstitial space to the intravascular compartment.

The effective oral dose of furosemide starts at 40 mg and that of bumetanide at 1 mg daily. Both drugs are classified as high ceiling diuretics, since increasing their dosage will increase the diuretic effects in congestive heart failure. The effective intravenous dose of furosemide begins at 10 mg while that of bumetanide is 1 mg. It is advisable to start with a conservative dosage of these diuretics and increase as necessary. Besides volume contraction, hypokalemia, hyponatremia, hyperuricemia, hyperglycemia, and metabolic alkalosis can occur with overvigorous diuretic therapy.

Vasodilation to Reduce Preload and Afterload

Congestive heart failure refractory to vigorous conventional treatment with digitalis and diuretics is not uncommon in clinical practice. Dramatic hemodynamic improvement can occur during the administration of vasodilator drugs (see Table 44-6) in patients with refractory left ventricular failure due to acute myocardial infarction, chronic ischemic heart disease, valvular heart disease, or cardiomyopathies.

Preload Reducers

In the failing myocardium, one of the initial responses is ventricular dilatation. This increases the fiber length and, in accordance with Starling's law of the heart (see Fig. 44-3), augments contractility by aligning more sites for actin and myosin to interact. However, increasing the volume of the ventricle also increases its intraventricular pressure. The heart must now expend more energy in maintaining that volume, since the left ventricular end-diastolic pressure has been increased. Unfortunately, with time the ventricle may dilate excessively, resulting in a loss of mechanical efficiency. By reducing the excessive volume returning to the heart (preload), this elevated volume and pressure may be decreased. The myocardial fibers may then be able to contract more efficiently, and they do not have to expend such large amounts of energy to maintain a given tension.

Preload can be reduced either by reducing blood volume or by dilating the veins, thus decreasing the volume returned to the heart at any given time. Volume can be reduced by the use of **diuretics** which decrease extracellular fluid volume and plasma volume. With plasma and blood volume decreased, the amount of blood returning to the heart in a given time is reduced.

Nitroglycerin and related agents are utilized primarily for their ability to dilate the venous circulation, thus reducing the volume of blood returned to the heart. By reducing the excessive intraventricular volume, the mechanical efficiency of the heart is improved at the same time the oxygen demand is reduced. In patients with widely dilated ventricles, the leaflets of the valves may not close tightly. This results in some backflow of blood and a reduction in the cardiac output. By reducing the blood return (with preload agents), the size of the ventricle may be reduced, and valves may again close tightly. This also may result in an increase in cardiac output. Interestingly, this has been postulated as a mechanism by which **morphine** may have beneficial circulatory effects. The clinical use of preload-reducing agents has led to the discovery that the diuretic **furosemide** has the effect of reducing plasma volume and also, following intravenous administration, a transient vasodilator effect, which may also reduce preload. Thus furosemide may be shown to decrease left ventricular end-diastolic pressure (left ventricular filling pressure) when that pressure is elevated from heart failure.

Afterload Reducers

The ability of the heart to pump blood is a function of the energy required during contraction to push blood through the aortic valve into the circulation. If the resistance behind the aortic valve is high (high afterload), the work necessary to pump blood during systole may be excessively high. Thus agents which reduce afterload may significantly enhance the ability of the heart to "unload" blood during systole. Agents utilized to reduce afterload are primarily those which dilate the arteriolar bed and in some dosages can be shown to cause hypotension. In general, the afterload-reducing agents are effective in improving cardiac hemodynamics if the left ventricular end-diastolic filling pressure is elevated (more than 15 mmHg).

TABLE 44-6 Vasodilators Used for the Treatment of Heart Failure*

GENERIC NAME	TRADE NAME	PRIMARY SITE OF ACTION	MODE OF ADMINISTRATION	DURATION OF ACTION
Phentolamine	Regitine†	Arterial	Continuous intravenous	Minutes
Phenoxybenzamine	Dibenzyline†	Arterial	Oral	Hours
Hydralazine	Apresoline‡	Arterial	Oral	Hours
Minoxidil	Lonetin‡	Arterial	Oral	Hours
Nitroprusside	Nipride‡	Arterial and venous	Continuous intravenous	Minutes
Trimethaphan	Arfonad‡	Arterial and venous	Continuous intravenous	Minutes
Prazosin	Minipress†	Arterial and venous	Oral	Hours
Nitroglycerin	Numerous brands§	Venous	Intravenous, sublingual, ointment, or patches	Minutes
Isosorbide dinitrate	Isordil, others§	Venous	Sublingual	Minutes to hours
Captopril	Capoten‡	Arterial	Oral	Hours
Nifedipine	Procadia§	Arterial	Oral	Hours

*Although all these drugs have been demonstrated to be effective vasodilators in the treatment of heart failure, not all have been approved for this use in the United States

†For pharmacology, see Chap. 14, and for use in shock, see Chap. 48.

‡For pharmacology and use in hypertension, see Chap. 40.

§For pharmacology and use in angina and myocardial infarction, see Chap. 43.

Source: E. Braunwald: "Heart Failure," in R. G. Petersdorf et al. (eds.), *Harrison's Principles of Internal Medicine,* 10th ed., New York: McGraw-Hill, 1983. Used by permission.

Parenteral Vasodilators

In dealing with acute failure of the pumping function complicating a myocardial infarction, vasodilator agents with quickly reversible hemodynamic effects are preferable. Intravenous sodium **nitroprusside, phentolamine,** and **nitroglycerin** are good examples; their hemodynamic effects are usually gone within minutes after stopping the drug. Significant hypotension during vasodilator therapy can be dangerous in the presence of myocardial ischemia if the arterial pressure is reduced below the critical pressure necessary to supply the coronary circulation. Patients on parenteral vasodilator therapy should be monitored in an intensive care unit. Parenteral vasodilator therapy can also be used in patients with refractory CHF, CHF with high blood pressure, and to evaluate patients who would be candidates for chronic vasodilator therapy.

Sodium Nitroprusside

Sodium nitroprusside (Nipride) was one of the first drugs evaluated for its effect on impedance (afterload) reduction. Sodium nitroprusside acts rapidly with direct stimulatory effects on the heart or inhibitory effects on the sympathetic nervous system. Nitroprusside appears to be particularly effective in congestive heart failure complicated by severe hypertension. It should be pointed out that where blood pressure is diminished (where mean arterial pressure is lower than 80 mmHg), nitroprusside can be hazardous. When using nitroprusside in the presence of ischemic heart disease, it is important to have enough aortic diastolic filling pressure to allow the diastolic coronary perfusion of the subendocardium.

The drug should be given using an infusion pump, with the dosage in CHF titrated to the patient's blood pressure and symptoms (usually starting at 0.5 μg/kg/min). With too-rapid blood pressure lowering, the patient will be more likely to demonstrate adverse reactions.

Phentolamine

Phentolamine (Regitene) is an α-adrenergic blocking agent that also has been used in refractory cardiac failure. Phentolamine appears to exhibit a greater dilator effect on the arterial than the venous side. Phentolamine is most useful in patients with low cardiac output without elevated left ventricular filling pressure. Reportedly it also has a positive inotropic effect, possibly secondary to its ability to increase the release of endogenous catecholamines.

Intravenous Nitroglycerin   Nitroglycerin is a potent venodilator with minimal effects on arterioles. The serum half-life is 1 to 3 min, which is useful for rapid titration of the patient. Treatment is usually started with a dose of 5 μg/min and then increased by 5 to 10 μg/min every 3 to 5 min. The maximum dose administered is usually 200 μg/min. The most common adverse effect is hypotension, which can usually be treated by stopping the infusion and administering volume expansion.

Oral Vasodilators

The following vasodilators have been used in the chronic therapy of congestive heart failure and related disorders: **nitrates, hydralazine, prazosin, minoxidil, captopril,** and **nifedipine.** These agents have been added to the more conventional therapeutic regimens in patients with refractory failure. In some patients the vasodilators lose their effectiveness during long-term therapy. This is often referred to as *vasodilator tolerance.* Hydralazine and minoxidil work predominantly by reducing afterload, while prazosin and captopril affect both preload and afterload (see Fig. 44-3). Combined therapy with these vasodilator agents and oral inotropic agents may indeed provide greater overall efficacy in the management of CHF in the future. The number of patients with refractory failure seems to be increasing due to the enhanced survival patterns of patients with acute cardiac events.

Nitrates   All the nitrate preparations have a similar mechanism of action but differ in their duration of action. The preparations most commonly used are oral **isosorbide dinitrate,** oral **sustained-release nitroglycerin,** and transdermal nitroglycerin preparations (**nitroglycerin patches** or **nitroglycerin ointment**).

Hydralazine   Hydralazine functions mainly as an afterload-reducing agent with some preload-reduction effect. The usual oral dose in the treatment of CHF is 75 to 100 mg qid although some patients may require larger doses. Patients on larger doses of hydralazine (greater than 400 mg/day) have the greatest risk for lupus-like syndrome.

Captopril   Captopril (Capoten) is the first angiotensin-converting enzyme inhibitor released for use in the United States. It provides a singular approach to afterload reduction by retardation of the production of the vasoconstrictor peptide angiotensin II. It is begun at small doses in the treatment of CHF (12.5 mg tid) and increased slowly to desired effect. The other vasodilators mentioned above consistently produce increased activity of the renin-angiotensin-aldosterone axis which may perpetuate CHF by increasing angiotensin II, which in turn disturbs peripheral circulatory hemodynamics and causes secondary hyperaldosteronism. This vasodilator tolerance with captopril may be somewhat prevented because of its pharmacologic action on the renin axis.

Prazosin   Prazosin is a postsynaptic α_1-adrenergic receptor blocker. The dose of prazosin is usually started at 1 mg at bedtime to prevent first-dose syncope. Ten to twenty percent of the patients may develop vasodilator tolerance which is not responsive to increasing the dose. In some cases, adding spironolactone may be helpful, but in many cases it is necessary to switch to a different vasodilator.

THERAPY OF ACUTE PULMONARY EDEMA

Acute pulmonary edema is a medical emergency requiring immediate therapy. Treatment should be directed at removing the precipitating causes of the acute cardiac decompensation, as well as the total constellation of changes responsible for it. The acronym MOST DAMP is utilized as a teaching tool to recall the therapeutic alternatives. It does not necessarily reflect the order of selection, and substitution of other agents with similar pharmacologic effects is sometimes made.

The *M* stands for **morphine sulfate,** which is best administered slowly by IV push. The dosage ranges from 4 to 8 mg given at a rate of 1 mg/min. The patient's blood pressure and heart rate need to be monitored closely following injection of the morphine. If hypotension or respiratory depression is going to occur, it will be evident within 15 or 20 min after the injection. Naloxone should be available in case of respiratory depression. Morphine sulfate has the following actions:

1. It depresses the responsiveness of the respiratory centers of the brainstem (pontine and medullary centers) to the increased Pa_{CO_2}, decreases responsiveness to electrical stimuli, and alters voluntary control of breathing.
2. It decreases the apprehension associated with the shortness of breath and dyspnea on exertion and decreases wakefulness by decreasing the sensitivity of the medullary center to CO_2.
3. It causes pooling of blood in the periphery by acting like an α-adrenergic blocking agent, particularly on the capacitance vessels, and decreases pulmonary artery pressure and basal metabolic rate, thereby decreasing left ventricular end-diastolic pressure.
4. It produces a delayed positive inotropic effect apparent in 15 to 30 min after intravenous administration.

The *O* is for **oxygen.** Oxygen may be administered to combat the hypoxia by mask, nasal catheter, or a positive-pressure breathing machine. A positive-pressure breathing machine causes an increase in intraalveolar pressure and thus reduces the rate of fluid transudation from the alveolar capillaries into the alveoli. It is important to remember that high concentrations of oxygen over a long time may have adverse effects and should be avoided when possible.

The *S* stands for "sit up." With the patient's head up and legs down, there is a decrease in venous return which results in some relief of the dyspnea. Edema fluid can accumulate in the subcutaneous tissues of the dependent part of the body rather than in the pulmonary vasculature. One danger to keep in mind at this point is that venous stasis may provide the setting for a later pulmonary embolus. Low-dose heparin therapy is advisable in most instances.

The *T* stands for tourniquets, which have largely been replaced by vasodilating drugs, such as **nitrates** (usually topically or intravenously), **nifedipine**, or **nitroprusside** (especially when blood pressure is elevated). If tourniquets are applied sufficiently tightly to occlude the venous return, approximately 500 to 800 mL of blood may be captured in the extremities. Normally the tourniquets are applied to three of the four extremities, and they are rotated every 15 min. These results can be achieved with a combination of nitrates and fast-acting loop diuretics. These agents must be monitored closely, and should be avoided in patients who are hypotensive or are known to be volume-depleted.

The *D* stands for digoxin, which is usually advocated; but since the onset and the maximal effects of digitalis occur long after the symptoms are controlled by other agents, digitalis is probably best used as a prophylactic agent against recurrence. In the patient with a rapid supraventricular arrhythmia who has not previously been digitalized, digitalis is probably indicated. If digitalis is not needed to treat the primary disease, it can be given safely in a less urgent situation. If the digitalizing dose is initiated during this period of time, it is important to administer it very slowly, since the peripheral vasoconstrictor effects may well cause a worsening of the pulmonary edema. In the absence of arrhythmias, the acute need for digitalis is debatable.

The *A* stands for **aminophylline**. The need for aminophylline has been dramatically reduced with the availability of loop diuretics. The loading dose of aminophylline is approximately 4 or 5 mg/kg and should be given slowly intravenously over about 15 to 30 min. The maintenance dose depends on the degree of failure and of liver function. The range is from 0.4 to 0.9 mg/kg/h. The dosage may be adjusted according to the serum levels obtained (the therapeutic range is from 10 to 20 μg/mL). Aminophylline is irritating regardless of route. It may cause burning and phlebitis at the IV site, pain on IM injection, and irritation of perianal areas when given by suppository (avoid IM and suppository routes). Rapid intravenous administration may cause bradycardia.

The *M* stands for mercurial diuretics, which are not used today (instead loop diuretics are used). Mercurial diuretics generally induce diuresis in 3 to 4 h, in contrast to the faster-acting **loop diuretics**, which have an onset of action of 15 to 30 min when given intravenously.

Finally, the *P* stands for phlebotomy (removal of blood from veins), which today is rarely necessary. Fast-acting loop diuretics induce a "bloodless phlebotomy" in a matter of minutes.

One final alternative, not included in the acronym, is afterload reduction, as previously discussed. This approach is particularly useful in dealing with the patient with acute myocardial infarction (when the mean arterial pressure is above 80 mmHg), cardiomyopathy, or other unresponsive forms of acute cardiac decompensation. This is usually accomplished acutely with **sodium nitroprusside**, with conversion to an oral agent if longer-term therapy is necessary.

NURSING PROCESS RELATED TO CONGESTIVE HEART FAILURE

The nursing process in congestive heart failure is discussed in relation to two groups of pharmacologic agents, the digitalis glycoside and the afterload-reducing agents (vasodilators plus loop diuretics). The nursing implications of other drugs employed in congestive heart failure are discussed elsewhere in this text. Diuretics are important therapeutic agents in CHF; the nursing process for these agents is covered in Chap. 23, "Edema."

Assessment

The initial nursing assessment of the patient in congestive heart failure serves as a baseline for evaluation of the subsequent response to therapy. In the acute setting, pertinent subjective data to record includes complaints of weakness, headaches, anorexia, nausea, dyspnea, hoarseness, orthopnea, paroxysmal nocturnal dyspnea, and palpitations. Vital signs are extremely important objective parameters to monitor, particularly the character and rate of the pulse and respiration. Signs of alteration in normal respiratory function include: cough, sputum production (document the character, consistency, and amount), increased respiratory rate, increasingly labored respirations, orthopnea, use of accessory muscles, and an irregular pulse. Another pertinent sign to assess and document is jugular venous distention. The patient should be at a 30° angle or greater to accurately assess jugular venous distention, which is usually an indication of central venous pressure. Auscultation of chest sounds will probably reveal rales which clear after vigorous coughing. Patients with congestive heart failure may also have extra heart sounds (S_3). Palpation and percussion of the abdomen will reveal tenderness of the liver from engorgement, hepatomegaly, splenomegaly, or ascites. Since weight is a sensitive indicator of fluid retention (10 to 20 lb of fluid can be retained in an adult without signs of edema), baseline and daily weights should be obtained. Dependent areas (the sacrum and posterior calves and thighs in the recumbent patient) should be assessed for edema. Baseline circumferential measurements of the calves (5 cm above the medial malleolus) and the abdomen (at the level of the umbilicus) are also good baseline parameters. Cognitive function (memory, orientation, judgment), peripheral pulses, and skin color and temperature should be checked for signs of peripheral perfusion. In the critical care setting, these observations may also be complemented with an ECG rhythm strip and measurements of central venous pressure and pulmonary artery and wedge pressure, as indicated by the severity of the failure.

The order for a cardiac glycoside necessitates further assessment. Appetite assessment is important, since anorexia is an early sign of **digitalis** toxicity. If the patient demonstrates prolongation of the PR interval or second- or third-degree heart block on ECG, this type drug is contraindicated. If the drug is given in first-degree block, as it may be when the benefits are expected to outweigh the disadvantages, the ECG is monitored for signs of increasing block. When the patient is elderly or has renal function impairment, the nurse should anticipate a lower dose of the digitalis preparation (usually digoxin). Electrolytes are also evaluated during digitalis therapy, since hypokalemia, hypercalcemia, or hypomagnesemia can predispose to toxicity. The potassium level is particularly important since so many patients are on concurrent diuretic therapy.

The apical pulse should be taken for a full minute and recorded on the medication record prior to each dose of digitalis preparation. This data should be integrated into the total assessment and not just ritually collected. Arrhythmias which cause a pulse deficit are those in which some beats heard apically are not of sufficient volume to be felt peripherally, such as atrial fibrillation or premature beats, and so this method may be used to evaluate for either therapeutic or adverse effects of the drug.

For the patient who is to receive an afterload-reducing agent including **amrinone**, the blood pressure and baseline pulse should be noted, and the drug should not be given in the presence of severe hypotension. A baseline platelet count is indicated prior to amrinone.

Management

Drug therapy is complemented by assisting the patient to rest and to assume a position that facilitates respiration. The administration of oxygen may also be beneficial. Nursing orders for a patient with congestive failure usually include monitoring of vital signs every 4 h, of intake and output, and of daily weight, and elevation of the head of bed (semi-Fowler's position is usually comfortable for these patients). Many patients tire easily and cannot consume enough calories and nutrients to meet their requirements. Thus, six small feedings or nutritional supplements are often indicated.

Utilization of the intravenously administered agents to improve cardiac output requires sophisticated hemodynamic monitoring with assessment of cardiac output, peripheral resistance, pulmonary artery pressures and other variables which can be monitored utilizing a balloon-tipped catheter (Swan-Ganz) within the pulmonary vasculature. In addition, if the patient's blood pressure is being significantly altered, it is wise to have an arterial catheter for continuous monitoring of pressure.

Intravenous administration of digitalis should be gradual,

the dose being given slowly over at least 5 min. *If the apical pulse taken prior to administration given by any route is less than 60 (or 70 to 110 in children, depending on age), unless otherwise stipulated, the drug should be withheld, and the physician notified.* Some physicians prefer to continue the medication even in the presence of low pulse. This low pulse may also indicate digitalis toxicity, and the nurse should assess the patient for other symptoms and signs.

The generic names of the digitalis preparations most commonly used are similar, digoxin and digitoxin, but their pharmacokinetics and maintenance dosage are quite different and should not be confused. Since the elixir and capsule forms are best absorbed, it may be the form of choice in some elderly people, but the patient should be observed for digitalis intoxication if the prescription is changed from tablet to elixir or capsule, since increased absorption may elevate plasma levels.

Digitalis preparations have a low therapeutic index and many institutions have a policy that all pediatric doses must be checked by two nurses prior to administration. During digitalization by the loading-dose method, the cardiac rhythm on the one-lead ECG monitor and vital signs are assessed frequently, and emergency resuscitation equipment should be available. While patients are on digitalis preparation, all ECGs should be labeled to show that the patient is on this drug.

This low therapeutic index is also the reason that teaching is so important for the patient who is to self-administer **digitalis** at home. The patient should be told the name and purpose of the drug. The importance of the drug and of taking it exactly as instructed must be emphasized. The patient should be warned of the dangers of discontinuing the drug when feeling better or of taking additional doses when not feeling well. Some patients may be taught to take their own pulse prior to administration of the drug and to withhold it if the pulse is lower than 60 or if the rhythm changes, but others will become more apprehensive if given this responsibility. The nurse must assess all patients carefully and secure the prescriber's agreement, when policy requires, before teaching the patient to regulate the drug in this manner. The patient should also be furnished with a written list of the signs of digitalis toxicity or of inadequate therapeutic effect, with indications of when the doctor should be called. The patient with heart failure should also be instructed about using a low sodium diet and in monitoring body weight for fluid retention. When an order for digitalis is received in the outpatient setting, the nurse should make sure that the patient is not already on the drug from another prescriber.

Both digitalis drugs and the afterload-reducing agents underline the principle that the nurse must know the therapeutic goal of therapy in order to give proper patient care. The digitalis drugs can be given for certain arrhythmias or for congestive heart failure, and the observations will vary according to the goal. Most of the afterload-reducing agents also have other uses besides heart failure. For example, isosorbide dinitrate (Isordil) and **nitroglycerin** can be given for angina as well as for their afterload effects. The nurse who is unaware of the purpose for which the drug is given may ask patients whether they have any chest pain, when in fact they have never had chest pain and the drug is being given for its afterload effects.

Evaluation

The observations listed under Assessment are repeated as frequently as indicated by the severity of the patient's condition and compared with the baseline information. The intake and output, as well as the daily weight, should be compared to the previous day so that the physician can be notified early if the patient is retaining fluid.

The nurse also needs to observe for the effects of teaching and for the adverse reactions specific to the drugs utilized, particularly at the time of the drug's peak effect. With **digitalis** preparations, the nurse should watch the ECG monitor for signs of toxicity. The common digitalis-induced arrhythmias are conduction defects (AV block) and ventricular disturbances (premature ventricular contractions). If the patient

is not on an ECG monitor, the nurse should check the pulse rate and regularity. Since the anorexia, nausea, and malaise that accompany intoxication are often confused with the influenza syndrome, critical evaluation of symptoms is necessary. The nurse must also be aware that digitalis intoxication may produce confusion and combativeness in the elderly patient.

Amrinone therapy requires monitoring of platelet count, chest pain (pleuritis or pericarditis), cardiac friction rub on auscultation (pericarditis), increased abdominal girth (ascites), blood pressure (for hypotension, especially if other hypotensive agents are used concurrently), and unexpected adverse effects, since this is a newly approved drug. The nurse must also assure that amrinone is mixed with a compatible IV solution.

If the patient develops angina while on digitalis, the physician should be notified. If the patient develops any other actual signs of digitalis intoxication, the drug should be withheld and the physician contacted. While assays for blood levels of drugs are useful, these should be interpreted in view of the clinical status of the patient.

CASE STUDY

R.B. is a 60-year-old widowed female who lives alone. Before retiring 14 years ago, she had worked as a department store clerk. She had had rheumatic fever at the age of 9 and subsequently developed valvular heart disease at 32 years of age. Two years prior to this admission a cardiac catheterization had been done which showed moderately severe mitral stenosis with slight mitral insufficiency. Secondary to left atrial hypertrophy, the patient had developed atrial fibrillation. Over the years she had developed significant subendocardial ischemia, and 5 years prior to this admission she had suffered a subendocardial infarction. Since then, she had had repeated episodes of congestive heart failure. During the 6 weeks prior to this hospital admission she had been taking digoxin (Lanoxin) 0.25 mg daily, furosemide (Lasix) 40 mg bid, and 25 meq of potassium supplement daily, along with a low-sodium diet. It had been extremely difficult to achieve control of the symptomatology with her current medication and diet. When attempts were made to improve her cardiac output by increasing the digoxin, she had to be hospitalized for digitalis toxicity. When the furosemide dose was increased, her intravascular volume became so depleted that she developed prerenal failure.

The reason for the patient's return to the clinic was that she had become increasingly short of breath over the previous week. At this time she found it difficult to breathe even when resting, while previously she had been able to walk several blocks without much problem. For some time she had found it necessary to sleep on two pillows. More

recently she had awakened repeatedly during the night, finding it difficult to catch her breath. On the morning of admission, she began coughing up some whitish frothy sputum.

Assessment

The patient's facial muscles were tense as she squirmed restlessly in her chair. While relating her symptoms of dyspnea, orthopnea, and paroxysmal nocturnal dyspnea to the nurse, she found it necessary to stop during the course of the conversation to catch her breath. Several times she answered questions inappropriately but was oriented to her surroundings. Her skin was cool and dusky in color. Sternocleidomastoid and abdominal accessory muscles were being utilized for respiration, with a rate of 26 per minute. Percussion was dull in the lung bases bilaterally; crackling and bubbling adventitious sounds were auscultated throughout both lung fields. Her heart rhythm was irregular, with a rate of 90 beats/min. S_1 and S_2 heart sounds were weak, and an S_3 sound was present. A grade II/VI systolic ejection murmur at the left sternal border and a grade II/VI diastolic murmur at the apex were auscultated. The jugular veins were distended at 4.5 cm above the sternal angle when she was sitting erect. Blood pressure in the right arm while sitting was 160/90. Peripheral pulse strength was normal except for bilateral weak posterior tibial and dorsalis pedis pulses. Pitting edema was present in the lower one-third of the lower extremities. The liver was enlarged, and a mild degree of ascites was present. Her weight was 69 kg.

The initial chest x-ray showed bilateral pleural fluid and a redistribution pattern of the pulmonary vasculature. Biventricular and left atrial enlargement were also present. A 12-lead ECG demonstrated atrial fibrillation, with a ventricular response of 82 beats/min. Initial blood chemistry showed normal electrolytes except for an elevated CO_2 (secondary to respiratory acidosis).

The nursing diagnosis was respiratory dysfunction, decreased cardiac output, and anxiety. This was compatible with the medical diagnosis of moderate pulmonary edema secondary to cardiac decompensation.

Management

As the importance of rest was explained, the patient was placed in her most comfortable position, which was upright orthopneic. Her head and shoulders were supported by the bedside table, and her legs rested on a chair. Oxygen was started at 3 L/min by nasal cannula. An intravenous line and Foley catheter were inserted. While being given furosemide 40 mg, following morphine sulfate 8 mg given slowly intravenously, she was informed that these medications would help to decrease her shortness of breath and thus allow her to rest. She was placed on a total fluid intake of 1200 mL/day. Sublingual isosor-

bide dinitrate [Isordil] was instituted by the physician at 5 mg q4h.

Evaluation

Mrs. B. responded favorably to lowering of the preload without any substantial drop in blood pressure or tachycardia, as would be expected with her elevated left ventricular end-diastolic pressure.

The first evening, the nursing staff monitored the patient frequently for any change in respiratory signs and symptoms. A few hours after admission to the cardiac care unit, her respiratory distress had lessened, although she felt exhausted. Her skin color had become pink. The bubbling adventitious noises in her lungs had decreased. She had passed 500 mL of urine following the initiation of therapy. She now changed to a semi-Fowler's position, with her feet elevated on the bed.

In the morning, the patient felt that she could breathe better; she was much more comfortable and had lost 1.8 kg. Her utilization of the respiratory accessory muscles had decreased to a minimum. The bubbling noises in her lungs were gone, although the crackling adventitious sounds were still present in the bases of both lung fields. Frequent deep breathing and coughing exercises brought up whitish sputum which was no longer frothy. The respiratory dysfunction was resolving.

REFERENCES

Awan, N. A., and B. M. Massie (eds.): "International Symposium: New Strategies in the Management of Severe, Chronic Heart Failure: Captopril," *Am Heart J,* **104:**1125–1228, 1982.

Braunwald, E.: "Mechanism of Contraction of Normal and Failing Heart," *N Engl J Med,* **277:**794, 1967.

——: "Mechanism of Contraction of Normal and Failing Heart," *N Engl J Med,* **277:**853, 1967.

——: "Mechanism of Contraction of Normal and Failing Heart," *N Engl J Med,* **277:**910, 1967.

——: "Mechanism of Contraction of Normal and Failing Heart," *N Engl J Med,* **277:**1012, 1967.

——: "Regulation of the Circulation," *N Engl J Med,* **290:**1124, pt. 1, 1974.

——: "Regulation of the Circulation," *N Engl J Med,* **290:**1420, pt. 2, 1974.

Campbell, C.: *Nursing Diagnosis and Intervention in Nursing Practice,* New York: Wiley, 1978.

Cohn, J. N., and J. A. Franciosa: "Vasodilator Therapy of Cardiac Failure," *N Engl J Med,* **297:**27–31, pt. 1, 1977.

——, and ——: "Vasodilator Therapy of Cardiac Failure," *N Engl J Med,* **297:**254–258, pt. 2, 1977.

Elenbaas, R. M., and J. O. Covinsky: "Approaches to the Management of Acute, Chronic, and Refractory Congestive Heart Failure," *J Contin Educ Pharm,* 1:11–39, 1979.

Iisalo, E.: "Clinical Pharmacokinetics of Digoxin," *Clin Pharmacokinet,* **2:**1–16, 1977.

Jelliffe, R. W.: "An Improved Method of Digoxin Therapy," *Ann Intern Med,* **69:**703, 1968.

——, et al.: "An Improved Method of Digoxin Therapy," *Ann Intern Med,* **73:**453, 1970.

Jones, D. A., C. F. Dunbar, and M. M. Jirovec: *Medical Surgical Nursing, A Conceptual Approach,* 2d ed., New York: McGraw-Hill, 1982.

Kannel, W. B., W. P. Castelli, P. M. McNamara, P. A. McKegg, and M. Feinleib: "Role of Blood Pressure in the Development of Congestive Heart Failure: The Framingham Study," *N Engl J Med,* **287:**781–787, 1972.

Katz, A. M.: "Congestive Heart Failure: Role of Altered-Myocardial Cellular Control," *N Engl J Med,* **293:**1183, 1975.

Kradjan, W. A., and M. A. Koda-Kimble: "Congestive Heart Failure," in B. S. Katcher, L. Y. Young, and M. A. Koda-Kimble (eds.), *Applied Therapeutics for Clinical Pharmacists,* San Francisco: Applied Therapeutics, 1983, pp. 161–216.

Meissner, J. E., and L. N. Gever: "Reducing the Risks of Digitalis Toxicity," *Nursing 80,* **10:**32–38, 1980.

Mungall, D. R., R. P. Robichaux, W. N. Perry, et al.: "Effects of Quinidine on Serum Digoxin Concentration: A Prospective Study," *Ann Intern Med,* **93:**689–693, 1980.

Nathan, M., S. A. Rubin, D. Siemienczuk, and H. J. C. Swan: "Effects of Acute and Chronic Minoxidil Administration on Rest and Exercise Hemodynamics and Clinical Status in Patients with Severe, Chronic Heart Failure," *Am J Cardiol,* **50:**960–966, 1982.

Packer, M.: "Selection of Vasodilator Drugs for Patients with Severe Chronic Heart Failure: An Approach Based on a New Classification," *Drugs,* **24:**64–74, 1982.

Schwartz, A.: "Abnormal Biochemistry in Myocardial Failure," *Am J Cardiol,* **32:**407, 1973.

Spotnitz, H. M.: "Structural Conditions in the Hypertrophied and Failing Heart," *Am J Cardiol,* **32:**398, 1973.

Wettrell, G., and K. E. Anderson: "Clinical Pharmacokinetics of Digoxin in Infants," *Clin Pharmacokinet,* **2:**17–31, 1977.

45

DISORDERS OF CARDIAC RHYTHM*

VINCENT C. SPERANZA
GILDA SAUL

LEARNING OBJECTIVES

Upon mastery of the contents of this chapter, the reader will be able to:

1. Describe the abnormalities in phase 4 and phase 0 that may result in cardiac arrhythmias.

2. Describe the role calcium plays in the normal electrophysiology of the heart.

3. List the factors that may precipitate arrhythmias.

4. Explain the mechanisms by which various drugs may induce tachyarrhythmias.

5. Describe the classification system for categorizing the different antiarrhythmic agents.

6. State the mechanism of action of the following drugs relative to electrochemical phases: quinidine, procainamide, disopyramide, lidocaine, phenytoin, propranolol, digitalis, bretylium, verapamil.

7. List the cardiovascular and noncardiovascular signs and symptoms of toxicity of quinidine and procainamide.

8. Give the indications for the following antiarrhythmic agents: quinidine, procainamide, disopyramide, lidocaine, phenytoin, propranolol, digitalis, bretylium, verapamil.

9. Identify the route of administration, therapeutic blood level and major toxicity of the following drugs: quinidine, procainamide, disopyramide, lidocaine, phenytoin, propranolol, digitalis, bretylium, verapamil.

10. Explain why lidocaine cannot be given orally.

11. Describe generally the advantages of investigational antiarrhythmics compared to available agents.

12. State the cautions for IV administration of antiarrhythmics.

13. Explain the rationale for combination therapy of antiarrhythmic agents.

14. List five aspects of assessment prior to administration of antiarrhythmic agents.

15. Write a care plan for treating a patient with a tachyarrhythmia on verapamil.

16. Write a discharge plan for a patient sent home on an antiarrhythmic agent.

17. Describe the evaluation of antiarrhythmic therapy for efficacy, adverse effects, and adequacy of patient education.

ELECTROPHYSIOLOGY OF THE HEART

Electrical conduction and arrhythmias are best understood if the events associated with conduction are first examined in an individual conducting fiber (Fig. 45-1). Conducting tissue has an electrical gradient created by the sodium potassium (Na^+-K^+) pump. This pump causes the concentration of potassium to be greater inside the myocardial fiber. Other electrolytes such as calcium (Ca^{2+}) and magnesium (Mg^{2+}) are also essential for normal conduction. A normal, slow leak of sodium into the myocardial fiber results in slow depolarization and is called phase 4 of the action potential. Phase 4 represents the ability of heart tissue to function without any outside stimulus, the property of *automaticity*.

When the electrical potential reaches the threshold potential, a rapid shift in sodium and potassium occurs that results in the formation of the electrical impulse referred to as phase 0 of the action potential. The impulse is then transferred to the surrounding fibers and conducted throughout the heart, the property of *conductivity*. The electrical impulse is associated with depolarization and subsequent muscular contraction.

The sinoatrial (SA) node usually depolarizes most rapidly and reaches the threshold potential first, making the SA node the pacemaker under normal conditions. Phases 1, 2, and 3 are associated with repolarization of the conducting fiber; the fiber is considered to be incapable of conduction until repolarization has occurred. The time during which

*The editors thank Michael E. Winter, Pharm. D., who contributed the chapter on this subject in the first edition.

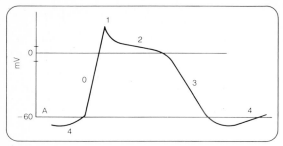

FIGURE 45-1

Action Potential for a Single Purkinje Fiber. Using an intracellular microelectrode, the following characteristics of the action potential can be identified: (*A*) Threshold, point at which fiber will depolarize. (*0*) Depolarization of fiber. (*1, 2,* and *3*) Repolarization of fiber. (*4*) Spontaneous slow depolarization back to *A,* caused by a slow leak of sodium (automaticity).

the fiber cannot conduct an impulse is referred to as the *refractory period.*

Ionic Basis of Membrane Activity

Resting transmembrane potential and membrane activity are based upon the concentrations of several ions (primarily sodium, potassium, and calcium) on either side of the membrane and the permeability of the membrane to these ions. The major route by which ions diffuse through membranes is through ion channels, protein molecules that span the membranes. The depolarization caused by the flow of sodium through sodium channels produces phase 0 of the action potential, leading to activation of the calcium channels and, more slowly, of the potassium channels. The plateau of the action potential (phases 1 and 2) reflects the inactivation of the sodium current, the activation and inactivation of the calcium channels and resultant calcium current, and the development of a repolarizing potassium current. (Since calcium currents are similar to sodium currents, some authors refer to calcium channels as *slow channels* and to sodium channels as *fast channels.*) Final repolarization (phase 3) results from complete inactivation of the calcium channels and increasing potassium permeability, which establishes the resting membrane potential.

Many drugs used to treat arrhythmias (e.g., **quinidine, procainamide, disopyramide, lidocaine, phenytoin,** etc.) are sodium channel blocking agents. Calcium is essential to muscle contraction (excitation-contraction coupling), as well as to electrical conduction. Thus, a new class of drugs called the calcium channel blockers (e.g., **verapamil, diltiazem, nifedipine**) are used to treat angina and arrhythmias.

Electrophysiology and the ECG

The sinoatrial (SA) node usually depolarizes most rapidly and reaches the threshold potential first, making the SA node the pacemaker under normal circumstances. The SA node triggers cardiac contraction at a frequency of 60 to 100 beats/min. The impulse spreads through the atria rapidly and enters the atrioventricular (AV) node, where conduction is normally slow. After passing through the AV node, the only conduction pathway between the atria and ventricles, the impulse propagates rapidly through the His-Purkinje system and then to the ventricles. This coordinated propagation of the impulse in the sequence is necessary for a hemodynamically effective cardiac contraction.

Each of the five major cardiac cell types (SA node, atrium, AV node, Purkinje, and ventricle) have a distinct action potential. The electrocardiogram (ECG) is the body surface manifestation of the combined depolarization and repolarization waves of the heart (Fig. 45-2).

ELECTROPHYSIOLOGIC CHANGES IN ARRHYTHMIAS

Disturbances in the normal action potentials of heart tissue can result in abnormal cardiac contractions or arrhythmias.

Disturbances in *automaticity* or phase 4, can result from a decrease or increase in the rate of rise of phase 0. For example, if the SA node, the normal pacemaker, begins to depolarize too rapidly, an increase in heart rate (tachycardia) will occur. If the rate of phase 4 in the SA node slows down

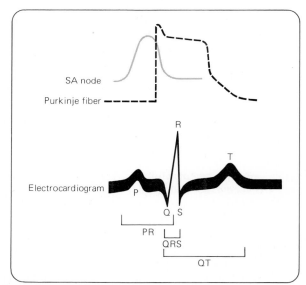

FIGURE 45-2

The Electrocardiogram Compared to the Action Potentials of Individual SA Node and Purkinje Fibers. The P wave reflects atrial activation, the QRS complex coincides with ventricular depolarization, and the T wave reflects ventricular repolarization. The PR interval indicates atrioventricular conduction time (usually 0.12 to 0.20 s), and the QT interval reflects the ventricular action potential duration.

TABLE 45-1   Factors That May Precipitate Arrhythmias

1. Electrolyte imbalances: hypocalcemia, hypomagnesemia, hypokalemia
2. Acid-base disorders
3. Hypoxia
4. Congestive heart failure (CHF)
5. Hyperthyroidism
6. Pericarditis
7. Ischemia or infarction
8. Pulmonary emboli
9. Drugs: digitalis glycosides, phenothiazines, tricyclic antidepressants, antiarrhythmic agents
10. Swanz-Ganz catheter, CVP lines, or pacing wires irritating the myocardium

sufficiently, other areas of the heart may reach the threshold potential first and thereby become *ectopic,* or abnormal, pacemakers. Rapid depolarization of other cardiac tissue independent of the SA node can also result in arrhythmias, as occurs when cardiac tissue is damaged or irritated.

Disturbances of conductivity result from changes in normal conduction velocity (phase 0). The slower the conduction velocity, the less likely it is that the electrical impulse (normal or abnormal) will be transmitted to the adjacent muscle fiber or tissue. Nonconduction of an impulse is usually referred to as conduction block and can be the result of direct damage to the tissue.

Automaticity and conductivity can be affected by drugs, electrolyte or acid-base imbalances, and injury to the heart or conduction system. Table 45-1 enumerates factors which may precipitate arrhythmias. Drugs of the digitalis class (**digoxin** and **digitoxin**) are arrhythmogenic. These drugs have a narrow therapeutic index; the difference between a therapeutic and toxic plasma level is small and subject to individual variation. Toxic levels of the cardiac glycosides inhibit the sodium-potassium pump, leading to conduction disturbances.

Phenothiazines (**chlorpromazine, thioridazine,** etc.) and tricyclic antidepressants (**imipramine, desipramine,** etc.) have varying effects on cardiac rhythm since they act both directly on the heart and indirectly on the cardiovascular system. One of the major complications of toxic plasma levels of both these drug classes is arrhythmias; for this reason patients with suspected drug overdose are routinely placed on an ECG monitor.

Identification of Arrhythmias

Arrhythmias are most frequently described by their rate, location, and/or conduction patterns. The rate may be slow (bradycardia), which is defined as a rate of less than 60 beats/min, or it may be rapid (tachycardia), which is a rate greater than 100 beats/min. Rapid rates may further be divided into the categories of *flutter* (250 to 350 beats/min) and *fibrillation* (greater than 400 beats/min).

The origin of the arrhythmia may be the SA node, the AV node, the bundle branches, or the ventricles. The conduction pattern may be interrupted at some point by a block. The block may be *complete,* indicating no conduction through that segment of the conducting system, or it may be *incomplete,* indicating slowed conduction.

Ventricular arrhythmias are generally more serious since the ventricles are responsible for the major pumping action of the heart.

Classification of Arrhythmias

The various types of arrhythmias can be broadly classified into conduction disturbances, disturbances of impulse formation, and combined disturbances of impulse formation and conduction (see Table 45-2).

Conduction disturbances are managed on a temporary basis with antiarrhythmic agents. When the underlying cause is identified and subsequently treated, the major conduction disturbances may resolve. If they persist, however, and are symptomatic, then pacemaker implantation may be indicated.

Disturbances of impulse formation are often a result of abnormalities of *automaticity,* and drugs such as **propranolol** and other β blockers, or **digoxin** excess. Since treatment of these disturbances is directed at removal of the underlying cause, specific drug treatment is rarely required.

Drug treatment does play a key role in the management of combined disturbances of conduction and impulse formation. The common disorder here is loss of normal pacemaker control. The AV node or junction is a useful anatomical dividing line for separating these arrhythmias. Arrhythmias originating in or above the AV node are referred to as supraventricular while those originating below the AV node are considered ventricular in nature.

TABLE 45-2   Classification of Arrhythmias

I. Conduction disturbances

    SA node block
    AV node block
    Bundle branch block

II. Disturbances of impulse formation

    Sinus bradycardia and tachycardia
    Premature atrial contractions
    Atrial tachycardia
    Premature ventricular contractions (PVCs)
    Ventricular tachycardia and flutter
    Ventricular fibrillation

III. Combination of disturbances of impulse formation and conduction

    Supraventricular tachycardias
    Atrial fibrillation and flutter
    Junctional tachycardias

CLINICAL PHARMACOLOGY AND THERAPEUTICS

A wide spectrum of drugs are currently available for the treatment of atrial and ventricular arrhythmias, and a number of investigational agents may soon be released.

One method of classification of antiarrhythmics is presented in Table 45-3. Table 45-4 summarizes the different electrophysiologic actions of the common antiarrhythmic agents.

Quinidine

Mechanism of Action Quinidine is the oldest and prototype antiarrhythmic agent; it is derived from the natural product, cinchona bark. Quinidine decreases automaticity, reducing the probability that ectopic foci will reach threshold before the SA node. The effect on automaticity is more pronounced on ectopic foci than on the SA node. Conduction velocity is decreased (diminished upstroke of phase 0 of the *fast* action potential). The refractory period is prolonged, lengthening the time during which the heart is unable to respond to stimuli; this reduces the likelihood of myocardial contraction from an ectopic focus. Quinidine also has an indirect vagolytic (atropine-like) effect which may enhance conduction though the AV node. This effect is significant, since in atrial fibrillation, reduced AV node

TABLE 45-3 Classification of Antiarrhythmic Drugs

TYPE	MECHANISM OF ACTION	DRUGS
I	Suppression of fast sodium current	Quinidine Procainamide (Pronestyl) Disopyramide (Norpace) Lidocaine (Xylocaine) Phenytoin (Dilantin) Lidocaine congeners: Mexilitene,* Tocainide, Encainide,* Aprindine*
II	β-Adrenergic blocking agents	Propranolol (Inderal)
III	Reduction of action potential duration disparity	Bretylium (Bretylol) Amiodarone (Cordarone)*
IV	Calcium channel blockers	Verapamil (Isoptin, Calan) Diltiazem (Cardizem)

*Investigational agents in the United States.

conductivity protects the ventricles from a rapid response. Reducing vagal tone with quinidine may result in a dangerously rapid ventricular rate.

Pharmacokinetics Quinidine is available as a number of different salts; the sulfate is the most commonly used. Although the particular salt chosen does not affect the phar-

TABLE 45-4 Electrophysiologic Actions of Antiarrhythmics Comparison Chart

CLASS*	DRUG	CONDUCTION VELOCITY	REFRACTORY PERIOD	AUTOMATICITY	AV NODAL CONDUCTION
I (Fast channel blockers)	Quinidine	↓↓	↑↑	↓↓	↑/↓
	Procainamide	↓↓	↑↑	↓↓	↑/↓
	Disopyramide	↓↓	↑↑	↓↓	↑
	Lidocaine				
	Normal tissue	○	↓	↓	○
	Ischemic tissue	↓↓	↑	↓↓	○
	Phenytoin				
	Normal tissue	○	↓	↓	↑
	Ischemic tissue	↓↓	↑	↓↓	↑
II (β Blockers)	Propranolol	↓	↓	↓	↓↓
III	Bretylium	○	↑↑	↑/○	↑/○
IV (Slow channel blockers)	Verapamil	○	○	○	↓↓
	Diltiazem	○	○	○	↓

Key: ↑ increase, ↓ decrease, ○ minimal or no effect, ↑/↓ variable
*Classification system adapted from B. N. Singh, J. T. Collett, and C. Y. C. Chew, "New Perspectives in the Pharmacologic Therapy of Cardiac Arrhythmias," *Prog Cardiovasc Dis*, 22:243–301, 1980.
  Source: Reprinted with permission from James E. Knoben and Philip O. Anderson (eds.): *Handbook of Clinical Drug Data*, 5th ed., Hamilton, IL: Drug Intelligence Publication, Inc., 1983.

macologic properties of the drug, it alters onset of action and perhaps bioavailability.

Peak plasma levels occur in approximately 1 to 4 h after oral administration. Since the estimated half-life is 6 to 8 h, 24 h is required to fully evaluate the efficacy of a given regimen.

Less than 20 percent of the drug is excreted unchanged in the urine. Liver failure or decreased hepatic blood flow which can result in congestive heart failure (CHF) may reduce the elimination of quinidine and result in accumulation and possible toxicity.

Although quinidine is seldom given intravenously, it can be administered safely in a coronary care unit with appropriate monitoring of ECG, heart rate, and blood pressure. Toxicities, primarily cardiac arrhythmias, previously reported with intravenous quinidine may have been caused by an excessive administration rate. Acute toxicity due to rapid infusion is a problem common to most antiarrhythmic agents.

Although used in the past, intramuscular administration is not recommended since severe pain and muscle damage may result.

Quinidine plasma levels are useful in maximizing therapeutic and minimizing toxic effects; the therapeutic range is 2 to 6 μg/mL in plasma.

Adverse Effects

Signs of quinidine toxicity are observed on ECG and include premature ventricular contractions (PVCs), ventricular tachycardia or fibrillation, and AV block. A QRS complex widening of greater than 50 percent results from decreased ventricular conduction velocity and is usually a sign of excessive quinidine plasma levels. Hypotension has been reported, but usually occurs only with IV or large oral doses. *Quinidine syncope,* or fainting spells, initially thought to result from hypotension caused by the drug's vasodilating effects, is actually hypotension caused by inadequate perfusion secondary to ventricular arrhythmias.

Nausea and diarrhea are frequently reported adverse effects of quinidine but rarely require discontinuance of therapy. *Cinchonism* may occur in up to 15 percent of patients treated with quinidine; symptoms of the syndrome include tinnitus, vertigo, blurred vision, headaches, and visual disturbances.

Salt forms of quinidine other than the sulfate are said to be more completely absorbed and may cause fewer gastrointestinal side effects. However, this has not been conclusively shown.

Rare cases of idiosyncratic and allergic reactions to quinidine have been reported. Reactions include rash, fever, hemolysis, thrombocytopenia, and hepatic dysfunction.

Drug Interactions

Quinidine has a number of drug interactions that must be considered. Since 75 to 90 percent or more of quinidine is bound to serum albumin, it may displace other drugs which are significantly albumin-bound resulting in enhanced therapeutic and possibly toxic effects. For example, **warfarin** (Coumadin) is significantly albumin-bound; addition of quinidine to a stable warfarin regimen may lead to an increased prothrombin time. Liver enzymes may be induced by a number of drugs including **phenytoin** (Dilantin), **phenobarbital, chloral hydrate** (Noctec), **glutethimide** (Doriden), and **methprylon** (Noludar). This enzyme induction may lead to enhanced quinidine metabolism with a resultant decrease in plasma levels.

The most significant interaction of quinidine is with **digoxin.** After 24 to 48 h of combined therapy, there may be a doubling of plasma digoxin levels with emergence of the signs and symptoms of digitalis toxicity. The mechanism of this interaction has not been completely elucidated but may result from a decrease in the number of or a displacement from myocardial digoxin binding sites or a diminished renal digoxin clearance. If the patient is maintained on digoxin, and quinidine is added to the regimen, plasma digoxin levels should be obtained in conjunction with appropriate patient monitoring.

Clinical Use

Quinidine is clinically employed in the treatment of both atrial and ventricular arrhythmias. It is considered the drug of choice for converting or preventing atrial fibrillation. Due to quinidine's vagolytic effects, however, prior digitalization is advisable to protect the ventricles from enhanced AV conduction.

Quinidine should be used cautiously in states of low cardiac output as a result of its direct depressant effects on the heart and conducting system and potential for inducing hypotension.

Preparations and Dosage

Quinidine is available in various salt forms for oral and parenteral administration. It is generally recommended that only quinidine sulfate or gluconate be prescribed. **Quinidine sulfate** (Cin-Quin, Quinoza, Quinidex) is available as tablets and capsules. **Quindine gluconate** (Quinaglute, Duraquin, Quinatime, Quin-Release) is available as extended-release tablets and for injection. It should be noted that the proportion of anhydrous quinidine base in the sulfate and gluconate preparations is 83 and 62 percent, respectively, so equivalent doses of quinidine gluconate will be higher than those of quinidine sulfate.

A test dose of 100 to 200 mg of quinidine sulfate is often administered to evaluate the possibility of an idiosyncratic reaction.

The usual adult dose is 1.0 to 2.4 g/day in four divided doses of quinidine sulfate or three divided doses of quinidine gluconate. Patients may be loaded with 200 mg administered every 2 to 3 h for five doses or until a therapeutic effect or toxicity is observed.

Intravenous administration (restricted to emergency use) is accomplished with 5 to 8 mg/kg of quinidine gluconate at a rate of 0.3 mg/kg/min or no faster than 16 to 25 mg/min.

The pediatric dose of quinidine sulfate is 30 mg/kg or

900 mg/m² of body surface administered in five divided doses. Pediatric parenteral dosage recommendations are not available from the manufacturer. Refer to Table 45-6 for complete dosing information.

Procainamide

Mechanism of Action The pharmacologic effects of procainamide (Pronestyl) are essentially identical to those of quinidine. It suppresses automaticity and slows conduction velocity; refractory period is prolonged and vagolytic activity is present. Occasionally procainamide may prove effective where quinidine has failed since the pharmacokinetics and patient response to both therapeutic and adverse effects are different.

Pharmacokinetics Oral absorption is efficient; 75 to 95 percent of an oral dose is bioavailable in most patients. Oral or intramuscular procainamide is rapidly absorbed with peak plasma levels occurring less than 60 min following administration.

The biologic half-life is about 3 to 4 h; therefore, the drug is usually administered every 4 h. Approximately 50 percent of procainamide is eliminated unchanged in the urine with the remainder metabolized by acetylation in the liver. Patients are classified as either slow or fast acetylators according to the rate at which N-acetyl procainamide (NAPA) is formed. Liver failure and CHF may decrease drug elimination, and dosage modifications should be considered in such patients.

The metabolite NAPA is a pharmacologically active antiarrhythmic agent. NAPA has a half-life of about 6 h in patients with normal renal function; the half-life is greatly prolonged in patients with renal failure requiring dosage adjustment.

Procainamide plasma levels are clinically employed in evaluating drug efficacy. The therapeutic plasma level of procainamide ranges from 4 to 10 µg/mL. NAPA plasma levels are also monitored and range from 9 to 20 µg/mL. Levels of procainamide greater than 12 µg/mL are commonly associated with toxicities.

Adverse Effects The myocardial toxicities of procainamide are very similar to those of quinidine. Caution should be used when administering procainamide in the presence of rapid atrial rates, as vagal blockade may result in greatly elevated ventricular rates. As with any antiarrhythmic agent, procainamide should not be administered when complete AV block is present since asystole may result. Ventricular arrhythmias are always problematic as it is difficult to distinguish whether too much or too little drug has been administered. A 30 percent widening of the QRS complex (indicating a significantly decreased ventricular conduction rate) may be interpreted as an indication to reevaluate therapy.

The most common adverse effects associated with procainamide include nausea, vomiting, and diarrhea. As with quinidine, hypotension has been reported with procainamide.

Procainamide has been associated with the development of systemic lupus erythematosus (SLE), a serious, though reversible, adverse effect occurring in about 30 percent of patients on chronic therapy. Positive antinuclear antibody (ANA) titers occur in most patients treated for longer than one year. Patients developing fever and joint pains should notify their physician since these symptoms may be prodromal to the development of SLE.

Miscellaneous adverse procainamide effects include mental changes (depression, giddiness, pyschosis), chills, fever, and skin rash.

Clinical Use As with quinidine, procainamide is effective in treating arrhythmias of atrial and ventricular origin. Some clinicians believe it is more successful in the treatment of ventricular arrhythmias, such as PVCs, flutter, and fibrillation than in the treatment of atrial arrhythmias.

Preparations Available and Dosage Procainamide (Pronestyl, Promine, Sub-Quin) is available as capsules, as tablets, and sustained-release tablets (Procan-SR; Pronestyl SR) and as an injectable drug.

The usual adult dose is 250 to 500 mg q3–4h. The average adult daily dose is 50 mg/kg/day, although this may vary from 1 to 9 g/day.

Therapy is generally initiated with low doses and then titrated upward. Plasma levels are monitored as is clinical response (resumption of normal cardiac rhythm).

In the elderly population, there is a general decrease in both hepatic and renal function permitting an increase in dosing interval to every 6 h. The sustained-release product

TABLE 45-5 Common Arrhythmias and Their Primary and Secondary Treatments of Choice

ARRHYTHMIA	PRIMARY TREATMENT	SECONDARY TREATMENT
Atrial flutter	Cardioversion	Digitalis
Atrial fibrillation	Cardioversion	Digitalis
Supraventricular tachycardia (SVT)	Vagotonic stimulation	Edrophonium Verapamil Propranolol Digitalis
Premature ventricular contractions (PVC)	Lidocaine	Procainamide Quinidine Disopyramide
Ventricular tachycardia	Cardioversion	Lidocaine Procainamide Bretylium
Ventricular fibrillation	Cardioversion Lidocaine	Bretylium

with a wax matrix formulation allows prolonged dosage intervals (every 6 h).

In life-threatening situations, where rapid termination of arrhythmia is necessary to maintain adequate cardiac output, a loading dose is administered to achieve immediate therapeutic plasma levels. This is usually accomplished intravenously at a carefully controlled rate. One regimen is to administer 1 to 2.5 g no faster than 20 to 25 mg/min; an alternative is to give 100 mg every 5 min until the arrhythmia is abolished (up to 1 g total dose) or until toxicity occurs. Blood pressure and ECG should be carefully monitored during administration. A maintenance infusion of 1 to 5 mg/min follows the loading dose; this rate should be decreased in renal or hepatic impairment or with decreased cardiac output. If hypotension is experienced, the patient should be placed in the Trendelenberg position until the blood pressure stabilizes.

Although pediatric dosing recommendations have not been established by the manufacturer, some clinicians suggest an oral daily dose of 50 mg/kg or 1.5 g/m^2 of body surface in four to six doses.

Disopyramide

Mechanism of Action   The pharmacologic activity of disopyramide (Norpace) on the myocardium is essentially equivalent to that of **quinidine** and **procainamide**: it reduces automaticity, conduction velocity, and prolongs the refractory period. It also has pronounced anticholinergic properties which account for many of its adverse effects.

Pharmacokinetics   Oral disopyramide is well absorbed (80 to 90 percent) with peak plasma levels occurring in 1 to 3 h. The biologic half-life is about 5 to 8 h. Although most (40 to 60 percent) of the drug is excreted unchanged in the urine, it is recommended that dosing adjustments be made in the presence of both renal and hepatic insufficiency. The therapeutic plasma level is 2 to 8 μg/mL; toxicity is generally associated with plasma levels greater than 9 μg/mL.

Adverse Effects   Disopyramide has numerous side effects, the majority of which are related to its anticholinergic activity; 30 percent of patients receiving the drug complain of dry mouth, urinary hesistancy and retention (especially in elderly men), constipation, dry eyes and throat, and nausea. Some effects are transient; others may necessitate dosage reduction or cessation of therapy.

Caution should be exercised in administering disopyramide to patients with preexisting left ventricular dysfunction since the drug's negative inotropic effect may precipitate CHF or hypotension in this patient population. Furthermore, the same cautions apply when disopyramide is used concomitantly with β **blockers** or **verapamil** due to their respective negative inotropic and additive cardiovascular effects.

Clinical Use   Disopyramide is effective in treating ventricular arrhythmias such as PVCs and episodes of ventricular tachycardia. The drug may also be of value in preventing atrial arrhythmias which have been unresponsive to quinidine.

Preparations and Dosage   Disopyramide is available as capsules (Norpace) and as a sustained-release preparation (Norpace CR). The usual adult maintenance dose is 150 mg every 6 h with a range of 400 to 800 mg/day. The sustained-release form is usually given in doses of 100 to 300 mg every 12 h. In patients weighing less than 50 kg or those with moderately impaired renal function or hepatic insufficiency, 100 mg every 6 h is recommended. Further dosage reduction is necessary in patients with declining renal function. When rapid control of ventricular arrhythmias is required, patients may be loaded with 300 to 400 mg of disopyramide. The safety and efficacy of disopyramide in pregnant women and children has not been established. Some clinicians recommend using 5 to 15 mg/kg/day in four divided doses. Dosage for children is individualized, but infants (<1 year) may require 10 to 30 mg/kg/day while those under 12 years of age average 10 to 20 mg/kg/day.

Lidocaine

Mechanism of Action   Lidocaine (Xylocaine) suppresses automaticity in the His-Purkinje system and suppresses spontaneous ventricular repolarization during diastole. It has little effect on AV nodal conduction and the specialized atrial conducting tissues are less sensitive to the effects of lidocaine than are those of the ventricles. In ischemic myocardial tissue, lidocaine decreases conduction velocity and increases the refractory period.

Pharmacokinetics   Although lidocaine is well absorbed from the gastrointestinal tract, it cannot be administered orally. The drug undergoes hepatic first-pass metabolism to such an extent that only 20 to 40 percent of an oral dose reaches the systemic circulation. Unfortunately, therapeutic plasma levels cannot be attained via this route, but toxicities appear. Two investigational congeners of lidocaine, **mexiletine** and **tocainide**, are minimally metabolized and have the advantage of oral administration.

Intravenous lidocaine has an initial rapid distribution phase (8 min) followed by a phase in which the drug is redistributed to less well perfused tissues. The redistribution phase (10 to 30 min) of lidocaine correlates with its brief duration of action following a single injection. It is apparent from these data that continuous IV infusion is the most logical regimen. To achieve instantaneous therapeutic plasma levels (1.5 to 6 μg/mL), a loading dose is administered concurrently with an infusion. Since the elimination half-life is approximately 100 min, it requires about 8 h to achieve approximate (95 percent) steady-state levels if an infusion is given without a loading dose.

The major route of elimination of lidocaine is via hepatic metabolism; less than 10 percent of a dose is excreted unchanged in the urine. Dosage adjustment is, therefore, unnecessary in renally compromised patients but mandatory in patients with liver disease, CHF, or any other disorder in which decreased liver perfusion is a problem. In these patients, the drug may accumulate resulting in elevated plasma levels and an increased risk of toxicity.

It is important to realize that while the pharmacologic effects of a single IV bolus terminate in a few minutes, toxicities resulting from excessive maintenance infusion (greater than 24 h) may take hours to subside. Minor toxicities are associated with levels of 6 to 9 μg/mL with more severe problems associated with levels greater than 9 μg/mL.

Adverse Effects With lidocaine, cardiovascular toxicities—hypotension, increased heart rate, negative inotropic effects—are rarely seen. AV block has been reported with excessive plasma levels.

The most common adverse effects of lidocaine are CNS depression, including dizziness, confusion, blurred vision, and psychosis. With plasma levels above 9 μg/mL, grand mal and focus seizures may occur.

Allergic reactions to lidocaine have been reported, but are quite rare.

Clinical Use Rapid onset of action following IV administration, relative safety, and lack of substantial adverse cardiovascular effects make lidocaine the drug of choice for ventricular arrhythmias especially in postmyocardial infarction patients. Lidocaine is most often used to control PVCs and ventricular tachycardia; supraventricular arrhythmias are less responsive to lidocaine.

Ventricular arrhythmias unresponsive to lidocaine may indicate suboptimal dosing. Plasma levels should be obtained and the dose maximized before alternative therapy is instituted.

Preparations and Dosage Lidocaine preparations intended for local anesthetic use, especially those containing epinephrine, should *never* be used for antiarrhythmic therapy.

Lidocaine is available as 1, 2, and 4% solutions for antiarrhythmic therapy as well as 0.4% premixed in dextrose 5% in water (2 g of lidocaine per 500 mL solution).

The initial bolus is 1 to 2 mg/kg injected over 1 to 2 min. An infusion is usually simultaneously initiated at a rate of 1 to 4 mg/min. If there is delay in the administration of the infusion, a second bolus may be required 10 to 20 min after the first dose. Pediatric patients may be loaded with a dose of 2 to 3 mg/kg administered over 5 to 10 min. This is fol-

lowed by an infusion of 30 to 50 μg/kg/min. The infusion is titrated to control the arrhythmia.

When a loading dose is administered and an infusion of constant rate simultaneously begun, plasma levels can be obtained and are interpretable in 20 min. If a constant infusion is initiated without administration of a loading dose, 6 to 8 h is necessary to allow the plasma level to equilibrate. Lidocaine infusions may be discontinued without tapering once the arrhythmia has been controlled since the drug pharmacokinetically tapers itself. Continuous monitoring for adverse CNS effects should accompany lidocaine infusion.

Phenytoin

Mechanism of Action Phenytoin (Dilantin) is used primarily as an anticonvulsant, but its effects on cell membrane potential and electrical conduction are useful in treating arrhythmias, both atrial and ventricular, especially those which are secondary to digitalis toxicity.

The drug depresses automaticity and decreases both action potential duration and effective refractory period in the Purkinje fibers. It has minimal effect on automaticity in the SA or AV nodes and has little effect on atrial tissue in general.

The pharmacokinetics and adverse effects of phenytoin are discussed in Chap. 33, "Neurologic Disorders."

Clinical Use Phenytoin, like lidocaine, is relatively ineffective in treating atrial fibrillation or flutter. It is more efficacious in the treatment of ventricular arrhythmias, especially those secondary to **digitalis** toxicity.

Preparations and Dosage Phenytoin (Dilantin, Ditan, Diphenylan) is available in capsules, chewable tablets, oral suspension, and parenteral injection. The usual adult loading dose to achieve therapeutic plasma levels ranges from 800 to 1200 mg. The loading dose may be administered orally or intravenously; however, the oral route is less reliable in achieving a rapid therapeutic effect. The pediatric IV loading dose is 2 to 5 mg/kg by slow infusion. This may be repeated in 15 to 30 min to a maximum dose of 600 mg. The oral dose is 5 to 10 mg/kg/day in two or three doses not to exceed 400 mg/day.

The rate of IV phenytoin administration must never exceed 50 mg/min due to the adverse effects associated with the diluent. During the administration period, the patient should be monitored for bradycardia, hypotension, and QRS widening.

Adult maintenance dosing varies, but averages 200 to 400 mg daily. Many patients are adequately controlled on once-daily dosing regimens, but some may require divided doses. If a patient is given a loading dose and placed on a maintenance regimen, a therapeutic plasma level can be attained within 24 h; plasma levels obtained at this time will facilitate evaluation of the dosage regimen.

Propranolol

Mechanism of Action   Propranolol (Inderal) has antiarrhythmic properties as a result of its β-adrenergic blocking and quinidine-like actions; it reduces automaticity and conduction velocity and decreases the refractory period of the Purkinje fibers. Atrioventricular nodal conduction is diminished in supraventricular arrhythmias. Generally, propranolol blocks the actions of norepinephrine (NE) and other endogenous or exogenous catecholamines on the heart.

The pharmacokinetics and adverse effects of propranolol are described in Chaps. 14 and 40. No correlation between plasma levels and antiarrhythmic effect has been observed.

Clinical Use   Although propranolol has been effective in the treatment of ventricular arrhythmias, it is clearly not the drug of choice. Propranolol has been used to control the ventricular rate in the presence of supraventricular tachycardia (SVT), including paroxysmal atrial tachycardia (PAT), especially in hyperthyroidism. The drug is effective in patients with SVT, either alone or in combination with other agents, especially when the arrhythmia is provoked by exercise or other situations resulting in catecholamine excess. In post MI patients, especially those suffering anterior wall infarction, there is the possibility that the drug may decrease mortality. **Oxyprenolol** (Trasicor) is the other β blocker with significant antiarrhythmic effects, although it is not yet approved for this use; it has FDA approval as an antihypertensive but was not marketed.

Preparations and Dosage   **Propranolol** (Inderal) is available as tablets and for IV administration. Patient response to a particular dose is variable and unpredictable; therefore, therapy is initiated at low doses and titrated upward until the desired therapeutic effect is achieved. The usual starting dose is 10 to 20 mg q6h. The sustained-release form (Inderal SA) is used for once-daily administration in comparable dosages. Each dose may be increased by 10 mg every 2 days until the ventricular rate drops to a satisfactory level or until toxicity is observed. If a dose of 480 mg/day or a plasma level of 100 ng/mL is ineffective, propranolol should be considered a therapeutic failure, and another agent should be substituted. Although the manufacturer has no specific pediatric dosing information, some clinicians recommend an oral dose of 1 to 4 mg/kg/day in 3 or 4 divided doses.

Intravenous administration should be reserved for life-threatening arrhythmias. Since the portal circulation is bypassed with IV administration, the IV dose is significantly less than commonly employed oral doses. Generally 1 mg is injected every 5 min at a rate no greater than 1 mg/min to a maximum of about 10 mg for the average adult. Alterna-

tively, a total dose of 0.1 mg/kg can be diluted in 5% dextrose in water and infused over 10 min. The pediatric IV dose is 0.05 to 0.1 mg/kg at a rate of 1 mg every 3 to 5 min.

Digitalis Glycosides

Mechanism of Action   The major use of a digitalis glycoside (**digoxin**, **digitoxin**) is as an inotropic agent in CHF. The drug's vagal stimulating effects make it useful in treating supraventricular arrhythmias, occasionally leading to conversion to normal sinus rhythm (NSR). Digitalis increases the effective refractory period in the AV node partly owing to a direct effect on the myocardium and partly owing to the vagotonic activity (stimulation of the vagus nerve) previously discussed. Reduction in the number of stimuli reaching the ventricles decreases the contraction rate, allowing adequate ventricular filling with resultant increased cardiac output.

Antiarrhythmic dosages are frequently higher than those employed in the management of CHF. The therapeutic endpoint is to control ventricular response, reducing the heart rate to below 100 beats/min. Digoxin (Lanoxin, others) is the most frequently used digitalis glycoside.

The pharmacokinetics and adverse effects of the digitalis glycosides are discussed in Chap. 44.

Clinical Use   The pharmacologic properties of the digitalis glycosides provide for the reduction of ventricular rate and alleviation of CHF, a major consequence of the arrhythmia; it is therefore the drug of choice for atrial fibrillation. If electrocardioversion from atrial fibrillation to flutter is instituted, digitalis should be discontinued 48 to 72 h before the procedure. Cardioversion in patients receiving digitalis products may result in refractory ventricular tachycardia or fibrillation.

The vagotonic properties of digitalis are therapeutically utilized in preventing paradoxical increases in ventricular rate caused by the vagal blocking effects of quinidine. Patients that are chemically cardioverted with digoxin and quinidine should be adequately anticoagulated prior to conversion to prevent embolus formation.

Preparations and Dosage   **Digoxin** (Lanoxin, others) is available as tablets, as elixir, and for injection.

Intravenous digoxin loading dose for antiarrhythmic activity is 13 to 15 $\mu g/kg$ in divided doses over 12 to 24 h at 6- to 8-h intervals. If the loading dose is administered orally, the dose must be adjusted for the percent oral absorption. Usual maintenance doses range from 0.125 to 0.5 mg/day for adults. Intramuscular administration is not recommended. In renally impaired patients, the maintenance doses must be decreased.

In children between 2 and 5 years of age, the oral loading dose is 30 to 40 $\mu g/day$; the IV dose is 80 percent of the oral

TABLE 45-6 Clinical Characteristics of Antiarrhythmic Agents

| DRUG(ROUTE) | HALF-LIFE | ELIMINATION | Dose | | Onset of Action | | THERAPEUTIC PLASMA LEVEL |
			INTRAVENOUS	ORAL	IV	PO	
Quinidine sulfate (PO, IM, IV)	6–8 h	70–90% excreted via hepatic metabolism. Urinary excretion pH-dependent	IV (as gluconate) 5–8 mg/kg at a rate of 0.3 mg/kg/min In CHF: 3.75–6 mg/kg	*Loading dose:* 200 mg q2–3h for 5 doses. *Maintenance dose:* 200–600 mg q6–8h	1–5 min	0.5–1 h	2–6 μg/mL
Procainamide (PO, IM, IV) (Pronestyl)	3–4 h	50% excreted unchanged in urine, the remainder metabolized to NAPA, an active metabolite	IV: 100 mg over 1 min *slowly,* repeat q5min to maximum 1 g *Maintenance:* 1.5–5 mg/min IM: 250–500 mg q4–8h	*Loading dose:* 1 g over 2 h in two divided doses (14 mg/kg). *Maintenance:* 20–50 mg/kg/day (1–9 g/day)	1–5 min	0.5–1 h	4–10 μg/mL NAPA: 9–20 μg/mL
Disopyramide (PO) (Norpace)	5–8 h	50% excreted unchanged in urine		*Loading:* 300–400 mg (14 mg/kg) *Maintenance:* 100–400 mg q6h; doses as high as 300–400 mg q6h should be reserved for patients with resistant arrhythmias		1 h	2–8 μg/mL
Lidocaine (IV, IM) (Xylocaine)	8-min distribution, 1.5 h	Primarily hepatic; clearance has a direct correlation with hepatic blood flow.	1–2 mg/kg, over 1 min, may repeat with 50–100 mg q5–10min to maximum 300 mg *Maintenance:* 1–4 mg/min infusion. IM: 4–5 mg/kg (200–300 mg)	Not recommended because of extensive hepatic metabolism	1–5 min IM: 15 min		1.5–6 μg/mL
Phenytoin sodium (IV, PO) (Dilantin)	8–60 h (average: 22 h)	Primarily hepatic	*Loading dose:* 100 mg q5min until effect is seen or to total of 1000 mg (approx. 12 mg/kg) Alternatively: 250 mg boluses q1h at max 50 mg/min to total of 1000 mg *Maintenance dose:* 200–400 mg/day	*Loading dose:* 14 mg/kg *Maintenance dose:* 200–400 mg/day	1–5 min	With loading dose 24 h	10–20 μg/mL

880

Drug	Half-Life	Metabolism/Elimination	Dosage	Onset	Duration	Therapeutic Level
Digoxin (IV, PO) (Lanoxin)	36 h	60–70% renal elimination	*Loading dose:* 13–15 µg/kg in divided doses over 12–24 h at intervals of 6–8 h *Maintenance:* 0.125–0.5 mg/day	15–30 min	4–6 h	0.5–2 ng/mL
Propranolol (IV, PO, Inderal)	3–6 h	Primarily hepatic; only 1–4% excreted unchanged in urine	1 mg q5min to maximum of 10 mg at a rate no faster than 1 mg/min. A total dose of 0.1 mg per kg can be diluted in 50–100 mL of D$_5$W and infused over 10 min	1–10 min	2–10 h	None definite, although β blockade is associated with plasma levels of 50–100 ng/mL.
Bretylium tosylate (IV, IM) (Bretylol)	5–10 h	70–85% excreted unchanged in urine	5–10 mg/kg can be given diluted with additional doses of 10 mg/kg q1–2h up to maximum of 30 mg/kg/day *IM:* 5–10 mg/kg q6h *IV infusion:* 1–2 mg/min; dilute in 50–100 mL of D$_5$W	20–60 min *IM:* 15–30 min		None established
Verapamil (IV, PO) (Isoptin, Calan)	3–7 h	Extensive hepatic metabolism, 3–4% excreted unchanged by kidneys. Active metabolite	5–10 mg (0.075 mg to 0.15 mg/kg) over 2 min (3 min if elderly); may repeat with 10 mg (0.15 mg/kg) if no response in 30 min *Constant infusion:* 0.005 mg/kg/min	1–15 min	30 min–1 h	0.08–0.3 µg/mL

dose. Pediatric patients usually require a larger dose of digoxin to achieve therapeutic effects. Oral and IV maintenance doses are 25 to 35 percent of the oral digoxin loading dose; maintenance doses in children under 10 years of age are given in two divided doses.

Bretylium

Mechanism of Action   Bretylium (Bretylol) was initially released as an antihypertensive agent but was found to have antiarrhythmic activity; it has since been approved for IV use in refractory ventricular arrhythmias. The mechanism of drug action is not completely understood. It appears to act by initially causing norepinephrine (NE) release from nerve terminals; release of NE in response to nerve stimulation is then inhibited, and uptake is blocked. This causes catecholamine depletion in the nerve terminals. It is thought that the mechanism of action may stem from the drug's ability to prolong action potential duration; however, this effect does not occur in atrial tissue.

Pharmacokinetics   Because bretylium is a quaternary ammonium compound, it is poorly absorbed following oral administration with only 15 to 20 percent of the drug reaching the systemic circulation. Since the drug is primarily excreted unchanged in the urine, dosage adjustment is required in patients with renal insufficiency.

After IV administration, pharmacologic effects may be delayed 20 to 60 min. The duration of effect is usually 6 to 12 h with a drug half-life of about 5 to 10 h. No therapeutic plasma level has been established. Both IM and IV routes are utilized.

Adverse Effects   Hypotension, usually orthostatic, is the most common adverse effect and occurs secondary to adrenergic blockade. A drop in arterial pressure, generally not greater than 20 mmHg, may occur; nausea and vomiting occur after rapid IV administration. Upon initial administration, blood pressure, heart rate, and myocardial contractility may increase presumably because of the initial catecholamine release.

Clinical Use   The drug is approved for the emergency treatment of recurrent ventricular tachycardia or fibrillation with a documented resistance to **lidocaine**, **procainamide**, and **phenytoin**. The drug has little, if any, effect on atrial arrhythmias.

Preparations and Dosage   Parenteral bretylium is available in ampuls. In the treatment of life-threatening ventricular arrhythmias, an IV bolus of 5 mg/kg over 5 to 10 min may be administered, with additional doses of 10 mg/kg repeated until the arrhythmia is terminated or until a total dose of 40 mg/kg has been given. Maintenance doses of 5 to 10 mg/kg, IV or IM, can be given every 6 h. Alternatively, a constant

infusion of bretylium in dextrose 5% in water may be administered at a rate of 1 to 2 mg/min.

An oral form is currently under investigation for the management of repeated episodes of ventricular tachycardia; 600 mg administered every 6 h has been effective.

Orthostatic hypotension is a dose-limiting adverse effect experienced with oral administration. The drug has been found to be effective in approximately 33 percent of ventricular arrhythmias that failed to respond to more traditional agents.

Verapamil

Mechanism of Action   Verapamil (Isoptin, Calan) a papaverine derivative, is the first of a new class of calcium channel blockers to be approved for intravenous use as an antiarrhythmic agent. Originally the drug was marketed for use primarily as an antianginal agent, but it was found to be valuable in the treatment of supraventricular tachyarrhythmias.

Verapamil inhibits the slow calcium currents that occur mainly during phase 2 of the action potential (plateau phase). It is the slow channels or currents that mediate the action potential of the SA and AV node via calcium influx. By blocking the slow calcium channels, verapamil prolongs AV nodal conduction and increases the refractory period of the AV as well as the SA node. This slows the ventricular response rate during a supraventricular tachyarrhythmia and may even convert to normal sinus rhythm (NSR). The drug is also a vasodilator, and it is useful in preventing both spontaneous and drug-induced coronary artery vasoconstriction which may precipitate angina.

The pharmacokinetics and adverse effects of verapamil are presented in Chap. 43.

Clinical Use   It is generally felt that IV verapamil is the drug of choice for reverting acute episodes of paroxysmal supraventricular tachycardia (PSVT) with a 90 percent success rate in some studies. Verapamil also slows ventricular response in both atrial fibrillation and flutter and, on occasion, converts patients to NSR. In acute episodes, verapamil is superior to digitalis due to its rapid onset of action. The role of oral verapamil as a prophylaxis against supraventricular tachycardia (SVT) in susceptible patients is currently under investigation.

Preparations and Dosage   Verapamil (Isoptin, Calan) is available as oral tablets and for IV use in ampuls. A commonly employed adult dose is 10 mg administered intravenously as a single bolus over 2 min. A repeat dose may be given in 30 min if no effect is seen. A constant infusion of 0.15 μg/kg/min may also be used. Oral dosing is usually initiated with 80 mg tid or qid, increasing at daily or weekly intervals until control is achieved.

Two other recently approved calcium channel blockers

include **nifedipine** (Procardia) and **diltiazem** (Cardizem). These agents are currently available for oral use and are approved exclusively for the treatment of angina pectoris. Nifedipine has limited effects on myocardial conduction; however, diltiazem has similiar properties to verapamil on cardiac tissue. The use of diltiazem in the treatment of supraventricular arrhythmias requires additional investigation.

Investigational Agents

Several agents are currently undergoing clinical trials for use as antiarrhythmic agents. Refer to Table 45-7 for more detailed information and clinical characteristics.

Aprindine, **mexiletine**, and **tocainide** are lidocaine congeners; these drugs are membrane stabilizers with electrophysiologic effects resembling those of quinidine, procainamide, disopyramide, and lidocaine. All three agents are available for oral administration and are useful in the treatment of ventricular arrhythmias; however only aprindine appears to be effective against atrial ectopy. Encainide, although structurally unrelated to other antiarrhythmic agents, has local anesthetic, membrane-stabilizing effects. The drug is effective in diminishing PVCs, preventing recurrent ventricular tachycardia and fibrillation in patients resistant to conventional agents.

Amiodarone (Cordarone) was originally developed for use in angina pectoris. The drug prolongs the action potential duration and refractory period; it also has some noncompetitive β-blocking effects. This agent has shown promise in a variety of supraventricular arrhythmias in patients refractory to standard agents.

Ethmozin is a phenothiazine derivative and has been shown effective against both atrial and ventricular arrhythmias.

Combination Therapy

The use of more than one antiarrhythmic agent at the same time in the treatment of cardiac arrhythmias is difficult to evaluate. In the event of a therapeutic failure, the ineffective drug is usually discontinued and another agent begun. Although procainamide can be effective where quinidine has failed, the selection of a drug with different electrophysiologic effects seems most reasonable. For example, when lidocaine fails to abolish either ventricular tachycardia or fibrillation, cardioversion will be instituted with concurrent administration of an additional therapeutic agent, e.g., bretylium, in difficult-to-convert ventricular arrhythmias. When using two agents of the same therapeutic class, the benefits of therapy must be weighed against the risks of possible additive adverse effects. Before adding a second agent, maximal doses of the first agent should be tried. Table 45-5 outlines the common arrhythmias and their primary and secondary treatments of choice. The clinical characteristics of the current and investigational antiarrhythmic agents, respectively, are given in Tables 45-6 and 45-7.

NURSING PROCESS RELATED TO ANTIARRHYTHMICS

Assessment

The health history may help identify not only the type of recurrent arrhythmia but the precipitating cause as well. Numerous symptoms are associated with arrhythmias including shortness of breath, palpitations, coughing, edema, syncope, and chest pain. Shortness of breath or cyanosis may result from poor cardiac output or pleural edema, preventing normal oxygen exchange. Syncope (fainting) or changes in mental status in general may be indicative of a marked decrease in cardiac output with resultant inadequate cerebral blood flow. Chest pain may be a symptom of myocardial infarction, or it may indicate a severe arrhythmia that has decreased cardiac output to the extent that the coronary arteries are poorly perfused, resulting in an anginal attack.

Allergies should always be investigated. If identified, specific details should be recorded, since there is cross-reactivity among the antiarrhythmics and other drugs.

Before administering drugs which affect the cardiovascular system, the nurse should always observe the patient carefully for therapeutic effects and symptoms of toxicity from previous doses. Knowledge of adverse effects and toxic symptoms of antiarrhythmic agents is essential. If the patient is not on an ECG monitor, the pulse should be taken for *one full minute* and recorded, noting the rate and quality of the rhythm; any changes from previous observations should also be noted. While this is usually done with patients on digitalis drugs, it should be routine with all antiarrhythmics.

Since several of these agents (**quinidine, procainamide, propranolol, lidocaine,** and **verapamil**) have the potential of causing hypotension, blood pressure should be obtained prior to drug administration. The drug may be withheld and the physician notified if the patient is hypotensive. Sometimes it is necessary, however, to weigh the adverse cardiovascular effects of the arrhythmia against those of the drug, to determine which will compromise circulation more.

Management

Since hypoxia and electrolyte imbalance may cause or contribute to the development of arrhythmia, management may involve oxygen administration and treatment of electrolyte abnormalities. In addition, situations which have been known to trigger arrhythmias should be avoided. The nurse and the patient should work together to devise a plan that will help patients identify these factors in their daily schedules.

Since constant plasma levels of these drugs may be necessary to control arrhythmias, the nurse should adjust dosage schedules according to pharmacokinetic parameters,

TABLE 45-7 Clinical Characteristics of Investigational Antiarrhythmic Agents

DRUG	ROUTE	HALF-LIFE	ELIMINATION	Dose INTRAVENOUS	Dose ORAL	Onset of Action IV	Onset of Action ORAL	THERAPEUTIC BLOOD LEVEL	SIDE EFFECTS	COMMENTS
Amiodarone (Cordarone)	IV, PO	15–45 days	Hepatic	5–10 mg/kg over 1–10 min	200–800 mg/day	5–10 min	4–6 h		Nausea, vomiting, constipation, blue-gray skin discoloration; Hypo- or hyperthyroidism; corneal microdeposits	Because of long half-life persistence of therapeutic effect is noted 30–45 days after cessation of therapy. Skin discoloration and microdeposits of cornea will reverse after cessation of therapy. Because of iodine moiety on drug molecule, aberration in thyroid function may occur.
Aprinidine (Fibocil)	IV, PO	30 h	Renal, hepatic	*Loading dose:* 300 mg, Infused as 25 mg bolus q2–3min, or constant infusion 5–15 mg/min	Dose 300–400 mg first day, 200–300 mg second day, 50–200 mg as a *maintenance dose,* or *load* on day 1: 100 mg q6h, then day 2: 75 mg q6h, with *maintenance:* 25–50 mg q8–12h.	5–10 min	2 h	1–3 mg/L	Neurologic: tremor, dizziness, ataxia, nystagmus, psychotic disturbances; rare: agranulocytosis, cholestatic hepatitis	Agranulocytosis although rare is serious and requires weekly WBC count during first few months of therapy. Reversible with prompt discontinuation of treatment.
Encainide	IV, PO	1.5–3.5 h	Primarily hepatic	0.6–0.9 mg/kg over 15 min as single injection	25–50 mg q4–6h; maximum of 240 mg/day	15 min	1.5 h		Dizziness, blurred vision, vertigo, paresthesia, leg cramps and metallic taste in mouth	Side effects are generally mild and respond to a slight decrease in dosage. The most severe adverse effect has been the initiation or exacerbation of arrhythmia in up to 10–15% of patients. Each patient therefore requires continuous ECG monitoring during initiation of therapy.

Drug	Route	Half-life	Metabolism/Excretion	Dosage (IV)	Dosage (PO)	Onset	Peak	Therapeutic level	Adverse effects	Comments
Ethmozin	IV, PO	4–13 h	Primarily hepatic	1–3 mg/kg *Loading dose,* although more work needs to be done to confirm IV dosing	75–150 mg q6h	5 min	2 h	0.5–1 mg/L	Nausea, pruritus, dizziness	Phenothiazine type, minimum effective dose appears to be 600 mg/day; up to 1200 mg/day have been administered.
Mexiletine (Mexitil)	IV, PO	8–14 h	Primarily hepatic; 8% excreted unchanged	100–250 mg over 5 min with continuous infusion of 1–3 mg/min	*Loading dose:* 400–600 mg; follow with 200–400 mg in 3 or 4 divided doses	5 min	1–2 h	0.5–2 mg/L	Nausea, vomiting, tremor, dizziness, nystagmus, blurred vision, confusion. Cardiac toxicities: hypotension, bradycardia, AV dissociation	A lidocaine congener, with similiar antiarrhythmic effects. May depress cardiac output in patients with preexisting left ventricular dysfunction.
Tocainide* (Tonocard)	IV, PO	10–17 h	Hepatic metabolism; 40% excreted unchanged	0.5–0.75 mg/kg/min for 15 min	*Loading dose:* 400–600 mg, *Maintenance:* 200–800 mg q8h	5–10 min	1.5 h	6–12 mg/L	Nausea, vomiting, lightheadedness, dizziness, tremor, blurred vision, paresthesias	A lidocaine congener developed for oral use; it escapes first-pass metabolism. Antiarrhythmic effects similar to lidocaine. Neurologic disturbances tend to be dose-related.

*Tocainide was approved for treatment of ventricular arrythmia in 1984.

giving the drug around the clock, if necessary, to maintain arrhythmia suppression.

Special care must be employed when antiarrhythmics are administered intravenously, since many of these agents can induce severe hypotension if given too rapidly or in too great a concentration. This is less common with **lidocaine** than with **procainamide, quinidine,** and **verapamil.** Drugs must be adequately diluted and then administered slowly according to the specific guidelines for each drug.

As with any chronic illness, patients must ultimately assume responsibility for their own care. Compliance is greatly increased when the patient understands the therapeutic regimen and rationale. Patients are frequently prescribed antiarrhythmics without comprehension of rationale, consequences of noncompliance, or possible adverse effects. Many patients believe their disease is "cured" if no immediate ill effects occur when the medication is discontinued. Frequently, arrhythmias require some triggering event; the absence of control may not be noted until the arrhythmia recurs, at which time medical aid may not be readily available.

The ability of patients to accept adverse drug effects is usually better if the causes are understood and especially if the effects are expected to be transient. Patients frequently fail to bring significant symptoms to the attention of health care professionals because they do not always make the association between the drug and the symptom.

When the patient is on the ECG monitor, information is available that may allow the nurse to identify the prodromes of lethal arrhythmias and react appropriately. On admission, a rhythm strip should be obtained to establish a base; subsequent strips obtained at specified times should be compared with the baseline strips. Lengthening of the QRS or PR intervals indicates conduction block which may be caused by the myocardial depressant effects of antiarrhythmic drugs. These changes should be reported; if the block is severe, the drug should be withheld. Appearance of abnormal beats may also herald drug toxicity. Signs of decreased perfusion (confusion, syncope, cold extremities, low urinary output) reveal whether cardiac function has been compromised. Arrhythmias may also precipitate congestive heart failure.

Recurrent premature ventricular contractions (PVCs) are a sign of ventricular irritability; they are often followed by ventricular tachycardia and/or fibrillation. Accordingly, PVCs are treated if they occur in excess of 5 or 6 per minute,

in runs, or back to back, or if the R wave of the PVC falls near the peak of the T wave of the previous beat. These events signify ventricular hyperirritability with possible resultant ventricular fibrillation. Usually it is the nurse who identifies this situation on the ECG monitor and administers IV lidocaine (according to protocol), first as a bolus and then as a drip. It is frequently necessary for the nurse to differentiate between PVCs and other arrhythmias which have a similiar appearance on ECG, such as PVCs with aberrant conduction (since these arrhythmias do not usually respond to lidocaine). The difference between the two is subtle. If the PVCs do not respond to the initial bolus, the nurse must decide whether the lack of response is due to misdiagnosis or whether additional dosage is required.

Evaluation

Evaluation involves the same parameters as assessment: monitoring pulse rate and rhythm, ECG monitoring (if available), obtaining blood pressure measurements, and observing the patient for adverse effects. The ECG pattern may also reveal changes in wave intervals that are characteristic of digitalis or quinidine toxicity. Most of the antiarrhythmic agents discussed here have been presented in the context of the hospitalized patient. The nurse must also be aware that these common drugs will be prescribed to the patient on an outpatient basis. The routine administration of these medications in the hospital setting is the ideal situation in which to educate the patient prior to discharge. Once the patient has been stabilized on a particular regimen in the hospital, it is important to note that the patient will most likely be discharged on the same or similiar dosing schedule at home.

Here the nurse plays a key role in teaching the patient when and how to take medication, pointing out some of the troublesome side effects that may occur, and finally showing the patient how to take his or her own pulse. Clear instruction from the nurse will raise the level of the patient's diligence in monitoring each medication carefully. If any problems with drug therapy arise at home, the patient should also be instructed to contact the physician immediately.

If the nurse can provide the patient with easy-to-follow instructions on the proper use and monitoring of this class of medications, it will help to alleviate the patient's anxiety and will prevent potential complications.

CASE STUDY

Mr. H.K., an 84-year-old male, was admitted with the chief complaint of retrosternal chest pain for 24 h prior to admission. He also experienced slight shortness of breath and palpitations. His ECG showed sinus rhythm with ST elevation in leads II, III, and AVF. His vital signs were: BP 160/90, pulse 86 and regular, temperature 37°C, respiratory rate 18. The patient had no previous cardiac history and had been in good health until this present hospitalization.

Assessment

At approximately 6 A.M. on the second day of hospital admission, the patient suddenly went into atrial fibrillation with a rate of 160. Blood pressure fell to 98/70. He was given verapamil 5 mg as an IV bolus gradually over 2 min. Within 2 or 3 min the heart rate decreased to 80. The patient's blood pressure remained at 90/70, and he became slightly diaphoretic. He was given dextrose 5% in normal saline at a rate of 100 mL/h. After 2 h his blood pressure gradually increased. After 3 h his blood pressure was 150/90; heart rate 84, with normal sinus rhythm. The IV was changed to 5% dextrose as a keep vein open (KVO).

Upon the patient's admission to the intensive care unit, the nurse took vital signs and obtained a baseline ECG monitor strip. The patient appeared alert and oriented. Upon auscultation his lungs had a few bibasilar rales. His heart rate was regular with typical S_1 and S_2 sounds. The patient had good pedal pulses. He had no complaints of chest pain at this time.

Management

Upon admission and every 2 h thereafter vital signs were taken and recorded. An ECG monitor strip was taken hourly. Temperature was recorded every 4 h. Upon the initial onset of rapid atrial fibrillation, blood pressure, apical rate, respiratory rate, and lung auscultation were taken and recorded every 15 min. During the administration of 5% dextrose and saline it was particularly important to monitor lung sounds and observe urinary output, being alert to the signs and symptoms of acute pulmonary edema.

When the patient's blood pressure, heart rate, and rhythm returned to within normal limits, vital signs were again taken every 2 h. Daily oral doses of digoxin 0.25 mg were given at 2 P.M. to allow the patient's physician to see and evaluate him each day before the dose was given. Apical pulse was counted and recorded before each daily dose of digoxin.

Evaluation

The patient remained in sinus rhythm with an acceptable rate in the 80s throughout his stay in the intensive care unit. He was diagnosed by ECG and serial enzyme studies as having had an acute inferior wall myocardial infarction.

REFERENCES

Anderson, J. L.: "Antiarrhythmic Drugs: Clinical Pharmacology and Therapeutic Uses," *Drugs,* 15:271–309, 1978.

Antman, E.: "Calcium Channel Blocking Agents in the Treatment of Cardiovascular Disorders: 1. Basic and Clinical Electrophysiological Effects," *Ann Inter Med,* 93:875–886, 1980.

Baky, S. H.: "Verapamil Hydrochloride: Pharmacological Properties and Role in Cardiovascular Therapeutics," *Pharmacotherapy,* 2:328–353, 1982.

Bauman, J. L.: "Cardiovascular Drugs," in J. E. Knoben and P. O. Anderson (eds.), *Handbook of Clinical Drug Data,* Hamilton, IL: Drug Intelligence Publications, 1983.

Benchimol, A.: "New Drugs for Treating Cardiac Arrhythmias," *Postgrad Med,* 69:77–84, 1981.

Bigger, T. J.: "Arrhythmias and Antiarrhythmic Drugs," *Adv Intern Med,* 18:251–257, 1972.

Canada, A. T.: "Amiodarone for Tachyarrhythmias: Pharmacology, Kinetics, and Efficacy," *Drug Intell Clin Pharm,* 17:100–104, 1983.

Federman, J.: "Antiarrhythmic Drug Therapy," *Mayo Clin Proc,* 54:531–542, 1979.

Gill, M. A.: "Cardiac Arrhythmias," in B. S. Katcher, L. Y. Young, and M. A. Koda-Kimble (eds.), *Applied Therapeutics for Clinical Pharmacists,* San Francisco: Applied Therapeutics, 1983.

Heger, J. J.: "New Antiarrhythmics Amiodarone and Encainide," *Drug Therapy (Hospital),* 7:65–73, 1982.

Henry, P. D.: "Comparative Pharmacology of Calcium Antagonists: Nifedipine, Verapamil, and Diltiazem," *Am J Cardiol,* 46:1047–1058, 1980.

Hotchkiss, R. S.: "A Pharmacologic Approach to Cardiac Arrhythmias: Traditional, New, and Potential Antiarrhythmic Agents," *Hosp Formul,* 17:1207–1218, 1982.

Josephson, M. E.: "Update on Quinidine, Procainamide, Disopyramide, and Verapamil," *Hosp Formul,* 13:896–905, 1978.

Keefe, D. L. D.: "New Antiarrhythmic Drugs: Their Place in Therapy," *Drugs,* 27:363–400, 1981.

Koch-Weser, J.: "Bretylium," *N Engl J Med,* 300:473–477, 1979.

Leonard, R. G.: "Calcium-Channel Blocking Agents," *Clin Pharm,* 1:17–33, 1982.

Nadenanee, K.: "Recent Advances in Drug Therapy of Cardiac Arrhythmias," *Hosp Formul,* 14:899–909, pt. 2, 1979.

Nies, A. S.: "Cardiovascular Disorders, Arrhythmias," in K. L. Melmon and H. F. Morelli (eds.), *Clinical Pharmacology: Basic Principles in Therapeutics,* 2d ed., San Francisco: Applied Therapeutics, 1978.

Rice, V.: "Calcium, the Heart, and Calcium Antagonists," *Crit Care Nurs,* 2:30–34, 1982.

Rodman, J.: "Progress in Arrhythmia Therapy," *Clin Pharm,* 2:307–311, 1983.

Rossi, L.: "Calcium Channel Blockers: New Treatment for Cardiovascular Disease," *Am J Nurs,* 83:382–386, 1983.

Sloskey, G. E.: "Amiodarone: A Unique Antiarrhythmic Agent," *Clin Pharm,* 2:330–340, 1983.

Stone, P.: "Calcium Channel Blocking Agents in the Treatment of Cardiovascular Diseases: 2. Hemodynamic

Effects and Clinical Applications," *Ann Intern Med,* 93:886–897, pt. 2, 1980.

"Treatment of Cardiac Arrhythmias," *Med Lett Drugs Ther,* 25:21–28, 1983.

Waxman, H. L.: "Verapamil for Control of Ventricular Rate in Paroxysmal Supraventricular Tachycardia and Atrial Fibrillation or Flutter," *Ann Intern Med,* 94:1–6, 1981.

Willett, G. A.: "Defining the Therapeutic Role of Verapamil," *Drug Therapy (Hospital),* 7:98–113, 1982.

Wulf, B. G.: "Mexiletine and Tocainide: Orally Active Congeners of Lidocaine," *Clin Pharm,* 2:340–346, 1983.

Zipes, D. P.: "New Antiarrhythmic Agents Amiodarone, Aprindine, Disopyramide, Ethmozin, Mexiletine, Tocainide, Verapamil," *Am J Cardiol,* 41:1005–1023, 1978.

CLINICAL PHARMACOLOGY & THERAPEUTICS IN NURSING SPECIALTIES

46

WOMEN'S HEALTH CARE

ELVIRA SZIGETI
ROSALIE SAGRAVES

LEARNING OBJECTIVES

Upon mastery of the content of this chapter, the reader will be able to:

1. Correlate the ovarian and uterine cycles with hormonal events.
2. State the effects of estrogens on the reproductive, hematologic, and metabolic physiology.
3. List at least six therapeutic uses for estrogens.
4. Indicate the adverse effects of estrogen medications.
5. List the routes by which estrogens are administered.
6. Outline teaching plans for women taking estrogens for birth control, menopause, or endometriosis.
7. Describe the reproductive and nonreproductive effects of progestogens.
8. List three clinical uses for progestogens.
9. Indicate the adverse effects of progestogen medications.
10. Compare the mechanism of action, effectiveness, and safety for each of the following methods of contraception to that of oral contraceptives: condom, diaphragm, rhythm method, sponge, intrauterine device, and spermicides.
11. State the indications for and adverse effects of spermicides.
12. Describe the adverse effects of oral contraceptives, including contraindications, drug interactions, and nursing process implications.
13. List the drug groups used to treat premenstrual disorders.
14. Describe the factors associated with toxic shock syndrome and the methods recommended to avoid its occurrence.
15. Explain the treatment of three types of vaginitis and the cautions related to use of douches in this condition.
16. Describe the general types of hormonal agents and durations of therapy for endometriosis.
17. State the indications for estrogen replacement in menopause.
18. List the drugs which may be of benefit in postmenopausal osteoporosis.
19. Explain the rationale for intermittent estrogen therapy or use of a progestogenic estrogen antagonist in menopause.
20. Describe three drugs used to treat infertility.
21. State the pharmacologic effects of prostaglandins on the uterus and gastrointestinal tract.
22. State the criteria for selection of an antihypertensive drug to treat hypertensive diseases of pregnancy.
23. State the indications, mechanism of action, and signs of drug toxicity of magnesium sulfate used to treat preeclampsia and eclampsia.
24. Identify the pharmacologic mechanism and adverse effects of β-sympathomimetic drugs used to prevent premature labor.
25. List two major oxytocics, and explain the nursing care associated with their use before and after delivery.
26. Explain how analgesics, sedatives, and anesthetics in labor and delivery can affect the mother, the fetus, and the progress of labor.
27. Explain the rationale and indications for the administration of RhoGAM.
28. Explain the pharmacologic mechanisms for stimulation and suppression of lactation.
29. Outline the nursing process related to vaginitis and dysmenorrhea, the use of prostaglandins in therapeutic abortion, in the treatment of preeclampsia or eclampsia with magnesium sulfate, in the prevention of preterm labor, and in lactation.

Historically, care of the childbearing woman has been an accepted nursing function. In recent years two factors have given impetus to the development of creative new models of women's health care as a clinical nursing specialty: (1) scientific advances in medicine, surgery, and pharmacology and (2) recognition that the health care needs of women are not adequately addressed in traditional health care settings. The renaissance of nurse midwifery, expansion of the role of the obstetric nurse, and development of related nurse practitioner specialties (e.g., family planning nurse practitioners, women's health care nurse practitioners) are responses to a growing awareness of the unique biophysical and psychosocial character of women.

MENSTRUAL CYCLE

An understanding of the female sexual cycle, or menstrual cycle, as a complex interplay among the limbic system, hypothalamus, pituitary, ovaries, and uterus is crucial to rational therapeutics in contraception, dysmenorrhea, therapeutic abortion, infertility, and other related disorders. Temporary derangements in ovulation and menstruation associated with emotional or environmental stimuli are thought to represent abnormalities in the limbic system or

other parts of the brain which control secretion of gonadotropin-releasing hormone (GnRH) from the hypothalamus: GnRH stimulates the secretion of follicle-stimulating hormone (FSH) and luteinizing hormone (LH) from the pituitary. FSH and LH, in turn, regulate events that promote ovarian output of estrogens and progestogens. The positive and negative feedback mechanisms (see Chap. 35) which orchestrate these hormones and their effects are complex and intricate. For example, high concentrations of progesterone inhibit FSH and LH release, but this effect is maximal only when adequate estrogen is present. Yet high levels of estrogen with low levels of progesterone exert a positive feedback on LH release.

The menstrual cycle may be divided into phases based on events in the ovary or uterus. The maturation of the ovum is the primary function of the *ovarian cycle,* whereas the preparation of the endometrium for implantation if fertilization occurs is the principal function of the *uterine cycle* (Fig. 46-1).

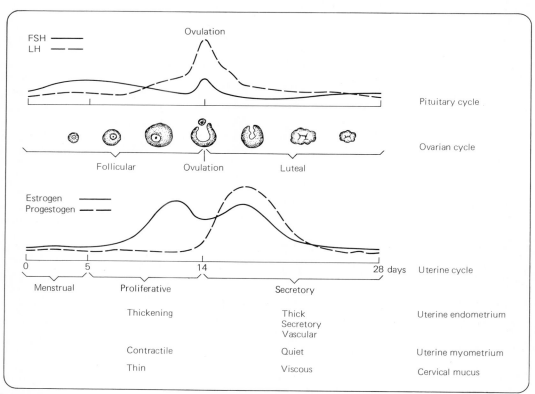

FIGURE 46-1

Temporal Relationship of Hormonal, Ovarian, and Uterine Events during the Menstrual Cycle. The proliferative uterine phase (late follicular phase, days 5–14) is dominated by FSH and ovarian estrogen, resulting in the thickening of uterine endometrium, thin cervical mucus, development of the follicle, and the LH surge. The LH surge stimulates ovulation (release of an ovum from the ruptured follicle). The secretory phase (luteal phase, days 15–28) is characterized by secretion of high levels of progesterone and estrogens from the corpus luteum (which develops from the ruptured follicle) and preparation of the uterus to receive the fertilized ovum. If fertilization does not occur to sustain hormonal levels, menstruation occurs (days 1–5).

Ovarian Cycle

The ovarian cycle may be divided into three phases:

1. The follicular or preovulatory phase
2. The ovulatory phase
3. The luteal or postovulatory phase

The *follicular phase* begins at the onset of menstruation and lasts approximately 14 days. It is the estrogen-dominated phase of the menstrual cycle. Low estrogen levels at the beginning of the follicular phase stimulate the release of follicle-stimulating hormone (FSH) from the anterior pituitary. FSH then stimulates several follicles to develop and mature within the ovary. As the follicles mature, estrogen is produced. Rising estrogen concentrations depress FSH secretion through negative feedback, while stimulating the release of luteinizing hormone (LH) from the anterior pituitary through a positive feedback mechanism. Toward the end of the follicular phase, all but one follicle will regress.

The *ovulatory phase* occurs on day 14 or 15 of the usual menstrual cycle. In response to a surge of LH triggered by high concentrations of estrogen, ovulation occurs with the release of the ovum and the formulation of the corpus luteum from the ruptured follicle.

The *luteal phase* encompasses the second half of the ovarian cycle and is progestogen-dominated. During this phase the corpus luteum secretes high levels of progesterone and estrogen until the corpus luteum regresses about day 26 of the menstrual cycle. When estrogen levels again drop to an extremely low level, the anterior pituitary will be stimulated to secrete FSH, and the cycle will begin again.

Uterine Cycle

The uterine cycle may be divided into three phases:

1. The menstrual phase
2. The proliferative phase
3. The secretory phase

The *menstrual phase* begins with the onset of menstruation, which usually corresponds to days 1 to 5 of the menstrual cycle. During this phase of the uterine cycle, the endometrium can no longer be maintained because of the decreasing hormonal levels and is sloughed.

The *proliferative phase* occurs between days 5 and 14 of the menstrual cycle, corresponding to the latter part of the ovarian preovulatory phase. During this estrogen-dominated phase, stromal cells, epithelial glands, and blood vessels of the endometrium proliferate. The endometrium may be 2- to 3-mm thick by day 14.

The *secretory phase* occurs between days 15 and 27 and corresponds to the postovulatory phase of the ovarian cycle. During this phase, progesterone is the dominant hormone. Glandular cells secrete small quantities of epithelial fluid while glycogen and lipid stores increase in stromal cells. The endometrial blood supply increases and the endometrium may be 4- to 6-mm thick prior to the beginning of the monthly menstrual flow. By day 25, if fertilization has not occurred, the corpus luteum declines and with it the levels of estrogen and progesterone. On day 28, an intense arterial spasm occurs in blood vessels leading to the mucosal layers of the endometrium. Hemorrhage and necrosis develop and the outer endometrial layers separate from the uterus. The tissue and blood are then expelled from the body as the menstrual flow. This process may be initiated under the influence of various *prostaglandins*.

If pregnancy occurs, the hormone output of the corpus luteum is maintained under the influence of human chorionic gonadotropin (HCG). Once the placenta matures, it sustains the hormonal needs of the developing embryo and fetus.

OVARIAN HORMONES

The ovary secretes steroid hormones, including estrogens, progestogens, and a nonsteroidal hormone, relaxin, which is believed to facilitate parturition. Although the ovary is the major source of the steroidal hormones, they are also formed in the testes, adrenals, and placenta.

Mechanism of Action Naturally occurring estrogens and progestogens are thought to act by the same mechanism as other steroids (see Chap. 35). Free steroids (i.e., those not bound to plasma proteins) interact with receptor proteins in cells and form a receptor-hormone complex which binds to the cell nucleus, stimulating messenger ribonucleic acid (mRNA) production. This results in the synthesis of specific proteins which stimulate physiologic processes characteristic of the steroid. Receptors for estrogens and progestogens are found in the female reproductive tract, breast, hypothalamus, and pituitary. Receptor distribution may differ in premenopausal and postmenopausal women.

Estrogens

The term *estrogen* refers to substances capable of inducing estrus, a sexual receptivity. This term has been expanded to include estrogens, metabolites of estrogens, and compounds which produce estrogenic uterine changes. In addition to naturally occurring steroidal estrogens from animal sources, synthetic steroidal estrogens and synthetic nonsteroidal estrogens are used therapeutically.

Estradiol is the most potent estrogen and the major secretory product of the ovary (Table 46-2). After estradiol is synthesized, it can be converted to estrone and estriol. During pregnancy the placenta synthesizes estrogens in a fashion similar to the ovary but in larger quantities.

Physiologic Effects In addition to sustaining the ovarian and uterine cycles, the estrogens result in the development and maintenance of the female sex organs. At puberty,

TABLE 46-1 Estrogen Preparations and Combinations

PREPARATION CONTENT	TRADE NAMES	DOSAGE FORM	INDICATIONS	USUAL DOSE
		Natural Conjugated Steroidal Estrogens		
Combined estrogens aqueous (mainly estrone)	Gynogen R.P.	IM injection	Abnormal uterine bleeding	2–5 mg daily for several days
			Estrogen deficiency, menopause	0.1–2 mg weekly
			Inoperable breast cancer	5 mg three or more times weekly
Estrogenic substance aqueous (mainly estrone)	Estaqua, Gynogen, others	IM injection	Severe menopause symptoms	0.1–0.5 mg two to three times weekly
			Female hypogonadism	0.1–2 mg weekly
Estrone aqueous	Theelin Aqueous, Estronol, others	See above	See above	See above
Estrogenic substance in oil	Gravigen in oil, Kestrin in oil	See above	See above	See above
Conjugated estrogens	Premarin Intravenous	IM or IV injection	Abnormal uterine bleeding	25 mg; repeat in 6–12 h if needed
	Premarin	Tablets	Menopause	1.25 mg/day cyclically
			Female hypogonadism	2.5–7.5 mg/day cyclically
			Osteoporosis	1.25 mg/day cyclically
			Prevent postpartum breast engorgement	3.75 mg q4h for 5 doses or 1.25 mg q4h for 5 days
	Premarin	Vaginal cream	Atrophic vaginitis	1 applicatorful 1–3 times weekly
Piperazine estrone sulfate (estropipate)	Ogen	Tablets	Menopause	0.625–5 mg/day cyclically
			Female hypogonadism	1.25–7.5 mg/day cyclically
		Vaginal cream	Atrophic vaginitis	1–2 applicatorfuls daily
Estradiol cypionate in oil	Depo-Estradiol Cypionate, depGynogen, others	IM injection	Menopause	1.5–5 mg q3–4 weeks
			Female hypogonadism	1.5–2 mg/month
Estradiol valerate in oil	Delestrogen, Valergen-10, Dioval, others	IM injection	Menopause, female hypogonadism	10–20 mg one time monthly
			Prevent postpartum breast engorgement	10–25 mg one dose
Esterfied estrogens	Menest, Estratab, others	Tablets	Menopause	0.3–3.75 mg/day cyclically
			Female hypogonadism	2.5–7.5 mg/day cyclically
			Inoperable breast cancer	10 mg tid
		Synthetic Steroidal Estrogens		
Ethinyl estradiol	Estinyl, Feminone	Tablets	Menopause	0.02–0.05 mg/day cyclically
			Female hypogonadism	0.05 mg 1–3 times/day cyclically
			Inoperable breast cancer	1 mg tid

TABLE 46-1   Estrogen Preparations and Combinations (*Cont.*)

PREPARATION CONTENT	TRADE NAMES	DOSAGE FORM	INDICATIONS	USUAL DOSE
Synthetic Steroidal Estrogens (Cont.)				
Quinestrol	Estrovis	Tablets	Menopause, female hypogonadism	100 µg/day for 7 days followed by 100 µg/week maintenance
Dienestrol	Ortho Dienestrol, DV, Estragard	Vaginal cream or suppository	Atrophic vaginitis	1–2 suppositories or 1–2 applicatorfuls of cream per day
				Maintenance: 1 applicator of cream or 1 suppository 1–3 times weekly
Synthetic Nonsteroidal Estrogen Analogs				
Diethystilbestrol (DES)	Stilbestrol	Tablets, enteric coated tablets	Menopause, female hypogonadism	0.2–0.5 mg/day cyclically
			Postcoital contraception	25 mg bid for 5 days within 72 h of exposure
			Inoperable breast cancer	15 mg/day
		Vaginal suppository	Atrophic vaginitis	1–2 per day
Chlortrianisene	Tace	Capsules	Menopause, female hypogonadism	12–25 mg/day cyclically
			Postpartum breast engorgement	12 mg qid for 7 days or 60 mg q6h for six doses or 72 mg bid for 2 days
Estrogens Combined with Sedatives				
Conjugated estrogens (0.045 mg) with meprobamate (400 or 200 mg)	Milprem-400, PMB-200, others	Tablet	Menopause	1 tablet tid cyclically
Esterified estrogens (0.2 or 0.4 mg) and chlordiazepoxide (5 or 10 mg)	Menrium 5-2, Menrium 5-4, Menrium 10-4	Tablets	Menopause	As above
Estrogens Combined with Androgens				
Estradiol valerate and testosterone ethanate or testosterone cypionate	Depotestosterone, Andro/Fem, Deladumone, others	IM injectable	Vasomotor spasms of menopause	Varies by product. Consult package insert
			Postpartum breast engorgement	As above. See section on lactation suppression
Ethinyl estradiol and fluoxymesterone	Halodrin	Tablets	As above	As above
Esterified estrogens and methyltestosterone	Estratest	Tablets	As above	As above
Diethylstilbestrol and methyltestosterone	Tylosterone	Tablets	As above	As above

estrogen causes the growth and development of the vagina, uterus, fallopian tubes, breasts, and external genitalia. Under the action of estrogen, the endometrium is prepared during the proliferative phase of the menstrual cycle, while the decline of estrogenic activity at the end of the secretory phase results in menstruation. The cervix, under estrogenic influence, produces a thin watery fluid which is attractive to spermatozoa. Estrogens also promote the distribution of fat to the hips, thighs, buttocks, and breasts, producing the female physique. The growth of the long bones that occurs with the pubertal spurt of growth and closure of the epiphyses is associated with estrogenic activity. The growth of axillary and pubic hair and the regional pigmentation of the nipples and areola are under the influence of both estrogens and androgens.

Metabolic effects of estrogens include sodium retention, water retention, increased serum levels of lipoproteins and triglycerides, and decreased cholesterol levels. Estrogens may also produce glucose intolerance in patients with diabetes mellitus or preclinical diabetes. The maintenance of the structure of the skin and blood vessels in women is under estrogenic control. Estrogens antagonize the effects of parathyroid hormone in the reabsorption of bone.

The composition and coaguability of blood is affected by estrogens, which increase the levels of γ_2-globulins such as thyroxine-binding globulin, corticosteroid-binding globulin, and sex hormone–binding globulin. By increasing levels of prothrombin and factors VII, IX, and X and by decreasing antithrombin activity, estrogens enhance blood clotting.

Therapeutic Uses Therapeutic uses for estrogens are outlined in Table 46-3 and are discussed in more detail under dysmenorrhea, oral contraception, and menopause in this chapter.

Pharmacokinetics Naturally occurring estrogens and their esters are readily absorbed from the gastrointestinal tract, skin, and mucous membranes. They are rapidly converted, during passage through the liver, into compounds with less estrogenic activity. They are primarily excreted renally as the inactive glucuronide and sulfate conjugates of estradiol,

estrone, and estriol, but also undergo enterohepatic recirculation. Estrogens are 50 to 80 percent bound to two plasma proteins, albumin and sex hormone–binding globulin.

Effects of *orally administered estrogens* can be prolonged by the administration of conjugated and esterified derivatives and synthetic estrogens which are readily absorbed from the gastrointestinal tract but are slowly metabolized. **Ethinyl estradiol** and **mestranol** are the synthetic estrogens contained in combination birth control pills. Mestranol is hepatically demethylated to ethinyl estradiol, the active compound. Peak serum concentrations of both are seen within 1 to 2 h following oral administration, with mestranol taking a slightly longer time to peak. The distribution half-life of ethinyl estradiol is 1 to 3 h with an elimination half-life of approximately 6 to 14 h. The major urinary metabolite of both is ethinyl estradiol glucuronide.

Injectable forms of naturally occurring estrogens in oil are relatively rapidly absorbed and inactivated when administered intramuscularly and must be dosed several times weekly. The effectiveness of *injected estrogens* may be prolonged by the use of esters (e.g., **estradiol cypionate**) which are more slowly absorbed after intramuscular administration and require dosing once per month.

Adverse Effects Many symptoms associated with estrogen therapy are similar to those seen in early pregnancy. The most common adverse effect associated with estrogen therapy is nausea. It is an unusual type of nausea that normally does not decrease eating. Dose-related anorexia, vomiting, and diarrhea may also occur. Other gastrointestinal problems include abdominal cramps, bloating, and possible cholestatic jaundice. There is an increased risk of endometrial cancer (approximately 5 to 15 times higher in estrogen users) in postmenopausal women on prolonged estrogen therapy. The risk of endometrial cancer also appears dose-related. Women using estrogens for menopausal symptoms should be on the lowest dose of estrogen that will control their symptoms, and they should be carefully monitored for adverse effects. Low doses of estrogen used in combination with progestogen for contraception are not associated with endometrial cancer.

The use of the estrogenic preparation **diethylstilbestrol** (DES) in pregnant women has been associated with the development of adenocarcinoma of the cervix in the daughters of women who took DES during pregnancy. Also, a high percentage of exposed women have vaginal adenosis. In male offspring of DES mothers, congenital anomalies including structural defects of the genitourinary tract and decreased semen levels have been reported. There may be an association between uterine exposure to female sex hormones and other congenital anomalies, including limb reduction defects and congenital cardiac defects. Estrogen and progestogen preparations have both been used to treat threatened or habitual abortion. Neither appear effective and the risks of using female sex hormones during pregnancy greatly outweigh the benefits.

TABLE 46-2 Relative Potency of Estrogens

ESTROGEN	EQUIVALENT DOSE*
Ethinyl estradiol	50 μg
Mestranol	80 μg
Conjugated estrogens	3.75 mg
17β-Estradiol	5 mg
Diethylstilbestrol	5 mg

*Determined by doses needed to suppress ovulation, stimulate vaginal cornification, cause endometrial proliferation, and stimulate cervical mucus ferning.

TABLE 46-3   Therapeutic Uses of Estrogens

INDICATION	COMMENTS
Contraception	Given orally in combination with progestogens.
Menopause	The symptoms of menopause can be relieved with the use of estrogen preparations, best given in cyclic pattern of 3 weeks on and 1 week off.
Atrophic vaginitis	Responds well to topically applied estrogens.
Dysmenorrhea	Relief of dysmenorrhea has been noted with the use of estrogen preparations. Presently they are given in the form of oral contraceptives.
Failure of ovarian development	Turner's syndrome responds well to the use of estrogens and given at the time of puberty will resemble physiologic development.
Neoplastic disorders	Estrogens alter the hormonal environment of tumors of the prostate and breast.
Suppression of postpartum lactation	Estrogens can decrease milk production in postpartum period.
Osteoporosis	It has been thought that estrogen may increase the bone density, especially in postmenopausal women. This effect has not been well documented, and it is still controversial.
Acne	Estrogens can be effective in suppressing acne in both sexes. Their usefulness in the male is limited by their adverse effects. In the female they may be given in the form of an oral contraceptive, but other methods for treatment are preferred.

Other adverse effects of estrogens including gallbladder disease, thromboembolism, myocardial infarction, liver tumors, and hypertension are extensively discussed in the sections on oral contraceptives and menopause. Women using estrogen therapy may have trouble tolerating contact lenses. Intramuscular introduction of estrogens has been associated with pain at the site of injection and sterile abscess formation.

Patient Education   When an estrogen-containing preparation is dispensed, a patient package insert (PPI) must also be dispensed. These inserts explain both adverse effects and contraindications for estrogen therapy. The use of PPIs does not reduce the obligation of the health care provider to explain both the uses and adverse effects of these agents to the client. Informed consent for estrogen therapy should always be obtained.

Preparations   Estrogens are available as vaginal, oral, and injectable products (Table 46-1). The combinations of estrogen with a sedative (e.g., **meprobamate, chlordiazepoxide**) in a single preparation is promoted for the treatment of the symptoms of menopause but is considered questionable therapeutics. Estrogens are also available in combination with progestogens for oral contraception and for the treatment of endometriosis and hypermenorrhea (see below). Also shown in Table 46-3 are the **estrogen-androgen** combinations which are marketed in parenteral and oral forms to treat severe vasomotor symptoms in menopause and postpartum breast engorgement.

Progestogens

Progestogens (progesterone and derivatives) are compounds which serve to prepare the uterus for reception and development of the fertilized ovum. Progesterone is secreted primarily by the corpus luteum during the luteal (secretory) phase of the menstrual cycle. Progestogens also serve as intermediates in the synthesis of estrogens, androgens, and corticosteroids. The ovarian progestogens include progesterone (the most abundant progestogen) and two others, 20α- and 20β-dehydroprogesterone. Small quantities of progesterone are also formed by the adrenal gland. The placenta serves as the primary source of progesterone during pregnancy.

Synthetic progestogens, 19-nortestosterone compounds, which possess progesterone-like activity are used orally. Progestogen compounds include **ethynodiol diacetate, norethindrone, norethindrone acetate, norethynodrel,** and **norgestrel.** The compounds possess not only varying progestational effects, but also various degrees of estrogenic, antiestrogenic, and androgenic activity. Table 46-4 compares the biologic effects of the progestogens. Thus, the selection of a progestogen or a combination oral contracep-

TABLE 46-4   Relative Biologic Effects of Progestogens in Common Use

PROGESTOGEN (AND SAMPLE TRADE NAMES*)	ESTROGENIC	ANTIESTROGENIC	ANDROGENIC	PROGESTATIONAL
Ethynodiol diacetate (Demulen, Ovulen)	+	+ +	+	+ +
Norethindrone (Norinyl 1 + 50, Ortho-Novum)	0	+	+	+
Norethindrone acetate (Loestrin, Norlestrin)	0	+ +	+ +	+
Norethynodrel (Enovid, Enovid-E)	+ +	0	0	±
Nogestrel (Lo-Ovral, Ovral)	0	+ + +	+ +	+ + +

Key: 0 = no activity;   ± = very slight;   + = moderate;   + + = strong;   + + + = very strong.
* Combination product containing the progestogen listed.

tive may depend on the biologic profile of the particular progestogen.

Physiologic Effects Progesterone prepares the uterus for the implantation of a fertilized ovum by the development of a secretory endometrium during the luteal phase of the menstrual cycle. The decline of progesterone released by the corpus luteum near the end of the menstrual cycle acts as a trigger for the start of menses. Progesterone also causes the production of scant, viscous cervical secretions. Tubal and uterine contractility are influenced by progesterone to favor implantation. During pregnancy, progesterone suppresses uterine contractility to maintain pregnancy. It may also have an effect on the immune system to prevent rejection of the developing fetus.

Estrogens and progesterone help in the development of the acini of the mammary glands in the breasts. However, lactation can only occur when the levels of progesterone and estrogen decrease at the time of birth. Progesterone given postpartum may suppress lactation.

Progesterone causes an increase in the basal temperature, approximately 1°F at midcycle, and may also act as a slight stimulant to respiration. It also appears to have a mild catabolic effect. Some progestogens (e.g., **norethidrone, norgestrel**) have antiestrogenic and androgenic activity. Progesterone affects carbohydrate metabolism, increasing insulin levels and decreasing response of blood glucose to insulin.

Therapeutic Uses Although primarily used in prevention of conception, progestogens are used in refractory or severe primary dysmenorrhea or premenstrual tension, dysfunctional uterine bleeding, endometriosis, galactorrhea, precocious puberty, and metastatic endometrial carcinoma. They are also used in testing estrogen levels and suppression of postpartum lactation. A more complete discussion of the uses of progestogens is presented in the sections of this chapter on these individual conditions.

Pharmacokinetics Progesterone is rapidly absorbed by any route and quickly inactivated in the liver to metabolites, which undergo conjugation to form glucuronides and sulfates. Progesterone, like estrogen, undergoes enterohepatic recycling. Although the serum half-life for progesterone is reported to be less than 90 min, its duration of effect is much longer. Small quantities of the hormone are stored in body fat. Fifty to sixty percent is renally eliminated, primarily as metabolites, with pregnanediol being the major metabolite. Twenty to thirty percent is eliminated in the feces as the parent compound or metabolites.

Little is known about the pharmacokinetics of synthetic progestogens. **Norethynodrel** and **norethindrone** are rapidly absorbed, resulting in peak concentrations 1 h after oral administration. **Norethindrone acetate** and **ethynodiol diacetate** undergo deacetylation in the gastrointestinal tract prior to absorption. **Norethynodrel** and **ethynodiol diacetate** are metabolized to norethidrone, which undergoes a complex metabolism resulting in renal elimination as various conjugates. **Norgestrel** is a totally synthetic progestogen, which undergoes metabolism similar to that for norethindrone. The progestogens and their metabolites undergo varying amounts of enterohepatic recycling and biliary excretion.

Adverse Effects Progestogens have been observed to cause breakthrough bleeding, amenorrhea, edema, weight gain, cholestatic jaundice, rash, pruritus, acne, and mental depression. Masculinization of female fetuses and congenital anomalies have occurred with intrauterine exposure to progestogens.

Progesterone injection has been associated with local irritation at the injection site. Large doses of progesterone injection (100 mg daily) can cause a catabolic effect and an increased loss of sodium and chloride. Hydroxyprogesterone caproate has been associated with allergic reactions. Additional adverse effects are discussed under oral contraception.

Preparations Progestogens are available as oral forms and parenteral liquids for intramuscular injection, as well as in oral forms combined with estrogens for the treatment of hypermenorrheas and endometriosis (Table 46-5). Estrogen-progestogen combinations for oral contraception (see below) generally contain lower doses of progestogens than those for endometriosis and hypermenorrhea.

NURSING PROCESS RELATED TO OVARIAN HORMONES

Perhaps more than with any other group of drugs, assessment and management of women who are to receive estrogens and progestogens involve psychosocial as well as physical components. Since sexual identity is an important part of one's psychologic being and the ovarian hormones are perceived as integral to female biology, use of these agents may have deeper implications than mere drug therapy to the patient. Further, the conditions treated with these agents and the goals of any therapy may be intimately interrelated with the woman's sexuality, values, self-image, and significant relationships. Since many of the women placed on these agents are not ill in a traditional medical sense but are seeking modification of usual physiologic processes such as menopause or fertility, a health (versus illness) orientation is important in delivery of care.

Table 46-6 outlines the nursing process relative to estrogens and progestogens.

BIRTH CONTROL

Nurses in all settings encounter patients, friends, and acquaintances who need information on contraception. Control of fertility is a highly personal matter, and nurses should be able to supply accurate and current information on birth control without personal bias.

Competent birth control counseling lies not in making decisions for people, but in providing the information they need to select the method that best suits their values, lifestyle, and relationships. The nurse should first assess how much the person or couple knows about reproductive physiology because many failures in birth control may be due to misconceptions about anatomy and physiology. The nurse should present the following information about each birth control method discussed: description, mechanism of action, advantages, disadvantages, and effectiveness. Once a method of contraception has been selected, the nurse should make sure the person understands both proper use of the method and what to do if problems occur. In Table 46-7, nonpharmacologic methods of birth control are compared to oral

contraceptives and spermicides, which are discussed in this chapter.

Oral Hormonal Contraception

It is estimated that approximately 80 million women worldwide use oral hormonal contraception. Oral contraceptives currently available include: conventional combination birth control pills (BCPs), progestin-only BCPs (minipills), and phasic BCPs (Table 46-8).

Mechanism of Action Estrogens in oral contraceptives help prevent pregnancy by several means:

1. They inhibit normal ovulatory patterns. Estrogen inhibits the hypothalamic control of LH and FSH release and may suppress the midcycle peak of LH and FSH, primarily LH. The preovulatory surge of estrogen and the postovulatory increase in progesterone may be blunted.

2. High doses of estrogens can inhibit the implantation of a fertilized egg.

TABLE 46-5 Progestogen Preparations and Combinations

PREPARATION CONTENT	TRADE NAMES	DOSAGE FORM	INDICATIONS	USUAL DOSE
		Progestogen Only		
Hydroxyprogesterone caproate in oil	Delalutin, Pro-Depo, others	IM injection	Amenorrhea or dysfunctional uterine bleeding	250–400 mg
Progesterone aqueous or in oil	Progelen aqueous, Femotrone in oil, others	IM injection	As above	5–10 mg/day for 6 to 8 days
Medroxyprogesterone acetate	Depo-Provera	IM injection	Endometrial carcinoma	400–1000 mg/week
	Provera, Amen, others	Tablet	Amenorrhea or dysfunctional uterine bleeding	5–10 mg/day for 5 to 10 days
Megestrol acetate	Megace	Tablet	Breast cancer or endometrial cancer	10–80 mg qid
Norethindrone	Norlutin	Tablet	Amenorrhea or endometriosis	5–30 mg/day
Progesterone	Progestasert	Intrauterine device	Contraception	Replaced yearly, releases 65 μg daily
Norethindrone acetate	Norlutate, Aygestin	Tablet	As above	2.5–15 mg/day
		Progestogen-Estrogen Combinations		
Norethynodrel and mestranol	Enovid 5, Enovid 10	Tablet	Endometriosis	5–20 mg norethynodrel daily
			Hypermenorrhea	5–30 mg norethynodrel per day cyclically
Norethidrone and mestranol	Ortho-Novum 2 mg, Norinyl 2 mg	Tablet	Hypermenorrhea	1 tablet/day cyclically

TABLE 46-6 Nursing Process with Ovarian Hormones

Assessment	Management	Evaluation
Perception of reason for medication, effect on lifestyle	How to take medication; on-off schedule; measures to help remember to take medication such as taking at time of some regular daily activity	Assess whether therapeutic goal has been achieved (e.g., contraception, menopausal symptom control, adequate replacement).
Understanding of reproductive anatomy and physiology	Importance of good health habits including diet, rest, exercise, yearly checkups	Checkups at least yearly should include pelvic exam, breast exam, blood pressure check, check for weight gain and edema, and any other factors that require special monitoring.
Menstrual and obstetric history	Potential side effects and measures to minimize or control them:	Note occurrence of any side effects:
Presence of factors that contraindicate use:	Nausea: Taking pill at bedtime; mastalgia and nausea usually decrease after several months.	Minor: Nausea, mastalgia, breakthrough bleeding, headache, libido change, missed menses
Cerebrovascular disease, estrogen-dependent neoplasm, thromboembolitic disorders present or past	Skin pigmentation: Wear hat and avoid exposure to sun.	Moderate: Vaginal infection, amenorrhea and difficulty conceiving after drugs discontinued (occurs most in those with irregular menses prior to use of medication), hirsutism, acne, increased skin pigmentation, weight gain
Adolescence prior to epiphyseal closure	Headache: Treat with mild analgesics; if migraines develop or become more severe after beginning to take estrogens, drug should be discontinued.	
Presence of factors that require use with caution and special monitoring:	Weight gain: Restrict salt or decrease calories; keep record of weight.	Severe: Hypertension, depression, jaundice and liver dysfunction, thrombophlebitis and other thromboembolitic disorders, gallbladder disease, retinal thrombosis, cervical cancer (in offspring if DES taken during pregnancy)
Conditions where sodium and water retention are undesirable such as CHF, renal failure, epilepsy	Hirsutism and acne: Use OTC preparations for hair removal and for cleaning and drying skin.	
Asthma	Vitamin B$_6$ and folate deficiencies: Maintain good diet or take vitamin supplements.	Carcinogenesis is presently being researched; may have protective effects on some organs and increase risk of cancer for others.
Liver disease	Should report any side effects, as these often can be controlled by change of dose or type of hormone	
Eczema	Contact physician immediately for loss or blurring of vision; menstrual irregularities; tenderness, swelling, or redness of an extremity	
Migraine		
Diabetes		
Hypertension		
Optic neuritis, retrobulbar neuritis	Estrogen therapy may alter lab tests for clotting and endocrine function.	
Recurrent depression		
Gallbladder disease	If more than one missed period with oral contraceptives, evaluate for pregnancy.	
Premenopausal over 35: check for risk factors for coronary artery disease especially smoking, but also hypertension, obesity, family history, and hypercholesterolemia	Assure that patient has given *informed consent* prior to use of these agents.	
Pregnancy		
Breast feeding		
Concurrent medication history		

3. Estrogens are also thought to increase the rate of ovum transport, thus further inhibiting implantation.

Progestogens may have contraceptive effects, because:

1. They create a thick, hostile cervical mucus which decreases sperm migration.

2. They change the characteristics of the cervical fluids and prevent capacitation (release of sperm from seminal fluids).

3. They may alter the time of tubular transport of the ovum to the uterus.

4. They inhibit implantation by altering the endometrium.

5. They may also inhibit ovulation.

Effectiveness The conventional combination pill (containing more than 50 μg of estrogen) is theoretically 100 percent effective when taken as directed. In actual clinical use it has a failure rate of less than 1 percent. Those containing less

TABLE 46-7 Comparison of Birth Control Methods

METHOD	MECHANISM OF ACTION	EFFICACY,* %	SAFETY†
Condom	Forms mechanical barrier.	80–97	Very high
Spermicides	Forms mechanical barrier, immobilizes and kills sperm.	70–96	High
Diaphragm with spermicide	Forms mechanical barrier.	80–97	Very high
Sponge with spermicide	Immobilizes and kills sperm, forms barrier.	80–96	Very high
Intrauterine device	Prevents implantation, dislodges implanted blastocyst, immobilizes sperm, stimulates prostaglandins, impairs uterine use of estrogens.	90–99	Low
Surgical sterilization	Removes or disrupts reproductive organs.	>99	High
Oral contraceptives	See text.		
Combination		98–99	Moderate
Phasic combinations		98–99	High
Minipill		97	High
Rhythm	Avoids intercourse during fertile periods	40–97	Very high
No contraception		20–40	Very high

*Percent of women using the method for one year who avoid pregnancy. Ranges often reflect the difference between actual effectiveness (low number) and theoretical effectiveness (high number).

†Incorporates the relative incidence and severity of adverse effects of the methods, but not the complications of pregnancy if the methods fail.

than 50 μg of estrogen are slightly less effective (range from 98 percent to more than 99 percent). The phasic combination pill is approximately 98 to 99 percent effective, which is similar to the minipills (progestin-only BCPs).

Combination Birth Control Pills

The conventional combination birth control pills contain set amounts of estrogen and progestogens which are taken during the first 21 days of a woman's cycle. Combination BCPs are also available in 28-day packets, with the last seven tablets being placebo or iron tablets. (Table 46-8 lists available combination products.) **Ethinyl estradiol** and **mestranol** are the estrogens used in combination BCPs, while the progestogen may be **ethynodiol diacetate, norgestrel, norethindrone, norethindrone acetate,** or **norethynodrel.** There appears to be no difference between the estrogens when used in equipotent doses, but the progestogens appear to differ in their progestogenic, estrogenic, antiestrogenic, and androgenic activity.

Before a woman is started on combination BCPs, a complete history and physical examination should be performed to determine whether there are any absolute or relative contraindications to their use. Table 46-9 lists both absolute and relative contraindications to combination BCPs, with most contraindications being associated with the estrogenic component.

Adverse Effects Combination BCPs, although an extremely effective method of birth control, are associated with numerous adverse effects, some of which may be life-threatening. Table 46-10 lists related adverse effects associated with BCPS.

Adverse effects may be classified as minor problems or serious complications. Minor problems include nausea, vomiting, weight gain, depression, fatigue, mild headaches, breakthrough bleeding, absence of withdrawal bleeding, glucose abnormalities, increased serum lipid concentration, increased monilia infections, and the development of chloasma (increased pigmentation on the forehead, under the eyes, and above the mouth which is worsened by sunlight). There may be worsening of a client's asthma, migraine headaches, epilepsy, renal disease, or hypertension—all of which are more severe than those cited above.

Although minor adverse effects are not serious or life-threatening, many women may discontinue BCPs because they are unable or do not wish to cope with them. The following are some of the commonly seen minor adverse effects associated with combination BCP usage.

TABLE 46-8   Oral Contraceptive Ingredients

BRAND NAME	ESTROGEN	PROGESTOGEN
Combination BCPs (>50 μg Estrogen per Tablet)		
Enovid-E Enovid 5 mg	Mestranol	Norethynodrel
Norinyl 1 + 80 Norinyl 2 mg Ortho-Novum 1/80 Ortho-Novum 2 mg	Mestranol	Norethindrone
Ovulen	Mestranol	Ethynodiol diacetate
Combination BCPs (50 μg Estrogen per Tablet)		
Demulen	Ethinyl estradiol	Ethynodiol diacetate
Norlestrin 1/50 Norlestrin 2.5/50	Ethinyl estradiol	Norethindrone
Norinyl 1 + 50 Ortho-Novum 1/50	Mestranol	Norethindrone
Ovcon-50 Ovral	Ethinyl estradiol Ethinyl estradiol	Norethindrone Norgestrel
Combination BCPs (<50 μg Estrogen per Tablet)		
Norlestrin 1.5/30 Loestrin 1/20	Ethinyl estradiol	Norethindrone acetate
LoOvral	Ethinyl estradiol	Norgestrel
Modicon Brevicon Norlestrin 1 + 35 Ortho-Novum 1/35 Ovcon-35	Ethinyl estradiol	Norethindrone
Progestogen-Only BCPs (The Minipill)		
Micronor Nor-Q.D.		Norethindrone
Ovrette		Norgestrel
Phasic Combination BCP		
Ortho-Novum 10/11 Ortho-Novum 7/7/7 Tri-Norinyl	Ethinyl estradiol	Norethindrone

Nausea and vomiting Usually nausea and vomiting occur early in therapy and may subside with time. These adverse effects are associated with the estrogenic component in the BCPs and may be reduced by the use of products containing 50 μg or less of estrogen. Other methods of reducing these problems include taking the BCP with food or at bedtime and supporting the client emotionally. Vomiting within 2 h of BCP ingestion may lead to decreased hormonal levels and decreased contraception, especially in women using low-dose estrogen-containing BCPs.

Absence of withdrawal bleeding Bleeding usually occurs during the 7 days of each cycle when the hormonal therapy is not given. Absence of withdrawal bleeding appears more frequently when combination BCPs containing less than 50 μg/tablet of estrogen are used. This problem probably results from the inhibition of the estrogenic proliferative effect on the endometrial lining, resulting in decreased or absent withdrawal bleeding. Once pregnancy has been ruled out, if the lack of withdrawal bleeding occurs during the first three cycles of combination BCPs, the client should continue her BCPs at the regularly scheduled time. The nonpregnant patient who continues to miss menstrual cycles may be started on a BCP with a lower progestogenic activity. If this fails, a higher estrogen containing preparation may be instituted.

Breakthrough bleeding Breakthrough bleeding or spotting that occurs early in the menstrual cycle is most fre-

TABLE 46-9   Contraindications to Combination Birth Control Pills

ABSOLUTE CONTRAINDICATIONS	RELATIVE CONTRAINDICATIONS
Thromboembolic disease (past or present)	Women over 35–40 years of age, nonsmokers
Cerebrovascular accident (past or present)	Women over 30 years of age, heavy smokers
Coronary artery disease or myocardial infarction (past or present)	Vascular or migraine headaches
Hepatic adenoma (past or present)	Hypertension
	Undiagnosed abnormal vaginal bleeding
Liver dysfunction	Varicose veins
Women over 35 years of age who are heavy smokers	Planned surgery, major injury to lower leg or casting of lower leg(s)
Malignancy of breast or reproductive system (past or present)	Diabetes, gestational diabetes, or positive family history for diabetes
Positive family history of breast or reproductive system cancer	Gallbladder disease
Pregnancy	Undiagnosed breast lumps, fibrocystic breast disease, or fibroadenomas of the breast
	Patients unable to comply with instructions, i.e., mentally retarded, alcoholic, young patient, or psychiatric patient
	Individuals suffering from the following problems may use the pill but must be monitored closely: asthma, epilepsy, depression, uterine fibromyomata, chloasma related to pregnancy, abnormal liver function.

quently associated with the use of BCPs which contain less than 50 μg of estrogen or contain the progestogen **norethindrone acetate** which has antiestrogenic activity. Breakthrough bleeding occurs primarily during the first three cycles of BCP usage. The major cause of this problem is decreased estrogenic support of the endometrium, although it might also be related to missed BCPs or a drug interaction (see below).

If this problem occurs beyond the initial 3 months of BCP usage, it may be resolved by increased compliance (what to do when doses are missed is described below under Preparations and Administration), taking the BCPs at the same time daily, or changing to one containing a progestogen with less antiestrogenic activity. Rarely will a BCP containing more estrogen be needed.

Depression A woman may complain of poor sleep, crying spells, irritability, fatigue, lethargy, or decreased libido while on BCPs. These symptoms of depression may be associated with estrogen excess or deficiency, progestogen excess, or possibly pyridoxine deficiency. If the patient wishes to continue using BCPs, a tablet containing low concentrations of both estrogen and progestogen might be used. Pyridoxine (25 to 50 mg daily) could be prescribed. (Pyridoxine is a cofactor in the metabolism of tryptophan to serotonin. One theory is that low concentrations of serotonin may be associated with depression.)

Weight gain Weight gain associated with BCP use may be acyclic or cyclic. The acyclic gain of weight appears associated with the progestogen. Usually the weight gain is minimal and may be controlled with diet and exercise. Changing to a lower progestogen dosage or to a progestogen with less anabolic activity may also be tried.

Cyclic weight gain is usually associated with excessive estrogenic activity which may cause sodium and water retention. Switching to BCPs with a lower estrogen concentration may be helpful.

Cardiovascular problems The risk of developing superficial or deep venous thrombosis or pulmonary embolism appears to be two to four times higher in combination BCP users as compared with nonusers. These complications appear to be estrogen-related and are associated with decreased antithrombin II and increased levels of various clotting factors. Long-term BCP users may have increased platelet aggregation as well as elevated platelet counts. Women with blood types A, AB, and B (especially A) have an increased risk for developing thromboemboli.

The risk of myocardial infarction (MI) in BCP users is two to four times that noted for nonusers, with the risk being three or four times greater in BCP users over age 35. Heavy smoking (>15 cigarettes daily) significantly increases the risk of MI in all age groups and quadruples the risk in the 40- to 44-year-old group. Other risk factors, including diabetes, hypertension, and hyperlipoproteinemia may synergistically increase the risk of MI in a woman on BCPs. Thus, the risk of MI outweighs the benefits of BCPs in women 35 to 45 years of age who are smokers or who have other risk factors for developing an MI. In nonsmoking women who are 35 to 45 years of age without risk factors for MI, the use of BCPs must be individually decided. All women above the age of 45 should not use BCPs as a contraceptive method because of adverse risk-to-benefit ratio.

The risk of MI appears associated with the estrogen concentration in BCPs and a decreased incidence should be associated with low-estrogen-containing products. Proges-

TABLE 46-10 Hormonal-Related Adverse Effects of Oral Contraceptives

Estrogen		Progestogen	
EXCESS	DEFICIENCY	EXCESS	DEFICIENCY
Breast tenderness, cyclical	Amenorrhea	Acne	Delayed onset of menses after last BCP
Chloasma	Atrophic vaginitis	Appetite increased	Heavy menstrual flow
Contact lens may fit poorly	Decreased libido	Breast tenderness	Late breakthrough bleeding
Cystic breast changes	Depression	Changes in libido	Weight loss
Edema	Dysparuria	Depression	
Headaches	Early and midcycle bleeding	Fatigue	
Hypermenorrhea	Hot flashes	Length of menstrual flow decreased	
Irritability	Irritability	Oily scalp and skin	
Leg cramps	Nervousness	Weight gain, noncyclical	
Leukorrhea			
Nausea and vomiting			
Vertigo			

togens, as well as estrogens, may be associated with the risk of cardiovascular disease, since some progestogens may increase serum concentrations of low-density lipoproteins (LDL). They also decrease levels of high-density lipoproteins (HDL); HDL appear protective against cardiovascular disease. When BCPs are initiated, a preparation low in both estrogen and progestogen content should be prescribed. The initiation or continued use of BCPs in women greater than 35 years of age should be done on an individual basis with caution and frequent monitoring.

Women who use BCPs are at a two to three times greater risk of developing hypertension (BP > 140/90) than nonusers. Hypertension associated with BCPs may develop slowly over months or years (typically between 3 months and 3 years) and may decrease slowly after BCPs are discontinued. Hypertension appears most likely associated with estrogen content, although it may be associated with certain progestogens. The mechansim for the development of hypertension may be associated with renin-angiotensin activity.

Breast disease There appears to be a lower incidence of benign breast disease in BCP users as compared to nonusers. No difference in the incidence of breast cancer is associated with BCP use.

Reproductive organ neoplasms There appears to be decreased risk of both ovarian and endometrial cancers in BCP users. BCPs may actually be beneficial. The relationship between cervical cancer and BCP usage is unclear.

Liver and biliary disease Benign liver tumors have an increased incidence in BCP users occurring at the rate of approximately two or three per 100,000 women-years. They are primarily seen in women who have taken high-dose estrogen-containing BCPs for 5 years or longer. Although liver tumors are usually benign, women may die from tumor rupture. Women who use BCPs are also at a two times greater risk of developing gallbladder disease that may require surgery.

Pregnancy Oral contraceptives should not be taken during pregnancy since the fetus may be at risk for teratogenicity. It is also recommended that patients should wait at least 3 months before trying to become pregnant after using BCPs, since there is an increased incidence of spontaneous abortion and teratogenic effects when pregnancy occurs sooner.

Drug Interactions. Antibiotics Antibiotics, including **ampicillin, chloramphenicol, neomycin, nitrofurantoin, phenoxymethyl penicillin, sulfamethoxypyridazine,** and **tetracycline** may decrease the enterohepatic recirculation of sex hormones by their effects on the gut flora and result in BCP failure. Although this drug interaction is debated, women using low-dose BCPs would be the most likely affected.

Rifampin is an antituberculosis medication which may induce the hepatic metabolism of estrogens resulting in decreased estrogen concentrations. This may decrease contraceptive control especially in women on low-estrogen-containing BCPs. The patient may need another medication rather than rifampin to treat her tuberculosis or may need an alternative birth control method.

Anticoagulants There are two potential drug interactions between BCPs and **warfarin**. Estrogens in BCPs may decrease the effectiveness of warfarin by decreasing antithrombin III activity or by increasing the concentrations of clotting factors.

Anticonvulsants **Carbamazepine, phenobarbital, phenytoin,** and **primidone** may include hepatic enzymatic metabolism of sex hormones, which may decrease the effectiveness of BCPs. Other methods of birth control should be considered in patients requiring anticonvulsants. Also, loss of seizure control, most likely associated with fluid retention, has been reported in women on BCPs and anticonvulsant therapy.

Preparations and Administration Most patients are initially started on combination BCPs with low estrogen concentrations (50 μg or less) which are balanced for estrogenic and progestogenic activity. Examples of these are Ortho-Novum 1/150 and Norinyl 1 + 50 (Table 46-11). Lower-dose estrogen BCPs containing 20 to 35 μg have been associated with higher incidences of breakthrough bleeding. The initiation of BCPs may also be selected according to a woman's estrogen-progesterone profile which is based on body build and menstrual cycle characteristics. Further dosage changes of BCPs may be individualized according to adverse effects associated with the use of particular BCPs.

Oral contraceptives should be started on day 5 after the menstrual period has begun, or on the first Sunday after the menstrual period starts. The pills should then be continued for 21 days (depending on the BCPs which are used), and then discontinued for 7 days. Preparations that contain 28 tablets have seven inert tablets included. This type of combination BCPs should be taken continuously. Oral contraceptive agents are best taken at the same time daily; preferably at night to avoid some of their adverse effects including nausea. A second method of birth control should be used during the first month of BCP usage.

If a client misses a BCP, she could take the missed tablet as soon as she remembers and also take that day's tablet at the regular time. If the client misses 2 days of BCPs, she should take two tablets as soon as she remembers and then two tablets the following day. (There might be some spotting, and an additional means of birth control should be used.) If the client misses three or more tablets, an alternate method of birth control must be used. When three tablets are missed, there is a good chance that ovulation will occur. The client should stop taking this package of BCPs and should wait 5 days and then start a new package. Another method of birth control must be used and should be continued for 14 days after restarting BCPs.

Progestogen-Only BCPs (Minipill)

Minipills contain only low concentrations of progestogen which act as an oral contraceptive by the mechanisms listed previously. By using only progestogen, some of the estrogen-related side effects may be avoided. However, the minipill is associated with spotting, breakthrough bleeding, and lack of withdrawal bleeding. If menstrual flow does not occur in 2 months, another method of contraception should be used after pregnancy has been ruled out.

Minipills are administered continuously starting on day 1 of the menstrual cycle. They should be taken at the same time daily. If the client misses a BCP, she should take it as soon as she remembers, and then take her tablet for that day at its usual time. If the patient misses two tablets, she should take only one as soon as she remembers, and her daily tablet at its regular time. Another nonhormonal method of contraception should be used for the next 14 days. The progestogen-only BCPs are listed in Table 46-8. An intrauterine device (Progestasert) which is replaced yearly and releases 65 μg progesterone daily is also available.

Phasic BCPs

Biphasic and triphasic BCPs contain concentrations of estrogen and/or progestogen which vary through the cycle to closely mimic the normal female menstrual cycle. The effectiveness of these BCPs is similar to that seen with conventional combination BCPs although the total monthly hormone dosage is lower.

Postcoital Pill (Morning-After Pill)

After unprotected coitus a postcoital pill can be given that will be effective in preventing pregnancy. The postcoital pill is especially useful after rape, incest, or where a client's mental or physical well-being is in jeopardy. Most postcoital pills contain high doses of estrogen alone or in combination with progestogens.

Diethylstilbestrol (DES) is an estrogen approved by the FDA for use in high doses as a morning-after pill. A DES dosage of 25 mg bid for 5 days should be initiated within 24 to 72 h after unprotected coitus. Its mechanism of action appears to be prevention of the implantation of an ovum. The failure rate is about 0 to 2.4 percent. Its most common adverse effects are nausea and vomiting. Although there is no current evidence that postcoital dosages of DES are carcinogenic to a fetus, abortion should be considered if DES therapy fails.

Vaginal Spermicidal Agents

Vaginal spermicidal agents, readily available without a prescription, include jellies, gels, creams, foams, and suppositories. Recently released is the spermicide-impregnated vaginal sponge. Some creams and jellies are specifically formulated to be used with diaphragms. These have lower concentrations of the spermicidal agent and have less spreading ability. Indications for spermicidal agents include use as contraceptive alone, with condoms or diaphragms, as a supplement to the rhythm method at midcycle, as a backup method during the first month of the use of BCPs or intrauterine device, when several BCPs are missed or the intrauterine device is expelled, and as an interim contraceptive after BCPs are stopped but before the woman wishes to become pregnant.

Mechanism of Action Spermicidal products are formulated to spread over the cervical os, forming a mechanical barrier. The inert base (i.e., foam, jelly, or cream) will hold

TABLE 46-11   Relative Estrogenic and Progestogenic Dominance of Oral Contraceptives

Estrogenic Dominance	Progestogenic Dominance		
	LOW	INTERMEDIATE	HIGH
HIGH	Enovid-E Norinyl 1 + 80 Ortho-Novum 1/80 Ortho-Novum 2 mg	Norinyl 2 mg	Enovid 5 mg
INTERMEDIATE	Brevicon Modicon Ovcon-35	Ovulen 0.5 Lo/Ovral* Norlestrin 1 + 35* Norinyl 1 + 50* Ortho-Novum 1/50* Ortho-Novum 1/35*	Ovulen Demulen
LOW	Ortho-Novum 10/11 Norinyl 1 + 35 Ortho-Novum 7/7/7 Tri-Norinyl	Norinyl 10 mg Nordette	Loestrin 1/20 Lestrin 1.5/30 Norlestrin 2.5/50 Ortho-Novum 10 mg Ovral Demulen 1/35

*Estrogenic and progestogenic effects are relatively balanced.

the spermicidal agent against the cervix while the spermicidal chemical immobilizes and kills the sperm.

Effectiveness Spermicidal agents theoretically have a 2.5 to 4 percent failure rate; but in actual practice, the failure rate is closer to 30 percent. The sponge, foams, and suppositories are more effective than creams, jellies, and gels when used alone for contraceptive purposes. For this reason many contraceptive experts do not recommend the use of the latter three types of vaginal spermicidal agents as sole agents in contraception. Vaginal spermicidal agents are most effective when used in conjunction with a condom or diaphragm.

Preparations and Administration The FDA advisory panel on nonprescription contraceptive agents has determined three nonionic surfactants (menfegol, octoxynol-9, and nonoxynol-9) to be safe and effective for use in vaginal spermicidal preparations. Specific preparations are listed in Table 46-12.

Future Birth Control Methods

The following are examples of current research in birth control methods. Some of these will probably be commercially available in the United States in the future.

Cervical caps are small diaphragm-like plastic caps that are placed over the cervix and held in place by suction. Their main advantage is their size (smaller than the conventional diaphragm). A major disadvantage, however, is the individualized fitting of the cervical cap. One new model has a one-way flap which allows for menstrual fluid escape. Cervical caps are approved for use in many European countries but have not received FDA approval for use in the United States. They are available as investigational agents from feminist health centers and other clinics.

Gossypol, a pigment from cotton plants, is being tested in Chinese men as a possible "male pill" or oral spermicidal agent which would kill sperm in the epididymis but would not affect spermatogenesis directly. Male fertility is reestablished several months after the gossypol is discontinued. Another possibility is the use of gossypol as a vaginal spermicidal agent. Also under investigation are long-acting progestogens as a female contraceptive. These include depot **medroxyprogesterone acetate** (DMPA) and **norethesterone enanthrate**, both given by injection every 2 to 3 months.

PERIMENSTRUAL SYMPTOMS

Premenstrual Syndrome (PMS)

The incidence of premenstrual syndrome ranges from 5 to 95 percent of women in their reproductive years with approximately 20 to 40 percent having significant physical and/or mental incapacitation on a temporary basis. Symptoms associated with premenstrual syndrome occur during the luteal phase of the menstrual cycle, usually commensing 2 or 3 days prior to menses with a symptom-free period of at least 1 week's duration following menses. The most common somatic symptoms include headache, abdominal swelling, enlarged and tender breasts, swollen ankles, and abdominal cramping. Tension, mood swings, and an inability to concentrate are common psychologic symptoms associated with premenstrual syndrome.

The pathogenesis of the premenstrual syndrome is currently unknown; there are many theories including estrogen excess, a progesterone deficiency at the beginning of menses, or an estrogen-progesterone imbalance. Other possible causes include vitamin A or vitmain B_6 deficiencies, hypoglycemia, elevated prolactin levels, vasopressin, gonadotrophins, endorphins, an underlying psychogenic disorder, or

TABLE 46-12 Vaginal Spermicides

DRUG	BRAND NAME	FORM	COMMENTS
Nonoxynol	Delfen, Koromex, Emko, Because	Foam	Adverse effects include irritation of vagina or penis. Possible association with congenital anomalies.
Nonoxynol	Ramses, Koromex II-A, Conceptrol Disposable, Gynol II*	Jelly	
Nonoxynol	Conceptrol, Ortho-Cream*	Cream	Spermicide should be used prior to intercourse, but within 1 h. Should be reapplied for each episode of intercourse. Should not douche until at least 6 h after intercourse. Suppositories require 10 min to dissolve.
Nonoxynol	Intercept, Encare, Semicid	Suppository	
Nonoxynol	Ramses Extra	Condom with spermicidal lubricant	
Nonoxynol	Today	Sponge	
Octoxynol	Koromex II,* Ortho-Gynol,* Koromex II*	Jelly	

*For use with a diaphragm.

fluid retention involving the renin-angiotensin system. Reid and Yen (1981) theorize that premenstrual tension is a multifactorial neuroendocrine problem, possibly involving aldosterone, dopamine, estrogen, prolactin, and vasopressin.

Clinical Pharmacology and Therapeutics

Because the etiology of premenstrual syndrome is unknown, specific therapy is not available. Treatment should be individualized to alleviate the symptoms experienced by a particular woman. Pain and discomfort associated with PMS may be alleviated by the use of aspirin or acetaminophen in analgesic doses (Chap. 17).

Combination birth control pills with progestogenic dominance may be tried if there are no contraindications for use in a particular patient (e.g., Norlestrin 1 mg, Demulin, Ovral; Table 46-11). Their use may alleviate symptoms in some but may exacerbate symptoms, especially fluid retention, in other women. The use of the minipill (progesterone-only birth control pill) and phasic combination birth control pills have not yet been evaluated for use in premenstrual syndrome.

The use of vitamin therapy for premenstrual syndrome appears no better than placebo therapy. One possible exception suggested by O'Brien (1982) is the use of **pyridoxine** (50 mg twice daily from day 14 until menses) if a woman is experiencing significant psychologic symptoms. **Benzodiazepines** and **meprobamate** have been used for severe anxiety, tension, and irritability associated with this syndrome. Severe depression may require antidepressant therapy. If benzodiazepines, meprobamate, or antidepressants are used for psychologic symptoms associated with premenstrual syndrome, the patient must be periodically evaluated for drug effectiveness and adverse effects.

Individuals experiencing edema, abdominal bloating, or increased weight may benefit from short-term diuretic therapy (2 or 3 days), but the therapeutic benefits must be cautiously weighed against potential side effects including electrolyte disturbances. Nonprescription menstrual products containing diuretics are available. (See related discussion under Dysmenorrhea.) Only a few good clinical trials have evaluated the effectiveness of diuretics in this syndrome. If diuretic therapy is needed, an aldosterone antagonist such as **spironolactone** (25 to 100 mg/day) or low doses of a thiazide diuretic (e.g., **hydrochlorothiazide**, 25 to 50 mg/day) should be considered. Diuretic therapy should be initiated 3 days prior to the expected menses. Patients suffering from premenstrual syndrome should also be advised to reduce dietary salt intake prior to their menses, which may help to decrease premenstrual edema.

Severe breast symptoms unrelieved by other therapeutic measures may be alleviated using **bromocriptine mesylate** (Parlodel) 5 mg at bedtime on days 10 to 26 of the menstrual cycle. Side effects most commonly associated with bromocriptine therapy include nausea, dizziness, syncope, and possible hypotension. Long-term therapy with high-dose brom-

ocriptine (20 to 100 mg daily) has been associated with pulmonary infiltrates and pleural effusions. Bromocriptine is further discussed in this chapter under Lactation suppression and in Chap. 33, "Neurologic Disorders."

Dysmenorrhea

Dysmenorrhea, pain at the time of menstruation, may be characterized by lower abdominal cramping, headaches, dizziness, nausea, vomiting, and backaches. In most cases, dysmenorrhea is most severe on the first day of the menstrual cycle and is incapacitating in a small percentage of women. Dysmenorrhea may be a symptom of an underlying pelvic problem (secondary dysmenorrhea) or may occur in the absence of any pelvic disease (primary dysmenorrhea). Increased concentrations of prostaglandins (which enhance uterine contractility) and their metabolites have been measured in the menstrual fluid, endometrium and peripheral circulation of women diagnosed as having primary dysmenorrhea. Therefore, the use of drugs which inhibit prostaglandin synthesis may decrease symptoms associated with dysmenorrhea. Many women with dysmenorrhea also suffer from the premenstrual syndrome.

Clinical Pharmacology and Therapeutics

After an anatomic cause for the dysmenorrhea has been ruled out, the treatment of dysmenorrhea is directed at the symptoms of pain and discomfort. The products most often used are analgesics such as aspirin or acetaminophen. Aspirin is an inhibitor of prostaglandin synthesis, while the effects of acetaminophen on prostaglandin synthesis are debated. Therapy with these agents should be started the day prior to the expected menses.

Many of the nonprescription, over-the-counter (OTC) preparations (Table 46-13) that are used for the treatment of dysmenorrhea also contain a diuretic in addition to the sample analgesics. The diuretics in OTC products are **caffeine**, **pamabron**, and **ammonium chloride** which have not been proved to be clinically effective. Many patients with symptoms of premenstrual edema respond well with low doses of thiazide diuretics (e.g., **hydrochlorothiazide**, 25 to 50 mg). The OTC preparations also contain antihistamines that are designed for their sedative effect, but these are usually present in doses one-third to one-eighth what is normally required for this effect. There are no supportive clinical data which show that these combination preparations are any more effective than the simple analgesics.

Patients whose symptoms are not relieved by nonprescription analgesics may be tested on one of the nonsteroidal anti-inflammatory agents (see Chap. 26). **Ibuprofen** (Motrin) and **mefenamic acid** (Ponstel) have been approved by the FDA for the treatment of primary dysmenorrhea. Many of the other agents have received favorable support of their efficacy in the treatment of primary dysmenorrhea in various clinical studies. Ibuprofen is available without prescription as Advil and Nuprin.

NURSING PROCESS RELATED TO PERIMENSTRUAL SYMPTOMS

Assessment

The history obtained from the woman with dysmenorrhea should include information about the type, duration, incidence, initial onset, and pattern of pain, as well as the measures which have been used to control the pain, how successful these measures have been, and whether any allergies are present, especially to aspirin. The amount of absenteeism from school or work caused by dysmenorrhea is also significant. Since women with dysmenorrhea often experience the premenstrual syndrome caused by fluid retention prior to menstruation, the nurse should ask the patient about backache, abdominal distention, breast tenderness, edema, headache, fainting, premenstrual weight gain, insomnia, irritability, and nervousness. The woman's knowledge about the physiology of menstruation and her attitude toward this physiologic function may be important. There is some indication that those who lack understanding about menstruation or who consider it to be a "curse" or "dirty" have a higher incidence of dysmenorrhea.

The assessment should include an analysis of total health habits including diet, rest and sleep, physical activity, and posture. Anemia, constipation, poor nutritional intake, sedentary occupations, overexertion, fatigue, and poor posture are correlated with primary dysmenorrhea.

The woman experiencing dysmenorrhea should undergo a thorough physical checkup, including a pelvic examination, to screen out tumors, endometriosis, and malpositioned uterus.

Management

The patient with dysmenorrhea is often a young woman seeking entry into the health care system as an adult for the first time. Empathy and understanding are necessary in the management of this patient since problems associated with sexuality and reproductive function are very personal. The young woman's experience at this time may influence future health-illness attitudes, patterns of usage of the health care system, and compliance. This is a good time to stress health habits which may improve her well-being and decrease the dysmenorrhea.

If the woman with dysmenorrhea is taught to drink a hot beverage, take a nonprescription analgesic as the symptoms begin, and lie down and rest for an hour while putting heat to the abdomen, the discomfort may be controlled. When nonprescription analgesics are no longer effective, nonsteroidal anti-inflammatory agents are prescribed. The patient should be well informed about the adverse effects of these agents. All patients should be discouraged from using medications prescribed for others or sharing their medications for dysmenorrhea with friends. Occasionally an analgesic containing **codeine** must be prescribed to control pain.

Decreasing caffeine consumption as well as alcohol, salt, and nicotine usage during the second half of the menstrual cycle often helps to minimize premenstrual tension.

Evaluation

Subjective reports by the patient provide the primary basis for evaluating the effectiveness of the management of dysmenorrhea. However, objective observation of weight gain, moods, absenteeism, and edema will aid in reviewing the treatment of both premenstrual tension syndrome and dysmenorrhea.

TOXIC SHOCK SYNDROME

Toxic shock syndrome (TSS) is an illness associated with use of internal sanitary products (tampons) during menstruation that occurs in young and otherwise healthy women. The syndrome is characterized by an abrupt onset of hypotension (a systolic blood pressure lower than 90 mmHg), fever (at least 38.8°C), and rash (most prominent on the palms of the hands and soles of the feet; it is diffuse erythematous, macular, and sunburnlike; it later desquamates). Other symptoms may include vomiting or diarrhea, myalgia, renal or he-

TABLE 46-13 Over-the-Counter Menstrual Products

TRADE NAME	Ingredients (mg)			
	ANALGESIC	DIURETIC	ANTIHISTAMINE	OTHER
Cope	Aspirin (421)	Caffeine (32)		Magnesium hydroxide (50), aluminum hydroxide (25)
Midol	Aspirin (454)	Caffeine (32.4)		Cinnemedrine HCl (14.2)
Pamprin	Acetaminophen (325)	Pamabron (25)	Pyrilamine maleate (12.5)	
Sunril Premenstrual	Acetaminophen (300)	Pamabron (25)	Pyrilamine maleate (12.5)	
Maximum Cramp Relief Formula	Acetaminophen (500)	Pamabron (25)	Pyrilamine maleate (15)	

patic insufficiency, thrombocytopenia, disorientation, and mucous membrane inflammation. These symptoms occur during the menstrual period or within 48 h afterward.

The federal Food and Drug Administration had made several recommendations to women who menstruate. To eliminate any risk of developing toxic shock syndrome, women should avoid the use of tampons entirely. Women who have not had toxic shock syndrome are at a very low risk of developing it and probably do not need to change their use of internal sanitary products. They must, however, change them four to six times each day. If a woman chooses to use tampons, she should alternate their use with sanitary napkins. Any woman developing the symptoms of toxic shock syndrome should seek medical care immediately and stop the use of tampons. Once a woman has had toxic shock syndrome, she is at a much higher risk of developing it again.

Clinical Pharmacology and Therapeutics

Since there is a strong association between TSS and the recovery of *Staphylococcus aureus* from vaginal cultures, it has been hypothesized that prolonged tampon use may promote vaginal colonization with this organism. Treatment is directed at the severe manifestations such as shock, renal or hepatic failure, and adult respiratory distress syndrome. Antibiotics are used; the *S. aureus* isolates are susceptible to those antibiotics generally used for the organism except for penicillin G and ampicillin. Corticosteroids have been employed, but their value in TSS has not been established.

VAGINITIS

Vaginitis is an inflammation of the vulva and vaginal epithelium, a manifestation of an underlying problem (irritation, allergy, or infection). It can occur at any age and affects most women at some time during their lives. The client may have an abnormal vaginal discharge (leukorrhea) with no other symptoms; but she may also present with itching, dyspareunia, or perineal irritation. The most common microorganisms causing vaginitis are *Candida albicans, Trichomonas vaginalis,* and *Gardnerella vaginale* (formerly *Haemophilus vaginalis*).

Clinical Pharmacology and Therapeutics

Douching, in most cases, is unnecessary; however, in the treatment of vaginitis, the use of a mild acetic acid (vinegar) douche may give symptomatic relief. Vinegar douche (¼% acetic acid) is prepared by using 2 tbsp (30 mL) of vinegar diluted in 1 L of water. If the itching and irritation associated with vaginitis are severe, they may be controlled by using a topical corticosteroid cream with or without antibacterial or antifungal agents.

Use of nonprescription feminine hygiene products (i.e., perfumed douches and deodorants) can aggravate or even cause vaginitis. These products contain a wide variety of astringents, antimicrobials, local anesthetics, antiseptics, proteolytic enzymes, counterirritants, and buffers. No studies have been conducted to substantiate the claims that these ingredients are beneficial or even to establish the optimum pH for such preparations. Nurses can inform women that these products are of questionable value and that they carry the risk of allergy or chemical irritation. When there are signs of infection, women should be advised to discontinue all such products and to seek the advice of a qualified practitioner, since the treatment of infection should be based on an accurate diagnosis of the causative organism and specific antimicrobial therapy.

Candida albicans Vaginitis   *Candida albicans* is found in the normal vaginal flora but factors such as broad-spectrum antibiotic therapy, corticosteroid therapy, oral contraceptive usage, pregnancy, cancer, and diabetes mellitus may predispose the patient to moniliasis (*Candida albicans* overgrowth). The client may complain of itching (which may be severe) and have a thick, white, cottage-cheese-like vaginal discharge and inflamed external genitalia.

To treat *Candida albicans vaginitis,* **nystatin** (Mycostatin) 100,000-U vaginal tablets may be inserted vaginally once or twice daily for 14 days (longer for persistent infections). The pregnant patient may need a 3-week course of therapy. If the woman is near term, therapy may be continued until delivery. Alternative antifungal agents (see Chap. 29 and Table 46-14) include **miconazole nitrate** (Monistat-7), **gentian violet**, and **clotrimazole** (Gyne-Lotrimin). Miconazole vaginal cream or clotrimazole vaginal preparations are now considered by most clinicians to be the treatment of choice for candidal vaginitis in nonpregnant women. Both of these agents appear to be as effective as nystatin when used nightly for 7 days, a shorter time course than usually required by nystatin. Gentian violet, used in concentrations of 0.5 to 1.0% as a cream, suppository, or gel, is also effective but has the disadvantage of staining clothes. A more acceptable dosage form of gentian violet is found in impregnated tampons (Genapex). These are inserted vaginally once or twice daily. In most cases a moist, warm environment favors the growth of *Monilia*. The client, therefore, should be warned against wearing tight-fitting, unventilated undergarments (e.g., nylon panties and panty hose).

Trichomonas vaginalis Vaginitis   *Trichomonas* is a sexually transmitted disease. The female client may complain of severe vulvar itching, a thin, greenish-white vaginal discharge, and an increased frequency of urination; but she may also be asymptomatic. The infection is diagnosed by finding motile flagellated trichomonads on a saline wet-mount slide. The treatment of the trichomonas infection is with **metronidazole** (Flagyl) given 500 mg orally bid for 5 days, or with 2 g orally at one time. The latter is useful for the noncompliant client. The male sexual partner should be treated with 250 mg of metronidazole bid for 10 days. The female should be instructed to refrain from sexual intercourse during treatment or the male should use a condom. The adverse effects of metronidazole include nausea, vomiting, and a metallic taste in the mouth. The patient should be warned against consuming alcohol as it may produce an disulfiram-like effect (nausea, flushing, dizziness). The drug should not be used during the first trimester of pregnancy, and it is secreted in breast milk.

Gardnerella vaginale Vaginitis *Gardnerella vaginale* is transmitted primarily by sexual contact and is the causative organism in 90 percent of nonspecific vaginitis. The female client may complain of vaginal itching, vaginal discharge (white to gray-green in color) with a foul odor, as well as pain on urination and with sexual intercourse.

Gardnerella is treated locally using a sulfonamide-con-

taining vaginal cream listed in Table 46-14. In many cases it may be necessary to use systemic antimicrobial agents such as ampicillin, 500 mg qid for 10 days, or **metronidazole**, 500 mg bid for 7 days. Both sexual partners may need treatment. Condoms should be used if intercourse is performed during treatment or if symptoms are present.

NURSING PROCESS RELATED TO VAGINITIS

The nursing process for vaginitis is outlined in Table 46-15.

TABLE 46-14 Vaginal Antimicrobials

INGREDIENT(S)	TRADE NAME	DOSAGE FORM	INDICATIONS	USUAL DOSE
Nystatin	Mycostatin, Nilstat, others	Vaginal tablets	Moniliasis (*Candida albicans* vulvavaginitis)	1 tablet (100,000 U) daily for 2 weeks
Miconazole nitrate	Monistat 7	Vaginal cream	As above	1 applicatorful at bedtime for 1 week
Clotrimazole	Gyne-Lotrimin, Mycelex G	Vaginal tablets, vaginal cream	As above	1–2 tablets or 1 applicatorful at bedtime for 1 to 2 weeks
Gentian violet	Genapax Hyva	Tampon Vaginal tablet	As above As above	1–2 each night As above
Sulfasoxazole	Koro-Sulf	Vaginal cream	*Gardnerella vaginale* vaginitis	1–2 applicatorfuls bid for 2 weeks
Sulfathiazole/sulfacetamide/ sulfabenzamide	Sultrin, Triple Sulfa, Trysul	Vaginal tablets, vaginal cream	As above	1 tablet or 1 applicatorful bid for 4 to 6 days
Sulfanilamide/amacrine*/ allantoin†	Cerves, AVC, Vagitrol, others	Vaginal suppositories, vaginal cream	As above	1 suppository or applicatorful of cream 1–2 times daily
Sulfasoxazole/amacrine*/ allantoin†	V.V.S., Vagilia, Cantri	Vaginal suppositories, vaginal cream	As above	1 suppository or applicatorful 1–2 times daily
Oxytetracycline/polymixin B	Terramycin with Polymixin B sulfate	Vaginal tablets	Mixed infections including gram-negative organisms and *Chlamydia trachomatis*	1 tablet twice daily
Oxyquinolone*/alkyl aryl sulfonate‡/amacrine*/copper sulfate§/sodium lauryl sulfate‡	Triva Jel	Vaginal gel	Mixed infections including *Candida albicans, Trichomonas vaginalis,* and *Gardnerella vaginale.*	1 applicatorful 1–2 times daily
Dienestrol¶/sulfanilamide/ amacrine*/allantoin†	AVC/Dienestrol	Vaginal suppositories, vaginal cream	Atrophic vaginitis	1 applicatorful or suppository 1–2 times daily

*Amacrine and oxyquinolone benzoate are antiseptics.
†Allantoin debrides necrotic tissue.
‡Alkyl aryl sulfonate and sodium lauryl sulfate are wetting agents.
§Copper sulfate is a weak antifungal.
¶Dienestrol is an estrogen.

TABLE 46-15 Nursing Process Related to Vaginitis

Assessment	Management	Evaluation
Amount, color, character of vaginal discharge; onset; associated burning or urinary frequency; pruritus, pain.	Teach public and patients about need to treat vaginitis early and vigorously to avoid chronicity.	Note appearance of new or changed rash or discharge (may indicate allergy to drug).
Objective observation of vulva for inflammation.	Teach clients names of drugs, side effects, and proper dosage; stress compliance.	Amount, color, character of vaginal discharge should return to normal with resolution of associated symptoms.
Pelvic examination may cause bleeding and pain.	Stress the use of condom for intercourse during treatment.	Ascertain if sexual partners have sought evaluation.
Client may need emotional support and a pad to protect clothing after vaginal exam.	Teach patient to use medications such as douches or vaginal inserts.	
	Discomfort from vulvar irritation may be decreased by sodium bicarbonate sitz baths or application of sterile lubricant (e.g., K-Y Jelly).	
	Sexual partners should be referred for evaluation and treatment since they may contract the disease.	
	May need pads to protect clothing with some medications (e.g., gentian violet).	

ENDOMETRIOSIS

Endometriosis is characterized by the growth of endometrial tissue outside the uterus. Usually these cells are located in the pelvic cavity, but they may also be found in other sites in the body. There are many theories concerning the etiology of endometriosis, including retrograde menstruation, direct extension from the endometrium, lymphatic masses, and surgical transplantation.

Abnormal bleeding associated with endometriosis varies from 16 to 33 percent and is usually dysfunctional. Hypermenorrhea, menorrhagia, or intermenstrual bleeding may be seen. Other signs and symptoms associated with endometriosis include infertility, pelvic pain, abdominal pain, dyspareunia, and dysmenorrhea. In more severe cases, endometrial tissue may infiltrate the upper third of the vagina and give the gross appearance of a pelvic mass.

Clinical Pharmacology and Therapeutics

Symptomatic Treatment The pain associated with endometriosis may be relieved by nonprescription analgesics (**aspirin** or **acetaminophen**), but it may also be necessary to add a narcotic analgesic (e.g., **codeine**) for severe pain. Women who desire to become pregnant should be encouraged to do so as soon as possible, since pregnancy is a "natural" way to receive hormonal therapy. However, it is unfortunate that many patients experiencing endometriosis are infertile as well. Further therapy depends on the age of the patient, the severity of the endometriosis, and the desire for pregnancy.

Surgery Surgery may be indicated for the improvement of fertility, for the relief of intractable pain, for the treatment of pelvic obstruction or acute abdomen associated with endometriosis, or as a definitive measure after childbearing is completed. Some patients will need hormonal therapy in conjunction with surgery. This may be of value to women whose endometriosis was not totally resolved by surgery. Hormonal therapy may decrease the extent of the endometriosis prior to a surgical procedure.

Hormonal Therapy The goal of hormonal therapy is a quiescent endometrium with no cyclical changes in hormonal levels. Therapeutic results should include amenorrhea and the cessation of bleeding from endometrial plaques. The use of either an **estrogen-progesterone** combination product or **danazol** (Danocrine) may be beneficial in the hormonal treatment of endometriosis.

Estrogen-Progestogen Combination Therapy Combination estrogen-progesterone products (Table 46-5) increase estrogen and progesterone concentrations which suppress FSH and LH. Decreased concentrations of these pituitary gonadotropins prevent the ovarian production of estrogens and progesterone. The patient undergoes a pseudopregnancy with cessation of bleeding when estrogen-progesterone combination products are used continuously rather than on a cyclical basis. Since endogenous hormones, unfortunately, may also directly stimulate the endometrium, several months of therapy is needed to overcome this effect and to achieve beneficial results.

Fertility rates following estrogen-progesterone therapy range from 45 to 55 percent in women desiring pregnancy. Rates may be increased when hormonal therapy is combined with corrective surgical procedures.

Dosage varies from 5 to 20 mg of **norethynodrel** daily with the dosage being individualized on the basis of breakthrough bleeding and adverse effects. The duration of therapy should be continuous for 6 months or longer, depending on the severity of the endometriosis.

Danazol.   Mechanism of action   Danazol (Danocrine) is a testosterone and is classified as a gonadotropin inhibitor. Although there are controversies as to its exact mechanism of action, danazol may inhibit the release of the pituitary gonadotropins LH and FSH. It may also directly inhibit ovarian hormone production and may affect estrogen receptors in endometrial cells, resulting in decreased estrogenic effects. Normal and ectopic endometrial cells have decreased activity and become atrophic. Anovulation and amenorrhea occur, producing a pseudomenopausal state.

Fertility rates following danazol therapy range between 30 and 70 percent. Danazol may be more effective than combination estrogen-progesterone products in relieving dysmenorrhea, menstrual problems, and dyspareunia associated with endometriosis, but further clinical studies are needed to clarify the effectiveness of danazol in endometriosis.

Pharmacokinetics   Danazol is excreted in the urine. Its half-life is about 29 h.

Adverse effects   Adverse reactions to danazol are primarily due to its androgenic effects which include acne, oily skin and hair, decreased breast size, hoarseness, deepening of the voice, weight gain, edema of the lower extremities, and clitoris enlargement. Flushing, sweats, and amenorrhea may be attributed to pituitary gonadotropin inhibition. Other adverse effects include dizziness, headaches, mood changes, nervousness, muscle spasms, vaginal dryness, and vaginal itching. Hepatic dysfunction has also been reported.

Androgenic-associated adverse effects may be dose-dependent. Fewer androgenic effects have been noted at doses of 400 mg daily compared to 800 mg daily. Low doses (200 mg) have been associated with breakthrough bleeding.

Dosage   Danazol (Danocrine) dosage varies between 200 and 800 mg daily with 200 mg twice daily being the usual starting dosage. Danazol therapy averages 6 months (range of 3 to 9 months). Symptoms associated with endometriosis may dissipate before 6 months, but the underlying pathology associated with endometriosis clears less quickly. If a contraceptive method is desired, the patient should use a nonhormonal contraceptive method during danazol therapy.

NURSING PROCESS RELATED TO ENDOMETRIOSIS

Assessment
Assessment of the amount, character, and onset of pain and hypermenorrhea should be recorded as baseline data. Evidence of fertility and dyspareunia are also noted.

Management
The nurse should encourage exercise and use of mild analgesics (**acetaminophen**) where needed. If the woman chooses pregnancy as the treatment modality, emotional support of the couple is indicated, since infertility can delay or eliminate the desired outcome. When ovarian hormones are prescribed, the nursing process outlined in Table 46-7 is appropriate.

Evaluation
Decreased menstrual abnormality and pain reveal the effectiveness of therapy. Not only must the adverse physical reactions to drug therapy be evaluated, but also the client's psychologic state. Maintenance of a positive self-image may be difficult for the client when **danazol** causes virilizing effects or low fertility prevents pregnancy.

THE CLIMACTERIC AND MENOPAUSE

The *climacteric* is that phase in the life cycle of a woman which marks the end of her reproductive years, usually between the fifth and sixth decade of life. It is characterized by waning ovarian function and decreased estrogen concentrations. *Menopause* is the actual cessation of menstruation which occurs between ages 40 and 57 with a median age of 51 years. It is a normal, physiologic process that lasts approximately two years in most women. Menopause is considered complete when a woman has not had a menstrual period for 12 months.

The exact mechanisms of the climacteric and menopause are not currently known. It appears that with aging, there is decreased ovarian production of estrogen and progesterone. In response to low hormonal concentrations, especially that of estrogen, FSH and LH secretion from the pituitary is increased. Although the circulating concentrations of FSH and LH are high, there appears to be decreased ovarian response to these pituitary hormones. Estrogen concentrations remain low postmenopausally, with estrone being the primary estrogen. Estrone is produced in the liver, adrenals, adipose tissue, and circulatory system rather than in the ovaries.

Menopausal symptoms associated with low estrogen concentrations include vasomotor instability, genital atrophy, osteoporosis, and decreased secondary sexual characteristics. Other *nonspecific symptoms* such as anxiety, irritability, headaches, dizziness, insomnia, depression, and fatigue may be indirectly related to decreased estrogen production or possibly to the psychologic stress associated with menopausal changes. Some of these symptoms may also be dependent on sociocultural influences.

Clinical Pharmacology and Therapeutics

Estrogen replacement should be used only for those menopausal symptoms which respond to estrogen therapy, that is, vasomotor instability, atrophic vaginitis, and probably osteoporosis. Nonspecific symptoms usually do not respond to estrogen therapy, but vomiting, headaches, dizziness, night sweats, and palpitations associated with hot flashes may decrease as the vasomotor instability subsides.

When symptoms are not estrogen-related or when estrogens are contraindicated, other medications may be used. Relief from hot flashes and sweats may be obtained with the administration of antianxiety agents such as **diazepam** (Valium) 2 to 5 mg two to four times daily or **chlordiazepoxide** (Librium) 5 to 10 mg three to four times daily. These agents are, however, usually reserved primarily for anxiety symptoms and do not replace the emotional support that many women need during the climacteric phase of their lives.

Vasomotor Instabilty

Between 75 and 80 percent of postmenopausal women suffer from *vasomotor instability* ("hot flashes"), but only 15 percent will seek medical attention for this problem. Approximately 37 to 50 percent of women who have had bilateral oophorectomy will also suffer from vasomotor instability. Hot flashes usually occur in the early postmenopausal period and last approximately one to two years. Therefore, **estrogen** therapy for 6 months to 2 years with gradual tapering as symptoms decrease usually alleviates this problem.

Atrophic Vaginitis

Genital atrophy, which may involve the fallopian tubes, uterus, cervix, vagina, and vulva, appears to progressively worsen as estrogen concentrations decline. *Atrophic vaginitis* is the most troublesome symptom. Regular sexual intercourse may decrease vaginal atrophy in most women. Oral and topical **estrogens** (Table 46-3) may also be used to decrease vaginal atrophy and to decrease the susceptibility to vaginal infection by preventing thinning of the vaginal epithelium. They also tend to restore vaginal pH toward premenopausal levels, which helps to prevent infection. Topical estrogens may be indicated to avoid the systemic effects, but since they are absorbed through the vaginal mucosa and overdosage can result in high serum estrogen

concentrations, proper administration must be emphasized to the patient. Also, continuous estrogen prophylaxis postmenopausally is not indicated, since genital atrophy usually does not occur until the sixth decade of life. When atrophic vaginitis occurs, daily topical treatment is usually necessary for only 1 to 4 months, but it may be needed thereafter on an intermittent basis (1 to 3 times weekly) to maintain the vaginal mucosa.

Osteoporosis

Osteoporosis is a group of bone disorders characterized by a reduction of bone mass below that required for adequate mechanical support. The disease is often asymptomatic and is detected incidentally on chest x-ray. The most common symptoms are pain in the back and deformity of the spine. Pain occurs as a result of collapse of the vertebrae, which can result in decreased height and dorsal kyphosis with cervical lordosis ("dowager's hump"). Acute pain usually abates within a few weeks after the collapse-fracture, but chronic aching may persist. While the disease is associated with aging, its cause is unknown but appears to be multifactorial. Women appear to have at least a three times greater loss of bone mass after age 50 than men. Small-framed Caucasian women who undergo menopause early are the most prone to developing osteoporosis. Osteoporosis makes many women susceptible to fractures, with hip fractures causing the deaths of approximately 15,000 women annually.

The administration of exogenous **estrogens** may decrease the development of osteoporosis in postmenopausal women, because they decrease urinary calcium excretion, rate of bone resorption, and increase circulating levels of the active form of vitamin D. Since estrogens cannot restore skeletal mass which has been previously lost, estrogen therapy must begin prior to the onset of osteoporosis and may be initiated at menopause. It also appears that estrogens must be used long-term for this effect, because termination of therapy will result in rapid bone demineralization. Estrogen therapy for osteoporosis is controversial. The risks and benefits of such therapy must be carefully weighed for each patient. In addition to the general adverse effects of estrogens, postmenopausal women on estrogens are at significantly increased risk for endometrial cancer (unless they have had hysterectomies) and for gallbladder disease.

Other drugs which have been approved or investigated for use in osteoporosis in conjunction with estrogens, include calcium preparations, vitamin D, fluoride, and thiazide diuretics. **Calcium salts** in doses of 1.0 to 1.5 g/day of elemental calcium decrease bone reabsorption and increase calcium retention in some patients. Addition of vitamin D in doses of 25,000 to 50,000 IV once or twice weekly may be useful in patients with malabsorption. Active metabolites of vitamin D such as **calcifediol** (Calderol) and **calcitriol** (Rocaltrol) may be even more effective if used every day in doses of 20 to 100 μg and 0.25 μg, respectively. Serum and urinary calcium should be monitored every 3 to 6 months in patients on calcium and vitamin D. **Fluoride,** which becomes incorporated into the bone structure and may also increase new bone formation, has been used in moderate doses of 25 mg/day (in conjunction with calcium and vitamin D). Results of fluoride therapy are variable, and high doses can result in ligamentous calcification, neurologic symptoms from bone overgrowth, and formation of poorly mineralized bone. Because they decrease calcium excretion, **thiazide diuretics** have also been investigated in treating osteoporosis. **Calcitonin** from salmon (Calcimar) has been extensively investigated for use in osteoporosis because it retards bone resorption (see Chap. 35, "Endocrine Disorders").

Dosage and Scheduling of Estrogens in Menopause

A wide variety of conjugated and unconjugated natural estrogens, as well as synthetic estrogens have been used to treat menopause (Table 46-3). In treating the symptoms of menopause, estrogens are usually administered cyclically for 21 to 25 days each month to patients who have not undergone a hysterectomy. While the patient is off estrogen therapy, concentrations decrease allowing the body to partially withdraw from estrogenic effects, which is thought to decrease the risk of endometrial cancer. Estrogen dosages also should be low enough to avoid withdrawal bleeding or spotting while off medication, but high enough to control menopausal symptoms.

The drug of choice for the treatment of postmenopausal symptoms is **conjugated estrogens** (Premarin) 0.625 to 1.25 mg daily. Suggested daily starting doses of other agents are **esterified estrogens,** 0.625 to 1.25 mg; **diethylstilbestrol,** 0.2 to 0.5 mg; **ethinyl estradiol,** 0.02 to 0.05 mg. The length of estrogen replacement therapy is dependent on the symptom requiring treatment (see above).

A truly estrogen-free interval may be unattainable because estrogens are stored in adipose tissue and released gradually. Therefore, progestogens may be given for possible antiestrogenic protective effects on the breast and the endometrium by physiologically blocking the stimulating effects of estrogens. Progestogens should be administered cyclically with estrogens for the last 5 to 10 days each month. **Medroxyprogesterone acetate,** 5 to 10 mg, or **norethindrone acetate,** 1 to 10 mg, may be used to deciduate and eventually slough the endometrial lining.

For the woman who has had a hysterectomy, there is less agreement about the need for cyclic estrogen therapy or for counteraction with a progestogen. If a patient is unable to take oral estrogen therapy daily, a long-acting estrogen (**chlorotrianisene,** 12 to 25 mg once daily) or an injectable estrogen, such as **estradiol valerate** in oil (10 to 20 mg every 4 weeks) or **estradiol cypionate** in oil (1 to 5 mg every 3 or 4 weeks), may be used. Since androgens are of little value in postmenopausal osteoporosis, fixed estrogen-androgen and estrogen-sedative combinations are rarely indicated in treating the symptoms of menopause.

NURSING PROCESS RELATED TO MENOPAUSE

Assessment

Since menopause has psychosocial as well as physical implications, the nurse should assess the meaning of the changes to the woman, her family, and friends as well as the actual physical manifestations. Concurrent life events that may contribute to the woman's psychosocial well-being should be considered. The woman's understanding of the physiology of menopause should be ascertained, since this may affect her reactions to the changes and compliance to the therapeutic approach.

Subjective data about the incidence and severity of symptoms including hot flashes and excessive perspiration and detailed information about other symptoms such as insomnia, headaches, nervousness, depression, and palpitations should be gathered. Further, painful intercourse, pruritus, and burning are signs of atrophic vaginitis which are parts of the syndrome. A thorough history and a physical examination, including laboratory, x-ray, and electrocardiogram (ECG) testing appropriate to the patient's symptoms, should be done to rule out organic and functional disorders. A maturation index performed on a smear taken from the wall of the vagina will indicate the patient's systemic estrogen status and give an indication of the potential effectiveness of replacement therapy.

Management

Emphasis on good health practices and an understanding attitude must underlie the approach to the treatment of the woman experiencing the climacteric. When the woman is coping poorly with the developmental changes of the life period, she may need to be referred for counseling.

Since overfatigue may aggravate the symptoms of menopause, physical activity and good nutrition must be balanced to ensure an overall sense of well-being. The need for a yearly physical examination with a Pap smear should be emphasized to the client and is most important if estrogens are prescribed. If replacement hormones are given after menopause, the client should be informed that the pseudomenstruation which occurs occasionally when the drug is withdrawn each month does not mean regained fertility and that bleeding should be reported to the physician or nurse for immediate evaluation or change in dosage.

The woman should be well informed of the potential dangers and advantages of hormone therapy. If the estrogen replacement therapy is to be discontinued, dosage should be gradually tapered to avoid eliciting menopausal symptoms.

The patient may need instruction on the method of application of hormone preparations used locally to treat atrophic vaginitis. She and her partner may require emotional support and reassurance that sexual function can continue to be satisfying for many years after menopause.

Evaluation

The degree of control of vasomotor symptoms is an important determinant of the effectiveness of therapy. Periodic weight checks and evaluation for peripheral edema will help in the detection of sodium and water retention. Yearly breast and pelvic examination with Pap smear is important for the maintenance of the patient's health.

INFERTILITY

Infertility can be defined as a failure to achieve conception during one or more years of intercourse without using any contraceptive measures. It is estimated that between 10 and 15 percent of couples in the United States are infertile. Infertility can be related to male factors in approximately 40 percent of the cases. Infertility in the female may be due to ovarian failure (10 to 15 percent), uterine pathology (20 to 30 percent), and cervical factors (5 percent). In 10 to 20 percent of infertile couples there is no definable cause of the infertility. Drugs to promote ovulation are useful in some cases of infertility.

Drugs Used to Stimulate Ovulation

The anterior pituitary secretes two gonadotropins, follicle-stimulating hormone (FSH) and luteinizing hormone (LH), which, along with estrogen and progesterone, affect ovulation and the functions of the corpus luteum. Another gonadotropin that is secreted by the placenta is human chorionic gonadotropin (HCG). Pharmacologic management of infertility involves the induction of ovulation by using agents which increase the levels of LH and FSH or simulate the effects of these hormones.

Clomiphene Citrate (Clomid)

Clomiphene is useful in women who are anovulatory with depressed gonadotropins but who have a functioning pituitary-ovarian system. Women who have withdrawal bleeding after a progestogen withdrawal test (a test for adequacy of estrogen output) will be more likely to ovulate in response to clomiphene therapy. Clomiphene has been useful in cases of dysfunctional uterine bleeding, oligomenorrhea, Stein-Leventhal syndrome, and secondary amenorrhea.

Mechanism of Action   Ovulation can occur in response to cyclic clomiphene therapy through increased production of the pituitary gonadotropins LH and FSH which stimulate the maturation of an ovarian follicle, ovulation, and the subsequent development and function of the corpus luteum. Clomiphene binds to estrogenic receptors in the cell, decreasing estrogenic effects. Estrogenic levels seem low, and the hypothalamus and pituitary respond by increasing the secretion of FSH and LH.

Pharmacokinetics   Clomiphene is readily absorbed after oral administration. It is excreted primarily in the feces and undergoes enterohepatic circulation.

Adverse Effects   Although no deleterious effects of clomiphene on the human fetus have been proved, clomiphene should be avoided if the patient is pregnant. To prevent its use in early pregnancy, the patient should monitor her basal body temperature (BBT) during therapy. An elevation in BBT without subsequent menstruation indicates pregnancy may have occurred.

Clomiphene can cause ovarian enlargement and cyst formation especially at high doses (100 to 200 mg daily) or with prolonged therapy. Ovarian enlargement and cysts usually regress spontaneously when the drug is discontinued. If an additional course of therapy is desired, lower doses should be used. Another complication of clomiphene therapy is an increased incidence of multiple births. The couple should be counseled about this possibility prior to therapy.

Ophthalmologic problems including blurred vision and scintillating scotomata (spots or flashes of light) appear dose-related. Other adverse effects include hot flashes similar to those experienced during menopause, nausea, vomiting, abdominal distention, skin rashes, breast discomfort, headaches, dizziness, vertigo, and abdominal uterine bleeding.

Dosage   Clomiphene citrate (Clomid) is usually started on the fifth day of the menstrual cycle, if present, as 50 mg daily for 5 days. If ovulation does not occur, the 5-day course may be repeated twice at monthly intervals using 100 mg daily. At the usual recommended doses, ovulation occurs in 70 percent and pregnancy in 30 percent of women using clomiphene. Investigationally, 5-day courses of up to 200 mg daily have been used on a monthly basis until pregnancy was achieved (or up to 5 to 9 cycles of therapy). Higher dosages have resulted in ovulatory rates of 96 percent and conception in 73 percent of women. **Estradiol benzoate** 1 mg IM has been used in conjunction with clomiphene in women who failed to ovulate after long-term, high-dose therapy.

Menotropins (Pergonal)

Menotropins or human postmenopausal gonadotropins (HMG), when given in sequence with HCG (see below), have proved effective in the treatment of functional anovulation such as primary amenorrhea, secondary amenorrhea, or polycystic ovaries, where primary ovarian failure has been excluded. The combination of HCG and HMG is also indicated for the stimulation of spermatogenesis in men with primary or secondary hypogonadotropic hypogonadism.

Mechanism of Action Human postmenopausal gonadotropin (HMG) is a purified preparation of gonadotropins obtained from the urine of postmenopausal women. It is standardized to contain 75 IU of FSH and 75 IU of LH. Treatment with HMG causes only follicular growth and maturation. For ovulation to occur, HCG must be given after HMG therapy.

Pharmacokinetics HMG is effective only if given by injection. The two components, LH and FSH, have biphasic half-lives. For LH these are 20 min and 4 h, while for FSH the half-lives are 4 h and 70 h. Little of the unchanged hormones is found in the urine, suggesting that they undergo extensive metabolism.

Adverse Effects Adverse effects in women include ovarian enlargement with or without pain, which usually subsides with the discontinuation of therapy. Hyperstimulation syndrome characterized by sudden ovarian enlargement occurs in 1.3 percent of women treated with HMG. It may occur with or without ascites and pleural effusions. If the syndrome occurs, therapy should be stopped and the patient hospitalized. Multiple births occur in 20 percent of the patients. Gynecomastia and erythrocytosis have been reported in men receiving HMG therapy.

Dosage The dosage of menotropins for functional anovulation must be individualized for each patient, but it is recommended that the initial dosage should be one ampul of menotropins (Pergonal) IM (containing 75 IU of FSH and 75 IU of LH) daily for 9 to 12 days. One day after the last dose of menotropins, 10,000 U of HCG should be given IM.

Therapy can be monitored by signs of estrogen activity that are indicative of follicular development. These changes include the appearance and volume of cervical mucus and spinnbarkheit elasticity and ferning of the cervical mucus. Indications of ovulation (without pregnancy) are related to progesterone production and can be monitored by a rise in basal body temperature (BBT), changes in cervical mucus pattern, vaginal cytology, increased elasticity of cervical mucus, increased urinary pregnanediol concentration, or menstruation after elevated BBT.

If ovulation occurs without pregnancy at the above dosage level, this dosage schedule should be continued for two more treatment cycles. If the patient is still not pregnant, the dosage may be doubled to two ampuls of HMG with the same dosage of HCG. This course of therapy may then be repeated for two more treatment cycles. If the patient is still not pregnant, no higher dosage schedule is recommended. When using this form of therapy, couples should be encouraged to have intercourse daily starting one day prior to HCG administration.

Human Chorionic Gonadotropin (HCG)

In addition to its use in the treatment of infertility, HCG is also used in the treatment of prepubertal cryptorchidism and has been used as adjunctive treatment of obesity. There is no evidence to support its effectiveness in the treatment of obesity.

Mechanism of Action HCG is a polypeptide hormone obtained from the placenta. It is composed of α and β subunits. The α subunit is similar to the α subunit of the pituitary hormones (FSH and LH) and thyroid-stimulating hormone (TSH). Its action is similar to that of LH, but it appears to have some FSH activity. In females it causes the corpus luteum to produce progesterone, while in males it causes the testes to produce androgens.

Pharmacokinetics HCG is effective only if administered by injection. It has a biphasic half-life of 1 and 23 h. A major portion of chorionic gonadotropins is excreted in the urine unchanged.

Adverse Effects Headaches, irritability, restlessness, depression, fatigue, edema, gynecomastia, and pain at the site of the injection have been reported with HCG usage. More severe adverse effects include sudden ovarian hyperstimulation, ascites, pleural effusion, arterial thromboembolism, and rupture of ovarian cysts. HCG and HMG should be administered by physicians experienced in fertility problems.

Dosage HCG is available under many trade names including Pregnyl, APL Secules, Chorex, Follutein, and Libigen. It is available as a lyophilized powder which must be reconstituted according to individual manufacturer's directions. When used in conjunction with HMG to stimulate ovulation, HCG 10,000 U is administered IM (see above).

NURSING PROCESS RELATED TO INFERTILITY

Table 46-16 outlines the nursing process in the pharmacologic treatment of infertility.

TABLE 46-16   Nursing Process in Pharmacologic Management of Infertility

Assessment	Management	Evaluation
Carry out a complete physical evaluation of both partners. Assess psychosocial status of the couple.	Patient education is very important: Advise when to take the drug and when coitus should occur. Discuss side effects of the drugs and the incidence of multiple births. Make sure the patient knows the signs of pregnancy (since fertility drugs are contraindicated in pregnancy) and is aware of the need for close medical supervision. Teach how to monitor basal body temperature (BBT). Tell the patient to avoid driving if vision blurred by clomiphene. Give written instructions. Support relationship between the physician and the couple.	Occurrence of pregnancy—evaluate for twins. Look at incidence and toleration of side effects. Evaluate psychologic response of couple to success or failure of therapy. Give pelvic exam to detect ovarian enlargement or cystic rupture.

TERMINATION OF PREGNANCY

Methods of termination of pregnancy include vacuum curettage, dilatation and curettage (D and C), hysterectomy, hysterotomy, intraamniotic injection of a hypertonic saline solution, and the use of prostaglandin compounds.

Prostaglandins

Prostaglandins are compounds with similar chemical structure, which fall into several main classes: PGA, PGB, PGG, PGD, PGE, and PGF. The prostaglandins of the E and F series are sometimes called the primary prostaglandins. They are the most prevalent, and the most research has been done with them. Most cells are capable of making prostaglandins from essential fatty acid precursors, most commonly arachidonic acid (see Chap. 26). The effects of the various prostaglandins are complex, affecting the reproductive organs, heart, clotting, intestinal secretion, blood vessels, and endocrine glands. Prostaglandins cause smooth muscle contraction. Prostaglandin E_1 and PGE_2 have a more potent uterine contraction effect than $PGF_{2\alpha}$. In contrast to oxytocin, they can induce labor if given at any time during pregnancy. Prostaglandins also cause luteolysis, which can terminate early pregnancy.

Mechanism of Action   Although prostaglandins are found in almost every cell, their role in reproduction physiology and pathology has not been clearly established. Even the mechanism by which they exert their effects is not clear.

Proposed mechanisms include a membrane-bound prostaglandin receptor, induction of changes in metabolic functions via a cycle adenosine monophosphate (cAMP), or a calcium-mediated system. Prostaglandins stimulate the uterus to contract enough to expel the products of conception.

Pharmacokinetics   Enzymes that catalyze the degradation of prostaglandins are prominent in the lung but are also present in the spleen, kidney, intestine, liver, and adipose tissue. Metabolism of prostaglandins is a two-step process. The first step, catalyzed by prostaglandin-specific enzymes, is rapid and results in an inactive metabolite. Degradation is completed by enzymes which catalyze the oxidation of most fatty acids.

Adverse Effects   The most common adverse reactions to prostaglandins are related to their smooth muscle stimulating effects, including nausea, vomiting, diarrhea, headache, and bronchial constriction. Other adverse effects include hyperpyrexia, anaphylaxis, decreased blood pressure, chills, dizziness, and abdominal cramping. Administration of prostaglandin E_2 as a suppository (**dinoprostone**) decreases the systemic effects. The abortion may also be complicated by blood loss, uterine infection, disseminated intravascular coagulation, perforation of the cervix, and hypovolemic shock.

Dosage and Preparations   Available preparations, indications, and recommended dosages are shown in Table 46-17.

Adjunctive Therapeutics

Laminaria

The laminaria, a small stick of compressed seaweed, is utilized to dilate the cervix. Placed through the endocervical canal, it is relatively painless to insert, is very effective, and dilates both the internal and external cervical os. It takes about 6 h to dilate the cervix, and use of a laminaria decreases the incidence of cervical tears.

There are two disadvantages to the use of a laminaria:

1. It requires an initial visit to insert it and a second visit to remove it and perform the abortion.
2. There is a higher incidence of endometriosis.

Oxytocin

Intravenous oxytocin (Pitocin, Syntocinon) is utilized to facilitate uterine contractions and may cause termination of pregnancy independent of other methods. It is commonly utilized with prostaglandin compounds and the D and C method. Oxytocin increases the incidence of cervical laceration, the drug cost of the procedure, and the potential for delivery of a live fetus.

NURSING PROCESS RELATED TO PHARMACOLOGIC TERMINATION OF PREGNANCY

Assessment

The nurse must take a complete history of the client who is to undergo an abortion, including dates of last menstrual period, previous pregnancies, history of previous surgeries, contraceptive history and future contraceptive plans, allergies including drugs, and current drug use. A complete physical examination including a pelvic exam should be performed. Laboratory data which must be obtained include a hemoglobin or hematocrit, Rh typing, and a gonorrhea screening. History of hypertension, epilepsy, clotting disorders, and asthma should be noted, as these may predispose the patient to the adverse effects of prostaglandins.

Management

As the decision to terminate a pregnancy is complex and emotionally draining for many women, preabortion counseling should be performed prior to therapeutic abortion. The environment in which the abortion takes place must be supportive, and the client should receive an explanation of the procedure and reports of its progression. She should be informed that the adverse effects of **prostaglandins**, such as nausea, vomiting, diarrhea, cramps, and headache are transient. Prophylactic antiemetics and antidiarrheic drugs may be given. The woman should remain supine for 10 min after a prostaglandin suppository is given to avoid expulsion. Since the physiology of abortion is analogous to delivery, especially in the second trimester, the woman will need similar nursing care including pain control, relief of anxiety, and protection from infection.

Verbal and written discharge instructions should be given. The client should be instructed that nothing is to be placed in the vagina until all bleeding is stopped. She should be encouraged to rest after the procedure and take it easy for several days.

The three most common complications of abortion include infection, retained products of conception or uterine blood clots, and excessive bleeding. The client must be instructed to contact the health care provider if she experiences cramping (from mild to severe), fever, increased vaginal discharge (ranging from bleeding to foul odor), and increased pelvic discomfort.

The client is to be instructed to discuss resumption of intercourse and methods of birth control with her health care provider. The method of birth control must be specific for the client and a method with which she can comply.

TABLE 46-17 Prostaglandins Used to Terminate Pregnancy

AGENT	TRADE NAME	DOSAGE FORM	INDICATIONS	USUAL DOSE
Dinoprostone (prostaglandin E_2)	Prostin E_2	Suppository	Termination of pregnancy in weeks 12–20; missed abortion or intrauterine death through week 28.	One 20-mg suppository high in the vagina. Repeat at intervals of 3–5 h.
Dinoprost tromethamine (prostaglandin $F_{2\alpha}$)	Prostin F_2 alpha	Intraamniotic injection	Termination of pregnancy in weeks 16–20.	40 mg.
Carboprost tromethamin	Prostin/15M	IM injection	Termination of pregnancy in weeks 13–20. Failure of abortion by another method.	250 μg; repeat at intervals of 1.5–3.5 h.

Evaluation

The prostaglandin should produce expulsion in 10 to 24 h. Vital signs should be monitored frequently during the procedure and every 2 to 4 h in the postoperative period. Extent of bleeding should be evaluated with a pad count. Respiratory distress, persistent hyperpyrexia, and convulsions should be reported to the physician immediately. The nurse should note the occurrence of gastrointestinal symptoms and the effectiveness of prophylaxis or treatment of these. If the woman has an Rh-negative blood type **Rh₀(D) immune human globulin (RhoGAM)** should be administered.

HYPERTENSIVE DISEASES OF PREGNANCY

There are many complications of pregnancy, but some of the most serious are the hypertensive diseases during pregnancy. Hypertension occurs in approximately 5 percent of all pregnancies. These may be classified as chronic hypertension, gestational hypertension, preeclampsia, and eclampsia. A pregnant woman with chronic hypertension may also have a superimposed preeclampsia. Although each hypertensive disease occurring in pregnancy results in an elevated blood pressure, treatment will vary with each hypertensive entity.

A pregnant woman is considered to have *chronic hypertension* when her blood pressure is 140/90 mmHg or greater prior to pregnancy and within the first 20 weeks of pregnancy. A woman is considered to have *gestational hypertension* when she initially develops blood pressure of 140/90 mmHg or greater during the first 20 weeks of pregnancy. Usually the patient with gestational hypertension does not have proteinuria.

Preeclampsia is characterized by the triad of edema, proteinuria, and elevated blood pressure. This type of hypertension is most common in primigravidas and is initially detected after the first 20 weeks of pregnancy. It may be divided into mild, moderate, and severe types, depending on the signs and symptoms of the patient. Mild preeclampsia should be considered in a patient who initially has blood pressure lower than 140/90 mmHg but who subsequently has diastolic pressure increases of 20 mmHg or more. (The blood pressure should be sustained over a 6-h period while the patient is at bed rest.) Moderate preeclampsia should be considered in a patient who has blood pressure between 140/90 mmHg and 160/110 mmHg, proteinuria, and edema of the lower extremities. A rise in the diastolic blood pressure of 20 mmHg or more or a systolic rise of 30 mmHg or more may also be seen in the patient with moderate preeclampsia. Severe preeclampsia must be suspected in a pregnant woman who has a blood pressure greater than 160/110 mmHg on two occasions over a 6-h period while she is at bed rest. The patient will also have a significant proteinuria and may have a headache, visual disturbances, epigastric pain, and hyperactive deep tendon reflexes. Edema of the face, hands, and lower extremities is usually present. Oliguria, pulmonary edema, hyperuricemia, and hemoconcentration may also occur.

In *eclampsia* the patient characteristically presents with hypertension, proteinuria, edema, and seizures. The seizures may occur prior to delivery and/or postpartum. The patient may also have hyperactive deep tendon reflexes, oliguria, and tachypnea. She may be combative, disoriented, or stuporous.

Chronic Hypertension

Clinical Pharmacology and Therapeutics

The therapy plan for the pregnant woman with chronic hypertension differs from that of the woman who develops hypertension during pregnancy. Blood pressure control on a continuous basis throughout pregnancy is extremely important in the chronic hypertensive woman. Drugs should be selected which have the least teratogenic potential but which maintain good uterine blood flow to prevent intrauterine growth retardation and fetal distress. Drug selection may also depend on the medications needed for blood pressure control prior to pregnancy. The patient should be on the least number of medications which will keep her blood pressure under reasonable control. **Methyldopa** (Aldomet) and **hydralazine** (Apresoline) present only minimal risks for the fetus, appear to maintain an adequate blood supply to the uterus, and have only minimal adverse effects for the mother.

Thiazide diuretics should be used cautiously during pregnancy because they deplete the intravascular volume which could result in decreased cardiac output and uterine blood flow. **Propranolol** is usually not recommended during pregnancy because it could decrease cardiac output and lower uterine blood flow. It also has been shown to decrease fetal heart rate. In addition to drug therapy, the patient will benefit from increased bed rest and a high-protein diet. Refer to Chap. 40, "High Blood Pressure," regarding the pharmacology and dosages of antihypertensives.

Preeclampsia

Clinical Pharmacology and Therapeutics

The therapy plan for the patient with mild or moderate preeclampsia may include hospitalization, bed rest in the lateral recumbent position, and sedation. **Phenobarbital** 60 to 180 mg, daily or **hydroxyzine** (Vistaril) 200 to 400 mg daily are most commonly used for sedation. Benzodiazepines, such as **diazepam** (Valium), should be avoided for sedation due to possible adverse fetal effects (see Chap. 7). The use of magnesium sulfate or antihypertensive agents often will not be required.

Treatment of severe preeclampsia is aimed at stabilizing the patient, controlling the hypertension, and terminating the pregnancy as soon as it is suitable for the mother and fetus. The therapy plan will include all measures employed in the care of the mild and moderate preeclampsia patients with the addition of antihypertensive drugs and **magnesium sulfate**. **Hydralazine** (Apresoline) and **methyldopa** (Aldomet) are the agents of choice in the patient with severe preeclampsia. **Diazoxide** (Hyperstat), commonly used intravenously in acute hypertension when diastolic pressures are 120 mmHg or greater, must be used cautiously in the pregnant woman because diazoxide may cause unpredictable blood pressure responses and may also stop labor (see Chap. 40). Regional anesthetics used during delivery may also lower blood pressure. The delivery of the fetus will resolve the preeclampsia state in the mother.

Magnesium Sulfate (MgSO₄) Magnesium sulfate is used for anticonvulsant and mild antihypertensive effects when a patient will be delivered in the next 24 h. It also serves as a uterine relaxant and may counteract uterine tetany associated with the administration of oxytocics. The mechanism of action is thought to be a blockade of neuromuscular transmission.

Pharmacokinetics Magnesium is excreted by the kidney and may reach toxic levels if renal function is impaired. Given intravenously, onset of magnesium sulfate is nearly immediate, and effects persist for about 30 min. The onset of action is 1 h, and the duration of effect is 3 to 4 h with IM administration. Effects correlate with serum levels; effective anticonvulsant levels range from 2.5 to 7.5 meq/L (normal plasma magnesium is 1.5 to 3.0 meq/L). Deep tendon reflexes begin to diminish around 4.0 meq/L, and levels of 10 meq/L are potentially lethal (absent deep tendon reflexes, respiratory paralysis, heart block).

Adverse effects High serum levels of magnesium can cause flushing, sweating, flaccid paralysis, depressed reflexes, hypotension, and central nervous system paralysis. Respiratory depression can result in death or in fetal or maternal morbidity. Effects on the newborn infant include weak cry, hyporeflexia, respiratory depression, and flaccidity. Long-term effects on the child are under investigation. Intravenous administration of **calcium** will reverse signs of magnesium toxicity. If possible, magnesium sulfate should be discontinued at least 2 h prior to delivery.

Dosage Intravenous solutions of 1 to 4 g in 250 mL are administered at rates no faster than 3 mL/min (approximately 12 to 48 mg/min). Intramuscular dosage is 1 to 5 g up to six times daily as required, given deep into a large muscle mass. The drugs should be withheld or discontinued if patellar tendon ("knee jerk") reflexes are absent.

Eclampsia

Clinical Pharmacology and Therapeutics

The eclampsia patient may need drug therapy for both seizures and hypertension. In addition to drug therapy, the patient may require an oral airway, oxygen, and suctioning,

if aspiration has occurred. **Diazepam** (Valium) or **amobarbital sodium** (Amytal sodium) may be administered by slow IV push. The usual diazepam dosage is 5 to 10 mg, while 250 mg of amobarbital sodium is administered slowly over 5 min. Additional medications for seizure control such as **phenobarbital** may be needed after initial diazepam or amobarbital sodium therapy. The eclampsia patient with seizures must be closely watched for respiratory depression. See Chap. 33, "Neurologic Disorders," for a complete discussion of drug therapy for the control of seizures. The patient may also need antihypertensive medications and magnesium sulfate which are discussed above, as well as induction of delivery, as soon as it is deemed reasonably safe for mother and fetus.

NURSING PROCESS RELATED TO ECLAMPTIC CONDITIONS

The nursing process in the treatment of preeclampsia and eclampsia with **magnesium sulfate** is outlined in Table 46-18.

LABOR AND DELIVERY

Prevention of Preterm Labor

Preterm or premature infants are those born before the 37th week of maternal amenorrhea. The morbidity of preterm infants is associated with many risk factors including socioeconomic status, maternal age, sex, birth order, birth weight, and gestational age. Of these, birth weight and gestational age appear most important. Prevention of preterm delivery may, therefore, improve infant outcome.

Currently there are many theories concerning the initiation of human parturition. Some factors associated with human parturition are increased estrogen levels, decreased progesterone levels, decreased progesterone-estradiol ratio, maternal and fetal prostaglandin levels, the number of uterine α and β receptors, uterine concentrations of cyclic guanosine 5'-monophosphate (cGMP) and cyclic adenosine-3'5'-monophosphate (cAMP), increased concentrations of free calcium in the myometrium, increased numbers of uterine oxytocin receptors, maternal catecholamine levels, uterine volume, and relaxin levels.

Tocolytic agents are pharmacologic agents that can inhibit uterine muscle contraction. The comparison of the capacity of these agents to prevent preterm labor is difficult because studies differ significantly as to patient selection criteria and definitions of successful outcome. None of the drugs currently used are uniformly successful in preventing preterm labor. Effectiveness appears most successful when cervical dilation is 4 cm or less at the initiation of therapy and when fetal membranes are intact. Most patients receiving pharmacologic therapy for preterm labor are in their 24th to 34th week of pregnancy. These agents may be used on a short-term basis or as maintenance therapy until the 37th week of pregnancy. Pharmacologic suppression of preterm labor may not be initiated if the membranes surrounding the fetus have ruptured. Fetal lung maturation may also be assessed by lecithin-sphingomyelin ratio (L/S ratio) or another method prior to the initiation of therapy and to determine when delivery is acceptable. Absolute contraindications to the inhibition of preterm labor include eclampsia or severe preeclampsia, intrauterine fetal death, chorioamnionitis, antepartum hemorrhage that requires immediate delivery, and fetal anomaly incompatible with life. Relative contraindications to pharmacologic intervention include maternal cardiac disease, uncontrolled maternal diabetes mellitus, fetal growth retardation, fetal distress not due to uterine contractions, or severe renal disease.

The β_2-sympathomimetic agents appear most effective for short- and long-term tocolytic therapy. Other possible tocolytic agents include the calcium channel blockers, ethanol, prostaglandin synthetase inhibitors, magnesium sulfate, and diazoxide.

β_2-Sympathomimetic Agents

Ritodrine, terbutaline, albuterol, metaproterenol, fenoterol, and **nylidrin** are β_2 sympathomimetics which have efficacy as tocolytic agents. **Isoxsuprine** (Vasodilan) is a sympathomimetic-like vasodilator which has also been used to decrease uterine contractions. **Ritodrine** (Yutopar) is the only drug in this class currently approved by the FDA for its tocolytic effects, although **terbutaline** (Brethine, Bricanyl) has been extensively studied and used in the United States. The wide use of terbutaline as a tocolytic has resulted from its effectiveness and low cost.

Stimulation of β_2 receptors in the uterus results in uterine relaxation. Uterine relaxation secondary to β_2-sympathomimetic therapy appears to result from a decreased myometrial cellular calcium concentration secondary to increased uptake of calcium by the sarcoplasmic reticulum of the cell. The decrease in free intracellular calcium concentrations prevents smooth muscle contraction.

Pharmacokinetics   Pharmacokinetic data for the β_2 sympathomimetics are currently unavailable for pregnant females. Intravenous ritodrine pharmacokinetic studies in nonpregnant females resulted in elimination half-life of 1.7 to 2.6 h. Oral bioavailability of ritodrine appears to be 30 percent. Pharmacokinetics of other β_2 agonists is discussed in Chap. 27.

Adverse Effects   The most common maternal adverse effects associated with the β_2 sympathomimetics include tachycardia, hypotension, hyperglycemia, hyperinsulinemia, hypokalemia, and lactic acidemia. Pulmonary edema has been reported in patients who were either concurrently

TABLE 46-18   Nursing Process in Treatment of Eclampsia with Magnesium Sulfate

Assessment	Management	Evaluation
Check daily weight, palpate for edema.	Nonpharmacologic treatment: Take measures to conserve energy (provide bed rest, decrease stress, give emotional support) and decrease stimuli (darken room; minimize pain which can provoke convulsions).	Check serum magnesium levels daily—keep levels lower than 7.5 meq/dL.
Monitor vital signs, mental status, deep tendon reflexes q1–4h.		Check patellar reflexes, vital signs, mental status qh with IV infusion; q2–4h with IM injection.
Withhold drug if knee jerk absent, respirations below 12, marked decrease in pulse, urine output below 30 mL/h.	Give IM injection deep in gluteal muscle by Z-track method; change needle after drawing up solution; massage after giving. A local anesthetic may be ordered to decrease pain of injection; divide large doses and give half in each buttock.	Check renal function, specific gravity, and serum creatinine.
Watch for signs of impending convulsions: restlessness, disorientation, epigastric pain, headache, and decreased pulse and respiration rate.		Evaluate length and strength of uterine contractions if labor occurs or is induced.
		Evaluate FHT and report fetal distress (patient should be maintained on a fetal monitor).
Monitor renal function: intake and output; urinalysis for protein, casts, RBCs, specific gravity; serum creatinine; should have indwelling urinary catheter if toxemia is severe.	Have calcium chloride (10%) and 20-mL syringe at bedside as an antidote for magnesium toxicity.	If convulsions occur, check for abdominal rigidity or vaginal bleeding (indicative of placental separation) and signs of labor.
	Since concomitant use of CNS depressants may cause excess depression, evaluate dosage carefully.	
Monitor fetal heart tones (FHT) for rate and regularity.		Check newborn for weak cry, hyporeflexia, respiratory depression, flaccidity.
	Arrange for equipment to resuscitate mother and newborn in case of emergency.	

on corticosteroids or who were fluid-overloaded. Angina pectoris has also been reported. Other adverse effects include tremors, nausea, vomiting, headaches, erythema, nervousness, restlessness, and anxiety.

Fetal and neonatal adverse effects include tachycardia, hypotension, hypocalcemia, and ileus. There is no evidence that exposure to ritodrine in utero causes differences in growth, psychomotor development, or physical abnormalities. While there may be high mortality rates in infants exposed in utero to **ritodrine**, **terbutaline**, or **isoxuprine**, the mortality rate might also be attributed to their average gestational age of 28 weeks or birth weight of 990 ± 71 g. Further studies are needed to determine if there are long-term fetal or neonatal effects.

Dosage   Table 46-19 lists usual dosage ranges for **ritodrine**, **terbutaline**, and **isoxuprine**. Intravenous administration of terbutaline and isoxuprine to decrease uterine contractions has not been approved by the FDA. Intraveneous ritodrine should be used within 48 h after preparation and should not be used if discolored, if it contains a precipitate, or if it has particulate matter. The intravenous dosage should be titrated slowly using an infusion pump until uterine contractions cease. Administration is best done in the left lateral position to minimize hypotension. The patient should be monitored carefully for adverse effects and to prevent fluid overload.

Other Agents

The use of calcium channel blocking agents such as **nifedipine** (Procardia) and **verapamil** (Calan, Isoptin) as possible tocolytic agents are currently being investigated. Decreased uterine contractions may result from direct calcium channel blockade in the myometrium.

Magnesium sulfate is a known calcium antagonist which decreases uterine contractions by its effects on uterine smooth muscle. A 4-g loading dose of magnesium sulfate may be given intravenously over 20 to 30 min followed by a constant infusion of 1 to 2 g/h using an infusion pump. It has not been a reliable uterine inhibitor for longer than 24 h or if the cervix is dilated to 1 cm or more. The mother and infant must be carefully monitored when magnesium sulfate is used (see above).

Although used for many years as a tocolytic, **ethanol** is now rarely used because of adverse effects including maternal nausea, vomiting, inebriation, and restlessness and possible neonatal depression. Prostaglandin synthetase inhibitors (nonsteroidal anti-inflammatory drugs; e.g., **indomethacin**) and **diazoxide** (Hyperstat IV) have been used experimentally as tocolytics, but they are not routinely used because of possible adverse maternal and fetal effects.

NURSING PROCESS RELATED TO PRETERM LABOR

Assessment

Prior to therapy with β_2 sympathomimetics, it is crucial to rule out any maternal conditions which contraindicate these agents or require special monitoring. The nurse should note any history of cardiac disease, hyperthyroidism, or diabetes

---

TABLE 46-19   Sympathomimetic Agents Used for the Treatment of Premature Labor

DRUG	INITIAL DOSE*	IV DOSAGE ADJUSTMENT*	THERAPY DURATION*	ORAL MAINTENANCE DOSAGE*
Ritodrine HCl† (Yutopar)	0.1 mg/min IV	Increase rate 0.05 mg/min q10min until contractions cease (usual dosage 0.15–0.35 mg/min IV).	12 h after contractions cease.	10 mg q2h for 1 day; 10–20 mg q4–6h thereafter.
Terbutaline SO₄ (Brethine, Bricanyl)	10 µg/min IV	Increase rate 5 µg/min q10min until 25 µg/min or contractions cease.	When contractions have ceased per monitor for 1 h, decrease rate by 5 µg/min q30min until the lowest effective dosage; stop 8 h after contractions cease.	0.25 mg SC q6h with 5 mg PO q8h for 3 days; then 5 mg PO q8h through week 36.
	0.25 mg SC qh		Until contractions cease.	5 mg PO q4h for 2 days; then 5 mg PO q6h.
Isoxsuprine HCl (Vasodilan)	0.25–0.5 mg/min IV	Increase rate q15min up to 0.75–1 mg/min IV.	24 h; gradually decrease IV rate.	10–20 mg PO q6h.

*Typical dosages; variations may be seen.
†FDA-approved as a tocolytic.

mellitus in the mother. Serious hemorrhage, cervical dilation more than 4 cm, greater than 80 percent effacement, and premature rupture of the membranes are obstetric parameters that require consideration prior to the decision to use β_2 sympathomimetics. If the woman has asthma, it should be ascertained what drugs she takes, as corticosteroids or concurrent use of β_2 sympathomimetics for bronchodilation can complicate therapy.

Management

The woman should be placed on bed rest; since aortocaval compression from the weight of the fetus can compound the hypotension which intravenous **ritodrine** and other β_2 sympathomimetics can cause, she should be encouraged to lie on her side. Maternal pulse and blood pressure should be closely monitored (at least every 15 min to 1 h), and her lungs should be auscultated for pulmonary edema every hour or at any sign of respiratory distress. Constant electrical monitoring of the fetus and uterine activity is advisable. In the case of maternal tachycardia ($>$100 beats/min) or diastolic hypotension, dosage of the β agonist should be reduced; persistent tachycardia or hypotension may indicate discontinuation of the drug. Sedative or depressant drugs should not be given if delivery appears imminent, as premature infants are sensitive to their effects. Longer-term therapy indicates laboratory evaluation for potassium levels and serum glucose.

Emotional support is crucial. Palpitations, tremulousness, and jitteriness can be caused by tocolytic therapy and can compound anxiety of the mother for the safety of the baby and for her own well-being.

Evaluation

The nurse must carefully monitor the effectiveness of the drug in eliminating contractions. Presence of fetal tachycardia or maternal tachycardia, hypotension, nausea, vomiting, arrhythmia, chest pain, or tremor should be noted, and dosage decreased accordingly. Equipment and personnel should be prepared for the delivery and care of a premature infant if therapy fails.

Stimulating Labor and Controlling Hemorrhage

Oxytocics are pharmacologic agents that have the ability to stimulate contractions of uterine smooth muscle. Of the many drugs that have oxytocic activity only **oxytocin**, the ergot alkaloids (**ergonovine maleate** and **methylergonovine maleate**), and certain prostaglandins are used clinically. Oxytocics are used to induce labor at or near term, to control postpartum hemorrhage, to increase uterine tone after delivery, and to induce therapeutic abortion after the first trimester.

Oxytocin

Physiological Effects It is known that uterine sensitivity to oxytocin increases as pregnancy progresses, but the role of endogenous oxytocin in labor initiation is, as yet, unresolved. It appears that labor stimulates oxytocin release rather than that oxytocin initiates labor. Oxytocin does appear to be extremely important in human parturition.

Mechanism of Action Exogenously administered oxytocin stimulates uterine smooth muscle contractions, resulting in uterine contractions like those seen in normal labor. As the amplitude of uterine contractions increases, dilation and effacement of the cervix follow.

Pharmacokinetics Oxytocin is not available for oral use, because it is destroyed by trypsin in the gastrointestinal tract. Therefore it can be administered only parenterally or intranasally.

When administered intravenously, oxytocin has an immediate uterine effect with uterine contractions increasing in frequency and duration over the next 60-min period. Effect usually lasts for 20 min following the termination of an intravenous infusion. The onset of action following intramuscular administration is about 5 min, with a duration of effect between 30 min and 1 h. Oxytocin for intranasal use is discussed in the section in this chapter on lactation stimulation. Oxytocin has a half-life of less than 5 min. It is hepatically metabolized and the inactive metabolites are renally eliminated.

Adverse Effects Nausea, vomiting, intestinal cramping, and premature ventricular contractions have been associated with oxytocin administration. Anaphylaxis has been reported. Oxytocin may also be associated with the development of cardiac arrhythmias and jaundice in neonates.

Prolonged intravenous administration of oxytocin at high doses in conjunction with overhydration may result in severe maternal water intoxication that might lead to convulsions, coma, and even death. Water intoxication has also occurred in women receiving oxytocin after undergoing hypertonic saline abortions. Cervical lacerations, uterine rupture, decreased uterine blood flow, and fetal morbidity have been associated with maternal hypersensitivity to oxytocin and excessive drug use.

Dosage and Preparations Oxytocin injection (Pitocin, Syntocinon) is a synthetic preparation containing 10 U/mL, with each unit being approximately equivalent to 2 μg of pure hormone. Although it may be administered either IM or IV, it most commonly is administered as a continuous intravenous infusion using an IV infusion pump. An oxytocin solution for IV administration may be prepared by aseptically adding 10 U of the drug to 1000 mL of dextrose 5% and 0.2% sodium chloride solution or another IV solution needed for a specific patient, yielding 10 mU (0.01 U) per milliliter.

The initial IV infusion rate of oxytocin for stimulation of labor is 1 to 2 milliunits per minute (mU/min). The dosage may be gradually increased every 15 to 30 min in 1- to 2-mU/min increments until uterine contractions are similar to normal labor. Rarely is it necessary to exceed an oxytocin dosage of 20 mU/min. During the oxytocin infusion, the mother and fetus should be closely monitored for significant fetal heart rate deceleration, prolonged maternal contractions, or other problems. If the necessity for oxytocin discontinuation occurs, serum concentrations will decrease rapidly because of its short half-life.

Postpartum uterine bleeding may be controlled by administering oxytocin IV at a rate of 20 to 40 mU/min. The infusion may be initiated after the infant and placenta have been delivered. Oxytocin for postpartum hemorrhage may also be administered IM. A dose of 10 U may be given by this route after the placenta has been delivered.

Ergot Alkaloids

Mechanism of Action Ergot alkaloids are potent stimulants of uterine activity which appears dose- and compound-related. Small doses increase both the frequency and force of uterine contractions followed by a period of normal uterine relaxation. Larger doses of ergot alkaloids result in very forceful and prolonged uterine contractions followed by an increased resting uterine tone. These effects are mediated through the activity of ergot alkaloids as partial agonists or antagonists at α-adrenergic, dopaminergic, and tryptaminergic receptor sites in uterine smooth muscle. Ergot alkaloids are effective in the prevention or treatment of postpartum bleeding due to urinary atony or subinvolution, but they should not be used to stimulate labor. **Ergonovine maleate** (Ergotrate Maleate) and its semisynthetic derivative, **methylergonovine maleate** (Methergine), are the ergot preparations of choice for oxytocic use because they have more potent effects on the uterus than the other ergot alkaloids.

Pharmacokinetics **Ergonovine maleate** is rapidly absorbed from the gastrointestinal tract, hepatically metabolized, and eliminated renally. Uterine contractions are seen within 15 min following oral administration, within 10 min after IM dosing, and immediately after IV administration.

Methylergonovine maleate has an onset of action which is quite rapid. Uterine contractions occur within 10 min after oral administration, within 5 min after IM administration, and immediately when used intravenously.

Adverse Effects The most common adverse effects are nausea and vomiting which may result from a direct effect on central nervous system emetic centers. Hypertension and headaches have been reported in association with regional anesthesia and IV oxytocic administration. Symptoms associated with ergot toxicity include vomiting, dizziness, hypo-

tension, hypertension, dyspnea, chest pain, diarrhea, numbness and tingling in the fingers and toes, muscle weakness, confusion, and unconsciousness. Hypercoagulability states and gangrene of the extremities have occurred from chronic ergotism secondary to overdosage or to an extreme susceptibility to ergot effects.

Dosage and Preparations Ergonovine maleate (Ergotrate Maleate) and methylergonovine maleate (Methergine) are available as tablets and in solution for parenteral administration. The IV dosage for both is 0.2 mg, but IV usage is usually reserved for emergency situations such as severe uterine hemorrhaging, since IV administration may be associated with hypertension and more frequent episodes of vomiting. When used intravenously, the medication should be given over 1 min with close monitoring of the maternal blood pressure.

An IM dosage of 0.2 mg may produce a rapid and lasting response. If needed to further decrease hemorrhaging, the dosage may be repeated at 2- to 4-h intervals. Oral doses of 0.2 to 0.4 mg of ergonovine may be used three to four times daily to promote involution of the uterus. Doses of 0.2 mg three to four times daily of methylergonovine orally may also be used.

Prostaglandins

The prostaglandins (PGE_1, PGE_2, and $PGE_{2\alpha}$), discussed in the section of this chapter on termination of pregnancy, have been used as oxytocics. The effects of the prostaglandins appear to be additive with other oxytocics, since they have different sites of action. Although oxytocin and ergonovine are presently in wider use clinically, prostaglandins may be used more extensively in the future.

NURSING PROCESS RELATED TO OXYTOCICS

Table 46-20 outlines the nursing process in the use of oxytocics in labor and postpartum.

Control of Pain during Labor and Delivery

Preparation of parents for childbirth and an increased utilization of regional anesthesia have resulted in a decreased need for obstetric analgesia. If analgesics or sedatives are needed during delivery, they should be employed judiciously to benefit the mother without harming the fetus. Administration of a narcotic analgesic to the mother may affect fetal heart rate patterns and reduce neonatal respiration; it may even have subtle effects on the neurobehavior of a neonate. Placental transfer of an analgesic such as **meperidine HCl**

(Demerol) may result in cord–maternal blood ratios of 0.75 to 1.0. The route and timing of medication administration will directly affect the amount of drug that will reach the fetus transplacentally prior to delivery. Therefore, it is important to avoid maternal narcotic or sedative administration, if possible, when the peak fetal effects of the drug will not have dissipated prior to delivery.

The administration of narcotic analgesics should be avoided, when possible, until the active phase of labor, since narcotics may slow labor progression. Prior to this phase of labor, the patient may benefit from the sedative effects of **secobarbital** (Seconal), **pentobarbital** (Nembutal), **promethazine** (Phenergan), or **hydroxyzine** (Vistaril). The mother and fetus should be closely monitored when obstetric anal-gesia is used. The narcotic antagonist **naloxone** (Narcan) must be available as well as equipment for resuscitation.

Narcotic Analgesics

Meperidine HCl (Demerol) and **alphaprodine HCl** (Nisentil) are commonly used for obstetric analgesia, due to their rapid onset of action, effective analgesia, and relatively short half-lives. Meperidine has an elimination half-life of approximately 3 h. Fetal serum concentrations occur within minutes after maternal administration. Peak fetal effects have been observed 1 to 3 h after IM maternal dosing or within the first hour after IV administration. Doses are usually 25 to 100 mg every 3 to 4 h.

TABLE 46-20 Nursing Process with Oxytocics (Intrapartal and Postpartal)

ASSESSMENT	MANAGEMENT	EVALUATION
	Labor and Delivery	
Contraindicated in unripe cervix (less than 2 cm or less than 30–40% effaced), overdistended uterus, predisposition to rupture (multiparous older primipara, prior cesarean birth), severe toxemia, fetal distress, cephalopelvic disproportion, abnormal presentation of the fetus.	Keep injectables in refrigerator, as they deteriorate with heat, light, age.	Prolonged use increases risk of severe side effects.
	As IV titration: oxytocin usually mixed in D₅W or Ringer's lactate with 10 U / 1000 mL and run at 10–40 drops / min. Rate is slowly increased and titrated for effect on frequency, duration, intensity of contraction. Rate is ordered by physician or by protocol. Use infusion pump for accurate rate. Should be piggybacked into main IV to allow rapid discontinuation.	Electronic monitoring of fetus and contractions best; otherwise monitor q15–30min.
Observe BP, FHT, contractions (length, strength, duration).		Stop or decrease dosage if contractions longer than 1 min or less than 2 min apart, as fetal hypoxia will occur.
		Monitor vital signs every 15–30 min, since bradycardia, arrhythmia, tachycardia, hypotension may occur.
	As buccal tablet (oxytocin): put in pouch between cheek and upper molars. Alternate pouches with each dose. If adverse reaction, spit out and rinse mouth.	May cause water intoxication, so keep accurate intake and output during labor and postpartum; also note lab values for hyponatremia and mental status.
	Can cause nausea and vomiting, diarrhea, cramps which can be treated by comfort measures or symptomatically with drugs.	Check on uterine bleeding (pad count) postpartum.
	May need much support and coaching since patterning of oxytocin-induced contractions may differ from natural ones.	Uterus becomes more sensitive to oxytocics with time, so dosage requirement may decrease over time. Sudden decrease in uterine contractions may indicate uterine tear, rupture, exhaustion: stop drug.
	Postpartum	
Check BP before each dose; hold if elevated.	Timing important: IV and IM often given immediately after detachment of placenta. If given before, it may prevent placental expulsion.	Check amount of bleeding, height and consistency of uterine fundus, pad count.
Contraindicated in preeclampsia, eclampsia, hypertension, sepsis. Use caution in renal and hepatic disease, peripheral vascular disease, coronary artery disease.		Evaluate effect on BP.
		May cause nausea and vomiting, cramps, epigastric distress, paresthesias, cold extremities, and claudication. Drug should be discontinued if discomfort is severe.

Usual obstetric doses of **alphaprodine HCl** (Nisentil) are 30 to 60 mg subcutaneously every 2 to 3 h or 10 to 30 mg IV every 2 h after cervical dilation has begun. Dosages should be individualized to the woman's needs, but excessive doses can cause convulsions. Maximum daily dose is 240 mg. Half-life of alphaprodine is 2 h with an onset of 2 to 30 min by the subcutaneous route or 1 to 2 min following IV administration. Duration of action of obstetric doses is approximately 1 to 2 h. (See Chap. 17 for the general pharmacology of narcotic analgesics.)

Anesthesia

Some clinicians and proponents of "natural childbirth" believe that anesthesia during childbirth can only have adverse effects on the fetus. Others, however, believe that maternal stress caused by pain and anxiety can cause fetal asphyxia and tachycardia and that anesthesia coupled with emotional support have benefits for both mother and fetus.

Physiologic changes in pregnancy have implications for anesthesia. Onset of inhalational anesthesia is more rapid due to pulmonary changes, and the margin of safety may narrow. Anesthetics used in obstetrics can increase the workload of the heart, which is already increased due to the demands of pregnancy and labor. Regurgitation during anesthesia is more common in the obstetric patient, and with the high acidity of gastric content, aspiration pneumonitis is a risk. Most anesthetic agents readily cross the placenta (except ester-type local anesthetics and most muscle relaxants). Of the amide-type local anesthetics, **bupivacaine** has a lower fetal–maternal blood ratio than **lidocaine** or **mepivacaine**. **Epinephrine** contained in local anesthetic agents can cause maternal hypotension (if absorbed in low doses) or hypertension and central nervous system effects (if inadvertently injected intravenously), as well as increased uterine contraction (accidental intravenous or myometrial injection).

Obstetric anesthesia can be local (perineal), regional, by intermittent inhalation (held by the mother), general (intravenous or inhalation), or dissociative anesthesia (using **ketamine**). Regional anesthesia, or conduction blockade, decreases the likelihood of fetal drug depression or maternal aspiration and allows the mother to be awake and to participate in the delivery, although voluntary effort may be diminished. Types of regional anesthesia include continuous lumbar epidural block, caudal block, spinal block, paracervical block, and pudendal block. The principles of anesthesia and the pharmacology of the anesthetic agents is discussed in Chap. 47.

NURSING PROCESS RELATED TO LABOR AND DELIVERY

The nursing process during labor and delivery is complicated by the fact that the nurse must be concerned with the well-being of both mother and infant. Obviously, it is important to eliminate the use of unnecessary medication, since all medications involve some risk, but the patient should not be deprived of the benefits of medication when these outweigh the risks.

Assessment

Assessment relative to pharmacotherapeutics in labor and delivery consists of the same parameters integral to any thorough collection of data on the woman in labor. These factors must be interpreted in light of the potential effects of any medications upon the progress of labor and upon maternal and fetal well-being. Information regarding past pregnancies and the course of the present pregnancy should be reviewed from the prenatal record or from a preadmission interview or questionnaire, since there might not be time to gather these data at the time of admission.

An important aspect of the initial assessment is the level of preparation of the mother for the labor and delivery experience. Those who are prepared through childbirth classes or comparable experiences may often require less analgesic, sedative, or antianxiety medication; many who are well prepared will require none of the agents. It is equally important to assess the patient's value system and feelings about pain and medication in childbirth. For some, the experience is viewed as one to be obliterated or dulled with medication, while others perceive it as a growth experience and may feel that they have failed if any medication is required. It is most important to ascertain what agreement has been reached between the midwife or physician and the patient regarding the use of medication during labor, since any unexpected deviations from this agreement will need to be explained. The presence of supportive people such as the husband or designated childbirth "coach" will also alter the need for medication. Subjective and objective assessment of the client's level of discomfort and anxiety should be made.

The vital signs of the mother, fetal heart tones (FHT), and progress of the labor (length, strength, and frequency of contractions) are important baseline observations performed by the nurse, as each of these can be altered by most of the medications used in labor and delivery. Determination of the degree of effacement and dilation of the cervix and position and presentation of the fetus are other important data to be considered.

Management

The nursing process associated with the oxytocics used during labor and delivery to induce or sustain uterine contractions is outlined in Table 46-20, while the specific implications of the various anesthetics for obstetrics are covered in Table 46-21.

An explanation of the reasons for medications and the method to be employed in administration (especially with anesthetics) is very important. The mother should know what sensations to expect; for example, with analgesics and sedatives she should know that she may experience drowsiness or dizziness. Bed rails should be raised and the call bell placed within easy reach. If ambulation is allowed, the client is instructed to ask for assistance if she gets up. The father or coach will need to be told that the mother may require more active or explicit coaching, since her responses can be dulled by the medication. It may be necessary to assure those who planned to avoid medication but later require it that their role in and control of labor and delivery need not be diminished and that they still have the right to feel pride in their accomplishments in labor. Reassurance should be given that the dosage and time of administration have been carefully selected to avoid threat to the mother and child and that both mother and fetus will be monitored. If a drug is given to decrease anxiety or to promote sleep, care should be taken that the environment is conducive to these reactions.

The nurse should be aware of the half-lives of any medication administered to the woman in labor. Since the infant does not have a well-developed enzyme systems to metabolize all medications, any drug must be administered sufficiently before delivery so that maternal enzyme systems can accomplish biotransformation of the drug, or the newborn may experience respiratory and generalized depression. Report by the delivery room nurse to the nursery should list the names of any drugs given during labor and the time they were given.

However, if central nervous system (CNS) depressant medications are given in excessive doses, the progress of labor may be delayed or stopped. Therefore the dosages of medication administered early in labor should be less than those used in the later, active phase. Smaller, more frequent doses given intravenously may be used in some situations so as not to alter the course of labor.

Evaluation

The effect of any medication upon maternal vital signs, fetal heart rate, and contractions should be ascertained every 15 to 30 min after the drug is given. It should be noted whether the drug accomplished the desired antianxiety, analgesic, or hypnotic effect. The nurse should watch for nausea which may be stimulated by these agents. There will be a need to assess other signs of the progress of labor besides pain, since the CNS depressants alter the response to pain, and the labor may appear to be progressing more slowly than is the case. The newborn should be assessed for depressed respiration at birth, and equipment for resuscitation should be available.

POSTPARTUM PERIOD

Prevention of Rh Sensitization

$Rh_o(D)$-negative, D^u-negative, women exposed to Rh-positive red blood cells during pregnancy, abortion, delivery, or through the transfusion of Rh-positive red blood cells may develop anti-$Rh_o(D)$ antibodies. Rh-positive infants subsequently born to these mothers may develop hemolytic disease of the newborn. This erythrocyte hemolysis may lead to congestive heart failure, anemia, edema, and ascites in the fetus. In severe cases the fetus may die in utero.

$Rh_o(D)$ Immune Globulin (RhoGAM)

An unsensitized (those having no serum anti-D antibodies) $Rh_o(D)$-negative, D^u-negative woman who delivers an $Rh_o(D)$-positive or D^u-positive infant, who aborts an Rh-positive fetus, or who has an ectopic pregnancy where the Rh status is unknown is a candidate for $Rh_o(D)$ immune human globulin. Amniocentesis or antepartum hemorrhage, where red blood cells might enter the maternal circulation, are also reasons for $Rh_o(D)$ immune human globulin usage. The preparation may be indicated also for accidental transfusion of Rh-positive whole blood, red blood cells or other blood components to an Rh_o-negative premenopausal woman.

Mechanism of Action $Rh_o(D)$ immune human globulin suppresses the immune response of the nonsensitized individual by interacting with the $Rh_o(D)$-positive or D^u-positive antigens. This prevents the formation of anti-Rh antibodies by Rh-negative individuals, so that subsequent exposure does not result in an immune response. However, $Rh_o(D)$ immune globulin is not 100 percent effective, and some patients develop anti-Rh antibodies several months after administration.

Adverse Effects Adverse effects include local tenderness and erythema at the site of administration. Temperature elevation may also occur. Plasma used in manufacturing this product is nonreactive for hepatitis B surface antigen.

Dosage and Preparations The standard $Rh_o(D)$ human immune globulin contains 300 μg of anti-D per vial and is available under various trade names (Gamulin Rh, HypoRho-D, RhoGAM). One vial should be administered intramuscularly (IM) after delivery, amniocentesis, abortion, or miscarriage or when dealing with an ectopic pregnancy at or beyond the 13th week of gestation. If it is felt that a large fetal-maternal transfusion has occurred, the Kleihauer-Betke test may be used to estimate the volume of Rh-positive red blood cells in the maternal circulation. The number of vials of $Rh_o(D)$ human immune globulin needed will be based on the test results. If antepartum prophylaxis is used, one vial of standard $Rh_o(D)$ immune human globulin is given at 28 weeks gestation and again within 72 h of delivery.

An $Rh_o(D)$ immune human globulin microdose contains 50 μg of anti-D per vial and is available under the trade names MICRhoGam and Mini-Gamulin Rh. One vial may be administered IM after amniocentesis, abortion, or miscarriage or with an ectopic pregnancy prior to the 12th week of gestation.

Both preparations should be administered IM within 72

TABLE 46-21 Nursing Management and Evaluation of Obstetric Anesthesia*

TYPE	MANAGEMENT	EVALUATION
	Local Anesthesia	
Local block	Used for episiotomy or repair lacerations.	Check for transient dizziness, headache, palpitations.
	Explain to patient that she may still feel pressure and tugging on surrounding tissues.	Take BP, pulse. Report any sudden changes.
		Check for anesthetic effects "wearing off."
	Regional Anesthesia	
Paracervical block	Anesthetizes the hypogastric plexus and ganglia for active phases of labor.	Anesthesia to dilating cervix lasts 1–2 h.
	Administration: Help client assume the lithotomy position. Explain that injection is through the vagina. Give emotional support during procedure. Patient may feel insertion of needle and tingling as anesthetic is injected.	Monitor FHT; fetal bradycardia should last no more than 5 min; if prolonged to 15–18 min, cesarean birth is indicated.
		Check maternal BP and mental status; sudden hypotension or convulsions may indicate systemic injection. Have resuscitation equipment available.
Pudendal block	Anesthetizes pudendal nerve plexus (innervates the perineum) for delivery and episiotomy repair.	Lasts about 1 h; takes 5–10 min to reach maximum effect; ineffective if not placed correctly. Skill of administration required.
	Administration: See procedure for paracervical block.	No effect on fetus.
	May diminish bearing-down reflex, which alters coaching needs and obliterates important cue of beginning of second stage.	Systemic injection has same implications as paracervical.
Caudal and epidural blocks	Caudal blocks anesthetize the sacral segments including the perineum and rectal areas and posterior lower extremities. Epidural block also anesthetizes more of the legs, buttocks, and inguinal areas.	May be one-time or intermittent injection; duration will vary.
		Check maternal BP; if patient is hypotensive, elevate feet for a few minutes and turn to side to take pressure off vena cava; may need an IV and O_2.
	Administration: Help patient to assume knee-chest or left lateral flexed position. Explain that the medication is inserted at lower back, and she may feel the needle insertion. Monitor vital signs q1min times 5 after test dose given. Give emotional support. Continue to monitor q1min times 5 min after every dosing.	Check FHT—drug or maternal hypotension may cause fetal distress which requires a cesarean birth.
		Evaluate for bladder distention since patient will not be aware of bladder fullness during labor or after until recovery is complete.
	Instruct not to attempt to walk after drug given. Lower extremities may be tingly and flushed; motor control is weak. During continuous epidural injection, woman should lie on her side.	Check effectiveness of anesthesia, and report diminished anesthesia during labor.
	During recovery, take precautions for postural hypotension.	Evaluate for recovery: check circulation, sensation, and motion of toes for return to normal and ability to maintain BP when sitting or standing.
	Diminished sensation will alter coaching needs.	

h of delivery, abortion, miscarriage, or amniocentesis. The injection should not be given to the infant.

Stimulation of Lactation

Lactation results from the coordination of the effects of many hormones, a process which begins early in pregnancy.

Estrogen, progesterone, and chorionic somatotropin prepare the breast for milk production, but the levels of these hormones decline rapidly after the delivery of the placenta. At this time prolactin output from the anterior lobe of the pituitary rises and acts on the epithelium of the alveoli of the breast to stimulate milk production. Prolactin release is under the control of two factors from the hypothalamus,

TABLE 46-21   Nursing Management and Evaluation of Obstetric Anesthesia* (*Cont.*)

TYPE	MANAGEMENT	EVALUATION
Regional Anesthesia (Cont.)		
Spinal and saddle blocks	Spinal block used primarily for cesarean birth; anesthetizes from just below diaphragm downward. Saddle block primarily anesthetizes sacral segments.	Monitor maternal BP administration throughout recovery; hypotension is not uncommon.
	For saddle block, the patient sits on edge of table with feet on stool. Give assistance and support as position is uncomfortable. Must remain sitting while anesthesia "sets." For spinal, position patient on side with knees and neck flexed. Nurse helps patient maintain the position.	Watch for change in the level of anesthesia. Observe respirations and be prepared to resuscitate.
		See section on recovery from epidural and caudal blocks.
	Keeping flat for a minimum of 8 h after delivery; good hydration may prevent spinal headache.	
	See epidural and caudal blocks.	
General Anesthesia		
Inhalation (intermittent)	Should be held by patient to avoid excess dosage. Support patient and assure her that she can fulfill this responsibility.	Observe for excessive drowsiness, as mask may not spontaneously drop.
		See section on recovery from general anesthesia.
	Inform anesthesiologist of any use of trichlorethylene, since anesthesia with closed system delivery machine is then contraindicated.	
	Help patient cope with labile emotions caused by nitrous oxide.	
General (IV and / or inhalation)	Keep patient NPO as long as possible before induction. Record time and amount of last food.	*Usual postanesthesia care:* turn on side during recovery and take measures to prevent aspiration— turn, cough, deep-breathe; assess for return of bowel and bladder function.
		Lack of balanced anesthesia may mean excessive nausea, vomiting, excitability.
		Give first dose of analgesia in reduced doses.
		Simultaneous combination of cyclopropane and oxytocin may cause arrhythmia, while with ergot it may cause postpartum hypertension.
		Check infant for depression—resuscitate as necessary.

* See Chap. 47 for general information. Nursing assessment is discussed in narrative.

prolactin-inhibiting factor (PIF), which is thought to be dopamine, and prolactin-releasing factor (PRF). Oxytocin, which initiates the letdown reflex, is releasing by suckling.

Prolactin secretion can be increased by drugs which act on the hypothalamus to suppress prolactin-inhibiting factor, such as phenothiazines, cimetidine (Tagamet), metoclopramide (Reglan), methysergide (Sansert), reserpine, clonidine (Catapres), and methyldopa (Aldomet). Only metoclopram-

ide, a potent stimulant of prolactin release, has been used investigationally to improve lactation. Doses of 30 to 45 mg/day in divided doses are used for this effect.

Infant suckling is the best stimulation for lactation. Nursing soon after birth initiates oxytocin-mediated uterine contractions and the induction of maternal milk production. Nursing in the delivery room following an uncomplicated vaginal birth may be helpful in establishing a good milk supply as well as helping in maternal-infant attachment.

Oxytocin Nasal Spray

Mechanism of Action   A woman who has an adequate milk supply, but who has difficulty with milk ejection (milk letdown) may benefit from the use of oxytocin nasal spray. Oxytocin stimulates mammary smooth muscle, the myoepithelium, to facilitate milk ejection.

Pharmacokinetics   The onset of action of oxytocin occurs within minutes following intranasal use with the duration of effect lasting approximately 20 min. The drug has a short half-life (1 to 6 min) and is eliminated unchanged via the renal system.

Adverse Effects   Adverse effects can include nausea, vomiting, intestinal cramping, uterine cramping, and cardiac arrhythmias. These are, however, rare and mild as compared to adverse effects seen on buccal or parenteral administration.

Dosage and Preparations   The usual dosage of oxytocin spray (Syntocinon) for milk ejection is one spray into one or both nostrils, 2 to 3 min before nursing or breast pumping. Oxytocin nasal spray contains 40 U/mL.

Suppression of Lactation

Pharmacologic agents may be used to suppress physiologic lactation in women who have decided not to breast-feed or who have had a stillbirth or undergone abortion. Drugs used for suppression of lactation may be classified as either nonhormonal (bromocriptine) or hormonal.

Bromocriptine

Mechanism of Action   Bromocriptine mesylate (Parlodel) is the most used nonhormonal drug for suppression of lactation. It is an ergot alkaloid derivative which reduces serum prolactin concentrations by directly inhibiting the release of prolactin from the anterior pituitary. Decreased prolactin concentrations lead to lactation suppression.

Pharmacokinetics   Bromocriptine is 28 percent absorbed from the gastrointestinal tract but only 6 percent reaches the systemic circulation because of hepatic first-pass effect. The drug is highly protein-bound; it is metabolized in the liver and is primarily eliminated as metabolites in bile (95 percent), with 5 percent eliminated renally. Bromocriptine has an elimination half-life of 45 to 50 h. Peak concentrations are observed in the serum from 1 to 3 h after oral ingestion. The onset of serum prolactin reduction occurs 2 h postingestion, with peak effects occurring 8 h postdose.

Adverse Effects   Adverse effects occur most frequently at the time bromocriptine is initiated. Those adverse effects associated with chronic use appear dose-related and rarely occur unless doses exceed 20 mg daily. Women using bromocriptine for lactation suppression usually have a lower incidence of adverse effects than individuals using the drug for other medical problems. One of the most commonly seen adverse effects is hypotension, which occurs in 30 percent of women postpartum. Supine diastolic blood pressure drops of 10 to 20 mmHg and systolic drops of 50 to 60 mmHg have been observed. Therefore, bromocriptine administration is not recommended until vital signs are stable postpartum and no sooner than 4 h after delivery. Since hypotension is most significant with the administration of the first dose, the initial dose is best taken while lying down. Blood pressures should be monitored during the first few days postpartum and should be monitored closely if the patient is receiving other medications that might also lower blood pressure. Other side effects include headaches, dizziness, nausea, vomiting, fatigue, syncope, diarrhea, and cramps.

Concurrent use of bromocriptine with **oral contraceptives** is not advised since oral hormones may interfere with the pharmacologic effects of bromocriptine. The first ovulation postpartum may occur earlier in women using bromocriptine; thus, nonhormonal contraception may need to be initiated. The administration of antihypertensive drugs concurrently must be done with caution and with possible dosage readjustment.

Dosage and Preparations   The usual dosage of bromocriptine for postpartum suppression of lactation is 2.5 mg orally twice daily for 2 weeks. Three weeks of therapy may be needed to prevent rebound lactation and breast engorgement.

Other Nonhormonal Agents

Other drugs that inhibit lactation by blocking prolactin secretion include **pyridoxine** (vitamin B_6), **levodopa**, and **monoamine oxidase inhibitors**. Because of side effects and the possible stimulation of gonadotropin secretion leading to early ovulation, levodopa and monoamine oxidase inhibitors are not used for lactation suppression. Pyridoxine, a mild lactation suppressant, is an ingredient found in many prenatal vitamins. It may have some effect on lactation when used postpartum. This should be kept in mind when prenatal vitamins are given to a nursing mother.

Hormonal Drugs

Mechanisms of Action   Hormones are used to suppress lactation by inhibiting the secretion of pituitary hormones. **Estrogens** may decrease the production of PIF, resulting in increased prolactin production. Estrogens, however, also have a direct lactation-inhibiting effect on the mammary gland. Therefore, hormonal suppression is effective only when started immediately after delivery or during end-stage labor. **Androgens** are ineffective in suppression of lactation but are effective in reducing pain and breast engorgement. Therefore, androgens combined with estrogens may be useful in lactation suppression.

Adverse Effects Androgenic virilization effects associated with estrogen-androgenic products rarely occur in the postpartum patient, but there is an increased risk of puerperal thromboembolism associated with high estrogen dosage. Other adverse effects associated with estrogen therapy are discussed above (in sections on ovarian hormones and oral contraception).

Dosages and Preparations **Estradiol valerate** 8 mg/mL in combination with **testosterone enanthate** 180 mg/mL (Deladumone OB) may be given as a single 2-mL injection prior to the onset of the second stage of labor to suppress lactation and prevent breast engorement in women who do not wish to breast-feed. Deladumone OB is very viscous and should be administered by the Z-tract method. Informed consent should be obtained prior to administration.

Chlorotrianisene (Tace) is a synthetic estrogen which has been used to prevent postpartum breast engorgement. A dosage of 72 mg twice daily for 2 days is usually effective in suppressing lactation and in preventing rebound breast engorgement.

NURSING PROCESS RELATED TO THE POSTPARTUM PERIOD

Assessment
The nursing process with oxytocics such as **ergonovine maleate** (Ergotrate), **oxytocin** (Pitocin, Syntocin), and **methylergonovine maleate** (Methergine) that are employed postpartum to support the process of involution and to prevent hemorrhage is outlined in Table 46-20. Implications for nursing care with the postpartum use of analgesics and hypnotics, with agents such as anticoagulants, anti-infectives, laxatives, and vitamins used to treat complications, and with drugs used to treat preexisting medical conditions are the same as the nursing process with these agents at other times with three important considerations: (1) if the mother is breast feeding, there is a potential for transfer of the drug to the infant (see Chap. 7); (2) lactation and involution may alter the normal homeostatic balance of the mother and require alteration of some drug dosages; and (3) there may be an additive effect between adverse drug effects and some common postpartal conditions, many of which can be prevented or minimized by nursing care. For example, **codeine** may increase the tendency toward constipation that is already common in the postpartum period, but a diet high in fiber and fluids should counteract this. Aspirin which is found in many analgesic preparations may increase bleeding and therefore should be avoided.

It is important to ascertain with certainty that the mother does not desire to breast-feed the neonate before any drug to suppress lactation is given. It is not unknown, particularly within some cultural groups, for mothers to plan to nurse the neonate after discharge from the hospital where they feel privacy and yet to bottle-feed the neonate while still in the hospital. The nurse should assess the mother's intentions regarding breast feeding based on cultural as well as stated needs.

Management
If for some reason the mother who has received one of the drugs to inhibit milk production does decide to breast-feed the neonate, the normal physiologic responses to the suckling of the neonate may overcome the effects of the drug. Furthermore, natural processes suppress lactation if the mother does not breast-feed, whether drugs are given or not. Application of ice, support with a bra or breast binder, and mild analgesics may be necessary if rebound breast engorgement occurs. Breasts should not be pumped as this will stimulate lactation. Symptoms should diminish within 36 to 48 h, even if medication has not been given.

Evaluation
To evaluate the effectiveness of the hormones given to suppress engorgement, the nurse should palpate the breasts for enlargement, warmth, and tenderness. Due to fluid retention and fluid shifts from hormonal effects, postpartum weight loss may be delayed. Patients receiving estrogens to suppress lactation should be evaluated for thrombophlebitis daily.

CONCLUSION

In dealing with the health of women, it is important to consider the woman within the context of her total health status and lifestyle. Many of her potential health problems will respond favorably to strong nursing support, meticulous health habits, and conservative management. Education of individuals and groups of women on sound psychologic and physical health habits, including the judicious and rational use of drugs, is the most important nursing function.

CASE STUDY

S.G., a 17-year-old previously healthy female, gravida 1, para 0, was admitted during the 37th week of gestation to the obstetric unit with a diagnosis of preeclampsia. She was treated with diet, bed rest, and magnesium sulfate to prevent eclamptogenic seizures. On her third postadmission day labor was induced with intravenous oxytocin and a 2750-g male was born 12 h later under pudendal block anesthesia.

As she was unmarried and had arranged to relinquish the child, S.G. was given Deladumone OB prior to delivery to suppress lactation.

The nursing process of this case will be presented in two parts in order to clarify the nursing process with the various agents used.

First Two Days—Toxemia

Assessment Upon admission it was noted that S.G., who was accompanied by her mother, was anxious. Her vital signs were BP 150/96; temperature, 37°C; pulse, 82; and respirations, 18. She was oriented, alert, and appropriate in her behavior. Her deep tendon reflexes were 3+. The urine contained a moderate amount of protein. She weighed 57.4 kg and reported a weight gain of 5 kg in the last week; edema of all extremities and face was noted. Fetal heart rate was 140. Laboratory studies revealed a blood urea nitrogen of 10 g/100 mL, and urine output for the first 24-h period was 2200 mL, showing adequate renal function.

She remained stable on bed rest in a quiet darkened room for the first 2 days. On the second evening a visitor who was a friend from school was heard to remark that S.G. seemed "spaced out" and "real touchy." The nurse noted inappropriate behavioral responses, complaints of headache and epigastric pain, and felt that it was probable that convulsions could occur.

Management The physician was notified of the data and assessment of the nurse. After examining the patient he agreed and ordered magnesium sulfate IM with an initial dose of 8 g followed by 4 g every 4 h, and made plans to begin induction as soon as the patient was stabilized. An indwelling catheter was inserted. The nurse obtained an order from the physician to add a local anesthetic to the injection since the pain of injection could stimulate seizures. The initial dose was divided into two injections, one administered into each buttock, while subsequent injections were alternated between the right and left gluteus medius muscles and massaged well to disperse the medication.

Nurses explained all procedures to the patient and spent as much time as possible with her, monitoring her urine output, fetal heart tones, vital signs, mental status, and reflexes, at least every hour before delivery and every 4 h for the first 48 h postpartally.

Evaluation S.G.'s blood pressure dropped transiently to 138/88 after the initial injection of magnesium sulfate. She became more sedated but demonstrated appropriate behavioral responses and was oriented, with knee jerk reflexes of 1+ to 2+. Fetal heart tones showed no fetal distress and her urine output was well over 100 mL every 2 h. No convulsions occurred. Her blood level of magnesium was 4.5 meq/L on the morning of the third day at which time she delivered.

Labor and Delivery

Assessment In addition to the data in the previous evaluation the nurse considered the results of the pelvic examination done by the intern the morning of the third day before initiating the oxytocin infusion. Since the exam revealed that the cervix was soft, 3 cm dilated, and 45 percent effaced, the fetal presenting part (vertex) was at −1 to 0 station, and there were no contraindicating factors, the induction of labor was begun.

Management The nurse started an IV of 5% dextrose in lactated Ringer's solution, 100 mL/h. To a second 1000 mL was added 10 U of oxytocin, which was piggybacked onto the main IV through an infusion pump at an initial rate of 10 gtt (drops)/min. This was gradually increased to 25 gtt/min over the next hour when contractions (as indicated by the electronic monitor) were strong, regular at every 3 min, and of about 45 s duration. Pain and nausea were treated with Demerol 50 mg and promethazine 25 mg given IM at 12 noon; the relatively low dose was given since the patient had received magnesium sulfate.

When S.G. was 8 cm dilated and 100 percent effaced, a pudental block anesthesia was administered with the patient in the lateral flexed position. No change in FHT or maternal vital signs was noted. Labor progressed well and the oxytocin was discontinued. Low forceps vaginal delivery of a male infant occurred at 2:37 P.M. After detachment of the placenta, the oxytocin drip was restarted briefly to prevent hemorrhage. Deladumone OB was given IM prior to delivery to suppress lactation.

Nursing staff remained with S.G. and her mother throughout most of the labor, assisting Mrs. G. to coach the patient during the contractions and monitoring the patient, the fetus, and the progress of the labor.

Evaluation The fetal heart rate, maternal vital signs, and uterine contractions were not altered significantly by the analgesic and anesthetic; although the patient's blood pressure did drop from 156/92 to 132/86 after the analgesic, this was considered therapeutic in the hypertensive patient. No excessive CNS depression was noted.

The oxytocic successfully induced an effective labor with no deleterious effects on the fetus. Nausea caused by this drug was controlled by the antiemetic.

The Apgar score of the newborn at 5 min was 6 (out of 10 possible); it was felt that there was some minor residual depression of the infant related to the drug therapy.

The IV and indwelling catheter were discontinued that evening and S.G. voided 400 mL at midnight. She showed a normal mental status and serum sodium, so it was felt the oxytocin had not caused water intoxication.

Throughout the postpartum period the nursing staff monitored for residual drug effects as well as toxemia and the complications of delivery. S.G. experienced no breast engorgement, was afebrile, and checks for calf tenderness and Homan's sign were negative, revealing that the Deladumone had been effective and without adverse effect.

One of the nurses on the unit taught a class on contraception and S.G. attended it. This was followed up by several private discussions with one of the staff nurses who noted that S.G. had a poor understanding of reproductive physiology initially but was eager and motivated to learn. S.G. and the nurse also spent considerable time talking about the patient's feelings of loss relative to the baby.

REFERENCES

Beck, W. W.: "Complications and Contraindications of Oral Contraception," *Clin Obstet Gynecol,* 24:893–900, 1981.

Bronson, R. A.: "Oral Contraception: Mechanism of Action," *Clin Obstet Gynecol,* 24:869–875, 1981.

Clark, R. B., and A. B. Seifen: "Systemic Medication During Labor and Delivery," in R. M. Wynn (ed.), *Obstetrics and Gynecology Annual,* New York: Appleton-Century-Crofts, 1983.

De Lia, J., and M. G. Emery: "Clinical Pharmacology and Common Minor Side Effects of Oral Contraceptives," *Clin Obstet Gynecol,* 24:879–891, 1981.

Dong, B. J., J. C. Eoll III, and M. A. Koda-Kimble: "Contraception," in B. S. Katcher, L. Y. Young, and M. A. Koda-Kimble (eds.), *Applied Therapeutics, The Clinical Use of Drugs,* 3d ed., San Francisco: Applied Therapeutics, 1983.

Droegemueller, W., and R. Bressler: "Effectiveness and Risks of Contraception," *Annu Rev Med,* 31:329–343, 1980.

Durand, J. L. and R. Bressles: "Clinical Pharmacology of the Steroidal Oral Contraceptives," *Adv Intern Med,* 24:97–126, 1979.

Fishburne, J. I.: "Systemic Analgesia During Labor," *Clin Perinatol,* 9:29–53, 1982.

Gilman, A. G., L. Goodman, and A. Gilman (eds.): *Goodman and Gilman's The Pharmacological Basis of Therapeutics,* 6th ed., New York: Macmillan, 1980.

Goldfien, A.: "The Gonadal Hormones and Inhibitors," in B.G. Kastrup (ed.), *Basic and Clinical Pharmacology,* Los Altos, CA: Lange Medical Publications, 1982.

Guyton, A. C.: *Textbook of Medical Physiology,* 6th ed., Philadelphia: Saunders, 1981.

Haesslein, H. C.: "Hypertensive Disease," in K. R. Niswander (ed.), *Manual of Obstetrics,* Boston: Little, Brown, 1980.

———: "Premature Labor," in K. R. Niswander (ed.), *Manual of Obstetrics,* Boston: Little, Brown, 1980.

Hammond, C. B., and W. S. Maxson: "Current Status of Estrogen Therapy for the Menopause," *Fertil Steril,* 37:5–25, 1982.

Hatcher, R. A., et al: *Contraceptive Technology 1982–1983,* 11th ed., New York: Irvington, 1982.

Hernandez, L: "Contraceptive Methods and Products," *Handbook of Nonprescription Drugs,* 7th ed., Washington: American Pharmaceutical Association, 1982.

Kastrup, E. K., et al. (eds.): *Facts and Comparisons,* St. Louis: Facts and Comparisons, 1984.

Katayama, K. P.: "Advances in Infertility," in R. M. Wynn (ed.), *Obstetrics and Gynecology Annual,* New York: Appleton-Century-Crofts, 1983.

Korberly, B. H., C. A. Sohn, and R. P. Tannenbaum: "Menstrual Products," *Handbook of Nonprescription Drugs,* 7th ed., Washington: American Pharmaceutical Association, 1982.

MacDonald, P. C.: "Estrogen Plus Progestin in Postmenopausal Women," *N Engl J Med,* 305:1644–1645, 1981.

Marx, G. F.: "Obstetric Anesthesia: Advances in the 1980's," *Clin Perinatol,* 9:3–27, 1982.

Miller, D. R., and S. G. Hoag: "Personal Care Products," *Handbook of Nonprescription Drugs,* 7th ed., Washington: American Pharmaceutical Association, 1982.

Mosher, B. A., and E. M. Whelan: "Postmenopausal Estrogen Therapy: A Review," *Obstet Gynecol Surv,* 36:467–475, 1981.

Niles, R. E.: "Normal Labor and Delivery," in K. R. Niswander (ed.), *Manual of Obstetrics,* Boston: Little, Brown, 1980.

O'Brien, P. M. S.: "The Premenstrual Syndrome: A Review of the Present Status of Therapy," *Drugs,* 24:140–151, 1982.

Raible, M. D.: "Pathophysiology and Treatment of Endometriosis," *Am J Hosp Pharm,* 38:1696–1701, 1981.

Reid, R. L., and S. S. Yen: "Premenstrual Syndrome," *Am J Obstet Gynecol,* 131(1):85–104, 1981.

Schnider, S. M.: "Choice of Anesthesia for Labor and Delivery," *Obstet Gynecol,* 58 (Suppl. 5):245–345, 1981.

Scott, D. B., and C. J. Sinclair: "Advances in Regional Anesthesia and Analgesia," *Clin Obstet Gynecol,* 9:273–289, 1982.

Souney, P. F., A. F. Kaul, and R. Osathanondh: "Pharmacotherapy of Preterm Labor," *Clin Pharm,* 2:29–44, 1983.

Tatum, H. J., and E. B. Tatum: "Barrier Contraception: A Comprehensive Overview," *Fertil Steril,* 36:1–12, 1981.

Utian, W. H.: "Analgesia and Anesthesia," in J. A. Pritchard and P. C. MacDonald (eds.), *Williams Obstetrics,* 16th ed., New York: Appleton-Century-Crofts, 1980.

———: "The Ovarian Hormones," in J. A. Pritchard and P. C. MacDonald (eds.), *Williams Obstetrics,* 16th ed., New York: Appleton-Century-Crofts, 1980.

———: "Estrogen Replacement in the Menopause," *Obstetrics and Gynecology Annual,* New York: Appleton-Century-Crofts, 1983.

47

SURGERY: DRUGS USED IN PERIOPERATIVE CARE

BARBARA GOULD SMITH

LEARNING OBJECTIVES

Upon mastery of the content of this chapter, the reader will be able to:

1. Define anesthesia, induction, emergence, and balanced anesthesia.
2. State the goal of preoperative preparation of the patient.
3. State the purpose of preoperative medications.
4. For each of the following organ systems, list how a preexisting disorder could complicate the surgical course: cardiovascular, respiratory, hepatic, gastrointestinal, endocrine, and renal.
5. Differentiate between local and general anesthesia.
6. State the mechanism of action of inhalational anesthetics.
7. Differentiate regional blockade, spinal blockade, caudal blockade, and epidural blockade.
8. Describe the flow of inhalational anesthetic from circuit to brain.
9. List the indications, adverse effects, and nursing implications of all the inhalational anesthetics in general.
10. Explain why halothane is generally used only once within a 6-month period for adult anesthesia.
11. Describe the phenomena of diffusion hypoxia and the second gas effect with nitrous oxide.
12. Compare nitrous oxide, halothane, enflurane, and isoflurane with respect to blood-gas partition coefficient, MAC, skeletal muscle relaxation, analgesia, respiratory and cardiac effects, and speed of induction and emergence.
13. Define blood-gas partition coefficient and MAC in relation to clinical effects of inhalational anesthetics.
14. List the indications for intravenous anesthetics.
15. Describe the pharmacokinetics of the ultrashort-acting barbiturates.

16. Describe ketamine, its indications, adverse effects, and nursing implications.
17. Explain neuroleptoanalgesia and neuroleptoanesthesia.
18. List five uses for local anesthetics.
19. List routes of administration of local anesthetics.
20. State the adverse effects of the local anesthetics.
21. Compare the metabolism of ester and amide local anesthetics and give an example of each.
22. Describe the functions of anesthetic adjuncts.
23. Explain the required dosage adjustments when phenothiazines or hydroxyzine are given with other sedating drugs, including fentanyl/droperidol (Innovar).
24. Describe at least two nursing actions for each step of the nursing process relative to the preoperative, intraoperative, and postoperative periods.

Surgical procedures performed prior to 1842 were done without anesthesia. Patients were given some type of opiate analgesic for the purpose of relieving pain, which unfortunately was not entirely successful. Shortly after the incision, consciousness was lost due to either pain or hemorrhage. Mortality was high. The success of a surgeon was not determined by skill, but by speed, since a shorter surgical time meant a greater chance for survival. With the discovery of ether the surgical experience changed radically. After 1846 when ether's anesthetic properties were established at Massachusetts General Hospital, the ability of the anesthetist to alleviate the pain of surgery enabled surgeons to broaden the scope and intricacy of surgical procedures. Although in these early years anesthetic techniques were not refined, the mortality rates during surgery dropped significantly.

Definitions

In order to understand the drugs used during the perioperative period, it is necessary to be familiar with certain terms and their definitions. *Anesthesia* is the loss of sensation of a single body part or of the total body. It may be induced by either a *local anesthetic* or by a *general anesthetic*. The anesthetic is administered by an anesthetist, either a physician (anesthesiologist) or a registered nurse (nurse anesthetist), who is trained in the administration and management of anesthesia.

General anesthesia is a nonarousable state of unconsciousness which is characterized by varying degrees of analgesia, amnesia, narcosis and skeletal muscle relaxation. It may be attained by the use of a single anesthetic or by the use of a combination of anesthetic agents, which is called a *balanced technique* or *balanced anesthesia*. The *induction* is the period from the start of a general anesthetic to the attainment of the state of anesthesia. Intubation (placement of a breathing tube into the trachea through either the mouth or the nose) is a usual procedure during induction. The time period during which the patient is awakening from a general anesthetic is known as the *emergence phase*.

The surgical experience is divided into three separate time periods.

1. The *preoperative period,* which begins upon admission to the surgical unit, has the goal of preparing the patient physiologically, psychologically, and legally for the operation. If the surgery is an emergency, rather than elective surgery, the preoperative period will be considerably abbreviated and only the most necessary preparations will be performed.

2. The *operative period* begins upon arrival to the operating room. This time is spent anesthetizing the patient and performing the operation.

3. The *postoperative period,* the final phase of the perioperative period, begins when the patient enters the recovery room. Here the patients are watched closely for signs of cardiorespiratory depression, and are treated for pain. The postoperative period may extend long after discharge from the hospital.

Generally, the nursing care provided during each perioperative period is done by a different group of nurses, and so continuity of care requires coordination of effort.

PREOPERATIVE PREPARATION OF THE PATIENT

Patients need to be in the best possible condition both physically and emotionally, since well-prepared patients will have a much smoother surgical course. Since many persons may contribute to the assessment of the patient, information that may have been missed by one member is likely to be obtained by another. For this reason it is necessary for all members of the team to do their own assessment and not gather their information based solely on another's data.

Preoperative Nursing Assessment

A thorough health history must be obtained including the patient's age, weight, nutritional status, and general health. Special emphasis should be placed on the patient's medication history (allergies, current medications including over-the-counter drugs, prior drug reactions) and previous hospitalizations and surgeries. It is important to review all organ systems with the patient, as he or she may have forgotten to mention a previous condition that is no longer of concern to the patient but may be of concern to the anesthetist.

During the preoperative period the nurse should gather baseline data about the patient's normal habits and physiologic functions, including tobacco, alcohol, or drug use—all of which may affect anesthetic management. Baseline vital signs are very important; the blood pressure and pulse should be noted at least three or four times to provide the anesthetist with a normal range for the individual. Normal bowel and bladder elimination patterns should also be noted. Many tests may be ordered and any abnormal results should be reported to the physician as soon as possible. For example, a low serum potassium may result in an intraoperative cardiac arrhythmia and should therefore be brought to the attention of the surgeon and anesthetist, so that corrective measures can be started immediately.

The nurse must also assess the emotional status of the patient as well as that of the family, since the emotional state of a patient, which may be influenced by the family, can affect the patient's reaction to the anesthetic. Highly apprehensive patients require more anesthetic, frequently have a stormy emergence from anesthesia, and experience a greater incidence of postoperative complications. The nurse should assess the patient's understanding of the illness, the operation, the reason for it, and any fears associated with it.

The Anesthetist's Assessment

The anesthetist will be very specific in gathering information about preexisting disorders, medications taken within the last year, and previous anesthetics. Disease and certain drugs increase the risk associated with surgery and anesthesia, and are factors in determining the type of anesthetic to be used. Information provided by the nurse may be of great benefit to the anesthetist.

Concomitant Medications

Patients scheduled for surgery are frequently taking prescription or nonprescription drugs for medical disorders. The operative risk for these patients is increased, as the drugs may interact unfavorably with the anesthetic, or may cause other problems during the surgical procedure. Previous drug orders may either be retained, changed to other agents or dosages, or discontinued during surgical procedures. For example, patients who are on pharmacologic doses of corticosteroids will need an increase in their dose prior to surgery to offset stress-induced needs for corticosteroids during the surgical period. Antihypertensive drugs are usually continued unchanged throughout the surgical procedure since the risk of high blood pressure is greater than the potential drug-drug interactions. Drugs like the **MAO inhibitors** are discontinued a few weeks prior to surgery due to the potential for an adverse interaction with the anesthetic and vasoactive drugs. Nurses involved in preoperative care must be aware of potential interactions between prescription or nonprescription drugs and anesthetic agents. Table 47-1 describes some potential drug-anesthetic interactions.

TABLE 47-1   Potential Drug-Anesthetic Reactions

DRUG	COMMENTS	DRUG	COMMENTS
Anticoagulant		*Corticosteroid*	
Warfarin	May increase bleeding during and after surgery.	Prednisone	Sudden withdrawal may cause adrenal cortical insufficiency; patients require a steroid boost to meet the stress of surgery.
Antimicrobial Drugs		*Drugs Acting on the Central Nervous System*	
Tetracyclines	Predispose to renal insufficiency after methoxyflurane anesthesia.	Anticonvulsants (phenytoin)	May enhance metabolism of inhalation anesthetics and diminish their effectiveness. Tapering off in too short a period before surgery may result in convulsions, and sudden cessation may lead to status epilepticus.
Kanamycin, streptomycin, gentamycin, neomycin, amikacin	Enhance neuromuscular block owing to an additive effect with nondepolarizing neuromuscular blocking agents.		
Cardiovascular Drugs		Monoamine oxidase inhibitors (tranylcypromine)	May cause hypertensive crises in conjunction with sympathomimetic amines. Potentiates analgesics, hypnotics, and anesthetics and may cause hypotension.
β-Adrenergic blockers (propranolol, nadolol)	Add to myocardial depression from general anesthesia, induce bronchospasm, and inhibit circulatory response. Continued in severe hypertension, arrhythmia, angina pectoris, or hyperthyroidism.		
		Phenothiazines (chlorpromazine)	May add to the hypotensive effects of sedatives, narcotics, and general anesthesia.
Digitalis glycosides (digoxin)	Digitalis intoxication and arrhythmias during general anesthesia should be watched for, although it may be advisable to continue therapy.	Levodopa	May cause hypotension and occasionally arrhythmias.
		Tricyclic antidepressants (imipramine, amytriptyline)	May cause hypotension and tachyarrhythmias.
Antiarrhythmic agents (quinidine, procainamide)	Aggravate myocardial depression, impair cardiac conduction, and cause peripheral vasodilation. May also potentiate neuromuscular blocking drugs.	*Hypoglycemic Agents*	
Diuretics (thiazides and furosemide)	May lead to hypovolemia, hypotension, and alterations in sodium and potassium balance.	Insulin	Dosage of insulin should be reduced just prior to surgery, but may need to be increased post-surgically.
Antihypertensive drugs (methyldopa)	May cause additive hypotensive effects or erratic blood pressure control.	Tolbutamide, other oral hypoglycemic agents	Preoperatively these patients should be placed on parenteral regular insulin.
Calcium channel blockers (verapamil, nifedipine)	Not yet formally studied. May increase a patient's resistance to anesthetically induced cardiac arrhythmias.	*Anti-inflammatory Antipyretic Agents*	
		Aspirin	May increase bleeding during and after surgery although some recent research refutes this.

Concomitant Diseases

Cardiovascular Disease   Disorders of the cardiovascular system pose serious problems to the surgical patient. Coronary artery disease is the most common cardiac disorder and is often associated with hypertension, congestive heart failure, and cardiac arrhythmias. These patients have a limited ability to increase the supply of oxygen to the heart during periods of increased demand, such as during stress. It is therefore imperative that the stress of the perioperative period be minimized. Good preoperative preparation, careful anesthetic management, and a smooth emergence make the surgical experience less stressful for these compromised patients.

Patients with congenital heart defects require special consideration for anesthetic care, aimed at minimizing any factors that may worsen an already serious problem.

Hepatic Disease   The liver is the major organ for detoxification of many drugs. If the liver is compromised, slow or incomplete metabolism of anesthetics may prolong their pharmacologic action. In patients with severe liver disease or impending hepatic failure, anesthesia with hepatotxic agents, such as the halogenated hydrocarbon **halothane**, is best avoided. Barbiturates and neuroleptic agents require competent hepatic activity for their normal metabolism, and patients with compromised livers will generally require decreases in dosage and an increase in the time interval between drug administrations to avoid toxicity.

Respiratory Disease   Any pulmonary disorder that affects the lung structure leads to failure of gaseous exchange and eventually to increased pulmonary artery pressures and cardiorespiratory failure. Two problems arise when these patients present for anesthesia:

1.   The uptake of inhalational anesthetics and oxygen may be decreased.
2.   These patients are more susceptible to respiratory depressant effect of many anesthetic and adjunct drugs.

Gastrointestinal Disorders   Diseases of the gastrointestinal system may compromise the hemodynamic state of the patient due to vomiting, fistula formation, obstruction, diarrhea, malabsorption, or peritonitis. These may cause complications such as dehydration and hypokalemia or other electrolyte imbalance, which should be corrected prior to surgery. A conservative, slow return of the body to normal homeostasis before any surgical intervention is most beneficial to the patient. Therapeutic regimens should be hurried only when acute surgical intervention is necessary.

Endocrine Disorders   Patients with endocrine disorders require special management prior to surgery. Consideration should be given to diabetes mellitus, adrenocortical insuffi-

ciency, pheochromocytoma, and hyper- or hypothyroidism. (See Table 47-1 and Chap. 35, "Endocrine Disorders.") Patients who are taking or have taken corticosteroids within the last year prior to surgery are at risk of developing sudden cardiovascular collapse from the stress of surgery and anesthesia. Generally a steroid supplement will be given to these patients preoperatively to prevent this potentially disastrous complication.

Renal Disease   Before any surgical procedure, it is important to have baseline data regarding the status and competency of the patient's renal function, since many anesthetic adjuncts, such as barbiturates and narcotics, use the kidney as a route of elimination. Thus, preexisting renal disease may prolong anesthesia.

Informed Consent

A preoperative visit allows for an exchange of information and an establishment of a rapport between the patient and anesthetist. During this visit patients are encouraged to ask questions and express their concerns or fears about the anesthetic. The anesthetist then informs the patient of the events to come during the next 24 h. Patients are instructed not to have anything by mouth for at least 8 h before surgery and are told that prior to being transported to the operating room they will receive a preoperative medication. Patients are informed that upon their arrival to the operating room an intravenous line will be started and monitoring equipment will be placed on them before the anesthetic is started. For children, this explanation is modified according to their age and ability to tolerate an intravenous line versus a mask induction. After the discussion of the anesthetic plan and associated risks, the patient or guardian is required to sign a consent form for the anesthetic. At this point, the patient is considered to be legally prepared for the anesthetic. A separate consent form may be required for the actual operation, and it is the surgeon who is legally required to discuss the procedure and risks of the surgery.

Preoperative Medications

The actual anesthetic begins with the preoperative medication which is given approximately 1 h before the scheduled surgical time. These drugs are administered according to the patient's age, sex, weight, general physical and emotional condition, and the type of operation to be performed, as well as the practitioner's personal preference.

The objectives of preoperative medications are: to allay the patient's apprehension, to provide analgesia for preoperative and postoperative pain, to provide amnesia, to dry secretions of the oral cavity and respiratory tract, to inhibit undesirable reflexes, to inhibit nausea and vomiting, and to facilitate the induction of anesthesia while reducing the amount of anesthetic required for surgery. The most common types of drugs used as premedicants are sedative-hypnotics, antihistamines, narcotics, antipsychotics, anxiolytics, and anticholinergic agents. Table 47-2, while not all inclusive, lists some commonly used premedicants and their usual dosages.

Sedative-Hypnotics

Barbiturates provide sedation and allay apprehension prior to surgery with minimal cardiorespiratory depression. An advantage of barbiturates as premedicants is that they rarely cause nausea and vomiting. Patients generally awaken more promptly from a general anesthetic when given a barbiturate than when given a narcotic. However, in the presence of pain, patients who have had barbiturates demonstrate a greater incidence of emergence delirium. **Pentobarbital** (Nembutal) and **secobarbital** (Seconal) are the barbiturates most frequently used for preoperative sedation. They may be administered either orally or intramuscularly.

Chloral hydrate may be used when it is advisable to avoid barbiturates due to a previous allergic or idiosyncratic reaction. Chloral hydrate is a safe and usually well-tolerated drug. As with barbiturates, delirium and excitement may develop in the presence of pain. It is usually administered orally to children or debilitated patients as a preoperative medication.

Antihistamines

Antihistamines have sedative, bronchodilating, antiemetic, antisialogogic (saliva drying), antiarrhythmic (through inhibition of reflex bradycardia), and ataractic (antianxiety) properties. **Hydroxyzine** (Vistaril) is a widely used antihistamine for preoperative sedation which causes minimal circulatory and respiratory depression. However, it potentiates other central nervous system depressants, such as narcotics and barbiturates. It may be administered orally or intramuscularly, and the dosage should be reduced when used in conjunction with other CNS depressant drugs.

Antipsychotics

Phenothiazines have been used as preoperative medications due to their sedative, antiemetic, antiarrhythmic, antihistaminic, and temperature-regulating properties. These are frequently given with narcotics or barbiturates to provide greater sedation. *The dosage of both drugs should be reduced when phenothiazines are given in combination with other sedative drugs.* Unlike the barbiturates, phenothiazines tend to prolong the recovery from anesthesia and may cause some cardiorespiratory depression. **Promethazine** (Phenergan) is the phenothiazine most commonly used for premedication.

TABLE 47-2 Preoperative Medications

MEDICATIONS	USUAL ADULT DOSAGE	USUAL CHILD DOSAGE
Sedative-Hypnotics		
Secobarbital (Seconal)	50–200 mg IM or PO	3–5 mg/kg IM or PO
Pentobarbital (Nembutal)	50–200 mg IM or PO	3–5 mg/kg IM or PO
Chloral hydrate (Noctec)	500–1000 mg PO	22.5 mg/lb PO; maximum single dose: 1000 mg
Antihistamines		
Hydroxyzine (Vistaril)	50–100 mg IM	0.6 mg/kg
Diphenhydramine (Benedryl)	50–100 mg IM	5 mg/kg/24h
Antipsychotics		
Promethazine (Phenergan)	20–50 mg IM	0.5 mg/lb IM, PO, PR
Droperidol (Inapsine)	1.25–5 mg IM	> 2 yr: 1–1.5 mg/25 lb IM
Anxiolytic		
Diazepam (Valium)	5–15 mg PO or IM	> 2 yr: 0.25 mg/kg
Lorazepam (Ativan)	1–4 mg IM or PO	Not for use in children at this time
Narcotics		
Morphine	6–15 mg IM	0.1 mg/kg IM
Meperidine (Demerol)	50–100 mg IM or SC	1–2 mg/kg IM or SC
Fentanyl (Sublimaze)	0.05–0.1 mg IM	Not used in children
Anticholinergics		
Atropine	0.4–0.6 mg IM	7–24 lb: 0.1–0.15 mg 24–65 lb: 0.2–0.3 mg 69–90 lb: 0.4 mg
Scopolamine	0.4–0.6 mg IM	Used infrequently in children
Glycopyrrolate (Robinul)	0.2 mg IM	0.002 mg/lb IM

Butyrophenones are antipsychotic drugs similar to phenothiazines. In addition to their sedative effect, they demonstrate some antiemetic properties and do not diminish cardiovascular stability, although they do possess some α-adrenergic blocking capabilities. Restlessness and extrapyramidal dyskinesia are the major adverse effects noted, which are especially prominent in children. **Atropine** is an effective reversal of the extrapyramidal dyskinesia. **Droperidol** (Inapsine) is the most widely used butyrophenone and is frequently combined with a narcotic to increase sedation.

Anxiolytics

The benzodiazepines are anxiolytic (antianxiety) drugs which allay apprehension and produce amnesia. They demonstrate a minimal effect on the cardiovascular system, but excessive doses may cause respiratory depression in susceptible patients (elderly or debilitated). **Diazepam** (Valium) is the drug of choice in treating and preventing convulsions, and is frequently administered as a premedicant. Another frequently used benzodiazepine for preoperative sedation is **lorazepam** (Ativan), which has a shorter half-life and is a more effective amnestic agent than diazepam.

Narcotics

Morphine is an effective analgesic with sedative properties. When administered preoperatively, it allows for a smoother induction of anesthesia and reduces the amount of anesthetic required. Respiratory depression, pupillary constriction, bronchial constriction, hypotension, biliary spasm, nausea and vomiting, and a slower recovery from anesthesia are adverse effects of morphine. Respiratory depression causes an increase in the P_{CO_2} which in turn dilates the cerebral vascular bed and in the susceptible individual will increase the intracranial pressure. For this reason narcotics are not administered to neurologically compromised patients.

Meperidine (Demerol) is also an effective analgesic, although its sedative capabilities are less than morphine. Patients receiving meperidine may experience respiratory depression, hypotension, and tachycardia. Although nausea and vomiting do occur with meperdine, the incidence is less than with morphine.

Fentanyl (Sublimaze) is a very potent synthetic narcotic. Its onset of action is more rapid than morphine, but its duration is much shorter. The effects of fentanyl are similar to those seen with other narcotics. **Sufentanil** (Sufenta) is a similar potent narcotic for use as an analgesic adjunct or primary anesthetic agent for major surgical procedures.

Anticholinergics

Atropine sulfate is given as a premedicant mainly for its antisialogogic properties and its ability to inhibit undesirable reflexes of the cardiovascular system. It produces minimal sedation, blurred vision, and dryness of the mouth about 15 min after injection. Systemic injection is not contraindicated in patients with glaucoma, since the intraocular pressure is not increased by the usual recommended dose. **Atropine** should be avoided in febrile patients as it inhibits sweating and the ability to dissipate heat.

Scopolamine has a greater antisialogogic and sedative effect than atropine, while its ability to prevent reflex bradycardia is less. There tends to be greater incidence of emergence delirium following the use of scopolamine. This adverse affect is easily reversed with 1 to 2 mg of **physostigmine**. It should also be avoided in the febrile patient.

Glycopyrrolate (Robinul) is a synthetic anticholinergic drug which does not cross the blood-brain barrier and therefore possesses no sedative properties. Its other properties are similar to atropine and scopolamine, including inhibition of the sweating mechanism for heat loss. For children this is the anticholinergic of choice.

Preoperative Nursing Management

To help minimize the dangerous effects of stress, it is often helpful to take the patient on a tour of the postoperative facilities, such as the intensive care unit or recovery room. Such activities have been found to decrease the incidence of postoperative complications. In many hospitals the operating room nurses make preoperative visits to patients on the day before surgery to assess the patient, to give the patient an opportunity to meet a staff person who will be in the operating room, and to allow the patient to ask questions.

Many of the complications of anesthesia and surgery are associated with the lungs and with the effects of immobilization. The preoperative period, when the patient is usually alert and pain-free, is an opportune time to teach the patient deep breathing and bed exercises.

Approximately 30 to 60 min before the surgery, as ordered or "on call," the nurse administers the preoperative medications. This is part of the total balanced anesthesia plan; therefore, it is vital that these drugs be given at the proper time. If a drug is not given at the time ordered, the nurse must clearly indicate this on the chart and on the preoperative checklist so that the anesthetist can make the appropriate adjustments. For proper absorption, parenteral preoperative medication should be given intramuscularly and no injection should exceed 2.5 mL in volume. If the medication order requires a larger volume than this, two injections should be given at different sites. Further, since many preoperative medications are physically or chemically incompatible, the nurse should check with the hospital pharmacy before mixing any two medications in one syringe and should never give any combination that is cloudy or shows a precipitate. For safety reasons the patient should not get out of bed after receiving the medications, since hypotension or drowsiness may cause a fall. After the medication is given, it is important that the patient relax and rest. The environment should be slightly darkened and quiet; relatives who remain at this time shoud be asked to sit quietly with the patient. The preparations preceding the surgery should be organized and should flow smoothly so that the patient does not become agitated from the commotion of nursing activities.

Preoperative Nursing Evaluation

Before the patient leaves for surgery the nurse should make a final evaluation. How well the patient slept the previous night should be evaluated and recorded. A final evaluation of the patient's anxiety level is also important. The nurse may evaluate the effect of the preoperative medication by taking vital signs at the time of the expected onset of action (usually about 20 min). This is important if the patient has developed respiratory difficulty, extreme depression of consciousness, a shocklike appearance, or other abnormal reaction. The nurse should clearly note that the vital signs reflect a postmedication determination, since some drop in blood pressure is expected, and this reading cannot be considered the preoperative baseline.

INTRAOPERATIVE CARE OF THE PATIENT

In the operating room the patient is cared for by the surgical team. The persons making up this team (the surgeon, anesthesiologist or nurse anesthetist, surgical assistants, scrub nurse or technician, and the circulating nurse) coordinate their efforts to make the patient's surgical experience as safe and pleasant as possible.

The *surgeon* heads the team and shares with the *anesthetist* the responsibility for the patient's life. While the surgeon performs the actual operation, the anesthetist administers the anesthetic, maintains an adequate oxygen–carbon dioxide exchange, administers all necessary fluids and medications, and continuously monitors the patient's vital signs. *Surgical assistants* are either surgeons, residents, or medical students. They assist the surgeon by retracting tissues, suctioning or sponging blood from the wound, and tying sutures.

Scrub nurses or technicians assist the surgeon during the operation by passing the instruments, sutures, and sponges as they are needed. It is the *circulating nurse* that actually runs the operating room. The circulator's job is one of continual assessment, so as to anticipate the needs of the other team members for the care of the patient. "Circulating" in the operating room requires a very quick and observant person as adverse circumstances may arise rapidly, requiring an immediate response.

Intraoperative Nursing Assessment

Assessment in the operating room begins as soon as the patient arrives. Patients are asked about allergies and medications and when they last had anything to eat or drink. Any important notations made by nurses on the preoperative unit should be brought to the attention of the surgeon and anes-

thetist. The chart should be checked for the operative permit which must be completed before an operation may proceed. This process of continual assessment enables the circulator to act quickly and efficiently to help ensure the safety and welfare of the patient.

All patients in the operating room are monitored regardless of the type of procedure being performed or the type of anesthetic (local, general, regional) being administered. During any procedure in which an anesthetist is present the standard monitoring equipment includes an electrocardiogram, a precordial or esophageal stethoscope, a thermometer, and a blood pressure cuff. Invasive monitoring techniques such as an arterial line, a central venous pressure line, and/or a Swan-Ganz pulmonary artery catheter may be used for very ill patients or complicated procedures with large fluid shifts. Patients should have at least one patent intravenous line before any type of anesthetic is given. Children are an exception to this rule. Frequently, the induction of anesthesia in children is by the inhalational route, after which an intravenous line is started.

General Inhalational Anesthetics

Mechanism of Action

Inhalational anesthetics are either gases or volatile liquids which are administered via the respiratory tract. The state of anesthesia can be achieved by a large number of agents, each with different chemical and physical properties. In order for the state of anesthesia to occur, the anesthetic must be delivered to the brain. The exact mechanism of action of anesthetic agents on the central nervous system is not precisely known. However, it has been postulated that the lipid solubility of an agent enhances its anesthetic action and that the more lipid-soluble an agent is, the more potent it is. There appears to be some type of alteration, either mechanical, biochemical, or neurophysiologic, of the cell membrane which then affects impulse transmission. By altering transmission within the central nervous system, a state of anesthesia is produced.

Dosing

Inhalational anesthetics are, as the name implies, administered by inhalation. The potency of the inhalational agents varies, and as such the required dosage of each agent to produce the same quantitative effect varies. The measure of potency for inhalational anesthetics is termed MAC, which is the *minimum alveolar concentration* of an anesthetic at one atmosphere of pressure that produces immobility in 50 percent of patients exposed to noxious stimuli (see Table 47-3).

Inhalational anesthetics are administered with oxygen and/or in combination with another anesthetic agent. The dosage of an agent is determined by its percentage of the total gas mixture that is delivered to the patient. For example, a mixture of anesthetic gases might contain 1% halothane, 60% nitrous oxide, and 39% oxygen, equaling a total of 100%. According to Dalton's law of partial pressures, each gas within the mixture exerts a pressure independent of the other gases. These pressures when added together equal the total pressure of the mixture, which at sea level would be 760 mmHg. Therefore, the percentage or concentration of an anesthetic within a gas mixture is proportional to its partial pressure or tension. Frequently when discussing the uptake and distribution of an inhalational anesthetic, the terms *concentration* and *tension* are used interchangeably.

Pharmacokinetics of Induction and Emergence

In order for an inhalational anesthetic to reach the target organ, the brain, it must first pass into the alveoli of the lungs, transfer to the blood, and eventually leave the blood and enter the brain. During the administration of an inhalational anesthetic a concentration gradient exists between the inspired concentration of the agent and its concentration within the alveoli. It is this gradient which is responsible for the diffusion of the agent into the alveoli, since diffusion occurs from an area of high partial pressure to one of a lower partial pressure. As the blood passes by the alveoli, another concentration gradient is established, and the agent diffuses from the alveoli into the blood. As the arterial blood carrying the agent circulates past the tissues, once again the process of diffusion occurs from an area of high concentration (blood) to one of low concentration (tissues). The concentration of this venous blood is now lower and, upon passing the alveoli again, more of the agent will diffuse from the alveoli into the blood, thus repeating the process. If the inspired concentration remains unchanged, eventually an equilibrium will be established between the inspired alveolar gas, blood, and tissue tensions.

Establishment of an equilibrium generally does not occur during the administration of an inhalational anesthetic, as the inspired tension is usually high for the induction, lower for maintenance, and zero for emergence. Diffusion is always occurring during an inhalational anesthetic, but the rate and direction of diffusion of the gas varies proportionally with the differences in partial pressures between the body compartments.

TABLE 47-3 Properties of Inhalational Anesthetics

ANESTHETIC	BLOOD-GAS PARTITION COEFFICIENT AT 37°C	BRAIN-BLOOD PARTITION COEFFICIENT AT 37°C	MAC, %
Halothane	2.30	2.6	0.75
Enflurane	1.80	2.6	1.68
Isoflurane	1.40	3.7	1.40
Nitrous oxide	.47	1.1	>100
Methoxyflurane	12.00	2.0	0.16

Factors Affecting Rate of Induction Many factors modify the rate of induction with an inhalational agent, and are listed below.

1. *Inspired tension.* The higher the inspired tension, the larger the difference between the partial pressures, and therefore, the faster the diffusion (induction) will occur.

2. *Pulmonary ventilation.* As the tidal volume is increased, the amount of gas inspired with each breath increases. This causes a more rapid rise in the alveolar tension, speeding the rate of induction. The rate of induction with highly soluble agents is minimally affected by ventilation (see below). Hyperventilation causes hypocapnea, a low carbon dioxide tension, resulting in constriction of cerebral vessels; this diminishes cerebral blood flow and may slow the rate of induction.

3. *Solubility.* The solubility or *blood-gas partition coefficient* of an inhalational anesthetic is the ratio of the amount of the agent in the blood phase to that in the gas phase in equal volumes at equilibrium. Agents of high solubility quickly pass from the alveoli into the blood, slowing the rate of rise of the alveolar tension and the rate of induction. Agents of lower solubility are associated with more rapid inductions as the alveolar tension rises rapidly and quickly saturates the blood. Figure 47-1 compares an agent of high solubility to one of lower solubility. In Table 47-3 the blood-gas partition coefficients of the most frequently used agents are listed. The brain-blood partition coefficient in Table 47-3 represents the affinity of the anesthetic for the brain. The higher the coefficient, the more readily the agent localizes in the brain, its site of action. Anesthetics with high brain-blood partition coefficients tend to cause slower recovery than those with low coefficients.

4. *Pulmonary perfusion.* In order for the agent to diffuse from the alveoli to the blood, blood flow through the pulmonary circuit must occur. The flow is determined by the volume of blood, the circulation time, and the patency of the pulmonary vessels.

5. *Tissue perfusion.* The greater the blood flow to the tissues the more rapid the uptake of the agent by the tissues. Some tissues receive a greater blood flow than others. Therefore, an equilibrium between the alveolar gas, blood, and tissue tension will be approached more rapidly in the well-perfused group than in the tissues receiving less blood flow. Tissue solubility of an agent is another factor which determines the rate of tissue uptake. Figure 47-2 illustrates the flow of inhalational anesthetics from the breathing circuit to the tissues.

Anesthetic Flow Cycle At the beginning of an inhalational anesthetic the alveolar tension rises rapidly at first and then more slowly as it approaches the inspired tension. This same phenomenon is seen with both blood and tissue compartment: an initial rapid rise in the tension, followed by a slower rise as equilibrium is approached. Figure 47-3 depicts

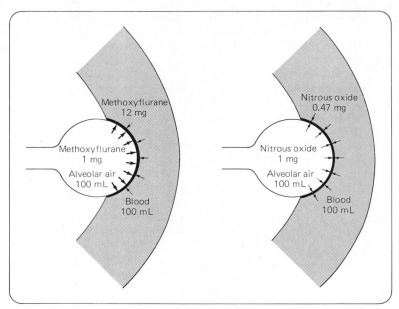

FIGURE 47-1

The Partition Coefficients for Two Anesthetics. At equilibrium the relative distribution of a gas into identical volumes of a gaseous phase (such as the alveolus) and a liquid phase (such as the blood) is characteristic of each anesthetic. This ratio is determined by the solubility characteristics of the anesthetic and is called the blood-gas partition coefficient. For methoxyflurane distributed between blood and air at 37°C, the ratio is 12:1; for nitrous oxide the ratio is 0.47:1. Thus the blood-gas partition coefficients of methoxyflurane and nitrous oxide are 12 and 0.47, respectively. Anesthetics with low blood-gas partition coefficients elicit a more rapid induction, so induction with nitrous oxide is more rapid than with methoxyflurane.

the uptake and distribution curves of some inhalational anesthetics. Note that all the curves have the same configuration. The steep portion of the curve represents alveolar uptake of the anesthetic. At the curved portion or "knee," equilibration between the well-perfused tissues and the blood is occurring. The final part of the curve represents the slower equilibration of anesthetic tension between the poorly perfused tissues and the blood.

Emergence from an inhalational anesthetic follows the same pathways as induction, but in reverse. The factors which affect the rate of induction also affect the rate of emergence. In other words, a slow induction means a slow emergence.

Adverse Reactions

Adverse effects of inhalational anesthetics are related to overdosage or underlying systemic disease. Most agents cause varying degrees of myocardial depression, which is of no consequence in a normal healthy patient. In a patient with a compromised cardiovascular system this myocardial depression may reduce the cardiac output to a level which is incompatible with life. Respiratory depression is another adverse effect caused by inhalational agents; without venti-

latory support, all patients are at risk of hypoxia and carbon dioxide retention. In patients with pulmonary disease, ventilatory support may even be required postoperatively due to this respiratory depression. Some of the agents used are metabolized in the liver and excreted in the urine. Hepatic and renal damage may be caused by general anesthetic agents, but is more likely to occur in patients who have some hepatic or renal insufficiency preoperatively. Another fairly common adverse effect is postoperative nausea and vomiting. Although this causes distress in the patient, its association with mortality is slight, unless the patient is too depressed from the anesthetic to protect the airway.

Medullary depression followed by cardiovascular collapse are the final stages of overdosage with all volatile anesthetics. Fortunately, today's monitoring techniques assist the anesthetist in evaluating anesthetic depth to prevent this sequela. If it should occur, the drug is discontinued immediately and supportive therapy initiated.

Depth of Anesthesia

Various observational and monitoring tools are used by the practitioner to evaluate the status of a patient receiving a general anesthetic. As patients progress from a state of alert-

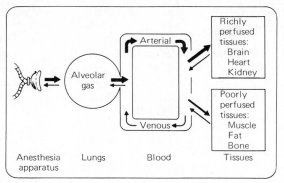

FIGURE 47-2

Flow of the Anesthetic Agent from the Apparatus to Lungs, Blood, and Tissues. Arrows represent relative transfer during induction stage when concentrations of the gas in the alveolus are high, resulting in a net transfer of anesthetic into the arterial circulation. Richly perfused tissue rapidly takes up anesthetic, while poorly perfused tissue accumulates the drug slowly. During recovery when the anesthetic apparatus is removed, the net drug flow is from the venous blood to the alveolus, where the drug is eliminated (exhaled). Anesthetic concentrations in highly perfused tissue fall rapidly during the recovery stage, but in poorly perfused tissue concentrations may actually rise, due to redistribution from well-perfused tissue, before declining slowly. *(From A. Goth, Medical Pharmacology, 7th ed., St. Louis: Mosby, 1974. Used by permission.)*

ness to an anesthetic sleep, they pass through certain sequential stages. These stages were first delineated under **ether** anesthesia, and were based on observed functional and physiologic depression of the central nervous system. Today, because the techniques and agents used are different, patients may pass through certain stages so quickly that the progression of central nervous system depression is not observable. In other cases, the use of anesthetic adjuncts may totally obliterate a physiologic parameter used to gauge anesthetic depth. For example, the concomitant use of a muscle relaxant paralyzes the muscles of respiration, and therefore the practitioner must assess the anesthetic depth using other signs. Table 47-4 delineates the stages of ether anesthesia and the signs that are used to judge depth of anesthesia. Although these stages are not completely accurate for other anesthetics, they may offer some guidelines to gauge anesthetic depth of all agents during induction, anesthesia, and recovery. With modern anesthetic techniques the most reliable indications that surgical anesthesia has been achieved are loss of the eyelid reflex and establishment of a respiratory pattern that is regular in rate and depth. Subsequently, the adequacy of the depth of anesthesia for the particular surgical situation is judged by the anesthetist mainly by changes of circulatory and respiratory status in response to stimulation.

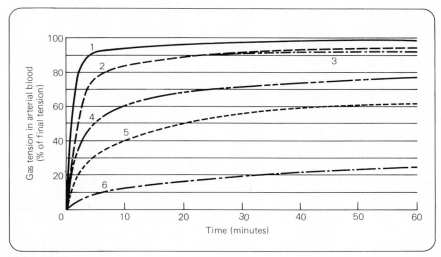

FIGURE 47-3

Time-Concentration Curves for Various Inhaled Anesthetics. 1, Ethylene; 2, nitrous oxide; 3, cyclopropane; 4, enflurane; 5, halothane; 6, methoxyflurane. The rate of the rise of tension in arterial blood of anesthetics administered at a constant inspired tension differs for each agent. As a result, the rate of induction differs. With nitrous oxide, where the curve rises sharply, the patient will be unconscious within 3 min. However, halothane or methoxyflurane, which have significant blood and tissue solubility, may require 30 min to several hours before surgical anesthesia is established. Thus, one anesthetic may be used for induction and another for maintenance. *(Modified from R. D. Dripps et al.: Introduction to Anesthesia: The Principles of Safe Practice, 6th ed., Philadelphia: W. B. Saunders, 1982. Used by permission.)*

Gaseous Anesthetics

Nitrous Oxide

Nitrous oxide is a colorless inert gas with a sweet odor and taste. It is stored in heavy metal cylinders under pressure in its liquid form. Under the usual conditions it is stable and does not react with soda lime (which is used for carbon dioxide absorption in the anesthetic circuit) or with other anesthetic agents. Although it is nonflammable, it does support combustion. Nitrous oxide does not irritate the respiratory tract or stimulate copious secretions. It is the most widely used inorganic gas for anesthesia. It also has the lowest blood-gas partition coefficient of all currently used anesthetics (see Table 47-3).

Indications and Dosing Nitrous oxide is an agent of marginal potency. Its limitation is its inability to produce surgical anesthesia when combined with oxygen in concentrations which maintain adequate tissue oxygenation. For this reason nitrous oxide is rarely used alone, although it is frequently used for dental procedures in subanesthetic concentrations of 35% or less. A mixture of 70% nitrous oxide with 30% oxygen is the highest concentration of nitrous oxide that may be used for maintenance anesthesia without causing tissue hypoxia. Nitrous oxide is a potent analgesic, as 40% in oxygen is equianalgesic to 15 mg of morphine. Generally it is used in combination with other drugs—either narcotics, hypnotics, muscle relaxants, or volatile inhalational agents—to produce surgical anesthesia. This combination technique (balanced anesthesia) provides anesthesia, muscle relaxation, analgesia, amnesia, and generally allows for a rapid emergence with postoperative comfort.

The use of nitrous oxide as an inhalational analgesic during the second stage of labor is of great value. Administration of 100% nitrous oxide during contractions and 100% oxygen between contractions provides safe levels of analgesic without interference of uterine contractions or maternal oxygen saturation.

Another technique which employs nitrous oxide as the

TABLE 47-4 Four Stages of Anesthesia

FROM	TO	PATIENT STATUS	NURSING ACTION
Stage I			
Beginning administration of gas or drug	Loss of consciousness	May appear inebriated, drowsy, dizzy.	Close OR doors; keep room quiet; stand by patient to assist, if necessary.
Stage II			
Loss of consciousness	Relaxation	May appear excited; may breathe irregularly; may move arms and legs or body; patient very susceptible to external stimuli (noise, being touched suddenly).	Be ready to restrain patient if needed; at patient's side, quiet and alert; assist anesthetist, if needed.
Stage III			
(Surgical anesthesia stage) relaxation	Loss of reflexes; depression of vital functions	Regular respiration, contracted pupils, eyelid reflexes disappear, jaw relaxed; auditory sensation lost during this stage.	Begin prep only when anesthetist indicates stage III has been reached and patient is under good control.
Stage IV			
(Danger stage) vital functions too depressed	Respiratory failure; possible cardiac arrest	Not breathing; little or no heartbeat or pulse.	If arrest occurs, react immediately to assist in establishing airway; provide cardiac arrest tray, drugs, syringes, long needles; assist surgeon with closed or open cardiac massage.

Source: J. Luckman and K. C. Sorenson: *Medical-Surgical Nursing—A Psychophysiological Approach,* Philadelphia: Saunders, 1980. Used with permission.

main anesthetic agent begins with a barbiturate induction, followed by a skeletal muscle relaxant and hyperventilation with 70% nitrous oxide and 30% oxygen to a carbon dioxide level of 25 torr. It is believed that the hyperventilation augments the analgesic properties of nitrous oxide. Patients receiving this type of anesthetic are minimally depressed and recover quite rapidly. However, there has been recall of surgical events by some patients with this anesthetic. In view of this fact, some type of supplement such as amnestic agents or potent inhalational agents should be used. After receiving low-dose supplementation, these patients still recover rapidly from the anesthetic.

Frequently, nitrous oxide is used as an adjuvant to the more potent inhalational anesthetics. As described below, the MAC of the potent inhalational anesthetics (**enflurane, isoflurane, halothane**) is reduced when nitrous oxide is added in 50 to 70% concentrations. Benefits of this technique are less cardiorespiratory depression with a more rapid recovery.

Pharmacokinetics   Nitrous oxide is primarily transported across the pulmonary epithelium. It does not undergo biotransformation and is eliminated unchanged primarily through the lungs, although a small amount diffuses out through the skin. When administered in high concentrations with oxygen, large amounts of nitrous oxide are taken up by the body within the first few minutes of induction. As it leaves the alveoli to enter the blood, a void is created within the alveoli which is rapidly filled as fresh gases flow in, thus augmenting the delivery of all gases to the body. This phenomenon is known as the *second gas effect,* and is due to its low solubility (blood-gas partition coefficient), which is very useful during induction as it increases the uptake of potent inhalational anesthetics and increases the alveolar oxygen concentration. The net effect is a more rapid induction and a reduced risk of hypoxia if high concentrations of nitrous oxide are used for induction. The reverse occurs when nitrous oxide is discontinued. It rapidly diffuses from the blood to the alveoli, resulting in a potentially dangerous decrease of oxygen in both the alveoli and the arterial blood. This is known as *diffusion hypoxia.* Administration by the anesthetist of 100% oxygen for approximately 5 min after discontinuing nitrous oxide will prevent its occurrence.

Adverse Reactions   Nitrous oxide is quite free of major toxicities. High concentrations cause a slight myocardial depression and increase the responsiveness of vascular smooth muscle to catecholamines. It also increases the amount of circulating norepinephrine. Its respiratory effect is minimal; there is a depression of the hypoxia response and a slight, if any, depression of the carbon dioxide response. There is no central nervous system toxicity and postoperative nausea and vomiting occurs only in 10 to 15 percent of patients. The greatest danger of nitrous oxide is its potential to cause diffusion hypoxia. Concentrations not greater than

70% and the administration of 100% oxygen after discontinuing nitrous oxide will avert tissue hypoxia.

Gaseous Anesthetics of Historical Interest

Cyclopropane   Cyclopropane is an alicyclic hydrocarbon which is the most potent of the gaseous anesthetics. It has a pleasant, sweet smell which is nonirritating in concentrations of less than 50%. Inductions with cyclopropane are smooth and rapid, owing to its high potency and low solubility. However, cyclopropane is a highly explosive agent, and for this reason it is no longer used.

Volatile Anesthetics

Halothane

Halothane (Fluothane) is a potent, highly soluble halogenated hydrocarbon. The MAC and the blood-gas partition coefficient of halothane are moderate relative to other agents (see Table 47-3). It is a clear, colorless, volatile liquid with a sweet, nonirritating odor. Halothane breaks down in ultraviolet light and spontaneously oxidizes. It is nonflammable in all concentrations in both air and oxygen.

Indications and Dosing   Induction with halothane is generally smooth and rapid, although it is somewhat slower than an induction with agents of lesser solubility. It is most popular as an induction agent for children, the usual induction dose being 2 to 4% in oxygen and nitrous oxide. Tracheal intubation may be performed with or without muscle relaxants, as halothane relaxes the masseter muscles, inhibits secretions, and blunts the laryngeal and pharyngeal reflexes. Rarely is it employed as an induction agent for adults, who usually prefer the intravenous route of induction.

Halothane is used to maintain anesthesia for almost all types of surgical procedures in concentrations of 0.4 to 1.0%. Respiratory depression occurs with all doses and is proportional to the depth of anesthesia. Ventilation, whether by mask or endotracheal tube, should be assisted or controlled, as carbon dioxide levels are extremely elevated with spontaneous ventilation during surgical anesthesia. Halothane does not produce skeletal muscle relaxation; therefore skeletal muscle relaxants must be administered with halothane for abdominal procedures.

Halothane is a potent smooth muscle relaxant. Even very low doses will depress uterine tone, which when used for dilatation and curettage or vaginal deliveries may increase bleeding and prolong labor. Vascular smooth muscle is also relaxed, which when added to the myocardial depression of halothane, may cause significant hypotension. Administration of fluids and surgical stimulation may help keep the blood pressure in an acceptable range in an individual with a healthy cardiovascular system. Adding **nitrous oxide** will enable the anesthetist to reduce the dose of halothane, which will also help maintain the blood pressure. Some surgical procedures require a hypotensive technique to improve visualization of the operative site and reduce blood loss. Halothane is frequently used for deliberate hypotensive cases, either alone or in combination with a vasodilator.

Pharmacokinetics Emergence from halothane is delayed due to its high solubility in blood and fat. About 60 to 80 percent of absorbed halothane is eliminated unchanged through the lungs within 24 h after administration is discontinued. Traces of halothane may be detected for days after the anesthetic is given. That which is not exhaled is either eliminated unchanged via skin and kidneys or is biotransformed in the liver to inactive metabolites and then excreted.

Adverse Reactions Halothane has been implicated as causing hepatic necrosis in a small percentage (1:10,000) of patients. Symptoms generally occur a few days to a couple of weeks after surgery and include fever, anorexia, nausea, and vomiting. Liver function tests reveal abnormalities characteristic of hepatitis. Mortality is high for these patients, approximately 50 percent. The incidence appears to be higher in patients receiving repeated administrations, and those who develop significant episodes of hypotension and/or hypoxia during surgery. For this reason halothane is not repeated in adults for a 6-month period. Halothane hepatitis does not affect children before the onset of puberty and in this age group halothane may be repeated within a 6-month period. Halothane's hepatotoxicity precludes its use in patients with evidence of preexisting hepatic disease.

Halothane has the potential to depress the myocardium and vascular smooth muscle. Arterial blood pressure, myocardial contractility, cardiac output, peripheral resistance, and cardiac rate may all be reduced by halothane. It is not recommended for patients with cardiovascular disease. Cardiac arrhythmias are common; there is a progressive depression of the pacemaker from the sinus node to the atrioventricular node. Ventricular arrhythmias are rare, but do occur during periods of light anesthesia, hypoxia, or respiratory acidosis. Sensitization of the myocardium to endogenous or exogenous catecholamines by halothane increases the likelihood of ventricular arrhythmias. Caution must be used during the administration of local anesthetics with **epinephrine** because of this sensitization, and the amount which can be coadministered is limited.

Respiratory depression with halothane is marked and generally requires assisted or controlled ventilation to prevent respiratory acidosis. Halothane does not have great analgesic properties and requires analgesic supplementation. It is contraindicated in patients with a personal or familial history of malignant hyperthermia, as it is known to be a trigger of this sometimes fatal disorder. Halothane is not used for intracranial procedures due to its vasodilating properties that increase cerebral blood flow, which in a susceptible patient may increase intracranial pressure.

Most patients demonstrate pyramidal tract signs and shivering during the recovery, although rarely do they complain of discomfort from it.

Enflurane

Enflurane (Ethrane) is a nonflammable halogenated ether. It is a clear, colorless liquid with a sweet yet pungent odor. Unlike halothane, it is chemically stable and is packaged without a preservative.

Indications and Dosing Enflurane is rarely used as an induction agent and is most often employed for maintenance of anesthesia. To achieve surgical anesthesia rapidly after induction with an intravenous agent, concentrations of 4 to 5% are required. Maintenance concentrations range between 1.5 to 3%. As with **halothane**, respiratory depression occurs requiring assisted or controlled ventilatory support during surgical anesthesia to maintain adequate oxygen–carbon dioxide exchange.

Enflurane has some skeletal muscle relaxant properties and potentiates nondepolarizing skeletal muscle relaxants. These properties make enflurane a good choice for most abdominal procedures. Frequently, nondepolarizing muscle relaxants and enflurane are used in combination which reduces the dosage of both, thus causing less depression and speeding the recovery.

Pharmacokinetics Approximately 80 percent of the enflurane administered to patients is eliminated unchanged by exhalation. The remainder is eliminated through other routes or is biotransformed in the liver by defluorination, producing a free inorganic fluoride ion.

Adverse Reactions Sensitization of the heart to catecholamines occurs with enflurane, but to a lessor degree than with halothane. **Epinephrine** should be administered judiciously with enflurane. Depression of contractility and vasodilation of vascular smooth muscle also occurs and is proportional to the dose. The drop in arterial blood pressure and the reduced cardiac output may in the susceptible individual induce myocardial ischemia. Enflurane should be administered with caution in patients with coronary heart disease.

High concentrations of enflurane in the presence of hypocapnea has produced seizure activity documented by EEG. During clinical practice the conditions necessary to initiate the seizures are rarely achieved. Due to its potential to induce seizures, enflurane is contraindicated in patients with a known history of a seizure disorder. Cerebral vasodilation also occurs with enflurane which may increase cerebral blood flow. In the neurologically compromised patient, an increase in cerebral blood flow will increase intracranial pressure, and may be fatal.

Enflurane is a potent respiratory depressant, and patients

require ventilatory support to maintain good oxygen–carbon dioxide exchange. Patients susceptible to malignant hyperthermia should not receive enflurane as it is known to trigger this disorder. As with halothane, enflurane diminishes uterine tone which limits its use for vaginal deliveries and gynecologic procedures on the uterus.

Biotransformation of enflurane to a free inorganic fluoride ion makes the use of enflurane potentially nephrotoxic. Fortunately renal damage after the use of enflurane is quite rare, since rapid execretion by the lungs limits the amount of enflurane available to be biotransformed. Still, enflurane should be avoided in patients with compromised renal function.

Isoflurane

Isoflurane (Forane) is a halogenated ether and is an isomer of enflurane. It is a clear, colorless liquid with a pungent ethereal odor. Like the other halogenated agents, it is nonflammable in all concentrations which may be used clinically. The MAC of isoflurane is between that of enflurane and halothane, while its blood-gas solubility coefficient is lower than both (see Table 47-3). Isoflurane is chemically stable, requires no preservatives, and is packaged in bottles.

Indications and Dosing Isoflurane is used for both inhalation inductions and maintenance of general anesthesia. Its low blood-gas solubility would be expected to result in a rapid rate of induction, as well as emergence, but the pungent odor limits the speed of induction, as patients frequently cough, breath-hold, and even develop laryngospasm. Adequate premedication and slowly increasing the inspired concentration may minimize these adverse reactions.

Isoflurane is a muscle relaxant, but since the concentration required to produce a desired degree of relaxation may be quite high, it is often administered with a nondepolarizing muscle relaxant. This reduces the amount of both agents required for the attainment of surgical anesthesia, which is beneficial in producing a less depressed patient and a more rapid recovery. Both **enflurane** and **isoflurane** potentiate nondepolarizing muscle relaxants; however, isoflurane also potentiates muscle relaxants of the depolarizing type.

Isoflurane depresses myocardial contractility equal to that seen with halothane, but less than enflurane at equipotent doses. Although there is a drop in stroke volume, the cardiac output remains unchanged due to an increase in heart rate. Giving increasing doses of isoflurane progressively decreases the total peripheral resistance and lowers the blood pressure. Because of this unique property of isoflurane, the depth of anesthesia can be determined by the degree of hypotension present. These cardiovascular effects reduce the oxygen demand of the heart and its workload, which may be of benefit in patients with impaired cardiovascular systems. However caution is advised when administering isoflurane to these patients, since it does cause reflex tachycardia due to vasodilation which may precipitate myocardial ischemia if they are unable to meet the increased oxygen demands.

Pharmacokinetics Isoflurane is taken up by and eliminated from the body rapidly because of its low blood-gas solubility. About 95 percent of that taken up is exhaled unchanged. Less than 0.2 percent is recovered as a urinary metabolite, substantially less than that found with **halothane**, **enflurane**, and **methoxyflurane**. Isoflurane's low solubility reduces the amount of time it persists in the body available for biotransformation.

Adverse Reactions Respiratory depression of isoflurane is similar to that caused by the other potent inhalational agents. The response to hypoxia and hypercarbia is diminished. Augmentation of ventilation during surgical anesthesia is required to maintain an adequate oxygen–carbon dioxide exchange. Uterine tone is depressed with isoflurane and for certain procedures may increase uterine bleeding. It does not produce convulsions like its isomer, **enflurane**. It does, however, decrease cerebral vascular resistance and increase cerebral blood flow, which elevates intracranial pressure in the susceptible individual. This occurs to a much greater degree with both enflurane and halothane than with isoflurane. As with the other potent agents, isoflurane may trigger the malignant hyperthermia reaction, and should not be administered to patients with a history of this disease.

Volatile Anesthetics of Historical Interest

Methoxyflurane Methoxyflurane (Penthrane) is the most potent of the halogenated hydrocarbons. Induction and emergence are prolonged due to its very high blood-gas partition coefficient. About half of the methoxyflurane absorbed is metabolized in the liver to a free inorganic fluoride ion. The concentration of the metabolite is dose-related, and it is extremely nephrotoxic in high concentrations. Like the other halogenated agents it is nonflammable in all concentrations used clinically. Its use is limited in modern practice because of its nephrotoxicity and high solubility.

Diethyl Ether Ether is another volatile anesthetic rarely used because of its high solubility and because it is flammable. As would be expected, induction and emergence are quite prolonged and are frequently characterized by increased salivation, vomiting, and laryngospasm.

Intravenous Anesthetics

Intravenous anesthetic agents are used to induce and maintain general anesthesia, amnesia, and hypnosis, as well as to supplement inhalational anesthetics. The administration of

IV agents differs from that of inhalational agents, as once they are injected there is no way to facilitate their removal from the body. The anesthetist can only support vital functions until the activity of the drug abates. While IV anesthetics are capable of inducing loss of consciousness and memory, their ability to abolish pain and its associated reflexes is variable, and these drugs frequently require analgesic supplementation.

Ultrashort-Acting Barbiturates

The most frequently used intravenous anesthetic agents are the ultrashort-acting barbiturates: **methohexital sodium**, **thiamylal sodium**, and **thiopental sodium**. Barbiturates are discussed in Chap. 22 as hypnotics and in Chap. 33 as anticonvulsants, and will only be discussed here as they function as general anesthesia. **Thiopental sodium** (Pentothal) is the most widely used of the three and is the prototype. Some of the differences and similarities of the ultrashort-acting barbiturates are shown in Table 47-5.

Indications and Dosing   Intravenous barbiturates are used when an intravenous induction is desirable in patients whose cardiovascular system is relatively stable. Induction is pleasant and rapid, the onset occurring within seconds of administration. Duration of a single induction dose is short, usually lasting for less than ½ h. Intravenous barbiturates may be used alone for very short procedures which are not extremely painful, as their analgesic properties are minimal and the duration of action is short. After the induction dose is administered, other IV agents such as narcotics, amnesics, and muscle relaxants, are administered to maintain anesthesia. Barbiturates are also used to induce anesthesia before the administration of an inhalational agent. Dosages of the most common agents are shown on Table 47-5.

Pharmacokinetics   Barbiturates have the ability to penetrate all body tissues; the rate of uptake by individual tissues is determined by regional blood flow. Tissues which are well-perfused, such as the brain, rapidly take up the drug and equilibrate with the blood concentration. As the barbiturate is slowly distributed to the poorly perfused tissues, the blood level drops. To maintain equilibrium, the drug progressively diffuses back into the blood from the well-perfused tissues. As this progressive redistribution phase occurs, the anesthetic activity of the barbiturate diminishes, and the patient begins to regain consciousness. In other words, recovery is not dependent on metabolism unless excessive or repeated doses of the barbiturate are given, which results in tissue saturation.

Adverse Reactions   Ultrashort-acting barbiturates produce varying degrees of respiratory depression depending on the dosage given and the patient's general status; thus depression may range from none at all to complete apnea. Laryngeal and pharyngeal reflexes may be hypersensitive and any stimulation of these structures before the stage of surgical anesthesia is reached may induce spasm. This is especially prominent in patients with reactive airway disease, such as asthma.

The circulatory actions of the ultrashort-acting barbiturates include an increase in total peripheral resistance and depression of myocardial contractility. A patient with cardiovascular disease may not tolerate this depressant action and may become hypotensive and even experience cardiovascular collapse. Barbiturates should not be given to patients with a history of acute intermittent porphyria, as the condition may be exacerbated, resulting in pain, weakness, and paralysis secondary to nerve demyelination. Extravenous injection may cause tissue sloughing, therefore the intravenous lines should be a large gauge type and should be checked for patency prior to induction to prevent this totally avoidable complication.

Etomidate

Etomidate (Amidate), a relatively new nonbarbiturate intravenous hypnotic agent, is classified as a carboxylated imidazole. It is a potent hypnotic with a short duration of action and a fairly wide margin of safety. It is approximately 25

TABLE 47-5   Ultrashort-Acting Barbiturates

	METHOHEXITAL SODIUM (BREVITAL)	THIAMYLAL SODIUM (SURITAL)	THIOPENTAL SODIUM (PENTOTHAL)
Percent solution	1	2–2.5	2–2.5
Induction dose	1 mg/kg	3–5 mg/kg	3–5 mg/kg
Onset of action	20–30 s	30–40 s	30–40 s
Duration of single dose	5–7 min	5–10 min	5–10 min
Metabolism	Complete, 10–15%/h	Complete, 10–15%/h	Complete, 10–15%/h
$t_{1/2}$ of single dose	3.5–6 h	3–8 h	3–8 h

times as potent as thiopental, although equally effective since it is used in smaller doses.

Indications and Dosing   Induction with etomidate in a patient with a healthy cardiovascular system elicits minimal cardiovascular effects. In patients with coronary heart disease, induction with etomidate causes slight mycardial depression. A transient drop in total peripheral resistance accompanied by reflex tachycardia is observed, but there is no alteration in the coronary perfusion pressure or myocardial oxygen consumption. Thus, etomidate may be used safely as an induction agent in the elderly or in patients with cardiovascular disease.

Etomidate produces little, if any, respiratory depression in the usual doses, which may be of benefit in short minor surgical or diagnostic procedures. Its short duration of action makes it a good agent for outpatient surgery, as recovery is speedy. The usual induction dose of etomidate is 0.2 to 0.3 mg/kg of body weight intravenously.

Pharmacokinetics   Sleep is induced within 30 to 60 s after injection of etomidate, and the duration of a single dose is 3 to 5 min. Etomidate is rapidly metabolized in the liver to inactive metabolites and does not undergo any significant tissue redistribution. The half-life of etomidate is 40 min. Within 24 h 75 percent of the metabolites are excreted in the urine.

Adverse Reactions   As etomidate is a safe and relatively nontoxic anesthetic, its adverse effects are minimal. Pain on injection is frequent, but may be minimized by avoiding the small veins on the dorsum of the hand for injection. The use of an intravenous narcotic just prior to induction has also been successful in diminishing the pain. Fortunately the pain on injection is not associated with thrombophlebitis. Postoperative nausea and vomiting is frequent.

The other major adverse effect is the development of myoclonus. This annoying, benign phenomenon is short-lived, usually lasting for less than 1 min and is self-limiting. Administration of **diazepam** or **fentanyl** prior to induction reduces the extent of the movement and may even totally abolish it.

Droperidol/Fentanyl

Innovar is the brand name for a precompounded combination of 2.5 mg of droperidol, and 0.05 mg/mL of fentanyl. This combination alone produces what is termed *neuroleptoanalgesia;* when **nitrous oxide** is added it becomes *neuroleptoanesthesia.* The terms are derived from the fact that **droperidol** is a butyrophenone neuroleptic and antipsychotic with effects similar to **haloperidol** (Haldol) (see Chap. 34) and **fentanyl** is a narcotic analgesic (see Chap. 17). Characteristics of neuroleptoanalgesia include a reduction in motor activity, relief from anxiety, and indifference to the surroundings; the patient is cooperative, responding appropri-

ately to commands. **Droperidol** (Inapsine) and **fentanyl** (Sublimaze) may be given separately or in the fixed combination as Innovar.

Indications and Dosing   Innovar is very useful for patients undergoing diagnostic procedures when cooperation and responsiveness are necessary. It is also of value for short, minor surgical procedures such as wound debridement and changes in dressing for the burn patient. Small doses of Innovar facilitate endotracheal intubation of conscious patients, who remain calm and cooperative during the procedure and have the ability to protect their own airway. Protection of the airway is very important in patients with full stomachs, as they easily regurgitate stomach contents.

Neuroleptoanesthesia is a safe anesthetic technique for the elderly or poor-risk patient. The cardiovascular system remains stable, except for a drop in blood pressure in the hypovolemic patient, and fluids will quickly correct this. Droperidol is generally given only for induction due to its long duration of action, while fentanyl is given as needed throughout the procedure. For skeletal muscle relaxation, a nondepolarizing muscle relaxant is given. Patients generally recover rapidly from this technique; consciousness is attained within a few minutes of discontinuing the nitrous oxide. Since droperidol is a potent antiemetic, nausea and vomiting are rare, but a few patients will complain of confusion or depression postoperatively.

Pharmacokinetics   Both droperidol and fentanyl are metabolized by the liver, and the metabolites are excreted in the urine. After IV or IM injection, onset of droperidol action is from 3 to 10 min, although the full effect may not be seen for 30 min. The duration of the sedation and tranquilizing effect is usually 2 to 4 h, although it may persist as long as 12 h. Onset of fentanyl action is 5 to 15 min, peaking within 30 min. Fentanyl has a very short half-life of 5 to 20 min, and the effect persists 1 to 2 h.

Adverse Reactions   Fentanyl is a potent narcotic. Its analgesic properties do not last as long as its respiratory depressant effects, which may persist for 3 to 4 h. Therefore patients may demonstrate some depression of respirations and still complain of pain. After receiving this combination, patients should not be left unattended as they may forget to breath and may literally need to be reminded. Fentanyl has a parasympathomimetic effect and may produce bradycardia and a slight hypotension even in usual dosages. It should not be given rapidly or in excessive doses as it may cause chest wall rigidity and inhibit respiration. This rigidity may be eliminated by the use of either a skeletal muscle relaxant or a narcotic antagonist. If a relaxant is used, the patient will require mechanical ventilation.

Droperidol has α-adrenergic blocking properties which in a hypovolemic patient may cause hypotension. Abrupt changes in posture should be avoided as severe hypotension could be precipitated. The extrapyramidal signs are more frequently seen in children than adults and are treated with 1 to 2 mg of **physostigmine**. Occasionally, patients receiving droperidol become confused and restless, although the incidence is reduced when patients also receive fentanyl. Droperidol potentiates narcotics; patients receiving postoperative analgesics should be closely watched for signs of respiratory depression. The usual dosage of a narcotic should be reduced at least to one-half of the normal dose for 12 h postoperatively.

Sufentanil

Sufentanil (Sufenta) is a potent narcotic analgesic that induces anesthesia in doses between 8 and 30 μg/kg. It is used in major surgical procedures such as cardiovascular surgery, neurological procedures in the sitting position, and other procedures where prolonged postoperative mechanical ventilation is anticipated. Sufentanil provides good myocardial and cerebral oxygen balance and, in higher doses, attenuates catecholamine release. In doses of 1 to 8 μg/kg, sufentanil can be used as an adjunct to nitrous oxide/oxygen anesthesia to provide hemodynamic stability. Maintenance doses are 10 to 50 μg/kg for stress and lightening of anesthesia. Children require 10 to 25 μg/kg administered with 100% oxygen for induction.

Benzodiazepines

Diazepam Diazepam (Valium) is a benzodiazepine with anticonvulsant, ataractic, amnestic, and central muscle relaxant properties. It is frequently used for the induction of anesthesia and as a sedative during local procedures. During induction, diazepam causes less hypotension than **thiopental**, and under certain conditions will actually improve left ventricular function. This property can be very beneficial in the poor-risk or elderly patient. Respiratory depression may occur with diazepam, but with careful titration of the drug, maximal sedation may be achieved with minimal respiratory depression. Diazepam is also useful for intubations or electrocardioversions when the patient is awake; the patients are relaxed, and recall is limited.

The pharmacology of diazepam is discussed in Chap. 34.

Midazolam Midazolam is a new benzodiazepine derivative still under investigation. Unlike other benzodiazepines it is a water-soluble salt, which makes it nonirritating upon intravenous injection and not associated with thrombophlebitis. Its onset of action is rapid, while its duration is short with a half-life of 1.3 to 2 h. It is about as potent as diazepam and produces similar effects. In animal studies, midazolam appears to maintain cardiovascular stability and to have no direct autonomic effects. It is being studied for its potential value as an induction agent and a maintenance agent of anesthesia for short procedures.

Ketamine

Ketamine (Ketalar) is an intravenous anesthetic which produces *dissociative anesthesia*. Patients receiving ketamine appear to be in a state of catalepsy; their eyes remain open and they may have nystagmus. There is an increase in skeletal muscle tone, and some patients move purposelessly, without relation to noxious stimuli. Other characteristics of ketamine include an increase in salivation, intact protective reflexes of the larynx and pharynx, cardiovascular stimulation (tachycardia and hypertension), and a high incidence of emergence reactions. These reactions range from a slight mood alteration to frank delirium. It is a potent analgesic, but has a minimal effect on visceral pain, requiring analgesic supplementation for thoracic and abdominal procedures.

Mechanism of Action Ketamine produces a functional and electrophysiologic dissociation between the limbic system and the thalamoneocortex, resulting in a dissociative state of anesthesia. The exact mechanism of this dissociation process is poorly understood. Depression of various stimulatory nuclei results in analgesia and a misperception of auditory and visual stimuli. This is thought to be the cause of the emergence reaction.

Indications and Dosing Ketamine is useful alone for short diagnostic procedures and superficial operations of short duration. It is used in both adults and children successfully. Occasionally it is used as an adjunct to regional anesthetic techniques, especially while the block is being administered. Acceptance of this procedure is generally good, and recall of the block is minimal.

The elderly or poor-risk patient is a good candidate for ketamine. Its cardiostimulatory properties are very beneficial in these patients, as a sudden drop in blood pressure may precipate a stroke or other severe reaction. Its use in hemorrhagic shock is controversial, since the cardiostimulatory properties are not as pronounced in patients in shock as in normovolemic patients. Occasionally ketamine may cause hypotension, since the cardiostimulatory effect are centrally mediated while ketamine exerts a direct depressant effect on the heart.

Ketamine can be used in patients with asthma since it appears to increase lung compliance and decrease airway resistance. Ketamine is also useful in patients who require high inspired oxygen tensions to maintain tissue oxygenation because 100% oxygen may be used.

In the past, ketamine was avoided in the obstetric patient due to a high incidence of emergence reactions and depression of newborns. However, these results were dose-related. Ketamine, in proper doses, provides good analgesia for the parturient patient without significantly depressing the newborn, rarely causing unpleasant recovery. In anesthetic doses, adequate surgical anesthesia is maintained, but emergence reactions are frequent. Increased bleeding does not occur because ketamine maintains uterine tone.

Administration may be achieved by the IV or IM route. The intravenous induction dose is 1 to 2 mg/kg of body weight given over 30 to 60 s. Onset of action occurs within 1 min, lasting for 5 to 10 min. Maintenance may be achieved with intermittent doses of 0.5 to 1 mg/kg administered approximately every 10 min. When given by IM injection the usual dosage is 3 to 5 mg/kg. Onset occurs within 5 min with a 12- to 15-min duration, and maintenance is generally by the IV route.

Pharmacokinetics   Distribution of a single dose of ketamine resembles that of **thiopental**. Its rapid onset of action is attributed to a high tissue solubility and rapid distribution to the well-perfused tissues such as the brain. Initial recovery is not due to metabolism but to redistribution of the drug to the lesser perfused tissues with a concomitant drop in the brain concentration. The half-life of the distribution phase is 7 to 11 min. Metabolism occurs in the liver, and the metabolites are excreted in the urine, the half-life being 2 to 3 h.

Adverse Reactions   Emergence reactions associated with ketamine may manifest themselves as either pleasant or unpleasant visual and auditory hallucinations. They may also manifest as irrational, confused, or excitatory behavior during the recovery phase. The incidence of these psychologic reactions is lower in children under age 15 years. Previously it was thought that providing a patient who had received ketamine with a quiet, dark environment for recovery would lessen the severity or totally abolish the psychic reaction. This has proved to be untrue. Explaining the emergence phenomenon preoperatively seems to lessen the incidence of these reactions. Concomitant administration of a benzodiazipine or an ultrashort-acting barbiturate is also helpful in diminishing or totally abolishing the reaction. **Lorazepam** is the most effective currently available benzodiazepine in preventing the psychic reaction.

Ketamine generally causes a rise in blood pressure and an increase in heart rate. These characteristics make the use of ketamine undesirable in patients with head trauma or impending cerebrovascular hemorrhage and in other clinical situations in which an elevated blood pressure may be undesirable or dangerous. This action of ketamine may, however, be an advantage in emergency situations when shock is present and when cardiovascular pressure and output must be maintained.

Other adverse effects with the agent are laryngospasm, cardiac arrhythmias, diplopia, nystagmus, an increase in intraocular pressure, clonic-tonic skeletal muscle movements (resembling seizures), and local pain or erythema at the injection site.

Local Anesthetic Agents

Local anesthetic agents are drugs that block nerve conduction when they are applied in sufficiently high concentration either to tissues containing nerve fibers or around the nerve fibers themselves. These agents act on all portions of the central and peripheral nervous systems and, as exemplified by the use of **lidocaine** for cardiac arrhythmias, suppress the excitable cells of other tissues as well. The degree to which a nerve may be blocked is dependent on the potency and concentration of the local anesthetic being used and on the specific characteristics of the nerve being blocked. As a rule, smaller unmyelinated nerves are blocked by lower concentrations than are the larger myelinated nerves. A general hierarchy of local anesthetic action may be graded in the following order: pain, temperature, touch, and deep pressure. In sufficient concentrations, local anesthetics will block all nerve impulse conduction, afferent and efferent. Thus, in sufficient concentrations these agents will induce a motor block as well as a sensory block.

Local anesthetics differ significantly from general (inhalation and IV) agents in that their focus of action may be chosen selectively and in that it is not necessary to produce unconsciousness in order to obtain analgesic or muscular paralysis in selected areas. These agents have many uses and routes of administration.

Regional or *conduction anesthesia* refers to an insensibility over a certain area due to the blocking of nerve pathways by a local anesthetic. Patients remain conscious during regional anesthesia. *Spinal block anesthesia* is produced by the injection of a local anesthetic into the cerebrospinal fluid of the subarachnoid space, which leaves the patient unable to move or to sense pain in the lower part of the body. *Epidural anesthesia* is similar to spinal anesthesia, as a loss of motor and sensory nerve function also occurs. However, with the epidural type the local anesthetic is injected just proximal to the spinal column between the vertebrae, in an area known as the epidural space. *Caudal anesthesia* is the injection of an anesthetic solution into the epidural space through the sacral hiatus (see Fig. 47-4). Topical application of a local anesthetic to the skin or eye produces relief of itching or gives local desensitization for a short test or procedure.

Mechanism of Action

Local anesthetics initially slow the generation and conduction of nerve impulses and, if used in sufficient concentrations, may totally block it. They also increase the threshold for electrical excitability of all cells. Blocking of the nerve action potential is due to the inhibition of the sodium and potassium ion flux across the cell membrane. The exact way the local anesthetics affect the cell membrane's permeability to sodium and potassium is not known.

Pharmacokinetics

Chemical composition of local anesthetics includes either an amide or an ester linkage. The difference in their chemical makeup does not affect their anesthetic capabilities but is the determining factor of their metabolism.

The ester-type anesthetics (Table 47-6) are metabolized by hydrolysis in the blood by plasma pseudocholinesterase and in the liver by cholinesterase. There are no esterases in the spinal fluid or epidural space, and so when these agents are used in spinal or epidural blocks, they must diffuse into the plasma before metabolism begins. Para-aminobenzoic acid (PABA) is one of the major metabolites of the esters, and

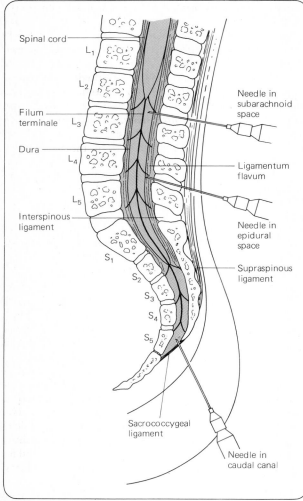

FIGURE 47-4

Regional Anesthesia Routes. Schematic diagram of lumbosacral anatomy, showing needle placement for subarachnoid, lumbar epidural, and caudal block. [*From S. M. Shnider, G. L. Levinson, and D. H. Ralson: "Regional Anesthesia for Labor and Delivery," in S. M. Shnider and G. L. Levinson (eds.), Anesthesia for Obstetrics, © 1979, Williams and Wilkins, Baltimore. Used by permission of the publisher and authors.*]

will occasionally cause an allergic reaction in some patients. PABA also interferes with the bacteriostatic action of sulfonamides and with biologic assay procedures for these anti-infective agents. Potency, toxicity, absorption, onset of action, and duration of effect differs among the various drugs, as described below for each agent.

The local anesthetics with an amide linkage (Table 47-7) are metabolized in the liver. Allergic reactions to the amides or their metabolites are rare. As with the esters, there are both quantitative and qualitative differences in their

potency, toxicity, systemic absorption, onset, and duration of action, as discussed below. The metabolites are excreted in the urine.

Toxicity of the local anesthetics is dependent on the rate at which they are absorbed systemically and on the rate of

TABLE 47-6 Ester Linkage Local Anesthetics

DRUG	COMMON USES	STRENGTH AND DOSES
Cocaine	Topical anesthesia of upper respiratory tract	1–10% solution; maximum dose 200 mg
Procaine (Novocaine)	Infiltration and peripheral nerve block	2–4% with or without epinephrine 1:100,000 or 1:200,000; maximum dose 1000 mg
	Caudal or epidural spinal	25 mL of a 1.5% solution 50–200 mg
Tetracaine (Pontocaine)	Infiltration and peripheral nerve block	0.1–0.25% solution with or without epinephrine; maximum dose 100 mg
	Caudal	30–35 mL of a 0.15–0.25% solution
	Spinal	10–20 mg with or without 0.2 mg of epinephrine
	Topical:	
	Eye	0.1 mL of a 0.5% solution
	Nose & throat	1 mL of 1–2% solution
	Damaged skin	0.5–1% ointment
Chloroprocaine (Nesicaine)	Infiltration and peripheral nerve block	1–2% with or without epinephrine 1:100,000 or 1:200,000; maximum dose 100 mg
Piperocaine (Metycaine)	Infiltration and peripheral nerve block	1–2% solution; maximum dose 750 mg
	Caudal	35 mL of 1.5% solution
	Spinal	30 mg/mL
	Topical	2–4% solution
Hexylclaine (Cyclaine)	Infiltration and peripheral nerve block	1–2% solution; maximum dose 500 mg
	Topical	5% solution; maximum dose 250 mg

metabolism. Local application of anesthetic to the mucosa of the oral cavity or respiratory tract will result in systemic absorption almost as rapid as an IV injection. Local anesthetics also enter the systemic circulation when injected for a regional blockade. The concomitant use of a vasoconstrictor such as **epinephrine** will slow the rate of absorption and will also prolong the duration of action. The slower the absorption, the less drug available to cause systemic toxicity. However, the most important factor in determining toxicity is the rate of destruction. Ester-type anesthetics are rapidly metabolized in the plasma, and therefore have a low rate of toxicity. On the other hand, the amides are more slowly metabolized in the liver; thus their potential for toxicity is greater. Liver disease prolongs the action and toxicity of the amides.

Protein binding of a local anesthetic in the blood, will prolong its duration within the circulation and may increase its potential for toxicity.

Chemical composition of local anesthetics is such that they possess both hydrophilic and lipophilic properties. Therefore they are soluble in water and lipids, both of which are necessary for anesthetic activity. Lipid solubility allows for absorption and transport to the site of action, while the water-soluble ionized form is necessary for the drug to exert its effect on the neural cell.

Indications

Topical   Local anesthetic agents may be applied to the skin, the mucous membranes, and the eye. Application may be for the relief of minor skin or mucous membrane pain or irritation, or it may be used to prevent pain. Thus, these drugs are used in ophthalmic procedures which require the cooperation of the patient or in procedures which are so minor that they do not warrant other forms of anesthesia. The preventive blockade of pain is also useful for the insertion of catheters or other localized invasive or painful techniques.

Blockade of Peripheral Nerves   Local anesthetics may be injected around peripheral nerve terminals (infiltration anesthesia) or into the sheaths of peripheral nerves. This technique allows for a relatively high degree of blockade in a localized area of the periphery. It is useful for painful injections, for minor surgical and dental procedures, and for surgical procedures on extremities. Administration of local anesthetics for this type of anesthesia is usually accomplished with intradermal, intraarticular, intrabursal, or in the case of Bier block, intravenous injections. Certain problems may be encountered in administering local anesthetics in this way. If the injection technique is poor, these agents may be introduced into the general circulation, which may lead to severe adverse reactions.

Spinal, Epidural, or Caudal Anesthesia   The level of anesthesia achieved by these techniques is dependent on the concentration of the anesthetic, its potency, the volume in which it is administered, the injection technique, and the patient's position. Spinal anesthesia is becoming more and more popular as an alternative to general inhalation anesthetic procedures when total anesthesia is neither necessary nor desirable. In many instances, patients may be premedicated with small doses of central nervous system depressants such as barbiturates, tranquilizers, or narcotics to keep them relaxed, yet awake.

These routes of administration must be used with great care. Blockade of the nerve trunks may produce marked hypotension. One problem associated with spinal or epi-

TABLE 47-7   Amide Linkage Local Anesthetics

DRUG	COMMON USES	STRENGTH AND DOSES
Lidocaine (Xylocaine)	Infiltration and peripheral nerve block	0.5–2% solution with or without epinephrine 1:100,000 or 1:200,000; mamimum dose with epinephrine 500 mg; maximum dose without epinephrine 300 mg
	Epidural	1–2% solution 30 mL with or without epinephrine 1:200,000
	Spinal	5% solution with 7.5% dextrose with or without 0.2 mg epinephrine; maximum dose 100 mg
	Topical	2–4% solution; 2% jelly
Dibucaine (Nupercaine)	Spinal	2.5–10 mg
	Topical	0.25–1% ointment or spray, 2.5 mg suppository
Prilocaine (Citanest)	Infiltration and peripheral nerve block	1–2% solution; maximum dose 500 mg
Bupivacaine (Marcaine)	Infiltration and peripheral nerve block	0.25–0.75% solution; maximum dose 200 mg
	Epidural and caudal	15–30 mL of a 0.25–0.75% solution
Etidocaine (Duranest)	Infiltration and peripheral nerve block	0.5–1.5% solution with or without 1:200,000 epinephrine; maximum dose 300 mg
	Epidural and caudal	0.5–1.5% solution

dural anesthesia is the inability to determine with accuracy the anesthetic level. If the drug inadvertently reaches the cervical cord, a respiratory arrest will ensue. Patients will require mechanical ventilation until the block wears off. Nausea and vomiting occasionally occur with spinal anesthesia, but may be controlled with antiemetics.

In patients who have spinal anesthesia affecting the limbs, there is a dramatic loss of proprioception in these areas. In the period of time before total dissipation of the local anesthetic, this may give the patient an uncomfortable sensation of phantom limb, similar to the feelings of the patient who has undergone amputation.

In addition to the pharmacologic side effects of spinal administration of local anesthetics, there are all of the inherent complications of any sort of lumbar puncture. Neurologic complications, trauma to the surrounding nerve tissues, headaches, and bacterial contamination are some possible problems. Headaches are extremely prominent if a dural puncture is accidentally made during the administration of an epidural injection, due to the relatively large gauge needle which is used.

Adverse Effects

With any technique of administering local anesthetics, unwanted side effects may develop in the circulatory, respiratory, or central nervous systems. Adverse effects in the central nervous system are of an excitatory or depressant nature and include restlessness, confusion, tremor, convulsions, and respiratory depression or paralysis. Toxic manifestations in the cardiovascular system are due to a direct depressant effect on the myocardium. These effects may be minor causing hypotension, or they may be severe enough to cause cardiac arrest. **Ultrashort-acting barbiturates** are given intravenously for the CNS manifestations, artificial ventilatory support for respiratory depression, and symptomatic therapy for other problems. The severity and incidence of these unwanted effects correlate with the blood levels of the local anesthetic.

Some local anesthetics can cause allergic reactions. Cross-sensitization does not occur between the amides and esters; thus, a patient allergic to **procaine** can be switched to **lidocaine**. In allergic patients it is good practice to do an intradermal skin test with any anesthetic agent prior to its use in order to identify potential allergic complications. Manifestations of these allergic problems include rashes, bronchospasms, and, possibly, anaphylaxis. The treatment of allergic responses to these agents includes the use of antihistamines and, if necessary, **epinephrine**.

Esters

Cocaine Cocaine is a benzoic acid ester which is used as a topical anesthetic for the nose, pharynx, larynx, and tracheobronchial tree. It has strong vasoconstrictor properties; thus it causes shrinkage of mucous membranes and reduces bleeding. It is sometimes used as a paste or "cocaine mud." The onset is immediate, and its duration is approximately 45 min. Cocaine is the standard to which other local anesthetics are compared for production of surface anesthesia.

Procaine Procaine (Novocaine) is an aminobenzoic acid ester which is employed for infiltration anesthesia, for peripheral nerve blocks, and for spinal, epidural, and caudal anesthesia. It is not effective as a topical anesthetic, but has been used intravenously to treat cardiac arrhythmias and experimentally, with limited results, to delay the aging process (as GH3 or Gerovital). The potential for toxicity is low, and it undergoes rapid hydrolysis in the blood. The onset of action occurs within 2 to 5 min and lasts generally for less than 1 h. **Epinephrine** may be added to increase its duration by slowing its absorption. Procaine is the standard by which the potency and toxicity of the other local anesthetics used for injection are compared.

Tetracaine Tetracaine (Pontocaine) is a PABA ester which is used for topical, ophthalmic, infiltration, peripheral nerve block, caudal, and spinal anesthesia. It is 10 times as potent and toxic as **procaine**, and is popular in use for spinal anesthetics. Onset of action occurs within 5 to 10 min, and it will provide anesthesia for about 2 h, although this may be increased by the addition of **epinephrine**.

Chloroprocaine Chloroprocaine (Nesacaine) is a halogenated analog of procaine and is used for infiltration, peripheral nerve block, caudal, and epidural anesthesia. It is twice as potent as **procaine**, undergoes rapid hydrolysis in the blood, and therefore is relatively low in toxicity. The onset of action is rapid with a short duration of action which may be prolonged with the addition of **epinephrine**.

Piperocaine Piperocaine (Metycaine) is a benzoic acid ester used for topical, infiltration, peripheral nerve block, spinal, and caudal anesthesia. It is less effective than **cocaine** as a topical anesthetic, and slightly more potent and toxic than **procaine** when used parenterally. Onset is immediate and the duration is about 1 h. Piperocaine is not used with **epinephrine**.

Hexylcaine Hexylcaine (Cyclaine) is a benzoic acid ester which is employed for topical, infiltration, and peripheral nerve block anesthesia. It too is slightly more toxic and potent than procaine. Parenteral onset occurs between 5 and 15 min with a duration of 1 to 1½ h. Topically it takes 2 to 3 min to start acting, and will last approximately 30 min. Reports of local irritation with skin necrosis and tissue sloughing after intradermal injection have decreased its use. It should not be used with **epinephrine**.

Amides

Lidocaine   Lidocaine (Xylocaine) is administered for topical, infiltration, peripheral nerve block, spinal, epidural, and caudal anesthesia. It is also administered intravenously to treat ventricular arrhythmias. As a topical agent it is less potent than **cocaine**, and as an injected anesthetic it is twice as toxic as **procaine** but more prompt, intense, and longer-lasting. It has a rapid onset, does not irritate tissues, and has a duration of greater than 1 h. It is a vasodilator; the addition of **epinephrine** will prolong its duration. Lidocaine is metabolized in the liver to active metabolites that have anesthetic properties and toxicities, particularly of the cardiovascular system (fibrillation and cardiac arrest).

Dibucaine   Dibucaine (Nupercaine) is a cinchoninamide derivative used for topical anesthesia for damaged skin or mucous membranes and for spinal anesthesia. It is the most potent and toxic of all the local anesthetics, and has a duration of about 3 h. Administered subcutaneously it generally causes tissue sloughing. It is not used with **epinephrine**.

Mepivacaine   Mepivacaine (Carbocaine) is an amide used for infiltration, peripheral nerve block, spinal, epidural, and caudal anesthesia. It is not an effective topical anesthetic. It has a rapid onset of action and lasts for about 2 h. Like **lidocaine**, mepivacaine produces vasodilation and as such is indicated for nerve blocks in areas of slight vascularity, e.g., fingers. The addition of epinephrine does not prolong its duration, but it is available for dental use with **levonordefin** as a vasoconstrictor. Its potency and toxicity are about equal to lidocaine.

Prilocaine   Prilocaine (Citanest) is an amide derivative used for infiltration and peripheral nerve block anesthesia. It is more potent and less toxic than procaine. High doses of prilocaine may cause methemoglobinemia, and for this reason is rarely used.

Bupivacaine   Bupivacaine (Marcaine) is an anilide derivative used for infiltration, peripheral nerve block, epidural, and caudal anesthesia. It is more potent and has a longer duration of action than does **lidocaine**, while it is equal in toxicity to **tetracaine**. In concentrations less than 0.57%, anesthesia occurs without a motor block.

Etidocaine   Etidocaine (Duranest) is the newest local anesthetic and is an amide. It is used for infiltration, perpheral nerve block, epidural, and caudal anesthesia. It has a long duration of action, between 4 and 6 h. Its toxicity is twice that of **lidocaine**, while it potency is four times greater. It is used with or without **epinephrine**.

Anesthetic Adjuncts

Several types of pharmacologic agents are used in conjunction with general or local anesthetic agents. These drugs may by used either to enhance one of the basic activities of the anesthetic agents or to provide an added pharmacologic dimension to the administration of anesthesia. For example, the general anesthetic **halothane** produces only a mild degree of skeletal muscle relaxation, which is not adequate for abdominal cases. Therefore, supplementation with a skeletal muscle relaxant (i.e., neuromuscular blocker) is required (see Chap. 16 and Table 47-8).

Patients who have received nondepolarizing skeletal muscle relaxants may have prolonged weakness unless the action of the relaxant is terminated. The action of these relaxants is reversed with anticholinesterase agents (e.g., **neostigmine**). Anticholinesterase agents allow acetylcholine to build up at the neuromuscular junction to overtake the competitive blockade of the nondepolarizing muscle relaxant, thus neuromuscular function returns. Without receiving a reversal agent, patients generally require postoperative ventilation.

The rationales for the use of the many different pharmacologic agents employed in the operating room as anesthetic adjuncts are numerous and complex. Usually, the basic pharmacology of the drugs will inherently show their usefulness during the anesthetic procedure. Table 47-9 outlines some of the adjunctive agents commonly used during and after the operative procedure. Those agents whose pharmacology is discussed in other parts of the text will only be mentioned here, and the reader is urged to review the basic mechanisms and indications for these drugs in light of their usefulness during the anesthetic procedure.

Intraoperative Nursing Management

Other than the nurse anesthetist, who has special education, the nurse is seldom involved in the administration of medications during the surgical procedure. However, the nurse does have responsibilities associated with these agents. Because of the excitability associated with stage II anesthesia, the nurse needs to make sure that quiet is maintained and that the patient is not touched until the anesthesiologist gives approval to do so. Because the blood pressure may purposely be maintained at a low level and because of the paralysis associated with anesthesia, the patient is prone to the formation of pressure sores; the nurse must ensure that the patient is positioned properly and that pressure points are adequately padded before the surgical drapes are applied.

Sometimes there is a tendency to adopt a false sense of security when local agents rather than general anesthetics are used. However, it should be remembered that there can be life-threatening complications to local anesthesia, and emergency drugs and equipment should be available. Since the part of the body that is anesthetized is insensitive, the nurse must protect the part from unnecessary trauma during and after surgery.

In spinal anesthesia the patient should not be moved until the anesthetic is "set," or the anesthetic could travel to the nerves associated with the muscles of respiration.

The patient who has received a general anesthetic must be moved from the operating table with care in a smooth, coordinated manner, since severe hypotension can develop if the patient is moved improperly while still under the influence of the anesthesia.

Intraoperative Nursing Evaluation

The ongoing evaluation of the patient's status is usually the responsibility of the anesthetist. The circulating nurse is in a position to assess the total picture of cardiorespiratory status, blood loss, and the progress of the surgery and to assist in emergency situations. In addition, some operating room nurses make a follow-up visit to the patient to see if any complications have occurred that may be attributable to the intraoperative period.

Frequently the nurse may be in attendance when a local anesthetic is used for a surgical procedure. The nurse then assumes the responsibility for evaluating the status of the patient by taking the vital signs, observing the respiratory status, and evaluating the neurologic status. In addition to the convulsions and shock that may occur if the local anesthetic is injected into or absorbed into the systemic circulation, a reaction known as *vasovagal syncope* often occurs just as the needle is withdrawn. It is thought to be caused by a massive vagal stimulation due to the patient's fear of the needle and sudden relief that the injection is over. If this occurs, the nurse should see that the patient is immediately placed in a flat position.

POSTOPERATIVE CARE OF THE PATIENT

The initial concern as the patient is received in the immediate postsurgical unit, whether it be recovery room, intensive care unit, or general duty unit, is to position the patient and obtain an immediate determination of the patient's status. Usually the anesthetist will accompany the patient to the recovery area and perform this initial determination of the vital signs and respiratory function.

TABLE 47-8   Neuromuscular Blocking Agents

DRUG	DOSAGE	ONSET	DURATION	DURATION OF RESIDUAL EFFECT
Nondepolarizing Agents				
Atracurium besylate (Tracrium)	0.4–0.5 mg/kg	Within 3–5 min	20–30 min	½–2 h
Tubocurarine	15–20 mg initially; 3 mg supplemental doses	3 min	30–40 min	2–4 h
Gallamine (Flaxedil)	1 mg/kg; 0.5–1 mg/kg supplemental	Within 1–2 min	20–40 min	
Pancuronium (Pavulon)	0.04–0.1 mg/kg initially; 1–2 mg supplemental doses	Within 3 min	30–40 min	2–4 h
Metocurine iodide	2–3 mg initially; 1–2 mg after 5 min; 0.3–1 mg supplemental	Within 3 min	20 min	2–4 h
Vercuronium bromide (Norcuron)	0.08 mg/kg; 0.01–0.015 mg/kg supplemental	Within 3 min	25–30 min	1–2 h
Depolarizing Agents				
Succinylcholine (Anectine, others)	Single IV dose 60–100 mg; 10–30 mg for short procedure; 0.5–5 mg/min IV infusion	Within 1 min	5–15 min	15 min
Decamethonium (Syncurine)	0.5–3 mg initially; 0.25–1.5 mg supplemental at 10–30 min	1 min	20–40 min	1–3 h

Postoperative Nursing Assessment

When the patient is situated and drainage tubes, respirators, oxygen, and other equipment are properly attached, the nurse will want to begin the assessment by getting the following information from the anesthetist, surgeon, or chart: the type and length of procedure performed, the surgical complications and pathologic findings, the amount of blood loss, the type and amount of anesthesia and adjuncts the patient received, the patient's general condition and particular complications to observe for, and the information the family has been given. The nurse writes this information down so that it can be included in the report given to the nurses when the patient is transferred from the recovery area along with a report of the recovery room course.

The nurse assesses the vital signs every 15 min in the recovery area, compares these to the preoperative baseline (since the blood pressure may have been maintained at a low level intraoperatively), and reports significant findings such as a systolic reading below 85 mmHg, a drop in the systolic reading of more than 20 mmHg, or a blood pressure that

TABLE 47-9   Intraoperative and Postoperative Anesthetic Adjuncts

DRUG CLASSIFICATION	AGENTS	USE IN ANESTHETIC PROCESS
Anticholinergics	Atropine, glycopyrrolate (Robinul), scopolamine	For antivagal activity, sedation, drying of oral secretions, treatment of bradycardia.
Benzodiazepines	Diazepam (Valium), lorazepam (Ativan)	To produce amnesia and reduce other anesthetic requirements; for sedation during local procedures.
Butyrophenones	Droperidol (Inapsine)	For its amnestic properties and for its antiemetic effect.
Narcotics	Fentanyl (Sublimaze), morphine, meperidine (Demerol), sufentanil (Sufenta)	As analgesic adjuncts for inhalational anesthetics. Given intraoperatively for postoperative analgesia.
Phenothiazines	Hydroxyzine (Vistaril), IM	For antiemetic effects and sedative effects.
Anticholinesterase agents	Neostigmine (Prostigmin), edrophonium (Tensilon)	To reverse the effect of skeletal muscle relaxants of the nondepolarizing type.
Narcotic antagonist	Naloxone (Narcan)	To reverse the actions of narcotics; given for the respiratory depression.
Respiratory stimulants	Doxapram (Dopram), ethamivan (Emivan), nikethamide (Coramine)	To reverse the respiratory depression of central nervous system depressants.
Vasopressors	Dopamine (Inotropin), epinephrine (Adrenalin), isoproterenol (Isuprel), metaraminol (Aramine), levarterenol (Levophed), phenylephrine (Neosynephrine), ephedrine	For sympathomimetic effects in treating low blood pressure during anesthesia.
Antiarrhythmics	Lidocaine (Xylocaine), verapamil, digoxin (Lanoxin), procainamide (Pronestyl)	To treat cardiac arrhythmias of ventricular and supraventricular origin.
β-Adrenergic blocking agent	Propranolol (Inderal)	To treat tachycardias unresponsive to fluid therapy and increased anesthetic concentrations.
Vasodilators	Nitroglycerin paste (Nitropaste), nitroprusside (Nipride), hydralazine (Apresoline)	To treat hypertensive episodes and to produce deliberate hypotension for certain procedures.
Coronary anti-ischemic agents	Nitroglycerin	To treat ischemic episodes by reducing preload and afterload.

continues to drop 5 to 10 mmHg over several successive readings. These criteria vary for infants and children. Bradycardia, tachycardia, or the appearance of an irregular pulse are also important to report. Restlessness; rapid, shallow respirations; shallow, slow respirations; or noisy respiration can be signs of respiratory distress. The nurse also evaluates the gag, cough, and lid reflexes every 15 min to gauge the recovery process and watches for irregular respiration, swallowing, and vomiting. Many types of sophisticated machinery may be used to monitor the patient, but the four basic concerns remain circulatory, respiratory, neurologic, and renal function, even when technology provides numerous assessment parameters. A knowledge of the specific characteristics of each anesthetic will help the nurse to identify the most important observational guidelines.

Generally, recovery from anesthesia proceeds in a reverse order from induction. Therefore, the nurse is able to gauge the progress of the recovery. Patients are ready to be transferred from the recovery area when they are fully awake and their color is good, when reflexes have returned to normal and they can move extremities on command, when they have been medicated for pain, when vital signs have been stable for 30 min to 1 h and there is no sign of excessive bleeding, and when all drains (urinary, wound, nasogastric, etc.) are functioning. After the anesthetist gives approval, the patient is transferred.

When patients have received a local anesthetic, it is still important to assess their circulatory status and the functioning of the affected areas. The nurse assesses the circulation for color, movement, sensation, and capillary refill in the extremities. Patients are not out of danger when they can wiggle their toes, since the autonomic nervous system is affected for longer than the voluntary nervous system, and circulatory collapse could still occur.

Once the patient has been transferred from the recovery area the nurse maintains ongoing assessment of the circulatory, respiratory, neurologic, and renal functioning, but the frequency of observation is progressively decreased as the patient remains stable. If there should be any significant abnormal finding, the nurse should contact the physician and should perform the determinations every 15 min. Later, the nursing assessment focuses upon the three most common anesthetic complications: pulmonary complications, infections, and thrombophlebitis.

Anesthesia, surgery, pain medication, and prolonged bed rest all contribute to the development of pulmonary complications, which are detected by changes in respiration (rate, character, cough, sputum), abnormal findings on auscultation (rales, rhonchi, consolidation), and laboratory results (WBC, differential, etc.). The temperature of the postsurgical patient should be monitored.

The nurse also monitors postoperatively for the return of gastrointestinal function. Many of the preoperative medications, as well as the surgical procedure itself, can contribute to intestinal atony, ileus, and constipation. Therefore, the nurse should assess for passage of flatus and for bowel sounds before the patient takes anything orally. In some settings the nurse advances the diet on the basis of these assessments without furthur orders from the physician. It is also important to assess for return of normal voiding and bowel habits in the postsurgical period.

Postoperative Nursing Management

During the recovery period a quiet atmosphere should be maintained, as patients may be excitable at times. Since vomiting is a reflex that may be elicited during the recovery period, the patient should be positioned to prevent aspiration, lying either on the side or, if the surgeon requires the patient to remain supine, with the head turned to the side. Suctioning equipment should be available at each bedside. It is also important to use safety rails or straps to protect the patient from falling off the bed or cart.

At times the patient will experience pain before the anesthetic effects have completely worn off, in which case less than a full dose of analgesic is given in the recovery room. Guidelines for the administration of analgesics are presented in Chap. 17, but several points particularly pertinent to the postoperative period should be emphasized:

1.   If the patient's vital signs or neurologic status are poor or unstable, the physician should be consulted before a narcotic analgesic is given.

2.   Nurses should not administer less than the ordered dose without consulting the physician, unless written hospital policies specifically approve this practice.

3.   Depending upon the type of surgery, patients will generally require regular parenteral analgesics for 24 to 72 h following major surgery, after which the required frequency of dosage begins to decrease and oral analgesics should begin to control pain. However, *there is no absolute "normal" pattern of analgesic requirement*, since the pain experience is highly individual.

4.   Narcotic analgesics should not be withheld postoperatively due to fear of causing narcotic dependence.

5.   Patients with prior drug abuse histories (including alcohol, sedatives, narcotics, etc.) require special management of analgesics in the perioperative period (as discussed in Chap. 49).

6.   The use of a neuroleptic agent such as **droperidol** in the preoperative or intraoperative period also requires special adjustment of the patient's postoperative medication. Generally the patient should receive only one-fourth to one-half the usual narcotic analgesic dose for up to 12 h after the neuroleptic, since these agents potentiate the action of narcotics. If **hydroxyzine** (Atarax, Vistaril) or phenothiazines [e.g., **Promethazine** (Phenergan)] are given concomitantly with narcotic analgesics, the dosages of both drugs should be lower than the usual recommended dose. Students and inexperienced nurses should seek assistance in the decision making about postoperative analgesic administration from a more experienced colleague.

Prevention of pulmonary complications and thrombophlebitis begins early in the postoperative period. The nurse in the recovery area begins the deep breathing, turning, coughing, and leg exercises as soon as the patient is alert enough, if these are not contraindicated. This will be effective if preoperative teaching was adequate. The period of suggestibility that may occur has been used effectively in getting patients to cough and in preventing postoperative urinary retention. Coughing and deep breathing excercises should be done every 1 to 2 h in the postoperative period for at least the first 24 h, and every 2 to 4 h for several days.

For some time after surgery the patient may have dryness of the mouth, caused by the parasympatholytic drugs and the atropine-like side effects of other drugs. Good oral care will minimize the discomfort of the dry mouth and should be given even in the recovery area. Further, the patient may feel cold or shiver, particularly after **halothane**, and the nurse should see that the patient is kept warm and dry. Overwarming should be avoided, but a warmed, soft blanket often contributes to patient comfort.

Normally the patient should void within 12 h after surgery if an indwelling catheter is not in place. The anesthetic or adjuncts may inhibit the voiding reflex, and the production of urine is decreased by the normal postoperative response to stress. Therefore, the nurse should assess the bladder for distention by percussion and palpation. Measures such as physiologic positioning (standing, for males, and sitting, for females), creating the sound of running water, or pouring warm water over the perineum may encourage voiding. If these fail, the physician may order pharmacologic measures or catheterization.

When the patient has had spinal anesthesia, the headache that is thought to be caused by a decrease in the cerebrospinal fluid pressure can be prevented or minimized by keeping the patient quiet and flat and by giving adequate fluids. If the anesthetic has been applied topically to the pharyngeal area, the nurse should see that the patient does not try to take food or fluids until the gag reflex is well reestablished.

Outpatient Surgery

Due to the expense and inconvenience of hospitalization, outpatient surgery is becoming a common procedure in which the patient returns to home or even to work the day of surgery. The same preoperative assessment of the patient will be accomplished, possibly during an office or clinic visit on a day prior to the surgery or on the day of surgery. Most of these procedures are done under local anesthesia, and the nurse may assume responsiblity for monitoring vital signs and patient status during the procedure, as well as during the recovery period. Extremely important are the instructions which the patient receives after the surgery. These should be written, as well as verbal, and should include a description or listing of

1. Expected course of recovery after surgery
2. Expected drainage and incision (if any) appearance
3. Dietary and activity restrictions
4. Symptoms and signs which signal that the physician should be contacted
5. Discomforts to be expected and how to control them
6. The time the patient should return for postoperative evaluation

Postoperative Nursing Evaluation

Evaluation in the postoperative period is concerned with pulmonary complications, thrombophlebitis, infections, and other complications. For example, the effectiveness of coughing and deep breathing exercises can be evaluated by auscultating for breath sounds before and after the procedures. Furthur, evaluation of the adequacy of postoperative assessment is important, i.e., were appropriate observations performed properly and with adequate frequency? Quality assurance programs, evaluating the procedures and the outcome for groups of surgical patients, have led to improved care of patients in all three phases, preoperative, intraoperative, and postoperative.

CASE STUDY

Mr. A.M., age 46, underwent surgery, an exploratory sternotomy, because of a mediastinal mass. The assessment and management by the recovery room nurse began even before the patient was brought to the recovery room. After reviewing the operative schedule, the recovery room nurse determined what equipment would probably be required, and placed it in the patient's cubicle. The nurse also checked the emergency drug supplies to see that these were available and made sure that the emergency equipment was in working order.

Mr. M. was brought to the recovery room by the anesthetist and the operating room nurse, who assisted the recovery room nurse in (1) attaching the indwelling urinary catheter to gravity drainage, (2) attaching the two chest tubes to suction at 20 cmH$_2$0 pressure and the nasogastric tube to low-pressure intermittent suction, and (3) establishing the monitor pattern on the bedside electrocardiograph monitor. Mr. M. was partially awake and an endotracheal tube was still in place: this was attached to oxygen at 40%. A subclavian catheter was attached to a central venous pressure apparatus, and both this and the peripheral IV lines were noted to be infusing well. The patient was kept supine since he had both a nasogastric tube and the endotracheal tube with an inflated balloon to occlude the trachea. The postoperative orders included: morphine sulfate 2 to 4 mg IV q3h PRN, acetaminophen suppository 600 mg q4h for temperature above 101°F, and blood gases and hemotocrit determinations immediately.

Assessment

After Mr. M. was settled, the anesthetist and recovery room nurse ascertained the following: blood pressure 100/70; apical pulse 70 with normal sinus rhythm on the ECG monitor; central venous pressure (CVP) 3 cmH₂0; respiratory rate 20 and not labored; temperature 37°C. The nurse obtained the following information from the anesthetist and the surgeon, who had just returned from talking to Mr. M.'s wife.

The surgical procedure was an exploratory sternotomy, bronchoscopy, and excision of a lymphoid mass. The diagnosis postsurgically was lymphoma. The physician had informed Mrs. M. of the diagnosis and prognosis, and planned to speak with the patient about this the next morning. The patient had received the following anesthetic agents during the operation: thiamylal (Surital) 300 mg and succinylcholine 100 mg for induction, followed by maintenance during the 3-h procedure with curare and a halothane-oxygen mixture. There had been a brief hypotensive episode during the surgery, and the surgeon asked that the nurse watch the urine output carefully.

The nurse anticipated that Mr. M. might have some residual muscle paralysis despite the fact that he was partially alert and the curare had been reversed. Further, the nurse anticipated that the patient might later exhibit shivering and superficial vasoconstriction from the halothane.

The patient had received preoperative teaching about deep breathing, coughing, and leg exercises and had toured the recovery room. His preoperative blood pressure baseline had been 130/80.

Over the next hour Mr. M. became more alert, responded to his name, coughed when the endotracheal tube was suctioned, experienced a return of the lid reflex, and could move all extremities on command. However, his blood pressure remained at 100 to 105/70, CVP at 3, pulse at 72, and urine output at 15 mL/h. Arterial blood gases and hematocrit were reported by the laboratory and were normal. The nurse contacted the anesthetist, who removed the endotracheal tube, continued the 40% oxygen by face mask, and ordered a unit of plasma protein fraction 5% (Plasmanate) to increase the blood pressure, CVP, and urine output.

Management

The nurse turned the patient to his left side, and oriented him to his surroundings. The plasma protein fraction 5% was infused IV. Making determinations every 15 min for 1 h, the nurse noted that Mr. M.'s blood pressure had stabilized at 126/78 and the CVP at 5 to 6 cmH₂0 and that the urine output had increased to 45 mL in an hour. The nurse had given Mr. M. oral care after the tube was removed. She kept him covered with a folded blanket. By splinting the incisional site, the nurse assisted him in coughing and deep breathing. However, because he was unable to perform the leg exercises because of pain at the incision site, the nurse administered morphine sulfate 2 mg IV.

The blood pressure dropped briefly after the morphine was given but returned to the previous level after 20 min and remained stable. The dressing remained dry and intact, the chest tubes drained a usual amount of sanguineous material, the nasogastric tube drained a small amount of bile-colored fluid, the IV sites were not inflamed nor infiltrated, and the IV infusions were running on schedule. Mr. M. was oriented as to time, place, and person. He could move all of his extremities, and he had a full return of all reflexes when the anesthetist approved his transfer to the intensive care unit. The recovery room nurse accompanied the patient and gave a report to the ICU nurse.

Evaluation

In evaluating the care, the recovery room nurse noted that such measures as maintaining a quiet environment, administering frequent oral care, administering morphine, covering the patient with the blanket, administering plasma protein fraction 5%, and helping the patient with coughing and deep breathing had been effective. This evaluation was based on the facts that Mr. M. had demonstrated no excitability; had stated he felt minimal discomfort from dry mouth; had experienced pain relief without any adverse effect on blood pressure or respiration; had maintained an adequate blood pressure, CVP, cardiac rhythm, respiratory status and urine output; had experienced minimal shivering, stating he felt warm enough; and had clear lungs on auscultation.

REFERENCES

Adriani, J.: *The Chemistry and Physics of Anesthesia*, Springfield, Ill.: Thomas, 1962.

Collins, V. J.: *Principles of Anesthesiology*, Philadelphia: Lea & Febiger, 1976.

Dripps, R. D., J. E. Eckenhoff, and L. D. Vandam: *Introduction to Anesthesia: The Principles of Safe Practice*, Philadelphia: Saunders, 1982.

Eger, E. I.: *Anesthesia Uptake and Action*, Baltimore: Williams and Wilkins, 1974.

———: "Isoflurane: A Review," *Anesthesiology*, 55:559–576, 1981.

Kaplan, J. A. (ed.): *Cardiac Anesthesia*, New York: Grune and Stratton, 1979.

Lebowitz, P. W. (ed.): *Clinical Anesthesia Procedures of the Massachusetts General Hospital*, Boston: Little, Brown, 1978.

Luckmann, J., and K. C. Sorenson (eds.): *Medical-Surgical Nursing: A Psychophysiological Approach*, Philadelphia: Saunders, 1980.

Marshall, B. E., and H. Wollman: "General Anesthetics," in A. G. Gilman, L. S. Goodman, and A. Gilman (eds.), *Goodman and Gilman's The Pharmacological Basis of Therapeutics*, 6th ed., New York: Macmillan, 1980.

Pakkanen, A., and J. Kanto: "Midazolam Compared with Thiopentone as an Induction Agent," *Scan Anesthesiol J*, 26:143–146, 1982.

Pieri, L., R. Schaffner et al.: *Pharmacology of Midazolam*, Pharmaceutical Research Department, Nutley, N.J.: F. Hoffmann-La Roche, 1982.

Ritchie, J. M. and N. M. Green: "Local Anesthetics," in A. G. Gilman, L. S. Goodman, and A. Gilman (eds.), *Goodman and Gilman's The Pharmacological Basis of Therapeutics*, 6th ed., New York: Macmillan, 1980.

Shea, J. H.: "Calcium Slow Channel Blockers: Physiology and Anesthetic Interactions," *Am Assoc Nurs Anesth J*, 50:564–568, 1982.

Smith, R. M.: *Anesthesia for Infants and Children*, St. Louis: Mosby, 1980.

Smith, T. C., L. H. Copperman, and H. Wollman: "History and Principles of Anesthesiology," in A. G. Gilman, L. S. Goodman, and A. Gilman (eds.), *Goodman and Gilman's The Pharmacological Basis of Therapeutics*, 6th ed., New York: Macmillan, 1980.

Snow, J. C.: *Manual of Anesthesia*, Boston: Little, Brown, 1977.

Steward, D. J.: *Manual of Pediatric Anesthesia*, New York: Churchill Livingstone, 1979.

Tornetta, F. J., S. Song, and A. D. Smoyer: "Etomidate: A Pharmacologic Profile of New Hypnotic," *Am Assoc Nurs Anesth J*, 48:517–525, 1980.

Wade, J. G., and W. C. Stevens: "Isoflurane: An Anesthetic for the Eighties?" *Anesth Anal*, 60:666–682, 1981.

White, P. F., W. L. Way, and A. J. Trevor: "Ketamine—Its Pharmacology and Therapeutic Uses," *Anesthesiology*, 56:119–136, 1982.

48

EMERGENCY AND INTENSIVE CARE*

SUZANNE L. HOWELL
THEODORE G. TONG
ROSS A. SIMKOVER
GRACE CARBONI RUGGIERO

Assessing and managing life-threatening emergencies such as cardiopulmonary arrest, shock, severe burns, or acute poisoning demand a most efficient and competent use of the nursing process. Assessment may mean *identifying which patients are at risk* for emergency problems. Some of these patients (and the associated risks) are the middle-aged man with chest pain and diaphoresis (post-myocardial infarction cardiac arrest), the elderly woman with a gram-negative urinary tract infection (septic shock), or the young child who has previously ingested a bottle of aspirin (repeated episode of poisoning). Carefully assessing patients, establishing baseline signs and symptoms, and identifying subtle changes and trends so that early therapy may be initiated can often mean the difference between restoring the patient to health or seeing progression to an irreversible state of shock or cardiopulmonary arrest.

DRUG THERAPY TECHNIQUES

LEARNING OBJECTIVES

Upon mastery of the content of this section, the reader will be able to:

1. Differentiate nursing process in emergency situations and situations in intensive care units from the appropriate process in less acute settings.

2. Explain the rationale for administering emergency and intensive care drugs only by the intravenous, endotracheal, or intracardiac routes.

3. Briefly describe the techniques of IV bolus, IV infusion, and endotracheal tube drug administration.

4. Explain titration of emergency and intensive care drugs.

Maintaining current knowledge and skill will allow the nurse to respond and act quickly, safely, and appropriately in a variety of emergency situations. By nature, an emergency is an acute and unscheduled situation, usually not allowing the nurse time to review procedure, to consult with someone else, or to check a drug reference. The nurse who practices in the emergency department or intensive care unit needs to be prepared to deal with emergencies as the rule rather than the exception. However, nurses in general care units, clinics, physicians' offices, schools, or any setting may, at some time, need to intervene in an emergency situation.

In some areas such as emergency rooms, intensive care units, or hospitals and clinics without physicians in immediate attendance, nurses may function in extended and expanded roles. They may initiate diagnostic and therapeutic management which in other circumstances would be the physician's responsibility. Even when working with a physician, however, a sound understanding of the rationale for drug therapy and medical management of cardiopulmonary arrest, shock, burns, and poisoning will greatly enhance the delivery of efficient and effective care.

When the emergency does occur, the immediate goal is the preservation and/or restoration of the patient's life. A management plan with specific predetermined steps should be initiated. The situation rarely allows for establishing goals with the patient, meeting other than immediate physiologic needs, and individualizing the initial plan of care. If the nurse has noted such things as a patient's drug allergies, current medications, and any medical conditions that were

*Ms. Howell wrote the sections on drug therapy techniques, cardiopulmonary arrest, shock, and burns. Drs. Tong and Simkover and Ms. Ruggiero contributed the section on poisoning and overdose.

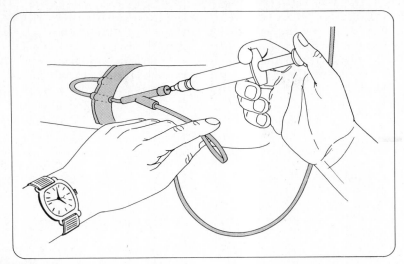

FIGURE 48-1

Drug Administration by IV Push. Careful timing is required when administering drugs by IV bolus. (*Courtesy of Larry Howell.*)

present prior to the emergency, anticipatory planning of how best to modify standard interventions is posssible.

The nurse has the responsibility for maintaining emergency equipment and supplies in the practice area. This means that all equipment is fully functional, all supplies are in the proper place, and all drugs are completely stocked and have not passed their expiration dates. Each member of the nursing staff needs to be thoroughly familiar with the standard procedures to be initiated in an emergency situation. Some of these procedures include how to summon additional assistance to the scene, how to begin CPR (cardiopulmonary resuscitation), and how to ensure that all necessary equipment and supplies are brought to the scene. During the emergency the dosages of all drugs and precise times given must be recorded. The nurse must be able to anticipate which drugs will be given and what equipment will be needed in order to have them immediately available. Time is of the utmost importance. Being thoroughly familiar with the expected effects of CPR and drug therapy facilitates evaluation and allows rapid adjustments in management to be made in order to restore and/or preserve life.

The critically ill patient who is recovering from cardiopulmonary arrest, or poisoning, or who is suffering from shock or severe burns frequently requires an unusually demanding type of nursing care on a one-to-one basis. The nursing process is ongoing and minute-to-minute with frequent changes in the patient's clinical status requiring rapid and accurate assessment, management, and evaluation. During these times the patient may waiver between life and death. The nurse must also have the knowledge and competence to explain treatments and progress to patients, even those whose responses are slow or absent.

ROUTES OF ADMINISTRATION

The route of choice for administering emergency and intensive care drugs is intravenous. During physiologic states of low blood flow, such as in cardiopulmonary arrest, shock, or severe burns, absorption and uptake of drugs administered orally, intramuscularly, or subcutaneously is slow and unpredictable.

Intravenous

The *intravenous (IV)* route provides for rapid action of the drug to be achieved while a precise adjustment of dosage is

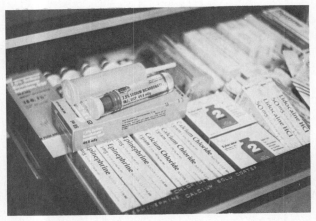

FIGURE 48-2

An Emergency Drug Drawer. Most emergency drugs are packaged in prefilled syringes. (*Photo by Larry Howell.*)

maintained. During an emergency, an intravenous infusion of 5% dextrose in water (D₅W) is begun in order to establish a route for administration of drugs. Since many of these drugs may cause tissue sloughing if allowed to infiltrate, a large peripheral vein (such as those of the antecubital fossa) and/or a central vein (such as the subclavian) are preferred sites.

Endotracheal

During some emergency situations it may be impossible to establish the intravenous route. Some of the drugs may then be given via an *endotracheal tube (ET)* or by the *intracar-diac (IC)* route. When using the ET route, drugs are more rapidly and efficiently absorbed when the dose is diluted with distilled water to a total volume of 5 to 10 mL. Following installation into the endotracheal tube, the drug is forced into the lower tracheobronchial tree and lungs by several rapid hyperventilations with a bag-valve device (e.g., Ambu).

Intracardiac

The IC route should be used only when all other routes have been tried. The technique is associated with complications and should only be performed by physicians experienced with the procedure.

INTRAVENOUS TECHNIQUES

Emergency drugs may be given intravenously by injection or infusion.

Intravenous Bolus

IV bolus (IV push or IV injection) is the administration of a relatively small amount of solution into the IV tubing by means of syringe over a time span of aproximately 1 to 10 min (see Fig. 48-1). Most of these drugs are available in a preloaded syringe form, making opening vials and mixing and diluting drugs (see Figs. 48-2 and 48-3) unnecessary.

Intravenous Infusion

Drugs prepared for IV infusion should be hung in tandem with the primary IV, thus allowing an IV line to remain open if the drug needs to be stopped. When drugs are to be given by IV infusion, they are usually diluted to provide a required dosage level for a rate of IV flow of less than 1 mL/min. In order to administer this small amount, an IV line with a *microdrop system* (60 gtt/mL) and an *infusion pump* are used. The infusion pump (such as IVAC) allows precise administration of very small volumes and prevents accidental rapid infusion (see Fig. 48-4).

Titrating Drugs

Most of the emergency and intensive care drugs have dosage ranges which are determined by *titration*. Titrating IV drugs is the process of dosing drugs according to the amount required to bring about the desired physiologic response; for example, titration of **norepinephrine** (Levophed) to maintain blood pressure, **lidocaine** to suppress ventricular ectopy, or **morphine sulfate** to relieve pain. It is the goal of dosage titration to use the smallest amount of the drug which achieves the therapeutic response while avoiding adverse effects. Parameters will be established in order to determine that the drug is creating a therapeutic effect that outweighs the harmful side effects. Specific dilutions for these drugs have been established by the drug company and/or hospital

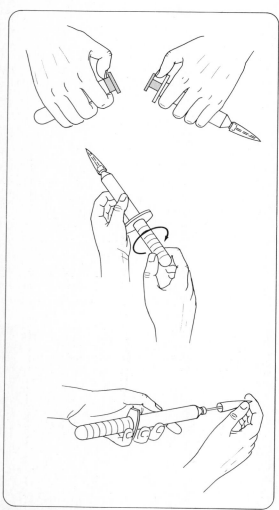

FIGURE 48-3

Preparing the Packaged Prefilled Syringe. (1) Remove protective caps, (2) insert vial into injector, using twisting motion, (3) remove needle cover. *(Courtesy of Larry Howell.)*

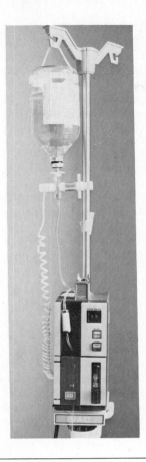

FIGURE 48-4

IVAC Infusion Pump Used for Accurate Control of IV Infusion Rate. *(Photo by Larry Howell.)*

committee. Formulas for dilution and administration rates should be prepared in advance and made readily available for use in emergency situations when calculation time is extremely limited. (See Case Study for example.) It is suggested that a formula for dilution be established for each drug which allows a rate of drops per minute to equal micrograms of drug per kilogram of body weight per minute (gtt/min = μg/kg/min). Precise doses per body weight should be calculated prior to need for any infant or child who is seriously ill or injured or in need of surgery.

Patients receiving emergency and intensive care drugs must be placed on cardiac monitors since all these drugs can precipitate arrhythmias, especially those of ventricular origin. The nurse must maintain a close watch on rates of many IV drugs and their effect on the patient in order to make immediate changes as necessary. Machines, computers, and specialized equipment do not replace the need for nurses to be highly competent in assessing the patient.

CARDIOPULMONARY ARREST

LEARNING OBJECTIVES

Upon mastery of the content of this section, the reader will be able to:
1. Define cardiopulmonary arrest.
2. List types of cardiopulmonary arrest.
3. Identify signs and symptoms of cardiopulmonary arrest.
4. Define basic life support (BLS) and advanced cardiac life support (ACLS).
5. Explain the rationale for the use of oxygen, sodium bicarbonate, epinephrine hydrochloride, calcium chloride, atropine sulfate, isoproterenol sulfate, lidocaine, procainamide, bretylium tosylate, and propranolol in the management of cardiopulmonary arrest.
6. Compare and contrast the management of ventricular fibrillation, ventricular asystole, and electromechanical dissociation (EMD).

MECHANISMS IN CARDIOPULMONARY ARREST

Cardiopulmonary arrest is defined as the abrupt cessation of cardiac and respiratory function. The underlying physiologic mechanisms involved may be (1) impaired cardiac electrical activity (lethal or nonperfusing arrhythmias), (2) impaired myocardial contractility (cardiac failure, hypoxia, acidosis), and/or (3) impaired venous return or cardiac output (hypovolemia, increased venous capacitance). These mechanisms alone or in combination give rise to three types of cardiopulmonary arrest:

1. Ventricular fibrillation
2. Ventricular asystole (ventricular standstill)
3. Electromechanical dissociation (EMD), also called cardiovascular collapse

Some causes of cardiopulmonary arrest include myocardial infarction, heart failure, drowning, airway obstruction, drug overdose, severe hemorrhage, electrocution, head trauma, and severe progressive shock.

ASSESSMENT AND DIAGNOSIS OF CARDIOPULMONARY ARREST

Regardless of the cause of cardiopulmonary arrest, the signs and symptoms are the same. The unconscious victim will have absence of pulses in the large arteries (carotid and femoral in adults and children; brachial in infants) and absence

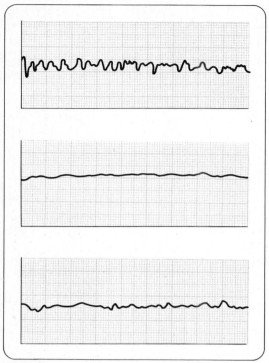

FIGURE 48-5

ECG Readings Taken during Cardiac Arrests. The uppermost reading is *ventricular fibrillation,* showing erratic, disorganized electrical activity. This activity may be further classified as fine or coarse fibrillation depending on the amplitude of the waves. The heart beats wildly without synchronized contractions and is unable to sustain an adequate cardiac output. Ventricular fibrillation is the most common cause of cardiopulmonary arrest in victims of sudden death, many of whom have no premonitory symptoms. The middle reading is *ventricular asystole* which looks like a "straight line" with only small deviations of baseline. There is little or no electrical activity and no myocardial contractions. The bottom reading is *electromechanical dissociation* (EMD), also known as cardiovascular collapse, resulting from severe myocardial contractile failure and profound shock. An absence of adequate cardiac output may be associated with normal or nearly normal ECG complexes.

of breathing. There will also be an absence of audible heart sounds and audible or palpable blood pressure. With increasing hypoxia, cyanosis and dilated pupils may rapidly develop. In cases of collapsed or unconscious persons, the adequacy or absence of breathing and circulation must be determined immediately so that emergency measures can be rapidly instituted. Optimally only seconds should intervene between recognition of an arrest and initiation of treatment. Biologic or brain death begins to occur within 4 to 6 min after cessation of cardiopulmonary function.

MANAGEMENT OF CARDIOPULMONARY ARREST

Cardiopulmonary Resuscitation (CPR)

Basic Life Support (BLS)

Basic life support incorporates the external support of circulation and respiration of the victim of cardiopulmonary arrest through cardiopulmonary resuscitation (CPR). If breathing alone is inadequate or absent, opening the airway or rescue breathing, or both, may be all that is necessary. If circulation is also absent, external chest compressions must be started in combination with rescue breathing. The outstanding advantage of CPR is that it permits the earliest possible treatment of cardiopulmonary arrest. CPR can and should by initiated by any person present when arrest occurs. Hospitals should require competence in CPR for all personnel.

Advanced Cardiac Life Support (ACLS)

ACLS includes CPR plus the use of adjunctive resuscitation equipment, establishment of an IV fluid line, cardiac monitoring, defibrillation, control of dysrhythmias, and postresuscitation care. ACLS requires the supervision and direction of a physician in person or a physician's standing orders. All nurses practicing in emergency departments or intensive care units must be competent in ACLS.

Drug Therapy in Cardiopulmonary Arrest

Drug therapy during cardiopulmonary arrest (see Table 48-1) is directed toward treating the specific cause of the arrest and restoring effective cardiac contraction. All cardiopulmonary arrest requires the sustained performance of CPR until effective spontaneous pulse and respirations are restored. Common to all forms of arrest is hypoxia which requires the administration of oxygen.

Ventricular Fibrillation The definitive therapy for ventricular fibrillation is *defibrillation* which is accomplished by delivering a high-voltage electric current to the heart through paddles placed directly on the chest wall. At the moment of electric shock, the myocardium is totally depolarized. This generally terminates fibrillation and allows the SA node to resume effective control of cardiac rate and rhythm. If ventricular fibrillation has not been terminated after two attempts with electric defibrillation, administration of **epinephrine** and **sodium bicarbonate** may enhance further attempts. Antiarrhythmic drugs should not be given early in the treatment of ventricular fibrillation because they often make electric defibrillation more difficult or produce asystole. After termination of fibrillation and an effective cardiac rate and rhythm has been restored, **antiarrhythmics** are usually given to stabilize cardiac function. The prognosis

TABLE 48-1   Drugs Used in Cardiopulmonary Resuscitation

DRUG	PHARMACOLOGIC EFFECTS	INDICATIONS	DOSAGE AND ADMINISTRATION	NURSING MANAGEMENT
Oxygen	Combats hypoxemia.	Absence of adequate spontaneous breathing.	100% concentration. *Spontaneous breathing:* 4–6 L/min via mask or nasal cannulae. *Assisted breathing:* 8–10 L/min via bag-valve mask (e.g., Ambu) or endotracheal (ET) tube.	Failure to adequately ventilate patient leads to build-up of CO_2 (hypercarbia) and respiratory acidosis. O_2 toxicity is not a concern since it does not occur with short-term exposure and hypoxic cellular damage is greater danger to patient.
Sodium bicarbonate	Combats metabolic acidosis due to lactic acid production during hypoxia-induced anaerobic metabolism.	Any absence of adequate cardiac or respiratory activity (unless arrest is very brief, e.g., 1–2 min).	*Initial dose:* 1 meq/kg (50–75 mL of prefilled syringe 1 meq/mL) by IV bolus. *Additional doses:* titrated with pH, arterial P_{CO_2} and base deficit; if blood gases unavailable, give ½ initial dose q10–15min during arrest. *Pediatric:* 1–2 meq/kg/per dose. Not to exceed 8 meq/kg/day.	Acidotic heart responds poorly to circulating and administered catecholamines leading to ↓ force of contraction and ↑ risk of ventricular fibrillation. Acidotic heart responds poorly to defibrillation. Avoid metabolic alkalosis causing tighter bond of O_2 to hemoglobin producing ↓ O_2 release to tissues. Avoid giving directly with catecholamines (causes inactivation) or calcium (forms precipitate). May cause hypernatremia.
Epinephrine (Adrenalin)	↑ Perfusion pressure. ↑ Amplitude of ventricular fibrillatory waves, increasing effectiveness of electrical defibrillation. Stimulates spontaneous or more forceful cardiac contractions. May restore cardiac electrical activity.	Ventricular fibrillation. Ventricular asystole. Electromechanical dissociation (EMD).	0.5–1.0 mg (5–10 mL of 1:10,000 solution) rapid IV bolus, endotracheal tube (ET), or intracardial (IC) route. Repeat dose q5min during cardiac arrest. *Pediatric:* 0.1 mL/kg (1:10,000 solution).	↓ Effectiveness in presence of acidemia. ↑ Myocardial O_2 consumption. May precipitate cerebral hemorrhage. Local infiltration causes tissue necrosis.
Calcium salts (chloride, gluconate, gluceptate)	Stimulates spontaneous or more forceful cardiac contractions. May restore orderly electrical cardiac rhythm.	Ventricular asystole. Electromechanical dissociation (EMD).	Calcium chloride: 5–7 mg/kg (2.5–5.0 mL of 10% solution) IV bolus. Calcium gluconate: 10–15 mL (4.8–7.2 meq). Calcium gluceptate: 5–7 mL (4.5–6.3 meq). May repeat q10min. *Pediatric:* calcium chloride: 0.3 mL/kg (slow IV bolus). May be given IC; ET method is controversial.	Calcium chloride has higher and more predictable levels of calcium ions making it drug of choice. Do not give to digitalized patient; may cause complete suppression of sinus impulse. Causes tissue sloughing if allowed to infiltrate. Slow IV injection (generally 1 mL/min or less).
Atropine sulfate	Accelerates cardiac rate. May allow resumption of pacemaker activity.	Asystole from complete heart block.	0.5 mg (0.1 mg/mL solution) IV bolus. May repeat dose q5min until desired heart rate (≤60 beats/min) is reached; not to exceed total dose of 2.0 mg. *Pediatric:* 0.01–0.03 mg/kg IV. May be given ET.	↑ Myocardial O_2 consumption. Ineffective in presence of hypoxia, acid-base imbalances, or electrolyte imbalances. May precipitate ventricular tachycardia or fibrillation.

TABLE 48-1 Drugs Used in Cardiopulmonary Resuscitation (*Cont.*)

DRUG	PHARMACOLOGIC EFFECTS	INDICATIONS	DOSAGE AND ADMINISTRATION	NURSING MANAGEMENT
Isoproterenol sulfate (Isuprel)	Stimulates spontaneous or more forceful cardiac contraction. Accelerates cardiac rate.	Asystole from complete heart block. Electromechanical dissociation (EMD).	2–20 μg/min continuous IV infusion titrated to heart rate ($\leq$60 beats/min) and rhythm. *Pediatric:* Begin at 0.1 μg/kg/min IV infusion (usual effect at 0.1–1.0 μg/kg/min). May be given ET.	↑ Myocardial O_2 consumption. Do not give to digitalized patient. May precipitate ventricular fibrillation.
Lidocaine (Xylocaine)	Suppresses ventricular ectopy.	Recurrent ventricular fibrillation. Ventricular fibrillation not terminated by electrical defibrillation.	50–100 mg (1 mg/kg) IV bolus (no faster than 50 mg/min) immediately followed by continuous IV infusion of 1–4 mg/min (20–50 μg/kg/min) titrated to ↓ PVCs/min and desired serum concentration. *Pediatric:* 1 mg/kg IV bolus followed by 30 μg/kg/min titrated IV infusion. May be given ET.	Drug of choice for suppression of ventricular ectopy. Avoid with complete heart block: may abolish ventricular pacemaker. Use with caution—if at all—in patients with known allergies to local anesthetics. Use only lidocaine which is labeled for cardiac use. ↓ Dosage in patients with liver disease, congestive heart failure, renal failure, shock, and >70 years of age. Side effects are primarily in CNS.
Procainamide (Pronestyl)	Suppresses ventricular ectopy.	Ventricular fibrillation not controlled by lidocaine or when lidocaine is contraindicated.	100-mg IV bolus q5min until dysrhythmia is suppressed or total of 1.0 g is given. *Caution:* IV bolus should not be given faster than 20 mg/min. Slow infusion if PR interval or QRS complex widens. Stop infusion if QRS widens by 50% or if hypotension develops. *Maintenance infusion:* 1–4 mg/min.	May precipitate complete heart block progressing to asystole. ↓ Dosage in patients with hepatic or renal dysfunction. Has more cardiovascular depressant effects than lidocaine. May cause profound hypotension if injected too rapidly.
Bretylium tosylate (Bretylol)	Suppresses ventricular ectopy.	Ventricular fibrillation not controlled by lidocaine or procainamide.	*Ventricular fibrillation:* 5 mg/kg rapid IV bolus; defibrillate; then 10 mg/kg repeated as necessary. *Recurrent or refractory ventricular tachycardia:* 5–10 mg/kg IV over 8–10 min. *Maintenance infusion:* 2 mg/min IV.	Avoid in presence of digitalis toxicity. Increase dosage interval in impaired renal function.
Propranolol (Inderal)	Suppresses ventricular ectopy.	Ventricular fibrillation not controlled by lidocaine.	1–3 mg slow IV bolus (not more than 1 mg/5 min while closely monitoring BP and ECG). May be repeated after 2 min to total of 3–5 mg. Thereafter, do not give drug in less than 4-h intervals.	Drug of choice for digitalis toxicity.

for successful resuscitation of the victim of ventricular fibrillation is generally good, especially if treatment was initiated within the first few minutes of arrest.

Ventricular Asystole This cause of cardiopulmonary arrest carries an extremely poor prognosis. Administration of **epinephrine** and **sodium bicarbonate** may restore electrical

activity and effective cardiac rhythm. If these fail, most authorities recommend giving **calcium chloride**. However, White (1982) condemns the use of calcium in asystole and suggests the use of a calcium channel blocker (e.g., **verapamil**) as the drug of choice. If these attempts are ineffective, **atropine** followed by **isoproterenol** or **epinephrine IC** may be tried. If ventricular asystole has resulted from complete heart block, a *temporary pacemaker* may be inserted after drug therapy has been given.

Electromechanical Dissociation (EMD)   The prognosis for successful resuscitation of the victim of EMD is poor. Drug therapy is **epinephrine, sodium bicarbonate, calcium chloride,** and **isoproterenol**. Since some form of profound shock is generally responsible for this condition, drug and non-pharmacologic therapies are initiated to promote stabilization.

CASE STUDY

Mr. B., aged 42, was admitted to the hospital for an elective hemorrhoidectomy. His preoperative laboratory studies and ECG were within normal limits. The history and physical examination revealed no evidence of heart disease, although Mr. B. was overweight, smoked heavily, and admitted that he got very little exercise. The evening before surgery, the nurse entered Mr. B.'s hospital room and found him lying unresponsive on the floor near his bed.

Assessment

After establishing that Mr. B. was unresponsive, the nurse immediately assessed for signs of breathing and palpated for presence of carotid pulse. Cardiopulmonary arrest was diagnosed by absence of spontaneous breathing and carotid pulse. The nurse also remembered that myocardial infarction is the most common cause of cardiopulmonary arrest.

Management

In such a situation the immediate goal is to prevent biologic death by initiating cardiopulmonary resuscitation. The nurse called for help and began basic life support. Another nurse responded to the call, alerted the cardiac arrest team, and brought the emergency equipment to the scene. While the first nurse continued rescue breathing and external chest compressions, the second nurse administered 100% oxygen by nasal cannula and attached Mr. B. to a cardiac monitor. Since the ECG pattern indicated ventricular fibrillation, the defibrillator machine was charged, and the paddles were lubricated. As soon as the cardiac arrest team arrived, CPR was briefly interrupted as the physician attempted defibrillation. The initial shock was unsuccessful, and another shock was repeated without success. CPR was resumed by another member of the arrest team. The patient had an endotracheal tube inserted and was ventilated with 100% oxygen by means of a bag-valve device. The second nurse initiated an IV infusion of D_5W to secure a route for administration of drugs. Emergency drugs were prepared by the first nurse. Epinephrine 1.0 mg IV and sodium

EVALUATION AND PROGNOSIS OF CARDIOPULMONARY ARREST

Advanced cardiac life support (ACLS) is continued until resuscitation effects have restored an effective cardiac rate and rhythm and an adequate blood pressure. The patient will then need continued intensive care to ensure adequate hemodynamic stabilization. The decision to terminate-unsuccessful resuscitative procedures is made by the physician. Efforts are continued as long as there is cardiovascular response.

bicarbonate 75 mL IV were given by rapid bolus (over approximately 1 min). The nurse did not allow these two drugs to mix in the IV tubing, because the epinephrine would be inactivated by the sodium bicarbonate. The second nurse then assumed responsibility for accurately recording all drugs with their dosages and precise times given. CPR was then interrupted and defibrillation was again attempted. This time Mr. B.'s ECG converted to a normal sinus rhythm and a spontaneous carotid pulse was palpated. Mr. B. was gaining consciousness and spontaneous breathing was gradually being resumed. To prevent ventricular arrhythmias, the physician ordered lidocaine to be administered. The first nurse administered lidocaine 100 mg IV bolus over a period of 2 min. A lidocaine infusion was prepared by adding 2 g to 500 mL of D_5W. The infusion was begun at 2 mg/min and was titrated to allow no more than 5 ventricular ectopic beats per minute. In establishing the IV rate, the nurse consulted the following standard dilution chart which had been prepared by the pharmacist and posted in the medication room (asterisk indicates initial dose for Mr. B.).

LIDOCAINE

DOSE DESIRED	mL PER MIN	MICRODROPS PER MIN
	2 g in 500 mL D_5W	
	(4 mg/mL)	
1 mg/min	0.25	15
2 mg/min*	0.5	30
3 mg/min	0.75	45
4 mg/min	1.0	60
	2 g in 1000 mL D_5W	
	(2 mg/mL)	
1 mg/min	0.5	30
2 mg/min	1.0	60
3 mg/min	1.5	90
4 mg/min	2.0	120

Mr. B. was stabilized and transferred to the intensive care unit. The first nurse gave a full report of Mr. B.'s cardiopulmonary arrest and subsequent resuscitation to the ICU nurse.

Evaluation

The initial goal had been to establish a diagnosis of cardiopulmonary arrest and prevent biologic death. The nurse was able to rapidly establish an accurate diagnosis and begin CPR within the first critical minutes. The second goal was to initiate advanced cardiac life support. The nurse began this management by summoning additional help, the emergency equipment and drugs, and the cardiac arrest team. The ECG established that the arrest was caused by ventricular fibrillation and specific definitive therapy was initiated to reverse this disturbance. After the cardiac arrest team arrived, the role of the nurse was to anticipate the medical management and give drug therapy as ordered by the physician. The third goal was to stabilize the patient's cardiopulmonary status through transfer to the intensive care unit. The nurse was aware of the potential complications (lethal ventricular arrhythmias) and observed the cardiac monitor carefully so that a therapeutic drug infusion was maintained. The ICU nurse assessed the psychosocial impact of resuscitation from cardiopulmonary arrest on Mr. B. and his family and used appropriate nursing measures to lessen anxiety and fear of a recurrent episode of "sudden death." Some of these measures included: giving explanations of all treatments, medications, and monitors used in care; showing sensitivity to the feelings of Mr. B. and his family; responding promptly when summoned by Mr. B. or his family; and providing appropriate psychologic weaning and support before removing any monitors on which Mr. B. had become dependent.

Mr. B. was diagnosed as having suffered an acute myocardial infarction. He was placed on a regimen of cardiac medications and discharged from the hospital in 3 weeks. Mr. B.'s prognosis is good if he continues a program of cardiac rehabilitation.

SHOCK

LEARNING OBJECTIVES

Upon mastery of the content of this section, the reader will be able to:

1. Define the process of shock.
2. Describe seven types of shock in terms of the underlying mechanisms responsible for each.
3. Identify eight signs and symptoms of shock in terms of their relationship to the body's compensatory mechanisms.
4. Explain how intravenous fluid therapy, respiratory support, and nonpharmacologic therapeutic devices support hemodynamic stabilization.
5. Explain the use of dopamine, dobutamine, vasopressors, isoproterenol, vasodilators, epinephrine, corticosteroids, potent diuretics, and cardiac glycosides in the management of shock.
6. List parameters for titrating the effects of sympathomimetic drugs.
7. Identify the evaluation of therapy for shock.

When either the cardiovascular or pulmonary system fails to function properly, the result is *inadequate oxygenation and tissue perfusion leading to tissue hypoxia,* which is the basic definition of shock. The body's ability to compensate for this condition is limited, and unless the process is reversed, cellular death occurs.

MECHANISMS IN SHOCK

Adequate tissue perfusion is dependent upon a balance between three mechanisms: (1) pumping action of the heart, (2) circulating blood volume, and (3) vasomotor tone to regulate the size of the vascular bed. Several types of shock can result from a disruption in any of these mechanisms (see Table 48-2).

ASSESSMENT OF SHOCK

Regardless of the cause of shock, the compensatory mechanisms result primarily from sympathetic stimulation which assists the body in "holding its own" against the stress of

TABLE 48-2   Mechanisms of Shock

Inadequate pumping action (*cardiogenic shock*)

Inadequate circulating blood volume (*hypovolemic shock*)

  Blood loss (*hemorrhagic shock*)

  Plasma loss (*burn shock* or other fluid shift)

  Fluid and electrolyte loss (vomiting, diarrhea, severe diuresis)

Vasomotor dysfunction (decreased arterial resistance, increased size of venous bed)

  Cell destruction from bacterial endotoxins (*septic shock*)

  Generalized antigen-antibody reaction causing release of vasoactive substances (*anaphylactic shock*)

  Abnormal dilation of blood vessels from spinal cord injury or spinal anesthesia (*neurogenic shock*)

tissue hypoxia until the underlying defects can be corrected. The compensatory mechanisms try to keep oxygenated blood flowing to vital organs, especially the heart and brain, while compromising oxygenation of all other organs. Obviously, shock must be assessed early in the compensatory stage in order to initiate therapy before irreversible organ damage occurs.

Some signs and symptoms are common to all types of shock. *Respirations* are initially rapid (10 to 12 respirations/min above the patient's normal) and shallow, with subjective feelings of air hunger, to compensate for metabolic acidosis due to lactic acid production during hypoxia-induced anaerobic metabolism. As compensatory mechanisms fail, breathing is slowed and progresses to complete respiratory failure. The *skin* is initially cool, clammy, and pale in response to peripheral vasoconstriction to shunt blood to vital organs. With increasing tissue hypoxia, cyanosis and diaphoresis develop. However, in early septic shock, the skin is warm, flushed, and dry due to vasodilation. *Heart rate* increases at least 20 beats/min above the patient's normal rate to maintain cardiac output and becomes weak and thready. Early in shock, systolic *blood pressure* rises due to compensatory peripheral vasoconstriction, but then will drop producing a narrowing pulse pressure. As the body fails to compensate, the systolic pressure drops to less than 90 mmHg, or 50 to 60 mmHg below the patient's normal. *Urinary output* decreases to less than 20 mL/h as blood is shunted away from the kidneys, although some forms of septic shock may have a very high urinary output. Assessment of the *sensorium* reveals initial restlessness and agitation, progressing to confusion, lethargy, and coma. The level of consciousness decreases as the brain becomes more hypoxic. As blood is shunted to vital organs, *body temperature* decreases. In early septic shock, the body temperature is increased due to bacterial infection. Body attempts to compensate for inadequate circulating blood volume result in subjective feelings of *thirst*.

MANAGEMENT OF SHOCK

Hemodynamic Stabilization

The morbidity and mortality due to shock are high and frequently little can be done to improve the patient's outcome. Despite therapeutic advances in the last several years, no highly effective drug or other therapy for treating severe shock has been developed. The objectives of the treatment of shock are the restoration of tissue perfusion and correction of the underlying cardiovascular defect.

Intravenous Fluid Therapy

Almost regardless of etiology, intravenous fluid therapy forms the base of management for most cases of shock. Careful fluid replacement should be adequate to restore vital organ perfusion, but not strain the heart to the point of congestive heart failure or pulmonary edema. The hourly urine output is a reflection of renal blood flow and a reliable index of volume replacement. Cuff measurement of peripheral blood pressure is not sufficient for the monitoring of the patient in shock and it does not give the true status of blood volume, and so *arterial blood pressure* should be monitored directly. *Central venous pressure (CVP)* monitoring indicates changes in blood volume and venous return to the right side of the heart. *Pulmonary artery wedge pressure (PAWP)* monitoring gives indications of left ventricular function and obtains a true status of blood volume.

Red blood cell replacement is the fluid of choice for treating hemorrhagic shock. Additional asanguineous fluids may supplement blood transfusion: *colloids* (human albumin, plasma protein fraction, dextran) and/or *crystalloids* (Ringer's lactate, normal saline, other balanced salt solutions) (see Chap. 24). Fluids used in burn shock will be discussed later in this chapter. Carefully monitored administration of crystalloids and/or colloids are required for hemodynamic stabilization in cardiogenic, septic, and anaphylactic shock states.

Respiratory Support

Adequate ventilation and oxygen therapy are necessary to correct hypoxia and acidosis. Respiratory therapy is guided by arterial blood gas (ABG) values.

Nonpharmacologic Therapeutic Devices

Several devices have been developed recently and have been shown to be of value in improving the hemodynamic status of certain shock victims. Adjunctive equipment is subject to regulation by the FDA Bureau of Medical Devices.

Medical Antishock Garments The garment consists of a one-piece double-layered fabric which fits on the patient similar to a pair of trousers. It has separate compartments that allow for inflation of compartments overlying each lower extremity and the abdomen. When external pressure is applied, the increasing central blood volume may result in improved heart, brain, and lung perfusion. The garment has been most effective in patients with hypovolemic shock. However, it has also been proved useful in supporting circulation in some cases of cardiogenic shock, although in this type of shock, it may aggravate pulmonary congestion.

Intraaortic Balloon Counterpulsation This device is indicated in cases of cardiogenic shock. A balloon on a catheter is surgically positioned in the descending thoracic aorta. The balloon inflates during diastole (increasing perfusion of the vital organs and myocardium) and deflates immediately before systole (decreasing the workload and metabolic needs of the heart).

Sympathomimetic Drug Therapy

The goal of treating shock with sympathomimetic drugs is to increase blood flow to critical organs with minimal adverse effects (see Table 48-3). There is no single standard drug regimen accepted or effective in treating shock. Rapidly changing advances in medical therapy, specific patient considerations, and physician preference may greatly vary clinical management. The nurse must consult with the physician before and frequently during sympathomimetic therapy. Because these drugs are extremely toxic and not for prolonged use, the nurse should ask the physician to communicate:

1. Desired speed of titration to achieve effective cardiac output
2. Maximum dose to be administered
3. The length of therapy

Mechanism of Action

The therapeutic mechanism of sympathomimetics in shock is a result of the stimulation of α, β_1, and β_2 receptors (see Table 48-4 and Chap. 13). The most important actions of sympathomimetic drugs are *positive inotropic* and *vasopressor*. Positive inotropism is increased force of cardiac contraction which is mediated by β_1 receptors. Vasopressor activity, resulting from α-receptor stimulation, increases total peripheral resistance. *Positive chronotropic* action (increased heart rate) is also β_1-mediated and generally is undesirable unless shock is being caused by nonperfusing bradycardia. Muscle vascular vasodilation is mediated by β_2 receptors, while dopaminergic effects include splanchnic and renal artery vasodilation. The hemodynamic effects of a drug are determined by the drug's effect on each type of receptor.

Dobutamine and low-dose **dopamine** are preferred in the treatment of heart failure without profound hypotension, because they increase cardiac output without markedly causing an increase in myocardial oxygen consumption. **Isoproterenol** is generally restricted to use with bradycardias because of its tendency to produce tachycardia and increasing myocardial oxygen consumption. Strong vasopressors are hazardous to use in the treatment of shock. Except in shock caused by vasomotor dysfunction, there is already much vasoconstriction causing decreased tissue perfusion. Vasopressors should not be used before volume deficits are corrected. Moderate to high-dose **dopamine** is the vasopressor of choice in unresponsive cardiogenic shock and in septic shock when blood pressure cannot be maintained with IV fluids. **Norepinephrine** and **metaraminol** may be used with profound hypotension. **Epinephrine** is advantageous in treating anaphylactic shock. The sympathomimetic drugs are often given in combination to produce the most beneficial effects. Table 48-5 outlines the use of these agents.

Pharmacokinetics

Dopamine, **epinephrine**, and **norepinephrine** are naturally occurring catecholamines, metabolized rapidly by monoamine oxidase (MAO) and catechol-o-methyltransferase (COMT) with only small amounts excreted unchanged in the urine. **Isoproterenol** is readily metabolized by the liver,

TABLE 48-3 Titration Guidelines for Sympathomimetic Drugs Used in Shock

ASSESSMENT PARAMETER	THERAPEUTIC GOAL	NURSING EVALUATION FOR ADVERSE EFFECTS OR INADEQUATE RESPONSE
Blood pressure Intraarterial pressure monitoring preferable Assess within 2–3 min after each increase in IV infusion flow rate	Systolic BP increased to 80–100 mmHg Increased pulse pressure	Extreme hypertension or hypotension depending on drug
Heart rate Cardiac monitor preferable	Heart rate $\geq$ 60 beats/min and $\leq$ 100 beats/min	Tachycardia Reflex bradycardia caused by norepinephrine and metaraminol
Heart rhythm Cardiac monitor preferable	Minimal ventricular ectopic beats	Arrhythmias, mainly ventricular
Urinary output Foley catheter with measurements made every 30–60 min	>30 mL/h	<20 mL/h
Peripheral perfusion Assess appearance of extremities	Skin of extremities warm, dry, flushed. Good capillary blood return in nailbeds.	Skin of extremities cold, clammy, pale. Decreased capillary blood return in nailbeds.

TABLE 48-4 Mechanisms of Sympathomimetic Drugs Used for Hemodynamic Stabilization*

DRUG	RECEPTORS STIMULATED	Hemodynamic Effect†					
		POSITIVE INOTROPIC	POSITIVE CHRONOTROPIC	PRESSOR (VASOCONSTRICTION)	VASODILATION	SYSTOLIC BP	DIASTOLIC BP
Dobutamine	β_1	+++	0	0	0	↑	↑
Dopamine (low dose)	β_2, dopaminergic	0	0	0	++‡	0	0
Dopamine (moderate dose)	β_1	+++	+	0	0	0	0
Dopamine (high dose)	β_1, α	+++	+	+++	0	↑	↑
Norepinephrine	α	++	++	+++	0	↑	↑
Metaraminol	α, β_1	+	+§	++	+	↑	↑
Isoproterenol	β_1, β_2	+++	+++	0	+++	↑	↓
Epinephrine	α, β_1, β_2	+++	+++	+++	++	↑	↑↓

*Actual clinical effect observed depends upon pretreatment status of patient.

†+ Mild effect; ++ moderate effect; +++ strong effect; 0 no effect; ↑ increase; ↓ decrease.

‡Dopaminergic activity results in increased renal and mesenteric blood flow.

§Reflex bradycardia may occur.

TABLE 48-5   Drugs Used for Hemodynamic Stabilization

DRUG	INDICATIONS	DOSAGE AND ADMINISTRATION	NURSING PROCESS IMPLICATIONS
		Sympathomimetics	
Dopamine (Intropin)	Cardiogenic shock. Septic shock. Any shock with decreased blood pressure, poor perfusion, decreased urinary output.	Continuous titrated IV infusion. *Low dose:* 2–5 μg/kg/min. *Moderate dose:* 5–20 μg/kg/min. *High dose:* >20 μg/kg/min. *Pediatric:* 2–10 μg/kg/min.	Urine output is good indicator of therapeutic effect. Onset 2–4 min, lasting 10 min. Rise in diastolic pressure indicates vasoconstriction and need to decrease infusion rate. Monitor peripheral perfusion of those with history of vascular occlusive disease (Raynaud's, frostbite, diabetic endarteritis). No CNS side effects. Avoid in patients with pheochromocytoma. At doses ≥ 10μg/kg/min, α effects (vasoconstriction) are predominant.
Dobutamine (Dobutrex)	Cardiac decompensation from myocardial infarction or congestive heart failure. Not effective in profound hypotension.	Continuous titrated IV infusion. *Low dose:* 0.5 μg/kg/min. *Usual dose range:* 2.5–10.0 μg/kg/min.	Monitor ECG and arterial pressure for tachycardia, ectopic beats, and exaggerated blood pressure response. May increase insulin requirements in diabetics. May be given with digitalis drugs.
Norepinephrine (levarterenol; Levophed)	Shock characterized by profound hypotension due to decreased systemic vascular resistance.	Continuous titrated IV infusion begun at 2–3 mL/min of 4 μg/mL solution. *Average maintenance dose:* 2–4 μg/min. *Pediatric:* begin at 0.1 μg/kg/min.	Monitor blood pressure at least every 2 min until desired blood pressure obtained, then at least every 5 min. Severely restricts tissue perfusion and may cause permanent kidney damage. Contraindicated in normal and near-normal blood pressures or hypovolemic states. May precipitate dangerous hypertension. Headache may indicate overdosage. May cause rebound vagal stimulation (bradycardia).
Metaraminol (Aramine)	Cardiogenic shock with profound hypotension. May be used to convert a cardiovascular compromising supraventricular tachycardia to normal sinus rhythm by causing reflex bradycardia from increasing blood pressure.	Continuous titrated IV infusion begun at solution concentration of 0.4 mg/mL of D₅W.	Monitor ECG, urine output, and sensorium because drug decreases renal and cerebral blood flow and causes ventricular irritability. Ineffective when used with patients with depleted catecholamine stores from prolonged metaraminol therapy or such conditions as chronic heart failure or reserpine therapy.

TABLE 48-5   Drugs Used for Hemodynamic Stabilization (*Cont.*)

DRUG	INDICATIONS	DOSAGE AND ADMINISTRATION	NURSING PROCESS IMPLICATIONS
		Sympathomimetics	
Isoproterenol (Isuprel)	Cardiogenic shock, particularly as caused from bradycardia due to heart block. Not effective in profound hypotension.	Continuous titrated IV infusion 0.5–5.0 μg/min. *Advanced shock:* up to 30 μg/min. *Pediatric:* begun at 0.1 μg/kg/min (usual effect 0.1–1.0 μg/kg/min).	Increases renal blood flow due to increased cardiac output. Should not be given to patients with ischemic heart disease or in those with normal to above-normal heart rates. If angina or heart rate >110 beats/min, decrease or discontinue infusion. Drug may produce extreme tachycardia leading to ventricular fibrillation. Large doses cause pooling of blood in skeletal muscles, causing severe hypotension. Do not give to patient with digitalis toxicity. May cause CNS side effects (tremors, dizziness, flushing, anxiety). Avoid giving simultaneously with epinephrine. May be given simultaneously with norepinephrine to lessen vasoconstriction in vital organs.
Epinephrine (Adrenalin)	Anaphylaxis; anaphylactic shock.	0.3–0.5 mg SC, IM, or IV depending on severity of reaction and hypotension. If there is profound drop in blood pressure and no vein can be found for injection, epinephrine may be given intralingually into the posterior ventral portion of the tongue. In order to increase and sustain arterial pressure and/or heart rate, epinephrine may be given by continuous titrated IV infusion begun at 1.0 μg/min, which may be increased to 3–4 μg/min (solution of 1.0 mg in 250 mL D_5W). *Pediatric:* begin at 0.1 μg/kg/min (usual effect $\geq$1.5 μg/kg/min).	Inhibits antigen-induced release of histamine to give rapid relief of hypersensitivity reactions. Do not use solution if it is brown, contains a precipitate, or is outdated. Evaluate for return of anaphylactic symptoms; repeat injection may be required. Do not give with other sympathomimetics. Monitor ECG for arrhythmias and arterial blood pressure during infusion.

TABLE 48-5 Drugs Used for Hemodynamic Stabilization (*Cont.*)

DRUG	INDICATIONS	DOSAGE AND ADMINISTRATION	NURSING PROCESS IMPLICATIONS
Arteriovenous Vasodilators			
Nitroprusside (Nipride, Nitropress)	Cardiogenic shock secondary to acute myocardial infarction.	Continuous titrated IV infusion. *Average initial dose:* 0.5–8.0 μg/kg/min, but 10.0 μg/min total dose may be adequate for pump failure. *Pediatric:* begun at 0.5 μg/kg/min (usual effect at 1–10 μg/kg/min).	Onset of action 30–60 s with 1–10 min duration after infusion discontinued. Monitor arterial blood gases (ABGs); metabolic acidosis is early and as a reliable sign of toxicity of the metabolite, cyanide. Toxicity more common in renal impairment. Protect IV bottle from light and dispose of solution if fluid is blue, green, or dark-red. Slow or discontinue temporarily if apprehension, headache, muscle twitching, palpitations, dizziness, or abdominal pain occur, which indicate too rapid reduction of blood pressure.
Nitroglycerin (Nitrol-IV, Nitrostat-IV, Tridil, Nitro-Bid IV)	Cardiogenic shock secondary to acute myocardial infarction.	50 μg IV bolus may be repeated every 3–5 min. Continuous titrated IV infusion begun at 5–20 μg/min and increased by 5–10 μg/min every 3–5 min. Must be diluted prior to administration by IV bolus or by continuous IV.	Use only with infusion set furnished and glass IV bottles. When titrating dose, decrease increments and prolong time intervals once a blood pressure response is noted. Slow or discontinue if PAWP falls during maintenance infusion.
Cardiac Glycosides			
Ouabain (G-strophanthin) Deslanoside (Cedilanid-D) Digoxin (Lanoxin)	Congestive heart failure. Cardiogenic shock.	Average digitalizing doses: ouabain 0.3–0.5 mg IV; deslanoside 0.8–1.6 mg IV in 1 or 2 doses; digoxin 0.75–1.0 mg IV.	Monitor ECG for ectopic beats, increasing block, bradycardia. Toxicity more common in renal impairment, hypokalemia, hypercalcemia. Nausea, vomiting, diarrhea, visual changes may indicate toxicity.
Narcotic/Vasodilator			
Morphine sulfate	Myocardial infarction. Acute pulmonary edema.	2–5 mg IV bolus given every 5–30 min titrated to relieve pain and anxiety without causing respiratory depression.	Given to relieve pain and anxiety and decrease O_2 consumption. Decreases venous return by vasodilation. Observe for respiratory depression, hypoxia.

TABLE 48-5   Drugs Used for Hemodynamic Stabilization (*Cont.*)

DRUG	INDICATIONS	DOSAGE AND ADMINISTRATION	NURSING PROCESS IMPLICATIONS
Loop Diuretics			
Furosemide (Lasix) Bumetanide (Bumex)	Cerebral edema following cardiac arrest. Acute pulmonary edema.	*Furosemide:* 40 mg IV bolus given slowly over 1–2 min. *Pediatric:* 1 mg/kg per dose IV bolus. *Bumetanide:* 0.5–1.0 mg IV over 1–2 min. May repeat every 2–3 h to maximum daily dose of 10 mg.	*Ototoxic:* Assess for tinnitus, hearing loss, vertigo. Monitor serum electrolytes, urea nitrogen, and CO_2. Bumetanide may be used in persons allergic to furosemide, since cross allergy is rare. Equivalent bumetanide dosage is approximately ¼₀ furosemide dosage.
Ethacrynate sodium (Edecrin)	Cerebral edema following cardiac arrest. Acute pulmonary edema.	50 mg IV bolus as initial dose; inject over 2–3 min.	(See furosemide.)
Corticosteroids			
Dexamethasone sodium phosphates (Decadron) Methylprednisolone sodium succinate (Solu-Medrol)	Severe shock with persistent unresponsive hypotension. Cerebral edema following cardiac arrest. Shock lung.	*Dexamethasone—Cerebral edema:* 10–20 mg IV bolus, followed by 4–10 mg repeated every 6 h. *Pediatric:* 0.2 to 0.3 mg/kg/24 h. *Methylprednisolone— Cerebral edema:* 60–100 mg IV bolus may be repeated every 6 h. *Shock lung:* 5–30 mg/kg IV bolus.	Stabilizes lysosomal membranes; vasodilator; facilitates pulmonary shunt closure; reduces cerebral inflammation. Monitor for hypertension, hypokalemia, edema, weight increase, hypoglycemia, ulcer disease, psychic derangements.
Bronchodilator			
Aminophylline	Anaphylaxis. Acute pulmonary edema.	*Loading dose:* IV infusion of 5–7 mg/kg in 250 mL D_5W over 20–30 min, maintenance doses based upon blood levels. Decrease loading dose if patient on chronic therapy with any theophylline.	Rapid-acting. Patient should be placed on cardiac monitor as too rapid administration may produce vagal response.

although 50 percent of an IV dose is excreted unchanged by the kidneys. **Metaraminol** and **dobutamine** are rapidly biotransformed to inactive metabolites.

Adverse Effects

Sympathomimetic drugs cause a predictable range of adverse effects when used to treat shock. Sinus or ventricular tachycardia and other arrhythmias are of particular concern, especially following myocardial infarction. Both hypotension and hypertension can occur, as can tachycardia and reflex bradycardia. Cardiac palpitations and angina secondary to cardiostimulation are reported. Central nervous system effects include anxiety, headache, nausea, vomiting, sweating, fear, facial flushing, mild tremors, and nervousness.

Since **MAO inhibitors, tricyclic antidepressants, guanethidine,** and **reserpine** alter synthesis, storage, and/or release of sympathomimetics, patients on these drugs require cautious administration and careful monitoring when sympathomimetics are taken concurrently. Of course, α and β **blockers** competitively antagonize the effects of sympathomimetics. Some **general anesthetics** sensitize the myocardium to the arrhythmogenic effects of sympathomimetics.

Most of the sympathomimetic drugs will cause local tissue necrosis if allowed to infiltrate. This hazardous effect may be minimized with the use of **phentolamine** (Regitine), an α receptor blocker. A solution of 5 to 10 mg phentolamine in 10 to 15 mL of normal saline may be locally infiltrated in the tissue. It may also be advantageous to add 5 mg of phentolamine to the catecholamine IV infusion. Further, small veins should be avoided for the infusion because gangrene can result.

Acid-base disturbances lessen the effectiveness of sympathomimetics. However, remember if giving sodium bicarbonate, it will inactivate catecholamines if mixed with them.

Patients should not be abruptly withdrawn from vasopressor therapy. Increasing IV fluid therapy may be useful in "weaning" patients in order to avoid rebound hypotension.

Vasodilator Therapy

Nitroprusside IV and nitroglycerin IV may be advantageous in treating cardiogenic shock resulting from myocardial infarction, although they are not recommended as initial therapy (see Table 48-5). They are used to increase cardiac output and not primarily to decrease venous return or improve systemic blood pressure. The patient must remain horizontal to obviate venous pooling and must be continuously monitored by an intraarterial pressure line. Increasing IV fluid therapy may be valuable during vasodilator therapy. Vasodilators may be given in combination with catecholamines for inotropic support. The effects of the drugs will be titrated against each other to achieve optimum vital signs,

urine output, peripheral perfusion, and blood pressure. The pharmacokinetics and adverse effects of these drugs are presented in Chap. 43.

Additional Drug Therapy

Long-term support with *digitalization* is advisable in cardiogenic shock. Other drugs used in the treatment of septic shock are *antibiotics*. A broad-spectrum combination of an aminoglycoside and a penicillin derivative or cephalosporin will give effective coverage until culture and sensitivity results are obtained. Antihistamines, such as **diphenhydramine** (Benadryl) 50 to 100 mg IM or IV, may be useful adjuncts in the treatment of anaphylactic shock.

EVALUATION OF THERAPY AND PROGNOSIS IN SHOCK

Indicators of successful therapy for the shock patient are improvement in cardiac output, oxygen saturation, arterial pH, and arterial blood gases. Cardiogenic shock most often occurs following an acute myocardial infarction. The mortality rate is 80 to 90 percent when treated aggressively. Septic shock carries a 30 to 50 percent mortality rate. Shock is very difficult to reverse. The aim of good nursing care is to identify patients at risk and prevent shock before it begins.

CASE STUDY

Ms. S., aged 58, was admitted to ICU after suffering an acute myocardial infarction (MI). Oxygen by nasal cannula was begun at 4 L/min. An IV infusion of D_5W was begun to keep her veins open for medication. Morphine sulfate IV was given in 2-mg increments titrated to relieve pain and anxiety. The cardiac monitor revealed a normal sinus rhythm with frequent PVCs. She was started on a constant lidocaine IV infusion at 2 mg/min. Ms. S.'s condition was listed as stable. She was alert and oriented, but anxious. Vital signs were: BP 110/60, pulse 76, respirations 18 and unlabored. On auscultation her heart sounds were normal and lungs were clear. Her skin was warm and dry. A Foley catheter was inserted to monitor hourly output.

Assessment

After the evening meal, the nurse found Ms. S. restless and unaware of her physical surroundings. Upon examining Ms. S., the nurse found her skin cool, clammy, and pale. Vital signs were: BP 100/66, pulse 98, respirations 26 and shallow. Chest auscultation revealed a ventricular diastolic gallop and rales at the base of either lung. Urinary output had also dropped to below 20 mL/h.

Cardiogenic shock was the probable diagnosis, since

cardiogenic shock occurs in about 15 percent of patients recovering from MI. Objectively, signs indicative of shock were clouded sensorium, decreasing blood pressure with narrowing pulse pressure, tachycardia, hyperventilation, decreased urinary output, and peripheral skin changes. Heart gallop and pulmonary rales indicated pump failure.

Management

The immediate goals were to maintain cardiac output, provide adequate tissue perfusion, and interrupt the shock process before complications from profound hypotension developed. The physician was notified immediately and arterial blood gases (ABGs) were obtained. The nurse anticipated that a positive inotropic drug or vasopressor might be required, and so another intravenous route using a large antecubital vein was secured. ABGs did reveal hypoxemia, with a P_{O_2} of 66 (normal at sea level is 80 to 100) and an oxygen saturation of 88 percent (normal is 90 to 95 percent). The pH was 7.36 (low-normal) and P_{CO_2} was normal at 40. The 100 percent oxygen flow rate was increased to 6 L/min.

The physician ordered a continuous IV infusion of dopamine to be started at 2.5 μg/kg/min to improve cardiac output and renal blood flow. Ms. S. weighed 110 lb, which the nurse converted to the 50-kg equivalent, using the ratio-proportion formula (see Chap. 3). The dose in milliliters per kilogram per minute (mL/kg/min) was ascertained from a standard dilution chart, a portion of which is reproduced below. (The asterisks indicate the ordered dose and dilution used.)

DOPAMINE

DESIRED DOSE, μg/kg/min	Flow Rate, mL/kg/min		
	400 mg IN 250 mL (1600 μg/mL)	200 mg IN 250 mL (800 μg/mL)	200 mg IN 500 mL (400 μg/mL)
2.0	0.00125	0.0025	0.005
*2.5	0.0015625	0.003125	*0.00625
3.0	0.001875	0.00375	0.0075
3.5	0.0021875	0.004375	0.00875
4.0	0.0025	0.005	0.01
4.5	0.0028125	0.005625	0.0125
.	.	.	.
.	.	.	.
.	.	.	.
20.0	0.0125	0.025	0.05

The nurse then calculated the volume in microdrops to be administered by the formula:

$$\text{Weight in kg} \times \text{mL/kg/min (from chart above)} \times \text{drop factor}$$

or

$$50 \times 0.00625 \times 60 = 18.75$$

After mixing 200 mg of dopamine into 500 mL D_5W in 0.45% saline, the nurse set the infusion pump to deliver 19 microdrops/min and continuously monitored blood pressure and urine output. Thirty minutes after the infusion began, the blood pressure dropped to 92/60, and there was no increase in urine output. The dose was gradually increased to 750 μg/min of dopamine (75 microdrops). Ms. S. did not respond favorably and developed tachycardia. The nurse immediately notified the physician.

One nurse was assigned to care for Ms. S, in order to decrease anxiety caused by lack of consistent support. The nurse provided simple explanations of the procedures being performed and maintained a calm manner in answering all of Ms. S.'s questions. When approaching the bedside to give a medication or to check equipment, the nurse remembered to keep her focus on the patient. Ms. S. said she thought she could face almost anything if the nurse stayed with her.

A Swan-Ganz catheter was inserted to measure pulmonary artery wedge pressure (PAWP) and give a more accurate measurement of left-sided heart function. An arterial pressure line was also inserted to allow precise minute-to-minute blood pressure readings to be taken. Ms. S.'s PAWP was 26 mmHg (normal is 4 to 12) indicating heart failure. The physician ordered the dopamine infusion to be discontinued and an IV infusion of dobutamine to be begun at 10 μg/kg/min. This dose was 500 μg/min for Ms. S. and was calculated as follows:

$$\text{Ordered dose} \times \text{weight in kg} = 10 \ \mu\text{g/kg/min} \times 50 \text{ kg}$$
$$= 500 \ \mu\text{g/min}$$

Since no standard dilution table was available on the unit for dobutamine, the IV was mixed by adding one vial of dobutamine (250 mg) to 500 mL of D_5W, which the nurse calculated contained 500 μg/mL (since there are 1000 μg/mg):

$$\frac{250 \text{ mg}}{500 \text{ mL}} = 0.5 \text{ mg/mL} = 500 \ \mu\text{g/mL}$$

The infusion pump was set to deliver 60 microdrops/min (60 microdrops = 1 mL = 500 μg dobutamine).

Within 1 h after the infusion was begun, vital signs were: BP 102/68, pulse 80, and respirations 20 and unlabored. PAWP was dropped to 20 mmHg, and urine output increased to 50 mL/h. Ms. S.'s sensorium was clearer, and her skin was warmer and dry. ABGs were: a P_{O_2} of 85 and oxygen saturation 92 percent.

Evaluation

The initial goal was to establish a diagnosis of beginning cardiogenic shock and to stop its progression. The nurse's early assessment and prompt action determined the selection of definitive therapy to alleviate shock. Ms. S.'s hemodynamic status had improved before she progressed to profound hypotension. By carefully monitoring the patient and the effects of drug therapy, the most effective intervention for Ms. S. had been found. Successful nursing measures to relieve psychosocial causes of anxiety had assisted in decreasing this potential source of increased oxygen demand. Dobutamine is a good choice of therapy to follow dopamine because of its ability to increase cardiac contractility without causing tachycardia. If Ms. S. had developed hypotension, dobutamine would have been ineffective and the use of a vasopressor might have severely decreased tissue perfusion. Because the nurse closely observed the patient, made rapid and accurate assessments to initiate and monitor therapy, Ms. S. was one of the 10 to 20 percent of victims who survive cardiogenic shock. The underlying cardiovascular defect, heart failure, was then successfully corrected through the use of a digoxin drug and Ms. S. made a full recovery.

BURNS

LEARNING OBJECTIVES

Upon mastery of the content of this section, the reader will be able to:

1. Describe the pathophysiology of major burn wounds in terms of fluid shifts and skin-loss derangements.
2. Describe the processes of assessing the burn injury during the emergency and acute phases.
3. Explain the rationale for the use of fluid resuscitation, systemic antibiotics, and topical wound therapy in the management of major burns.
4. Compare and contrast the advantages, disadvantages, and nursing process considerations in the use of the common topical drugs used to treat burn wounds.
5. Identify indicators of successful therapy for major burns during the emergency and acute phases.

Over 2 million Americans suffer burn injuries each year. Approximately 12,000 of these victims eventually die, making burn injuries the third leading cause of death in the United States. A severe burn is one of the most physically and psychologically devastating types of trauma that can occur. It is appropriately termed a *pansystemic injury* because all other organs are required to take over the role of the injured skin. Burns may be classified as thermal, chemical, electrical, or radiation injuries.

PATHOPHYSIOLOGY OF MAJOR BURNS

A major burn is considered to be one that injures approximately 20 to 30 percent of the total body surface area (TBSA). Pathophysiologic derangements following major burns result from fluid shifts and loss of normal skin functions.

Fluid Shifts When a burn injury occurs, the capillaries are damaged and capillary permeability is increased. With an increase in permeability, both crystalloid and colloid fluids pass freely and rapidly from the intravascular space into the interstitial space. In major burns, up to 50 percent of the plasma portion of the circulating blood volume may be lost from the critical vascular compartment resulting in hypovolemia and *burn shock*.

Loss of Protection from Infection A major function of the skin is protection against infection. The tissue killed by burning (eschar) separates from the underlying viable tissue by the process of liquefaction. This leaves a large open wound highly susceptible to *gram-positive, gram-negative,* and *fungal* infections. Infection causes delayed wound healing, contractures, septicemia, prolonged hospitalization, and one-half of the deaths from burn injuries.

Other Skin-Loss Derangements With severe burns the body is unable to properly regulate body temperature and fluid loss from open wounds, creating a state of hypermetabolism. Loss of large areas of skin also causes problems with excretion, sensation, production of vitamin D, and body image.

ASSESSMENT OF BURNS

Severity of Injury

The burn injury is obvious, but the patient must be thoroughly assessed for other injuries. Problems with airway, breathing, and circulation remain top priorities for assessment and immediate management. Burn injuries will not render the patient unconscious. The problem may be anoxia (likely from smoke inhalation), cardiovascular accident (CVA), head injury, or a multitude of other possibilities. The severity of the burn injury is related to five factors:

1. Extent of burn
2. Depth of burn
3. Age of patient
4. Past medical history
5. Part of body burned

Extent of Burn As a general rule, mortality increases with the TBSA burned. There are two methods currently used to estimate the size of the burn injury. In the "rule of nines" the adult body is divided into areas equal to multiples of 9 percent. Berkow's method of calculation and the Lund and Browder scale are more accurate, especially in children, since they take into account differences in body proportions. A quick and easy method of determining body surface area is to use the palm of the adult hand as approximately 1 percent of the TBSA.

Depth of Burn The preferred terms for determining depth of burn are *partial-thickness* and *full-thickness*. Partial-thickness wounds may be superficial or deep, injuring or destroying the epidermis, but only damaging the dermis. These burns have reddened areas which blanch and refill with pressure, moist areas, and large blisters, and are very painful. Partial-thickness wounds heal completely by reepithelialization in about 2 or 3 weeks. Full-thickness burns destroy the epidermis, dermis, and often underlying subcutaneous tissue and muscle. These wounds are dry and anesthetic. They may be white, charred, brown and leathery, or red without ability to blanch and refill. Full-thickness wounds will heal by granulation and require autografting.

Age The mortality increases when patients are at the ends of the age continuum. Children under the age of 4 have a poor response to infection. There is exacerbation of latent degenerative processes, particularly arteriosclerotic, in persons over 60 years of age.

Past Medical History   Mortality from burn injuries particularly increases in persons with diabetes mellitus, cirrhosis of the liver, or any respiratory or cardiac disease.

Part of the Body Burned   Respiratory problems are likely to develop in burns of the head, neck, or chest. Burns of the perineum are in danger of severe infection. Crippling deformities are likely to occur when the face, hands, or feet are burned.

Assessment for Infection

Sepsis can be a catastrophic complication from burn injuries. Partial-thickness burns may be converted to full-thickness as the result of infection. Accurate nursing assessment is the key to preventing morbidity and mortality from sepsis.

General signs of infection in a burn wound are redness around the wound edge, swelling, purulent drainage, increased wound pain, bad odor, soupiness, or rapid separation of eschar. The most common organisms infecting burn wounds are group A *streptococcus, Staphylococcus aureus, Klebsiella, Pseudomonas aeruginosa, Serratia,* and *Candida albicans.* Quantitative microorganism counts from wound biopsies are more accurate for determining sepsis than swab cultures. Antibiotic sensitivities of the cultured organism should also be obtained.

PHARMACOLOGIC MANAGEMENT OF BURNS

Fluid Resuscitation

After airway assessment, fluid replacement becomes the most critical aspect of burn management in the emergency phase. Patients with more than 15 to 20 percent TBSA burns require fluid resuscitation. Although there are many formulas for types and amounts of fluids to be used, the American Burn Association has agreed upon one formula (Parkland formula) which has demonstrated most successful resuscitation. The IV fluid of choice to be used in the first 24 h is **Ringer's lactate.** The amount of fluid to be given is 2 to 4 mL/kg of body weight for each percent of body surface area burned. For example, a person weighing 70 kg with a 50 percent burn would require 14,000 mL of fluid. Half the fluid is given in the first 8 h after injury, one-fourth during the second 8 h, and the remaining fluid in the third 8 h.

The most accurate index of adequate fluid resuscitation is urine output, which should average 1 mL/kg/h. Urine output should be assessed every 30 to 60 min, and IV fluid rate adjusted accordingly about every 2 h.

Antibiotics

Intravenous antibiotic therapy is generally initiated early in the management of burn injuries and should be guided by routine blood cultures and sensitivity testing (see Table 48-6).

Topical Wound Therapy

Topical agents are the critical line of defense against wound infection (see Table 48-7). Therapy begins immediately after initial cleansing and debridement of the burn wound. The goals of topical therapy are to control infection, promote healing, and increase the patient's comfort. The physician must specify the area to be treated with the topical agent as full-thickness, partial-thickness, or graft site. Each may require different treatment.

TABLE 48-6   Course of Burn Infection and Its Treatment

TIME COURSE	MOST COMMON ORGANISM	AGENT OF CHOICE*	USUAL ROUTE(S)
Initial 0–7 days	β-Hemolytic streptococcus	Penicillin G or derivative	IV
Autolytic: 8–21 days	*Staphylococcus aureus*	Penicillinase-resistant penicillins†	IV, IM, PO
		Erythromycin	PO, IV
		Novobiocin	PO
Granulating: 22–30 days	*Pseudomonas aeruginosa*	Gentamicin, other aminoglycosides	IV, IM
		Third-generation cephalosporins‡	IV, IM
		Carbenicillin, ticarcillin, pipercillin	IV, IM
		Colistin sulfate	IV
Grafting: 31 days to coverage	β-Hemolytic streptococcus	Penicillin G or derivative	IV
		Chloramphenicol	PO, IV
	Yeast	Ketoconzole	PO
		Amphotericin B	IV

*Based on blood or wound culture and sensitivity reports.

†Penicillinase-resistant penicillins include: methicillin (IM, IV), nafcillin (IM, IV, PO), oxacillin (IM, IV, PO), cloxacillin (PO), dicloxacillin (PO).

‡Third-generation cephalosporins include cefoperazone, cefotaxine, moxalactam, ceftizoxime.

Source: Modified from J. Luckmann and K. C. Sorensen (eds.): *Medical-Surgical Nursing: A Psychophysiologic Approach,* 2d ed., Philadelphia: W. B. Saunders Co., 1980. Used with permission.

TABLE 48-7   Topical Drugs Used to Treat Burn Wounds

DRUG	PHARMACOLOGIC EFFECTS	ADVANTAGES	DISADVANTAGES	NURSING PROCESS
Silver sulfadiazine (Silvadene Cream)	Antibacterial, binds to bacteria cell membrane and interferes with DNA. Broad-spectrum against gram-negative and gram-positive bacteria, as well as yeast. Prevents and treats wound sepsis with deep partial-thickness and full-thickness wounds.	Does not cause electrolyte imbalance or kidney disease. Long-lasting action (up to 48 h). Has long shelf life. Delays eschar separation less than many other topical drugs. Fast, painless, easy to apply. Increases ROM due to softening of eschar.	May cause rash, burning, and pruritus. Not consistently effective against large burns (> 60% TBSA). Not consistently effective against some bacteria and yeasts. May depress granulocyte formation. Absorbed into eschar less than other topical drugs.	Cream is easily applied directly to burn wound with sterile gloved hand or applied to sterile gauze and then directly to burn wound. Removed completely with water (usually hydrotherapy tanking prior to reapplication). Assess for signs of wound infection, such as soupiness. Do not use with topical proteolytic enzymes because silver may inactivate enzyme. Do not use in patients with history of kidney disease. Assess for toxic symptoms: nausea and vomiting, oliguria, anuria, hematuria, cyanosis, anemia, leukopenia, granulocytopenia, mental changes, jaundice, skin rashes.
Mafenide acetate (Sulfamylon)	Bacteriostatic against many gram-negative and gram-positive organisms such as P. aeruginosa, S. aureus, Aerobacter aerogenes. Penetrates eschar to prevent and treat bacterial wound invasion.	Effective against Pseudomonas. Has long shelf life. Penetrates thick eschar. Excellent treatment for electrical burns. Relatively nontoxic.	May cause rash, hyperpnea, metabolic acidosis. Causes burning and stinging lasting 15–60 min after application. Tends to slow eschar separation. May promote superinfection. Inhibits epithelial proliferation and may delay healing if used after wound is free of infection.	Cream is easily applied directly to burn wound with sterile gloved hand or applied to sterile gauze and then directly to burn wound. Remove completely with debridement prior to reapplication. Use with caution, if at all, in patients with history of sulfa drug allergy, respiratory, or kidney disease. Assess patient for signs and symptoms of metabolic acidosis: hyperpnea, acid-base and electrolyte imbalances. Use analgesics and emotional support for managing painful drug therapy.

TABLE 48-7   Topical Drugs Used to Treat Burn Wounds (*Cont.*)

DRUG	PHARMACOLOGIC EFFECTS	ADVANTAGES	DISADVANTAGES	NURSING PROCESS
Silver nitrate	Antimicrobial. Bacteriostatic solution effective in reducing surface bacteria.	Inexpensive. Reduces evaporative water loss from burn wounds. Produces more rapid debridement of eschar (from frequent dressing changes) and earlier readiness for grafting.	Since it does not penetrate eschar and only penetrates wound 1–2 mm, it acts only on surface organisms. Stings on application. Stains everything it comes in contact with. May cause hyponatremia, hypochloremia, hypocalcemia, hypokalemia, hypomagnesemia.	Solution is easily applied: after initial care, wound is covered with 8 to 10 layers of sterile gauze (not fine mesh), then saturated with warm solution every 2 h. Check serum electrolytes daily. Use analgesia and emotional support for managing painful drug therapy.
Povidone-iodine (Betadine)	Microbicidal against gram-negative and gram-positive organisms, yeast, fungi, viruses, protozoa.	Effective against many infections not well controlled by silver sulfadiazine. Several dosage forms available (solution, foam, ointment). Long shelf life.	May cause metabolic acidosis due to elevated serum iodine levels. Crusts may form if wounds are not properly cleaned. May cause rash and burning when applied. Stains clothing and linen. ROM may be impaired with bulky dressings.	Foam or ointment is easily applied to burn wound with sterile gloved hand. If solution is used, keep dressings moist. Do not use in patients with sensitivity to iodine. Check serum electrolytes and serum iodine levels frequently. Thoroughly cleanse wound in hydrotherapy tank.
Gentamicin sulfate (Garamycin)	Broad-spectrum antibiotic, effective against many organisms not responding to other topical antibiotics.	Effective against *Pseudomonas*. Painless application. Available as cream or ointment.	May develop resistant organism strains. May cause ototoxicity and nephrotoxicity.	Cream is rapidly absorbed and should not be applied beneath occlusive dressings because topical effects are quickly lost. Ointment is absorbed at slower and more constant rate and may be used under light dressings. Use with caution in patients with decreased renal function. Monitor serum creatinine and creatinine clearance studies before treatment and weekly during treatment.
Sodium hypochlorite (Dakin's solution)	Bactericidal.	Aids in debriding wounds. Aids in drying wounds that have become soupy.	Dissolves blood clots. May inhibit clotting. May cause skin irritation.	Dressings should be changed every 4–12 h. Carefully assess wound site for signs of irritation.

TABLE 48-7 Topical Drugs Used to Treat Burn Wounds (*Cont.*)

DRUG	PHARMACOLOGIC EFFECTS	ADVANTAGES	DISADVANTAGES	NURSING PROCESS
Nitrofurazone (Furacin)	Broad-spectrum antibacterial. Inhibits enzymes necessary for bacterial metabolism.	Available as cream, solution, water-soluble powder. Effective against *S. aureus* and some antibiotic-resistant organisms. Not absorbed systemically. Low incidence of sensitivity. Does not cause pain or maceration.	In rare instances, may cause contact dermatitis.	Assess patient carefully for signs of allergic reaction or evidence of superinfection. Turns urine a reddish color.
Bismuth tribromphemate (Xeroform) (on petroleum jelly gauze)	Nonantiseptic preparation. Debrides and protects donor site. Protects graft.	Conforms to wound. Nontoxic and nonsensitizing. Long shelf life.	Neither antiseptic nor antimicrobial. May stick to wound so that removal is very painful.	Apply carefully so that gauze sheets don't overlap. Assess patient carefully for signs of infection. Use analgesia and emotional support for managing painful drug therapy.
Scarlet red (red dye in oil base on gauze)	Nonantiseptic preparation.	Promotes healing and protects donor site. Long shelf-life	May cause systemic effects. Irritates skin and causes pain when patient moves. Stains clothing and temporarily stains skin.	Applied to donor sites at time of harvest; leave until site heals and scarlet red gauze sloughs. Assess closely for signs of infection beneath gauze. If site needs to be dried, use heat lamp for a few minutes every 4 h.
Sutilains ointment (Travase)	Proteolytic enzyme. Digests necrotic tissue. Facilitates removal of eschar and purulent exudate.	Aids initial debridement, before patient can tolerate surgical debridement. Easily applied.	Causes mild, transient pain on application. May cause paresthesia, bleeding, dermatitis. Requires refrigeration. Increases fluid loss. Nonbactericidal.	Dressings must be kept moist at all times. Patient must be stable enough for surgery after a few days so that debrided wounds can be covered with membranes or grafted. Assess patient closely for signs of infection. Do not use on more than 15% of total burn surface at one time. Do not use with Silvadene, iodine, Furacin, or silver nitrate. Use with Sulfamylon, gentamicin. Change dressings every 8 h.

TABLE 48-7   Topical Drugs Used to Treat Burn Wounds (*Cont.*)

DRUG	PHARMACOLOGIC EFFECTS	ADVANTAGES	DISADVANTAGES	NURSING PROCESS
Fibrinolysin and desoxyribonuclease, combined (bovine) (Elase)	Proteolytic enzymes. Digests necrotic tissue. Facilitates removal of eschar and purulent exudate.	Long shelf life. Does not require refrigeration.	Preparation must be immediately before application. Causes itching and burning.	Wait for physician to debride any thick, dry eschar before application. Assess patient closely for signs of infection. Change dressings daily. Do not use with patients allergic to bovine materials.

Subeschar Clysis   A valuable adjunct to effective topical therapy is subeschar clysis. The technique involves the injection of antibiotic solutions directly into the tissues beneath the burn eschar, permitting high concentrations to be used. Subeschar clysis is often used in burns of greater than 40 percent TBSA.

Chloramine-T-Glycerine Dressings   This investigational topical agent has shown much promise. Use of the solution suggests that it is excellent for wound cleansing, stimulation of granulation tissue, preparing wounds for split-thickness skin grafting, and maintaining heavily contaminated skin grafts. There seems to be no skin or granulation tissue injury, allergic responses, or metabolic or electrolyte disturbances (Figgie et al., 1982).

Tetanus Immunization

Burn wounds are highly contaminated, and eschar promotes growth of tetanus organisms. Tetanus toxoid is administered to all burn patients upon admission. If it has been more than 10 years since the patient has received immunization, tetanus immune globulin (human) is also administered.

Analgesics

During the first few hours after burn injury, narcotics should be used cautiously in order not to depress level of consciousness or depress respiration. **Morphine sulfate** may be given in small (2 to 4 mg) IV increments titrated in amounts just sufficient to relieve pain and anxiety.

EVALUATION OF THERAPY AND PROGNOSIS IN BURNS

Emergency Phase

This phase includes approximately the first 2 to 4 days immediately following a major burn injury. Management during this time is directed toward life-saving measures, the most important of which are correction of any respiratory distress and fluid resuscitation from burn shock. During this time, evaluation and revision of the management is continuous and fast-paced. Evaluation is based on maintaining therapy that prevents the occurrence of cardiopulmonary distress and shock discussed earlier in this chapter. Prognosis is favorable if the patient's hemodynamic status is maintained.

Acute Phase

This phase includes the entire time required to resurface all areas of full-thickness skin loss, which may take weeks to many months. It is important for the nurse to remember that the patient is acutely, not chronically, ill and requires intensive nursing care. Mortality and morbidity are high during this time particularly due to the complications from sepsis. Evaluation focuses on whether the burn wounds heal with healthy granulation tissue to facilitate grafting and/or early closure. Prognosis is favorable once the burn wound has been reduced to less than 20 percent of the body surface.

CASE STUDY

Ms. J., aged 19, had sustained scald injuries over her anterior chest and abdomen, and the anterior surface of her left arm and leg (approximately 30 percent TBSA). At the scene of the injury her wet clothes had been removed. She was wrapped in a clean, dry blanket and rushed to a nearby emergency department. In the emergency department, an airway was secured and fluid resuscitation was begun with Ringer's lactate. Because her left arm was edematous from the burn, a large-bore IV catheter was inserted in her right antecubital vein.

Since Ms. J. weighed 50 kg, she needed to receive 6000 mL fluid in the first 24 h following her injury. A Foley catheter was inserted to monitor urine output. Vital signs were: BP 130/90, pulse 80, and respirations 18. Tetanus toxoid 0.5 mL IM was administered. Ms. J. was taken to the hydrotherapy room for a full body cleansing. The physician ordered that after the bathing, her burns were to be covered with silver sulfadiazine cream (Silvadene). She was admitted to the burn unit. Several days later, after hemodynamic status had been stabilized, Ms. J. was taken to the operating room. A split-thickness graft was harvested from her right thigh and placed on a clean granulating area of her abdomen. The areas of full-thickness burn on her chest were surgically debrided and covered with pigskin (temporary graft). The donor site on her right thigh was covered with scarlet red–impregnated gauze dressings and the remaining burns were covered with silver sulfadiazine and dressed. Ms. J. was then returned to the burn unit.

Assessment

During the acute phase following burn injury, the nurse remembered that Ms. J. was especially susceptible to wound infection. The nurse made frequent and careful assessments of Ms. J., including vital signs and neurologic status. The burn wounds were carefully assessed each day after the dressings were removed in hydrotherapy. The nurse assessed Ms. J.'s ability to tolerate the discomfort of daily dressing changes and wound debridement. Approximately 20 min before each trip to hydrotherapy, Ms. J. would show signs of intense anxiety such as hyperventilation, cool and clammy skin, and increased agitation. She told the nurse that the experience was like "being a prisoner who is sent off to the torture chamber." Ms. J. admitted to having great difficulty with situations in her life over which she could have no control. The nurse also learned that needlepoint was Ms. J.'s favorite means of relaxation.

On her seventh day after burn injury, the nurse noticed that the wounds on her left thigh were becoming reddened around the edges, developing soupiness, and had a purulent drainage. Also the wounds on the left arm were not debriding well. The nurse notified the physician immediately and wound biopsies were made. Several hours later, Ms. J. became restless and unaware of her surroundings. The nurse examined her and found that vital signs were: temperature 38.5°C, pulse 100, respirations 24 and shallow. The physician was summoned immediately and wound and blood cultures were obtained. A diagnosis of wound and systemic infection was made.

Management

Based upon microscopic examination showing gram-positive cocci and a negative β-lactamase assay, the physician ordered a course of IV penicillin G, 500,000 U/8 h. Silver sulfadiazine therapy to the left thigh and arm was discontinued. Povidone-iodine (Betadine) ointment was ordered to be applied to thigh burns and petroleum-jelly-impregnated gauze treated with bismuth tribromphenate (Xeroform) was applied to the arm burns daily using strict aseptic technique.

Ms. J. was ordered to have morphine sulfate 10 mg IM q3–4h PRN for pain relief. The nurse explained that the drug would be administered to Ms. J. approximately 20 min before the hydrotherapy session. Ms. J. was taught that the drug would decrease her discomfort and allow her to have more control by alleviating much of the anxiety caused by her anticipation of pain. The nurse discussed the debridement procedure with Ms. J., and together they made some plans. Ms. J. chose to work on a simple needlepoint project for diversion on some days, and on others she chose to assist in the debriding and control the speed of the procedure. Ms. J. was also given the option of canceling a session once per week.

Evaluation

The primary goal during the acute phase of burn recovery is to prevent and control infection. The nurse made rapid and accurate assessments of the patient's wounds and systemic response. Specific definitive antibiotic therapy was immediately begun. Subsequent culture and sensitivity reports confirmed that the infecting organism was β-hemolytic streptococcus sensitive to penicillin G.

The approach in topical burn therapy is to initiate a new treatment if one is not effective. Betadine is often effective against many infections not well controlled by silver sulfadiazine. The goals of topical burn therapy are to assist in debriding wounds with multiple dressing changes and to promote the growth of viable healing tissue. When the body has been completely resurfaced with skin, the acute phase has ended, and prognosis for full recovery is good.

Pain control during topical burn therapy may be difficult to achieve. Within 1 week, the nurse was able to see a very significant decrease in Ms. J.'s anxiety prior to hydrotherapy sessions. Ms. J. said that the ability to control the experience was of great benefit to her. By the end of the third week of these nursing measures, Ms. J. was able to use only 5 mg PO of diazepam 30 min prior to leaving for hydrotherapy. She did not choose to cancel any of the sessions.

POISONING AND OVERDOSE

LEARNING OBJECTIVES

Upon mastery of this section, the reader will be able to:

1. Identify the probable class of agent involved in an overdose, given the signs, symptoms, and other diagnostic clues.

2. Describe the appropriate treatment for overdose from opiates, sedative-hypnotics, organophosphate insecticides, cyanide, amphetamines, petroleum distillates, and corrosives.

3. Identify situations in which the following can be used as specific antidotes: naloxone, atropine, pralidoxime, physostigmine, dimercaprol, deferoxamine.

4. Give two examples of situations in which emesis is not recommended in the management of the poisoned patient.

5. Identify the most effective methods of retarding or preventing absorption of ingested substances.

6. Identify two effective cathartics in the treatment of ingested poisons.

7. Discuss the efficacy, toxicity, and indications for syrup of ipecac.

8. Discuss the purpose and efficacy of forced diuresis, alteration of urine pH, and dialysis for the treatment of drug or chemical ingestion.

INCIDENCE AND CAUSE

The accidental or intentional ingestion of commonly used and accessible household products, chemicals, plants, and drugs is a problem of epidemic proportions in the United States today. Once considered to be a problem among children only, poisoning now involves individuals of all ages, particularly young adults.

The National Clearinghouse for Poison Control Centers processed more than 160,000 reported cases of poison ingestion in 1982; this figure is probably a gross underestimation, since many patients are treated for poisoning in facilities and by physicians not associated with a poison control center. One estimate is that 2 to 3 million cases of toxic ingestion and overdose occur each year, accounting for more than 5000 deaths.

Accidental poisonings involving young children are complex events. The age of highest risk is 2 to 3 years. In over half the cases, the offending agent, chemical, or drug was not in its original container when the child came in contact with it. Household products in particular are in constant use and are out of their original packaging when they are accidentally taken by children. The risk of repeated ingestion is also significantly greater for the child with a history of previous ingestion than for one without such a history. The

"accidental" poisoning of a child may be a case of child abuse or intentional neglect.

The most common agents involved in poisonings of children are aspirin, insecticides, plants, soaps, detergents, bleaches, solvent cleansers, and nonprescription cold medicines. While the accidental ingestion of aspirin has been declining in percentage of total poisonings and in actual numbers since 1972, the incidence for other substances has increased significantly.

Persons who have misused and abused drugs and chemicals, intentionally or otherwise, are frequently seen and cared for in the emergency room. The agents most commonly misused or abused in those poisonings are sedative-hypnotic drugs such as **diazepam** (Valium), **alcohol** in combination with drugs, and the **barbiturates**. The opiates (**heroin, methadone**) and **aspirin** are the other major agents involved in such overdoses. Statistics on the causes of acute overdose deaths reveal that opiates, alcohol in combination with drugs, barbiturates and other sedative-hypnotics, **propoxyphene** (Darvon), and the antidepressant drug **amitriptyline** (Elavil) are the most lethal.

There is growing concern now for the exposures to toxic and hazardous materials that occur at the workplace and surrounding environment. The increasing frequency of these incidents should raise the possibility of occupational or environmental cause when an illness of uncertain etiology, or one known to have an association with environmental factors, is diagnosed (see Chap. 49).

ASSESSMENT AND CLINICAL FINDINGS IN POISONING

Decisions for the initial management of the poisoned or overdosed patient are best made when the ingested agent has been identified, but often this cannot be done immediately. A drug history is frequently confused and unreliable. Thus, physical examination of the patient may yield the only information upon which a presumptive identification of the toxic agent can be made. Signs and symptoms that are recognized and associated with a particular drug overdose or toxic ingestion allow for a rapid presumptive diagnosis and early initiation of appropriate treatment.

Signs and Symptoms

Tables 48-8 and 48-9 list the signs and symptoms associated with drugs and toxic agents frequently involved in poisoning and overdoses. It should be noted that ingestions often involve mixtures of multiple drugs and chemicals, so that the physical findings may be complex, confusing, and even clinically misleading. Details given in an overdose or toxic incident are often incomplete, incorrect, and unreliable, particularly when an illicit substance or drug is involved. The dilemma of how to treat the patient is complicated also by problems caused from adulterants and other contaminants

TABLE 48-8 Signs and Symptoms of Commonly Overdosed Drugs and Toxic Agents*

AGENT	SIGNS AND SYMPTOMS	AGENT	SIGNS AND SYMPTOMS
Acetaminophen	Anorexia, nausea, vomiting; delayed-onset symptoms (48–72 h) of jaundice, hypoglycemia, encephalopathy, and hepatic failure	Hydrocarbons	Pulmonary edema, lipid pneumonia, tinnitus, convulsions, diplopia, ventricular fibrillation
Antifreeze	Metabolic acidosis, hypocalcemia, oxalate crystals in urine, renal failure, delirium, no odor	Iron	Diarrhea, coma, bloody vomiting, radiopacity on x-ray, hypotension
		Isopropyl alcohol	Severe gastritis, acetonemia with normoglycemia
Arsenic	Garlicky breath, vomiting, profuse diarrhea; symptoms may be delayed up to 12 h	Lead	Severe abdominal pain, increased blood pressure, milky vomitus, convulsions, muscle weakness, metallic taste, anorexia, encephalopathy
Atropine	Fever, flushing, dilated pupils, hallucination, dry skin, decreased secretions, mild tachycardia, disorientation		
		Lithium	Tremor, seizures, polyuria, delayed CNS toxicity
Belladonna	Fever, flushing, dilated pupils, hallucinations, dry skin, decreased secretions, mild tachycardia, disorientation	Mercury	Stomatitis, gingivitis, colitis, nephrotic syndrome, acute renal failure, metabolic acidosis
		Methyl alcohol	Occurrence in alcoholic patient, hyperventilation, decreased vision
Boric acid	Red skin, blue-green diarrhea, severe acidosis, convulsions, coma	Mushrooms	Nausea, vomiting, hallucinations (*muscaria* type), delayed liver failure and renal failure (*phalloides* type)
Bromide	Drowsiness, coma, ataxia, mimic alcoholic hallucinosis, increased pigmentation, dementia, ache, psychosis, hyperchloremia		
		Nitrites	Postural hypotension, flushing, methemoglobinemia (chocolate-colored blood, cyanosis)
Caffeine	Vomiting, extreme miosis, visual disturbances, hypertension, tachycardia, glycosuria, acetonuria, salivation, muscle twitching	Organophosphates	Miotic pupils, cramps, bronchorrhea, salivation, lacrimation, urination, diarrhea, bradycardia
Carbon monoxide	Headache, confusion, seizures, red skin, coal-gas odor, bullae, cyanois, retinal hemorrhages	Paraquat	Oropharynx burning, headache, vomiting, diarrhea, acute renal failure, pleural effusion
Clonidine	Miosis, hyper- or hypotensive, decreased pulse, no response to naloxone	Phenothiazines	Postural hypotension, hypothemia, miosis, tremor, dystonic disorder, radiopacity on x-ray of abdomen, increased QT interval on ECG
Cyanide	Bitter-almond odor on breath, convulsions, coma, abnormal ECG, lactic acidosis		
Digitalis	Visual disturbances, delirium, abnormal ECG, nausea, vomiting	Propoxyphene	Seizures, miosis, coma, pulmonary edema, erratic response to narcotic antagonist
Ethchlorvynol	Deep coma, pungent aromatic odor, lowered pulse and blood pressure, pink gastric aspirate		
		Salicylates	Hyperventilation, vomiting, fever, bleeding, acidosis, tinnitus
Fluoride	Decreased serum potassium and magnesium, tetany	Strychnine	Stiff neck, status epilepticus
		Scopolamine	Tachycardia, decreased secretions, urinary retention, dilated pupils, hallucinations, confusion, dry skin, fever
Gasoline	Distinctive odor, choking, pulmonary infiltrates, feeling of lightness, transitory visual hallucinations		
Glutethimide	Dilated pupils, coma, prolonged respiratory depression, laryngeal spasms	Tricyclic antidepressant	Ileus, supraventricular arrhythmia, convulsions, response to physostigmine, radiopacity on x-ray, coma, cardiac conduction disturbances

*For drugs of abuse, refer to Chap. 49.

TABLE 48-9 Commonly Observed Signs and Symptoms of Poisoning and Toxic Overdose

SIGN OR SYMPTOM	AGENT	SIGN OR SYMPTOM	AGENT
	Neurologic		*Pulse Rate*
Ataxia	Alcohol, barbiturates, bromide, carbon monoxide, phenytoin, hallucinogens, heavy metals, organic solvents, phenothiazines, tricyclic antidepressants	Slow	Narcotics, digitalis, sedative-hypnotics, β blockers, clonidine, organophosphates
Tremor	Theophylline, lithium, alcohol withdrawal	Rapid	Alcohol, amphetamines, atropine, salicylates
			Respiration
Convulsions and muscle twitching	Alcohol, amphetamines, antihistamines, chlorinated hydrocarbons and organophosphate insecticides, cyanide, isoniazid, lead, plants (e.g., hemlock), methaqualone, salicylates, strychnine, barbiturate withdrawal, phenothiazines, phencyclidine, theophylline	Rapid rate	Amphetamines, cocaine, methanol, carbon monoxide, petroleum distillates, salicylates, barbiturates (early)
		Slow rate	Alcohol, narcotics, barbiturates (late)
		Paralysis	Organophosphate insecticides, nicotine, botulism
Dystonia	Phenothiazines, PCP, haloperidol	Wheezing and pulmonary edema	Narcotics, petroleum distillates, organophosphates, respiratory irritants
Coma and drowsiness	Alcohol, atropine, scopolamine, antihistamines, barbiturates and other sedative-hypnotics (e.g., chloral hydrate), narcotics, salicylates, antipsychotics (e.g., phenothiazines), antidepressants, propoxyphene		*Mouth*
		Salivation	Mushrooms, organophosphates, mercury, arsenic, corrosives, strychnine
Confusion	Many agents include alcohol, anticholinergics, CNS stimulants, hallucinogens, antihistamines, isoniazid, levodopa, propranolol, digitalis, solvent abuse	Dry	Atropine, belladonna, amphetamines, narcotics, antihistamines, Jimson weed (stramonium)
		Gum discoloration	Lead, arsenic, mercury
	Eye		*Breath Odor*
		Alcohol	Ethanol
Pinpoint pupils (miosis)	Narcotics, organophosphates, propoxyphene, mushrooms (muscarinic type), barbiturates (occasionally), physostigmine, pilocarpine	Garlicky	Arsenic, phosphorus, organophosphate insecticides
		Bitter almonds	Cyanide
		Acetone	Isopropyl alcohol, methanol, phenol
Dilated pupils (mydriasis)	Amphetamines, antihistamines, atropine, barbiturates (coma), belladonna, cocaine, LSD, methanol, opiate withdrawal, tricyclic antidepressants, glutethimide; dilated, fixed pupils do not rule out possibility of opiates in a comatose patient and may be the result of anoxia or mixed overdose	Pungent	Ethchlorvynol
		Violets	Turpentine
		Wintergreen	Methyl salicylate
		Pearlike	Chloral hydrate
		Other	Ammonia, gasoline, kerosene, petroleum distillate
			Gastrointestinal
Nystagmus	Barbiturates, sedative-hypnotics (e.g., benzodiazepines, meprobamate), phenytoin, phencyclidine, alcohol	Emesis (often with hematemesis)	Caffeine, corrosives, boric acid, heavy metals, iron, salicylates, theophylline, phenol, isopropyl alcohol
Visual disturbance	Botulism, methanol, organophosphates, alcohol, atropine, belladonna	Abdominal colic	Arsenic, lead, heavy metals, organophosphate insecticides, mushrooms, narcotic withdrawal
Hallucinations	Alcohol, cocaine, LSD, PCP, MDA, mescaline	Diarrhea	Arsenic, iron, mushrooms, organophosphates, boric acid, food poisoning
		Constipation	Narcotics, lead, anticholinergics

TABLE 48-9 Commonly Observed Signs and Symptoms of Poisoning and Toxic Overdose (*Cont.*)

SIGN OR SYMPTOM	AGENT	SIGN OR SYMPTOM	AGENT
	Metabolic		*Skin Color*
Acidosis	Salicylates, methanol, ethylene glycol, oxalic acid, isoniazid, carbon monoxide, cyanide	Jaundice	Acetaminophen (delayed), arsenic, carbon tetrachloride, mushroom (delayed)
Hypoglycemia	Ethanol, insulin, hypoglycemics, isopropyl alcohol	Cyanosis	Cyanide, amyl nitrite, nitrites, strychnine, carbon monoxide, asphyxiant gases, hypoxemia
	Skin	Red and flushed	Alcohol, antihistamines, atropine, carbon monoxide, boric acid
Purpura	Salicylates, snake and spider bites		
Sweating	Amphetamines, atropine, alcohol, LSD, cocaine, barbiturates, mushrooms, organophosphate insecticides, salicylates		*Other*
		Hypothermia	Sedatives, alcohol, phenothiazines, opiates, hypoglycemia, exposure
Needle marks	Narcotics, amphetamines, phencyclidine, "street drugs"	Hyperthermia	Salicylates, amphetamine, anticholinergics, tricyclic antidepressants, CNS stimulants, cocaine, intractable convulsions
Bullae	Barbiturates, carbon monoxide		
		Hyperpnea	Metabolic acidosis, salicylates, CNS stimulants

in these areas. The adverse effects of unconventional treatment administered by misinformed accomplices in resuscitation attempts should also be suspect when dealing with emergencies that substance abusers experience.

Temporal Factors

Common signs and symptoms associated with a poison may not occur concurrently, and, in some cases, the level of intoxication dictates whether signs and symptoms will apppear at all. Unlike the onset of a therapeutic response to a drug, the time of onset of symptoms following poisoning or overdose is difficult to predict. Some symptoms, such as hepatotoxicity, have a delayed onset following ingestion or exposure to certain toxic materials or drugs. Delay in absorption can be caused by drugs that delay stomach emptying time and produce symptoms of toxicity much later than the usual anticipated time of onset. In contrast, products in solution are more rapidly absorbed than solid formulations, and so toxic symptoms may occur earlier. The onset of symptoms for contact irritants and inhaled vapors may be variable, but generally such symptoms are evident within 2 to 4 h following exposure. An abdominal x-ray examination may supply useful clues to the identity of the material ingested, since some agents (such as phenothiazines, tricyclic antidepressants; heavy metals such as iron, lead and arsenic; halides such as chloride and iodine, chloral hydrate, and enteric coated tablets) are radiopaque.

Assessment Parameters

The first consideration in the care of the poisoned or overdosed patient is to ensure support of vital functions. Then, the degree of impairment of neurologic, cardiovascular, cardiac, and pulmonary functions must be thoroughly assessed to determine the cause and severity of the toxic reaction. Arterial blood gases should be monitored closely, particularly if the patient is comatose or unresponsive, to detect hypoxia from respiratory depression and unsuspected acid-base derangements. Examination of the mouth, breath, skin, pupils, and vital signs may yield important clues as to the probable causative agent. The head should be examined for possible bleeding or other signs of trauma. Unusual neurologic signs suggesting subdural injury or intracranial lesions should be noted, as well as swelling, rigidity, etc. A search for causes of coma or seizures, excluding drugs or toxins, should be made. Shock, sepsis, hypothermia, hyperthermia, hyperglycemia, or hypoglycemia, and other metabolic derangements should be ruled out. A chest x-ray may show pulmonary edema. The electrocardiogram may show irregular cardiac rhythms and rates or conduction defects. Urinalysis may reveal crystals or myoglobinuria.

Toxicologic Analysis

Toxicologic information aids in confirming a presumptive diagnosis and gives some further guidance in formulating a treatment plan. In most cases, toxicologic analysis plays a small but important role in the diagnosis and determination of inherent toxicity or lethality of poisoning from certain drugs and toxic substances. Qualitative results from screening procedures for the commonly overdosed drugs (**aspirin, barbiturates, phenothiazines,** and **opiates**) are reliable and readily available and are particularly useful when the poisoned patient is unconscious or when a history is unattainable. If a sample of the suspected drug is not available, appropriate specimens of blood or urine should be obtained from the patient for toxicologic examination. Residual material from the stomach is the ideal source of toxicologic examination if the drug was ingested. Much lower concentrations are found in the blood or urine, because of incomplete absorption and high tissue affinity. Whether or not a toxic dose or a toxic drug product is detected, treatment must be carefully tailored to fit the symptoms of poisoning or overdose.

MANAGEMENT OF POISONING

The basic treatment for acute poisoning is to provide supportive treatment (maintenance of airway, provision for fluid and electrolyte balance) and symptomatic care. The airway must be kept unobstructed and cleared of secretion or aspirated material. Overzealous use of nonspecific and questionably effective modes of treatment often will produce more harm than the poison itself. Removal of still-unabsorbed material from the stomach as a means of minimizing further absorption is useful after acute ingestion of drugs or other materials, contraindications notwithstanding. For some poisons, specific antidotes are available. Promotion of elimination of the absorbed drugs may be effective in some poisonings.

Minimizing Absorption of the Poison

The initial treatment of the patient who has ingested a toxic substance is to remove the material from the stomach as quickly as possible. The two methods used are *emesis* and *gastric lavage*. Neither method has been universally accepted as superior, although emesis is generally preferred. However, vomiting may be hazardous if the airway is not protected or if corrosive materials (lye, mineral acids, or other caustic substances) have been ingested. Contraindications to the induction of emesis also include pronounced central nervous system depression, coma, loss of gag reflex, ingestion of convulsants, and any instance where activated charcoal has already been given.

Emesis

To be effective, evacuation of the stomach should be initiated soon after the ingestion. Most authorities recommend that the stomach be emptied if the patient is seen within 4 h of the ingestion. Nevertheless, on occasion, emesis has proved useful even after delays of 9 to 10 h. Emptying the stomach in **aspirin** overdose or in patients who have ileus (following atropine-like drug ingestions) have been shown to be beneficial even though as much as 6 to 8 h have elapsed since the ingestion took place. The patient should be carefully supervised when an emetic is being administered (see Table 48-10) to ensure an open airway and to protect against aspiration. Spontaneous emesis should not be assumed to be sufficient to preclude induction of emesis where ingestion of drugs and toxins has occurred. Introduction of a finger, spoon, or other objects into the throat to induce emesis should never be advised.

Lavage

If emesis cannot be induced or is contraindicated, lavage should be started to dilute and remove unabsorbed materials (particularly when phenothiazines, antihistamines, or tricyclic antidepressants are involved). Following ingestion of strong corrosives such as a mineral acids or alkali, the gastrointestinal tract may easily be perforated by the lavage tube; therefore lavage is contraindicated. Lavage should also not be used following ingestion of **strychnine**. The use of lavage following ingestion of petroleum distillates (kerosene, lighter fluid) is controversial, since there is a risk of aspiration and pneumonitis. However, if an inflatable cuff and endotracheal tube are properly placed to protect the airway, gastric lavage can be safely performed when large amounts of petroleum products have been ingested.

Proper lavage technique and selection of correct lavage solution is essential. The patient should be positioned on the left side with head down to minimize the risk of aspiration. Lavage should continue, with fluids given in small (20 to 30 mL) amounts, until no solid material returns. The total amount of lavage fluid given should not be less than 2 L for a child and 2 to 5 L for an adult. Avoid distending the stomach. At completion of lavage, activated charcoal (usually 30 g) can be instilled and allowed to remain in the stomach. Gastric samples should be saved for laboratory toxicology.

Absorbents

Activated charcoal can rapidly inactivate many poisons if given before much of the poison has been absorbed. It is effective for virtually all chemicals and drugs, especially **aspirin, tricyclic antidepressants, barbiturates, phenothiazines,** and **propoxyphene,** except **cyanide, lithium, ferrous sulfate,** mineral acids, and caustic alkali. Burnt toast or the "universal antidote" should not be given, since neither is efficacious. Activated charcoal is usually given orally or by nasogastric tube as 6 to 8 heaping tablespoons in 8 oz of water or 4 to 6 oz of 70% sorbitol. Given after emesis has been successfully induced by **syrup of ipecac,** activated charcoal may be indicated. There are no known contraindications or adverse effects from activated charcoal. Repeated administration every 2 to 4 h of the activated charcoal dose as long as bowel sounds are heard is particularly helpful for absorbing ingested materials which undergo appreciable enterohepatic recirculation or reabsorption (i.e., **barbiturates, phenytoin, phenycyclidine,** etc.) or sustained-release dosage forms.

TABLE 48-10 Commonly Used Emetics

EMETIC	COMMENTS
Syrup of ipecac	Emetic of choice, often effective. Onset of vomiting is delayed (10 to 30 min) after oral administration. Doses in children, 10–20 mL; adults 30 mL. Dose can be repeated once in 15–30 min if no response. Give with sufficient volume of fluids (1–2 glasses of water). No more than two doses should be given. Children under the age of 1 should receive ipecac under the direct supervision of a physician or qualified health professional, and emesis should not be induced at home. Systemic toxicity is rare, although drowsiness, diarrhea, dizziness, faintness, hypotension, and minor ECG changes have been reported. Ipecac is effective in inducing emesis following so-called "antiemetic" drug ingestion of phenothiazines, tricyclic antidepressants, antihistamines, anticholinergics, or combinations of these drugs. Nearly 95 percent respond with emesis following a single and repeated dose.
Apomorphine	Very effective given intramuscularly or subcutaneously. It is a *narcotic* and its respiration-depressing and emetic effects can be reversed by a narcotic antagonist (e.g., naloxone). Onset of action is immediate. *Not* to be used in comatose patients or patients with central nervous system depression. Solution must be freshly prepared and should not be used if it is discolored. Recommended subcutaneous (SC) dose for adults, 5–6 mg; for children, 0.07 mg/kg. Doses should *not* be repeated. Dose of naloxone to reverse narcotic effects is 0.01 mg/kg IV, IM, or SC. Use apomorphine with *extreme caution.*
Mustard water	Not effective.
Salt water	Not effective. Can be dangerous, since it has caused severe electrolyte abnormalities (hypernatremia). Should not be used.
Copper sulfate, zinc sulfate	Sometimes effective. Should not be used because of their toxicity, which can cause hemolysis and hepatic damage.

Cathartics

Cathartics may be useful in removing material by speeding up the transit time of gastrointestinal contents, although there is little evidence to prove their efficacy. Most frequently used are saline cathartics (e.g., **sodium sulfate** or **magnesium sulfate**), although **milk of magnesia** (magnesium hydroxide) may also be used. Magnesium salts should not be used if the ingested poison is nephrotoxic or if the patient has severe electrolyte disturbance or renal failure. Cathartics may cause further injury to the intestine if given following ingestion of corrosives. In young children, avoid unintended dehydration from excessive or repeated administration of cathartics. The usual adult dose is 30 mL of a 10% **magnesium sulfate** solution (Epsom salt) given orally. **Mineral oil** or stimulant cathartics, such as **castor oil**, should *not* be used.

Fluids

Fluids given orally are useful since they can dilute or neutralize ingested poisons, especially those which can produce local irritability or corrosiveness. Water is, in most cases, satisfactory. Oral fluids can be given if the patient is alert, with a gag reflex present. Petroleum distillates are best diluted with milk and water. Milk should not be used after ingestion of paradichlorobenzene (mothballs), since it may increase absorption. Corrosives and caustic materials should be neutralized with milk and water. When acids are ingested, carbonates and bicarbonates must be avoided, since they will react to liberate carbon dioxide and cause distention. For drug ingestions, diluents (fluids to dilute the poison) should *not* be given, since absorption may be enhanced as a result of tablet or dissolution or increased transit of stomach contents into the lower gastrointesinal tract.

Decontamination

Certain chemicals, in particular the organophosphate insecticides, can be absorbed through the skin and mucous membranes. Contaminated clothing must be removed and the underlying area thoroughly washed with copious amounts of water and soap.

For inhalation, skin, and ocular exposures, removal of the patient from the toxic environment followed with thorough decontamination and first-aid treatment is necessary. Eyes should be flushed with copious amounts of water for 15 to 20 min. Neutralizers are not used. The tears should be checked with pH paper following irrigation if either an acid or caustic was involved. A careful ophthalmologic examination of the eye is indicated afterwards.

Specific Antidotes

There are relatively few specific antidotes of significant clinical utility, considering the vast array of drugs and toxic substances involved in poisonings and toxic overdoses; however, organophosphate insecticides, methanol, cyanide, and the opiates do have specific antidotes, and these substances must be identified immediately so that the appropriate antidote can be given (Table 48-11). The antidote must be given *promptly* if it is to be effective. Other poisons with specific antidotes are rarely involved in overdoses. It should be reemphasized that *overzealous or inappropriate use of an antidote may complicate the initial injury,* causing another form of poisoning. Sensible selection and careful use of drugs and therapeutic measures for support and symptomatic relief are likely to be more beneficial than an antidote in the majority of poisoning cases.

Removal of Drugs and Poisons by Other Methods

Diuresis

When significant amounts of an ingested drug or poison have been absorbed, forced diuresis may be helpful in promoting elimination of the substance if it is excreted in the urine. Excretion may be enhanced by giving fluids or osmotic diuretics such as mannitol. **Mannitol** is administered intravenously in a dose of 1.5 g/kg in 20% solution up to a maximum dose of 100 g/day. Adequate hydration is necessary with mannitol therapy, and careful records must be made of intake and output levels to avoid drastic changes in fluid and electrolyte balance. Forced diuresis should not be used in the presence of renal insufficiency, pulmonary edema, heart failure, or shock.

Alkalinization

The concomitant use of osmotic diuresis and alkalinization of the urine is quite effective for enhancing renal elimination of some drugs such as barbiturates and salicylates (weak acids). Alkalinization can be achieved with an infusion of 1 to 2 meq/kg of **sodium bicarbonate** or **sodium lactate. Acetazolamide** (Diamox) should *not* be used since, in addition to alkalinizing the urine, it produces metabolic acidosis. The rate of bicarbonate administration is determined by urinary and arterial blood pH. Potassium depletion from alkalinization should be carefully monitored, using serum potassium levels and electrocardiography.

Acidification

Acidification of the urine along with osmotic diuresis can increase the elimination of some drugs such as amphetamines (weak bases). **Ammonium chloride,** at a dose of 75 mg/kg/day in four divided doses (children) or 1 or 2 g q10h (adults) given orally or intravenously as a 2% solution, is used to produce this acidification; the goal is to produce a urine pH of 5 or less. However, this should be used with care since it may further aggravate underlying metabolic acidosis from the overdose. Other adverse effects from acidification attempts include hypokalemia and hyponatremia. Patients who experience muscular hyperactivity, rigidity, or seizures

should not have their urines acidified for purposes of promoting drug elimination (e.g., PCP) since myoglobin deposition would enhance the possibility of myoglobinuric renal failure.

Hemodialysis or Peritoneal Dialysis

The general indications for dialysis include the presence of a dialyzable drug or poison in potentially lethal concentrations; the presence of a drug or poison which can be converted to a more toxic metabolite (ethylene glycol, methanol); situations in which supportive measures are inadequate to prevent serious complications from the overdose; and liver failure, renal failure, or acute tubular damage and shock. Poisons or drugs that are bound to tissues or plasma proteins are not removed sufficiently by dialysis. Many drugs and toxins on lists of dialyzable agents are, in fact, not dialyzable, e.g., **etchlorvynol, glutethimide,** and mushroom poisons. Dialysis is useful for removing **salicylates, methanol, chloral hydrate, ethylene glycol,** and **bromides.** Lipid dialysis and column Amberlite hemoperfusion, recently introduced, have been shown to increase clearance of certain drugs (**barbiturates** and **glutethimide**) from the blood.

Peritoneal dialysis is less effective than hemodialysis for removing drugs or poisons but is much simpler to perform and more readily available. Following dialysis or perfusion, drug concentrations in the blood may often "rebound" as redistribution between the peripheral to body compartments takes place; the result often seen will be a patient who unexplainably relapses into a toxic state seen prior to treatment.

General Care of the Poisoned or Overdosed Patient

The general care of the poisoned or overdosed patient does not differ greatly from the care of any critically ill comatose patient. Supportive care should be the major focus of attention. Fluid and electrolyte balance, care of the urinary and intravenous catheter sites, and preventive skin care must be maintained. Administration of adequate fluids is important to correct deficits, maintain balance, or replace losses during treatment. Respiratory care must be particularly vigorous, as pulmonary complications are a leading cause of death in hospitalized overdosed patients. Atelectasis, pulmonary edema, arrhythmias, deep vein thrombosis, pneumonias, and urinary tract infections are common complications that develop in these patients during the hospital course. Convulsions are another problem encountered. Hypoxia, hypoglycemia, or metabolic abnormalities may be the underlying cause, and treatment must be directed at these disturbances. Central nervous system (CNS) stimulants should *never* be given to depressed or comatose patients, because their effects are unpredictable, and they can produce excitation and convulsion.

Anticonvulsant treatment with CNS depressants carries the inherent risk of increasing the depression already pres-

TABLE 48-11 Specific Antidotes

ANTIDOTE	POISON	COMMENTS
Naloxone (Narcan)	Narcotic drugs, propoxyphene, pentazocine, diphenoxylate methadone	A specific antagonist of narcotics. *Adults:* 2.0 mg (5 mL) IV, IM, SC, may be repeated every 2–3 min for two or three doses. Larger doses may be needed to reverse effects of overdose with methadone and propoxyphene. Since duration of antagonism may be shorter than narcotic's effect, repeated doses may be needed.
Atropine sulfate	Anticholinesterases, organophosphates, physostigmine, carbamates	Test dose 2 mg (for children, 0.05 mg/kg) IV or IM until symptoms of atropinism, repeated q10–15min, with cessation of secretions the desired therapeutic endpoint.
Pralidoxime (2-PAM)	Anticholinesterases, organophosphates, physostigmine	Used for organophosphate poisoning *after* atropine. *Adults:* 1 g IV slowly, which may be repeated q8–12h as needed. *Pediatric:* 250 mg.
Ethanol	Methanol, ethylene glycol (antifreeze)	Antidote for methanol poisoning. Ethanol (10% IV–50% PO) is infused 1 mL/kg initially and repeated q2–3h to maintain ethanol blood level of 100 mg/100 mL. Dose may have to be increased or given by continuous infusion. Methanol metabolism to its toxic products is blocked and is eliminated unchanged. Constant monitoring of blood alcohol required. Glucose must be included in ethanol infusion. Monitor serum glucose levels also. Can maintain treatment for 2–3 days in methanol and 3–5 days for ethylene glycol poisoning.
Sodium nitrite, sodium thiosulfate, amyl nitrite	Cyanide	Antidote for a rapid and lethal poison. Nitrites cause methemoglobin, which has greater affinity for cyanide than oxyhemoglobin. *Adults:* sodium nitrite 3% (10 mg/kg) IV over 5 min. Sodium thiosulfate 25% (50 mL) IV over 10 min. Reduced doses for children. Amyl nitrite is inhaled for 15–30 s (there is a commercially available cyanide kit made by Eli Lilly).
Physostigmine salicylate	Anticholinergic and atropine agents, tricyclic antidepressants	Used to reverse seizures and cardiac toxicity (supraventricular tachycardia) from atropine, anticholinergic drugs, and tricyclic antidepressants. *Adults:* 1 mg IV slowly (usually 0.5 mg given first); then wait for changes in symptoms (decreased heart rate, decreased convulsions, improved mental status). *Maximum initial doses:* 4 mg (adults); 2 mg (children). Effects are transient (30–60 min), lowest effective dose may be repeated when symptoms return. Conduction abnormalities from excess tricyclic antidepressant or anticholinergic activity, preexisting heart disorder, may be aggravated by physostigmine. Phenothiazines in "mixed" overdose with tricyclics may produce complex cardiac problems that physostigmine may worsen. Reverse physostigmine effects (i.e., sinus bradycardia, cardiac standstill, cholinergic excess) with atropine. Give 0.5 mg of atropine for every 1 mg of physostigmine.

TABLE 48-11   Specific Antidotes (*Cont.*)

ANTIDOTE	POISON	COMMENTS
Deferoxamine (Desferal Mesylate)	Iron salts	If poisoning is severe, 15 mg/kg/h in IV *after* blood has been drawn for serum iron and iron-binding determinations. Urine will usually become characteristically red in color. Lavage solution of 1–5% of bicarbonate solution to chelate iron in stomach can be given. Deferoxamine may be discontinued at 24 h or sooner, depending on what the serum iron levels are and on when urine color returns to normal.
Dimercaprol (BAL)	Arsenic, lead	Antidote for arsenic forms complex that competes for arsenic with enzyme systems. 3–5 mg/kg q4h IM for first 2 days, then 2.5–3 mg/kg q6h IM for 2 days, then q12h for 1 week. When urine arsenic level falls below 50 mg/24 h, antidote may be stopped. Monitor blood pressure. Adverse effects of BAL can include fever, flushing, myalgia, hypotension or hypertension, pulmonary edema.
Diphenhydramine (Benadyl)	Phenothiazines, haloperidol	For dystonic-extrapyramidal reactions; give 25–50 mg IV.
Penicillamine	Copper, lead, mercury	Dose: 100 mg/kg/day up to 1 g/day in divided oral doses up to 5 days. Avoid in patients with penicillin allergy. Monitor for proteinuria.
Calcium disodium edetate (CaEDTA)	Lead	Antidote (along with BAL) for lead intoxication. Given 50–75 mg/kg/day IM or IV in 3–6 divided doses up to 5 days in cases of encephalopathy or blood levels of 100 mg/100 mL or more. Lower doses can be given where no encephalopathy and lower blood lead levels. Stop when urine returns to nontoxic levels. Push fluids to maintain output. Complicatons: mostly renal tubular necrosis, and so fluids must be maintained in adequate quantities.
Methylene blue	Nitrites	Antidote for methemoglobinemia from nitrites, nitrates. Give 0.1–0.2 mL of 1% (1 mg/kg) slowly. Do not give if patient has G6PD deficiency.

ent in the overdosed patient. Intravenous **diazepam** or **phenytoin** must be given with caution during episodes of seizure. In tricyclic antidepressant or anticholinergic drug overdoses, **physostigmine** may be carefully given intravenously before conventional anticonvulsants such as **diazepam** or **phenytoin** are used. Use of vasopressors (**dopamine, levarterenol, metaraminol,** or **isoproterenol**) may be initiated cautiously after considering the need for them; hypotension may be adequately managed with fluids alone. Vasopressors may reverse severe shock, but urinary output must be closely monitored since it may be diminished even further by them.

Table 48-12 summarizes the major consideration in caring for patients who are poisoned or overdosed with various agents.

POISONOUS PLANTS

Among the more frequent causes of accidental ingestion involving young children are plants, particularly of the indoor varieties commonly found in the home. Adults are occasionally poisoned when they consume plants which contain toxic substances under the mistaken impression that they are edible. Exposure to toxic plants may produce symptoms ranging from dermatitis and local mucous membrane irritation to gastrointestinal upset, systemic symptoms, and even death on very rare occasions (Table 48-13). It is estimated that perhaps 10 percent of victims of plant ingestions develop symptoms; fewer than 0.5 percent experience symptoms serious enough to require hospitalization. In cases of

TABLE 48-12 Major Treatment Considerations in Poisoned or Overdosed Patients

AGENT	COMMENTS	TREATMENT CONSIDERATIONS
Sedative-hypnotics (Valium, Librium, Tranxene, Serax, Ativan, Xanax, Dalmane, phenobarbital, Nembutal, Seconal, Noctec, Doriden, Noludor, Placidyl, Quaalude, and various others)	Central nervous system depression, coma, hypotension, hypoxia, and respiratory and cardiac failure are seen. Withdrawal with hyperirritability and serious, life-threatening seizures can occur 16–24 h following discontinuance. Simultaneous ingestion with other depressants (alcohol) is common. In severe acute sedative-hypnotic overdose, prolonged absence (24 h) of brain activity and function may be reversible with favorable outcome. Nonbarbiturate sedative-hypnotics (chloral hydrate, glutethimide, meprobamate, methylprylon, ethchlorvynol) produce a clinical picture similar to barbiturates (secobarbital, pentobarbital, amobarbital, phenobarbital). They may be much more toxic than barbiturates, and duration of coma much longer. Benzodiazepines (diazepam, chlordiazepoxide, flurazepam) are often involved in overdoses. While inherent lethality is low when they are taken alone, combination with alcohol and other sedative-hypnotics greatly increases risk.	Treatment is supportive. Forced diuresis and alkalinization of urine to remove drug may be beneficial in long-acting barbiturate overdose. In view of the number of overdoses involving barbiturates, there is a remarkably high recovery rate. Respiratory assistance, rehydration, management of hypotension, and maintenance of adequate urine output are important treatment considerations. Do *not* use respiratory stimulants in an attempt to arouse overdosed patients from coma. The effects from these drugs are unpredictable and can produce seizures. The effectiveness of forced diuresis and dialysis is insignificant for most nonbarbiturate hypnotics because of their protein binding and affinity for lipids. The use of resin hemoperfusion systems may prove effective for severe barbiturate overdoses with prolonged coma as more experience with this method is gained. If physical dependence on sedative-hypnotics is established, treatment for withdrawal should be closely supervised and carried out in a hospital setting.
Ethanol	Severe hypoglycemia may occur in children following ingestion of large quantities. Mouthwashes, OTC prescription cough and cold preparations, perfumes, and colognes are common sources of ethanol ingestion in children. Varying degrees of intoxicated behavior are seen. Ethanol should always be suspected as a contributory cause in acute overdoses when the patient appears to have ingested agents with CNS depressant effects.	Treatment is supportive and symptomatic. Convulsions associated with hypoglycemia are seen and can be treated with glucose and diazepam.
Aspirin	In acute overdose, peak salicylate levels may not occur until 6–10 h after ingestion. Severity of overdose estimated on basis of blood salicylate level and interval between ingestion and measurement. Metabolic acidosis, which will enhance salicylate distribution to the brain, should be avoided. Hyperventilation, tinnitus, fever, acidosis, hypoglycemia are symptoms often seen in mild to moderately severe overdose. Serum salicylate levels, electrolytes, blood gases and pH, renal and cardiac function must be monitored.	Removal of aspirin by emesis or lavage has been successful even 10 h after ingestion. Activated charcoal can be a useful adjunct to treatment. Alkalinization of urine promotes elimination of salicylates. Administration of potassium and fluids can facilitate attempts at alkalinization of urine.

TABLE 48-12 Major Treatment Considerations in Poisoned or Overdosed Patients (*Cont.*)

AGENT	COMMENTS	TREATMENT CONSIDERATIONS
Acetaminophen (Tylenol, Datril, and various others)	Commonly available and widely promoted over the counter; seen increasingly and frequently in overdoses. Can be a serious liver toxin in acute overdose.	Treatment of choice is prevention of further absorption of drug. Supportive care required and close monitoring for 3–5 days with particular attention to liver function and symptoms of jaundice and to impending ecephalopathy. *N*-Acetylcysteine is now being used investigationally in its treatment (see Chap. 17).
Narcotics [propoxyphene (Darvon), pentazocine (Talwin), diphenoxylate (Lomotil), codeine, and various others]	Opiate overdose patients classically present with pinpoint pupils (unless anoxia has caused dilation), areflexia, respiratory depression, and cyanotic, clammy pallor. Immediate cardiopulmonary resuscitation provided if needed, with protection of airway, vital functions. Opiate-dependent user may experience severe abstinence syndrome during recovery from acute overdose, or this may be precipitated by use of narcotic antagonist.	Comatose patient with small pupils, bradycardia, depressed respiratory function, and hypotension should be given narcotic antagonist. Naloxone is drug of choice and will reverse symptoms if overdose involves opiate. Commonly used narcotics such as heroin have relatively short half-lives, while methadone and propoxyphene have much longer half-lives; hence repeated administration of antagonist over 24–36 h may be required. Supportive treatment is important and consists mainly of assisting ventilation and oxygenation, supporting blood pressure, maintaining circulation and airway.
Tricyclic antidepressants (Elavil, Endep, Aventyl, Vivactil, Tofranil, Norpramin, Pertofrane, Sinequan, and various others)	Cardiovascular effects are complex and often serious. Supraventricular tachycardias, premature ventricular contractions, ventricular tachycardia, and quinidine-like myocardial toxicity (e.g., bradycardia, heart block) are seen. Other serious symptoms include ileus, hypothermia, convulsions.	Basic approach to treatment is supportive and symptomatic. Forced diuresis and dialysis not effective in removing drug because of protein binding and large tissue distribution. ECG monitoring and vital signs for at least 48–72 h. Physostigmine may reverse CNS and cardiac toxicity but should only be used when coma, convulsions, or supraventricular tachycardias occur. Emesis or lavage followed by activated charcoal should be used as early as possible unless contraindicated. Convulsions intractable to physostigmine can be controlled with diazepam IV. Quinidine and procainamide are contraindicated since they may worsen conduction defects. In severe overdose with tachyarrhythmia and heart block, cardiac pacing may be reasonable approach before physostigmine or other antiarrhythmics are used (e.g., lidocaine, phenytoin). Monitor arterial pH to keep greater than 7.45. Newer compounds (Asendin, Ludiomil) with antidepressant activity comparable to tricyclics in an overdose appear to produce more central stimulation activity, seizures, than cardiovascular and cardiac effects.

TABLE 48-12 Major Treatment Considerations in Poisoned or Overdosed Patients (*Cont.*)

AGENT	COMMENTS	TREATMENT CONSIDERATIONS
Phenothiazines (Thorazine, Mellaril, Stelazine, Trilafon), thioxanthenes (Navane), butyrophenone (Haldol), dibenzoxazepines (Loxitane)	Number of cases increasing among children and adults. Four common clinical syndromes: hypotension, arrhythmias, dystonic reactions, and atropism. Other effects include quinidine-like effects on ECG, dry mouth, hypothermia, ileus, and seizures. Although dilated pupils are commonly found, constricted pupils may be seen in more severely poisoned patients. Phenothiazines are radiopaque.	Dystonic reactions seen occasionally; diphenhydramine 50 mg IV is given. Repeated (2–3) doses may be needed since phenothiazine is longer-acting than diphenhydramine. Hypotension often can be treated by expanding circulatory volume or placing patient in Trendelenburg position. Cardiac depressant effect can be reversed with phenytoin or, in more severe circumstances, with cardiac pacemaker.
Organophosphate insecticides (Parathion, Malathion, Diazinon, Methyl Parathion)	Poisoning can occur from ingestion and absorption through the skin. Five important physical signs are characteristic: salivation, lacrimation, urination, defecation, and constriction of pupils. Response to large amounts of atropine confirms diagnosis.	2-Pralidoxime (2-PAM) should be used in organophosphate poisoning unresponsive to atropinization. Blood should be drawn for estimation of cholinesterase in red cells before 2-PAM is given. Thorough decontamination must be carried out.
Hydrocarbons, petroleum distillates	Vomiting and diarrhea often experienced. CNS depression can occur. Aspiration pneumonitis a serious complication. Chemical pneumonitis has occurred even after intravenous injection of hydrocarbon material (lighter fluid). Inhalation may cause euphoria, headache, nausea. Chronic inhalation may result in hepatic and renal damage.	Emesis before CNS depression occurs, followed by cathartics, may provide some protection against absorption and major toxicities (hepatic, etc.). Avoid emesis of product with low viscosity. Lavage is reserved for patient with absent gag reflex, coma, or convulsion and *must* be preceded by intubation with cuffed endotracheal tube. Corticosteroid use in these circumstances is controversial. Treatment is supportive and symptomatic.
Corrosives	Concentrated solutions of caustic material can cause burns of esophagus that characteristically progress from inflammatory phase to necrosis and constriction. *Sources:* liquid and crystalline corrosives, Clinitest tablets, certain household bleaches, dentifrices, electric-dishwasher soaps.	Immediate treatment is dilution with copious amounts of water. Emesis and lavage should be avoided. Olive oil, vinegar, juices should *not* be given. Patient should be evaluated by esophagoscopy and possible surgical follow-up.
Methanol	Ingestion (usually as substitute for ethanol) is highly toxic. May be 6–30 h symptom-free period, followed by abdominal pain and muscle weakness. Hyperventilation and profound metabolic acidosis are seen. Toxic products may produce blindness. Other clinical effects include anorexia, acidosis, nausea, vomiting, dizziness, headache, muscle weakness, and malaise.	Blood methanol level should be determined. Methanol level greater than 50 mg / 100 mL is an indication for hemodialysis.

TABLE 48-12   Major Treatment Considerations in Poisoned or Overdosed Patients (*Cont.*)

AGENT	COMMENTS	TREATMENT CONSIDERATIONS
Ethylene glycol (antifreeze)	Ingestion usually due to use as substitute for ethanol. Metabolism by alcohol dehydrogenase to oxalic acid produces renal damage with significant renal tubular necrosis and failure; ethanol can inhibit this reaction. Urine should be examined for oxylate crystals.	Renal status should be evaluated and hemodialysis begun in severe poisoning (marked acidosis, electrolyte abnormalities, renal failure).
Household products	Cleaning agents, bleaches, solvents, and cosmetics constitute the largest group of toxins available in the home. Many products relatively nontoxic, at least in amounts usually ingested. See Table 48-14.	All soaps and detergents can cause gastrointestinal irritation. Other toxic manifestations range from none (bar soaps) to severe mucous membrane damage, hypocalcemia, (electric-dishwasher detergents), shock. Treatment of severe intoxication should include immediate dilution and supportive care. Many liquid general-purpose cleaners and polishes contain petroleum distillates, and ingestion should be treated as hydrocarbon ingestion. Ammonia intoxication can be caused by exposure to its vapors, which can be decontaminated, or by ingestion, which should be treated as corrosive ingestion. Most bleaches are generally only moderately toxic and will not cause esophageal burns or strictures. Sodium perborate is highly toxic and management requires removal, support of vital functions, and control of seizures if they occur. Common household solvents, such as acetone, have effects similar to ethanol when ingested except for more CNS depression. Treatment is supportive care, decontamination, and minimization of further absorption.
Mushrooms	Number of cases of mushroom poisoning rising as a result of increasing popularity of wild mushroom consumption. Most nonlethal poisonous mushrooms produce symptoms (e.g., GI disturbance, cholinergic activity, hallucinations) soon after ingestion and recovery occurs within 24 h, whereas those known to cause life-threatening reactions produce symptoms 6–24 h after ingestion. Symptoms of more toxic species occur characteristically in three stages: GI effects during first 6–24 h; a 24- to 48-h period of symptom remission; finally, 3 to 4 days after ingestion, hepatocellular damage and renal impairment.	Treatment primarily supportive. Induction of emesis beneficial if done soon after ingestion. Numerous forms of therapy have been used, but none have been shown to be more effective than supportive care.

TABLE 48-13 Some Common Poisonous Plants

COMMON NAME	TOXIC PARTS	SIGNS AND SYMPTOMS
Castor bean	All parts	Nausea, vomiting, burning in mouth and throat.
Precatory bean	Seeds	Nausea, vomiting, burning in mouth and throat.
Jequirity bean	Seeds	Nausea, vomiting, burning in mouth and throat.
Dieffenbachia	Stem and leaf	Burning of mouth, tongue, lips; may affect breathing. Sap in eye causes inflammation.
Philodendron	Stem and leaf	Burning of mouth, tongue, lips; may affect breathing. Sap in eye causes inflammation.
Oleander	All parts; sap, leaves, and seeds	Nausea, vomiting, blurred vision, headache, irregular pulse, arrhythmias.
Foxglove	All parts, especially leaves and seeds	Nausea, vomiting, blurred vision, headache, irregular pulse, arrhythmias.
Jimson weed	All parts	Intense thirst, urinary retention, dry mouth, rapid and weak pulse, hyperpyrexia, delirium, seizure.
Lantana	Berries (unripe)	Muscle weakness, lethargy, cyanosis, circulatory collapse.
Daffodil	Bulbs	Gastrointestinal upset, vomiting, diarrhea.
Narcissus	Bulbs	Gastrointestinal upset, vomiting, diarrhea.

plant ingestions, the history is seldom precise or helpful. The report is often vague: "red berries from a bush." The common name given to a plant is often a misnomer; the botanical name is unknown or unobtainable in most instances.

POISON CONTROL CENTERS AND INFORMATION ASSISTANCE

Poison control centers are available in many communities on a 24-hour-a-day basis to give poison information and treatment referral assistance to consumers and health professionals. A center should be staffed with specialists who have available comprehensive resources and up-to-date information on the toxicity of prescription and nonprescription drugs, substances of abuse, household products, plants, chemicals, and other hazardous materials which are most often involved in poisonings. In cases of poisoning, the nurse can assist the poison center by being prepared to give the following details:

Identity, if known, of the suspected poison

Approximate quantity taken, injected, inhaled, or exposed to

The time the poisoning occurred

Signs, symptoms, or complaints that the victim may be showing or showed at the time of initial evaluation

Treatment that has already been given

With this information, the poison center specialists should be able to assess the severity, risk, and probable outcome of an incident; the center will also be better able to recommend the next step. A list of poison control centers and their telephone numbers is shown inside the rear cover of this textbook.

EVALUATION AND FOLLOW-UP OF POISONING

Frequently, the first contact with a poisoned patient or with a problem involving poison takes place over the telephone, whether it is a minor ingestion or serious emergency. The nurse, in a physician's office, clinic, or emergency department, is very often the medical professional that must obtain basic information from the caller. The initial evaluation should ascertain the product name or substance, ingredients, amount ingested, and current symptoms. Caution must be taken here since nearly one-half of the time, histories at this point are incorrect either as to the agent, amount, or time of ingestion! Inquire also whether the patient has any underlying illnesses and whether any treatment or antidote has already been given. Evaluation of severity must consider whether there is any immediate or potential danger from the ingestion or exposure. On all occasions, the caller's phone number and address is important to obtain since follow-up of the initial evaluation and assessment of patient status will often be necessary. In a critical situation, the location of the patient is needed in order to dispatch emergency assistance. Some ingestions may be safely managed at home. If an ingestion is managed at home, appropriate follow-up must be done. The patient or responsible party must be given clear and simple instructions of what signs or symptoms should be seen if the patient becomes symptomatic. If a patient is referred to an emergency facility for evaluation and treatment, nursing and medical personnel at that facility should be alerted and given details of the case in advance of the patient's arrival.

If the ingestion is *clearly* nontoxic (refer to Table 48-14) and without symptoms, it is helpful to offer poison prevention hints over the phone in addition to reassurance. Loca-

TABLE 48-14   Some Common Nontoxics*

Antacids	Lipstick
Antibiotics	Magic markers
Ballpoint pen inks	Makeup
Birth control pills	Model clay
Bubble bath soaps	Newspaper
Candles	Pencils
Chalk	Putty
Crayons	Rubber cement
Drying packets (Silica)	Shampoo
Diaper rash ointments	Shaving creams and lotions
Deodorants	Soap and soap products
Glues and pastes	Sweetening agents
Hand lotions and creams	Thermometers
Incense	Toothpaste
Indelible markers	Water colors
Ink	

*When taken in small amounts.

tions considered unsafe for storage of hazardous substances, such as drain and household cleansers, dishwashing supplies, paints and thinners, pesticides and herbicides, automobile care products, medicines, and cosmetics, could be pointed out. These products should be stored in their original containers and out of children's reach. Factors that contribute to accidental ingestions around the home include:

1. Poisonous products not put away immediately after their use
2. Empty containers improperly discarded

3. Any stressful situation or change in the household's routine (holiday or vacation preparations, illness, visitors)

The most common poison emergencies involve medication, especially over-the-counter medications. If there are particular problems in the home, it is often useful to schedule the patient for further discussion or a visit by a public health nurse. Multiple ingestions are sometimes the result of child neglect or abuse; when this situation is suspect, appropriate referral is critical. If a parent has become hysterical over a minor problem, such as the child chewing on a cake of soap, it may be more helpful to reassure and calm the parent first, and then make a follow-up call for further discussion. If efforts to calm or reassure the anxious caller are unsuccessful, he or she should be referred to a physician or to an emergency facility for evaluation. There are several other circumstances where attempting management of the ingestion or exposure at home is not appropriate:

1. When a child under 1 year of age is involved
2. When a rapid-acting drug, caustic, or corrosive has been taken
3. When a suicide attempt has been made involving either an adult or adolescent
4. When the history given is complicated, confusing, or inconsistent

Whenever any of these circumstances is described in a poisoning or overdose situation, the caller should be referred to an emergency facility or to a physician.

CASE STUDY

Mrs. P. arrives at the emergency room with Albert, her 3-year-old grandson. Mrs. P. stated that the child had probably gotten into some prescription medication during a visit to her house. He may have ingested an unknown quantity of several of the medications that belonged to his grandfather. On the way to the emergency room, Albert vomited once in the car; several tablets were seen in the vomitus. Mrs. P. thinks the child may also have experienced a seizure. This seizure has occurred once, lasting for about 1 min.

Assessment

The emergency room nurse joined Mrs. P. and the child in the examining room to make the initial assessment. Albert was lying on the examining table conscious, although very lethargic. There was an occasional clonic jerking movement of his arms and legs. A slight tremor of the extremities was also noted. The child was warm and not sweating. Vital signs were: temperature 37.5°C, pulse 90, respirations 25, BP 80/50. His pupils were 6 mm in diameter, equal-sized, and reactive to light. The abdomen

appeared distended, and no bowel sounds were heard on auscultation. As the nurse assessed Albert, she inquired of Mrs. P. whether she had any idea what type of medication might have been ingested by the child and whether she had brought along the medication bottles. Mrs. P. replied that her husband had lots of pills in their bedroom drawer and that the child was found with many of them spread all over the floor. The grandfather had been depressed, having recently been diagnosed to have parkinsonism and had been on medication since that time. A number of vitamins were also found and may have been taken as well. Mrs. P. had not thought to bring any bottles since no one was sure what the child had taken. The vomitus did contain several tablets that appeared to be vitamin tablets.

From the hypotension, atropine-like symptoms (dry mouth, dilated pupils, ileus), and dystonia described by the grandmother, the nurse suspected that a drug with anticholinergic effects, such as an antidepressant, might be involved. The nurse asked whether there was any iron in the vitamins that the child may have taken. The grandmother now remembers the vitamins did contain iron since she had bought them several years ago to correct an anemic condition.

The concerned grandmother mentions that, "fortunately," she remembered to administer a solution of salt water to the child to induce vomiting. She asked the nurse whether this was the right thing to do.

Management

The nurse requested the physician to come to the examining room quickly and had other nurses bring the emergency cart into the room. The nurse placed the child in Trendelenburg position for the hypotension and started an IV. Another nurse was asked to attach the child to an electrocardiogram and begin monitoring. The x-ray technician was called to arrange a flat plate on the abdomen since the tablets may be radiopaque. The child was not allowed to have any fluid by mouth because of the ileus. The nurse drew venous blood for electrolyte and glucose level determinations; vital signs, neurologic status, and respiratory signs were monitored carefully since not only had the poisoning not been definitely identified but several drugs could have been ingested simultaneously. As the physician arrived, the nurse reported the data to her. The x-ray revealed at least 10 radiopaque tablets, and the physician ordered lavage, which the nurse performed. Six tablets were recovered from the procedure. The gastric material was tested for presence of blood. It was positive. The remainder was saved for toxicologic screen. Activated charcoal in a 70% sorbitol slurry was then given. The child was transferred to the pediatric intensive care unit. Determination of serum iron was immediately done. Analysis of the stomach contents subsequently indicated that the poisoning had been iron and amitriptyline (Elavil). The serum sodium was also found to be elevated possibly from the well-meaning but incorrect use of the home remedy for emesis.

Evaluation

The initial goal had been to stabilize the patient, get a history from witnesses, and then identify the poison in this complex case. The nurse had been able to make several important contributions based on her ability to observe for signs and symptoms and had then initiated supportive treatment. The lavage had limited success in removing the poison. The charcoal was given in repeated fashion every 6 h over the next 24 h. Deferoxamine was administered intravenously to chelate the iron. The chelation was discontinued 24 h later when the child's urine no longer showed the characteristic red-orange color denoting the presence of excess-free iron. The child did not develop any further cardiac or neurologic symptom throughout his hospitalization. The nurse was aware of the potential complications and observed carefully and prepared for their possible occurrence. The signs and symptoms subsided over the next 72 h, and the child recovered without complications.

REFERENCES

Barrows, J. J.: "Shock Demands Drugs," *Nursing 82,* **12**:34–41, 1982.

Comer, J. B.: *Pharmacology in Critical Care,* Bethany, Conn.: Fleschner, 1981.

Crumlish, C. M.: "Cardiogenic Shock: Catch It Early!" *Nursing 81,* **11**:34–41, 1981.

Done, A. K.: "Poisoning from Common Household Products," *Pediatr Clin North Am,* **17**:569–581, 1970.

Donegan, J. H.: *Cardiopulmonary Resuscitation: Physiology, Pharmacology and Practical Application,* Springfield, Ill.: Thomas, 1982.

Dyer, C.: "Burn Care in the Emergent Period," *J Emerg Nurs,* **6**:9–16, 1980.

Figgie, H. H., et al.: "Chloramine-T—Glycerin Dressings for Burns," *J Burn Care Rehab,* **3**:223–225, 1982.

Giving Cardiovascular Drugs Safely (Nursing Skillbook), Springhouse, PA: Springhouse Intermed, 1980.

Goldfrank, L. R. (ed.): *Toxicological Emergencies: A Comprehensive Handbook in Problem Solving,* New York: Appleton-Century-Crofts, 1982.

Greenberg, M. I., et al.: "The Use of Endotracheal Medication for Cardiac Arrest," *Top Emerg Med,* **1**:29–40, 1979.

Hills, S. W., and J. J. Birmingham: *Burn Care,* Bethany, CT: Fleschner, 1981.

Kastrup, E. K. (ed.): *Facts and Comparisons,* Philadelphia: Lippincott, 1984.

Kenner, C. V., et al.: *Critical Care Nursing: Body-Mind-Spirit,* Boston: Little, Brown, 1981.

Kurth, C. L.: "Hemodynamic Monitoring and Specialized Equipment," in R. C. Sanderson and C. L. Kurth (eds.), *The Cardiac Patient: A Comprehensive Approach,* 2d ed., Philadelphia: Saunders, 1983.

Letz, G., T. G. Tong, and K. R. Olson: "Acute Toxic Exposures," in H. D. Watts (ed.), *Handbook of Medical Treatment,* 17th ed., Greenbrae, MA: Jones, 1983.

McIntyre, K. M., and A. J. Lewis (eds.): *Textbook of Advanced Cardiac Life Support,* Dallas: American Heart Association, 1981.

Manoguerra, A., and L. Weaver: "Poisoning with Tricyclic Antidepressant Drugs," *Clin Toxicol,* **10**:149–158, 1977.

"Nursing Care of Patients in Shock: 1. Pharmacotherapy (Programmed Instruction)," *Am J Nurs,* **82**:943–964, 1982.

Okun, R.: "Treatment of Sedative Drug Overdose," *Clin Toxicol,* **6**:13–21, 1973.

Peterson, R. G., and B. H. Rumack: "Toxicity of Acetaminophen Overdose," *J Am Coll Emerg Physicians,* 7:202–205, 1978.

Purcell, J. A.: "Shock Drugs: Standardized Guidelines," *Am J Nurs,* 82:965–974, 1982.

Rogove, H. J.: "Pathophysiology of Cardiac Arrest," *Top Emerg Med,* 1:17–27, 1979.

Rumack, B. H., and R. G. Peterson: "Poisoning," in C. H. Kempe, H. R. Silver, and D. O'Brien (eds.), *Current Pediatric Therapy,* 6th ed., Los Altos, CA: Lange, 1980.

——, and A. R. Temple (eds.): *Management of the Acutely Poisoned Patient,* New York: Science, 1977.

Schofferman, J., and T. Yamauchi: "Overdose: The Early Treatment," *West J Med,* 123:160–163, 1975.

Schumann, L., and S. Gaston: "Commonsense Guide to Topical Burn Therapy," *Nursing 79,* 9:34–39, 1979.

Smith-Collins: "Dobutamine: A New Inotropic Agent," *Nursing 80,* 10:62–66, 1980.

"Standards and Guidelines for Cardiopulmonary Resuscitation (CPR) and Emergency Cardiac Care (ECC)," *JAMA,* 244 (Suppl.):453–509, 1980.

Temple, A. R.: "Pathophysiology of Aspirin Toxicity with Implications for Management," *Pediatrics,* (Suppl.), 62:873–876, 1978.

Tong, T. G.: "Poisoning and Its Treatment: 1. Incidence and Clinical Signs of Poisoning and Toxic Overdose," *Nurse Pract,* 2:35–36, 1976.

——: "Poisoning and Its Treatment: 2. Treatment of Poisoning and Toxic Overdose," *Nurse Pract,* 2:29–32, 43, 1977.

Walraven, G., and M. Kavanaugh: "Cardiac Arrest: A Review of the Resuscitation Process," *Top Emerg Med,* 1:115–126, 1979.

White, B. C.: "Pharmacology of Resuscitation," in A. L. Harwood (ed.), *Cardiopulmonary Resuscitation,* Baltimore: Williams and Wilkins, 1982.

Worrell, C. L.: "The Management of Organophosphate Intoxication," *South Med J,* 68:335–339, 1975.

Zweng, D., and B. C. Galt: "Intravenous Medications Commonly Used in the Emergency Department," *J Emerg Nurs,* 7:234–236, 1981.

49

COMMUNITY HEALTH CARE*

JOAN K. MAGILVY
THEODORE G. TONG
JAMES R. BONK
ROSS A. SIMKOVER

Community health nurses are actively involved in promotion and protection of the health of their community; nursing practice in this setting involves several roles related to drug therapy and preventing exposure to chemical toxicants. Historically, community or public health nurses have been concerned with the epidemiology of communicable diseases and environmental health problems such as sanitation and housing. They have traditionally made health promotion home visits to young childbearing families as well as to older persons with chronic or terminal diseases. In addition to these activities, today's community health nurses also practice in primary care clinics where they administer immunizations to infants and young children. During outbreaks of communicable diseases, they are part of the investigation team, and may participate in community-wide surveillance programs in addition to holding special immunization clinics. Prevention, education, and treatment of accidental poisoning (see Chap. 48) and drug abuse and misuse are also important health protective roles.

The environment in which the public lives and works is another major emphasis. Community health nurses are often involved in health promotion and protective programs related to environmental pollution. In school and occupational health settings, nurses are concerned with the health of students and workers, especially focusing on occupational toxicants and hazards in the workplace. Community health nursing practice can include health promotion and protective activities aimed at individuals across the life span, in various groups, and in the community at large. Immunizations, environmental and occupational health hazards, and drug abuse are the specific community health nursing topics discussed in this chapter.

---

*The sections on immunization and environmental and occupational health were written by Dr. Magilvy; Drs. Tong, Bonk, and Simkover collaborated on the section on drug abuse.

IMMUNIZATION

LEARNING OBJECTIVES

Upon mastery of the content of this section, the reader will be able to:

1. Define active and passive immunity.
2. Differentiate between the two general types of antigen used to induce artificial active immunity.
3. Name seven recommended active immunizations for infants and children and the usual combinations used.
4. List at least three precautions and contraindications associated with routine active immunization.
5. List three main types of passive immunization and give examples of the uses of each.
6. Explain the hazard associated with the use of serum of animal origin.
7. Give examples of high-risk patients who should receive passive immunization.
8. Explain the nursing process related to routine immunization of children and adults and of those about to travel abroad.

Immunization can safely and effectively prevent or control many acute childhood or adult diseases. The ultimate goal of immunization programs is to eradicate the preventable communicable diseases. Vaccines are now available to prevent diphtheria, pertussis, tetanus, poliomyelitis, measles, mumps, and rubella, yet nearly 10 percent of the children in the United States remain unprotected against these diseases. The federal government, along with state and local organizations, has developed programs aimed at increasing the level of immunization in this country. Nurses working in local and state health departments, schools, and other community settings are part of a major interdisciplinary effort to implement these programs. Just as smallpox has been virtually eliminated in its natural state, it is hoped that the other diseases will become more of historical than of clinical significance.

Although immunization biologicals used today have been improved to be as safe and effective as possible, they are not without risk. Some vaccines may not be totally protective, while others may cause adverse reactions. The goal in development of vaccines today and for the future is to achieve the highest degree of safety and protection possible. New vaccines and immunization products are continually being developed; during the 1970s and 1980s, several new vaccines for influenza, pneumonia, hepatitis, chicken pox, and herpes have been released for clinical trials or public distribution. Much research effort and money is being spent on developing immunizations for numerous diseases where treatment is unavailable or ineffective. Genetic engineering principles are being applied for further development of vaccines. Removing the disease-producing portions of DNA within an infectious microbe is one such research technique. Other research is focused on the antigen portion of an organism, using surface antigens or even synthesizing antigens for vaccine production. Production and storage of presently used vaccines are being investigated to increase effectiveness, reduce costs, and decrease the occurrence of adverse effects.

Although most nurses are not involved in the production and research aspects of immunization technology, there are several related issues with which nurses are actively concerned. In many states it is required that immunization be documented in order for a child to attend school. Nurses working in school and in well-child clinic settings must serve in an educative role with parents and school officials, as well as be responsible for maintaining accurate records. Immunization clinics in most health departments are run by nurses. Nurses also administer immunizations in private health care practices. Each nurse must be aware of vaccines in current use, dosages, storage requirements, and adverse effects. Because of occasional reports in the news media of untoward effects of vaccination, such as those which triggered the pertussis vaccine controversy (see below), or because of restrictions imposed by certain religious, philosophical, or other convictions, some parents may consider withholding immunizations from their children. Nurses must be prepared to counsel these families and must keep informed about current ethical and legal issues related to the immunization field.

TYPES OF IMMUNITY

The human body can protect itself from many foreign disease-causing stimuli. Immunity can be acquired through either natural or artificial means. When an individual has a disease and is not protected by a natural resistance to it, the body produces specific antibodies to attack the foreign antigen; the individual remains resistant to that specific antigen in the future. This process of immunity is called *natural active immunity.* Medical research has also devised means of developing immunities artificially and safely, referred to as *artificial acquired immunity.*

There are two major types of artificial immunity, active and passive. In *active immunity,* the body is stimulated to develop resistance by being injected with specific antigens, causing the production of antibodies, as well as the cellular response of the lymphocytes. This form of immunity can be achieved with bacterial or viral agents that have been altered or modified in order to eliminate the pathogenicity of the organism.

When a large supply of antibodies is needed in the blood immediately in order to combat an infection or when there is not enough time for the body to develop active immunity, natural or artificial, the patient can be *passively immunized* by receiving ready-made or preformed antibodies. In passive immunity, the patient usually has already been exposed to the disease, but has not received vaccination prior to that exposure. The antibody given passively will prevent or modify the disease in that individual. A *natural passive immunity* is also possible. Infants receive this type of immunity from their mothers by transfer through the placenta or from breast milk. This natural passive immunity lasts only a short time into infancy. In passive immunity the individual's body manufactures no antibodies. For this reason, passive immunity does not last long, and as blood cells are replaced, eventually the antibodies are lost.

Artificial active immunity is usually considered to be a safer and more effective method of immunization. It has a longer duration and has fewer adverse effects than passive immunizations, since animal serum or strong antitoxins are often used in the passive immunity agents. Active immunity is thus produced by an individual's own body either through contracting an infectious disease or receiving artificial active immunizations such as *vaccines* and *toxoids.* Booster doses are often given to reactivate the antibody production. Passive immunity is a less effective protective immunity, producing an immediate, short-lived effect with potentially dangerous side effects.

Passive Immunity

Administration of antibodies from an immune subject may provide temporary protection. Passive immunization consists of antibodies (immunoglobulins) taken from serum from either human or animal sources; thus these immunoglobulins are often called *serums.* Three types of preparations are available:

1. Standard human immune serum globulin (ISG) or gamma globulin, for general use
2. Special human ISG with a known antibody content for specific illnesses
3. Animal antiserums or antitoxins

Generally, passive immunization lasts for only 1 to 6 weeks. It is not always effective, and it may even cause adverse reactions, such as fever and malaise.

Indications

Passive immunization has several indications:

1. For persons who are unable to form antibodies (e.g., with immune-deficient diseases, such as agammaglobulinemia)
2. To prevent disease or infection when there is not sufficient time for active immunity (e.g., preexposure to a disease)
3. For treatment of certain specific diseases (e.g., tetanus, rabies)
4. For treatment of conditions such as snakebite and of persons who are immunosuppressed (e.g., chemotherapy or transplant patients)

Whenever possible, human serum is preferred over animal serum, because of prevalence of hypersensitivity reactions from the latter. The half-life of antibodies from human serum is also longer in humans, allowing for smaller dosages given over a longer period of time.

Adverse Effects

Two types of serum reaction may be seen, an acute *anaphylactic reaction* (manifested by urticaria, dyspnea, cyanosis, vasomotor collapse, loss of consciousness) and *serum sickness*, either of which may occur in patients who are injected with serum for the first time, or more frequently, in those previously injected with serum. Serum sickness is dose-related, with manifestations of urticaria, adenopathy, arthritis, and fever. The reaction may occur a few hours to several days after a second injection of serum or about 7 to 12 days after a first injection. *Anaphylaxis* is treated with an immediate subcutaneous or intramuscular dose of **epinephrine** 1:1000 (0.01 mL/kg), which may be repeated intravenously if no response is seen immediately. Serum sickness is treated symptomatically with **aspirin** or **acetaminophen, antihistamines,** or **corticosteroids.**

Preparations and Administration

Products for passive immunization are referred to as *biologicals;* since many have special storage requirements, package directions should be consulted. Administration of these products is by intramuscular injection (except the new IV form of human ISG). Immunization should be given as soon as possible after exposure. Patients should be questioned about previous injections with the serum as well as tested for hypersensitivity to animal sera. Active immunization with live vaccines (e.g., polio, measles, etc.) should not be given within 2 to 3 months of passive serum immunization or

immunity will not develop. Tetanus is an exception to this situation; active immunization should be given at the same time as the toxoid is administered. Several products for passive immunity are discussed in more detail below.

Human Gamma Globulin (Immune Serum Globulin, ISG)

ISG is an antibody-rich fraction of pooled plasma from normal donors. Advantages over plasma include greater freedom from hepatitis virus, concentration of the antibodies into a small volume for intramuscular use, and stable antibody content, which allows storage for several years. ISG is usually given intramuscularly, administered with an 18- or 20-gauge needle, frequently in the buttocks. If more than 5 mL is to be administered (in practice, the dose is often 10 mL or more), the dose should be divided and injected into several sites. Peak blood levels are attained in about 2 days, and the half-life in circulation is 20 to 25 days.

A preparation of pooled ISG is now available for intravenous use. **Immune globulin intravenous** (Gamimmune) is an expensive preparation used for patients needing immediate high levels of antibodies, and for whom intramuscular administration is contraindicated. Research is also progressing on an ISG preparation to be used in a subcutaneous pump.

The value of ISG is clearly documented for (1) measles prophylaxis or modification, (2) viral hepatitis type A (infectious hepatitis) prophylaxis or modification, and (3) antibody deficiency diseases. ISG may be useful for prevention of rubella in the first trimester of pregnancy, for prevention or modification of viral hepatitis type B (serum hepatitis) after accidental inoculation, with life-threatening bacterial infections in conjunction with antibiotics, and in prophylaxis of infections in premature infants.

Specific Human Immune Serum Globulins

Special human ISGs are derived from the sera of hyperimmunized persons or those convalescing from specific infections. Because of their higher specific antibody concentrations, they are useful in several disorders in which normal ISG is of little or no benefit. **Human tetanus immune globulin,** for example, is used for the prophylaxis and treatment of tetanus. For prophylaxis or treatment of vaccinial complication of smallpox vaccination, **human vaccinia immune globulin** may be used. **Human varicella-zoster immune globulin** is for prevention or modification of varicella or zoster. **$Rh_o(D)$ immune globulin** has been employed to prevent erythroblastosis fetalis in subsequent Rh-positive offspring (see Chap. 46) or sensitization to incompatible whole blood inoculation. **Rubella immune globulin** will prevent rubella in exposed individuals except fetuses of exposed mothers. **Human rabies immune globulin,** a preparation to prevent rabies in exposed individuals, must be combined with rabies immunization to be effective. **Human hepatitis B immune globulin** is used for prophylaxis in exposed individuals who have not already produced the antibody.

Other Products Available   See Table 49-1 for a list of commonly used passive immunizations. In addition to those in the table, the following clinically effective products are available: **antilymphocyte serum globulin** (ALG) for use as an adjunct to immunosuppression in organ transplant, **human varicella zoster immune globulin** (VZIG) for immunodeficient children, **black widow spider antivenin, coral snake antivenin, crotalid** (pit viper) **antivenin,** and **ABE polyvalent antitoxin** for the treatment of botulism and definite exposure to botulism. Not recommended due to doubtful efficacy are gas gangrene antitoxin, pertussis immune globulin, and mumps immune globulin.

Active Immunity

Sources of active immunization agents are microorganisms or products of microorganisms such as toxoids or polysaccharides (parts of a bacterium). The goal of active immunization is to mimic a natural infection using low-risk vaccine preparations to stimulate an immunologic response by the recipient. This response involves formation of antibodies or the development of cell-mediated immunity that may last a lifetime for some diseases or provide only partial protection for others. For some diseases, a single dose of vaccine is sufficient for immunization, while for others a series of doses with one or more periodic booster doses are required. Indications, doses, schedules of immunizations, and products and techniques of administration are important variables to be considered for successful immunization.

There are two types of preparations of infectious microorganisms: a *live, attenuated preparation* is often used with viruses, while a *killed, inactivated preparation* is used with some viruses and most bacteria. Pertussis is an example of a killed bacterial agent; tetanus toxoid and diphtheria are examples of detoxified bacterial products. Examples of viral agents include live attenuated products such as measles and inactivated agents such as influenza.

Each type of preparation has certain advantages and dis-

TABLE 49-1   Commonly Used Products for Passive Immunization

PRODUCT	INDICATION	DOSE
Diphtheria antitoxin (equine)	Diphtheria; nonimmune contacts should have active immunization.	20,000–120,000 U IM, depending on duration and severity of disease.
Immune globulin intramuscular (human) (Gamastan, Gammar)	Hepatitis A: Should be given to those with close household contact and to those traveling to endemic area. Will modify but not prevent disease.	0.02 mL/kg IM after exposure. Protects about 2 months.
	Hepatitis non-A non-B: Immunize those with parenteral exposure to serum from patients with hepatitis.	IM 0.06 mL/kg can be repeated in 25–30 days
	Measles: Give as soon as possible after exposure (although active immunization is usually effective up to 48 h after exposure)	0.25 mL/kg IM after exposure. For immunocompromised give 0.5 mL/kg
	Poliomyelitis: Give to exposed nonimmunized individuals.	0.15 mL/kg IM
	Hypogammaglobulinemia: Goal is to have 200 mg/100 mL of circulating IgG levels	Initial dose 1.2 mL/kg followed by 0.6 mL/kg every 3–4 wks
Hepatitis B immune globulin (human) (Hyper-Hep, H-BIG, Hep-B-Gammagee)	Nonimmune close contacts (parenteral serum or mucous membrane exposure) if negative for anti-HB-s Ag antibody. Regular immune globulin may also be effective.	0.06 mL/kg IM within 7 days of exposure. Reimmunize 25–30 days after exposure.
Rabies immune globulin (RIG) (human), antirabies serum (ARS) (equine)	Exposure to scratch or bite of carnivores, unless the animal's brain has been found to be rabies-free. Rabies vaccine (active killed virus) must also be given.	20 IU/kg; up to half of dose infiltrated into wound site and remainder given IM. 40 IU/kg of ARS should be used only when RIG is not available.
Tetanus immune globulin (human) (Hyper Tet, others)	Tetanus: Give prophylactically for major or contaminated wound for persons with less than two doses toxoid in past (or less than three doses if tetanus-prone wound).	Prevention: children 4 U/kg; adult 250–500 U/kg. Treatment: 3000–6000 U/IM

advantages. Live attenuated products most often produce long-lasting immunity. They stimulate the resistance accomplished by a natural infection and can sometimes be given orally as well as parenterally. These preparations, however, can lead to an increased risk of the disease when the attenuated organism reverts to virulence (e.g., polio). A mild form of the actual disease is sometimes required to induce immunity, and there could be a risk of the recipient becoming a carrier. Occasionally an attenuated agent may change and cause a new type of the disease. These agents are also labile and are difficult to store.

Inactivated, or killed, agents cause little risk of the disease; they are less labile, and can be stored or shipped easier, and may be highly purified (e.g., toxoids). Their disadvantages include:

1. The immunity is often short-lived, requiring reimmunization.
2. Occasionally the desired protection is not accomplished, or reinfection or carrier states can occur.
3. They can be toxic (e.g., pertussis, influenza).
4. They usually require parenteral administration.

Indications for Infants and Children

Active immunization of infants and children has been implemented to prevent disease and maintain health. Recommendations for immunization schedules and vaccine use in the United States are made by two independent groups, the Advisory Committee on Immunization Practices (ACIP) of the U.S. Public Health Service and the American Academy of Pediatrics (AAP). These recommendations are generally quite similar. The recommendations for the active immunization schedule are presented in Table 49-2. It is important to remember that these are recommendations, not rules, which must be constantly evaluated and modified (e.g., if there is a measles epidemic in the community, the measles immunization might become the priority, with other routine immunization delayed for a month or two).

General contraindications (see Nursing Process section) and specific contraindications established by the AAP (see specific preparations) should be noted. Special precautions for children receiving immunosuppressive therapy, children with neurologic disorders, those in institutions, and other special circumstances are discussed in detail in the *Report of the Committee on Infectious Diseases* (AAP, 1982).

Recommendations for children not immunized in infancy are outlined in Table 49-3. Prescribers may choose to alter the sequence of these schedules if specific infections are prevalent at a given time. Simultaneous administration of DTP, MMR, and TOPV has proved effective without increasing the incidences of adverse effects. Other antigen vaccines should not be administered simultaneously since one virus could theoretically interfere with the development of immunity to another.

Indications for Travel

Recommendations for travel to foreign countries change frequently. Current recommendations are listed in Table 49-4. Travelers should check with their local health department or state health department for the latest requirements.

Adverse Effects

Adverse effects occasionally occur in reaction to an intrinsic property of a vaccine antigen or some component of the vaccine. Reactions are usually mild to moderate and do not tend to have permanent sequelae. Examples of these milder adverse effects can include fever or local irritation (especially after immunization with DTP), a rash and fever after administration of live measles virus vaccine, and tenderness and induration following vaccination for cholera or typhoid. Allergic or hypersensitivity reactions can occur to the constituents of a vaccine, for example, chicken or duck egg media used to culture a virus can sometimes cause allergic reactions to these products.

More severe adverse reactions to active immunizations are rare, but can be life-threatening. They are thought to be

TABLE 49-2 Recommended Schedule for Active Immunization of Normal Infants and Children

AGE	IMMUNIZATIONS
2 months	DTP,* TOPV†
4 months	DTP, TOPV
6 months	DTP, TOPV‡
1 year	Tuberculin skin test
15 months	Measles,§ rubella,§ mumps
1½ years	DTP, TOPV
4–6 years	DTP, TOPV
14–16 years	Td¶ and thereafter every 10 years

*DTP: Diphtheria and tetanus toxoids combined with pertussis vaccine.

†TOPV: Trivalent oral poliovirus vaccine. This recommendation is suitable for breast-fed as well as bottle-fed infants.

‡A third dose of TOPV may be considered optional except in areas of high endemicity, e.g., some areas of southwestern United States.

§May be given at 1 year as measles-rubella or measles-mumps-rubella combined vaccines.

¶Td is the combined tetanus and diphtheria toxoids (adult type) for those over 6 years of age, in contrast to diphtheria and tetanus (DT), which contains a larger amount of diphtheria antigen. *Tetanus toxoid at time of injury:* for clean, minor wounds, no booster dose is needed by a fully immunized child unless more than 10 years has elapsed since the last dose. For contaminated wounds, a booster dose should be given if more than 5 years has elapsed since the last dose.

Source: Compiled from CDC: *Morbidity and Mortality Weekly Report,* **32**(1), January 14, 1983, and *Report of the Committee on Infectious Diseases,* 19th ed., Evanston, IL: American Academy of Pediatrics, 1982.

TABLE 49-3 Primary Immunization for Children Not Immunized in Infancy

1 Through 6 Years of Age	
First visit	DTP, TOPV, Tuberculin test
1 month later	Measles, rubella, mumps (MMR or singly) if child is over 15 months of age
2 months later	DTP, TOPV
4 months later	DTP, TOPV*
6 to 12 months later or preschool	DTP, TOPV
Age 14–16 years	Td—continue every 10 years
7 Years of Age and Over	
First visit	Td, TOPV, measles, rubella, mumps
2 months later	Td, TOPV
6 to 12 months later	Td, TOPV
10 years after third Td	Td—continue every 10 years

*A third dose of TOPV may be considered optional except in areas of high endemicity.

Source: Compiled from CDC: *Morbidity and Mortality Weekly Report,* **32**(1), January 14, 1983, and *Report of the Committee on Infectious Diseases,* 19th ed., Evanston, IL: American Academy of Pediatrics, 1982.

due either to intrinsic properties of the agent or to some idiosyncratic characteristic of the recipient. Examples of serious adverse effects include an encephalomyelitis associated with the pertussis vaccine (see discussion in section on pertussis administration below) and paralytic poliomyelitis after administration of TOPV. Guillain-Barré syndrome has occurred with various viral immunizations, and it occurred in relatively large numbers following the nationwide administration of the swine flu vaccine. Central nervous system reactions (such as convulsions) can also occur shortly after the administration of a dose of antigen. However, it must be noted that the occurrence of adverse effects following vaccination is not sufficient proof that the vaccine caused the symptoms; further investigation is always indicated. When CNS reaction occurs, further immunization should be delayed until the child reaches at least 1 year of age and evidence of any active cerebral irritation has subsided.

Preparations and Administration

Vaccines are available as those that contain a single separate antigen and in combination containing two or more antigens. Combination vaccines are composed of antigens that are safe and effective when given simultaneously. They are advantageous if there is a threat of concomitant exposure or if it is possible that the child will be inaccessible for further

immunization. Further, these combinations prevent the need for multiple injections. The gluteus medius muscle of the buttock is not recommended for routine immunizations. The site should be selected based on the volume of material to be injected and the size of the muscle in the child; the anterolateral aspect of the thigh, for example, is the largest muscle in an infant and is therefore the preferred site. For an older child, the deltoid muscle of the upper arm would be of sufficient mass for injection there. During primary immunizations, each injection should be given in a different site.

Storage Vaccines are also biologicals and have storage specifications and expiration dates. Storage for most vaccines must be at cold temperatures, usually from 2 to 8°C

TABLE 49-4 Immunization for Foreign Travel*†

VACCINE	COMMENT
Cholera	One dose or booster required for entry into Asia, Middle East, or Africa. Full immunization requires two initial doses, 6-month duration of effect.
Hepatitis A (ISG)	Immune serum globulin (ISG) recommended for travel to Africa, Asia, Central America, rural Mexico, Philippines, southern Pacific islands, South America. Repeat every 6 months during exposure.
Plague	Recommended for persons who must be in known plague areas; Mongolia, southwestern Russia, central China, Brazil, Saudi Arabia, Vietnam, Nepal, Java, southern India, Bolivia, Peru, South Africa. Boosters every 6 months, although increased reactivity with subsequent injections.
Rabies	For residence and work in areas where rabies is prevalent in domestic and wild species. Primary vaccination of three doses with boosters as needed to maintain adequate antibody titers.
Typhoid	For travel to areas where typhoid is endemic. Initial series of two doses with boosters at least every 3 years.
Yellow fever	For travel in endemic areas of Africa and South America. Certificate of vaccination required for entry into several countries. Boosters every 10 years.

*Check with local health department for latest requirements and recommendations.
†Diphtheria, tetanus, pertussis, and polio immunization should also be current for all travel.

TABLE 49-5 Products for Active Immunization

VACCINE	INDICATIONS	TYPE	Immunization Schedule PRIMARY	Immunization Schedule BOOSTER	ROUTE OF ADMINISTRATION
Bacterial Vaccines and Toxoids					
BCG vaccine (Bacillus Clamette-Guerin)	Persons with negative skin tests and repeated exposure to sputum-positive cases of tuberculosis.	Live	One dose; repeat if skin test after 2 months is negative	None.	Intradermal
Cholera vaccine	See Table 49-4.	Killed	Two doses a week or more apart.	Every 6 months.	SC, IM
Diphtheria toxoid (available as DTP, DT, Td, and diphtheria alone)	See Tables 49-2, 49-3, and text.	Toxoid	Three doses 4 weeks or more apart with one dose a year later.	Single dose anytime after 10 years.	IM
Meningitis vaccines: meningococcal polysaccharide, group A (Menomune A); meningococcal polysaccharide vaccine, group C (Menomune-C); groups A & C (Menomune A/C, Meningovax AC); meningococcal polysaccharide vaccine, groups A, C, Y, and W-135 (Menomune A/C/Y/W135)	For epidemic situations, military installations, family contacts. Children less than 2 years should receive Group A only.	Polysaccharide	One dose.	None (?)	SC
Pertussis vaccine (available as DTP and pertussis alone)	See Tables 49-2, 49-3, and text. Not usually recommended beyond age 6.	Killed	Three doses 4 or more weeks apart plus one dose 1 year later.	None.	IM
Plague vaccine	See Table 49-4.	Killed	Three doses.	Three boosters every 6 months, then every 1–2 years.	IM
Pneumococcal polyvalent vaccine (Pneumovax, Pnu-Immune)	High risk for serious pneumococcal disease.	Polysaccharide	One dose.	Every 5 years.	SC or IM
Tetanus toxoid (available as DTP, DT, Td or tetanus alone)	See Tables 49-2, 49-3, and text.	Toxoid	Three doses 4 weeks or more apart.	Single dose anytime after 10 years; for wound give booster if more than 5 years since immunization or booster.	IM
Typhoid vaccine	Travel (see Table 49-4), household exposure, and epidemics.	Killed	Two doses 4 weeks apart.	Every 3 years.	SC or intradermal

Viral Vaccines

Vaccine	Indications	Type	Primary schedule	Booster	Route
Hepatitis B vaccine (Heptavax-B)	High-risk patients, occupations, and lifestyles.	Killed virus protein	First dose at elected day. Second dose 1 month later. Third dose 6 months later.	One booster after about 5 years.	IM
Influenza virus vaccine [Fluogen (split virus), Fluzone (whole virus)]	Given by November to high-risk patients. Composition varies by epidemiologic situation.	Killed	One dose except children (<13 years; use split virus only) who require two doses.	Every 1–3 years.	IM
Measles (available combined with mumps and rubella with rubella only and alone)	See Tables 49-2, 49-3, and text. Nonimmune exposed patients within 48 h of exposure.	Live	One dose at 15 months or later.	None	SC
Mumps (available with measles and rubella, with rubella, and alone)	See Tables 49-2, 49-3, and text.	Live	One dose.	None	SC
Poliovirus vaccine, live, oral, trivalent (TOPV, Sabin) (Orimune)	See Tables 49-2, 49-3, and text.	Live	Two doses 6–8 weeks apart, followed by third dose 8–12 months later, and then on entering school.	None	Oral
Poliomyelitis vaccine (IPV, Salk)	Immunocompromised persons.	Killed	Three doses at 4- to 6-week intervals, followed by one dose 6–12 months later.	Every 2–3 years	SC
Rabies vaccine human diploid cell cultures (HDCV) (Imunovax, WYVAC)	Preexposure for high-risk occupation: veterinarians, animal handlers, forest rangers. Postexposure treatment for those scratched or bitten by carnivore.	Killed	Preexposure three doses 1 week apart; postexposure 5 or 6 doses. Given with rabies immune globulin.	Based on antibody titers	IM, SC
Rubella vaccine (available with measles and mumps, with measles, with mumps, and alone)	See Tables 49-2, 49-3, and text.	Live	One dose after 15 months of age.	None	SC
Smallpox vaccine (Dryvax)	Not recommended. Only for individuals at special risk.	Live			
Yellow fever	See Table 49-4.	Live	One dose.	10 years	SC

and they usually must not be frozen. Refrigerators in some clinics, nursing units, and other settings may be too warm or too cold. Vaccines with exceptional storage requirements include live oral poliovirus vaccine (stored in a freezer at or below $-10°C$) and liquid smallpox (stored below $0°C$). Those vaccines which must be reconstituted may be active for a limited time after reconstitution, such as reconstituted live measles vaccine, which can be stored refrigerated up to 8 h. For further information on storage of active and passive immunization products, see information packed with the product or consult a formulary.

Information about the products used in active immunization, doses, and administration are listed in Table 49-5. Each product will be discussed briefly below.

Trivalent Oral Polio Vaccine (TOPV) This vaccine is administered orally, and contains types 1, 2, and 3 of live, attenuated poliovirus. It should be stored in a freezer and used within 7 days of being opened. TOPV is usually administered prior to giving injections (e.g., DTP) in infants and small children to enhance cooperation and to decrease the possibility of expulsion of the dose or aspiration due to crying. Care should be taken not to contaminate the dropper while administering the vaccine into the side of the infant's mouth when TOPV is prepared in a multiple-dose bottle. In some rare cases, TOPV has been associated with paralysis. Poliovirus of the vaccine type is present in the stools of recipients for several weeks following immunization, and the virus could be transmitted to an immunocompromised individual. Therefore, immunologically normal siblings or other close contacts of an individual with an immune deficiency should not receive TOPV.

Diphtheria, Tetanus, Pertussis (DTP) The DTP vaccine is a combination of diphtheria and tetanus toxoids with pertussis vaccine. It is usually given to establish the initial immunity for infants and young children and requires three doses repeated at 2-month intervals with booster doses given 1 year and 4 to 6 years after the initial series. See Tables 49-2 and 49-3 for details. These products can also be given as DT (full doses of diphtheria and tetanus toxoids), Td (a full dose of tetanus toxoid with a reduced dose of diphtheria toxoid), or each product can be given separately. Older children and adults most commonly receive Td, since the pertussis vaccine can cause adverse effects in adults.

Tetanus vaccine is used in wound management. When a patient presents with a new puncture wound, severe burns, or other traumatic injury and has had at least two tetanus immunizations from the primary series, a booster is necessary only if the most recent immunization was not within 5 years. If the treatment of the wound was delayed over 24 h or if the patient has had less than two tetanus immunizations, tetanus immune globulin (human product) is given (250 U IM). Tetanus immune antitoxin (500 U IM) is given if the tetanus immune globulin is unavailable. Tetanus toxoid is also given to those without two prior tetanus immunizations. The horse-serum product (antitoxin) can cause a severe reaction, and its administration and effect should be monitored by the physician.

The DTP immunization is preferably given into the lateral thigh muscle of the infant. Instructions to parents after the DTP immunization are important. They should be told that the child may develop a fever within 24 to 48 h after the immunization and that they should use **acetaminophen** or **aspirin** for fever, administering it q4–6h. The acetaminophen can be used prophylactically if the infant had a reaction to prior DTP injections. The lump at the site of the injection may persist for several months but will eventually resolve. In one out of 7000 children a more serious reaction may develop, which would include severe fever, shock, encephalopathy, convulsions, and long periods of crying. These reactions are due to the pertussis vaccine (see below).

When a DTP immunization is to be given, the infant's reaction to the prior dose should be assessed. If it was severe, the prescriber may want to decrease the dose and increase the number of injections (not recommended) or switch to DT only. The child's temperature should be taken before immunization, since DTP should not be given in the presence of febrile illness. However, if the compliance history and health care values would indicate that the child might not return at a subsequent appointment, the child with a minor upper respiratory infection can be immunized. If a convulsive episode occurs, DT should be used instead of DTP, and pertussis immunization should not be repeated if thrombocytopenia develops after a DTP injection.

Measles, Mumps, Rubella (MMR) The MMR vaccine is a combination of live attenuated viruses of measles, mumps, and rubella. These vaccines are also available separately and in paired combinations. The combination MMR or individual vaccines are injected subcutaneously, usually in the upper arm. Tuberculosis skin testing should be performed before giving a measles immunization since the latter can cause a false-positive tuberculosis reaction, and may even activate latent tuberculosis. Specific contraindications to the use of measles, rubella, and mumps live attenuated vaccines, for example, are pregnancy, malignant diseases (leukemia, lymphoma, others), impaired cell-mediated immunity, immunosuppressed patients, severe febrile illness, and recent administration of immune serum globulin, plasma, or blood. The reaction to the MMR vaccine develops within 7 to 10 days. It may manifest as lethargy and high fever of 24 to 48 h durations and is treated symptomatically with fluids and **acetaminophen**.

Neither rubella nor mumps immunization will give any benefit after exposure to the disease, but measles vaccine, if given within 48 h of exposure, will be effective in preventing the disease. The exact details of exposure should be assessed; if given with 48 h of exposure, the measles vaccine will be effective protection. Those seeking medical intervention more than 48 h after exposure are given measles immune globulin (MIG) or standard immune serum globulin (ISG), either of which affords 3 months protection. The measles immunization (live, attenuated measles virus vaccine) should be administered after that time, since ISG or MIG interferes with the vaccine's effectiveness. The measles vaccine is usually not given until the child is 15 months of age, although in epidemic situations it is given to younger infants, who should then be reimmunized after they are 15 months old.

A measles vaccine used during the 1960s was of the killed-virus type. Persons immunized with this product are not only *not protected,* but also may develop atypical measles. Reimmunization of those who received this killed virus is imperative. Approximately 12 to 20 percent of measles vaccines suffer potency failure from improper storage and refrigeration, so some immunized persons may develop the disease. Extreme care in storage of this drug is indicated.

Women of childbearing age should be instructed to use contraception for 2 months after the rubella immunization. The most significant problems associated with rubella infection are the congenital abnormalities that occur if the infection occurs during pregnancy. To prevent these abnormalities, all children from 15 months of age to puberty and all women of childbearing age should be immunized.

NURSING PROCESS RELATED TO IMMUNIZATION

Assessment

The basis for assessment should include the patient's immunization history and the history of the diseases involved. Gathering these data may be difficult when the patient or the parent of the young patient has not kept written records. This may occur when an adult has moved away from the place in which immunizations were received, when a parent has taken a child to one or more different clinics or physician's offices for immunizations, or when parents or adult patients have not realized the necessity to maintain these records.

When written records are misplaced, the parents may confuse the immunization histories of several children. Adult patients or parents may forget this information, leading to inaccurate, uncertain, or incomplete data. Analyzing the reliability of the informant is therefore important in the immunizaton history. Adults may find their records accessible through military, camp, or school records. Parents can be encouraged to write to obtain their children's records from physicians or clinics whenever possible. Community health nurses and school nurse practitioners must be especially alert to the immunization status of children in their caseloads and encourage families to keep accurate records.

A parent might ask about the necessity of MMR immunization if a child has had one of the diseases, or has recently been exposed. Since the clinical symptoms of measles, rubella, and mumps are easily confused with those of other disorders, it is often hard to ascertain from the history whether someone has had these diseases or to which entity children have been exposed. However, parents should understand that administration of the immunization will do no harm to a child who has already had the disease or who has been exposed to the disease.

Several other considerations are important during the assessment process. A child or adult should be checked for febrile illness prior to administering any immunizations; immunizations should be deferred during an acute febrile illness. The nurse should also assess for other conditions which would contraindicate some immunizations: pregnancy, leukemia, lymphoma, other generalized malignant diseases, impaired cell-mediated immunity, immunosuppressive therapy, and recent administration of immune serum globulin, plasma, blood, tuberculin testing, and other recent immunizations of any type. Allergies must also be considered. Animal antisera or antitoxins, as well as some constituents of vaccines, may cause allergic or even anaphylactic reactions; history of any allergies and information about prior experiences with passive and active immunization reactions should be discussed with the parent or adult patient.

Management

Educating parents and the public on the recommended immunizations is an important nursing function. Parents who may feel that the immmunizations commonly given are for diseases that no longer exist or that are "simple childhood diseases" may not be motivated to seek immunization for their children. Understanding the risks of contracting these diseases and their potential sequelae is important. Parents should also know what the normal childhood immunizations are, rather than merely calling them all "baby shots."

Recent controversy surrounding the risks and benefits of the pertussis vaccine has prompted many parents to deny their children this immunization due to fear of death or permanent brain damage. The nurse should be prepared to discuss this situation with the parents. The Public Health Service ACIP reported that although local and mild reactions to this vaccine occur frequently, recent studies indicated that a debatable causal relationship between pertussis vaccine and permanent brain damage and an extremely low incidence of this side effect or death. The ACIP further estimated a 70-fold increase in pertussis cases and a fourfold increase in deaths if the pertussis immunization program was interrupted. The disease itself can be a serious illness, resulting in many major complications and possible death. The Public Health Service ACIP therefore strongly recommends routine immunization of infants and young children against pertussis (PHS, 1982; Centers for Disease Control, 1982).

Parents should not assume that a child over 18 months

old will not need further immunizations until school age, since disease patterns, available products, or recommended immunization may change. Parents should also be taught the importance of written immunization records. Included in the record should be the date of immunization, where it was obtained, the type of immunization, the specific variety (including lot number, if possible), and a description of any reactions that occurred. Parents should be informed that they should ask for and record the name of the immunization, such as Sabin TOPV, or Schwarz measles, in case future research should have implications for those receiving a certain drug or type.

The nurse should be aware that the immunization procedure may be more frightening for parents than for children. On sensing the parents' anxiety, children may also become anxious; time spent reassuring both parents and children is well spent. While good visualization and stability of the injection site are necessary, an infant often objects more to restraint than to the actual injection. Relaxation of the child is desirable, as tense, straining muscles will increase the pain and bleeding. Many infants respond well if the injection is administered while they are held over the parent's shoulder (as though being burped). Another useful position is to have an older infant sit across the parent's lap, with the child's legs held between the parent's legs, and the parent hugging the upper body of the child (see Fig. 49-1). Infants and children do not respond well to being held down on a hard examining table for their immunizations. Parents should also know the common symptoms of reaction to the immunization, their proper management, and the appropriate time to call the health care provider.

Evaluation

The nursing assessment and management with regard to immunization are evaluated on patient compliance with sug-

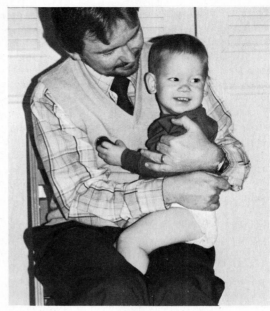

FIGURE 49-1

Suggested Position for Anterolateral Thigh Immunization. Positioning the toddler across the parent's thigh with his legs held between the parent's legs permits good visualization of the site, as well as stabilization and comfort of the child.

gested immunization schedules and on whether the patient develops the disease. The patient or parent's knowledge of indications and importance of immunizations should also be evaluated, as well as his or her ability to give an accurate immunization history and provide written records.

CASE STUDY

The T.L. family had three children living at home, Connie, 17; Kevin, 5; and Michael, 2 months. A notice was sent home from school stating that there was an epidemic of measles (rubeola or "hard measles" or "seven-day measles") among the children in the elementary school. Parents were encouraged to make sure that all children had received immunization for both measles and rubella. Mrs. L. called the community health nurse at the health department clinic to find out whether the children were protected. She also asked whether Michael should be given his first DTP immunization, as she had heard that the pertussis portions could cause serious side effects.

Assessment

Since the L. family was new to the area, the nurse questioned Mrs. L. about the children's immunization history, which she was able to supply from the written record she had maintained on each child. Connie had received the

killed-virus type of immunization for measles as an infant but had neither been vaccinated for rubella or mumps, nor ever had these illnesses. Kevin had received the MMR combination at 15 months of age, and Michael had not yet begun his initial immunization series.

Analyzing the children's records, the nurse felt that Connie was not protected against rubella, measles, or mumps. Kevin was completely protected. Because Michael was not exposed to other children outside the home, and as MMR immunizations are not usually given to children under 12 months, Michael should not need this immunization. However, the nurse strongly recommended that Michael receive his first DTP and TOPV vaccines.

Management

The nurse asked the mother to bring Michael and Connie to the clinic, where Connie would receive the MMR vaccine, and Michael would receive the DTP and TOPV. Mrs.

L. agreed to come and asked to discuss Michael's DTP with the nurse at that time.

Before administering the vaccine to Connie, the nurse explained to her that the rubella vaccine was potentially harmful to unborn babies if given to a pregnant woman or if the woman becomes pregnant within 2 months. Connie stated that she was currently having normal menses and was not sexually active. The necessity for contraception should she have intercourse in the next 2 months was indicated.

The nurse took Michael's temperature and, finding it normal, discussed the importance of the DTP immunization for Michael. The potential side effect of permanent brain damage from the pertussis immunization is felt to be of extremely low incidence by the ACIP and the AAP. The increased possibility of contracting pertussis, with its potential for severe side effects or death if Michael were not immunized, was stressed to the mother. She decided to immunize Michael with his first DTP at this time; the TOPV was also given.

Evaluation

No adverse effects of the immunizations or evidence of the diseases in the children were ever noted. Mrs. L. brought Michael to the clinic at 4 and 6 months of age for his second and third DTP and second TOPV vaccines, and at 15 months for the MMR immunization. An immunization record was started for Michael and was updated at each visit.

ENVIRONMENTAL AND OCCUPATIONAL HEALTH

LEARNING OBJECTIVES

Upon mastery of the content of this section, the reader will be able to:

1. Identify some of the major sources of environmental health hazards.
2. List the common routes of entry of hazardous environmental agents.
3. Discuss at least one example of an air polluting agent and its effect on human health.
4. Describe how pesticides and other chemicals can endanger water and food sources.
5. Identify populations at risk for specific environmental and occupational health hazards.
6. List several strategies for nursing involvement and occupational health issues.

The environment in which we live and work can have a profound impact on the quality of our life and health. Agents in the environment and work setting that can be toxic or hazardous to human tissues enter the body by inhalation, percutaneous absorption, ingestion, and sensory organ channels. Principal environmental health hazards are listed in Table 49-6. Each agent can impact human health, leading to acute conditions such as accidents, poisoning, respiratory, or skin diseases and chronic health conditions such as cancer and cardiovascular, genetic, respiratory, or neurologic diseases (see Table 49-7). Because chemical toxicants alter physiologic function, the resultant health problems may be considered *drug-induced diseases* (see Chap. 6).

AIR POLLUTION

Nearly 80 percent of the American population resides in urban areas where pollution from toxic gases and particulates can most directly affect health. Air pollution is often divided into two categories, based on type of chemical reaction involved. *Reducing type pollution* (smog) is characterized by incomplete combustion of coal combined with cool temperatures and fog, producing sulfur dioxide and smoke. The *oxidizing or photochemical air pollution* is characterized by hydrocarbons, nitrogen oxides, and photochemical oxidants. In these reactions inversion layers of polluted air over a city can sometimes occur due to the reaction of intensive sunlight on automobile exhaust and to meteorologic temperature differences. During inversion episodes, people with respiratory and cardiac diseases are at a high health risk. Research shows that carbon monoxide, sulfur oxides (including sulfur dioxide and sulfur-containing aerosols), and nitrogen oxides (including nitrous oxide and nitrite aerosols) account for 98 percent of air pollution.

Carbon Monoxide

The major pollutant, carbon monoxide (CO), is a colorless, odorless gas resulting from incomplete combustion of organic matter. In addition to automobile emissions, other sources of exposure to CO include inadequate furnace venting and cigarette smoking. Inhalation of CO leads to an increase in carboxyhemoglobin (COHb) concentration in the blood, which markedly decreases the capacity of hemoglobin to carry oxygen and to dissociate available oxyhemoglobin. Carbon monoxide toxicity first affects the central nervous system; as the blood becomes increasingly saturated, coma, convulsions, depressed cardiac and respiratory function, and death result.

Sulfur Dioxide

The combustion of sulfur-containing fossil fuels results in the respiratory irritant, sulfur dioxide (SO_2), which can cause

TABLE 49-6 Principal Environmental Health Hazards

GENERAL CATEGORY	SPECIFIC EXAMPLES
Air pollutants	Particulate or dust, sulfur dioxide (SO_2), ozone (O_3), hydrocarbons, carbon monoxide (CO), nitrogen oxides (NO_x), hydrogen sulfide (H_2S), mercaptans (RSH) and sulfides, carcinogens and heavy metals.
Water pollutants	Pathogenic bacteria, viruses, amoeba and other protozoa; mercury and other heavy metals; organic compounds (oxygen depleting); toxic substances—nitrite (NO_2^-), cyanide (CN^-); excess nutrients such as phosphate (PO_4^{3-}) and nitrate (NO_3^-), which cause algal blooms (eutrophication).
Industrial and occupational pollutants	*Physical:* Noise, thermal, cold, radiation. *Carcinogens:* asbestos, β-naphthylamine, soot, radium, radon, nitrosamines, benzo[a]pyrene. *Dusts:* Silica, cotton, sugar cane, coal dust. *Metals:* Beryllium (Be), lead (Pb), cadmium (Cd), mercury (Hg), arsenic (As), nickel (Ni), manganese (Mn), copper (Cu), etc. *Gases:* Halogens [chlorine (Cl_2), bromine (Br_2), and fluorine (F_2)], halogen acids [hydrogen fluoride (HF), hydrogen chloride (HCl), hydrogen bromide (HBr)], sulfur oxides (SO_x), nitrogen oxides (NO_x), ozone (O_3). *Organic toxins and solvents:* Carbon tetrachloride (CCl_4), benzene (C_6H_6), and other organic solvents. *Neurotoxins:* Parathion and other organophosphate insecticides.
Ecopoisons	Mercury, DDT, PCBs,* and other chlorinated hydrocarbons, petroleum (in water).
Food toxins	Produced by *Clostridium botulinum, Salmonella,* and *Staphlyococcus.*
Solid wastes	Organics, nonmetabolizable toxic substances, and heavy metals.

*Polychlorinated biphenyls.

Source: Reprinted with permission from Norman M. Trieff: *Environment and Health,* Ann Arbor: Ann Arbor Science Publishers, Inc., 1980.

bronchial constriction on inhalation. Some SO_2 in the atmosphere is partially converted to sulfuric acid and several sulfates; these chemicals can also cause bronchial constriction, especially when combined with atmospheric conditions such as fog and suspended particulates. Higher levels of SO_2 pollution have been associated with increased occurrence of respiratory infections and acute bronchitis. People with congenital or chronic pulmonary and cardiac diseases and those who smoke are especially at risk from SO_2 and particulate pollution.

Nitrogen Dioxide

Adverse health effects are also caused by nitrogen dioxide (NO_2). NO_2 is thought to penetrate membranes in the alveolar capillaries and, when it is converted there to nitric acid, it can cause pulmonary edema. At low concentrations, NO_2 causes lower respiratory illnesses. Silo fillers' disease (an occupational poisoning from NO_2 and CO inhalation), pulmonary edema, and bronchiolitis obliterans may result from acute high-level exposure to NO_2.

Thus, air pollutants can cause a variety of acute pulmonary diseases and exacerbate chronic conditions. Other notable examples include pulmonary fibrotic diseases from inhalation of asbestos or silicone particles. Another significant and potentially lethal health effect of many air pollutants, especially the particulates, is cancer. Asbestos, for example, has been positively linked with bronchial cancer and with mesothelioma, a rapidly fatal malignancy. These diseases can occur as long as 20 to 30 years after exposure.

WATER POLLUTION

Toxic agents found in water can be caused by such human-produced chemicals as industrial wastes and pesticides or biologic pollutants such as sewage which contains bacteria and viruses. Water pollution can affect health directly through ingestion or skin contact or indirectly through chemical contamination of human food sources. Water pollution may also be a major cause of carcinogenesis and mutagenesis (birth defects).

Chemical water pollutants include pesticides, petroleum products, and inorganic compounds. Another chemical pollutant, acid rain, occurs as rain droplets pass through the atmosphere, acquiring or reacting with chemicals such as nitrogen oxides, ammonia, and sulfur oxides. These reactions can produce acids such as sulfuric acid droplets that can destroy plants, trees, roads, bridges, and aquatic life.

Cardiovascular diseases and cancer are two serious health problems which have been linked to chemical water pollution. Ingestion of biologically polluted water causes diseases such as shigellosis, typhoid fever, and hepatitis. Seafood and crops irrigated with polluted water can become contaminated and spread disease to animals or to humans ingesting them. Skin contact with contaminated water is another health concern.

Pesticides are often a major contaminant of water and food supplies; insecticides, rodenticides, fungicides, herbicides, and fumigants are all types of pesticides. Incidents involving polychlorinated biphenyls (PCBs) and polybrominated biphenyls (PBBs) illustrate the dangers of these chemicals. PCBs have been found in human tissues and breast milk. Accidental PBB contamination of cattle feed has led to growth deformities in the cattle and high tissue levels of PBBs in humans. The toxic effects of DDT are also well documented, including CNS disturbances and possible carcinogenesis.

TABLE 49-7   Major Health Manifestations of Principal Pollutants in Large Doses

MANIFESTATION	POLLUTANT*	MANIFESTATION	POLLUTANT*
Aging (premature)	Ozone; PAN; other oxidants, radiation	Dermatitis	Nickel, chromium, arsenic, formaldehyde, organophosphates
Alopecia (loss of hair)	Lead, arsenic, radiation	Emphysema	Most respiratory pollutants
Anemia	Lead, molybdenum, vanadium	Eye irritation	Ozone, PAN, formaldehyde, nitrogen oxides, acrolein, ammonia
Asthma			
Allergic	Fungi, pollen; TDI, cobalt, epoxy resins, respiratory pollutants	Fever	Manganese, zinc, boron, other metals
Nonallergic	Fungi, pollen; TDI, cobalt, epoxy resins, respiratory pollutants	Fibrosis (scarring) of lungs	Quartz, silica, selenium, cobalt, iron
Ataxia	Manganese, fluorides	Gastroenteritis	Lead, mercury, fluorides, arsenic, zinc, selenium
Bone disease	Strontium, fluorides		
Brain involvement	Boron, carbon monoxide, lead, mercury, zinc	Hypertension, arteriosclerosis	Cadmium, barium, organophosphates, carbon monoxide
Bronchitis	Irritating gases	Headaches	Lead, fluoride, carbon monoxide
Cancer		Kidney disease	Lead, mercury, selenium, cadmium
Abdomen	Nickel carbonate	Leukemia	Atomic explosions, radionuclides
Bones	Strontium	Liver disease	Molybdenum, selenium, chlorinated hydrocarbons
Gallbladder	Nitrosamines		
Lungs	Asbestos, beryllium, nickel carbonate benzo[a]pyrene	Melanosis (dark skin)	Arsenic
Nose, sinuses	Selenium, nickel carbonate, chromium, strontium	Mesothelioma	Asbestos
Skin	Arsenic	Myalgia (muscle weakness and pain)	Fluorides, lead
Testicles	Cadmium	Mutagenic agents	Chlorinated hydrocarbons, lead, arsenic, cadmium, radionuclides, mercury
Coronary heart disease	Carbon monoxide, cadmium, hydrogen sulfide		
Cyanosis	Nitrites, carbon monoxide	Nasal irritation (septum)	Nickel, chromium, arsenic, selenium
Dental caries	Selenium	Visual reduction	Ozone, selenium, fluoride

*PAN = peroxyacetyl nitrate (photoactivated air pollutant); TDI = toluene diiodocyanate
Source: Reprinted with permission from George L. Waldbott: *Health Effects of Environmental Pollutants,* 2d ed., St. Louis: Mosby, 1978.

Another important environmental hazard is ionizing radiation. Naturally occurring radioactive materials found in water, soil, and air account for nearly half of the ionizing radiation to which the public is exposed. Another 45 percent of radiation comes from medical and dental diagnostic and treatment materials while only 5 percent comes from nuclear power production, industry and consumer products. Ionizing radiation can cause cancer, genetic defects, and tissue damage.

OCCUPATIONAL HEALTH PROBLEMS

Each occupational environment exposes its workers to a variety of chemical toxicants. Environmental lung diseases represent a major occupational health concern. Depending on the type of work environment, many different agents can affect the worker's respiratory health status, causing acute and chronic lung infections, obstructive ventilatory disorders, and cancer. Some examples of hazardous agents and their sequelae include silicates (silicosis), carbon and coal dusts (black lung disease), and bacteria (e.g., tuberculosis, anthrax). Some common hazardous agents in the workplace are listed in Table 49-8.

Occupational Hazards during Pregnancy

Increasingly, women are working outside their homes and are employed in nearly every occupation. Many women work well into their third trimester of pregnancy, exposing themselves and their developing fetuses to a variety of chemical toxicants and ionizing radiation. Even their husbands' occupations may affect conception and the health of the fetus. Vinyl chloride (used in the plastics industry), lead, and hydrocarbons (used in many industries) can cause reproductive failure in both men and women. Birth defects have been linked to many chemical toxicants, for example, anesthetic gases; an increased incidence of birth defects has occurred in families of men, as well as women, working in operating rooms.

Three types of compounds have been found to affect reproductive function: mutagens, teratogens, and carcinogens. Mutagens cause a change in genetic material and can lead to miscarriage, congenital defects, mental retardation, and other abnormalities. Teratogens are toxic agents which affect fetal development after conception, and carcinogens induce cancer which often occurs many years after prenatal exposure to the agent [e.g., diethylstilbestrol (DES) can cause cervical cancer in women whose mothers took this drug during their pregnancy]. Major occupational toxicants that have known or suspected effects on reproduction include: toluene, mercury, carbon tetrachloride, chloromethyl ether, nearly all pesticides, and chlorinated hydrocarbons. Atomic particles, ionizing radiation, and microwaves can be hazardous to persons employed in nuclear industries, the health fields, computer and word processing, and other occupations. Other potential hazards during pregnancy include inhaled chemicals such as ozone, asbestos, carbon monoxide, and anesthetic gases. Hair dyes and other cosmetology agents, chemicals used in painting, arts and crafts, dry cleaning, the textile industry, electronics, and a variety of manufacturing industries are all potential hazards to pregnant women and their offspring.

The Health Professions

People employed in the health professions are exposed daily to numerous occupational hazards. Examples include mercury (used by dental personnel), anesthetic gases, radioisotopes, x-rays, infectious diseases, hexachlorophene, chloromethyl ether, and toluene. Inhalation or skin contact with these agents, or exposure to ionizing radiation can have carcinogenic effects on the worker and possible mutagenic or teratogenic effects on a fetus. Some unique health hazards to which health care workers are exposed, in addition to infections and higher risk for disease, include withdrawal angina caused by handling nitroglycerin and an increased risk of fetal deaths in pregnant anesthetists. Antineoplastic agents are also thought to have deleterious effects on the health of nurses and other health care professionals handling these substances. All antineoplastic agents should be prepared in a biohazard hood and, in general, in the pharmacy, where personnel have the requisite training and equipment.

TABLE 49-8 Some Common Hazardous Agents in the Workplace

CAUSATIVE AGENT	CONDITION CAUSED
Dust: SiO_2, carbon, beryllium, asbestos, cotton, moldy grain	Pneumoconiosis: occupational pulmonary disabling disease due to inhalation of dusts
Chemical irritants	Industrial dermatosis
Noise	Noise-induced hearing loss
Chemical agents	Acid or alkaline burns, ocular damage
Metal fumes: Zn, Sn, etc.	Metal fume fever
Heavy metal poisoning: Pb, Cd, etc.	Neurologic cardiac toxicity
Organic solvent inhalation: chlorinated hydrocarbons	Liver and kidney involvements
Carcinogenic agents: Benzo[a]pyrene, β-naphthylamine, radium, radon	Tumors

Source: Reprinted with permission from Norman M. Trieff: *Environment and Health,* Ann Arbor: Ann Arbor Science Publishers, Inc., 1980.

NURSING PROCESS RELATED TO ENVIRONMENTAL AND OCCUPATIONAL HEALTH

Assessment

Identification of toxic environmental agents is the first step toward prevention of their adverse health effects. Local and state governments are working to reduce the vulnerability of their citizens to these substances by enacting monitoring programs and passing laws to regulate emisssions, sewage disposal, and use of pesticides. Community health nurses often participate in surveillance programs in which health appraisals identify chronic illnesses and toxic effects in humans.

Nurses working in occupational health settings must become familiar with principles of toxicology and epidemiology and identify rapid sources of information about occupational diseases such as the National Institute for Occupational Safety and Health (NIOSH) publication *Occupational Diseases, A Guide to Their Recognition* (1977). An accurate history and physical of workers and safety surveillance are also essential to the occupational health nursing role. Nurses in every setting, however, should incorporate a thorough occupational history into the health history, being especially aware of this issue with women clients of childbearing age.

Management

Agencies of the federal govenment such as the Environmental Protection Agency, the Department of Health and Human Services, and the National Cancer Institute are involved in regulatory as well as research activities related to environmental health hazards. Nurses serve on regulatory boards and commissions, undertake research investigations, and participate in special health care delivery projects in their communities. Likewise, occupational health nurses are involved at the local, state, and national levels in policy making, legislative, and research activities related to occupational health hazards. Occupational health nurses are also involved in health promotion and protection activities within their industries. For example, the nurse might counsel a pregnant worker to change her work site to decrease the risk of exposure to mutagenic or teratogenic agents or radiation.

Nurses practicing in community settings including public health and home health agencies, schools, and industries must be aware of these health hazards and work toward some definitive interventions to protect the health of all individuals within the community. Public education, health education, health screening, and political involvement in community health issues, however, may be the most powerful roles nurses can take in the management of environmental health hazards.

Evaluation

Occupational and environmental health programs are generally of such a broad scope that evaluation research studies must be undertaken to appraise their effectiveness, In some settings the nurse maintains records and/or performs this research. Nurses must also be apprised of private and governmental studies and consult these resources for information on the effectiveness of education, screening, and pollution control programs.

DRUG ABUSE

LEARNING OBJECTIVES

Upon mastery of this section, the reader will be able to:

1. Define tolerance, psychologic dependence, physical dependence, abstinence syndrome.
2. Name the primary pharmacologic actions of alcohol.
3. Give specific effects of alcohol on various organ systems, particularly from its chronic consumption.
4. Give five major criteria for the diagnosis of alcoholism.
5. List the advantages and disadvantages of using various sedative-hypnotic drugs in the management of the chronic alcoholic patient and the alcoholic patient in withdrawal.
6. Give six major manifestations of the acute alcohol withdrawal phenomenon.
7. Describe specific nursing interventions that can be implemented to assist an acutely intoxicated or withdrawing patient from alcohol.
8. Describe the unique pharmacokinetics of the benzodiazepine drugs when given to alcoholic patients.
9. Describe the behavioral and physiologic effects of alcohol in a nonalcoholic person at a given blood level of alcohol.
10. Describe the importance of taking an accurate alcohol intake history for patients known or suspected to be alcohol-dependent.
11. Describe the role of disulfiram in the management of chronic alcoholism.
12. Describe the disulfiram-alcohol reaction.
13. Give at least four specific examples of alcohol-drug interactions.
14. List major nutritional deficiencies associated with chronic alcoholism.
15. Describe two major neurologic effects of chronic excessive use of alcohol and describe their treatment.
16. Explain the general management of acute narcotic intoxication.
17. Describe the role of narcotic antagonists in the treatment of an acute narcotic drug overdose.
18. Describe the role of methadone in the detoxification process for opiate dependency.
19. Describe the major manifestations of the opiate withdrawal syndrome and tell how they differ from the manifestations of alcohol and barbiturate withdrawal.
20. Explain the use of nonnarcotic symptomatic medical management of the opiate withdrawal syndrome.
21. Give specific examples of the pathologic effects of chronic use of opiates on various organ systems and the medical complications from drug abuse.
22. Give at least three specific examples of medically useful drugs that pose a significant risk for abuse and dependency.
23. List specific examples of the most widely abused sedative-hypnotic drugs.
24. Characterize sedative-hypnotic drug dependency and the detoxification process involved in its treatment.
25. Describe the use of nicotine resin complex in tobacco withdrawal.
26. Give three examples of prescription drugs that are often sought in the polydrug abuse or misuse circumstance.
27. Give at least three specific examples of widely used or available psychedelic and hallucinogenic drugs.
28. Explain the general principles in the management

of "bad trips" from psychedelic and hallucinogenic drugs.

29. Characterize the clinical manifestations of amphetamine abuse.

30. Describe the treatment of toxic reaction and withdrawal symptoms from amphetamine abuse.

31. Characterize the clinical effects of cocaine.

32. Describe the treatment of toxic reactions from overdose with cocaine.

33. Outline the nursing process related to addictive disorders.

The recognition and management of the acute toxic effects or withdrawal reactions of alcohol, opiates, depressants, stimulants, hallucinogens, and other consciousness-altering substances is frequently complicated by the presence of complex physiologic and psychologic disturbances. The diagnosis and treatment of acute drug intoxication or withdrawal syndrome is often begun on the basis of clinical impressions without a clear idea of the agent(s) responsible. This section directs attention to the symptoms of drug-dependent disorders, briefly reviews the pharmacology of substances of abuse and misuse, and discusses the management and care of acute toxic and withdrawal effects of these drugs, mindful of the critical role of nurses in this effort.

In this chapter, alcohol and other addictive and mind-altering drugs are treated separately. This should *not* be construed as indicating that they are different in any significant way. While there are differences in social attitudes toward drinking and drug abuse, many features of alcohol and "hard drugs" are remarkably similar. Many drug abuse encounters involve a multiplicity of substances in addition to alcohol; therefore, their similarities and differences should be appreciated and understood by those who are involved in the diagnosis, treatment, care, and rehabilitation of drug-dependent patients. The purpose of this section is to facilitate the attempt at becoming more aware of these concerns.

TERMINOLOGY

What is *drug dependence* and how is it recognized? Drug dependence has three aspects: *psychologic dependency, physical dependency,* and *tolerance.* Psychologic dependency involves the compulsive use of and craving for a drug. Physical dependency is characterized by a series of physiologic events that occur when the drug is discontinued, including the withdrawal or abstinence syndrome. Tolerance develops when the continued use of a drug is required and increasing doses are needed to produce the same effect.

While the most important feature of addictive disorders is the psychologic dependency, it is the least understood of the three factors. A person can be made physically dependent on a drug but addiction or abuse may not be deter-

mined until behavioral effects secondary to psychologic dependence are present. Many persons consume alcoholic beverages, but relatively few (approximately 10 percent) develop physical and psychologic dependency on alcohol. With narcotics and the sedative-hypnotic drugs, the risk of physical and psychologic dependence and addiction is much greater. When patients are detoxified, the physical symptoms of dependence (withdrawal syndrome and tolerance) are quickly reversed. In the drug-dependent person, this process will have little if any effect on the psychologic dependence.

ALCOHOL (ETHANOL, ETHYL ALCOHOL)

Alcohol is the most misused drug in the United States today. Estimation of the incidence of alcoholism in the United States ranges from 10 to 15 million persons. It is a condition far more common than generally perceived, with only 3 to 5 percent of the country's alcoholic population classified as the "skid row" or public inebriate type. Alcoholics come from all levels of our society; the majority are found in the working and homemaking population, and the problems related to alcohol abuse and alcoholism are increasing. The economic costs associated with the misuse of alcohol are estimated to exceed $40 billion a year. Alcoholism is a true *illness,* but years may go by before recognizable pathologies develop. It can considerably shorten the life span and has recently been shown to have teratogenic effects. Certain individuals such as adolescents, women, and the elderly may experience major medical complications from the chronic use of alcohol in much less time than other persons. Alcoholism is a treatable illness when diagnosed in its early stages. Alcoholism is a diagnosis not easily made by the health practitioner, since the early clues and findings for this condition are subtle at best. The situation is further complicated by the acknowledged higher incidence of alcoholism among health professionals when compared to other occupations. Subconscious denial that this problem exists may be contributing to this oversight and the relatively little importance often given to its recognition and treatment by the physician, nurse, or other practitioners involved. In general, the prevailing attitude in the United States toward excessive alcohol consumption can be described as confused, ignorant, and often ambivalent.

Alcohol is a dependency-producing drug, since those persons who abuse it generally experience physical and psychologic dependency and tolerance. It is a psychoactive drug which can be characterized pharmacologically as a sedative-hypnotic. While able to provide anxiety relief and sedation at one dose level, it produces sleep and central nervous system depression at higher levels.

Alcohol is present in a variety of popular beverages: beer and ale are products of the fermentation of cereals and are 3 to 6% alcohol; wine is the result of the fermentation of yeast on sugars present in fruits and contains 11 to 12%

alcohol; brandy is produced from the distillation of wine products and usually contains 40% alcohol; hard liquors are the distillates of fermented products such as grain, available as gin, rye, bourbon, and vodka, and contain approximately 40 to 50% alcohol by volume (commonly expressed by a proof number that is twice the alcohol concentration by volume).

Pharmacokinetics

Alcohol is fully absorbed by the stomach and proximal small intestine in 30 to 120 min after ingestion. Absorption is direct, by simple (passive) diffusion, and alcohol distributes itself freely in body tissues and fluids. The concentration of alcohol in the brain rapidly approaches that in the blood following completed absorption. Factors that modify alcohol absorption are volume, dilution, rate of ingestion, and presence of food in the stomach. Interestingly, carbonation increases the absorption of alcohol. Alcohol also crosses the placenta and may be found in the milk of lactating mothers.

While most drugs are known to be metabolized or cleared from the body in a fixed percentage of the dose taken (first-order pharmacokinetics), alcohol is unique in that it is eliminated from the blood in a fixed amount over time (zero-order pharmacokinetics). In a 70-kg (approximately 150-pound) person, the rate of alcohol metabolism approximates 7 g/h. At this rate of metabolism, the blood alcohol level will decline at a rate of 15 mg/100 mL/h. An average "shot" of distilled spirit, 86-proof, contains about 15 g of ethyl alcohol; since body water approximates 65 percent of body weight in a 70-kg person, the blood alcohol content following one shot will be 15 g/50 L, or 30 mg/dL, with 50 L being the approximate volume of total body water calculated from the percentage of weight. If one "shot" is taken in one swallow, it will take approximately 2 h for the blood alcohol level to return to zero. A 70-kg person would have a blood alcohol concentration of 100 mg/mL (the amount legally defined as intoxification in most states) after drinking, within 1 h, any of the following: five 12-oz cans of beer; or four 4-oz glasses of table wine; or five 1-oz shots of distilled spirits; or three 3-oz martinis; or four 8-oz mixed highballs.

The liver is the main site of oxidation of ethyl alcohol. The alcohol is oxidized by alcohol dehydrogenase to acetaldehyde, which subsequently is oxidized by aldehyde dehydrogenase to acetate, or acetyl coenzyme A. This enters the Krebs cycle to form carbon dioxide and water or to participate in protein and fat synthesis. Both oxidizing enzymes are responsible for converting nicotinamide adenine dinucleotide (NAD) to NADH, which has been thought to contribute to the many metabolic abnormalities (e.g., hyperlipidemia, ketosis, hyperlactacidemia, hyperuricemia) associated with chronic alcohol ingestion. Acetaldehyde, the first metabolite of ethanol, may be more slowly metabolized in alcoholics and has been implicated in the pathogenesis of alcohol-induced tissue toxicity.

Intoxication and Blood Alcohol Concentration

The relationship between blood ethyl alcohol concentration and clinical signs and symptoms of intoxication are variable and depend on rate of ingestion, amount consumed, alterations in absorption, metabolism, excretion, and chronicity of exposure (Table 49-9). As a consequence of tolerance, higher blood alcohol concentrations may be required in alcoholics to produce clinical effects as compared with occasional drinkers.

The diagnosis of alcoholism is difficult since there is little agreement on the definition of alcoholism. The clinical signs and subtleties of the condition are varied and without reliable parameters. Much depends on the experience and motivation of the observer in deciding whether a patient is suffering from alcoholism or not. Although not absolute, the criteria established by the National Council on Alcoholism (NCA) can serve as a convenient starting point for the diagnosis of alcohol dependence (Table 49-10).

Medical Complications

Alcoholics have an alarmingly high incidence of diseases and disorders. Alcohol affects almost every organ system in the body. The more important and known medical complications and pathologic consequences from excessive alcohol consumption are summarized in Table 49-11.

The *lethal dose* of alcohol is variable. In adults, it is 5 to 8 g/kg of body weight. In children, it is approximately 3 g/kg of body weight. The ratio of therapeutic to toxic doses of alcohol is about 1:5—low by comparison with some of the other sedative-hypnotics. **Diazepam** (Valium) and **chlor-**

TABLE 49-9 Blood Ethanol Concentrations and Clinical Effects in the Nontolerant Drinker

BLOOD ETHANOL, mg/mL	CLINICAL EFFECTS
20–99	Slight changes in mood and feelings, progressing to muscular incoordination, impaired sensory function, personality and behavioral changes (talkative, noisy, morose)
100–149	Marked mental impairment, boastful, remorseful, combative, incoordination, clumsiness and unsteadiness in standing or walking (ataxia), prolonged reaction time, gross intoxication
150–199	Decreased pain sensation, slurred speech, muscle incoordination, drowsiness, stupor
200–299	Acute intoxication, marked decrease in response to stimuli, incoordination, nausea, vomiting, diplopia, marked ataxia, stupor
300–399	Hypothermia, severe dysarthria, amnesia, stage 1 anesthesia, hypotension, tachycardia
400–700	Coma, respiratory failure, and death

TABLE 49-10 Summary of Diagnostic Criteria of Alcoholism

Major Criteria

(Definitive, obligatory; it is sufficient for the diagnosis of alcoholism that any of these criteria can be fulfilled)

Physiologic conditions:
Use of alcohol results in withdrawal symptoms upon cessation of drinking, e.g., gross tremor, hallucinations, seizures, delirium tremens.

Use of alcohol results in tolerance, i.e., blood level of 150 mg/100 mL without apparent intoxication, a level of 300 mg/100 mL or more at any time or a history of regular ingestion of one-fifth distilled spirits or 2 quarts fortified wine or 3 quarts table wine or twenty-three 12-oz bottles of beer or equivalent in one day for a 180-lb person.

Clinical conditions:
Use of alcohol results in diagnosable alcohol-related organ damage, e.g., alcoholic hepatitis or alcoholic cerebellar generation.

Behavioral conditions:
Blatant and indiscriminate use of alcohol continued in spite of medical and social contraindications, e.g., alcohol-related organ damage or social and psychologic disruption.

Minor Criteria

(Probable: Strong suspicion of alcoholism if several criteria are present)

Physiologic and clinical conditions:
Use of alcohol results in amnesia ("blackout periods"), fatty liver in absence of other possible causes, pancreatitis with cholelithiasis, chronic gastritis, peripheral neuropathy, alcoholic myopathy, or cardiomyopathy.

Behavioral conditions:
Constant and repetitive use of alcohol results in drinking alone and surreptitious use of alcohol; spouse complains about drinking; the person admits to drinking more than peers, outbursts of rage and suicidal gestures while drinking; loss of interest in activities not directly associated with drinking; failure of repeated attempts at abstinence; "skid-row" social behavior.

Minor Criteria

(Possible: Manifestations are common in many persons but are not in themselves strong indicators of alcoholism; suspicion should be aroused and further evidence sought)

Physiologic and clinical conditions:
Patient presents with unexplained hypoglycemia, lactic acid and uric acid elevation, potassium and chloride depletion, SGOT elevation, EEG abnormalities, hyperreflexia or hyporeflexia, hematologic abnormalities (anemia), beriberi, scurvy, pellagra, decreased immune response, or increased incidence of infections.

Behavioral conditions:
Patient presents with unexplained depression, paranoia, frequent accidents, major family disruptions, job loss, increasing interpersonal difficulties; chooses employment that facilitates or encourages drinking; gulps drinks.

diazepoxide (Librium), for example, have a ratio of therapeutic to toxic doses of approximately 1:7000.

Management of Acute Alcohol Abstinence (Withdrawal) Syndrome

Acute abstinence or minor withdrawal syndrome is a common problem experienced by the alcoholic when alcohol is discontinued or the blood alcohol level decreases; *delirium tremens* (DTs, major withdrawal) is the most severe form. The severity of the withdrawal syndrome cannot always be predicted on the basis of quantity or duration of alcohol ingestion. While most patients experience only minor symptoms, it is difficult to rule out the possibility that progressively more severe and even life-threatening withdrawal reactions may occur. The early physiologic and behavioral effects of acute alcohol abstinence (8 to 36 h after cessation of drinking) includes tremors ("shakes"), increased blood pressure, pulse, respiration rate, temperature, intermittent hallucinations, seizures ("rum fits"), sleep disturbance, and sweating. Major withdrawal syndrome or delirium tremens,

TABLE 49-11 Medical Complications of Alcohol

ACUTE INGESTION	CHRONIC ALCOHOLISM
Fluid and electrolyte abnormalities	Increased morbidity and mortality
Hypoglycemia or hyperglycemia	Liver disease:
	Alcoholic hepatitis
	Alcoholic cirrhosis
Acute fatty liver	Portal hypertension
	Ascites
Encephalopathy	Esophageal varicies
Acute gastritis	Gastrointestinal problems:
	Peptic ulcer
Malabsorption diarrhea	Pancreatitis
	Malabsorption
Myopathy	
	Cardiomyopathy
Injuries: burns, skeletal injury, hypothermia	Chronic myopathy
	Immune impairment and infection
Fetal alcohol syndrome	Hematologic diseases:
	Thrombocytopenia
	Anemia
	Leukopenia
	Neurologic:
	Polyneuropathy
	Cerebellar degeneration
	Organic brain syndrome (dementia)
	Wernicke's disease
	Korsakoff's psychosis
	Skin disorders
	Fetal alcohol syndrome

which occur 3 to 5 days after cessation of drinking, is characterized by profound disorientation and frightening hallucinations, marked agitation and excitation, fever, tachycardia, severe diaphoresis, severe tremors, marked sleep disturbances, and other major life-threatening complications. Polydrug abuse is common in the chronic alcoholic. Withdrawal from barbiturates and opiates may be further complications encountered.

Patients with delirium tremens are seriously ill and should be considered to be a medical emergency. Although the mortality rate for this condition has decreased during the past 50 years, deaths from DTs still occur (variously estimated at 7 to 15 percent), particularly in those patients with underlying or associated diseases such as pancreatitis or cirrhosis.

It should not be taken for granted that intoxicated or bizarre behavior in alcoholics is an effect of alcohol alone; hypoglycemia may be a contributing problem, and glucose may be needed.

Drug Therapy During Alcohol Withdrawal

The object of detoxification is to remove alcohol from the body with as few withdrawal symptoms as possible. This process involves the substitution of a long-acting sedative-hypnotic drug for a shorter-acting one, alcohol. In carefully conducted studies of the effectiveness of such drugs in treating withdrawal syndrome, little value over placebo is shown. The major benefit of the antianxiety agents may accrue to the staff as the patient is made more manageable.

Benzodiazepines The sedative-hypnotic drugs of the benzodiazepine group (e.g., diazepam, chlordiazepoxide, etc.) are longer-acting and safer when compared with other sedative-hypnotic drugs (e.g., barbiturates, paraldehyde, etc.). They do not produce gastritis, and they also have antiseizure properties. They are used also because of the convenient dose forms available. The usual therapeutic end-point is to produce a calmed but awake patient by using whatever doses are required.

The pharmacokinetics of the benzodiazepines in patients undergoing alcohol withdrawal or in patients with mild liver impairment are of clinical interest. In alcoholic cirrhosis, the elimination of **diazepam** (Valium) from the body is presumably decreased because of decreased clearance by the liver and increased tissue distribution. Since the major metabolites of diazepam, **chlordiazepoxide** (Librium) and **clorazepate** (Tranxene), are also psychoactive, accumulation of effects during chronic administration of this drug should be evaluated in patients with cirrhosis. There is no evidence to suggest that any one of the benzodiazepines is a better choice for use of detoxification than any other. **Oxazepam** (Serax) is similar to the other benzodiazepines in its effectiveness in alcohol withdrawal. Because it is metabolized to an inactive product, this drug has been given to patients with hepatic disorders. The relatively slow oral absorption and the lack of parental dose forms of oxazepam has limited its popularity for use in alcohol detoxification.

Dosage requirements of these drugs for detoxification are quite variable. The usual range for **diazepam** (Valium) is 15 to 200 mg given in divided doses during the first 24 h, but a few cases require up to 1000 mg or even more. It should be remembered that withdrawing alcoholics may require a higher sedative-hypnotic drug dose than other agitated patients, probably because of tolerance and decreased sensitivity. Because dosage requirements are variable, no fixed dose schedule can be predicted for a given patient. In mild to moderate withdrawal syndrome, an initial oral diazepam dose of 20 mg can be given, followed by 10 to 20 mg q2–3h. Elderly patients should receive 10 mg initially. Regular orders for repetitive doses should be discouraged. The patient should be reevaluated and drug requirements reassessed every few hours until initial sedation is achieved, then at least daily during the maintenance phase. In severe withdrawal, intravenous diazepam is given in a dose of 10 to 30 mg until the patient is calm. Then a maintenance regimen of 10 to 20 mg as needed during the day and for sleep can be given. Intramuscular administration of diazepam or chlordiazepoxide should be avoided because of its slow and erratic absorption. The risks of hypotension and respiratory depression should always be assessed when sedative-hypnotic drugs are given simultaneously. Attempts at complete eradication of withdrawal symptoms should be avoided since this usually infers overmedication.

Drugs of Doubtful Value

Phenothiazines The major tranquilizers [e.g., **chlorpromazine** (Thorazine)] have not been shown to be more effective than the sedative-hypnotics in the treatment of acute alcohol abstinence. They can result in increased incidence of seizures, extrapyramidal effects, and postural hypotension.

Phenytoin Phenytoin (Dilantin) has been advocated for routine use in alcohol withdrawal to prevent seizures. However, there is no evidence that the drug actually prevents seizures associated with alcohol abstinence.

Paraldehyde The difficulty in administering paraldehyde, its variability in dose-response, and the current recommended use of safer drugs (e.g., benzodiazepines) should make for less use of this drug in treating alcohol withdrawal. A major complication from the metabolism of paraldehyde is metabolic acidosis, which can further complicate an already altered acid-base status.

Antihistamines Antihistamines such as **hydroxyzine** (Atarax, Vistaril) have sometimes been recommended and used in alcohol withdrawal. Therapeutic benefits are only equivocal, however.

TABLE 49-12   Nursing Management Related to Alcohol Withdrawal Syndromes

NURSING DIAGNOSIS	GOAL	NURSING ACTIVITIES
Impending minor (acute) or major (delerium tremens; DTs) withdrawal syndrome	Detect changes in vital signs that indicate increase in agitation or of complicating conditions associated with withdrawal	Check vital signs hourly for first 4 h after admission, then q4h for 24 h, then tid. If pulse reaches 100 or more and blood pressure exceeds 150/90 in the absence of concurrent illnesses, drugs with a cross-tolerance to alcohol (benzodiazepines) may be ordered. Assess duration of drinking episode, time of last drink, amount, nature of past withdrawal experience, and presence of other illnesses or acute conditions to determine potential severity of withdrawal reaction. Explain procedures to client.
Agitation, anxiety, fatigue, insomnia, and belligerence due to CNS stimulation in withdrawal	Promote decreased psychomotor agitation; rest and relaxation; adequate sleep; decreased feelings of anxiety	Maintain a quiet, orderly, calm environment. Eliminate extraneous noises. Inform client of procedures and what is happening to him/her. Talk in a quiet reassuring manner. Use consistent approach. Keep lighting even and bright enough to minimize the creating of shadows but not so bright as to cause glare. Administer sedating medications promptly as ordered. Evaluate their effectiveness. Do not undersedate. If necessary, transfer to a more secure ward.
Potential malnutrition related to gastric distress, nausea, and poor eating habits	Attain client status of absence of nausea or gastric distress, retention of food and liquids, regular intake of meals	Bland foods, high-protein, high-carbohydrate, low-fat diet is usually best. Provide frequent small feedings. Administer antiemetic medication and antacids for gastric distress as ordered. Evaluate effectiveness of medications. Administer vitamin B preparations as ordered.
Potential seizures	Prevent seizures associated with withdrawal; no occurrence of seizure activity	Administer anticonvulsant medications as ordered. Evaluate effectiveness. Observe seizure precautions especially if patient has past history of seizure activity during withdrawal. Initiate measures to assist patient during and after a seizure.
Perceptual ability greatly decreased from hallucinations and delirium (symptoms of delirium tremens)	Promote orientation to reality by controlling environmental stimuli and decreasing possibility of distortion; no symptoms of DTs	Observe for such symptoms of impending or current DTs as increased tremors, fever, elevated pulse and blood pressure, excitement, anxiety, increased disorientation, hallucinations, rigidity, and convulsions. Provide isolation, physical protection, and restraint as needed (transfer to more secure unit if needed). Maintain quiet and calm environment. Administer medication as ordered and evaluate effectiveness. Minimize number of people in contact with patient. Remain with patient during this time, orient to surroundings, talk slowly in modulated tones, and move deliberately.
Guilt associated with alcoholic behavior pattern	Promote decreased sense of guilt and interest in treatment	Interact with patient in a nonjudgmental and accepting manner, even with relapses. Maintain contact at regular specified times. Discuss with patient and significant others the available treatment programs and facts about alcoholism after the withdrawal period (refer to others for this information if necessary).

Fructose Solutions of 10% and 40% fructose given intravenously, increase the rate of ethanol elimination and decrease the duration of intoxication. However, side effects (e.g., lactic acidosis, hyperuricemia, fructose intolerance, gastrointestinal discomfort) make the use of fructose in acute alcohol intoxication less than desirable.

NURSING PROCESS RELATED TO ACUTE ALCOHOL WITHDRAWAL

Refer to Table 49-12 for an overview of the nursing management of the acute abstinence syndrome.

Alcohol-Drug Interactions

Since approximately 70 to 80 percent of adults consume alcoholic beverages, it is almost inevitable that medications either prescribed by a physician or bought over the counter will be taken concomitantly with alcohol or while alcohol is still in the body. Worsening of a patient's condition or failure to respond to drug therapy is almost always assumed to be due to exacerbation of the disease state; the concomitant use of alcohol is seldom considered as a contributing factor. Alcohol is not found only in alcoholic beverages; many common prescriptions and readily available nonprescription preparations also contain significant amounts of alcohol (Table 49-13). Often these preparations are sources of the alcohol which interacts with prescribed medications to produce uptoward effects in the unsuspecting patient (Table 49-14).

Management of Chronic Alcoholism

Detoxification is often completed in 7 to 10 days, but it may take many months for the physiologic processes to return to normal. In managing the chronic alcoholic, the goal is to achieve and maintain sobriety or to prolong periods of sobriety, giving the patient the opportunity to cope with the cause(s) of the excessive drinking. It is commonly thought that alcoholism is primarily a manifestation of underlying psychiatric problems, and while the patient continues to drink, most methods of treatment and of dealing with those problems will not succeed.

There are various types of treatment facilities that provide care for the chronic alcoholic. The most effective alcohol treatment facilities offer coherent organization, aggressive intake and follow-up procedures, in addition to a wide selection of carefully constructed treatment options. Examples of types of alcohol treatment facilities include: community alcohol centers, alcoholism inpatient treatment programs, aversion-conditioning hospitals, halfway houses, alcoholism outpatient clinics, and rehabilitation programs

in businesses and industries. Alcoholics Anonymous (AA) is not a treatment facility but provides a means of regaining lost social esteem and social status, while providing a framework for resocialization and the development of a new ideology of life in a structured approach (called the "12 Steps and Traditions"). AA operates best in collaboration with other treatment facilities, rather than as an intrinsic part of treatment programs. Alanon and Alateen are based on the AA approach, but are geared for family members and significant other persons associated with an individual who is an alcoholic. In some parts of the country, there are groups modeled after AA principles called Alatots which are for children who come from alcoholic homes. Nurses need to be aware of what alcoholism treatment facilities are available in the community so that appropriate referrals can be made.

Disulfiram

Disulfiram (Antabuse) interferes with the metabolism of alcohol, producing alcohol intolerance. When given alone, disulfiram is relatively nontoxic, but causes a highly unpleasant reaction if alcohol is consumed or absorbed through the skin. The intensity and duration of symptoms of this reaction are related to the disulfiram dosage, the amount of alcohol consumed, and individual sensitivity. The patient on

TABLE 49-13 Alcohol Content of Some Common Nonprescription and Prescription Preparations

Cough and cold remedies	Mouthwashes
Vicks 44 (10%)	Listerine (25%)
Romilar CG (10%)	Scope (18%)
Pertussin-Plus (25%)	Colgate 100 (70%)
Nyquil (25%)	Astring-O-Sol (70%)
Dristan (12%)	Cepacol (14%)
Robitussin-CF, DM, PE (1.4%)	Lavoris (5%)
Bactalin (14%)	Pentacresol 1:1000 (30%)
Comtrex (20%)	Vitamins and tonics
CoTylenol Cold (7.5%)	Gevrabon (18%)
CoTylenol, Children's (8.5%)	Geritol (12%)
Halls Cough (22%)	Gevizol (15%)
Quiet-Nite (25%)	Gerix (20%)
Terpin hydrate (42%)	Geritonic (20%)
Bronchodilators (elixirs)	Other
Elixophyllin (20%)	Paregoric tincture (45%)
Brondecon (20%)	Propadrine (16%)
Asbron (15%)	Belladonna tincture (67%)
Theolixir (20%)	Kaon elixir (5%)
Oraphyllin (20%)	Benadryl elixir (14%)
Isuprel Compound (19%)	Donnagel suspension (4%)
Lufyllin (20%)	Tinctures (40–50%)
	Elixirs (20–30%)

TABLE 49-14   Summary of Selected Alcohol-Drug Interactions

DRUGS INTERACTING WITH ALCOHOL	MECHANISM	EFFECT	SIGNIFICANCE
Disulfiram	Inhibits intermediate metabolism of alcohol	Abdominal cramps, headache, flushing, vomiting, confusion, hypotension, or hypertension	Major
Warfarin (Coumadin)	Metabolism enhanced	Diminished anticoagulant effect with *chronic* alcohol abuse	Moderate
	Metabolism reduced	Increased anticoagulant effect with *acute* alcohol intoxication	Moderate
Antihistamines	Additive	Increased CNS depression	Moderate
Anticonvulsants	Metabolism enhanced	Diminished anticonvulsant effect with *chronic* alcohol intoxication	Moderate
	Metabolism reduced	Increased anticonvulsant effect with *acute* alcohol intoxication	Moderate
Isoniazid (INH)	Metabolism enhanced	Diminished isoniazid effect in chronic alcohol abuse	Moderate
Antidiabetic Agents Sulfonylureas, tolbutamide (Orinase), chlorpropamide (Diabinese), acetohexamide (Dymelor)	Additive	Hypoglycemic effect increased	Moderate
	Metabolism enhanced	Decreased effect in chronic alcohol abuse	Moderate in chronic alcoholic
	Accumulation of acetaldehyde, increase in prostaglandins, enkephalins	Antabuse-like reaction	Moderate
Insulin	Interferes with hepatic gluconeogenesis	Increased hypoglycemic effects	Moderate, but major if liver damage
Antihypertensives Methyldopa (Aldomet), reserpine, guanethidine (Ismelin), hydralazine (Apresoline), prazosin (Minipres)	Additive	Sedation	Minor
	Additive	Postural hypotensive effect increased	Minor to moderate
Analgesics Meperidine (Demerol), morphine, methadone, other narcotics	Additive	Increased CNS depression with acute alcohol intoxication; increased effect also if cirrhotic	Major
Aspirin	Additive	Increased GI bleeding, occult blood loss, and damage to gastric mucosa	Mild to moderate

TABLE 49-14 Summary of Selected Alcohol-Drug Interactions (*Cont.*)

DRUGS INTERACTING WITH ALCOHOL	MECHANISM	EFFECT	SIGNIFICANCE
Sedative-Hypnotics Barbiturates (phenobarbital, pentobarbital, secobarbital); nonbarbiturates (ethclorvynol, meprobamate, glutethimide); benzodiazepines	Additive	Increased CNS depression with acute alcohol intoxication	Major
Chloral hydrate	Competition for metabolic pathway; additive	Increased CNS depression	Major
Antipsychotics Chlorpromazine (Thorazine, etc.)	Additive	Impaired coordination and judgment, also increased CNS depression	Moderate
Tricyclic Antidepressants Amitriptyline (Elavil, Triavil), imipramine (Tofranil), nortriptyline	Additive	Possible increase in sedation, also additive to anticholinergic effects of tricyclics	Major
Nitroglycerin	Additive	Hypotension potentiated, may cause cardiovascular collapse	Major

disulfiram who ingests alcohol may present with flushed, scarlet appearance; as the vasodilation continues, headache and hypotension, and occasionally hypertension, occur. Patients may also have respiratory difficulty, nausea, vomiting, blurred vision, and vertigo. The reaction may be produced by as little as 7 mL of alcohol and can last from 30 min to several hours. Although the disulfiram-alcohol reaction is usually short-lived and without sequelae, death can occur.

Mechanism of Action Disulfiram blocks the metabolism of alcohol by inhibiting the enzyme aldehyde dehydrogenase. This results in a buildup of the metabolite acetaldehyde which causes the alcohol-disulfiram reaction (see Fig. 49-2).

Pharmacokinetics Disulfiram is rapidly absorbed from the GI tract; it achieves full pharmacologic action in approximately 12 h. Disulfiram is eliminated slowly, with approximately 20 percent remaining in the body after a week.

Adverse Effects Although it is relatively safe, disulfiram can cause elevation of blood pressure and acne-form eruptions, fatigue, tremor, restlessness, reduced sexual activity, and a garlicky or metallic taste in the mouth. Disulfiram has also been shown to retard the metabolism of **oral anticoagulants, isoniazid**, and other drugs. There are reports of anti-

dotal treatment of the disulfiram-alcohol reaction with vitamin C, iron, or antihistamines; the results of these treatment modes are not definitive. Supportive measures such as placing the patient in Trendelenberg position, administration of oxygen, fluids, and electrolytes, are more beneficial than the unproven use of questionable antidotes.

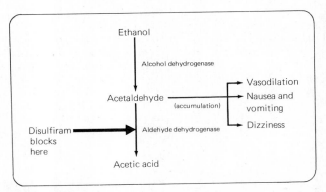

FIGURE 49-2

Metabolic Pathway of Ethanol. The mechanism of disulfiram action is inhibition of aldehyde dehydrogenase, resulting in accumulation of acetaldehyde. This causes the clinical symptoms of the alcohol-disulfiram reaction.

Dosage and Administration The usual initial dosage of disulfiram is 250 to 500 mg/day for 5 to 7 days, after which the dosage may be reduced to 125 to 250 mg/day.

Sedative-Hypnotic Drugs

Sedative-hypnotic and antianxiety agents have a high abuse potential in the alcoholic population. There is no evidence to support outpatient use of psychotropic drugs in the treatment of alcoholism. The use of placebo for relief of anxiety may be worthwhile when basic behavioral problems are dealt with concomitantly.

Tricyclic Antidepressants

Tricyclic antidepressants should be considered for patients in need of therapy for chronic and severe depression only after careful evaluation and selection. Tricyclic antidepressant drugs are dangerous in overdose amounts, and too frequently they provide a convenient means of attempting suicide for the depressed alcoholic patient.

Propranolol (Inderal)

Theoretically, a β-adrenergic blocking drug such as propranolol would be beneficial in preventing the adrenergic overactivity that occurs during alcohol withdrawal. However, because propranolol can precipitate congestive heart failure, asthmatic attacks, or peripheral vascular insufficiency, and can mask the symptoms of hypoglycemia, benefits from its use should be carefully weighed against the risks before it is used in acute alcohol withdrawal syndrome.

Lithium Carbonate

It has been suggested that lithium carbonate may prevent the progress of primary alcoholism; this still awaits confirmation. Lithium may also be an effective ancillary medication in treating the alcohol withdrawal syndrome.

Behavioral Therapies

Aversive conditioning and behavioral modification have also been utilized to help the patient abstain from alcohol. With any of these methods, there is little empirical data on the effectiveness of these approaches. More research is needed therefore to determine their usefulness in assisting the alcoholic to maintain sobriety.

NURSING PROCESS RELATED TO CHRONIC ALCOHOLISM

The nursing process related to disulfiram therapy in the treatment of chronic alcoholism is shown in Table 49-15.

OPIATES

Opiate abusers fall into the categories of "street addicts," methadone-maintained patients, infants of addicted mothers, physicians, nurses, and other health professionals, and a "new wave" of middle-class heroin users. The risk of physiologic and psychologic dependency on narcotics (heroin,

TABLE 49-15 Nursing Process Related to Disulfiram (Antabuse)

ASSESSMENT	MANAGEMENT	EVALUATION
Assess for informed consent, motivation, social stability, understanding of use. Pregnancy, heart disease, mental illness, suicidal ideation, serious liver impairment, uncontrolled epilepsy, and diabetes are contraindications.	Effect begins within 12 h and lasts for a week following discontinuation. Metallic taste may cause anorexia; good oral hygiene may decrease taste. Tell patient to avoid alcohol; give list of OTC drugs containing alcohol (Table 49-13); instruct to avoid body and shave lotions, colognes, mouthwashes, and alcohol sponges. Phenytoin (Dilantin) may cause interactions and dosage adjustment may be necessary for either drug; careful observation indicated. Fluid intake, nutrition, hygiene should be encouraged. Family member or other should observe patient take dose. Concurrent psychotherapy or behavioral therapy should be used. Close patient–care provider relationship is important. Give with caution concurrently with other CNS depressants; may potentiate their effects. Patient should carry appropriate ID for this drug. Instruct client and family members what to do in case of reaction.	Check for adverse effects (usually transient, lasting 2 weeks), drowsiness, fatigue, impotence, acneform eruption, metallic taste. Nausea and vomiting, dizziness, hypertension, flushed face, and red eyes in alcohol ingestion reaction. Take vital signs and observe when these symptoms occur.

morphine, methadone, meperidine, hydromorphone) is great. The central nervous system and analgesic effects of heroin depend on its conversion to morphine in the body. One of the most significant effects produced by opiates is *respiratory depression*. This effect is usually dose-dependent, particularly in the nonnarcotic-tolerant or nondependent person.

The potential for addiction is greatest for heroin because of its marked *euphoriant* properties and rapid onset of action. While heroin is usually cited as the common "street" form of opiate abused, many other drugs (Table 49-16) can be obtained either licitly or illicitly. Chronic administration of heroin over a period of a few weeks will cause *tolerance*.

The rate at which tolerance develops is a function of the size of the dose and the frequency of administration. Tolerance does not develop equally to all effects of the narcotics; even persons highly tolerant of heroin will continue to experience pupillary constriction and constipation from it. Tolerance for heroin and other opiates disappears following complete withdrawal. This can result in unintentional acute intoxication from heroin if the "usual" dose is taken after weeks or months of abstinence.

Acute Intoxication

Clinical Findings

Acute overdose with narcotics produces a stuporous or comatose patient with fixed pinpoint pupils and depressed res-

---

TABLE 49-16 Opiates and Related Compounds

Natural Opium and Derivatives
  Opium
  Tincture of opium
  Paregoric (camphorated opium tincture)
  Morphine
  Codeine
Meperidine and Congeners*
  Meperidine, pethidine (Demerol)
  Anileridine (Leritine)
  Diphenoxylate (Lomotil)
  Fentanyl (Innovar, Sublimaze)
  Loperamide (Imodium)
Semisynthetic Derivatives
  Heroin (diacetylmorphine)
  Hydromorphone (Dilandid)
  Oxymorphone (Numorphan)
  Hydrocodone (various)
  Oxycodone (Percodan, Tylox, Percocet)
Methadone and Congeners
  Methadone (Dolophine)
  L-Acetylmethadol (LAAM)
  Propoxyphene (Darvon)
Others
  Pentazocine (Talwin)
  Butorphanol (Stadol)
  Nalbuphine (Nubain)

*Congener: Member of same pharmacologic group.

---

piration. Hypotension, bradycardia, pulmonary edema, and hypothermia may also be experienced. While pinpoint pupils are well characterized as an opiate effect, mydraisis may develop when hypoxia or asphyxia intervenes. Other causes of small-to-pinpoint pupils should be considered in the differential diagnosis, e.g., cerebellar infarction of the pontine angle, organophosphate poisoning, heat stroke, **pilocarpine** eye drops, drug overdose with either clonidine or a phenothiazine.

The exact amount of morphine that is toxic or lethal differs greatly between the nontolerant and the opiate-tolerant. The lethal dose of morphine may be as much as 1000 mg in the narcotic-tolerant person. Toxic and lethal dosage levels may be drastically reduced by concomitant use of alcohol and other psychotropic agents, e.g., **barbiturates, phenothiazines,** or **tricyclic antidepressants**. The content of heroin in "street buys" may vary. Heroin in its origin is in the form of **morphine**; to reach the illicit market, it is converted by acetylation to diacetyl morphine in illegal laboratories. This heroin eventually courses through many "dealers" and is progressively diluted or "cut" to a product that might yield only 1/20 to 1/100 of the original opiate content. The heroin content can range from zero to 85 percent in a "bag" or "balloon" (West Coast variety) containing 100 to 150 mg of material, usually adulterants, including procaine, quinine, talc, flour, cornstarch, baking soda, lactose, or mannitol.

Management with Narcotic Antagonists

A narcotic antagonist is used in acute opiate intoxication. **Naloxone** (Narcan) is the drug of choice, since it is a "pure" antagonist and safe, without agonist or respiratory-depressant effects. The dose is 0.01 mg/kg; 0.8 mg is the usual adult dose given intravenously. Much larger doses have been required occasionally for acute propoxyphene or pentazocine overdoses. This may be repeated after 15 min if needed or whenever signs of intoxication reappear. The narcotic antagonists will reverse the apnea and the coma caused by **heroin, morphine, codeine, meperidine, propoxyphene, methadone, pentazocine,** and other related drugs. The peak effect of naloxone takes place within 1 to 2 min and the duration of action may be 2 to 3 h. **Nalorphine** (Nalline) or **levallorphan** (Lorfan) are narcotic antagonists that have agonist properties which may worsen respiratory depression. They should be avoided in coma or respiratory depression where the cause is unclear. The duration of propoxyphene, methadone, and pentazocine action is longer than that of the other opiates—12 to 24 h—and so the acute intoxication must be observed carefully for the need to readminister the shorter-acting narcotic antagonists. In these situations, it may be convenient to infuse naloxone in a dose sufficient to produce an antagonistic effect, usually 0.8 to 1.2 mg/h. However, it is not uncommon to precipiate with antagonists an opiate withdrawal syndrome in the opiate-dependent patient, resulting in a combative patient or one who leaves the treatment facility against medical advice before attention can be given to accompanying illnesses. A balance must be maintained between the persistent opiate effects and abstinence.

Because patients who receive naloxone occasionally vomit, comatose patients should be carefully intubated to prevent aspiration. The most important consideration in the opiate-overdosed patient is monitoring and mechanical support of respiration and blood pressure, since changes in neurologic, cardiovascular, and respiratory status can occur suddenly. If depressed respiration fails to respond to administration of naloxone, intubation and assisted ventilation must be performed. Often, before an acutely overdosed patient is seen in the emergency room, resuscitative efforts have been made by the victim's friends or associates. Cold water baths; intramuscular or intravenous administration of milk; and salt water and ice placed on the face, breast, and genitalia have all been employed, presumably in the hope that such measures would arouse the narcotic-overdosed patient from unconsciousness.

Severe acute overdoses and deaths have occurred when "bags" or "balloons" of heroin are swallowed to escape apprehension; the danger of this action when the heroin is accidently released from the container and absorbed should not be overlooked. A narcotic antagonist should be readily available in such cases. Since narcotic antagonists may precipitate the withdrawal syndrome, the patient should be observed closely (Table 49-17). If it is possible that the opiate or other drugs have been ingested orally, the usual measures of emesis in a conscious patient or of intubation and gastric lavage in the unconscious person should be taken. **Activated charcoal** and **cathartic** should then be given.

Narcotic Abstinence or Withdrawal Syndrome

Clinical Findings

When the usual dose of heroin or other narcotic is withheld from a physically dependent person, a predictable sequence of responses will occur. The severity of these withdrawal responses depends on the degree of tolerance, the duration of chronic use, and the usual dose of the drug. The symptoms of narcotic abstinence syndrome (Table 49-17) usually begin 8 to 12 h after the last dose, reaching their peak about 40 to 60 h later. The symptoms may be as mild as those of the common cold, or they may be the more severe type known as "cold turkey" withdrawal. The symptoms of abstinence are unpleasant but not life-threatening. Withdrawal symptoms of concurrent dependencies, such as for alcohol or other CNS depressants, can produce life-threatening complications and should be carefully distinguished from those purely related to opiates.

Management with Methadone

The current method relies on the substitution of **methadone** for heroin or other opiates, with gradual dose reduction until a stabilized dose is reached or withdrawal is complete.

Detoxification refers to medically supervised withdrawal with the aid of methadone from a condition of physical dependence on opiates. The time required to complete this process varies from several days to weeks, usually 21 days. The amount of time will usually depend on individual level and severity of addiction, regardless of whether detoxification is conducted in a hospitalized or outpatient basis. Methadone is an addicting narcotic and is used only when addiction to heroin is definitely established. Fatalities have occurred from overdoses with methadone in nontolerant persons. Side effects from methadone include excessive sweating, constipation, sedation, nausea, decreased libido, drowsiness, and "nodding." Because of its slow metabolism, a single daily dose of methadone is sufficient. Failure to continue treatment will lead to an abstinence syndrome that is milder—usually some muscle ache and nasal congestion— but more prolonged than heroin withdrawal. Other medically supervised detoxification options include administration of **morphine**, withdrawing the patient "cold turkey," or the administration of **propoxyphene** (Darvon), **propranolol** (Inderal), or **clonidine** (Catapres).

Maintenance is the use of methadone as an oral substitute for opiates on a continuing basis. A patient addicted to opiates for more than 2 years is eligible for methadone maintenance if physical dependence can be demonstrated. Maintenance treatment is permitted to be undertaken only by an FDA-approved methadone maintenance program. Problems with methadone maintenance are not medical but administrative. Because of the possibility of illicit diversion of the drug, patients must take their methadone under supervision, usually on a daily basis.

The daily dose of methadone is started at 10 and 20 mg/ day, depending on the level of tolerance, and is stabilized at a dose of 60 to 80 mg, reached in 10-mg increments until the tolerance level is reached. A single daily dose is given in solution for oral ingestion. Methadone is less likely than other opiates to produce euphoria or sedation, and tolerance is rapidly developed. At a dose of about 40 mg/day, the craving for opiates disappears; at higher doses, approximately 80 mg, the "blockading" effect becomes prominent so that little or no effect is experienced from the use of additional opiates.

TABLE 49-17 Symptoms of Narcotic Abstinence Syndrome

Dilated pupils	Vomiting
Elevation of pulse rate	Diarrhea
Elevation of blood pressure	Dehydration
Elevation of temperature	Weakness
Elevation of respiratory rate	Chills
Muscle aches	Rhinorrhea
Irritability	Lacrimation
Twitching	Gooseflesh
Tremulousness	Yawning
Nausea	Restlessness

A long-acting methadone-like drug, L-acetyl methadone (LAAM), has received limited clinical use. LAAM can be given only once every 3 days instead of daily.

Medical Complications of Narcotic Dependence

In addition to toxic and withdrawal reactions, numerous medical complications occur in narcotic addicts (Table 49-18). *Abnormal liver function* is common, probably as a result of repeated use of unsterile hypodermic equipment, exposure to toxic adulterants, and excessive use of alcohol. Acute hepatitis of either serum or viral type is a frequent reason for hospitalization of addicts.

TABLE 49-18   Some Common Medical and Surgical Complications from Intravenous Drug Abuse

Skin	Abscesses, cellulitis, edema, emboli, excoriation, jaundice, macules, nodules, purpura, "tracks," ulcers.
Lymph nodes	"Addict's lymphadenopathy," lymphatic hyperplasia.
Eyes	Emboli from talc and cornstarch, quinine amblyopia, scleral icterus.
Mouth	Poor dental hygiene.
Pulmonary	Infections secondary to aspiration, bronchiectasis, atelectasis, septic emboli, tuberculosis, pulmonary hypertension, decreased vital capacity, asthma, noncardiogenic pulmonary edema.
Cardiovascular	Arrhythmias, endocarditis complicated by systemic and pulmonary emboli, vasculitis, gangrene.
Hematologic	Anemia, hemolysis, malaria.
Neurologic	Subarachnoid hemorrhage, neuropathies, meningitis, central and peripheral emboli, nerve damage.
Gastrointestinal	Hepatomegaly, hepatitis, splenic abscess, portal hypertension, constipation, bowel obstruction, hemorrhoids.
Genitourinary	Heroin nephropathy, vasculitis, glomerulonephritis secondary to hepatitis or infection, myoglobinuria from muscle destruction, acute tubular necrosis, amenorrhea, gonorrhea, syphilis.
Extremities	Phlebitis, edema, arthritis, rhabdomyolysis, tetanus.
Immunologic	False positive VDRL, rheumatoid factor, hypergammaglobulinemia, serologic abnormalities. Intravenous drug use has been associated with an increased risk for acquired immunodeficiency syndrome (AIDS).

Acute bacterial endocarditis is another frequent complication of intravenous drug abuse. *Staphylococcus aureus* is the most common infecting organism followed by *streptococci*, gram-negative bacilli (*Pseudomonas* and *Serratia*), and fungi (*Candida*). Recurrent episodes of endocarditis are frequent, often resulting in heart valve damage. Treatment with antibiotics is often complicated by resistant infective organisms. Fever and leukocytosis are frequent findings on hospital admission of addicts. Often, there is no other evidence of an infectious process. *Splenomegaly* secondary to septic embolization and infarction from the bacterial or fungal endocarditis is common.

Pulmonary complications may be secondary to embolic pneumonia, bacterial pneumonia, pulmonary fibrosis from injection of foreign-body emboli (e.g., starch, cotton fibers, or talc) or foreign-body granulomas. Increasing abuse of **methylphenidate** (Ritalin) and **pentazocine** (Talwin) among heroin users has resulted in greater numbers of embolic complications in this group following intravenous administration of tablets containing talc and other diluents. Pulmonary edema is not uncommon in the overdosed addict.

Tetanus is a serious infectious complication of illicit intravenous drug use. It is frequently secondary to "skin popping" and is often fatal. Protection from *Clostridium tetani* is afforded by immunization with tetanus toxoid.

Cellulitis and *skin abscess* are often seen at sites of injection; *Staphylococcus aureus* is the most frequent offending organism. This is often seen in "skin poppers" or subcutaneous users of heroin.

The Hospitalized Narcotic-Dependent Patient

Management of hospitalized patients who are dependent on opiates requires skill and patience. It is usual to continue their dependence by placing them on methadone until the acute phase of their illness has resolved. Attempts to withdraw opiate dependents from opiates during an acute medical or surgical illness often will complicate the management of the problem and are unlikely to be successful.

Because of an unreliable history and possible exaggeration or feigning of discomfort, the addict should be given methadone only *after* physical symptoms of abstinence syndrome are seen. Presence of fresh needle "tracks" and a urinalysis showing the presence of morphine on admission may serve as evidence of addiction. A modest dose (5 to 10 mg) of methadone can then be given to prevent withdrawal symptoms.

It is unusual for an opiate-dependent patient, not already being maintained on methadone, to require more than a total of 10 to 20 mg of methadone given in divided doses daily in order to deal with withdrawal symptoms while hospitalized. The dose of methadone is often not revealed to the patient. The drug is given in solution with juice to be taken orally.

Patients on methadone maintenance rapidly develop tolerance to the analgesic effects of methadone. The addition of short-acting opiate analgesics, e.g., **morphine** or **meperidine**, in the usual doses (10 to 15 mg of morphine or 50 to 100 mg of meperidine) will relieve pain in these patients.

When a patient mentions being enrolled in a methadone maintenance program, it is important to contact the program or the patient's counselor, nurse, or physician to ascertain the maintenance dose of methadone being given because addicts have a tendency to exaggerate their needs. Lack of communication with the program before treatment with methadone may result in unintentional methadone overdose. Addicted patients unable to take methadone orally may be given it either intramuscularly or subcutaneously.

Often, the illness or concomitant treatment of the hospitalized methadone-maintained patient will necessitate readjustment of the methadone dosage. Titration of the usual methadone dose must be anticipated where the underlying illness involves the liver, pulmonary, or central nervous system or where large amounts of opiate analgesics are required.

On leaving the hospital, the patient can make one of several choices: to enroll in a methadone program, to be detoxified, or simply to be discharged. Federal Food and Drug Administration prerequisites for eligibility in a methadone maintenance program must be met and the waiting period may extend for several months. The most convenient alternative is to be detoxified while still in the hospital. Detoxification can be carried out by a daily or every-second-day reduction of 20 percent of the total methadone dose, keeping the withdrawal symptoms at a tolerable level. If a partially detoxified patient elects to be discharged, the dose of methadone being given should be revealed. This is accomplished with a warning about the decreased opiate tolerance to the amount of heroin used prior to hospitalization.

Nonnarcotic Technique of Heroin Withdrawal

The nonnarcotic technique of withdrawal involves treating the symptoms with a variety of nonnarcotic medications. The GI symptoms of vomiting, diarrhea, and stomach cramps are treated with atropine-like drugs such as **scopolamine**. Sleeping medications, such as **flurazepam** (Dalmane), are occasionally needed with nonnarcotic withdrawal because of insomnia. **Propoxyphene** (Darvon) has been used as part of symptomatic therapy and is reported to be effective in large doses (600 to 1400 mg/day) as the only drug in the management of heroin withdrawal symptoms. This appears to be most useful in mild opiate dependence. Although not classified as an opiate, its weak cross-tolerance with narcotics suggests its usefulness in withdrawal. Sedatives, such as **diazepam** (Valium), may be useful in controlling the irritability and apprehension which commonly accompany withdrawal from opiates. **Clonidine** (Catapres), a drug therapeutically used to lower blood pressure, has also been reported to successfully ameliorate the abstinence

symptoms experienced following methadone withdrawal. The success of this drug, given in divided doses totaling 10 to 20 $\mu g/kg/day$ to reduce symptoms of opiate withdrawal, and the striking similarity of the narcotic and clonidine overdoses have led to speculations that naloxone might be effective in reversing the toxic effects of clonidine. However, results from situations where this has been attempted have been equivocal.

Naltrexone (Trexan) is a narcotic antagonist similar to naloxone, which works by competitively blocking opiate receptors. Because of its long half-life, it is used as an adjunct in the rehabilitation of opiate-dependent persons. The duration of naltrexone blockade is illustrated by studies which show it blocks the effects of 25 mg of heroin given IV 96% at 24 h, 86% at 48 h, and 47% at 72 h. Naltrexone suppresses the desire to return to opiate use and blocks analgesia, euphoria, physiologic changes, physical dependence, and tolerance. It is effective orally, and sustained-release dosage forms are under investigation. Average dosage range is 50 to 150 mg/day, although doses of 800 mg/day have been used. Maintenance programs employ 100-mg doses on Monday and Wednesday and 150 mg on Friday. The New Drug Application for this drug was marked approvable by the FDA in the fall of 1984.

BARBITURATES AND OTHER CNS DEPRESSANTS

Acute Intoxication or Drug Overdose

Barbiturates and other sedative-hypnotic drugs ("downers") produce their effects through generalized depression of the central nervous system: lowered blood pressure, depressed respiration and tendon reflexes, and slurred speech. There may be nystagmus on lateral gaze. Ataxia and coma occur. In intoxication with **methaqualone** (Quaalude), hyperirritability, seizures, and hyperactive reflexes may also occur. Hypoxia, acidosis, and sepsis often will complicate the hypotension following an acute CNS-depressant overdose. Arrhythmias may result from hypotension, hypoxia, acidbase and/or electrolyte disturbances. Pulmonary edema suggests narcotics, sedative-hypnotic and/or salicylate overdose. Cross-tolerance and cross-dependence exist among most drugs in the CNS-depressant group. Acute intoxication from the combined use of alcohol and the barbiturates is a frequent problem. Many of the drugs in this group produce a serious withdrawal syndrome which can be lifethreatening.

Management of Acute Intoxication

The goals of management are to treat the physical effects and to get the patient to admit to the problem. If patients are treated in the emergency room and released, the nurse should ensure that someone accompanies them home since withdrawal symptoms can appear later and may be serious.

The basic treatment in acute sedative-hypnotic intoxication is to maintain and support vital functions and may include use of the mechanical respirator, dialysis, ECG monitoring, and intensive nursing care. CNS stimulants have *no* place in the treatment of the sedative-hypnotic overdose. In treatment, three major problems are encountered:

1. *Pneumonia* is the leading cause of morbidity and mortality, regardless of the duration or cause of the coma.
2. *Overhydration* in the severely obtunded patient is poorly tolerated and may contribute to pulmonary edema.
3. Complications from *unnecessary therapeutic maneuvers* only compound the difficulties.

It is important that barbiturate abusers recognize that there are still alternatives open to them and that only they can make the choice. The nurse must be firm while not confronting patients or encroaching on their power to make decisions. If they feel forced to do something, they will resist. Since these patients often resent intrusion, initiating a trusting relationship may be difficult.

Abstinence Syndrome

Clinical Findings
Unlike withdrawal from narcotics, abstinence from barbiturates and other sedative-hypnotic drugs may be associated with postural hypotension, cardiovascular collapse, seizures, and even death. Mild symptoms such as insomnia, weakness, and tremulousness can appear within 24 h after the last dose was taken. Major symptoms of withdrawal, which usually develop after the second or third day, include agitation, delirium, psychosis, convulsions, and high fever. These symptoms should be considered signs of severe withdrawal syndrome with hospitalization required.

Major signs of physical dependence have been demonstrated with **secobarbital** or **pentobarbital** when taken at doses of 600 to 800 mg daily for 30 to 60 days. The withdrawal or abstinence syndrome has been described for almost every sedative-hypnotic drug, including the antianxiety drugs: **meprobamate** (Miltown), **diazepam** (Valium), and **chlordiazepoxide** (Librium). The dosage and time required to produce the major signs of withdrawal have not been as well established for these drugs as for secobarbital and pentobarbital.

Management (Detoxification)
The most successful technique for detoxifying barbiturate-dependent persons involves the substitution of **phenobarbital** for the addicting drug, with subsequent withdrawal of the phenobarbital. Phenobarbital produces smaller changes or fluctuations in barbiturate blood level to afford protection against the development of withdrawal symptoms. Phenobarbital has an additional advantage in that it does not normally produce the euphoria or "high" experienced with the shorter-acting barbiturates; this is why the shorter-acting

agents are more frequently abused. All sedative-hypnotics can be withdrawn by the phenobarbital technique because of the cross-tolerance among them.

The patient's history of barbiturate addiction and estimated daily intake should be a guide to initiating therapy. The dose of phenobarbital can be calculated by substituting 30 mg of phenobarbital for each 100 mg of pentobarbital or secobarbital or for each 400 mg of meprobamate which the patient has been taking. The daily dose, which may be as much as 600 to 700 mg of phenobarbital, is given in three to four divided doses and the patient is observed for signs of intoxication. The presence of toxic symptoms (ataxia, stupor, etc.) requires omission of a dose and adjustment of the daily dose accordingly. **Phenytoin** (Dilantin), given to protect against seizures from barbiturate withdrawal, has not been demonstrated to be effective.

When the daily quantity of barbiturate is unclear or unknown before detoxification treatment is begun, a test dose of 200 mg of **pentobarbital** (Nembutal) can be given. Experience with the unreliable histories of patients regarding daily intake suggests that this is often the preferred method. If mild withdrawal symptoms are present in 2 to 3 h, another 200 mg can be given. If the patient is asleep or mildly intoxicated from this dose, the degree of tolerance to the barbiturates is probably not significant. If withdrawal symptoms are moderate or severe, another 200- to 300-mg dose of pentobarbital can be given and periodically repeated until the level of tolerance is determined (when the patient falls asleep or develops symptoms of barbiturate intoxication).

After stabilization with phenobarbital is achieved, the total daily dose of phenobarbital is decreased 30 mg each day. The withdrawal schedule should permit gradual reduction of dosage, with signs of intoxication or withdrawal symptoms used as the basis for adjustment. The most successful detoxification takes place in the supervised inpatient setting. Occasionally, patients requiring detoxification have mixed addictions, usually of the opiate-sedative type. In these cases, the patient is maintained on sufficient amounts of methadone until detoxification from the sedative-hypnotic drug(s) is completed. The methadone is then withdrawn over the following week.

THE RECREATIONAL DRUG USER

When a modest amount of a psychoactive substance is taken for its pleasure-producing effects, for experimental reasons, or out of curiosity, the pattern of use is characterized as "casual" or "recreational." Readily available and inexpensive, alcohol and tobacco are the most frequently used socially acceptable licit sources of psychotropic activity.

The recreational drug users have traditionally been adolescents or young adults, although other age groups are becoming increasingly involved. They are found equally among males and females, and they come from all racial, socioeconomic, and occupational backgrounds. The early

1980s witnessed significant changes in the trends of both licit and illicit psychoactive substance use. There is historic precedent in this country to expect a cyclic pattern of depressant-drug abuse to be followed by stimulant-drug abuse. The current interest in stimulant drugs such as cocaine, "freebase," the "look-alike" over-the-counter diet and cold preparations involving phenylpropanolamine, ephedrine, and caffeine suggest that a return to heavy-depressant-type drug abuse is likely to take place in the near future. An estimate of the current prevalence of licit and illicit recreational drug use is difficult. In most instances, this casual type of drug use has not been equated inevitably with any specific character disorder. No direct consequence on the physical, psychologic, or social adjustment of the user is apparent, unlike the circumstance with the opiate- or depressant-"dependent" or -habituated individual who has a repetitive and excessive need for an increasing amount of drug or drugs to produce the desired psychomimetic experience. This typical impression may certainly change as the nature and pattern of "recreational" drug use evolve during the 1980s.

Although they still are a major problem of concern, the use of **phencyclidine** (PCP) and **lysergic acid** (LSD) has experienced a leveling off and even a decline in some communities. There are, however, a growing number of users of **isobutyl nitrite**, **nitrous oxide**, and volatile solvents which signals a renewed interest in the psychotropic effects of inhalants by the subculture of recreational drug user. Despite our focus on the individual pharmacology and toxicology of the various psychomimetic agents involved in recreational drug use and drug abuse, attention must also be given to the psychologic, social, environmental, and personal factors which are integral parts of the drug-taking scene when patients who are "high" require attention and care.

CENTRAL NERVOUS SYSTEM STIMULANTS

Amphetamines

Amphetamines ("uppers") are widely abused for their CNS-stimulant effects. The symptoms of amphetamine intoxication include elevated blood pressure, arrhythmia, hyperactive tendon reflexes, dilated pupils, dry mouth, sweating, fever, and in severe intoxication, confusion, paranoid ideation, and aggressive behavior. **Methamphetamine** (Desoxyn) and **methylphenidate** (Ritalin) are similar to the **dextroamphetamines** (Dexedrine) and have similar effects (Table 49-19).

Amphetamines are occasionally used to increase alertness, to relieve depression and fatigue, and to treat obesity. Tolerance for amphetamine-like drugs can develop rapidly, over a few days, weeks, or months. Eventually, hundreds of times the ordinary dose can be tolerated.

"Snorting" (inhaling) or injecting the amphetamine provides a rapid "high" and an intense "rush" or "flash." Methamphetamine ("speed") is the most frequently abused stimulant that is injected intravenously. Methylphenidate use in this manner, however, is rapidly becoming as widespread because of its greater availability. During a "speed run," repeated injections are continued for days or weeks. As much as 1000 mg may be injected in a single dose and 5000 to 8000 mg over a 24-h period.

The taking of antacids with amphetamine can greatly prolong the stimulant effects experienced. Antacids decrease the renal clearance of amphetamine by causing the urine pH to become more alkaline. Another pattern of amphetamine abuse is "speedballing" in which an amphetamine, usually methamphetamine, is injected together with heroin. Methylphenidate (Ritalin) tablets are being used intravenously with increasing frequency although they are considered less desirable than methamphetamine; as much as 500 to 800 mg is injected daily for the stimulant effects.

During an amphetamine "run," the subject will be hostile, overactive, and impulsive. Prolonged periods of paranoid ideation (usually ideas of being persecuted), poor impulse control, and poor judgment are common. Inexplicable and bizarre behavior has been associated with amphetamine abuse. After a few days or weeks of a "speed run," the patient is so exhausted or delusional that "crashing" occurs. The withdrawal syndrome from amphetamine is characterized by long periods of sleep, marked depression and suicidal thoughts, apathy, complaints of aches and pains, and hunger. Often the depression is so severe that it may initiate another "run." "Overamped" describes the condition that occurs after the dose of amphetamine has been increased too rapidly; it is characterized by consciousness, without the ability to move or speak. Extremely rapid pulse, increased temperature and blood pressure, and chest pain are experienced. Severe agitation, sleeplessness, tachycardia, arrhythmias, elevated blood pressure, fever, and hallucinations occur when nontolerant persons overdose acutely with amphetamines.

Abrupt withdrawal from amphetamines produces only a few and somewhat mild symptoms of abstinence, e.g., fatigue, muscle aches, depression, hunger, and apathy. Seizures are not a potential complication of amphetamine withdrawal, unlike sedative-hypnotic withdrawal. It is not necessary to withdraw amphetamine gradually. Treatment of

TABLE 49-19 Common Signs and Symptoms of Amphetamine Intoxication

Restlessness	Paranoid
Anxiety	Delusional thought
Tremor	Visual hallucinations
Muscle tension	Auditory hallucinations
Repetitious body movement	Physical malnutrition
Facial grimacing	Needle tracks and abscesses
Dystonia	Hypertensive crisis
Temporary amnesia	Cardiac arrhythmias

the acute amphetamine intoxication is primarily support of vital functions. Maintaining a quiet room during withdrawal is important since stimulation can cause panic. On the other hand, staff and visitors should be warned not to whisper around the patient, and it is most helpful for the nurse to maintain some distance and to keep conversation uncomplicated and concrete. Suicide precautions are also indicated during the withdrawal period. **Chlorpromazine** (Thorazine) and other phenothiazines should not be given to treat mental or physiologic disturbances caused by amphetamine reactions. **Diazepam** (Valium) can be given orally or intravenously for sedation if any is required.

Medical Complications of Chronic Amphetamine Abuse

Abuse of methamphetamine can produce a systemic necrotizing angiitis and generalized spasm of the cerebral blood vessels. Infrequently, cerebral hemorrhages and cardiac arrhythmias may occur. Malnutrition and cachexia are common complications of amphetamine abuse. A syndrome of severe abdominal pain mimicking acute appendicitis is occasionally seen. The risk of impulsive self-destructive behavior and activity is great in the chronic amphetamine abuser. During the withdrawal phase, when depression is usually most intense, careful observation of the patient is important. Unfortunately, long-term management of the chronic amphetamine abuser is difficult, and relapse is frequent.

Cocaine

Cocaine is an alkaloid of the evergreen shrub *Erythroxylum coca*, which is cultivated in the upper Andes of Peru and Bolivia. Illegally imported cocaine as the hydrochloride salt enters the United States in varying degrees of purity up to 95 percent. It is subdivided by being diluted with adulterants (or "stepped on") by each dealer in the chain of distribution until it reaches the user. Mannitol, lactose, glucose, inositol are sugars used along with a variety of commercial synthetic local anesthetics such as **lidocaine**, **procaine**, and **tetracaine** to "cut" the cocaine. Less common adulterants are caffeine, **benzocaine**, **amphetamine**, **heroin**, **phencyclidine**, and **quinine**.

One "line" of street cocaine contains between 5 and 10 mg, depending on the purity. One "coke spoonful" (one sniff) contains slightly less. "Freebasing" or smoking of the pure cocaine base usually involves a single "hit" or dosage of a "tenth" (100 mg) to "fifteenth" (65 mg) of a gram. Freebase or base cocaine is a colorless, odorless, transparent crystalline material almost totally insoluble in water but freely soluble in diethyl ether. The melting point of freebase is 98°C.

The action of cocaine depends on the site and route of administration and is markedly affected by individual variability. Cocaine's pharmacologic action as a local anesthetic can be characterized as one with high efficacy and toxicity; as a potent CNS stimulant, it is of rapid onset and relatively short duration of action accompanied by a low margin of safety.

Acute Reactions

Clinical Findings The effects of cocaine (which is usually inhaled but sometimes injected intravenously) are similar to those of intravenous amphetamine except that the duration of action is briefer and the onset of the effect quicker (Table 49-20). Ingested cocaine is well absorbed. However, this method of administration is infrequent because it is usually done unintentionally or unknowingly, since the desired onset of effects is more delayed than when inhaled or injected. Children who ingest cocaine can become acutely symptomatic, presenting with tachycardia, hyperpyrexia, hypotension and hypertension, and seizures.

Large doses of cocaine may cause cardiac arrhythmias and cardiovascular and respiratory complications. Because cocaine is expensive and also has a local anesthetic effect, it is often adulterated with **benzocaine** or **procaine**, two drugs

TABLE 49-20 Summary of Physiologic and Psychologic Effects of Cocaine*

Physiologic Effects	
Heart rate increase	Increase in blood pressure
Dilation of pupils	Tightening of sphincters
Mobilization of epinephrine	Rise in body temperature
Slowing of digestion	Increased capacity for muscular activity
Appearance of stereotypic movements: "picking," "stroking," bruxism, tics	Vomiting
	Sweating
Dry throat	Hypertension
Dizziness	Increase in respiratory rate followed by depressed rate
Hyperreflexia	
Clonic-tonic convulsions	Central respiratory depression
Cheyne-Stokes respiration	Local inflammation
Hypoxia	Perforation of nasal mucosa and septum
Ventricular arrhythmias	
Ischemic necrosis	

Psychologic Effects	
"Rush"	Euphoria
Paranoia	Restlessness/irritability
Agitation/hostility/apprehension	Excitement
Fully alert	Withdrawn/confusion
Delirium	

*Depends on external environment.

noted for their cardiac and anesthetic effects. Chronic abusers of cocaine often manifest psychotic and paranoid behavior, along with striking changes in affect. Whether the cocaine is inhaled or injected, once under the influence of the drug the user may be considered dangerous; this is in sharp contrast to the narcotic-dependent individual who may be dangerous when he or she does not possess the drug.

When freebase cocaine is taken, onset of euphoric and stimulant effect is rapid with an intensity similar to that following intravenous administration. The duration of action is extremely short, leading to repeated use. The potential for overdose is great in users of freebase because the pattern of use often involves rapid escalation of the frequency and quantity of cocaine smoked.

In acute cocaine intoxication, hyperventilation precedes a later respiratory depression. In severe cases, the "caine" reaction, characterized by clonic-tonic convulsions and cardiovascular and respiratory collapse, can take place. Deaths following intranasal, intravenous, and oral administration of cocaine have resulted from respiratory arrest, cardiac and cardiovascular failure, and seizures. Strenuous physical exertion combined with use of cocaine have high morbidity; cases of "sudden death," possibly from cardiac arrhythmias, have been described after use of freebase cocaine along with physical exertion.

Management Treatment includes supportive care (cooling blanket, fluids) and maintenance of vital functions (airway, blood pressure, etc.). A sedative drug such as **diazepam** (Valium) can be given if the toxic psychosis is severe. Electrocardiographic monitoring for arrhythmias should be considered in severe cocaine intoxication or reactions. Seizures are treated by **diazepam**, **phenytoin**, or **phenobarbital**. Tachyarrhythmias have been managed successfully with low doses (1 to 2 mg) of intravenous **propranolol**. There are descriptions of dramatic control by propranolol for the profound sympathetic overstimulation with hypertension.

HALLUCINOGENS

A variety of chemicals, both synthetic (e.g., **phencyclidine**, or PCP, and **lysergic acid diethylamide**, or LSD) and natural (e.g., psilocybin) are taken for their hallucinogenic effects, with a wide range of perceptual or psychologic and physiologic effects (Table 49-21).

The earliest symptom of LSD ingestion is pupillary dilation, even when only small doses are taken. The physiologic and cardiovascular symptoms have a rapid onset; the sensory, psychologic, and cognitive effects, which are highly variable, generally occur 30 to 60 min after ingestion. The anxiety or panic reaction is often the cause of a "bad trip" which is not entirely dose-related. The user's personality and experience with LSD and environmental factors play an important part in it.

The "flashback" experience is an acute but transient recurrence of the LSD experience in the absence of subsequent use. Flashbacks may occur many months or a year after the LSD experience. It has been suggested that these are triggered by stress or anxiety or by the use of other centrally acting drugs. Withdrawal of LSD or other hallucinogens produces no physical symptoms.

"Bad trips" from PCP are a problem often requiring emergency care. PCP is sold alone or in combination with a variety of other drugs. Often it is discovered in samples sold on the street as "pure" THC (tetrahydrocannabinol), LSD, psilocybin, or mescaline. The symptoms of PCP reaction differ in several respects from the effects of other hallucinogenic agents and include disorientation, hallucination, agitation, and rigid and purposeless motor hyperactivity. In low doses, PCP produces effects that resemble alcohol intoxication with anxiety, disorientation, and visual and perceptual disturbances. Mental status varies from euphoria to confusion, hostility, and depersonalization. During recovery from PCP overdose, episodes of dystonic posturing and involuntary movement of the extremities are frequent, with striking manifestations such as catatonia-like opisthotonic posture, torticollis, and facial grimacing. Recovery is usually rapid although some reports of massive PCP overdoses have

TABLE 49-21 Symptoms of Hallucinogenic Reactions

Sensory

Altered perception of color, objects, size, and shape
Distortion of time, direction, and distance
Synesthesias, e.g., "seeing sounds," "hearing colors"

Psychologic

Depersonalization and loss of body image
Anxiety, panic, depression
Mood alterations
Paranoid ideation
Hallucinations (when sufficiently large doses are taken)

Cognitive

Impaired memory, recall, attention
Reduced mental performance
Difficulty with problem solving

Physiologic

Dilated pupils	Coma
Tremor	Elevated temperature
Piloerection ("gooseflesh")	Nausea
Sweating	Vomiting
Dizziness	Hunger
Weakness	Tachycardia
Paresthesias	Bleeding (in massive LSD
Ataxia	overdoses; thought to be evidence of platelet dysfunction)
Blurred vision	dence of platelet dysfunction)
Hyperreflexia	Clonic movements of muscles
Elevated blood pressure	Blood pressure decline (in
Hyperactivity	severe overdoses)

described symptoms lasting several weeks. Mental status may take several days to weeks to return to normal.

Certain other popular hallucinogens are anticholinergic substances found in both prescription and nonprescription medications. **Trihexyphenidyl** (Artane) and **benztropine** (Cogentin) are prescribed often for the treatment of the extrapyramidal effects that accompany the use of phenothiazine-type drugs. These drugs are often obtained for illicit purposes through false representation by feigning symptoms of extrapyramidal disorders. Antiparkinson drugs can cause CNS stimulation ranging from mild symptoms to a toxic delirium. High doses of anticholinergic drugs, resulting in a toxic psychosis, are characterized by euphoria, confusion, hallucination, and paranoia. Anticholinergic agents occasionally misused for their CNS effects include over-the-counter drugs containing **scopolamine** that are marketed as sleep aids.

Management of Hallucinogenic Reactions

Adequate supportive care, reduction of sensory stimulation, and reassurance ("talking down" by helping the patient to redefine the bad experiences) are the keys to successful management of the "bad trip." In cases of acute PCP reactions, sensory deprivation is most important in order to avoid further exacerbation of the symptoms. The agitated and excited patient should be protected from self-inflicted injuries with soft restraints, used only when absolutely needed. Phenothiazine drugs, such as **chlorpromazine**, should not be given since their hypotensive and possible seizure-producing effects outweigh any benefit. The benzodiazepines (e.g., **diazepam** or **chlordiazepoxide**) can be useful in the severely agitated patient.

MARIJUANA

Marijuana comes from the hemp plant *Cannabis sativa*, which contains numerous psychoactive substances (cannabinols). The psychoactive substances are present in highest quantity in the flowering tops of the plant and in hashish, which is the resin from the flowering plant secreted by the plant in hot, dry weather. The cannabinols include cannabidol, cannabinolic acid, the most potent form Δ-tetrahydrocannabinol (Δ^9 THC), and many others. The amounts of the psychoactive agents vary, depending upon the type of plant, the location and method of cultivation, and the strength of heat and sun.

Effects   The exact effects of marijuana and hashish are difficult to quantify since there are numerous variables including the occasional presence of other nonpsychoactive cannabinoids and varying different factors such as dose, route of administration, setting, and previous experience of the user. Basically, the effects are euphoric, sedative, and hallucinogenic. It is often legally classified as a narcotic, but

pharmacologically, it is not and does not fall into conventional categories of CNS stimulants or depressants or of hallucinogens. It is uncertain whether marijuana can cause significant physical dependence or tolerance, even after continuous use. It has been claimed by many users to have a "reverse tolerance" effect in which, after use of the drug, it takes less to get the same effect. There are persons who use marijuana daily and feel they need it for its psychologic effects, although the majority of marijuana is smoked by casual users.

Tolerance to the effects of marijuana can be shown experimentally where large doses are given over a prolonged period of time. Insomnia, anorexia, irritability, sweating, and excessive dreaming has been observed following cessation of high-dose chronic THC or cannabis ingestion. There may be a distortion of time and space with little effect on reaction time except in higher doses. The libido is said by many to be enhanced, leading to the claim that it is an aphrodisiac. In group settings, laughter may be uncontrolled and prolonged. Appetite and appreciation for food may be enhanced. Also, it can cause dry mouth, thirst, increase in heart rate, reddening of conjunctivae. Individuals who smoke marijuana are usually less hostile and aggressive than those who drink alcohol. Most users of marijuana use doses which produce the desired euphoric effect. In this circumstance, tolerance and dependence is not experienced at these doses.

Pharmacokinetics   The average marijuana cigarette (joint) is said to contain between 0.1 and 3.0 percent Δ^9 THC. When this is smoked, not more than 50 percent is absorbed. The THC that is absorbed is extensively bound to body tissues, particularly to lipids like those in the brain. It is rapidly metabolized by the liver and lung. Because of its extensive distribution in the tissues, THC is released from the tissues in small amounts over weeks or longer. THC slows gastric emptying and gastric transit; therefore, its own absorption when taken orally and the absorption of other drugs and gastrointestinal contents will be delayed. The onset of action when inhaled is between 10 and 30 min and may last for 2 to 3 h. When ingested orally, its effect or onset of action is slower (30 min to 1 h or longer). It may not peak until 2 to 3 h, and may last for up to 3 to 5 h.

Adverse Effects   There is a growing collection of clinical knowledge concerning the chronic long-term effects of marijuana. For the occasional user (especially low-potency preparations), the adverse effects appear to be minimal. The adverse effects appear to be dose-related and highly individualized. Responses are often influenced by the expectation of the user. The higher dose's adverse effects may include a state of acute paranoia, a dissociative state, and, less commonly, acute psychotic reactions. Other adverse effects include an amotivation syndrome and a sense of alteration in time and space, which may cause perceptual problems especially when driving. Marijuana was also supposed to lead to "harder drugs," but this has never been proved. Some users have claimed that after prolonged use in high doses it produces a mild withdrawal syndrome (nervousness and sleepiness).

Management of the Overdose The management of an overdose of marijuana is principally supportive. Emesis or lavage may be indicated particularly if a large amount was ingested or if a young child was involved. Respiratory support is seldom necessary; fluids and placement in a supine position should be helpful where orthostatic hypotension is experienced. Where a panic reaction or toxic psychosis is encountered, reduction of unnecessary stimulation and calm and reassuring verbal support are often effective and all that is needed. In agitated psychosis, parenteral administration of **diazepam** or **haloperidol** can be considered.

TOBACCO

The impact of tobacco abuse is one of the major contemporary problems facing health professionals. The overall mortality for all male cigarette smokers exceeds nonsmokers by 70 percent. The mortality ratio increases with the amount smoked, but former cigarette smokers experience a declining overall mortality ratio as the years of discontinuance increase.

Smoking is one of the three major independent risk factors contributing to fatal and nonfatal myocardial infarction and sudden cardiac death in adult men and women. Smoking cigarettes is a major risk factor for morbidity from arteriosclerotic peripheral vascular disease and atherosclerosis of the aorta and coronary arteries. Although cigarettes do not cause chronic hypertension, smoking acts synergistically to increase the risk of heart disease in the presence of hypertension.

Cigarette smoking has been causally related to lung cancer in both men and women. The risk is increased by number of cigarettes smoked per day, duration of smoking, age of initiation of smoking, degree of inhalation, and "tar" and nicotine content of cigarettes smoked. Cigarette smoking is also a causative factor in the development of cancer of the larynx, of the oral cavity, and of the esophagus. It has been associated with cancer of the kidney in men and related to pancreatic cancer.

Tobacco products may serve as vectors for illness by becoming contaminated with toxic agents found in the workplace. Smoking may produce additive or synergistic pathology as with coal dust and asbestos, respectively. Cigarette smoking is significantly associated with the incidence of peptic ulcer disease and also increases the risk of death from peptic ulcer disease. Cigarette smoking alters the pharmacodynamic and pharmacokinetic actions of some drugs.

Nicotine

Nicotine pharmacology is complex and unpredictable because of the variety of neuroeffector sites where it may act and also because this agent has both stimulant and depressant actions. Nicotine causes the release of catecholamines which increase heart rate and blood pressure, cardiac output, stroke volume, oxygen consumption, coronary blood flow, and possible arrhythmias. Nicotine is also responsible for increased mobilization and utilization of free fatty acids, hyperglycemic effects, and decreased patellar reflex response. A common factor of all tobacco use is the action of the addictive agent, nicotine, on the body. Most habitual tobacco users require the nicotine effect approximately every 20 to 30 min throughout the waking hours. Nicotine is known to stimulate the release of several neurotransmitters, some of which have been associated with the hypothalamic reward system, so discontinuation of the smoking habit is complicated by psychologic and physical dependence on nicotine. Nicotine chewing gum (Nicorette), coupled with a stop-smoking program, is showing promise in this regard.

Nicotine Resin Complex (Nicorette)

The mechanism of nicotine gum in the cessation of tobacco use is the provision of an alternative source of nicotine to help alleviate tobacco withdrawal. This allows the smoker to concentrate on overcoming the psychologic and social factors that support the habit.

Pharmacokinetics The nicotine in the gum, bound to an ion exchange resin, is released by chewing, and release increases with vigorous chewing. Blood levels of nicotine achieved with the chewing gum show less pronounced peaks and troughs than blood levels after smoking. Swallowing the agent does not produce significant blood levels. Nicotine is metabolized by the liver with 20 percent excreted unchanged in the urine.

Adverse Effects Nicotine chewing gum is contraindicated in pregnancy, recent myocardial infarction, angina, vascular occlusive disease, and arrhythmias. Local adverse effects include mechanical injury from chewing, jaw ache, and eructation from swallowing air. Systemic side effects include nonspecific gastrointestinal distress, nausea and vomiting, dizziness, light-headedness, and hiccoughs.

Dosage and Administration Each piece of gum contains 2 mg of nicotine. Initially, patients are told to chew one piece immediately whenever they have the urge to smoke. The gum should be chewed slowly over 30 min. Most patients require 10 pieces of gum daily for the first month. The maximum daily dose of 30 pieces should not be exceeded. Therapy beyond 6 months with this prescription drug has not been well studied and is, therefore, not recommended.

NURSING PROCESS RELATED TO DRUG DEPENDENCY

While medications often play a life-saving role in the treatment of addictive disorders or allow the dependent individual to benefit from a therapeutic milieu, support system, or psychotherapy, nurses should recognize that drug dependency is never cured by drug therapy alone. There probably is no other type of therapeutic situation where the nurse's approach has such a profound effect on patient outcome. The nurse will encounter the alcoholic or other drug-dependent patient in every setting—clinics, emergency room, intensive care, general medical and surgical units, obstetrics, community health settings—not only in the psychiatric setting. While there is no *one* correct approach to dependent persons, a few principles are presented here that can guide the nurse who is caring for them in any setting.

Assessment

Data is collected about the drug-dependent person in three major areas: history of drug use, physical effects or compli-

cations resulting from the use, and psychosocial data. An accurate drug history is valuable but not always attainable, since multiple-drug abuse is the rule rather than the exception. The addict may not be able to give information because of confusion or coma, lack of knowledge about the content of street drugs, or fear of legal reprisal; the alcoholic may not admit to an addiction problem or may tend to understate the extent of alcohol use. If the patient is unable to provide such information, then secondary sources need to be consulted (family members, friends, previous hospital records). All drugs, including alcohol use, prescription drugs, OTC drugs, and street drugs, and the extent of use of each should be recorded because of the potential of drug-drug or drug-disease interaction during detoxification. The drug history should be incorporated into every assessment the nurse performs. Knowledge of common street terms (Table 49-22) will aid this assessment.

The manner in which the history is taken will not only affect the quality of the data but can influence the outcome of therapy or even determine whether the patient will seek assistance once the acute problem is resolved. Therefore, it is vitally important for nurses to be aware of their own attitudes and beliefs concerning drug use and abuse. So often

TABLE 49-22   Glossary of Common Street Terms Referring to Drugs of Abuse and Their Use*

Acid	LSD; can also refer to any psychedelic drug	Love drug	Methaqualone
Angel dust	Phencyclidine	Ludes	Methaqualone
Bag	A packet of drug	Meth	Methamphetamine
Bang	To inject drugs	Mainline	To inject a drug into a vein
Blotter	LSD	Mary Jane	Marijuana
Brick	A kilogram of marijuana in bulk	Mod	Stuporous, lethargic drug state
C	Cocaine	OD	Overdose
Candy	Cocaine	Pop	To inject drugs subcutaneously; to swallow a drug
Ciba	Methylphenidate	Peace pill	Phencyclidine
Coke	Cocaine	Rocket fuel	Phencyclidine
Cartwheels	Benzedrine	Reds	Secobarbital
Chippy	An occasional user of drugs	Rush	Rapid onset of drug euphoria
Cold turkey	Abrupt withdrawal from drug use	Scag	Heroin
Cube	LSD	Smack	Heroin
Cop	To buy drugs	Snow	Cocaine
Crystal	Phencyclidine; can also refer to amphetamines	Splash	Methamphetamine
Crank	Methamphetamine	Speed	Methamphetamine; can also refer to any stimulant
Dope	Any drug; generally refers to marijuana	Stuff	Any drug, usually heroin
Downer	Depression; a barbiturate	Strung out	To be out of drugs and craving; sick on drugs
Fix	An injection of drugs; heroin	Tracks	Needle marks from injections
Goofer	Sedative	Trip	Hallucinations; drug experience
Gun	Hypodermic needle	Turn on	To use drugs
Grass	Marijuana	Up, uppers	Drug-exhilarated; stimulant
Hit	To inject a drug successfully into a vein	Weed	Marijuana
Hype	A user who injects drugs into a vein	Window glass, window pane	LSD
Hog	Phencyclidine		
Joint	Marijuana cigarette	Zen	LSD
Juice	Alcohol	Zonked	Highly intoxicated by a drug
Junk; junkie	Heroin; heroin addict		

*Some terms are used interchangeably and must therefore be considered in their context.

these factors influence how the questions are presented and how the patients react and respond. "Why" and "how" questions and "should" statements are to be avoided and the focus placed on what, where, when, who, and how much. The focus needs to be on simple, direct, and open questions without a judgmental or confronting tone.

The multiple physical effects or complications of alcohol and drug use are often overlooked and the patient's complaints discounted as symptoms of withdrawal. A thorough health history and review of systems, as well as a physical examination, should be done initially and each physical complaint should be explored thoroughly with special attention to manifestations of common complications. Examples of psychosocial data to gather include place and type of residence, employment, relations with significant other individuals, religious affiliation, the manner in which a typical day is spent, and the effect the addiction has had on each of the above factors. The nurse should also assess for depression or other emotional problems and for the patient's view of the problems.

Recognition of alcoholism or other drug dependency in patients admitted to the hospital for other medical reasons is imperative if optimal care is to be given. Should the patient begin to experience withdrawal during anesthesia or should DTs be misdiagnosed, the results can be disastrous. The nurse should be alerted to assess for alcoholism in patients who appeared to be intoxicated when admitted, who have diseases commonly associated with chronic alcoholism, who have predictable mood swings, with tremor, nausea, and vomiting, or who are irritable in the morning before having access to alcohol (which may be hidden in toiletries or brought in by family or friends). Another useful indicator is failure to respond to standard doses of sedatives and hypnotics. While the severity of the alcohol withdrawal syndrome cannot be predicted with certainty, the nurse should identify those patients in whom the duration or quantity of alcohol ingestion indicates high risk of a severe reaction. An increase in vital signs may herald a severe alcohol withdrawal reaction, in contrast to an overdose of CNS depressants, in which all vital signs decrease. The vital signs of these patients should, therefore, be taken frequently.

Management

Manipulation of the environment can be effective in acute abstinence syndromes from drugs or alcohol, particularly when a patient is hallucinating. The nurse's assurance that the hallucinations are an effect of the drug will often augment the patient's sense of security. A well-lighted room with hall, closet, and bathroom doors closed to avoid shadows and to shut out excessive noise is appropriate. The number of people in contact with the patient should be minimized. Someone should remain with the patient, and those who care for him should talk slowly in modulated tones, referring to concrete items in the environment, and should move deliberately.

Hypoglycemia has been found in both drug and alcohol withdrawal syndromes and may be one cause of agitation and anxiety. Good nutrition, adequate fluids, and appropriate exercise and positioning are important nursing responsibilities.

To avoid manipulation by the patient during the withdrawal period, health care workers must be firm and consistent. Some clinicians feel that the nurse's approach should be one of unconditional friendliness rather than confrontation, so that the patient can gain confidence that the nurse will give physical and emotional support (including medications) and will not withdraw this support if the patient fails to meet expectations.

Evaluation

Avoidance of preventable complications of drug intoxication and addiction, prompt reversal of treatable complications, successful abstinence from the agent, recognition of the addiction, and control of the life disruption caused by it are the criteria used to evaluate the management of addiction. Success must be based on the evaluation of progress toward individualized patient goals.

CASE STUDY

G.L. is a 56-year-old male who was admitted as an inpatient to a 5-week alcoholism treatment program. The program consisted of individual and group counseling, therapeutic community, assertiveness training, lectures, and films on alcoholism. Although not a central component of the program, the client's participation in Alcoholics Anonymous (AA) was highly recommended along with the use of disulfiram. After completion of the program, the client took up residence in subsidized housing for the elderly. He was discharged on disulfiram (Antabuse) 250 mg and hydrochlorothiazide 50 mg bid for control of his high blood pressure.

Assessment

The psychiatric nurse therapist was assigned as the primary therapist for G.L. while he was an inpatient and for follow-up sessions. The following assessment was completed.

G.L. was born and raised in a large east coast city. He came from a small family and described his relationship with family members as close while he was growing up. Presently, only one sibling is alive and he still keeps in contact with her. His mother died when he was 14 years old, and his father died 11 years ago from lung cancer;

more recently, a brother died of unknown causes. There is no parental history of alcoholism; however, G.L. described his brother and an uncle as persons who could "really hold their drinks." G.L., married for nearly 15 years, has been a widower for the past 5 years. He has one daughter and grandchild living in another state. He does not keep in contact with them. He has spent the past several years traveling across the country, working various part-time jobs. At the time of admission, he was looking forward to settling down in one spot "for a while."

G.L. began using alcohol when he was 15 years old. His involvement with alcohol soon led to the use of heroin. He described himself as being addicted to heroin in addition to being a dealer of heroin for several years. G.L. was using and dealing heroin when he was married and working as a maintenance man in an urban hospital. He tried to keep his "problem" a secret from his family and work associates. He decided to get out of the business due to the increased risks involved. A year after his wife's death, G.L. did successfully complete a detoxification treatment program for heroin and was maintained on methadone for several years. When he was using heroin, his alcohol consumption was very low. However, alcohol became a problem for him when he began the methadone maintenance program. G.L. described himself as a binge drinker. He drank anything that he could find and would drink up to one-fifth per day on occasion. He related that he has been hospitalized several times for alcohol-related problems during the past 3 years; he has had several periods of sobriety lasting anywhere from 1 month to 3 months. G.L. did not stop drinking until a week prior to admission to the program. The main reasons for seeking help centered around health problems, specifically, high blood pressure and ill health.

G.L.'s medical history includes a past history of tuberculosis at age 12 and a fractured skull with subdural hemorrhage that occurred 10 years ago. No residual side effects from these problems were noted at the time of admission. G.L.'s lab reports and physical and mental health status exams were all within normal limits except for his high blood pressure.

Management

During treatment, the major emphasis was focused on teaching G.L. about alcoholism and its effects on all aspects of his life. Individual sessions focused on setting up goals to assist G.L. to develop alternate support systems, to build trust relationships with others, to express and deal with feelings of loss, to learn how to utilize leisure time better, and to maintain sobriety. G.L. was also interested in doing volunteer work at the hospital and in the community and in taking adult education classes for self-enhancement. Appropriate referrals were made in the community for him in these areas. During the 5-week program, G.L. was involved in the group, lectures, and discussion sessions. He was also actively involved in AA meetings. G.L. chose to take disulfiram and began taking it 2 weeks before discharge. He was told about the common side effects of the drug and about which drugs, food, and toiletries to avoid.

G.L. was also referred to the hypertension clinic for his elevated blood pressure which was successfully brought under control by hydrochlorothiazide 50 mg bid. He was advised to have his blood pressure measured periodically since the addition of disulfiram to his therapy may contribute to a slight increase in pressure. He was also seen by the dietitian for a nutritional evaluation and education on what foods were necessary to good nutrition and which should be avoided for control of his high blood pressure.

Evaluation

G.L. successfully completed the 5-week alcoholism program. Since discharge, he has been actively involved in attending AA meetings at the treatment unit and in the community plus the treatment unit's after care group which meets once a week. He has also been involved in doing volunteer work at the hospital and in helping elderly individuals in his apartment complex. He is also preparing to take a course in typing through one of the community colleges.

G.L. did experience a period of feeling "more tired than usual" after discharge. This was attributed to the use of disulfiram. These symptoms subsided after 2 or 3 weeks. At this time, he continues to take Antabuse and experiences no side effects. He also continues to attend the hypertension clinic twice a month and continues to be compliant with his medication regimen. G.L. relates feeling good (physically and emotionally), keeping himself busy, and maintaining his sobriety.

REFERENCES

Immunization

Alper, J.: "Vaccine Research Gets New Boost," *High Technology*, 58–63, April 1983.

Brown, M. W.: "What You Should Know about Communicable Diseases and Their Immunizations: A Guide for Nurses in Ambulatory Settings," *Nursing*, 5:70–72, September 1975; 5:56–60, October 1975; 5:55–60, November 1975.

Centers for Disease Control: *Pertussis and Pertussis Vac-*

cine, Center for Prevention Services, Atlanta, Apr. 14, 1982.

———: *Health Information for International Travel,* Superintendent of Documents, Washington: U.S. Government Printing Office, 1983.

Control of Communicable Diseases in Man, Washington: American Public Health Association, 1980.

Johnson, R. J., and R. J. Ellis: "Immunobiologic Agents and Drugs Available from the Center for Disease Control," *Ann Intern Med,* **81:**61, 1974.

Koplan, J. P., S. C. Schoenbaum, M. C. Weinstein, and D. W. Fraser: "Pertussis Vaccine—An Analysis of Benefits, Costs and Risks," *N Engl J Med,* **301:**906–911, 1979.

Mills, J.: "Vaccines, Immune Globulins and Other Complex Biologic Products," in B. G. Katzung (ed.), *Basic and Clinical Pharmacology,* Los Altos, CA: Lange, 1982.

Public Health Service: *Talk Paper, Pertussis Vaccine,* Washington: Food and Drug Administration, Apr. 20, 1982.

Report of the Committee on Infectious Diseases, 19th ed., Evanston, IL: American Academy of Pediatrics, 1982.

Rosenberg, H., and P. Y. Yih: "Update on Pediatrics Immunization," *U.S. Pharmacist,* **3:**36–50, October 1978.

Environmental and Occupational Health

D.H.E.W.: *Human Health and the Environment—Some Research Needs,* Washington: U.S.D.H.E.W., Public Health Service, National Institute of Environmental Health Sciences, 1977 (DHEW Public No. NIH 77-1277).

———: *Healthy People—The Surgeon General's Report on Health Promotion and Disease Prevention,* Washington: U.S.D.H.E.W., Public Health Service, 1979 [DHEW (PHS) Pub. No. 79-55071].

Dix, H. M.: *Environmental Pollution,* Chichester, U.K.: Wiley, 1981.

Environmental Protection Agency: *The Quality of Life Concept, A Potential New Tool for Decision Makers,* Washington: The Environmental Protection Agency, Office of Research and Monitoring, Environmental Studies Division, 1973.

Greenberg, J.: "Implications for Primary Care Providers of Occupational Health Hazards on Pregnant Women and Their Infants," *J Nurse Midwife,* **25:**21–30, July–August 1980.

Klassen, C. D.: "Nonmetallic Environmental Toxicants: Air Pollutants, Solvents and Vapors, and Pesticides," in A. G. Gilman. L. S. Goodman, and A. Gilman (eds.), *Goodman and Gilman's The Pharmacological Basis of Therapeutics,* 6th ed., New York: Macmillan, 1980.

Marrack, D.: "Water and Health," in N. M. Trieff (ed.), *Environment and Health,* Ann Arbor, MI: Ann Arbor Science, 1981.

NIOSH: *Occupational Diseases: A Guide to Their Recognition,* rev. ed., U.S. Dept. Health, Education and Welfare, Public Health Service, Center for Disease Control, National Institute for Occupational Safety and Health, June 1977 (DHEW - NIOSH Public No. 77-181).

Reist, P. C.: "Air Pollution," in L. L. Jarvis, *Community Health Nursing: Keeping the Public Healthy,* Philadelphia: Davis, 1981.

ReVelle, C. and P. ReVelle: *Sourcebook on the Environment,* Boston: Houghton Mifflin, 1974.

Severs, R. K.: "Air Pollution and Health," in N. M. Trieff (ed.), *Environment and Health,* Ann Arbor, MI: Ann Arbor Science, 1981.

Spath, D. P., and J. Crook: "Water Pollution," in L. L. Jarvis, *Community Health Nursing: Keeping the Public Healthy,* Philadelphia: Davis, 1981.

Trieff, N. M.: "Contemporary Occupational Health Problems," in N. M. Trieff (ed.), *Environment and Health,* Ann Arbor, MI: Ann Arbor Science, 1981.

Drug Abuse

Abramowicz, N. (ed.): "Diagnosis and Management of Reactions to Drug Abuse," *Med Lett Drug Ther,* **19:**1–3, 1977.

American Medical Association Council on Scientific Affairs: "Marijuana, Its Health Hazard and Therapeutic Potentials," *JAMA,* **246:**1823–1825, 1981.

Becker, C. E.: "The Clinical Pharmacology of Alcohol," *Calif Med,* **113:**37–45, 1970.

———, R. L. Roe, and R. A. Scott: *Alcohol as a Drug: A Curriculum on Pharmacology, Neurology and Toxicology,* New York: Medcom, 1974.

Blose I.: "The Relationship of Alcohol to Aging and the Elderly," *Alcoholism: Clin Exper Res,* **2:**17–21, 1978.

Bode, J.: "Factors Influencing Ethanol Metabolism in Man," in R. Thurman, T. Yonetani, J. Williamson, and B. Chance (eds.), *Alcohol and Aldehyde Metabolizing Systems,* New York: Academic, 1974, pp. 457–468.

Bradley, L.: "Avoiding a Crisis: The Assessment," *Am J Nurs,* **82:**12, 1865–1871, December 1982.

Burch, G. E., and T. D. Giles: "Alcoholic Cardiomyopathy: Concept of the Disease and Its Treatment," *Am J Med,* **50:**141–145, 1971.

Burkwalter, P. K.: *Nursing Care of the Alcoholic and Drug Abuser,* New York: McGraw-Hill, 1975.

Clark, P., and L. Kricka: *Medical Consequences of Alcoholism,* New York: Wiley, 1980.

Cohen, S.: "Amphetamine Abuse," *JAMA,* **231:**414–415, 1975.

Cohn, L.: "The Hidden Diagnosis," *Am J Nurs,* **82:**12, 1862–1871, December 1982.

Detzer, E., A. S. Carlin, and B. Muller: "Detoxifying the Barbiturate Addict: Hints for the Psychiatric Staff," *Am J Nurs,* **76:**1306–1307, 1976.

Diagnostic Distribution of Admissions to Inpatient Services of State and County Mental Hospitals, Mental Health Statistical Note No. 138, Rockville, MD: National Institute of Mental Health, 1975.

Distasio, C., and M. Nawrot: "Methaqualone," Am J Nurs, 73:1922–1925, 1973.

Ditzler. J.: "Rehabilitation for Alcoholics," Am J Nurs, 76:1722–1775, 1976.

Eichner, E. R.: "The Hematologic Disorder of Alcoholism," Am J Med, 54:621–630, 1973.

Ellinwood, E. M., and S. Ghen: "Amphetamine Abuse," Science, 171:420, 1971.

Estes, N. J., and M. E. Heinemann (eds.): Alcoholism Development, Consequences, and Interventions, 2d ed., St. Louis: Mosby, 1982.

———, D. Smith, K. Julio, and M. E. Heinemann: Nursing Diagnosis of the Alcoholic Person, St. Louis: Mosby 1980.

Fultz, J. L., and E. C. Senay: "Guidelines for Management of Hospitalized Narcotic Addicts," Ann Intern Med, 82:815–818, 1975.

Gay, G. R.: "Clinical Management of Acute and Chronic Cocaine Poisoning," Ann Emerg Med, 11:562–572, 1982.

Green, H. G.: "Infants of Alcoholic Mothers," Am J Obstet Gynecol, 118:713–716, 1974.

Greenblatt, D. J., and M. Greenblatt: "Which Drug for Alcohol Withdrawal?" J Clin Pharmacol, 12:429–431, 1972.

Hadden, J., K. Johnson, S. Smith, L. Price, and E. Giardina: "Acute Barbiturate Intoxication: Concepts of Management," JAMA, 209:893–899, 1969.

Heineman, E., and N. Estes: "Assessing Alcoholic Patients," Am J Nurs, 76:785–789, 1976.

Inaba, D. S.: "Oral Methadone Maintenance Techniques in the Management of Morphine-Type Dependence," JAMA, 219:1618, 1972.

———, G. R. Gay, G. A. Whitehead, J. A. Newmeyer, and D. Bergin: "The Use of Propoxyphene Napsylate in the Treatment of Heroin and Methadone Addiction," West J Med, 121:106–111, 1974.

Jones, B., and M. Jones, "Women and Alcohol: Intoxication, Metabolism, and the Menstrual Cycle," in M. Greenblatt and M. Schuckitt (eds.), Alcoholism Problems in Women and Children, New York: Grune and Stratton, 1976.

Khantzian, E. G., and G. J. McKenna: "Acute Toxic and Withdrawal Reactions Associated with Drug Use and Abuse," Ann Intern Med, 90:361–372, 1979.

Krajick-Weist, J., M. G. Lindeman, and M. Newton: "Hospital Dialogues," Am J Nurs, 82:1874–1877, December 1982.

Kurose, K., T. N. Anderson, W. N. Bull, H. M. Gibson, P. Grubb, N. Kreptz, A. S. Nagvi, and M. Smith: "A Standard Care Plan for Alcoholism," Am J Nurs, 81:1001–1006, May 1981.

Lewis, L. W.: "The Hidden Alcoholic: A Nursing Dilemma," Nursing, 5:20–30, 1975.

Lieber, C. S.: "Hepatic and Metabolic Effects of Alcohol (1966 to 1973)," Gastroenterology, 65:821–846, 1973.

———: "Liver Adaptation and Injury in Alcoholism," N Engl J Med, 288:356–362, 1973.

———: "Alcohol and Malnutrition in Pathogenesis of Liver Disease," JAMA, 233:1077–1082, 1975.

Louria, D. B., and E. A. Wolfson: "Medical Complications of Drug Abuse," Drug Ther, 2:35–44, 1972.

Mendelson, J. H.: "Biological Concomitants of Alcoholism," N Engl J Med, 283:24–31, 1970.

———, and M. K. Mello (eds.): The Diagnosis and Treatment of Alcoholism, NNeeew Yooork: MMccccGraw-Hill, 1979.

National Council on Alcoholism: "Criteria for Diagnosis of Alcoholism," Ann Intern Med, 77:249–258, 1973.

National Institute on Alcohol Abuse and Alcoholism: Second Special Report to the U.S. Congress on Alcohol and Health from the Secretary of Health, Education and Welfare, Waashington, June 1974.

———: Fourth Special Report to the U.S. Congress on Alcohol and Health from the Secretary of Health and Human Services, Washington, January 1981.

Nelson, K.: "The Nurse in a Methadone Maintenance Program," Am J Nurs, 73:870–874, 1973.

Parker, W. J.: "Alcohol-Drug Interactions," J Am Pharm Assoc, 10:664–665, 1970.

Pillari, G., and J. Narus: "Physical Effects of Heroin Addiction," Am J Nurs, 73:2105–2108, 1973.

Schuckit, M.: "Geriatric Alcoholism and Drug Abuse," Gerontologist, 17:168–174, 1979.

———, and P. Pastor: "The Elderly as a Unique Population: Alcoholism," Alcoholism: Clin Exper Res, 2:31–38, 1978.

Seixas, F. A.: "Alcohol and Its Drug Interactions," Ann Intern Med, 83:86–92, 1975.

———, K. Williams, and S. Eggleston (eds.): "Medical Consequences of Alcoholism," Ann NY Acad Sci, 252:5–399, 1975.

Sellers, E. M., and H. Kalant: "Alcohol Intoxication and Withdrawal," N Engl J Med, 294:957–961, 1976.

Smith D. E., and D. R. Wesson: "A New Method of Barbiturate Dependence," JAMA, 213:294–295, 1970.

Szara, S.: "Clinical Pharmacology of Cannabis: Scientific and Nonscientifffic CConnstraints," iin M. C. Brrrraauude and SS. Szara (eds.), Pharmacology of Marijuana, New York: Raven, 1976, pp. 27–33.

Thompson, W. I., A. D. Johnson, and W. C. Maddrey: "Diazepam and Paraldehyde for Treatment of Severe Delirium Tremens," Ann Intern Med, 82:175–180, 1975.

Viamontes, J. A.: "Review of Drug Effectiveness in the Treatment of Alcoholism," Am J Psychiatry, 128:120–121, 1972.

Vourakis, C., and G. Bennett: "Angel-Dust—Not Heaven Sent," *Am J Nurs,* **79:**649–653, April 1979.

Wesson, L., G. R. Gay, and D. E. Smith: "Treatment Techniques for Narcotic Withdrawal with Special Reference to Mixed Narcotic-Sedative Addiction," *J Psychedelic Drugs,* **4:**118–122, 1971.

White, A. G.: "Medical Disorders in Drug Addicts: 200 Consecutive Admissions," *JAMA,* **223:**1469–1471, 1973.

Williams, N.: "Alcohol Problems in Elderly Compounded by Many Factors," *NIAAA Information & Feature Service,* IFS No. 103, Dec. 31, 1982.

Yowell, S., and C. Brose: "Working with Drug Abuse in the ER," *Am J Nurs,* **77:**82–85, 1977.

INDEX

Boldfaced page numbers refer to main discussions of drugs.
Italicized page numbers refer to illustrations and tables.